Present Knowledge in Food Safety

A Risk-Based Approach Through The Food Chain

Present Knowledge in Food Safety

A Risk-Based Approach Through The Food Chain

Edited by

Michael E. Knowles, PhD

Lucia E. Anelich, PhD

Alan R. Boobis, OBE PhD

Bert Popping, PhD

ELSEVIER

ACADEMIC PRESS
An imprint of Elsevier

ILSI

Academic Press is an imprint of Elsevier
125 London Wall, London EC2Y 5AS, United Kingdom
525 B Street, Suite 1650, San Diego, CA 92101, United States
50 Hampshire Street, 5th Floor, Cambridge, MA 02139, United States
The Boulevard, Langford Lane, Kidlington, Oxford OX5 1GB, United Kingdom

ISBN: 978-0-12-819470-6

For Information on all Academic Press publications
visit our website at https://www.elsevier.com/books-and-journals

Publisher: Nikki Levy
Acquisitions Editor: Nina Bandeira
Editorial Project Manager: Mariana Kuhl
Production Project Manager: Sruthi Satheesh
Cover Designer: Christian Bilbow

Typeset by MPS Limited, Chennai, India
Transferred to Digital Printing 2023

Dedication

We dedicate this first edition of *Present Knowledge in Food Safety* to the global food safety community, who continue to seek the best science, interpret that science for the good of people worldwide, and persist in countering unscientific food safety information with evidence-based approaches to safer food. We also dedicate this edition to our own scientific mentors and colleagues who have persuaded and occasionally pushed us in the direction of the highest quality food safety science. In particular, we dedicate this work to the late John Milner, former chair of the ILSI Publications Committee, who conceived the idea for this publication and created the foundation upon which it was built.

Contents

Section IV
Changes in the chemical composition of food throughout the various stages of the food chain: manufacture, packaging and distribution

Section VII
Changes in pathogenic microbiological contamination of food throughout the various stages of the food chain post-processing

Section X
Safety assessment of genetically modified organisms and other biological alterations

Section XI
Food safety: risk perception and communicating with the public

List of contributors

Amie Adkin Risk Assessment Unit, Food Standards Agency, London, United Kingdom

Timothy E.H. Allen MRC Toxicology Unit, University of Cambridge, Cambridge, United Kingdom

Felipe Alves de Almeida Department of Nutrition, Federal University of Juiz de Fora (UFJF), Governador Valadares, Brazil

Lucia E. Anelich Anelich Consulting, Pretoria, South Africa

Mark Arnold Department of Epidemiological Sciences, APHA Weybridge, Addlestone, United Kingdom

Sandrine Auger MICALIS Institut, Univerisité Paris-Saclay, INRAE, AgroParisTech, Jouy en Josas, France

Tessa Avermaete Sustainable Food Economies Research Group, KU Leuven, Belgium

Craig Baker-Austin Centre for Environment, Fisheries and Aquaculture (CEFAS), Weymouth, United Kingdom

Forrest L. Bayer Bayer Consulting and UW Imaging, LLC, Atlanta, GA, United States

Kiran N. Bhilegaonkar ICAR—Indian Veterinary Research Institute, Regional Centre, Pune, Maharashtra, India

Xiaoyu Bi Exponent, Inc., Washington, DC, United States

W. Marty Blom Netherlands Organisation for Applied Scientific Research TNO, Utrecht, The Netherlands; University Medical Center Utrecht, Utrecht, The Netherlands

Alan R. Boobis National Heart and Lung Institute, Imperial College London, London, United Kingdom

Marija Boskovic Faculty of Veterinary Medicine, University of Belgrade, Belgrade, Serbia

Hans Bouwmeester Division of Toxicology, Wageningen University, Wageningen, The Netherlands

Gary Bowering Independent Science Communicator, Wellington, New Zealand

Ioannis S. Boziaris Lab of Marketing and Technology of Aquatic Products and Foods, Department of Ichthyology and Aquatic Environment, School of Agricultural Sciences, University of Thessaly, Volos, Greece

Christopher J. Breen Food and Agriculture Organization of the United Nations (FAO), Office of Climate Change, Biodiversity, and the Environment (OCB), Rome, Italy

Hugo Brouwer Division of Toxicology, Wageningen University, Wageningen, The Netherlands

Ian Brown Oxford University Hospitals, Oxford, United Kingdom; The Institute of Food, Nutrition and Health, University of Reading, Reading, United Kingdom

Robert L. Buchanan Center for Food Safety and Security Systems, Department of Nutrition and Food Science, University of Maryland, College Park, MD, United States

Elna M. Buys Department of Consumer and Food Sciences, Faculty of Natural and Agricultural Sciences, University of Pretoria, Pretoria, South Africa; Department of Consumer and Food Sciences, University of Pretoria, Hatfield, South Africa

Jane M. Caldwell Caldwell Food Safety LLC, Springfield, MO, United States

Elena Canellas University of Zaragoza, Campus Rio Ebro, Zaragoza, Spain

Deisy Guimarães Carneiro Department of Microbiology, Federal University of Viçosa (UFV), Viçosa, Brazil

Karin Carstensen Woolworths South Africa (Pty) Ltd, Cape Town, Western Cape, South Africa

Brayan R.H. Cervantes-Huamán Area of Human Nutrition and Food Science, Departament de Ciència Animal i dels Aliments, Facultat de Veterinària, Universitat Autònoma de Barcelona, Barcelona, Spain

Roger Clemens Department of Regulatory and Quality Science, School of Pharmacy, University of Southern California, Los Angeles, CA, United States

Luca Cocolin Department of Agriculture, Forest and Food Sciences, University of Turin, Grugliasco, Italy

Samuel M. Cohen Department of Pathology and Microbiology, University of Nebraska Medical Center, Omaha, NE, United States

David Coles School of Natural and Environmental Sciences, Newcastle University, Newcastle upon Tyne, United Kingdom

Alessia Cossettini Dipartimento di Scienze AgroAlimentari, Ambientali e Animali, Università di Udine, Udine, Italy

Natália Cruz-Martins Faculty of Medicine, University of Porto, Porto, Portugal; Institute for Research and Innovation in Health (i3S), University of Porto, Porto, Portugal; TOXRUN – Toxicology Research Unit, University Institute of Health Sciences, Polytechnic and University Cooperative (CESPU), Gandra, Portugal

György Csikó Department of Pharmacology and Toxicology, University of Veterinary Medicine, Budapest, Hungary

Michelle Danyluk Department of Food Science and Human Nutrition, Citrus Research and Education Center, Institute of Food and Agricultural Sciences, University of Florida, Lake Alfred, FL, United States

Wageh Sobhy Darwish Food Control Department, Faculty of Veterinary Medicine, Zagazig University, Zagazig, Egypt

Barbara De Coninck Crop Biotechnics, KU Leuven, Belgium

Christina A. Mireles DeWitt Seafood Research and Education Center, Coastal Oregon Marine Experiment Station, Department of Food Science and Technology, College of Agricultural Sciences, Oregon State University, Astoria, OR, United States

B.C. Dlamini Department of Biotechnology and Food Technology, Faculty of Science, University of Johannesburg, Johannesburg, South Africa

John Doe School of Pharmacy and Biomolecular Sciences, Liverpool John Moores University, Liverpool, United Kingdom

Simon Douglas Kelly Food Safety and Control Laboratory, Joint FAO/IAEA Centre of Nuclear Techniques in Food and Agriculture, Department of Nuclear Sciences and Applications, International Atomic Energy Agency, Vienna International Centre, Vienna, Austria

Eleonora Dupouy Food Systems and Food Safety Division (ESF), Food and Agriculture Organization of the United Nations (FAO), Rome, Italy

Gerhard Eisenbrand Food Chemistry and Toxicology, University of Kaiserslautern, Heidelberg, Germany; University of Kaiserslautern, Germany (Retired), Heidelberg, Germany

James A. Elegbeleye Department of Consumer and Food Sciences, Faculty of Natural and Agricultural Sciences, University of Pretoria, Pretoria, South Africa; Department of Consumer and Food Sciences, University of Pretoria, Hatfield, South Africa

Pablo Estévez Biomedical Research Center (CINBIO), Department of Analytical and Food Chemistry, University of Vigo, Vigo, Spain

Ricardo Franco-Duarte Centre of Molecular and Environmental Biology (CBMA), Department of Biology, University of Minho, Braga, Portugal

Leonardo Luiz de Freitas Department of Microbiology, Federal University of Viçosa (UFV), Viçosa, Brazil

Nigel French New Zealand Food Safety Science and Research Centre, School of Veterinary Science, Massey University, Palmerston North, New Zealand

Lynn J. Frewer School of Natural and Environmental Sciences, Newcastle University, Newcastle upon Tyne, United Kingdom

Yuqi Fu Center for Alternatives to Animal Testing (CAAT), Johns Hopkins Bloomberg School of Public Health, Baltimore, MD, United States

Shoji Fukushima Japan Bioassay Research Center, Hadano, Kanagawa, Japan

Ana Gago-Martinez (Gago) Biomedical Research Center (CINBIO), Department of Analytical and Food Chemistry, University of Vigo, Vigo, Spain

Alejandro Dorado Garcia Food and Agriculture Organization of the United Nations (FAO), Rome, Italy; Animal Production and Health Unit (NSA), Rome, Italy

Steven M. Gendel Gendel Food Safety LLC, Silver Spring, MD, United States

Anne Gerardi GFSI at the Consumer Goods Forum, Paris, France

Anuradha Ghosh Biology Department, Pittsburg State University, Pittsburg, KS, United States

Milica Glisic Faculty of Veterinary Medicine, University of Belgrade, Belgrade, Serbia

Samuel Benrejeb Godefroy Food Risk Analysis and Regulatory Excellence Platform (PARERA), Institute of Nutrition and Functional Foods (INAF), Québec, QC, Canada; Department of Food Sciences, Faculty of Agriculture and Food Sciences, Laval University, Quebec City, QC, Canada

Nigel J. Gooderham Department of Metabolism, Digestion and Reproduction, Imperial College London, London, United Kingdom

Gerard Govers Geography and Tourism, KU Leuven, Belgium

Tomasz Grenda Department of Hygiene of Animal Feedingstuffs, National Veterinary Research Institute, Pulawy, Poland

F. Peter Guengerich Department of Biochemistry, Vanderbilt University School of Medicine, Nashville, TN, United States

Sandrine Guillou SECALIM, INRAE, Oniris, Nantes, France

Steve Gutsell Unilever Safety and Environmental Assurance Centre, Colworth Science Park, Sharnbrook, United Kingdom

Muriel Guyard-Nicodème ANSES – Ploufragan-Plouzané-Niort Laboratory, Ploufragan, France

Nabila Haddad SECALIM, INRAE, Oniris, Nantes, France

Ndaindila N.K. Haindongo Food and Agriculture Organization of the United Nations (FAO), Office of Climate Change, Biodiversity, and the Environment (OCB), Rome, Italy

Christie L. Harman Flavor and Extract Manufacturers Association, Washington, DC, United States

Thomas Hartung Center for Alternatives to Animal Testing (CAAT), Johns Hopkins Bloomberg School of Public Health, Baltimore, MD, United States; University of Konstanz, CAAT-Europe, Konstanz, Germany

A. Wallace Hayes College of Public Health, University of South Florida, Tampa, FL, United States

Graham Head Bayer Crop Science, Chesterfield, MO, United States

Stephen S. Hecht Masonic Cancer Center and Department of Laboratory Medicine and Pathology, University of Minnesota, Minneapolis, MN, United States

Jeljer Hoekstra RIVM, The National Institute for Public Health and the Environment, Bilthoven, The Netherlands

Louwrens Hoffman Centre for Nutrition and Food Sciences, Queensland Alliance for Agriculture and Food Innovation, The University of Queensland, Gatton, QLD, Australia

Olivier Honnay Ecology, Evolution and Biodiversity Conservation, KU Leuven, Belgium

Geert Houben Netherlands Organisation for Applied Scientific Research TNO, Utrecht, The Netherlands; University Medical Center Utrecht, Utrecht, The Netherlands

Jan Jetten Ex-TNO, Zeist, The Netherlands

Shan Jin School of Natural and Environmental Sciences, Newcastle University, Newcastle upon Tyne, United Kingdom; Faculty of Business and Law, University of Portsmouth, Portsmouth, United Kingdom

Karen Job The Food Brain Consultancy, Melbourne, VIC, Australia

Snehal Kadam Institute of Bioinformatics and Biotechnology, Savitribai Phule Pune University, Pune, India

Shraddha Karanth Department of Nutrition and Food Science, University of Maryland, College Park, MD, United States

Agnes Karmaus Integrated Laboratory Systems, LLC, Morrisville, NC, United States

Manos Karvounis Agroknow, Maroussi, Greece

Fumiko Kasuga National Institute for Environmental Studies, Tsukuba-City, Japan

Karishma S. Kaushik Institute of Bioinformatics and Biotechnology, Savitribai Phule Pune University, Pune, India

Marc C. Kennedy Fera Science Ltd, York Biotech Campus, York, United Kingdom

John G. Keogh Henley Business School, University of Reading, Henley-on-Thames, United Kingdom

Wannes Keulemans Crop Biotechnics, KU Leuven, Belgium

Nida Khan Nash FintechX, Esch-sur-Alzette, Luxembourg

Michael E. Knowles Kavakia-Rachi, Veria, Greece

Dimitra Kogiannou Institute of Marine Biology, Biotechnology and Aquaculture, Hellenic Centre for Marine Research, Anavyssos, Greece

Serhii Kolesnyk L.I. Medved's Research Center of Preventive Toxicology, Food and Chemical Safety, Ministry of Health, Kyiv, Ukraine; University of Basel, Department of Pharmaceutical Sciences, Division of Molecular and Systems Toxicology, Basel, Switzerland

Rahul P. Kolhe KNP College of Veterinary Science, MAFSU, Shirwal, Maharashtra, India

Timm Konold Department of Pathology and Animal Sciences, APHA Weybridge, Addlestone, United Kingdom

Zoi Kotsiri Environmental and Microbiology Unit, Department of Public Health, Medical School, University of Patras, Patras, Greece

Matt Krug Southwest Florida Research and Education Center, Institute of Food and Agricultural Sciences, University of Florida, Immokalee, FL, United States

Krzysztof Kwiatek Department of Hygiene of Animal Feedingstuffs, National Veterinary Research Institute, Pulawy, Poland

Youngjoo Kwon Department of Food Science and Biotechnology, Ewha Womans University, Seoul, South Korea

Francesca Latronico Food and Agriculture Organization of the United Nations (FAO), Rome, Italy; Joint Centre for Codex Standards and Zoonotic Diseases (CJW), Rome, Italy

José M. Leao Biomedical Research Center (CINBIO), Department of Analytical and Food Chemistry, University of Vigo, Vigo, Spain

Jeffrey T. LeJeune Food and Agriculture Organization of the United Nations (FAO), Rome, Italy; Food Systems and Food Safety Division (ESF), Rome, Italy

Wenjing Li School of Natural and Environmental Sciences, Newcastle University, Newcastle upon Tyne, United Kingdom; School of Economics and Management, Huazhong Agricultural University, Wuhan, P.R. China

Matthew J. Linman Flavor and Extract Manufacturers Association, Washington, DC, United States

Rebeca López-García Logre International Food Science Consulting, Mexico City, Mexico

Thomas Luechtefeld Center for Alternatives to Animal Testing (CAAT), Johns Hopkins Bloomberg School of Public Health, Baltimore, MD, United States; ToxTrack Inc., Baltimore, MD, United States

Bernadene Magnuson Health Science Consultants Inc, Collingwood, Canada

Louise Manning Sustainable Agri-food Systems, Lincoln Institute for Agri-food Technology, University of Lincoln, United Kingdom

Nikos Manouselis Agroknow, Maroussi, Greece

Marisa Manzano Dipartimento di Scienze AgroAlimentari, Ambientali e Animali, Università di Udine, Udine, Italy

Marco Marin MICALIS Institut, Univerisité Paris-Saclay, INRAE, AgroParisTech, Jouy en Josas, France

María Salomé Mariotti Escuela de Nutrición y Dietética, Facultad de Medicina, Universidad Finis Terrae, Santiago, Chile

Jaime Martinez-Urtaza Centre for Environment, Fisheries and Aquaculture (CEFAS), Weymouth, United Kingdom; Department of Genetics and Microbiology, Faculty of Biosciences, Autonomous University of Barcelona, Barcelona, Spain

Lynn M. McMullen Department of Agricultural, Food and Nutritional Science, University of Alberta, Edmonton, AB Canada

Cronan McNamara Creme Global Ltd., Dublin, Ireland

Angel Medina Environment and Agrifood Theme, Cranfield University, Cranfield, United Kingdom

N.N. Mehlomakulu Department of Consumer and Food Sciences, Faculty of Natural and Agricultural Sciences, University of Pretoria, Pretoria, South Africa

Jyotigna M. Mehta ADAMA Agricultural Solutions, Reading, United Kingdom

Marjolein Meijerink Netherlands Organisation for Applied Scientific Research TNO, Utrecht, The Netherlands

J. David Miller Department of Chemistry, Carleton University, Ottawa, ON, Canada

E.N. Clare Mills Division of Immunity, Infection and Respiratory Medicine, School of Biological Sciences, Manchester Academic Health Sciences Centre, Manchester Institute of Biotechnology, Manchester, United Kingdom

Stephen C. Mitchell Department of Metabolism, Digestion and Reproduction, Imperial College London, London, United Kingdom

Angelo Moretto Department of Cardio-Thoraco-Vascular and Public Health Sciences, University Hospital, Padua, Italy

Desmond T. Mugadza Department of Food Science and Nutrition, Midlands State University, Gweru, Zimbabwe

Keya Mukherjee Food Systems and Food Safety Division (ESF), Food and Agriculture Organization of the United Nations (FAO), Rome, Italy

Francis Z. Naab School of Natural and Environmental Sciences, Newcastle University, Newcastle upon Tyne, United Kingdom

Hanspeter Naegeli Institute of Veterinary Pharmacology and Toxicology, University of Zurich, Zurich, Switzerland

Maristela S. Nascimento University of Campinas, Campinas, Brazil

Ivan Nastasijevic Institute of Meat Hygiene and Technology, Belgrade, Serbia

Maarten Nauta National Food Institute, Technical University of Denmark (DTU), Kgs. Lyngby, Denmark; Statens Serum Institut, Copenhagen S, Denmark

Lev Neretin Food and Agriculture Organization of the United Nations (FAO), Office of Climate Change, Biodiversity, and the Environment (OCB), Rome, Italy

Cristina Nerín University of Zaragoza, Campus Rio Ebro, Zaragoza, Spain

Victor Ntuli Department of Biology, National University of Lesotho, Maseru, Lesotho

Elena G. Olson Department of Animal and Dairy Sciences, University of Wisconsin-Madison, Madison, WI, United States

John O'Brien The Food Observatory, UK and Nutrition Innovation Centre for Food and Health, School of Biomedical Sciences, Ulster University, Coleraine, United Kingdom

Sakshi Painuli Department of Biotechnology, Graphic Era University, Dehradun, India

Efstratia Panteleli Environmental and Microbiology Unit, Department of Public Health, Medical School, University of Patras, Patras, Greece

Mihalis Papakonstantinou Agroknow, Maroussi, Greece

Foteini F. Parlapani Lab of Marketing and Technology of Aquatic Products and Foods, Department of Ichthyology and Aquatic Environment, School of Agricultural Sciences, University of Thessaly, Volos, Greece

Ewelina Patyra Department of Hygiene of Animal Feedingstuffs, National Veterinary Research Institute, Pulawy, Poland

Franco Pedreschi Departamento de Ingeniería Química y Bioprocesos, Pontificia Universidad Católica de Chile, Santiago, Chile

Sandrine Pigat Creme Global Ltd., Dublin, Ireland

Bert Popping FOCOS GmbH – Food Consulting Strategically, Alzenau, Germany

Morten Poulsen National Food Institute, Technical University of Denmark (DTU), Kgs. Lyngby, Denmark

Abani K. Pradhan Department of Nutrition and Food Science, University of Maryland, College Park, MD, United States; Center for Food Safety and Security Systems, University of Maryland, College Park, MD, United States

Peter Pressman Saba University School of Medicine, Saba, Dutch Caribbean; Polyscience Consulting, Chatsworth, CA, United States

Mykola Prodanchuk L.I. Medved's Research Center of Preventive Toxicology, Food and Chemical Safety, Ministry of Health, Kyiv, Ukraine

Monika Przeniosło-Siwczyńska Department of Hygiene of Animal Feedingstuffs, National Veterinary Research Institute, Pulawy, Poland

Ans Punt Wageningen Food Safety Research, Wageningen, The Netherlands

Alfons Ramel Faculty of Food Science and Nutrition, University of Iceland, Reykjavik, Iceland

Abderahman Rejeb University of Rome Tor Vergata, Rome, Italy

Katherine Rich New Zealand Food & Grocery Council, Wellington, New Zealand

Steven C. Ricke Department of Animal and Dairy Sciences, University of Wisconsin-Madison, Madison, WI, United States

Ivonne M.C.M. Rietjens Division of Toxicology, Wageningen University, Wageningen, The Netherlands

George Rigos Institute of Marine Biology, Biotechnology and Aquaculture, Hellenic Centre for Marine Research, Anavyssos, Greece

Carolina Ripolles-Avila Area of Human Nutrition and Food Science, Departament de Ciència Animal i dels Aliments, Facultat de Veterinària, Universitat Autònoma de Barcelona, Barcelona, Spain

Francesco Rizzotto MICALIS Institut, Univerisité Paris-Saclay, INRAE, AgroParisTech, Jouy en Josas, France

Célia Fortuna Rodrigues TOXRUN – Toxicology Research Unit, University Institute of Health Sciences, Polytechnic and University Cooperative (CESPU), Gandra, Portugal; LEPABE – Laboratory for Process Engineering, Environment, Biotechnology and Energy, ALiCE-Associate Laboratory in Chemical Engineering - Faculty of Engineering, University of Porto, Porto, Portugal

José Juan Rodríguez-Jerez Area of Human Nutrition and Food Science, Departament de Ciència Animal i dels Aliments, Facultat de Veterinària, Universitat Autònoma de Barcelona, Barcelona, Spain

Martin Rose Manchester Institute of Biotechnology, University of Manchester, Manchester, United Kingdom

Thomas J. Rosol Department of Biomedical Sciences, Heritage College of Osteopathic Medicine, Ohio University, Athens, OH, United States

Joyjit Saha Citrus Research and Education Center, Institute of Food and Agricultural Sciences, University of Florida, Lake Alfred, FL, United States

Tor Savidge Department of Pathology and Immunology, Baylor College of Medicine, Houston, TX, United States; Department of Pathology, Texas Children's Microbiome Center, Texas Children's Hospital, Houston, TX, United States

Eyassu Seifu Department of Food Science and Technology, Botswana University of Agriculture and Natural Resources, Gaborone, Botswana

Prabhakar Semwal Department of Biotechnology, Graphic Era University, Dehradun, India

Thulani Sibanda Department of Consumer and Food Sciences, University of Pretoria, Hatfield, South Africa; Department of Applied Biology and Biochemistry, National University of Science and Technology, Bulawayo, Zimbabwe

Sik Yu So Department of Pathology and Immunology, Baylor College of Medicine, Houston, TX, United States; Department of Pathology, Texas Children's Microbiome Center, Texas Children's Hospital, Houston, TX, United States

Susana Socolovsky Pentachem Consulting Group, Buenos Aires, Argentina

Giannis Stoitsis Agroknow, Maroussi, Greece

Katelynn Stull Citrus Research and Education Center, Institute of Food and Agricultural Sciences, University of Florida, Lake Alfred, FL, United States

Marta H. Taniwaki Institute of Food Technology, Campinas, Brazil

Sean V. Taylor Flavor and Extract Manufacturers Association, Washington, DC, United States

Lesa A. Thompson Regional Representation for Asia and the Pacific, World Organisation for Animal Health (WOAH), Tokyo, Japan

Zeynal Topalcengiz Department of Food Engineering, Faculty of Engineering and Architecture, Muş Alparslan University, Muş, Turkey

George T. Tzotzos Bioinformatics researcher, Vienna, Austria

Michaela van den Honert Centre for Food Safety, Department of Food Science, University of Stellenbosch, Matieland, South Africa

Femke L.N. Van Oijen Division of Toxicology, Wageningen University, Wageningen, The Netherlands

Maria Cristina Dantas Vanetti Department of Microbiology, Federal University of Viçosa (UFV), Viçosa, Brazil

Apostolos Vantarakis Environmental and Microbiology Unit, Department of Public Health, Medical School, University of Patras, Patras, Greece

Paula Vera University of Zaragoza, Campus Rio Ebro, Zaragoza, Spain

Jasmina Vidic MICALIS Institut, Univerisité Paris-Saclay, INRAE, AgroParisTech, Jouy en Josas, France

Priya Vizzini Dipartimento di Scienze AgroAlimentari, Ambientali e Animali, Università di Udine, Udine, Italy

Rosemary H. Waring School of Biosciences, University of Birmingham, Birmingham, United Kingdom

Qinglong Wu Department of Pathology and Immunology, Baylor College of Medicine, Houston, TX, United States; Department of Pathology, Texas Children's Microbiome Center, Texas Children's Hospital, Houston, TX, United States

Khaldoon Zaid-Kaylani InCube Mobility Solutions, Oakville, ON, Canada

Tjitske Anna Zwart Sustainable Food Economies Research Group, KU Leuven, Belgium

About the editors

Michael E. Knowles, PhD

Dr. Michael E. Knowles is a pharmacist and medicinal chemist who spent the first half of his career with the UK Ministry of Agriculture, Fisheries and Food, where he became the chief scientist (Fisheries & Food) and head of the Food Science Group. In that position he was a member of the Advisory Committee on Pesticides, the Committee on Veterinary Medicines, and chair of the Steering Group on Chemical aspects of Food Surveillance. The second half of his 44-year career was spent with The Coca-Cola Company, where he became the vice president of Global Scientific & Regulatory Affairs, from which he retired in 2013. As a graduate of the University of Nottingham, Dr. Knowles is a fellow of several scientific societies; past global president of the ILSI and chair of the ILSI Europe Board; a liveryman of the Society of Apothecaries, London; and a freeman of the City of London. His scientific publications are mainly in the area of food safety, and he is joint founding editor of the journal Food Additives and Contaminants. He is a former chair of the Food Group of the UK Society of Chemical Industry (SCI), former chairman of the Board of the European Technology Platform's "Food for Life," a former governing council member of the International Union of Food Science & Technology, and chair of its membership committee and various other committees dealing with food safety and regulatory affairs in EU food and drink associations.

Lucia E. Anelich, PhD

Professor Lucia Anelich has a PhD in microbiology and is currently the managing director of her own food safety training and consulting business, Anelich Consulting, which she started in 2011. Prior to that, she spent 5 years at the Consumer Goods Council of South Africa where she established and headed up a food safety body for the food industry, a first for the country, until 2010. Before joining the CGCSA, she spent 25 years in academia at the Tshwane University of Technology where she was the head of Department of Biotechnology and Food Technology and associate professor. She is a member of the International Commission on the Microbiological Specifications for Food (ICMSF), fellow of the International Academy of Food Science and Technology, past chair of the Scientific Council of IUFoST, immediate past chair of the Food Hygiene Committee of the South African Bureau of Standards, and immediate past president of the South African Association for Food Science and Technology. She is an adjunct professor at the Central University of Technology, South Africa and is currently a food safety expert for the African Union (AU) and a member of the advisory group establishing the AU Food Safety Authority.

Alan R. Boobis, OBE PhD

Alan Boobis is an Emeritus professor of toxicology at Imperial College London. He was a professor of biochemical pharmacology and director of the Toxicology Unit (supported by Public Health England and the Department of Health) at the Imperial College until June of 2017, when he retired after over 40 years at the college. His main research interests lie in mechanistic toxicology, drug metabolism, mode of action, and chemical risk assessment. He has published approximately 250 original research papers (h-index of 80). He is a member of several national and international advisory committees, the Committee on Toxicity (chair), the WHO Study Group on Tobacco Product Regulation, Joint FAO/WHO Expert Committee on Food Additives (veterinary residues), and Joint FAO/WHO Meeting on Pesticide Residues. He has been a member of the UK Advisory Committee on Pesticides, Committee on Carcinogenicity, the European Food Safety Authority (EFSA) Panel on Food Contaminants, and the EFSA Panel on Plant Protection Products and their Residues. He is a member and a past chair of the Board of Trustees of the International Life Sciences Institute (ILSI) and a member of the Board of Directors and has served as the vice president of ILSI Europe and has served as a member and chair of the Board of Trustees of the Health and Environmental Sciences Institute (HESI). He sits on several international scientific advisory boards, in both the public and private sectors. Awards include honorary fellow of the British Toxicology Society, fellow of the British Pharmacological Society, the BTS John Barnes Prize Lectureship, honorary membership and Merit Award of EUROTOX, the Royal Society of Chemistry

Toxicology Award, the Society of Toxicology Arnold J. Lehman Award, the Toxicology Forum Philippe Shubik Distinguished Scientist Award, and Officer of the British Empire (OBE).

Bert Popping, PhD

Dr. Bert Popping is an independent consultant and managing director of the strategic food consulting company FOCOS. He previously worked as chief scientific officer and director of Scientific Development and Regulatory Affairs for multinational contract laboratories. Dr. Popping has more than 20 years of experience in the food testing industry and has authored over 50 publications on topics related to food safety, food authenticity, food analysis, validation, and regulatory assessments. He also edited one book in this field. He is member of the editorial board of the Journal of Food Additives and Contaminants and the Journal of Food Analytical Methods. He serves on the Thought Leaders Advisory Committee of AOAC International and on panels of several other international organizations. He is an active member of numerous national and international organizations, including USP, CEN, ISO, BSI, and several governmental method working groups. He also chairs a recently established working group on emerging and future technology developments and their impact on food industry and consumers. In addition, Dr. Popping serves on the Board of Directors of AOAC International.

Foreword

Information about the safety of foods is critical to safeguard human health and well-being and to promote better food safety practices from farm to table. The dissemination of timely and relevant food safety and nutrition information is the mission of the International Life Sciences Institute (ILSI), and we're pleased to present the first edition of *Present Knowledge in Food Safety*.

A brand-new publication in 2022, *Present Knowledge in Food Safety* was launched with the goal of providing readers with current information addressing the many areas of food production and processing that are impacted by food safety concerns. Reflecting the global relevance of food safety, the authors encompass a variety of countries and are internationally recognized in the food safety arena.

ILSI is a worldwide nonprofit organization that seeks to foster science for the public good and collaboration among scientists, all governed by ILSI's core principles of scientific integrity. With 14 entities worldwide, 38 scientific publications, and 173 workshops in 2021, ILSI is a world leader in creating public–private partnerships that advance science and achieve positive, real-world impact for the betterment of public health.

We trust that this new publication will be a valuable resource for researchers, health professionals, educators, and advanced food microbiology and toxicology students. ILSI is proud of this contribution made by the authors and editors in advancing the field of food safety.

Kerr Dow
ILSI Board of Trustees

Michael Doyle
ILSI Board of Trustees

Preface

We are honored to edit the first edition of *Present Knowledge in Food Safety: A Risk-Based Approach Through The Food Chain*. The underlying concepts we adopted for the book are exposure-led risk assessment (wherever feasible) and management of changes in chemical, physical, and microbiological composition of food at all key stages of production from "farm to consumption."

Within this framework, the book has taken a holistic approach to food safety and identifies "critical control points" from the contributions of experts in their relevant fields: pre- and postharvest, slaughter, fishing and aquaculture; manufacture, packaging, and consumption; novel technologies; public understanding and communications of risk; hazard versus risk-based regulations and their impact on availability and trade; and, of course, the consequences of climate change on security and safety. The applications of the latest science and future developments in toxicology, including allergenicity and analysis, which improve reliability and predictability are also reviewed.

This food-chain approach, introducing new scientific ideas at each stage, is intended to stimulate reviews of established methodologies and recent research. It will also further the research agenda for improving food safety evaluation and management, and ultimately consumer protection.

In addition to print volumes, to make this first edition of *Present Knowledge in Food Safety: A Risk-Based Approach Through The Food Chain* as accessible and continuously relevant as possible, it is available in electronic formats. We hope this volume will be a valuable reference and resource for researchers, educators, advanced students of food safety, health professionals, and policy-makers.

Michael E. Knowles
Veria, Greece

Lucia E. Anelich
Pretoria, South Africa

Alan R. Boobis
London, United Kingdom

Bert Popping
Alzenau, Germany

Acknowledgments

The production of this new book on food safety, with its holistic approach through the food chain, required a commitment to its concept and a major application of time and effort by a large team of people. We would like to thank the authors of all chapters for contributing their respective expertise in a way that collectively meets the objectives of the book. Further, this first edition of *Present Knowledge in Food Safety* would not have been produced without the unremitting support, work, and guidance of James Cameron and Allison Worden of the International Life Sciences Institute, for which we are deeply grateful. The completion of a project of this size would not have been possible without the continuing forbearance of family, colleagues, and friends throughout its long gestation period and we owe them a deep debt of gratitude.

Section I

Changes in the chemical composition of food through the various stages of the food chain: plants before harvest

Chapter 1

Natural toxicants in plant-based foods, including herbs and spices and herbal food supplements, and accompanying risks

Ivonne M.C.M. Rietjens[1] **and Gerhard Eisenbrand**[2]

[1]*Division of Toxicology, Wageningen University, Wageningen, The Netherlands,* [2]*University of Kaiserslautern, Germany (Retired), Heidelberg, Germany*

Abstract

Our modern food chain may contain natural toxins from plants, either due to their natural presence in the plant-derived food or in the raw material used for food production or because these constituents are added during the regular production process, or present as contaminants. The present chapter presents an overview of situations where natural toxins from plants may raise concern, illustrated by examples of relevant structural features, toxic modes of action, their safety or risk assessment, and potential regulations related to their occurrence in the modern food chain. It is concluded that the safety concerns in part arise from the fact that botanicals and botanical preparations are considered food and thus a priori not subject to premarket evaluation and/or quality control for their safety in use. The chapter ends with a discussion presenting existing data gaps and research directions.

Keywords: Natural toxins; plant-based foods; mode of action; risks and regulation

1.1 Introduction

Plant-based foods are part of our daily diet in the form of fruits and vegetables, but also as herbs and spices, herbal teas and/or botanical food supplements and in specific cases even as herbal medicines. For some of these food categories, the estimated intakes are increasing because of the presumed beneficial health effects, a vegetarian diet, and/or the fact that botanicals and botanical preparations are generally accepted by consumers as 'natural' or "safe." This presumption of safety applies to a large number of plant-based foods, in part relying on a history of safe use, so that many botanical food constituents are generally regarded as safe at normal dietary intake. However, this does not hold for all plant-based foods since in some cases they may contain natural toxins of potential concern for human health. Plants synthesize secondary metabolites, so-called phytochemicals, as a defense mechanism against herbivores, insects, and pathogens.[1] Some of these plant constituents may raise a health concern in situations where consumers can be exposed to exceedingly high levels of intake. The present chapter presents an overview of situations where natural toxins from plants may raise concern, illustrated by examples of relevant structural features, toxic modes of action, their safety or risk assessment, and potential regulations related to their occurrence in the modern food chain. It is concluded that the safety concerns in part arise from the fact that botanicals and botanical preparations are considered food and thus a priori not subject to premarket evaluation and/or quality control for their safety in use. The chapter ends with a discussion presenting existing data gaps and research directions.

1.2 Risk and safety assessment of natural toxins from plants

At the current state-of-the-art, risk and safety assessment of the use of botanicals and botanical preparations in food is not harmonized around the world. In a study comparing the regulatory framework for botanical food supplements in the EU, the USA, Australia, Canada, New Zealand, India, Japan, and China it was concluded that national

Present Knowledge in Food Safety. DOI: https://doi.org/10.1016/B978-0-12-819470-6.00066-4

approaches towards regulation of for example botanical food supplements differ significantly.[2] However, national authorities are increasingly considering the implementation of intensified scrutiny for such products. This is in part due to human case studies reporting adverse health effects and the fact that some plant-based foods and/or their constituents may raise a concern for human health. Adverse effects of natural toxins from plant-based foods may arise under various conditions, as exemplified in some more detail below. Conditions and examples discussed include improper food handling so that levels of natural toxins present in plants may reach levels of concern, use of botanicals containing natural toxins as famine food, the occurrence of sensitive individuals in the population, use of food supplements or herbal teas containing constituents of concern, accidental switching of varieties and/or replacement of innocuous botanicals with toxic plants, abuse of botanical preparations and/or adulteration with pharmaceutical substances.

1.3 Situations where natural toxins from plants may raise concern: Improper food handling [toxic proteins, glycoalkaloids (GAs), quinolizidine alkaloids (QAs)]

Processing and preparation of plant-based foods can be an essential step to reduce levels of natural toxins. On the other hand, inadequate storage conditions may result in increased levels of natural plant toxins. This implies that improper food handling can be the cause of exposure to toxic levels of botanical constituents of concern. Examples of botanical constituents that could pose a concern for human health because of improper food handling include toxic proteins, GAs (solanines), and QAs. In the subsequent sections on famine food and sensitive individuals, there are additional examples including cyanogenic glycosides and furocoumarins (FCs).

1.3.1 Toxic proteins

1.3.1.1 Toxic proteins: relevant structural features

Toxic proteins are generated in plants as a defense mechanism against herbivores and microbes. Especially, lectins, inhibitors of proteolytic enzymes including trypsin and chymotrypsin, and ribosome-inactivating proteins (RIPs) have been associated with toxic effects on human health.[3] Lectins are present in plants of the *Leguminoseae*, *Solanaceae*, and *Gramineae* families, including chickpeas, mung beans, and soybeans. Nowadays, there are about 500 lectins commercially available. Toxic examples are Concanavalin A, soy hemagglutinin, kidney-bean agglutinin, black bean agglutinin, and Lima bean agglutinin.[3]

RIPs are another example of toxic proteins occurring in plant-based foods that require proper food processing to avoid adverse effects. More than 100 RIPs with varying degrees of toxicity have been isolated from different plants and bacteria.[4] Based on their structure, RIPs are grouped into different classes. Type I RIPs are polypeptides carrying an A domain which is the site of N-glycosidase activity. Type II RIPs carry, in addition to an A domain a B domain with lectin-binding properties, fused to the A domain by disulfide bonds. These properties facilitate entry into the cell, thus making Type II particularly cytotoxic. Examples are ricin from the castor oil plant, *Ricinus Communis*, and abrin isolated from the seeds of *Abrus precatorius* (jequirity or rosary pea).[3,4]

1.3.1.2 Toxic proteins: toxic mode of action and adverse effects

Lectins are inhibitors of serine protease enzymes reducing the activity of these enzymes in the digestion of proteins and carbohydrates, resulting in anti-nutritional effects. Interaction of the lectins with the gut epithelial cells can also cause gastrointestinal and immune distress, while the lectins may also cause agglutination of red blood cells.[3,5] Most of these toxic plant proteins can be detoxified by heat treatment, which implies that insufficient heating may result in adverse health effects.

RIPs catalyze the removal of a signal adenine from rRNA at the eukaryotic 60S ribosome by their N-glycosidase activity resulting in irreversible inhibition of protein synthesis.[4]

1.3.1.3 Toxic proteins: risk assessment

EFSA reported an oral LD_{50} of ricin up to 20–30 mg/ kg bw.[6] This LD_{50} upon oral exposure is about 1000 fold higher than the LD_{50} of 22 μg /kg bw in humans exposed via injection or inhalation. This difference is ascribed to the destruction of the constituents in the gastrointestinal tract upon oral exposure.[6] Ricin has also been classified as a potential biological warfare agent and a likely source of bioterrorism.[4] For abrin an estimated human fatal dose of 0.1–1 mg/kg bw has been reported and cases resulting in death after accidental poisoning due to both improper food handling and/or intentional poisoning have been reported.[7]

EFSA evaluated the risks of ricin because of the potential use of castor seed in animal feed. Upon this evaluation, EFSA concluded that RIPs are unlikely to become an issue in the modern food chain because the EU feed producers do not use castor seed meal as feed for livestock, and also because exposed animals are sensitive to ricin so they would be affected and are expected to not enter the food chain.[6]

1.3.2 Glycoalkaloids

1.3.2.1 Glycoalkaloids: relevant structural features

The second group of plant-based toxins that provide an example of food safety concerns upon improper food handling is the groups of glycoalkaloids (GAs) present in plants of the *Solanaceae*, or nightshade family, including potato (*Solanum tuberosum*), tomato (*Solanum lycopersicum*) and eggplant (*Solanum melongena).* Fig. 1.1 presents the structure of examples of GAs including α-solanine and α-chaconine (from potatoes), tomatine (from tomatoes), and solasonine (from eggplant), with the corresponding aglycones being solanidine, tomatidine, and solasodine. The GAs are usually concentrated in a 1.5 mm layer under the skin and this implies that peeling will remove a large part (50%–95%) of the GAs.[8] GAs are hardly affected by food processing (baking, cooking, and frying) but their content is influenced by the type of cultivar and original total GA content, by light, mechanical injury and storage.[8]

1.3.2.2 Glycoalkaloids: toxic mode of action and adverse effects

Adverse effects that occur upon α-solanine and α-chaconine poisoning include gastrointestinal disturbances like vomiting, diarrhea, and usually severe abdominal pain and, when the constituents are consumed at high dose levels, also neurological disorders including drowsiness and apathy, confusion, weakness, and visual disturbances.[8,9] The adverse effects may also include fever, rapid and weak pulse, low blood pressure, and rapid respiration.[8]

The underlying mode of action relates to the inhibition of acetylcholinesterase, the enzyme required for the degradation of the neurotransmitter acetylcholine.[8]

1.3.2.3 Glycoalkaloids: risk assessment

Health-based guidance values for solanine like an acute reference dose (ARfD) or tolerable daily intake (TDI) have not been defined. The maximum safe acute oral dose of total potato GAs has been estimated to be about 1 mg/kg bw, the acute toxic dose between 2 and 5 mg total GAs/kg bw, while a dose between 3 and 6 mg total GAs/kg bw may be lethal.[8] The Federal Institute for Risk Assessment (BfR) has derived a No Observed Adverse Effect Level (NOAEL) which is defined as the highest dose at which no adverse health effect would be expected, of 0.5 mg/ kg bw/day.[10] The BfR and also JECFA[11] concluded that GA levels found in normally grown potatoes (50–100 mg/kg potatoes), would not result in intake levels of concern. However, potatoes that have been exposed to light, mechanical injury, and started to green, can have concentrations of 1000 mg/kg or more.[8,12] Thus proper handling of this plant-based food is essential to make sure the GA level in potatoes for human consumption remains at a safe level.

α-Tomatine is considered to be 20 times less toxic than the GAs found in potatoes. This is illustrated by the fact that Peruvians were reported to consume tomatoes with an α-tomatine content of 500–5000 mg/kg dry weight without experiencing adverse health effects and the fact that no poisoning in humans due to consumption of tomatoes has been reported.[13,14]

1.3.3 Quinolizidine alkaloids

1.3.3.1 Quinolizidine alkaloids: relevant structural features

QAs are another example of botanical constituents that may become a concern upon improper handling of plant-based foods. Especially QAs in plants from the genus lupinus raise a concern.

The most common QAs are sparteine and lupanine, 13α-hydroxylupanin, α-isolupanine, and anagyrine (Fig. 1.2). The Australia New Zealand Food Authority (ANZFA, now called FSANZ Food Standards Australia New Zealand) indicated that anagyrine is absent in lupin cultivars for human use.[15,16]

Bitter and sweet lupin varieties vary in their QA content. The QA level may amount to > 10,000 mg QAs /kg dry matter and < 500 mg/kg dry matter in bitter and sweet lupin respectively.[17] Seeds (also referred to as

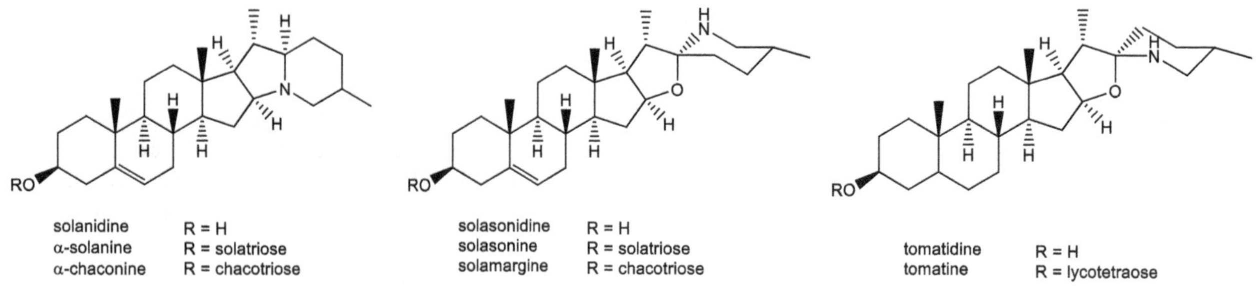

FIGURE 1.1 Chemical structures of glycoalkaloids.

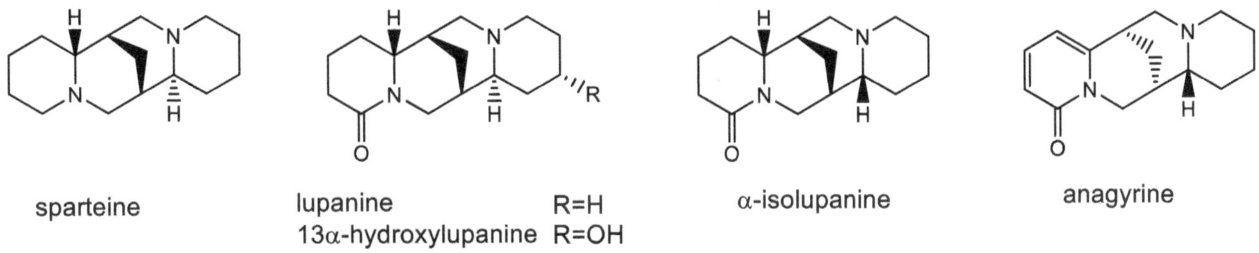

FIGURE 1.2 Chemical structures of quinolizidine alkaloids.

beans) from bitter lupins, also known as European lupins, are consumed in Southern Europe. Before consumption, the QA level in these seeds is reduced through a debittering process involving extensive soaking or washing with water followed by cooking.[18] De-bittered lupin seeds contain QAs at levels of approximately 500 mg/kg.[15] Australian lupin varieties, resulting from plant breeding programs, and known as sweet lupins, contain much lower QA levels.[15] The mean total alkaloid content of Australian sweet lupin (*L. angustifolius*) seeds amounts to 130–150 mg/kg.[15] Human exposure to QAs mainly results from the use of lupin flour from these low QA varieties to partly substitute wheat floor in preparation of bakery products, or to replace soybean flour, and/or from lupin-based meals, pasta, pastries, cakes, biscuits and others.[8,15,16]

1.3.3.2 Quinolizidine alkaloids: toxic mode of action and adverse effects

Some case studies of acute toxicity of QAs in humans have reported adverse effects because of consumption of bitter lupin flour containing 100 times the allowed QA level.[19] Moreover, poisoning cases after ingestion of raw or inadequately cooked lupin seeds have been reported,[20,21] as well as a case resulting from drinking half a liter of water used for de-bittering of lupin seeds.[22] Even some cases with fatal outcomes were reported in children after consumption of nondebittered lupin seeds.[23,24] Acute lupin toxicity leads to an anticholinergic syndrome resulting in agitation, blurry vision, tachycardia, mydriasis, dry mouth, urinary retention, delirium, and even death.[20,21,23] These adverse effects of QAs have been ascribed to the blocking of the nicotinic cholinergic receptor and a weak antagonistic effect on the muscarinic cholinergic receptor.[22]

1.3.3.3 Quinolizidine alkaloids: risk assessment

The Australia New Zealand Food Authority (ANZFA) concluded that a daily dose of 0.35 mg lupin alkaloids/kg bw can be tolerated in human adults without adverse effects. An uncertainty factor of 10 was applied to account for uncertainties in the data and interindividual human variation, and a provisional TDI for humans of 0.035 mg lupin alkaloids/kg bw/day was established.[15] Koleva et al. concluded that a daily intake of 0.125 mg lupin alkaloids/kg bw/day would not be a safety concern, based on a NOAEL of 12.5 mg/kg bw/day from subchronic toxicity studies in rats and a safety factor of 100.[8]

Given that the seeds of modern cultivars (i.e., 'sweet lupins' of *L. angustifolius*) contain <200 mg alkaloids/kg, this would imply a daily consumption of 10.7–37.2 g of sweet lupin seeds to be tolerable. This calculation underlines that control of QA levels and adequate debittering of lupin seeds and/or flour used for food purposes is essential.

1.4 Situations where natural toxins from plants may raise concern: Famine food (cyanogenic glycosides, lathyrogens)

Periods of famine due to a shortage of food may provide situations in which ingestion of toxins present in plant-based foods may cause adverse health effects. To illustrate this, two important groups of toxins will be discussed in more detail, including the cyanogenic glycosides and lathyrogens.

1.4.1 Cyanogenic glycosides

1.4.1.1 Cyanogenic glycosides: relevant structural features

Cyanogenic glycosides can be present in more than 2600 plant species, including up to 26 economically important crops.[25] They include compounds like amygdalin (present in bitter almonds and apricot kernels), dhurrin (present in sorghum), linamarin and lotaustralin (both present in cassava), linustatin and neolinustatin (both present in linseed), prunasin (present in *Prunus* species) and its diastereoisomer sambunigrin (present in the elderberry plant *Sambucus nigra*, but not in its ripe berries) (Fig. 1.3).

Cyanogenic glycosides all contain a cyano (CN) moiety in their structure which results in the production of hydrogen cyanide (HCN) upon their metabolic conversion. Hydrolysis may be catalyzed by β-glucosidases liberated upon the destruction of the plant tissue, or by the

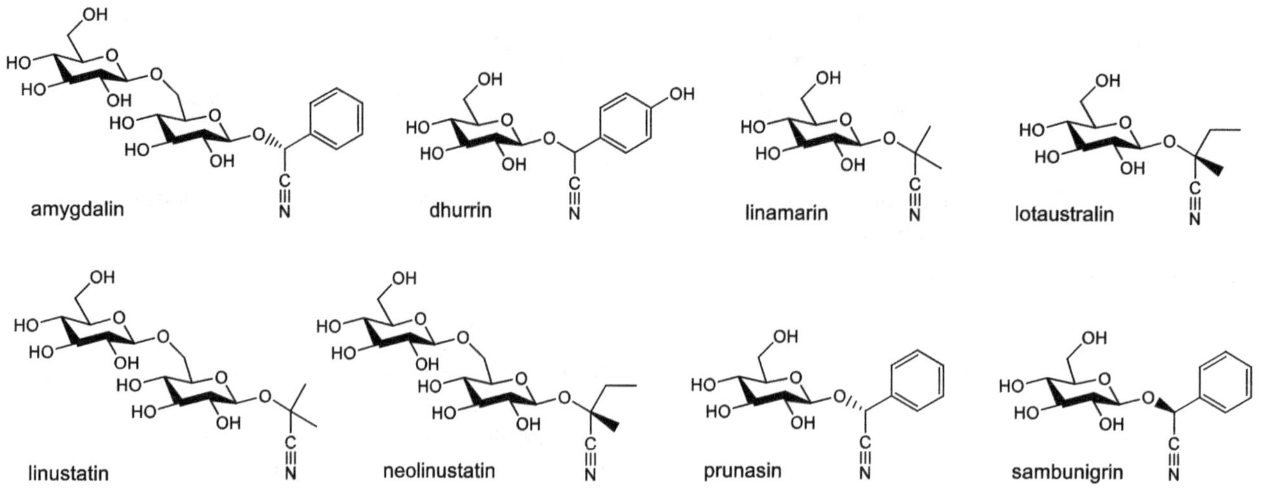

FIGURE 1.3 Chemical structures of cyanogenic glycosides.

intestinal microflora upon oral intake.[25] The HCN formed from cyanogenic glycosides raises health concerns.

Linamarin is present in the roots of cassava (*Manihot esculenta*) at levels of 10–1120 mg HCN (free and bound)/kg, and also in Lima bean seeds (*Phaseolus lunatus*) at levels of 100–3000 mg HCN (free and bound)/kg.[25] Dhurrin is naturally present in sorghum, and amygdalin in seeds of apples and pears, and the leaves, fruit, and seeds of black cherry, almond, cherry, plum, peach, and apricot trees at levels up to 300–4000 mg HCN (free and bound)/kg.[25,26] Linseed may contain linustatin and neolinustatin at levels up to 100–300 mg HCN (free and bound)/kg.[25]

Cassava is one of the most drought-tolerant crops that can be successfully grown on marginal soils and gives reasonable yields where many other crops do not grow well. Cassava is also a major staple food in the developing world. The more toxic varieties of cassava are a "food security crop" in times of famine or food insecurity.

Other food items that may contain cyanogenic glycosides are almonds and/or marzipan-containing confectionery and baked goods. These may contain levels up to 40 mg/kg, with raw marzipan paste containing levels of up to 50 mg/kg HCN (free and bound)/kg.[26]

1.4.1.2 Cyanogenic glycosides: toxic mode of action and adverse effects

Cyanogenic glycosides are an example of plant-based food toxins of potential concern from use as a famine food and also because of improper food handling. Cassava must be cooked properly to release and detoxify the cyanide before consumption. The cyanide causes adverse effects via binding to cytochrome oxidase in the mitochondrial electron transport chain, thereby disturbing ATP production or even blocking cellular respiration. Especially the central nervous system is sensitive to this adverse effect because of its high dependence on energy supply via oxidative phosphorylation.[25] Detoxification of HCN in humans proceeds via conversion to thiocyanate (historic name rhodanide) (SCN^-) by the enzyme rhodanase. Of note, thiocyanate is well known to inhibit iodide uptake in the thyroid, causing or aggravating goiter.

1.4.1.3 Cyanogenic glycosides: risk assessment

In their evaluation of cyanogenic glycosides, EFSA established an ARfD of 20 μg/kg bw for cyanide.[27] Acute cyanide toxicity can cause headache, tightness in the throat and chest, muscle weakness, nausea, vomiting, giddiness, headache, palpitations, hyperpnoea, then dyspnea, bradycardia, unconsciousness, and violent convulsions, followed by death.[25,27] Chronic exposure to linamarin from cassava has been reported to cause malnutrition, diabetes, congenital malformations, neurological disorder, and myelopathy.[28] Exposure to linamarin via consumption of cassava has also been proposed as the cause of Konzo, a form of tropical myelinopathy with sudden onset of spastic paralysis.[29] Goiter may occur when cyanogenic glycosides are present at a level of 10–50 mg/kg in food.[30] So far a TDI as a health-based guidance value for chronic exposure to cyanide has not been established.

Also in Europe cases of adverse health effects linked to exposure to cyanogenic glycosides have been reported resulting from the consumption of apricot kernels containing amygdalin as snacks. Life-threatening conditions and even death were reported after consumption of bitter apricot kernels or bitter almonds.[25] Levels as high as 2750 mg cyanide/kg kernels, reported in the Rapid Alert System for Food and Feed (RASFF) portal would imply that consumption of already 1 kernel by a 70 kg adult gives rise to exposure at the level of the ARfD of 20 μg/kg bw for cyanide. In line with this estimation, EFSA in its opinion on the acute health risks related to the presence of cyanogenic glycosides in raw apricot kernels and products derived from raw apricot kernels concluded that the ARfD for cyanide would be exceeded by the consumption of one small kernel by a toddler and consumptions of 3 small or one large kernel by an adult.[27] Despite this, raw apricot kernels are marketed as a snack in portions of 100 g. In addition on the internet cancer patients are advised to consume 10–60 kernels a day. Meanwhile in many countries supplements containing amygdalin (also called laetrile or vitamin B17), promoted as an alternative drug to treat cancer, are illegal. The use of these supplements containing amygdalin at 500 mg per capsule would result in exposure equal to 400 μg/kg bw cyanide for a 70 kg adult, thereby substantially exceeding the ARfD.

Although case studies of acute toxicity resulting from consumption of apricot kernels as a snack or consumption of insufficiently detoxified fresh cassava roots have been reported,[25] longer-term use of cassava as a "food security crop" in times of famine or food insecurity also raises health concerns with respect to chronic adverse health effects of this class of plant-based food toxins. Especially in periods of drought and famine, it may be expected that adequate maceration of the cassava roots for detoxication before consumption becomes an issue.

Some regulations on levels of cyanide in food have been installed. These include a ban on products containing amygdalin, including apricot kernels, as free-over-the-counter products.[25] Furthermore, HCN shall not be added as such to food, while the level of naturally occurring HCN is restricted to a maximum of 5 mg/kg for canned stone fruits, 50 mg/kg for "nougat, marzipan or its substitutes or similar products", and 35 mg/kg for alcoholic beverages. A maximum level of 10 mg/kg is established for edible cassava flour products.[25]

1.4.2 Lathyrogens

1.4.2.1 Lathyrogens: relevant structural features

Lathyrogens are toxins present in certain legumes of the genus *Lathyrus, especially Lathyrus sativus* (also known as *grass pea*) and to a lesser degree *Lathyrus cicera, Lathyrus ochrus*, and *Lathyrus clymenum*.

1.4.2.2 Lathyrogens: toxic mode of action and adverse effects

The toxin, β-oxalyl-L-α,β-diaminopropionic acid (ODAP, also known as β-*N*-oxalyl-amino-L-alanine, or BOAA) causes neurotoxicity by acting as a structural analog of the neurotransmitter glutamate.[31] The adverse effects include paralysis, reflected by a lack of strength in the lower limbs or an inability to move the lower limbs. The disease is also called neurolathyrism.[31] Consumption of *Lathyrus odoratus* seeds (*sweet peas*) causes osteolathyrism, resulting from an effect of the toxin beta-aminopropionitrile on the formation of cross-connections between collagen and elastin, resulting in weakness of the connective tissue including skin, bones, and blood vessels.[32]

1.4.2.3 Lathyrogens: risk assessment

In spite of knowledge of how to detoxify Lathyrus, by soaking the peas with water and cooking,[33] drought conditions can lead to fuel and water shortages preventing these necessary detoxification steps from being taken. Excessive consumption of these *Lathyrus* seeds may be caused especially by a lack of alternative food sources. Lathyrism can also be caused by food adulteration. *Lathyrus sativus* L. is mentioned in the EFSA compendium of botanicals that have been reported to contain toxic, addictive, psychotropic, or other substances of concern.[34] The EFSA compendium also indicates that there is little information on the toxic dose for humans but that Ludolph and Spencer[35] suggest a toxic dose of BOAA of 15–150 mg/kg bw/day estimated to amount to an accumulated dose of 1.35–13.5 g/kg bw over a typical latent period of 90 days.

1.5 Situations where natural toxins from plants may raise concern: Sensitive individuals (allergens, fava glucosides, and FCs)

Natural toxins from plants may also raise concern for specific, vulnerable subgroups in the population. This is obvious for plant-based food allergens against which consumers may be sensitized. There are, however, also other examples of plant-based toxins that pose a risk to specific subgroups within the populations. Two examples to be discussed in some more detail are fava glycosides and FCs.

1.5.1 Allergens

Plant-based allergens in food that raise concern include allergens from cereals containing gluten, peanuts, soy, tree nuts, celery mustard sesame, and lupin. These all belong to the 14 major food allergens requiring adequate labeling by law. These plant-based toxins are discussed in more detail in Chapter 52, and therefore not discussed to a further extent in this section, but they do represent an example of natural plant toxins that raise a concern for specific subgroups in the population. Risk management of

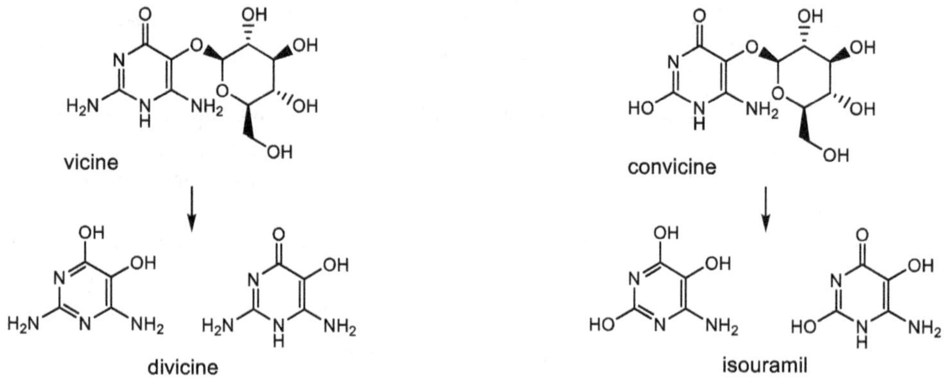

FIGURE 1.4 Chemical structure of vicine and convicine and their hydrolysis to divicine and isouramil showing the two possible tautomeric forms of the aglycones.

this class of toxins is achieved by adequate and obligatory food labeling.

1.5.2 Fava pyrimidine glycosides

1.5.2.1 Fava pyrimidine glycosides: relevant structural features

Fava pyrimidine glycosides from fava beans (*Vicia faba*) include compounds like vicine and convicine (Fig. 1.4) which are known to cause favism, a hemolytic response of the red blood cells.

1.5.2.2 Fava pyrimidine glycosides: toxic mode of action and adverse effects

Favism is observed especially in subjects with a genetic predisposition because of a defect in the gene for glucose-6-phosphate dehydrogenase (G6PD).[36] It is a heritable X chromosomal-recessive disease, prevailing in about 10% of South-Sahara Africans and the Mediterranean area, but also in certain South East Asian regions. One reason for this prevalence in specific populations was supposed to result from enhanced resistance against Malaria infections brought about by the G6PD-gene defect. G6PD is important for maintaining adequate levels of NADPH, relevant for maintaining the glutathione (GSH) status in red blood cells, especially for regeneration of reduced glutathione by GSH reductase, requiring NADPH as the cofactor. Deficient G6PD and resulting NADPH and GSH deficiency, make red blood cells more sensitive to oxidative challenges.

Upon consumption of fava beans, the fava glycosides vicine and convicine are hydrolyzed by the intestinal microflora to their respective aglycons, divicine, and isouramil (Fig. 1.4), which are facilitating high levels of free radical generation via redox cycling.[37] The ROS production and the resulting oxidative stress result in GSH oxidation.

1.5.2.3 Fava pyrimidine glycosides: risk assessment

In healthy individuals, oxidized glutathione can be efficiently reduced by glutathione reductase at the cost of NADPH, and ROS production is not a problem. However, in individuals with a deficiency for G6PD, this GSH regeneration is hampered. In consequence, GSH is depleted and ROS levels in the red blood cells are enhanced, resulting in hemolytic anemia. Favism has been reported in 35 countries with over 3000 cases, involving especially children.[38] The data indicate that favism occurs especially in areas where the frequency of G6PD deficiency is relatively high and fava beans (also known as broad beans) are a popular food item. This includes southern Europe, the Middle East, and Southeast Asia but not, for example, northern Germany, where fava beans are grown but G6PD deficiency is rare, or West Africa, where G6PD deficiency has a high prevalence but fava beans are not grown.

Food safety with respect to this health concern is best guaranteed by assuring that G6PD deficient and thus sensitive subjects refrain from fava bean consumption.

1.5.3 Furocoumarins

1.5.3.1 Furocoumarins: relevant structural features

Furocoumarins (FCs) are natural constituents of foods, especially from carrot plants (*Apiaceae*, *Umbelliferae*), legume plants (*Fabaceae*), and citrus plants (*Rutaceae*), including food items like celery, parsnip, carrots, and various citrus fruits and juices thereof.[39] They are formed particularly under stress conditions such as microbial infections.[25] Depending on the position of the furan ring with respect to the coumarin ring, FCs are divided into linear psoralene-type FCs, including 8-methoxypsoralene (8-MOP) and 5-methoxypsoralene (5-MOP), and angular angelicin-type FCs (Fig. 1.5).

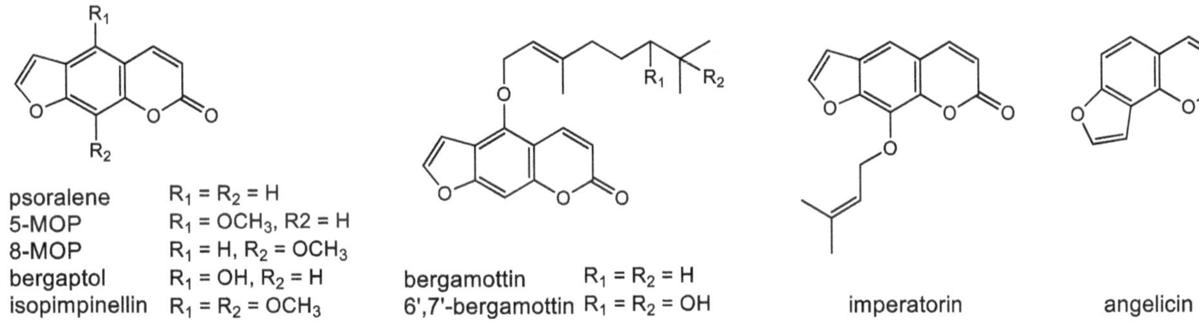

FIGURE 1.5 Chemical structure of furocoumarins.

1.5.3.2 Furocoumarins: toxic mode of action and adverse effects

In combination with UVA FCs may trigger phototoxicity due to their activation to reactive intermediates that interact with cellular target molecules such as proteins and nucleic acids resulting in skin lesions, mutagenicity, or even carcinogenicity.[40,41] The FCs 8-MOP and psoralen have been classified as class 1 human carcinogens when they are combined with UV light.[42] Both, 5-MOP and 8-MOP are genotoxic. In a 2-year study with 8-MOP in rats, even the lowest tested dose of 37.5 mg/kg bw/day was nephrotoxic and carcinogenic.[41] However, a conclusive estimation of the carcinogenic risk to humans was not considered feasible, due to the complexity of the influencing factors, particularly the levels of exposure, the metabolism, its modulation, and the influence of light.[41] Relative potency factors for the photogenotoxicity of a range of FCs indicate differences in potency.[43]

Some human volunteer studies reported acute toxicity effects after oral intake of FCs in combination with sunlight or UVA light.[40] The phototoxicity effects relate to adverse effects on the skin including erythemas, oedemas, and blisters observed in human volunteers exposed to oral doses of 50 mg 8-MOP and exposed to sunlight or exposed via consumption of 450-gram celery resulting in an estimated intake of 45 mg FCs, followed by about 30 min UVA exposure.[40,44] Human thresholds for occurrence of phototoxic effects of 14 mg 8-MOP (0.23 mg/kg bw) and of 15 mg 8-MOP equivalents (0.25 mg/kg bw) were reported.[44,45] Adverse effects are especially observed in specific subgroups of the population in which FC exposure is combined with exposure to UVA or sunlight, such as psoriasis patients or patients with other skin diseases. Oral therapeutic doses of FCs may amount to 0.5–0.6 mg 8-MOP/kg bw or 1.2 mg 5-MOP/kg bw in combination with UVA, exceeding these thresholds.

Another adverse effect related to FC exposure relates to their potential to inhibit cytochromes P450 including CYP1A, CYP2B, and CYP3A enzymes. This may result in untoward food-drug interactions such as the ones ascribed to the inhibition, especially of CYP3A enzymes by bergamottin and analogs present in grapefruit juice. Because this may affect drug metabolism it may lead, for instance, to increased maximum plasma levels and prolonged half-lives, potentially resulting in adverse health effects.[46]

1.5.3.3 Furocoumarins: risk assessment

The Senate Commission on Food Safety (SKLM) of the German Research Foundation (DFG) performed a risk assessment of FCs in foods, considering data on exposure, metabolism, kinetics, toxicity, carcinogenicity, reproductive and developmental toxicity, as well as the effects of these substances on xenobiotic metabolism.[40,41] FC levels in fruits and vegetables may depend on cultivation and storage conditions, with high levels reported for inappropriately stored samples of celery and parsnip infected by microorganisms.[40] Microbiologically infected parsnips may contain concentrations of 570–2500 mg/kg.[40] The average concentration in retail parsnips amounts to values between 20 and 124 mg/kg.[40] Consumption of such microbiologically infected celery or parsnip roots, may lead to intakes of more than 100 mg per person, equivalent to 1.67 mg/kg bw for a 60 kg person which exceeds the human threshold of 0.23–0.25 mg/kg bw. Intake from a normal diet has been estimated to be substantially lower, amounting to values that vary from 0.56 to 1.45 mg/person which is equivalent to 0.010–0.024 mg/kg bw for a 60 g person.[40,41] Based on these average intake estimates, the SKLM concluded that the consumption of typical quantities of plant-derived foods that potentially contain FCs, including flavored soft drinks, does not present a significant risk regarding phototoxic effects when these foods are appropriately stored or processed.[40,41]

Thus FCs present an example of plant-based food constituents that may raise concerns upon improper food handling for specific individuals, including especially patients under UVA treatment and or high consumers of celery and parsnips, because there is a risk for significant increases in FC concentrations, depending on the storage, processing and production conditions.

1.6 Situations where "normal" dietary intake of natural toxins from plant-based foods may raise concern

In contrast to situations where improper food handling raises levels of natural toxins to values that raise concern, or when especially sensitive individuals are at risk, there are also situations where "normal" dietary intake of natural toxins from plant-based foods may pose a risk to the general population. Especially use of herbal teas and plant-based food supplements, considered to be food in the European regulation,[2] may result in intake levels that raise a concern. Examples of plant-derived toxins for which this holds are glucosinolates, allylalkoxybenzenes, and pyrrolizidine alkaloids (PAs).

1.6.1 Glucosinolates

1.6.1.1 Glucosinolates: relevant structural features

Glucosinolates are found in cruciferous vegetables (Brassicceae) like broccoli, cauliflower, Brussels sprouts, kale, and cabbage but also in rapeseed, important for edible oil production, where the press cake is going into animal feed. In these plants over 120 different glucosinolates have been found, including aliphatic, aromatic, and indolic glucosinolates (Fig. 1.6).[47]

1.6.1.2 Glucosinolates: toxic mode of action and adverse effects

Glucosinolates need activation via hydrolysis to isothiocyanates (ITCs) and other metabolites by myrosinases, enzymes that are liberated upon damage of the plant tissues (Fig. 1.6).

Because ITCs have been related to beneficial health effects, including chemopreventive and chemotherapeutic effects, functional foods and food supplements based on ITC containing plants or containing ITCs as isolated compounds, have been developed. However, the electrophilic reactivity of ITCs, considered to induce beneficial effects, at the same time may bring about adverse effects, such as potential genotoxicity by the formation of DNA adducts. Beneficial effects relate to the induction of the Kelch-like ECH-associated protein 1 (Keap1)-nuclear factor erythroid 2-related factor 2 (Nrf2)-antioxidant response element (ARE) pathway, also called the electrophile

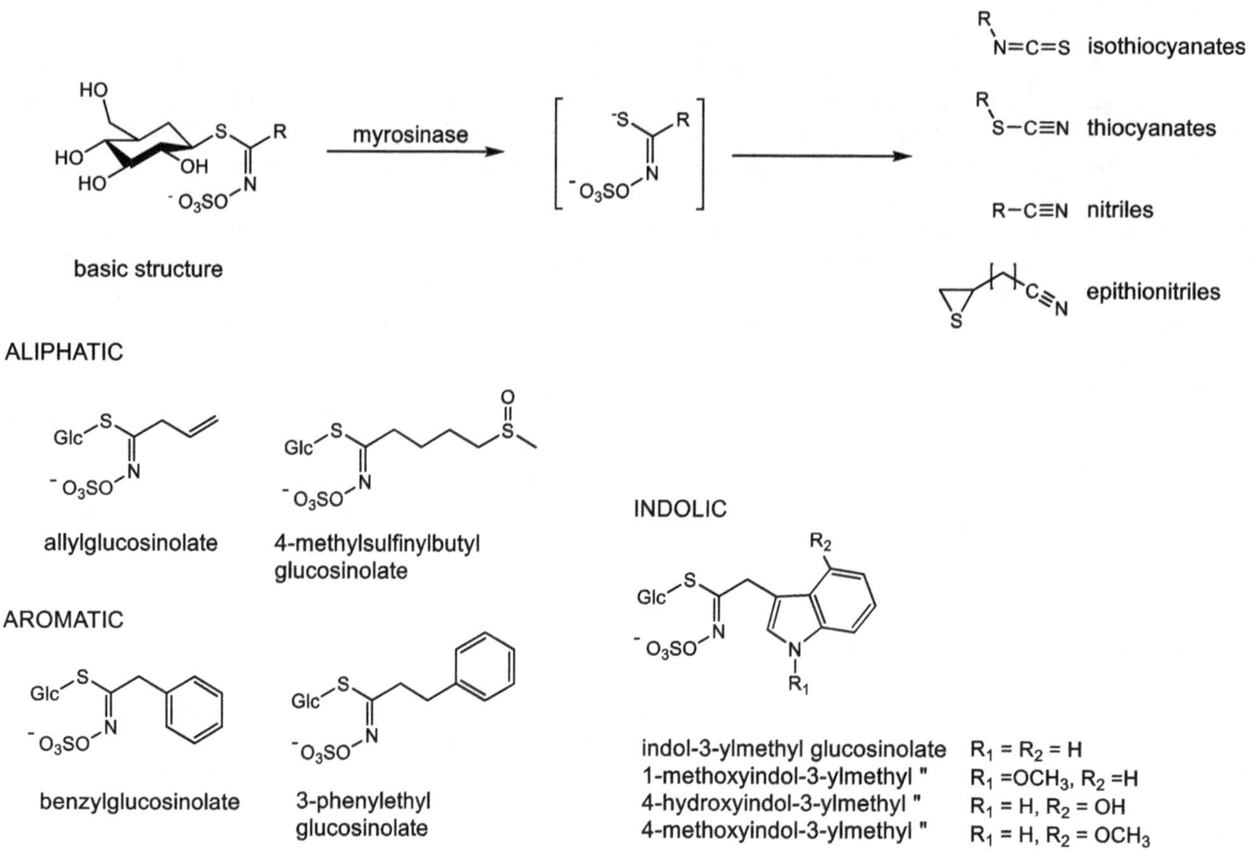

FIGURE 1.6 Chemical structure of aliphatic, aromatic, and indolic glucosinolates, and their bioactivation to isothiocyanates, thiocyanate, nitriles, and epithionitriles upon conversion by myrosinase.

responsive element (EpRE) dependent pathway. Induction of Nrf2 mediated gene expression results in increased levels of enzymes involved in protection against oxidative and electrophilic stress and Keap1-Nrf2-EpRE/ARE has been considered a critical anti-cancer pathway in chemoprevention.[48] Regular daily (co)exposure to ITCs may prevent the formation of DNA adducts by well-known food-borne carcinogens like aflatoxin B1, and PhIP (2-amino-1-methyl-6-phenylimidazo[4,5-b]pyridine).[49] Likewise, oxidative DNA damage, such as the formation of 8-oxo-7,8-dihydro-2-deoxyguanosine (8-oxodG) upon exposure to 2-nitropropane can be counteracted.[49] However, ITC mediated DNA adduct formation in *Salmonella typhimurium* exposed to brassica tissue homogenates and/or pure glucosinolates in the presence of myrosinase has also been reported.[50] Moreover, the mechanism underlying the potent genotoxicity, both, in bacterial and in mammalian cells of 1-methoxy-3-indolylmethyl glucosinolate has been described.[51]

1.6.1.3 Glucosinolates: risk assessment

The actual risk-benefit balance related to daily and/or irregular consumption of these bioactive plant-derived constituents remains to be established. There is agreement that beneficial effects, such as reducing cancer risk, appear attributable to glucosinolate-derived degradation products like ITCs and indoles, formed by the hydrolytic action of plant myrosinase and/or glucosidases deriving from the human microbial flora. The same decomposition products appear, however also responsible for detrimental effects, encompassing antinutritive and especially genotoxic activities of ICTs. Although the relevance of genotoxic activities to human health is not known yet, a qualitative comparison of the benefit and risks of broccoli consumption suggested the benefit from intake in modest quantities and processed forms outweigh the potential risks.[52] For other preparations (fortified broccoli-based dietary supplements, diets with extraordinary high daily intake, consumption as a raw vegetable) further studies, both for potential risks and beneficial effects appear required.[52]

1.6.2 Alkenylbenzenes including allylalkoxybenzenes and 1-propenylalkoxybenzenes

1.6.2.1 Alkenylbenzenes: structural features

Some botanicals raise a concern in the modern food chain because they contain naturally occurring substances that are genotoxic and carcinogenic. Examples can be found in the group of alkenylbenzenes containing compounds like the allylalkoxybenzenes estragole, methyleugenol, elemicin, safrole, myristicin, and apiole (Fig. 1.7). Safrole, estragole, and methyleugenol are genotoxic and hepatocarcinogenic in experimental animals.[53,54] For methyleugenol, DNA adducts have also been detected in the liver samples of human subjects.[55,56]

High levels of these constituents can be found in several herbs and spices and their essential oils. Safrole, methyleugenol, and/or estragole are constituents of for example nutmeg (*Myristica fragrans*), star anise (*Illicium verum*), and cinnamon (*Cinnamomum*), tarragon (*Artemisia dracunculus*), sweet basil (*Ocimum basilicum*), and fennel (*Foeniculum vulgare*). Myristicin occurs in nutmeg (*M. fragrans*), elemicin in nutmeg (*M. fragrans*), parsley (*Petroselinum crispum*), sassafras (*Sassafras albidum*), and apiole in parsley (*P. crispum*).[57] The compounds are present in the herbs but also in their essential

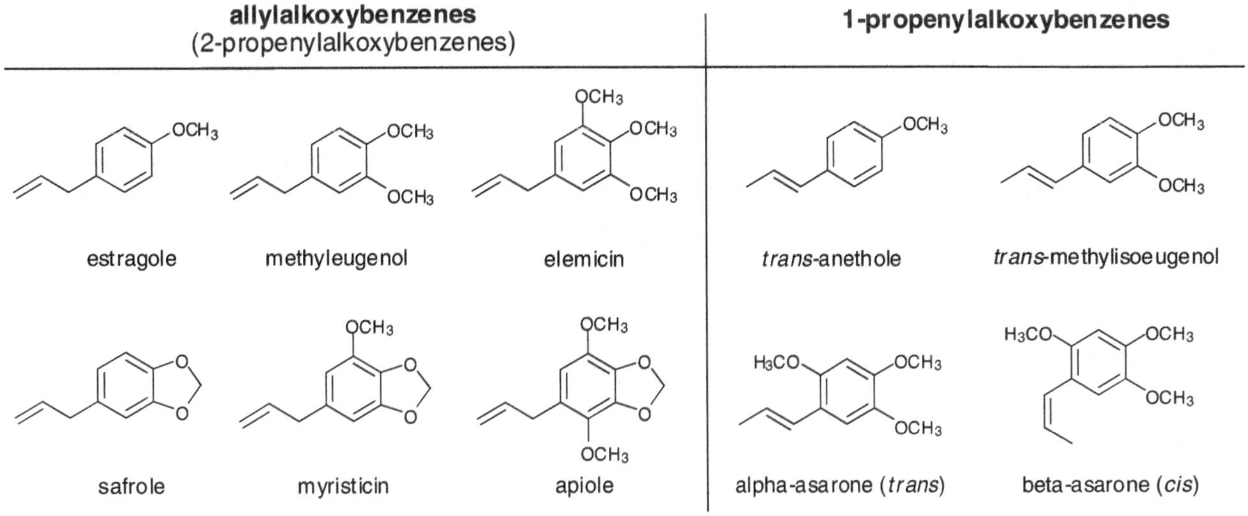

FIGURE 1.7 Chemical structures of allylalkoxybenzenes (2-propenylalkoxybenzenes) and 1-propenylalkoxybenzenes.

oils as well as in food products derived from these plants such as basil-based pesto sauce, some cola drinks, and herbal food supplements.[25,57]

The group of alkenylbenzenes also contains a series of 1-propenylalkoxybenzenes including *trans*-anethole, alpha- and beta-asarone, and *trans*-methylisoeugenol (Fig. 1.7). Alpha-asarone is a constituent of plants of the genus *Acorus* (e.g., *Acorus calamus* and *Acorus gramineus*), hazelwort (*Asarum europaeum*), and some peppers (e.g., *Piper sarmentosum*). Beta-asarone is found in hazelwort and *A. calamus*.[58] The SCF[58] estimated the daily exposure to beta-asarone from the use of Calamus oil in food including alcoholic beverages to amount to levels up to 115 μg/person/day equal to 2 μg/kg bw/day for a 60 kg person.

1.6.2.2 Alkenylbenzenes: toxic mode of action and adverse effects

Bioactivation of allylalkoxybenzenes to DNA reactive metabolites proceeds by cytochrome P450 (P450) mediated 1′-hydroxylation followed by sulfotransferase (SULT) mediated formation of the 1′-sulfooxy metabolite (Fig. 1.8).[57,59]

Evidence for the carcinogenicity of these allylalkoxybenzenes comes especially from rodent bioassays that reveal increased incidences of hepatocellular adenomas and carcinomas at high dose levels.[59–61]

For the 1-propenylalkoxybenzenes the liver is also the target organ for toxicity. *Trans*-anethole was reported to induce liver carcinogenicity when given at high dietary dose levels to female Sprague Dawley rats,[62] and alpha- and beta-asarone induced hepatocellular carcinomas in male C57BL/6 J × C3H/HeJ F1 mice.[59] Data on induction of leiomyosarcomas in the intestine of male rats by beta-asarone revealed a $BMDL_{10}$ of 9.6–21.5 mg/kg bw/day.[63] Similar tumors were found in rats treated with calamus oils.[58]

In contrast to the mode of action underlying the carcinogenicity of allylalkoxybenzenes, for *trans*-anethole, a nongenotoxic mode of action may apply. This is assumed to proceed via the formation of anethole-1′,2′-epoxide, which may induce hepatotoxicity and eventually regenerative hyperplasia (references[57,64,65] and therein). Although *trans*-anethole was reported to induce the formation of DNA adducts, identified by ^{32}P-post labeling in turkey fetal egg livers,[66] a nongenotoxic mode of action for *trans*-anethole is favored, supported by negative results in several in vitro and in vivo genotoxicity studies.[57]

This is also supported by the mode of action underlying the bioactivation and resulting carcinogenicity of alpha- and beta-asarone. It is different from that of safrole, methyleugenol, and estragole since there appears to be no role for SULT mediated bioactivation as shown for estragole and safrole.[59,67–69] This difference originates from the different positions of the double bond in the side chain in the 1′-propenylalkoxybenzenes and the allylalkoxybenzenes (Fig. 1.7). And although DNA reactivity of the side-chain epoxides of alpha- and beta-asarone was observed in vitro,[70] beta-asarone tested negative in an in vivo micronucleus test in the bone marrow of mice exposed orally.[71] Given the putative pivotal role of the epoxide metabolites in the toxicity of these 1-propenylalkoxybenzenes, it is of interest to note that the allylalkoxybenzenes are also converted to epoxide metabolites that appeared to be DNA-reactive in vitro. However, the accumulation of the respective DNA adducts in vivo appeared to be minimal because of the swift detoxification of the respective epoxides by epoxide hydrolases and/or glutathione *S*-transferases.[72–75]

For *trans*-methylisoeugenol data on carcinogenicity are not available, but it was previously concluded that the rate of DNA adduct formation was very low, both in vitro in rat hepatocytes and in vivo in mice[72,76,77] Furthermore, epoxidation of its side-chain is a minor metabolic pathway so a genotoxic mode of action seems to be rather unlikely.[25]

1.6.2.3 Alkenylbenzenes: risk assessment

The scientific committee on food (SCF) concluded that safrole, estragole, and methyleugenol are genotoxic and carcinogenic indicating restrictions for use in food.[78–80] As a result, in Europe the use of estragole, methyleugenol, and safrole as flavoring substances in foodstuffs is prohibited since 2008, and only as naturally occurring constituents maximum levels of these are allowed for a few food categories.[81] In the United States the GRAS (generally recognized as safe) status of methyleugenol is no longer supported[82] and the use of safrole has already been prohibited since 1960.[25] More details on the risk and

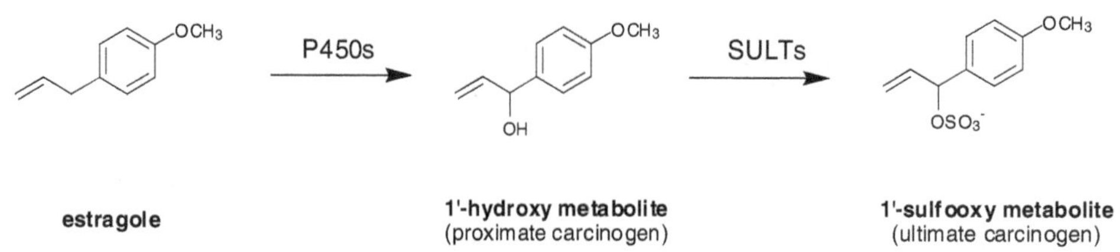

FIGURE 1.8 Bioactivation of alkenylbenzenes to the ultimate carcinogenic 1′-sulfooxymetabolite by cytochromes P450 (P450s) and sulfotransferases presented using estragole as the model compound.

safety evaluation of flavors and their constituents added for flavoring purposes to food, including taste and flavor modifiers, is provided in Chapter 14.

For some allylalkoxybenzenes $BMDL_{10}$ values have been defined (for an overview see Ref.[25]), to be used for risk assessment of these food-borne plant constituents using the so-called Margin of Exposure (MOE) approach. Reported $BMDL_{10}$ values amount to 3.3 mg/kg bw/day for estragole, 1.9 mg/kg bw/day for safrole[63] and 15.3 mgkg bw/day for methyleugenol, a value recently updated by model averaging to 22.2 mg/kg bw/day.[83]

The exposure from all sources was estimated by the SCF to sum up to 4.3–8.7 mg/person/day (0.06 and 0.12 mg/kg bw/day) for estragole,[78] to 13–36 mg/person/day (0.19 and 0.53 mg/kg bw/day) for methyleugenol,[79] and to 0.3–0.5 mg/person/day (0.004–0.007 mg/kg bw/day) for safrole.[80] By reference to the above $BMDL_{10}$ levels, these intake estimates would result in MOE values lower than 10 000, thus entailing a priority for risk management, as recommended by EFSA.[84] However, given the regulatory restrictions in use,[81] the currently estimated exposures are probably substantially lower than previously estimated by the SCF, resulting in substantially higher MOE values, and therefore a lower concern for human health.

Given that liver toxicity and carcinogenicity of the 1′-propenylalkoxybenzenes proceeds by a nongenotoxic mode of action, via hepatotoxicity and regenerative hyperplasia, a safe level of daily exposure can be established. However, health-based guidance levels for safe daily exposure of these 1′-propenylalkoxybenzenes have so far not been established. In the EU the use of beta-asarone as a food flavoring substance is not allowed, while a maximum level of 1 mg/kg exists for naturally occurring beta-asarone in alcoholic beverages.[81] The use of alpha-asarone as a flavoring substance is not regulated in the EU while In the US and Canada the addition of *A. calamus*, calamus oil, or calamus extracts is prohibited.[25]

1.6.3 Pyrrolizidine alkaloids

1.6.3.1 Pyrrolizidine alkaloids: structural features

PAs are another group of naturally occurring plant toxins that raise a concern. PAs are produced by plants of the families Boraginaceae (e.g., genus *Heliotropium*, *Symphytum*, *Trichodesma*), Asteraceae (alternate name: Compositae) (e.g., genus *Senecio*, *Eupatoria*, *Tussilago*), and Fabaceae (alternate name: Leguminosae) (e.g., genus *Crotalaria*).[25] More than 660 PAs and PA *N*-oxides have been identified from an estimated 6000 plants.[85] Especially 1,2-unsaturated PAs are hepatotoxic and considered genotoxic carcinogens, thus posing a potential risk to human health.[25] Depending on the type of esterification the PAs can be divided into monoesters, open diesters, and cyclic diesters (Fig. 1.9). A recent evaluation of the food chain revealed the presence of 1,2-unsaturated PAs at relatively high levels especially in honey, teas, herbal infusions, and food supplements.[86] Based on occurrence data, EFSA considered especially 17 PAs relevant for monitoring in food and feed.[86,87] These PAs include intermedine, lycopsamine, intermedine-N-oxide, lycopsamine-N-oxide, senecionine, senecivernine,

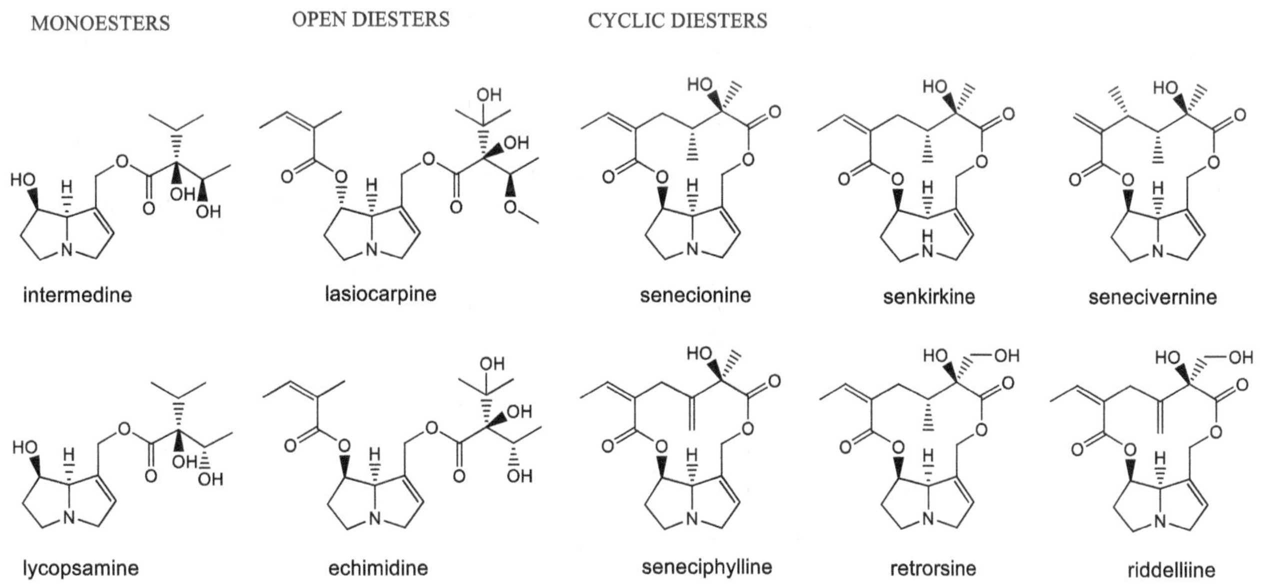

FIGURE 1.9 Chemical structures of 1,2-unsaturated pyrrolizidine alkaloids subdivided by the type of esterification into monoesters, open diesters, and cyclic diesters.

senecionine-N-oxide, senecivernine-N-oxide, seneciphylline, seneciphylline-N-oxide, retrorsine, retrorsine-N-oxide, echimidine, echimidine-N-oxide, lasiocarpine, lasiocarpine-N-oxide and senkirkine (Fig. 1.9).[86]

1.6.3.2 Pyrrolizidine alkaloids: toxic mode of action and adverse effects

Generally, PAs can be metabolized via three metabolic pathways. These include esterase-mediated hydrolysis resulting in the formation of necines and necic acids, and the N-oxygenation pathway mediated by cytochromes P450 and flavin-containing monooxygenase (FMO) resulting in the formation of PA N-oxides. These two pathways are considered detoxification pathways because the metabolites formed have relatively higher water solubility and are rapidly excreted via the urine compared to their parent compounds.[88] A third pathway is the bioactivation pathway catalyzed by cytochromes P450 and resulting in the formation of a pyrrolic ester via hydroxylation at the C-3 or C-8 position of the necine base followed by dehydration.[88,89] This metabolite can be further metabolized via hydrolysis to the formation of a racemic compound called (±) 6,7-dihydro-7-hydroxy-1-hydroxymethyl-5H-pyrrolizine (DHP). Due to the electrophilic nature of the pyrrolic esters and DHP, these metabolites are chemically and biologically reactive and form adducts with cellular components such as proteins, glutathione, and DNA.[88,89] The pyrrolic esters and DHP were generally considered to be detoxified by reacting with glutathione (GSH) to form 7-GS-DHP or 7,9-diGSH-DHP and 9-GS-DHP.[89–91] However, it was found that 7-GS-DHP also produced DHP-DNA adducts in incubations of rat and human liver microsomes in the presence of calf thymus DNA and upon incubation with HepG2 cells, indicating that 7-GS-DHP adducts can be reactive metabolites of PAs leading to DNA adduct formation.[92] In humans, CYP 3A4 is identified as the main enzyme for the bioactivation pathway of PAs.[89,93,94]

Adverse effects caused by 1,2-unsaturated PAs relate to acute and chronic liver toxicity including carcinogenicity.[88] Human case reports in consequence of treatment with herbal medicines and infusions and/or outbreaks of human poisoning due to exposure to PAs from *Crotalaria, Heliotropium, Symphytum* or *Senecio species* have been documented.[8,25] Herbal preparations including teas and food supplements, containing levels of PAs that raise a health concern are currently found on the market.[86,95]

Acute human poisoning with 1,2-unsaturated PAs results in acute hepatic veno-occlusive disease (VOD) and is associated with high mortality.[25] Chronic exposure to low levels of PAs, may result in chronic VOD reflected by cirrhosis of the liver and also effects on other organs.[8] With respect to carcinogenicity lasiocarpine, riddelliine, and monocrotaline have been classified by the IARC in group 2B (possibly carcinogenic to humans), and isatidine, retrorsine, and senkirkine in group 3 (not classifiable).[96–98]

1.6.3.3 Pyrrolizidine alkaloids: risk assessment

Several regulatory bodies have advised against the consumption of comfrey or comfrey-containing products [99,100] and in some countries, maximum residue levels for PAs have been established. For example, in the Netherlands, a maximum level of 0.1 μg PAs/100 g of food has been suggested.[101] EFSA concluded that 1,2-unsaturated PAs may act as genotoxic carcinogens in humans, and established a $BMDL_{10}$ of 237 μg/kg bw per day for riddelliine based on a two-year carcinogenicity study in rats[102] as the most suitable point of departure in a MOE approach for risk assessment.[86]

Based on available risk assessments it can be concluded that dietary exposure to PAs may occur at levels that raise a concern, especially for subpopulations that consume relatively large amounts of specific PA-containing foods such as, for example, (herbal) teas.[86,103]

Given that the source of PAs in (herbal) teas made from non-PA producing plants may be related to co-harvesting of PA-producing plants, risk management actions are indicated.

1.7 Situations where natural toxins from plants may raise concern: Switching varieties [grayanotoxins (GTXs), anisatin, and aristolochic acids (AAs)]

Accidental or erroneous replacement of botanicals with toxic plants presents another situation where natural toxins from plants may raise a concern in the modern food chain.[104] Examples of toxins that caused adverse health effects because of this situation are aristolochic acids (AAs) and anisatin. Another example where the use of the wrong plant variety may lead to health concerns relates to the grayanotoxins. These three examples of natural toxins from plants will be discussed in this section.

1.7.1 Grayanotoxins

1.7.1.1 Grayanotoxins: structural features

GTXs (Fig. 1.10), represent a group of naturals plant toxins present in plants of the Ericaceae family, particularly the *Rhododendron*, *Pieris*, *Agarista*, and *Kalmia* genera.[105] Honeys derived from these plants may raise a health concern because of considerable levels of GTXs that have been detected in honeys derived from GTX-containing plants.[105]

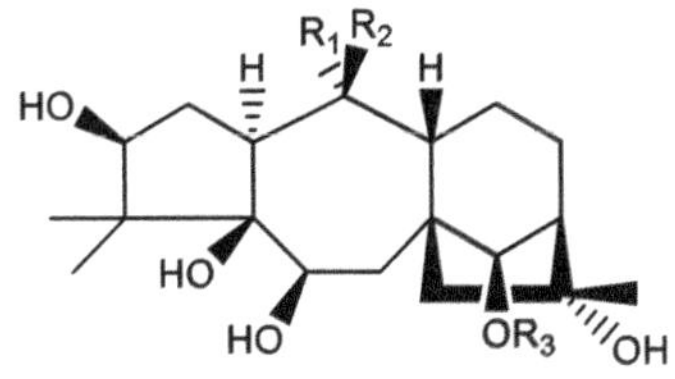

grayanotoxin I — $R_1 = OH, R_2 = CH_3, R_3 = COCH_3$
grayanotoxin II — $R_1R_2 = {=}CH_2, R_3 = H$
grayanotoxin III — $R1 = OH, R_2 = CH_3, R_3 = H$

FIGURE 1.10 Chemical structure of grayanotoxins.

1.7.1.2 Grayanotoxins: toxic mode of action and adverse effects

Honey containing GTXs is known as "mad honey." Mad honey poisoning has been frequently reported in the Eastern Black Sea region of Turkey, but may also occur when honey from that region is imported into other regions.[25] Especially feeding infants with "mad honey" is considered of concern. Thus this group of plant toxins presents another example of a toxin that is especially of concern for sensitive or vulnerable subgroups within the population. Although consumption of honey is contraindicated for infants under one year of age, "mad honey" poisoning in a 5-month-old infant has been reported.[106]

The dose of rhododendron honey reported to cause adverse health effects varies between 5 and 180 g.[25] GTxs are neurotoxins that act by binding to voltage-dependent sodium channels, thereby interfering with the transmission of the action potential.[105,107] The resulting adverse health effects include dizziness, nausea, vomiting, salivation, perspiration, and weakness, followed by diarrhea, paresthesia, blurry vision, and typically hypotension and bradycardia.[25,107] Higher dose levels may result in complete atrioventricular block, convulsions, and loss of consciousness, and/or life-threatening cardiac complications.[25,107,108]

1.7.1.3 Grayanotoxins: risk assessment

The BfR concluded that poisoning through honey is only expected in regions where GTX-containing plants dominate the vegetation and that especially rhododendron honeys from regions of the Turkish Black Sea coast could contain GTXs levels that may raise a health concern.[109]

1.7.2 Anisatin

1.7.2.1 Anisatin: structural features

Anisatin (Fig. 1.11) is a neurotoxin present in Japanese star anise (*Illicium anisatum*) but not in the Chinese star anise (*I. verum*) which is used for preparing tea.

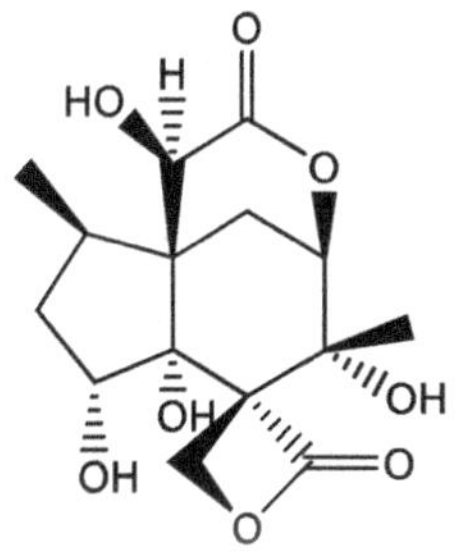

FIGURE 1.11 Chemical structure of anisatin.

1.7.2.2 Anisatin: toxic mode of action and adverse effects

In September 2001 in The Netherlands, more than 60 persons showed nausea and vomiting, after drinking a herbal tea called star mix tea, with 22 persons being hospitalized due to tonic-clonic seizures.[110] The adverse effects were ascribed to anisatin present in the tea due to accidental use of Japanese star anise instead of the nontoxic Chinese star anise. Several studies[111,112] reported that in the emergency department of Miami Children's Hospital over a 2-year period, 7 infants with signs and symptoms of star anise intoxication were seen who were given star anise tea to treat infant colic. These authors also reported the contamination of Chinese star anise with Japanese star anise, pointing at a need for stricter federal regulation.

Anisatin is a noncompetitive gamma-amino butyric acid (GABA)-antagonist that can cause tonic-clonic seizures.[113]

1.7.2.3 Anisatin: risk assessment

Consumption of *I. verum* is considered safe. However given the risk of erroneous switching of varieties and the fact that in infants relatively small quantities may be sufficient to produce adverse neurological effects,[111,112] use of star anise in children should be discouraged.[30]

1.7.3 Aristolochic acids

1.7.3.1 Aristolochic acids: structural features

A final example of adverse human health effects resulting from (accidental) switching of botanical varieties relates to the unintentional exposure to AAs. After the intake of a Chinese herb-based weight loss preparation, in Belgium over 100 young women suffered from kidney damage, developing in several patients into cancer of the kidneys and the urinary tract. In these herbal preparations, *Stephania tetranda* was mistakenly replaced by *Aristolochia fanchi*,[114] likely because both plants are used under the same name "Fangji" in Chinese folk medicine.[114,115]

Aristlochia fanchi, like other plants from the *Aristolochiaceae* family, contains AAs.[115,116] AAs occur

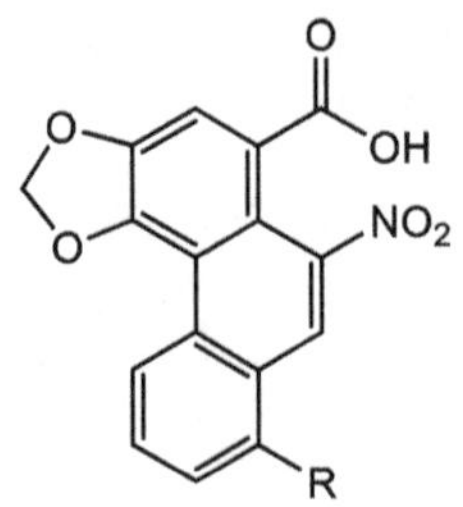

aristolochic acid I R = OCH_3
aristolochic acid II R = H

FIGURE 1.12 Chemical structure of aristolochic acid I and II.

as a mixture of related nitrophenanthrene carboxylic acids, including aristolochic acid I (AAI) and aristolochic acid II (AAII) (Fig. 1.12).[117]

1.7.3.2 Aristolochic acids: toxic mode of action and adverse effects

AAs require reductive metabolic activation by cytochromes P450 and/or NAD(P)H:quinone:oxidoreductase to become reactive and form DNA adducts.

Due to the supposed beneficial properties of *Aristolochia* species, AA-containing preparations have been developed as pharmaceutical preparations,[118–120] until studies proved that AAs were carcinogenic in rats.[121] AAs are nephrotoxic and carcinogenic. Studies conducted over the years have associated AAs with Chinese Herb Nephropathy and Balkan Endemic Nephropathy, later known as Aristolochic Acid Nephropathy (AAN).[122] Similar cases have been described in other countries including Spain, Japan, France, the United Kingdom, and China.[123]

1.7.3.3 Aristolochic acids: risk assessment

IARC concluded that herbal preparations with *Aristolochia* spp. are carcinogenic to humans (Class I).[117] In several countries the presence of AAs and their derivatives in food including herbal preparations is limited or prohibited.[124] Meanwhile, international Food and Medicine Authorities have published lists of traditional herbal preparations suspected to contain AAs. Despite the limitations and bans, targeted sampling strategies demonstrated that herbal preparations containing AAs are still on the market, resulting in exposures that raise a concern for human health.[103,124,125]

1.8 Situations where natural toxins from plants may raise concern: Abuse [tropane alkaloids (TAs), opium alkaloids, delta-9-tetrahydrocannabinol (THC)]

Another situation where natural toxins from plants may raise concern relates to situations of abuse, and/or use of plants because of hallucinogenic constituents, to induce changes in perception or emotional state of mind. The use of these so-called "herbal highs" is an emerging trend originating from South America or Asia where these herbal ingredients have traditionally been used since ancient times.[126,127] The present chapter deals only with these herbal constituents as far as they become relevant for the modern food chain, describing TAs, opium alkaloids, and delta-9-tetrahydrocannabinol.

1.8.1 Tropane alkaloids

1.8.1.1 Tropane alkaloids: structural features

TA-containing plants are found in numerous families such as *Solanaceae*, *Erythroxylaceae*, *Convolvulaceae*, *Brassicaceae*, and *Euphorbiaceae*.[128] TAs of relevance in the food chain include (−)- and (+)-hyoscyamine (the racemic mixture of these being known as atropine), (−)-scopolamine (also known as (−)-hyoscine), and cocaine (Fig. 1.13).[25] Cocaine is a constituent of coca leaf. Under strict regulations, decocainized coca leaf extracts are being used in some soft drinks.

1.8.1.2 Tropane alkaloids: toxic mode of action and adverse effects

Several TAs (e.g., scopolamine) are hallucinogenic and some are powerful anticholinergic drugs (e.g., atropine, hyoscyamine, scopolamine). Intoxications by TAs have been reported, resulting from accidental exposure and/or from abuse of TA-containing plants such as *Datura stramonium* because of their hallucinogenic effects.[128,129] Several case studies have been reported, generally related to contamination of raw materials with Datura seeds.[8] The biological effects of atropine, hyoscyamine, and scopolamine result from their antagonistic action on muscarinic acetylcholine receptors.[130] The adverse effects reported upon high intake of these plant toxins include dryness of the mucosa of the upper digestive and respiratory tract, constipation, pupil dilatation and disturbance of vision, photophobia, hypotension, bradycardia or tachycardia, arrhythmias, nervousness, and, at higher dose levels, hypertension, restlessness, irritability, disorientation, ataxia, seizures and respiratory distress.[25]

1.8.1.3 Tropane alkaloids: risk assessment

Concerns over the presence of TAs in the modern food chain result mainly from the presence of seeds of *Datura* spp. plants, containing high concentrations of hyoscyamine and scopolamine, as impurities in animal feed.[6,131] However, it has been concluded that carry-over into animal products does not raise a concern.[129] Exposure of both animals and humans rather results from the use of herbal teas, herbal preparations (e.g., traditional Chinese or Ayurvedic preparations), and/or, by mistaking fruits of belladonna (deadly nightshade) with blueberries or blackberries (either fresh or dried) and edible flowers.[129]

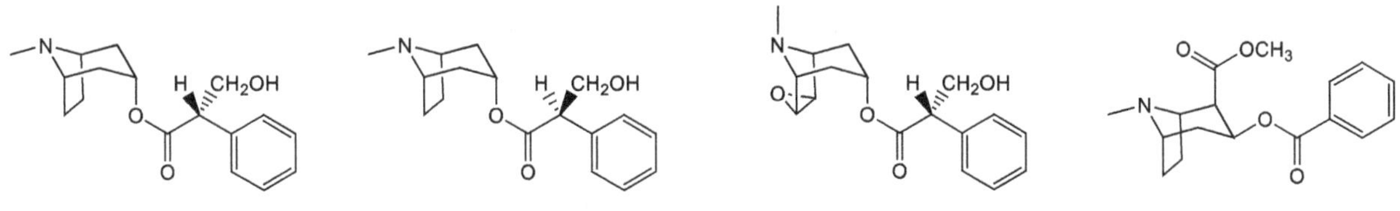

(-)-hyoscyamine (+)-hyoscyamine scopolamine = (-)-hyoscine cocaine

FIGURE 1.13 Chemical structure of tropane alkaloids.

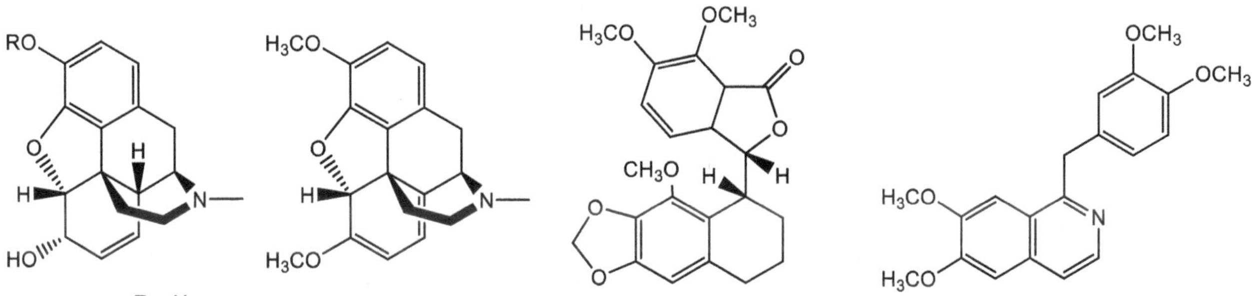

morphine R = H
codeine R = CH_3 thebaine noscapine papaverine

FIGURE 1.14 Chemical structure of opium alkaloids.

Contamination has also been found in buckwheat, soybean, and linseed. In September 2003, in Slovenia, contamination of buckwheat flour with seeds from *D. stramonium* resulted in cases of domestic food poisoning with TAs.[132] Adamse and Van Egmond concluded that buckwheat-based products such as buckwheat-based flour, buckwheat groats grains, buckwheat kernels, or roasted buckwheat grains, also known as "kasha" in Eastern European cuisine, are products that should be monitored to prevent accidental exposure of humans to TAs, from for example Datura seeds.[129]

Based on a human volunteer study with a mixture of (−)-hyoscyamine and (−)-scopolamine a NOAEL of 0.16 μg/kg bw, expressed as the sum of (−)-hyoscyamine and (−)-scopolamine, was established.[133] EFSA derived an ARfD of 0.016 μg/kg bw for the sum of (−)-hyoscyamine and (−)-scopolamine (group ARfD) and concluded that for toddlers, this group ARfD can be exceeded through the consumption of cereal products.[134] The BfR agreed with this conclusion; within the EU maximum levels of 1 μg atropin/kg and 1 μg scopolamine/kg have been established for processed cereal-based foods and baby foods for infants and young children, containing millet, sorghum, buckwheat, or their derived products.[25]

1.8.2 Opium alkaloids

1.8.2.1 Opium alkaloids: structural features

Opium alkaloids are present in the latex of *Papaver somniferum* (opium poppy). So far around 50 different alkaloids have been isolated from opium with the main alkaloids being morphine, codeine, thebaine, noscapine (also called narcotine), and papaverine (Fig. 1.14).[25] The opium alkaloids may end up in food when the seeds, potentially contaminated with latex, are used to produce an edible oil or to prepare cakes or desserts.

1.8.2.2 Opium alkaloids: toxic mode of action and adverse effects

Morphine acts by activation of the opioid receptors in the central and peripheral nervous system and the gastrointestinal tract resulting in pharmacological effects, but also upon acute poisoning in adverse effects, including miosis, respiratory depression, and unconsciousness (coma).

1.8.2.3 Opium alkaloids: risk assessment

For adults, doses of 200 mg of morphine may be acutely lethal.[135] Case studies reporting adverse effects upon consumption of commercially available poppy seeds, for instance in the form of desserts have been reported.[25] BfR recommended a 'provisional daily upper intake level' for morphine of 6.3 μg/kg bw/day which should not be exceeded during one meal or several meals distributed over the day.[136,137] Based on this health-based guidance value a provisional guidance value for morphine in poppy seeds was derived.[136] EFSA established an ARfD of 10 μg morphine equivalents/kg bw and concluded that this ARfD can be exceeded during a single serving by some consumers, particularly children, across the EU.[138]

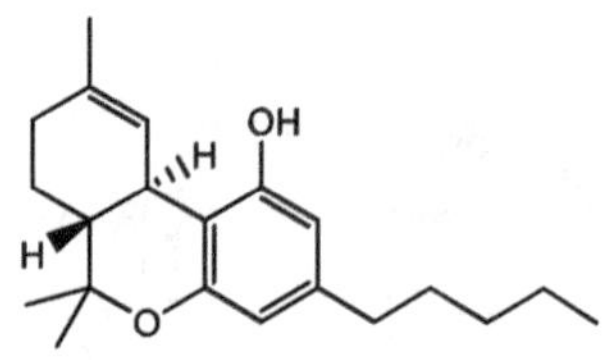

delta-9-tetrahydrocannabinol (THC)

FIGURE 1.15 Structure of delta-9-tetrahydrocannabinol.

1.8.3 Delta-9-tetrahydrocannabinol

1.8.3.1 Tetrahydrocannabinol: structural features

Delta-9-tetrahydrocannabinol (THC) (Fig. 1.15) is the main psychoactive substance found in *Cannabis sativa*, the cannabis or hemp plant.

In the form of marijuana or hashish, the plant provides a "recreational drug",[139] especially the plants containing THC.[25] The hemp varieties allowed for cultivation in the European Union may not exceed 0.2% THC (EU Regulation 1307/2013).

Hulled hemp seeds, hemp seed oil, hemp seed flour, or extracts of parts of the hemp plant may be used as food ingredients.[140,141]

1.8.3.2 Tetrahydrocannabinol: toxic mode of action and adverse effects

Intake of THC contaminated hemp seed oil used for the preparation of a salad has been reported to result in nausea, vomiting, dizziness, and perceptual disturbances.[142] THC acts by binding to the cannabinoid receptor CB 1, located mainly in the central nervous system, and to the peripheral CB 2 receptor.[139,143]

1.8.3.3 Tetrahydrocannabinol: risk assessment

It is recommended that the daily intake of THC with hemp containing food should not exceed 0.001–0.002 mg/kg bw/day and based on these maximum intake levels, THC guidance values of maximum contents of 0.005 mg/kg for nonalcoholic and alcoholic beverages, 5 mg/kg for edible oils, and 0.150 mg/kg for all other foods were derived.[25]

EFSA issued an opinion on the safety of hemp (*Cannabis* genus) for use as animal feed indicating that THC and metabolites with psychoactive properties may be excreted via milk.[144] EFSA also established an ARfD of 1 μg THC/kg bw and estimated that exposure to THC from the consumption of milk and dairy products may amount to levels between 0.001 and 0.03 μg/kg bw per day in adults, and 0.006 and 0.13 μg/kg bw per day in toddlers.[145] This resulted in the conclusion that exposure to THC via consumption of milk and dairy products, resulting from the use of hemp seed-derived feed materials is unlikely to pose a health concern. EFSA could not conclude on the possible risks to public health from exposure to THC via consumption of animal tissues and eggs because of a lack of data on possible transfer from feed to these food products.[145]

1.9 Adulteration with pharmaceutical substances

A final situation to consider that raises concerns for natural plant constituents in foods relates to adulteration. In these examples, problems arise from the adulteration of herbal preparations with drugs or drug-related nonapproved compounds to make sure the herbal preparations will have the required effect. An example in this field is the adulteration of herbal preparations for the treatment of erectile dysfunction with PDE-5 inhibitors like sildenafil (the active ingredient of Viagra), tadalafil (Cialis), and vardenafil (Levitra) and even with nonapproved structural analogs.[146,147] Reported side effects of the approved PDE-5 inhibitors include headache, facial flushing, nasal congestion, and dyspepsia.[148] PDE-5 inhibitors are contra-indicated in patients using antihypertensive nitrate medication, patients with hypotension, or patients using α-adrenergic blockers or CYP3A4 inhibitors.[147,149,150] Their combined intake can synergistically promote increased relaxation of smooth muscle cells, resulting in a drastic reduction of systemic blood pressure.[149,151–153] Such a sudden drop in blood pressure (hypotension) may lead to cardiovascular effects in vulnerable people, with extreme cases resulting in sudden shock and eventually death.[150]

Another example of adulteration of herbal food preparations in the food chain relates to the presence of active pharmaceutical ingredients in herbal weight loss preparations.[154] Although these adulterations represents an important concern for plant-based food supplements, the topic is not discussed in further detail because these concerns do not relate to natural plant constituents.

1.10 Discussion including existing data gaps and research directions

Taking it all together it becomes clear that our modern food chain may contain natural toxins from plants, either due to their natural presence in the plant-derived food or the raw material used for food production, or because these constituents are added during the regular production process, or present as contaminants. Whether these constituents raise a concern will depend on the levels of exposure and thus on their level of occurrence in the respective food and its consumption. Health-based guidance values for these natural constituents are by no means always available, often due to substantial data gaps in the available toxicological databases. Where health-based guidance values like ARfDs or TDIs are available, risk assessment may be hampered by a lack of adequate exposure data. In most cases, information on the potential adverse effects resulting from natural toxins in plant-based food relies on human case reports showing adverse health effects. Estimated exposure levels linked to the adverse effects reported are often inaccurate since they are generally based on levels detected in the relevant food item and on personal consumption data. Nevertheless, several situations can be envisaged where natural toxicants in plant-based foods, including herbs and spices and herbal food supplements, may be present at levels that raise a concern and present a risk for the consumer. Such situation may include (1) improper food handling, resulting in adverse effects by inadequately high exposure to natural toxins in plants (2) use of botanicals containing natural toxins as famine food, (3) exposure of sensitive/vulnerable individuals in the population, (4) use of food supplements or herbal teas containing herbal constituents of concern, (5) accidental replacement of botanicals with toxic plants, (6) abuse of herbal preparations and/or (7) adulteration with pharmaceutical substances. The compounds of concern include neurotoxins, enzyme inhibitors, compounds causing oxidative stress or inhibiting ATP production, and also genotoxic or nongenotoxic carcinogens. Depending on the situation raising the concerns, different risk management options and recommendations for research addressing data gaps emerge.

For use of toxic plant varieties as famine food clearly, alternative food sources and improved food security will be essential to avoid adverse human health effects. Consumer education can also be expected to support the mitigation of adverse health effects resulting from improper food handling. Other actions should include improved quality control and perhaps even a premarket risk assessment of botanicals and botanical preparations to reveal data gaps. A further issue is that for instance individual genotoxic and carcinogenic PAs or allylalkoxybenzenes do not occur in isolation. Botanicals and botanical preparation from plants containing these compounds usually contain more than one of these constituents of concern.[85,95] This points to a need for the evaluation of combined exposure which requires the definition of relative potency factors (REPs). "Interim REP" factors have been defined already for PAs[155] but were considered not to be robust enough to be taken into account in the risk assessment of combined exposure.[156]

Moreover, concomitant intake of different herbal preparations resulting in exposure to constituents of concern from different categories may be relevant, given that use of different preparations may be common practice for people using herbal supplements.[157] In addition, the use of herbal supplements together with other dietary sources of constituents of concern may have to be considered, exemplified by exposure to allylalkoxybenzenes from aggregate intake of herbs and spices, vegetables, teas, and/or traditional medicines. In all these cases potential interactions of constituents of concern remain to be elucidated, as well as potential matrix effects on bioavailability and/or toxicity of the ingredients of concern. These should be considered on a case-by-case basis.

Risk assessment of chronic effects of natural plant toxins is often based on an assumed lifetime exposure scenario. However, the use of such preparations may often be for only a limited time such as during periods of illness or famine. This will require adequate adjustment of risk assessment, especially when deriving an MOE relating to exposure to genotoxic carcinogens via less-than-lifetime use of herbal preparations. For example, intake of a herbal preparation for 2 weeks every year during a lifetime instead of during a whole lifetime, could be assessed according to Haber's rule ($D \times T = \text{constant}$), if there is evidence that the adverse effect accumulates linearly. Exposure would in this case be 26 times lower, resulting in MOE values 26 times higher than what would be calculated assuming daily lifetime exposure.[158]

A future key issue will be how to ascertain quality control throughout the whole food chain. This needs to start already with exact and proven botanical identity and nomenclature of the plants used, characterization of geographic origin and harvest, processing, composition, storage, packaging, and distribution to mention but a few key issues. However, since at present botanical preparations are considered food, the producer is responsible for the safety in use, and premarket evaluation generally is not required. The lack of adequate quality control brings about enhanced health risks to the consumer as exemplified in this review by teas from non-PA producing plants, but containing unacceptable high levels of PAs,[85] honeys containing GTXs,[105] herbal supplements containing allylalkoxybenzenes, AAs, and/or PAs at levels that result in MOE values below 10.[95] This applies as well to adulteration by pharmaceutical ingredients, including unapproved analogs of drugs,[146,147,154] apricot kernels with levels of amygdalin that make the intake of 1–3 kernels already a risk for an adult consumer,[27] and reported case studies on switching of harmless varieties for toxic ones. Furthermore many botanical preparations especially teas and plant food supplements are sold over the internet where adequate quality control is mandatory (but not applied), as exemplified by an illegal sample containing amygdalin, labeled as a vitamin (vitamin B17). It can be concluded that the regulations and import controls on supplements, traditional medicine, and so-called "health foods" and their constituents require scrutiny, especially given the increased consumer interest.

Lastly, often data required to perform an adequate risk assessment and to support risk management actions are inadequate or even absent, as exemplified by PAs where data on the carcinogenicity upon oral dosing of only a few congeners are available, and reliable exposure estimates are scarce. Many natural plant constituents of concern today can be adequately analyzed and quantified in complex botanical matrices, as required to perform an exposure assessment. Yet, despite highly advanced analytics, exposure assessments are often compromised by a lack of data on dietary intake of botanical preparations and/or by the fact that not even directions for use are given on the labels of some plant food supplements.[95] In such cases biomonitoring might be considered to better quantify actual exposure.

In conclusion, the presence of natural toxicants in plant-based foods, in the food chain of both developing and developed countries at levels that may raise a concern for human health cannot be excluded at present as a result of marketing botanicals and botanical preparations, including herbal food supplements

In addition to ascertaining quality throughout the whole food chain as outlined above, improved education of producers, retailers, and consumers may provide the path to improvement.

References

1. Wittstock U, Gershenzon J. Constitutive plant toxins and their role in defense against herbivores and pathogens. *Curr Opin Plant Biol.* 2002;5(4):300–307. Available from: https://doi.org/10.1016/s1369-5266(02)00264-9.
2. Low TY, Wong KO, Yap ALL, De Haan LHJ, Rietjens IMCM. The regulatory framework across international jurisdictions for risks associated with consumption of botanical food supplements. *Compr Rev Food Sci Food Saf.* 2017;16(5):821–834. Available from: https://doi.org/10.1111/1541-4337.12289.
3. Wu WB, Sun R. Toxicological studies on plant proteins: a review. *J Appl Toxicol.* 2012;32(6):377–386. Available from: https://doi.org/10.1002/jat.1780.
4. Walsh MJ, Dodd JE, Hautbergue GM. Ribosome-inactivating proteins potent poisons and molecular tools. *Virulence.* 2013;4 (8):774–784. Available from: https://doi.org/10.4161/viru.26399.
5. Soetan KO, Oyewole OE. The need for adequate processing to reduce the anti-nutritional factors in plants used as human foods and animal feeds: a review. *Afr J Food Sci.* 2009;3(9):223–232.
6. EFSA. Ricin (from *Ricinus communis*) as undesirable substances in animal feed1 scientific opinion of the panel on contaminants in the food chain. *EFSA J.* 2008;726:1–38.
7. Dickers KJ, Bradberry SM, Rice P, Griffiths GD, Vale JA. Abrin poisoning. *Toxicol Rev.* 2003;22(3):137–142. Available from: https://doi.org/10.2165/00139709-200322030-00002.
8. Koleva II, van Beek TA, Soffers AEMF, Dusemund B, Rietjens IMCM. Alkaloids in the human food chain – natural occurrence and possible adverse effects. *Mol Nutr Food Res.* 2012;56(1): 30–52. Available from: https://doi.org/10.1002/mnfr.201100165.
9. McMillan M, Thompson JC. Outbreak of suspected solanine poisoning in schoolboys: examination of criteria of solanine poisoning. *Q J Med.* 1979;48(190):227–243.
10. BfR Table potatoes should contain low levels of glycoalkaloids (solanine) BfR Opinion No 010/2018, 2018.
11. JECFA JFWECoFA Solanine and chaconine. In: Toxicological evaluation of certain food additives and naturally occurring toxicants prepared by the 39th meeting of the JECFA, WHO Food additives series 30. 1993. World Health Organization, Geneva 1993.
12. Friedman M, McDonald GM. Postharvest changes in glycoalkaloid content of potatoes. *Adv Exp Med Biol.* 1999;459:121–143.
13. Friedman M. Tomato glycoalkaloids: role in the plant and in the diet. *J Agric Food Chem.* 2002;50(21):5751–5780. Available from: https://doi.org/10.1021/jf020560c.
14. Friedman M. Analysis of biologically active compounds in potatoes (*Solanum tuberosum*), tomatoes (*Lycopersicon esculentum*), and jimson weed (*Datura stramonium*) seeds. *J Chromatogr A.* 2004;1054(1-2):143–155. Available from: https://doi.org/10.1016/j.chroma.2004.04.049.
15. ANZFA Lupin alkaloids in food, a toxicological review and risk assessment. Technical report series no. 3. 2001, pp. 1–21. Technical report series no 3:pp 1-21.
16. Reinhard H, Rupp H, Sager F, Streule M, Zoller O. Quinolizidine alkaloids and phomopsins in lupin seeds and lupin containing food. *J Chromatogr A.* 2006;1112(1-2):353–360. Available from: https://doi.org/10.1016/j.chroma.2005.11.079.
17. Gremigni P, Wong MTF, Edwards NK, Harris D, Hamblin J. Potassium nutrition effects on seed alkaloid concentrations, yield and mineral content of lupins (*Lupinus angustifolius*). *Plant Soil.* 2001;234(1):131–142. Available from: https://doi.org/10.1023/a:1010576702139.
18. Joray ML, Rayas-Duarte P, Mohamed A, van Santen E. Coated lupin bean snacks. *J Food Qual.* 2007;30(2):267–279. Available from: https://doi.org/10.1111/j.1745-4557.2007.00120.x.
19. Pingault NM, Gibbs RA, Barclay AM, Monaghan M. Two cases of anticholinergic syndrome associated with consumption of bitter lupin flour. *Med J Aust.* 2009;191(3):173–174. Available from: https://doi.org/10.5694/j.1326-5377.2009.tb02732.x.
20. Di Grande A, Paradiso R, Amico S, Fulco G, Fantauzza B, Noto P. Anticholinergic toxicity associated with lupin seed ingestion: case report. *Eur J Emerg Med.* 2004;11(2):119–120. Available from: https://doi.org/10.1097/01.mej.0000124515.82084.c9.
21. Litkey J, Dailey MW. Anticholinergic toxicity associated with the ingestion of lupini beans. *Am J Emerg Med.* 2007;25(2):215–217. Available from: https://doi.org/10.1016/j.ajem.2006.08.004.
22. Marquez RL, Gutierrezrave M, Miranda FI. Acute-poisoning by lupine seed debittering water. *Vet Hum Toxicol.* 1991;33(3):265–267.
23. Daverio M, Cavicchiolo ME, Grotto P, Lonati D, Cananzi M, Da Dalt L. Bitter lupine beans ingestion in a child: a disregarded cause of acute anticholinergic toxicity. *Eur J Pediatr.* 2014;173(12):1549–1551. Available from: https://doi.org/10.1007/s00431-013-2088-2.
24. Pilegaard K, Gry J. *Alkaloids in Edible Lupin Seeds: A Toxicological Review and Recommendations.* Copenhagen: Nordic Council of Ministers; 2008.
25. Dusemund B, Rietjens IMCM, Cartus A, Schaefer B, Lampen A. Plant-derived contaminants in food. Occurrence, effects and risk assessment. *Bundesgesundheitsblatt-Gesundheitsforschung-Gesundheitsschutz.* 2017;60(7):728–736. Available from: https://doi.org/10.1007/s00103-017-2561-6.

26. EFSA. Opinion of the scietific panel on food additives, flavourings, processing aids and materials in contact with food (AFC) on a request from the commission related to hydrocyanic acid. *EFSA J.* 2004;105:1–28.
27. EFSA. Acute health risks related to the presence of cyanogenic glycosides in raw apricot kernels and products derived from raw apricot kernels. *EFSA J.* 2016.
28. Baumeister RGH, Schievelbein H, Zickgrafrudel G. Toxicological and clinical aspects of cyanide metabolism. *Arzneimittel-Forschung/Drug Res.* 1975;25(7):1056–1064.
29. Tylleskar T, Banea M, Bikangi N, Cooke RD, Poulter NH, Rosling H. Cassava cyanogens and konzo, an upper motoneuron disease found in Africa. *Lancet.* 1992;339(8787):208–211. Available from: https://doi.org/10.1016/0140-6736(92)90006-o.
30. Rietjens IMCM, Martena MJ, Boersma MG, Spiegelenberg W, Alink GM. Molecular mechanisms of toxicity of important food-borne phytotoxins. *Mol Nutr Food Res.* 2005;49(2):131–158. Available from: https://doi.org/10.1002/mnfr.200400078.
31. Ravindranath V. Neurolathyrism: mitochondrial dysfunction in excitotoxicity mediated by L-beta-oxalyl aminoalanine. *Neurochem Int.* 2002;40(6):505–509. Available from: https://doi.org/10.1016/s0197-0186(01)00121-8.
32. Kristanc L, Kreft S. European medicinal and edible plants associated with subacute and chronic toxicity part II: plants with hepato-, neuro-, nephro- and immunotoxic effects. *Food Chem Toxicol.* 2016;92:38–49. Available from: https://doi.org/10.1016/j.fct.2016.03.014.
33. Getahun H, Lambein F, Vanhoorne M, Van der Stuyft P. Neurolathyrism risk depends on type of grass pea preparation and on mixing with cereals and antioxidants. *Trop Med Int Health.* 2005;10(2):169–178. Available from: https://doi.org/10.1111/j.1365-3156.2004.01370.x.
34. EFSA. EFSA Compendium of botanicals that have been reported to contain toxic, addictive, psychotropic or other substances of concern. *EFSA J.* 2009;7(9):281.
35. Ludolph AC, Spencer PS. Toxic models of upper motor neuron disease. *J Neurol Sci.* 1996;139(Suppl):53–59.
36. Mager J, Glaser G, Razin A, Izak G, Bien S, Noam M. Metabolic effects of pyrimidines derived from fava bean glycosides on human erythrocytes deficient in glucose-6-phosphate dehydrogenase. *Biochem Biophys Res Commun.* 1965;20(2):235. Available from: https://doi.org/10.1016/0006-291x(65)90352-9.
37. Ho HY, Cheng ML, Chiu DTY. Glucose-6-phosphate dehydrogenase – beyond the realm of red cell biology. *Free Radic Res.* 2014;48(9):1028–1048. Available from: https://doi.org/10.3109/10715762.2014.913788.
38. Luzzatto L, Arese P. Favism and glucose-6-phosphate dehydrogenase deficiency. *N Engl J Med.* 2018;378(1):60–71. Available from: https://doi.org/10.1056/NEJMra1708111.
39. Wagstaff DJ. Dietary exposure to furocoumarins. *Regul Toxicol Pharmacol.* 1991;14(3):261–272. Available from: https://doi.org/10.1016/0273-2300(91)90029-u.
40. Eisenbrand G. Toxicological assessment of furocoumarins in foodstuffs. *Mol Nutr Food Res.* 2007;51(3):367–373. Available from: https://doi.org/10.1002/mnfr.200600270.
41. SKLM Toxicological assessment of furocoumarins in foodstuffs. 2006. Available at [accessed July 2016]: <http://www.dfg.de/download/pdf/dfg_im_profil/reden_stellungnahmen/2006/sklm_furocoumarine_en_2006.pdf>.
42. IARC. *Monographs on the evaluation of carcinogenic risks to humans. Overall Evaluations of Carcinogenicity: An Updating of IARC Monographs.* Volumes 1–42. Lyon, France: World Health Organization; 1987. Supplement 7.
43. Raquet N, Schrenk D. Application of the equivalency factor concept to the phototoxicity and -genotoxicity of furocoumarin mixtures. *Food Chem Toxicol.* 2014;68:257–266. Available from: https://doi.org/10.1016/j.fct.2014.03.014.
44. Schlatter J, Zimmerli B, Dick R, Panizzon R, Schlatter C. Dietary-intake and risk assessment of phototoxic furocoumarins in humans. *Food Chem Toxicol.* 1991;29(8):523–530. Available from: https://doi.org/10.1016/0278-6915(91)90044-8.
45. Brickl R, Schmid J, Koss FW. Pharmacokinetics and pharmacodynamics of psoralens after oral administration: considerations and conclusions. *Natl Cancer Inst Monogr.* 1984;66:63–67.
46. Evans AM. Influence of dietary components on the gastrointestinal metabolism and transport of drugs. *Ther Drug Monit.* 2000;22(1):131–136. Available from: https://doi.org/10.1097/00007691-200002000-00028.
47. Textor S, Gershenzon J. Herbivore induction of the glucosinolate-myrosinase defense system: major trends, biochemical bases and ecological significance. *Phytochem Rev.* 2009;8(1):149–170. Available from: https://doi.org/10.1007/s11101-008-9117-1.
48. Hayes JD, McMahon M, Chowdhry S, Dinkova-Kostova AT. Cancer chemoprevention mechanisms mediated through the Keap1-Nrf2 pathway. *Antioxid Redox Signal.* 2010;13(11):1713–1748. Available from: https://doi.org/10.1089/ars.2010.3221.
49. IARC IARC handbooks of cancer prevention. Volume 9 Cruciferous vegetables, Isothiocyanates and Indoles(Lyon), 2004.
50. Baasanjav-Gerber C, Monien BH, Mewis I, et al. Identification of glucosinolate congeners able to form DNA adducts and to induce mutations upon activation by myrosinase. *Mol Nutr Food Res.* 2011;55(5):783–792. Available from: https://doi.org/10.1002/mnfr.201000352.
51. Glatt H, Baasanjav-Gerber C, Schumacher, et al. 1-Methoxy-3-indolylmethyl glucosinolate, a potent genotoxicant in bacterial and mammalian cells: mechanisms of bioactivation. *Chem Biol Interact 30.* 2011;192(1-2):81–86. Available from: https://doi.org/10.1016/j.cbi.2010.09.009).
52. Latte KP, Appel KE, Lampen A. Health benefits and possible risks of broccoli, an overview. *Food Chem Toxicol.* 2011;49:3287–3309.
53. SCF EC. *Opinion of the Scientific Committee on Food on estragole (1-Allyl-4-methoxybenzene).* Belgium: Health and Consumer Protection Directorate-General Brussels; 2001.
54. SCF EC. *Opinion of the Scientific Committee on Food on methyleugenol (4-Allyl-1,2-dimethoxybenzene).* Belgium: Health and Consumer Protection Directorate-General Brussels; 2001.
55. Herrmann K, Schumacher F, Engst W, et al. Abundance of DNA adducts of methyleugenol, a rodent hepatocarcinogen, in human liver samples. *Carcinogenesis.* 2013;34(5):1025–1030. Available from: https://doi.org/10.1093/carcin/bgt013.
56. Tremmel R, Herrmann K, Engst W, et al. Methyleugenol DNA adducts in human liver are associated with SULT1A1 copy number variations and expression levels. *Arch Toxicol.* 2017. Available from: https://doi.org/10.1007/s00204-017-1955-4.
57. Rietjens IMCM, Cohen SM, Fukushima S, et al. Impact of structural and metabolic variations on the toxicity and carcinogenicity

of hydroxy- and alkoxy-substituted allyl- and propenylbenzenes. *Chem Res Toxicol.* 2014;27(7):1092–1103. Available from: https://doi.org/10.1021/tx500109s.

58. SCF Opinion of the scientific committee on food on the presence of beta-asarone in flavourings and other food ingredients with flavouring properties. 2002. Available at [accessed July 2016]: http://ec.europa.eu/food/fs/sc/scf/out111_en.pdf.
59. Wiseman RW, Miller EC, Miller JA, Liem A. Structure-activity studies of the hepatocarcinogenicities of alkenylbenzene derivatives related to estragole and safrole on administration to preweanling male C57BL/6J × C3H/HeJ F1-mice. *Cancer Res.* 1987;47(9):2275–2283.
60. Miller EC, Swanson AB, Phillips DH, Fletcher TL, Liem A, Miller JA. Structure-activity studies of the carcinogenicities in the mouse and rat of some naturally-occurring and synthetic alkenylbenzene derivatives related to safrole and estragole. *Cancer Res.* 1983;43(3):1124–1134.
61. NTP NTP Toxicology and Carcinogenesis Studies of Methyleugenol (CAS No. 93-15-2) in F344/N Rats and B6C3F1 Mice (Gavage Studies), NTP Report Series 491, National Toxicology Program, Research Triangle Park, NC. 2000. Available at [accessed July 2016]: <http://ntp.niehs.nih.gov/ntp/htdocs/LT_rpts/tr446.pdf>.
62. Truhaut R, Lebourhis B, Attia M, Glomot R, Newman J, Caldwell J. Chronic toxicity carcinogenicity study of trans-anethole in rats. *Food Chem Toxicol.* 1989;27(1):11–20. Available from: https://doi.org/10.1016/0278-6915(89)90086-0.
63. Van den Berg SJPL, Restani P, Boersma MG, Delmulle L, Rietjens IMCM. Levels of genotoxic and carcinogenic ingredients compounds in plant food supplements and associated risk assessment. *Food Nutr Sci.* 2011;2:989–1010.
64. Newberne PM, Carlton WW, Brown WR. Histopathological evaluation of proliferative liver lesions in rats fed trans-anethole in chronic studies. *Food Chem. Toxicol.* 1989;27:21–26.
65. Gorelick NJ. Genotoxicity of trans-anethole in vitro. *Mutat. Res.* 1995;326:199–209.
66. Kobets T, Duan JD, Brunnemann KD, Etter S, Smith B, Williams GM. Structure-Activity Relationships for DNA Damage by Alkenylbenzenes in Turkey Egg Fetal Liver. *Toxicol. Sci.* 2016;150:301–311.
67. Berg K, Bischoff R, Stegmuller S, Cartus A, Schrenk D. Comparative investigation of the mutagenicity of propenylic and allylic asarone isomers in the ames fluctuation assay. *Mutagenesis.* 2016;31(4):443–451. Available from: https://doi.org/10.1093/mutage/gew007.
68. Cartus AT, Schrenk D. Metabolism of the carcinogen alpha-asarone in liver microsomes. *Food Chem Toxicol.* 2016;87:103–112. Available from: https://doi.org/10.1016/j.fct.2015.11.021.
69. Cartus AT, Stegmuller S, Simson N, et al. Hepatic metabolism of carcinogenic beta-asarone. *Chem Res Toxicol.* 2015;28(9):1760–1773. Available from: https://doi.org/10.1021/acs.chemrestox.5b00223.
70. Cartus AT, Stegmuller S, Berg K, Schrenk D. Metabolism, mutagenicity, and DNA adduct formation of the naturally occurring alkenylbenzene beta-asarone. *Naunyn-Schmiedeb Arch Pharmacol.* 2016;389(1):S10–S10.
71. AshaDevi S, Subramanian B, Premikumar K-a. In vivo genotoxic studies of beta-asarone in mice bone marrow. *Int J Drug Dev Res.* 2014;6:128–132.
72. Cartus AT, Herrmann K, Weishaupt LW, et al. Metabolism of methyleugenol in liver microsomes and primary hepatocytes: pattern of metabolites, cytotoxicity, and DNA-adduct formation. *Toxicol Sci.* 2012;129(1):21–34. Available from: https://doi.org/10.1093/toxsci/kfs181.
73. Guenthner TM, Luo G. Investigation of the role of the 2 ',3 '-epoxidation pathway in the bioactivation and genotoxicity of dietary allylbenzene analogs. *Toxicology.* 2001;160(1-3):47–58. Available from: https://doi.org/10.1016/s0300-483x(00)00456-x.
74. Luo G, Guenthner TM. Metabolism of allylbenzene 2',3'-oxide and estragole 2','-oxide in the isolated-perfused rat-liver. *J Pharmacol Exp Ther.* 1995;272(2):588–596.
75. Luo G, Qato MK, Guenthner TM. Hydrolysis of the 2',3'-allylic epoxides of allylbenzene, estragole, eugenol, and safrole by both microsomal and cytosolic epoxide hydrolases. *Drug Metab Dispos.* 1992;20(3):440–445.
76. Cartus AT, Merz KH, Schrenk D. Metabolism of methylisoeugenol in liver microsomes of human, rat, and bovine origin. *Drug Metab. Dispos.* 2011;39:1727–1733.
77. Herrmann K, Engst W, Meinl W, Florian S, Cartus AT, Schrenk D, Appel KE, Nolden T, Himmelbauer H, Glatt H. Formation of hepatic DNA adducts by methyleugenol in mouse models: drastic decrease by Sult1a1 knockout and strong increase by transgenic human SULT1A1/2. *Carcinogenesis.* 2014;35:935–941.
78. SCF Opinion of the Scientific Committee on Food on Estragole (1-Allyl-4-methoxybenzene). Health and Consumer Protection Directorate-General. Directorate C, Scientific Opinions, Brussels, Belgium, 2001.
79. SCF Opinion of the Scientific Committee on Food on Methyleugenol (4-Allyl-1,2-dimethoxybenzene). Health and Consumer Protection Directorate-General. Directorate C, Scientific Opinions, Brussels, Belgium, 2001.
80. SCF Opinion of the Scientific Committee on Food on the Safety of the Presence of Safrole (1-Allyl-3,4-methylene Dioxy Benzene). Health and Consumer Protection Directorate-General. Directorate C, Scientific Opinions, Brussels, Belgium, 2001.
81. EU Regulation (EC) No 1334/2008 of the European Parliament and of the Council of 16 December 2008 on flavourings and certain food ingredients with flavouring properties for use in and on foods, 2008. Available at [accessed Februrary 2015]: <http://eur-lex.europa.eu/LexUriServ/LexUriServ.do?uri = OJ:L:2008:354:0034:0050:en:PDF>.
82. Gooderham NJ, Cohen SM, Eisenbrand G, et al. The safety evaluation of food flavoring substances: the role of genotoxicity studies. *Crit Rev Toxicol.* 2020;. Available from: https://doi.org/10.1080/10408444.2020.1712589.
83. Suparmi S, Ginting AJ, Mariyam S, Wesseling S, Rietjens IMCM. Levels of methyleugenol and eugenol in instant herbal beverages available on the Indonesian market and related risk assessment. *Food Chem Toxicol.* 2019;125:467–478. Available from: https://doi.org/10.1016/j.fct.2019.02.001.
84. EFSA. Opinion of the scientific committee on a request from EFSA related to a harmonized approach for risk assessment of substances which are both genotoxic and carcinogenic. *EFSA J.* 2005;282:1–31.
85. Bodi D, Ronczka S, Gottschalk C, et al. Determination of pyrrolizidine alkaloids in tea, herbal drugs and honey. *Food Addit Contam Part A Chem Anal Control Expo Risk Assess.* 2014;31(11):1886–1895. Available from: https://doi.org/10.1080/19440049.2014.964337.

86. Knutsen HK, Alexander J, Barregard L, et al. Risks for human health related to the presence of pyrrolizidine alkaloids in honey, tea, herbal infusions and food supplements. *EFSA J.* 2017;15(7). Available from: https://doi.org/10.2903/j.efsa.2017.4908.
87. Bodi D, Ronczka S, Gottschalk C, et al. Determination of pyrrolizidine alkaloids in tea, herbal drugs and honey. *Food Addit Contam Part A Chem Anal Control Expo Risk Assess.* 2014;31(11):1886–1895.
88. EFSA. Scientific opinion on pyrrolizidine alkaloids in food and feed. *EFSA J.* 2011;9:2406. Available from: http://ehtpa.eu/pdf/2406.pdf.
89. Fu PP, Xia QS, Lin G, Chou MW. Pyrrolizidine alkaloids—genotoxicity, metabolism enzymes, metabolic activation, and mechanisms. *Drug Metab Rev.* 2004;36(1):1–55. Available from: https://doi.org/10.1081/dmr-120028426.
90. Chen M, Li L, Zhong D, Shen S, Zheng J, Chen X. 9-Glutathionyl-6,7-dihydro-1-hydroxymethyl-5H-pyrrolizine is the major pyrrolic glutathione conjugate of retronecine-type pyrrolizidine alkaloids in liver microsomes and in rats. *Chem Res Toxicol.* 2016;29(2):180–189. Available from: https://doi.org/10.1021/acs.chemrestox.5b00427.
91. EFSA. Scientific opinion on pyrrolizidine alkaloids in food and feed. *EFSA J.* 2011;9(11).
92. Xia Q, He X, Ma L, Chen S, Fu PP. Pyrrolizidine alkaloid secondary pyrrolic metabolites construct multiple activation pathways leading to DNA adduct formation and potential liver tumor initiation. *Chem Res Toxicol.* 2018;31(7):619–628. Available from: https://doi.org/10.1021/acs.chemrestox.8b00096.
93. Li N, Xia QS, Ruan JQ, Fu PP, Lin G. Hepatotoxicity and tumorigenicity induced by metabolic activation of pyrrolizidine alkaloids in herbs. *Curr Drug Metab.* 2011;12(9):823–834. Available from: https://doi.org/10.2174/138920011797470119.
94. Miranda CL, Reed RL, Guengerich FP, Buhler DR. Role of cytochrome P450IIIA4 in the metabolism of the pyrrolizidine alkaloid senecionine in human liver. *Carcinogenesis.* 1991;12(3):515–519.
95. Prinsloo G, Steffens F, Vervoort J, R IMCM. Risk assessment of herbal supplements containing ingredients that are both genotoxic and carcinogenic. *Crit Rev Toxicol.* 2019;49:567–579.
96. WHO (World Health Organization), 1983. IARC Monographs on the Evaluation of the Carcinogenic Risk of Chemicals to Humans. 1983, Vol. 31.
97. WHO (World Health Organization), 1987. IARC Monographs on the Evaluation of Carcinogenic Risks to Humans. 1987, Vol. 1 to 42, Supplement 7.
98. WHO (World Health Organization), 2002. IARC Monographs on the Evaluation of Carcinogenic Risks to Humans. 2002, Vol. 82.
99. BfR (Bundesinstitut für Risikobewertung, Federal Institute for Risk Assessment), 2007. Salad mix contaminated with groundsel containing pyrrolizidine alkaloids. BfR Opinion No. 028/2007. Available at [accessed July 2016]: http://www.bfr.bund.de/cm/349/salad_mix_contaminated_with_groundsel_containing_pyrrolizidine_alkaloids.pdf.
100. COT, Committee on Toxicity of Chemicals in Food, Consumer Products and the Environment, COT Statement on Pyrrolizidine Alkaloids in Food, Food Standard Agency, UK, 2008.
101. Van Engelen JGM, Van Egmond HP, Speijers GJA, 1997. Pyrrolizidine Alkaloiden (Pyrrolizidine Alkaloids). Centrum voor Stoffen en Risicobeoordeling (Centre for Substances and Risk Assessment), CSR rapport 05666A00. Rijksinstituut voor Volksgezondheid en Milieu (National Institute of Public Health and the Environment): The Netherlands.
102. NTP. Toxicology and carcinogenesis studies of riddelliine (CAS No. 23246-96-0) in F344/N rats and B6C3F1 mice (gavage studies). Natl Toxicol Program Tech Rep Ser. 2003;508:1-280.
103. Chen L, Mulder PPJ, Louisse J, Peijnenburg A, Wesseling S, Rietjens IMCM. Risk assessment for pyrrolizidine alkaloids detected in (herbal) teas and plant food supplements. *Regul Toxicol Pharmacol.* 2017;86:292–302. Available from: https://doi.org/10.1016/j.yrtph.2017.03.019.
104. Stegelmeier BL, Brown AW, Welch KD. Safety concerns of herbal products and traditional Chinese herbal medicines: dehydropyrrolizidine alkaloids and aristolochic acid. *J Appl Toxicol.* 2015;35(12):1433–1437. Available from: https://doi.org/10.1002/jat.3192.
105. Jansen SA, Kleerekooper I, Hofman ZLM, Kappen I, Stary-Weinzinger A, van der Heyden MAG. Grayanotoxin poisoning: 'mad honey disease' and beyond. *Cardiovasc Toxicol.* 2012;12(3):208–215. Available from: https://doi.org/10.1007/s12012-012-9162-2.
106. Bilir O, Ersunan G, Yavasi O, Kalkan A. Mad honey-related intoxication in an infant: a case report. *J Emerg Med Case Rep.* 2016; 7(4). Available from: https://doi.org/10.5152/jemcr.2016.1476.
107. Koca I, Koca AF. Poisoning by mad honey: a brief review. *Food Chem Toxicol.* 2007;45(8):1315–1318. Available from: https://doi.org/10.1016/j.fct.2007.04.006.
108. Gunduz A, Durmus I, Turedi S, Nuhoglu I, Ozturk S. Mad honey poisoning-related asystole. *Emerg Med J.* 2007;24(8):592–593. Available from: https://doi.org/10.1136/emj.2006.045625.
109. BfR (Bundesinstitut für Risikobewertung, Federal Institute for Risk Assessment), 2010. Cases of poisoning through grayanotoxins in rhododendron honey originating from the Turkish Black Sea Region. BfR Opinion No. 043/2010. Available at [accessed July 2016]: http://www.bfr.bund.de/cm/349/cases_of_poisoning_through_grayanotoxins_in_rhododendron_honey_originating_from_the_turkish_black_sea_region.pdf.
110. Johanns ESD, van der Kolk LE, van Gemert HMA, Sijben AEJ, Peters PWJ, de Vries I. An epidemic of epileptic seizures after consumption of herbal tea. *Ned Tijdschr Geneeskd.* 2002;146(17):813–816.
111. Ize-Ludlow D, Ragone S, Bruck IS, Bernstein JN, Duchowny M, Garcia Peña BM. Neurotoxicities in infants seen with the consumption of star anise tea. *Pediatrics.* 2004;114(5):e653–e656.
112. Ize-Ludlow D, Ragone S, Bernstein JN, Bruck IS, Duchowny M, Pena BMG. Chemical composition of Chinese star anise (*Illicium verum*) and neurotoxicity in infants. *JAMA.* 2004;291(5):562–563. Available from: https://doi.org/10.1001/jama.291.5.562.
113. Kakemoto E, Okuyama E, Nagata K, Ozoe Y. Interaction of anisatin with rat brain gamma-aminobutyric acid(A) receptors: allosteric modulation by competitive antagonists. *Biochem Pharmacol.* 1999;58(4):617–621. Available from: https://doi.org/10.1016/s0006-2952(99)00129-x.
114. Vanherweghem JL, Depierreux M, Tielemans C, et al. Rapidly progressive interstitial renal fibrosis in young-women: association with slimming regimen including chinese herbs. *Lancet.* 1993;341(8842):387–391. Available from: https://doi.org/10.1016/0140-6736(93)92984-2.
115. Vanhaelen M, Vanhaelenfastre R, But P, Vanherweghem JL. Identification of aristolochic acid in chinese herbs. *Lancet.*

1994;343(8890). Available from: https://doi.org/10.1016/s0140-6736(94)90964-4. 174-174.

116. Hashimoto K, Higuchi M, Makino B, et al. Quantitative analysis of aristolochic acids, toxic compounds, contained in some medicinal plants. *J Ethnopharmacol.* 1999;64(2):185–189. Available from: https://doi.org/10.1016/s0378-8741(98)00123-8.

117. IARC. *IARC Monographs on the Evaluation of Carcinogenic Risks to Humans.* vol 82. World Health Organization; 2002:68–128.

118. EMEA The European Agency for the Evaluation of Medicinal Products, Position paper on the risks associated with the use of herbal products containing Aristolochia species, 2000. <http://www.emea.eu.int/pdfs/human/hmpwp/002300en.pdf>.

119. Stiborová M, Frei E, Arlt VM, Schmeiser HH. Metabolic activation of carcinogenic aristolochic acid, a risk factor for Balkan endemic nephropathy. *Mutat Res.* 2008;658(1):55–67.

120. Zhang H, Cifone M, Murli H, Erexson G, Mecchi M, Lawlor T. Application of simplified in vitro screening tests to detect genotoxicity of aristolochic acid. *Food Chem Toxicol.* 2004;42 (12):2021–2028.

121. Mengs U, Lang W, Poch J-A. The carcinogenic action of aristolochic acid in rats. *Arch Toxicol.* 1982;51(2):107–119.

122. Grollman AP, Scarborough J, Jelakovic B. Aristolochic acid nephropathy: an environmental and iatrogenic disease. *Adv Mol Toxicol.* 2009;3:211–227.

123. Arlt VM, Schmeiser HH, Pfeifer GP. Sequence-specific detection of aristolochic acid-DNA adducts in the human p53 gene by terminal transferase-dependent PCR. *Carcinogenesis.* 2001;22(1): 133–140. Available from: https://doi.org/10.1093/carcin/22.1.133.

124. Martena MJ, van der Wielen JCA, van de Laak LFJ, Konings EJM, de Groot HN, Rietjens IMCM. Enforcement of the ban on aristolochic acids in Chinese traditional herbal preparations on the Dutch market. *Anal Bioanal Chem.* 2007;389(1):263–275. Available from: https://doi.org/10.1007/s00216-007-1310-3.

125. Abdullah R, Diaz LN, Wesseling S, Rietjens IMCM. Risk assessment of plant food supplements and other herbal products containing aristolochic acids using the margin of exposure (MOE) approach. *Food Addit Contam Part A Chem Anal Control Expo Risk Assess.* 2017;34(2):135–144. Available from: https://doi.org/10.1080/19440049.2016.1266098.

126. Arunotayanun W, Gibbons S. Natural product 'legal highs'. *Nat Product Rep.* 2012;29(11):1304–1316. Available from: https://doi.org/10.1039/c2np20068f.

127. Graziano S, Orsolini L, Rotolo MC, Tittarelli R, Schifano F, Pichini S. Herbal Highs: review on psychoactive effects and neuropharmacology. *Curr Neuropharmacol.* 2017;15(5):750–761. Available from: https://doi.org/10.2174/1570159x14666161031144427.

128. EFSA. Tropane alkaloids (from Datura sp.) as undesirable substances in animal feed. Scientific opinion of the panel on contaminants in the food chain. (EFSA-Q-2003-063) Adopted on 9 April 2008. *EFSA J.* 2008;691:1–55.

129. Adamse P, Van Egmond HP Tropane Alkaloids in Food. 2010. RIKILT Institute of Food Safety. Report no. 2010.011. 2010. Available at <https://edepot.wur.nl/160741.1-24>.

130. Brown JH, Taylor P. In: Brunton LL, Lazo JS, Parker KL, eds. *Goodman & Gilman's The Pharmacological Basis of Therapeutics.* 11th Edn. New York: McGraw-Hill. *Med Publ Div.* 2006:183–200.

131. EFSA (European Food Safety Authority). Tropane alkaloids (from Datura sp.) as undesirable substances in animal feed. Scientific Opinion of the Panel on Contaminants in the Food Chain. (EFSA-Q-2003-063) Adopted on 9 April 2008. *EFSA Journal.* 2008;691:1–55.

132. Perharic L. Mass tropane alkaloid poisoning due to buckwheat flour contamination. *Clin. Toxicol.* 2005;43:413.

133. Perharic L, Juvan KA, Stanovnik L. Acute effects of a low-dose atropine/scopolamine mixture as a food contaminant in human volunteers. *Journal of Applied Toxicology.* 2013;33:980–990.

134. EFSA (European Food Safety Authority). EFSA CONTAM Panel (EFSA Panel on Contaminants in the Food Chain). Scientific Opinion onTropane alkaloids in food and feed. *EFSA Journal.* 2013;11(10):3386. 113.

135. Frohne, D. and Pfänder, H.J., 2004. Giftpflanzen. 5. Auflage, Wissenschaftliche Verlagsgesellschaft, Stuttgart.

136 BfR (Bundesinstitut für Risikobewertung, Federal Institute for Risk Assessment), 2006. BfR recommends provisional daily upper intake level and a guidance value for morphine in poppy seeds. BfR Health Assessment No. 012/2006. Available at [accessed July 2016]: http://www.bfr.bund.de/cm/349/bfr_recommends_provisional_daily_upper_intake_level_and_a_guidance_value_for_morphine_in_poppy_seeds.pdf.

137. Dusemund B, Appel K-E, Lampen A. BfR risk assessment of alkaloids as ingredients and contaminants of food: Quinine, opium alkaloids, and senecio pyrrolizidine alkaloids. In: DFG Senate commission on Food safety (SKLM), ed. *Risk Assessment of Phytochemicals in Food.* Weinheim: Wiley-VCH Verlag; 2010:1382–1390. see: chrome-extension://efaidnbmnnnibpcajpcglclefindmkaj/https://eur-lex.europa.eu/legal-content/EN/TXT/PDF/?uri = CELEX:32013R1307.

138. EFSA. Update of the scientific opinion on opium alkaloids in poppy seeds. *EFSA J.* 2018;16(5):5243.

139. Hager, ROM, Stramonii Semen, Springer Verlag, Heidelberg 2006.

140. Taschan H. Hanfhaltige Lebensmittel: Psychedelische Lebensmittel, neuartige Lebensmittel oder Rauschmittel? *Verbraucherdienst.* 1999;44:144–148.

141. BgVV (Bundesinstitut für gesundheitlichen Verbraucherschutz und Veterinaermedizin, Federal Institute for Consumer Health Protection and Veterinary Medicine), 2000. BgVV recommends guidance values for THC (tetrahydrocannabinol) in hemp containing food. Press release 07/2000, 16.03.2000, Germany. Available at [accessed July 2016]: http://www.bfr.bund.de/en/presseinformation/2000/07/bgvv_recommends_guidance_values_for_thc__tetrahydrocannabinol__in_hemp_containing_foods-1309.html.

142. Meier H, Vonesch H-J. Cannabis-Intoxikation nach Salatgenuss. *Schweiz. Med. Wochenschr.* 1997;127:214–218.

143. Brunton LL, Lazo JS, Parker KL, eds. *Goodman & Gilman's The Pharmacological Basis of Therapeutics.* 11th ed. New York: McGraw-Hill. *Med Publ Div* 2006.

144. EFSA. Scientific Opinion on the safety of hemp (Cannabis genus) for use as animal feed. *EFSA J.* 2011;9(3):41.

145. EFSA. Scientific Opinion on the risks for public health related to the presence of tetrahydrocannabinol (THC) in milk and other food of animal origin. *EFSA J.* 2015;13(6):4141. 125.

146. Gilard V, Balayssac S, Tinaugus A, Martins N, Martino R, Malet-Martino M. Detection, identification and quantification by H-1 NMR of adulterants in 150 herbal dietary supplements marketed for improving sexual performance. *J Pharm Biomed Anal.* 2015;102:476–493. Available from: https://doi.org/10.1016/j.jpba.2014.10.011.

147. Reeuwijk NM, Venhuis BJ, de Kaste D, Hoogenboom LAP, Rietjens IMCM, Martena MJ. Sildenafil and analogous phosphodiesterase type 5 (PDE-5) inhibitors in herbal food supplements sampled on the Dutch market. *Food Addit Contam Part A Chem Anal Control Expo Risk Assess*. 2013;30(12):2027–2034. Available from: https://doi.org/10.1080/19440049.2013.848294.
148. Gresser U, Gleiter CH. Erectile dysfunction: comparison of efficacy and side effects of the PDE-5 inhibitors sildenafil, vardenafil and tadalafil - review of the literature. *Eur J Med Res*. 2002;7(10):435–446.
149. Cheitlin MD, Hutter AM, Brindis RG, et al. Use of sildenafil (Viagra) in patients with cardiovascular disease. *Circulation*. 1999;99 (1):168–177.
150. Langtry HD, Markham A. Sildenafil: a review of its use in erectile dysfunction. *Drugs*. 1999;57(6):967–989. Available from: https://doi.org/10.2165/00003495-199957060-00015.
151. EMA. *Withdrawal Assessment Report for Viagra*. London: European Medicines Agency; 2008.
152. Kloner R. Erectile dysfunction and hypertension. *Int J Impot Res*. 2007;19:296–302.
153. Torfgard KE, Ahlner J. Mechanisms of action of nitrates. *Cardiovasc Drugs Ther*. 1994;8:701–717.
154. Reeuwijk NM, Venhuis BJ, de Kaste D, Hoogenboomc R, Rietjens IMCM, Martena MJ. Active pharmaceutical ingredients detected in herbal food supplements for weight loss sampled on the Dutch market. *Food Addit Contam Part A Chem Anal Control Expo Risk Assess*. 2014;31(11):1783–1793. Available from: https://doi.org/10.1080/19440049.2014.958574.
155. Merz KH, Schrenk D. Interim relative potency factors for the toxicological risk assessment of pyrrolizidine alkaloids in food and herbal medicines. *Toxicol Lett*. 2016;263:44–57. Available from: https://doi.org/10.1016/j.toxlet.2016.05.002.
156. EFSA. Risks for human health related to the presence of pyrrolizidine alkaloids in honey, tea, herbal infusions and food supplements. *EFSA J*. 2017;15(7):4908. Available at. Available from: https://efsa.onlinelibrary.wiley.com/doi/epdf/10.2903/j.efsa.2017.4908.
157. Lieberman HR, Marriott BP, Williams C, et al. Patterns of dietary supplement use among college students. *Clin Nutr*. 2015;34(5): 976–985. Available from: https://doi.org/10.1016/j.clnu.2014.10.010.
158. Felter SP, Conolly RB, Bercu JP, et al. A proposed framework for assessing risk from less-than-lifetime exposures to carcinogens. *Crit Rev Toxicol*. 2011;41(6):507–544. Available from: https://doi.org/10.3109/10408444.2011.552063.

Chapter 2

Soil, water, and air: potential contributions of inorganic and organic chemicals

Wageh Sobhy Darwish[1] **and Lesa A. Thompson**[2]

[1]*Food Control Department, Faculty of Veterinary Medicine, Zagazig University, Zagazig, Egypt,* [2]*Regional Representation for Asia and the Pacific, World Organisation for Animal Health (WOAH), Tokyo, Japan*

Abstract

Environmental pollution by inorganic and organic chemicals in soil, water, and air is a global problem, with several deleterious effects. These chemicals find their way into plant foods and agricultural crops via absorption and uptake from the environment. Ingestion of such contaminated food sources by animals and humans may lead to various toxicological implications. In this chapter, the potential sources for contamination of soil, water, and air by organic and inorganic chemicals—including heavy metals, pesticides, plastics, antimicrobials, and other industrial chemicals—are reported. Furthermore, recent publications screening the occurrence of these chemicals in the environment are reviewed. Suggested preventive measures and remediation approaches toward such chemicals are discussed. Some reports describing uptake of the chemicals by plant foods and agricultural crops are also reviewed. Finally, potential human health risks associated with consumption of foods contaminated by inorganic and organic chemicals are further outlined.

Keywords: Organic chemicals; inorganic chemicals; soil; water; air; plant foods; human health risks; remediation approaches; food safety

2.1 General introduction

Contamination of the environment by various inorganic and organic chemicals is not only a potentially serious problem for the animals and plants living therein, but it is also a great issue for human health. This chapter explores several of the more common chemicals in this category, outlining their presence in soil, water, and air—important sources of contamination for food (Fig. 2.1). The possible risks to human health from these chemicals and how to undertake health risk assessments are discussed, along with strategies for remediation and reduction of environmental contamination. In the future, targeted scientific research and policy implementation are vital to reduce these risks.

2.2 Heavy metals

2.2.1 Introduction

Heavy metals are a group of inorganic chemicals characterized by their persistence in the environment and their bioaccumulative and biomagnification nature. The terms heavy metals or metalloids were given to these chemicals because of their high atomic number or high density in the environment. The most common metals with public health significance introduced into the environment are lead (Pb), cadmium (Cd), arsenic (As), mercury (Hg), copper (Cu), zinc (Zn), nickel (Ni), and chromium (Cr). Environmental pollution with heavy metals is a problem of global interest.[1] Heavy metals are released into the environment via weathering of metal-bearing rocks, volcanic eruptions, and anthropogenic activities, leading to potentially serious adverse effects on human health. Numerous studies have been conducted worldwide to investigate the sources of contamination by heavy metals. Here, the sources of contamination of air, water, and soil with heavy metals; recent studies on their incidence; and possible remediation approaches will be summarized.

2.2.2 Sources of heavy metal contamination

2.2.2.1 Air

Air is polluted with heavy metals mainly through anthropogenic activities including both agricultural and

Present Knowledge in Food Safety. DOI: https://doi.org/10.1016/B978-0-12-819470-6.00037-8

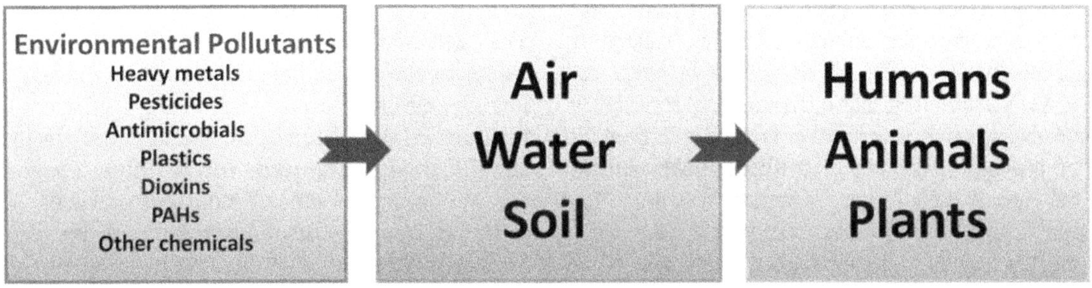
Environmental Pollutants
Heavy metals
Pesticides
Antimicrobials
Plastics
Dioxins
PAHs
Other chemicals
Air
Water
Soil
Humans
Animals
Plants

FIGURE 2.1 Diagrammatic indication of air, water, and soil as possible sources for transmission of environmental pollutants to humans, animals, and plants.

industrial processes. Furthermore, air contamination with heavy metals can be accelerated by the release of dust and particulate matter (PM). Important sources include automobile exhausts, release from electroplating, petrochemical and ceramic factories, burning of fossil fuels, airports, volcanic eruptions, forest fires, and wind-blown dust.[2,3] Some metals such as Hg are evaporated into the environment. Major elements involved in air pollution include Pb, Cd, and Hg.[4]

2.2.2.2 Water

Metals can manage to enter into water bodies via industrial and anthropogenic activities such as direct release of industrial wastes into aquatic streams. The release of metals from the soil into water bodies via irrigation water is another source. Similarly, the direct release from drainage systems into water streams contributes to the metal load in the water.[5] Water can also be contaminated with heavy metals through water pipes made from certain metals such as copper and lead.[6,7] Release of metals from water containers into the water itself represents another source.[8]

2.2.2.3 Soil

Soil can be contaminated with different heavy metals via various sources including the weathering of rocks releasing their corresponding metals into the soil. Anthropogenic activities are considered major routes for soil contamination by heavy metals, including activities such as mining and milling cycles, and direct disposal of metals to recycling sites.[9,10] Plant fertilizers involve the direct addition of some trace elements (such as phosphate, Zn, selenium, Cu, and sulfur) for the healthy growth of plants; toxic metals such as Pb and Cd can be found as impurities in these fertilizers.[11,12] Spraying of pesticides constitutes another source for contamination of soil by heavy metals, as several pesticides contain heavy metals in their ingredients: copper-containing fungicides, lead arsenate used for the control of some parasites, and arsenic-containing compounds used for livestock production and sometimes added directly into the grazing lands.[13,14] Heavy metals also act as ingredients for painting materials and cement manufacture, and subsequently can contaminate the soil after disposal of some painting waste or building materials. Animal excreta, manure and sewage sludge are added to increase the fertility of the agricultural lands and soils; these materials may contain metals excreted by the animals.[15,16] Wastewater and direct disposal of drainage water and effluents into soil or arable land might contaminate the soil with various heavy metals.[17] Some lands are even irrigated with wastewater and effluents. Soil can be contaminated with metals from airborne sources and rain; some metals such as Hg, Pb, Cd, and As are volatilized or released from vehicles into the environment, particularly near highways and airports,[18,19] and can find their way via the air to settle into soil.[20,21] Some metals are released into adjacent soil during manufacture of petrochemicals, textiles, electroplating factories, and pharmaceuticals.[22,23]

2.2.3 Incidence

2.2.3.1 Air

Determination of heavy metals in the ambient atmosphere is of particular importance for public health; therefore metal load in the air and fine particles have been estimated worldwide. For instance, Gharaibeh et al.[3] reported that Pb, Fe, Cu, Ni, Mn, and Zn were detected at high concentrations during the summer season in Irbid city, Jordan. Furthermore, Tan et al.[2] recorded high concentrations of Zn, Mn, Cu, As, Cd, and Pb in the PM collected from Foshan city, a ceramics manufacturing center located in southern China. Similarly, Pb, Cr, Cd, Zn, Mn, As, Fe, Cu, and Ni were detected in PM samples in the vicinity of secondary smelting operations in Ile-Ife, Nigeria.[24] Collectively, Suvarapu and Baek[25] reported that Cr, Pb, Cd, Ni, and As receive major attention worldwide. In addition, Goddard et al.[4] detected antimony and barium in air quality samples around the United Kingdom.

2.2.3.2 Water

Water represents a major pathway for heavy metals to reach animals and humans. For instance, laboratory animals were exposed to toxic metals as Pb and Cd leached from water bottle components into the animals' drinking water.[8] In Egypt, toxic metals such as Pb, Cd, Ni, and As were detected in drinking water introduced into quail farms.[6,7] High levels for toxic metals and trace elements were recorded in drinking water in the provinces of Punjab and Khyber Pakhtunkhwa, Pakistan; the chronic daily intake for humans was in the following order: Cr > Ni > Mn > Cu > As > Pb > Co > Cd.[26] Furthermore, Chen et al.[27] detected Cd, Cr, Pb, and As in drinking water in Xigu District, Lanzhou, China, although levels were within standard limits. In addition, Dong et al.[28] evaluated the heavy metal load in a main drinking water source in Dalian, China; six metals, namely Cu, Zn, Cd, Ni, As, and Hg, were detected, with only Hg exceeding the Chinese standard limits.

2.2.3.3 Soil

Relatively high levels of heavy metals are recorded in soil worldwide. For instance, Różański et al.[19] studied the impact of highway traffic on the total content and bioavailability of Zn, Cu, Ni, Cd, Cr, and Pb in nearby soils in Poland. They recorded moderate and high bioavailability for Cd and Pb, respectively. Likewise, a study by Massas et al.[18] monitored heavy metal distribution in soils close to Athens International Airport in Attica, Greece. They recorded higher concentrations of high potential availability of Pb, Mn, Cu, and Ni in the study area. In Brazil, do Nascimento et al.[29] evaluated the heavy metal content in soils from the southwestern Brazilian Amazon. They detected Cd, Cr, Cu, Fe, Mn, Ni, Pb, and Zn at variable concentrations. Several studies investigate the metal load in soil and the factors affecting it. Cai et al.[30] found higher levels for Cd, Pb, Zn, Ni, Cu, and Hg in the agricultural soils of Gaogang Town, China. They concluded that agricultural practices, industrial practices, and traffic activities were the main sources of Cd, Pb, Hg, and Zn. Similarly, Xiao et al.[22] investigated the distribution of heavy metals and their potential availability in vegetable fields around electroplating factory outlets and irrigated by the factory wastewater in Guangzhou, China. They concluded that the potential availability of heavy metals in soil was positively correlated with Mn oxides in soil and, therefore, that Mn oxides can enhance the potential availability of heavy metals (Table 2.1).

2.2.4 Remediation and preventive measures

There is limited information about possible remediation technologies for the removal of heavy metals from air. However, prevention of major sources of contamination will help reduce metal load entering the atmosphere. The use of electric-powered vehicles will reduce the release of the metals from vehicle exhausts. The increase in cultivation of agriculture belts around cities and nearby mining fields will help filter air and additionally act as indicators for the air pollution.[31]

TABLE 2.1 Incidence of heavy metal contamination in soil, water, and air as reported in some countries.

Source	Metal	Place of study	References
Air	Pb, Fe, Cu, Ni, Mn, and Zn	Jordan	3
Air	Zn, Mn, Cu, As, Cd, and Pb	China	2
Air	Pb, Cr, Cd, Zn, Mn, As, Fe, Cu, and Ni	Nigeria	24
Air	Cr, Pb, Cd, Ni, and As	Worldwide	25
Air	Antimony, barium	United Kingdom	4
Water	Cd, Cr, Pb, and As	China	27
Water	Pb, Cd, As, and Ni	Egypt	6,7
Water	Cr, Ni, Mn, Cu, As, Pb, Co, and Cd	Pakistan	26
Water	Cu, Zn, Cd, Ni, As, and Hg	China	28
Water	Pb, Cd	United States	8
Soil	Mn	China	22
Soil	Cd, Pb, Zn, Ni, Cu, and Hg	China	30
Soil	Cd, Cr, Cu, Fe, Mn, Ni, Pb, and Zn	Brazil	29
Soil	Cd and Pb	Poland	19
Soil	Pb, Mn, Cu, and Ni	Greece	18

Removal of heavy metals from water sources is a major concern worldwide. The scientific community has developed several physical and chemical methods for this process including: membrane filtration technologies,[32] electrocoagulation,[33] redox methods,[34] and chemical precipitation.[35] Adsorption is considered an environmentally friendly method for the removal of heavy metals from water. This method can be employed using a variety of substances such as activated carbon,[36] pomegranate seeds,[37] maize hull,[38] tree ash,[39] clay mineral,[40] and carbon nanotubes.[41]

Heavy metal removal from soil depends on some conventional techniques such as adsorption, electrodialysis, precipitation, and ion exchange. Bioremediation is another technique used to convert harmful substances like heavy metals into less harmful ones; this process can be introduced into the soil via in and ex situ techniques. In situ techniques include use of (1) the bioventing method, whereby supply of oxygen into soil enhances growth of beneficial microorganisms; (2) the biostimulation method, where supply of some nutrients stimulates growth of the beneficial organisms; and (3) the bioattenuation method with passive remediation of the soil.[42] Ex situ techniques include use of (1) bioreactors which change soil pH and aeration levels, (2) the biopile process involving excavation of contaminated soil with nutrients, (3) the windrow process with continuous turning and irrigation of piled soil, and (4) land farming by specific plants that can assist in absorption of some heavy metals.[43]

2.3 Pesticides

2.3.1 Introduction

Pesticides are a group of large and diverse organic chemicals that are intentionally applied into the environment to control various pests. The group contains several categories including insecticides, herbicides, fungicides, and rodenticides. Exposure to pesticides can have severe adverse health effects on humans and untargeted animal species. This attracts the attention of public health, food safety, environmental and policy sectors. A well-known example that stimulated public health awareness was Rachel Carson's book *Silent Spring* (1962), which placed the spotlight on the adverse effects of pesticides on untargeted species, birds in particular. This book had a significant effect on the international environment movement and for creation of the US Environmental Protection Agency (US EPA) in 1970. Several classes of pesticides are characterized by their persistent nature and their stability in the environment, sometimes for decades, for example dichlorodiphenyltrichloroethane (DDT). The release of pesticides into air, water, and soil represents a major route for contamination of human foods and subsequent potentially severe adverse health effects if contaminated foods are ingested. In this section, the sources of contamination of air, water and soil with pesticides, examples of some recent reports on the incidence of such contamination, and possible remediation strategies will be discussed.

2.3.2 Sources of contamination

2.3.2.1 Air

Use of pesticides made from petroleum-based hydrocarbons led to the entry of hydrocarbon mixtures into the air in agricultural lands.[44] Spraying of crops is a major source for contamination of air with various pesticides such as insecticides and herbicides.[45] The soil-air exchange of pesticides accounts for their cross-contamination as in the case of volatilization of pesticides such as organochlorine pesticides (OCPs), particularly in agricultural lands.[46] Indoor and outdoor spraying of insecticides is also used to control insects such as mosquitoes, which act as vectors for human diseases such as malaria.[1]

2.3.2.2 Water

Spilling of pesticides into surrounding water streams is considered one port of entry for mixtures of hydrocarbons into water sources.[44] Pesticides can be deposited into water streams after aerial spraying for control of crop pests.[45] In addition, Bidleman et al.[47] reported the exchange of OCPs between water, soil, and air. The direct addition of herbicides to control unwanted plants growing in rivers and lakes represents a source for contamination of water with certain classes of pesticides. Drainage of wastewater from irrigated pesticide-contaminated soils is a potential source for contamination of water streams. In other words, pesticides may leach from irrigation of plants into groundwater and surface water.[48] The direct release of wastes from pesticide factories into water bodies is an additional source of water contamination.

2.3.2.3 Soil

Spilling of pesticides into surrounding soil is a major route of entry for soil contamination by hydrocarbon mixtures.[44] Spraying of pesticides at low levels over agricultural crops may inadvertently be transferred for long distances by wind and deposited over soil causing contamination of soil at a distant site.[45] Air–soil exchange of pesticides is also reported as a source for cross-contamination via deposition of sprayed pesticides into soil matrices.[46,49] Soil may act as a sink for persistent organic pesticides such as OCPs.[50] Certain herbicides and rodenticides are also directly added to soil for control of unwanted plants and rodents.

2.3.3 Incidence

The occurrence of pesticides in air, water, and soils from selected studies around the world is reported in Table 2.2.

2.3.3.1 Air

Several studies have investigated the occurrence of pesticides in the air and atmosphere worldwide. For instance,[51] reported levels of herbicides, OCPs, and organophosphates (OPPs) in the atmosphere across Canadian agricultural regions. Aliyeva et al.[52] detected high levels of OCPs including DDTs in air samples surveyed across Azerbaijan. Similarly, Ma et al.[53] recorded high levels of DDTs in air samples monitored over one year in the center of China. Furthermore, Mai et al.[54] detected high levels of OCPs in air from the North Sea region of Europe. Aslam et al.[55] recorded high levels of DDTs and (Hexachlorocyclohexane) HCHs in filter dust from indoor air-conditioners in Lahore city, Pakistan.

2.3.3.2 Water

Water can be contaminated with various pesticides. For instance, atrazine, tebuconazole, and diethyltoluamide were detected in surface water in Argentina.[56] Sultana et al.[57] detected neonicotinoid pesticides including thiamethoxam, clothianidin, and imidacloprid in raw water from agricultural regions of southern Ontario, Canada. Furthermore, a study by Sjerps et al.[58] recorded high levels of two neonicotinoids (acetamiprid and thiamethoxam) in groundwater and surface water sources used for drinking water production in the Netherlands. Elfikrie et al.[48] detected insecticides including imidacloprid, propiconazole, and buprofezin in surface water collected from Tanjung Karang, Selangor, Malaysia. In addition, the herbicides bromobutide and bentazone, commonly used in rice cultivation, were detected in high concentrations in treated drinking water in Japan.[59]

2.3.3.3 Soil

Růzicková et al.[50] observed that industrial soils from the Czech Republic were heavily polluted with DDTs as a result of previous pesticide production. Chakraborty et al.[46] reported high levels of DDTs and endosulfans in soils collected from several cities in India (New Delhi, Agra, Kolkata, Mumbai, Goa, Chennai, and Bangalore). Pokhrel et al.[49] reported air–soil exchange of OCPs in tropical Nepali cities; additionally, the study recorded high concentrations of OCPs including DDT, endosulfans, and hexachlorobenzene. Ma et al.[53] recorded high levels of OCPs, and HCHs in soil from urban, rural, and forestry locations in the Hami region of Xinjiang, China. Furthermore, Gereslassie et al.[60] detected high levels of OCPs in the soil samples collected from central China.

TABLE 2.2 Incidence of pesticide contamination in air, water, and soil as reported in some countries.

Source	Pesticides	Place of study	References
Air	Herbicides, OCPs, OPPs	Canada	51
Air	DDTs	Azerbaijan	52
Air	DDTs	China	53
Air	OCPs	Europe	54
Air	DDTs, HCHs	Pakistan	55
Water	Atrazine, tebuconazole, and diethyltoluamide	Argentina	56
Water	Thiamethoxam, clothianidin, and imidacloprid	Canada	57
Water	Acetamiprid and thiamethoxam	The Netherlands	58
Water	Imidacloprid, propiconazole, and buprofezin	Malaysia	48
Water	Bromobutide and bentazone	Japan	59
Soil	DDTs	Czech Republic	50
Soil	DDTs and endosulfans	India	46
Soil	DDTs and endosulfans	Nepal	49
Soil	OCPs and HCHs	China	53
Soil	OCPs	China	60

DDT, dichlorodiphenyltrichloroethane; *HCH*, hexachlorocyclohexane; *OCPs*, organochlorine pesticides; *OPPs*, organophosphates.

2.3.4 Remediation and preventive measures

The most effective methods for reduction of pesticide load in the environment require effective multisectoral collaboration, including public, environment, food safety, water and soil sectors. Continuous monitoring and surveillance programs to study the current situation of pesticide contamination globally are highly recommended. Over and above this, it is suggested to: use pesticides with a short half-life and easy degradation, avoid unnecessary massive usage of pesticides, ban pesticides with high toxicity and persistent nature, have a registration process for pesticides with periodical screening, isolate contaminated lands and soils, and reduce aerial use. Proper application of pesticides will reduce unnecessary use. Additionally, proper storage and disposal of pesticides and/or their containers is necessary to reduce accidental release into the environment. Irrigation management and proper drainage to control the runoff of pesticides from the soil into groundwater are important. Using environmentally friendly pesticides is also advisable. Looking to the future, finding alternatives such as natural bioactive compounds or using biological control methods for the control of plants, insects, or rodents should be prioritized. Establishment of green barriers may also impede drift movement of pesticides.[1,61]

2.4 Antimicrobials

2.4.1 Introduction

A number of pharmaceutical agents, collectively known as Pharmaceuticals and Personal Care Products as Pollutants (PPCPs), can contaminate the environment. A specific concern is those PPCPs which are antimicrobials. These include agents that act against bacteria (antibiotics), fungi (antifungals), viruses (antivirals), and parasites (antiparasitics). These agents are vital in modern-day times to treat a huge range of pathogens and have transformed the healthcare of people and animals, and contribute to food security and food safety. Unfortunately, their widespread use and oftentimes poor disposal have resulted in contamination of the environment.

An associated problem faced globally is that of antimicrobial resistance (AMR), which continues to increase. Overuse and misuse of antimicrobials have accelerated emergence and spread of AMR.[62,63] Back at the beginning of the 21st century, the Institute of Medicine estimated that infections from antibiotic-resistance bacteria bore an annual cost to the United States of USD 4–5 million.[64] These costs include those attributable to mortality, morbidity, care time, diagnosis, and treatment. About 700,000 people died due to AMR infections around the world in 2016 but this is estimated to rise to 10 million a year by 2050.[65,66]

2.4.2 Sources of contamination

The major sources of antimicrobial contamination in the environment are from (1) contaminated human and animal waste (urine and feces), (2) improper disposal of unused antimicrobial agents, and (3) use on crops to reduce certain pathogens. As such, antimicrobials may be contaminants of sewage outflows and rubbish disposal from humans, but may also originate from use of the agents in livestock, farmed fish, or crop cultivation. The resulting contamination may include the primary antimicrobials and also potentially active breakdown products.

2.4.2.1 Air

In general, air is not considered a major point of environmental contamination by antimicrobials, although there is the possibility that contaminated dried manure particles or such like may be carried in the air. Antimicrobial resistant pathogens may certainly be transported via air.

2.4.2.2 Water

Water may become contaminated by running through soil which is contaminated as mentioned above. Additionally, industrial effluent from pharmaceutical manufacturing plants or medicated (animal) feed plants may be contaminated by antimicrobials. Antimicrobials may be deliberately added to water sources. For example, they may be used in domestic aquaculture farming (e.g., fish and shrimp) to treat or prevent infections. These farming systems are very rarely discrete, and contiguous waterways will also be contaminated.

2.4.2.3 Soil

Antimicrobials can contaminate soil from several sources. Improper disposal of unused antimicrobials into general waste can result in soil contamination at landfill sites, or wherever the waste is disposed. This is a source of antimicrobial access to the environment including wildlife for which the compounds were not intended. Animals which have been given antimicrobials will excrete some of these compounds and their metabolic breakdown products in urine and feces onto pastures. Both animal and human manure may be used as fertilizer and thus contaminate crops. In some instances, waste materials in human sewage may be sedimented in treatment plants and then used as fertilizers on land, or dumped at land or sea.

In some countries, it is not uncommon for people to dispose of unused antimicrobials via toilet systems. In this fashion, the antimicrobials will contaminate the sewage system. Despite various treatments of sewage, antimicrobials or their breakdown products may remain active even after these processes.

TABLE 2.3 Examples of studies on antimicrobials detected in the environment.

Source	Key point	References
Water	Surface water and tap water may contain antimicrobials and multidrug-resistant bacteria, even after wastewater treatment	67
Water	Well water may be contaminated by multiple antimicrobials	68
Water	Antimicrobials used in (salmon) aquaculture may result in widespread dissemination of both agents and AMR	69
Water	Tap water and even bottled water may contain antimicrobials	70
Soil	Antibiotics can be taken up from the environment into edible crops	71
Soil	Different antimicrobials have different sorption behaviors in soils, for example, florfenicol is highly mobile in soils and may contaminate water	72
Soil	Fluoroquinolones are abundant in agricultural resources and in soil	73
Soil	There can be seasonal variation in contamination of peri-urban areas	74

AMR, antimicrobial resistance.

2.4.3 Incidence

Recent publications have identified and monitored antimicrobials in the environment (Table 2.3). Their presence appears to be ubiquitous in soil and water.

2.4.4 Remediation and preventive measures

Guidelines to be followed for appropriate use of antimicrobials can be found for both human and veterinary health, according to the Global Action Plan on Antimicrobial Resistance[62] and the OIE Strategy on Antimicrobial Resistance and the Prudent Use of Antimicrobials,[63] respectively. Due to the serious risks associated with AMR, it is vital for antimicrobial selection to consider WHO's list of critically important antimicrobials (WHO CIA list[75]) and the OIE list of antimicrobials of veterinary importance.[76] National *legislation* (and associated implementation) should cover sale and distribution of antimicrobials, with prescriptions from licensed medical doctors and veterinarians required for purchase. For manufacturing or processing units, including medicated feed merchants, national legislation should include measures for limiting environmental contamination from industrial outfall, with strict monitoring to ensure limits are not exceeded. In countries where antimicrobials are well regulated, their use will be lower and thus so will environmental contamination. Therefore the most important strategy to reducing environmental contamination by antimicrobials is to support good stewardship of these agents in human, animal, and environmental sectors—promoting effective legislation to control prescribing, use, and disposal of antimicrobials. Implementation of legislation necessarily includes effective monitoring by governments of antimicrobial production, sale, and use, and surveillance of AMR in the environment.

Monitoring of samples from people, animals, and the environment for organisms resistant to various antimicrobials should be conducted. Various international guidelines are available for laboratories monitoring AMR, including those testing animal products for human food. The Global Antimicrobial Resistance Surveillance System (GLASS), launched by WHO in 2015, promotes a standardized approach for human priority pathogens.

Hand in hand with this is the need to *educate* both private and public sectors on the risks of misusing antimicrobials and disposing of them inappropriately. All sectors should be targeted with awareness programs on the possible consequences of misuse and antimicrobial contamination in the environment, and necessary remediation to reduce AMR. Medical and veterinary professionals should be educated on use of antimicrobials and able to provide sound advice to others—using the compounds appropriately, and giving advice on completion of courses prescribed and disposal of unused medicines.

A specific measure to reduce environmental contamination relates to manure. Pretreatment by anaerobic digestion has been shown to degrade some contaminants, for example 87%–95% of AMR genes by activated carbon with microwave pretreatment.[77] Even the physical action of managed composting resulted in partial removal of antimicrobials and resistant genes.

To reduce the use of antimicrobials, some *alternatives* are available and others are under development. WHO principles of infection prevention and control (IPC) and water sanitation and health (WASH) have been designed to prevent infections, starting with the simple act of hand hygiene and further including other preventative measures. Development of vaccinations for numerous pathogens have enabled great reductions, including in livestock and aquaculture, and remains a key focus of research into alternatives to reduce the dependence of animal sectors on antimicrobials.

Improving biosecurity when introducing new stock and choosing alternatives to antimicrobials for health control measures can greatly reduce the contamination levels. In 2017 Norway produced more than half of the total world production of Atlantic salmon. This rising production and a series of infectious diseases toward the latter part of the 20th century led to a massive increase in antibiotic use in the farmed fish. Production of a number of effective vaccines in combination with biosecurity and regulatory improvements led to a drop in use of antibiotics in the country.

The cross-sectoral implications of antimicrobial contamination in the environment and the risks of AMR have assured that this problem is being tackled in a One Health manner, with multisectoral collaboration between human health, animal health, and environmental sectors. AMR is now recognized by governments and international organizations as a major health threat globally in the 21st century. Left unchecked, the potential economic implications and effects of AMR on human and animal health are massive. Contamination of the environment by antimicrobials and their breakdown products is the main driver for increasing AMR. Stricter control measures regarding sale and use of antimicrobials are key means to reducing antimicrobial contamination. In conjunction with this, it is vital for healthcare stakeholders to work together on alternative methods of tackling pathogens causing disease—including development of vaccines, improving sanitary standards throughout the human population, and increasing biosecurity measures for livestock.

2.5 Plastics

2.5.1 Introduction

Plastics are a large group of natural or synthetic compounds that can be molded into different shapes. The extensive use of plastics worldwide combined with their low biodegradation and difficulty in recycling had resulted in the emergence of widespread environmental pollution with plastics. This problem has attracted the world's attention because of the severe adverse effects of plastics on the entire environment, and animal and human health. In this section, the sources, examples for occurrence of plastics in air, water, and soil, and suggested remediation and prophylactic measures will be discussed.

2.5.2 Sources of contamination

2.5.2.1 Air

The incineration of plastic waste in open fields constitutes a major source for air pollution by plastics and plasticizers. Domestic and industrial release of plastic waste directly into the open air is another source for transfer of plastic residues into the atmosphere.[78] The release of microplastics (MPs) from house dust into indoor and outdoor air is an additional source for contamination.[79]

2.5.2.2 Water

Surface water, groundwater, and water streams can all be contaminated by plastics including MPs from various sources. Of these, direct release by plastic factories of their waste into water streams is a significant source. Plastic waste disposal by the public directly into water streams, especially in developing countries, is another major source. Biological fragmentation of plastics in water bodies by aquatic biota is considered a significant source for aquatic contamination by MPs. Thermal fragmentation of plastics by ultraviolet (UV) from sunlight is an additional mechanism whereby water bodies may be contaminated by MPs. Wastewater treatment plants may transfer the residues from plastics into surface or groundwater.[78] MPs in rain is another source for transfer of plastics from the air into water bodies.[80]

2.5.2.3 Soil

The direct dumping of plastic waste by the public and other industrial activities represents the major source for soil contamination by plastics. Incineration of plastics in the open field is another notable source for soil contamination by plastics. Thermal fragmentation of plastics by UV in sunlight is considered a source for slow release of MPs to soil.[78] Erosions and abrasions of synthetic rubber car tires contribute significantly to soil contamination by plastics. Plastic in rain is an additional source for transfer of plastics from air to soil. Plastic recycling plants may release high concentrations of plastics—particularly those released from personal care products, bottle water, and plastic shopping bags—to the surrounding environment, including to soil.[81] Lastly, some organisms such as earthworms and mites can contribute to the formation of MPs and breakdown of large plastics molecules, and the transfer of these chemicals into deep layers of soil.[82]

2.5.3 Incidence

Several studies have been conducted worldwide to investigate the incidence of plastics (including MPs) and plasticizers in air, water, and soil as indicated in Table 2.4.

2.5.3.1 Air

Fromme et al.[83] reported the occurrence of plasticizers in air and dust samples from German daycare centers. Takeuchi et al.[84] detected plasticizers including phthalates and adipates in indoor air samples from the living rooms

TABLE 2.4 Incidence of plastic contamination in air, water, and soil as reported in some countries.

Source	Plastic type	Place of study	References
Air	Plasticizers	Germany	83
Air	Phthalates and adipates	Japan	84
Air	Plasticizers	United States	85,86
Air	Phthalates	Thailand	87
Air	Phthalates	China	88
Water	Phthalates	Iran	89
Water	MPs	Thailand	90
Water	MPs	United Kingdom	91
Water	MPs	China	92
Water	MPs	China	79
Soil	Phthalates	South Korea	85,86
Soil	MPs	Mediterranean Sea	93
Soil	MPs	China	94
Soil	MPs	Italy	95
Soil	Polyethylene, polystyrene, and polyvinyl chloride	France	96

MPs, microplastics.

of 21 dwellings in 11 prefectures across Japan, with compounds mainly present as particles smaller than 2.5 μm and therefore likely able to reach the deepest parts of lungs after inhalation. Likewise, Kim et al.[85,86] investigated the occurrence of plasticizers in indoor air and dust collected from various microenvironments in the Albany area of New York State in the United States. They detected high levels of plasticizers in sampled bulk air, vapor phase, and dust. Furthermore, Promtes et al.[87] reported the presence of phthalates in the indoor home environment in Bangkok, Thailand. In addition, Wang et al.[88] detected phthalates in plastic agricultural greenhouse air in Shaanxi Province, China, at 5305 ng/m^3; this level was higher in winter compared to summer.

2.5.3.2 Water

Abtahi et al.[89] detected phthalates in water resources, bottled water, and tap water in Tehran, Iran. Kankanige and Babel[90] demonstrated the presence of smaller-sized MPs in single-use (Polyethylene) PET-bottled water in Thailand. Johnson et al.[91] characterized MPs in eight water treatment works in England and Wales. In China, Tong et al.[92] reported high levels of MPs in tap water. Similarly, Zhang et al.[79] recorded high levels of MPs in the water bodies of rivers at a range of 3.9–7900 items/m^3.

2.5.3.3 Soil

Kim et al.[85,86] demonstrated the toxicity of phthalates on multiple soil species in a study conducted in South Korea. High levels of MPs were recorded in soils collected from the Northwestern Mediterranean Sea.[93] Li et al.[94] separated MPs from the soil and sewage sludge in China. Additionally, Piehl et al.[95] recorded large MPs (1–5 mm) within beach sediments at the Po River Delta, northeast Italy, with high tendency to accumulate polystyrene. Wahl et al.[96] isolated nanoplastics (20–150 nm) from three major plastic families (polyethylene, polystyrene, and polyvinyl chloride) in a soil amended with plastic debris in France.

2.5.4 Remediation and preventive measures

There is an urgent need to maintain monitoring and surveillance studies to understand the scenarios for the occurrence of plastics in the environment. Communication between scientists and decision makers is endorsed to solve the environmental pollution problem, particularly with plastics. Prevention and/or reduction of disposal of plastic waste either at domestic or industrial levels will indeed reduce the contamination level in the environment. Preventing or minimizing the use of single-use plastic containers in shopping and other daily activities will help reduce their disposal into the environment. Legislations to ban sources of plastic release into the environment have been introduced in the European Union, Canada, and United States,[97] and similar approaches are greatly needed worldwide. Biodegradation of plastics with organisms like certain bacteria and fungi is considered a safe and reliable plan to reduce the emission of MPs into the environment.[98] Plastic manufacturers are requested to clearly identify reuse and recycle policies of their products. Improvement in incineration fields for plastic waste should be applied for better isolation and to avoid cross-contamination of the environment. Training and educational courses should be introduced for the public and other stakeholders to reduce the release of plastic waste into the environment.

2.6 Other industrial chemicals

2.6.1 Introduction

In this section the sources, state of occurrence, and possible remediation and preventive measures for other industrial-released chemicals such as polycyclic aromatic hydrocarbons (PAHs), dioxins [polychlorinated dibenzo-*p*-dioxins], polychlorinated dibenzofurans, and dioxin-like (Polychlorinated biphenyls) PCBs (dl-PCBs) will be discussed. These environmental chemicals are of global interest, as several are listed as persistent organic pollutants in the Stockholm Convention, and have severe adverse health effects on humans and animals in addition to deleterious effects on the environment.[1]

2.6.2 Sources of contamination

2.6.2.1 Air

PAHs and dioxins are released into the air via many anthropogenic activities such as waste incineration, fuel and wood combustion, and in the metal industry. In addition, natural sources include volcanic eruptions and forest fires.[99] PAHs are also released in tobacco smoking, in burning of rice straw, and during barbecuing of meat.[6,7]

2.6.2.2 Water

Surface or groundwater can be contaminated with PAHs and dioxins near metal smelting. In the case of contamination in the atmosphere, rain may collect and deposit these contaminants to water streams. Erosions from contaminated soils may enter groundwater. In addition, direct release of chemical waste from factories into water streams represents a source for water contamination.[100] PAHs have been reported in leachate from cigarette butts into water.[101]

2.6.2.3 Soil

PAHs and dioxins are hydrophobic chemicals that have high tendency to accumulate in soil for decades. These chemicals may be found due to human activities such as in soil near waste incineration sites. Burning of rice straw, metal smelting sites, and coal manufacturing also contribute to accumulation of PAHs and dioxins in soil. Air–soil exchange of PAHs and dioxins represent a major source for deposition from contaminated air into soil. Volcanic eruptions and forest fires help in buildup of these chemicals into soil.[100,102]

2.6.3 Incidence

Several surveillance studies conducted worldwide address the occurrence of industrial chemicals such as PAHs, dioxins, and dioxin-like compounds. Some reports of contamination of air, water and soil with such contaminants are introduced in Table 2.5.

2.6.3.1 Air

Gune et al.[105] detected high levels of PAHs in air samples collected from the south-west coast of India. Wang et al.[106] reported that total concentrations of PAHs in the air of Dalian, China, ranged from 6.37 to 124 ng/m^3 with

TABLE 2.5 **Incidence of contamination with PAHs, dioxins, and dioxin-like compounds in air, water, and soil as reported in some countries.**

Source	Contaminants	Place of study	References
Air	Dioxins	Hong Kong	103
Air	Dioxins and PCBs	Spain	104
Air	PAHs	India	105
Air	PAHs	China	106
Water	Dioxins	Japan	107
Water	PAHs	China	108
Water	PAHs	China	100
Water	PAHs	China	109
Soil	Dioxins	United States	102
Soil	PAHs	China	108
Soil	PAHs	China	110
Soil	PAHs	China	106
Soil	PAHs	India	105
Soil	PAHs	Sweden	111

PAHs, polycyclic aromatic hydrocarbons.

an average of 23.1 ± 26.6 ng/m^3. Choi et al.[103] demonstrated the presence of dioxins in air sampled in Hong Kong. López et al.[104] detected both dioxins and dioxin-like PCBs in ambient air samples collected from both industrial and urban areas in the Valencian Region, Spain.

2.6.3.2 Water

Li et al.[108] detected 15 priority PAHs in water samples from the Aojiang River and its estuary in China. Furthermore, Wu et al.[100] recorded high levels of 16 priority PAHs in shallow groundwater at a metal smelting area in Southeastern China. Similarly, Zhang et al.[109] recovered high levels of 16 priority PAHs in drinking water from different administrative level cities throughout mainland China. Regarding dioxins, Minomo et al.[107] reported high levels in Ayase River, an urban river in Japan.

2.6.3.3 Soil

Verbrugge et al.[102] recorded high concentrations of dioxins in surface soil surrounding pentachlorophenol-treated utility poles on the Kenai National Wildlife Refuge, Alaska, USA. Li et al.[108] detected 15 priority PAHs in soil and sediment samples from the Aojiang River waterway in Wenzhou, China. In addition, Xiao et al.[110] detected PAHs of high and low molecular weight in forest soils from urban and rural areas in the Pearl River Delta of Southern China. Wang et al.[106] reported total concentrations of PAHs in soil from Dalian, China, ranging from 42.8 to 28,600 ng/g with an average of 2580 ± 5730 ng/g. In India, Gune et al.[105] reported the occurrence of PAHs in soil surrounding a coal-fired thermal power plant on the south-west coast. Furthermore, Dreij et al.[111] detected 21 PAHs, 11 oxygenated PAHs, and 7 methylated PAHs in soils collected from 25 urban parks in Stockholm City, Sweden.

2.6.4 Remediation and preventive measures

Dioxins, PAHs, and other industrial chemicals have severe deleterious effects on the environment. In this regard, scientific efforts should be directed to find appropriate solutions for this global problem. As dioxins and PAHs are released from incinerators for medical, industrial, and other wastes; therefore it is mandatory to use the best available technology to control incinerators and to follow best environmental practices to prevent cross-contamination and emission of such chemicals. Prevention of release from various sources causing environmental pollution with PAHs and dioxins will indeed help in reducing the environmental load. In addition, decontamination processes including photochemical degradation and GeoMelt technology should be followed.[112] Dias-Ferreira et al.[113] introduced the electrodialytic remediation method for dioxins in fly ash to control air pollution. Further, Chang et al.[114] suggested that thermal oxidation and pyrolysis for remediation of dioxins from sediment, pyrolysis is the preferred method. Microbial degradation using aerobic bacteria from the genera *Sphingomonas*, *Pseudomonas*, and *Burkholderia* has been introduced as a reliable method for attenuation of dioxins in the environment.[115] Soil washing with mixed anionic and nonanionic surfactants has been reported to be an efficient method for removal of PAHs from contaminated soil.[116]

In general, continuous monitoring, surveillance studies, and remediation trials are highly recommended to update our knowledge and the data available on environmental pollution and remediation of such industrial chemicals. Additionally, collaboration and cross-talks between all sectors concerned with environmental pollution, food safety, public health, and decision makers are necessary to save our environment.

2.7 Uptake of environmental pollutants from air, water, and soil to plant foods

Plant foods might absorb considerable concentrations of environmental chemicals via absorption from contaminated air, water, and soil, and subsequently find their way into animal and human bodies if these are ingested (Table 2.6). For instance, Chen et al.[117] reported translocation of Cd, Cu, Zn, and Pb from contaminated soils into corn, rice, and wheat near a zinc smelter in Guizhou Province, China. Furthermore, Darwish et al.[6,7] concluded that contamination of poultry feed with heavy metals such as Pb, Cd, As, and Ni is possible from use of contaminated crops in the manufacture of poultry feed in Egypt. Okra, pumpkin, tomato, potato, eggplant, spinach, and cabbage from Faisalabad, Pakistan, were found to be highly contaminated with toxic metals such as Pb, Cd, As, and Hg.[118] Plant foods and agricultural crops were found to be contaminated with pesticides such as OCPs in many African countries.[119] OCPs, OPPs, carbamates, and acaricides were detected in tomatoes, chili, and eggplants in Nepal,[120] and also in onions, tomatoes, cabbage, and watermelons freshly produced in Tanzania.[121] There is a clear lack of information available on contamination of agricultural crops and plant foods by plastics. In a recent report by Oliveri et al.[122] found that apple and carrot had the highest accumulation pattern for MPs among certain tested fruits and vegetables from Italy. Two personal care products with antimicrobial activities, triclocarban (TCC) and triclosan (TCS), were found to be taken up by eleven food crops grown in hydroponic nutrient media in a study conducted in the United States.[123] Furthermore, Pan and Chu[67] reviewed the uptake of antimicrobials by edible

TABLE 2.6 Uptake of environmental chemicals from air, water, and soil to plant foods and agriculture crops.

Group	Examples	Involved plants or crops	Location of study	Reference
Heavy metals	Cd, Cu, Zn, and Pb	Corn, rice, wheat	China	117
	Pb, Cd, As, and Ni	Corn	Egypt	6,7
	Pb, Cd, As, and Hg	Okra, pumpkin, tomato, potato, eggplant, spinach, cabbage	Pakistan	118
Pesticides	OCPs	Agricultural crops	Africa	119
	OCPs, OPPs, and acaricides	Tomatoes, chili, eggplants	Nepal	120
	OCPs, OPPs, carbamates, and acaricides	Onions, tomatoes, cabbage, watermelons	Tanzania	121
Plastics	MPs	Apple, carrot	Italy	122
Antimicrobials	TCC and TCS	Various crops	United States	123
	Antimicrobials	Edible crops	China	67
Industrial chemicals	PAHs	Plant foods	China	108
	Dioxins	Alfalfa, maize, apple, basil, beet pulp pellets containing molasses	Poland	124

MPs, Microplastics; *OCPs*, organochlorine pesticides; *OPPs*, organophosphates; *PAHs*, polycyclic aromatic hydrocarbons; *TCC*, triclocarban; *TCS*, triclosan.

crops in China. Plant foods can accumulate PAHs through absorption from air, as reported in Wenzhou, China.[108] Of note, Piskorska-Pliszczynska et al.[124] reported that plant-derived animal feed—including alfalfa, maize, apple, basil, and beet pulp pellets containing molasses—in Poland contained considerable concentrations of dioxins and dioxin-like compounds.

2.8 Human health risk assessment

2.8.1 Introduction

Common health problems that may be associated with various inorganic and organic chemicals have been reviewed elsewhere. Identification of symptoms may give a clinical or toxicologist field worker some indication of potential hazardous contaminants that may be involved in a particular situation (Table 2.7). However, these are rarely pathognomonic for a specific contaminant, and individual or group testing may be required to differentiate the cause of ill health. In other situations, it may be useful to proactively search for ill effects in a population if a contamination situation has been detected by environmental surveillance.

2.8.2 Individual or group health assessments

In certain situations, it becomes necessary to assess the health of either individuals or a section of a population. The approach to these may be somewhat different.

2.8.2.1 Individual

If an individual either has a history of possible exposure to contaminants (e.g., a worker in the chemical industry) and/or shows clinical signs that are suspicious for toxic effects, they may undergo testing for levels of a specific agent in body samples. Such tests will vary depending on the suspected toxin. For some contaminants, they are easily tested from a sample, such as Pb levels in blood. Although there is no "safe" level of Pb, higher levels are considered more serious; a blood Pb level above 5 μg/dL (0.24 μmol/L) is considered elevated. For other contaminants, it may be challenging for laboratory analysis to detect or may require specialist equipment, such as for pesticides.

In cases of an ill individual, general health tests may also be conducted—for example urinalysis for kidney function, blood tests for liver, kidney or immune system function, and/or mental health assessments for cognitive function. Biological markers may be useful to detect exposure to contaminants, for example DNA or protein adducts, mutation, or chromosomal aberrations. A specific example of a biomarker is urinary arsenic, which may enable estimation of the dose over time. Biochemical or molecular markers may be used to indicate disease.

2.8.2.2 Group

If several people within a population are showing similar signs of ill health, it may be appropriate to test them all individually as above. However, if an environmental

TABLE 2.7 Possible effects on human health associated with various environmental contaminants.

Group	Examples	Possible health effects
Pesticide	Chlorpyrifos	Neurological symptoms
	DDTs	Neurological symptoms; endocrine disruption
	DDTs and other OCPs	Infertility and fetal malformation
Heavy metal	Arsenic	Dermal, respiratory, nervous, mutagenic and carcinogenic effects
	Cadmium	Renal dysfunction; associated with a high risk of lung and breast cancer; osteomalacia and osteoporosis
	Lead	Effects on the nervous system and red blood cells; reduced cognitive development and intellectual performance; death in children
	Mercury	Cardiovascular, reproductive, developmental, neural, renal, and immune toxicity; carcinogenic
	Nickel	Dermal effects; lower body weight; fetotoxicity
Dioxins and dioxin-like compounds	Doxins	Language delay; disturbances in mental and motor development
Antimicrobial	Macrolides	Hypersensitivity and anaphylactic shock
	Quinolones	Drug-resistant pathogens
	Sulfonamides	Nephropathy
	Tetracyclines	Impaired intestinal flora
	Antimicrobial resistance	Transfer of resistant genes between pathogens
Industrial chemicals	Various	Dermal irritation; ocular, respiratory, and reproductive toxicity; carcinogenic
Plastics	Various	Ocular, respiratory, hepatic, dermal, reproductive, cardiovascular, and gastrointestinal effects; carcinogenic; teratogenic

DDT, dichlorodiphenyltrichloroethane; *OCPs*, organochlorine pesticides.
Source: Adapted from Thompson LA, Darwish WS. Environmental chemical contaminants in food: review of a global problem. *J Toxicol.* 2019;2019:2345283.

contamination is suspected, such as the case of ingestion of contaminated plant foods or agricultural crops with environmental pollutants such as heavy metals or pesticides, it is often necessary to assess many population members to screen for toxicity even before symptoms of illness are present. The focus of such an investigation is likely to be on a specific test to measure levels of a toxin in body samples to ascertain the exposure of the general population. It is important to sample sufficient members of a population to draw general conclusions about exposure.

2.8.3 Health risk assessment

For certain contaminants, a limit has been defined above which clinical signs of toxicity are likely to occur. For many of these agents, acute exposure toxicity levels may vary from longer term exposure—whereby a lower dose over a longer time may accumulate within the body and lead to ill effects. For this reason, it can be useful to consider both acute and long-term exposures when performing a risk assessment of environmental contaminants. The US EPA has developed references for many contaminants.[125]

2.8.3.1 Acute exposure

This method usually considers once-in-a-lifetime short-term exposures and refers to the general population, without considering potentially significant differences such as age or gender. This is more important when considering accidental exposure to a highly concentrated source, for example ingestion of a volume of pesticide. However, in certain instances, high levels may be present in the environment and could lead to acute ill health. The no-observed-adverse-effect level is frequently reported, or lowest-observed-adverse-effect level at which there are biologically significant adverse effects. For certain substances, minimal risk levels (MRLs) have been determined by the Agency for Toxic Substances and Disease

Registry (ATSDR), covering oral or inhaled exposure. These may be represented as acute or short-term values. The US EPA defines acute exposure as <24 h, short-term as 24 h to 30 days, and longer term as >30 days up to approximately 10% of a human life span (using 70 years as the average life span).

2.8.3.2 Long-term exposure

For many toxic contaminants, the effects relate to conditions that may be difficult to link directly to one agent. For example, reproductive health effects, carcinogenicity, or immunotoxicity may be seen with several of the contaminants discussed in this chapter. In this case, it can be useful to consider the likely daily exposure and consider how that may remain in a person's body over time, potentially increasing if bioaccumulation occurs. Chronic or repeated exposure is defined by the US EPA as more than approximately 10% of a human life span. There is also an ATSDR intermediate MRL (covering a period between 15 and 364 days). Subchronic and chronic toxicity studies may be used to obtain levels for longer exposures, and may relate to laboratory testing undertaken on animals over the course of their lifetime—to evaluate toxicities such as cardiovascular, reproductive, neurological, immune system or carcinogenic effects. The reference dose (*RfD*) is the estimate of the daily oral exposure likely to be without appreciable risk of deleterious effects during a lifetime. RfD is usually used in US EPA noncancer health assessments. The reference concentration (RfC) is a similar estimate for inhalation exposure.

Using these estimates for toxicity levels, a human health *risk assessment* can be determined for the potential adverse health effects from exposure. This therefore considers scientific information regarding the hazard of the environmental agents, the dose–response relationship, and the exposure assessment. *Risk* is usually expressed in values between 0 (certain that no harm will occur) and 1 (certain that harm will occur). For those contaminants known to have carcinogenic effects, a specific health risk assessment is conducted using calculations linked to lifetime exposure.[126] Particularly in cancer risk assessment, age of children at the time of exposure may be important as there may be critical periods of exposure for certain toxicities. Finally, it is important to correlate human exposure for each contaminant with particular food items. For instance, exposure to heavy metals is usually linked to the ingestion of fish with a high trophic level in the food chain. Human exposure to pesticides is mostly linked to ingestion of contaminated plant foods and agricultural crops, while human exposure to antimicrobials is associated with consumption of livestock and poultry products. Human exposure to plastics is linked to ingestion of contaminated fish and shellfish. Lastly, human exposure to PAHs and dioxins is mostly associated with heat-treated meat and meat products.

References

1. Thompson LA, Darwish WS. Environmental chemical contaminants in food: review of a global problem. *J Toxicol*. 2019;2019:2345283. Available from: https://doi.org/10.1155/2019/2345283. Jan 1.
2. Tan JH, Duan JC, Ma YL, et al. Source of atmospheric heavy metals in winter in Foshan, China. *Sci Total Environ*. 2014;493:262–270. Available from: https://doi.org/10.1016/j.scitotenv.2014.05.147. Sep 15.
3. Gharaibeh AA, El-Rjoob AW, Harb MK. Determination of selected heavy metals in air samples from the northern part of Jordan. *Environ Monit Assess*. 2010;160(1–4):425–429. Available from: https://doi.org/10.1007/s10661-008-0706-7.
4. Goddard SL, Williams KR, Robins C, Brown RJC. Determination of antimony and barium in UK air quality samples as indicators of non-exhaust traffic emissions. *Environ Monit Assess*. 2019;191(11):641. Available from: https://doi.org/10.1007/s10661-019-7774-8.
5. Adesiyan IM, Bisi-Johnson M, Aladesanmi OT, Okoh AI, Ogunfowokan AO. Concentrations and human health risk of heavy metals in rivers in Southwest Nigeria. *J Health Pollut*. 2018;8(19):180907. Available from: https://doi.org/10.5696/2156-9614-8.19.180907. Sep 10.
6. Darwish WS, Atia AS, Khedr MHE, Eldin WFS. Metal contamination in quail meat: residues, sources, molecular biomarkers, and human health risk assessment. *Environ Sci Pollut Res Int*. 2018;25(20):20106–20115. Available from: https://doi.org/10.1007/s11356-018-2182-0.
7. Darwish WS, Ikenaka Y, Nakayama S, Mizukawa H, Thompson LA, Ishizuka M. β-carotene and retinol reduce benzo[a]pyrene-induced mutagenicity and oxidative stress via transcriptional modulation of xenobiotic metabolizing enzymes in human HepG2 cell line. *Environ Sci Pollut Res Int*. 2018;25(7):6320–6328. Available from: https://doi.org/10.1007/s11356-017-0977-z.
8. Nunamaker EA, Otto KJ, Artwohl JE, Fortman JD. Leaching of heavy metals from water bottle components into the drinking water of rodents. *J Am Assoc Lab Anim Sci*. 2013;52(1):22–27.
9. Kabata-Pendias A, Pendias H. *Trace Metals in Soils and Plants*. 2nd ed. Boca Raton, FL: CRC Press; 2001.
10. Pierzynski GM, Sims JT, Vance GF. *Soils and Environmental Quality*. 2nd ed. London: CRC Press; 2000.
11. Lasat MM. Phytoextraction of metals from contaminated soil: a review of plant/soil/metal interaction and assessment of pertinent agronomic issues. *J Hazard Subst Res*. 2000;2:1–25.
12. Raven PH, Berg LR, Johnson GB. *Environment*. 2nd ed. New York, NY: Saunders College Publishing; 1998.
13. Jones LHP, Jarvis SC. The fate of heavy metals. In: Green DJ, Hayes MHB, eds. *The Chemistry of Soil Processes*. New York, NY: John Wiley & Sons; 1981:593.
14. McLaughlin MJ, Hamon RE, McLaren RG, Speir TW, Rogers SL. Review: a bioavailability-based rationale for controlling metal and metalloid contamination of agricultural land in Australia and New Zealand. *Aust J Soil Res*. 2000;38(6):1037–1086.
15. United States Environmental Protection Agency (US EPA). *A Plain English Guide to the EPA Part 503 Biosolids Rule. USEPA Rep. 832/R-93/003*. Washington, DC: US EPA; 1994.

16. Weggler K, McLaughlin MJ, Graham RD. Effect of chloride in soil solution on the plant availability of biosolid-borne cadmium. *J Environ Qual*. 2004;33(2):496–504.
17. Bjuh J. Trace *Metals in Soils Irrigated with Waste Water in a Periurban Area Downstream Hanoi City, Vietnam*, Seminar Paper, Institutionen for markvetenskap, Sveriges lantbruksuniversitet (SLU), Uppsala, Sweden; 2007.
18. Massas I, Gasparatos D, Ioannou D, Kalivas D. Signs for secondary buildup of heavy metals in soils at the periphery of Athens International Airport, Greece. *Environ Sci Pollut Res Int*. 2018; 25(1):658–671. Available from: https://doi.org/10.1007/s11356-017-0455-7.
19. Różański S, Jaworska H, Matuszczak K, Nowak J, Hardy A. Impact of highway traffic and the acoustic screen on the content and spatial distribution of heavy metals in soils. *Environ Sci Pollut Res Int*. 2017;24(14):12778–12786. Available from: https://doi.org/10.1007/s11356-017-8910-z.
20. United States Environmental Protection Agency (US EPA). *Report: Recent developments for in situ treatment of metals contaminated soils*. Office of Solid Waste and Emergency Response, U.S. Environmental Protection Agency; 1996.
21. Smith LA, Means JL, Chen A, et al. *Remedial Options for Metals-Contaminated Sites*. Boca Raton, FL: Lewis Publishers; 1995.
22. Xiao L, Guan D, Chen Y, et al. Distribution and availability of heavy metals in soils near electroplating factories. *Environ Sci Pollut Res Int*. 2019;26(22):22596–22610. Available from: https://doi.org/10.1007/s11356-019-04706-0. Epub 2019 Jun 4. PMID: 31165447.
23. Sumner ME. Beneficial use of effluents, wastes, and biosolids. *Commun Soil Sci Plant Anal*. 2000;31(11–14):1701–1715.
24. Ogundele LT, Owoade OK, Hopke PK, Olise FS. Heavy metals in industrially emitted particulate matter in Ile-Ife, Nigeria. *Environ Res*. 2017;156:320–325. Available from: https://doi.org/10.1016/j.envres.2017.03.051. Jul.
25. Suvarapu LN, Baek SO. Determination of heavy metals in the ambient atmosphere. *Toxicol Ind Health*. 2017;33(1):79–96. Available from: https://doi.org/10.1177/0748233716654827.
26. Hussain S, Habib-Ur-Rehman M, Khanam T, Sheer A, Kebin Z, Jianjun Y. Health risk assessment of different heavy metals dissolved in drinking water. *Int J Environ Res Public Health*. 2019;16(10):1737. Available from: https://doi.org/10.3390/ijerph16101737.
27. Chen YF, Sun SW, Duan XL, et al. Refined assessment of exposure and health risks of heavy metals in water for the children in Xigu District. *Lanzhou Huan Jing Ke Xue*. 2020;41(1):262–272.
28. Dong W, Zhang Y, Quan X. Health risk assessment of heavy metals and pesticides: a case study in the main drinking water source in Dalian, China. *Chemosphere*. 2020;242:125113. Available from: https://doi.org/10.1016/j.chemosphere.2019.125113. Mar.
29. do Nascimento CWA, Lima LHV, da Silva FL, Biondi CM, Campos MCC. Natural concentrations and reference values of heavy metals in sedimentary soils in the Brazilian Amazon. *Environ Monit Assess*. 2018;190(10):606. Available from: https://doi.org/10.1007/s10661-018-6989-4. Sep 24.
30. Cai LM, Wang QS, Wen HH, Luo J, Wang S. Heavy metals in agricultural soils from a typical township in Guangdong Province, China: occurrences and spatial distribution. *Ecotoxicol Environ Saf*. 2019;168:184–191. Available from: https://doi.org/10.1016/j.ecoenv.2018.10.092. Jan 30.
31. Bahadoran M, Mortazavi SN, Hajizadeh Y. Evaluation of Anticipated Performance Index, biochemical, and physiological parameters of *Cupressus arizonica* Greene and *Juniperus excelsa* Bieb for greenbelt development and biomonitoring of air pollution. *Int J Phytoremediat*. 2019;21(5):496–502. Available from: https://doi.org/10.1080/15226514.2018.1537251.
32. Figoli A, Cassano A, Criscuoli A, et al. Influence of operating parameters on the arsenic removal by nanofiltration. *Water Res*. 2010;44:97–104.
33. Zhang C, Jiang Y, Li Y, Hu Z, Zhou L, Zhou M. Three-dimensional electrochemical process for wastewater treatment: a general review. *Chem Eng J*. 2013;228:455–467.
34. Zou Y, Wang X, Khan A, et al. Environmental remediation and application of nanoscale zero-valent iron and its composites for the removal of heavy metal ions: a review. *Environ Sci Technol*. 2016;50:7290–7304.
35. Grimshaw P, Calo JM, Hradil G. Cyclic electrowinning/precipitation (CEP) system for the removal of heavy metal mixtures from aqueous solutions. *Chem Eng J*. 2011;175:103–109.
36. Jusoh A, Shiung LS, Noor M. A simulation study of the removal efficiency of granular activated carbon on cadmium and lead. *Desalination*. 2007;206:9–16.
37. Ghaneian M, Bhatnagar A, Ehrampoush M, et al. Biosorption of hexavalent chromium from aqueous solution onto pomegranate seeds: kinetic modeling studies. *Int J Environ Sci Technol*. 2017;14:331–340.
38. Ghasemi SM, Mohseni-Bandpei A, Ghaderpoori M, et al. Application of modified maize hull for removal of Cu (II) ions from aqueous solutions. *Environ Prot Eng*. 2017;43:93–103.
39. Sanchooli Moghaddam M, Rahdar S, Taghavi M. Cadmium removal from aqueous solutions using saxaul tree ash. *Iran J Chem Eng*. 2016;35:45–52.
40. Jiang M, Jin X, Lu X, Chen Z. Adsorption of Pb(II), Cd(II), Ni(II) and Cu(II) onto natural kaolinite clay. *Desalination*. 2010; 252:33–39.
41. Taghavi M, Zazouli MA, Yousefi Z, Akbari-adergani B. Kinetic and isotherm modeling of Cd (II) adsorption by L-cysteine functionalized multi-walled carbon nanotubes as adsorbent. *Environ Monit Assess*. 2015;187:682.
42. Kapahi M, Sachdeva S. Bioremediation options for heavy metal pollution. *J Health Pollut*. 2019;9(24):191203. Available from: https://doi.org/10.5696/2156-9614-9.24.191203.
43. Fomina M, Gadd GM. Biosorption: current perspectives on concept, definition and application. *Bioresour Technol*. 2014;160:3–14. Available from: https://doi.org/10.1016/j.biortech. May.
44. Woodrow JE, Gibson KA, Seiber JN. Pesticides and related toxicants in the atmosphere. *Rev Environ Contam Toxicol*. 2019;247: 147–196. Available from: https://doi.org/10.1007/398_2018_19.
45. Bradford DF, Stanley KA, Tallent NG, et al. Temporal and spatial variation of atmospherically deposited organic contaminants at high elevation in Yosemite National Park, California, USA. *Environ Toxicol Chem*. 2013;32(3):517–525. Available from: https://doi.org/10.1002/etc.2094.
46. Chakraborty P, Zhang G, Li J, Sivakumar A, Jones KC. Occurrence and sources of selected organochlorine pesticides in the soil of seven major Indian cities: assessment of air-soil exchange. *Environ Pollut*. 2015;204:74–80. Available from: https://doi.org/10.1016/j.envpol.2015.04.006. Sep.

47. Bidleman TF, Leone AD, Falconer RL, et al. Chiral pesticides in soil and water and exchange with the atmosphere. *Sci World J.* 2002;2:357–373. Available from: https://doi.org/10.1100/tsw.2002.109. Feb.
48. Elfikrie N, Ho YB, Zaidon SZ, Juahir H, Tan ESS. Occurrence of pesticides in surface water, pesticides removal efficiency in drinking water treatment plant and potential health risk to consumers in Tengi River Basin, Malaysia. *Sci Total Environ.* 2020;712:136540. Available from: https://doi.org/10.1016/j.scitotenv.2020.136540. Apr 10.
49. Pokhrel B, Gong P, Wang X, Chen M, Wang C, Gao S. Distribution, sources, and air-soil exchange of OCPs, PCBs and PAHs in urban soils of Nepal. *Chemosphere.* 2018;200:532–541. Available from: https://doi.org/10.1016/j.chemosphere.2018.01.119. Jun.
50. Růzicková P, Klánová J, Cupr P, Lammel G, Holoubek I. An assessment of air-soil exchange of polychlorinated biphenyls and organochlorine pesticides across central and southern Europe. *Environ Sci Technol.* 2008;42(1):179–185. Available from: https://doi.org/10.1021/es071406f.
51. Yao Y, Harner T, Blanchard P, et al. Pesticides in the atmosphere across Canadian agricultural regions. *Environ Sci Technol.* 2008; 42(16):5931–5937. Available from: https://doi.org/10.1021/es800878r.
52. Aliyeva G, Kurkova R, Hovorkova I, Klánová J, Halsall C. Organochlorine pesticides and polychlorinated biphenyls in air and soil across Azerbaijan. *Environ Sci Pollut Res Int.* 2012; 19(6):1953–1962. Available from: https://doi.org/10.1007/s11356-012-0944-7.
53. Ma ZL, Mao XX, Ding ZY, et al. Residual levels in air, soil and soil-air exchange of organochlorine pesticides in Hami region of Xinjiang and its potential ecological risk. *Huan Jing Ke Xue.* 2013;34(3):1120–1128.
54. Mai C, Theobald N, Hühnerfuss H, Lammel G. Persistent organochlorine pesticides and polychlorinated biphenyls in air of the North Sea region and air-sea exchange. *Environ Sci Pollut Res Int.* 2016;23(23):23648–23661. Available from: https://doi.org/10.1007/s11356-016-7530-3.
55. Aslam I, Mumtaz M, Qadir A, et al. Organochlorine pesticides (OCPs) in air-conditioner filter dust of indoor urban setting: implication for health risk in a developing country. *Indoor Air.* 2020;. Available from: https://doi.org/10.1111/ina.12772. Nov 28.
56. De Gerónimo E, Aparicio VC, Bárbaro S, Portocarrero R, Jaime S, Costa JL. Presence of pesticides in surface water from four sub-basins in Argentina. *Chemosphere.* 2014;107:423–431. Available from: https://doi.org/10.1016/j.chemosphere.2014.01.039. Jul.
57. Sultana T, Murray C, Kleywegt S, Metcalfe CD. Neonicotinoid pesticides in drinking water in agricultural regions of southern Ontario, Canada. *Chemosphere.* 2018;202:506–513. Available from: https://doi.org/10.1016/j.chemosphere.2018.02.108. Jul.
58. Sjerps RMA, Kooij PJF, van Loon A, Van Wezel AP. Occurrence of pesticides in Dutch drinking water sources. *Chemosphere.* 2019;235:510–518. Available from: https://doi.org/10.1016/j.chemosphere.2019.06.207. Nov.
59. Kamata M, Matsui Y, Asami M. National trends in pesticides in drinking water and water sources in Japan. *Sci Total Environ.* 2020;744:140930. Available from: https://doi.org/10.1016/j.scitotenv.2020.140930. Nov 20.
60. Gereslassie T, Workineh A, Atieno OJ, Wang J. Determination of occurrences, distribution, health impacts of organochlorine pesticides in soils of Central China. *Int J Environ Res Public Health.* 2019;16(1):146. Available from: https://doi.org/10.3390/ijerph16010146.
61. Langenbach T, Caldas LQ. Strategies for reducing airborne pesticides under tropical conditions. *Ambio.* 2018;47(5):574–584. Available from: https://doi.org/10.1007/s13280-017-0997-4. Epub 2017 Dec 14. PMID: 29243054; PMCID: PMC6072638.
62. World Health Organization (WHO). *Global Action Plan on Antimicrobial Resistance.* <https://www.who.int/antimicrobial-resistance/publications/global-action-plan/en/>; 2015 Accessed 27.12.20.
63. World Organisation for Animal Health (OIE). T*he OIE Strategy on Antimicrobial Resistance and the Prudent Use of Antimicrobials.* <https://www.oie.int/fileadmin/Home/eng/Media_Center/docs/pdf/PortailAMR/EN_OIE-AMRstrategy.pdf>; 2016 Accessed 27.12.20.
64. McGowan Jr JE. Economic impact of antimicrobial resistance. *Emerg infect Dis.* 2001;7(2):286.
65. Friedman ND, Temkin E, Carmeli Y. The negative impact of antibiotic resistance. *Clin Microbiol Infect.* 2016;22(5):416–422.
66. O'Neill J. *Tackling drug-resistant infections globally: final report and recommendations the review on antimicrobial resistance chaired by Jim O'Neill.* <https://amr-review.org/sites/default/files/160525_Final%20paper_with%20cover.pdf>; 2016 Accessed 28.12.20.
67. Pan M, Chu LM. Fate of antibiotics in soil and their uptake by edible crops. *Sci Total Environ.* 2017;599–600:500–512.
68. Rath S, Fostier AH, Pereira LA, et al. Sorption behaviors of antimicrobial and antiparasitic veterinary drugs on subtropical soils. *Chemosphere.* 2019;214:111–122.
69. Riaz L, Mahmood T, Khalid A, et al. Fluoroquinolones (FQs) in the environment: a review on their abundance, sorption and toxicity in soil. *Chemosphere.*. 2018;191:704–720.
70. Zhao F, Yang L, Chen L, et al. Soil contamination with antibiotics in a typical peri-urban area in eastern China: seasonal variation, risk assessment, and microbial responses. *J Environ Sci (China).* 2019;79:200–212.
71. Giebułtowicz J, Tyski S, Wolinowska R, et al. Occurrence of antimicrobial agents, drug-resistant bacteria, and genes in the sewage-impacted Vistula River (Poland). *Environ Sci Pollut Res Int.* 2018;25(6):5788–5807.
72. Maran NH, Crispim BD, Iahnn SR, Araújo RP, Grisolia AB, Oliveira KM. Depth and well type related to groundwater microbiological contamination. *Int J Environ Res Public Health.* 2016; 13(10):1036.
73. Millanao AR, Barrientos-Schaffeld C, Siegel-Tike CD, et al. Antimicrobial resistance in Chile and The One Health paradigm: dealing with threats to human and veterinary health resulting from antimicrobial use in salmon aquaculture and the clinic. *Rev Chil. Infectol.* 2018;35(3):299–308.
74. Wang H, Wang N, Wang B, et al. Antibiotics in drinking water in Shanghai and their contribution to antibiotic exposure of school children. *Environ Sci Technol.* 2016;50(5):2692–2699.
75. World Health Organization (WHO). *WHO List of Critically Important Antimicrobials WHO CIA List 6th Revision Released in 2019.* Geneva: WHO. <https://www.who.int/foodsafety/publications/antimicrobials-sixth/en/>; 2019 Accessed 27.12.20.

76. World Organisation for Animal Health (OIE). *OIE List of Antimicrobial Agents of Veterinary Importance*. OIE Int Committee. <https://www.oie.int/fileadmin/Home/eng/Our_scientific_expertise/docs/pdf/AMR/A_OIE_List_antimicrobials_July2019.pdf>; 2019 Accessed 27.12. 20.
77. Congilosi JL, Aga DS. Review on the fate of antimicrobials, antimicrobial resistance genes, and other micropollutants in manure during enhanced anaerobic digestion and composting. *J Hazard Mater*. 2020;405:123634. Available from: https://www.sciencedirect.com/science/article/abs/pii/S0304389420316204.
78. Karbalaei S, Hanachi P, Walker TR, Cole M. Occurrence, sources, human health impacts and mitigation of microplastic pollution. *Environ Sci Pollut Res Int*. 2018;25(36):36046–36063. Available from: https://doi.org/10.1007/s11356-018-3508-7.
79. Zhang Z, Zulpiya M, Chen Y. Current research and perspective of microplastics (MPs) in soils (dusts), rivers (lakes), and marine environments in China. *Ecotoxicol Environ Saf*. 2020;202:110976. Available from: https://doi.org/10.1016/j.ecoenv.2020.110976. Oct 1.
80. Brahney J, Hallerud M, Heim E, Hahnenberger M, Sukumaran S. Plastic rain in protected areas of the United States. *Science*. 2020;368(6496):1257–1260. Available from: https://doi.org/10.1126/science.aaz5819.
81. Duis K, Coors A. Microplastics in the aquatic and terrestrial environment: sources (with a specific focus on personal care products), fate and effects. *Environ Sci Eur*. 2016;28:2.
82. Rillig MC, Ziersch L, Hempel S. Microplastic transport in soil by earthworms. *Sci Rep*. 2017;7:1362.
83. Fromme H, Lahrz T, Kraft M, et al. Organophosphate flame retardants and plasticizers in the air and dust in German daycare centers and human biomonitoring in visiting children (LUPE 3). *Environ Int*. 2014;71:158–163. Available from: https://doi.org/10.1016/j.envint.2014.06.016. Oct.
84. Takeuchi S, Tanaka-Kagawa T, Saito I, et al. Differential determination of plasticizers and organophosphorus flame retardants in residential indoor air in Japan. *Environ Sci Pollut Res Int*. 2018;25(8):7113–7120. Available from: https://doi.org/10.1007/s11356-015-4858-z.
85. Kim D, Cui R, Moon J, Kwak JI, An YJ. Soil ecotoxicity study of DEHP with respect to multiple soil species. *Chemosphere*. 2019;216:387–395. Available from: https://doi.org/10.1016/j.chemosphere.2018.10.163. Feb.
86. Kim UJ, Wang Y, Li W, Kannan K. Occurrence of and human exposure to organophosphate flame retardants/plasticizers in indoor air and dust from various microenvironments in the United States. *Environ Int*. 2019;125:342–349. Available from: https://doi.org/10.1016/j.envint.2019.01.065. Apr.
87. Promtes K, Kaewboonchoo O, Kawai T, et al. Human exposure to phthalates from house dust in Bangkok, Thailand. *J Environ Sci Health A Tox Hazard Subst Environ Eng*. 2019;54(13):1269–1276. Available from: https://doi.org/10.1080/10934529.2019.1637207.
88. Wang X, Zhang Y, Huang B, et al. Atmospheric phthalate pollution in plastic agricultural greenhouses in Shaanxi Province, China. *Environ Pollut*. 2021;269:116096. Available from: https://doi.org/10.1016/j.envpol.2020.116096. Jan 15.
89. Abtahi M, Dobaradaran S, Torabbeigi M, et al. Health risk of phthalates in water environment: occurrence in water resources, bottled water, and tap water, and burden of disease from exposure through drinking water in Tehran, Iran. *Environ Res*. 2019;173:469–479. Available from: https://doi.org/10.1016/j.envres.2019.03.071. Jun.
90. Kankanige D, Babel S. Smaller-sized micro-plastics (MPs) contamination in single-use PET-bottled water in Thailand. *Sci Total Environ*. 2020;717:137232. Available from: https://doi.org/10.1016/j.scitotenv.2020.137232. May 15.
91. Johnson AC, Ball H, Cross R, et al. Identification and quantification of microplastics in potable water and their sources within water treatment works in England and Wales. *Environ Sci Technol*. 2020;54(19):12326–12334. Available from: https://doi.org/10.1021/acs.est.0c03211.
92. Tong H, Jiang Q, Hu X, Zhong X. Occurrence and identification of microplastics in tap water from China. *Chemosphere*. 2020;252:126493. Available from: https://doi.org/10.1016/j.chemosphere.2020.126493. Aug.
93. Constant M, Kerhervé P, Mino-Vercellio-Verollet M, et al. Beached microplastics in the Northwestern Mediterranean Sea. *Mar Pollut Bull*. 2019;142:263–273. Available from: https://doi.org/10.1016/j.marpolbul.2019.03.032. May.
94. Li Q, Wu J, Zhao X, Gu X, Ji R. Separation and identification of microplastics from soil and sewage sludge. *Environ Pollut*. 2019;254(Pt B):113076. Available from: https://doi.org/10.1016/j.envpol.2019.113076.
95. Piehl S, Mitterwallner V, Atwood EC, Bochow M, Laforsch C. Abundance and distribution of large microplastics (1–5 mm) within beach sediments at the Po River Delta, northeast Italy. *Mar Pollut Bull*. 2019;149:110515. Available from: https://doi.org/10.1016/j.marpolbul.2019.110515. Dec.
96. Wahl A, Le Juge C, Davranche M, et al. Nanoplastic occurrence in a soil amended with plastic debris. *Chemosphere*. 2021;262:127784. Available from: https://doi.org/10.1016/j.chemosphere.2020.127784. Jan.
97. Rochman CM, Cook A-M, Koelmans AA. Plastic debris and policy: using current scientific understanding to invoke positive change. *Environ Toxicol Chem*. 2016;35:1617–1626.
98. Lwanga EH, Thapa B, Yang X, et al. Decay of low-density polyethylene by bacteria extracted from earthworm's guts: a potential for soil restoration. *Sci Total Environ*. 2018;624:753–757.
99. Dopico M, Gómez A. Review of the current state and main sources of dioxins around the world. *J Air Waste Manag Assoc*. 2015;65(9):1033–1049. Available from: https://doi.org/10.1080/10962247.2015.1058869.
100. Wu C, Zhu H, Luo Y, Wang J. Concentrations and potential health hazards of polycyclic aromatic hydrocarbon in shallow groundwater of a metal smelting area in Southeastern China. *Sci Total Environ*. 2016;569–570:1561–1569. Available from: https://doi.org/10.1016/j.scitotenv.2016.06.250. Nov 1.
101. Dobaradaran S, Schmidt TC, Lorenzo-Parodi N, et al. Polycyclic aromatic hydrocarbons (PAHs) leachates from cigarette butts into water. *Environ Pollut*. 2020;259:113916. Available from: https://doi.org/10.1016/j.envpol.2020.113916. Apr.
102. Verbrugge LA, Kahn L, Morton JM. Pentachlorophenol, polychlorinated dibenzo-p-dioxins and polychlorinated dibenzo furans in surface soil surrounding pentachlorophenol-treated utility poles on the Kenai National Wildlife Refuge, Alaska USA. *Environ Sci Pollut Res Int*. 2018;25(19):19187–19195. Available from: https://doi.org/10.1007/s11356-018-2269-7.

103. Choi MP, Ho SK, So BK, Cai Z, Lau AK, Wong MH. PCDD/F and dioxin-like PCB in Hong Kong air in relation to their regional transport in the Pearl River Delta region. *Chemosphere*. 2008; 71(2):211–218. Available from: https://doi.org/10.1016/j.chemosphere.2007.09.060.
104. López A, Coscollà C, Hernández CS, Pardo O, Yusà V. Dioxins and dioxin-like PCBs in the ambient air of the Valencian Region (Spain): levels, human exposure, and risk assessment. *Chemosphere*. 2021;267:128902. Available from: https://doi.org/10.1016/j.chemosphere.2020.128902. Mar.
105. Gune MM, Ma WL, Sampath S, et al. Occurrence of polycyclic aromatic hydrocarbons (PAHs) in air and soil surrounding a coal-fired thermal power plant in the south-west coast of India. *Environ Sci Pollut Res Int*. 2019;26(22):22772–22782. Available from: https://doi.org/10.1007/s11356-019-05380-y.
106. Wang Y, Bao M, Zhang Y, et al. Polycyclic aromatic hydrocarbons in the atmosphere and soils of Dalian, China: source, urban-rural gradient, and air-soil exchange. *Chemosphere*. 2020;244:125518. Available from: https://doi.org/10.1016/j.chemosphere.2019.125518. Apr.
107. Minomo K, Ohtsuka N, Nojiri K, Matsumoto R. Influence of combustion-originated dioxins in atmospheric deposition on water quality of an urban river in Japan. *J Environ Sci (China)*. 2018;64:245–251. Available from: https://doi.org/10.1016/j.jes.2017.06.027. Feb.
108. Li J, Shang X, Zhao Z, Tanguay RL, Dong Q, Huang C. Polycyclic aromatic hydrocarbons in water, sediment, soil, and plants of the Aojiang River waterway in Wenzhou, China. *J Hazard Mater*. 2010;173(1–3):75–81. Available from: https://doi.org/10.1016/j.jhazmat.2009.08.050.
109. Zhang Y, Zhang L, Huang Z, et al. Pollution of polycyclic aromatic hydrocarbons (PAHs) in drinking water of China: composition, distribution and influencing factors. *Ecotoxicol Environ Saf*. 2019;177:108–116. Available from: https://doi.org/10.1016/j.ecoenv.2019.03.119.
110. Xiao Y, Tong F, Kuang Y, Chen B. Distribution and source apportionment of polycyclic aromatic hydrocarbons (PAHs) in forest soils from urban to rural areas in the Pearl River Delta of Southern China. *Int J Environ Res Public Health*. 2014; 11(3):2642–2656. Available from: https://doi.org/10.3390/ijerph110302642.
111. Dreij K, Lundin L, Le Bihanic F, Lundstedt S. Polycyclic aromatic compounds in urban soils of Stockholm City: occurrence, sources and human health risk assessment. *Environ Res*. 2020;182:108989. Available from: https://doi.org/10.1016/j.envres.2019.108989. Mar.
112. Takeda N, Takaoka M. An assessment of dioxin contamination from the intermittent operation of a municipal waste incinerator in Japan and associated remediation. *Environ Sci Pollut Res Int*. 2013;20(4):2070–2080. Available from: https://doi.org/10.1007/s11356-012-1412-0.
113. Dias-Ferreira C, Kirkelund GM, Jensen PE. The influence of electrodialytic remediation on dioxin (PCDD/PCDF) levels in fly ash and air pollution control residues. *Chemosphere*. 2016;148: 380–387. Available from: https://doi.org/10.1016/j.chemosphere.2016.01.061. Apr.
114. Chang MB, Hsu YC, Chang SH. Removal of PCDD/Fs, PCP and mercury from sediments: thermal oxidation vs pyrolysis. *Chemosphere*. 2018;207:10–17. Available from: https://doi.org/10.1016/j.chemosphere.2018.05.037. Sep.
115. Field JA, Sierra-Alvarez R. Microbial degradation of chlorinated dioxins. *Chemosphere*. 2008;71(6):1005–1018. Available from: https://doi.org/10.1016/j.chemosphere.2007.10.039.
116. Shi Z, Chen J, Liu J, Wang N, Sun Z, Wang X. Anionic-nonionic mixed-surfactant-enhanced remediation of PAH-contaminated soil. *Environ Sci Pollut Res Int*. 2015;22(16):12769–12774. Available from: https://doi.org/10.1007/s11356-015-4568-6.
117. Chen F, Dong ZQ, Wang CC, Wei XH, Hu Y, Zhang LJ. Heavy metal contamination of soils and crops near a zinc smelter [Chinese]*Huan Jing Ke Xue*. 2017;38(10):4360–4369. Available from: https://doi.org/10.13227/j.hjkx.201704140.
118. Iqbal SZ, Ullah Z, Asi MR, et al. Heavy metals in selected vegetables from markets of Faisalabad, Pakistan. *J Food Prot*. 2018;81(5):806–809. Available from: https://doi.org/10.4315/0362-028X.JFP-17-256.
119. Thompson LA, Darwish WS, Ikenaka Y, Nakayama SM, Mizukawa H, Ishizuka M. Organochlorine pesticide contamination of foods in Africa: incidence and public health significance. *J Vet Med Sci*. 2017;79(4):751–764. Available from: https://doi.org/10.1292/jvms.16-0214.
120. Bhandari G, Zomer P, Atreya K, Mol HGJ, Yang X, Geissen V. Pesticide residues in Nepalese vegetables and potential health risks. *Environ Res*. 2019;172:511–521. Available from: https://doi.org/10.1016/j.envres.2019.03.002. May.
121. Kapeleka JA, Sauli E, Sadik O, Ndakidemi PA. Co-exposure risks of pesticides residues and bacterial contamination in fresh fruits and vegetables under smallholder horticultural production systems in Tanzania. *PLoS One*. 2020;15(7):e0235345. Available from: https://doi.org/10.1371/journal.pone.0235345.
122. Oliveri Conti G, Ferrante M, Banni M, et al. Micro- and nano-plastics in edible fruit and vegetables. The first diet risks assessment for the general population. *Environ Res*. 2020;187:109677. Available from: https://doi.org/10.1016/j.envres.2020.109677. Aug.
123. Mathews S, Henderson S, Reinhold D. Uptake and accumulation of antimicrobials, triclocarban and triclosan, by food crops in a hydroponic system. *Environ Sci Pollut Res Int*. 2014;21 (9):6025–6033. Available from: https://doi.org/10.1007/s11356-013-2474-3.
124. Piskorska-Pliszczynska J, Malagocki P, Pajurek M. Levels and trends of PCDD/Fs and DL-PCBs in Polish animal feeds, 2004–2017. *Food Addit Contam Part A Chem Anal Control Expo Risk Assess*. 2019; 36(3):447–463. Available from: https://doi.org/10.1080/19440049.2019.1576926.
125. United States Environmental Protection Agency (US EPA). *A Review of the Reference Dose and Reference Concentration Processes*. Washington, DC: Risk Assessment Forum, U.S. Environmental Protection Agency. <https://www.epa.gov/sites/production/files/2014-12/documents/rfd-final.pdf>; 2002. Accessed 27.12.20.
126. United States Environmental Protection Agency (US EPA). *Guidelines for Carcinogen Risk Assessment*. Washington, DC: Risk Assessment Forum, U.S. Environmental Protection Agency. <https://www.epa.gov/sites/production/files/2013-09/documents/cancer_guidelines_final_3-25-05.pdf>; 2005 Accessed 27.12.20.

Chapter 3

Agrochemicals in the Food Chain

Rosemary H. Waring[1], Stephen C. Mitchell[2] and Ian Brown[3,4]

[1]*School of Biosciences, University of Birmingham, Birmingham, United Kingdom,* [2]*Department of Metabolism, Digestion and Reproduction, Imperial College London, London, United Kingdom,* [3]*Oxford University Hospitals, Oxford, United Kingdom,* [4]*The Institute of Food, Nutrition and Health, University of Reading, Reading, United Kingdom*

Abstract

Agrochemicals include herbicides, insecticides, and fungicides and improve both the quality and quantity of agricultural produce. Residues of pesticides in foodstuffs are common and are analyzed by national or supra-national organizations in rolling programs; the results are then published. The main modes of action for pesticides are via dysregulation of either neuronal pathways or energy supply. Because these metabolic routes are often shared to some extent with mammals, pesticides may also affect human populations when their residues are ingested. Possible areas of concern include potential for endocrine disruption, the "cocktail effect" where multiple residues are present in a product at the same time, and alterations to the gastrointestinal microbiome. In particular, chronic exposure to cleaning agents and disinfectants may disrupt the bacterial profile in the gut. The long-term effects, if any, of pesticides on human health might be elucidated using "omics" techniques with human cell lines.

Keywords: Pesticides; mode of action; residues; food; microbiome

3.1 Introduction

The term "agrochemicals" includes a wide range of compounds with varied structures; all that they have in common is that they are used at some stage in growing crops or in food preparation. Examples include curing agents, fertilizers, pesticides, desiccants, growth regulators, fumigants, and biological agents such as insect endocrine disrupters and inhibitors of chitin synthesis. Some agrochemicals such as copper sulfate, found in Bordeaux mixture, have "organic" status, although they are not necessarily nontoxic and may bioaccumulate. However, they are not usually analyzed in a wide range of foods and data are therefore scarce. Nitrate and nitrite ions are used as curing agents to inhibit the growth of microorganisms, particularly *Clostridium botulinum*, in processed meats. They occur naturally in foodstuffs, particularly green leafy vegetables, and in groundwater as runoff from nitrates used as crop fertilizers. Input from these various sources means that dietary levels can be high. The ions are potentially precursors of carcinogenic nitrosamines but also promote cardiovascular health; the situation is complex and the risk/benefit ratio has recently been reviewed.[1] Of all the classes of agrochemicals, pesticide residues have been of most concern and methods for their detection and determination in plant or food matrices are routinely available. Pesticides are used to maximize the output of a specific crop and include herbicides, which remove competing plants, insecticides, which reduce the numbers of insects eating the crop, and fungicides, which improve the keeping qualities of the crop. Without this input from exogenous chemicals, much of the food grown in the world today would never reach harvest. Given that the world population is 7.8 billion (10^9) and increasing, the considered and appropriate use of pesticides must play a major part in improving the global food supply both in quantity and quality.

3.2 In vivo metabolism of agrochemicals

Agrochemicals fall into the general category of "xenobiotics," compounds which may enter the body but which are not part of the endogenous metabolic pathways. Once internalized in food, the biological fate of any xenobiotic depends on its polarity. Compounds which are highly charged, such as the quaternary ammonium compounds (QACs), are not absorbed across the lipophilic membranes lining the gut wall unless there is a specific protein transporter. Consequently, they are excreted unchanged. However, most compounds are absorbed, at least to some extent, from the gastrointestinal tract and are carried by the systemic blood circulation into all the organs,

Present Knowledge in Food Safety. DOI: https://doi.org/10.1016/B978-0-12-819470-6.00006-8

including the liver. Here, they are acted on by enzyme systems which convert them to more polar compounds. As the major excretion route is via urine and these products are more water-soluble than the parent compound, they are readily removed from the body via the kidneys. Compounds such as the fat-soluble organochlorine insecticide DDT (dichlorodiphenyltrichloroethane), which are difficult to transform into more polar metabolites, are sequestered in adipose tissue and have long half-lives in vivo (~6 years). Small amounts of these nonpolar compounds can be excreted in bile and then evacuated in fecal material. However, modern pesticides are usually formulated so that they can be metabolized to polar compounds and then clear the body by the urinary route within 72 h. A long-term body burden of pesticide residues is therefore now unlikely. The metabolic pathways that make these transformations possible are traditionally divided into "Phase 1" and "Phase 2" enzyme systems. In Phase 1, the compound is metabolized, usually by a microsomal membrane-bound enzyme complex, cytochrome P450. This carries out several reactions, particularly hydroxylation, which have the effect of making the metabolite more polar than its parent compound and hence more water-soluble. Excretion and detoxification are made more rapid by Phase 2 enzymes which link either the parent compound or its Phase 1 metabolites to water-soluble groups. Generally, glucuronic acid or sulfate derivatives are formed; these are usually pharmacologically inactive and removed from the body in urine via the kidneys.

3.3 Regulation of agrochemicals

Agrochemical residues in food, whether herbicides, insecticides, or fungicides, should be as low as practically possible, preferably below some statutorily agreed standardized level of detection of the nation state. This level in the United Kingdom and European Union (EU) is designated the "Maximum Residue Level" or MRL. Pesticide levels in food and drink are unlikely to be zero but may be reported as "below the level of detection (LOD)" (analytical methods are now so sensitive the "undetected" level usually needs to be stated as "less than 0.01 mg/kg"). This is known as an agreed limit of determination and will be reported as "below the LOD." The foodstuff is therefore considered satisfactory for a lifetime's consumption, although occasional exceedances of LODs or even MRLs can occur without the product being unsafe.

When introducing a new agrochemical to the market, manufacturers need to overcome a number of hurdles before the new product is licensed for use. The first of these is its effectiveness in controlling the pest without significant toxicity to nontarget organisms, including beneficial insects, aquatic life and all animals including humans. The new product must also offer a significant advantage when compared with whatever else is available on the market since testing is expensive and time-consuming. Standard toxicological methods are used to determine the levels of agrochemicals that can be considered safe for a lifetime's consumption, irrespective of individual age or food intake.

Agrochemicals that might end up as residues in the food are tested at different levels in repeated dose studies in two mammalian species, including rats. Generally a sigmoid "dose-response" relationship is obtained and the dose threshold where there is no detectable response of the test species is determined. This is known as the "No Observed Effect Level," often abbreviated to the "NOEL" and is essential for setting regulatory exposure limits such as the "Acceptable Daily Intake" (ADI) which measures chronic toxicity. Where agrochemicals might find their way into food, an adjustment factor (usually 100-fold) is built into the ADI. This allows for species differences since rats and humans are not metabolically identical. It also allows for the variability in individual human response because both Phase 1 and Phase 2 enzymes, which are largely genetically controlled, have different activities within the population. Therefore, for the majority of agrochemicals the ADI becomes the NOEL in (mg/kg)/day divided by 100. For agrochemicals where the margin of safety needs to be greater, the dividing factor may then be up to 1000, and this higher denominator will be used where there could be a number of agrochemical residues with similar modes of action (MOA), (i.e., cholinesterase inhibitors). These safety factors allow for exceedances that may occur where application rates are not strictly adhered to or when certain storage or weather conditions have not been optimal.

The WHO definition of an ADI is therefore an estimate of the amount of a substance in food or drinking water that can be consumed over a lifetime without presenting an appreciable risk to health. In addition to the above regulatory levels, the Acute Reference Dose (ARfD) reflects acute toxicity and covers short-term exposures to agrochemicals that are known to have some recognized toxicological effect at a particular dose. It is an estimate of a substance in food or drinking water that can be ingested over a short period of time, usually during one meal or one day, without appreciable health risk to the consumer. This is always higher than the ADI.

To ensure that the above standards are met, an MRL is established and then set in law at the highest level of agrochemical that the relevant regulatory body would expect to find in a crop that has been treated in accordance with good agricultural practice (GAP). If a food has a higher level of residue than the MRL, it does not automatically mean that it is unsafe to eat, although it may show that the farmer has not used the pesticide properly and has not demonstrated GAP. Some pesticides may be permitted for use in the country of export but not for use in the EU, and so the MRL may be set at the default level, which will be the LOD.

There is a Europe-wide surveillance program for agrochemicals in food. Under the European Community Regulation (EC) No. 396/2005, the EU Member States monitor pesticide residue levels in food samples and submit the monitoring results to the European Food Safety Authority (EFSA). EFSA provides annual reports with comparison of the monitoring results on organic and conventionally produced food samples. For example, samples (28,912 conventional and 1940 organic foods) were taken in the framework of the EU-coordinated control programs in the reference periods 2013, 2014, and 2015. Overall, 44% of the conventionally produced food samples contained one or more quantifiable residues, while in organic food the frequency of samples with measurable pesticide residues was lower (6.5%). The MRL exceedance rate for conventional and organic foods amounted to 1.2% and 0.2% of the samples tested, respectively.

The equivalent committee in the United Kingdom is the Expert Committee on Pesticide Residues in Foods (PRiF) which also produces detailed annual reports. All exceedances of agrochemicals in food are examined and the wholesaler or retailer is notified. To ensure that food is safe for consumers, the "Rapid Alert System for Food and Feed" (RASFF) enables information to be shared efficiently between its members, (EU Member State national food safety authorities, the Commission, EFSA, ESA, United Kingdom, Norway, Liechtenstein, Iceland, and Switzerland). Vital information exchanged through RASFF can lead to products being urgently recalled from the market.[2] Nevertheless, given that only a small percentage of foods can be sampled, compared with the total available, some inappropriately high levels of pesticides must slip through the regulatory net. To partly address these problems, regulatory agencies usually place added emphasis on testing products which have previously been problematic.

3.4 Agrochemicals commonly found as residues in foodstuffs

In 2019, 96,302 samples of different foods from all the EU Member States were analyzed for pesticide residues.[3] For 2019, 96.1% fell below the MRL and 3.9% (4.5% in 2018) exceeded this level, of which 2.3% (2.7% in 2018) were noncompliant, exceeding the MRL after the taking the measurement uncertainty into account. Those pesticides most noted for MRL exceedances included chlordecone, chlorpyrifos, nicotine, dithiocarbamates, dimethoate, glyphosate, flonicamid, chlormequat, mepiquat, and ethephon. EFSA has concluded that if at least 683 samples/food item were monitored, then an MRL exceedance rate above 1% could be estimated with a margin of error of 0.75%. Because different foods are sampled each year, it is not always possible to make comparisons and of course the number of samples analyzed is very small compared with the total amount of food that is actually eaten so the reports only give a snapshot of pesticide levels in foodstuffs. EFSA also noted that 11.3% of samples were of unknown origin, reducing the traceability. Despite the existence of a coordinated framework of EU-approved pesticides, some EU-nonapproved pesticides were found in commodities produced in EU territory (Table 3.1). This unauthorized use suggests that some producers have retained or obtained pesticides which were previously available commercially and considered efficacious.[4] EU-nonapproved pesticides exceeding the legal limits were also found in samples coming in from countries outside the EU (Table 3.2).

Fat-soluble persistent organic pollutant (POP) residues such as DDT, chlordecone (Kepone), and hexachlorobenzene

TABLE 3.1 European Union (EU)-unauthorized pesticides present in samples from EU Member States in 2018.

Pesticide	Foodstuff
Omethoate	Aubergines
Bitertanol, carbendazim, flusilazole	Broccoli
Dieldrin, chlorfenapyr	Melons
Chlorfenapyr, triadimefon	Sweet peppers
Carbendazim, omethoate, acephate	Table grapes
Carbendazim, fenitrothion	Wheat
Iprodione	Virgin olive oil

TABLE 3.2 European Union (EU)-unauthorized pesticides exceeding the legal limits present in samples from non-EU countries in 2018.

Pesticide	Foodstuff
Carbofuran, chlorfenapyr	Aubergines
Carbendazim	Bananas
Isocarbophos, bromopropylate, diazinon, fenthion	Grapefruit
Carbaryl, fenitrothion, carbofuran, propiconazole	Sweet peppers
Acephate, carbendazim	Table grapes

TABLE 3.3 Pesticides detected over the maximum residue levels in 2018 in the United Kingdom.

Pesticide	Fruit/vegetable	Country
Chlorfenapyr, dithiocarbamates, Fipronil, cyhalothrin	Uri dolols beans	Malaysia
Dimethoate, fenpropathrin, lufenuron	Yard long beans	Malaysia
Dimethoate, acephate, flusilazole, methamidophos, fipronil, monocrotophos	Guar beans	India
Phosphamidon	Hyacinth beans	India
Flubendiamide, permethrin	Blackberries	Mexico
Fosetyl	Blueberries	Ukraine
Clothianidin, cyromazine	Ginger	China
Captan	Grapes	Chile
Procymidone	Lentils	United Kingdom[b]
Chlormequat, 2-phenylphenol	Mushrooms[a]	United Kingdom[b]
Chlorfenapyr, oxamyl, chlorothalonil, thiacloprid	Okra	Honduras
Emamectin, diafenthiuron, flonicamid, diuron, propargite, nitenpyram		India
Thiacloprid, abamectin		Jordan
Chlorfenapyr		Vietnam
Thiabendazole	Eddoes	Spain
Ethephon	Peppers	Poland

[a]*The carry-over use of cereal straw as a substrate for cultivating fungi was thought to explain the presence of pesticides found in cultivated mushrooms.*
[b]*Not necessarily the country of origin but the country where the final packaging was done.*

were found in some samples of animal origin such as chicken eggs and bovine fat. Although these chemicals are no longer in use as pesticides, they are very persistent in the environment and occur in fat-rich foods as historical contaminants since they still occur in soils even though use of the chemicals stopped many years previously. Acute risk was identified for dithiocarbamates, especially mancozeb and ziram, while chronic risk was identified for metiram and ziram; a comprehensive review of dithiocarbamate MRLs was therefore proposed.

In comparison, in the United Kingdom in 2020, 2460 samples of food and drink in the UK supply chain were tested for pesticide residues (there are 371 methods in the analytical suite).[5] Of these, 58.46% had no residues, while 2.52% of the samples exceeded the MRL (after allowing for uncertainty measurement). Those residues detected in foods are listed in Table 3.3.

In 2019 in the United Kingdom, different fruits/vegetables were sampled so the results are not easily comparable but acephate, captan, flonicamid, methamidophos, monocrotophos, dimethoate, fenpropathrin, and procymidone were present above the MRLs, while the seven most frequently found pesticides above the LOQ (limit of quantification - defined as the minimum concentration of the analyte that can be determined with precision and accuracy) but below the MRLs were chlormequat, imazalil, fludioxonil, boscalid, thiabendazole, pyrimethanil, and imidacloprid. There are trends in pesticide use but organophosphates occur in most residue lists. Processing factors may reduce the levels of pesticides in food as it is finally consumed and health risk assessments for different populations have used modeling approaches to allow for this.[6] Technology for decontamination of foodstuffs includes cold plasma,[7] ozone/lactic acid,[8] and electrolyzed water[9]; these have been reported as having no negative effects on the sensory properties of the treated foods (Table 3.2).

3.5 Types of agrochemicals and modes of action

As can be seen from the list below, agrochemicals fall into many different classes and MOA. Some sets, such as the pyrethrins, contain many compounds, while in other classes only one pesticide is currently in commercial use. Clearly, successful pesticides must have a large margin of toxicity between the target organism and other creatures. This is often achieved by size differentials since fungi or insects are so much smaller than the rest of the natural world that very small amounts of pesticide may disrupt their metabolism while having little or no effect on anything larger. Nevertheless, beneficial insects, such as bees, may be near the relevant size range and fish, with fewer detoxication pathways, may also be susceptible. Ideally, a pesticide acts on a specific pathway, such as chitin synthesis, which does not occur in mammals. However, because the main metabolic routes are generally common to all organisms, "crossover" can occur to cause toxicity in nontarget life forms. Generally, most pesticides are formulated to affect target organisms in two main ways. They either disrupt ion channels, altering the functioning of the central nervous system (CNS) and nerves and muscles in the peripheral nervous system or they dysregulate energy/growth metabolism. If more than one application of a pesticide is considered warranted, then those chosen should be selected to have different MOA. Some of the more important mechanisms of action are discussed below although some pesticides are either nonspecific or have actions which have not yet been identified (Table 3.3).

3.5.1 Cleaning/disinfecting agents

Cleaning/sterilizing agents such as chlorates and disinfectants such as the QACs are widely used in food preparation and on surfaces to limit contamination by bacteria. This reduces spoilage but may leave residues on the final product.

Sodium chlorate is a widely used nonselective herbicide while the chlorate ion (ClO_3^-) is generated as a byproduct when drinking water is disinfected. It can be found as a result of the complex chemical interaction of ozone with chloride ions in neutral or alkaline solution and is commonly formed when water is treated with chlorine dioxide (ClO_2) as a disinfectant. Authorization of chlorate for pesticide use was withdrawn in the EU so that the default MRL for foods is 0.01 mg/kg. This has led to problems since if routinely disinfected water is used in preparation of foodstuffs such as fruits or vegetables, then chlorate residues may be left in excess of the default MRL. For example, when irrigation water treated with chlorine dioxide was used on spinach and lettuce, chlorate accumulated in the vegetables up to 0.99 mg/kg-1.[10,11] A study in 2016 which measured chlorate in drinking water taken from 39 sampling points across Europe found that the levels ranged from <0.003 to 0.803 mg/L with a mean of 0.145 mg/L. Analysis of more than 3400 food samples (dairy products, meats, fruits, vegetables) found that 50.5% contained chlorate above the MRL[12] and a more recent investigation of chlorate in drinking water found that 69% of 284 samples contained chlorate above the level of 0.01 mg/L.[13] Ingestion of trace amounts of chlorate from water and foods, particularly leafy vegetables, must therefore be relatively common. The ion has a range of effects in vivo—it is a renal toxin in rats, causing damage to the enzymes of the brush border membranes with increased generation of hydrogen peroxide, DNA fragmentation, and increased DNA-protein cross-linking. Oral dosage of chlorate in rats also caused significant intestinal DNA damage, probably via production of reactive oxygen species (ROS).[14]

QACs are cationic detergents, surface-active substances with the general structures of $R_1R_2R_3R_4N^+$ which occur as salts, usually with chloride ions. They are often used as nonspecific biocides, pesticides, and disinfectants. Where the QACs have long alkyl chains as "R" groups, the compounds are effective antimicrobial agents, interacting with the cytoplasmic membranes of bacteria and the plasma membranes of yeasts to disorganize the lipid/protein layers. This allows leakage of cell contents and autolysis of the organism with binding to intracellular targets such as DNA. QACs are often used in personal care products such as hand sanitizers and in the dairy industry to disinfect surfaces and treat milking equipment, milk storage tankers, and ice cream machines. Where hygiene practices are inadequate, traces of these biocides may contaminate foodstuffs, particularly dairy products. QACs are often marketed as mixtures with different "R" groups and depending on the formulation, may be active against noro-viruses. DDAC (mostly didecyldimethylammonium chloride, C10, with small amounts of the C8 and C12 congeners) is a commonly used QAC, which seems to be relatively nontoxic to man, although there have been suggestions that its use might cause neural tube defects in rodents.[15] Benzalkonium chloride (BAC, a mixture of alkylbenzyldimethylammonium chlorides with alkyl chain lengths of C8, C10, C12, C14, C16, and C18, particularly C12 and C14) has largely replaced cetrimide in antibacterial soaps and its widespread use and presence in the environment in wastewater treatment plants and waterways has led to concerns about the development of antibiotic resistance. Tolerance to BAC has been reported for *Listeria monocytogenes* which is commonly found in food processing factories. BACs can potentially also affect mammalian membrane structure by generating ROS, while their presence in the gastrointestinal tract exacerbated inflammation in mice by disrupting intestinal barrier function and increasing the circulating levels of bacterial toxins.[16]

3.5.2 Pesticides

3.5.2.1 Neurotoxins

3.5.2.1.1 GABA-gated chloride channel antagonists

Fipronil is a highly fluorinated phenylpyrazole derivative that displays broad-spectrum insecticidal activity with a wide application both in crop protection and veterinary practice. It is no longer approved for use on crops or animals which enter the food chain but remains available for veterinary use and may occur as a residue in foods after inappropriate handling. Fipronil interferes with the functioning of the insect nervous system by blocking γ-aminobutyric acid (GABA) receptors, and displays a higher toxicity to insects owing its greater affinity for chloride channels that are both GABA-gated and glutamate-gated (the latter are absent in mammals). This noncompetitive binding reduces the frequency and time of ion channel opening and suppresses the insect receptor activity.[17] It is metabolized quite rapidly, primarily to its sulfone and other metabolites which bind to organic soil particles.

3.5.2.1.2 Chloride channel activators

Avermectins, milbemycins, and spinosyns

Abamectin is a natural bacterial fermentation product of the soil actinomycete, *Streptomyces avermitilis*. It contains a mixture of compounds differing slightly in structure and known as avermectin B1a and B1b. These are 16-membered macrocyclic lactone derivatives and are usually attached to sugar residues.[18] Chemical modifications of these original structures have produced a range of products known collectively as avermectins, which possess an altered spectrum of activity, improved efficiency, and a longer duration of action. They find use as insecticides and in the treatment of both internal and external parasitic infections, usually in livestock and domestic animals (cats and dogs), although ivermectin is used in man.

They function by binding to the invertebrate-specific glutamate-gated chloride channels in the membranes of nerve and muscle cells of the target species causing an influx of chloride ions with ensuing hyperpolarization and subsequent paralysis.[19] Binding also occurs to the GABA receptors and they may have other interactions.[20] Milbemycins are a group of closely related 16-membered macrocyclic lactones isolated from *Streptomyces hygroscopicus*[21] and the spinosyns, 12-member ring macrolides, are obtained from *Saccharopolyspora spinosa*.[22] The milbemycins operate, like the avermectins, by opening the glutamate-sensitive chloride channels, whereas the spinosyns mainly function as allosteric nicotinic acetylcholine receptor (nAChR) agonists although they may have secondary effects on GABA receptors.[23] Synthetic versions such as spinetoram are now available; all have very complex structures and are used to control codling moths, thrips, and other pests of grapes, apples, pears, and apricots. Currently they are not UK-approved.

These large molecules are hydrophobic, having a high lipid solubility and are concentrated in adipose tissues. In mammals and man, they are released slowly, being excreted in the bile and eliminated via the gastrointestinal tract.[24,25] This seems to be a general pattern for these macrolide compounds.

They are rapidly degraded in the environment after application, with eventual decomposition to carbon dioxide.[26] Incubation with liver microsomes gives hydroxylation products.

3.5.2.1.3 Sodium channel modulators

1. Pyrethrins

   Natural pyrethrins have insecticidal activity and are produced by the flowers of pyrethrums (*Chrysanthemum cinerariaefolium* and *Chrysanthemum coccineum*). They have good "knock down" effects on insects but are rapidly degraded under field conditions so synthetic versions, "pyrethroids," have been developed. These are more resistant to degradation by light and air but also have higher mammalian toxicity—examples are permethrin, cypermethrin, deltamethrin, fenvalerate, cyfluthrin, flumethrin, and etofenprox. Pyrethroids do not necessarily have common chemical structures, although many contain a three-membered cyclopropane ring derivative like the naturally occurring chrysanthemic acid. However, they all have the same MOA, prevention of the closure of the voltage-gated sodium channels in the axonal membranes. When the channels are kept in the open state, the nerves cannot repolarize and the organism is paralyzed. Pyrethroids are often combined with the synergist piperonyl butoxide which inhibits the cytochrome P450 enzymes which control the detoxication pathways.[27] Other metabolic routes include glucuronidation; pyrethroids are more toxic to cats and fish which have low capacity for formation of glucuronide derivatives. Pyrethroids have relatively low acute toxicity to mammals generally, including humans, as they bind less efficiently to the sodium channels and are poorly absorbed via the skin; levels in vivo usually reflect inhalation from insecticidal aerosol sprays or ingestion from residues on food. Transfer of pyrethroid residues into food seems to be relatively low; there was a leaching efficiency of 2.2%–3.4% from treated tea leaves to the final infusion[28] and there were no residues of cypermethrin in meat from cattle given a topical application as an insecticide.[29] Pyrethroid intake in Norway was estimated as being well below the ADI.[30] However, this parameter may not pick up subtle effects occurring in humans rather than rodents and chronic effects of pyrethroids are of growing importance. The compounds are endocrine disrupters which can damage male and female fertility via complex mechanisms[31,32] and affect fetal development in rodents.[33] Pyrethroids are of course neurotoxic and may cause low-level nonlethal effects in mammals. Exposure to deltamethrin caused behavioral changes in adolescent mice[34] while prenatal exposure to pyrethroids was associated with attention-deficit/hyperactivity disorder–related traits at 2–4 years of age in the Odense Child Cohort.[35]

2. DDT

   DDT opens Na^+ channels and, like other chlorinated POPs, is no longer approved for food use but is still used in Asia to control mosquitoes and may contaminate crops when used in error. It also occurs at low levels in fat-rich foods (meat, butter) from areas of high historical use since the soil half-life is ~30 years.

3.5.2.1.4 Voltage-dependent sodium channel blockers

Indoxacarb is an oxadiazine which nearly irreversibly blocks open/inactivated but not resting Na + channels. This dysregulates neuronal firing, causing death. Insect sodium channels are more sensitive to indoxacarb when compared to mammals making it some 103 times more neurotoxic to insects.[36] Resistance to indoxacarb seems to be due to increased levels of the glutathione-S-transferase and cytochrome P450 enzymes which presumably control the detoxication pathways.[37] Surfactants such as the quaternized ammonia compounds increase its toxicity to Lepidoptera pests but also to aquatic organisms such as *Daphnia magna*.

3.5.2.1.5 Acetylcholinesterase inhibitors

1. Organophosphates

   Organophosphorus pesticides are a major group of insecticides that once had the largest share of the market and have been used extensively around the planet. They are systemic in plants, active in the soil and vapor phase against both endoparasites and ectoparasites and used against a wide range of crop (and animal) pests.[38] There are many compounds that fall within this classification but the more noteworthy include, azamethiphos, azinphos-methyl, chlorpyrifos, diazinon, dichlorvos, fenitrothion, malathion, parathion, phosmet, terbufos, and tetrachlorvinfos.

   These compounds are phosphorylating agents (transfer of phosphate group) and covalently bind to the side-chain hydroxyl group of a serine residue within the active site of acetylcholinesterase (AChE). This enzyme is crucial for removing the neurotransmitter, acetylcholine, from cholinergic nerve endings. Once inactivated, acetylcholine accumulates within the synaptic cleft. With this build-up, the ion channel of the cholinergic synapse remains in a permanently open configuration allowing sodium ions to continue to pass, resulting in sustained membrane depolarization, incessant neuronal firing, muscle convulsions, and eventual death.[39]

   Although it is difficult to generalize, two of the substituents on the phosphorus atom are usually simple alkyl groups with the third linked via a labile bond and designated as a "leaving group." This detaches via hydrolysis during enzyme phosphorylation. Metabolism of these compounds is extensive and dependent upon the initial structure. Hydrolysis that splits the molecule is often the principal detoxification route and decreases or abolishes biological activity. Insects have much lower capacity to undertake this reaction which explains the relative selectivity in species toxicity.

   Some organophosphorus compounds also possess fungicidal and herbicidal properties. Compounds such as ediphenphos, iprobenfos, pyrazophos, and tolclofos-methyl, interfere with the construction of membrane components, and act as general phospholipid biosynthesis inhibitors, particularly targeting phosphatidylcholine formation.

2. Carbamates

   Carbamates ($ROC(=O)NR_2$) are a class of insecticides derived from carbamic acid (NH_2COOH) by replacing the hydrogen atom of the carboxyl group with an organic moiety to form an ester. Substitution also occurs at the nitrogen atom. Examples include aldicarb, bendiocarb, benfuracarb, carbaryl, carbofuran, carbosulfan, ethiofencarb, fenobucarb, oxamyl, methomyl, and trimethacarb. Most show systemic activity, being able to be taken in via the roots and distributed throughout the plant where they reach insecticidal concentrations. They also act as contact poisons being absorbed directly through the insect cuticle.

Like the organophosphorus insecticides, they act at the serine hydroxyl group within the active site of AChE. This carbamoylation of the AChE enzyme is slowly reversible, unlike organophosphates. Hydrolysis with subsequent decarbamolyation of the enzyme and its reactivation does occur but requires hours rather than the microseconds found for the normal functioning of AChE. Consequently, carbamoylated AChE accumulates and the insect shows a sequence of hyperactivity, loss of coordination, and convulsive movements, followed by paralysis and eventual death (carbamate intoxication syndrome). Fenoxycarb possesses a carbamate component within its side chain but acts as an insect growth regulator preventing immature insects from reaching maturity by mimicking insect juvenile hormone (JH). It therefore operates through a different mechanism not involving AChE.

Most carbamates are rapidly degraded in the soil, mainly by microbial metabolism, the compounds being hydrolyzed and forming bound residues. Biotransformation reactions include hydroxylation, epoxidation, *N*-dealkylation, and sulfoxidation with glucuronic acid conjugation or sulfonation in mammals and glycosides in plants. Rates of hydrolysis are probably faster in mammals than plants and insects, which may explain the potential selective toxicity. Combinations of carbamate and organophosphorus insecticides are often used together to achieve synergistic effects, eradicating a wide range of pests including some which may have developed compound-specific resistance.

3.5.2.1.6 Nicotinic acetylcholine receptor agonists

Neonicotinoids, butenolides, and sulfoximines

Nicotine has been widely used for centuries. The application of aqueous infusions of tobacco leaves ("tobacco wash") to control insect pests dates back to the 17th century. However, its volatility, rapid degradation in light and air, its narrow range of insecticidal activity, its toxicity to mammals, and its relatively high cost of production led to a search for alternatives. A group of compounds similar in structure to nicotine and known as neonicotinoids ("neonics") were developed and became available during the 1990s.[40] Over the ensuing years the popularity of this class of insecticide increased dramatically until these pesticides were amongst the most extensively used worldwide. Flupyradifurone and sulfoxaflor are recent additions to the range but are usually referred to as butenolides and sulfoximines, respectively. Currently many neonicotinoids are either banned or have restricted use because they have been found to affect pollinating insects such as bees.[41]

The neonicotinoids function by acting selectively on nAChRs located within the CNS of insects. These agonists produce an overstimulation which blocks the receptor, eventually causing paralysis and death. The enzyme, AChE, which normally hydrolyzes the endogenous neurotransmitter, acetylcholine, is unable to break down the neonicotinoid molecules and their binding is irreversible. The high inbuilt selectivity for insect receptors resulting from subtle conformational differences in binding site interactions vastly decreases any associated toxicity to vertebrates, in contrast to nicotine itself.[42] Their relatively poor penetration of the mammalian blood–brain barrier helps to offset any potential toxicity, although insects also possess simpler protective neural barriers.

Most neonicotinoids are nonvolatile solids that are water-soluble and show good systemic activity in plants. Translocation around the plant via the xylem ensures that they reach sap-sucking and chewing insects and their transfer into pollen deters insect feeding. They are also widely employed for seed treatment. In soils many neonicotinoids degrade relatively quickly within a few weeks (e.g., acetamiprid), whereas some may persist for many months or even years (e.g., imidacloprid).[43]

In living systems these compounds are extensively metabolized and usually break down into smaller, more water-soluble, products. Ring cleavage and conjugation reactions occur as does linkage with glutathione and further modification to yield *N*-acetylcysteine and S-methyl metabolites. Glucosides and gentiobiosides (glucose disaccharide) have been detected in plants with condensations of unidentified endogenous plant components.[43,44]

3.5.2.1.7 Nicotinic acetylcholine receptor channel blockers

Cartap is degraded into nereistoxin which has a longer residual period. Risk assessment studies on the use of cartap during tea planting showed that nereistoxin was the main residue in tea made after the manufacturing process, with transfer rates of $\sim 100\% \pm 20\%$.[45] Cartap is increasingly used for self-harm in India and causes neuromuscular weakness which can result in respiratory failure.

3.5.2.1.8 Octopamine receptor agonists

Amitraz is a nonsystemic triazapentadiene pesticide possessing insecticidal and acaricidal properties. It also has insect repellent effects and has been used in veterinary practice to remove mites. If used on domestic animals, it can potentially enter the human food chain if strict hygiene is not employed.

The molecule appears to have several biological effects, its major MOA being thought to be as an agonist on octopamine receptors. Octopamine acts as the insect equivalent of noradrenaline, operating throughout the insect brain, in all sense organs and important ganglia.[46] Gross interference is thus fatal. Amitraz is also an agonist acting at α-adrenergic receptors, a class of G-protein-coupled receptors, within the CNS and peripheral tissues. Stimulation usually elicits a sympathetic response and increased nervous activity. At relatively high concentrations it inhibits the effects of the enzyme monoamine oxidase, while in vitro studies have shown it to inhibit the synthesis of prostaglandin E2 from arachidonic acid.[47]

Biotransformation occurs rapidly in both plants and animals, with the generation of many metabolites as would be expected for a multinitrogen-containing molecule. Complete degradation of the molecule to carbon dioxide has also been observed.[48] Any Amitraz that falls to the ground as runoff from plant applications and other processes is rapidly broken down in the soil and totally degraded within a few days.

3.5.2.1.9 Ryanodine receptor modulators

Ryanodine is a natural diterpenoid originally used as an insecticide. This had high affinity for the aptly named ryanodine receptor, a group of intracellular calcium channels found in muscle and neuronal tissue. These receptors mediate the release of Ca^{2+} ions from the sarcoplasmic and endoplasmic reticula into the cytoplasm, an essential step in muscle function. Controlled calcium flow is also essential for neuron transmitter release and for signal transduction processes occurring in many other cell types. Interference with this process by activation of these receptors and disruption of the Ca^{2+} balance leads to lethargy, paralysis, and death. Recent research has led to the development of the phthalic acid diamides, including flubendiamide, and the anthranilic acid diamides cyantraniliprole and chlorantraniliprole. These have particularly high activity against Lepidoptera and chewing insects and are potent activators of insect ryanodine receptors. They are active both by ingestion and contact and owing to their unusual MOA they can potentially be used to eradicate insects that have become resistant to other pesticides. The ryanodine receptors in insects are different from those in mammals both in protein sequence and intrinsic sensitivity. This makes them highly efficient and selectively toxic toward insects while enhancing mammalian safety.

In livestock the metabolism of these compounds is extensive, with oxidation, hydroxylation, formation of a variety of cyclic metabolites, and conjugation. These insecticides when applied to the soil move upward into the growing plant. Following seed-coating treatment or foliar application of chlorantraniliprole, there was systemic translocation throughout the leaves and plant; metabolism was limited with the parent compound being the major residue.[49]

3.5.2.1.10 Selective feeding blockers—Kir channel inhibition

Flonicamid is a pyridine carboxamide which is active against a variety of aphids, whiteflies, and thrips. It is more effective when ingested than on contact and is believed to block the Kir (inward-rectifying K^+) channels at nanomolar concentrations.[50] Insects stop eating and starve to death, possibly because the chordotonal organ system is particularly affected, so altering their sense of balance. However, salivary and renal excretion are also blocked, so flonicamid has multifactorial effects.

3.5.2.2 Energy metabolism modulators

3.5.2.2.1 Uncouplers of oxidative phosphorylation

1. Fludioxonil is a widely used phenylpyrrole fungicide, often applied postharvest to fruit and vegetables, particularly tomatoes, to minimize losses from gray mold (*Botrytis cinerea*). Its MOA is not fully understood, although it is known to act as an uncoupler in mitochondria from bumblebees (*Bombus terrestris*).[51] Its potential to disrupt endocrine and neurological systems has led to suggestions that it may impact human health.[52] It is relatively insoluble in water; only 9.8% of residues on chrysanthemum flowers used for traditional herbal teas actually entered the infusions so the health risk was considered low in comparison with other pesticides.[53]
2. Inhibition of electron transfer in mitochondria—strobilurins and oudermansins.

The first compounds, known as strobilurin A and B, were isolated from a species of Basidiomycetes fungus, *Strobilurus tenacellus*, also referred to as the "pinecone cap," a native to Asia and Europe.[54] Further strobilurins have been obtained from other saprobic wood-rotting fungi, such as *Oudemansiella mucida* ("porcelain mushroom").[55] The compounds are part of a larger group of quinone outside inhibitors and work by obstructing electron transfer between cytochromes b and c in the mitochondria after binding to the ubihydroquinine oxidation center of the bc_1 complex. The (*E*)-β-methoxyacrylate moiety is the toxicophore.[56] The fungi themselves are naturally resistant as specific amino acid alterations in the sequence of their cytochrome b reduce strobilurin binding to the target site center Q_p of the cytochrome bc_1 complex. Resistance may also reflect other factors such as efficient efflux transporters and alternative respiration pathways. To overcome initial problems of photolability and high vapor pressure, the structures of the natural compounds were chemically altered to give synthetic products which were more suitable for agricultural usage[57] and today they are amongst the world's leading fungicides.

As a general rule, strobilurins are easily degraded in biological and environmental systems and have similar metabolic fates.[58] Cleavage of the molecule and aromatic ring hydroxylation leads to phenolic derivatives that may undergo conjugation. Many minor metabolites have been reported.[59] Whilst on the leaf surface the compounds are susceptible to photoisomerism and photodegradation; mandestrobin (a recent synthetic strobilurin derivative) has a photolysis half-life of around 2–4 days.[60]

3.5.2.2.2 Mitochondrial complex electron transport inhibitors

Tolfenpyrad and rotenone both inhibit Complex 1 of the respiratory chain, while succinate dehydrogenase inhibitors (SDHIs) bind to the ubiquinone-binding site of Complex II, decreasing ATP (adenosine 5′-triphosphate) production; they are an essential group of fungicides for controlling gray mold caused by *B. cinerea* in many crops including tomatoes. One of the main SDHIs is boscalid, which is effective against spore germination and germ tube elongation and is widely used, although resistance now occurs worldwide. In zebra fish, boscalid is a neurodevelopmental toxin, inducing oxidative stress.[61] It also causes liver and kidney damage in adult fish, affecting carbohydrate and lipid metabolism with increases in hexokinase, glycogen, and insulin, and decreases in acetyl CoA and triglycerides in the liver.[62] Fluopyram is a more recent introduction and has nematocidal activity as well as fungicidal properties. It is effective against the southern root knot (*Meloidogyne incognita*) and reniform (*Rotylenchulus reniformis*) nematodes which damage tomatoes and other crops, particularly in the United States. Complex III inhibitors also exist, bifenazate being currently the most commonly used. Inhibitors of mitochondrial ATP synthase, such as propargite and organotin compounds, act as energy depressors for all life forms.

3.5.2.3 Insect growth dysregulation

Many insecticides have relatively specific MOA where they target the various stages of insect growth. Insects start as eggs which hatch to form larvae. These pass through various stages (instars), increasing in size by molting and shedding the old skin each time, until they reach the pupa stage and then the adult or imago. The moves through the larval stages are controlled by 20-hydroxyecdysone and the presence of JH (juvenile hormone). Once JH is no longer synthesized, the program to form the adult insect is switched on. Compounds which dysregulate this process may be molting disruptors such as hexythiazox and cyromazine or ecdysone receptor agonists (methoxyfenozide, etoxazole) or JH mimics (methoprene, fenoxycarb). Chitin, a polymer of *N*-acetylglucosamine, is the main component of insect exoskeletons and the cell walls of fungi. Both buprofenazine, an acaricide and insecticide controlling whiteflies and leafhoppers, and benzoylureas such as chlorfluazuron inhibit its synthesis, blocking formation of the adult insect. In general, inhibitors of chitin synthesis also have some fungicidal activity. Once the adult insect is formed, the *Bacillus thuringiensis* protein toxins, which are microbial insect midgut membrane disruptors, can be effective, although residues are rarely found on foodstuffs and are readily hydrolyzed in the mammalian gut.

3.5.2.4 Fungicides

3.5.2.4.1 Inhibitors of lipid/steroid/sterol synthesis

1. Conazoles

   The suffix, "conazole," is applied to a cluster of synthetic organic molecules that are employed to treat fungal contamination and infestation in plants and animals. Their chemical structures include a five-membered azole ring and they may be categorized into two subgroups: those containing an imidazole moiety (e.g., miconazole, ketoconazole) in which the ring contains two nitrogen atoms, and the later-developed triazoles (e.g., propiconazole, bromuconazole) in which three nitrogen atoms are present. Currently, the triazole derivatives, which are the most potent,[63] and their second-generation modifications are the most widely used conazole fungicides.[64]

   These pesticides work by interfering with the synthesis of ergosterol, the most abundant sterol in fungal cell membranes. Its presence is crucial in regulating the overall integrity, fluidity, and permeability of the plasma membrane, as well as maintaining the correct functioning of membrane-bound enzymes.[65] Azoles inhibit the cytochrome P450 catalyzing the vital demethylation step in the formation of ergosterol (CYP51; lanosterol 14-α-demethylase)[66] and mutations in the *ERG11* gene which codes for this particular isozyme have been shown to bestow fungal resistance.[67] Some azoles also affect C22-sterol desaturase (Δ^{22}-desaturase; CYP61) activity as well as influencing the action of other enzyme systems.[68]

   Generally, azoles are lipophilic weak bases and easily penetrate cells, some having a systemic action in plants. However, although passage into the fungal cell may occur by passive diffusion, substantially more of the compound appears to enter via facilitated diffusion being assisted by protein carriers and membrane channels.[69] Azoles are rapidly adsorbed onto soil particles and may remain within the environment for several months before being degraded to carbon dioxide.

   Azoles are extensively metabolized in mammals, generating a larger array of metabolites when compared to plants. Following oral dosing of bromuconazole to rats, 59 metabolites were detected, cyproconazole administration provided 34 metabolites and no unchanged compound was excreted after oral intake of prochloraz.[70] Metabolism is dominated by cytochrome P450–mediated reactions. Usually the ring structures are separated from each other and the molecule broken down into smaller units with subsequent oxidative degradation. Such metabolites exist freely or may be further conjugated, usually as glucuronides and sulfates in mammals and as glucosides in plants.[71]

2. The chiral fungicide imazalil is an androgen receptor antagonist which has been linked to endocrine disruption in mice and human fetal testis explants.[72] Like other azoles, it synergizes the effect of pyrethroid insecticides by inhibiting their cytochrome P450 (CYP)-dependent detoxication pathways. It was originally designed to inhibit the fungal CYP isozyme lanosterol-14-demethylase (CYP51) but also inhibits CYP1 and CYP19 (aromatase) in mammals. In mice, chronic exposure to low doses of imazalil (0.1 mg/kg) induced hepatotoxicity and affected the pathways for bile acid secretion.[73] Imazalil residues in food are common; a study of the French ELFE cohort of pregnant women identified the compound as giving the highest dietary exposures of the 284 pesticides

assessed.[74] A Canadian study on 4727 Quebecois, which evaluated the health risks and benefits of eating fruits and vegetables with pesticide residues, considered that the chronic health risks were low although uncertainties remained.[75] Nevertheless, imazalil contributed most to the noncancer risks and the authors of the study recommended that there should be a focus on reducing exposure to the compound.

3. Tetronic and tetramic acid derivatives such as spiromesifen, spirodichlofen, and spirotetramat are inhibitors of acetyl CoA carboxylase. They block lipid synthesis and are used as acaricides to control mites, aphids, earwigs, and whitefly on soft fruit, tomatoes, and cucumbers.

3.5.2.4.2 Inhibitors of methionine synthesis

Pyrimethanil (PYM) is a pyrimidine-based fungicide, which is used both pre- and postharvest against molds, powdery mildew, and rusts on fruit and potatoes. Although it has a low acute toxicity, it is of toxicological concern because it has antiandrogenic properties. In human volunteers about 80% of an oral dose was metabolized to 4-hydroxypyrimethanil which was then mainly excreted in urine as glucuronide and sulfate conjugates. Biomonitoring of PYM in Swedish populations found nearly 50% of urine samples from environmentally exposed individuals contained 4-OH PYM, while the corresponding value for occupational exposure was 96%.[76] When 200 blood samples from an environmentally exposed population in the Jiangsu province of China were analyzed, again PYM was found in more than 50%.[77] PYM residues on food can carry through processing to the final product; 22.4% of wine samples contained the compound at concentrations of $>10\,\mu m/L$.[78] Cyprodinil (CYL) has a similar structure and MOA and is metabolized to hydroxylated metabolites which are excreted in urine as glucuronides and sulfates. Like PYM, it is sprayed on grapes as a fungicide then may be carried through into the wine; 6.8% of samples of international wines, which were analyzed by antibody-based assays, contained CYL residues.[78] CYL is an activator of the aryl hydrocarbon receptor and also acts on the estrogen receptor so could disrupt endocrine pathways. Both PYM and CYL reduce cellular ATP in neuronal cell lines, probably via toxic effects on the mitochondrial membrane potential and cause oxidative stress in vitro.[79]

3.5.2.4.3 Multisite action

The protectant fungicide captan is a phthalimide derivative which significantly reduces brown rot caused by *Monilinia fructicola* on peaches in the preharvest fruit ripening period. It is also active against apple diseases such as apple scab (*Venturia inaequalis*) and bitter rot (*Colletotrichum* spp.) and is believed to have multisite action. Toxicity from captan causes oxidative stress and effects on cell membranes; this may underlie the reported link between captan exposure and age-related macular degeneration (AMD) since one of the factors in AMD is thought to be damage from oxygen free radicals.[80] Although it is considered relatively nontoxic to mammals, it is a potential inhibitor of human CYP19A1 (aromatase) and has been associated with the development of multiple myeloma in North American farmers.[81] Exposure to captan induces DNA base alterations and replicative stress in mammalian cell lines[82] so it may be genotoxic in man.

Iprodione, which is no longer approved in the EU because of its carcinogenic and endocrine-disrupting potential, acts as a fungicide by inhibiting DNA and RNA synthesis in germinating fungal spores. It also inhibits NADH (nicotinamide adenine dinucleotide) cytochrome c reductase and glutathione synthesis, leading to formation of ROS. It is toxic to honey bees and other pollinators.

Thiabendazole is a systemic fungicide with a benzimidazole structure which is used to control molds and storage diseases such as rot. Generally, it is used as a postharvest agent, acting against *Aspergillus* and *Fusarium* spp. It is applied in a wax matrix to banana skins and citrus fruit and is also widely used as an anthelmintic in both livestock and man, as it controls round worm and hook worm. It binds to β-tubulin, probably isotype 1, preventing polymerization of microtubules.[83] In rats it caused loss of hepatic mitochondrial membrane potential and activated both the mitochondrial and death receptor pathways of apoptosis.[84] Data from the French national birth cohort (ELFE) explored the relationship between residues of 64 pesticides and their metabolites in hair taken from 311 women who gave birth in 2011 and the measurements of their neonates at birth. Thiabendazole was statistically significantly associated with reduced head circumference and with reduced birthweight in boys.[85] Carbendazim, which no longer has EU approval, is also a benzimidazole fungicide which inhibits β-tubulin assembly in mitosis and disrupts spermatogenesis in mammals. These findings should be interpreted with caution until they are replicated by other studies but suggest pesticide residues affecting mitosis may have small but measurable effects on fetal growth and development.

3.5.2.5 Herbicides

3.5.2.5.1 Cell walls/growth regulation

Gibberellins are plant hormones which stimulate development of all plant organs, increasing cell division and elongation and inhibiting root growth. Generally, when cereals are grown, the plant that puts its energy into producing long stems will have smaller and fewer seeds. As the seeds are the commercially important part of the crop, growth regulators can be used to inhibit gibberellins and so produce shorter stems with better seed production. This in turn improves harvesting as plants with shorter thicker stems are less likely to "lodge," lying flat after wet and windy weather. Lodging makes the cereal more difficult and expensive to collect and quaternized nitrogen compounds are often used to try to limit damage from the weather at harvest time. Chlormequat is an alkylating agent and sprout suppressant which is widely used on cereal crops and on vegetables. It causes developmental toxicity in mammals; mepiquat acts similarly but is less effective. Like chlormequat, it has endocrine-disrupting potential and has been suggested to cause hypospadias and atrial septal defects.[86] As both mepiquat and chlormequat are used on plants just before harvest, their residues are frequently found as contaminants in the food chain. Paraquat is very toxic to man and mammals and was banned from use in the EU in 2007. However, paraquat levels over the EU maximum limits were found in 60% of wheat and barley samples from France and its overseas territories in the period 2012–2016.[87] This suggests that unauthorized use is still occurring, possibly from previously stored product. Although it is strongly polar, paraquat is readily absorbed from the gastrointestinal tract, probably via the spermine transporter since the two compounds have similar charges and configurations. It rapidly causes release of ROS which disrupt the provision of energy via the mitochondrial oxidative phosphorylation pathway and fatally damage the lungs, liver, and kidney so that patients die from multiple organ failure. Paraquat has frequently been used as a vehicle for suicide but has also caused many unintentional deaths when stored in beverage bottles. It is a neurotoxin and long-term spraying with paraquat, like other pesticides, is associated with the development of Parkinson's disease (PD).[88] Diquat is a nonselective contact and preharvest desiccant and defoliant which, like paraquat, is toxic to man and mammals, particularly causing kidney damage.[89] Similarly, it disrupts mitochondrial bioenergetics and generates ROS, while chronic exposure is again linked with PD.[90] Its use within the EU is now banned (04/02/2020).

3.5.2.5.2 Ripening

The volatile gas ethylene blocks the action of auxins, plant hormones which stimulate the elongation of cells in plant stems. It stimulates ripening of fruit and is produced naturally by the plant. Synthetic chemicals which are ethylene precursors are used to speed up and synchronize the pre- and postharvest ripening of soft fruit, particularly grapes and tomatoes, with bananas and pineapples. Ethephon, which breaks down to give ethylene, phosphate, and chloride, is widely used for this purpose, and residues are frequently found on treated produce. At high doses (200 mg/kg) the compound is a reproductive toxin in rats.[91]

3.5.2.5.3 Dysregulation of plant metabolism

Glyphosate is a systemic broad-spectrum herbicide which is very widely used to control weed infestations in commercial crops. It is also used preharvest as a desiccant to dry leaves and stems, thus making the final collection of the produce much easier. Glyphosate is active in plants which are growing at the time of spraying and works by disrupting the shikimic acid pathway which is largely plant-specific, although it is present and necessary for growth in some bacteria and fungi. The sodium salt is also a plant growth regulator and improves crop ripening. Glyphosate residues in small amounts can be found in foods, particularly those made from cereals, and trace amounts of glyphosate and its metabolite aminomethylphosphonic acid have been found in urine from volunteers eating a conventional diet.[92] In a review of human studies,[93] the urinary glyphosate levels for environmental exposure ranged from 0.16 to 7.6 ng/L. Numerous risk assessments have been carried out by national and international agencies since it was suggested that glyphosate might be carcinogenic. Although IARC (International Agency for Research on Cancer) had reclassified the compound in 2015 as category Type 2A (probable human carcinogen), in 2017 the European Chemical Agency (ECHA) concluded that glyphosate was toxic to eyes and to aquatic life but that the pure compound was not a carcinogen. However, it is normally formulated with a range of surfactants and these mixtures appear to be more toxic than the parent chemical itself, particularly the "Roundup" formulation containing polyethoxylated tallow amine (POEA).[94,95] The many toxicological studies that have been carried out on glyphosate and its mixtures have all been criticized for failures in study design and inadequate interpretation of the results, so the exact situation is still unclear. Measured and estimated systemic exposures to glyphosate in humans were less than the ADIs and ARfDs (Acute Reference Doses).[96] Nevertheless, Davoren and Schiestl[94] who reviewed the topic recommended that the chronic reference dose levels should be reduced to 0.175 mg/kg/day and that future research on glyphosate should include studies on the commercially formulated material and focus into its effects on the microbiome (since the compound can affect bacterial metabolic pathways) and possible nonmonotonic (nonlinear) effects on systemic inflammation and endocrine disruption.

3.6 Potential points of concern for agrochemical residues in the food chain

3.6.1 The "cocktail effect"

Pesticides undergo rigorous testing for toxic effects but always as single entities. They are never tested in combination with the various chemicals which are added as carriers to the formulation to improve spraying properties or "wettability." Similarly, most fruit and vegetables are treated with more than one pesticide over the course of the growing season and some have many residues at the point of sale. This is particularly the case for soft fruit, salad vegetables, and tomatoes; typical results from the fourth quarter report of the PRiF show that samples of grapes collected between September and November 2020 contained between 2 and 17 different pesticide residues. This reflects the fact that the samples were made up from grapes from several suppliers. All values were below the MRLs and were not expected to affect health; however, it is not clear whether the combined presence of these very small amounts could give additive, subtractive, or synergistic effects. This problem has been referred to as the "cocktail effect," and it has been studied in depth. Metabolomic analysis of tissues from rats and offspring that had been fed a mixture of eight pesticides (representative of the main environmental exposure in Brittany) suggested development of oxidative stress with impaired glucose and lipid metabolism.[97]Chronic dietary exposure to pesticide residues was analyzed in the French ELFE cohort of pregnant women where statistically significant cumulative risk was suggested for neurochemical effects related to high intakes of organophosphate insecticides.[74] It is generally assumed that compounds with the same MOA would be additive but there are currently no clear conclusions for combinations of compounds with different MOA (which is usually the case). EFSA (European Food Safety Authority) has published various reports on the topic[98–100]; the cumulative dietary risk characterization of pesticides that have chronic effects on the thyroid was assessed using probabilistic modeling, with monitoring data collected by EU Member States. It was concluded (with varying degrees of certainty) that this cumulative exposure did not exceed the threshold for regulatory consideration[98]; given the varying consumption data available for different populations, the certainty was least for Dutch children (85%–90% vs 99% for adult populations). A similar article focused on modeling any potential neurological effects.[99] Again, probabilistic modeling of cumulative assessment exposures and monitoring data were combined, and then used to determine the risk of AChE inhibition and functional alterations of the motor division. Similar conclusions to the thyroid study were reached with varying degrees of certainty; the cumulative exposure did not reach the threshold for regulatory consideration, although the certainty for some child populations was less (80%) than that for the adult populations (99%). The pesticide exposure appears to be too low for any effects to become manifest, at least in the short term, although several studies have suggested that professional pesticide crop sprayers, who presumably have higher exposure levels, may be more susceptible to PD.[88]

Reduced synthesis of cellular energy has been linked with neurodegenerative problems and Alzheimer's disease (AD) and this correlates with the high energy requirements of the brain where any chronic reduction in metabolism could have long-term consequences. These would be more likely if residues contained two or more pesticides that reduced ATP synthesis by different mechanisms, for example, neonicotinoids (inhibition of Complex 1) with chlorfenapyr (disruption of the proton gradient). *In vitro,* combinations of pyrimethanil, cyprodinil, and fludioxonil reduced cellular ATP in human neuronal cell lines[79] so *in vivo* effects may occur. Clearly, combinations with pesticides where the MOA was not relevant to humans, such as chitin synthesis inhibitors, would be less of a risk. Unfortunately, there are no good animal models for PD or AD so that this hypothesis is not testable, although possibly metabolomic techniques might provide answers for the future. A diet with a wide range of constituent foods could avoid chronic dosage with the same combinations of pesticides.

3.6.2 Endocrine disruption

Many pesticides also affect the endocrine systems as "endocrine disruptors" (EDs), dysregulating hormonal function. They may do this by altering steroid synthesis or degradation, by acting as agonists or antagonists at steroid receptors or by affecting signaling pathways. The androgen and estrogen systems may be involved so that pesticides act as feminizing or sometimes masculinizing agents or thyroid function may be dysregulated. Biosystems such as fish and amphibians can be affected but mammalian responses are clearly more relevant to humans. As part of the regulatory requirements, pesticides are routinely tested in rodents, particularly rats, which seem to be susceptible to dietary and environmental EDs. However, despite a large amount of research effort, it is not clear whether EDs can affect human beings and if they do, at what levels these responses would occur. Generally, unlike rodents, humans seem resistant to ED action; diethylstilboestrol is an estrogen agonist which has major effects on rats but relatively few problems were seen in many women who were prescribed large amounts for long periods of time.[101] Nevertheless, when human cell lines were used as test systems, low-level combinations of EDs which acted at different points in the hormone pathways gave similar responses to those given by higher levels of single EDs.[102] This may suggest that if foodstuffs contain small traces of several different pesticides, as is often the case, then there might be a cumulative effect. The situation is complex and made difficult both by the lack of data and the use of rodents as test animals when their reproductive systems are unlike those in humans. Further, potential alterations in the endocrine pathways may have subtle effects on neurodevelopment or the immune system and these are difficult to model in rodents.

3.6.3 Effects on the microbiome

The human gut microbiome is an aggregate of microbiota consisting of bacteria with archaea, fungi, especially yeasts, and viruses. This microbial community is thought to contain 500–1000 species of bacteria but just a few phyla, Firmicutes and Bacteroidetes being predominant. Many of these microorganisms are difficult or impossible to culture but new technologies, where DNA or RNA is directly extracted from stools, have allowed identification of the gut microbiota. DNA isolation and amplification of the 16S ribosomal RNA gene or shotgun sequencing now allow the characterization of bacterial species that was previously impossible. In humans, the gut microbiome is shaped early in life depending on a variety of factors including diet, type of delivery at birth, and antibiotic use. It remains relatively stable in adult life but differs between individuals depending on lifestyle, cultural factors, and diet.[103] Recently it has become clear that the microbiome acts as an endocrine organ[104] and that dysregulation of its constituent communities is linked with chronic health problems. In a review on this topic, an altered microbiome was linked with immune responses, metabolic syndrome and Type 2 diabetes, with obesity and with inflammatory bowel disease.[105] The gut/brain axis has been extensively investigated and it is now clear that hormones and metabolites released by the microbiome[106,107] can affect the functioning of the CNS[108]; for example, adolescent patients with depression have altered ratios of bacterial species[109] as do children with autism.[110] The various compounds produced by the microbiome, such as the short-chain fatty acids, also affect the immune system.[111] As chemical compounds in the gastrointestinal tract can alter the ratios of the constituent bacterial species, this raises the possibility that pesticide residues in the food chain could potentially change the microbiome simply by being present in the gut contents. This is more likely as pesticides are formulated to have biocidal activity at very low levels. While acute ingestion of tiny amounts of such chemicals would probably not cause changes, chronic ingestion of specific compounds might be sufficient to affect the microbiome over a period of months or years. In this context, cleaning agents such as DDAC, which are designed to be effective against enteric bacteria, particularly *Escherichia coli*, might be able to disrupt the gut microbial communities.[112] This is problematic because the quaternized nitrogen compounds are ubiquitous and as they are used to clean surfaces as well as disinfect food, the total daily intake may be far greater than analysis of the diet alone would suggest. Although the compounds themselves would be rapidly excreted, they might leave an altered microbiome which could in turn be a factor in chronic ill health. Some pesticides have already been identified as affecting the microbiome in mammals; the effects of organophosphates on microbiota have been reviewed.[113] In rats, the gut flora are known to be modulated by the organophosphate metabolite diethyl phosphate which enriched opportunistic pathogens,[114] while chlorpyrifos affected bacteria involved in regulating the endocrine system and the immune response.[115] In mice, aldicarb, a carbamate insecticide, enhanced gut bacterial pathogenicity and disturbed brain metabolism,[116] while imazalil[73] and penconazole altered the ratios of the microflora.[117] In humans, *in vitro* studies with intestinal epithelial TC7 cells suggested that when in combination with other environmental contaminants, pesticides promoted an inflammatory state in the gut and altered the profiles of volatile organic compounds.[118] In reviews of the effects of single and combined toxic exposures on the gut microbiome,[105,118–120] it was concluded that there should be more concentration on exposure to real-life mixtures of pesticides with other toxicants. This is a complex topic, made more difficult by the individual variation occurring in human gut microbiomes, but there is enough evidence to flag up an area of potential concern.

3.7 Conclusions and potential areas for further study

Agrochemicals are found in trace amounts in many foodstuffs. Despite findings of low levels of exposure to a variety of pesticide residues in food, there is so far little evidence of adverse health effects in the general population. Risk/benefit assessments should weigh the potential for both crop losses and harmful effects of microbial toxins against the possibility of unintended biological effects. Future investigations should focus on potential disruption of the endocrine, neurodevelopmental, and gut microbiome systems. The impact of low-level exposure to combinations of pesticides and other environmental contaminants should be considered. These should be studied in vitro in human cell lines using metagenomic, transcriptomic, and metabolomic techniques to improve the chances of identifying "unknown unknowns."

References

1. Kalaycioglu Z, Erim FB. Nitrate and nitrites in foods: worldwide regional distribution in view of their risks and benefits. *J Agric Food Chem.* 2019;67(26):7205–7222.
2. Piglowski M. The intra-European Union food trade with the relation to the notifications in the rapid alert system for food and feed. *Int J Environ Res Public Health.* 2021;18(4):0208.

3. Cabrera LC, Pastor PM. The 2019 EU report on pesticide residues in food. *EFSA J.* 2021;19(4):6491.
4. Boucaud-Maitre D, Rambourg MO, Sinno-Tellier S, et al. Human exposure to banned pesticides reported to the French Poison Control Centers 2012–2016. *Environ Toxicol Pharmacol.* 2019;69:51–56.
5. Expert Committee on Pesticide Residues in Food (PRiF), *Annual report 2020: Food Standards Agency*; 2020:1–49.
6. Jankowska M, Lozowicka B, Kaczynski P. Comprehensive toxicological study over 160 processing factors of pesticides in selected fruit and vegetables after water, mechanical and thermal processing treatments and their application to human health risk assessment. *Sci Total Environ.* 2019;652:1156–1167.
7. Gavahian M, Sarangapani C, Misra NN. Cold plasma for mitigating agrochemical and pesticide residue in food and water: similarities with ozone and ultraviolet technologies. *Food Res Int.* 2021;141:110138.
8. Pounraj S, Bhilwadikar T, Manivannan S, et al. Effect of ozone, lactic acid and combination treatments on the control of microbial and pesticide contaminants of fresh vegetables. *J Sci Food Agric.* 2021;101(8):3422–3428.
9. Liu Y, Wang J, Zhu X, et al. Effects of electrolyzed water treatment on pesticide removal and texture quality in fresh-cut cabbage, broccoli and color pepper. *Food Chem.* 2021;353:129408.
10. Lopez-Galvez F, Gil ML, Meireles A, et al. Demonstration tests of irrigation water disinfection with chlorine dioxide in open field cultivation of baby spinach. *J Sci Food Agric.* 2018;98(8):2973–2980.
11. Lopez-Galvez F, Andujar S, Marin A, et al. Disinfection byproducts in baby lettuce irrigated with electrolysed water. *J Sci Food Agric.* 2018;98(8):2981–2988.
12. Kettlitz B, Kemendi G, Thorgrimsson N, et al. Why chlorate occurs in potable water and processed foods: a critical assessment and challenges faced by the food industry. *Food Addit Contam Part A Chem Anal Control Expo Risk Assess.* 2016;33(6):968–982.
13. Constantinou P, Louca-Christodoulou D, Agapiou A. LC-ESI-Ms/Ms determination of oxyhalides (chlorate, perchlorate, and bromate) in food and water samples and chlorate on household water treatment devices along with perchlorate in plants. *Chemosphere.* 2019;235:757–766.
14. Ali SN, Arif H, Khan AA, et al. Acute renal toxicity of sodium chlorate: redox imbalance, enhanced DNA damage metabolic alterations and inhibition of brush border membrane enzymes in rats. *Environ Toxicol.* 2018;33(11):1182–1194.
15. Hrubec TC, Melin VE, Shea CS, et al. Ambient and dosed exposure to quaternary ammonium disinfectants causes neural tube defects in rodents. *Birth Defects Res.* 2017;109(14):1166–1178.
16. Sanidad KZ, Yang H, Wang W, et al. Effects of consumer antimicrobials benzalkonium chloride, benzethonium chloride and chloroxylenol on colonic inflammation and colitis-associated colon tumorigenesis in mice. *Toxicol Sci.* 2018;163(2):490–499.
17. Narahashi T. Neurophysiological effects of insecticides. In: Krieger R, ed. *Haye's Handbook of Pesticide Toxicology.* 3rd ed. Amsterdam: Academic Press; 2010:799–817.
18. Fisher MH, Mrazik H. Chemistry. In: Campbell WC, ed. *Ivermectin and Abamectin.* New York: Springer-Verlag; 1989:1–23.
19. Yates DM, Wolstenholme AJ. An ivermectin-sensitive glutamate-gated chloride channel subunit from *Dirofilaria immitis. Int J Parasitol.* 2014;34(9):1075–1081.
20. Bloomquist JR. Chloride channels as tools for developing selective insecticides. *Arch Insect Biochem Physiol.* 2003;54(4):145–156.
21. Takiguchi Y, Mishima H, Okuda M, Terao M. Milbemycins, a new family of macrolide antibiotics: fermentation, isolation and physico-chemical properties. *J Antibiot.* 1980;33:1120–1127.
22. Sparks T, Crouse GD, Durst G. Natural products as insecticides: the biology, biochemistry and quantitative structure-activity relationships of spinosyns and spinosoids. *Pest Manag Sci.* 2001;57(10):896–905.
23. Watson GB, Chouinard SW, Cook KR, et al. A spinosyn-sensitive *Drosophila melanogaster* nicotinic acetylcholine receptor identified through chemically induced target site resistance, resistance gene identification, and heterologous expression. *Insect Biochem Mol Biol.* 2010;40(5):376–384.
24. Roberts TR, Hutson DH. Macrocylic insecticides. In: Roberts TR, Hutson DH, Lee PW, Nicholls PH, Plimmer JR, Robert MC, eds. *Metabolic Pathways of Agrochemicals: Part 2: Insecticides and Fungicides.* Cambridge: Royal Society of Chemistry; 1999:79–104.
25. Canga AG, Prieto AMS, Liébana MJD, Martinez NF, Vega MS, Vieitez JJG. The pharmacokinetics and interactions of ivermectin in humans – a mini review. *AAPS J.* 2008;10(1):42–46.
26. Sadakane S, Tanaka K, Muraoka E, Ando M. Metabolic fates of milbemycin A_3 and A_4 in rats. *J Pestic Sci.* 1992;17(3):147–154.
27. Matsuo N. Discovery and development of pyrethroid insecticides. *Proc Jpn Acad Ser B Phys Biol Sci.* 2019;95(7):378–400.
28. Yang J, Luo F, Zhou L, et al. Residue reduction and risk evaluation of chlorfenapyr residue in tea planting, tea processing and tea brewing. *Sci Total Environ.* 2020;738:139613.
29. Ferre DM, Jotallan PJ, Lentini V, et al. Biomonitoring of the hematological, biochemical and genotoxic effects of the mixture cypermethrin plus chlorpyrifos applications in bovines. *Sci Total Environ.* 2020;726:138058.
30. Rousis NI, Gracia-Lor E, Reid MJ, et al. Assessment of human exposure to selected pesticides in Norway by wastewater analysis. *Sci Total Environ.* 2020;723:138132.
31. Wang Q, Shen JY, Zhang R, et al. Effects and mechanisms of pyrethroids on male reproductive system. *Toxicology.* 2020;438:152460.
32. Wang H, He Y, Cheng D, et al. Cypermethrin exposure reduces the ovarian reserve by causing mitochondrial dysfunction in granulosa cells. *Toxicol Appl Pharmacol.* 2019;379:114693.
33. Singh D, Irani D, Bhagat S, et al. Cypermethrin exposure during perinatal period affects fetal development and impairs reproductive functions of F1 female rats. *Sci Total Environ.* 2020;707:135945.
34. Zhang J, Liu H, Lou L, et al. Exposure to deltamethrin in adolescent mice induced thyroid dysfunction and behavioural disorders. *Chemosphere.* 2020;241:125118.
35. Dalsager L, Fage-Larsen B, Bilenberg N, et al. Maternal urinary concentrations of pyrethroid and chlorpyrifos metabolites and attention deficit hyperactivity disorder (ADHD) symptoms in 2–4 year-old children from the Odense Child Cohort. *Environ Res.* 2019;176:108533.
36. Gwaltney-Brown SM. Atypical topical spot-on products. In: Peterson ME, Talcott PA, eds. *Small Animal Toxicology.* 3rd ed. St. Louis: Elsevier Saunders; 2013:741–754.
37. Zhang S, Zhang X, Shen J, et al. Cross-resistance and biochemical mechanisms of resistance to indoxacarb in the diamond back moth *Plutella xylostella. Pestic Biochem Physiol.* 2017;140:85–89.

38. Voss G, Neumann R, Kobel W. Economy-society-environment: how fit are organophosphorus insecticides? In: Eto M, Casida JE, eds. *Progress and Prospects of Organophosphorus Agrochemicals*. Fukuoka: Kyushu University Press; 1995:31–41.
39. Chowdhary S, Bhattacharyya R, Banerjee D. Acute organophosphorus poisoning. *Clin Chem Acta*. 2014;431:66–76.
40. Ohno I, Tomizawa M, Durkio KA, Naruse Y, Casida JE, Kagabu S. Molecular features of neonicotinoid pharmacophore variants interacting with the insect nicotinic receptor. *Chem Res Toxicol*. 2009;22(3):476–482.
41. Ihara M, Matsuda K. Neonicotinoids: molecular mechanisms of action, insights into resistance and impact on pollinators. *Curr Opin Insect Sci*. 2018;30:86–92.
42. Tomizawa M, Casida JE. Molecular recognition of neonicotinoid insecticides: the determinants of life or death. *Acc Chem Res*. 2009;42(2):260–269.
43. Roberts TR, Hutson DH. Neonicotinoids. In: Roberts TR, Hutson DH, Lee PW, Nicholls PH, Plimmer JR, Robert MC, eds. *Metabolic Pathways of Agrochemicals: Part 2: Insecticides and Fungicides*. Cambridge: Royal Society of Chemistry; 1999:105–126.
44. Casida JE. Neonicotinoid metabolism: compounds, substituents, pathways, enzymes, organisms, and relevance. *J Agric Food Chem*. 2011;59:2923–2931.
45. Dai J, Jiang C, Gao G. Dissipation pattern and safety evaluation of cartap and its metabolites during tea planting, tea manufacturing and brewing. *Food Chem*. 2020;314:126165.
46. Farooqui T. Review of octopamine in insect nervous systems. *Open Access Insect Physiol*. 2012;4:1–17.
47. Yim GK, Holsapple MP, Pfister WR, Hollingworth RM. Prostaglandin synthesis inhibited by formamidine pesticides. *Life Sci*. 1978;23(25):2509–2515.
48. Roberts TR, Hutson DH. Miscellaneous insecticides. In: Roberts TR, Hutson DH, Lee PW, Nicholls PH, Plimmer JR, eds. *Metabolic Pathways of Agrochemicals: Part 2: Insecticides and Fungicides*. Cambridge: The Royal Society of Chemistry; 1999:729–733. Part 2.
49. Pes MP, Melo AA, Stacke RS, et al. Translocation of chlorantraniliprole and cyantraniliprole applied to corn as seed treatment and foliar spraying to control *Spodoptera frugiperda* (Lepidoptera: Noctuidae). *PLoS One*. 2020;15(4):e0229151. Available from: https://doi.org/10.1371/journal.pone.0229151.
50. Ren M, Niu J, Hu B, et al. Block of Kir channels by flonicamid disrupts salivary and renal excretion of insect pests. *Insect Biochem Mol Biol*. 2018;99:17–26.
51. Syromyatnikov MY, Kokina AV, Lopatin AV, et al. Evaluation of the toxicity of fungicides to flight muscle mitochondria of bumblebee (*Bombus terrestris*). *Pestic Biochem Physiol*. 2017;135:41–46.
52. Brandhorst TT, Klein BS. Uncertainty surrounding the mechanism and safety of the post-harvest fungicide fludioxonil. *Food Chem Toxicol*. 2019;123:561–565.
53. Jiang M, Zhang W, Zhang T, et al. Assessing transfer of pesticide residues from chrysanthemum flowers into tea solutions and associated health risks. *Ecotoxicol Environ Saf*. 2020;187:109859.
54. Anke T, Oberwinkle F, Steglich W, Schramm G. The strobilurins – new antifungal antibiotics from the basidiomycete *Strobilurus tenacellus* (Pers. ex Fr.) Sing. *J Antibiot*. 1977;30(10):806–810.
55. Anke T, Hecht HJ, Schramm G, Steglich W. Antibiotics from basidiomycetes. IX. Oudemansin, an antifungal antibiotic from *Oudemansiella mucida* (Schrader ex Fr.) Hoehnel (Agaricales). *J Antibiot*. 1979;32(11):1112–1117.
56. Erkel G. Non-β-lactam antibiotics. vol. 10, Industrial Applications (Hofrichter M, ed) In: Esser K, ed. *The Mycota. A Comprehensive Treatise on Fungi as Experimental Systems for Basic and Applied Research*. 2nd ed. Berlin, Heidelberg: Springer; 2010:123–149.
57. Sauter H. Strobilurins and other complex III inhibitors. In: Krämer W, Schirmer U, Jeschke P, Witschel M, eds. *Modern Crop Protection Compounds*. Weinheim: Wiley-VCH Verlag GmbH; 2012:587–627. Section 15.2.
58. Jewess P, Lee P, Nicholls P, Plimmer J. Strobilurin analogues. In: Roberts T, Hutson D, eds. *Metabolic Pathways of Agrochemicals. Part 2; Insecticides and Fungicides*. Cambridge: Royal Society of Chemistry; 1999:1327–1342.
59. Joseph RSI. Metabolism of azoxystrobin in plant and animals. In: Brooks GT, Roberts TR, eds. *Pesticide Chemistry and Biosciences: The Food Environment Challenge*. Cambridge: The Royal Society of Chemistry; 1999:265–278.
60. Adachi T, Suzuki Y, Nishiyama Y, Kodaka R, Fujisawa T, Katagi T. Photodegradation of strobilurin fungicide mandestrobin in water. *J Agric Food Chem*. 2018;66(32):8514–8521.
61. Wang H, Meng Z, Liu F, et al. Characterisation of boscalid-induced oxidative stress and neurodevelopmental toxicity in zebrafish embryos. *Chemosphere*. 2020;238:124753.
62. Qian L, Zhang J, Chen X, et al. Toxic effects of boscalid in adult zebrafish (*Danio rerio*) on carbohydrate and lipid metabolism. *Environ Pollut*. 2019;247:775–782.
63. Davis JL, Papich MG, Heit MC. Antifungal and antiviral drugs. In: Riviere JE, Papich MG, eds. *Veterinary Pharmacology and Therapeutics*. 9th ed. Ames: John Wiley & Sons; 2009: 1013–1052.
64. Shulka PK, Singh P, Yadav RK, Pandey S, Bhunia SS. Past, present and future of antifungal drug development. Topics in Medicinal Chemistry In: Saxena A, ed. *Communicable Diseases of the Developing World*. 29. New York, Cham: Springer; 2016: 125–162.
65. Hof H. A new, broad spectrum azole antifungal: posaconazole – mechanism of action and resistance, spectrum of activity. *Mycoses*. 2006;49:2–6.
66. Vanden Bossche H, Ausma J, Bohets H, et al. The novel azole R126638 is a selective inhibitor of ergosterol synthesis *in Candida albicans*, *Trichophyton* spp. and *Microsporum canis*. *Antimicrob Agents Chemother*. 2004;48:3272–3278.
67. Marichal P, Kaymans L, Willemsens S, et al. Contribution of mutations in the cytochrome-P450 14α-demethylase (Erg11p, cyp51p) to azole resistance in *Candida albicans*. *Microbiology*. 1999;145:2701–2713.
68. Loose DS, Kan PS, Hirst MA, Marcus RA, Feldman D. Ketoconazole blocks adrenal steroidogenesis by inhibiting cytochrome P450-dependent enzymes. *J Clin Investig*. 1983;71(5): 1495–1499.
69. Esquivel BD, White TC. Accumulation of azole drugs in the fungal plant pathogen *Magnaporthe oryzae* is the result of facilitated diffusion influx. *Front Microbiol*. 2017;8:1320. Available from: https://doi.org/10.3389/fmicb.2017.01320.
70. Laignelet L, Rivière JL, Le Huguenot JC. Metabolism of an imidazole fungicide (prochloraz) in the rat after oral administration. *Food Chem Toxicol*. 1992;36(7):575–583.

71. Roberts TR, Hutson DH. Azoles and analogues. In: Roberts TR, Hutson DH, Lee PW, Nicholls PH, Plimmer JR, Robert MC, eds. *Metabolic Pathways of Agrochemicals: Part 2: Insecticides and Fungicides*. Cambridge: Royal Society of Chemistry; 1999: 1011–1104.
72. Gaudriault P, Mazaud-Guittot S, Lavoue V, et al. Endocrine disruption in human fetal testis explants by individual and combined exposures to selected pharmaceuticals, pesticides and environmental pollutants. *Environ Health Perspect*. 2017;125(8):087004.
73. Jin C, Luo T, Fu Z, et al. Oral imazalil exposure induces gut microbiota dysbiosis and colonic inflammation in mice. *Chemosphere*. 2016;160:349–358.
74. de Gavelle E, de Lauzon-Guillain B, Charles MA, et al. Chronic dietary exposure to pesticide residues and associated risk in the French ELFE cohort of pregnant women. *Environ Int*. 2016;92–93:533–542.
75. Valcke M, Bourgault MH, Rochette L, et al. Human health risk assessment on the consumption of fruits and vegetables containing residual pesticides: a cancer and non-cancer risk/benefit perspective. *Environ Int*. 2017;108:63–74.
76. Faniband M, Ekman E, Littorin M, et al. Biomarkers of exposure to pyrimethanil after controlled human experiments. *J Anal Toxicol*. 2019;43(4):277–283.
77. Chang C, Chen M, Gao J, et al. Current pesticide profiles in blood serum of adults in Jiangsu Province of China and a comparison with other countries. *Environ Int*. 2017;102:213–222.
78. Esteve-Turrillas FA, Agullo C, Abad-Somovilla A, et al. Fungicide multiresidue monitoring in international wines by immunoassays. *Food Chem*. 2016;196:1279–1286.
79. Coleman MD, O'Neil JD, Woehrling EK, et al. A preliminary investigation into the impact of a pesticide combination on human neuronal and glial cell lines in vitro. *PLoS One*. 2012;7(8): e42768.
80. Montgomery MP, Postel E, Umbach DM, et al. Pesticide use and age-related macular degeneration in the Agricultural Health Study. *Environ Health Perspect*. 2017;125(7):077013.
81. Presutti R, Harris SA, Kachuri L, et al. Pesticide exposures and the risk of multiple myeloma in men: an analysis of the North American Pooled Project. *Int J Cancer*. 2016;139(8):1703–1714.
82. Inoue T, Kinoshita M, Oyama K, et al. Captan-induced increase in the concentrations of intra cellular Ca^{2+} and Zn^{2+} and its correlation with oxidative stress in rat thymic lymphocytes. *Environ Toxicol Pharmacol*. 2018;63:78–83.
83. Tyden E, Skarin M, Andersson-Franko M, et al. Differential expression of beta tubulin isotypes in different life stages of *Parascaris* spp after exposure to thiabendazole. *Mol Biochem Parasitol*. 2016;205(1–2):22–28.
84. Seide M, Marion M, Mateescu MA, et al. The fungicide thiabendazole causes apoptosis in rat hepatocytes. *Toxicol In Vitro*. 2016;32:232–239.
85. Beranger R, Hardy EM, Binter AC, et al. Multiple pesticides in mothers' hair samples and children's measurements at birth: results from the French national birth cohort (ELFE). *Int J Hyg Environ Health*. 2020;223(1):22–33.
86. Rappazzo KM, Warren JL, Davalos AD. Maternal residential exposure to specific agricultural pesticide active ingredients and birth defects in a 2003–2005 North Carolina birth cohort. *Birth Defects Res*. 2019;111(6):312–323.
87. Francesquett JZ, Rizzetti TM, Cadaval Jr TRS, et al. Simultaneous determination of the quaternary ammonium pesticides paraquat, diquat, chlormequat and mepiquat in barley and wheat using a modified quick polar pesticides method, diluted standard solution, addition calibration and hydrophilic interaction liquid chromatography coupled to tandem mass spectrometry. *J Chromatogr A*. 2019;1592:101–111.
88. Perrin L, Spinosi J, Chaperon L, et al. Pesticides expenditures by farming type and incidence of Parkinson disease in farmers: a French nationwide study. *Environ Res*. 2021;197:111161.
89. Magalhaes N, Carvalho F, Dinis-Oliveira RJ. Human and experimental toxicology of diquat poisoning: toxicokinetics, mechanisms of toxicity and clinical features and treatment. *Hum Exp Toxicol*. 2018;37(11):1131–1160.
90. Pouchieu C, Piel C, Carles C, et al. Pesticide use in agriculture and Parkinson's disease in the AGRICAN cohort study. *Int J Epidemiol*. 2018;47(1):299–310.
91. Abd Eldaim MA, Tousson E, El Sayed IET, et al. Ameliorative effects of *Saussurea lappa* root aqueous extract against Ethephon-induced reproductive toxicity in male rats. *Environ Toxicol*. 2019;34(2):150–159.
92. Conrad A, Schroter-Kermani C, Hoppe HW, et al. Glyphosate in German adults – time trend (2001–2015) of human exposure to a widely used herbicide. *Int J Hyg Environ Health*. 2017;220(1): 8–16.
93. Guillezeau C, van Gerwen M, Shaffer RM, et al. The evidence of human exposure to glyphosate. *Environ Health*. 2019;18(1):2.
94. Davoren MJ, Schiestl RH. Glyphosate-based herbicides and cancer risk: a post-IARC decision review of potential mechanisms, policy and avenues of research. *Carcinogenesis*. 2018;39(10): 1207–1215.
95. Meftaul IM, Venkateswarlu K, Dharmarajan R, et al. Controversies over human health and ecological impacts of glyphosate: is it to be banned in modern agriculture? *Environ Pollut*. 2020;263(Pt A):114372.
96. Solomon KR. Estimated exposure to glyphosate in humans via environmental, occupational and dietary pathways: an updated review of the scientific literature. *Pest Manag Sci*. 2020;76(9):2878–2885.
97. Bonvallot N, Canlet C, Blas-Y-Estrada F, et al. Metabolome disruption of pregnant rats and their offspring resulting from repeated exposure to a pesticide mixture representative of environmental contamination in Brittany. *PLoS One*. 2018;13(6): e0198448.
98. Chatzidimitriou E, Mienne A, Pierlot S, et al. Assessment of combined risk to pesticide residues through dietary exposure. *EFSA J*. 2019;17(S2):e170910.
99. Craig PS, Dujardin B, Hart A, et al. Cumulative dietary risk characterisation of pesticides that have chronic effects on the thyroid. *EFSA J*. 2020;18(4):6088.
100. Craig PS, Dujardin B, Hart A, et al. Cumulative dietary risk characterisation of pesticides that have acute effects on the nervous system. *EFSA J*. 2020;18(4):6087.
101. Harris RM, Waring RH. Diethylstilboestrol – a long-term legacy? *Maturitas*. 2012;72:108–112.
102. Waring RH, Ramsden DB, Jarratt PDB, et al. Biomarkers of endocrine disruption: cluster analysis of effects of plasticisers on Phase 1 and Phase 2 metabolism of steroids. *Int J Androl*. 2012;35(30): 415–423.

103. Inda ME, Broset E, Lu TK, et al. Emerging Frontiers in Immunology. *Trends Immunol.* 2019;40(10):952–973.
104. Li R, Li Y, Zheng D, et al. Gut microbiota and endocrine disorder. *Adv Exp Med Biol.* 2020;1238:143–164.
105. Roca-Saavedra P, Mendes-Vilabrille V, Miranda JM, et al. J Food additives, contaminants and other minor components: effects on human gut microbiota – a review. *J Physiol Biochem.* 2018;74:69–83.
106. Chen Y, Wu G, Zhao Y. Gut microbiota and alimentary tract injury. *Adv Exp Med Biol.* 2020;1238:11–22.
107. Schirmer M, Garner A, Vlamakis H, et al. Microbial genes and pathways in inflammatory bowel disease. *Nat Rev.* 2019;17(8): 497–511.
108. Cryan JF, O'Riordan KJ, Sandhu K, et al. The gut microbiome in neurological disorders. *Lancet Neurol.* 2020;19(2):179–194.
109. Simkin DR. Microbiome and mental health, specifically as it relates to adolescents. *Curr Psychiatry Rep.* 2019;21(9):93.
110. Saurman V, Margolis KG, Luna RA, et al. Autism spectrum disorder as a brain-gut-microbiome axis disorder. *Dig Dis Sci.* 2020;65 (3):818–828.
111. Pekmez C, Dragsted LO, Brahe LK. Gut microbiota alterations and dietary modulation in childhood malnutrition-the role of short chain fatty acids. *Clin Nutr.* 2019;38:615–630.
112. Harrison KR, Kappell AD, McNamara PJ. Benzalkonium chloride alters phenotypic and genotypic antibiotic resistance profiles in a source water used for drinking water treatment. *Environ Pollut.* 2020;257:113472.
113. Roman P, Cardona D, Sempere L, et al. Microbiota and organophosphates. *Neurotoxicology.* 2019;75:200–208.
114. Yang F, Li J, Pang G, et al. Effects of diethyl phosphate, a non-specific metabolite of organophosphorus pesticides on serum lipid, hormones, inflammation and gut microbiota. *Molecules.* 2019;24(10).
115. Li JW, Fang B, Pang GF, et al. Age- and diet-specific effects of chronic exposure to chlorpyrifos on hormones, inflammation and gut microbiota in rats. *Pestic Biochem Physiol.* 2019;159:68–79.
116. Gao B, Chi L, Tu P, et al. The carbamate aldicarb altered the gut microbiome, metabolome and lipidome of C57BL/6J mice. *Chem Res Toxicol.* 2019;32(1):67–79.
117. Meng Z, Liu L, Jia M, et al. Impacts of penconazole and its enantiomers exposure on gut microbiota and metabolic profiles in mice. *J Agric Food Chem.* 2019;67(30):8303–8311.
118. Tsiaoussis J, Antoniou MN, Koliarakis I, et al. Effects of single and combined toxic exposures on the gut microbiome: current knowledge and future directions. *Toxicol Lett.* 2019;312: 72–97.
119. Groh KJ, Geueke B, Muncke J. Food contact materials and gut health: implications for toxicity assessment and relevance of high molecular weight migrants. *Food Chem Toxicol.* 2017; 109:1–18.
120. Utembe W, Kamng'ona AW. Gut microbiota-mediated pesticide toxicity in humans: methodological issues and challenges in the risk assessment of pesticides. *Chemosphere.* 2021; 271:129817.

Chapter 4

Mycotoxins: still with us after all these years

J. David Miller
Department of Chemistry, Carleton University, Ottawa, ON, Canada

Abstract
This chapter discusses the mycotoxins of greatest importance to human and animal health including aflatoxin, fumonisin, deoxynivalenol, zearalenone and ochratoxin. For each toxin, the fungi concerned, their management through the value chain as well as the basis for their regulation are discussed. Despite the passage of more than 60 years since the isolation and characterization of the first of these toxins, aflatoxin, the challenges have in some ways become greater because of genetic change in the fungi, unanticipated effects of crop breeding and most of all climate change.

Keywords: Mycotoxins; food; feed; toxicology; toxigenic fungi; health

4.1 Introduction

The term "mycotoxicosis" was first used just over six decades ago by researchers in the former USSR. During World War II, scientists there were trying to understand the deaths of large numbers of horses from exposure to contaminated straw due to *Stachybotrys chartarum* toxins, and, the deaths of large numbers of Russians from eating overwintered grain contaminated by T-2 toxin, Alimentary Toxic Aleukia.[1,2] Mycotoxins are secondary metabolites of Ascomycetes known to make humans and animals sick. By convention, the definition excludes mushroom toxins.[3] Largely ignored until aflatoxin was discovered in 1962, most of the focus was on animal diseases including stachybotryotoxicosis and the consumption of grain infected by a variety of fungi in storage including "moldy corn toxicosis" from *Aspergillus flavus*, Alimetary Toxic Aleukia, and facial eczema in sheep from *Pithomyces chartarum* metabolites.[4] By the late 1960s a long list of fungi had been associated with metabolites or extracts that were associated with animal diseases.[5–7] Other than ergotism and the consumption of abused grain, the idea that fungal metabolites could have a material effect on human health was not firmly recognized until the mid-1970s into the 1990s.[1]

As implied, laboratory cultures of the fungi that grow on grains or nuts almost invariably result in extracts that are toxic in some in vitro assay. This has resulted in the relatively recent trend to label virtually any fungal metabolite, a "mycotoxin." For many years there were four important mycotoxins, aflatoxin, deoxynivalenol, zearalenone, and ochratoxin A.[8] With the discovery of fumonisin, there are five agriculturally important fungal toxins in commercial agriculture worldwide: deoxynivalenol (replaced in some areas by nivalenol), zearalenone, ochratoxin A (OTA), fumonisin, and aflatoxin.[9,10] This is based on extensive analytical results (e.g., Refs. 11–13) and detailed information on the distribution of fungi on staple crops.[14,15]

Mycotoxin-producing fungi in crops have been historically divided into two groups: field and storage fungi.[16] Field fungi include those which invade and produce their toxins before harvest. The second group which become a problem after harvest are known as storage fungi. Invasion by fungi before harvest is governed primarily by plant-fungus and other factors such as insect and bird damage as well as too much or too little water. Growth by fungi postharvest is governed by crop (nutrients), physical factors (temperature, moisture), and storage insects. Four types of toxigenic fungi can be identified in grains and oilseeds: (1) plant pathogens such as *Fusarium graminearum* and related species; (2) fungi that produce their mycotoxins on senescent or stressed plants, such as *Fusarium sporotrichioides*, *F. verticillioides*, *A. flavus*, and *A. parasiticus*; (3) fungi that colonize the plant in the field and predispose the crop to mycotoxin contamination in storage, such as *A. flavus*; and (4) fungi that are found in the soil or decaying plant material that occurs on the

Present Knowledge in Food Safety. DOI: https://doi.org/10.1016/B978-0-12-819470-6.00009-3

developing kernels in the field and later proliferate in storage if conditions permit, for example, *Penicillium verrucosum*.[9,15]

In considering the topic of mycotoxins in crops and foods, there are two worlds: the fully developed market economies and the developing world. The investments required to keep exposures to the important fungal toxins within the tolerable daily intakes involve significant expense. In the United States and Canada, sampling costs are on the order of $US 7/ha. Although >20,000 official tests are done, private sector labs conduct testing on 20–50 times more samples.[17] Large bioethanol plants are another major user of mycotoxin testing because the toxins are concentrated 3–5 times in the Distiller's Dried Grain with Solubles (DDGS; Ref. [18] and references cited therein). Sampling and analyses represent a cost to the North American agri-food sector of >$200 million in a good year and much more in bad years.[17]

The economic consequences to a region suffering periodic high mycotoxin years are enormous. Chronic problems with mycotoxins will cause farmers to shift away from the affected crop and plant other commodities. If a region is seen to be an unreliable source of a food crop meeting quality standards, the value chain will move to regions that can.[19] Contamination of wheat by deoxynivalenol in the small grain areas of the upper Midwest United States has resulted in a cumulative impact of upwards of $3 billion.[20,21] In these regions, farmers moved away from susceptible small grains to maize, soy, and canola.[21] Similar losses were experienced in the wheat-growing areas of Ontario and Manitoba.[22] The last serious aflatoxin contamination in the US corn crop resulted in economic losses in excess of $1 billion.[23] Contamination of DDGS can also result in important economic losses in bad years,[24] since the DDGS needs to be blended before incorporating into animal feed or destroyed. The economic impact of mycotoxins is felt across a wide spectrum of commodities other than cereals from dried fruits,[25,26] wine and grape juice,[27] coffee,[28,29] to spices.[30,31]

In Africa as well as parts of Latin America and East Asia, more than 500 million people are exposed to aflatoxin and fumonisin at multiples, sometimes orders of magnitude of safe levels. This results in enormous losses in human life and animal productivity.[32–36] In addition, where there are export opportunities to nearby Europe, these are essentially precluded because of mycotoxin contamination and production capacity in the present-day value chain. Although this is often cast in terms of economic losses in the billions, the value chain would need improvements in both capacity and quality before it might be realized.[37–39] The private sector in the middle economies in these regions has an incentive to improve the value chain for the commodities they purchase.[40,41] Uplifting the whole food system will improve the domestic supply and is necessary to prevent the highly contaminated materials from being consumed by the poorest—which it mostly is now.[42] As capacity is improved, where global demand exceeds supply, export markets could be developed.

4.2 Compounds of minor public health significance

There are a number of mycotoxins that are known to affect human and/or animal health and that are of lesser public health significance. The most important of these less common toxins is T-2/HT-2 toxins which can be a problem areas particularly when it rains during harvest during cool wet years[43,44] notably in northern Europe.[45] These toxins are mainly produced by *F. sporotrichioides* but are also produced by *Fusarium langsethiae* in northern Europe in small grains including oats.[45,46] In contrast, T-2/HT-2 toxins are uncommon in export grains and feed in Canada[47,48] and essentially never occur in food in the United States or Canada (e.g., Refs. 49,50). There is more exposure to T-2/HT-2 toxins in Europe but generally below the European Food Safety Agency (EFSA) Tolerable Daily Intake.[51,52] Unless the grain is left in the field wet in the fall and then harvested, colonization by the fungus tends to be of the lemmae. Thus after milling, T-2/HT-2 are found in the chaff and dusts rather than the flour (e.g., Refs. 53,54). In oats, about half of the T-2/HT-2 was found in small kernels.[55]

Known for centuries, ergot alkaloids seldom now appear in meaningful concentrations in food in North America or Europe because ergot sclerotia are efficiently removed during milling. There are some data suggesting that ergot is getting more common again in parts of Europe[56] and western North America.[57] Regardless, grading standards for the presence of ergot bodies in grains have existed in the United States and Canada for more than a century. Today these vary somewhat by jurisdiction.[58] Removal of the sclerotia before milling means the majority of food products made from wheat or rye may contain traces of ergot alkaloids but without material public health impact.[59–62]

Over the past 50 years, there has been an astonishing convergence of dietary patterns worldwide. Consumption of cassava, sorghum, millet, and sweet potatoes (crops important in Africa) has declined, having been replaced with cereals and oilseeds. Soy and oilseeds along with wheat, rice, and maize increased in both relative and absolute terms in national food supplies.[63–65] The change has been particularly dramatic in Africa where maize and groundnuts, both New World crops and highly susceptible to mycotoxins, are widely consumed. In 1950 by far the major source of dietary starch in sub-Saharan Africa was sorghum and millet (40%), followed by cassava (30%) and then maize (15%).[66] Commercial production of peanuts for export began in the early 19th century. Among the early difficulties was convincing local populations to grow groundnuts instead of millet.[67] The shift to maize and groundnuts has had a major role in increasing aflatoxin and fumonisin exposures in Africa.[35] The indigenous crops, sorghum and millet are less prone to aflatoxin contamination.[35,68] Along with these toxins, maize can also be a material source of zearalenone and deoxynivalenol.[69]

Thus from a public health perspective, exposure to all the five important toxins is by far from cereals and, for aflatoxin, also some oilseeds (see, e.g., Ref. 70). Thus the remainder of this chapter will focus on issues around the five mycotoxins in cereals and some oilseeds. This is where the largest public health impact costs to society, and serious ongoing threats lie.

4.3 Toxins from *Fusarium graminearum* and related species

F. graminearum, *Fusarium culmorum*, or *Fusarium asiaticum* can cause Fusarium Head Blight or Gibberella ear rot when there is rain at anthesis or silk emergence, respectively, under warm, but not hot, conditions.[71–73] *F. culmorum* is associated with cooler growing conditions.[43] In 1983 the two dominant chemotypes of *F. graminearum* were reported.[74] Strains from the Americas produced deoxynivalenol via the 15-acetyl deoxynivalenol precursor (15ADON) and those from Japan, China, and Europe mainly via 3-acetyl deoxynivalenol (3ADON) precursor.[75] This recognition prompted genetic studies by United States Department of Agriculture scientists who determined that *F. graminearum* comprises a number of clades. *F. gramineaurm sensu stricto* and *F. asiaticum* are the most common.[76]

For decades, the populations of *F. graminearum* and related species were genetically stable on a continental basis. Isolates of *F. graminearum* from wheat or corn in the Americas were of the 15ADON chemotype and those from elsewhere were generally of the 3ADON chemotype.[75,77] Thirty years ago, *F. culmorum* was the dominant species in cooler wheat-growing areas in western Europe. As the climate has warmed, this taxon has been replaced by *F. graminearum*,[78,79] most of which are of the 15ADON genotype.[80] *F. culmorum* strains in Europe remain 3DON producers.[75,80,81]

Unfortunately, this long pattern of general species and genetic stability has been disrupted. In the United States and Canada, two "new" chemotypes have appeared .[82] *F. graminearum* strains from the new world have been collected, which produce deoxynivalenol, the "new" trichothecene 3NX, and/or both deoxynivalenol and 3NX.[77,83–85] Identifying these changes have been hampered by an overdependence on using genetic markers to assess chemotype. Desjardins[86] warned against conflating the terms "genotype" and chemotype, that is, the chemicals that may occur in the crop. At least in some populations of *F. graminearum*, the commonly used PCR probes can misclassify chemotype[77,85] (see also Ref. 87). Similar broad genetic changes are evident in China, South America, and Europe[10,80,88,89] but the impact on chemotype is poorly understood.[77] *Fusarium* species have a demonstrated, considerable variation in toxin profiles resulting from recombination. The OECD Report "Challenges for agricultural research" noted the need for monitoring of populations of toxigenic fungi to follow these changes.[90]

4.3.1 Toxins

Deoxynivalenol was discovered from cultures of *F. graminearum* strains isolated from grain that made people sick in Japan. Exposures sufficient to make people sick were not uncommon in China and India, as well as other countries in Asia and the Soviet Union in the past.[1,91] The primary symptoms were nausea and vomiting. Swine is the most sensitive domestic animal, and humans have comparable or somewhat greater sensitivity to deoxynivalenol.[91] As noted above contamination of small grains and maize by deoxynivalenol is a chronic problem except in dryland wheat production. Prior to 30 years ago, exposure to DON in parts of Europe was much greater than the current TDI (e.g., Refs. 92–94). This is because most wheat in the United States and Canada is produced in areas not prone to Fusarium Head Blight; thus comparably exposures were much lower.[95] The introduction of regulations in Europe have greatly reduced exposure.[96] Nonetheless, there are other parts of the world where this still remains an issue. Exposures in China three decades ago were much higher than that in Europe and North America, resulting in prevalence of acute toxicoses.[97] Despite enormous strides in the management of Fusarium Head Blight grains in China,[89] a material fraction of the population is exposed to deoxynivalenol above the Provisional Maximum Tolerable Daily Intake (PMTDI).[98]

Because this is a high human exposure toxin, and because it cannot be eliminated, there is a comprehensive understanding of its toxicology.[10,99] The Joint Expert Committee on Food Additives and Contaminants of the FAO and WHO (JECFA) PMTDI is based on weight reduction in a two-year study in male and female B6C3F1 mice.[100]

Aside from being toxic to humans and animals, deoxynivalenol is a virulence factor in the disease process in small grains and maize.[101] Thirty years ago, the ability of Fusarium Head Blight–tolerant wheat to conjugate with a sugar was recognized.[102] This helps to protect the plant from invasion by this necrotrophic pathogen since deoxynivalenol-3-glucoside does not affect plant cell membranes or protein synthesis.[103–105] The gene that codes for the enzyme responsible of adding the sugar is linked to a QTL associated with *F. graminearum* tolerance in wheat.[106]

At the time of the original report,[102] the concentration of deoxynivalenol glucoside in Canadian grains in eastern Canada was modest. By the early 2000 researchers in Austria demonstrated that genotypes of wheat grown in that part of the world when infected by *F. graminearum* could have very high concentrations of deoxynivalenol glucoside.[107] Wheat cultivars from Europe tend to have high relative amounts of deoxynivalenol-3-glucoside, approaching 100% of that of the deoxynivalenol in the grain.[108] The limited data on wheat in the United States suggest the relative values are somewhat lower.[109] It appears that genotypes of barley in Canada and the United States tend to have lower to comparable relative amounts of deoxynivalenol glucoside[110,111] to those in Europe.

Deoxynivalenol glucoside is much less toxic than the native toxin in the mink emesis model and has modest bioavailability in rats.[112,113] However, the sugar is cleaved off by the gut microbiome in both humans and pigs.[114–116] A practical outcome of this is that a high percentage of children in Europe are over the TDI (e.g., Refs. 117,118). For this reason, (EFSA) added deoxynivalenol-3-glucoside to the TDI that applies in Europe.[96]

Although DON, 3ADON, 15ADON, NX, and deoxynivalenol-3-glucoside can be measured by LC-MS/MS, the situation with commonly used ELISA kits is problematic. The available kits do not respond to NX and response is idiosyncratically variable for the compounds other than DON.[119–121] There is an additional problem namely, where the *F. graminearum* genotype 15ADON dominates (much of the United States and Canada, and parts of Europe), the major glycoside can be 15ADON3 glucoside, which is not being measured.[17,122]

The trichothecene nivalenol can occur in grains affected by a relatively uncommon *F. graminearum* chemotype albeit more common in Asia.[10] The toxicity of nivalenol is comparable to deoxynivalenol.[99,123,124] EFSA and the Food Safety Commission of Japan set TDIs for nivalenol.[125,126] The 'new' trichothecene toxins 3NX and NX have been demonstrated in corn in Ontario 1–7% of the DON concentration.[85] As with other trichothecenes, 3NX and NX inhibit peptidyl transferase in vitro and NX demonstrated comparable immunomodulatory and pro-inflammatory potential to DON in immortalized cell lines.[127,128] However, studies involving a relevant animal tissue, porcine jejunal explants, 10 μm to NX resulted in cell vacuolization, a damaged epithelial barrier and high loss of villi. A comparison of whole transcriptome profiling after exposure to NX, DON and 3ANX indicated that the three toxins affected cell proliferation, differentiation, apoptosis and growth, and particularly immune and pro-inflammatory responses. However, NX was more potent than DON or its acetylated precursor 3NX.[129] In the murine anorexia model described by Wu et al.,[113] NX was 2x more potent than DON IP and 25 x more potent by the oral route (Wu, personal communication).

The other important toxin of *F. graminearum* and related species, zearalenone is a potent estrogen analog. This toxin was isolated from maize that had caused uterotrophic activity in pigs.[1] Zearalenone efficiently binds to both mammalian estrogen receptors.[10] There is some evidence that zearalenone exposure affects reproductive health in young women from studies in China, Italy, and the United States.[130–132] The PMTDI is based on study in swine.[133] Estimated exposures to zearalenone in Europe based on dietary surveys were below the PMTDI.[133,134] As with deoxynivalenol, zearalenone can be conjugated by plants[108] but there is no evidence that these result in material increases in exposure to the parent compound.

4.3.2 Management

Assessing the quality of grain coming into the country elevators can be quickly done by taking samples of the load and counting Fusarium Damaged Kernels. This is rapid, inexpensive, and quite effective but the relationship changes from year to year as wheat cultivars are replaced.[135,136] At the country elevator level, taking representative samples is a challenge. A simple procedure to collect a representative sample is to collect dust in the air as the load is being dumped into the elevator.[137–139] As with all mycotoxins, consideration must be given to the size and number of samples to obtain a reliable analytical result.[48] Another strategy that has been proposed is to measure deoxynivalenol in wheat dockage, which was significantly correlated to that in the whole grain.[140]

A great deal is known about the impact of milling and baking on deoxynivalenol in flour and baked products. Depending on grain processing method, there are significant reductions in deoxynivalenol concentration from the cleaned grain.[46,141–144] However, deoxynivalenol concentrations are higher, sometimes materially higher in the bran compared to the flour.[46,141]

The impact of milling on deoxynivalenol in maize is broadly similar in both wet and dry milling processes.[145,146] Because zearalenone is a less common as the dominant mycotoxin in crops because of climate change,[147] there are few modern studies on the impact of milling on this toxin. However, as with deoxynivalenol, this toxin is similarly reduced during wet and dry milling of maize[148] and wheat.[145,149,150]

An enormous effort has been made to develop management practices to limit the possibility of contaminated small grains entering the food value chain. Although some progress has been made in breeding tolerant cultivars, so far these have not been widely adopted because of yield penalties in the context that Fusarium Head Blight is periodic. The grower gets no benefits from a lower yielding yet tolerant cultivar in most years. However, practical benefits have been obtained by continuously excluding the most susceptible cultivars from recommended varieties each year (e.g., Refs. 151,152). Aside from this, management of Fusarium Head Blight is achieved in the field by monitoring for conditions that are known to favor disease and toxin accumulation and allowing the judicious use of fungicides.[71,152–154] In areas of chronic contamination in the United States and Canada, a six-step process has evolved since the early 1980s (Ref. 153 and references therein), which is effective. This includes (1) selecting tolerant varieties to Fusarium Head Blight each year, (2) using toxin prediction systems allowing appropriate use of fungicides in the event of an elevated risk, (3) assessing the quality of grains coming to country elevators by one of several means to allow diversion of the contaminated grains to feed or other uses, (4) cleaning prior to milling, (5) processor specifications, and (6) surveillance by governments.

Although moisture and temperature at silk emergence are important variables for the occurrence *F. graminearum* disease in maize (Gibberella ear rot), prediction models have proven to be more difficult to develop.[71,155] One reason for this is that major epidemics of ear rot can occur late in the season if rain precludes harvest.[73]

4.4 Toxins from *Fusarium verticillioides* and related species

Maize affected by Fusarium kernel rot has long been associated with a variety of disparate disease outcomes in domestic animals, notably equine species.[1] The primary toxin responsible for these disparate toxicosis, fumonisin B1 was discovered because of concerns of elevated rates of esophageal cancer associated with the consumption of maize affected by Fusarium kernel rot in the former Transkei in South Africa.[156] There are limited epidemiology data from the southern United States and northern Italy from the past, suggesting that consumption of corn containing fumonisin is associated with neural tube birth defects.[157–159]

Fumonisins are among the most prevalent mycotoxins in maize including in the United States and southern Europe.[11,13,160–162] In much of Africa as well as parts of central and South America, fumonisin exposures are substantial.[34,35] These are produced by *F. verticillioides*, *Fusarium proliferatum*, *Fusarium fujikuroi*, and a number of uncommon species.[163,164] Fumonisin can contaminate rice from infection by *F. proferatum* and *F. fujikuroi*.[165] In some parts of the world, fumonisin B2 can occur in wheat infected by *F. proliferatum*.[166]

As noted, most fumonisin exposure results from the consumption maize affected by the disease Fusarium kernel rot caused mainly by *F. verticillioides*. This species or *F. proliferatum* can be isolated from virtually all maize kernels including those that are healthy.[91,167] Fumonisin accumulates in stressed or senescing kernel tissue under warm and dry conditions after silking.[167] Insect damage increases fumonisin concentrations.[168,169] Maize genotypes containing the Bt protein have reduced amounts of fumonisin compared to non-Bt genotypes.[168,170] The use of Bt maize is a proven intervention to reduce fumonisin contamination in affected areas.[35]

4.4.1 Toxins

There are a four naturally occurring fumonisins in maize. Usually fumonsin B1 is by far dominant, followed by FB2, FB3, and FB4.[15,34] In corn-producing areas in South America, FB2 produced by *F. proliferatum* can be the dominant fumonisin.[10,171] Albeit not contributing much to human exposure, FB2 and B4 from *Aspergillus niger* can occur in raisins and other dried fruits, and can be found in wine.[10]

FB1 is toxic to the liver in all species and the kidney in a range of laboratory and farm animal species. FB1 and other fumonisins inhibit ceramide synthase in all species including humans. This is the underlying the mechanism of toxicity and pathogenesis of fumonisin-related diseases.[34,159,172,173] The JECFA TDI is based a study of liver toxicity in male transgenic mice and renal toxicity in a 90-day rat study.[34,174]

In high human exposure areas, fumonisin is associated with child stunting and based on animal data, plausibly could increase the risk of birth defects.[34]

4.4.2 Management

As noted above, the use of Bt maize is the only useful intervention to reduce fumonisin concentrations, although it is important to ensure that the hybrids that are planted are within their area of adaptation.[167] The complexity of sampling to obtain a reliable analytical result for shelled corn for fumonisin is similar to other *Fusarium* toxins.[175] As with the other *Fusarium* mycotoxins, after milling, fumonisins are concentrated in bran and fines.[176–179]

4.5 Toxins from *Aspergillus flavus*, *Aspergillus parasiticus*, and related species

Famously, the discovery of aflatoxin was motivated by the deaths of large numbers of turkeys in the United Kingdom in 1960. However, the first human fatality from consumption of highly contaminated food was documented in Africa by 1967[180] followed by many other case reports in India and parts of Asia.[1,34] Aflatoxin is produced by many species of *Aspergillus*, but *A. flavus* dominates on maize and almonds worldwide and *A. parasiticus* is most common on groundnuts.[181] In the case of Brazil nuts in South America, a number of apparently uncommon species are responsible for aflatoxin contamination.[181] *A. flavus* contamination of groundnuts was first recognized to cause alfatoxicosis in domestic animals[1] and is the most important species affecting crops. Most toxigenic strains of *A. flavus* produce aflatoxin B1 and B2 on maize and *A. parasiticus* produces aflatoxin B1, B2, G1, and G2. *A. flavus* is a cosmopolitan species, whereas *A. parasiticus* is associated with peanuts in the Americas.[182] Three decades ago, *A. parasiticus* (and aflatoxin G1 and G2) were uncommon outside the Americas.[183] Groundnuts are new world plants and the movement of genotypes around the world has resulted in *A. parasiticus* being detected more often in groundnuts in parts of Africa and in Asia (e.g., Refs. 184–186).

Although *A. flavus* and *A. parasiticus* are among the most studied fungi, their sexual stages were discovered only a decade ago.[187–189] Studies of the ability to produced aflatoxin in *A. flavus* and *A. parasiticus* demonstrated that in cooler wet areas, atoxigenic strains predominate, and toxigenic strains predominate in warm dry areas. Both qualitative and quantitative variation in aflatoxin chemotypes (B1, B2, G1, G2), *o*-methyl sterigmatocystin, and cyclopiazonic acid are seen in sexual strains.[190,191] That is, sexuality generates novel toxin chemotypes.[192] In the United States, there are three genetic populations, one of which produces more aflatoxin and is prone to genetic recombination.[193,194]

To the extent climate change has increased the area under maize and groundnut cultivation favorable for aflatoxin production, there is an increased risk of evolving chemotypes and aflatoxin producing potential in *A. flavus*.[195] As with the Fusarium head blight species above, there is a need for continuous monitoring of the population genetics of *A. flavus*.[90]

4.5.1 Management

There is an immense literature on the management of aflatoxin in all manner of affected commodities. However, most human exposure is from maize and groundnuts and similarly, the largest global economic impact by far is associated with these crops.[196] *A. flavus* infection of corn or peanuts results from airborne or insect-transmitted spores grow into the ear in drought and temperature stressed plants. Insect kernels are damaged by the fungus and accumulate aflatoxin. Similarly with groundnuts, drought, nutrient, or temperature stressed plants are more susceptible to damage by *A. flavus* or *A. parasiticus*.[10,15] Studies of the impact of Bt on aflatoxin accumulation in maize have been mixed. However, if the correct Bt transgene combination for the insect population in the region is present in the maize under conditions favorable to aflatoxin accumulation, reductions may be seen.[197] In support of this, a recent analysis of data from the serious aflatoxin contamination problem in the 2012 maize crop demonstrated that Bt reduced insurance claims for aflatoxin contamination.[198]

In the United States, there are two registered atoxigenic *A. flavus* products that can be used to reduce aflatoxin on maize when conditions warrant.[199] US State Extension scientists recommend that farmers use atoxigenic strains to control aflatoxin in maize if the farm is in an area where aflatoxin is an annual threat. Unless the conditions are favorable for aflatoxin accumulation in maize, no economic advantage will accrue.[200] In addition, there are recent data that suggest the need for the use of atoxigenic *A. flavus* strains that match the genetic structure of the endemic population.[201] Expansion of the use of biocontrol requires increased attention to the ability for the introduced strains to undergo genetic change.[35] Concerns include the potential for introduced strains to produce other mycotoxins, notably cyclopiazonic acid, as well as reproductive and genetic stability.[35,202,203]

Studies in the United States have shown that usually insect damage and *A. flavus*-infested kernels are randomly distributed in ears.[204] These generally few kernels on a cob have very high aflatoxin contents compared to the very low regulatory values. This is an important reason why the sampling of maize for aflatoxin to obtain preliminary results in the field[205] and in a lot of shelled maize[206,207] is a challenge.

In temperate climates, highly evolved procedures for preventing aflatoxin development in storage emerged decades ago.[204,208] In subtropical environments, the infection process involves systemic infection from the field making preventing aflatoxin in storage more challenging than in temperate climates.[10,15]

Managing contamination by aflatoxin in commercial groundnut production requires a number of preharvest strategies including managing drought stress, soil nutrition, and crop rotation, among other agronomic factors. The economic benefit of the use of atoxigenic strains for biological control in groundnuts in the United States remains unclear.[209] Management at harvest involves removal of damaged kernels from shelled lots by screening, kernel sizing, and color sorting and providing appropriate storage conditions. This is very effective.[209,210]

In the fully developed market economies, commercial milling operations and ethanol plants require maize entering the value chain meets FDA or European Union (EU) regulations; thus there are few modern studies of milling. As with the other mycotoxins discussed, the majority of the toxins end up in bran and germ and the feed grade materials.[150,211,212]

4.5.2 Toxins

There are many detailed reviews of the toxicology of aflatoxins but the most thorough treatment is the monograph of the 83rd JECFA.[36,174] At the time of drafting the monograph on aflatoxins, there were 11,000 scientific publications in PubMed on aflatoxin, almost twice the number available at the time of drafting 49th JECFA monograph 20 years ago. In 2017 the database of the American Chemistry Society recorded 28,000 publications on aflatoxin. Considering every journal possible, the total number may have approached 160,000. Arguably, aflatoxins are among the most studied biochemicals on the planet.

Aflatoxin B1, the most toxic of the aflatoxins, causes a variety of adverse effects in domestic and laboratory animals. Naturally occurring mixtures of aflatoxins were classified as group 1 human carcinogens and aflatoxin B1 is also a group 1 human carcinogen. There is inadequate evidence for the human carcinogenicity of aflatoxin M1, the metabolite of aflatoxin B1 found in human and animal milk.[15,36] Aflatoxin exposure causes ~25% of liver cancer worldwide but particularly in Africa (40%) and Asia (27%).[213] Although aflatoxin is a potent chemical carcinogen, exposure in people seropositive to hepatitis B are at greater risk. This alters the response to the hepatocarcinogenic viruses. The rates of liver cancer in hepatitis B positive populations are an order of magnitude greater when exposed to aflatoxin. In high human exposure areas, aflatoxin is associated with child stunting and fatalities. The JECFA evaluation of aflatoxins is based on human data, although a somewhat similar estimate would be derived using the best available rodent data.[36]

Aflatoxin exposure also results in fatalities mainly in children and there is sufficient evidence that aflatoxin exposure results in child stunting in high exposure areas.[35,36]

Where there is high human exposure to both aflatoxin and fumonisin, there is an additional concern. FB1 is a potent mutagen and DNA-reactive carcinogen while FB1 is an effective cancer promoter with a nongenotoxic mechanism of action. Coexposures in relevant animal models are additive or synergistic; thus coexposure is likely to enhance hepatoxicity and hepatocarcinogenicity in humans.[174,214]

4.6 Ochratoxin-producing *Penicillium* and *Aspergillus* species

Ochratoxin was discovered in a laboratory strain of *Aspergillus ochraceus* in 1965. The toxin was not reported as a natural contaminant until 1969 in the United States, the following year in Canada and in 1973 in Denmark. It was a major cause of porcine nephrosis in Denmark and other northern European countries.[215–217] After 50 years of study, there is little evidence for ochratoxin as causing human disease.[218, 219] The sole example of a document human health consequence is a case report after putative very high occupational exposures to contaminated material. Di Paolo et al.[220] reported a case of acute renal failure in a farmer who spent 8 h in a disused granary. This was believed to be due to inhalation of ochratoxin which was isolated from the wheat debris in the grain store. The researchers were able to demonstrate acute kidney failure in laboratory animals exposed to moldy wheat in their cages.

Many species of fungi produce ochratoxin A.[10] However, in cereals, *P. verrucosum* is the sole producer of this storage toxin.[9] Another dietary source of ochratoxin is coffee where the main producers are species closely related to *A. niger* and species related to *Aspergillus ochraceus*, depending on the environment. The production occurs from failures to dry the beans quickly after harvest.[181,221,222] Most strains of *A. niger* can also produce fumonisin B2. Both of these toxins are present in commercial coffee sold in Europe and Canada at low levels.[28,223,224] However, in economically poorer countries, ochratoxin concentrations in coffee are often higher.[29,225]

From the early detection, ochratoxin was uncommon in cereals in the United States and Canada (e.g., Refs. 226,227). However, in Europe and the United Kingdom, a high percentage of cereal samples were contaminated, often at quite high concentrations even at the retail level.[158,228] This reflects important differences between the weather conditions in cereal production areas in the United States and Canada, and Europe, with respect to ochratoxin accumulation. In Western United States and Canada, it is usually dry at harvest and it is rather cold in the winter (e.g., Refs. 229,230).

Infestation of some kernels by the ochratoxin-producing fungus *P. verrucosum* occurs from anthesis. Normally, a few percent of surface-disinfected wheat and barley kernels collected at harvest in the United Kingdom, Denmark, and Sweden were contaminated by *Penicillium aurantiogriseum* and *P. verrucosum*.

However, the absolute level of preharvest infestation can be quite high and varies according to agronomic factors of the farm and from year to year.[9,231–233] In the United States and Canada, generally, *Penicillium*-contaminated kernels are typically less than 1% (e.g., Refs. 43,234,235). Regardless, at harvest, the combine further spreads the spores.[236]

4.6.1 Management

Because the growing and storage conditions in the northern hemisphere are so different between much of Europe and the cold drier wheat-growing areas in the United States and Canada, best management practices and risk factors are necessarily different. Greatest protection against the accumulation of ochratoxin in storage comes from harvesting the crop when it is ready to dry and ensuring that the farm has sufficient capacity to rapidly dry the day's harvest before putting it into storage. Grain stores need to be designed to suit the climate. Residual pockets of grain and debris are highly contaminated by storage fungi, and the bins and augers should be cleaned before filling.[237–241] In north temperate Europe, continued attention to cooling and drying is recommended to prevent ochratoxin contamination.[237,240] In practice, these conditions are hard to maintain through the northern European value chain and monitoring for ochratoxin is needed.[242]

In the cold cereal-growing areas of the United States and Canada, continued aeration needs to be carefully done to avoid mixing warm and cold air during rapid temperature changes. In addition, condensation from downspouts and improperly vented bins can also create pockets of mold and toxin formation.[216,238] Monitoring of cereals-based foods in the United States and Canada indicate ochratoxin contamination is generally uncommon.[50] In contrast to the EU,[243] neither country has a specific regulation on this toxin.[218,244]

The complete colonization of a nutrient source with massive sporulation is called the "*Penicillium* growth pattern."[245] In the case of *P. verrucosum* on wheat, ochratoxin A concentrations in single contaminated wheat kernels can reach 5 mg/kg.[246] This means that 10 kernels in 10,000 can push the lot over the limit in the European Economic Community, if it ends up in the subsample. Based on a large dataset collected in Canada, a sampling curve for small grains was not developed until a few years ago.[247] As noted by Walker,[248] prevention of contamination at source is the most effective public health measure, not sampling.

The impact of milling on ochratoxin is less well studied than the other toxins discussed. Milling reduces ochratoxin into the flour and with some other mycotoxins, the majority of toxin in the raw grain is in the screenings into the bran and fractions that might be used for feed or disposed.[249–251] When the raw grain has lower versus higher concentrations of OTA, scouring is beneficial.[251]

4.6.2 Toxins

The last International Agency for Research on Cancer (IARC) evaluation of ochratoxin determined it to be a possible human carcinogen.[158] In 1995 the JECFA established tolerable weekly intake of 100 ng/kg bw per week.[252] In reaching this conclusion, "the Committee noted the large safety factor applied to the NOEL for nephrotoxicity in deriving the tolerable weekly intake, which corresponds to a factor of 1500 applied to the NOEL for carcinogenicity in male rats, the most sensitive species and sex for this end-point." The difference in approaches to the risk assessments between JECFA and EFSA arises from differing opinions whether the rodent carcinogenicity occurs through a thresholded mechanism or not.[248] Prevention of contamination at source is considered to be the most effective public health measure.

4.7 Key issues for the next decade

Nearly six decades after the discovery of aflatoxin, the issue of mycotoxins seems an old story. Perspectives on the problem vary depending on your position in the value chain, whether in academia or when on panels setting international standards for trade and for global public health.

Exposure assessment: In the fully developed market economies, the needs of public health are largely being met. However, as noted, there is a concern about children being exposed above the PMTDI to deoxynivalenol particularly in some parts of Europe because of the high prevalence of deoxynivalenol-3-glucoside in cereals affected by Fusarium Head Blight (e.g., Refs. 118,253). This is further complicated by the fact that the majority of *F. graminearum* strains in western Europe are of the 15 ADON genotype.[80] This may result in a portion of the exposure results from 15ADON3 glucoside.[17,122] At least in some areas, these data strongly indicate that the traditional way of estimating exposure to deoxynivalenol, that is commodity surveys and probabilistic modeling,[254] is not adequate, especially for children. Regardless of the glucosides, Chen et al.[255] suggest that in some areas the existing regulations for deoxynivalenol may not be sufficiently protective. Addressing these concerns will require more reliable biomonitoring capacity and focus.

UNEP[256] noted the high prevalence of mycotoxins in staple crops in developing countries. In such countries the need for cost-effective biomonitoring to assess exposure is acute. Although some have argued for the creation of central laboratories (e.g., Ref. 257), this is probably not feasible or even immediately useful compared to other investments.[35] As described above, limiting mycotoxin exposure is not done by surveillance but the action of very large numbers of people through the value chain. The challenge is to make it cheaper to assess exposure to the aflatoxin DNA adduct in serum and urinary fumonisin, deoxynivalenol, deoxynivalenol glucuronides, and zearalenone and zearalenols using labeled standards. Current analyses of these compounds can only be reliably done in a few laboratories and involve expensive technology and highly qualified staff (e.g., Ref. 69).

Climate and crop convergence: A major factor affecting population exposure to mycotoxins relates to the fact that essentially all countries have converged on a small number of cereal and oil seed crops.[64,65] Even in the United States, crop diversity peaked six decades ago and now is at levels seen in the mid-19th century.[258] As noted, in Africa, there was a profound shift from a more diverse food system prior to the 1960s to one where maize and nuts supply most calories.[1,35] All the cereals and most oil crops are susceptible or highly susceptible to mycotoxin accumulation under permissive conditions. Some climate changes trigger accumulation of toxins in crops: depending on crop, too much or too little water, or, changing the timing of seasonal rainfall events increases the risk of mycotoxin accumulation.[147,256,259] In addition, changing climate has moved the five important mycotoxins into new areas lacking the capacity to manage them during epidemic years. From a governance perspective the critical necessity is the capacity to do the necessary chemical analyses and manage the issue with the least economic damage.[147, 260]

A recent example of a lack of capacity and foresight was the appearance of maize produced within the European Economic Community that was highly contaminated by aflatoxin. This resulted in the loss of milk from cows fed the maize in a number of countries before the problem was detected.[261] It had been assumed that aflatoxin could not be a problem in Europe but was an issue for imported food only.[262] This event fostered a realization that climate had increased the risk for aflatoxin and steps needed to be taken to develop better sampling and management capacity.[261–263] A second example was a serious Fusarium Head Blight epidemic in durum wheat in dryland areas of Western Canada and Northwestern United States in 2016. These areas have been largely free of serious problems with Fusarium Head Blight since the introduction of small grains to the region but this is changing. Canadian farmers lost $1 billion farm gate value because of the epidemic in this area in 2016.[48,264] In contrast to areas that have had chronic problems for decades with Fusarium Head Blight (e.g., Ontario), the capacity to predict and mitigate the damage had not been developed.

Focus: The five important mycotoxins discussed here have been known as natural contaminants for between 30–55 years. For all these compounds there is unambiguous evidence of an impact on domestic animal health. For four of them, aflatoxin, deoxynivalenol, fumonisin, and zearalenone there is unambiguous to good evidence of an impact on human health. The best evidence is that exposure to these compounds is a major economic and, in some regions, a clear and present threat to public health and animal welfare. These old problems have not been solved and it seems important to maintain focus on improved exposure characterization and management.

The increase in availability of sensitive analytical methods has unsurprising led to literally thousands of papers containing data on fungal metabolites in foods and feeds in modest concentrations (e.g., Ref. 265). Absence of toxicology data and "possible synergistic effects" are increasingly invoked as arguments for more investment in studies of dozens of fungal metabolites in food and feed. While there are many voices suggesting coexposures to generally minor amounts of many other fungal compounds is a public health hazard, this remains implausible. Aside from analytical data, these claims are supported by a plethora of in vitro studies using techniques not validated for regulatory purposes. Even for what they are, there are almost always methodological and statistical flaws (e.g., Ref. 266). Bliss[267] articulated statistical methods to assess interactions of poisons using mathematical approaches still in use. He noted that the "mixture cannot be assessed from that of the individual ingredients but depends upon a knowledge of their combined toxicity when used in different proportions" in a relevant animal model. In the once case where the JECFA has affirmed both additivity and synergistic interactions in two mycotoxins, fumonisin and aflatoxin, three necessary criteria have been defined: (1) use of relevant animal models, (2) experiments bracketing a broad dose range of both compounds, and (3) mechanistic plausibility.[214] This is consistent with the approaches that have evolved for the combined therapies of pharmaceutical drugs.[268]

After six decades, the many successes in reducing exposures in the fully developed economies have been achieved at great cost requiring ongoing attention to the five most important mycotoxins.

References

1. Pitt JI, Miller JD. A concise history of mycotoxin research. *J Agric Food Chem*. 2017;65:7021–7033.
2. Eppley RM, Bailey WJ. 12, 13-Epoxy-Δ9-trichothecenes as the probable mycotoxins responsible for stachybotryotoxicosis. *Science*. 1973;181(4101):758–760.
3. Bennett JW, Klich M. Mycotoxins. *Clin Microbiol Rev*. 2003; 16:497–516.

4. Forgacs J, Carll WT. Mycotoxicoses. *Adv Vet Sci.* 1962;7: 873–882.
5. Krogh P. The pathology of mycotoxicoses. *J Stored Prod Res.* 1969;5:259–264.
6. Brook PJ, White EP. Fungus toxins affecting mammals. *Ann Rev Phytopathol.* 1966;4:171–192.
7. Rodricks JV. *Mycotoxins and Other Fungal Related Food Problems. Am Chem Soc Series 149.* Washington, DC; 1976.
8. Ciegler A, Bennett JW. Mycotoxins and mycotoxicoses. *Bioscience.* 1980;30:512–515.
9. Miller JD. Fungi and mycotoxins in grain: implications for stored product research. *J Stored Prod Res.* 1995;31:1–6.
10. Miller JD. Mycotoxins in food and feed: a challenge for the 21st century. In: Li D-W, ed. *Biology of Microfungi.* Cham: Springer International Publishing; 2016:469–493.
11. Lee HJ, Ryu D. Worldwide occurrence of mycotoxins in cereals and cereal-derived food products: public health perspectives of their co-occurrence. *J Agric Food Chem.* 2017;65:7034–7051.
12. Eskola M, Kos G, Elliott CT, Hajšlová J, Mayar S, Krska R. Worldwide contamination of food-crops with mycotoxins: validity of the widely cited 'FAO estimate' of 25%. *Crit Rev Food Sci Nutr.* 2020;60:2773–2789.
13. Gruber-Dorninger C, Jenkins T, Schatzmayr G. Global mycotoxin occurrence in feed: a ten-year survey. *Toxins.* 2019;11(7):375.
14. Pitt JI, Hocking AD. *Fungi and Food Spoilage.* vol. 519. New York: Springer; 2009.
15. Pitt JI, Wild CP, Baan RA, et al. *Improving Public Health Through Mycotoxin Control.* International Agency for Research on Cancer Scientific Publications Series, No. 158. Lyon, France; 2012: 151 pp.
16. Meronuck R. The significance of fungi. *Plant Dis.* 1987;71: 287–291.
17. Renaud JB, Miller JD, Sumarah MW. The mycotoxin testing paradigm: challenges and opportunities for the future. *J AOAC Int.* 2019;102:1681–1688.
18. Schaafsma AW, Limay-Rios V, Paul DE, Miller JD. Mycotoxins in fuel ethanol co-products derived from maize – a mass balance for deoxynivalenol. *J Sci Food Agric.* 2009;89:1574–1580.
19. Miller JD, Schaafsma AW, Bhatnagar D, et al. Mycotoxins that affect the North American Agri-Food sector: state of the art and directions for the future. *World Mycotoxin J.* 2014;7:63–82.
20. Nganje WE, Kaitibie S, Wilson WW, Leistritz FL, Bangsund DA. *Economic impacts of Fusarium head blight in wheat and barley: 1993–2001* (No. 1187-2016-93545). Fargo, ND: North Dakota State University; 2004: 62 pp.
21. Wilson W, Dahl B, Nganje W. Economic costs of Fusarium head blight, scab and deoxynivalenol. *World Mycotoxin J.* 2018;11: 291–302.
22. Schaafsma AW. *Economic changes imposed by mycotoxins in food grains: case study of deoxynivalenol in winter wheat. Mycotoxins and Food Safety.* Boston, MA: Springer; 2002:271–276.
23. Mitchell NJ, Bowers E, Hurburgh C, Wu F. Potential economic losses to the US corn industry from aflatoxin contamination. *Food Addit Contam A.* 2016;33:540–550.
24. Wu F, Munkvold GP. Mycotoxins in ethanol co-products: modeling economic impacts on the livestock industry and management strategies. *J Agric Food Chem.* 2008;56:3900–3911.
25. Scott PM, Trucksess MW. Prevention of mycotoxins in dried fruit, other fruit products, and botanicals. *ACS Symp Ser.* 2009;1031:17–35.
26. Trucksess MW, Scott PM. Mycotoxins in botanicals and dried fruits: a review. *Food Addit Contam.* 2008;25:181–192.
27. Welke JE. Fungal and mycotoxin problems in grape juice and wine industries. *Curr Opin Food Sci.* 2019;19:7–13.
28. Bessaire T, Perrin I, Tarres A, Bebius A, Reding F, Theurillat V. Mycotoxins in green coffee: occurrence and risk assessment. *Food Control.* 2019;96:59–67.
29. Khaneghah AM, Fakhri Y, Abdi L, Coppa CFSC, Franco LT, de Oliveira CAF. The concentration and prevalence of ochratoxin A in coffee and coffee-based products: a global systematic review, *meta*-analysis and *meta*-regression. *Fungal Biol.* 2019;123: 611–617.
30. Iha MH, Trucksess MW. Management of mycotoxins in spices. *J AOAC Int.* 2019;102:1732–1739.
31. Kabak B, Dobson AD. Mycotoxins in spices and herbs – an update. *Crit Rev Food Sci Nutr.* 2017;57:18–34.
32. Logrieco AF, Miller JD, Eskola M, et al. The Mycotox Charter: increasing awareness of, and concerted action for, minimizing mycotoxin exposure worldwide. *Toxins.* 2018;10:149.
33. Atherstone C, Grace D, Lindahl JF, Kang'ethe EK, Nelson F. Assessing the impact of aflatoxin consumption on animal health and productivity. *Afr J Food Agric Nutr Dev.* 2016;16: 10949–10966.
34. Riley RT, Edwards SG, Aidoo K, et al. Fumonisins. In: *Safety Evaluation of Certain Contaminants in Food: Prepared by the Eighty-Third Meeting of the Joint FAO/WHO Expert Committee on Food Additives (JECFA).* WHO Food Additives Series, No. 74; 2018a: 415–571.
35. Wild C, Miller JD, Groopman JD. *Mycotoxin Control in Low and Middle Income Countries.* IARC Working Group Report #9. Lyon, France: International Agency for Research on Cancer; 2015: 70 p. ISBN 978-92-832-2510-2.
36. Doerge DR, Shephard GS, Adegoke GO, et al. Aflatoxins. In: *Safety Evaluation of Certain Contaminants in Food: Prepared by the Eighty-Third Meeting of the Joint FAO/WHO Expert Committee on Food Additives (JECFA).* WHO Food Additives Series, No. 74; 2018: 3–279.
37. Rios LD, Jaffee S. *Barrier, Catalyst, or Distraction? Standards, Competitiveness, and Africa's Groundnut Exports to Europe.* Washington DC: The World Bank; 2008. Agriculture and Rural Development Discussion Paper 39.
38. Coulibaly O, Hell K, Bandyopadhyay R, Hounkponou S, Leslie JF. Economic impact of aflatoxin contamination in sub-Saharan Africa. In: Leslie JF, Bandyopadhyay R, Visconti A, eds. *Mycotoxins: Detection Methods, Management, Public Health and Agricultural Trade.* Cambridge: CABI; 2008:67–76.
39. Emmott A. *Market-led Aflatoxin Interventions: Smallholder Groundnut Value Chains in Malawi.* Focus 20, Brief 8. Washington, DC: IFPRI; 2013.
40. Kussaga JB, Jacxsens L, Tiisekwa BP, Luning PA. Food safety management systems performance in African food processing companies: a review of deficiencies and possible improvement strategies. *J Sci Food Agric.* 2014;94:2154–2169.
41. Agbai VA. *Is Ghana Equipped to Benefit from the European Partnership Agreements? A Qualitative Multi-stakeholder Study Of Opportunities and Barriers Faced by Ghanaian Fresh Fruit and Vegetable Exporters to the EU.* MSc Thesis. University of Applied Sciences, Berlin; 2018.

42. Magamba K, Matumba L, Matita G, et al.) Aflatoxin risk management in commercial groundnut products in Malawi (Sub-Saharan Africa): a call for a more socially responsible industry. *J Consum Prot Food Saf.* 2017;12:309–316.
43. Miller JD. Epidemiology of *Fusarium graminearum* diseases of wheat and corn. In: Miller JD, Trenholm HL, eds. *Mycotoxins in Grain: Compounds Other than Aflatoxin.* St. Paul, MN: Eagan Press; 1994:19–36.
44. Miller JD, Culley J, Fraser K, et al. Effect of tillage practice on Fusarium head blight of wheat. *Can J Plant Pathol.* 1998;20: 95–103.
45. Hjelkrem AGR, Aamot HU, Brodal G, et al. HT-2 and T-2 toxins in Norwegian oat grains related to weather conditions at different growth stages. *Eur J Plant Pathol.* 2018;151:501–514.
46. Edwards SG, Dickin ET, Macdonald S, et al. Distribution of *Fusarium* mycotoxins in UK wheat mill fractions. *Food Addit Contam A.* 2011;28:1694–1704.
47. Shi H, Schwab W, Yu P. Natural occurrence and co-contamination of twelve mycotoxins in industry-submitted cool-season cereal grains grown under a low heat unit climate. *Toxins.* 2019;11:160.
48. Tittlemier SA, Chan J, Gaba D, et al. Revisiting the sampling, sample preparation, and analytical variability associated with testing wheat for deoxynivalenol. *World Mycotoxin J.* 2019;12:319–332.
49. Lombaert GA, Pellaers P, Roscoe V, Mankotia M, Neil R, Scott PM. Mycotoxins in infant cereal foods from the Canadian retail market. *Food Addit Contam.* 2003;20:494–504.
50. Zhang K, Flannery BM, Oles CJ, Adeuya A. Mycotoxins in infant/toddler foods and breakfast cereals in the US retail market. *Food Addit Contam B.* 2018;11:183–190.
51. Arcella D, Gergelova P, Innocenti ML, Steinkellner. Human and animal dietary exposure to T-2 and HT-2 toxin. *EFSA J.* 2017; 15(8):e04972.
52. EFSA. Scientific opinion on the risks for animal and public health related to the presence of T-2 and HT-2 toxin in food and feed. *EFSA J.* 2011;9(12):2481.
53. Lancova K, Hajslova J, Kostelanska M, et al. Fate of trichothecene mycotoxins during the processing: milling and baking. *Food Addit Contam.* 2008;25:650–659.
54. Pascale M, Haidukowski M, Lattanzio VMT, Silvestri M, Ranieri R, Visconti A. Distribution of T-2 and HT-2 toxins in milling fractions of durum wheat. *J Food Prot.* 2011;74:1700–1707.
55. Brodal G, Aamot HU, Almvik M, Hofgaard I. Removal of small kernels reduces the content of Fusarium mycotoxins in oat grain. *Toxins.* 2020;12(5):346.
56. Krska R, Crews C. Significance, chemistry and determination of ergot alkaloids: a review. *Food Addit Contam.* 2008;25:722–731.
57. Menzies JG, Turkington TK. An overview of the ergot (*Claviceps purpurea*) issue in western Canada: challenges and solutions. *Can J Plant Pathol.* 2015;37:40–51.
58. MacDonald SJ, Anderson WAC. *A Desk Study to Review Current Knowledge on Ergot Alkaloids and Their Potential for Contamination to Cereal Grains.* Research Review No. PR575. Sand Hutton: Fera Science Ltd.; 2017.
59. Malysheva SV, Larionova DA, Diana Di Mavungu J, De Saeger S. Pattern and distribution of ergot alkaloids in cereals and cereal products from European countries. *World Mycotoxin J.* 2014;7:217–230.
60. Scott PM. Ergot alkaloids: extent of human and animal exposure. *World Mycotoxin J.* 2009;2:141–149.
61. Scott PM, Lombaert GA, Pellaers P, Bacler S, Lappi J. Ergot alkaloids in grain foods sold in Canada. *J AOAC Int.* 1992;75: 773–779.
62. EFSA. Human and animal dietary exposure to ergot alkaloids. *EFSA J.* 2017;15(7):e04902.
63. Khoury CK, Achicanoy HA, Bjorkman AD, et al. Origins of food crops connect countries worldwide. *Proc R Soc B Biol Sci.* 2016;283(1832):20160792.
64. Martin AR, Cadotte MW, Isaac ME, Milla R, Vile D, Violle C. Regional and global shifts in crop diversity through the Anthropocene. *PLoS One.* 2019;14(2):e0209788.
65. Khoury CK, Bjorkman AD, Dempewolf H, et al. Increasing homogeneity in global food supplies and the implications for food security. *Proc Natl Acad Sci U S A.* 2014;111:4001–4006.
66. Miracle MP. *Maize in Tropical Africa.* Madison, WI: University of Minnesota Press; 1966:109–113.
67. Brooks GE. Peanuts and colonialism: consequences of the commercialization of peanuts in West Africa, 1830–70. *J Afr Hist.* 1975;16:29–54.
68. Bandyopadhyay R, Kumar M, Leslie JF. Relative severity of aflatoxin contamination of cereal crops in West Africa. *Food Addit Contam.* 2007;24:1109–1114.
69. Collins SL, Walsh JP, Renaud JB, et al. Improved methods for biomarker analysis of the big five mycotoxins enables reliable exposure characterization in a population of childbearing age women in Rwanda. *Food Chem Toxicol.* 2020;147:111854.
70. Abrunhosa L, Morales H, Soares C, et al. A review of mycotoxins in food and feed products in Portugal and estimation of probable daily intakes. *Crit Rev Food Sci Nutr.* 2016;56:249–265.
71. Schaafsma AW, Hooker DC. Climatic models to predict occurrence of *Fusarium* toxins in wheat and maize. *Int J Food Microbiol.* 2007;119:116–125.
72. Stack RW, McMullen MP. Head blighting potential of *Fusarium* species associated with spring wheat heads. *Can J Plant Pathol.* 1985;7:79–82.
73. Sutton JC. Epidemiology of wheat head blight and maize ear rot caused by *Fusarium graminearum. Can J Plant Pathol.* 1982;4:195–209.
74. Miller JD, Taylor A, Greenhalgh R. Production of deoxynivalenol and related compounds in liquid culture by *Fusarium graminearum. Can J Microbiol.* 1983;29:1171–1178.
75. Miller JD, Greenhalgh R, Wang YZ, Lu M. Trichothecene mycotoxin chemotypes of three *Fusarium* species. *Mycologia.* 1991;83:121–130.
76. O'Donnell K, Kistler HC, Tacke BK, Casper HH. Gene genealogies reveal global phylogeographic structure and reproductive isolation among lineages of *Fusarium graminearum*, the fungus causing wheat scab. *Proc Natl Acad Sci U S A.* 2000;97:7905–7910.
77. Crippin T, Renaud JB, Sumarah MW, Miller JD. Comparing genotype and chemotype of *Fusarium graminearum* from cereals in Ontario, Canada. *PLoS One.* 2019;14(5):e0216735.
78. Van der Fels-Klerx HJ, De Rijk TC, Booij €JH, et al. Occurrence of *Fusarium* head blight species and *Fusarium* mycotoxins in winter wheat in the Netherlands in 2009. *Food Addit Contam A.* 2012;29:1716–1726.
79. Bilska K, Jurczak S, Kulik T, et al. Species composition and trichothecene genotype profiling of Fusarium field isolates recovered from wheat in Poland. *Toxins.* 2018;10:325.

80. Pasquali M, Beyer M, Logrieco A, et al. A European database of *Fusarium graminearum* and *F. culmorum* trichothecene genotypes. *Front Microbiol*. 2016;7:406.
81. Vogelgsang S, Beyer M, Pasquali M, et al. An eight-year survey of wheat shows distinctive effects of cropping factors on different Fusarium species and associated mycotoxins. *Eur J Agron*. 2019;105:62–77.
82. Valverde-Bogantes E, Bianchini A, Herr JR, Rose DJ, Wegulo SN, Hallen-Adams HE. Recent population changes of *Fusarium* head blight pathogens: drivers and implications. *Can J Plant Pathol*. 2020;42:315–329.
83. Varga E, Wiesenberger G, Hametner C, et al. New tricks of an old enemy: isolates of *Fusarium graminearum* produce a type A trichothecene mycotoxin. *Environ Microbiol*. 2015;17:2588–2600.
84. Aitken A, Miller JD, McMullin DR. Isolation, chemical characterization and hydrolysis of the trichothecene 7α-hydroxy, 15-deacetylcalonectrin (3ANX) from *Fusarium graminearum* DAOMC 242077. *Tetrahedron Lett*. 2019;60:852–856.
85. Crippin T, Limay-Rios V, Renaud JB, Schaafsma AW, Sumarah MW, Miller JD. *Fusarium graminearum* populations from corn and wheat in Ontario, Canada. *World Mycotoxin J*. 2020;13(3):355–366.
86. Desjardins AE. Natural product chemistry meets genetics: when is a genotype a chemotype? *J Agric Food Chem*. 2008;56:7587–7592.
87. Villafana RT, Ramdass AC, Rampersad SN. Selection of *Fusarium* trichothecene toxin genes for molecular detection depends on TRI gene cluster organization and gene function. *Toxins*. 2019;11:36.
88. Zhang H, Zhang Z, Van der Lee T, et al. Population genetic analyses of *Fusarium asiaticum* populations from barley suggest a recent shift favoring 3ADON producers in southern China. *Phytopathology*. 2010;100:328–336.
89. Qiu J, Xu J, Shi J. *Fusarium* toxins in Chinese wheat since the 1980s. *Toxins*. 2019;11:248.
90. Hornok L. *Major trends in mycotoxin research. Challenges for Agricultural Research*. OECD Publishing; 2011:177–188. Available from: http://doi.org/10.1787/9789264090101-16-en.
91. Miller JD. Mycotoxins in small grains and maize: old problems, new challenges. *Food Addit Contam*. 2008;25:219–230.
92. Larsen JC, Hunt J, Perrin I, Ruckenbauer P. Workshop on trichothecenes with a focus on DON: summary report. *Toxicol Lett*. 2004;153:1–22.
93. Pieters MN, Freijer J, Baars BJ, Fiolet DC, van Klaveren J, Slob W. *Risk assessment of deoxynivalenol in food: concentration limits, exposure and effects. Mycotoxins and Food Safety*. Boston, MA: Springer; 2002:235–248.
94. Snijders CHA. Fusarium head blight and mycotoxin contamination of wheat, a review. *Neth J Plant Pathol*. 1990;96:187–198.
95. Kuiper-Goodman T. Prevention of mycotoxicoses through risk management and risk assessment. In: Miller JD, Trenholm HL, eds. *Mycotoxins in Grain*. Eagan Press; 1994:439–469.
96. EFSA. Risks to human and animal health related to the presence of deoxynivalenol and its acetylated and modified forms in food and feed. *EFSA J*. 2017;15(9):e04718.
97. Luo XY. *Outbreaks of moldy cereals poisoning in China. Issues in Food Safety*. Washington DC: Toxicology Forum; 1988:56–63.
98. Sun J, Wu Y. Evaluation of dietary exposure to deoxynivalenol (DON) and its derivatives from cereals in China. *Food Control*. 2016;69:90–99.
99. Pestka JJ. Deoxynivalenol: mechanisms of action, human exposure, and toxicological relevance. *Arch Toxicol*. 2010;84:663–679.
100. JECFA. *Deoxynivalenol*. Geneva: World Health Organization; 2011. 72nd Joint FAO/WHO Expert Committee on Food Additives and Contaminants. WHO Food Additives Series, No. 63.
101. Proctor RH, Desjardins AE, McCormick SP, Plattner RD, Alexander NJ, Brown DW. Genetic analysis of the role of trichothecene and fumonisin mycotoxins in the virulence of *Fusarium*. *Eur J Plant Pathol*. 2002;108:691–698.
102. Miller JD, Arnison PG. Degradation by suspension cultures of the *Fusarium* head blight resistant cultivar Frontana. *Can J Plant Pathol*. 1986;8:147–150.
103. Miller JD, Ewen MA. Toxic effects of deoxynivalenol on ribosomes and tissues of the spring wheat cultivars Frontana and Casavant. *Nat Toxins*. 1997;5:234–237.
104. Boutigny AL, Richard-Forget F, Barreau C. Natural mechanisms for cereal resistance to the accumulation of *Fusarium* trichothecenes. *Eur J Plant Pathol*. 2008;121:411–423.
105. Cossette F, Miller JD. Phytotoxic effect of deoxynivalenol and Gibberella ear rot resistance of corn. *Nat Toxins*. 1995;3:383–388.
106. Lemmens M, Scholz U, Berthiller F, et al. The ability to detoxify the mycotoxin deoxynivalenol colocalizes with a major quantitative trait locus for Fusarium head blight in wheat. *Mol Plant Microbe Int*. 2005;18:1318–1324.
107. Berthiller F, Dall'Asta C, Schuhmacher R, Lemmens M, Adam G, Krska R. Masked mycotoxins: determination of a deoxynivalenol glucoside in artificially and naturally contaminated wheat by liquid chromatography– tandem mass spectrometry. *J Agric Food Chem*. 2005;53:3421–3425.
108. Zhang Z, Nie D, Fan K, et al. A systematic review of plant-conjugated masked mycotoxins: occurrence, toxicology, and metabolism. *Crit Rev Food Sci Nutr*. 2020;60:1523–1537.
109. Simsek S, Ovando-Martínez M, Ozsisli B, Whitney K, Ohm JB. Occurrence of deoxynivalenol and deoxynivalenol-3-glucoside in hard red spring wheat grown in the USA. *Toxins*. 2013;5:2656–2670.
110. Schwarz PB, Qian SY, Zhou B, et al. Occurrence of deoxynivalenol-3-glucoside on barley from the upper midwestern United States. *J Am Soc Brew Chem*. 2014;72:208–213.
111. Tucker JR, Badea A, Blagden R, Pleskach K, Tittlemier SA, Fernando WG. Deoxynivalenol-3-glucoside content is highly associated with deoxynivalenol levels in two-Row barley genotypes of importance to Canadian barley breeding programs. *Toxins*. 2019;11(6):319.
112. Nagl V, Schwartz H, Krska R, et al. Metabolism of the masked mycotoxin deoxynivalenol-3-glucoside in rats. *Toxicol Lett*. 2012;213:367–373.
113. Wu W, Zhou HR, Bursian SJ, et al. Comparison of anorectic and emetic potencies of deoxynivalenol (vomitoxin) to the plant metabolite deoxynivalenol-3-glucoside and synthetic deoxynivalenol derivatives EN139528 and EN139544. *Toxicol Sci*. 2014;142:167–181.

114. Mengelers M, Zeilmaker M, Vidal A, De Boevre M, De Saeger S, Hoogenveen R. Biomonitoring of deoxynivalenol and deoxynivalenol-3-glucoside in human volunteers: renal excretion profiles. *Toxins*. 2019;11:466.

115. Gratz SW, Duncan G, Richardson AJ. The human fecal microbiota metabolizes deoxynivalenol and deoxynivalenol-3-glucoside and may be responsible for urinary deepoxy-deoxynivalenol. *Appl Environ Microbiol*. 2013;79:1821–1825.

116. Gratz SW, Currie V, Richardson AJ, et al. Porcine small and large intestinal microbiota rapidly hydrolyze the masked mycotoxin deoxynivalenol-3-glucoside and release deoxynivalenol in spiked batch cultures in vitro. *Appl Environ Microbiol*. 2018;84: e02106–e02117.

117. Deng Y, You L, Nepovimova E, et al. Biomarkers of deoxynivalenol (DON) and its modified form DON-3-glucoside (DON-3G) in humans. *Trends Food Sci Technol*. 2021;110:551–558.

118. Heyndrickx E, Sioen I, Huybrechts B, et al. Human biomonitoring of multiple mycotoxins in the Belgian population: results of the BIOMYCO study. *Environ Int*. 2015;84:82–89.

119. Nguyen NT, Varga E, Maragos C, Baumgartner S, Adam G, Berthiller F. Cross-reactivity of commercial and non-commercial deoxynivalenol-antibodies to emerging trichothecenes and common deoxynivalenol-derivatives. *World Mycotoxin J*. 2019;12: 45–53.

120. Ruprich J, Ostrý V. Immunochemical methods in health risk assessment: cross reactivity of antibodies against mycotoxin deoxynivalenol with deoxynivalenol-3-glucoside. *Cent Eur J Public Health*. 2008;16:34–37.

121. Tangni EK, Motte JC, Callebaut A, Pussemier L. Cross-reactivity of antibodies in some commercial deoxynivalenol test kits against some fusariotoxins. *J Agric Food Chem*. 2010;58:12625–12633.

122. Renaud JB, Sumarah MW. Data independent acquisition-digital archiving mass spectrometry: application to single kernel mycotoxin analysis of *Fusarium graminearum* infected maize. *Anal Bioanal Chem*. 2016;408:3083–3091.

123. Sugita-Konishi Y, Nakajima T. *Nivalenol: the mycology, occurrence, toxicology, analysis and regulation. Mycotoxins in Food, Feed and Bioweapons*. Springer; 2010:253–273.

124. Wu W, Bates MA, Bursian SJ, et al. Comparison of emetic potencies of the 8-ketotrichothecenes deoxynivalenol, 15-acetyldeoxynivalenol, 3-acetyldeoxynivalenol, fusarenon X. *and nivalenol. toxicological sciences*. 2013;131(1):279–291.

125. EFSA. Scientific opinion on risks for animal and public health related to the presence of nivalenol in food and feed. *EFSA J*. 2013;11(6):3262.

126. FSCJ. *Risk Assessment Report Deoxynivalenol and Nivalenol (Mycotoxin)*. Risk Assessment Report—Veterinary Medicines FS/ 872/2010. Food Safety Commission of Japan; 2010.

127. Varga E, Wiesenberger G, Woelflingseder L, et al. Less-toxic rearrangement products of NX-toxins are formed during storage and food processing. *Toxicol Lett*. 2018;284:205–212.

128. Woelflingseder L, Gruber N, Adam G, Marko D. Pro-Inflammatory Effects of NX-3 toxin are comparable to deoxynivalenol and not modulated by the co-occurring pro-xxidant aurofusarin. *Microorganisms*. 2020;8(4):603.

129. Pierron A, Neves M, Puela S, et al. Intestinal toxicity of the new type A trichothecenes, NX and 3ANX. *Chemosphere*. 2021;288 132415.

130. Massart F, Saggese G. Oestrogenic mycotoxin exposures and precocious pubertal development. *Int J Androl*. 2010;33:369–376.

131. Bandera EV, Chandran U, Buckley B, et al. Urinary mycoestrogens, body size and breast development in New Jersey girls. *Sci Total Environ*. 2011;409:5221–5227.

132. Deng F, Tao FB, Liu DY, et al. Effects of growth environments and two environmental endocrine disruptors on children with idiopathic precocious puberty. *Eur J Endocrinol*. 2012;166:803–809.

133. EFSA. Scientific opinion on the risks for public health related to the presence of zearalenone in food. *EFSA J*. 2011;9(6):2197.

134. De Ruyck K, Huybrechts I, Yang S, et al. Mycotoxin exposure assessments in a multi-center European validation study by 24-hour dietary recall and biological fluid sampling. *Environ Int*. 2020;137:105539.

135. Tittlemier SA, Gaba D, Chan JM. Monitoring of *Fusarium* trichothecenes in Canadian cereal grain shipments from 2010 to 2012. *J Agric Food Chem*. 2013;61:7412–7418.

136. Tittlemier SA, Arsiuta J, Mohammad U, et al. Variable relationships between *Fusarium* damage and deoxynivalenol concentrations in wheat in western Canada in 2016. *Can J Plant Pathol*. 2020;42:41–51.

137. Limay-Rios V, Schaafsma A. Relationship between mycotoxin content in winter wheat grain and aspirated dust collected during harvest and after storage. *ACS Omega*. 2021;6:1857–1871.

138. Reichel M, Staiger S, Biselli S. Analysis of *Fusarium* toxins in grain via dust: a promising field of application for rapid test systems. *World Mycotoxin J*. 2014;7:465–477.

139. Sanders M, De Boevre M, Dumoulin F, et al. Sampling of wheat dust and subsequent analysis of deoxynivalenol by LC-MS/MS. *J Agric Food Chem*. 2013;61:6259–6264.

140. Tittlemier SA, Sobering D, Bowler K, et al. By-products of grain cleaning: an opportunity for rapid sampling and screening of wheat for mycotoxins. *World Mycotoxin J*. 2015;8:45–53.

141. Scudamore K. Fate of *Fusarium* mycotoxins in the cereal industry: recent UK studies. *World Mycotoxin J*. 2008;1:315–323.

142. Stadler D, Lambertini F, Woelflingseder L, et al. The influence of processing parameters on the mitigation of deoxynivalenol during industrial baking. *Toxins*. 2019;11:317.

143. Stuper-Szablewska K, Szablewski T, Buśko M, Perkowski J. Changes in contents of trichothecenes during commercial grain milling. *LWT Food Sci Technol*. 2016;69:55–58.

144. Young JC, Fulcher RG, Hayhoe JH, Scott PM, Dexter JE. Effect of milling and baking on deoxynivalenol content of eastern Canadian wheats. *J Agric Food Chem*. 1984;32:659–664.

145. Trigo-Stockli DM, Deyoe CW, Satumbaga RF, Pedersen JR. Distribution of deoxynivalenol and zearalenone in milled fractions of wheat. *Cereal Chem*. 1996;73:388–391.

146. Hazel CM, Patel S. Influence of processing on trichothecene levels. *Toxicol Lett*. 2004;153:51–59.

147. Miller JD. Changing patterns of fungal toxins in crops: challenges for analysts. *J AOAC Int*. 2016;99:837–841.

148. Ryu D, Jackson LS, Bullerman LB. *Effects of processing on zearalenone. Mycotoxins and Food Safety*. Boston, MA: Springer; 2002:205–216.

149. Schwake-Anduschus C, Proske M, Sciurba E, Muenzing K, Koch M, Maul R. Distribution of deoxynivalenol, zearalenone, and their respective modified analogues in milling fractions of naturally contaminated wheat grains. *World Mycotoxin J*. 2015;8:433–443.

150. Brera C, Catano C, de Santis B, et al. Effect of industrial processing on the distribution of aflatoxins and zearalenone in corn-milling fractions. *J Agric Food Chem.* 2006;54:5014–5019.
151. Snijders CHA. Resistance in wheat to *Fusarium* infection and trichothecene formation. *Toxicol Lett.* 2004;153:37–46.
152. Xia R, Schaafsma AW, Wu F, Hooker DC. Impact of the improvements in Fusarium head blight and agronomic management on economics of winter wheat. *World Mycotoxin J.* 2020;13: 1–18.
153. Bianchini A, Horsley R, Jack MM, et al. DON occurrence in grains: a North American perspective. *Cereal Foods World.* 2015;60:32–56.
154. Janssen EM, Mourits MCM, van der Fels-Klerx HJ, Lansink AO. Pre-harvest measures against *Fusarium* spp. infection and related mycotoxins implemented by Dutch wheat farmers. *Crop Prot.* 2019;122:9–18.
155. Dalla Lana F, Madden LV, Paul PA. Natural occurrence of maize *Gibberella* ear rot and contamination of grain with mycotoxins in association with weather variables. *Plant Dis.* 2021;105:114–126.
156. Marasas WFO. Discovery and occurrence of the fumonisins: a historical perspective. *Environ Health Perspect.* 2001;109 (S2):239–243.
157. Missmer SA, Suarez L, Felkner M, et al. Exposure to fumonisins and the occurrence of neural tube defects along the Texas–Mexico border. *Environ Health Perspect.* 2006;114: 237–241.
158. IARC. IARC Monographs on the evaluation of carcinogenic risks to humans: some naturally occurring substances, food items and constituents, heterocyclic aromatic amines and mycotoxins. *IARC Monogr.* 1993;56:391–392. International Agency for Research on Cancer.
159. Voss KA, Riley RT. Fumonisin toxicity and mechanism of action: overview and current perspectives. *Food Saf.* 2013;1(1). 20130006.
160. Munkvold GP, Arias S, Taschl I, Gruber-Dorninger C. *Mycotoxins in corn: occurrence, impacts, and management. Corn.* AACC International Press; 2019:235–287.
161. Berardo N, Lanzanova C, Locatelli S, Laganà P, Verderio A, Motto M. Levels of total fumonisins in maize samples from Italy during 2006–2008. *Food Addit Contam B.* 2011;4:116–124.
162. Cano-Sancho G, Ramos AJ, Marín S, Sanchis V. Occurrence of fumonisins in Catalonia (Spain) and an exposure assessment of specific population groups. *Food Addit Contam A.* 2012;29:799–808.
163. Rheeder JP, Marasas WF, Vismer HF. Production of fumonisin analogs by *Fusarium* species. *Appl Environ Microbiol.* 2002;68: 2101–2105.
164. Suga H, Kitajima M, Nagumo R, et al. A single nucleotide polymorphism in the translation elongation factor 1α gene correlates with the ability to produce fumonisin in Japanese Fusarium fujikuroi. *Fungal Biol.* 2014;118:402–412.
165. Uegaki R, Tohno M, Yamamura K, Tsukiboshi T. Changes in the concentration of fumonisins in forage rice during the growing period, differences among cultivars and sites, and identification of the causal fungus. *J Agric Food Chem.* 2014;62:3356–3362.
166. Cendoya E, Chiotta ML, Zachetti V, Chulze SN, Ramirez ML. Fumonisins and fumonisin-producing *Fusarium* occurrence in wheat and wheat by products: a review. *J Cereal Sci.* 2018; 80:158–166.
167. Miller JD. Factors that affect the occurrence of fumonisin. *Environ Health Perspect 109.* 2001;(suppl 2)321–324.
168. De la Campa R, Hooker DC, Miller JD, Schaafsma WA, Hammond BG. Modelling effects of environment, insect damage and BT genotypes on fumonisin accumulation in maize in Argentina and the Philippines. *Mycopathologia.* 2005;159: 539–552.
169. Parsons MW, Munkvold GP. Associations of planting date, drought stress, and insects with *Fusarium* ear rot and fumonisin B1 contamination in California maize. *Food Addit Contam.* 2010;27:591–607.
170. Cappelle KM, Munkvold GP, Wolt JD. *Meta*-effect of insect resistant maize on fumonisin B1 in grain estimated by variance-weighted and replication-weighted analyses. *World Mycotoxin J.* 2019;12:141–151.
171. Ramirez ML, Pascale M, Chulze S, Reynoso MM, March G, Visconti A. Natural occurrence of fumonisins and their correlation to *Fusarium* contamination in commercial corn hybrids growth in Argentina. *Mycopathologia.* 1996;135:29–34.
172. Riley RT, Torres O, Matute J, Gregory SG, Ashley-Koch AE, Showker JL. Evidence for fumonisin inhibition of ceramide synthase in humans consuming maize-based foods and living in high exposure communities in Guatemala. *Mol Nutr Food Res.* 2015;59:2209–2224.
173. Riley RT, Merrill AH. Ceramide synthase inhibition by fumonisins: a perfect storm of perturbed sphingolipid metabolism, signaling and disease. *J Lipid Res.* 2019;60:1183–1189.
174. JECFA. *Fumonisin.* Geneva: World Health Organization; 2017. 83rd report of the Joint FAO/WHO Expert Committee on Food Additives and Contaminants. WHO Technical Report Series, No.1002.
175. Whitaker TB, Hagler WM, Johansson AS, Giesbrecht FG, Trucksess MW. Distribution among sample test results when testing shelled corn lots for fumonisin. *J AOAC Int.* 2001;84:770–776.
176. Bennett GA, Richard JL. Influence of processing on *Fusarium* mycotoxins in contaminated grains. *Food Technol.* 1996;(50) 235–238.
177. Pietri A, Zanetti M, Bertuzzi T. Distribution of aflatoxins and fumonisins in dry-milled maize fractions. *Food Addit Contam A.* 2009;26:372–380.
178. Ryu D, Bianchini A, Bullerman LB. Effects of processing on mycotoxins. *Stewart Postharvest Rev.* 2008;4:1–7.
179. Vanara F, Scarpino V, Blandino M. Fumonisin distribution in maize dry-milling products and by-products: impact of two industrial degermination systems. *Toxins.* 2018;10(9):357.
180. Serck-Hanssen A. Aflatoxin-induced fatal hepatitis. *Arch Environ Health.* 1970;20:729–731.
181. Taniwaki MH, Pitt JI, Magan N. *Aspergillus* species and mycotoxins: occurrence and importance in major food commodities. *Curr Opin Food Sci.* 2018;23:38–43.
182. Horn BW. Ecology and population biology of aflatoxigenic fungi in soil. *J Toxicol Toxin Rev.* 2003;22:351–379.
183. Pitt JI, Hocking AD, Bhudhasamai K, Miscamble BF, Wheeler KA, Tanboon-Ek P. The normal mycoflora of commodities from Thailand. 1. Nuts and oilseeds. *Int J Food Microbiol.* 1993;20: 211–226.
184. Dadzie MA, Oppong A, Ofori K, et al. Distribution and genetic diversity among *Aspergillus flavus* isolates across three

agro-ecologies essential for maize cultivation in Ghana. *Plant Pathol.* 2019;68:1565–1576.
185. Okun DO, Khamis FM, Muluvi GM, et al. Distribution of indigenous strains of atoxigenic and toxigenic *Aspergillus flavus* and *Aspergillus parasiticus* in maize and peanuts agro-ecological zones of Kenya. *Agric Food Security.* 2015;4(1):14.
186. Mohammed A, Chala A, Dejene M, et al. *Aspergillus* and aflatoxin in groundnut (*Arachis hypogaea* L.) and groundnut cake in Eastern Ethiopia. *Food Addit Contam B.* 2016;9:290–298.
187. Horn BW, Ramirez-Prado JH, Carbone I. Sexual reproduction and recombination in the aflatoxin-producing fungus *Aspergillus parasiticus. Fungal Genet Biol.* 2009;46:169–175.
188. Horn BW, Ramirez-Prado JH, Carbone I. The sexual state of *Aspergillus parasiticus. Mycologia.* 2009;101:275–280.
189. Horn BW, Moore GG, Carbone I. Sexual reproduction in *Aspergillus flavus. Mycologia.* 2009;101:423–429.
190. Olarte RA, Horn BW, Dorner JW, et al. Effect of sexual recombination on population diversity in aflatoxin production by *Aspergillus flavus* and evidence for cryptic heterokaryosis. *Mol Ecol.* 2012;21:1453–1476.
191. Olarte RA, Worthington CJ, Horn BW, et al. Enhanced diversity and aflatoxigenicity in interspecific hybrids of *Aspergillus flavus* and *Aspergillus parasiticus. Mol Ecol.* 2015;24:1889–1909.
192. Moore GG, Elliott JL, Singh R, et al. Sexuality generates diversity in the aflatoxin gene cluster: evidence on a global scale. *PLoS Pathog.* 2013;9(8):e1003574.
193. Drott MT, Fessler LM, Milgroom MG. Population subdivision and the frequency of aflatoxigenic isolates in *Aspergillus flavus* in the United States. *Phytopathology.* 2019;109:878–886.
194. Drott MT, Satterlee TR, Skerker JM, et al. The frequency of sex: population genomics reveals differences in recombination and population structure of the aflatoxin-producing fungus *Aspergillus flavus. mBio.* 2020;11(4).
195. Moore GG. Sex and recombination in aflatoxigenic Aspergilli: global implications. *Front Microbiol.* 2014;5:32.
196. Wu F. Mycotoxin risk assessment for the purpose of setting international regulatory standards. *Environ Sci Technol.* 2004;38:4049–4055.
197. Pruter LS, Brewer MJ, Weaver MA, Murray SC, Isakeit TS, Bernal JS. Association of insect-derived ear injury with yield and aflatoxin of maize hybrids varying in Bt transgenes. *Environ Entomol.* 2020;113:2950–2958.
198. Yu J, Hennessy DA, Wu F. The impact of Bt corn on aflatoxin-related insurance claims in the United States. *Sci Rep.* 2020;10(1): 1–10.
199. Abbas HK, Accinelli C, Shier WT. Biological control of aflatoxin contamination in US crops and the use of bioplastic formulations of *Aspergillus flavus* biocontrol strains to optimize application strategies. *J Agric Food Chem.* 2017;65:7081–7087.
200. Isakeit T, Allen T, Chilvers M, et al. Using atoxigenics to manage aflatoxin. <https://cropprotectionnetwork.org>; 2016.
201. Lewis M, Carbone I, Luis J, et al. Biocontrol strains differentially shift the genetic structure of indigenous soil populations of *Aspergillus flavus. Front Microbiol.* 2019;10:1738.
202. Moore GG. Practical considerations will ensure the continued success of pre-harvest biocontrol using non-aflatoxigenic *Aspergillus flavus* strains. *Crit Rev Food Sci Nutr.* 2021;1–18.
203. Gell RM, Horn BW, Carbone I. Genetic map and heritability of *Aspergillus flavus. Fungal Genet Biol.* 2020;144:103478.
204. Payne GA, Widstrom NW. Aflatoxin in maize. *Crit Rev Plant Sci.* 1992;10:423–440.
205. Brera C, De Santis B, Prantera E, et al. Effect of sample size in the evaluation of "in-field" sampling plans for aflatoxin B1 determination in corn. *J Agric Food Chem.* 2010;58:8481–8489.
206. Whitaker TB, Dickens JW, Monroe RJ. Variability associated with testing corn for aflatoxin. *J Am Oil Chem Soc.* 1979;56:789–794.
207. Johansson AS, Whitaker TB, Hagler WM, Giesbrecht FG, Young JH, Bowman DT. Testing shelled corn for aflatoxin, part I: estimation of variance components. *J AOAC Int.* 2000;83: 1264–1269.
208. Widstrom N. The aflatoxin problem with corn grain. In: Sparks DL, ed. *Advances in Agonomy.* vol. 56. San Diego: Academic Press; 1996:219–280.
209. Jordan D, Brandenburg R, Payne G, Akromah R, Appaw W, Ellis W. *Preventing mycotoxin contamination in groundnut cultivation. Achieving Sustainable Cultivation of Grain Legumes.* vol. 2. Burleigh Dodds Science Publishing; 2018:203–234.
210. Dorner JW. Management and prevention of mycotoxins in peanuts. *Food Addit Contam.* 2008;25:203–208.
211. Bennett GA, Anderson RA. Distribution of aflatoxin and/or zearalenone in wet-milled corn products: a review. *J Agric Food Chem.* 1978;26:1055–1060.
212. Park DL. *Effect of processing on aflatoxin. Mycotoxins and Food Safety.* Boston, MA: Springer; 2002:173–179.
213. Liu Y, Wu F. Global burden of aflatoxin-induced hepatocellular carcinoma: a risk assessment. *Environ Health Perspect.* 2010; 118:818–824.
214. Riley RT, Hambridge T, Alexander J, et al. Co-exposure of fumonisins with aflatoxins. In: *Safety Evaluation of Certain Contaminants in Food: Prepared by the Eighty-Third Meeting of the Joint FAO/WHO Expert Committee on Food Additives (JECFA). WHO Food Additives Series*, No. 74; 2018b: 879–948.
215. Krogh P, Hald B, Pedersen EJ. Occurrence of ochratoxin A and citrinin in cereals associated with mycotoxic porcine nephropathy. *Acta Pathol Microbiol Scand B.* 1973;81:689–695.
216. Limay-Rios V, Miller JD, Schaafsma AW. Occurrence of *Penicillium verrucosum*, ochratoxin A, ochratoxin B and citrinin in on-farm stored winter wheat from the Canadian Great Lakes Region. *PLoS One.* 2017;12(7):e0181239.
217. Van der Merwe KJ, Steyn PS, Fourie L, Scott DB, Theron JJ. Ochratoxin A, a toxic metabolite produced by *Aspergillus ochraceus* Wilh. *Nature.* 1965;205(4976):1112–1113.
218. Bui-Klimke TR, Wu F. Ochratoxin A and human health risk: a review of the evidence. *Crit Rev Food Sci Nutr.* 2015;55: 1860–1869.
219. Haighton LA, Lynch BS, Magnuson BA, Nestmann ER. A reassessment of risk associated with dietary intake of ochratoxin A based on a lifetime exposure model. *Crit Rev Toxicol.* 2012;42:147–168.
220. Di Paolo N, Guarnieri A, Loi F, Sacchi G, Mangiarotti AM, Di Paolo M. Acute renal failure from inhalation of mycotoxins. *Nephron.* 1993;64:621–625.
221. Pitt JI, Taniwaki MH, Cole MB. Mycotoxin production in major crops as influenced by growing, harvesting, storage and processing, with emphasis on the achievement of Food Safety Objectives. *Food Control.* 2013;32:205–215.

222. Taniwaki MH, Pitt JI, Copetti MV, Teixeira AA, Iamanaka BT. Understanding mycotoxin contamination across the food chain in Brazil: challenges and opportunities. *Toxins*. 2019;11(7):411.
223. Lombaert GA, Pellaers P, Chettiar M, Lavalee D, Scott PM, Lau BY. Survey of Canadian retail coffees for ochratoxin A. *Food Addit Contam*. 2002;19:869–877.
224. Nielsen KF, Ngemela AF, Jensen LB, De Medeiros LS, Rasmussen PH. UHPLC-MS/MS determination of ochratoxin A and fumonisins in coffee using QuEChERS extraction combined with mixed-mode SPE purification. *J Agric Food Chem*. 2015;63:1029–1034.
225. Taniwaki MH. *An update on ochratoxigenic fungi and ochratoxin A in coffee. Advances in Food Mycology*. Boston, MA: Springer; 2006:189–202.
226. Andrews RI, Thompson BK, Trenholm HL. A national survey of mycotoxins in Canada. *J Am Oil Chem Soc*. 1981;58: A989–A991.
227. Prior MG. Mycotoxins in animal feedstuffs and tissues in Western Canada 1975 to 1979. *Can J Comp Med*. 1981;45:116–119.
228. Richardson EA, Flude P, Patterson DP, Mackenzie DR, Wakefield E. Ochratoxin A in retail flour. *Lancet*. 1978;312 (8104):1366–1367.
229. Abramson D, Sinha RN, Mills JT. Mycotoxin formation in HY-320 wheat during granary storage at 15 and 19% moisture content. *Mycopathologia*. 1990;111:181–189.
230. Kuruc JA, Schwarz P, Wolf-Hall C. Ochratoxin A in stored US barley and wheat. *J Food Prot*. 2015;78:597–601.
231. Lillehoj EB, Elling F. Environmental conditions that facilitate ochratoxin contamination of agricultural commodities. *Acta Agric Scand*. 1983;33:113–128.
232. Lund F, Frisvad JC. *Penicillium verrucosum* in wheat and barley indicates presence of ochratoxin A. *J Appl Microbiol*. 2003;95: 1117–1123.
233. Elmholt S. Ecology of the ochratoxin A producing *Penicillium verrucosum*: occurrence in field soil and grain with special attention to farming system and on-farm drying practices. *Biol Agric Hortic*. 2003;20:311–337.
234. Clear RM, Patrick SK. Prevalence of some seedborne fungi on soft white winter wheat seed from Ontario, Canada. *Can Plant Dis Surv*. 1993;73:143–149.
235. Dhungana B, Ali S, Byamukama E, Krishnan P, Caffe-Treml M. Incidence of *Penicillium verrucosum* in grain samples from oat varieties commonly grown in South Dakota. *J Food Prot*. 2018;81:898–902.
236. Flannigan B. Primary contamination of barley and wheat grain storage fungi. *Trans Br Mycol Soc*. 1978;71:37–42.
237. Anon. *The UK Code of Good Storage Practice to Reduce Ochratoxin A in Cereals*. Food Standards Agency, UK; 2007.
238. Anon. *Preventing Ochratoxin in Stored Small Grains*. Toronto: Food & Consumer Products Association of Canada. <https://www.fcpc.ca/Industry-Resources>; 2018.
239. Fleurat-Lessard F. Integrated management of the risks of stored grain spoilage by seedborne fungi and contamination by storage mould mycotoxins – an update. *J Stored Prod Res*. 2017;71: 22–40.
240. Magan N, Aldred D. Post-harvest control strategies: minimizing mycotoxins in the food chain. *Int J Food Microbiol*. 2007;119: 131–139.
241. Tuite JF, Christensen CM. Grain storage studies. XXIII. Time of invasion of wheat seed by various species of *Aspergillus* responsible for deterioration of stored grain, and source of inoculum of these fungi. *Phytopathology*. 1957;47:265–268.
242. Magan N, Aldred D, Baxter ES. Good postharvest storage practices for wheat grain. In: Leslie JF, Logrieco A, eds. *Mycotoxin Reduction in Grain Chains*. Wiley-Blackwell; 2014:258–267.
243. EFSA. Opinion of the Scientific Panel on contaminants in the food chain CONTAM. related to ochratoxin A in food. *EFSA J*. 2006;4(6):365.
244. Kolakowski B, O'Rourke SM, Bietlot HP, Kurz K, Aweryn B. Ochratoxin A concentrations in a variety of grain-based and non–grain-based foods on the Canadian retail market from 2009 to 2014. *J Food Prot*. 2016;79:2143–2159.
245. Wicklow DT. The mycology of stored grain: anecological perspective. In: Jayas DS, White NDG, Muir W, eds. *Stored Grain Ecosystems*. New York: Marcel Dekker; 1994:197–249.
246. Nowicki T, Roscoe M. An alternative to slurry mixing to minimise sample preparation variance for determination of ochratoxin A in wheat. *World Mycotoxin J*. 2010;3:147–156.
247. Whitaker TB, Slate AB, Nowicki TW, Giesbrecht FG. Variability and distribution among sample test results when sampling unprocessed wheat lots for ochratoxin A. *World Mycotoxin J*. 2016;9:163–178.
248. Walker R. *Risk assessment of ochratoxin: current views of the European Scientific Committee on Food, the JECFA and the Codex Committee on Food Additives and Contaminants. Mycotoxins and Food Safety*. Boston, MA: Springer; 2002:249–255.
249. Osborne BG, Ibe F, Brown GL, et al. The effects of milling and processing on wheat contaminated with ochratoxin A. *Food Addit Contam*. 1996;13:141–153.
250. Schaarschmidt S, Fauhl-Hassek C. The fate of mycotoxins during the processing of wheat for human consumption. *Compr Rev Food Sci Food Saf*. 2018;17:556–593.
251. Scudamore KA, Banks J, MacDonald SJ. Fate of ochratoxin A in the processing of whole wheat grains during milling and bread production. *Food Addit Contam*. 2003;20:1153–1163.
252. Benford D, Boyle C, Dekant W, et al. *Ochratoxin A. Safety Evaluation of Certain Mycotoxins in Food*. Geneva: WHO; 2001:281–415. WHO Food Additive Series 47.
253. Solfrizzo M, Gambacorta L, Visconti A. Assessment of multi-mycotoxin exposure in southern Italy by urinary multi-biomarker determination. *Toxins*. 2014;6(2):523–538.
254. Lambe J. The use of food consumption data in assessments of exposure to food chemicals including the application of probabilistic modelling. *Proc Nutr Soc*. 2002;61:11–18.
255. Chen C, Turna NS, Wu F. Risk assessment of dietary deoxynivalenol exposure in wheat products worldwide: are new codex DON guidelines adequately protective? *Trends Food Sci Technol*. 2019;89:11–25.
256. UNEP. *UNEP Frontiers 2016 Report: Emerging Issues of Environmental Concern*. Nairobi: United Nations Environment Programme; 2016: 54–62.
257. Pitt JI, Boesch C, Whitaker TB, Clarke R. A systematic approach to monitoring high preharvest aflatoxin levels in maize and peanuts in Africa and Asia. *World Mycotoxin J*. 2018;11:485–491.
258. Hijmans RJ, Choe H, Perlman J. Spatiotemporal patterns of field crop diversity in the United States, 1870–2012. *Agric Environ Lett*. 2016;1(1):160022.

259. Wu F, Bhatnagar D, Bui-Klimke T, et al. Climate change impacts on mycotoxin risks in US maize. *World Mycotoxin J.* 2011;4:79–93.
260. Balbus JM, Boxall AB, Fenske RA, McKone TE, Zeise L. Implications of global climate change for the assessment and management of human health risks of chemicals in the natural environment. *Environ Toxicol Chem.* 2013;32:62–78.
261. De Rijk TC, Van Egmond HP, Van der Fels-Klerx HJ, et al. A study of the 2013 Western European issue of aflatoxin contamination of maize from the Balkan area. *World Mycotoxin J.* 2015;8:641–651.
262. Battilani P, Toscano P, Van der Fels-Klerx HJ, et al. Aflatoxin B 1 contamination in maize in Europe increases due to climate change. *Sci Rep.* 2016;6:24328.
263. Moretti A, Pascale M, Logrieco AF. Mycotoxin risks under a climate change scenario in Europe. *Trends Food Sci Technol.* 2019;84:38–40.
264. Haile JK, N'Diaye A, Walkowiak S, et al. Fusarium Head Blight in durum wheat: recent status, breeding directions, and future research prospects. *Phytopathology.* 2019;109:1664–1675.
265. Streit E, Schwab C, Sulyok M, Naehrer K, Krska R, Schatzmayr G. Multi-mycotoxin screening reveals the occurrence of 139 different secondary metabolites in feed and feed ingredients. *Toxins.* 2013;5(3):504–523.
266. Alassane-Kpembi I, Schatzmayr G, Taranu I, Marin D, Puel O, Oswald IP. Mycotoxins co-contamination: methodological aspects and biological relevance of combined toxicity studies. *Crit Rev Food Sci Nutr.* 2017;57:3489–3507.
267. Bliss CI. The toxicity of poisons applied jointly. *Ann Appl Biol.* 1939;26:585–615.
268. Vlot AH, Aniceto N, Menden MP, Ulrich-Merzenich G, Bender A. Applying synergy metrics to oncology combination screening data: agreements, disagreements and pitfalls. *Drug Discov Today.* 2019;24:2286–2298.

Section II

Changes in the chemical composition of food throughout the various stages of the food chain: animal and milk production

Chapter 5

Occurrence of antibacterial substances and coccidiostats in animal feed

Ewelina Patyra, Monika Przeniosło-Siwczyńska and Krzysztof Kwiatek

Department of Hygiene of Animal Feedingstuffs, National Veterinary Research Institute, Pulawy, Poland

Abstract

The production, processing, and marketing process in the food chain starting at the stage of primary production and ending with households, that is, after traveling all the way "from farm to fork," it is exposed to various risks for food producers and consumers. This chapter presents the legal requirements for the production of feed, the presence of antimicrobial substances and coccidiostats in feed, and the problem of contamination of feed with antibacterial substances. The influence of antimicrobial substances on the possibility of the development of drug-resistant microorganisms, the possible transfer of these compounds to the natural environment, the possibility of residual antibacterial substances in food of animal origin, and the techniques enabling their determination in feed were described. The chapter concludes with a future perspective to reduce the use of antimicrobial substances in the food chain and challenges to the development of new analytical methods to control antimicrobial substances in feed and food.

Keywords: Antibiotics; coccidiostats; antibiotic growth promoters; cross-contaminations; antimicrobial resistance; feed; medicated feed; analytical methods; EU legislation

Chapter points

1. The use of antibiotics and coccidiostats in feed is an attempt to protect animal health against bacterial diseases.
2. The use of antibiotics and coccidiostats in medicated feed leads to contamination of nontarget feed with these substances.
3. Ingestion of low concentrations of antibacterial substances by animals may lead to toxic reactions and selection of drug-resistant microorganisms.
4. Antimicrobial substances pollute the natural environment by introducing excrements from slaughter animals for plant cultivation.
5. It is necessary to control the presence of antimicrobial substances in nontarget feed and to implement appropriately sensitive and reliable analytical methods.

5.1 Introduction

Unintended contaminants or residues in animal feed have the potential to transfer to human food derived from such contaminated animals and present a risk to consumers' health. Examples of such sources are environmental, for example, polychlorinated biphenyls (PCBs), heavy metals; agrochemicals, for example, pesticides, hormones; microbiological, for example, mycotoxins; biological, for example, prions bovine spongiform encephalopathy (BSE); and veterinary medicines, for example, cross-contamination during manufacture. Transfer factors for a wide range of chemical classes have been proposed for such unintended "additions to human food" have been proposed as a part of risk assessment.[1] However, the regulated use of additives and veterinary medicines in animal feed for specific purposes is not considered "unintended" and is controlled to ensure there is no unacceptable risk to human health through consumption of derived animal products.

To address all the unintended and legitimate, regulated substances in animal feed and their consequences for risks to human health within this chapter is clearly impossible. The presence of certain antimicrobial veterinary drugs in human food is a current and increasing concern to public health given the increasing incidence of microbial resistance to human antimicrobial drugs, and therefore this chapter will focus on the use of such veterinary medicines in animal feed, their purpose, controls, and future developments.

In January 2000 the European Union (EU) European Commission (EC) presented a White Paper on Food Safety[2] highlighting the need to improve transparency and

Present Knowledge in Food Safety. DOI: https://doi.org/10.1016/B978-0-12-819470-6.00031-7

safety along the entire food chain—it coined the term "farm to fork," which signaled the responsibilities of all stakeholders at each link in the food chain. Hazards should not be present in food at levels which present unacceptable risks for consumers. To ensure this international bodies such as FAO, WHO Codex Alimentarius, and European Food Safety Authority (EFSA), together with national bodies, such as United States Food and Drug Administration/United States Department of Agriculture/Environmental Protection Agency, carry out risk assessments and propose limits for such undesirable substances at key stages of the food chain.

One such key stage is the production of animal feed, especially medicated feed, a "critical control point" Hazard analysis and critical control points (HACCP) in the food chain and the regulatory limits set are essential for quality control in feed production including transfer into the environment, and the sophisticated analytical methodology is required to provide the sensitivity need for quality assurance for regulated substances and undesirable contaminants.

5.2 Antibacterial drugs in feed

5.2.1 Antimicrobials in feed

Antibiotics as feed additives started to be used at the turn of the 1940s and 1950s, when it was discovered quite by accident that adding streptogramin to feed for chickens increased their weight gain. Shortly thereafter, in 1949, a similar effect was also observed in chickens after administration of digestate containing small amounts of chlortetracycline production of *Streptomyces aureofaciens*.[3] This type of stimulating effect on weight gain was also confirmed in further studies with pigs and cattle.[4–6] These observations formed the basis for the widespread introduction of antibiotics in animal nutrition as growth promoters in animal production. Several antibiotics have been in use as growth promoters of farm animal ever since.[4]

The use of feed antibiotics was an attempt to protect farm animals against disturbances in the microbiological balance of the digestive tract. The use of bactericidal properties of antibiotics against Gram-positive bacteria allowed for the elimination of chronic intestinal infections, thereby increasing the efficiency of animal production.[3,7–10] Subsequent tests confirmed that the presence of an antibiotic in the feed improves the weight gain of the animals as well as the degree of feed conversion by better absorption of nutrients in the intestinal villi.[11] The observations carried out showed that the administration of antibiotics in the feed improves the growth of slaughter animals by about 4%–8%, and increases the feed conversion by 2%–5%.[12] They also inhibit absorption from the intestine of toxins in the feed which can have adverse effects on the health of the animals. The growth-promoting effect of antibiotics might stem from their ability to suppress harmful organisms. It is also suggested that animals reared in unhygienic environments always bear some latent infections, which trigger a cascade of events in their immune system.[13]

The use of antibiotics as feed additives has been a hallmark of modern animal husbandry, but this widespread practice is not without criticism. In the early years, all antibiotics were allowed for use, although some did not enhance growth and many were too expensive.[4] After a certain period of their use, it was noticed that excessive, often unjustified use, as well as inadequate dosage and nontherapeutic use have become the cause of many problems. The most important of these turned out to be the phenomenon of drug resistance and the constantly growing number of microbial species resistant to the antibiotics used, which posed a significant threat to the effectiveness of these drugs in the treatment of infectious diseases.[13]

The first discussions on the use antibiotics as growth promoters began in the late 1960s and resulted in the "Swann Report," which was issued in the United Kingdom. This report contained a proposal to limit and organize the use of antibiotics as feed additives. The report also recommended limiting their use in animal husbandry and pointed out, interalia, attention to the need to separate the so-called feed antibiotics, for exclusive use in veterinary medicine and available only with the prescription of a veterinarian, and also paid attention to the possibility of the development of drug-resistant microorganisms. This report also formed the basis for the EU legislation in Directive 70/524,[14] in which a list was published of allowable additives with their maximum and minimum dosages, withdrawal period from slaughter, and animal species in which the product may be used.[15] The directive was later implemented in the national legislation of the various EU Member States. These recommendations led to the withdrawal in 1972–74 of antibiotics such as penicillin, streptomycin, and tetracyclines as stimulants in many European countries. As a result, in 1986, a complete ban on the use of antibiotic growth promoters (AGPs) in farm animals was introduced in Sweden. Since 1997 this and several other antibiotics such as bacitracin, virginiamycin, tylosin, spiramycin, avoparcin, avilamycin, olaquindox, and carbadox have been forbidden in EC Member States for their use as feed additives. A similar ban was issued in Norway in 1995 due to reports of the emergence of vancomycin resistance among *Enterococcus* strains. Denmark soon followed suit, gradually phasing out AGPs used in animal nutrition since 1999. Opponents of such a solution argued that the consequence of abandoning the use of antibiotic growth promoters (AGPs) would be an increase in the use of chemotherapeutic agents for therapeutic purposes, which, unlike AGPs, easily penetrate the intestinal wall and are absorbed into the animal's body.[16]

In 2003 the European Parliament and the Council adopted Regulation No. 1831/2003 on feed additives which, as of 1 January 2006, completely prohibited the use of AGPs other than histomonostats and coccidiostats in the feeding of farm animals. Currently, in all EU Member States, the only legal route for administering antibacterial substances in feed is the so-called medicated feed.

5.2.2 Coccidiostats in feed

Coccidiostats are pharmacologically active molecules employed since 1940, to prevent and inhibit parasitic protozoa of the Phylum Apicomplexa and the genus *Eimeria*, referred to as coccidia, causing a very contagious disease of the gastrointestinal tract in many farmed animals.[17,18] These agents are used to treat intensively reared species including poultry, sheep, cattle, pigs, and rabbits. Coccidiosis represents a major disease in poultry, causing diarrhea, poor weight gain, poor feed conversion, and in some cases death. In the United States, annual losses due to coccidiosis in poultry are estimated at $127 million, so it is more financially viable to administer coccidiostats as feed additives to broiler chickens for almost their entire life rather than treating coccidiosis therapeutically.[19] Coccidiostats are authorized as feed additives for target animal species according with Regulation (EC) No. 1831/2003[20] of the European Parliament and of the Council of September 22, 2003 on additives for use in animal nutrition and can be categorized as naturally occurring polyether ionophores produced by Streptomycetaceae bacterial family, such as monensin, narasin, lasalocid, salinomycin, semduramicin, and maduramicin, or as synthetic coccidiostats such as halofuginone, robenidine, nicarbazin, decoquinate, and diclazuril. Each coccidiostat has individual toxicological characteristics which are based on molecular mechanisms of action that effect transmembrane ion transport in the case of the ionophoric compounds. The synthetic (nonionophoric) compounds represent a very heterogenous group of molecules which have partially unknown mechanisms of action.[21]

The production, manufacture, and marketing of coccidiostats, premixes with coccidiostats, and feed with coccidiostats are regulated by the Directive No. (EC) 95/69[22] of December 22, 1995 and in Article 10 of the Regulation No. (EC) 183/2005.[23] The authorization of coccidiostats as feed additives is based on studies that demonstrate safety of their use in relation to the target species at the highest proposed levels of incorporation in feed or water and at multiples of that level to establish a margin of safety.

5.3 Medicated feed production

Antimicrobial substances in feed may be administered only as medicated feed, which, according to the definition of Regulation (EU) 2019/4[24] of the European Parliament and of the Council of December 11, 2018, means feed ready for direct feeding to animals without further processing, consisting of a homogeneous mixture of at least one veterinary medicinal product or product intermediate and feed materials or feed compound. While there is a great deal of variability in feed regulations and animal production systems between countries, the majority of veterinary drugs added to feed are antimicrobials and coccidiostats.[25]

Medicated feed is usually manufactured by commercial feed mills regulated and inspected by competent authorities. However, some countries authorize on-farm production of medicated feed.[26] Specifics of veterinary drug approval and use in animal feed vary greatly between countries and regions. For example, in all EU member countries the use of veterinary drugs and medicated feed requires a prescription by an authorized veterinarian and must be done according to the label directions.[26] Medicated feed containing antimicrobial veterinary medicinal products shall be used in accordance with Article 107 of Regulation (EU) 2019/4, except as regards paragraph 3 thereof, and shall not be used for prophylaxis (Article 17 of Regulation (EU) 2019/4). In the United States, extralabel use of veterinary drugs in feed is prohibited by the Animal Medicinal Drug Use and Clarification Act.[27] But otherwise this is done in Canada, where off-label use of drugs in feed is allowed as long as this is done with a veterinarian's prescription.[28] However, in many countries around the world, the use of veterinary drugs in animal feed can take place with little or no veterinary supervision. Veterinary drugs such as antibiotics and coccidiostats must be used according to specific instructions. Compounds authorized for use in animal feed must be of appropriate quality, proven to be effective, and safe for animals that consume the feed, feed factory employees, and the environment. The EC launched a public consultation on the delegated act establishing the draft criteria for the designation of antimicrobials to be reserved for the treatment of certain infections in humans. The EC will use these criteria to establish a list of antimicrobials to be reserved for use in humans as part of its legislation on veterinary medicinal products. Interested stakeholders have until April 23, 2021 to respond to the consultation.

5.3.1 Cross-contamination during feed production, transport, and storage

Feed business operators can produce a wide range of feeds for different target animals in one facility, containing different types of ingredients, such as veterinary medicinal products and feed additives. The production of different types of feed on the same production line may lead to the presence of traces of the active substance on that line, which will end up in the first production batches of the next feed. This transfer of trace amounts of an active ingredient from one production batch to another is called "cross-contamination." So, according to the Regulation (EU) 2019/4, cross-contamination means contamination of nontarget feed with an active substance from the earlier use of premises or equipment. Cross-contamination can occur during the production, processing, storage, or transport of feeds, when the same equipment is used for feeds containing different ingredients both at the production plant and on the farm.

During feed manufacturing, veterinary drugs may be carried over from medicated feed to nonmedicated feed.[29] Carryover of a veterinary drug can occur during feed processing, handling, delivery, or storage. The type of drug, number of species exposed, and feed production and delivery systems determine the hazards associated with drug carryover.[30] Carryover may lead to serious adverse effects on human and animal health depending on the drug and the quantity and distribution of the feed that was contaminated.[31–34] In order to protect animal health, human health, and the environment, a maximum level for cross-contamination of active substances in nontarget feed should be established based on a scientific risk assessment carried out by the EFSA, in cooperation with the European Medicines Agency, and taking into account good manufacturing practice and principles such as "As Low As Reasonably Achievable" (ALARA). Even low-level carryover of veterinary drugs may be sufficient to cause residues in the edible tissues or products (e.g., eggs or milk) from animals consuming feed containing carryover drug residues.[31,32,35–43] Even if such residues are not an animal health or food safety concern, they may cause trade issues.[44] Residues of veterinary drugs can be present in feed when ingredients of animal origin (terrestrial and aquatic) are used, but this is not considered a significant source of drug carryover.[45,46] There are a number of causes of unwanted drug carryover in medicated feed.[47] Significant amounts of drug or medicated feed may remain in any part of the feed manufacturing and distribution system and contaminate subsequent batches of feed. Residual medicated feed can remain in mixers, surge bin conveyors and elevators, bin and bulk feed trucks. Leaking connections can cross from feed mill equipment, packaged feed, and feed storage containers on-farm, the most contaminated sampling site was the production line, and most of the positive samples were collected from a batch of nonmedicated feed produced immediately following processing of the medicated feed.[48] The type of feed and the composition of the veterinary drug are important factors determining the amount of carryover.[49] The electrostatic properties of some drugs, particularly those in powder form such as the sulfonamides and coccidiostats, cause them to adhere to equipment surfaces, making it very difficult to completely clean equipment between batches of feed.[25,36,50] Some manufacturers have responded to this problem by producing granular preparations with reduced electrostatic properties, and this has reduced but not completely eliminated problems with carryover of these drugs.

Thus feed cross-contamination can take place in a feed mixing plant where different feeds are produced on the same production line and pass through the main mixer. Several studies have shown that a completely contamination-free production of premixes and compound feeds in existing multiproduct plants is impossible in practice. Various process parameters and physiochemical characteristics of the product act together to determine the residual amount remaining in the circuit and hence the rate of cross-contamination from one feed batch to the subsequent batches in the same production line. High dusting potential, low product moisture, adherence due to electrostatic charge, as well as environmental conditions contribute to cross-contamination. An accumulation of feed material in filters and incomplete or inappropriate cleaning can lead to cross-contamination of these compounds into the next production batch. Also a high electrostatic loading potential, as well as higher product moisture can cause adhesions inside production plants and can result in cross-contamination.

The potential for cross-contamination from carryover of veterinary drugs occurs at different points throughout the production line, such as the main mixer, the surge bin, the bucket elevator, the holding bins, the pellet mill, the pellet cooler, and the holding bins, before loading onto the delivery trucks.[25,47,49]

Lynas et al.[51] reported that chlortetracycline was most frequently indentified contaminating antimicrobial, being detected in 15.2% of supposedly CTC-free feedingstuffs tested. The majority of the contaminating CTC concentrations were between 0% and 1% of the most frequent therapeutic inclusion rate in finished feeds (300 mg/kg). Przeniosło-Siwczyńska et al.[52] also found the presence of tetracycline antibiotics in many nonmedicated feed samples. Of the 186 tested feed samples, in 42 samples of nonmedicated feed, the authors confirmed the presence of tetracyclines. Doxycycline and chlortetracycline were found in a total of 31 (73.8%) samples. The levels of antibiotics ranged from 0.3 to 5 mg/kg. Low levels of contamination suggest cross-contamination during manufacturing in the feed mill or on the farm. Moreover, two feed samples contained doxycycline together with tylosin at concentrations of 7.9 and 10.9 mg/kg and 3.7 and 0.4 mg/kg, respectively, indicating either the illegal use of the antibiotics or cross-contamination. Kennedy et al.[29] investigated the occurrence of cross-contamination in poultry feed where monensin was the major coccidiostat for fattening chickens. Monensin, at levels in excess of 5% of the authorized dose for target animals (here approximately 110 mg/kg), was present in 22.5% of 40 samples of feed for nontarget animals. The prepelleting bins and the pelleting die were identified as the most likely reservoirs of contamination, and feed handling at the mill was changed accordingly. Subsequently, the number of feed batches containing more than 5% of the therapeutic dose of monensin dropped from 22.5% to 2.5%. The possible mechanisms by which cross-contamination nicarbazin at a feed mill may occur were explored by McEvoy.[25] The author examined three sequential batches of 3 tons each of nicarbazin-free feed produced after a batch which had contained nicarbazin at the statutory level of 125 mg/kg. Sampling was performed both before and after pelleting of the feed. It was observed that the first batch of feed produced after feed with nicarbazine contained 3.4 mg/kg of this substance before pelleting. Higher concentrations of nicarbazin up to 7.2 mg/kg were determined in the feed were found postpelleting—after 8 tons had passed through.

Cross-contamination may take place during the transport and unloading of the feed in the bin of the delivery truck during successive loading of feed into the same bin (intra-bin contamination). It may also take place in the transfer system, when traces of previously transported medicated feed remain in the conveyor screws and cross-contaminate the nonmedicated feed subsequently delivered to a farm.[47] To minimize the risk during feed delivery, the use of new trucks, the use of back bins to reduce the length of the circuit, and the careful flushing or cleaning after delivery are possible risk reduction measures.[47]

Cross-contamination is also possible at the farm level, where carryover of veterinary drugs can occur when nonmedicated feed is stored in close proximity to, or subsequently to, medicated feed. Cross-contamination may also occur during the distribution of the feed on the farm.[47] Raising the awareness of farmers and farm workers on safe feed handling is essential to avoid cross-contamination at the farm level that may adversely affect human and animal health and trade.

Currently, for antimicrobial substances in nonmedicated feed, they must not be present and there are no maximum level (ML) set for them. According to the Regulation of the European Parliament and of the Council 2019/4, maximum levels of cross-contamination of nontarget feeds with antimicrobial active substances and methods of their analysis in feed are to be indicated by January 28, 2023.

For coccidiostats maximum carryover levels in nontarget feeds have been established by Commission Regulation (EU) No. 574/2011.[53] For the purpose of enabling the feed manufacturer to manage unavoidable carryover, a carryover rate of approximately 3% of the authorized maximum content should be considered acceptable as regards feed for less sensitive nontarget animal species, while a carryover rate of approximately 1% of the authorized maximum content should be considered acceptable for feed intended to sensitive nontarget animal species and feed used for the period before slaughter. The carryover rate of 1% should also be considered acceptable for cross-contamination of other feed for target species to which no coccidiostats are added, and as regards nontarget feed for "continuous food-producing animals," such as dairy cows or laying hens, where there is evidence of transfer from feed to food of animal origin. The established limits for 11 coccidiostats are presented in Table 5.1.

TABLE 5.1 Maximum levels of coccidiostats in nontarget feeds due to unavoidable carryover in feeds.

Coccidiostat	1% carryover level for nontarget feeds (mg/kg)	3% carryover level for nontarget feeds (mg/kg)
Diclazuril	0.01	0.03
Decoquinate	0.40	1.20
Halofuginone	0.03	0.09
Lasalocid	1.25	3.75
Maduramicin	0.05	0.15
Monensin	1.25	3.75
Nicarbazin	1.25	3.75
Narasin	0.70	2.10
Robenidine	0.70	2.10
Semduramicin	0.25	0.75
Salinomycin	0.70	2.10

The carryover of 1% applies to feeds for sensitive species, continuous food-producing animals, and target species for the period before the slaughter; 3% carryover applies to feeds for all other nontarget species and categories of animals.

5.3.2 Toxicity to nontarget animal species

While there are clear examples of drugs that are toxic to animal species for which they are not approved or contraindicated to be mixed with other drugs, carryover of veterinary drugs and subsequent feed to food transfer is most significantly an international trade issue. Feed mixing errors and ingestion of feed formulated for other species are the most common means by which poisonings from man-made materials occur. There are many scientific reports on the toxic effects of low concentrations of tiamulin on nontarget animals when they are used with ionophore antibiotics. Ionophore feed additives and antibacterial agents are especially toxigenic to horses. Effects of ionophores in horses include clinical, clinicopathologic, and pathologic changes associated with cardiac, muscular, and neurologic tissues involvement. The acute effects of ionophores, however, can result in long-term cardiac dysfunction. Antibacterial effects are associated with changed microbial populations in the digestive tract that results in bacterial toxin liberation.[55] There are reports of interaction between ionophores and dihydroquinolone antioxidants, tiamulin, macrolide antibiotics, chloramphenicol, and sulfonamides. Tiamulin and macrolide antibiotics have been shown to inhibit the cytochrome P450 activity of several species, which may be involved in enhancing toxicity. Additionally, the interaction of tiamulin and monensin in pigs is minimized by concurrent administration of vitamin E and selenium. Meingassner et al.[56] concluded that tiamulin reduced metabolic degradation and extraction of monensin in chickens and led to an overdosing effect. Sakar et al.[57,58] demonstrated that tiamulin caused muscle damage reflected by the increasing level of related enzymes in blood serum in pigs, while administered with narasin or monensin, but withdrawal of both drugs reduced the enzymes to normal levels within a few days. Histological and ultrastuctural examination of muscle tissues in broiler after administration of lasalocid, monensin, maduramicin, salinomycin, or narasin with tiamulin revealed myopathies and cardiomyopathies.[59] Studies by Frigg et al.[60] indicate that sulfonamides increase the toxicity of monensin. Also the coadministration of chloramphenicol, erythromycin, oleandomycin, and furazolidone with monensin gave similar results. Therefore it is important to establish maximum levels of cross-contamination for nontarget feeds and control of feed contaminations with antibiotics and coccidiostats to protect animal health.

5.4 Antimicrobial residues in food derived from animals

For some time, increasing attention has been paid to the risk to consumers posed by chemical contaminants or residues in animal feed.[1]

Until very recently, concerns about residues revolved around allergic reactions and the possible adverse effects on the flora of the human gastrointestinal tract. In general, allergy to substances in food are rare, although there were confirmed cases of allergic reactions in sensitized individuals provoked by penicillin residue in milk,[61] hypersensitivity, cases of chronic urticaria, or fatal blood dyscrasia triggered by chloramphenicol residue in food. The adverse effect of antibiotic residues on the bacterial flora of the human intestinal tract is linked to selection for resistance or transfer of resistance. There is some scientific information on the point that most resistant enterobacteria in the human gut of untreated individuals come from bacterial contamination of raw foods.[61]

In many countries, governmental authorities have established monitoring programs to determine antibiotic levels in foods, as well as the maximum residue levels (MRLs).[62] EC[26] defines residues as "pharmacologically active substances (whether active principles, recipients, or degradation products) and their metabolites which remain in foodstuffs obtained from animals to which the veterinary medicinal products in question has been administered." After being administered to an animal body, most of the drugs are metabolized and excreted. In general, most of the parent product and its metabolites are excreted in urine and a lesser extent via feces. However, after excretion, a portion of the drugs may persist in milk, eggs, and meat for a certain period of time as residues.[63]

In animals, antibiotics are usually administered via feed, water, or parenterally. All routes of administration may result in residues of these drugs appearing in the tissues and organs of animals or be transferred to their products, that is milk, eggs, and honey. The presence of residues of veterinary drugs is believed to be the result of noncompliance with the withdrawal periods necessary for elimination of the drug from the animal's body, inappropriate drug administration, dosing inconsistent with the indications or their use in animal species for which they are not intended. Another reason for the presence of antibiotic residues is their arbitrary administration by breeders, without the supervision of a veterinarian, as well as accidental contamination of the feed, for example, after the production of medicated feed. Another reason for the presence of residues of antibacterial substances in food of animal origin may be uneven mixing of the medicinal premix with feed components, which affects the uptake of excessive doses of drugs by animals, mistakenly introducing another drug substance and deliberately or accidentally exceeding the drug dose.

One of the most frequently used groups of antibacterial substances in the production of medicated feed are tetracyclines. Their abuse in animal husbandry may cause allergic and toxic reactions in both animals and humans, and the acquisition of resistance to these antibiotics by pathogenic microorganisms.[64] In studies carried out in Germany by Vockel et al. in 2000–02, residues of tetracycline antibiotics were found in 58% of the samples tested. Among the identified substances there are, among others chlortetracycline, oxytetracycline, and tetracycline.[65] Piątkowska et al.[66] describes a case where illegally used antibiotics, that is Lasalocid, doxycycline, and enrofloxacin in laying hens. All of these therapeutic substances were banned for use in these animals. The reason for the presence of doxycycline and enrofloxacin in eggs was their use in the poultry watering system. Doxycycline is characterized by high ability to bind to proteins, including egg white, which always entails huge economic losses. All eggs in which the presence of antibiotic is found must be transferred for disposal.[66] In addition, tetracycline antibiotics, as well as other substances with amine groups (other drugs, natural food ingredients, plant protection products), have potential interactions with nitrates (III) and (V). This combination may lead to the formation of *N*-nitro compounds, showing a strong carcinogenic effect. Numerous studies indicate that most of the analyzed *N*-nitrosamines can cause cancer of the liver, esophagus, and nasal cavity. The carcinogenic effect occurs after prior activation in the course of metabolic processes, resulting in the formation of an active metabolite initiating the neoplastic process.[67] For example, Segato et al.[41] conducted studies in order to obtain information on the transfer of doxycycline to chicken tissues, when feed contaminated by this antibiotic at the level of 4 mg/kg is administered to poultry. Under the accepted experimental conditions, doxycycline achieved mean concentrations in each tissue (muscle, liver, kidney) lower than the determined MRL, but the analyte was present. This study showed the role played by feed; in the absence of withdrawal period contaminating drugs can pose a risk to the consumers due to the occurrence of residues. McEvoy et al.[37,68] fed concentrates containing sulfadiazine, sulfadimidine, or chlortetracycline at levels (250 mg/kg) normally used for treatment of pigs and poultry to dairy cattle for 21 days. Peak levels of sulfonamides in milk were in the range around 100 μg/L, which is the European MRL value for sulfonamides.[69]

In addition to tetracycline derivatives, other antibiotics, such as chloramphenicol and fluoroquinolones, were found in the meat of farm animals. This phenomenon applies in particular to aquaculture, mainly shrimp and salmon, conducted in South Asia and South America.[65]

The reason for the detection of fluoroquinolones in farm animals is their large-scale use in aquaculture, that is shrimp farms or salmon farms, and the increase in their use in farms of poultry, pigs, cattle, and companion animals (dogs, cats). Undoubtedly, this leads to an increase in resistance to fluoroquinolones, which is confirmed, among others, by epidemiological data from the United States.[65] Although fluoroquinolone antibacterial substances are not authorized in EU countries for use in feed and feed materials for farm animals, there are cases of low concentrations of these chemotherapeutic agents in feed. Due to inadequate practice, these drugs may not be effective at managing infections in humans.

Several publications provide research results for egg and milk contamination with coccidiostats. For example, van Rhijn et al.[70] investigated the excretion of nicarbazin into dairy milk after administration of feeds containing nicarbazin at concentrations of 1, 5, and 12.5 mg/kg. Some body fat samples were also analyzed after the completion of the study. No nicarbazin was detected by the authors, indicating that carryover of nicarbazin from feed to milk is not a very likely process. Similarly, Bagg et al.[71] was unable to find detectable monensin residue in lactating Holsteins receiving up to 4865 mg monensin per day. Depletion studies on the coccidiostats toltrazuril and halofuginone were described by Mulder et al.,[72] showing that these drugs (and ponazuril, a metabolite of toltrazuril) preferentially partitioned into the yolk. Chickens given a medicated feed containing 3 mg/kg halofuginone exhibited a maximum egg concentration of 450 μg/kg, with rapid depletion once treatment was terminated.

Excessive and unjustified use of antibacterial substances (antibiotics, sulfonamides, and quinolones) and coccidiostats in the treatment of livestock diseases may lead to the formation of resistant microorganisms of the antibacterial substances and to the presence of their residues in food of animal origin. The presence of antibiotic residues in food materials is considered to be a problem for human health, as some of these residues are associated in some cases with allergic reactions, imbalance of intestinal microbiota, and development of antibacterial resistance.

5.5 Antimicrobial resistance

In general, antimicrobial resistance (AMR) is the capacity of a microorganism to resist the growth inhibitory or killing activity of an antimicrobial beyond the normal susceptibility of the specific bacterial species.[73] Antimicrobials comprise antibiotics, as well as any substances that have a growth inhibiting or killing effect on microorganisms. The discovery of antibiotics was a real breakthrough in the treatment of bacterial diseases, and their introduction to treat infectious diseases revolutionized medicine. However, after more than 70 years of antibiotic therapy, both in human and veterinary medicine, we encounter more and more infections that are difficult to treat or refrain from conventional therapy. This is mainly due to the constant increase in the presence of antibiotic-resistant microorganisms in the environment. The widespread use of antibiotics in human medicine, as well as in veterinary medicine and in animal production and other areas of agriculture, has resulted in increasing antibiotic resistance among pathogenic bacteria, which has created a major threat to the effectiveness of these drugs in the treatment of infectious diseases. Changes in the types of bacterial resistance to antimicrobial drugs result from the emergence of new mechanisms or from the ever-increasing selection of bacteria as a result of the extensive use of antibiotics. It should be emphasized that AMR is a natural biological phenomenon that is influenced by many factors, including human activity. The selective environmental pressure associated with the widespread and inadequately controlled use of antibiotics enables the adaptation and survival of bacteria bearing antibiotic resistance genes. One of the important ways of transferring antibiotic-resistant bacteria is direct contacts between healthy animals and animals carrying antibiotic-resistant bacteria and the environment (soil, water) contaminated with these bacteria. Moreover, food can be contaminated with antimicrobial-resistant bacteria and/or AMR genes in several ways. A first way is the presence of antibiotic-resistant bacteria on food selected by the use of antibiotics during agricultural production,[73] because, as is known modern food animal production uses large amounts of antibiotics for disease control. This provides favorable conditions for selection, spread, and persistence of antimicrobial-resistant bacteria capable of causing infections in animals and humans. Unlike in human medicine, antibiotics in food-producing animals are used for three different purposes: (1) treatment of bacterial infections, (2) prevention and control, and (3) in feed to promote growth.[54] Due to concerns over AMR, the use of antimicrobials for growth promotion has been greatly reduced.

Various scientific studies support the hypothesis of a link between the use of antibiotics during animal production and AMR of human pathogens. Especially, the use of subtherapeutic doses in healthy animals for prophylaxis and growth promotion, coupled with imprecise dosages given to ill and healthy animals (by delivery of antibacterials through feed or water), facilitates AMR through selection.

In antimicrobial treatment of animals, some practices may exert greater selective pressures for resistance than others. There are considerable evidences that antimicrobial use in animals selects for resistance in commensals and in zoonotic enteropathogens. For instance, feeding animals growth promoters, which entails exposing bacteria to sublethal concentrations of drugs over long periods, would appear conducive to selecting and maintaining resistant organisms. Many in-feed medications are administered at comparatively low concentrations to animals for weeks and often for years in successive generations of animals. Such uses of subtherapeutic drugs lead to development of resistance; considerable selection pressure may be applied when animals are treated in that way. Moreover, many antimicrobials are administered at higher doses in feed or water to herds or flocks for prophylactic or metaphylactic purposes.

Several studies describe by Cogliani et al.[74] established a direct relation between the low-doses and nontherapeutic administration of antibiotics in farm animals and the emergence and spread of resistance genes. It is also proved that the antibiotic resistance patterns in humans is determined by the same mechanism as in animals and that the dissemination of the resistance genes occurs from the food chain to the intestinal flora of humans but also via direct contact with animals.[75]

The role of antimicrobial use as a selective pressure for the emergence and maintenance of resistance in bacterial populations has been widely recognized.[76] The study conducted by Gibbons et al. provided data on the occurrence of AMR of fecal *Escherichia coli* isolates from pig farms as a consequence the use of four antimicrobial classes in-feed (penicillins, aminoglycosides/aminocyclitols, trimethoprim-sulfonamides, and tetracyclines). The study revealed that the use of sulfonamide and tetracycline antimicrobials on farms was a predictor of resistance to members of their respective antimicrobial classes. But more importantly, the use of related aminocyclitol antibiotic spectinomycin was a predictor of resistance to gentamicin, a critically important antibiotic in human medicine.

In animals AMR in zoonotic enteropathogens (e.g., *Salmonella*, *Campylobacter*, *Yersinia*, and some strains of *E. coli*, such as serotype O157:H7) and commensals (e.g., enterococci, most generic *E. coli*) is of special concern to human health, because these bacteria are most likely to be transferred through the food chain to humans, or resistance genes in commensal bacteria may be transferred to the zoonotic enteropathogens.[77]

The concern about resistance in enterococci and the emergence of vancomycin-resistant enterococci (VRE) was roused after detection of vancomycin-resistant Enterococcus *faecium* in pigs and poultry being fed an antibiotic called avoparcin, a growth promoter chemically related to the glycopeptide antibiotic vancomycin. This finding provoked the debate about role of animal use of avoparcin in the development of VRE in man. There is strong evidence that one type of the (vanA) developed in animals fed avoparcin.[78,79] Transfer of resistant bacteria to humans from animals fed with avoparcin has also been described.[78–80]

Other types of antibiotic resistance reported in enterococcal isolates from animals include resistance to the macrolide-lincosamide-streptogramin group, to tylosin[81] and to virginiamycin. For example, the use of animal feed supplemented with tylosin resulted in the development of erythromycin-resistant streptococci and staphylococci not only in the animals but also in their caretakers.[82] Whereas, bacteria resistant to streptogramin, quinupristin, and dalfopristin were found in turkeys that had been given virginiamycin.[83]

Thus, in feeding experiments it has been shown that the use of enrofloxacin, tetracycline, and tylosin in different concentrations will select for resistance among both intestinal and skin bacteria.[81]

Antibiotics in feed can spur the spread of resistance by promoting new genetic mutations as well as by promoting the transfer among gut bacteria of resistance genes through phages.

Several potential risks arise from cross-contamination of negative feeds, both to animals and to consumers:

1. Unexpected antibiotics in feedingstuffs could interact with other medical agents administered to animals. Therefore a therapeutic failure might be observed associated with economic losses for the producer.
2. A mixture of medicated and nonmedicated feeds could prompt subtherapeutic concentrations of antimicrobials in feed, creating an ideal scenario for the induction and transfer of antibiotic-resistance mechanisms. In this way, these antimicrobials could become ineffective against animals' pathologies and the resistance mechanisms could even be spread, contributing to reduce effectiveness of human medical treatments.
3. Moreover, these unintentional antimicrobials in feed could enter the food chain (eggs, milk, meat, etc.) since withdrawal times will not be followed. Researchers have proved that low levels of cross-contamination (2 mg of sulfonamides/kg of feed) can be significantly involved in the presence of residues in animal tissues. In certain circumstances, residues of antimicrobials above MRL could even be found in foods of animal origin. The detection of these illegal products by control mechanisms (self-management plans, official controls, analysis in industries) could give rise to considerable economic losses for the producer and legal issues. In the worst case scenario, these contaminated foods could elude control barriers, reaching the consumer and could be linked to allergic reactions of toxicity in sensitized individuals. However, it is generally assumed that their main risk is the development of antibiotic resistance mechanisms in human pathogens.

Unfortunately, antibiotics are used not only in medicine and to treat food animals, but also to prevent animals from diseases and to promote their growth (AGPs). These applications and misuse of antibiotics have resulted in the development and spread of antibiotic resistance, which causes treatment failures. This has important consequences for public health, as resistance genes can be passed on to people. The magnitude of the problem is illustrated by the fact that more than 25,000 people in the EU Member States die each year from infections caused by antibiotic-resistant bacteria. The EC launched a public consultation on the delegated act establishing the draft criteria for the designation of antimicrobials to be reserved for the treatment of certain infections in humans. The EC will use these criteria to establish a list of antimicrobials to be reserved for use in humans as part of its legislation on veterinary medicinal products. Interested stakeholders have until April 23, 2021 to respond to the consultation.

5.6 Antimicrobial drugs: impact on the environment

Antibiotics are not completely metabolized in the bodies of animals; a high percentage of administered drugs is discharged into water and soil through animal manure, sewage sludge, and biosolids.[84] After administration of antibiotics between 30% and 90% of the initial dose given is excreted as active metabolites or as nonmetabolized form. Therefore high concentrations of antibiotics and/or their metabolites can be present in urine or feces.[85] In general, a high percent of the initial dose administrated is excreted unchanged (more than 60%); therefore in general, antimicrobials are excreted by human and animals as active and/or inactive metabolites.[86] For example, *N*4-acetylosulfonamides which are the metabolites of sulfonamides are less active compared to the parent drugs. On the other hand, ciprofloxacin is the metabolite of enrofloxacin which is also antimicrobially active.[87]

Livestock feces and liquid manure are used as land fertilizers for its high levels of phosphorus, nitrogen, and organic matter that can improve the physical and chemical properties of soil and provide essential nutrients to plants.[88] Application of manure as fertilizer is a common practice in many countries including EU countries. Residues of antibiotics excreted and present in the animal manures/feces enter to the environment either by spreading of livestock wastes onto agricultural fields as fertilizer or in the form of sludge after manure collection and storage. Antibiotics present in manures/feces can be a risk for human and the environment.[85] The problem of environmental pollution with antibacterial substances present in organic fertilizers (liquid manure, pig, and poultry feces) is becoming more and more recognizable in the world. In recent years, researchers have published several papers demonstrating that antibiotics in feces derived from slaughtered animals are present in high concentrations. In China, organic fertilizers from chickens were analyzed. Researchers found high concentrations of enrofloxacin and norfloxacin of 1420 and 225 mg/kg, respectively. In 2007 Martinzez-Carballo and colleagues examined pig droppings in Austria, in which they found the presence of antibiotics from the tetracycline group in amounts of several dozen grams per kilogram of feces (tetracycline—23 mg/kg, oxytetracycline—29 mg/kg, and chlorotetracycline—46 mg/kg).[89] The lack of information on the concentration of antibiotic residues in manure applied to agricultural land, with or without processing, are necessary to conduct an adequate environmental risk assessment of veterinary drugs.[88] According to Berendsen and coworkers[90] analyzing antibiotics in animal feces can help to have knowledge on the dispersion of antibiotics in the environment and their ecotoxicological effects. The study may provide an answer on the emergence of bacterial resistance in the intestines of animals, and thus be a valuable source of information on the relationship between antibiotic residues and bacterial resistance.

Scientists have long been aware of potential problems from the presence of antibiotics in soil. Determined antibiotic concentrations in soil matrices have ranged from a few nanograms to milligrams per kilogram of soil. The highest concentrations are usually found in areas treated with manure or used for livestock. The concentrations of oxytetracycline and chlortetracycline in some agricultural lands may reach extremely high levels. In studies conducted by Hamscher et al.[91] in Germany in the years 2000–01, they confirmed the presence of tetracyclines in the soil at a concentration of up to 300 μg/kg of soil, indicating that this class of antibiotics used worldwide is persistent and can accumulate in the soil after fertilization with manure from intensive animal husbandry. The conducted research did not show any evidence that these compounds move to deeper layers of the earth or groundwater due to the strong sorption of this group of drugs in the soil. In Italy and the United States of America, field studies have confirmed the presence of tetracyclines in soil following the application of slurry. In a study by researchers from Turkey, all samples of soil fertilized with slurry from pig farms showed the presence of oxytetracycline at the maximum concentration of 500 μg/kg of soil. On the other hand, in the studies conducted by Huang et al.[92] in agricultural areas of China, including two groups of chemotherapeutic agents (fluoroquinolones and tetracyclines) in soils fertilized with slurry obtained from pig farms, tetracycline, oxytetracycline, chlortetracycline, ciprofloxacin, enrofloxacin, and ofloxacin were found. The highest concentrations were reported for enrofloxacin (637.3 μg/kg) and chlortetracycline (2668.9 μg/kg).

Elevated concentrations of antibacterial substances in the soil selects for preferential outgrowth of antibiotic-resistant bacteria, which results in changes to antibiotics sensitivity of entire microbial populations.[93–96] Even very low concentrations of antibacterial substances in the soil creates conditions for genetic changes in bacterial genomes and transfer of antibiotic resistance genes and associated mobile genetic elements, such as plasmids, transposons, and genomic islands, between and among microbial populations.[97–99] Autochthonous bacteria in soil may also represent a reservoir of resistance genes in the environment that can be transferred to the bacteria that colonize the human body.[100] Moreover, soil microorganisms perform many vital processes and participate in the maintenance of soil health and quality. Many microorganisms act as biological control agents by inhibiting the growth of pathogens. The high antimicrobial activity of antibiotics in soil should differentially inhibit the growth of soil microorganisms and thus influence the soil microbial community composition, which may result in alterations of the ecological functionality of the soil. Antibacterial substances can also influence nitrification and/or denitrification rates for bacteria in soil. For example, sulfadimethoxine inhibited soil nitrification. A study by DeVries et al.[101] revealed that low doses of sulfamethoxazole, sulfadiazine, narasin, or gentamicin inhibited denitrification. Antibacterial substances may also change the turnover rate of iron in soil. For example, sulfadiazine and monensin blocked Fe(III) reduction in soil.[102] Antibacterial substances can also influence the inhibition of enzyme activity in soil. It may be related to inhibition of growth or death of sensitive microorganisms in soil.[103] Environmental antibacterial substances pollution from food production animals is a problem that is expected to gain more attention because the use of antibiotics in these animals is one of the ways of environmental pollution, and animal feces should also be investigated prior to their introduction into farmland and soil in which have been introduced in animal feces to limit the transfer of antimicrobial substances to the environment.

5.7 Analytical methodology

Chromatographic methods play a dominant role in the study of antimicrobial substances in feed. One of the first methods used for detection and determination of antibacterial substances was thin layer chromatography (TLC). This method is characterized by high specificity and simplicity, but does not allow the analysis of low concentrations of antibiotics in feed. TLC was used in the 1980s and 1990s for the simultaneous determination of several antibiotics belonging to one chemical group in feed[104,105] Liquid chromatography plays an important role in determining the presence of antimicrobial substances in feed. Since the 1980s, ultraviolet (UV) and fluorescent detectors have been used.[106–108] Then diode array detectors were introduced into the analytical technique, giving greater possibilities of identifying the tested compounds, as they allow to distinguish substances based on their UV spectra. However, the greatest possibilities are offered by the combination of chromatographic techniques with mass spectrometry. The introduction of tandem mass spectrometry, that is the MS-MS system, significantly increases the sensitivity of analytical methods and facilitates the confirmation of the presence of analytes.[109] One of the most sensitive techniques is high-resolution mass spectrometry (HRMS), used for confirmation purposes.[110] Hence, in recent years there has been an increasing number of studies on methods for the determination of antibiotics in feed, based on the technique of liquid chromatography with mass spectrometry.[111,112]

In scientific literature we can find some chromatographic methods for analyzing antibiotics in feeds such as fluoroquinolones[113], macrolides,[114] tetracyclines,[115–117] sulfonamides,[118] and phenicols[119,120] but multiclass residue methods for the analysis of antimicrobial agents in nontarget feed are still rare because of the analytical challenges that have to be overcome. These challenges are based on the complex composition of feed matrices and the several chemical groups (physical—-chemical properties) of the different veterinary drugs.[110,112,121] Only few methods can be found in the scientific literature that allow the analysis of over a dozen or several dozen antibacterial substances at carryover level in nontarget feeds. One of these methods was developed by Boscher et al.[112] who reported a methodology for the analysis of 33 analytes from 14 groups of antibiotics (including tetracyclines, quinolones, penicillins, ionophore coccidiostats, macrolides, and sulfonamides) with the use high-performance liquid chromatograph - tandem mass spectrometry with quantification limits ranging from 3 to 65 μg/kg for all analyzed antibacterial substances. Also in 2010 Cronly et al.[121] published another multiclass method that employ HPLC-MS/MS for the confirmation of 14 prohibited medicinal additives in pig and poultry feed (including sulfonamides, nitroimidazole, coccidiostats, oligosaccharides, macrolides, streptogramins, phenicols, carbadox, and dinitolimide). Patyra et al.[122] published a method for the determination of residues of 11 antibacterial substances from different therapeutic classes (β-lactams, lincosamides, fluoroquinolones, macrolides, pleuromutilins, and sulfonamides) in animals. For the extraction of antibacterial substances from feed samples, authors used 0.1% formic acid in acetonitrile. Separation of the analytes was performed on biphenyl column with a gradient of 0.1% formic acid in acetonitrile and 0.1% formic acid in Milli-Q water. Borras et al.[111] developed another multiclass method which also employs HPLC-MS/MS for the identification of amphenicols, quinolones, sulfonamides, benzimidazoles, coccidiostats, polipeptides, macrolides, lincosamides, tetracyclines, nitrofurans, pleuromutilin, and trimethoprim in animal feeds with quantification limits ranging from 0.2 to 238.1 μg/kg. On the other hand, Kaklamanos et al.[110] published a protocol for analyzing 48 antibacterial agents in pig feeds (quinolones, sulfonamides, tetracyclines, coccidiostats, macrolides, and lincosamides) employing HPLC coupled to orbitrap mass spectrometry.

Several screening and/or confirmation methods have been developed to quantify coccidiostats in meat, eggs, and feed samples. An ELISA screening test has been set up for coccidiostats in eggs and muscle,[123] and individual methods have been developed to quantify halofuginone, robenidine, diclazuril, lasalocid sodium, nicarbazin, or narasin in feed by HPLC—UV spectrofluorimetry.[124–126] Many works have also led to multiresidue methods allowing quantification of several coccidiostats, with LC—MS/MS as an analytical tool[39,40,127–129]

Moretti et al.[127] developed a method for the determination of 11 regulated coccidiostats including the ionophore antibiotics lasalocid, maduramicin, monensin, narasin, salinomycin, and semduramicin and the chemical coccidiostats decoquinate, diclazuril, halofuginone, nicarbazin, and robenidine in animal feed. The analytes were determined by LC—MS/MS in the positive or negative electrospray ionization mode. Samples were extracted with methanol and concentrated up before filtering through a 0.22 μm filter. The method performance characteristics were estimated in the relevant application field from 0.003 to 200 mg/kg. A method by Vincent et al. allowed for the analysis of the six ionophore coccidiostats by LC—MS/MS. Purification was done by solid phase extraction and quantification was by matrix-matched standards or by standard addition.[129] Cronly et al.,[130] for the determination of 11 coccidiostats, proposed extraction of coccidiostats from feed sample with water and acetonitrile with the addition of anhydrous magnesium sulfate and sodium chloride. The extract then undergoes a freezing out step before being diluted and injected onto the LC—MS/MS system. Pietruk and coworkers in 2015 a published method also for determination 11 coccidiostats in feed; they used 1% ammonium solution in methanol and performed liquid chromatograph - tandem mass spectrometry (LC-MS/MS) analysis.

Due to increasing sensitivity of analytical methodology the analytical limits of detection and quantification of veterinary drug residues are continuously being lowered. That means that more and more substances which could not be detected a few years ago can now be detected at lower concentrations. The development and implementation of new analytical methods are an important aspect in order to protect animal and human health and environment, and they should be constantly improved and developed, depending on the analytical capabilities of laboratories conducting research in the field of safety of the entire food chain.

5.8 Research gaps and future directions

The food system, from production to consumption and waste, has a big impact on the environment, health, and food safety. With the so-called "farm-to-fork strategy" presented on May 20, 2020, the EC intends to build a sustainable EU food system ensuring food security and protecting animals, people, and the environment. In this respect, the setting of limits has been a significant progress cross-contamination of feed with coccidiostats, which has been regulated by the EU Commission Regulation No. 574/2011.[53] It is expected that such legislation will also be introduced for nontarget contamination of feed with antibiotics, sulfonamides and quinolones, as the term "zero tolerance" is now in place for antibiotics in feed, which is difficult to achieve for feed mills producing medicated feed and feed without antibiotics on the same technological lines.

It is known that, as a result of the excessive and inappropriate use of antibiotics, especially in the animal husbandry process (antibiotics for prophylaxis and as growth promoters), and insufficient infection control practices in the treatment of both humans and animals, AMR has become a serious threat. Therefore an important aspect in the protection of animal and human health is the release of antibacterial substances for exclusive use in human and veterinary medicine. This is to protect public health and to reduce the selection of antibiotic-resistant microorganisms.

The Draft European Parliament Resolution on the European One Health Action Plan to combat AMR aims to reduce the use of antimicrobial substances by 50% by 2030, maintaining the effectiveness of treating infections in humans and animals, reducing the occurrence and spread of AMR, as well as faster development and availability of new effective antimicrobials, both inside and outside the EU.

In addition, further progress is needed in the development of new, reliable, and sensitive analytical methods for the determination of the presence of antimicrobial substances in feed and food of animal origin in order to control compliance with the established limits for feed and food contamination with these substances.

References

1. Leeman WR, Van Den Berg KJ, Houben GF. Transfer of chemicals from feed to animal products: the use of transfer factors in risk assessment. *Food Addit Contam.* 2007;24(1):1–13.
2. Commission of the European Communities. *White Paper on Food Safety*. Brussels; 12 January 2000.
3. Jukes TH, Stokstad LR, Taylor RR, Combs TJ, Edwards HM, Meadows GB. Growth promoting effect of aureomycin on pigs. *Arch Biochem.* 1950;26:324–330.
4. Butaye P, Devriese LA, Haesebrouck F. Antimicrobial growth promoters used in animal feed: effects of less well known antibiotics on Gram-positive bacteria. *Clin Microbiol Rev.* 2003;16(2):175–188.
5. Gustafson RH, Bowen RE. Antibiotic use in animal agriculture. *J Appl Microbiol.* 1997;83:531–541.
6. Jukes TH, Williams WL. Nutritional effects of antibiotics. *Pharmacol Rev.* 1953;5:381–420.
7. Stokstad ELR, Jukes TH. Further observation on the "Animal Protein Factor.". *Exp Biol Med.* 1950;73:523–528.
8. Dibner JJ, Richards JD. Antibiotic growth promoters in agriculture: historic and mode of action. *Poult Sci.* 2005;84:634–643.
9. Pejsak Z, Truszczyński M. Konsekwencje zakazu stosowania antybiotykowych stymulatorów wzrostu. *Życie Wet.* 2006;81:236–239.
10. Phillips J, Casewall M, Cox T, et al. Does the use of antibiotics in food animals pose a risk to human health? A critical review of published data. *J Antimicrob Chemother.* 2004;53:28–52.
11. Bedford MR. Removal of antibiotic growth promoters from poultry diets: implications and strategies to minimise subsequent problems. *World Poult Sci J.* 2000;56(4):347–365.
12. Ewing WN, Cole DJA. *The Living Gut: An Introduction to Microorganisms in Nutrition*. Dungannon: Context; 1994.
13. Chattopadhyay MK. Use of antibiotics as feed additives: a burning question. *Front Microbiol.* 2014;5. Available from: https://doi.org/10.3389/fmicb.2014.00334.
14. Council Directive of 23 November 1970 concering additives in feeding-stuffs (70/524/EEC). *Official Journal of the European Communities;* 1970.
15. Swann Report. Use of antibiotics in animal husbandry and veterinary medicine. HC Deb 20 November; 791: 1525–1531; 1969.
16. Corpet DE. Microbiological hazard for humans of antimicrobial growth promotor use in animal production. *Rev Med Vet.* 1996;147:851–862.
17. Clarke L, Fodey TL, Crooks SR, et al. A review of coccidiostats and the analysis of their residues in meat and other food. *Meat Sci.* 2014;97:358–374.
18. Annunziata L, Visciano P, Stramenga A, et al. Determination of regulatory ionophore coccidiostat residues in feedstuffs at carry-over levels by liquid chromatography-mass spectrometry. *PLoS One.* 2017;12:e0182831. Available from: https://doi.org/10.1371/journal.pone.0182831.
19. Chapman HD. Milestones in avian coccidiosis research: a review. *Poult Sci.* 2014;93:501–511.
20. European Commission. Regulation (EC) No 1831/2003 of the European Parliament and of the Council of 22 September 2003 on additives for use in animal nutrition. <https://eur-lex.europa.eu/legal-content/EN/TXT/?uri = CELEX%3A32003R1831>; 2003.
21. Roila R, Branciari R, Staccini B, et al. Contribution of vegetables and cured meat to dietary nitrate and nitrite intake in Italian population: safe level for cured meat controversial role of vegetables. *Ital J Food Saf.* 2018;7:7692. Available from: https://doi.org/10.4081/ijfs.2018.7692.
22. Council Directive 95/69/EC of 22 December 1995 laying down the conditions and arrangements for approving and registering certain establishments and intermediaries operating in the animal feed sector and amending Directives 70/524/EEC, 74/63/EEC, 79/373/EEC and 82/471/EEC. <https://eur-lex.europa.eu/legal-content/EN/ALL/?uri = celex:31995L0069>;1995.
23. European Commission. Regulation (EC) No 183/2005 of the European Parliament and of the Council of 12 January 2005 laying down requirements for feed hygiene. <https://eur-lex.europa.eu/legal-content/EN/ALL/?uri = CELEX%3A32005R0183>; 2005.
24. European Commission. Regulation (EU) 2019/4 of the European Parliament and of the Council of 11 December 2018 on the manufacture, placing on the market and use of medicated feed, amending Regulation (EC) No 183/2005 of the European Parliament and of the Council and repealing Council Directive 90/167/EEC; 2018.
25. McEvoy JDG. Contamination of animal feedingstuffs as a cause of residues in food: a review of regulatory aspects, incidence and control. *Anal Chim Acta.* 2002;473:3–26.
26. European Commission Directorate General for Health and Consumers Evaluation of the EU Legislative Framework in the Field of Medicated Feed; 2010.
27. Davis JL, Smith GW, Baynes RE, Tell LA, Webb AI, Riviere JE. Update on drugs prohibited from extralabel use in food animals. *J Am Vet Med Assoc.* 2009;235(5):528–534.

28. Grignon-Boutet R, Ireland MJ, Adewoye L, Mehrotra M, Russell S, Alexander I. Health Canada's policy on extra-label drug use in food-producing animals in Canada. *Can Vet J.* 2009;49(7):689–693.
29. Kennedy D, Smyth WG, Hewitt SA, McEvoy JD. Monensin carry-over into unmedicated broiler feeds. *Analyst.* 1998;123(12):2529–2533.
30. Harner JP, Herrman TJ, Falk J, Behnke K. *Avoiding Drug Carryover During Feed Processing and Delivery.* Manhattan, KS: Kansas State University Extension Beef Cattle Resource Committee. <www/iowabeefcenter.org/bch/AvoidingDrugCarryover.pdf>; 1996.
31. Pietruk K, Olejnik M, Posyniak A. Coccidiostats in milk: development of a multi-residue method and transfer of salinomycin and lasalocid from contaminated feed. *Food Addit Contam A.* 2018;35(8):1508–1518.
32. Vandenberge V, Delezie E, Huyghebaert G, Delahaut P, Daeseleire E, Croubels S. Residues of sulfadiazine and doxycycline in broiler liver and muscle tissue due to cross-contamination of feed. *Food Addit Contam A.* 2012;29(2):180–188.
33. Doonan GR, Brown CM, Mullaney TP, Brooks DB, Ulmanis EG, Slanker MR. Monensin poisoning in horses – an international incident. *Can Vet J.* 1989;30(2):165–169.
34. Association of American Feed Control Officials (AAFCO). *AAFCO Feed Inspector's Manual.* Champaign, IL: AAFCO. <http://www.aafco.org/Portals/0/SiteContent/Publications/AAFCO_Feed_Inspectors_Manual_7th_ed.pdf>; 2017.
35. Danaher M, Shanahan C, Butler F, et al. Risk-based approach to developing a national residue sampling plan for testing under European Union regulation for veterinary medicinal products and coccidiostat feed additives in domestic animal production. *Food Addit Contam A Chem Anal Control Expo Risk Assess.* 2016;33(7):1155–1165.
36. Dorne JL, Fernandez-Cruz ML, Bertelsen U, et al. Risk assessment of coccidostatics during feed cross-contamination: animal and human health aspects. *Toxicol Appl Pharmacol.* 2013;270(3):196–208.
37. McEvoy JD, Mayne CS, Higgins HC, Kennedy DG. Transfer of sulphamethazine from contaminated dairy feed to cows' milk. *Vet Rec.* 1999;144(17):470–475.
38. Mitchell JM, Griffiths MW, McEwen SA, McNab WB, Yee AJ. Antimicrobial drug residues in milk and meat: causes, concerns, prevalence, regulations, tests, and test performance. *J Food Prot.* 1998;61(6):742–756.
39. Olejnik M, Szprengier-Juszkiewicz T, Jedziniak P. Distribution of semduramicin in hen eggs and tissues after administration of cross-contaminated feed. *Food Addit Contam A.* 2014;31(8):1393–1398.
40. Olejnik M, Szprengier-Juszkiewicz T. Deposition and depletion of decoquinate in eggs after administration of cross-contaminated feed. *Food Addit Contam A.* 2015;32(7):1124–1128.
41. Segato G, Benetti C, Angeletti R, Montesissa C, Biancotto G. Doxycycline and sulfadimethoxine transfer from cross-contaminated feed to chicken tissues. *Food Addit Contam A.* 2011;28(7):860–868.
42. Tkacikova S, Kozarova I, Macanga J, Levkut M. Determination of lasalocid residues in the tissues of broiler chickens by liquid chromatography-tandem mass spectrometry. *Food Addit Contam A.* 2012;29(5):76176–76179.
43. Vandenberge V, Delezie E, Huyghebaert G, et al. Residues of sulfadiazine and doxycycline in egg matrices due to cross-contamination in the feed of laying hens and the possible correlation with physicochemical, pharmacokinetic and physiological parameters. *Food Addit Contam A.* 2012;29(6):908–917.
44. Heberer T, Lahrssen-Wiederholt M, Schafft H, et al. Zero tolerances in food and animal feed – are there any scientific alternatives? A European point of view on an international controversy. *Toxicol Lett.* 2007;175(1–3):118–135. Available from: https://eur-lex.europa.eu/legal-content/EN/TXT/?uri = CELEX%3A32019R0004.
45. Pinotti L, Bellagamba F, Paratte R, Savoini G, Dell'orto V. Detection of cross-contamination in feedstuffs: presence of constituents of animal origin. *Vet Res Commun.* 2003;27(suppl 1):655–658.
46. FAO and IFIF. Good practices for the feed industry – implementing the codex alimentarius code of practice on good animal feeding. In: *FAO Animal Production and Health Manual*, No. 9. Rome; 2010.
47. Filippitzi ME, Sarrazin S, Imberechts H, Smet A, Dewulf J. Risk of cross-contamination due to the use of antimicrobial medicated feed throughout the trail of feed from the feed mill to the farm. *Food Addit Contam A.* 2016;33(4):644–655.
48. Annunziata L, Visciano P, Stramenga A, et al. Investigation of nonionophoric coccidiostat residues in feed as a consequence of carryover. *J Food Prot.* 2018;81(3):482–489.
49. Stolker AA, Manti V, Zuidema T, et al. Carry-over of veterinary drugs from medicated to non-medicated feeds in commercial feed manufacturing plants. *Food Addit Contam A.* 2013;30(6):1100–1107.
50. Kennedy DG, Cannavan A, Mccracken RJ. Regulatory problems caused by contamination, a frequently overlooked cause of veterinary drug residues. *J Chromatogr A.* 2000;882(1–2):37–52.
51. Lynas L, Currie D, McCaughey WJ, McEvoy JDG, Kennedy DG. Contamination of animals feedingstuffs with undeclared antimicrobial additives. *Food Addit Contam.* 1998;15(2):162–170.
52. Przenioslo-Siwczyńska M, Patyra E, Grelik A, Chyłek-Purchała M, Kozak B, Kwiatek K. Contamination of animal feed with undeclared tetracyclines—confirmatory analysis by liquid chromatography–mass spectrometry after microbiological plate test. *Molecules.* 2020;25(9). Available from: https://doi.org/10.3390/molecules25092162.
53. Commission Regulation (EU) No 574/2011 of 16 June 2011 amending Annex I to Directive 2002/32/EC of the European Parliament and of the Council as regards maximum levels for nitrite, melamine, *Ambrosia* spp. and carry-over of certain coccidiostats and histomonostats and consolidating Annexes I and II thereto Text with EEA relevance. <https://eur-lex.europa.eu/legal-content/EN/TXT/?uri = CELEX:32011R0574>; 2011.
54. Schwarz S, Chaslus-Dancla. Use of antimicrobials in veterinary medicine and mechanisms of resistance. *Vet Res.* 2001;32:201–225.
55. Hall JO. Toxic feed constituents in the horse. *Vet Clin North Am Equine Pract.* 2001;17(3):479–489.
56. Meingassner JG, Schmook FP, Czok R, Mieth H. Enhancement of the anticoccidial activity of polyether antibiotics in chickens by tiamulin. *Poult Sci.* 1979;58:308–313.
57. Sakar D, Belèiæ Z, Blagoviæ S, Pompe-Gotal J. Narasin toxicity in pigs and its incompatibility with tiamulin. *Vet Arch.* 1991;5:269–281.

58. Sakar D, Pompe-Gotal J, Belèiæ Z, Blagoviæ S, Kanižaj V. Effect of therapeutic level of tiamulin on higher toxicity of monensin in weaned pigs. *Vet Arch.* 1991;2:67–82.
59. Madej JA, Mazurkiewicz M, Kuryszko J, Gawel A. Histological and ultrastructural examination of muscles in broilers administered tiamulin together with ionophoric anticoccidials. *Arch Vet Pol.* 1993;33:5–17.
60. Frigg M, Broz J, Weber G. Compatibility studies of ionophore anticoccidials with various antibiotics and chemotherapeutics in broiler chicks. *Arch Geflügelkd.* 1983;47:213–220.
61. Barton MD. Antibiotic use in animal feed and its impact on human health. *Nutr Res Rev.* 2000;13:279–299.
62. Ramirez A, Gutierrez R, Diaz G, et al. High-performance thin-layer chromatography-bioautography for multiple antibiotic residues in cow's milk. *J Chromatogr B.* 2003;784(2):315–322.
63. Sachi S, Ferdous J, Sikder MH, Hussani SMAK. Antibiotic residue in milk: past, present and future. *J Adv Vet Anim Res.* 2019;6 (3):315–332.
64. Patyra E, Kwiatek K. Stosowanie i kontrola laboratoryjna tetracyklin w paszach leczniczych. *Pasze Przem.* 2015;3–4:66–73.
65. Mersch-Sundermann V, Stein J. Szkodliwe działanie zanieczyszczeń żywności i pozostałości występujących w produktach spożywczych. In: Bronkowska M, red. nauk., *Wybrane Zagadnienia z Zakresu Toksykologii Żywności Oraz Wpływu Pokarmu na Farmakoterapię.* Wrocław: MedPharm Polska; 2016: 121–142.
66. Piątkowska M, Gbylik-Sikorska M, Olszewska Miw. Stosowanie nielegalnych antybiotyków w wodzie na fermie niosek jaj konsumpcyjnych – opis przypadku. *Pasze Przem.* 2015;2:28–33.
67. Gertig H. Interakcje leków ze składnikami pożywienia. In: Gertig H, Przysławski J, red., *Bromatologia. Zarys Nauki o Żywności i Żywieniu.* Warszawa: Wydawnictwo Lekarskie PZWL; 2007: 271–272.
68. McEvoy JDG, Higgins HC, Mayne CS, Kennedy DG. Transfer of sulfadiazine from contaminated diary feed to cows' milk. In: *Proceedings of the Euroresidue IV.* Veldhoven, The Netherlands; May 8–10, 2000; 753–757.
69. Kan CA, Petz KM. Residues of veterinary drugs in eggs and their distribution between yolk and white. *J Agric Food Chem.* 2000;48 (12):6397–6403.
70. van Rhijn HJ, Yedema ESE, Beek WMJ, Kan CA, Sebec LBJ. Investigation into the excretion of nicarbazin in cows milk after administration of feeds containing low-levels of nicarbazin. In: *Proceedings of the Euroresidue IV Conference.* Veldhoven, The Netherlands; May 8–10, 2000.
71. Bagg R, Vessie GH, Dick CP, Duffield T, Wilson JB, Aramini JJ. Milk residues and performance of lactating dairy cows administered high doses of monensin. *Can J Vet Res.* 2005;69(3):180–185.
72. Mulder PPJ, Balzer-Rutgers PB, Brinke PEM, et al. Deposition and depletion of the coccidiostats toltrazuril and halofuginone in eggs. *Anal Chim Acta.* 2005;529(1–2):331–337.
73. Verraes C, Van Boxstael S, Van Meervenne E, et al. Antimicrobial resistance in the food chain: a review. *Int J Environ Res Public Health.* 2013;10:2643–2669.
74. Cogliani C, Goossens H, Greko C. Restricting antimicrobial use in food animals: lessons from Europe. *Microbe.* 2011;6:274–279.
75. Kemper N. Veterinary antibiotics in aquatic and terrestrial environment. *Ecol Indic.* 2008;8(1):1–13.
76. Gibbons JF, Boland F, Egan J, Fanning S, Markey BK, Leonard FC. Antimicrobial resistance of faecal *Escherichia coli* isolates form pig farms with different durations of in-feed antimicrobial use. *Zoonoses Public Health.* 2016;63:241–250.
77. McEwen SA, Fedorka-Cray PJ. Antimicrobial use and resistance in animals. *Clin Infect Dis.* 2002;34:93–106.
78. Collignon P. Vancomycin-resistant enterococci and use of avoparcin in animal feed: is there a link? *Med J Aust.* 1999;171:144–146.
79. Witte W. Selective pressure by antibiotic use in livestock. *Int J Antimicrob Agents.* 2000;(suppl 1)19–24.
80. Wegener HC, Madsen M, Nielsen P, Aarestrup FM. Isolation of vancomycin-resistant *Enterococcus faecium* from food. *Int J Food Microbiol.* 1997;35:57–66.
81. Aarestrup FM. Association between the consumption of antimicrobial agents in animal husbandry and the occurrence of resistant bacteria among food animals. *Int J Antimicrob Agents.* 1999;12(4):279–285.
82. Khachatourians GG. Agricultural use of antibiotics and the evolution and transfer of antibiotic-resistant bacteria. *CMAJ.* 1998;159:1129–1136.
83. Peters J, Mac K, Wichmann-Schauer H, Klein G, Ellerbroek L. Species distribution and antibiotic resistance patterns of enterococci isolated from food of animal origin in Germany. *Int J Food Microbiol.* 2003;88:311–314. Available from: https://doi.org/10.1016/S0168-1605(03)00193-4.
84. Cycoń M, Mrozik A, Piotrowska-Seget Z. Antibiotics in the soil environment-degradation and their impact on microbial activity and diversity. *Front Microbiol.* 2019;10(338). Available from: https://doi.org/10.3389/fmicb.2019.00338.
85. Zhao L, Dong YH, Wang H. Residues of veterinary antibiotics in manures from feedlot livestock in eight provinces in China. *Sci Total Environ.* 2010;408:1069–1075.
86. Boxall ABA, Fogg LA, Blackwell PA, et al. *Veterinary medicines in the environment. Reviews of Environmental Contamination and Toxicology.* New York: Springer; 2004:1–99.
87. Berendsen BJA, Lahr J, Nibbeling C, et al. The persistence of a broad of antibiotics during calve, pig and broiler manure storage. *Chemosphere.* 2018;204:267–276.
88. Qian M, Wu H, Wang J, et al. Occurrence of trace elements and antibiotics in manure-based fertilizers from the Zhejiang Province of China. *Sci Total Environ.* 2016;559:174–181.
89. Martinez-Carballo E, Gonzalez-Barreiro C, Scharf S, Gans O. Environmental monitoring study of selected veterinary antibiotics in animal manure and soils in Austria. *Environ Pollut.* 2007;162:56–62.
90. Berendsen BJA, Wegh RS, Memolink J, Zuidema T, Stolker LAM. The analysis of animal faeces as a tool to monitor antibiotic usage. *Talanta.* 2015;132:258–268.
91. Hamscher G, Sczesny S, Hoper H, Nau H. Determination of persistent tetracycline residues in soil fertilized with liquid manure by high-performance liquid chromatography with electrospray ionization tandem mass spectrometry. *Anal Chem.* 2002;74:1509–1518.
92. Huang X, Liu C, Li K, et al. Occurrence and distribution of veterinary antibiotics and tetracycline resistance genes in farmland soils around swine feedlots in Fujian Province, China. *Environ Sci Pollut Res.* 2013;20:9066–9074.
93. Binh CTT, Heuer H, Gomes NCM, et al. Short-term effects of amoxicillin on bacterial communities in manured soil. *FEMS Microbiol Ecol.* 2007;62:290–302. Available from: https://doi.org/10.1111/j.1574-6941.2007.00393.x.

94. Atashgahi S, Sánchez-Andrea I, Heipieper HJ, van der Meer JR, Stams AJM, Smidt H. Prospects for harnessing biocide resistance for bioremediation and detoxification. *Science*. 2018;360: 743–746. Available from: https://doi.org/10.1126/science.aar3778.
95. Halling-Sorensen B, Jacobsen A-M, Jensen J, Sengelov G, Vaclavik E, Ingerslev F. Dissipation and effects of chlortetracycline and tylosin in two agricultural soils: a field-scale study in southern Denmark. *Environ Toxicol Chem*. 2009;24(4):802–810.
96. Ma J, Lin H, Sun W, Wang Q, Yu Q, Zhao Y. Soil microbial systems respond differentially to tetracycline, sulfamonomethoxine, and ciprofloxacin entering soil under pot experimental conditions alone and in combination. *Environ Sci Pollut Res*. 2014;21: 7436–7448. Available from: https://doi.org/10.1007/s11356-014-2685-2.
97. Tang X, Lou C, Wang S, Lu Y, Liu M, Hashmi MZ. Effects of long-term manure applications on the occurrence of antibiotics and antibiotic resistance genes (ARGs) in paddy soils: evidence from four field experiments in south of China. *Soil Biol Biochem*. 2015;90:179–187. Available from: https://doi.org/10.1016/j.soilbio.2015.07.027.
98. Grenni P, Ancona V, Barra Caracciolo A. Ecological effects of antibiotics on natural ecosystems: a review. *Microchem J*. 2018;136:25–39. Available from: https://doi.org/10.1016/j.microc.2017.02.006.
99. Keen PL, Patrick DM. Tracking change: a look at the ecological footprint of antibiotics and antimicrobial resistance. *Antibiotics*. 2013;2:191–205. Available from: https://doi.org/10.3390/antibiotics2020191.
100. Zhou Y, Niu L, Zhu S, Lu H, Liu W. Occurrence, abundance, and distribution of sulfonamide and tetracycline resistance genes in agricultural soils across China. *Sci Total Environ*. 2017; 599–600:1977–1983. Available from: https://doi.org/10.1016/j.scitotenv.2017.05.152.
101. DeVries SL, Loving M, Li X, Zhang P. The effect of ultra low dose antibiotics exposure on soil nitrate and N_2O flux. *Sci Rep*. 2015;5:16818. Available from: https://doi.org/10.1038/srep16818.
102. Toth JD, Feng Y, Dou Z. Veterinary antibiotics at environmentally relevant concentrations inhibit soil iron reduction and nitrification. *Soil Biol Biochem*. 2011;43:2470–2472. Available from: https://doi.org/10.1016/j.soilbio.2011.09.004.
103. Marx M-C, Kandeler E, Wood M, Wermbter N, Jarvis SC. Exploring the enzymatic landscape: distribution and kinetics of hydrolytic enzymes in soil particle-size fractions. *Soil Biol Biochem*. 2005;37:35–48. Available from: https://doi.org/10.1016/j.soilbio.2004.05.024.
104. Gafner JL. Identification and semiquantitative estimation of antibiotics added to complete feeds, premixes, and concentrates. *J AOAC Int*. 1999;82:1–8.
105. Markaksis PK. Determination of tetracyclines in animal feeds in the presence of other drugs by thin-layer chromatography and microbiological method. *J AOAC Int*. 1996;79:375–379.
106. Garandos-Chinchilla F, Sanchez J, Garcia F, Rodríguez C. A novel green chemistry method for nonaqueous extraction and high-performance liquid chromatography detection of first-, second-, and third-generation tetracyclines, 4-epitetracycline, and tylosin in animal feeds. *J Agric Food Chem*. 2012;60:7121–7128.
107. Khan NH, Roets E, Hoogmartens J, Vanderhaeghe H. Quantitative analysis of chlortetracycline and related substances by high-performance liquid chromatography. *J Pharm Biomed Anal*. 1989;7:339–353.
108. Khan NH, Roets E, Hoogmartens J, Vanderhaeghe H. Quantitative analysis of oxytetracycline and related substances by high-performance liquid chromatography. *J Chromatogr A*. 1987;405:229–245.
109. Xu JZ, Ding T, Wu B, Yang WQ, Zhang XY. Analysis of tetracycline residues in royal jelly by liquid chromatography-tandem mass spectrometry. *J Chromatogr B*. 2008;868:42–48.
110. Kaklamanos G, Vincent U, von Holst C. Analysis of antimicrobial agents in pig feed by liquid chromatography coupled to orbitrap mass spectrometry. *J Chromatogr A*. 2013;1293:60–74.
111. Borras S, Companyo R, Guiteras J, Bosch J. Multiclass method for antimicrobial analysis in animal feeds by liquid chromatography-tandem mass spectrometry. *Anal Bioanal Chem*. 2013;405:8475–8486.
112. Boscher A, Guignard C, Pellet T, Hoffman L, Bohn T. Development of a multi-class method for the quantification of veterinary drug residue in feedingstuffs by liquid chromatography-tandem mass spectrometry. *J Chromatogr A*. 2010;1217:6394–6404.
113. Patyra E, Kwiatek K. Determination of fluoroquinolones in animal feed by ion pair high-performance liquid chromatography with fluorescence detection. *Anal Lett*. 2017;50:1711–1720. Available from: https://doi.org/10.1080/00032719.2016.1249876.
114. Gonzalez de la Huebra MJ, Vincnet U. Analysis of macrolide antibiotics by liquid chromatography. *J Pharm Biomed Anal*. 2005;39 (3–4):376–398.
115. Przeniosło-Siwczyńska M, Patyra E, Chyłek-Purchała M, Kozak B, Kwiatek K. Occurrence of tetracyclines in feedingstuffs – results of a two-year study within the official control of feed. *Bull Vet Inst Pulawy*. 2015;59:527–532.
116. Gavilán RE, Nebot C, Veiga-Gómez M, et al. A confirmatory method based on HPLC-MS/MS for the detection and quantification of residue of tetracyclines in nonmedicated feed. *J Anal Methods Chem*. 2016;. Available from: https://doi.org/10.1155/2016/1202954.
117. Patyra E, Kwiatek K. Development and validation of multi-residue analysis for tetracycline antibiotics in feed by high performance liquid chromatography coupled to mass spectrometry. *Food Addit Contam A*. 2017;34(9):1553–1561.
118. Patyra E, Przeniosło-Siwczyńska M, Kwiatek K. Determination of sulfonamides in feeds by high-performance liquid chromatography after fluorescamine precolumn derivatization. *Molecules*. 2019;24(3):452. Available from: https://doi.org/10.3390/molecules24030452.
119. Gavilán RE, Nebot C, Patyra E, Vazquez B, Miranda JM, Cepeda A. Determination of florfenicol, thiamfenicol and chloramfenicol at trace levels in animal feed by HPLC–MS/MS. *Antibiotics*. 2019;8(2):59.
120. Patyra E, Kwiatek K. Quantification and analysis of trace levels of phenicols in feed by liquid chromatography–mass spectrometry. *Chromatographia*. 2020;83:715–723.
121. Cronly M, Behan P, Foley B, et al. Development and validation of a rapid multi-class method for the confirmation of fourteen prohibited medicinal additives in pig and poultry compound feed by liquid chromatography–tandem mass spectrometry. *J Pharm Biomed Anal*. 2010;53:929–938.
122. Patyra E, Nebot C, Gavilán RE, Cepeda A, Kwiatek K. Development and validation of multi-residue and multi-class

method for antibacterial substances analysis in non-target feed by liquid chromatography–tandem mass spectrometry. *Food Addit Contam A*. 2018;35(3):467–478.

123. Huet A-C, Morier L, Daeseleire E, Fodey T, Elliott C, Delahaut P. Screening for the coccidiostats halofuginone and nicarbazin in egg and chicken muscle: development of an ELISA. *Food Addit Contam A*. 2005;22(2):128–134.
124. Thalmann A, Wagner K, Tomassen M, Driessen J, De Jong J. Liquid chromatographic method to determine narasin in feedingstuffs and premixtures: development, validation, and interlaboratory study. *J AOAC Int*. 2004;87(6):1278–1286.
125. De Jong J, Stoisser B, Wagner K, et al. Determination of maduramicin in feedingstuffs and premixtures by liquid chromatography: development, validation, and interlaboratory study. *J AOAC Int*. 2004;87(5):1033–1041.
126. European Commission. Commission Regulation, 2009/152/EC laying down the methods of sampling and analysis for the official control of feed; 2009.
127. Moretti S, Fioroni L, Giusepponi D, Pettinacci L, Saluti G, Galarini R. Development and validation of a multiresidue liquid chromatography/tandem mass spectrometry method for 11 coccidiostats in feed. *J AOAC Int*. 2013;96(6): 1245–1257.
128. Turnipseed SB, Roybal JE, Pfenning AP, Gonzales SA, Hurlbut JA, Madson MR. LC/MS confirmation of ionophores in animal feeds. *J AOAC Int*. 2001;84(3):640–647.
129. Vincent U, Chedin M, Yasar S, von Holst C. Determination of ionophore coccidiostats in feedingstuffs by liquid chromatography–tandem mass spectrometry: part I. Application to targeted feed. *J Pharm Biomed Anal*. 2008;47(4–5): 750–757.
130. Cronly M, Behana P, Foleya B, Malone E, Shearan P, Regan L. Determination of eleven coccidiostats in animal feed by liquid chromatography–tandem mass spectrometry at cross contamination levels. *Anal Chim Acta*. 2011;700(1–2): 26–33.

Chapter 6

Residues relating to the veterinary therapeutic or growth-promoting use and abuse of medicines

György Csikó

Department of Pharmacology and Toxicology, University of Veterinary Medicine, Budapest, Hungary

Abstract

Medicines in livestock production are inevitable as they are essential for treatment or prevention of diseases, and improvement of growth and productivity. Furthermore, drugs are crucial for the economical production of food, and they may ensure higher food safety. Improper or illicit medicine uses, dosing failures, among others, can lead to the formation of drug residues in edible tissues and other foodstuffs with animal origin. Rules introduced in the last few decades support the authorization of good-quality and efficient veterinary drugs. At the same time, they should be safe for treated animals, operators, and environment, as well as for food consumers. The production of drug residue–free food of animal origin requests well-established and controlled medicine administration in food-producing animals. This chapter deals with the legal ways of medicine authorization and administration, and the role of authorities, veterinarians, and farmers in drug residue–free food production, and presents further perspectives on this topic.

Keywords: Human food safety; veterinary medicines; drug residues; withdrawal period; abuse of medicines

6.1 Introduction, general terms, and significance of the topic

Food products of animal origin are important protein sources for human beings. Improving livestock production is a central concern because of the constantly increasing demand in human nutrition. The worldwide average meat consumption is estimated at 42.9 kg per capita, with industrial countries consuming about 76.1 kg, twice the quantity in developing countries (33.6 kg). However, it has been predicted that the consumption of meat and meat products will double globally by 2050. Chickens can be raised at remarkable rates of weight gain and great metabolic efficiency to yield lean white meat. Laying hens provide a useful protein source in the eggs they produce. Cattle and sheep are significant sources of meat and milk for human consumption. Currently more than 109 million tons of pork are produced annually in the world; accordingly pork is an important source of meat.[1–3] Considering differences in food consumption patterns, besides the traditional food-producing species, so called minor food-producing animal species are also significant (Table 6.1). For instance, rabbit production has gained increasing significance recently, which leads to the growing importance of health promotion in rabbit herds. Demand for honey products is growing, and also Salmonidae and other fish species have become popular too.

Foods produced from minor species can be important on the one hand to provide more food and on the other hand to make better use of agricultural production sites. It is highly important to produce good-quality meat, milk eggs, and honey with high food safety and free from illegal drug residues in large-scale production.

During the growing period animals are exposed to numerous adverse factors, including inflammation or bacterial, viral, and parasitic pathogens, which will lead to decreased weight gain and impaired general condition. Medicinal products are frequently applied in food-producing animals to cure or to prevent disease conditions, and to maintain economical production in livestock. The global animal medicine market reached a value of nearly $38 billion in 2019, having grown at a compound annual growth rate of 11.7% since 2015. North America was the largest region in the animal medicine market, accounting for 47.1% of the global market in 2019. It was followed by Asia-Pacific, Western Europe, and then the other regions.[4] When overall sales of antibiotics, in tons

Present Knowledge in Food Safety. DOI: https://doi.org/10.1016/B978-0-12-819470-6.00028-7

TABLE 6.1 Major and minor food-producing animal species in the European Union (EU) and in the United States (according to European Medicines Evaluation Agency and Food and Drug Administration).

Major food-producing species for MRLs	*Cattle* (dairy, meat animals) *Sheep* (meat animals) *Pig* *Chicken* (including laying hens) *Turkey* (in United States but not in EU) *Salmonidae*
Minor food-producing species for MRLs	*Other ruminants* (bovidae, caprinae, and their milk) (deer, reindeer) *Dairy sheep* *Other avian species and their eggs* *Other fish species* *Other mammalian species* (horse, rabbit, dromedary) *Honey bees*

MRLs, maximum residue limits.

of active ingredient, split by tablets (used mainly, in companion animals) and all other pharmaceutical forms (used mainly in food-producing animals) are compared, approximately 100 times more active substance has been applied in the livestock, during this period, that is 68.6 tons versus 6703 tons, respectively.[5]

The most frequently applied veterinary drugs in food-producing animals are antibiotics (tetracyclines, beta lactams, macrolides, aminoglycosides, etc.) and antiparasitics (ionophores, benzimidazoles, avermectines, milbemycins, antiprotozoals, etc.). Other drug classes frequently used for the treatment of livestock are antiinflammatory drugs, antifungals, anesthetics and analgesics, hormones, antiseptics, and immunological products, among others. In livestock, parallel with the medicines, disinfectants, insecticide, and pesticide products are used in the environment of the animals to control epidemics or vectors spreading infections. These and other chemical feed additives (e.g., antioxidants) can accumulate in food from animal origin and may present the same food residue challenges as veterinary medicines. These latter categories are discussed elsewhere in different sections of this book.

There are many aspects of medicine use in veterinary practice; the main accepted uses are therapeutic, prophylactic, or metaphylactic administrations. Other subsidiary purposes of drug applications are for diagnostic and euthanasic uses.

Therapeutic medicine use could be causative (e.g., antibiotic treatment in order to kill pathogenic bacteria or slow their growth) or symptomatic (e.g., mitigate diarrhea or fever). In many cases, veterinarians use both of them in the same time. With respect to the number of treated animals, it could be considered individual therapy or group medication. Individual drug therapy is applied in the small animal veterinary praxis; however, it is also used in the treatment of horses, cattle, and swine. In exceptional cases, high-value breeding poultry could also be treated in the above-mentioned way. Group (mass) medication occurs in case of farm animals (most frequently, poultry, swine) and fish. In mass medication, the drug is mixed into the feed or given via drinking water. The use of medicines to prevent disease is termed drug-prophylaxis; a case-specific administration of preventive medicine (antibiotics, antiparasitics, etc.) to animals in livestock production or to an individual patient (e.g., an animal could be treated with antibiotics after surgery or injurious trauma). For many decades it was not uncommon for veterinarians to give antibiotics to animals that were not currently ill, but where there was a high risk of cross-infection. In livestock, group administration of antibiotics was often applied in case of transporting or moving young animals, and in preventing respiratory and intestinal maladies when animals have been subjected to severely stressful conditions.

The term metaphylaxis refers to the administration of the product at the same time to a group of clinically healthy (but presumably infected) in-contact animals, to prevent them from developing clinical signs, and to prevent further spread of the disease. The presence of the disease in the group/flock must be established before the product is used. A metaphylaxis claim will always have to be combined with a treatment claim. In other words, metaphylaxis means the mass medication of a group of clinically healthy animals within the population in advance of an expected outbreak of disease. However, in the same population from the disease afflicted individuals are treated with the same medicine. However, use of antibiotics should never be intended to replace the need for good management practices.

Antibiotic medicinal products should not be used for prophylaxis other than in exceptional cases only for the administration to an individual animal. Antimicrobial medicinal products should be used for metaphylaxis only when the risk of spread of an infection or of an infectious disease in a group of animals is high and where no appropriate alternatives are available. Such restrictions should allow the decrease of prophylactic and metaphylactic use in animals toward representing a smaller proportion of the total use of antimicrobials in animals.[a]

Growth promotion is a special use of medicine in veterinary praxis. Substances such as hormones, beta-2 adrenergic agonists, and antimicrobial growth promoters (AGPs) have widely been used for many decades to increase growth performance and to alter composition of foodstuffs (e.g., fat–protein ratio). The use of hormonally active growth promoters ("hormones") in farm animals can increase the production of veal and beef significantly, for example, by up to 15%. However, in different parts of the world the regulations regarding the use of such hormones differ sharply. In the European Union (EU) there exists a total ban on such use in contrast to the United States where the use of some hormones is authorized under strict conditions.[6] AGPs may improve the average daily weight gain by 4% in broiler chickens, 17% in piglets, and 7% in beef cattle, and feed efficiency by 4%, 9%, and 7%, respectively; furthermore AGPs may reduce the mortality rate by 50%.[7] However, AGPs are prohibited to use in food animal production since 2006 in the EU, 2016 in the United States, and 2017 in Canada.[8,9]

The routes of drug administration are classified as external or internal medicine use. The first type means the administration of drugs on skin, outer mucosal parts, and hoof, and with rare exception the application leads to local effect of the active agents. The internal medicine administration is further divided as enteral [per os (PO), rectal] and parenteral drug use [e.g., intravenous (IV), intramuscular (IM), or subcutaneous (SC) injections]. In comparison to external treatment the effect of internally applied medicines is frequently systemic, affecting the deeper tissues and body organs. In veterinary medicine there are some unique application routes such as intramammary and intrauterine drug uses. Table 6.2 summarizes the important characteristics of the most frequent drug administration routes in animals.

During the medicine applications animals can be treated individually or in smaller or larger groups. The individual treatment often needs more time and human labor compared to group medication; however, the former type is considered to be more precise regarding dosage. However, mass medication (in group drug application) often needs less time and work; therefore it is frequently applied in livestock. Although drenching and multiple injecting are suitable drug deliveries in big populations, these routes need individual handling and fixing of animals, which is unnecessary when medicated drinking water or medicated feed is administered. Because of individual differences in water and feed intake, only medicines with a high therapeutic index [the ratio of LD50 (in 50% of animals' lethal dose) and ED50 (in 50% of animals' effective dose)] are safe to give via drinking water or feed to animals. Acute phase reaction of diseases or altered body condition, among others, may influence the water and feed consumption of animals. In this manner, huge individual differences may occur in medicine uptake within the treated flock. These factors may result in underdose or overdose in certain individuals in the animal population.[10,11] Furthermore, homogenous mixing of medicated feed or water is essential to ensure safety and efficacy of these administration forms.

Water-soluble medicines can be applied via the drinking water of the population. This is one of the accepted routes to administer veterinary medicinal products (VMPs) to the animals orally. In veterinary practice, besides the liquid dose forms such as solutions and emulsions, large amount of water-soluble powders or granules are authorized to prepare medicated drinking water. When the active substance is nonwater-soluble, it may be mixed into the feed of animals. Medicated feed is a frequent way to provide medication in food-producing animals. Depending on given situations, this can be the most effective way for a farmer to cure their livestock. Just like in case of medicated drinking water, medicated feed can be prepared by farmers, animals' owners by using suitable pharmaceutical dose forms (solid powders,

TABLE 6.2 Comparison of main routes of drug applications.

Route	Advantages	Disadvantages
Per Os	Convenient, cheap, no need for sterilization, variety of dose forms (fast/slow release, coated tablets, liquids, gels)	Variability due to physiology, feeding, disease Intractable patients (*neophobia*) First-pass effect
Intramuscular	More consistent absorption than PO or subcutaneous (SC) Certainty of administration (e.g., to unconscious, vomiting patients) Depot or sustained effect is possible	Pain, tissue irritation Muscle damage, discoloring Dose cannot be recovered
Subcutaneous	Can be given by the owner Vasoconstrictor can be added to prolong effect at site of interest	Variability, more autonomic control over blood flow (than muscle), dehydration, heat, cold, stress, and so on Tissue irritation
Topical	Easy, painless application (e.g., mass medication of cattle) If skin therapy—reduced systemic effects/enhanced skin effects	Toxic skin reactions Variable blood flow to skin Patients groom themselves (may lead to oral absorption)

granules, pellets or liquid, semiliquid forms) and methods (mixing, top dressing, or spraying). As a legal based category, medicated feed can only be produced by authorized feed mixers (feed mills). According to definition, medicated feed is a homogenous mixture of medicinal premixes, other VMPs or coccidiostats, histomonostats, and suitable feeding-stuffs. Only VMPs for which this route of administration has been approved by the authority may be included in the feed. Medicinal premixes are special veterinary dose forms, there are many shapes, such as pellet feed, powder feed, liquid feed, and so on, and the only authorized way of their use is inclusion into the feed. Many of the premixes, the antibiotic containing ones always are, according to the standard term, prescription-only medicines (POMs). Feed mixers are allowed to incorporate medicines into the animals feed, typically according to a special order form (prescriptions for medicated feedstuff, PMFs). Coccidiostats or histomonostats and certain anthelmintic (deworming) agents can be incorporated into the feed without PMF. As final product, medicine containing feed is delivered to animal owners or farmers, and the whole amount must be used for feeding until the indicated expiry date. No further sale or trade of the product is allowed. Medicated feed is used mainly but not exclusively in larger populations of food-producing animal species such as poultry, swine, and fish. To a lesser extent, medicated feed is permitted in ruminant species as well.

Rarely can medicated feed be applied in hobby and pet species too (e.g., horses, dogs, pigeons, and game birds) and feeding this type of medicated feed to food-producing animals has to be strictly avoided, because it may contain active ingredients (e.g., metronidazole, ronidazole, nitrofurans) that are prohibited to use in animals raised for human consumption.[b]

After the discovery of the first antimicrobials from the 1950s, medicated feed has been the preferred method of administering antibiotics and growth promoters for decades in food-producing livestock. Later, antiparasitic drugs and, from the late 1970s, ionophore coccidiostats were also used effectively through feed. As a result of recent restrictions on the use of antibiotics and a total ban on growth promotion, the legal use of medicated feed is becoming limited in animals.[13] On the one hand, medicines can be added to feed only if they are authorized for administration via feed. Alternatively, in group medication, preventive and metaphylactic administration can only be allowed if there are no other methods, including immunization, available to prevent the disease condition. In other words, the purpose of the medicine usage should be the individual treatment of the animals, rather than the preventive administration with mass medication. Consequently in this way the unnecessary overuse of the antibiotics can be prevented and the development and spreading of antimicrobial resistance (AMR) can be decreased. Development of AMR is a natural phenomenon but certain human and veterinary actions accelerate its emergence and spread, which has global impact on successful chemotherapy in both animals and humans.[14] Prudent use of antimicrobials is the optimal selection (most appropriate active substance) and dosing of drug (dose size, frequency, and duration). Another important argument for the limitation of the use of medicated feed is increasing the food safety. It is postulated that the antimicrobial drug residues in food may increase the emergence and spread of AMR in humans.

Following the administration of medicines, regardless of the route of administration, the utilized drug molecules and their metabolites are present in different tissues, including the edible ones. According to definition they are collectively called a "drug residue." With few rare exceptions these drug residues are continuously eliminated from body. Drug molecules are generally first metabolized in the liver with the help of CYP450 and other types of enzyme-mediated processes (e.g., oxidation, reduction, conjugation). This is characteristic for lipophilic agents; hydrophilic molecules may remain unchanged. The parent (unchanged) molecules and their metabolically transformed derivatives (metabolites) are excreted mainly with urine and bile (Fig. 6.1). Other bodily excretion routes such as milk, honey, and eggs can contain significant concentration of these residual substances.[15]

After shorter or longer time period—depending on several factors such as type and characteristics of the drug molecules, applied dose and formulation, species, age and gender of animals, and so on—the drug level drops under the maximal acceptable level (*maximum residue limit, MRL*, see later). Diseases of liver or kidneys may decrease the clearance (speed of elimination rate) critically. Another significant delaying factor of drug elimination could be the concomitant use of other medicines or feed additives. If the VMP is not absorbed or is converted into harmless products, drug residue formation would not be a significant concern. Unfortunately, this is not usually the case. Drugs or their metabolites persist often in edible tissues or in other animal products (eggs, milk, honey) for several hours or days, sometimes for couple weeks or months. During this period foodstuffs are not suitable for human consumption, because they may cause harmful effects to human beings. Residual drug content in foods could, depending on the level, potentially harm human consumers in several ways including acute and chronic toxicity, allergic reaction, and genotoxicity. Chronic toxicity related to drug residues might, if present at significant levels, have mutagenic, teratogenic, or carcinogenic potential. Although it is frequently postulated, there is inconclusive evidence that antibiotic residues transferred

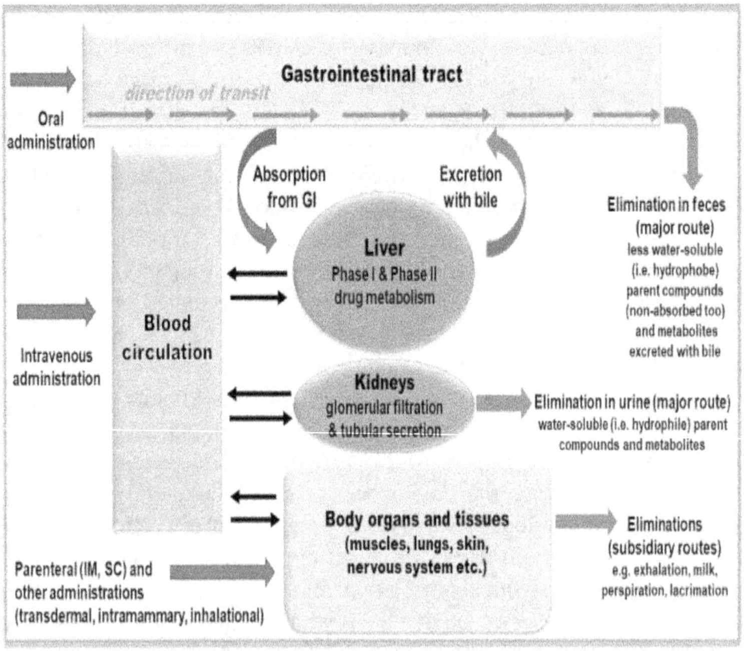

FIGURE 6.1 Main utilization and elimination pathways of the medicinal substances in animals. *Back and forth* arrows represent the two-way transport of medicines between the tissues/organs and blood.

to humans through food might set up a biological milieu that favors the emergence of altered microbiota within a host. Nevertheless, consumption of antibiotic residue containing animal products may pose health risk to consumers due to development of antibiotic-resistant bacteria.[2,3]

6.2 Authorization process and legal uses of veterinary medicines

The potential human health risk from drug residues in food can be decreased by appropriate regulatory steps. To avoid the drug residues in human food, the administration of medicines in food-producing animals must be limited and strictly controlled. This should include applying rules regarding to authorization, production, selling, and using of veterinary medicines in livestock.

6.2.1 Types of medicines used in veterinary practice

Medicinal product (also referred to as medicine, pharmaceutical drug, or simply drug) is a substance used to diagnose, cure, treat, or prevent disease.[c] In livestock production the growth promotion had been another accepted use for decades. Recently authorized medicinal products are forbidden to use for this purpose. Therefore the significance of veterinary complementary products and feed additives (pre- and probiotics, phytotherapeutics, water acidifiers, enzymes, etc.) is continuously increasing.[16,17] Drug therapy (pharmacotherapy) is an important part of the medical field. Ingredients in medicines are classified as "active substance" or "excipient." Active substance means any substance or mixture of substances intended to be used in the manufacture of a VMP that, when used in accordance with its instructions, has a desired biological effect. Excipient means any constituents of a VMP other than an active substance or packaging material.

According to their origin, the next categories of substances in medicines could be distinguished ingredients from:

- plant sources (e.g., from leaves, flowers, roots, seed, and bark of plants)
- human or animal sources (e.g., hormones, antibodies isolated from blood or other tissues of animals)
- mineral sources (e.g., salts, kaolin)
- microbiological sources (e.g., antibiotics produced by fungi or bacteria)
- chemical synthetic and semisynthetic (partly synthetic) sources
- products manufactured by recombinant DNA technology (e.g., vaccines, antibodies)

Based on their authorization procedure and ways of legal supply (trade of them), substances used in the treatment and disease prevention are different. In the veterinary praxis, as in human medicine, medicinal products may be grouped as "real medicines" and "complementary substances and other categories." From the viewpoint of the healthcare of the animals these two groups are separated only didactically (Fig. 6.2).

The former group (real medicines) includes two major types of drugs. These are the nonlicensed medicines and

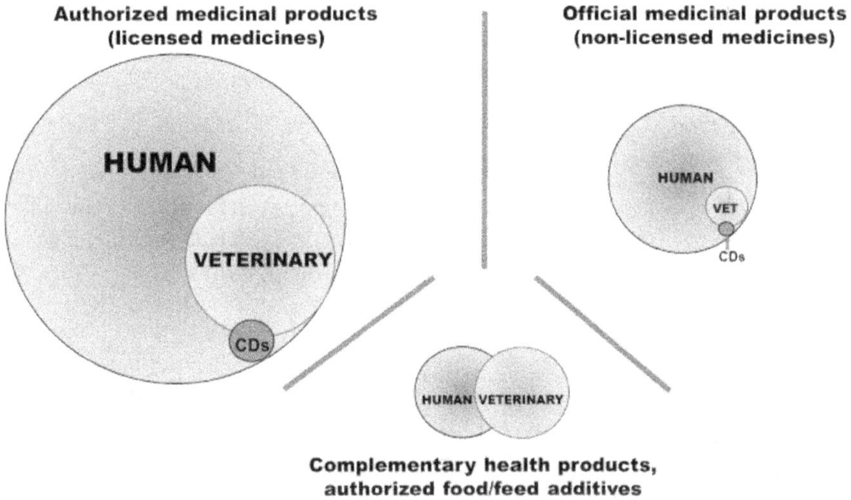

FIGURE 6.2 Classification of substances administered/prescribed by veterinary practitioners. Circle sizes approximately correlate with the number of available products. Both licensed and nonlicensed human drugs may be supplied for the treatment of animals (see details in the text); therefore circles are overlapping each other. *CDs*, controlled drugs such as narcotics, anesthetics, and sedatives.

the licensed medicines. The nonlicensed drugs are frequently referred as official drugs. They are more traditional (historical), and these substances are listed in national or international pharmacopoeias [European Pharmacopoeia, British Pharmacopoeia, U.S Pharmacopoeia, International (World Health Organization, WHO) Pharmacopoeia, etc.]. Pharmacopoeias are accepted standards for medicinal materials and include all ingredients (active substances and excipients) that are allowed to use in pharmacy for instance during the preparation of occasionally made, individual drugs (also see Section 6.2.4). The substances are listed in pharmacopoeias according to alphabetical order of their nonproprietary names. Besides these, many other types of official substances such as blood products, herbal remedies, immunobiological drugs (serums, vaccines), and radiotherapeutics are also presented in detailed manner.

The "international nonproprietary name (INN)" or "common name" of substances is recommended by the WHO and can be identical or closely related to each other in the different pharmacopoeias. This name is also referred to as generic or official name. In the British Pharmacopoeia, U.S Pharmacopoeia, International (WHO) Pharmacopoeia the INN names are English. European Pharmacopoeia uses the English common names and their Latinized version at the same time. Those substances, which are official only for veterinary use, are distinguished with a term "For veterinary use only" and/or they are separated in an exclusive chapter (British Pharmacopoeia). In certain rare cases the substances included into pharmacopoeias may be supplied in their pure form (official drugs). With the combination of the official drugs (i.e., active ingredients and excipients) occasionally prepared (magistral) formulations may be prepared (see also "cascade" in Section 6.2.4). They are supplied by pharmacist to owners, often based on the written order or prescription of practitioners. British Pharmacopoeia contains descriptions of so-called formulated preparations as well. These are medicinal formulations of determined composition and quality.

Licensed products are human licensed medicines or veterinary licensed medicines. The description and information about these recent drug products are available in websites of medicine authorities. The name of the licensed medicines can be an invented name, which cannot be confused with the common name, or the common scientific name followed by trademark "®" or the name of the marketing authorization holder. Veterinary medicines, also known as medicinal products for veterinary use, veterinary drugs, or VMPs, are substances or combinations of substances to treat, prevent, or diagnose disease only in animals. Veterinary medicines are strictly forbidden to use in human beings; however, veterinarians are allowed to order (i.e., prescribe) or use licensed human medicinal products in animals according to special circumstances (see cascade in Section 6.2.4).

The use of complementary health product, feed additives (e.g., vitamin premix, microelement premix, complete premix, pre- and probiotics, etc.), biocides (e.g., pesticides, rodenticides) and disinfectants is significant in daily medical practice and in livestock husbandry. Feed-premixes, biocides, and other products such as herbal remedies, probiotics, prebiotics, and healthcare products could be counted as major aiding factors in animal framing. Strategic use of them controls microbial diseases, parasites, and vectors in the environment of animals and human beings. Lack of use of these agents can lead to less healthy populations and significant economic losses in animal husbandry.

The medicines are classified according to their supplying rules: prescription or nonprescription drugs. These legal categories are often distinguished with special terms or abbreviations such as POM or Rx (symbol of POM) and general sales list (GSL) medicine or over-the-counter drugs, respectively. In this point of view, a more detailed classification of VMPs has been introduced in United Kingdom.[d] This includes the next categories:

1. Prescription-only medicine—veterinarian (POM-V)
   (*may only be supplied by legally authorized veterinary surgeon or a pharmacist in accordance with a prescription from a veterinary surgeon*)
2. Prescription-only medicine—veterinarian, pharmacist, suitably qualified person (SQP) (POM-VPS)
   (*may only be supplied by a veterinary surgeon, a pharmacist, or a SQP and must be in accordance with a prescription from one of those persons*)
3. Nonfood animal—veterinarian, pharmacist, SQP (NFA-VPS)
   (*may be supplied without prescription, but only by a veterinary surgeon, a pharmacist, or an SQP*)
4. Authorized veterinary medicine—GSL (AVM-GSL)
   (*there are no restrictions on the supply of these products*)

"Veterinary prescription" means a document issued by a veterinarian for a VMP or a medicinal product for human use for its use in animals. Pharmacists (i.e., authorized medicine traders) are not allowed to supply POM/Rx preparations to owners of animals or farmers without valid, genuine prescription of a veterinarian with practice authorization. Furthermore, POMs or premixes cannot be mixed into the medicated feed unless previously medicated feedstuff prescription was issued by a veterinary practitioner. Medicinal products containing narcotic or psychotropic substances, products intended for administration following a diagnosis or clinical assessment by a veterinary surgeon must be classified POM/Rx. Over and above, when granting the marketing authorization the relevant authority must classify the following as POM (POM-V and POM-VPS in United Kingdom); products for food-producing animals, products in respect of which special precautions must be taken in order to avoid any unnecessary risk to the target species, the person administering the products to the animal, and the environment, products that may cause effects that impede or interfere with subsequent diagnostic or therapeutic measures. Products containing a new active substance will usually be categorized as POM. The pharmacist or veterinarians—if they are authorized traders—should use their specialist knowledge to check that the prescription matches their own understanding of the product. If they have any concerns about the prescription, they should contact the prescribing veterinarian before supplying the medicine. In case of forgery and mistake of document, suppliers must refuse to supply against a prescription.

6.2.2 Types of directorates/authorities

In the EU there are four different routes (national, centralized, mutual recognition, and decentralized) for obtaining marketing authorizations of veterinary medicines, and drugs can be authorized at national or international level. The national or international authorities are also responsible for presentation of data about the products to the public.

Nationally authorized products: Applications are submitted to the national competent authority. For instance, this authority is the Veterinary Medicines Directorate (VMD) in the United Kingdom, Federal Office of Consumer Protection and Food Safety (BVL) in Germany, or French Agency for VMPs (ANMV) in France, and many other national offices. Marketing authorization granted under this national procedure is only valid in that particular country, for example, United Kingdom, Germany, or France, accordingly. This procedure does not involve any other member state.

Centrally authorized products (CAPs): The centralized procedure is used when an applicant wants to market a product throughout the EU. CAPs are evaluated by the European Medicines Evaluation Agency Committee for Medicinal Products for Veterinary Use (EMEA/CVMP) and issued by the European Commission—therefore they are assessed and approved at community level involving all member states. The authorization is pan-European and allows marketing and sale in all member states. The centralized procedure is compulsory for certain biotechnology products and may be requested for other innovative products.

Mutually recognized products: These products are assessed and approved involving at least two member states via a mutual recognition procedure, where the product is already authorized in at least one member state and an authorization is sought in one or more other member states. In this case, the reference member state has authorized the product and submits their evaluation to the other concerned member states.

The decentralized procedure also results in a mutually recognized product. The decentralized route may be used if the product is not authorized in any member state and the applicant would like authorization in several or all member states. This may occur where the centralized procedure is not mandatory, or the product is not eligible for centralized procedure, or where optional—the applicant does not wish to use the centralized procedure.

Regulation (EC) No 1831/2003 lays down a procedure for the authorization of feed additives. Applications for authorization are submitted to the European Commission. The Commission then ensures that member states are informed and forwards the applications to the European Food Safety Authority (EFSA).

In the United States, the FDA (US Food and Drug Administration) carries the responsibility for both authorization of veterinary medicines [FDA/Centre for Veterinary Medicine (CVM)] and animal food based on

TABLE 6.3 Major regulatory authorities of the veterinary medicines.

Country/region	Description/activities	Website address
Australia	*Australian Pesticides and Veterinary Medicines Authority (APVMA)* Registration of all agricultural and veterinary chemical products into the Australian marketplace. This website contains information on all approved animal products and their labels as well as summaries of adverse drug reactions (ADRs).	http://www.apvma.gov.au
Canada	*Health Canada* *Veterinary Drugs Directorate (VDD)* Evaluates and monitors the safety, quality, and effectiveness, sets standards, and promotes the prudent use of veterinary drugs administered to food-producing and companion animals. Information on regulations, ADRs, and antimicrobial resistance.	https://www.canada.ca/en/health-canada.html
European Union	*European Medicines Evaluation Agency Committee for Medicinal Products for Veterinary Use (EMEA/CVMP)* Information on veterinary medicines, vaccines, and biocides. Presentation of scientific guidelines, European Public Assessment Reports (EPARs) and pharmacovigilance reports.	https://www.ema.europa.eu/en/committees
European Union	*European Food Safety Authority (EFSA)* Based on the EFSA opinion, the European Commission decides whether to authorize or deny the authorization of the feed additives. Proposal for the establishment of maximum residue limits for feed additives.	http://www.efsa.europa.eu/
International	*VICH International Cooperation on Harmonization of Technical Requirements for Registration of Veterinary Medicinal Products* Provides efficacy and pharmacovigilance guidelines.	http://vichsec.org/
United Kingdom	*Veterinary Medicines Directorate (VMD)* Information on veterinary products, legislation, ADRs, Veterinary Medicines Regulations, 2013, and many useful links.	https://www.gov.uk/government/organisations/veterinary-medicines-directorate
United States	*Food and Drug Administration (FDA)* *Centre for Veterinary Medicine (CVM)* Regulates the manufacture and distribution of drugs that will be given to animals. Database of all approved products (Green Book), information on ADRs as well as Freedom of Information (FOI) summaries.	http://www.fda.gov/cvm
United States	*US Department of Agriculture (USDA)* Regulates animal vaccines and bacterins.	http://www.aphis.usda.gov
United States	*US Environmental Protection Agency (EPA)* Regulates topically applied external parasiticides.	http://www.epa.gov/pesticides

the regulations of Federal Food, Drug, and Cosmetic Act. CVM home page contains a searchable database of all FDA-approved animal drugs and approved food additives are listed in Title 21 of the Code of Federal Regulations. FDA works together with American Feed Control Officials (AAFCO) in the area of animal food regulation. AAFCO is responsible for the enforcement of state laws regulating the safe production and labeling of animal food, including livestock and poultry feed and pet food. FDA's current veterinary feed directive (VFD) regulation established requirements relating to the distribution and use of VFD drugs and animal feeds containing such drugs. This amendment is intended to improve the efficiency of FDA's VFD program while protecting human and animal health.

Table 6.3 summarizes the authorities and their major activities regarding to authorization veterinary medicines and feed additives in Europe, United States, Australia, and Canada.

6.2.3 Authorization of the veterinary medicines and feed additives at national and international level

Regulatory evaluation of submissions in support of a new animal drug is a multidisciplinary activity, involving chemists, toxicologists, environmental scientists, clinically trained veterinarians, and sometimes epidemiologists and other skills. The different drug authorities around the world work to support the development and authorization of safe, effective, and quality VMPs for food-producing and companion animals, ensuring their availability and guaranteeing the highest level of public health, animal health, and environmental protection. At the EU level, the European Medicines Agency (EMA) is responsible for the scientific evaluation and monitoring of medicines. In EU-wide authorization procedures are in place since the mid-1990s and the system is supported by the EMA. The EU regulates the manufacture, placing on the market and use of medicated feed, which is a specific type of feed as well. The current legal framework for VMPs and medicated feed, Directive 2001/82/EC, Regulation (EC) No 726/2004 and Directive 90/167/EEC have been replaced by Regulation (EU) 2019/6[19] on VMPs and Regulation (EU) 2019/4 on medicated feed; the new regulations will apply from January 28, 2022. The law governing VMPs in the EU sets standards to ensure adequate health protection. Based on the principle of marketing authorization by the EU or by the national competent authorities, it also promotes the functioning of the internal market, with measures to encourage innovation. These also include harmonized provisions for the manufacture, wholesale, and advertising of VMPs.

In the United States, FDA's CVM approves and regulates new animal drugs upon the regulatory bases of "The Federal Food, Drug, and Cosmetic Act." CVM is made up of six offices that work together to approve new animal drugs and monitor the drugs after they are on the market. The Office of New Animal Drug Evaluation is the "pre-approval office," meaning that it is the lead office for reviewing the information about a new animal drug before it is approved.

In the United Kingdom, the Veterinary Medicines Regulation provides for legislative requirements concerning the manufacture, classification, supply, marketing, and use of veterinary medicines. In the United Kingdom, the national competent authority and independent regulator is the VMD.

The new VMPs are authorized by Australian Pesticides and Veterinary Medicines Authority (APVMA) in Australia and by Health Canada Veterinary Drugs Directorate (VDD) in Canada.

Regulatory authority requires that before any new animal health product can be marketed, it must be proved through rigorous testing that it is both safe and effective and meets the quality criteria. Only when the independent regulator is satisfied on all three criteria can a marketing authorization be considered, which may then be used to legally place a VMP on the market in accordance with the regulations in force.

In a *1993 Food and Agriculture Organization (FAO)* publication, these quality, safety, and efficacy terms were defined as follows:

- Quality means that medicines must be manufactured with appropriate quality control procedures, in premises that are inspected and licensed; the ingredients must be of appropriate purity, in the correct proportions and correctly processed; the containers must be robust with secure closures; and the labeling must be accurate and informative.
- Safety is interpreted widely, to include the animal being treated and in-contact animals; the user, including the veterinarian, farmer, or pet owner administering the medicine; the consumer of livestock products from treated animals; and the environment.
- Efficacy means that the medicines must be effective against the diseases, in the species of animals, at the dose rate, frequency and duration of treatment, and by the route of administration claimed by the manufacturer.

All authorized veterinary medicines available for animals must undergo a strict regulatory approval process, before they gain a Marketing Authorization (MA) or license for sale and supply. Scientific studies by animal medicine companies, and subsequent evaluation by independent regulatory authorities, ensure that each authorized VMP meets the required standard of safety, efficacy, and quality. This ensures that animal medicines are safe to use, they are efficacious (effective), and they meet quality criteria.

The development of a new veterinary product containing a new active ingredient is a costly, time-consuming, and difficult process. In case of a generic veterinary product, the cost and the time interval of the drug development can be reduced. Generic veterinary products are such products in which the quality and quantity composition of constituents (active ingredient, vehicle, etc.) and the pharmaceutical dose form are essentially same to a medicinal product (reference) authorized in the Member State of EU. In this case, the results of toxicological, pharmacological, and residue tests, preclinical and clinical trials are not required. However, these properties of the new and reference products should be compared by a bioequivalence study. Toxicological, pharmacological, pharmacokinetic, target animal safety, clinical and environmental toxicity studies should be performed by the same special regulations and test methods in all the Member States of EU.

Fig. 6.3 introduces the most important steps and study types of veterinary medicine research and development.

The special regulations are ensured by the principles of good laboratory practice (GLP) regulated by directive 2004/10/EC on the harmonization of laws, regulations and administrative provisions relating to the application of the principles of GLP and the verification of their applications for tests on chemical substances. According to the type of the investigations, different guidelines can be used. Organization for Economical Cooperation and

PRE-AUTHORIZATION STUDIES

- PRE-CLINICAL PHASE

  PHARMACOLOGICAL INVESTIGATIONS evaluation of drug mechanisms and pharmacodynamic activities

  TOXICITY STUDIES

  - toxicological studies

    single-dose toxicity (acute toxicity)

    repeated-dose toxicity (subacute, subchronic, chronic (long-term))

    dermal toxicity

  - special toxicological studies

    reproductive toxicity (teratogenicity)

    genotoxicity (mutagenicity, carcinogenicity)

  SAFETY STUDIES TO

  target animal

  human beings: food-consumer (food safety), user/operator

  environment (air, soil, aquatic decomposition)

  PHARMACOKINETIC STUDIES and/or BIOEQUIVALENCE STUDIES

  DRUG RESIDUE STUDIES

- CLINICAL PHASE *in vitro* and *in vivo* studies (big number of real clinical cases from animal population)

POST-AUTHORIZATION STUDIES

- PHARMACOVIGILANCE Post-Authorization Safety Studies

FIGURE 6.3 Phases and major study types of the development of veterinary medicines (The various pharmaceutical studies, for instance tests on quantity and quality of the ingredients and final products, stability test of the ingredients, intermediates and finalized products are not detailed in this figure).

Development (OECD) guidelines are recommended for testing of the physical-chemical properties, health effects, toxicological properties, and environmental fate (e.g., degradation, accumulation), and effects on biotic system of chemicals and medicinal products. Today the recommendations by the European Committee and the EMA can also be used (*Eudralex volumes: The rules governing medicinal products in the European Community*).

Besides, VICH guidelines (International Cooperation on Harmonization of Technical Requirements for Registration of Veterinary Medicinal Products) are recommended for investigations of the properties, effects, and efficacy of VMPs. During the development of them account was taken of OECD guidelines and of national/regional guidelines, and the current practices for evaluating the safety of veterinary drug residue in human food in the EU, Japan, the Unites States, Australia, New Zealand, and Canada.

The different test guidelines are found at the following home pages:

OECD guidelines:

http://www.oecd.org/env/ehs/testing/oecdguidelines-forthetestingofchemicals.htm

VICH guidelines:

http://www.vichsec.org/en/guidelines2.htm

Eudralex volumes:

http://ec.europa.eu/health/documents/eudralex/index_-en.htm

For all authorized veterinary medicines, there is an ongoing process of safety and efficacy monitoring—called pharmacovigilance—that ensures the continued safe use of effective medicines.

In the EU there are two types of authorizations of feed additives. The first type is, when authorizations issued to a holder of authorization (zootechnical additives, coccidiostats, and histomonostats, as well as additives produced from genetically modified organisms) The second type is, if authorizations not issued to a holder of authorization for substances' technological additives, sensory additives, and "nutritional additives." The applicant must send to EFSA a copy of the application and the complete dossier (applicant's name and address, a description of the method of production, manufacturing and intended uses of the additive, proposed conditions for placing the additive on the market, the safety and efficacy studies, etc.). EFSA is responsible for conducting the risk assessment based on the dossier submitted by the applicant. The applicant must also send samples of the additive to the EU Reference Laboratory for analysis. EFSA may, if necessary, ask for further information to the applicant during the assessment procedure. Additives intended for use in animal nutrition must receive a favorable opinion before being granted authorization for their use and placing on the market. Within six months of receipt of an application, the EFSA gives an opinion based on the information provided by the applicant. Based on the EFSA opinion, the European Commission decides whether to authorize or deny the authorization of the additive. The officer's opinion must include information on the specific conditions or restrictions relating to handling, monitoring requirements following placing on the market, and use of the additive, including the animal species and categories of animals for which the additive is to be used: information on specific additional requirements for labeling of the additive, and, where appropriate, a proposal for the establishment of MRLs in the relevant foodstuffs of animal origin. The evaluation report prepared by the Community Reference Laboratory on the method of analysis of the additive should be included in the opinion. The European Commission prepares a draft implementing Regulation to grant or deny the authorization. The Commission is assisted in the procedure by the Member States within the Standing Committee on Plants, Animals, Food and Feed—section Animal Nutrition. Authorizations are valid for 10 years throughout the EU and the European Economic Area (EEA).

6.2.4 Proper handling and uses, according to label versus off-label use, cascade concept

Current relevant regulations and legislation relating to VMPs strictly determine the proper legal mode of handling and using the products. Rules cover the aspects of handling the drugs by traders, veterinary practitioners, and users (farmers), and include general instructions on proper storage, order, and application. The accepted way of the handling and destruction of unused stuffs and packages are determined as well.

In general terms, the use of the drug should be consistent with the labeled directions unless compelling reasons direct alternative use. *Extra-label (off-label) drug use* (ELDU) of veterinary drugs often refers to use of a drug in an animal that is not in accordance with the approved labeling. Extra-label use may arise from use of an animal drug, a drug approved for use in humans or occasionally prepared preparations (see Section 6.2.1) and includes:

- use for indications not listed in the labeling
- use in unauthorized physiological state (e.g., pregnancy, lactation)
- use at dosage levels, frequencies, or routes of administration not listed in the labeling
- use of human medicine in different animal species

Veterinary medicines are mainly authorized to use in major food-producing animals, because it is more profitable. Over and above the availability of medicines intended to use in minor food-producing species, for example dairy sheep, goats, and waterfowls is critically low in more economically developed countries as well. In addition, there is a constant need for off-label use of human products, as no equivalent amount of product is available for animal species (Fig. 6.2). Generally, in EU extra-label use is limited to situations when the health of an animal is threatened or suffering, or death may result from failure to treat, and no approved animal drug is available that is considered likely to be effective. Where there is no authorized VMP in a Member State (MS) for an indication concerning a food-producing animal species, the animals may exceptionally be treated with the following medicinal product:

- a VMP authorized in the relevant MS or in another MS for use in the same or in another food-producing animal species for the same indication, or for another indication;
- a VMP authorized under this Regulation in the relevant MS for use in a non-food-producing animal species for the same indication;
- a medicinal product for human use authorized in accordance with Directive 2001/83/EC or Regulation (EC) No 726/2004;
- a veterinary medicine prepared extemporaneously (official, magistral, occasionally formulated medicines, see Section 6.2.1) in accordance with the terms of a veterinary prescription.

This above introduced ranking of medicines is often mentioned as "Cascade." Veterinarians are bound by regulations to select and use medicines according to this ranking for the administration in animals. Food-producing animals may only be treated under the Cascade with medicines listed in the table of allowed substances (Table 6.1) in Commission Regulation EU No 37/2010. Medicines containing pharmacologically active substances listed in Table 6.2[e] of the same regulation are strictly banned to use in food-producing individuals of the different animal species.

FDA recognizes the professional judgment of veterinarians and permits the ELDU of drugs by veterinarians under certain conditions. Before prescribing or dispensing an approved animal drug or approved human drug for an extra-label use in food animals, the veterinarian must:

- Make a careful diagnosis and evaluation of the conditions for which the drug is to be used;
- Establish a substantially extended withdrawal period (WP) prior to marketing of milk, meat, eggs, or other edible products supported by appropriate scientific information, if applicable;
- Institute procedures to assure that the identity of the treated animal or animals is carefully maintained; and

- Take appropriate measures to assure that assigned time frames for withdrawal are met and no illegal drug residues occur in any food-producing animal subjected to extra-label treatment.

Extra-label use of drugs may only take place within the scope of a valid veterinarian–client–patient relationship and such use must be accomplished in accordance with an appropriate medical rationale. Extra-label use of an approved human drug in a food-producing animal is not permitted if an animal drug approved for use in food-producing animals can be used in an extra-label manner for the particular use. ELDU is prohibited if any residue exceeds established safe level, safe concentration, or tolerance. FDA may prohibit the extra-label use of an approved animal drug or approved human drug or class of drugs in food-producing animals if FDA determines that an acceptable analytical method has not been established or cannot be established, or the extra-label use of the drug or class of drugs presents a risk to the public health.

Any drug prescribed and dispensed for extra-label use by a veterinarian or dispensed by a pharmacist on the order of a veterinarian must bear or be accompanied by labeling information adequate to assure the safe and proper use of the drug.

6.3 Preventing drug residues in food with animal origin

The administration of VMPs in livestock may leave drug residues in the foodstuffs obtained from treated or diagnosed animals. *These residues comprise pharmacologically active substances, excipients or degradation products, and their metabolites*. Some of these substances could be harmful to humans while consuming that contaminated foodstuffs.

To protect human health, the European Parliament and Council laid down uniform rules to ensure consumer protection against potentially harmful effects of residues in foodstuffs of animal origin. Similar rules were applied by the governments of different countries (United States, Australia, Canada, Japan, etc.) and internationally by FAO. These rules provide for a science-based establishment of *maximum residue limits (MRL)* for VMPs. The MRL is the maximum accepted concentration of a residue of a pharmacologically active substance which may be permitted in food of animal origin. Ideally, national MRLs are brought into alignment with international MRLs as these are developed by the Codex Alimentarius Commission.[14]

6.3.1 Control of drug residues in foodstuffs, maximum residue limits concept

The appropriate MRL value for each medicinal substance used in food animal practice is the significant step in controlling drug residue levels to those which do not cause harm to consumers. Moreover, MRL has to be considered during the determination of WP of VMPs prior the authorization procedure. To determine the WP, regulatory authorities must employ a scientific process that includes establishing the MRL for that medicine. Therefore medicine authorities like EMA, FDA, and at international level FAO make publicly available the MRL values of the different veterinary agents in their websites (Table 6.3). Establishing MRLs requires information relating to drug usage, including the recommended dose and frequency of application; pharmacokinetic and metabolic studies in experimental and food-producing animals; residue depletion studies in target animals; a description of the method of analysis for detecting and quantifying the residues, including the marker residue; and studies designed to assess the impact of residues of antimicrobial agents on food processing.

During establishment of MRL firstly a No Observed (Adverse) Effect Level (NO(A)EL) is identified through toxicological studies using the active substance. These studies include single- and repeat-dose toxicity tests, reproductive-, genotoxicity, and carcinogenicity tests. Immunotoxicity, neurotoxicity, and potential effects on human gut microbiota should also be considered. The NO(A)EL is the highest dose of active ingredient that does not cause adverse effects. This figure is then divided by an "uncertainty" or "safety factor," for example, by 100–1000 to determine the acceptable daily intake (ADI). The ADI is the amount of the residue that is considered safe for an individual to eat every day for their lifetime taking into account a number of safety factors. In deriving MRLs it shall be assumed that the consumer will eat a standard food basket of animal-derived products every day. It consists of 0.3 kg meat, 0.05 kg fat (0.09 fat + skin in case of poultry), 0.1 kg liver, 0.05 kg kidney, 1.5 kg milk, and 0.1 kg eggs. With the help of appropriate MRL consumer safety shall be ensured by keeping the total amount of residues in the standard food basket below the ADI.[f]

No MRL has to be determined for substances with little or negligible adverse effect, or for agents with zero percentile utilization by standard administration routes.

6.3.2 Determination of withdrawal period after administration of medicines

Based on the definition of on European regulation on VMPs:

> *"**withdrawal period**" means the minimum period between the last administration of a veterinary medicinal product to an animal and the production of foodstuffs from that animal which under normal conditions*

of use is necessary to ensure that such foodstuffs do not contain residues in quantities harmful to public health.[g]

In other words, following this time period, the foodstuffs contain only traces of these potentially harmful contaminants, far below the accepted MRL value (see previous section). Regarding to WP analogous definitions have been introduced by other federal or national regulations (e.g., FD&C act in United States, Food and Drug Act in Canada, Food and Medicine regulation in Australia) or internationally by FAO WHO.[20] When animals were medicated with VMPs farmers are not allowed to send animals to slaughter or collect milk, eggs for human consumption before WP elapsed. The determination of WP is primarily based upon the product information details, label, and summary of product characteristics (SPC). The established value is acceptable exclusively when medicine usage has been strictly based on the "product literature" of the medicinal product. These publicly available WPs are based upon the research conducted by the medicine companies, more closely on the results of pharmacokinetic and residue studies. During the marketing authorization the officers critically evaluate the research documents. The WP values proposed in the documentation of the new VMP will only be accepted if they are based on reliable studies performed in accordance with the latest guidelines on, inter alia, "residue depletion studies" and "GLP." The WP can be calculated by taking into account the rate of residue depletion, to below the MRL, in all edible tissues and food products. The terminal elimination of a drug from tissues, the residue depletion, in most cases follows a one-compartment model. The first-order kinetic equation for this terminal elimination is

$$C_t = C_0 \times \mathrm{e}^{-ke \times t}$$

where C_t is the concentration at time t, C_0 is the fictitious concentration at $t = 0$, and k_e is elimination rate constant.

The plot of lnC versus time need to be linear. This indicates that the model for residue depletion is applicable. In this way linear regression analysis can be applied for the calculation of WPs. It should be confirmed that the variances of the log-transformed concentrations of the different slaughter days are homogeneous. Commonly used tests preferred by EMA for homogeneity of variances are Hartley's test and Cochran's test. The FDA recommends Bartlett's test. WPs are determined as the time when the upper one-sided tolerance limit (95% or 99%) with a given confidence (95%) is below the MRL. If this time point does not make up a full day, the WP is to be rounded up to the next day. The FDA recommends calculating the 99th percentile of the population with a 95% confidence level by a procedure which requires the noncentral t-distribution.[21]

This above calculation together with the detailed presentation of residue depletion studies have to be included to the registration documentation of the new VMP. Sponsors typically submit to regulatory authorities a description of, and validation data for, the method used to quantify the residue and marker residue in residue depletion studies. At the end of registration procedure, the established and accepted WP will appear in the product literature (SPC, label text, inserted package leaflet) and in the public assessment report. For the veterinary drugs containing substances, for what no MRL has to be established "zero" (nil) days withdrawal time can be established and published.

According to drug "Cascade" veterinarians must choose a medication what has been authorized to use in given target food-producing animal species consistently to label instructions. There are situations where no suitable authorized VMP is available. This frequently happens to individuals of minor food-producing species.[22,23] There are cases where VMP is not available for a given age, disease, and so on. In these ELDU situations (see above), by way of exception, veterinarians are allowed to prescribe other medicinal products (veterinary licensed medicine for other disease, species,[h] human licensed drug, nonlicensed medicines), as it was detailed in Section 6.2.4. To minimize the risk of appearance of drug residue in food the European authority declared the following minimum WPs (Table 6.4).

In a general sense, the determination of the WP is always the responsibility of the veterinarian who has prescribed or administered the medicinal product to the food-producing animals. In other words, authorities establish only the minimum duration of WP. Based on the judgment of responsible veterinarians the minimum duration may be accepted or extended. Veterinary professionals upon the examination of the actual circumstances have right to determine longer WP than the supposed shortest value. There are several factors which may influence the pharmacokinetic characteristics of the applied VMPs. Among the others; older age, diseases, decreased function of liver and kidneys, drug interactions can prolong the drug elimination from the edible tissues of the food-producing animals (see Section 6.1). If veterinary practitioners determine a shorter WP than enough, it will increase the risk associated with drug residues that remain in the tissues of treated animals at the time of slaughter. (for more details see section 6.4.)

6.3.3 Responsibilities of authorities, veterinary practitioners, and farmers in prevention of formation of drug residues in food

The administration of animal medicines and medicated feed for food-producing animals are strictly controlled by

TABLE 6.4 Establishing withdrawal period (WP) for medicinal products used outside the terms of the marketing authorization.

Category of food obtained from terrestrial species	Minimum duration of the WP following the use of medicinal products		
	Authorized for other food-producing animals	Not authorized for food-producing animals	With zero WP in other species
Meat and offal of food-producing animals (mammals and birds)	Longest WP multiplied by factor 1.5	28 days[a]	1[b] day
Milk	Longest WP multiplied by factor 1.5	7 days	1 day
Eggs	Longest WP multiplied by factor 1.5	10 days	Not indicated

Nonterrestrial species	Minimum duration of the WP following the use of medicinal products			
	Authorized for other aquatic species	Authorized for terrestrial food-producing animals	Not authorized for food-producing animals	with zero WP in other species
Aquatic species (fish)	Longest WP multiplied by factor 1.5 and expressed as degree-days	Longest WP multiplied by factor 50 expressed as degree-days, but not exceeding 500 degree-days	500 degree-days	25 degree-days

Degree-days = the cumulative sum of the mean daily water temperature in Celsius degrees.
[a]*If medicine is included to the "List of substances essential for the treatment of Equidae" (Commission Regulation No 122/2013), in Equidae the WP will be six months.*
[b]*If the medicinal product is used in a different taxonomic family.*

the European law and by the national regulations in United States, United Kingdom, Australia, Canada, and so on. The responsibility, for ensuring our food from animal origin does not contain residues above the statutory limit, is shared by all those involved in the farm animal sector. Veterinarians, Pharmacists, SQPs in the United Kingdom, and professional keepers of animals, including farmers, all have well-defined function in this. Using animal medicines in proper way and responsibly is a fundamentally important step in providing our food safety. Veterinary surgeons may be subject to legislative sanction if found responsible for causing illegal residues in food.

According to regulations veterinary treatments should be given appropriately—in terms of authorized route of administration, dose and duration of treatment—and WPs should be observed for animals and their animal products such as milk, eggs, and honey. Moreover, farmers should apply medicines in food-producing animals by or under the supervision of a licensed veterinarian. To ensure consumers are provided with safe food from animals when medicines are used, farmers and veterinarians must observe the WP for all medicines. Basically, all licensed veterinary medicine dispensed for animals have to be administered according to label. In the label (product literature) clear instructions are given not only about the dosing but also the duration of WP of VMPs. However, in certain rare individual cases, to reduce the unnecessary suffer of animals VMPs may be used not according to label, or other medicine categories may be chosen along the "Cascade" ranking. The term off-label (ELDU) is defined when a veterinarian prescribes a drug in a way that is not specifically indicated on the label. This can include a different dosing size, different ailment than what the drug is labeled to treat, a different treatment regimen, as well as a different species that is not explicitly stated on the label of VMP, or using human licensed and nonlicensed medicines. The ELDU is accepted and regulated by law (see details in Section 6.2.4). It cannot be overemphasized that the off-label medicine application always requests special scientific knowledge and veterinarians are entirely responsible toward farmers and authorities. The veterinarian has assumed the responsibility for making clinical judgments regarding the health of the patient and the need for medical treatment and the client's owner has agreed to follow the veterinarian's instructions. Furthermore, veterinarians are readily available for follow-up evaluation in the event of adverse reactions or failure of the treatment regimen (pharmacovigilance system).

On farms, there is a legal requirement to record all veterinary medicines obtained and used in food-producing animals or any types of treatment of the food-producing animals. In other words, requirements on farm include the recording of all medicines bought and administered. Regarding to the recent European regulations records shall include: date of the first administration of the medicinal product to the animals; name of the medicinal product; quantity of the medicinal product administered; name or company name and permanent address or registered place of business of the supplier; evidence of acquisition of the medicinal products they use; identification of the animal or group of animals treated; name and contact details of the prescribing veterinarian; WP even if such period is zero; duration of treatment.

In the framework of the drug residue monitoring in 2017, 28 EU Member States reported the results for 708,880 samples, based on requirements for sampling laid down in Council Directive 96/23/EC and in Commission Decision 97/747/EC. Based on Article 31 of Regulation EC 178/2002, the European Commission (EC) requested the assistance of the EFSA to collect data and report to European Council. The examined residues are classified into two groups A and B. Substances in group A are hormones and hormonally active substances, beta-agonists and prohibited medicines listed in Table 6.2.[i] Group B includes antibiotics (B1), antiparasitics, other drugs (B2), as well as other substances and environmental "contaminants" (B3). The report summarizes the results with the help of 42 tables. There were 1273 of noncompliant samples out of the 360,293 targeted samples in 2017. The overall frequency of noncompliant samples (0.35%) was comparable to the previous 10 years (0.25%–0.37%).[24]

In the United Kingdom, when veterinary medicines are administered to farm animals, the safety of food from these animals and their products (e.g., meat, milk, eggs) is monitored through a statutory residue surveillance scheme. The VMD oversees a statutory residue surveillance scheme that analyzes samples from animal foodstuff and publishes results annually. The annual reports contain, in table format, the type of examined samples (i.e., muscle, kidneys, milk, eggs, etc.), the name of chemicals detected, and their concentrations. The name of the used medicine, the geographical region, and a relatively detailed description on the circumstances leading to drug residue in food are also given (https://www.gov.uk/government/collections/residues-statutory-and-non-statutory-surveillance-results).

The surveillance reports from the VMD show that the vast majority of samples tested are compliant. This provides assurance that the regulatory control measures and actions are safeguarding the food from animals.

In the United States, the CVM's Division of Compliance is responsible for reviewing violative residues reported to the Agency by the USDA's Food Safety and Inspection Service. The residues are ranked using a Risk Model to ensure Federal and/or State investigation of the residues of greatest public health concern for which assignments are issued (https://www.fda.gov/animal-veterinary/compliance-enforcement/drug-residues).

6.4 Reasons for the drug residues in food of animal origin

Since the last few decades each medicinal substance must be investigated on a species-by-species basis to guarantee the effective and safe use of drugs. This includes the food safety considerations as well for each target animal species. Good practice in the use of veterinary drugs is defined as the official recommended or authorized usage, including WPs, approved by national authorities, of veterinary drugs under practical conditions.[25] Legal base of animal treatments and medicine use is also well declared by recent regulations and directives in developed countries. The veterinarians calculate drug doses on the basis of a fixed dose recommended on a product label or in a textbook, expecting that the recommended dose will give a described drug response and safety. It is expected that the "average" dose of drug will achieve "average" blood and tissue concentrations and "average" responses in "average" patients. Recommended dose may give a response that differs markedly from that which is expected: (either a small response is seen or side effects or toxicity occur) and may lead to accumulation of medicines in meat and other food products. Both the relative and absolute overdosing of VMPs can lead to drug residues. Certain disease conditions or infection request the application of higher dose or longer duration of the use of medicines than it is indicated in the authorized label. In such cases veterinarians should apply longer WP than the requested minimum.[26,27] The determination of appropriate withholding time is considerably more difficult, when the dose of VMDs should be extrapolated in ELDU for minor food-producing animal species.[28] When the suggested dose of VMPs is applied to animals, disease conditions may prolong the elimination and accordingly the tissue depletion of medicines. Typically, the decreased kidney or liver clearance can be responsible for the delayed elimination; however, other diseases or infections may sustain the excretion of drugs as well.[29,30] For instance, older age and drug interactions due to concomitant medicine use, as well as any external or internal factor which inhibit the standard rate of drug metabolism, may critically delay the depletion of residues.[31] Unintended administration to nontarget animals, due to mistake or inattention, can cause problems, for example, broiler feed containing ionophores can cause residue in eggs of laying hens. The application tools of medicines (e.g., syringes, drench guns) or feed mixing equipment should thoroughly be cleaned to avoid the cross-contamination with other drugs. The above examples were the most common causes of drug residues in food found during official investigations.[j] Once the veterinarians use a medicine or farmers administer a drug under the control of practitioners in food-producing animals, the WP has to be determined and recorded into the food animal treatment record. One of three copies of this record should be kept in farm, where the animals are reared. The prescriptions of medicines intended for use in food-producing animals contain the WP in written form as well. Based on this information, the farmers/owners of food animals should apply the given withholding period. One of the most frequent errors in this system is, when the animal owners ignore the WP. In other words, the animals are sent to slaughter, or eggs and milk are collected for human consumption earlier than the WP has been finished. The most frequent reason of the ignorance of this rule is the economic losses due to the decreased production (i.e., longer rearing period) and extra costs of the disposal of the residue containing milk and eggs.

Drug residues in food are often derived from illegal drug administration. Simply, it could happen because of illegal supply or use of an authorized veterinary medicine, for example, POM/Rx medicine, without veterinary prescription or control. Further aspects of the illegal veterinary medicine use include counterfeit, falsified, and unregistered products and unapproved parallel imports. In some regions, mainly in developing countries, using illegal veterinary medicines is a significant and growing problem. The amount of the supplied falsified medicines can be almost equal to that of the legal medicines.[32,33] The widespread use of illicit drugs in certain regions could lead to a complete collapse in food safety.

6.5 Conclusions and further perspectives

The importance of food safety includes the reduction of drug residues in our food supply and cannot be overemphasized. European, US, UK, and so on regulatory controls on veterinary medicines cover activities in the discovery, research, and development phases, through authorization of medicines and extend throughout the postauthorization phase. Pharmacovigilance and the monitoring and evaluation of adverse events allow for the ongoing improvement of the safety profile of medicines on the market. The classification of authorized veterinary medicines and the "Cascade" of the medicine use designate the supply and distribution of these agents. Strict controls on medicines for food-producing animals, including record keeping and observance of WPs, ensure the safety from residues of veterinary medicines in food from treated animals. Official guidelines, concept papers relating to the development, and supply of VMDs are continuously reviewed and renewed. Besides other reasons (drug safety and efficacy), the continuous improvement of food safety is a major motivation of these amendments. Therefore suitable analytical procedures (e.g., high-performance liquid chromatography, enzyme-linked immunosorbent assay, biosensors) are requested. In general, methods and equipment intended for use in these studies have to be specific and sensitive enough, and these characteristics are continuously developing.[3] Furthermore, currently only healthy animals should be used in drug research and development. In other words, the pathophysiological conditions are different in experimental and clinically treated animals. As it was detailed in previous sections, disease conditions, especially that of the kidneys and liver, may prolong the elimination of medicines. This can lead to the establishing of a too short WP. Therefore the determination of actual WP always has to be based on the personal decision of the licensed veterinarians, according to multiple factors. Farmers should respect the established longer WP, regardless of their knowledge of the minimal WP. For better understanding and cooperation, the continuous education of professionals (i.e., veterinarians and farmers) is essential with the help of postgraduate trainings and sharing information on websites of regulatory and professional organizations. Residue surveillance annual reports of VMD (United Kingdom) introduce the most common reasons of the presence of medicine residues in foodstuffs. Since these reports are publicly available, knowledge of resolved cases can help avoid further drug residue problems (see Section 6.3.3). Dissemination of this type of reporting method would be helpful for all veterinary practitioners and farmers. According to current practice, authorities in other countries usually only publish the number of noncompliance cases, but not the reasons of the presence of drug residue in food.

A total ban on AGPs and recent radical restrictions on the use of antimicrobials prophylactically/metaphylactically in economically developed countries will lead to a huge reduction in the amount of drug used in animal husbandry (WHO, 2017). It may result in a lower probability of remaining drug residues in non-imported (produced in internal market) food with animal origin.

In the last few decades, the trend for so-called "chemical-free" food has led to increased demand for food from organic production primarily, because of its increased cost, in economically developed countries. Organic agricultural systems have already proved able to produce food with high quality standards.[34,35] Such choices are not generally available in the majority of less-developed countries, where it is much more important to have enough food which is safe and of equivalent high nutritional quality, which should be the primary goal to improve overall diets. On the other hand, less-intensive agriculture, animal husbandry, lower pesticide and drug use in these regions indicate lower probability of forming residues. Notably, organic agriculture is also gaining importance in a number of developing countries including China, Egypt, India, Philippines, Sri Lanka, and Uganda.[36,37] Organic (bio) food products come from farms that do not administer medicines and chemical feed additives. The feed used in these farms should also be organic products, obtained from the same or other organic farms. Ethno-veterinary practices play a significant role in maintaining or restoring animal health in several regions of the world, especially in areas where livestock is a main source of income for rural people. Ethno-veterinary preparations are often obtained from herbs and their use does not cause drug residues.[3] Development and breeding of disease resistant livestock could be a great help to reduce the use of drugs. Organic producers are required to obtain special certification based on standards set by the government in order to sell organic food. The full licensing system and continuous monitoring of these organic farms is a prerequisite to guarantee the production of drug-free food of animal origin.

Endnotes

[a]EC Regulation 2019/6.

[b]Commission Regulation (EU) No 37/2010[12] (Table 6.2).

[c]EC Regulation, 2019/6.

[d]The Veterinary Medicines Regulations, 2013, United Kingdom.[18]

[e]Commission Regulation EU No 37/2010.[12]

[f]Commission Regulation (EU) 2018/782.

[g]EC Regulation 2019/6.

[h]FDA, Animal Medicinal Drug Use Clarification Act of 1994 (AMDUCA).

[i]Commission Regulation EU (European Union) No 37/2010.[12]

[j]https://www.efsa.europa.eu/en/supporting/pub/en-1578; https://www.gov.uk/guidance/residues-surveillance.

References

1. Jha R, Berrocoso JD. Review: dietary fiber utilization and its effects on physiological functions and gut health of swine. *Animal.* 2015;9:1441–1452.
2. National Research Council (US) Committee on Drug Use in Food Animals. *The Use of Drugs in Food Animals: Benefits and Risks.* Washington DC: National Academies Press; 1999.
3. Falowo A, Akinmoladun O. *Veterinary Drug Residues in Meat and Meat Products: Occurrence, Detection and Implications.* Intechopen; 2019.
4. Research and Markets. *Animal Medicine Global Market Opportunities and Strategies to 2023*; 2020: 1–460.
5. EMA and ESVAC. *Sales of veterinary antimicrobial agents in 31 European countries in 2017* (European Surveillance of Veterinary Antimicrobial Consumption). European Medicines Agency; 2019.
6. Stephany RW. Hormones in meat: different approaches in the EU and in the USA. *APMIS Suppl.* 2001;S357–S363. discussion S363–S354.
7. Teillant A, Brower CH, Laxminarayan R. Economics of antibiotic growth promoters in livestock. *Annu Rev Resour Econ.* 2015;7:349–374.
8. Omonijo FA, Ni L, Gong J, Wang Q, Lahaye L, Yang C. Essential oils as alternatives to antibiotics in swine production. *Anim Nutr.* 2018;4:126–136.
9. Garcia, JF, Diez, MJ, Sahagun, AM, et al. The online sale of antibiotics for veterinary use. *Animals.* 2020;10.
10. Gruys E, Toussaint MJM, Niewold TA, Koopmans SJ. Acute phase reaction and acute phase proteins. *J Zhejiang Univ Sci B.* 2005; 6:1045–1056.
11. Lin L, Wong H. Predicting oral drug absorption: mini review on physiologically-based pharmacokinetic models. *Pharmaceutics.* 2017;9:41.
12. Commission Regulation (EU) No 37/2010 on the pharmacologically active substances and their classification regarding maximum residue limits in foodstuffs of animal origin. <https://eur-lex.europa.eu/legal-content/EN/TXT/?uri = CELEX%3A32010R0037>.
13. Krasucka D, Mitura A, Cybulski W, Kos K, Pietroń W. Tiamulin hydrogen fumarate–veterinary uses and HPLC method of determination in premixes and medicated feeding stuffs. *Acta Pol Pharm.* 2010;67:682–685.
14. Crawford, LM. The impact of residues on animal food products and human health. *Rev Sci Tech OIE (France).* 1985; 4:669–685.
15. Toutain P-L, Ferran A, Bousquet-Mélou A. Species differences in pharmacokinetics and pharmacodynamics. In: Cunningham F, Elliott J, Lees P, eds. *Comparative and Veterinary Pharmacology.* Berlin, Heidelberg: Springer; 2010:19–48.
16. Palocz O, Gal J, Clayton P, et al. Alternative treatment of serious and mild *Pasteurella multocida* infection in New Zealand White rabbits. *BMC Vet Res.* 2014;10:276.
17. Palócz O, Szita G, Csikó G. Alteration of avian hepatic cytochrome P450 gene expression and activity by certain feed additives. *Acta Vet Hung.* 2019;67:418–429.
18. The Veterinary Medicines Regulations. <http://www.legislation.gov.uk/uksi/2013/2033/schedule/3/part/1/made>; 2013.
19. Regulation (EU) 2019/6 of the European Parliament and of the Council of 11 December 2018 on veterinary medicinal products and repealing Directive 2001/82/EC. <https://eur-lex.europa.eu/eli/reg/2019/6/oj>.
20. JECFA. *Scientific Guidelines for the Preparation of Veterinary Drug Residue Monographs, Working Papers and Related Summary Documents for Joint FAO/WHO Expert Committee on Food Additives (JECFA) Drafting Experts and Reviewers Assigned by FAO.* FAO JECFA Secretariat; 2016.
21. EMEA. *Guideline on Determination of Withdrawal Periods for Edible Tissues.* EMA/CVMP/SWP/735325/2012; 2018.
22. Macrì A, Purificato I, Tollis M. Availability of veterinary medicinal products for food producing minor animal species in the Mediterranean area. *Ann Ist Super Sanita.* 2006;42:422–426.
23. FDA. *Sec. 615.115 Extralabel Use of Medicated Feeds for Minor Species Compliance Policy Guide*; 2016.
24. EFSA (European Food Safety Authority). Report for 2017 on the results from the monitoring of veterinary medicinal product residues and other substances in live animals and animal products. *EFSA Support Publ.* 2019;16(5):1578E. 88 pp.
25. Codex Alimentarius Commission. *Procedural Manual.* World Health Organization and Food and Agriculture Organization of the United Nations; 2008.

26. Lees P, Toutain P-L. The role of pharmacokinetics in veterinary drug residues. *Drug Test Anal*. 2012;4:34–39.
27. Wang W, Chen H, Yu B, Mao X, Chen D. Tissue deposition and residue depletion of melamine in fattening pigs following oral administration. *Food Addit Contam A*. 2014;31:7–14.
28. Baynes RE, Payne M, Martin-Jimenez T, et al. Extralabel use of ivermectin and moxidectin in food animals. *J Am Vet Med Assoc*. 2000;217:668–671.
29. Kandeel M. Pharmacokinetics and oral bioavailability of amoxicillin in chicken infected with caecal coccidiosis. *J Vet Pharmacol Ther*. 2015;38:504–507.
30. van Miert A. Influence of febrile disease on the pharmacokinetics of veterinary drugs. *Ann Rech Vet*. 1990;21(suppl 1):11s–28s.
31. Reeves PT. Drug residues. In: Cunningham F, Elliott J, Lees P, eds. *Comparative and Veterinary Pharmacology*. Berlin, Heidelberg: Springer; 2010:265–290.
32. Kingsley P. Inscrutable medicines and marginal markets: tackling substandard veterinary drugs in Nigeria. *Pastoralism*. 2015;5:2.
33. Rowan T. *Illegal Veterinary Medicines Impact and Effective Control*. Health for Animals, Global Animal Medicines Association; 2017: 1–51.
34. Hamzaoui-Essoussi L, Zahaf M. *Production and distribution of organic foods: assessing the added values. Organic Farming and Food Production*. Intechopen; 2012:145.
35. Lairon D. Nutritional quality and safety of organic food. A review. *Agron Sustain Dev*. 2010;30:33–41.
36. Semos A. *Organic Production, Organic Food and the Role of Agricultural Policy*. Aristotle University of Thessaloniki; 2003.
37. Tandon A, Dhir A, Kaur P, Kushwah S, Salo J. Behavioral reasoning perspectives on organic food purchase. *Appetite*. 2020;154:104786.
38. Wilds, N., 2017. Corrosion under insolation. in: Trends in Oil and Gas Corrosion Research and Technologies (ed. M. El-Sherik), 409-429, Woodhead Publ., Sawston, UK, 2017.
39. WHO guidelines on use of medically important antimicrobials in food-producing animals. Geneva: World Health Organization; 2017. Licence: CC BY-NC-SA 3.0 IGO.

Further reading

Animal Medicines Training Regulatory Authority (AMTRA). Information on the regulatory of SQPs. <http://www.amtra.org.uk/>.

EMA Committee of Medicinal Products for Veterinary Use (CVMP). <http://ema.europa.eu/ema/index.jsp?curl = pages/about_us/general/general_content_000262.jsp>.

EU Legislation for the pharmaceutical sector, including medicinal products for veterinary use. <https://ec.europa.eu/health/documents/eudralex/index_en.html>.

European Medicines Agency (EMA). Veterinary medicines regulatory information. <http://www.ema.europa.eu/ema/index.jsp?curl = pages/regulation/landing/veterinary_medicines_regulatory.jsp&mid = >.

FDA approved animal drug products. <https://animaldrugsatfda.fda.gov/adafda/views/#/search>.

IFAH-Europe – Regulatory affairs, bringing veterinary medicines to market. <http://www.ifaheurope.org/regulatory-affairs/bringing-veterinary-medicines-to-market.html>.

Manufacturing authorisations for veterinary medicines, VMD guidance. <http://www.gov.uk/guidance/manufacturing-authorisations-for-veterinary-medicines>.

NOAH compendium of datasheets. <http://noahcompendium.co.uk/Compendium/Overview/-21789.html>.

Regulation (EU) 2017/625 of the European Parliament and of the Council of 15 March 2017 on official controls and other official activities performed to ensure the application of food and feed law, rules on animal health and welfare, plant health and plant protection products, amending Regulations (EC) No 999/2001, (EC) No 396/2005, (EC) No 1069/2009, (EC) No 1107/2009, (EU) No 1151/2012, (EU) No 652/2014, (EU) 2016/429 and (EU) 2016/2031 of the European Parliament and of the Council, Council Regulations (EC) No 1/2005 and (EC) No 1099/2009 and Council Directives 98/58/EC, 1999/74/EC, 2007/43/EC, 2008/119/EC and 2008/120/EC, and repealing Regulations (EC) No 854/2004 and (EC) No 882/2004 of the European Parliament and of the Council, Council Directives 89/608/EEC, 89/662/EEC, 90/425/EEC, 91/496/EEC, 96/23/EC, 96/93/EC and 97/78/EC and Council Decision 92/438/EEC (Official Controls Regulation) Text with EEA relevance. <https://eur-lex.europa.eu/legal-ontent/en/TXT/?uri = CELEX:32017R0625>.

Reporting of adverse events to the VMD. <https://vmd.defra.gov.uk/AdverseReactionReporting/Default.aspx>.

The Veterinary Products Committee (VPC). <http://www.gov.uk/government/organisations/veterinary-products-committee/about>.

Veterinary Medicines Directorate (VMD) product information database. <http://www.vmd.defra.gov.uk/ProductInformationDatabase/>.

Veterinary Medicines Directorate (VMD) Veterinary Pharmacovigilance information. <http://www.gov.uk/guidance/veterinary-pharmacovigilance-your-responsibilities>.

Veterinary Pharmacovigilance in the United Kingdom. VMD annual review 2018. <https://www.gov.uk/government/publications/veterinary-medicines-pharmacovigilance-annual-review-2018-summary>.

VMD Enforcement Strategy. <https://www.gov.uk/government/uploads/system/uploads/attachment_data/file/447830/Enforcement_Strategy.pdf>; 2015.

VMD guidance for marketing authorisations for veterinary medicines. <http://www.gov.uk/guidance/marketing-authorisations-for-veterinary-medicines>.

VMD residue surveillance information <http://www.gov.uk/guidance/residues-surveillance>.

VMD retail of veterinary medicines guidance. <http://www.gov.uk/guidance/retail-of-veterinary-medicines>.

VMD wholesale dealers authorisation (WDA) guidance. <http://www.gov.uk/guidance/apply-for-a-veterinary-medicine-wholesale-dealers-authorisation-wda>.

Section III

Changes in the chemical composition of food throughout the various stages of the food chain: fishing and aquaculture

Chapter 7

Marine biotoxins as natural contaminants in seafood: European perspective

Pablo Estévez, José M. Leao and Ana Gago-Martinez (Gago)

Biomedical Research Center (CINBIO), Department of Analytical and Food Chemistry, University of Vigo, Vigo, Spain

Abstract

The proliferation of harmful algal blooms is a natural phenomenon in the marine environment of relevant impact in seafood safety. The marine biotoxins resulting from this natural contamination can accumulate in seafood causing different kinds of food poisoning in humans. The implementation of surveillance programs to monitor the presence of marine biotoxins, in order to protect public health, has been intensified in the European Union (EU) over the last few decades. The transition from mouse bioassay to instrumental analytical methods, typically liquid chromatography coupled to different detection modes, has been a key achievement, allowing the reliable identification, quantification, and even confirmation of the different toxin analogs involved in the contamination, contributing to the risk characterization associated to these toxic compounds. Three different toxin groups, lipophilic, amnesic, and paralytic are currently regulated in the EU; however, future challenging needs are coming which are demanding the attention of the scientists working in this field, in particular the ones related to the appearance of emerging toxins, which are being detected in certain coastal areas of Europe, as a consequence of the climate change, among other factors, representing a potential and additional seafood safety risk.

Keywords: Marine biotoxins; emerging marine biotoxins; seafood safety climate change; Europe

7.1 Introduction

The massive proliferation of marine phytoplankton is a natural phenomenon of relevant socioeconomic impact in coastal areas where the shellfish or in general seafood industry is an important economic resource. The phenomenon is commonly known as harmful algal blooms (HABs), and although has been widely evaluated and discussed over decades, the specific conditions are not yet entirely understood. Nevertheless, changes in the temperature, salinity, or nutrients have been identified as some of the responsible factors for HABs. Additional factors (e.g., climate change or the transport of nonnative species in ballast waters) might be linked to the increase in the frequency and persistence of HABs and their detection in regions where they were absent previously.[1,2]

Marine biotoxins are secondary metabolites produced during HABs. The role of these compounds in HABs is not clear; some authors suggest that they act as a defense mechanism over other species,[3] but there are still some unknowns and controversy regarding the particular role of some marine biotoxins, and even on the potential precursors present in algae which might cause their occurrence in seafood. The consumption of seafood containing marine biotoxins might cause food poisonings in humans. Most of these food poisonings are linked to the consumption of seafood such as shellfish, specifically bivalve mollusks and filter-feeding species, but they can also be present in fish which have accumulated marine biotoxins.[4–6] Over the last decades, efforts have focused on the monitoring of marine biotoxins in seafood worldwide. The development and validation of reliable analytical methodologies with the ability to identify the compounds responsible for the contamination have led to the performance of toxicological studies and the establishment of regulatory limits protecting public health. The occurrence and toxic profile of the main marine biotoxins have been successfully identified, controlling their presence in seafood and the food safety of these products. However, emerging marine biotoxins have been detected in seafood from areas where they were not present before. This issue opens a new challenge to the marine biotoxin community, making necessary the constant monitoring of seafood to evaluate the spread and/or prevalence of marine biotoxins.

This chapter is focused on providing an updated overview of the main marine biotoxins affecting seafood and endangering public health and general aspects regarding

Present Knowledge in Food Safety. DOI: https://doi.org/10.1016/B978-0-12-819470-6.00044-5

the analytical methods available for their monitoring. The chapter includes updated and summarized information regarding the main marine biotoxins that are emerging in the European coasts.

Paralytic shellfish toxins (PSTs), lipohilic toxins (LTs) including okadaic acid (OA) and its derivatives, dinophysistoxins (DTXs) considered as the typical diarrhetic shellfish poisoning (DSP toxins), azaspiracids (AZAs), yessotoxins (YTXs), and amnesic shellfish toxins (ASTs) including domoic acid (DA), and isomers are the most common marine biotoxins causing food poisonings after the consumption of seafood, in particular bivalve mollusks and clearly related to the proliferation of HABs. Generally, a principal compound or main analog is responsible for the toxic effect, and additional analogs or congeners might be present contributing to the total toxicity which is typically expressed in equivalents by using toxicity equivalence factors that have been used to evaluate the individual toxicity.[7]

7.1.1 Paralytic shellfish poisoning

Paralytic shellfish poisoning (PSP) is a neurotoxic poisoning caused by the consumption of contaminated seafood. PSP toxins have been detected worldwide in marine bivalves and gastropods but they can be also present in crabs and fish. The main symptoms related to PSP intoxications are ataxia, respiratory depression or failure, tachycardia, and heart paralysis. There is no antidote for these toxins and treatment is the medical assistance performing a gastric lavage if the puke is not spontaneous. Initially, the toxins associated with this food poisoning were the saxitoxins (STXs). However, further research identified more than 21 additional toxic compounds causing PSP.[8] These toxins are mainly produced by dinoflagellates of the genera *Gymnodinium* and *Alexandrium*, and they are characterized for being polar and soluble in solvents such as water.[9]

Saxitoxin (STX) is a tetrahydropurine with two guanidine functional groups and a diol group.[10] These toxins share the same ring structure with variations in the substitution in R1, R2, R3, and R4, resulting in different chemical and toxicological properties. Depending on the substituent present in R4, PSP toxins can be classified as carbamate, sulfocarbamate, and decarbamate (Fig. 7.1). These compounds can be bioconverted between each other due to the structural relations they have. STX is the most potent PSP toxin congener and the concentration of these toxins are referred to this compound being the regulatory limit in the European Union (EU) established in 800 μg STX · 2HCl eq/kg.[11]

7.1.2 Diarrhetic shellfish poisoning

DSP is a food poisoning related to the consumption of contaminated seafood producing gastrointestinal symptoms. Professor Takeshi Yasumoto and his research group identified in the 1980s the correlation between the dinoflagellate *Dinophysis fortii* and this food poisoning.[12,13] The main toxins responsible for DSP are OA and dinophysistoxins (DTXs).

DSP cases have been identified worldwide in regions such as Japan, Spain, Italy, Canada, United States, or Chile. The toxic profile of the DSP cases can vary, OA, DTX1, DTX2, and DTX3 being the main responsible for the contamination. These compounds are cyclic polyethers with a lipophilic nature, heat-stable, and soluble in solvents such as acetone or chloroform, and they can be acylated with saturated and unsaturated fatty acids (Fig. 7.2). The acylated metabolites of these compound also show a toxic activity and it has been suggested that they are metabolic products produced in the digestive gland of seafood.[14] OA and DTX1 act as potent inhibitors of the phosphatase protein 1 and 2A (PP1 and PP2A) and the regulatory limit established in the EU for DSP toxins is 160 μg OA eq/kg.[11]

Pectenotoxins (PTXs) and yessotoxins (YTXs) were initially included in this group despite showing a different symptomatology; PTXs are hepatotoxic, and YTXs are cardiotoxic.[15,16] The reason of the inclusion of PTXs and YTXs in this group was due to the presence of these toxins with OA and DTXs in bivalve mollusks and their lipophilic nature, which cause their coextraction and their intraperitoneal injection in mouse producing a toxic effect. However, PTXs and YTXs are considered a different group.

PTX-2 was the only analog detected in dinoflagellate cultures of *D. fortii* and *Dinophysis acuta*.[17,18] The additional PTX analogs were only detected in seafood and might be the result of biotransformations. PTXs are macrocyclic polyethers with a lactone ring structurally different to OA or YTXs (Fig. 7.2). The toxicity of PTXs in humans has been controversial and widely discussed over the last few years; also the fact of PTXs being always present together with OA was a reason to justify that the seafood safety would be ensured and, therefore, the deregulation of YTX in the EU legislation has been effective since 2021.[19]

YTXs are produced by dinoflagellates species *Protoceratium reticulatum* and *Gonyaulax polyedra*.[20,21] These species are prevalent in numerous coastal areas and they adapt to several conditions such as temperature, salinity, pH, or nutrients. YTX and analogs are disulfated polycyclic polyethers with an unsaturated side chain (Fig. 7.2).[22] The human toxicity of YTX has also been under debate and the conclusions led to the decision of including a modification of the EU legislation including a less restrictive regulatory level.[23]

7.1.3 Azaspiracid shellfish poisoning

The azaspiracids (AZAs) were the compounds identified as responsible for the azaspiracid shellfish poisoning (AZP).[24]

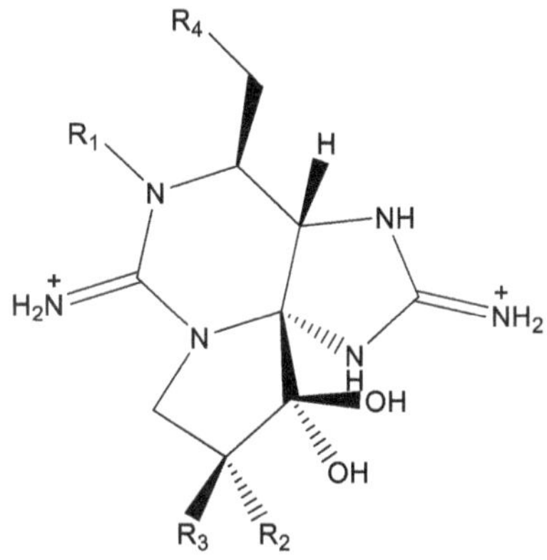

R1	R2	R3	*Carbamoyl* **R4 = -** OCONH2-	*N-sulfocarbamoyl* **R4 = -** OCONHSO3-	*Decarbamoyl* **R4 =** -OH
H	H	H	STX	GTX5	dcSTX
H	H	OSO3-	GTX2	C1	dcGTX2
H	OSO3-	H	GTX3	C2	dcGTX3
OH	H	H	NEO	GTX6	dcNEO
OH	H	OSO3-	GTX1	C3	dcGTX1
OH	OSO3-	H	GTX4	C4	dcGTX4

FIGURE 7.1 Paralytic shellfish poisoning toxins structures.

AZP was first reported in the Netherlands and associated with the consumption of mussels from Ireland. The symptoms observed in this outbreak were similar to those observed in the DSP (nausea, diarrhea, and vomiting) but including neurotoxic symptoms such as paralysis or respiratory distress.[25] AZP has been detected in areas such as England, Norway, or Spain. In contrast with other marine biotoxins which are mostly present in the mussel hepatopancreas, AZAs are characterized for being present equally in all organs. There are more than 20 analogs of AZA, and these compounds are produced by species *Azadinium spinosum*.[26] They are characterized for having a cyclic amine, a tri-spiro-assembly, and a carboxylic acid group. The regulatory limit established in the EU for these compounds is 160 μg AZA1 eq/kg (Fig. 7.3).

The current EU legislation includes diarrhetic toxins, yessotoxins, and azaspiracids in the group of lipophilic toxins due to their common lipophilic character which also allows their determination using multianalyte methods using the same conditions for an efficient extraction from the contaminated matrix.

7.1.4 Amnesic shellfish poisoning

Amnesic shellfish poisoning (ASP) was first identified in Prince Edward Islands (Canada) in 1987 associated with the consumption of seafood.[27] The symptoms included the loss of memory, confusion, and also diarrhea and vomiting. The DA was identified as responsible for the ASP. DA is an analog of the glutamic acid and it was isolated from phytoplanktonic species of *Pseudonitzschia*.[28] This compound is soluble in water and its structure depends on the pH. Despite the identification of more than five analogs, the DA is the principal compound

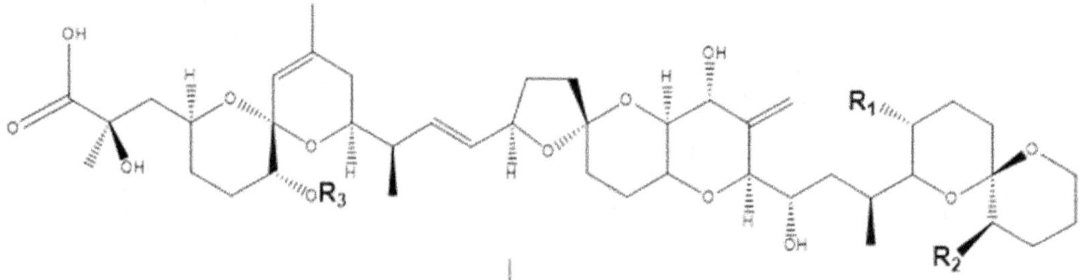

R1	R2	R3	Compound
CH_3	H	H	Okadaic acid (OA)
CH_3	CH_3	H	Dinophysistoxin-1 (DTX1)
H	CH_3	H	Dinophysistoxin-2 (DTX2)
H/ CH_3	H/ CH_3	Acyl	Dinophysistoxin-3 (DTX3)

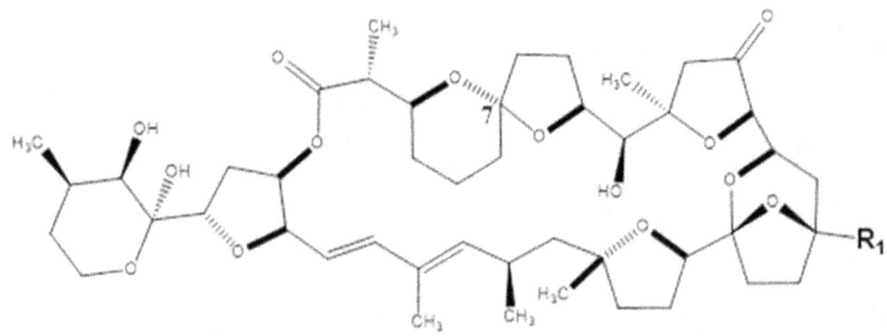

Compound	R1	C7
PTX-1	CH_2OH	R
PTX-2	CH_3	R
PTX-3	CHO	R
PTX-4	CH_2OH	S
PTX-5	CH_2OH	R
PTX-6	COOH	R
PTX-7	COOH	S
PTX-8	CH_2OH	S
PTX-9	COOH	S
PTX-10	CH_2OH	R

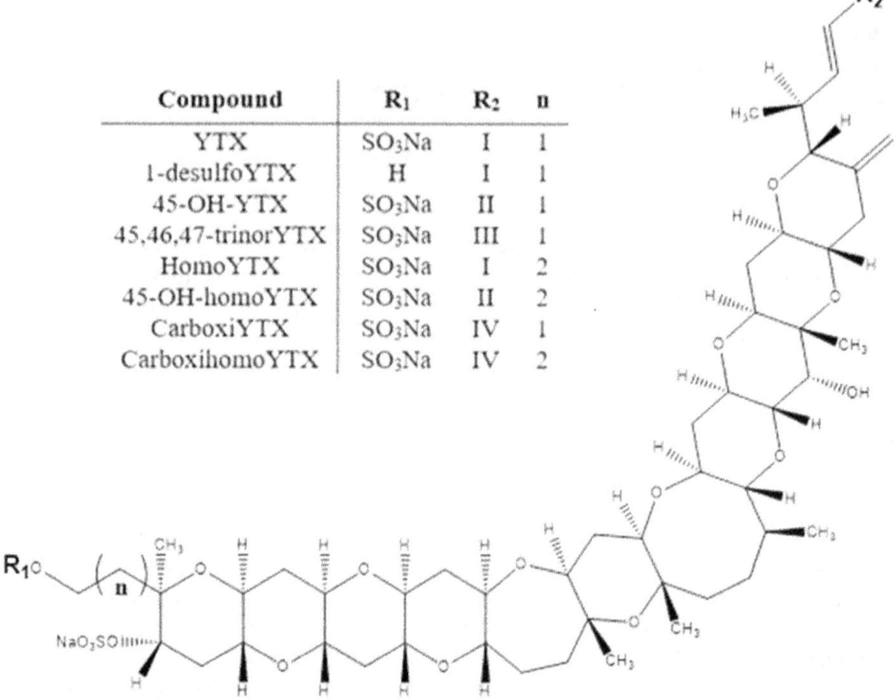

Compound	R1	R2	n
YTX	SO_3Na	I	1
1-desulfoYTX	H	I	1
45-OH-YTX	SO_3Na	II	1
45,46,47-trinorYTX	SO_3Na	III	1
HomoYTX	SO_3Na	I	2
45-OH-homoYTX	SO_3Na	II	2
CarboxiYTX	SO_3Na	IV	1
CarboxihomoYTX	SO_3Na	IV	2

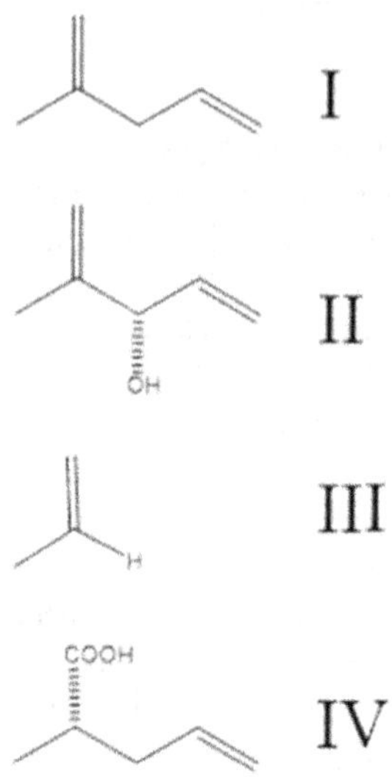

FIGURE 7.2 Diarrhetic shellfish poisoning (OA, dinophysistoxins) toxins, pectenotoxins (PTXs), and yessotoxins (YTXs) structures.

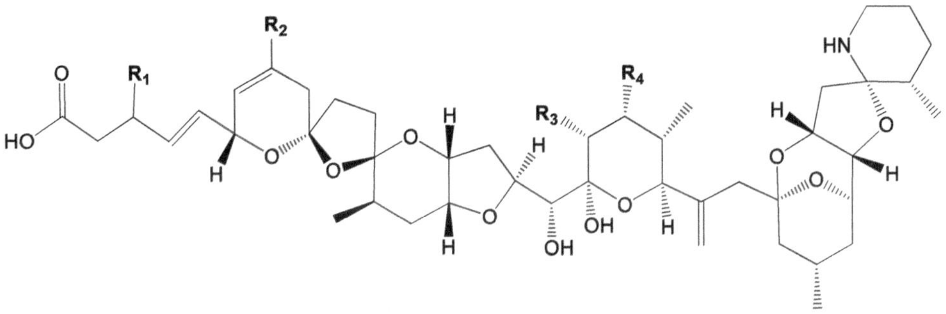

FIGURE 7.3 Azaspiracid shellfish poisoning toxins structures.

Compound	R1	R2	R3	R4
AZA1	H	H	CH3	H
AZA2	H	CH3	CH3	H
AZA3	H	H	H	H
AZA4	OH	H	H	CH3
AZA5	H	H	H	OH

present in both phytoplankton and seafood (Fig. 7.4). The regulatory limit established in the EU for the sum of DA and epi-domoic acid (epi-DA), DA C5′-diastereomer, is 20 mg/kg.

7.2 Analytical methods

Over the last decades, the proliferation of marine phytoplankton and the subsequent contamination of seafood with marine biotoxins have drawn the attention of the authorities. The identification and quantification of the compounds responsible for these contaminations is crucial to protect public health, allowing the establishment of regulatory limits to minimize the impact of marine biotoxins not only in human health but also in the local economy. Since the first identification of the compounds responsible for food poisoning after the consumption of seafood, scientists have been focusing their efforts on the development of reliable analytical methods. The advancement in the isolation and structural elucidation of marine biotoxins, the availability of reference materials of these compounds, and the technological improvements have led to the development of numerous detection methods for marine biotoxins.

The biological methods were the first methods used in the monitoring of marine biotoxins in seafood. Feeding tests in several animals such as mongoose or cats were initially used due to their simplicity but they were rapidly substituted because they are cumbersome and not quantitative. Mouse bioassay (MBA) is the bioassay most widely used. MBA consists of the intraperitoneal (i.p.) injection in mice of the semipurified extract of seafood. Mice are observed and it can be obtained a semiquantitative value through the relationship between dose and time to death. MBA was applied for the detection of numerous toxins such as ciguatoxins (CTXs) and tetrodotoxins (TTXs), and to date is the official method for the monitoring of PSP toxins in seafood.[29] MBA was also widely used in the monitoring of other regulated toxins such as DSP, ASP, or AZA toxins.[30] However, this method has some disadvantages such as the lack of specificity which can give false positives or negatives, or ethical issues related to animal welfare.

In the last decades, alternative methods such as immunoassays or cell-based assays have been developed and applied to the monitoring of marine biotoxins in seafood.[31,32] Immunoassays have the advantage of showing a high sensitivity and specificity while cell-based assays are more suitable to *screening* process due to their high sensitivity and limited specificity which relies on the interaction of the toxin with specific receptors of the cell. However, the applicability of these methods is limited and further improvements are needed.

The chromatographic methods are considered the most adequate detection methods for the monitoring of marine biotoxins in seafood. The selectivity provided by the chromatographic separation of the different toxins coupled to the sensitivity of detectors such as fluorescence (FLD) ultraviolet (UV), or mass spectrometry (Ms) allow the reliable identification, confirmation, and quantification.

Liquid chromatography (LC)-FLD is used for the monitoring of PSP toxins after their derivatization to

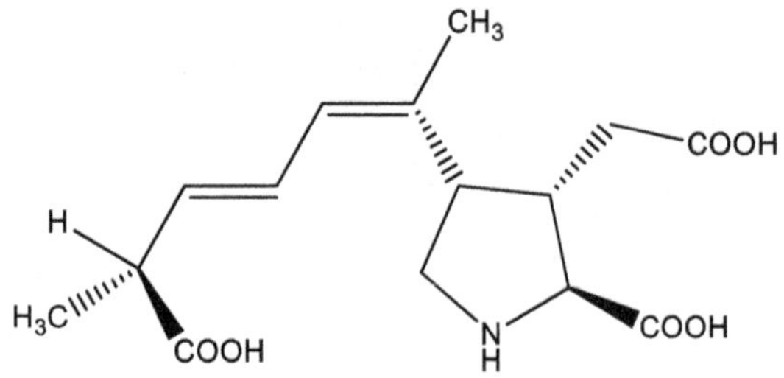

Domoic acid

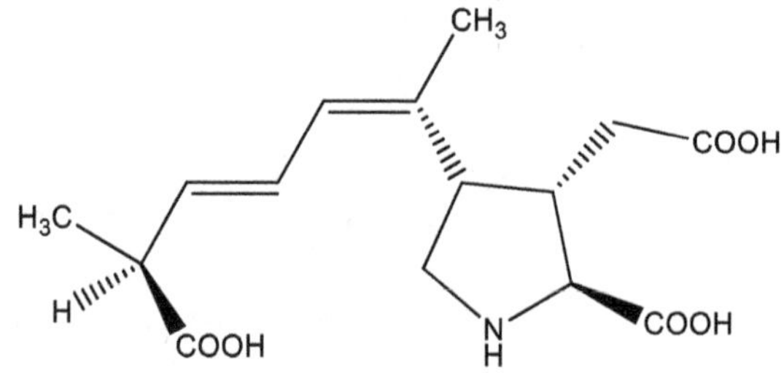

Isodomoic G (C5′-diastereomer)

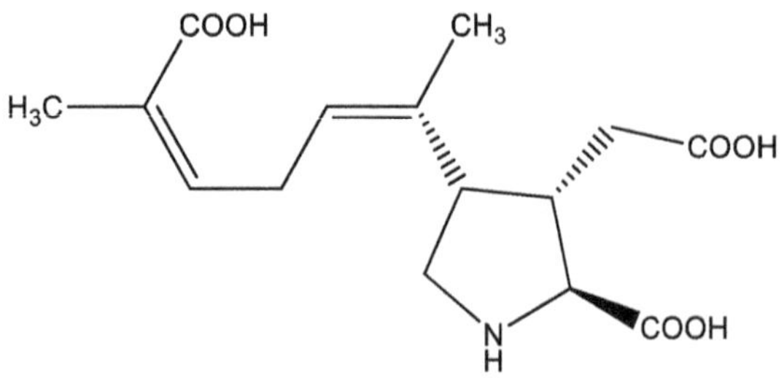

Isodomoic A

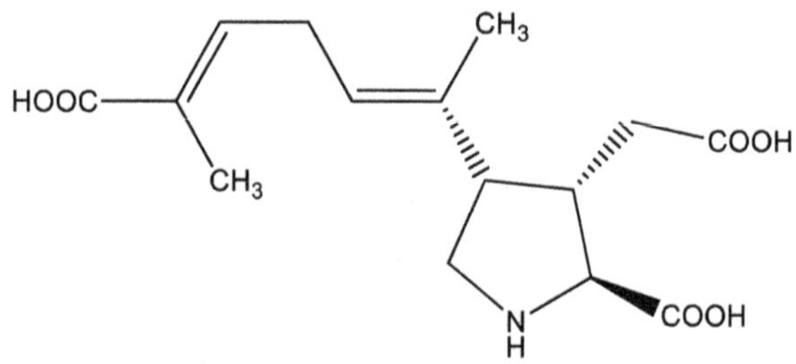

Isodomoic B

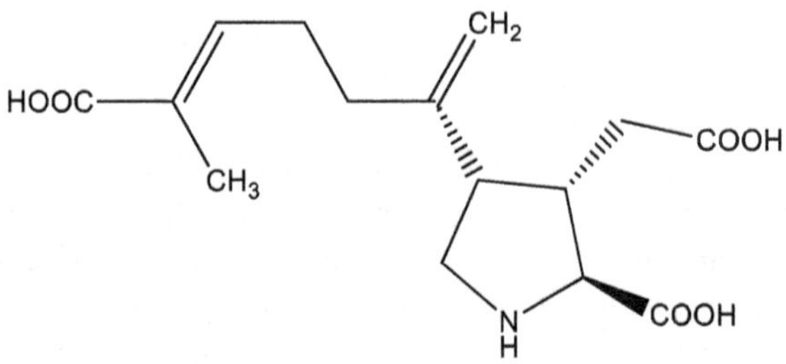

Isodomoic C

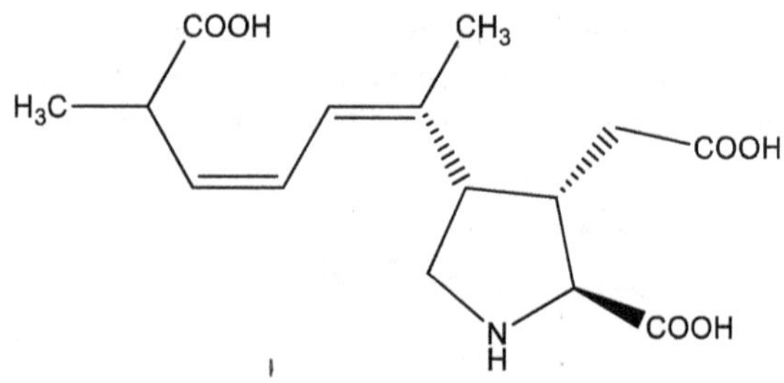

Isodomoic D

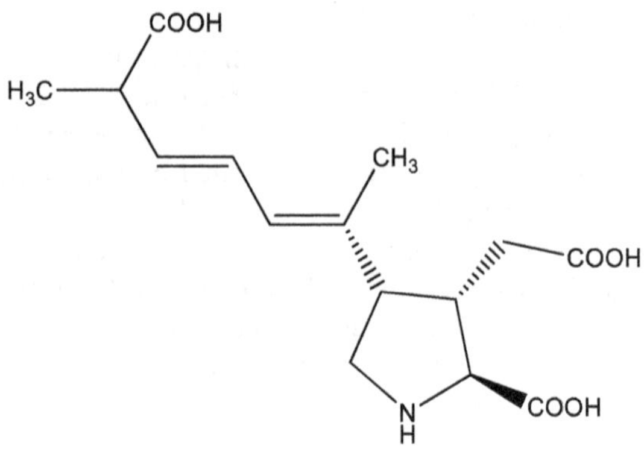

Isodomoic E

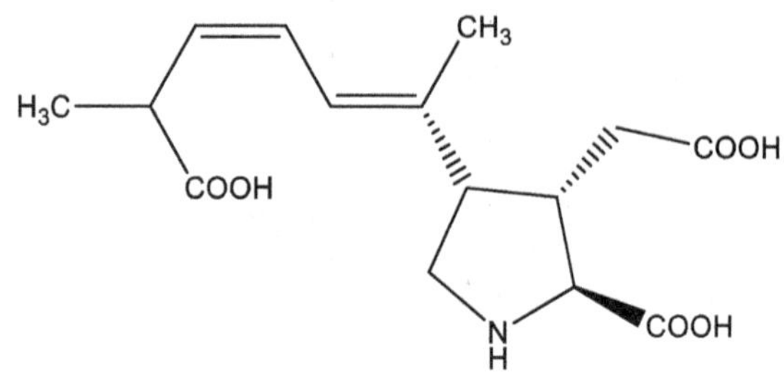

Isodomoic F

FIGURE 7.4 Amnesic shellfish poisoning toxins structures.

obtain fluorescence properties. This method provides a sensitive and selective monitoring of these compounds while the derivatization process through oxidation can be performed precolumn or postcolumn.[33,34] On the other hand, ASP toxins are commonly analyzed by LC-UV.[35] The improvements in the Ms technology triggered their application to the monitoring of marine biotoxins. LC-Ms and LC coupled to tandem mass spectrometry (LC-Ms/

MS) allowed the sensitive confirmation of the toxins by the monitoring of their mass-to-charge ratio and their fragmentation. Consequently, LC-Ms/MS has been established as official method in the EU for the monitoring of the lipophilic toxins DSP, YTXs, PTXs, and AZAs.[36] Additionally, LC-Ms/MS has been applied to monitoring of PSP toxins and also emerging marine biotoxins such as CTXs, TTXs, or cyclic imines (CIs).[37–39] More recently, LC coupled to high-resolution mass spectrometry (LC-HRMS) has also been applied to the monitoring of marine biotoxins.[40,41] LC-HRMS has the advantage of monitoring the exact mass of the toxins comparting the theoretical and the experimental isotopic pattern. However, the sensitivity provided by these instruments is lower compared to LC-Ms/MS instruments.

Reference materials are needed to implement instrumental methods and in particular the chromatographic methods to be able to identify, quantify, and even confirm the toxins involved in the contamination. Also, in the case of complex matrix such as fish or shellfish, previous steps of sample pretreatment might be needed to remove interfering compounds of the matrix which can affect the performance of the method. Solid phase extraction is the most common sample pretreatment procedure to selectively remove the interferences and also useful for toxin concentration to satisfy the sensitivity requirements.

7.3 Transition from biological to chemical methods

MBA was a practical tool for marine biotoxins control which has been used for several years despite its disadvantages. Important efforts have been carried out over the last years to replace the MBA by instrumental methods; the transition from animal tests to chemical methods has been challenging and it is not only justified by ethical issues and by the protection of animal welfare, but also to look for efficient and sensitive reliable methodologies with ability for identification, quantitation, and even confirmation of the toxin analogs involved in the seafood contamination. According to this, multitoxin chromatographic methods have been selected as the analytical option using different detection modes. LC-Ms/MS has been developed and validated for the analysis of LTs.[42,43] This method has been the first method included in the EU legislation as a replacement of the MBA being the method that initially established the transition from MBA.

LC-FLD with pre or postcolumn oxidation[33,34] have been also proposed for monitoring PSTs; the original methods were internationally validated, becoming official methods of analysis (OMA AOAC 2005.06 and OMA AOAC 2011.02). Recently the precolumn LC-FLD has been accepted as reference method to be included in the EU legislation for the control of PSTs in seafood.[33] The current situation in the EU legislation is, therefore, marked by the total replacement of the MBA by chromatographic methods with different detection modes: LC-UV for ASP toxins, LC-Ms/MS for LTs, and LC-FLD for PSP toxins.

7.4 Emerging toxins: incidence and present challenges for their control

The improvements in the development of more sensitive analytical methods as well as key factors such as climate change and global warming, with the increased interest of the scientific community in marine biotoxins, have triggered the detection of emerging toxins in regions where they were not present before.[44] The factors related to the detection of emerging marine biotoxins are not clear. Climate change, globalization, the increase in tourism, and the transport of nonnative species in ballast water all over the world might be the cause of the spread and prevalence of these toxins over the last decades.

Human poisonings related to the consumption of seafood contaminated with marine biotoxins make important the study of these natural contaminants to protect human health. The presence of emerging marine biotoxins in seafood entails a challenge for scientists mainly due to the lack of harmonized detection methods and reference materials of these compounds which would allow their reliable identification, quantification, and confirmation.

Consequently, in 2006 as requested by the European Commission (EC), the European Food Safety Authority (EFSA) published a series of scientific opinions including both regulated and emerging marine biotoxins which may be a risk for public health.[45–49] The objective of the EFSA opinions was to control the presence of marine biotoxins to assess if they may be a future concern.

Among the emerging marine biotoxins of special concern in the EU, which are occurring in places where they have never been reported before, can be included: CIs, palytoxin (PTX or PLTX), brevetoxins (PbTx), ciguatoxins (CTXs), and tetrodotoxins (TTXs) (Fig. 7.5).

7.4.1 Cyclic imines

The CIs include a group of toxins produced by dinoflagellates and accumulated in bivalve mollusks: gymnodimine (GYMs), spirolides (SPXs), pinnatoxins (PtTXs), prorocentrolides, and spiroprorocentrimines. GYMs are associated with species of *Karenia selliformis*, while SPXs are produced by species of *Alexandrium ostenfeldii* and *Alexandrium peruvianum*, and PnTXs by *Vulcanodinium rugosum*.[50–54] All these macrocyclic compounds have a common CI from 4- to 6-member ring, which is the biological active group of CIs (Fig. 7.5).[55] The toxicological

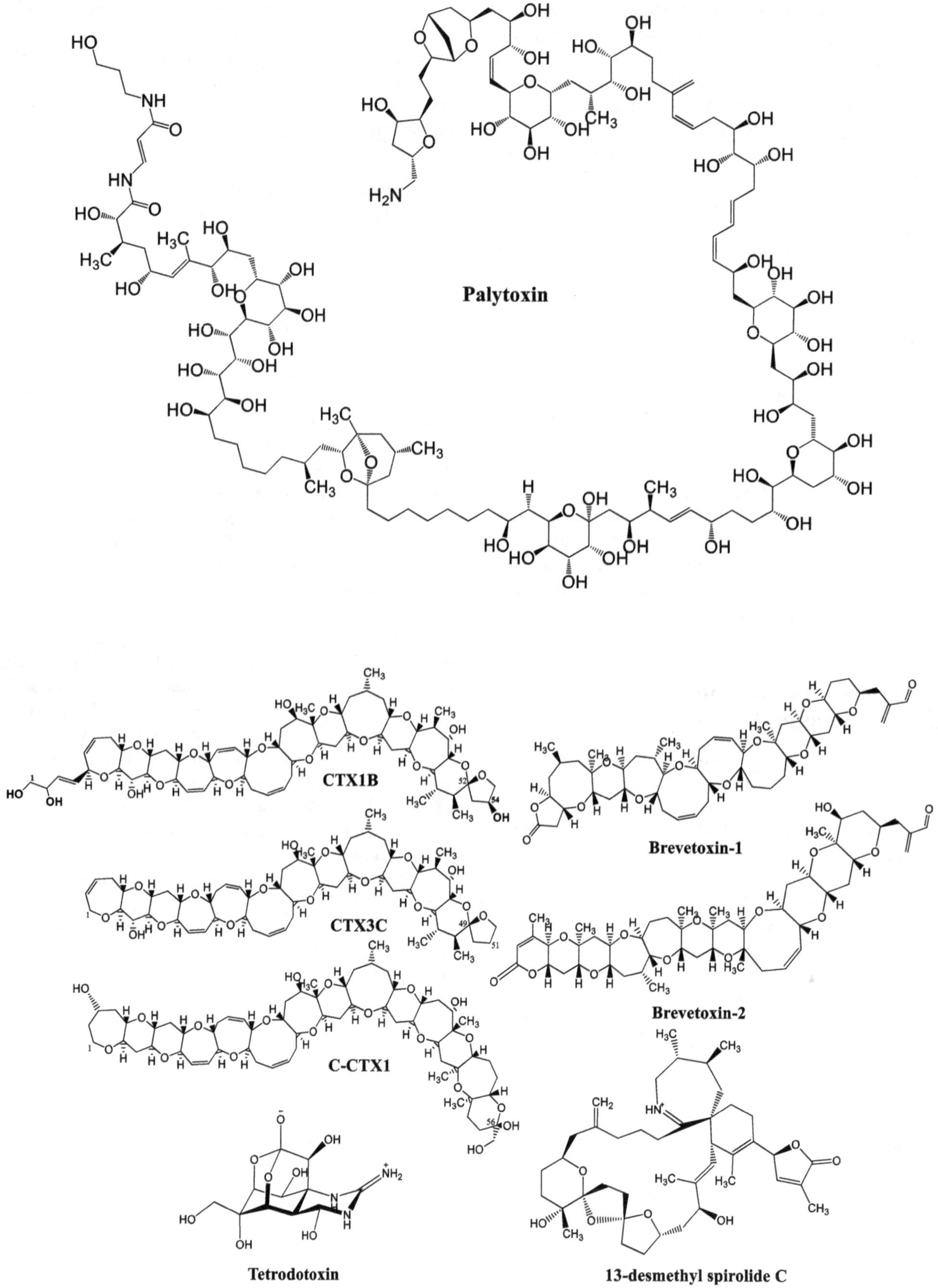

FIGURE 7.5 Structures of the main emerging marine biotoxins.

studies showed that these compounds can endanger public health due to their neurotoxic effect through the interaction with nicotinic receptors of acetylcholine.[56] However, no food poisoning related to CIs have been reported till date.

Most of the CIs were identified in the 1990s. GYMs were reported for the first time in New Zealand, SPXs in Canada, and PnTXs in Japan.[57–59] However, in recent years these toxins have been detected in regions of the European waters. CIs were detected in Galician mussels (Northwest Spain),[60,61] in the Mediterranean Sea in mussels and clams from Ingril, a French Mediterranean lagoon,[62] and more recently in mussels farmed in the Adriatic Sea (Italy).[63] Therefore the EFSA published a public opinion including the need of obtaining more occurrence data as well as the development and optimization of confirmatory methods of LC-Ms/MS for the detection of these compounds.[47]

7.4.2 Palytoxins

Palytoxins (PlTXs) are a group of marine biotoxins which can be present in corals of the genus *Palythoa* and are produced by dinoflagellate species of *Ostrepsis*. PlTXs were first reported in Hawaii and Japan but now they can be detected worldwide. Blooms of *Ostrepsis* spp. have been detected in several regions of Europe such as Spain, France, Greece, and Italy.[64–66] This can result in a risk due to the possible contamination of shellfish and further consumption causing poisoning in humans.

PlTXs are complex and large polyhydroxylated compounds with lipophilic and hydrophilic regions and stable to temperature (Fig. 7.5).[67,68] There are several analogs of PlTXs such as ostreocin-D, ovatoxin-A, homopalytoxin, bishomopalytoxin, neopalytoxin, deopalytoxin, and 42-hydroxypalytoxin. However only PlTX and ostreocin-D were structurally elucidated and are considered the principal responsible for the contamination.[69]

There are no regulatory limits for these compounds due to the lack of occurrence data.[48] PlTXs is one of the most potent toxins by intraperitoneal injection, with symptoms such as ataxia, drowsiness, weakness, myalgia, and even death. Fatalities are rare, but they have been reported in Philippines, Brazil, and Japan.[70] The toxicity of PlTX is dependent of the route of administration, being much less toxic after the oral than intraperitoneal injection.[71,72] Due to the limited toxicological data, the EFSA was only able to derive an acute reference dose (ARfD) of 0.2 μg/kg b.w. for the sum of PlTx and ostreocin-D.[48]

Traditionally MBA has been used for the detection of PlTXs, but the ethical issues related to animal welfare as well as the lack of specificity made necessary the development of additional detection methods. Cell-based assays provided high sensitivity for these compounds, but additional toxins can interfere in these assays and, therefore, these results must be confirmed with chemical analysis such as LC-FLD or LC-Ms/MS.[73,74] Therefore it is critical to increase the commercial availability of standards and reference materials of PlTXs to develop, optimize, and validate these detection methods.

7.4.3 Brevetoxins

Brevetoxins (PbTXs) are a group of marine biotoxins produced by dinoflagellate species of *Karenia brevis*. PbTXs are cyclic polyethers, lipid soluble, and can accumulate in shellfish and fish causing neurotoxic shellfish poisoning (NSP).[75] The main symptoms of NSP are nausea, diarrhea, paralysis, paresthesia, seizures, or coma. Despite of the severity of these symptoms, no persistent or fatalities have been reported.

PbTXs have been reported in fish and shellfish from the Caribbean Sea and New Zealand.[76,77] PbTXs can be classified into two groups depending on their backbone (type A and B) (Fig. 7.5). Brevetoxin-2 (PbTX-2) (type B) is the principal compound present in *K. brevis* and with brevetoxin-1 (PbTX-1) (type A) can accumulate in fish and shellfish giving rise to several toxic analogs resulting from metabolization.[78] The toxicological data are limited and, therefore, no regulatory limits have been established in EU.[46]

The public opinion of the EFSA published in 2010 stated that an ARfD should be established.[46] However, the lack of occurrence data and the limited data on acute and chronic toxicity hampered the comment on the risk associated with PbTXs in the European coasts. PBTXs have been recently detected in mussels from the French Mediterranean coast; thus efforts are necessary to increase surveillance programs to monitor these compounds and to obtain occurrence data.[79] As a consequence of the detection of PbTXs on the European coasts, the French Agency for Food, Environmental and Occupational Health & Safety (Anses) proposed a guidance level of 180 μg PbTX-3 eq/kg.[80]

As for most of the marine biotoxins, the MBA was initially used to detect PbTXs. However, the poor specificity and ethical concerns, as well as the lack of efficiency in the extraction process of PbTXs by following the standard MBA protocol, triggered the use of alternative detection methods. In vitro assays as well as immunoassays showed their ability to detect PbTX-like compounds but they need further development.[32,81] LC-Ms/MS seem the best approach to monitor these compounds with adequate sensitivity and specificity obtaining a quantitative value of the specific PbTXs responsible for the contamination.[82] However, the development of this method is limited by the lack of certified reference materials.

7.4.4 Ciguatoxins

Ciguatoxins (CTXs) are cyclic polyethers with a ladder-shaped structure and stable to temperature (Fig. 7.5).[83] These complex toxins are produced by dinoflagellates of the genera *Gambierdiscus* and *Fukuyoa* and they can be accumulated mostly in fish.[84] The consumption of fish contaminated with CTXs produce a food poisoning called ciguatera poisoning (CP). CP is endemic in tropical and subtropical regions of the world such as French Polynesia in the Pacific Ocean, the Caribbean Sea, or the Indian Ocean. Depending on the geographical region where they are present and their chemical structure they can be classified as Pacific, Indian and Caribbean CTXs (P-, I-, and C-CTXs) (Fig. 7.5). The symptoms of CP include neurological, gastrointestinal, and cardiovascular.[85]

Recent reports showed that CP is expanding worldwide affecting regions where they were not present before. From 2004 until now, numerous cases of CP were reported in the Canary Islands (Spain) and Madeira archipelago (Portugal) related to the consumption of fish.[86] Consequently, in 2010 the EFSA Panel on Contaminants in the Food Chain (CONTAM Panel) assessed the risk associated with the consumption of fish containing CTXs. There are no regulatory limits for CTXs in the EU being forbidden by the regulation to place on the market products containing CTXs. The toxicological studies for CTXs are limited and, therefore, it was not possible to establish an ARfD. Based on case reports and on MBA the Food and Drug administration (FDA) established a security level of 0.1 μg/kg for C-CTX1 and 0.01 μg/kg for CTX1B.[87] Additional occurrence data are needed to be able to propose regulatory limits for these compounds. The main limitation in the field of CP is the lack of standards and reference materials, the low concentration of the toxins presents in fish (<1 μg/kg), the complexity of the matrix, and the lack of harmonized methodologies with adequate sensitivity and specificity.[88]

Concerning the detection methods for CP, cell-based assays such as Neuroblastoma-2a (N2a), where the composite toxicity of the sample is evaluated, are commonly used in the analysis of these compounds. Despite of the high sensitivity provided by this method their specificity is limited by the detection of CTX-like compounds activators of voltage-gated sodium channels (VGSCs).[32,89] Therefore LC-Ms/MS is considered the best detection method due to its sensitivity and specificity confirming selected CTXs responsible for CP.[90,91]

7.4.5 Tetrodotoxins

Tetrodotoxins (TTXs) are a group of potent neurotoxins commonly associated to species of pufferfish. These hydrophilic, nonprotein low molecular–weight marine biotoxins consist of a heterocyclic compound with a guanidinium moiety connected to an oxygenated backbone possessing a 2,4-dioxa-adamantane structure with hydroxyl groups (Fig. 7.5).[92] TTXs are produced by bacteria and there are identified more than 25 analogs of TTXs with toxic activity which can be present not only in fish but also in marine bivalves and gastropods.[93] The main symptoms produced by the consumption of seafood containing TTX are lingual and perioral numbness, paresthesia, incoordination, hypotension, bradycardia, cardiac dysrhythmias, and unconsciousness. Death can be caused by both respiratory failure and cardiac collapse.[94] As mentioned above TTX is generally associated with the pufferfish in Japan. However, TTX has also been detected in bivalve mollusks from Japan and New Zealand.[95,96] More recently, TTXs have been detected for the first time in marine bivalves and gastropods from the European coasts.[97–99] Consequently, the EFSA published a public opinion requesting for more occurrence data and established a recommended level of 44 μg TTX/kg.[45]

Among the detection methods for TTX, MBA was one of the first approaches used to monitor TTX. This method was quickly substituted to more ethics and specific alternative methods such as surface plasmon resonance or ELISA.[100,101] Furthermore, the mechanism of action of TTX as blocker of sodium channels is used in the cytotoxicity assay of N2a to evaluate the composite toxicity produced by the possible presence of TTX-like compound in the sample.[32] This method showed a high sensitivity and is considered a good screening approach to monitor TTX-like compounds. However, the most adequate detection method to monitor TTX is LC-Ms/MS due to the higher sensitivity and specificity provided by the mass spectrometric detection.[102,103] Hydrophilic interaction LC (HILIC) allows the effective separation of the TTX during the LC-Ms/MS analyses. Consequently, the European Union Reference Laboratory for Marine Biotoxins (EURLMB) proposed an HILIC-Ms/MS method for the monitoring of TTX, which was interlaboratory validated and transferred to the EU National Reference Laboratories.[104]

7.5 Future perspectives

The future perspective of the marine biotoxins present in seafood relies on three principles interconnected:

1. Increase the availability of standards and reference materials of marine biotoxins to develop, optimize, and validate analytical methods and also to perform toxicological studies establishing regulatory limits and protecting public health.
2. Transition from biological to chemical methods and development of quantitative multianalyte methodologies based on LC-Ms/MS and LC-HRMS.

3. Deeper insight into the emerging marine biotoxins, monitoring their spread and prevalence and impact on public health.

References

1. Hallegraeff GM. Ocean climate change, phytoplankton community responses, and harmful algal blooms: a formidable predictive challenge1. *J Phycol*. 2010;46:220–235.
2. Visciano P, Schirone M, Berti M, Milandri A, Tofalo R, Suzzi G. Marine biotoxins: occurrence, toxicity, regulatory limits and reference methods. *Front Microbiol*. 2016;7:1051.
3. Bagnis R, Berglund F, Elias PS, van Esch GJ, Halstead BW, Kojima K. Problems of toxicants in marine food products. 1. Marine biotoxins. *Bull World Health Organ*. 1970;42:69–88.
4. Ciminiello P, Fattorusso E. Bivalve molluscs as vectors of marine biotoxins involved in seafood poisoning. In: Cimino G, Gavagnin M, eds. *Molluscs: From Chemo-ecological Study to Biotechnological Application*. Berlin, Heidelberg: Springer; 2006:53–82. ISBN 978-3-540-30880-5.
5. James KJ, Carey B, O'Halloran J, van Pelt FNAM, Škrabáková Z. Shellfish toxicity: human health implications of marine algal toxins. *Epidemiol Infect*. 2010;138:927–940.
6. Landsberg JH. The effects of harmful algal blooms on aquatic organisms. *Rev Fish Sci*. 2002;10:113–390.
7. EFSA. Marine biotoxins in shellfish – summary on regulated marine biotoxins. *EFSA J*. 2009;7:1306.
8. Onodera H, Satake M, Oshima Y, Yasumoto T, Carmichael WW. New saxitoxin analogues from the freshwater filamentous cyanobacterium *Lyngbya wollei*. *Nat Toxins*. 1997;5:146–151.
9. Oshima Y, Blackburn SI, Hallegraeff GM. Comparative study on paralytic shellfish toxin profiles of the dinoflagellate *Gymnodinium catenatum* from three different countries. *Mar Biol Int J Life Ocean Coast Waters*. 1993;116:471–476.
10. Schantz EJ, Ghazarossian VE, Schnoes HK, et al. Structure of saxitoxin. *J Am Chem Soc*. 1975;97:1238–1239.
11. Regulation EC 853/2004; 2004.
12. Yasumoto T, Murata M, Oshima Y, Sano M, Matsumoto GK, Clardy J. Diarrhetic shellfish toxins. *Tetrahedron*. 1985;41: 1019–1025.
13. Yasumoto T, Oshima Y, Sugawara W, et al. Identification of *Dinophysis fortii* as the causative organism of diarrhetic shellfish poisoning. *Nippon Suisan Gakkaishi*. 1980;46:1405–1411.
14. Torgersen T, Miles CO, Rundberger T, Wilkins AL. New esters of okadaic acid in seawater and blue mussels (*Mytilus edulis*). *J Agric Food Chem*. 2008;56:9628–9635.
15. Burgess V, Shaw G. Pectentoxins – an issue for public health: a review of their comparative toxicology and metabolism. *Environ Int*. 2001; 27:275–283.
16. Alfonso A, De la Rosa L, Vieytes MR, Yasumoto T, Botana LM. Yessotoxin, a novel phycotoxin, activates phosphodiesterase activity: effect of yessotoxin on cAMP levels in human lymphocytes. *Biochem Pharmacol*. 2003;65:193–208.
17. Miles CO, Wilkins AL, Munday R, et al. Isolation of pectenotoxin-2 from *Dinophysis acuta* and its conversion to pectenotoxin-2 seco acid, and preliminary assessment of their acute toxicities. *Toxicon*. 2004;43:1–9.
18. Draisci R, Lucentini L, Giannetti L, Boria P, Poletti R. First report of pectenotoxin-2 (PTX-2) in algae (*Dinophysis fortii*) related to seafood poisoning in Europe. *Toxicon*. 1996;34:923–935.
19. Commission Implementing Regulation (EU) 2021/1709; 2021.
20. Satake M, MacKenzie L, Yasumoto T. Identification of *Protoceratium reticulatum* as the biogenetic origin of yessotoxin. *Nat Toxins*. 1997;5:164–167.
21. Draisci R, Ferretti E, Palleschi L, et al. High levels of yessotoxin in mussels and presence of yessotoxin and homoyessotoxin in dinoflagellates of the Adriatic Sea. *Toxicon*. 1999;37:1187–1193.
22. Murata M, Kumagai M, Lee JS, Yasumoto T. Isolation and structure of yessotoxin, a novel polyether compound implicated in diarrhetic shellfish poisoning. *Tetrahedron Lett*. 1987;28:5869–5872.
23. Commission Regulation (EU) No 786/2013; 2013.
24. Satake M, Ofuji K, Naoki H, et al. Azaspiracid, a new marine toxin having unique spiro ring assemblies, isolated from Irish mussels, *Mytilus edulis*. *J Am Chem Soc*. 1998;120:9967–9968.
25. Twiner MJ, Rehmann N, Hess P, Doucette GJ. Azaspiracid shellfish poisoning: a review on the chemistry, ecology, and toxicology with an emphasis on human health impacts. *Mar Drugs*. 2008;6: 39–72.
26. Tillmann U, Elbrächter M, Krock B, John U, Cembella A. *Azadinium spinosum* gen. et sp. nov. (Dinophyceae) identified as a primary producer of azaspiracid toxins. *Eur J Phycol*. 2009; 44:63–79.
27. Perl TM, Bédard L, Kosatsky T, Hockin JC, Todd ECD, Remis RS. An outbreak of toxic encephalopathy caused by eating mussels contaminated with domoic acid. *N Engl J Med*. 1990;322: 1775–1780.
28. Fritz L, Quilliam MA, Wright JLC, Beale AM, Work TM. An outbreak of domoic acid poisoning attributed to the pennate diatom *pseudonitzschia australis*. *J Phycol*. 1992;28:439–442.
29. Regulation EC 2074/2005; 2005.
30. Yasumoto T, Oshima Y, Yamaguchi M. Occurrence of a new type of shellfish poisoning in the Tohoku district. *Nippon Suisan Gakkaishi Jpn Ed*. 1978;44:1249–1255.
31. Llamas NM, Stewart L, Fodey T, et al. Development of a novel immunobiosensor method for the rapid detection of okadaic acid contamination in shellfish extracts. *Anal Bioanal Chem*. 2007; 389:581–587.
32. Manger RL, Leja LS, Lee SY, et al. Detection of sodium channel toxins: directed cytotoxicity assays of purified ciguatoxins, brevetoxins, saxitoxins, and seafood extracts. *J AOAC Int*. 1995;78: 521–527.
33. Lawrence JF, Niedzwiadek B, Menard C, et al. Quantitative determination of paralytic shellfish poisoning toxins in shellfish using prechromatographic oxidation and liquid chromatography with fluorescence detection: collaborative study. *J AOAC Int*. 2005;88: 1714–1732.
34. Oshima Y. Postcolumn derivatization liquid chromatographic method for paralytic shellfish toxins. *J AOAC Int*. 1995;78:528–532.
35. Quilliam MA, Xie M, Hardstaff WR. Rapid extraction and cleanup for liquid chromatographic determination of domoic acid in unsalted seafood. *J AOAC Int*. 1995;78:543–554.
36. EU-Harmonised Standard Operating Procedure for determination of lipophilic marine biotoxins in molluscs by LC-MS/MS; 2011.
37. Dell'Aversano C, Hess P, Quilliam MA. Hydrophilic interaction liquid chromatography-mass spectrometry for the analysis of

paralytic shellfish poisoning (PSP) toxins. *J Chromatogr A*. 2005;1081:190–201.

38. Boundy MJ, Selwood AI, Harwood DT, McNabb PS, Turner AD. Development of a sensitive and selective liquid chromatography-mass spectrometry method for high throughput analysis of paralytic shellfish toxins using graphitised carbon solid phase extraction. *J Chromatogr A*. 2015;1387:1–12.
39. Yogi K, Sakugawa S, Oshiro N, Ikehara T, Sugiyama K, Yasumoto T. Determination of toxins involved in ciguatera fish poisoning in the pacific by LC/MS. *J AOAC Int*. 2014;97:398–402.
40. Zendong Z, McCarron P, Herrenknecht C, et al. High resolution mass spectrometry for quantitative analysis and untargeted screening of algal toxins in mussels and passive samplers. *J Chromatogr A*. 2015;1416:10–21.
41. Dom I, Biré R, Hort V, Lavison-Bompard G, Nicolas M, Guérin T. Extended targeted and non-targeted strategies for the analysis of marine toxins in mussels and oysters by (LC-HRMS). *Toxins (Basel)*. 2018;10.
42. Braña-Magdalena A, Leão-Martins JM, Glauner T, Gago-Martínez A. Intralaboratory validation of a fast and sensitive UHPLC/MS/MS method with fast polarity switching for the analysis of lipophilic shellfish toxins. *J AOAC Int*. 2014;97:285–292.
43. McNabb P, Selwood AI, Holland PT. Multiresidue method for determination of algal toxins in shellfish: single-laboratory validation and interlaboratory study. *J AOAC Int*. 2005;88:761–772.
44. Gerssen A, Gago-Martínez A. Emerging marine biotoxins. *Toxins (Basel)*. 2019;11.
45. EFSA Panel on Contaminants in the Food Chain. Risks for public health related to the presence of tetrodotoxin (TTX) and TTX analogues in marine bivalves and gastropods. *EFSA J*. 2017;15:e04752.
46. EFSA Panel on Contaminants in the Food Chain. Scientific Opinion on marine biotoxins in shellfish – emerging toxins: brevetoxin group. *EFSA J*. 2010;8:1677.
47. EFSA Panel on Contaminants in the Food Chain (CONTAM). Scientific Opinion on marine biotoxins in shellfish – cyclic imines (spirolides, gymnodimines, pinnatoxins and pteriatoxins). *EFSA J*. 2010;8:1628.
48. EFSA Panel on Contaminants in the Food Chain. Scientific Opinion on marine biotoxins in shellfish – palytoxin group. *EFSA J*. 2009;7:1393.
49. EFSA Panel on Contaminants in the Food Chain. Scientific Opinion on marine biotoxins in shellfish – emerging toxins: ciguatoxin group. *EFSA J*. 2010;8:1627.
50. Cembella AD;, Lewis NI, Quilliam MA. The marine dinoflagellate *Alexandrium ostenfeldii* (Dinophyceae) as the causative organism of spirolide shellfish toxins. *Phycologia*. 2000;39:67–74.
51. Touzet N, Franco JM, Raine R. Morphogenetic diversity and biotoxin composition of *Alexandrium* (Dinophyceae) in Irish coastal waters. *Harmful Algae*. 2008;7:782–797.
52. Miles CO, Wilkins AL, Stirling DJ, Mackenzie AL. Gymnodimine C, an isomer of gymnodimine B, from *Karenia selliformis*. *J Agric Food Chem*. 2003;51:4838–4840.
53. Rhodes L, Smith K, Selwood A, et al. Dinoflagellate *Vulcanodinium rugosum* identified as the causative organism of pinnatoxins in Australia, New Zealand and Japan. *Phycologia*. 2011;50:624–628.
54. Nézan E, Chomérat N. *Vulcanodinium rugosum* gen. nov., sp. nov. (Dinophyceae): a new marine dinoflagellate from the French mediterranean coast [*Vulcanodinium rugosum* gen. et sp. nov. (Dinophyceae), un nouveau dinoflagellé marin de la côte méditerranéenne française]. *Cryptogam Algol*. 2011;32:3–18.
55. Hu T, Curtis JM, Walter JA, Wright JLC. Characterization of biologically inactive spirolides E and F: identification of the spirolide pharmacophore. *Tetrahedron Lett*. 1996;37:7671–7674.
56. Munday R. Toxicology of cyclic imines: Gymnodimine, spirolides, pinnatoxins, pteriatoxins, prorocentrolide, spiro-prorocentrimine, and symbioimines. In: *Seafood and Freshwater Toxins: Pharmacology, Physiology, and Detection*. Boca Raton: CRC Press; 2008.
57. Hu T, Curtis JM, Oshima Y, et al. Spirolides B and D, two novel macrocycles isolated from the digestive glands of shellfish. *J Chem Soc Chem Commun*. 1995;2159–2161.
58. Seki T, Satake M, Mackenzie L, Kaspar HF, Yasumoto T. Gymnodimine, a new marine toxin of unprecedented structure isolated from New Zealand oysters and the dinoflagellate, *Gymnodinium* sp. *Tetrahedron Lett*. 1995;36:7093–7096.
59. Uemura D, Fukuzawa S, Chou T, et al. Pinnatoxin A: a toxic amphoteric macrocycle from the Okinawan bivalve *Pinna muricata*. *J Am Chem Soc*. 1995;117:1155–1156.
60. Otero P, Miguéns N, Rodríguez I, Botana LM. LC–MS/MS analysis of the emerging toxin Pinnatoxin-G and high levels of esterified OA group toxins in Galician commercial mussels. *Toxins (Basel)*. 2019;11.
61. Moreiras G, Leão JM, Gago-Martínez A. Analysis of cyclic imines in mussels (*Mytilus galloprovincialis*) from Galicia (NW Spain) by LC-MS/MS. *Int J Environ Res Public Health*. 2020;17.
62. Hess P, Abadie E, Hervé F, et al. Pinnatoxin G is responsible for atypical toxicity in mussels (*Mytilus galloprovincialis*) and clams (*Venerupis decussata*) from Ingril, a French Mediterranean lagoon. *Toxicon*. 2013;75:16–26.
63. Bacchiocchi S, Siracusa M, Campacci D, et al. Cyclic imines (CIs) in mussels from North-Central Adriatic Sea: first evidence of Gymnodimine A in Italy. *Toxins (Basel)*. 2020;12.
64. Fraga M, Vilariño N, Louzao MC, et al. First identification of palytoxin-like molecules in the Atlantic coral species *Palythoa canariensis*. *Anal Chem*. 2017;89:7438–7446.
65. Gladan ŽN, Arapov J, Casabianca S, et al. Massive occurrence of the harmful benthic dinoflagellate *Ostreopsis* cf. *ovata* in the eastern Adriatic sea. *Toxins (Basel)*. 2019;11.
66. Aligizaki K, Katikou P, Nikolaidis G, Panou A. First episode of shellfish contamination by palytoxin-like compounds from *Ostreopsis* species (Aegean Sea, Greece). *Toxicon*. 2008;51:418–427.
67. Moore RE, Scheuer PJ. Palytoxin: a new marine toxin from a coelenterate. *Science*. 1971;172:495–498.
68. Moore RE, Bartolini G. Structure of palytoxin. *J Am Chem Soc*. 1981;103:2491–2494.
69. Ukena T, Satake M, Usami M, et al. Structure elucidation of Ostreocin D, a palytoxin analog isolated from the dinoflagellate *Ostreopsis siamensis*. *Biosci Biotechnol Biochem*. 2001;65:2585–2588.
70. Alcala AC, Alcala LC, Garth JS, Yasumura D, Yasumoto T. Human fatality due to ingestion of the crab *Demania reynaudii* that contained a palytoxin-like toxin. *Toxicon*. 1988;26:105–107.
71. Sosa S, Del Favero G, De Bortoli M, et al. Palytoxin toxicity after acute oral administration in mice. *Toxicol Lett*. 2009;191:253–259.

72. Ito E, Yasumoto T. Toxicological studies on palytoxin and ostreocin-D administered to mice by three different routes. *Toxicon*. 2009; 54:244–251.
73. Tartaglione L, Mazzeo A, Dell'Aversano C, et al. Chemical, molecular, and eco-toxicological investigation of *Ostreopsis* sp. from Cyprus Island: structural insights into four new ovatoxins by LC-HRMS/MS. *Anal Bioanal Chem*. 2016;408:915–932.
74. Klijnstra MD, Gerssen A. A sensitive LC-MS/MS method for palytoxin using lithium cationization. *Toxins (Basel)*. 2018;10.
75. Nakanishi K. The chemistry of brevetoxins: a review. *Toxicon*. 1985;23:473–479.
76. Abraham A, Flewelling LJ, El Said KR, et al. An occurrence of neurotoxic shellfish poisoning by consumption of gastropods contaminated with brevetoxins. *Toxicon*. 2021;191:9–17.
77. Ishida H, Nozawa A, Totoribe K, et al. Brevetoxin B1, a new polyether marine toxin from the New Zealand shellfish, *Austrovenus stutchburyi*. *Tetrahedron Lett*. 1995;36:725–728.
78. Abraham A, Wang Y, El Said KR, Plakas SM. Characterization of brevetoxin metabolism in *Karenia brevis* bloom-exposed clams (*Mercenaria* sp.) by LC-MS/MS. *Toxicon*. 2012;60:1030–1040.
79. Amzil Z, Derrien A, Terre Terrillon A, et al. Monitoring the emergence of algal toxins in shellfish: first report on detection of brevetoxins in French Mediterranean mussels. *Mar Drugs*. 2021;19.
80. Arnich N, Abadie E, Amzil Z, et al. Guidance level for brevetoxins in French shellfish. *Mar Drugs*. 2021;19.
81. Tang J, Hou L, Tang D, et al. Magneto-controlled electrochemical immunoassay of brevetoxin B in seafood based on guanine-functionalized graphene nanoribbons. *Biosens Bioelectron*. 2012; 38:86–93.
82. McNabb PS, Selwood AI, Van Ginkel R, Boundy M, Holland PT. Determination of brevetoxins in shellfish by LC/MS/MS: single-laboratory validation. *J AOAC Int*. 2012;95:1097–1105.
83. Yasumoto T. The chemistry and biological function of natural marine toxins. *Chem Rec*. 2001;1:228–242.
84. Yasumoto T, Nakajima I, Bagnis R, Adachi R. Finding of a dinoflagellate as a likely culprit of ciguatera. *Nippon Suisan Gakkaishi*. 1977;43:1021–1026.
85. Lewis RJ, Holmes MJ. Origin and transfer of toxins involved in ciguatera. *Comp Biochem Physiol C*. 1993;106:615–628.
86. Estevez P, Castro D, Pequeño-Valtierra A, et al. An attempt to characterize the ciguatoxin profile in *Seriola fasciata* causing ciguatera fish poisoning in Macaronesia. *Toxins (Basel)*. 2019;11.
87. Dickey RW, Plakas SM. Ciguatera: a public health perspective. *Toxicon*. 2010;56:123–136.
88. Estevez P, Castro D, Pequeño-Valtierra A, Giraldez J, Gago-Martinez A. Emerging marine biotoxins in seafood from European coasts: incidence and analytical challenges. *Foods*. 2019;8.
89. Castro D, Manger R, Vilariño O, Gago-Martínez A. Evaluation of matrix issues in the applicability of the neuro-2a cell based assay on the detection of CTX in fish samples. *Toxins (Basel)*. 2020;12.
90. Estevez P, Castro D, Leao JM, Yasumoto T, Dickey R, Gago-Martinez A. Implementation of liquid chromatography tandem mass spectrometry for the analysis of ciguatera fish poisoning in contaminated fish samples from Atlantic coasts. *Food Chem*. 2019;280:8–14.
91. Estevez P, Sibat M, Leão-Martins JM, Reis Costa P, Gago-Martínez A, Hess P. Liquid chromatography coupled to high-resolution mass spectrometry for the confirmation of Caribbean ciguatoxin-1 as the main toxin responsible for ciguatera poisoning caused by fish from European Atlantic coasts. *Toxins (Basel)*. 2020;12.
92. Chau R, Kalaitzis JA, Neilan BA. On the origins and biosynthesis of tetrodotoxin. *Aquat Toxicol*. 2011;104:61–72.
93. Yotsu-Yamashita M, Abe Y, Kudo Y, et al. First identification of 5,11-dideoxytetrodotoxin in marine animals, and characterization of major fragment ions of tetrodotoxin and its analogs by high resolution ESI-MS/MS. *Mar Drugs*. 2013;11:2799–2813.
94. Noguchi T, Ebesu JSM. Puffer poisoning: epidemiology and treatment. *J Toxicol Toxin Rev*. 2001;20:1–10.
95. Kodama M, Sato S, Sakamoto S, Ogata T. Occurrence of tetrodotoxin in *Alexandrium tamarense*, a causative dinoflagellate of paralytic shellfish poisoning. *Toxicon*. 1996;34:1101–1105.
96. McNabb PS, Taylor DI, Ogilvie SC, et al. First detection of tetrodotoxin in the bivalve *Paphies australis* by liquid chromatography coupled to triple quadrupole mass spectrometry with and without precolumn reaction. *J AOAC Int*. 2014;97:325–333.
97. Gerssen A, Bovee THF, Klijnstra MD, Poelman M, Portier L, Hoogenboom RLAP. First report on the occurrence of tetrodotoxins in bivalve mollusks in The Netherlands. *Toxins (Basel)*. 2018;10.
98. Vlamis A, Katikou P, Rodriguez I, et al. First detection of tetrodotoxin in Greek shellfish by UPLC-MS/MS potentially linked to the presence of the dinoflagellate *Prorocentrum minimum*. *Toxins (Basel)*. 2015;7:1779–1807.
99. Leão JM, Lozano-Leon A, Giráldez J, Vilariño Ó, Gago-Martínez A. Preliminary results on the evaluation of the occurrence of tetrodotoxin associated to marine *Vibrio* spp. in bivalves from the Galician Rias (Northwest of Spain). *Mar Drugs*. 2018;16.
100. Yakes BJ, Deeds J, White K, DeGrasse SL. Evaluation of surface plasmon resonance biosensors for detection of tetrodotoxin in food matrices and comparison to analytical methods. *J Agric Food Chem*. 2011;59:839–846.
101. Stokes AN, Williams BL, French SS. An improved competitive inhibition enzymatic immunoassay method for tetrodotoxin quantification. *Biol Proced Online*. 2012;14:3.
102. Yotsu-Yamashita M, Jang J-H, Cho Y, Konoki K. Optimization of simultaneous analysis of tetrodotoxin, 4-epitetrodotoxin, 4,9-anhydrotetrodotoxin, and 5,6,11-trideoxytetrodotoxin by hydrophilic interaction liquid chromatography–tandem mass spectrometry. *Forensic Toxicol*. 2011;29:61–64.
103. Bane V, Hutchinson S, Sheehan A, et al. LC-MS/MS method for the determination of tetrodotoxin (TTX) on a triple quadruple mass spectrometer. *Food Addit Contam Part A*. 2016;33:1728–1740.
104. Determination of Tetrodotoxin by HILIC-MS/MS. European Union Reference Laboratory for Marine Biotoxins. <https://www.aesan.gob.es/en/CRLMB/docs/docs/metodos_analiticos_de_desarrollo/HILIC-LCMSMS_SOP_for_TTX_in_mussels.pdf>; Accessed 08.07.21.

Chapter 8

Pollutants, residues and other contaminants in foods obtained from marine and fresh water

Martin Rose
Manchester Institute of Biotechnology, University of Manchester, Manchester, United Kingdom

Abstract

Food has been harvested from the seas and rivers for many thousands of years, and provides a valuable source of nutrition. Perhaps one of the biggest changes seen relatively recently over the past few decades is large increase in aquaculture. Farming fish helps to address in part issues around overfishing. Pollution from agriculture, industrial activity and domestic sources can all end up having an impact on rivers and ultimately the Oceans from where it can be distributed globally. Water is critical not only for foods harvested from rivers and seas, but is critical for all farming and food producing activity.
In addition to consumption of conventional products such as fish and shellfish, products such as algae are gaining popularity in the West, while they have been consumed in Asia as a traditional and nutritious food for generations.
Chemical contaminants include residues of agricultural products such as veterinary medicines and pesticides, persistent organic pollutants such as dioxins, polychlorinated biphenyls, polyfluorinated alkylated substances, brominated flame retardants, heavy metals and arsenic. More visible signs of pollution have been attracting media attention in recent years in terms of plastic waste, and the micro- and nanoplastic fragments associated with this type of pollution is subject of much on-going research.
Risks associated with these contaminants need to be assessed but should be balanced against the benefits associated with the vitamins, nutrients, and other beneficial components of seafood. In addition to risks to humans associated with foods harvested from aquatic environments, it is important to consider the risks to the environment associated with pollution sources to ensure a sustainable future.

Keywords: Fish; seafood; risk assessment; residues and contaminants; aquaculture

Chapter points

1. Food has been harvested from the seas and rivers for many thousands of years, and provides a valuable source of nutrition.
2. Aquaculture has increased dramatically over the past few decades, and helps to address in part issues around overfishing.
3. Pollution from agriculture, industrial activity and domestic sources can all end up having an impact on rivers and ultimately the Oceans and is a global issue.
4. Water is critical not only for foods harvested from rivers and seas, but is critical for all farming and food producing activity.
5. Products such as algae are gaining popularity in the West, while they have been consumed in Asia as a traditional and nutritious food for generations.
6. Chemical contaminants include residues of agricultural products such as veterinary medicines and pesticides, persistent organic pollutants (POP) such as dioxins, polychlorinated biphenyls (PCB), polyfluorinated alkylated substances, brominated flame retardants (BFR), heavy metals and arsenic.
7. Micro- and nanoplastic fragments associated with plastic waste has recently started to gain mainstream attention.
8. Risks associated with chemical contaminants need to be assessed but should be balanced against the benefits associated with the vitamins, nutrients, and other beneficial components of seafood.
9. Environmental risk assessment is a useful tool to assess the health of an ecosystem.

8.1 Introduction

The Old Testament of the Bible records that the Israelites ate a variety of fresh and saltwater fish, and this is backed up by both archeological and textual evidence. There is similar evidence in art and culture of the importance of fish and seafood in the diet from around the world

Present Knowledge in Food Safety. DOI: https://doi.org/10.1016/B978-0-12-819470-6.00040-8

including from ancient Greece, China, Japan, indigenous American population, and in medieval Europe. The river Nile was known to be a plentiful source of fish in ancient times,[1] and fresh and dried fish were a staple food for much of the population. The Egyptians had implements and methods for fishing and these are illustrated in tomb scenes, drawings, and papyrus documents. Some representations hint at fishing being pursued as a pastime (Fig. 8.1).

The practice of fishing and the consumption of seafoods is an ancient practice, dating back many centuries to at least the Upper Paleolithic period (between 50,000 and 10,000 years ago).[2] Isotopic analysis of the skeletal remains of a Tianyuan human, a 40,000-year-old modern human from eastern Asia, has shown that freshwater fish was regularly consumed in that period.[3] Shell heaps, discarded fish bones, cave paintings, and other archeology features show that sea foods were important for survival and consumed in significant quantities (https://www.york.ac.uk/archaeology/middens/index.htm).

There are various religious doctrines surrounding the consumption of fish and seafood. In Islam, the Shafi'i, Maliki and Hanbali traditions allow the eating of shellfish, while the Shi'ite tradition (Ja'fari) and the Hanafi do not permit it in Sunni Islam. The Jewish laws of Kashrut forbid the eating of shellfish and eels. The King James bible indicates that it is acceptable to eat finfish, but that shellfish and eels are an abomination and should not be eaten. Could it be that some of these doctrines were put in place to protect the population from some of the dangers associated with the consumption of seafood? Admittedly, if that was the case, then it is more likely to have arisen due to microbiological rather than chemical contamination issues.

All that are in the waters: all that... hath not fins and scales ye may not eat *(Deuteronomy 14:9–10) and are "an abomination" (Leviticus 11:9–12).*

As the global population has expanded, many of the recent problems associated with fish and shellfish consumption, center around the practice of overfishing, that is, taking more fish than the ecosystem can replenish. The number of overfished stocks globally has tripled in the last 50 years, and it is estimated that currently one-third of the world's fisheries are currently overfished (Food and Agriculture Organization of the United Nations). The term "bycatch" is related to overfishing and describes the capture of unwanted sea life while fishing for a different species (https://www.worldwildlife.org/threats/overfishing). This can result in the needless loss of billions of fish, along with hundreds of thousands of sea turtles, cetaceans and other species. The damage done by overfishing affects not only the marine environment, but extends to the billions of people who rely on fish for protein, and to those for whom fishing is their main source of income (Fig. 8.2).

Water conflict is a term describing a conflict between countries, states, or groups over the rights to access water resources.[4,5] The United Nations recognizes that water disputes result from opposing interests of water users, public or private (https://www.un.org). Historically, fisheries have been the main sources of question, as nations expanded and claimed portions of oceans and seas as territory for "domestic" commercial fishing. Certain lucrative areas, such as the Bering Sea, have a history of dispute; in 1886 Great Britain and the United States clashed over sealing fisheries.[6]

It is generally recognized that fish and shellfish are good sources of many vitamins and minerals. Oily fish, such as salmon and sardines, is also particularly high in

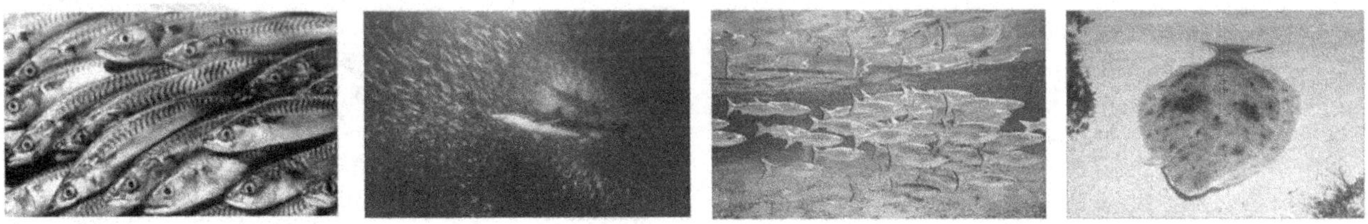

FIGURE 8.1 Fish from the sea.

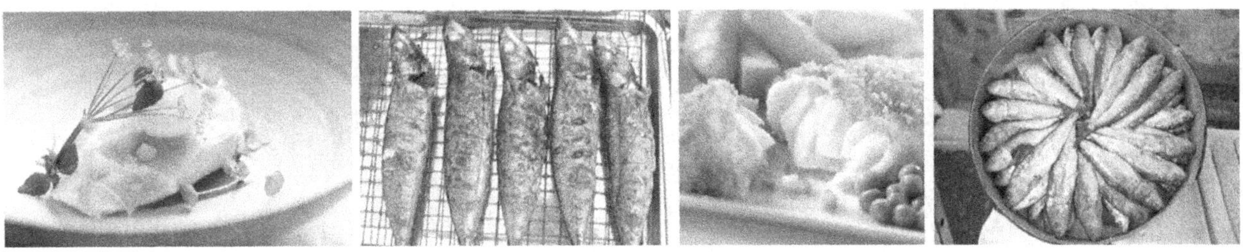

FIGURE 8.2 Fish as food.

long-chain omega-3 fatty acids, which support cardiac health. For example, in the United Kingdom, government advice is that "a healthy, balanced diet should include at least two portions of fish a week, including one of oily fish." However, such sources of advice also often contain words of caution. The advice from the UK Government above, continues with specific caution for pregnant women: "Eating fish is good for your health and the development of your baby. However, pregnant and breast-feeding women should avoid some types of fish and limit the amount they eat of some others. This is because of the levels of mercury and pollutants that some fish can contain."

During the last half century or so, as environmental concerns have moved up the political agenda, there has been some visible and obvious improvements in water quality. These have been focused on actions that have obvious public impact and include cleaner beaches, reduced raw sewage input into water streams and other actions. There has also been some less obvious progress with the implementation of polluter pays policies to give disincentives for industries to pollute waterways. The impact of these policies is clearly noticed in cities and at beaches where, for example, the Thames in London has changed in the last 50 years from a river that was essentially dead and devoid of life to one where dolphins, salmon, porpoises, other wildlife including even whales can be found.

Within the EU, the Marine Strategy Framework Directive encourages collaboration and coordination between member countries in order to reduce pollution inputs and improve the sustainability of marine ecosystems. Under the directive, one of the descriptors for good environmental status involves the reduction of fish and seafood contamination, including compliance with regulated maximum contaminant levels or other relevant standards.

Several of the United Nations sustainable development goals (SDGs) (https://sdgs.un.org/) are directly related to food from aquatic sources, namely zero hunger, clean water, and sanitation, life below water, and most of the SDGs are in some way related to the topic.

The remaining sections of this chapter discusses different water systems, the pollutants and contaminants that are viewed as most important to wildlife and food production, the types of food that can be harvested from these waters, and the impact on the environment (Fig. 8.3).

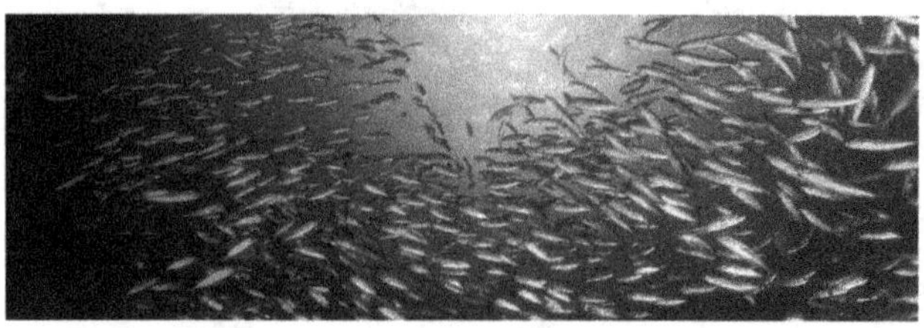

FIGURE 8.3 Fish are often found in large shoals.

8.2 Main text

8.2.1 Water systems

8.2.1.1 Freshwater (rivers, lakes, etc.) versus marine environments

Perhaps the most significant difference between inland and marine waters in terms of pollutants is the fact that inland systems contain much smaller volumes of water. Pollutants within a river, lake or pond that may originate as run-off from agricultural farm land, or as a result of the direct or indirect discharge of industrial waste, will therefore typically be present at a much higher concentration. When the river empties into a sea, the pollutant level will be vastly diluted in comparison. Of course, this is a generalization, and some remote streams, rivers and even large lakes in pristine environments will be relatively clean, whereas some seas, especially those where water flow is restricted or where rivers from relatively large or polluted land masses enter into them, such as the Baltic, will harbor relatively high levels of pollutants.

8.2.1.2 Aquaculture and farmed fish versus wild fish

For both wild and farmed fish, contaminants, nutrients and other constituents present in water or food /feed, whether intentionally or unintentionally, can be either metabolized and excreted (typical for products such as veterinary drugs added to commercial fish feed). Other contaminants such as the POP (e.g., dioxins, PCBs, BFR and organo-fluorine PFAS compounds) may bioaccumulate in fish.[7] The bioaccumulation of toxic contaminants by farmed fish, bivalves, crustaceans and molluscs can in some circumstances be sufficiently significant to result in concerns for human health. The contaminant concentration in farmed fish and shellfish depends on various factors such as the species, the capture season, the origin, the development state, and the tissue, and the levels vary within species and between species in both wild and farmed fish (Fig. 8.4).[8,9]

Fish farming (aquaculture) is defined as the rearing or cultivation of aquatic organisms using techniques designed to increase the production of those organisms beyond the natural capacity of the environment.[10] Marine

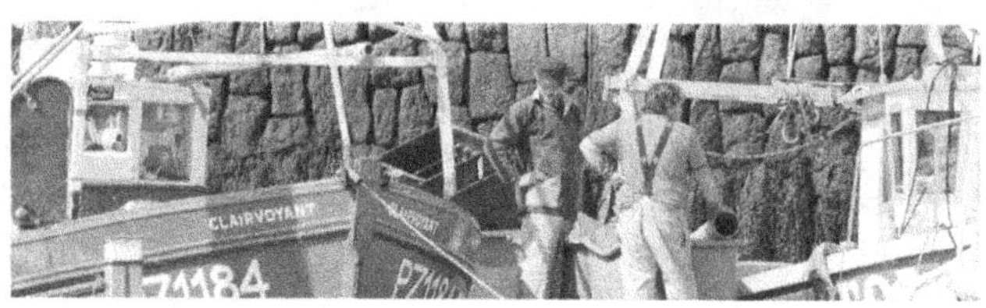

FIGURE 8.4 Commercial fishing is often carried out by small businesses at a local level.

aquaculture usually occurs in cages on the seafloor or suspended in the water column, and the species most produced are oysters, clams, mussels, shrimp and salmon; freshwater aquaculture usually occurs in ponds or recirculating aquaculture tanks, and the species most produced are catfish, trout, tilapia, and bass.[11] Aquaculture usually involves intensive methods where large numbers of fish are kept in close proximity. They are usually fed with commercial feed which can be formulated for optimal nutrition and can also be medicated to support a healthy fish community and to prevent disease. This results in greater control over production and exposure for the produce, but increases the likelihood that residues may exist in the food. Wild fish is less likely contain residues of agricultural products (veterinary medicines, pesticides, etc.) but there is less control over all aspects of production including geographical restrictions of where the fish may have been and control over diet.

Aquaculture can take place in either extensive or intensive systems, defined according to the density of the fish. Extensive systems are generally those where organisms grow in lagoons or brackish waters and importantly are naturally fed, while in intensive systems, fish are given special feeds. Semiintensive systems also exist when the natural diet is supplemented with special feeds.[12]

It has been reported that some residues and contaminants such as pesticides, polybrominated biphenyl ethers (PBDE) and PCB are generally found at higher concentrations in farmed fish than in wild fish (salmon, catfish, turbot, and sea bass),[13] but there is a need for the standardization of sampling procedures before a robust comparison of wild and farmed fish can be made.[8]

World aquaculture production in 2012 reached over 90 million tons including 67 million tons of fish and seafood for human consumption. Almost 90% of global aquaculture production is in Asia and China alone accounts for around two thirds. Europe accounted for less than 5% of the total global aquaculture production in 2012.[14]

Aquaculture can be a valuable food supply in addition to the important economic benefits it brings to many countries, but it can result in environmental problems such as pollution of the surrounding waters with nutrients, solid wastes and chemicals (e.g., antibiotics) that are used for disease control in the aquaculture tanks. These pollutants may not only be problematic in environmental terms, but may also result in chemical contaminants in the fish, the amount being related to the concentration in the water used and duration of exposure. The ingredients of commercial animal feeds themselves can be responsible for food safety risks in aquaculture in addition to pollutants in the water. Major animal feed contaminants are veterinary drug residues, POPs, pesticides, metals and mineral salts (mercury, lead, cadmium, hexavalent chromium, arsenic, and selenium).[15] Both the ingredients used in making feeds, and the quality of waters can be considered to be important critical factors contributing to chemical contaminants in foods produced in aquaculture (Fig. 8.5).[16]

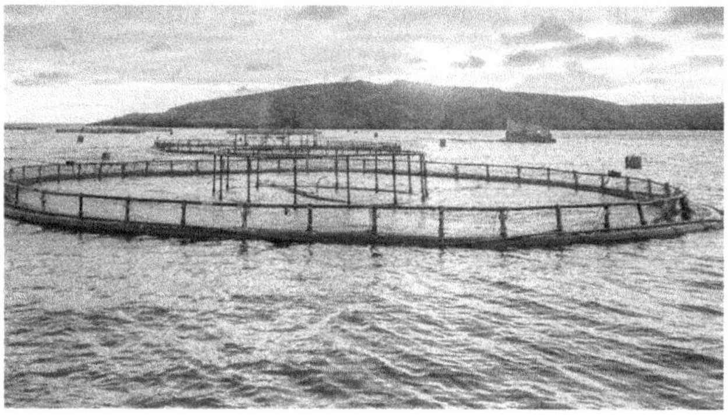

FIGURE 8.5 Aquaculture.

8.2.2 Risk assessment

Although biological hazards are more likely to result in a higher short-term risk for the health of the consumer, chemical hazards are generally perceived as representing the top safety issue. Chemical hazards can be broadly divided into residues of agricultural chemicals used in food production, such as pesticides and veterinary medicines, and contaminants of chemicals that arise either as result of natural processes (e.g., mycotoxins) from industrial or anthropogenic activity (e.g., PCBs, dioxins, flame retardants, PFAS), or as a result of the geology of the region where the food is produced (e.g., lead, arsenic). It was Paracelsus (1493–1541) who is credited to have been the first to state that whether or not a substance is poisonous depends only on the dose ("*sola dosis facit venenum*," or only the dose makes the poison). In more recent years, various food safety agencies around the world have established formal risk assessment processes to determine the scale of the risks associated with the hazards. The risk assessment process consists of an evaluation of the nature of the hazard (hazard identification and characterization) combined with an assessment of the exposure of the population to the hazard. The hazard characterization is evaluated against the exposure assessment in a process termed risk characterization to give an overall assessment of the scale of the risk to the population. This risk assessment process is fully science and evidence based.[17] Risk managers balance the risk assessment with economic, social, and political considerations before taking measures to minimize the risk (risk management). It is also important to consider that fish is a very important source of nutrients and as such is a highly valuable food source, and risks of consumption should be balanced against benefits.

8.2.3 Pollutants, residues, and contaminants

8.2.3.1 Veterinary medicines and pesticides

Pesticides are widely used in commercial terrestrial agriculture for the production of food. When applied to the land, excess pesticides are inevitably transported via wind or washed following rainfall into streams and rivers that eventually flow into the seas. So even though pesticides are not normally used in aquaculture, they can be present in water and therefore in foods produced as a result of pollution of waterways for both aquaculture and wild fish stocks. Similarly, medicines used to treat terrestrial farm animals can be excreted onto farm lands and end up in waterways as with pesticides, and human pharmaceuticals can also be present in wastewaters as a result of water entering the system as outflow from waste water treatment plants.

Some chemicals normally classed as pesticides can be intentionally used in fish farming, for example, to control lice in salmon. But when they are used in this way to treat an animal, they are classed as a veterinary medicine.

In terrestrial and aquatic animal production systems, veterinary medicines are used for disease prevention (vaccines), as therapeutants (antimicrobial agents and antiparasitics) and for husbandry purposes (anesthetics for handling, hormones to enhance reproduction and production, and disinfectants). Whereas there are only a few main species of animals farmed in terms of terrestrial animals, in aquaculture the number and diversity of species cultured is large with over 500 species of finfish, crustaceans, amphibians, molluscs, other invertebrates, seaweeds. There is a lack of information on efficacy and safety for many species, and the relatively small production levels for some species often results in limited interest by pharmaceutical companies to invest in costly product development and registration.[18]

In aquaculture, as in other animal production sectors, veterinary medicines are used mainly to prevent and treat disease. In aquaculture, antimicrobial agents are typically applied either mixed in medicated feed or used as bath treatments. Populations of aquatic animals requiring antimicrobial treatment typically contain some individuals that are healthy and feeding well, and others that are infected and may show clinical signs of disease, including reduced feeding. In aquaculture, the most common practice is a group-medication procedure that endeavors to treat diseased animals while medicating others in the group to prevent disease, known as metaphylactic treatment. Antimicrobial agents can be used as growth promoters in land-based agriculture, where low doses antimicrobial agents improve growth and feed utilization by decreasing the gut mass and increasing absorption of nutrients.[19] These effects have not been reported in aquatic animals, and the practice is not common in aquaculture.[20]

The enormous growth in aquaculture that has been seen globally over the past 30 years would not have been possible without the use of veterinary medicines. As in other veterinary applications, antimicrobial agents used in aquaculture are also important for human medicine. There are no antimicrobial agents that have been specifically developed for aquaculture use, and due to the high development costs and limited potential for returns on investment, this is unlikely to change.

The use of veterinary medicines has increased in the aquaculture industry as the understanding of their use in health management and biosecurity has developed. However, veterinary medicines have not always been used in a responsible manner, and there have been a number of cases where imports have been rejected due to the presence of residues (e.g., ref.[21]). Since 2001, the presence of the antimicrobial chloramphenicol in shrimp has caused much concern,[22] resulting in a slowdown of imports and consequent economic losses for producers and their governments. As a result, many authorities have introduced changes or strengthened national regulations on the use of antimicrobial agents.

Using veterinary medicines is likely to remain an important tool for controlling aquatic animal diseases, but there is increasing recognition of the limitations. The emergence of vaccines has dramatically reduced dependence on antimicrobial agents in some sectors of aquaculture. In other cases, rather than providing a solution, the use of veterinary medicines may complicate health management by triggering toxicity, resistance, residues and occasionally, public health and environmental consequences. In addition, the efficacy of some veterinary medicines under the conditions found in certain aquatic environments is questionable, both with respect to efficacy and with respect to the potential environmental and socio-economic costs of unpredicted impacts.

Maintaining animal health under culture conditions requires the availability of effective antimicrobial agents to increase population survival rates, reduce effects resulting from infections, and improve feed conversion ratios. There is no doubt that the use of veterinary medicines, enhances aquaculture food production in terms of quantity. Rather than further restrictions, more judicious use of veterinary medicines by producers, better enforcement of current regulations by government and improved health extension support to the farmers would result in a more prudent and responsible use of veterinary medicines in aquaculture development.[18]

8.2.3.2 Benefits of using veterinary medicines in aquaculture

The primary benefit of the use of veterinary medicines in aquaculture, as in the commercial livestock and poultry sectors, is to support the development of intensive, industrial-scale food production systems. They are needed to achieve the greatest production outputs for society and the most financial gains for investors through increasing the efficiency of production by minimizing the resources (land, water, feeds, etc.) required to produce a unit of aquatic food. The use of veterinary medicines is essential to modern agricultural production (including aquaculture), through improved on-farm biosecurity and husbandry (e.g., via the use of vaccines and disinfectants) and for the treatment of diseases that lead to reduced production (e.g., reduced growth, lower feed conversion ratios and decreased survival). In addition, veterinary medicines are indispensable for the treatment of epizootic disease outbreaks having the potential to cause mass mortalities, the failure of individual aquaculture enterprises and the occasional collapse of entire industries. Veterinary medicines have proved particularly useful in aquaculture situations involving topics including new species' culture development where it may take time to gain a full understanding of important pathogens to a new species, failure of preventive measures such as vaccination and good husbandry, emerging and re-emerging infectious disease, changes in culture and environmental conditions including climate change and warmer sea temperatures, and changes in animal welfare standards may make it important to use veterinary medicines for the wellbeing of the infected animals.

8.2.3.3 Concerns surrounding excessive-use of veterinary medicines

Concerns can be broken down into four main categories: (1) disease diagnostics issues; (2) human and animal health issues resulting from misuse; (3) environmental/ecological issues; and (4) legislative and enforcement issues.

Disease diagnostics issues center around the need for aquaculture practitioners to have rapid diagnoses of pathogens before using veterinary medicines. For antimicrobial agents in particular, there is also the need to ensure that the antibiotic selected will be effective against the pathogen causing the disease outbreak.

The main concern around human and animal health issues is the development of resistance in bacteria associated with human disease. Antimicrobial resistance (AMR) and residues of banned substances in animal products is increasingly being recognized as an important issue. AMR may arise either directly via enrichment of these bacteria in the aquaculture environment or indirectly via the enrichment for genes that encode such resistance, and which may subsequently be transferred to bacteria associated with human disease. Another principal concern is the degree that residues in aquaculture products may affect human health by either exerting a selective pressure on the dominant intestinal flora, favoring the growth of microorganisms with natural or acquired resistance, promoting, directly or indirectly, the development of acquired resistance in pathogenic enteric bacteria, impairing colonization resistance or by changing metabolic enzyme activity of the intestinal microflora. The risk to human health due to the presence of antimicrobial residues in food products is evaluated as part of the authorization procedure for veterinary drugs. If present in concentrations above the established maximum residue limit, residues can present an hazard to consumers of fish and shellfish produced in aquaculture. Some of the most publicized toxic effects of residues are those caused by chloramphenicol and by residues leading to drug allergies.

Environmental and ecological concerns relating to the use and misuse of veterinary medicines include the release of medicines into the aquatic environment through leaching from unconsumed feeds, intentional or unintentional release of effluent waters from aquaculture facilities, and the presence of residues in fecal materials. Impacts on local ecosystems are in general poorly studied but include concerns about accumulation of residues in sediments and impacts of drugs and chemicals on natural biota, including possible development of AMR in aquatic bacteria.

Legislative and enforcement issues relate to the need for countries to have in place appropriate policies and well-conceived legislation and regulations covering the use of veterinary medicines in aquaculture, including aspects such as procedures for registering medicines used, licensing of aquatic animal health professionals, extra-label use, and record keeping by all involved. Countries must also have the trained workforce and infrastructure necessary to enforce legislation and regulations, with appropriate penalties for noncompliance.[18]

8.2.4 Persistent organic pollutants

8.2.4.1 The Stockholm Convention

POPs are organic chemical substances that possess a particular combination of physical and chemical properties such that, once released into the environment, they remain intact for exceptionally long periods of time (many years), become widely distributed throughout the environment as a result of natural processes involving soil, water and air, they accumulate in the fatty tissue of living organisms including humans, and are found at higher concentrations at higher levels in the food chain, and they are toxic to both humans and wildlife.

They arise as a result of releases to the environment over the past several decades mainly due to industrial and other human activities. This extensive contamination of the environment and living organisms includes many foodstuffs, especially fish and seafood, and has resulted in the sustained exposure of many species, including humans, for periods of time that span generations, resulting in both acute and chronic toxic effects.

Most POPs are lipophilic, that is, they are not soluble in water, but are readily absorbed in fatty tissue, where concentrations can become magnified by upto 70,000 times the background levels. Fish, predatory birds, mammals, and humans are high up the food chain and so absorb the greatest concentrations. POPs can be found in people and animals in all regions of the globe, including those living in remote regions such as the Arctic, far away from major sources.

Specific effects of POPs can include cancer, allergies and hypersensitivity, damage to the central and peripheral nervous systems, reproductive disorders, and disruption of the immune system. Some POPs are also considered to be endocrine disrupters, which, by altering the hormonal system, can damage the reproductive and immune systems of exposed individuals as well as their offspring; they can also have developmental and carcinogenic effects.

The Stockholm convention on POPs is a global treaty to protect human health and the environment from exposure to POPs (http://www.pos.int). Initially, in 2001, twelve POPs were recognized by the Convention and came from 3 categories: (1) Pesticides: aldrin, chlordane, DDT, dieldrin, endrin, heptachlor, hexachlorobenzene, mirex, toxaphene; (2) Industrial chemicals: hexachlorobenzene, PCBs; and (3) By-products: hexachlorobenzene; polychlorinated dibenzo-p-dioxins and polychlorinated dibenzofurans (PCDD/PCDF), and PCBs. In 2009 an additional 17 classes falling in the same broad three categories were added to the list, including some BFR such as PBDEs. Perfluorooctane sulfonic acid (PFOS), its salts and perfluorooctane sulfonyl fluoride (from the group of perfluorinated alkyl substances, or PFASs, sometimes called "forever chemicals") were also added at this time. PFOS is both intentionally produced and an unintended degradation product of related anthropogenic chemicals. The current intentional use of PFOS is widespread and includes: electric and electronic parts, fire-fighting foam, photo imaging, hydraulic fluids and textiles. PFOS is still produced in several countries, and as restrictions on its use increase, industry is changing to shorter chain alternatives that still possess some of the same characteristics in terms of persistence, bioaccumulation and toxicity.

Some PFASs are extremely persistent and have substantial bioaccumulations and biomagnifying properties, although they do not follow the classic property of other POPs in terms of partitioning into fatty tissues. Instead, they bind to proteins in the blood and the liver, resulting in bioaccumulation as for the other POPs, and thus when considering their properties of toxicity and persistence (including long-range transport), they also fulfill the criteria of the Stockholm Convention.

8.2.4.2 Persistent organic pollutants in fish and seafood

The primary source of POPs in fish and seafood products produced from aquaculture is from feed, whereas for wild seafood the primary source is directly from anthropogenic sources such as industrial pollution or as a result of using materials that contain POPs either directly or as contaminant by-products. These chemicals can be released into the environment through water run-off from industrial or farm land into streams and rivers (and eventually the sea), air deposition, wastewater discharge from industrial processes, or from leaching from landfills. To characterize their influences in biota, studies examining levels and trends of POPs from invertebrates to vertebrates from several regions (the Arctic, North America, Asia and Europe) have been conducted. Over several decades, such studies have helped elucidate the accumulation, possible sources, metabolic fate, as well as the potential health effects of these compounds in aquatic biota. The trophic transfer of these compounds via bioaccumulation and biomagnification can result in higher concentrations in top predators, and a wide range of toxic effects (e.g., endocrine disruption, developmental and reproductive effects, and immunotoxicity) have been reported in diverse species, especially those occupying high trophic levels, for example, marine mammals, predatory fish, and oily fish. For many contaminant-stressed populations, the added stress of climate change is exacerbating the problem, causing shifts in food webs and increasing both the distribution and toxicity of POPs in coastal and oceanic environments.[23,24]

Fish and seafood make the largest contribution to dietary exposure from POPs for many consumers.

8.2.5 Metal(oid)s in fish

Various metals are present in the aquatic environment as a result of geochemical processes and anthropogenic industrial sources. Fish are able to accumulate metals from the aquatic environment and in aquaculture can uptake them through feeds. Metal ions when dissolved in waters are absorbed through the gills and other permeable body surfaces, and metals bound to solid particles are ingested, and then detached from their carrier particles in the digestive system and subsequently absorbed through the gut epithelium. Levels of metals in muscle tissue are significantly lower than in liver. Elements such as Fe, Zn, Cu, Co, Mn, Cr, Se and Ni are essential for the normal metabolism in fish, but a high accumulation can cause an increase in mortality and can lead to lot of deformities in rainbow trout (*Oncorhynchus mykiss*) and growth reduction of European sea bass (*Dicentrarchus labrax*) as well as mortality, deformation, and low hatching success for carp (*Cyprinus carpio*) larvae.

Some of the toxic effects of heavy metals include impaired renal (Pb, Cd, Hg) and liver (Pb and Cd) function, decreased cognitive function (Pb, Hg), impaired reproductive capacity (Cd, Pb), hypertension (Cd), neurological changes (Hg, Pb), teratogenic effects (Hg), and cancers (Cd). In terms of human health concerns, mercury and arsenic are probably the most important elements in terms of exposure from consuming fish and seafood.

Mercury can be of great concern in the aquatic environment, mainly for fish and shellfish, which can concentrate the metal in their bodies, mostly in the organic form of methyl mercury. The toxicity of methyl mercury is higher than its inorganic form due to the high solubility of methyl mercury in lipids and its low elimination rate from the organism, resulting in bioaccumulation. The consumption of contaminated fish and other seafood containing bioaccumulated organic mercury is the main pathway for human exposure. Methyl mercury can cause severe neurological damage to humans, in the form of physical lesions manifested as tingling and numbness of fingers and toes, loss of coordination, difficulty in walking, or tremors.[7]

In contrast to the situation with terrestrial systems, organisms from marine ecosystems have a particular facility to convert inorganic arsenic into organic arsenic compounds, and to accumulate arsenic in these organic forms, and more than 70 organic arsenic compounds have been identified in the marine environment. Arsenobetaine is by far the predominant arsenic-containing compound in marine animals, whereas arsenosugars dominate the arsenic content of marine algae. The reasons why arsenic occurs at such high levels in marine organisms is still unknown, but it is possibly due to the fact that arsenic shares a similar chemistry with phosphorus and nitrogen (all are group 15 elements). Marine algae have been reported to take up arsenate from seawater via the same processes designed to take up essential phosphate, and the potentially toxic arsenate is then detoxified by transformation into organic arsenic compounds, primarily arsenosugars. The biosynthesis of arsenobetaine is less certain but its accumulation by marine animals may be related to its structural similarity to glycine betaine.

8.2.6 Eutrophication

Eutrophication is the enrichment of surface waters with plant nutrients, which can occur naturally, but is more usually associated with anthropogenic sources of nutrients, such as those used in agriculture. The "trophic status" of lakes is an important consideration in lake management, and is a term used to describe the relationship between the nutrient status of a lake and the growth of organic matter within the lake. Eutrophication is the process of change from one trophic state to a higher one as a result of the presence of nutrients. Agriculture is a major factor in eutrophication of surface waters, and although both nitrogen and phosphorus contribute to eutrophication, classification of trophic status usually focuses on that nutrient which is limiting, usually phosphorus. When farm land is treated with fertilizers, they can eventually make their way into rivers, lakes and oceans, fertilizing blooms of algae that deplete oxygen and leave "dead zones" downstream. In the extreme, this can result in areas where fish or typical sea life has difficulty to survive.[25]

Harmful algal bloom species can flourish as a result of eutrophication, and have the capacity to produce toxins that are dangerous to humans. Algal toxins are observed in marine ecosystems where they can accumulate in shellfish and more generally in seafood, reaching levels that may be a concern for human as well as animal health. Examples include paralytic, neurotoxic, and diarrhoic shellfish poisoning. Finfish can also be a vector for toxins, as in the case of ciguatera, where it is typically predator fish whose flesh is contaminated with the toxins originally produced by dinoflagellates. Consumption of such contaminated fish by humans can result in symptoms including gastrointestinal and neurological effects.

8.2.7 Microplastics and nanoplastics

Around 70%–80% of plastics that arrive in the oceans are transported there via rivers. Most of this material arises from industry, agriculture and from effluent discharged from waste water treatment plants.[26,27] It has also been found that fibers and microplastics can be generated when clothes are washed, and it has been estimated that a standard 5 kg washload of polyester fabrics may release up to 6,000,000 microfibers, most of which (> 95%) are retained in the biosolids from the treatment plant. These biosolids is often used on agricultural land and during this process, the microplastics can be scattered by the wind or transported by rainwater drainage back into river systems until they eventually reach the sea.

Marine-source plastic litter comes from shipping, oil and gas platforms, leisure activities and fishing (e.g., discarded nets), although it is also recognized that a large proportion of microplastics found are as a result of wear from pneumatic tyres. Much marine plastic debris is composed of particles that have similar sizes and appearance to organisms such as zooplankton and can therefore be regarded as food by marine life. As fish and shellfish are a major source of protein for many of the world's population, plastic particles may easily enter the human food supply by this route. At the top of the marine food chain, North Sea fish and Atlantic cod from Newfoundland have been found to have low particle counts, but most estuarine fish from a South American river had plastic debris inside the gut, suggesting that freshwater fish are more vulnerable to pollution by microplastics. Sampling near the river Thames in London, United Kingdom, showed that upto 75% of European flounder, which are bottom feeders, had MPs in the gut as opposed to 20% of European smelt which are predators of other fish. Zooplanktivorous fish such as anchovy, pilchard, and herring had microplastic contamination with particles found in the liver. Fish at the top of the food chain and living in the sea rather than rivers is generally less polluted. Fish tend to accumulate microplastics in their gills, liver and gut, which may not be relevant to human consumption since these tissues are not usually consumed.

Microplastics seem to be more readily taken up by filter feeders, probably because they are of the same order of magnitude in size as their preferred diet. Blue mussels exposed to nanoplastics (30–100 nm) had a high degree of intestinal uptake; adsorption of nanoplastics onto green algae and subsequent movement through the aquatic food chain via zooplankton to fish has also been demonstrated. Analysis of soft tissues from commercially grown blue mussels and the giant Pacific oyster gave microplastic levels of 36 ± 7 and 47 ± 16 particles/100 g wet weight, respectively. Like other shellfish, these are eaten whole and it has been estimated that European shellfish consumers could potentially ingest 11,000 microplastic particles/year although it should be borne in mind that many consumers only rarely consume fish and so exposure would be lower for a large group of the population. Using the blue mussel as a test organism, 10 μm was the upper limit for translocation into the circulatory system, and so this seems like a useful indicator of size that may be relevant for human ingestion (Fig. 8.6).

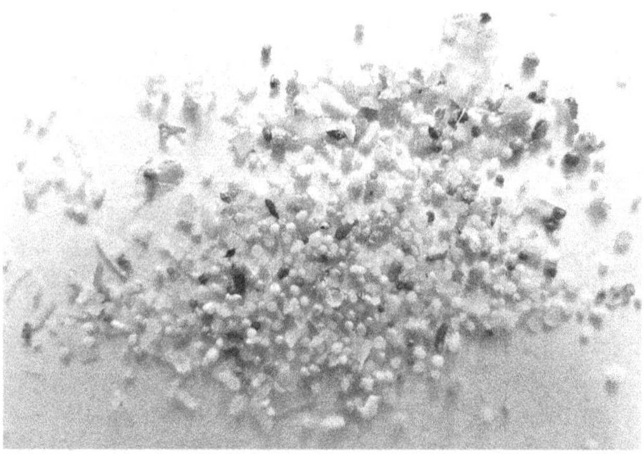

FIGURE 8.6 Microplastics pollution.

8.2.7.1 Adsorption of pollutants

Small plastic particles have a high surface to volume ratio and some have the potential to adsorb other marine contaminants, such as the hydrophobic POPs (e.g., dioxins, PCBs, BFR), potentially concentrating them onto "mats" of microplastics. These can subsequently aggregate and act as "sinks" for a range of chemicals at higher concentrations than normally found. POPs may cause a wide range of toxicological responses such as cancer and endocrine disruption (see earlier). Additionally, marine plastic debris is often visual and detracts from tourism, the leisure industry and commercial fishing. When plastic debris collects, this has been termed the "plastisphere" and has been proposed as a vector for spreading harmful algal blooms and fecal indicator organisms.

Given that many sewage plants release partly-treated effluent into coastal areas of the sea, where pollution is common, this has the effect of concentrating pathogenic species and making the spread of disease more likely. This potential combination of both microbial and chemical agents onto plastic must increase the risk to consumers, especially when contaminated fish, crustaceans or shellfish are consumed.

8.2.8 Foods produced

8.2.8.1 Fish, shellfish, and other animal species

One of the largest differences between animal foods produced in the terrestrial environment when compared to the aquatic one is the vast number of species that can be and are widely consumed in terms of fish and shellfish when compared with only a handful of species that make up the vast majority of terrestrial animals that are used for food.[18] This is slowly changing to some extent as aquaculture is responsible for producing an increasingly large proportion of foods from aquatic systems, and relatively few species are commercially farmed.

For fish, food safety issues can be related to characteristics associated with the species. Oily or fatty fish are associated with higher concentrations of lipophilic contaminants such as POPs including dioxins, PCBs, BFR, legacy pesticides (e.g., DDT, etc.). Toxic metals and other elements such as mercury and arsenic bioaccumulate up the food chain (as do POPs) and are therefore found in higher concentrations in predatory fish such as shark, swordfish, merlin, etc. Both pelagic (top feeders) and benthic (bottom feeders) fish can be contaminated by the foods they eat and by direct uptake from the water, but the differences here are likely to be more variable according to specific local environmental conditions, although benthic fish will be more affected by any pollution in sediments.[28]

Many shellfish have a different metabolism to other animal species and are filter feeders. Species of filter feeders include oysters, clams, and other shellfish, and this process helps to remove excess nitrogen from waters by incorporating it into their shells and tissue as they grow.[29] Polycyclic aromatic hydrocarbons (PAHs) accumulate in filter feeding shellfish whereas most other animal species are able to metabolize this class of contaminant. PAHs are important in terms of toxicity since they form a large class of several hundred compounds, some of which are known to be genotoxic carcinogens. They are normally associated with combustion and can also be found in burnt (charred) or smoked foods.[30]

Sea mammals include cetaceans such as porpoises, dolphins and whales, pinnipeds such as phocid seals and otarids, sea otters, and sirenians such as manatees and dugongs. As top predators, these species accumulate high body burdens of POPs and other bioaccumulative contaminants, and can transfer these to their offspring via placental and lactational transfer. While there have been studies largely as environmental indicators of pollution, it should be borne in mind that such species are consumed by some human population groups. Similarly reptiles such as sea turtles have been used as sentinels of contamination and as such contaminant levels are widely reported, and again both turtles and their eggs are consumed by some communities. Eggs of gulls and other marine birds are fairly widely consumed and contaminants will have a direct relationship with the fish and food they consume.[24]

8.2.8.2 Plant foods: seaweeds, algae, etc

Seaweed has long been regarded as a staple food in Asia, and has seen a significant rise in popularity amongst European consumers over the last decade. Shifts towards a plant based more sustainable diet and also the perception of seaweed as a health food are likely to see this increase further.[31] It has been estimated that by 2050, as much as 0.1% of our oceans will be used for seaweed production, producing fifteen times more food of this type than current production.

There are currently no specific regulations covering the safety and quality of seaweed outside Asia.

The reputation as a "superfood" is associated with seaweed containing high concentrations of vitamin B_{12}, dietary fiber, omega-3 fatty acids, polyphenols, sulfated polysaccharides and pigments that are all associated with health benefits. It is also known that seaweeds can bioaccumulate minerals and trace elements from their surrounding waters. While many of these are also beneficial, some such as lead, mercury, and arsenic are known to be toxic in at least some of the forms in which they are found. Iodine is beneficial at a certain level, and is in fact essential for thyroid hormone synthesis, but high levels can trigger thyroid gland disfunction. The European Food Safety Authority (EFSA) recommends an upper level for iodine intake of 600 μg per day for adults, meaning that the high concentrations of iodine found in some species of seaweed can result in dietary exposure exceeding this amount even when only small amounts of seaweed are consumed. Mercury, lead, cadmium, and arsenic have no beneficial effect and can be harmful in small amounts. Lead has been classified as a possible carcinogen and neurotoxic properties, and arsenic is a class I carcinogen.

Different types of seaweed have different properties in terms of bioaccumulation. Environmental factors such as geographical location, pollution status of water, season, etc. can also have an impact on the amount of elements found within seaweed. Hijiki seaweed can contain so much arsenic that regulatory authorities have recommended that it is not consumed.[32]

In 2018, the European Commission advised member states to monitor elements in seaweed with a view that limits may be needed, depending upon the results of evaluation by EFSA (Fig. 8.7).

8.2.9 Environmental considerations

8.2.9.1 Environmental risk assessment

Environmental risk assessment is a process used to assess the health of an ecosystem and the wider environment. This can have a direct impact on the safety of food produced within the system, in particular with respect to fish and seafood. Whereas a conventional human health risk assessment for exposure to hazardous compounds within food (as discussed earlier) will address the safety of foods by combining an evaluation of the nature of hazards within the foods with an estimate of exposure, an environmental risk assessment will take a more holistic view of the whole ecosystem. An environmental risk assessment can consider a wide array of bioaccumulation markers and biomarkers, which can be used to demonstrate exposure to and effects of environmental contaminants.[33]

Fish bioaccumulation markers may be applied in order to investigate the aquatic behavior of environmental contaminants, as bioconcentrators to identify certain substances with low water levels and to assess exposure of aquatic organisms, normally to evaluate the threat imposed to them, rather than to consumers of species that may be used as food. To predict the fate of xenobiotic substances with simple partitioning models, toxicokinetics, metabolism, biota-sediment accumulation factors (BSAFs), organ-specific bioaccumulation and bound residues need to be taken into account. Even highly complex models do not fully predict bioaccumulation in fish, and so it is important to support an assessment with analytical data. Fish bioaccumulation markers that give a good

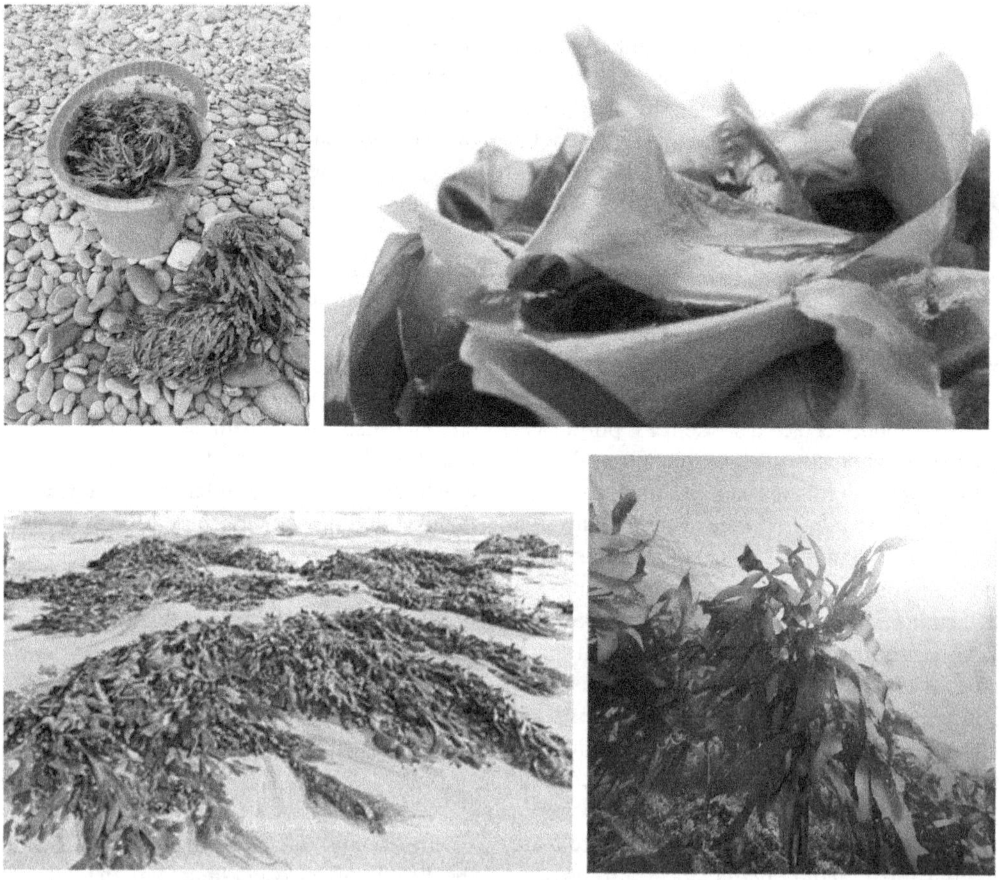

FIGURE 8.7 Algae and seaweed.

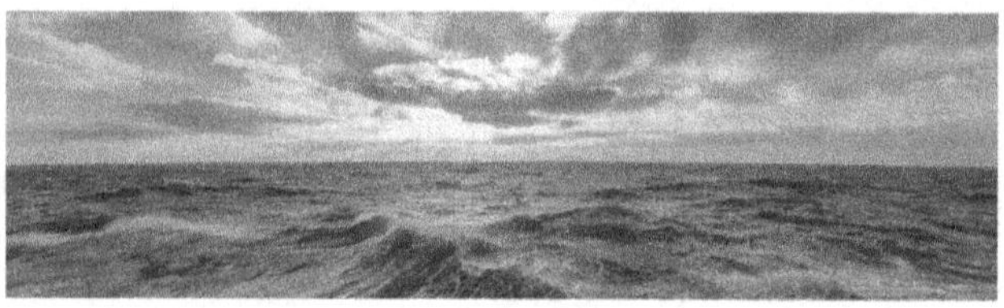

FIGURE 8.8 Environmental risk assessment.

indication of environmental health are body burdens of POPs, like dioxins, PCBs, BFRs, and DDT. Easily biodegradable compounds, such as PAHs and chlorinated phenols, do not tend to accumulate in fish tissues in quantities that reflect the exposure (Fig. 8.8).

8.2.10 Water-table contamination: arsenic in rice as a case study

The focus of this chapter is contaminants in fish and seafood. But it is important to realize that all foods produced rely on water. One particular example of contamination resulting from problems associated with water supply is the production of foods in areas where arsenic is found in the geological make-up of the region.[34]

Arsenic is naturally present in the groundwater in a number of countries, most notably in South Asia. Contaminated water used for drinking, food preparation and irrigation of food crops poses a threat to public health due to the toxic properties of arsenic (especially in its inorganic form) mentioned in the section on metal(oids) in fish above.

Prior to the 1970s, Bangladesh had one of the highest infant mortality rates in the world associated with microbial contamination of the water supply. Ineffective water purification and sewage systems as well as periodic monsoons and flooding contributed to these problems. In order to help, UNICEF and the World Bank advocated the use of wells to tap into deeper groundwater, and millions of wells were constructed. Infant mortality and diarrheal illness were reduced by fifty percent as a result of this initiative. However, with over 8 million wells constructed, it was found that the water from the wells was contaminated with arsenic, coming from the underground sediment of the Ganges Delta, with approximately one in five exceeding the government's drinking-water standard. A 2007 study found that over 137 million people in more than 70 countries are probably affected by arsenic poisoning of drinking water. Since this time, significant progress has

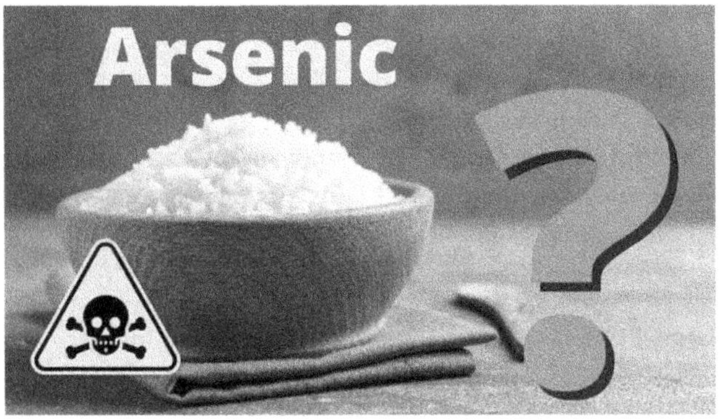

FIGURE 8.9 Arsenic in rice.

been made since and the number of people exposed to arsenic exceeding the Bangladesh drinking-water quality standard has decreased significantly. Since the contamination of water is widespread, the issue affects many foods and drinking water in the region. Since rice from that region is a valuable export crop, concerns about arsenic in rice have a global impact (Fig. 8.9).

8.2.11 Risk substitution

There are water-related health risks associated with all forms of water supply. In reducing one water-related health risk another may be substituted, sometimes of greater magnitude. In Bangladesh, a consequence of reducing the risk from microbial contamination of drinking water was the inadvertent substitution of a risk from arsenic. In developing an emergency response to the arsenic crisis, the potential for risk substitution from other hazards must be considered. Water supply options should be selected within an overall risk management framework of Water Safety Plans. In selecting options, it is important that a consistent approach is adopted in evaluating all risks.

The hazards that may substitute for arsenic include: microbial hazards (pathogens), toxins derived from cyanobacteria in surface water, and chemical contaminants from pollution, but the concept of risk substitution is more general and should always be taken into account by risk managers when trying to address contamination issues.

8.3 Research gaps and future direction

8.3.1 Risk-benefit analysis and personalized medicine

Often high concentrations of chemicals that give rise to health concern (PCBs, dioxins) are found in similar species with high nutrient value (Vit-D, omega fatty acids, etc).

While conventional risk assessment procedures designed to assess the risk of hazards to protect human health are well established, and environmental risk assessment is also to some extent established, an evaluation of risks and benefits is much less commonly undertaken. Yet this is critically important with regard to consumption of fish and seafood. Contaminants such as POPs are associated with oily fish, and these species are also known to contain high levels of Vitamin D and omega-3 fatty acids. To recommend a reduction in consumption of oily fish in low-light countries may result a serious consequence of Vitamin D deficiency, especially in winter months. Avoidance of oily fish may be advised in order to reduce the risk of exposure to carcinogenic pollutants. However, this may result in a decrease in protection against heart disease offered by omega-3 fatty acids. While this advice may be good for an individual with a high cancer risk, who has a fit and healthy lifestyle and genetic make up to suggest a low risk from heart disease, it may not be the best advice for an individual with a low cancer risk but a greater risk from heart disease. Public health advice designed to protect the wider population may be good for most, but may be harmful to certain individuals and should be done with great caution. The topics of risk-benefit analysis and personalized medicine are important future research needs.

8.3.2 Risk assessment of mixtures

Chemical contaminants are rarely found in isolation. Most risk assessments and control limits enforced by regulatory authorities are established for individual contaminants or contaminant classes and do not consider the effect of mixtures. There is some progress in this field but it is largely confined to the assessment of risk of compounds with a similar mode of toxic action, for example dioxins and dioxin-like PCBs which all interact with the AhH receptor. Some attempts to conduct risk assessments for endocrine disrupters have also been made. But often the classes of contaminants that are found together have quite distinctive modes of action and it is not clear how to assess the risks, say, arsenic, mercury, dioxins, and polyfluorinated alky substances, all of which are frequently found together in fish. Mechanisms to address the assessment of such mixtures should be made high priority to help to protect human and environmental health.

8.3.3 Microplastics and nanoplastics

Microplastics and nanoplastics were discussed earlier in this chapter. Research in this area is still very much in its infancy and there are some major challenges ahead. Methods are needed to establish the types of plastics that may make up a mixture to which species are exposed, how to assess the toxicity, the overall absorption and bioavailability, the impact of adsorption of chemical pollutants on the surface of particles and many other topics.

8.3.4 Algae

Algae as a source of food is gaining recognition as a valuable commodity to exploit. Research is needed to fully explore the possibilities for using this wide range of plant materials in food products and ingredients while ensuring the safety of foods that are produced.

8.3.5 Climate change and impact of flooding

Rising sea temperatures can have an impact on many factors including the distribution of mercury between its inorganic form and the more toxic methyl mercury.[35] Mercury is methylated to produce methyl mercury in aquatic environments by microbiotic and chemical mechanisms. Warmer oceans facilitate the methylation of mercury. The subsequent uptake of methyl mercury in fish and mammals has been estimated to increase by 3%–5% for each 1°C rise in water temperature, thus increasing the potential for human exposure via consumption of fish.

Flood events can transport dioxins, heavy metals and hydrocarbons from a contaminated area to a noncontaminated one. This was evidenced in the transfer of dioxins from contaminated soil deposited onto floodplains following flooding of the Elbe and Mulde rivers in central Europe in 2002 and in two river systems in the United Kingdom that flow through urban and industrial areas.[36] Elevated dioxin levels were found subsequently in milk from cows grazing the floodplains compared with barn fed or control pastures, demonstrating that allowing animals to graze on contaminated areas can represent a potential threat to food quality.

The floodwaters resulting from hurricane Katrina illustrated the potential for chemical contamination from a variety of sources including leakage from damaged sewage treatment plants, oil refineries, chemical plants, storage facilities, poorly managed hazardous waste sites or mobilization from one contaminated area to another. Elevated levels of arsenic, lead, and PAH were detected in a proportion of the 1800 sediment and soil samples collected and analyzed by the USEPA following the hurricane in 2005. The highest concentrations of arsenic were considered likely to have resulted from herbicide use in the vicinity. Localized PAHs found near a landfill site were indicative of landfill spillage and elevated levels of lead comparable to historical concentrations are thought to reflect the potential for flood events to mobilize environmental chemicals from one site to another.[37]

8.3.6 Cross boundary management/ considerations

Many major rivers form borders between countries or run through many countries during their course. This can result in pollution being transported between countries with different regulatory regimes and approach to environmental regulation, thus resulting in heightened tensions.[38] Building of dams for water or using river water for irrigation can result in supply problems downstream. Increasing populations and demands on water supply has resulted in predictions that water may be the source of international tensions and disputes in future. Agreement at an international level on how to manage such tensions and disputes may be important to mitigate droughts and conflict.

References

1. Feidi. Fisheries history: gift of the Nile: the fisheries of Egypt, whose source is the River Nile, have always played a significant role, both in ancient and present times. <https://web.archive.org/web/20061110185510/http://www.icsf.net/jsp/publication/samudra/pdf/english/issue_28/art01.pdf>; 2001 Accessed 24.05.21.
2. National Geographic News. African bone tools dispute key idea about human evolution. Available from <http://www.accuca.conectia.es/ngnov801.htm>; 2001 Accessed 24.05.21.
3. Yaowu Hu Y, Hong Shang H, Haowen Tong H, et al. Stable isotope dietary analysis of the Tianyuan early modern human. *Proc Natl Acad Sci U S A*. 2009;106(27):10971–10974.
4. Kameri-Mbote P. Water, conflict, and cooperation: lessons from the Nile river Basin" (PDF). Navigating peace. Woodrow Wilson International Center for Scholars (4). Archived from the original (PDF) on 2010-07-06. <http://www.wilsoncenter.org/topics/pubs/NavigatingPeaceIssue4.pdf>; 2007 Accessed 24.05.21.
5. Tulloch J. "Water conflicts: fight or flight?" Allianz. Archived from the original on 2008-08-29. <https://archive.ph/20080829171957/http:/knowledge.allianz.com/en/globalissues/climate_change/natural_disasters/water_conflicts.html>; 2009 Accessed 24.05.21.
6. Columbia Electronic Encyclopedia. 6th ed. Columbia University Press, Copyright © 2007.
7. Justino CIL, Duarte KR, Freitas AC, Panteleitchouk TSL, Duarte AC, Rocha-Santos TAP. Contaminants in aquaculture: overview of analytical techniques for their determination. *TrAC Trends Anal Chem*. 2016;80:293–310.
8. ESFA. Opinion of the scientific panel on contaminants in the food chain on a request from the European Parliament related to the safety assessment of wild and farmed fish. *EFSA J*. 2005;236: 1–118.
9. Håstein T, Hjeltnes B, Lillehau A, Skare JU, Berntssen M, Lundebye AK. Food safety hazards that occur during the production stage: challenges for fish farming and the fishing industry. *Rev - Int Epizoot*. 2006;25:607–625.
10. European Council. Council Directive 2006/88/EC on animal health requirements for aquaculture animals and products thereof, and on the prevention and control of certain diseases in aquatic animals. *J Eur Union*. 2006;L 328. Available from: http://eur-lex.europa.eu/legal-content/EN/TXT/PDF/?uri = CELEX:32006L0088& from = EN.
11. NOAA fisheries. What is aquaculture? National Oceanic and Atmospheric Administration. <http://www.nmfs.noaa.gov/aquaculture/what_is_aquaculture.html>; 2016.

12. Creti P, Trinchella F, Scudiero R. Heavy metal bioaccumulation and metallothionein content in tissues of the sea bream Sparus aurata from three different fish farming systems. *Environ Monit Assess*. 2010;165:321–329.
13. Cole DW, Cole R, Gaydos SJ, et al. Aquaculture: environmental, toxicological, and health issues. *Int J Hyg Environ Health*. 2009;212:369–377.
14. FAO. *The State of World Fisheries and Aquaculture Opportunities and Challenges*. Rome: Food and Agriculture Organization of the United Nations; 2014. Available from: http://www.fao.org/3/a-i3720e.pdf.
15. Tacon AGJ, Metian M. Aquaculture feed and food safety. The role of the Food and Agriculture Organization and the Codex Alimentarius. *Ann N Y Acad Sci*. 2008;1140(2008):50–59.
16. Cirillo T, Fasano E, Esposito F, Amorena M, Cocchieri RA. Occurrence of NDL-PCBs, DL-PCBs, PCDD/Fs, lead and cadmium in feed and in rainbow trout (Oncorhynchus mykiss) farmed in Italy. *Food Addit Contam Part A Chem Anal Control Expo Risk Assess*. 2014;31:276–287.
17. Benford D. Risk assessment of chemical contaminants and residues in food. In: Rose M, Fernandes A, eds. *Chapter 8 in Persistent organic pollutants and toxic metals in food*. Cambridge: Woodhead Publishing; 2013. ISBN 978-0-85709-245-8.
18. FAO. Aquaculture development. 8. Recommendations for prudent and responsible use of veterinary medicines in aquaculture. FAO Technical Guidelines for Responsible Fisheries. Rome; 2019:No. 5. Suppl. 8.
19. Hernández SP. Responsible use of antibiotics in aquaculture. FAO Fisheries Technical Paper. no. 469. Rome: FAO; 2005:97.
20. Smith P. Antibiotics in aquaculture; reducing the use and maintaining the efficacy. In: Austin B, ed. *Infectious Diseases in Aquaculture*. Woodhead: Cambridge; 2012.
21. Koonse B. A summary of the United States Food and Drug Administrations' Food Safety Program for Imported Seafood; one country's approach. *Foods*. 2016;5(2):31. Available from: https://doi.org/10.3390/foods5020031 (Published online 2016 Apr 29).
22. Hanekamp JC, Frapporti G, Olieman K. Chloramphenicol, food safety and precautionary thinking in Europe. *Environ Liabil*. 2003;11(6):209–221.
23. Rose M. Dioxins and dioxin-like compounds in food and feed. In: Alaee M, ed. *Dioxin and Related Compounds: Special Volume in Honor of Otto Hutzinger (The Handbook of Environmental Chemistry)*. 49. Switzerland: © Springer International Publishing; 2016, ISBN: 978-3-319-23888-3 (Print) 978-3-319-23889-0 (Online). Available from: http://rd.springer.com/chapter/10.1007/698_2016_461.
24. She J, Ip HSS, Guan Y, et al. Levels, trends, and health effects of dioxins and related compounds in aquatic biota. In: Alaee M, ed. *Dioxin and Related Compounds: Special Volume in Honor of Otto Hutzinger (The Handbook of Environmental Chemistry)*. 49. Switzerland: © Springer International Publishing; 2016:153–202. 2016, Published online: 16 March 2016.
25. Ongley ED. Control of water pollution from agriculture - FAO irrigation and drainage paper 55. GEMS/Water Collaborating Centre. Canada Centre for Inland Waters. Burlington, Canada: Food and Agriculture Organization of the United Nations. Rome; 1996.
26. Alimi OS, Budarz JF, Hernandez LM, Tufenkji N. Microplastics and nanoplastics in aquatic environments: aggregation, deposition, and enhanced contaminant transport. *Environ Sci Technol*. 2018;52:1704–1724.
27. Waringa RH, Harrisa RM, Mitchell SC. Plastic contamination of the food chain: a threat to human health? *Maturitas*. 2018;115 (2018):64–68.
28. Zhihua L, Panton S, Marshall L, et al. Spatial analysis of polybrominated diphenylethers (PBDEs) and polybrominated biphenyls (PBBs) in fish collected from UK and proximate marine waters. *Chemosphere*. 2018;195:727–734. Available from: https://doi.org/10.1016/j.chemosphere.2017.11.114.
29. Mill A, Rushton S, Murray A, Rose M. PAH contamination in shellfish: modelling to estimate exposure. *Ecotoxicology*. 2012;21 (2):393–408.
30. Rose M, Holland J, Dowding A, et al. Investigation of the formation of PAHs in foods prepared in the home to determine the effects of frying, grilling, barbecuing, toasting and roasting. *Food Chem Toxicol*. 2015;78:1–9.
31. Holdt SL. DTU in New Food Magazine. Vol 24, Issue 1. 2021.
32. Rose M, Lewis J, Langford N, et al. Arsenic in seaweed—forms, concentration and dietary exposure. *Food Chem Toxicol*. 2007;45: 1263–1267.
33. van der Oost R, Beyer J, Vermeulen NPE. Fish bioaccumulation and biomarkers in environmental risk assessment: a review. *Environ Toxicol Pharmacol*. 2003;13:57/149.
34. Howard G. Arsenic, drinking-water and health risk substitution in arsenic mitigation: a discussion paper. A report prepared for the Arsenic Policy Support Unit, Local Government Division, Government of Bangladesh. World Health Organization. Geneva; 2003.
35. Thomson B, Rose M. Environmental contaminants in foods and feeds in the light of climate change. *Qual Assurance Saf Crop Foods*. 2011;3:2–11.
36. Lake IR, Foxall CD, Lovett AA, et al. Effects of river flooding on PCDD/F and PCB levels in cows' milk, soil, and grass. *Environ Sci Technol*. 2005;39(23):9033–9038.
37. Briceño H, Miller G, Davis III SE. Relating freshwater flow with estuarine waterquality in the southern everglades mangrove ecotone. *Wetl Off Sch J Soc Wetl Sci*. 2013;. Available from: https://doi.org/10.1007/s13157-013-0430-0. ISSN 0277-5212 Wetlands DOI.
38. Brack W. Solutions for present and future emerging pollutants in land and water resources management. Policy briefs summarizing scientific project results for decision makers. *Environ Sci Eur*. 2019;31:74.

Chapter 9

Antimicrobial drugs in aquaculture: use and abuse

George Rigos and Dimitra Kogiannou
Institute of Marine Biology, Biotechnology and Aquaculture, Hellenic Centre for Marine Research, Anavyssos, Greece

Abstract
Aquaculture, the most dynamic food sector, is continuously growing to meet the challenge of the increasing demand for animal protein and health benefits of fish consumption. Intensification of production, introduction of new farmed species, and other unpredicted factors may create animal welfare problems, resulting inevitably in higher risks of disease outbreaks and thus increasing use of antimicrobials mainly in top-producing countries. Residues of antimicrobials in farmed animals have received much attention in recent years because of growing food safety and public health concerns, especially in regions where imports of aquatic food are necessary to cover unmet local demand. Development of antimicrobial drug resistance, hypersensitivity reaction, possible carcinogenicity, and disruption of normal intestinal flora are the most crucial concerns for consumers. Several legislative directives and control systems have been implemented to regulate use of antimicrobials and protect consumers from unwanted side effects. Along with the encouragement for modern husbandry and biosecurity practices, increased prevention and prudent chemical use at a farm level, international organizations and national governments should enforce rigid monitoring of antimicrobials and promote further measures to reduce potential human health risks.

Keywords: Aquaculture; antibacterials; drug; residues; veterinary; legislation; surveillance; hazard; resistance; public health; food safety

9.1 Introduction

9.1.1 Importance of aquaculture globally to meet consumer demand for fish

Human society must successfully meet the enormous challenge of producing food for a population reaching over 9 billion by the middle of the 21st century, without neglecting the necessity of moving to sustainable production and adapting to the adverse impacts of climate change.[1] Among the main animal farming sectors, fish production will play a leading role in facing this challenge, especially in developing regions, which suffer most from poverty and hunger. Global fish production peaked at about 171 million tons in 2016, with aquaculture representing almost half of its volume.[1] Forecasting for aquaculture production is being more optimistic for fish farming as opposed to fisheries, where stable or even reduced catches are expected. Indeed, aquaculture is the most dynamic food sector compared to other major food production industries, although it no longer enjoys the accelerated growth gained in the previous decades. Aquaculture displayed comparable production figures to the main land-based livestock sectors (Fig. 9.1). Global aquaculture production in 2016 included around 80 million tons of fish and 30 million tons of aquatic plants. Farmed/fish production is led by finfish production

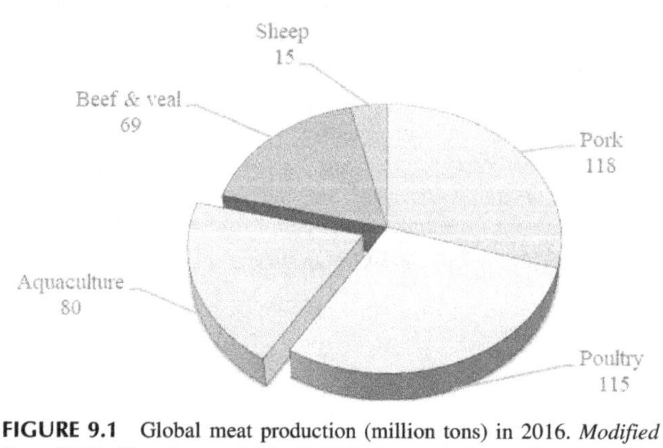

FIGURE 9.1 Global meat production (million tons) in 2016. *Modified from FAO.* The State of World Fisheries and Aquaculture 2018 – Meeting the Sustainable Development Goals. *Rome: FAO; 2018; https://www.statista.com/statistics/237632/production-of-meat-worldwide.*

Present Knowledge in Food Safety. DOI: https://doi.org/10.1016/B978-0-12-819470-6.00027-5

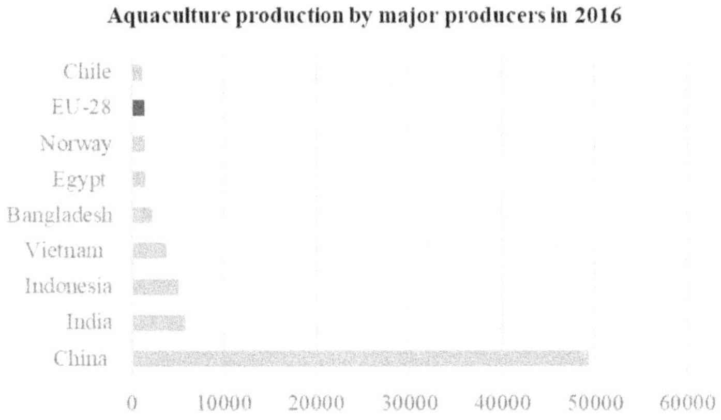

FIGURE 9.2 Aquaculture production (million tons) by major producers in 2016. *Modified from FAO.* The State of World Fisheries and Aquaculture 2018 – Meeting the Sustainable Development Goals. *Rome: FAO; 2018.*

(54.1 million tons), followed by mollusks (17.1 million tons), crustaceans (7.9 million tons), and other aquatic animals (<1 million tons). Asia dominates aquaculture production, with China being by far the leading producer of farmed fish in 2016, providing more than 60% of global fish supply. Other major producers are also from Asia, including India, Indonesia, Vietnam, and Bangladesh (Fig. 9.2). Egypt and Chile are the leading aquaculture producers in Africa and America, respectively, while Norwegian aquaculture alone slightly exceeds the respective European Union (EU)-28 production (Fig. 9.2).[1]

Global demand for fish products is continuously increasing as reflected by the average annual increase in global food fish consumption (3.2%), as compared to the corresponding meat from all terrestrial animals combined (2.8%).[1] Fish consumption nowadays accounts for almost 20% of the animal protein consumed globally. Annual per capita fish consumption is unequal, ranging from 2 to 50 kg, between different global regions, where developing countries have a higher share of fish protein in their diets compared to those in developed countries.

9.1.2 European Union—the world's biggest importer of aquaculture products

Although EU aquaculture sector production reached 1.4 million tons of seafood in 2016 (https://ec.europa.eu/fisheries/cfp/aquaculture_en), EU is by far the world's biggest importer of aquatic products (http://www.eumofa.eu/), with demand considerably exceeding local production. Consumption of seafood in the EU is estimated to be around 24 kg per capita in 2017 (https://www.seafoodsource.com/news/supply-trade/european-markets-importing-exporting-more-seafood-products). Given that seafood production has currently limited space for further regional growth, EU self-sufficiency for seafood has remained at values below 50% during the last decade, revealing a disappointing trade profile in fisheries and aquaculture products, and thus an increasing dependence on imported products. The EU imports of both fisheries and aquaculture products were dependent on nearly 150 countries around the world, although a majority of the total value was sourced from only few countries, such as Norway, China, and Ecuador (https://ec.europa.eu/fisheries/press/eu-fish-market-2019-edition-out-everything-you-wanted-know-about-eu-market-fish-and-seafood_en). Shrimps are currently the leading imported products in terms of value, ahead of salmon and cod whilst tuna, cod, salmon, and pollack are now the main species consumed in the EU. Despite the EU market's global strength, following a strong period of growth in consumption in the last decade, consumption dropped by 5% between 2008 and 2010 and has since remained stable. Of the seafood consumed in the EU 75% is derived from fisheries, but consumption of farmed products has been decreased by 5%. Concerning seafood trade trends, EU imports from third-countries increased by 4% in volume and 2% in value over the previous year, reaching an almost 6 million tons dependence (ec.eumofa.eu).

Import rules for these products are harmonized among EU countries. For non-EU countries the European Commission (EC) is the negotiating partner that defines import conditions and certification requirements. Also, for most countries with existing trade, the EC negotiates on behalf of the Member States. Moreover, EC has developed the European Market Observatory for Fisheries and Aquaculture (EUMOFA) as a market intelligence tool in the EU fisheries and aquaculture sector (https://www.eumofa.eu). Its tasks include increasing market transparency and efficiency, analyzing EU markets dynamics and supporting policy-making. The EUMOFA enables direct monitoring of volumes, values, and prices of fisheries and aquaculture products, from the first sale to retail stage, including imports and exports. General rules for fishery products imports into the EU are subjected to official certification, which is based on the recognition of the competent authority of the non-EU country by the EC. This formal recognition of the reliability of the competent authority is a prerequisite for a candidate country to be authorized for EU exports. All bilateral negotiations and other relevant aspects concerning imports of fishery products must be undertaken by the national competent authority (The EU fish market, 2017). The eligibility importing criteria selected for aquaculture edible products have been established by EC and stated below (https://ec.europa.eu/food/sites/food/files/safety/docs/ia_trade_import-cond-fish):

- Exporting countries must have a competent authority, which is responsible for official controls throughout the production chain. The authorities must be empowered, structured, and resourced to implement effective inspection and guarantee credible public health and animal health attestations in the certificate to accompany fishery products that are destined for the EU.
- The national authorities must also guarantee that the relevant hygiene and public health requirements are met. The hygiene legislation contains specific requirements on the structure of vessels, landing sites, processing establishments, and on operational processes, freezing, and storage. These provisions are aimed at ensuring contamination of the product during processing.
- In the case of aquaculture products, a control plan on heavy metals, contaminants, residues of pesticides, and veterinary drugs must be in place to verify compliance with EU requirements. A suitable control plan must be designed by the competent authority and submitted to the EC high standards and at preventing any for initial approval and yearly renewal.
- Inspections by the Commission's Food and Veterinary Office are necessary to confirm compliance with the above requirements. Such an inspection mission is the basis of establishing confidence between the EC and the competent authority of the exporting country.

9.1.3 Strategies to reduce import dependence of aquaculture products in European Union: farming of new fish species

The EU self-sufficiency ratio in seafood products, which measures the capacity of EU Member States to meet demand from their own production, showed a decreasing profile from 47.4% to 46.0% (2015), reflecting that more of the consumed fisheries and aquaculture products were supplied through imports from non-EU countries than through EU catches or aquaculture production. It furthered declined to 43% in 2017 (https://ec.europa.eu/fisheries/press/eu-fish-market-2019-edition-out-everything-you-wanted-know-about-eu-market-fish-and-seafood). Imported volumes of seafood are thus increased approaching 6 million tones. In 2016 the volume increase was only 3%, while the growth observed in value terms was 9% (The EU fish market, 2017). The EU trade balance deficit reached a negative peak of more than €20 billion. In 2017 aquaculture production in the EU reached a 10-year high of 1.37 million tons with a value of more than €5 billion. Its value almost doubled in those 10 years, due to the increased production of high value species, such as salmon, European seabass, and bluefin tuna, and to the strong price increase of some major species, including salmon, European seabass, gilthead seabream, oyster, and clams. Although slightly less than in 2016, the 2017 consumption of farmed products in the EU was 2% above its decade average. Consumption of fish and seafood in the EU was estimated at 24.4 kg per capita in 2017. On average, EU citizens ate 0.5 kg less compared to the previous year. More than 25% of fish and seafood products imported in the EU originate from Norway, Sweden, and Denmark; the main entry points for Norwegian products into the internal market allow the imports to reach other Member States' markets.

One of the potential strategies to reduce import dependence of aquaculture products in EU is the farming of new fish species. This direction may compensate for increased import dependence of seafood of often questionable quality, in parallel with market stagnation of some established farmed fish species in the EU. European aquaculture constitutes a safe, healthy, and potentially sustainable source of aquatic products and increase in local farmed fish production will be a partial solution to create independence to a certain degree from seafood imports. This strategy could be of special importance since fisheries production, as in other areas of the world, is not expected to enjoy its increasing pattern in the EU. Culture of fast grower species such as greater amberjack and meager with increased commercial value and tremendous potential production could be pioneers in raising seafood production in the EU (http://www.diversifyfish.eu). Both species are still considered as niche products, although European meager production has already reached several thousand tons.[2] Greater amberjack on the other hand has been baptized as the "Mediterranean salmon" and it could soon easily be one of the leaders in EU aquaculture production if specific barriers (diseases, survival, etc.) are solved.

9.1.4 Disease a limiting factor for aquaculture necessitates the use of more and new drugs

Diseases are functional disruptions which can have serious effects on living organisms especially if numerous individuals are confined in small areas, such as the environments of intensive production systems. Treatment of ill-farmed animals is essential to confront disease and return the production enterprises to a profitable pattern.

During the 20th century, the use of veterinary drugs in farm animals was rapidly expanded and included nontherapeutic applications. By the turn of the 21st century it was estimated that half of the global production of antibiotics was being used in farm animals (http://www.who.int/mediacentre/news/releases/2011), while more recently, global antibiotic use for animal farming even exceeded that of human consumption.[3] Antimicrobials play a major role in modern livestock production for prevention and treatment of diseases and even growth promotion. Administration of antibiotics in food animals has been uncontrolled in many countries due to weak regulations and poor management practices.[4] Alarming projections stressed that growing meat consumption, mainly in developing countries, will be associated with an almost 70% increase of antibiotic use in livestock in the coming decades.[3] Nowadays, increase in animal production has largely been accomplished through modernization of the farming practices but also via intensification of existing systems, resulting inevitably in higher risks of disease outbreaks and, thus, increased use of antimicrobials.

In aquaculture medicine, use of therapeutics for prevention is not recommended and is actually prohibited for growth stimulation. The global rise in production and demand for aquaculture products has been paralleled with the promotion of several microbial diseases, resulting, thus, in increasing dependence on antimicrobials with often undesired impacts. Human welfare mainly related to the accumulation of drug residues in the products directed for consumption as well as environmental pollution are the main associated concerns.[5] The economic cost due to the incidence of diseases in aquaculture has been catastrophic on some occasions, and thus the need of effective therapeutic tools is paramount. It has been estimated that the annual cost solely due to parasites in aquaculture is >US$ 1 billion[6] and US$ 6 billion due to all diseases.[7] For example, sea lice infestations generate average damage of almost US$ 0.5 per kilogram of harvested Atlantic salmon in Norwegian farms.[8] Salmonid rickettsial septicemia, one of the most important disease problems in the Chilean salmon farming industry, has caused serious losses (>US$ 100 million) in the past.[9] The same industry has suffered a 30% production crash during the last decade, mainly attributed to infectious salmon anemia and to the sea lice.[10] In Bangladesh, one of the major aquaculture producers globally, the overall average economic loss due to fish diseases has been yearly calculated as high as BDT 24,870 (US$ 293) per ha.[11] In China, the leader in the aquaculture industry, it is estimated that diseases are responsible for losses accounting to 15%–20% of production annually, which implies an economic loss of 5–7 billion Yuan (~US$ 0.7–1 billion).[12]

Pharmaceuticals in aquatic medicine are represented by a wide range of compounds used mainly for therapeutic purposes such antibiotics, antivirals, antifungals, and antiparasitic substances. Unfortunately, pharmaceuticals have not always been used in a responsible manner in the aquaculture industry. The urgency of the farmer's response to an outbreak often results in ill-informed decision-making based on a rushed diagnosis and possible use of inappropriate drugs. Chemicals have been used in fish farming for more than 100 years; however, intensive efforts to register fish toxicants only commenced in the 1950s to late 1970s.[13] Misuse of drugs has been associated with increased microbial resistance, thus necessitating the application of new therapeutics. Novel diseases have been also emerged. Sadly, in most cases, the battle in intensive fish farming appears to be in favor of the pathogen.

Current levels of antimicrobial use in aquaculture worldwide are not easy to monitor because different countries have different distribution and registration systems.[4] In developed countries, the effective use of vaccines, better management and implementation of biosecurity programs has led to a substantial reduction to the use of antibacterial compounds against bacterial pathogens. In Norway for example, consumption of antibacterials has been reduced to 0.36 mg/kg fish produced in 2014, which during the 1990s ranged from 1.2 to 11 mg/kg fish produced.[14] The impact, however, of sea lice on salmonid aquaculture has led to the search for additional therapeutic tools mainly in Norway and the total use of antiparasitics is not in accordance with the reduced pattern of antibacterial use.[15] Indeed, although in recent years, several strategies involving physical and biological measures have been employed in addition to chemical approaches, the amount of chemical antisea lice agents used has been actually increased from 1992 to 2015 but decreased in 2016 and 2017.[15]

Detailed and accurate information on the use of aquaculture chemotherapeutics in Asian aquaculture, where the leading producing counties exist, is relatively limited and in most cases is based on surveys rather than official governmental monitoring.[16] The latter survey reports the outcomes on the use of chemical products in numerous grow-out aquaculture farms in four major producer countries such as China, Thailand, Bangladesh, and Vietnam. Sixty different veterinary medicinal ingredients were recorded, including 26 antibiotics, 19 disinfectants, and 15 parasiticides, a much larger list in comparison with those registered in EU (Table 9.1). Interestingly, shrimp farms in China, Thailand, and Vietnam showed an overall decrease in the use of antibiotic treatments. The amount of total chemical use was estimated to be close to <19 kg per average ton of harvested shrimp in China and Thailand,[16] with parasiticides contributed a considerable portion of the total therapeutics applied.

TABLE 9.1 List of registered antimicrobials for use in aquaculture (European Union and Norway).

Compound	Dosing schedule	MRL (μg/kg edible tissue)	Source
Antibacterials			
Oxytetracycline, chlortetracycline	75 mg/kg, 10 days	100	17
Flumequine	12 mg/kg, 5 days	600	18
Oxolinic acid	10–30 mg/kg, 5–7 days	100	19
Sulfadiazine, sulfamethazine	25 mg/kg, 5 days	100	20
Trimethoprim	5 mg/kg, 5 days	50	21
Amoxicillin, ampicillin	80 mg/kg, 10 days	50	22
Florfenicol	10–15 mg/kg, 10 days	1000	23
Parasiticides			
Formalin	100–200 ppm, 60 min	0	http://mri.cts-mrp.eu/, ES/V/0184/001/MR
Emamectin benzoate	50 μg/kg/d, 7 days	100	24
Azamethiphos	0.1–0.2 ppm, 60 min	0	25
Cypermethrin	5 ppm, 60 min	50	26
Deltamethrin	2–10 ppm, 30 min	10	27
Diflubenzuron	3 mg/kg/d, 14 days	1000	28
Teflubenzuron	10 mg/kg/d, 7 days	500	29
Hydrogen peroxide	30–100 ppm, 30–60 min	0	Nonchemical
Lufenuron	10 mg/kg/day, 7 days	1350	under EMA consideration
Hexaflumuron	2 ppm, 60–120 min	500	under EMA consideration

EMA, European Medicines Agency; *MRL*, maximum residue limit.

9.1.5 General use of veterinary drugs

9.1.5.1 Global and aquaculture levels

Livestock production is one of the fastest growing agricultural sectors, and for health and productivity to be maintained, the use of veterinary drugs is inevitable. The pharmaceuticals used globally in food animals comprise a broad variety of chemical compounds' classes including vaccines, antimicrobials, antiparasitics, and β-agonists. Specifically, the common antibacterials used in livestock production include tetracyclines, penicillins, streptomycin, sulfonamides, tylosin, aminoglycosides, β-lactams, macrolides, lincosamides, and quinolones.

Until recently, the global average annual consumption of antimicrobials per kilogram of animal produced was estimated at >100 mg/kg[30] and this consumption was surprisingly twice that of humans.[31] In detail, according to the study of Van Boeckel et al.,[32] in 2013, the global consumption of all antimicrobials in food animals was estimated at 131,109 tons (100,812 to 190,492 tons) and is projected to almost double in volume by 2030 (from 150,848 to 297,034 tons). Globally, China is by far the largest user of veterinary drugs in livestock production (318 mg/population correction unit—PCU—which takes into account the animal population as well as the weight of each particular animal at the time of treatment with antibiotics), followed by United States and Brazil. On the other hand, considerably low consumption levels were found for Norway (8 mg/PCU).[3]

In United States, the key observations of Food and Drug Administration (FDA)'s recently published report regarding antimicrobial use[33] include:

Domestic sales and distribution of medically important antimicrobials approved for use in food-producing animals is:

- increased by 9% from 2017 through 2018
- decreased by 38% from 2015 (the year of peak sales) through 2018
- decreased by 21% from 2009 (the first year of reported sales) through 2018
- tetracyclines increased by 12% from 2017 through 2018.

Of the 2018 domestic sales and distribution of medically important antimicrobials approved for use in food-producing animals, tetracyclines accounted for 66%, penicillins for 12%, macrolides for 8%, sulfas for 5%, aminoglycosides for 5%, lincosamides for 2%, cephalosporins for 1%, and fluoroquinolones for >1%. The highest percent of chemicals (42%) was intended for use in cattle, 39% in swine, 11% in turkeys, 4% in chickens, and 4% in other species

In the EU, in the recently published ninth European Surveillance of Veterinary Antimicrobial Consumption report, data on the sales of veterinary antimicrobial agents from 31 European countries in 2017 were presented.[34] The main observations of the aforementioned report are summarized below:

- A large difference in the sales for 2017, expressed as mg/PCU, was observed between the countries with the highest and lowest sales (range: 3.1–423.1 mg/PCU).
- Of the overall sales of antimicrobials in the 31 countries in 2017, the largest amounts, expressed as mg/PCU, were accounted for by tetracyclines (30.4%), penicillins (26.9%), and sulfonamides (9.2%). Overall, these three classes accounted for 66.5% of total sales in the 31 countries.
- Pharmaceutical forms suitable for group treatment, that is, premixes accounted for 28.8%; oral powders for 9.9%; and oral solutions for 50.7%, accounted for 89.4% of the total sales.
- For the 25 countries which provided sales for all years between 2011 and 2017, an overall decline in sales (mg/PCU) of 32.5% was observed (from 162.0 mg/PCU in 2011 to 109.3 mg/PCU in 2017).

In the aquaculture sector, as a consequence of the intensification of the culture systems and of the diversification of both the species cultured and the culture methods employed, that pathogens will flourish is inevitable. Disease agents such as viruses, bacteria, fungi, and parasites have caused serious problems in major producing countries in the past.

A variety of compounds is used in aquaculture and categorized as antimicrobials, disinfectants, pesticides, hormones, anesthetics, probiotics and prebiotics, pigments, minerals, and vitamins. Similar to livestock production sector, the aforementioned compounds are used in aquatic animal health management, soil and water management, improvement of natural aquatic productivity, live transportation, feed formulation, manipulation of reproduction, growth promotion, and so on.

In aquaculture, the ideal approach to maintain fish health and welfare would be to prevent the introduction of disease agents so vaccine usage would seem preferable compared to chemical agents; however, this is not always the case. Therefore the use of chemotherapeutics is inevitable to control the impact of a disease. Unfortunately, statistical data regarding the use of chemicals in global aquaculture is relatively limited with a few exceptions (e.g., Norway, United Kingdom, United States, Chile, etc.). This is due for several reasons: (1) different countries have different distribution and registration systems,[4] and thus the requirement for the use of veterinary drugs among countries differs; (2) the scarcity of them specifically developed for use in aquaculture,[35] (3) the diversity of species and culture systems, (4) the unconsolidated nature of production in many regions, and (5) the often unregulated use of chemicals that are labeled and registered for use in aquaculture production.[36]

9.2 Main text

9.2.1 Aquatic animal diseases

9.2.1.1 OIE database in aquatic animal diseases

The need to combat animal diseases at global level has led to the creation of the Office International des Epizooties (OIE) almost a century ago (https://www.oie.int/). In the turn of the 21st century, OIE was renamed as the World Organization for Animal Health, keeping though its historical acronym. The OIE is the intergovernmental organization responsible for improving animal health that has been recognized as a reference organization by the World Trade Organization (WTO), having currently a total of 182 Member Countries (https://www.oie.int/). Among other production systems, OIE has produced the Aquatic Animal Health Code (Aquatic Code) which provides standards for the improvement of aquatic animal health worldwide as well as for the welfare of farmed fish and the use of antimicrobials. The sanitary measures in the Aquatic Code should be used by the Competent Authorities of importing and exporting countries for the prevention, early detection, reporting, and control of pathogenic agents in aquatic animals (amphibians, crustaceans, fish, and mollusks) and to prevent their spread via international trade in aquatic animals and their products, while avoiding unjustified sanitary barriers to trades. The objective of listing notifiable diseases (Table 9.2) is to support Member Countries by providing information needed to take appropriate action to prevent the transboundary spread of important diseases of aquatic animals.

9.2.1.2 Alien farmed fish species may result in new pathogens being introduced locally

Aquatic diseases can emerge from established farmed animals, but also might be triggered by novel pathogens being introduced by alien farmed fish species. As many as 27 alien species, of which 20 are freshwater, have been intentionally introduced into Europe for aquaculture and related activities.[37] Accordingly, three variables have been considered to assess their negative ecological

TABLE 9.2 OIE-listed diseases for aquatic farmed animals.

Disease	Infectious agent	Susceptible species
1. Fish		
Viral		
Epizootic hematopoietic necrosis	Ranavirus	Redfin perch (*Perca fluviatilis*) and rainbow trout (*Oncorhynchus mykiss*)
Infectious hematopoietic necrosis	Rhabdovirus	Pacific salmons including chinook (*Oncorhynchus tshawytscha*), sockeye (*Oncorhynchus nerka*), chum (*Oncorhynchus keta*), pink (*Oncorhynchus* gorbuscha), amago (*Oncorhynchus rhodurus*), masou (*Oncorhynchus masou*), and coho (*Oncorhynchus kisutch*), and Atlantic salmon (*Salmo salar*)
Spring viremia of carp	Rhabdovirus	Common carp (*Cyprinus carpio carpio*) and koi carp (*C. carpio koi*), crucian carp (*Carassius carassius*), silver carp (*Hypophthalmichthys molitrix*), bighead carp (*Aristichthys nobilis*), grass carp, *white amur* (*Ctenopharyngodon idella*), goldfish (*Carassius auratus*), ide (*Leuciscus idus*), and tench (*Tinca tinca*)
Viral hemorrhagic septicemia	Novirhabdovirus	Isolated from 82 different fish species. Most susceptible is rainbow trout
Infectious salmon anemia	Orthomyxovirus	Atlantic salmon
Red sea bream iridoviral disease	Iridovirus	41 fish species
Koi herpesvirus disease	Herpesvirus	Common carp, koi carp, Ghost Carp (*Cyprinus Carpio Albino*), and hybrids of these varieties
Parasitic		
Gyrodactylosis	*Gyrodactylus salaris*	Mainly Atlantic salmon
Oomycetic		
Epizootic ulcerative syndrome	*Aphanomyces invadans*	76 fish species
2. Mollusks		
Viral		
Withering syndrome	Xenohaliotis californiensis	Abalone (*Haliotis* spp.)
Viral ganglioneuritis	Herpesvirus	Abalone
Parasitic		
Bonamiosis	*Bonamia exitiosa*	*Ostrea chilensis*, *Ostrea angasi*, and *Ostrea edulis*
	Bonamia ostreae	Oysters such as European flat oyster (*O. edulis*), *Argentinian oyster* (*Ostrea puelchana*), *southern mud oyster* (*O. angasi*), and dredge oyster (*O. chilensis*)
Marteliosis	*Marteilia refringens*	European flat oyster, blue mussel (*Mytilus edulis*), and Mediterranean mussel (*Mytilus galloprovincialis*)
Perkinsosis	*Perkinsus marinus*	Eastern oyster (*Crassostrea virginica*), Pacific oyster (*Crassostrea gigas*), suminoe oyster (*Crassostrea ariakensis*), mangrove oyster (*Crassostrea rhizophorae*), Cortez oyster (*Crassostrea corteziensis*), soft-shell clam (*Mya arenaria*), and Baltic macoma (*Macoma balthica*)
	Perkinsosis olseni	Sydney cockle (*Anadara trapezia*), New Zealand cockle (*Austrovenus stutchburyi*), Palourde clam (*Tapes decussatus*), Japanese cockle (*Tapes philippinarum*), maxima clam (*Tridacna maxima*), crocus clam (*Tridanca crocea*), clam (*Pitar rostrata*), Pacific oyster (*C. gigas*), Suminoe oyster (*C. ariakensis*), Kumamoto oyster (*C. sikamea*), black-lip pearl oyster

(Continued)

TABLE 9.2 (Continued)

Disease	Infectious agent	Susceptible species
		(*Pinctada margaritifera*), Akoya pearl oyster (*Pinctada martensii*), black-lip abalone (*Haliotis rubra*), smooth Australian abalone (*Haliotis laevigata*), staircase abalone (*Haliotis scalaris*), and whirling abalone (*Haliotis cyclobates*)
3. Crustaceans		
Viral		
Taura syndrome	Taura syndrome virus (Dicistroviridae)	Pacific white shrimp (*Penaeus vannamei*) and Pacific blue shrimp (*Penaeus stylirostris*)
White spot disease	Nimaviridae viruses	All decapod crustaceans from marine and brackish or freshwater sources
Yellowhead disease	Yellowhead virus (*Roniviridae*)	Black tiger prawn (*Penaeus monodon*), white Pacific shrimp (*P. vannamei*), kuruma prawn (*Penaeus japonicus*), white banana prawn (*Penaeus merguiensis*), Pacific blue prawn (*P. stylirostris*), white prawn (*Penaeus setiferus*), red endeavor prawn (*Metapenaeus ensis*), mysid shrimp (*Palaemon styliferus*), and Antarctic krill (*Euphausia superba*)
Infectious hypodermal and hematopoietic necrosis	Infectious hypodermal and hematopoietic necrosis virus	Black tiger prawn, Pacific white shrimp, Pacific blue shrimp (*P. stylirostris*) and Pacific blue prawn
Infectious myonecrosis	Infectious myonecrosis virus (totivirus)	Pacific white shrimp
White tail disease	RNA virus	Giant freshwater prawn (*Macrobrachium rosenbergii*)
Oomycetic		
Crayfish plague	*Aphanomyces astaci*	Noble crayfish (*Astacus astacus*), white clawed crayfish (*Austropotamobius pallipes*), stone crayfish (*Austropotamobius torrentium*), and the Turkish crayfish (*Astacus leptodactylus*)
Bacterial		
Necrotizing hepatopancreatitis	Intracellular rickettsia-like organism (α-proteobacterium)	Pacific white shrimp (*Litopenaeus vannamei*), western blue shrimp (*Litopenaeus stylirostris*), Atlantic white shrimp (*Litopenaeus setiferus*), northern brown shrimp (*Farfantepenaeus aztecus*), and yellowleg shrimp (*Farfantepenaeus californiensis*)

impacts: (1) their distribution across Europe (including non-EU Member States), (2) evidence of their environmental impact in the wild and lastly and more importantly, and (3) evidence of being vectors of nontarget alien species pathogens. Alien crayfish have been blamed, for example, for the spread of crayfish plague in local crustaceans.[37] Peeler et al.[38] have reviewed the effects of nonnative aquatic animals' introductions on disease emergence in Europe. They stressed that enteric red mouth disease and infectious hematopoietic necrosis of salmonids have invaded European aquaculture with the import of live fish and eggs, respectively. Oysters have been also affected by diseases introduced with nonnative species.

The movement of alien aquaculture species across Europe and the possible dispersal of alien pathogens from introduction of nonendemic fish species in the region is mainly controlled by EU Regulation 304/2011, amending Council Regulation 708/2007, which concerns the use of alien species in aquaculture. Aquaculture animals and products, from both the EU and from non-EU countries, must fulfill similar health requirements before they can be moved across national borders. The animal health conditions governing the placing on the market of aquaculture animals and products are defined in Council Directive 2006/88/EC. This Directive has been regularly amended to update the current legislation from new scientific knowledge. Due to the fact that fish health status varies across the territory of the EU, the movement regulations are based on the concept of approved disease-free zones for nonexotic diseases (Table 9.3) listed in Part II of Annex IV to Directive 2006/88/EC. The Directive describes the criteria for the granting, suspension, restoration, and withdrawal of approval of such zones and farms

TABLE 9.3 Aquatic diseases listed as exotic in Annex IV to Directive 2006/88/EC.

Animals	Diseases	Susceptible species
Fish	Epizootic hematopoietic necrosis	Rainbow trout and redfin perch
	Epizootic ulcerative syndrome	Genera: *Catla, Channa, Labeo, Mastacembelus, Mugil, Puntius,* and *Trichogaster*
Mollusks	*Bonamia exitiosa*	Australian mud oyster and Chilean flat oyster
	Perkinsus marinus	Pacific oyster and Eastern oyster
	Mikrocytos mackini	Pacific oyster, Eastern oyster, Olympia flat oyster, and European flat oyster
Crustaceans	Taura syndrome	Gulf white shrimp, Pacific blue shrimp, and Pacific white shrimp
	Yellowhead disease	Gulf brown shrimp, Gulf pink shrimp, Kuruma prawn, black tiger shrimp, Gulf white shrimp, Pacific blue shrimp, and Pacific white shrimp

as well as certification requirements for movement into disease-free zones and farms. It also contains rules governing import from non-EU countries. Based on the Directive, aquatic diseases are divided into exotic and nonexotic diseases. The first group is considered exotic in the EU and animals infected are destroyed as soon as possible to prevent transmission of the disease. Nonexotic diseases are important endemic diseases that should be eradicated in the long term. Where aquatic animals are suspected of being infected or are actually infected with an exotic disease, movement of the animals is allowed only with authorization from the authorities.

9.2.2 Legislation governing use of veterinary chemicals in aquaculture in European Union, United States, and elsewhere

9.2.2.1 Concepts of acceptable daily intake, maximum residue limit and withdrawal time

After various pharmacological, toxicological, microbiological, and other tests undertaken to demonstrate the safety of the substance are completed, the first major stage in the process of safety evaluation is the establishment of the acceptable daily intake (ADI). ADI is an estimate by the joint Food and Agriculture Organization (FAO)/WHO Expert Committee on Food Additives (JECFA) of the amount of a veterinary drug, expressed on a body weight basis that can be ingested daily over a lifetime without appreciable health risk. The basis ADI calculation is the no observed (adverse) effect level (NOEL) or, in certain cases the lowest observed (adverse) effect level with respect to the most sensitive parameter in the most sensitive appropriate test species, or in some cases, in humans. An uncertainty factor—often called a safety factor—is then applied to take into account the inherent uncertainties in extrapolating animal toxicity data to human beings and to take account of variations within the human species. The ADI concept is not applicable to substances for which it is not possible to determine a NOEL because they demonstrate nonthreshold effects (such as genotoxicity and delayed neurotoxicity). In such cases, an alternative approach to safety evaluation may be applied on a case by case basis, having regard to all the data available. Since the ADI is related to body weight, an arbitrary average human BW is defined at 60 kg (average value for all age groups in the European population). The ADI expressed on a μg or mg per kg body weight basis is therefore multiplied by 60 to give the total amount of residue, which can be ingested by an individual. The safe concentration for each edible tissue using the ADI will be calculated by FDA as follows: Safe concentration = [ADI (μg/kg/day) × 60 kg]/(grams consumed/day). Since accurate consumption profiles are difficult to be estimated, and there are substantial variations between individual consumers and between groups of consumers, arbitrarily high fixed values are used to ensure the protection of the majority of consumers. Alternatively, the Temporary ADI (TADI) is used by JECFA when data are sufficient to conclude that use of the substance is safe over the relatively short period of time required to generate and evaluate further safety data, but are insufficient to conclude that use of the substance is safe over a lifetime. A higher-than-normal safety factor is used when establishing a TADI and an expiration date is established by which time appropriate data to resolve the safety issue should be submitted to JECFA.

Several parameters have been globally established to regulate the use of antimicrobials in animal production including aquaculture. Maximum Residue Limit for veterinary drugs (MRL or MRLVD) is the maximum concentration of residue resulting from the use of a veterinary drug (expressed in mg/kg or μg/kg on a fresh weight basis) that is recommended by the Codex Alimentarius Commission to be legally permitted or recognized as acceptable in or on a food. The MRLs for veterinary drugs are established through the Codex Committee on Residues of Veterinary Drugs in Foods (CCRVDF) in

Codex Alimentarius last amended in 2018.[39] MRL establishment is based upon a risk assessment of the joint FAO/WHO JECFA. Albeit efforts have been made to harmonize MRL worldwide under the aegis of WTO and the Codex Alimentarius, MRLs still vary between geographical locations which might be related to the differences found in risk assessment. In fact, MRLs in a particular animal product may differ from one country to another depending on the local food safety regulatory agencies and drug usage patterns but most developing countries have yet to develop their own MRLs. In Europe, the main legislative documents regarding veterinary chemicals are Regulation 726/2004 and Directive 2001/82. Directive 2001/82/EC,[40] amended by Commission Directive 2009/9/EC[41] and by Regulation 470/2009,[42] is the safety net that foodstuffs of animal origin do not contain drug residues which can induce undesirable effects on human health from a toxicological, pharmacological, or microbiological point of view. The primary purpose of this law is the safeguarding of public health. Furthermore, Regulation 726/2004[43] lays down the procedures for the authorization and supervision of medicinal products for human and veterinary use as well as the structure and mission of the EMEA (European Agency for the Evaluation of Medicinal Products). The European Medicines Agency's (EMA), Committee for Medicinal Products for Veterinary Use is responsible for preparing the opinion of the Agency on issues concerning the evaluation of the quality, safety, and efficacy of veterinary drugs and the recommendation of the MRL of veterinary chemicals that can be accepted in foodstuffs of animal origin. Regulation 470/2009[42] lays down the Community rules and procedures for the establishment of MRLs of pharmacologically active substances in foodstuffs of animal origin, repealing Council Regulation No 2377/90[44] and amending Directive 2001/82/EC of the European Parliament and of the Council and Regulation 726/2004 of the European Parliament and of the Council.[43] In Article 14 of the aforementioned legislation, the pharmacologically active substances are classified into (1) substances with a defined MRL, (2) substances with a provisional MRL, (3) substances that do not require MRL, and (4) substances whose use is forbidden in food-producing animals. Finally, in the Commission Regulation 37/2010[45] the classified pharmacologically active substances with respect to MRL, for reasons of ease of use, are listed in one Annex in alphabetical order. In the United States, the FDA under the Federal Food, Drug, and Cosmetic Act (FFDCA) is the responsible agent who establishes tolerances for veterinary drugs. Limitations are published in the Code of Federal Regulation.[46] The FDA also prohibits the usage of some drugs under the 21 Code of Federal Regulation for extra-label animal and human uses in food-producing animals. In Canada, the Health Canada's Veterinary Drugs Directorate sets the limits for veterinary drugs residues found in foods and also prohibits the use of specific chemicals in animals intended for human consumption.[47,48] In China, the Ministry of Agriculture issued a National Food Safety Standard on Maximum Residue Limits for Veterinary Drugs in Foods (GB 31650-2019), which took effect on April 1, 2020.[49] The aforementioned standard replaces portions from Announcement No. 235 of the Ministry of Agriculture and Rural Affairs, published in December 2002. Additionally, the prohibited veterinary drugs and other chemicals in food animals are listed in the National Standard No 193.[50]

Another parameter regulating the use of antimicrobials is withdrawal time (WT) or withholding time. WT is defined as the period of time between the last administration of a drug and the collection of edible tissue or products from a treated animal that ensures the contents of residues in food comply with the MRL for this veterinary drug. The establishment of an MRL allows the setting of a withdrawal period of the drug. In most food-animal species withdrawal periods are defined in days, but with fish the EU requires data to be presented from trials conducted at least two water temperatures relevant to the proposed conditions of use. If depletion of residues is found to be temperature-dependent, then a withdrawal period in degree-days will be set, making the withdrawal period a function of temperature and time. If the data do not indicate a temperature effect on depletion, then a day-based withdrawal can be accepted.[51] Additionally, for meat of fish, when no specific withdrawal period is defined, a withdrawal period of 500-degree days has to be respected. According to the FDA "the WT is determined when the tolerance limit on the residue concentration is at or below the permitted concentration. A tolerance limit provides an interval within which a given percentile of the population lies, with a given confidence that the interval does contain that percentile of the population. FDA will use the 99th percentile of the population and the 95% confidence level."[52] In Europe, EMA recently issued documentation that provides a standard approach to be used across the EU in the analysis of residue depletion data for the purpose of establishing withdrawal periods for edible tissues.[53]

Admittedly, the number of medicines that can be used "on label" in aquaculture is extremely low and only very few pharmaceutical antibacterial-based products have been licensed at different national level for specific use against fish diseases. The differences between countries (even at EU country-level) regarding licensed products are also an add-on problem. If no licensed medicine for fish are available in a country but available in other EU countries, then it is also possible to use another legal mechanism known as "importation and use of veterinary medicines under exceptional circumstances." In these cases, it is possible to apply to the responsible national authorities for a particular import authorization. Unfortunately, given the lack of specific licensed medicines for finfish, this mechanism becomes common instead of exceptional and requires additional bureaucratic efforts.

The scarcity of specific "on label" medicines, also problematic for other animal species, such as the so-called "minor species," has also been alleviated by the "prescribing cascade" mechanism. EU regulations (90/676; 19/6; 19/4) provide a "prescribing cascade" to support the use of medicines authorized for other farmed animals, when no suitable compound has been licensed to treat diseases in fish. In such cases, a minimum standard withdrawal period is imposed, corresponding to 500-degree days in fish in order to ensure consumer safety, and is enforced by an established MRL, which is derived from toxicity testing data.

9.2.2.2 Hazard analysis and critical control point approaches

The hazard analysis and critical control point (HACCP) system, which is science-based and systematic, identifies specific hazards and measures for their control to ensure the safety of food. HACCP is a tool used to assess hazards and establish control systems that focus on prevention rather than relying mainly on end-product testing. This tool can be applied throughout the food chain from primary production to final consumption and its implementation should be guided by scientific evidence of risks to human health. As well as enhancing food safety, implementation of HACCP can provide other significant benefits. In addition, the application of HACCP systems can aid inspection by regulatory authorities and promote international trade by increasing confidence in food safety.

Agriculture experts believed that the application of HACCP would have been difficult at the "farm level." On the contrary, HACCP system has been proven suitable and has been applied for almost 30 years in aquaculture sector. According to Jensen and Martin,[54] the first exposure of the US aquaculture community to HACCP occurred during 1989 and 1990 when three Aquaculture Application Workshops were conducted by the National Fisheries Institute in cooperation with the National Marine Fisheries Service (NMFS). The first HACCP Regulatory Model for Aquaculture was published and released by NMFS in 1991. There, participants of the International Conference on Quality Assurance in the Fish Industry held in Denmark agreed that HACCP was a superior method of fish inspection and that the HACCP concept should be applied in the fish industry to cover food safety, plant/ food hygiene, and economic fraud issues.[55] During the Second International Conference on Fish Inspection and Quality Control held in Washington, DC, United States, in 1996, participants affirmed that HACCP-based programs were in the process of being implemented on a global scale. Urged on by this International Conference, governments as well as the aquaculture industry alike continued their efforts to give a high priority to the full implementation of HACCP-based systems.[56]

The development of an HACCP plan for an aquaculture facility requires the collaboration of a team of experts from several disciplines related to public health and aquaculture, for example, public health specialists, veterinarians (food inspectors and fish pathologists), aquaculturists, and fishery extension workers. Such HACCP plans and HACCP-based regulations, regarding the safety of fish and fish products, including products from aquaculture, are applied by a large number of countries globally. Specifically, HACCP systems are being put into practice in aquaculture at various levels but mainly in the sectors of high-valued farmed species such as salmon in Norway, Canada, Ireland, United States, New Zealand, United Kingdom, and Chile; shrimp in Thailand, Ecuador, Australia, Cuba, Brazil, and Central American countries, and United States; trout in European countries, Argentina, Peru, and Brazil; catfish in United States; crawfish in United States; and bullfrogs in Brazil.

HACCP-based system can be apparently applied without difficulty to intensive cultural commercial aquaculture ventures; however, in small-scale, subsistence aquaculture systems, where fish are mainly farmed for domestic consumption under minimal inputs, knowledge, and assistance, application of an effective HACCP-based system poses considerable difficulties. Therefore the design and implementation of HACCP systems should be considered following careful evaluation of the feasibility of applying such a control system to a particular aquaculture system, the risks associated with the systems components and procedures, and the identification of the correct and appropriate critical control points.[57]

As mentioned above, the HACCP system has for years been widely adopted in the fisheries sector. EU rules on food safety and food standards are complex and subject to regular changes as International and European standards, commercial factors, scientific knowledge, food and food inspection technology, and known hazards are all in constant development. New hygiene rules were adopted in April 2004 (providing for primary responsibility for food safety on the food business operator, registration or approval for certain food establishments, and general implementation of procedures based on the HACCP principles) which have generally been welcomed by the aquaculture industry.[58] Additionally, both the General and Fisheries Directives[59,60] have a requirement for the use of HACCP or HACCP-based principles. In the United

States, HACCP has been mandatory for the fisheries sector by 1997. Specifically, on December 18, 1995, FDA published as a final rule 21 CFR 123, "Procedures for the Safe and Sanitary Processing and Importing of Fish and Fishery Products" that requires processors of fish and fishery products to develop and implement Hazard Analysis Critical Control Point (HACCP) systems for their operations.The regulation became effective on December 18, 1997. The agency also published the "Fish and Fishery Products Hazards and Controls Guide" ("the Guide") in September, 1996, to assist processors in the development of their HACCP plans, and to provide information to help them identify hazards that may be associated with their products and formulate control strategies for those hazards. The guide was developed to coincide with the issuance of the final regulation.

9.2.2.3 Surveillance programs and national control systems

One of the major health concerns in addition to the presence of harmful veterinary residues in aquaculture products is the development of antimicrobial resistance. Admittedly, the relationship between antibiotic use in food animals and antibiotic resistance in human and animal pathogens has been postulated as a contributing not causative factor.[61] In the aquaculture sector, development of antimicrobial resistance is more pronounced in countries where aquaculture medicine is heavy and uncontrolled, since bacteria in the aquatic environment share a large assortment of mobile genetic elements and antimicrobial resistance genes with a wide range of terrestrial bacteria.[62]

To monitor trends in resistance and allow for timely corrective action and evaluation of interventions, WHO[63] suggested:

- a surveillance system for the usage of antibiotics in people and food animals and
- an integrated (among the public health, food, and veterinary sectors) surveillance system to monitor antibiotic resistance in selected food-borne bacteria.

A surveillance system for the usage of antibiotics in aquaculture requires data to be collected on a regularly and reported as weight of active substance per animal species and antibiotic class. In addition the data should be further assorted regarding their therapeutic use and reported by route of administration. Typically, the data on overall use could be obtained from the pharmaceutical industry, wholesalers, pharmacies, and tariff declarations, for countries without a pharmaceutical industry or wholesalers, which depend on the distribution system for antibiotics used in animals in each country.[63] In cases where collecting detailed data for an entire country is difficult, they could be collected through surveys in a representative area by a statistically robust sampling scheme probably from sources such as the records of veterinary practitioners and producers. The usage data should be combined with data on animal population size and ideally with data on animal health status in order to reflect the need for using different kinds of antibiotics.

As an example, the US cage salmon aquaculture industry was the first food animal industry to report monthly antimicrobial use at the farm level to the government.[64] Norway, Chile, Canada, and Scotland have also produced comprehensive reports on salmon production and veterinary drug use.[65–68] To date most countries, however, do not have a surveillance system of antibiotic use and different methodologies are used for presenting those data. This could explain the variability of information and lack of reliable data; therefore EMA has worked on the development of a harmonized approach to surveillance of antibiotic usage in animals in the EU.[63] The surveillance of antibiotic resistance in zoonotic and commensal bacteria in different food animal reservoirs and aquaculture products is a prerequisite for understanding the development and dissemination of antibiotic resistance, providing relevant risk assessment data, and implementing and evaluating targeted interventions. This surveillance entails specific and continuous data collection, analysis, and reporting that quantitatively monitor temporal trends in the occurrence and distribution of resistance to antibiotics.[63]

As in most regions, EU Member States have a responsibility to monitor the use of veterinary medicines in food-producing animals, to ensure that produce from these animals do not contain residues that could be harmful to consumers. It is a requirement to implement surveillance monitoring in accordance with the Residues Directive (Directive 96/23/EC) and to have in place national plans for the monitoring of certain chemical substances and residues in a range of all food producing species and related products. The specifications for the harmonized surveillance of antibiotic resistance in food animals have been recently documented by EFSA (European Food safety Authority).[69] Other agencies such as European Surveillance of Veterinary Antimicrobial Consumption (ESVAC), European Centre for Disease Prevention and Control (ECDC), and EMA are also part of the European Surveillance System (TESSy) in order that the EU Commission can manage the public health risk of antimicrobial resistance and to evaluate the impact of interventions.[70]

A policy publication has evaluated EU sampling strategies for the detection of veterinary drug residues in aquaculture species.[71] This communication examined the existing EU sampling schedule for aquaculture products and evaluated its possible application in a global context.

The UK statutory sampling data were the main subject of evaluation in the study and the findings confirmed the effectiveness of the directive; however, it was mentioned that the methodology might lead to unnecessary sampling. Concerning examination of aquaculture imports, evaluation of the Rapid Alert System for Food and Feed database using process control charts and statistical modeling suggested that the sampling protocol is effective but not sufficiently flexible for the range of existed aquaculture practices.

Indeed, as aquaculture enterprises and markets continue to develop, the challenge will be to develop efficient sampling strategies for residue surveillance that are flexible, reactive, and relevant to different farm animals and practices. Presently there is no consensus agreement regarding sampling regimens for veterinary residues for countries exporting to the EU. While Directive 96/23/EC may be applied within the EU region, it does not entertain global acceptance. Therefore Directive 96/23/EC should not be considered a suitable replacement for CODEX sampling protocols, which provide alternative global sampling strategies for food animals.

In addition to surveillance programs, national food control systems (NFCS) are a group of elements organized and arranged in a way that they can act as a whole to protect consumers' health. The principal objectives of NFCS have been determined by FAO and WHO[72] and Codex Alimentarius.[73] Food control systems need to be up-to-date, which means that they need to adapt to today's food production and distribution practices. Thus principles and guidelines for NFCS should focus on the entire chain, that is, production, packing, storage, transport, handling, and sale of foods within national borders. Since a great part of food products is intended to be consumed outside a country, properly designed import and export control systems, as part of the overall NFCS, are essential. Principles and Guidelines for National Food Control Systems are published by Codex Alimentarius (CAC/GL 82-2013), serving as guidance to countries. This document allows countries to be flexible on how to best design their food control system and implement specific control measures; therefore identical NFCS cannot be found. According to Lupin,[74] the EU has adopted the most comprehensive food safety control system in the world with the most stringent legislation and regulation toward food safety. Furthermore, the EC regulations No. 178/2002[75] and No. 854/2004,[76] and No. 882/2004,[77] set the objectives of a general food law and give the conditions required for an effective national implementation.

Different inspection programs in imported aquatic products have in most cases revealed residues of registered antibacterials above legal levels or the presences of banned compounds. For example, national statutory surveillance schemes on residues of veterinary medicines in food carried out annually in the United Kingdom (http://www.gov.uk/government/statistics/residues-of-veterinary-medicines-in-food), have shown the illegal use of antimicrobials. These included increased levels of emamectin and presence leucomalachite green (biotransformation product of banned malachite green) in local farmed salmon. An earlier Canadian surveillance study revealed that Canadian consumers during the period of 1993–2004 were exposed to low concentrations of some prohibited veterinary drugs via the consumption of certain imported farmed fish and shrimp.[78] Sadly, metabolites of furazolidone, nitrofurazone and furaltadone, leucomalachite green, and even chloramphenicol were found in the examined aquatic products. In a Japanese survey, it was reported that the number of violations regarding veterinary drugs in imported food has increased largely, and most of them were attributed to chloramphenicol and nitrofurans in seafood from Asian countries.[79] Lastly, Love et al.[80] presented veterinary drug violations among four inspecting bodies (EU, United States, Canada, and Japan), using government-collected data from the period of 2000 to 2009. Most drug violations were detected in species that are commonly farm-raised in Asian such as shrimp and prawns, catfish, crab, tilapia, and eel. Chilean salmon was also among the most commonly found violated aquatic products. Vietnam had the greatest number of violations among exporting countries. Nitrofurans and chloramphenicol represented the dominant drug violations in farmed crustacean tested, while in farmed fish, top illegal findings consisted of malachite green, nitrofurans, and chloramphenicol.

9.2.3 Public/consumer health issues

Antimicrobials used in aquaculture are commonly applied to combat aquatic microbial pathogens via the feed or less frequently directly to the water (baths in cages, tanks, raceways) and seldom by injection (broodstock). These practices are inevitably responsible for chemical pollution into the environment due to released antimicrobials after the completion of the therapy as well as from metabolic and fecal products and uneaten medicated feed particles. Such chemical releases from aquaculture facilities can contribute to increased risk of antibacterial resistance development in environmental compartments which at the end may affect human welfare. More importantly as related to consumer health and irrespective of the route or purpose of administration, antimicrobials can accumulate as residues in tissues of the aquaculture products, before they are being excreted from the fish body compartment. The occurrence of residues in farmed aquatic organisms is most likely when these animals are harvested for human consumption after medication, before the necessary withdrawal period elapses. Antimicrobial residues can also occur in fish when the drugs are administered outside of the labeled recommendations or suggested dosing schedules. Extra-label usage of antimicrobials in aquaculture is practicing though the "cascade" system mentioned above but is required to be supervised by veterinarians to minimize risk. Illegal chemotherapeutics can be also found as fish residues. Consumption of such "polluted" products may result in many health problems in humans including allergic reactions, toxicity side effects, disruption of normal intestinal flora, and lastly and perhaps more importantly, development and propagation of antimicrobial resistance.

1. Allergic reactions could also arise in sensitive consumers when the aquaculture products have increased levels of antimicrobials (above MRL). A notable proportion of the general population may have allergic sensitivity to these substances mainly due to prior medical treatments rather than being exposed to dietary residues. Indeed, cases of proven allergy to such substances in food are extremely rare, based on clinical and laboratory proof of an immunological reaction, whereas there are less well-substantiated reports blaming antibiotics. Clearly, any exposure to a chemical will carry at least a notional risk of causing harm, which could be a reversible functional deviation, or a permanent and rarely even life-threatening disease.[81] The factors highlighted to determine the nature and magnitude of the risk, are the properties of the substances, the level of exposure and the constitution of the exposed individual as related to the genetic background. Such cases are usually related to high medications along with short exposure, whereas any risk from residues in food would probably represent prolonged ingestion of small amounts. However, it is still worth analyzing the evidence from recorded medical cases if dietary veterinary residues were associated with a possible disorder.
2. Possible carcinogenic and mutagenic effects to consumers may be linked to the presence of illegal toxic compounds, occasionally detected in aquacultured products. Perhaps the most hazardous agent is chloramphenicol, which has been banned for use in livestock, but its detection through monitoring programs in farmed aquatic products from Asia is not uncommon.[82] Chloramphenicol has been extensively used in human medicine in the past such as eye drops and topical cream due to its powerful broad spectrum antimicrobial activity.[82] However, chloramphenicol is known to exert many side effects in humans such as allergic reactions and gastrointestinal disorders,[83] but more importantly, may lead to an increased risk of developing cancer and in very low concentrations may trigger aplastic anemia, a disease that causes bone marrow to stop producing red and white blood cells and could be fatal. Chloramphenicol is thus not allowed for use in the treatment of animals for food production in the EU and elsewhere and may not be used in the production of food of animal origin, which is imported into the EU. Actually, in 2002, the EU imposed a 30-month ban on shrimp imports from China because of illegal chloramphenicol antibiotic use, and in 2006 the United States rejected shrimp imports from China because of repeated chloramphenicol contamination,[84] both of which caused a huge economic impact on China's aquatic production industry. The Chinese government also has banned the use of chloramphenicol in aquatic species, but chloramphenicol residues are frequently detected in aquatic products by the government enforcement departments.

   Monitoring programs carried out in EU or in North America on imported aquaculture products have also indicated the presence of other illegal drugs. Particularly, a Canadian survey revealed that local consumers are exposed to low concentrations of banned veterinary residues via the consumption of certain fish and shrimp.[78] Nitrofurans (e.g., furazolidone, furaltadone), another group of hazardous antimicrobials for consumers, were included in the detected drugs in addition to chloramphenicol. Nitrofurans belong to a family of antibacterials, which have broad-spectrum antimicrobial activities and can be used in both human and veterinary medicine. Due to concerns about potential carcinogenicity of the drug residues and their potential to cause harmful effects on human health, the EU banned their use in food-producing animals in 1995,[85] but residues continue to be found in imported shrimp because of their ready availability and high efficacy in veterinary therapy.
3. Disruption of the normal intestinal flora could be associated to antibacterial consumption in humans.[86] The bacteria that usually live in the intestine act continuously to protect against pathogen infection, which could cause diseases. Antibacterials might reduce the total number of these beneficial bacterial communities or selectively kill some important species. Consequently, antimicrobials might adversely affect a wide range of intestinal flora and subsequently cause gastrointestinal disturbance and imbalance. This disturbance can cause bacterial overgrowth and emergence of resistant microorganisms, which may lead to serious infections and encourage transfer of resistance factors among bacteria. As in the case of allergic reactions, this abnormality mainly refers to high and prolonged medication for therapeutic reasons rather than to residues resulting from food consumption. There is little scientific information on the effect of antimicrobial residues on the bacterial flora

of the human intestinal tract, because human studies have mainly been carried out at therapeutic dose levels and not at the residue range concentrations.[87]

4. Chiefly, among the major health concerns related to the presence of veterinary residues in aquacultured products, is the potential development of antimicrobial resistance. Antibacterial resistance, especially that induced by use of chemicals in livestock production, poses a global challenge with serious economic damage and devastating effects on public health.[70] There is increasing evidence for a direct relationship between antibacterial use in farmed animals and the emergence of resistance both in human and animal pathogens.[61] Even more, there are alarming signs that antibacterial use in aquaculture has also a potential to select for antimicrobial-resistant bacteria in the aquatic environment.[62,88,89] Particularly, aquaculture systems contain high numbers of diverse bacteria, which exist in combination with the current and past use of different antibacterials. Such production systems have been actually blamed as genetic hotspots for gene transfer.[90] The associated risk for development and transfer of antimicrobial resistance via the measures of aquatic medicine is mainly related to the release of uneaten medicated diet, undigested food, and fish excreta containing unabsorbed and secreted drug metabolites, which can remain in the water and sediment near farming sites for an extensive period. Development of antimicrobial resistance could be more apparent in farming sites in countries where aquaculture medicine usage is heavy, prophylactic, and uncontrolled, since bacteria in the aquatic environment share a large assortment of mobile genetic element and antimicrobial resistance genes with a wide range of terrestrial bacteria.[62] Indeed, there is strong laboratory proof of horizontal gene transfer between bacteria in the aquatic environment and human pathogens.[91] As a result of horizontal gene transfer, the genetic materials originating from the aquatic ecosystem may be inserted into the genome of terrestrial bacteria, bridging the aquatic and land counterparts and eventually affecting the treatment of human diseases in some cases.[62] Indeed, many aquatic bacteria harbor a large variety of mobile genetic elements and resistance determinants such as plasmids, integrons, and transposons that can readily recombine and promote the emergence of new genetic combinations.[62,92]

In addition to dissemination of antimicrobial-resistant bacteria via the aquatic environment, excessive use of antimicrobials in aquaculture may affect human health via the dietary route if residues exceed certain levels.[88] Specifically, contamination of fish products for human consumption with antimicrobial residues at doses higher than MRL, are often. When such products are accidentally and repeatedly eaten, they can potentially select for antimicrobial-resistant bacteria.[88,89] Furthermore, bacterial strains carrying resistance determinants in aquaculture products, which may include human pathogenic bacteria, could eventually spread resistance genes, thereby increasing the risk of spreading antimicrobial resistance from aquaculture to the consumer.[93–95]

In addition to the farmed aquatic products, caution should be also paid to the consumption of wild animals from the vicinity of aquaculture sites with possible chemical pollution,[96] since antimicrobials can reach these animals via uneaten medicated feed, metabolic products, and excreta of farmed fish. The potential bridging of aquatic and human pathogen genetic backgrounds leads to emergence of new antimicrobial-resistant bacteria, resulting to a possible dissemination of antimicrobial resistance genes into human populations. Efforts to prevent antimicrobial overuse and ensure prudent use in aquaculture must include education of all stakeholders about its detrimental effects on the welfare of fish, aquatic ecosystem, and consumers. The absolute contribution of aquaculture to the emergence of antimicrobial-resistant human infections needs to be fully determined and clarified as to its past occurrence. For example, the cholera pandemic in Ecuador during the 1990s, which was characterized by the emergence of multiresistance strains of *Vibrio cholerae*, was blamed on the use of antimicrobials in Ecuadorian shrimp farms. However, this hypothesis was finally rejected based on the available knowledge concerning the epidemic and the emergence of resistance.[97] In the absence of thorough prophylaxis, even increase in the list of new antimicrobials will not be possibly sufficient alone to prevent a crisis in the treatment of bacterial infectious diseases in both human and veterinary populations.[98]

9.2.4 Analytical techniques to identify drug residues

The need of sensitive and rapid advanced analytical techniques to detect and quantify drug residues of pharmacologically active compounds, in foodstuffs of animal origin, has become mandatory. Admittedly, there is also an urgent need for cheap, portable, and fast analytical methods enabling screening followed by confirmatory analysis.

The Commission Decision 2002/657/EC[99] reported the technical guidelines and performance criteria for method validation for the control of the different residues.

According to EU guidelines, screening methods should be used to detect the presence of a substance or class of substances at the level of interest prior to confirmatory analysis. Screening analysis allows testing of large number of samples faster, thus excluding compliant samples from further analysis. Additionally, according to 2002/657/EC, the confirmatory methods for organic residues or contaminants should provide information on the chemical structure of the analyte suggesting that only chromatographic separation coupled with spectrometric detection is suitable as confirmatory methods. It should be noted, however, that under certain conditions, fluorescence and ultraviolet-visible detectors might also be used for confirmation.[99]

The decision limit (CCα) and the detection capability (CCβ) were introduced to 2002/657/EC, having replaced the formerly used limits of detection and quantification.[99] CCα is the concentration at and above which can be concluded with an error probability of α (5%) that a sample is noncompliant (positive), while CCβ is the smallest content of the substance that may be detected, identified, and/or quantified in a sample with an error probability of β. The concept of the minimum required performance limit for banned substances, which corresponds to the minimum content of an analyte in a sample that has to be detected and confirmed and constitutes the lowest level that can be reliably considered nonzero, was also introduced to this legislation document. Furthermore, 2002/657/EC introduced a system of identification points (IPs) for Ms (mass spectrometry) detection.[99] In detail for confirmation of substances belong to A group, a minimum of four IPs are needed, while for substances belong to B group, a minimum of three.[99]

For years, the applied analytical methods mainly focused on the extraction and determination of a single class of analyte, which apparently was not time- and cost-efficient. When food safety issues are concerned, designing methods that allows increased number of samples tested per day and multiresidue analysis are of high importance.

In recent years, analytical instrumentation has been significantly advanced. In particular, fast scanning and sensitive high resolution mass spectrometry (HRMR) instruments (resolution ≥20,000 FWHM, full width at half maximum), for example, (Q)TOF-Ms (Quadrupole Time of Flight Mass Spectrometer), FT (Fourier-transform) ion cyclotron resonance-Ms, and FT Orbitrap-Ms combined with recent developments in chromatographic systems like ultra-high-performance liquid chromatography and columns allow the introduction of new analytical methods. Therefore the residue testing laboratories can now apply considerable faster, multiresidue and multiclass screening and confirmatory methods that include simplified sample preparation procedures, which offer advantages such as simplicity, high sample throughput, and reduced costs. These methodologies, also called dilute-and-shoot or QuEChERS which stands for quick, easy, cheap, effective, rugged, and safe, are being used for some time now; however, the criteria for performance assessment has not been established yet.

Due to the progress in the analytical methodologies, more detailed criteria should be introduced than those documented in 2002/657/EC in order to define clearly the requirements for a reliable confirmation with LC-HRMS technologies.[100] Therefore it has been proposed that the performance and validation criteria should be revised on a regular basis, for example, every 5 years.[101]

9.3 Research gaps and future directions

Aquaculture has become an increasingly important industry for production of finfish, crustaceans, and shellfish for human consumption. Relative to the livestock sector, aquaculture is, however, highly diverse involving the farming of some hundred species. The big diversity of farmed aquaculture species translates into a greater number of pathogens, which may cause disease. The use of antimicrobials in aquaculture to confront disease outbreaks, even as a last resort, is inevitable and may result in deposition of residues in edible portions of aquaculture products. Registered antibacterials at concentrations above legal limits and illegal presence of banned compounds may pose an unacceptable risk to public health. To minimize the risk, strict procedures should be enforced locally, including prudent and responsible use of antimicrobials under veterinary supervision, provided that prevention has failed and proper diagnostic management was undertaken. Optimization of treatment regimens using modern pharmacokinetic data is advised to reduce total antibacterial use and enhance efficacy, safety, and risk of selecting resistant organisms.

Several preventive strategies, including genetic selection, dietary manipulation, functional diets, vaccination, probiotics, immune-stimulants, and phage therapy, should be applied when possible to reduce therapeutic use. Biosecurity measures and high level of husbandry practices at the farm level must also be mandatory to eliminate disease outbreaks. Alternative strategies and preventive compounds mentioned above are gaining increasing interest because of their safe status, ease of application, lack of authorization in most cases, and wide acceptance. Although the application of these alternatives to aquaculture medicine is very promising mainly at small scale, further clinical studies are needed to gain more insight about their mechanisms of actions and to evaluate their impact on the environment and host welfare. Vaccination covers only a small list of aquaculture pathogens and thus new research effort should be devoted to this direction.

At the farm level, record keeping of antimicrobial use is still poor in most top producing countries, thus limiting the ability to establish a comprehensive antimicrobial database for aquaculture at regional or country level. Such databases are vital to identify local sources in which antimicrobials are improperly used and to direct the necessary management efforts. Specific guidelines on prudent antibacterial use should be developed and communicated. Risk assessment approaches for preventing diseases and spread of antibacterial resistance in farming sites need to be established. Identifying the potential link between antimicrobial use in aquaculture and antimicrobial resistance in the terrestrial environment is also of critical importance for both environments. Also, at regional level, governments should ensure the appropriate production and sale of antimicrobials in a controlled manner. Government controls on drug use and compliance with both legislation and agreed codes of practice are important factors if appropriate antimicrobial use is to be permitted. However, the lack of strict regulations or law enforcement in many low income, top-aquaculture-producing countries has induced reductions of drug residues in seafood exported to high-income countries because of the latter's governmental controls. Even though this is an important mechanism to control drug use, it only applies to internationally traded products and occasionally leaves production directed for domestic consumption largely unregulated. Communication and education strategies that emphasize the multibeneficial aspect of prudent drug use by all stakeholders, but with main emphasis on farmers, should be established. Eventually, a thorough global mapping of drug use in aquaculture enterprises would be the ideal accomplishment for controlling safety in and from aquatic farmed products.

To avoid the necessity of importing high volumes of seafood with unknown or questionable safety, new research should be directed toward fast grower species and close farming systems, in order to increase local aquaculture production in conditions where environmental and chemical control is well regulated. This increased local aquaculture production will not only reduce dependence on imports and thereby minimize the risk of consuming unsafe products, it would also allow government inspection resources to be more focused at those areas of higher risk to protect public health and allow increased surveillance programs, with improvements in sampling methodology, to be applied. Ensuring the same high levels of food safety in imported aquaculture products compared to those domestically produced is paramount for consumer confidence, public health, and efficient and effective use of governmental resources.

References

1. FAO. *The State of World Fisheries and Aquaculture 2018 – Meeting the Sustainable Development Goals*. Rome: FAO; 2018.
2. FEAP. *Annual Report Federation of European Aquaculture Producers*; 2017.
3. Van Boeckel TP, Brower C, Gilbert M, et al. Global trends in antimicrobial use in food animals. *Proc Natl Acad Sci U S A*. 2015;112:5649–5654.
4. Okocha RC, Olatoye IO, Adedeji OB. Food safety impacts of antimicrobial use and their residues in aquaculture. *Public Health Rev*. 2018;39:21.
5. Rigos G, Troisi GM. Antibacterial agents in Mediterranean Finfish farming: a synopsis of drug pharmacokinetics in important Euryhaline fish species and possible environmental implications. *Rev Fish Biol Fish*. 2005;15:53–73.
6. Shinn A, Pratoomyot J, Bron J, Paladini J, Brooker E, Brooker A. Economic impacts of aquatic parasites on global finfish production. Glob Aquac Advocate. 2015: 58–61.
7. World Bank. *World Bank Reducing Disease Risk in Aquaculture*. Washington DC: World Bank; 2014.
8. Abolofia J, Asche F, Wilen J. The cost of lice: quantifying the impacts of parasitic sea lice on farmed salmon. *Mar Resour Econ*. 2017;32.
9. Figueroa J, Cárcamo J, Yañez A, et al. Addressing viral and bacterial threats to salmon farming in Chile: historical contexts and perspectives for management and control. *Rev Aquac*. 2019;11: 299–324.
10. Shinn A, Pratoomyot J, Bron J, Paladini G, Brooker E, Brooker A. Economic costs of protistan and metazoan parasites to global mariculture. *Parasitology*. 2015;142:196–270.
11. Bagum N, Monir M, Khan MH. Present status of fish diseases and economic losses due to incidence of disease in rural freshwater aquaculture of Bangladesh. *J Innov Dev Strategy*. 2013; 7:48–53.
12. Li X, Li J, Wang Y, et al. Aquaculture industry in China: current state, challenges, and outlook. *Rev Fish Sci*. 2011;19:187–200.
13. Schnick R. Use of chemicals in fish management and fish culture. In: Smith D, Gingerich W, Beconi-Barker M, eds. *Xenobiotics in Fish*. Kluwer/Plenum Press; 1999:1–14.
14. Norwegian Veterinary Institute (NVI). *Use of Antibiotics in Norwegian Aquaculture*. Report 22. Oslo: Norwegian Veterinary Institute; 2016.
15. Hannisdal R, Nøstbakken OJ, Hove H, Madsen L, Horsberg TE, Lunestad BT. Anti-sea lice agents in Norwegian aquaculture; surveillance, treatment trends and possible implications for food safety. *Aquaculture*. 2020;521:735044.
16. Rico A, Phu TM, Satapornvanit K, et al. Use of veterinary medicines, feed additives and probiotics in four major internationally traded aquaculture species farmed in Asia. *Aquaculture*. 2013; 412–413:231–243.
17. EMEA. *Oxytetracycline, Tetracycline, Chlortetracycline*. Summary Report (3). EMEA/MRL/023/95. Committee for Veterinary Medicinal Products/The European Agency for the Evaluation of Medicinal Products; 1995.
18. EMEA. *Flumequine (Extension to All Food Producing Species)*. Summary Report (4). EMEA/MRL/823/02-FINAL. Committee for Veterinary Medicinal Products/The European Agency for the Evaluation of Medicinal Products; 2002.

19. EMEA. *Oxolinic Acid (Extension to All Food Producing Species).* EMEA/MRL/41090/2005-FINAL. Summary Report (5). Committee for Veterinary Medicinal Products/The European Agency for the Evaluation of Medicinal Products; 2005.
20. EMEA. *Sulphonamides.* Summary Report (2). EMEA/MRL/026/95. Committee for Veterinary Medicinal Products/The European Agency for the Evaluation of Medicinal Products; 1995.
21. EMEA. *Trimethoprim.* Summary Report (2). EMEA/MRL/255/97-FINAL. Committee for Veterinary Medicinal Products/The European Agency for the Evaluation of Medicinal Products; 1997.
22. EMEA. *Penicillins.* Summary Report. EMEA/MRL/Revision 1. Committee for Veterinary Medicinal Products/The European Agency for the Evaluation of Medicinal Products; 2008.
23. EMEA. *Florfenicol (Extension to All Food Producing Species).* Summary Report (6). EMEA/MRL/822/02-FINAL. Committee for Veterinary Medicinal Products/The European Agency for the Evaluation of Medicinal Products; 2002.
24. EMEA. *Emamectin.* Summary Report (1). EMEA/MRL/546/99-FINAL. Committee for Veterinary Medicinal Products, The European Agency for the Evaluation of Medicinal Products Veterinary Medicines Evaluation Unit; January 1999.
25. EMEA. *Azamethiphos.* Summary Report (2). EMEA/MRL/527/98-FINAL. Committee for Veterinary Medicinal Products, The European Agency for the Evaluation of Medicinal Products, Veterinary Medicines Evaluation Unit; January 1999.
26. EMEA. *Cypermethrin (Extrapolation to All Ruminants).* Summary Report (4). EMEA/MRL/890/03-FINAL. Committee for Veterinary Medicinal Products, European Medicines Agency Veterinary Medicines and Inspections Unit; June 2004.
27. EMEA. *Deltamethrin (Extrapolation to All Ruminants).* Summary Report (4). EMEA/MRL/893/03-FINAL. Committee for Veterinary Medicinal Products, European Medicines Agency Veterinary Medicines and Inspections Unit; June 2004.
28. European Medicines Agency (EMA) *Diflubenzuron. Salmonidae.* MRL Summary Opinion. EMA/CVMP/259781/2015. Committee for Medicinal Products for Veterinary Use, EMA; May 8, 2015.
29. EMEA. *Teflubenzuron.* Summary Report (1). EMEA/MRL/221/97-FINAL. Committee for Veterinary Medicinal Products, The European Agency for the Evaluation of Medicinal Products Veterinary Medicines Evaluation Unit; May 1997.
30. Vishnuraj MR, Kandeepan G, Rao KH, Chand S, Kumbhar V. Occurrence, public health hazards and detection methods of antibiotic residues in foods of animal origin: a comprehensive review. *Cogent Food Agric.* 2016;2(1):1235458.
31. Aarestrup F. Get pigs off antibiotics. *Nature.* 2012;486(7404): 465–466.
32. Van Boeckel TP, Glennon EE, Chen D, et al. Reducing antimicrobial use in food animals. *Science.* 2017;357(6358):1350–1352.
33. FDA. *Antimicrobials sold or distributed for use in food-producing animals*; 2019.
34. EMA. *European Surveillance of Veterinary Antimicrobial Consumption. Sales of Veterinary Antimicrobial Agents in 31 European Countries in 2017. Trends from 2010 to 2017.* Ninth ESVAC Report. (EMA/294674/2019); 2019.
35. Boison JO, Turnipseed SB. A review of aquaculture practices and their impacts on chemical food safety from a regulatory perspective. *J AOAC Int.* 2015;98(3):541–549.
36. Henriksson PJ, Rico A, Troell M, et al. Unpacking factors influencing antimicrobial use in global aquaculture and their implication for management: a review from a systems perspective. *Sustain Sci.* 2018;13(4):1105–1120.
37. Savini D, Occhipinti–Ambrogi A, Marchini A, et al. The top 27 animal alien species introduced into Europe for aquaculture and related activities. *J Appl Ichthyol.* 2010;26:1–7.
38. Peeler EJ, Oidtmann BC, Midtlyng PJ, Miossec L, Gozlan RE. Non-native aquatic animals introductions have driven disease emergence in Europe. *Biol Invasions.* 2011;13:1291–1303.
39. Codex Alimentarius. *Maximum Residue Limits (MRLs) and Risk Management Recommendations (RMRs) for Residues of Veterinary Drugs in Food.* CAC/MRL 2-2018; 2018.
40. EC. European Parliament and Council Directive 2001/82/EC, of 6 November 2001. Official Journal of the European Communities, L 311; 2001: 67–128.
41. EC. Commission Directive 2009/9/EC, of 10 February 2009. Official Journal of the European Union, L 44; 2009: 10–61.
42. EC. European Parliament and Council Regulation (EC) 470/2009, of the 6 May 2009. Official Journal of the European Union, L 152; 2009: 11–22.
43. EC. European Parliament and of the Council Regulation (EC) No. 726/2004, of 31 March 2004. Official Journal of the European Union, L 50; 2004: 1–32.
44. EEC. Council Regulation 2377/90 of 26 June 1990. Official Journal of the European Communities, L 224; 1990: 1–8.
45. EC. Commission Regulation (EU) 37/2010, of 22 December 2009. Official Journal of the European Union, L 15; 2009: 1–72.
46. CFR. US Food and Drug Administration Code of Federal Regulation Title 21. <https://www.accessdata.fda.gov/scripts/cdrh/cfdocs/cfCFR/CFRSearch.cfm>; 2019.
47. Health Canada. List of banned drugs. <https://www.canada.ca/en/health-canada/services/drugs-health-products/veterinary-drugs/list-banned-drugs.html>; 2005.
48. Health Canada. List of maximum residue limits (MRLs) for veterinary drugs in foods. <https://www.canada.ca/en/health-canada/services/drugs-health-products/veterinary-drugs/maximum-residue-limits-mrls/list-maximum-residue-limits-mrls-veterinary-drugs-foods.html>; 2017.
49. U.S. Department of Agriculture (USDA). *China Publishes Maximum Residue Limits for Veterinary Drugs in Food*; 2019.
50. U.S. Department of Agriculture (USDA). *List of Veterinary Drugs Banned for Use for Food Animals in People's Republic of China*; 2011.
51. Subasinghe R., Alderman D. *Basic Overview of the Regulatory Procedures for Authorisation of Veterinary Medicines with Emphasis on Residues in Food Animal Species.* Unpublished Document. FAO Fishery Department; 2002.
52. FDA. *General Principles for Evaluating the Human Food Safety of New Animal Drugs Used in Food-Producing Animals*; 2018.
53. European Medicines Agency (EMA). *Guideline on Determination of Withdrawal Periods for Edible Tissues.* EMA/CVMP/SWP/735325/2012. Committee for Medicinal Products for Veterinary Use, EMA; September 13, 2018.
54. Jensen GL, Martin RE. The impacts of federal Food Safety Initiatives on the aquaculture producer-processor HACCP juncture. In *Proceedings of the Twenty-First Annual Meeting of the Seafood Science and Technology Society of The Americas Held Jointly with*

the Atlantic States Fisheries Technology Society. Florida Sea Grant College Program. Gainesville, FL; 1997.

55. Codex Alimentarius. *Hazard Analysis and Critical Control Point (HACCP) System and Guidelines for Its Application.* Annex to CAC/RCP 1-1969, Rev. 3; 1997.
56. dos Santos CAL. Hazard analysis critical control point and aquaculture. In: Jahnke ML, Garrett ES, Reilly A, Martin RE, Cole E, eds. *Public, Animal and Environmental Health Issues*. New York: Wiley Interscience; 2002:103–119.
57. World Health Organization, & Joint FAO/NACA/WHO Study Group on Food Safety Issues Associated with Products from Aquaculture. *Food Safety Issues Associated with Products from Aquaculture: Report of a Joint FAO/NACA/WHO Study Group* (vol. 883). World Health Organization; 1999.
58. EC. Regulation (EC) No 852/2004 of the European Parliament and of the Council of 29 April 2004 on the Hygiene of Foodstuffs. Official Journal of European Union. 2004; 1–54.
59. Council Directive 91/493/EEC of 22 July 1991 Laying Down the Health Conditions for the Production and the Placing on the market of fishery products. Official Journal L, 268(24/09), 0015-0034; 1991.
60. Council Directive 93/43/EEC of 14 June 1993 on the hygiene of foodstuffs. Official Journal of the European Communities. OJ L 36, 175.
61. Feiyang M, Shixin X, Zhaoxin T, Zekun L, Lu Z. Use of antimicrobials in food animals and impact of transmission of antimicrobial resistance on humans, Bio. health. 2021;3:32–38
62. Cabello F, Godfrey H, Tomova A, et al. Antimicrobial use in aquaculture re-examined: its relevance to antimicrobial resistance and to animal and human health. *Environ Microbiol*. 2013;15:1917–1942.
63. WHO. *Tackling Antibiotic Resistance From a Food Safety Perspective in Europe*. World Health Organization Regional Office for Europe; 2011.
64. Love DC, Fry JP, Cabello F, Good CM, Lunestad BJ. Veterinary drug use in United States net pen Salmon aquaculture: implications for drug use policy. *Aquaculture*. 2020;518:734820.
65. BCSFA. Sustainability Progress Report: Salmon Aquaculture 2016. In BC Salmon Farmers Association, ed.; 2016.
66. Seafood Watch. Atlantic Salmon: Scotland marine net pens. In Monterey Bay Aquarium, ed.; 2017.
67. SERNAPESCA. SERNAPESCA, National Fisheries and Aquaculture Service; 2018.
68. Simonsen G, A Urdahl, A Astrup, K Larsen, F Width-Gran. *Usage of Antimicrobial Agents and Occurrence of Antimicrobial Resistance in Norway*. Tromso, Oslo: Norwegian Veterinary Institute; 2016: 142 pp.
69. EFSA. Technical specifications on harmonised monitoring of antimicrobial resistance in zoonotic and indicator bacteria from food-producing animals and food. *EFSA J*. 2019;17(6):e05709.
70. Ferri M, Ranucci E, Romagnoli P, Giaccone V. Antimicrobial resistance: a global emerging threat to public health systems. *Crit Rev Food Sci Nutr*. 2017;57(13):2857–2876.
71. Morris DJ, Gray AJ, Kay JF, Gettinby G. EU sampling strategies for the detection of veterinary drug residues in aquaculture species: are they working? *Drug Test Anal*. 2012;4(suppl 1):1–9. Available from: https://doi.org/10.1002/dta.1350.
72. FAO and WHO. *Assuring Food Safety and Quality: Guidelines for Strengthening National Food Control Systems*. Rome: FAO and WHO; 2003.
73. Codex Alimentarius. *Principles and Guidelines for National Food Control Systems*. CAC/GL, 82-2013; 2013.
74. Lupin HM. Introduction to the analysis of regulations and texts of interest to safety of fish products from aquaculture. *Cah Options Médit*. 2000;51:23–30.
75. EC. Regulation No 178/2002 of the European Parliament and of the Council of 28 January 2002 laying down the general principles and requirements of food law, establishing the European Food Safety Authority and laying down procedures in matters of food safety. Official Journal of the European Communities, L 31, 2002: 1–24.
76. EC. Regulation No. 854/2004 of the European Parliament and of the Council of 29 April 2004 laying down specific rules for the organization of official controls on products of animal origin intended for human consumption. Official Journal of the European Communities, 226(83); 2004: 25–26.
77. EC. Regulation No. 882/2004 of the European Parliament and of the Council of 29 April 2004 on official controls performed to ensure the verification of compliance with feed and food law, animal health and animal welfare rules. Official Journal of the European Communities, L 191; 2004.
78. Tittlemier SA, Van de Riet J, Burns G, et al. Analysis of veterinary drug residues in fish and shrimp composites collected during the Canadian Total Diet Study, 1993–2004. *Food Addit Contam*. 2007;24:14–20.
79. Yamamoto M, Toda M, Sugita T, Tanaka K, Uneyama C, Morikawa K. Studies on the results of monitoring of veterinary drug residues in food products of animal origin in Japan and other countries. *Kokuritsu Iyakuhin Shokuhin Eisei Kenkyusho Hokoku*. 2009;127:84–92 (In Japanese).
80. Love DC, Rodman S, Neff RA, Nachman KE. Veterinary drug residues in seafood inspected by the European Union, United States, Canada, and Japan from 2000 to 2009. *Environ Sci Technol*. 2011;45:7232–7240.
81. Dayan AD. Allergy to antimicrobial residues in food: assessment of the risk to man. *Vet Microbiol*. 1993;35:213–226.
82. Bakar M, Morshed A, Islam F, Karim R. Screening of chloramphenicol residues in chickens and fish in Chittagong city of Bangladesh. *Bangladesh J Vet Med*. 2014;11:173–175.
83. Mehdizadeh S, Kazerani H, Jamshidi A. Screening of chloramphenicol residues in broiler chickens slaughtered in an industrial poultry abattoir in Mashhad, Iran. *Iran J Vet Sci Technol*. 2010;1:25–32.
84. Disdier A-C, Marette S. The combination of gravity and welfare approaches for evaluating non-tariff measures. *Am J Agric Econ*. 2010;92:713–726.
85. Vass M, Hruska K, Fránek M. Nitrofuran antibiotics: a review on the application, prohibition and residual analysis. *Vet Med*. 2008; 53:469–500.
86. Elvers KT, Wilson VJ, Hammond A, et al. Antibiotic-induced changes in the human gut microbiota for the most commonly prescribed antibiotics in primary care in the UK: a systematic review. *BMJ Open*. 2020;2020(10):e035677. Available from: https://doi.org/10.1136/bmjopen-2019-035677.
87. Kyuchukova R. Antibiotic residues and human health hazard – review. *Bulg J Agric Sci*. 2020;26(3):664–668.
88. Cabello F. Heavy use of prophylactic antibiotics in aquaculture: a growing problem for human and animal health and for the environment. *Environ Microbiol*. 2006;8:1137–1144.

89. Sapkota A, Sapkota AR, Kucharski M, et al. Aquaculture practices and potential human health risks: current knowledge and future priorities. *Environ Int.* 2008;34:1215–1226.
90. Watts J, Schreier H, Lanska L, Hale M. The rising tide of antimicrobial resistance in aquaculture: sources, sinks and solutions. *Mar Drugs.* 2017;15:158.
91. Lupo A, Coyne S, Berendonk T. Origin and evolution of antibiotic resistance: the common mechanisms of emergence and spread in water bodies. *Front Microbiol.* 2012;3:18.
92. Sørum H. Chapter 6 – Antibiotic resistance associated with veterinary drug use in fish farms. In: Lie Ø, ed. *Improving Farmed Fish Quality and Safety*. Woodhead Publishing; 2008:157–182.
93. Chiu T-h, Kao L-Y, Chen M-L. Antibiotic resistance and molecular typing of *Photobacterium damselae* subsp. *damselae*, isolated from seafood. *J Appl Microbiol.* 2012;114:1184–1192.
94. Gauthier DT. Bacterial zoonoses of fishes: a review and appraisal of evidence for linkages between fish and human infections. *Vet J.* 2015;203:27–35.
95. Ryu S-H, Park S-G, Choi S-M, et al. Antimicrobial resistance and resistance genes in Escherichia coli strains isolated from commercial fish and seafood. *Int J Food Microbiol.* 2012;152:14–18.
96. Han QF, Zhao S, Zhang XR, Wang XL, Song C, Wang SG. Distribution, combined pollution and risk assessment of antibiotics in typical marine aquaculture farms surrounding the Yellow Sea, North China. *Environ Int.* 2020;138:105551.
97. Smith M. Antimicrobial use in shrimp farming in Ecuador and emerging multi-resistance during the cholera epidemic of 1991: A re-examination of the data, *Aqua.* 2007;271:1–7.
98. Cabello F, Godfrey H, Buschmann AH, Dölz HJ. Aquaculture as yet another environmental gateway to the development and globalisation of antimicrobial resistance. *Lancet Infect Dis.* 2016;16:e127–e133.
99. EC. Commission Decision 2002/657/EC of 12 August 2002 implementing Council Directive 96/23/EC concerning the performance of analytical methods and the interpretation of results. Official Journal of the European Union, L 221; 2002: 8–35.
100. Marazuela MD. *Determination of veterinary drug residues in foods by liquid chromatography-mass spectrometry: basic and cutting-edge applications. Liquid Chromatography.* Elsevier; 2017:539–570.
101. Vanhaecke T, Pauwels M, Vinken M, Ceelen L, Rogiers V. Towards an integrated in vitro strategy for repeated dose toxicity testing. *Arch. of tox.* 2011;84:365–6. https://doi.org/10.1007/s00204-011-0711-4.

Section IV

Changes in the chemical composition of food throughout the various stages of the food chain: manufacture, packaging and distribution

Chapter 10

Manufacturing and distribution: the role of good manufacturing practice

Michael E. Knowles
Kavakia-Rachi, Veria, Greece

Abstract
This chapter discusses the use of good manufacturing practice (GMP) in the production of safe food through changes in chemical composition in the manufacturing and distribution processes. To achieve this the use of hazard analysis and preventative controls are essential which require a wide variety of data sources covering ingredients that may contain agrochemical residues, veterinary drug residues, environmental contaminants, allergens, and cross-contamination additives and processing aids, flavors, heat-produced contaminants and addition of chemicals for food crime and fraud. In-factory potential hazards from equipment, cleaning and sanitizing agents, process water together with physical hazards from ingredients and workers, and the need for automatic foreign body detection and prevention. The numerous data sources within this book are referenced at progressive stages of manufacture and are supplemented by recent complementary publications. The use of "big data" and AI/ML together with "blockchain" methodologies as developing technologies to aid hazard analysis and preventative controls together with the need to need to consider emerging chemical risks from existing and new sources are discussed. Finally, the broad impact of climate change on sources of chemical contamination and the concomitant impact on hazard analysis and risk assessment are discussed.

Keywords: GMP; hazard analysis; sources of chemicals; new technologies; AI/ML; blockchain; climate change; food safety and integrity

10.1 Introduction

Good manufacturing practice (GMP) has two complementary and mutually interdependent components: the manufacturing operations and the quality control/quality assurance (also known as "food control") systems. Both of these components must be well designed and effectively implemented and the same must apply to their respective managements. A full explanation of what this means is not just management competence but also involves up to date knowledge of current and emerging quality issues, food safety hazards, and best practices in terms of food science and technology relating to the ingredients, processes, packaging, and products concerned, including awareness and understanding of current regulatory controls. For a full explanation of these basic requirements of GMP see as an example the guidelines produced by the UK Institute of Food Science & Technology (IFST), namely "Food & Drink—Good Manufacturing Practice: A Guide to its Responsible Management"[1] and the US FDA Food Safety Modernisation Act (FSMA)—Final Rule For Preventative Controls For Human Food.[2] The latter is an example of a national Regulation that contains specific and explicit actions within GMP that must be implemented to ensure the production of safe food which complies with national regulations.

Both of these GMP Guidance documents will be used in this chapter to illustrate the specific requirements needed to ensure the safe management and control of changes to the chemical composition of the finished foodstuff as delivered to the consumer.

Therefore the manufacture and production of food in its final or near-final state above for sale to the consumer, whether it be "pre- or postfarm gate in small or large food businesses," should, and in some jurisdictions is legally required, to follow these comprehensive GMP Guidelines, which collectively ensure to the fullest extent possible, it's safety, integrity, quality, and compliance with all relevant local regulations. However, the theme of this chapter is "the change in the chemical composition of food" (food being entirely chemical in its composition at all stages of its production[3]) during manufacture, distribution, and storage either through deliberate addition of permitted substances for specific technological and/or organoleptic

Present Knowledge in Food Safety. DOI: https://doi.org/10.1016/B978-0-12-819470-6.00049-4

reasons or from its ingredients or adventitiously from sources within the manufacturing facility or during distribution.

Both the above Guidance Documents require a food business to have a "food safety culture" or "food safety plan" which includes "hazard analysis and risk-based preventative controls" or "hazard analysis critical control points (HACCP)" to be identified and implemented to ensure that any changes in the chemical composition do not pose an unacceptable health risk. HACCP is of course used to control any microbiological risks during manufacture.

As they are central to the theme of this chapter they will be discussed in detail, along with the sources of information necessary for effective HACCP, in the following sections of the chapter. It should also be understood that all stakeholders in the food chain have a responsibility to undertake their hazard analyses and controls and that the food manufacturer is made aware of any contamination, including permitted residues, in the chemical composition of the ingredient being supplied is within regulatory and/or acceptable safe levels in accompanying documentation.

10.2 Hazard analysis and critical control points and preventive controls

Whilst HACCP is generally thought of in terms of microbiological hazards it is equally applicable to all other hazards including chemical (including radiological hazards) and physical hazards, as will be discussed in detail in this chapter.

It is mandatory in some jurisdictions to "conduct a hazard analysis and to identify critical control points (CCPs) of known or reasonably foreseeable chemical hazards" and even if not a regulatory requirement, compliance with GMP requires that it be done. Not only is GMP essential to ensure the safety of the manufactured food but it also helps provide a reasonable defense in cases of accidents and food recalls.

It is also necessary to develop "recall plans" in case of accidents or other issues which demand a recall of products from the market to protect public health.

The following is based on the FDA GMP requirements[2] and illustrates the steps needed to be taken into consideration:

1. *Requirement for hazard analysis.*
   a. You must conduct a hazard analysis to identify and evaluate, based on experience, illness data, scientific reports, and other information,(*particularly information from suppliers—author's note)* known or reasonably foreseeable hazards for each type of food manufactured, processed, packed, or held at your facility to determine whether there are any hazards requiring a preventive control.
   b. The hazard analysis must be written regardless of its outcome.
2. *Hazard identification.* The hazard identification must consider:
   a. Known or reasonably foreseeable hazards that include:
      i. Biological hazards, including microbiological hazards such as parasites, environmental pathogens, and other pathogens; (*these will not be discussed in this chapter—author's note*)
      ii. Chemical hazards, including radiological hazards, substances such as pesticide and drug residues, natural toxins, decomposition, unapproved food or color additives, and food allergens; and
      iii. Physical hazards (such as stones, glass, and metal fragments); and
   b. Known or reasonably foreseeable hazards that may be present in the food for any of the following reasons:
      i. The hazard occurs naturally;
      ii. The hazard may be unintentionally introduced; or
      iii. The hazard may be intentionally introduced for purposes of economic gain. (e.g., *fraud —author's note*)
3. *Hazard evaluation.*
   a. The hazard analysis must include:
      i. An evaluation of the hazards identified in paragraph (b) of this section to assess the severity of the illness or injury if the hazard were to occur and the probability that the hazard will occur in the absence of preventive controls.
      ii. The hazard evaluation required by paragraph (c)(1)(i) of this section must include an evaluation of environmental pathogens whenever a ready-to-eat food is exposed to the environment before packaging and the packaged food does not receive a treatment or otherwise include a control measure (such as a formulation lethal to the pathogen) that would significantly minimize the pathogen.
   b. The hazard evaluation must consider the effect of the following on the safety of the finished food for the intended consumer:
      i. The formulation of the food;
      ii. The condition, function, and design of the facility and equipment;
      iii. Raw materials and other ingredients;
      iv. Transportation practices;
      v. Manufacturing/processing procedures;
      vi. Packaging activities and labeling activities;
      vii. Storage and distribution;
      viii. Intended or reasonably foreseeable use;
      ix. Sanitation, including employee hygiene; and

x. Any other relevant factors, such as the temporal (e.g., weather-related) nature of some hazards (e.g., levels of some natural toxins).

10.3 Preventive controls and recall plans

1. You must identify and implement:
   a. Preventive controls to provide assurances that any hazards requiring a preventive control will be significantly minimized or prevented and the food manufactured, processed, packed, or held by your facility will not be adulterated under section 402 of the Federal Food, Drug, and Cosmetic Act or misbranded under section 403(w) of the Federal Food, Drug, and Cosmetic Act.
   b. Preventive controls required by paragraph (a)(1) of this section include:
      i. Controls at CCPs, if there are any CCPs; and
      ii. Controls, other than those at CCPs, are also appropriate for food safety.
2. Preventive controls must be written.
3. Preventive controls include, as appropriate to the facility and the food:
   a. *Process controls.* Process controls include procedures, practices, and processes to ensure the control of parameters during operations such as heat processing, acidifying, irradiating, and refrigerating foods. Process controls must include, as appropriate to the nature of the applicable control and its role in the facility's food safety system:
      i. Parameters associated with the control of the hazard; and
      ii. The maximum or minimum value, or combination of values, to which any biological, chemical or physical parameter must be controlled to significantly minimize or prevent a hazard requiring a process control.
   b. *Food allergen controls.* Food allergen controls include procedures, practices, and processes to control food allergens. Food allergen controls must include those procedures, practices, and processes employed for:
      i. Ensuring protection of food from allergen cross-contact, including during storage, handling, and use; and
      ii. Labeling the finished food, including ensuring that the finished food is not misbranded under section 403(w) of the Federal Food, Drug, and Cosmetic Act.
   c. *Sanitation controls.* Sanitation controls include procedures, practices, and processes to ensure that the facility is maintained in a sanitary condition adequate to significantly minimize or prevent hazards such as environmental pathogens, biological hazards due to employee handling, and food allergen hazards. Sanitation controls must include, as appropriate to the facility and the food, procedures, practices, and processes for the:
      i. Cleanliness of food-contact surfaces, including food-contact surfaces of utensils and equipment;
      ii. Prevention of allergen cross-contact and cross-contamination from unsanitary objects and from personnel to food, food packaging material, and other food-contact surfaces and from raw product to processed product.
   d. *Supply-chain controls.* Supply-chain controls include the supply-chain program as required by subpart G of this part.
   e. *Recall plan.* Recall plan as required by § 117.139.
   f. *Other controls.* Preventive controls include any other procedures, practices, and processes necessary to satisfy the requirements of paragraph (a) of this section. Examples of other controls include hygiene training and other current GMP.

10.4 Potential sources of chemical hazards during manufacture and distribution*

1. Ingredients

   'Provenance and authenticity is an integral part of the IFST GMP Guidelines and essential for hazard analysis and may be required as part of the regulatory and additional information which must be included on labels and in contractual agreements with suppliers. External standards, such as those developed by GFSI and discussed in Chapter 70 also provide additional information and reassurance in this context.

   The ingredient–related chemical hazards which may need to be considered, depending on information from the above sources and the scientific literature, are:

   1. Plants before and after harvest: intrinsic natural toxicants in plants, herbs, and spices, are described in Chapter 1 and may give rise to concern, such as toxic proteins, for example, lectins, glycoalkaloids, quinolizidine alkaloids, cyanogenic glycosides, and lathyrogens, fava pyrimidine glycosides furocoumarins, glucosinolates, alkenylbenzenes, pyrrolizidine alkaloids and also guides exposure and risk assessment that requires appropriate adjustment for the formula and likely consumption of the manufactured foodstuff. In addition, information is also presented on accidental or erroneous switching of varieties of plants that have given rise to adverse health effects due to plant toxicants in the wrong plant variety.

Finally, the deliberate use of plants that contain pharmacologically –active substances, such as tropane and opium alkaloids and THC particularly in herbal preparations needs to be monitored. Further information on natural toxicants has been developed and published by EFSA.[4]

2. Environmental contamination from soil, water, and air, such as heavy metals, for example, lead, cadmium, pesticides phthalates, PCBs, and dioxins, related to the geographical origins of the plant material are described in Chapter 2. The effects of processing on their concentration in the final food also require hazard analysis and possible preventative actions. Further, the impact which climate change will have on the occurrence and diversity of, for example, industrial chemicals in water, is an emerging phenomenon needing to be taken into account and is discussed in Chapters 21 and 72.

   Pesticide residues which include insecticides, herbicides, and fumigants are common residues that may exceed their MRLs and hence be of particular risk to public health, as described in Chapter 3. Compliance with local regulations or those of the country to which the final food is to be marketed must be checked.

   All the above are discussed in detail in Section I of this Book with appropriate references as an additional in-depth resource.

   In some situations, radiological hazards may be incorporated into plants through local water which is high in natural radionuclides, such as radium-226 and—228 and uranium. In addition, ingredients that are sourced from areas that have been subject to atmospheric contamination from a nuclear accident, such as Chernobyl (Ukraine) or Fukushima (Japan) where cesium-137 levels may be above the usual background levels should be checked and each shipment monitored by the supplier with appropriate documentation.

3. Ingredients derived from meat and milk: residues from veterinary drug usage, especially antimicrobial drug residues from feed or direct treatment of the animals is described in Section II. The use of these substances is controlled by regulation and compliance must be indicated by the supplier on each shipment.

4. Ingredients from fish or shellfish: the uptake of pollutants from the aqueous environment in which they grow together with residues from veterinary drugs used in aquaculture are discussed in Section III. Again veterinary residues are subject to regulatory limits and conformity must be shown in suppler documentation. Similarly, some of the common contaminants from seawater are regulated, such as heavy metals and compliance must be indicated by suppliers. New contaminants, such as micro- and nanoplastics are reviewed in Chapter 40—see also paragraph 5 below.

5. Allergens: The presence of a substance belonging to the main group of common allergens—crustacea (and mollusks); egg; fish; milk (dairy); peanuts; tree nuts (e.g., brazil, almonds, cashews, walnuts, pecans, hazelnuts); soy; wheat – must be clearly labeled on the final product. Certain other substances, for example, lactose, sulfite, and some food colors, can cause intolerant reactions in some consumers and similarly, their presence must be indicated on the final food label.[1,2] Chapter 48 discusses this issue in detail.

6. Direct addition: the use of all food additives and processing aids, as required by the formula of the foodstuff being manufactured, must be in complete compliance with local regulations or those of the country to which it is destined for sale. Similarly, for the addition of flavorings, their addition must comply with the regulations of the country of sale including the levels of any "biologically active substance" present in the flavoring extract. These are discussed in Chapters 11 and 12 respectively.

2. Cross-contamination

   This is a general requirement of all food manufacturing processes to ensure integrity, safety, and legal compliance of the final product but it is of particular importance regarding food allergens. Inadvertent contamination of food by an allergen that is not a declared component, ie. not labeled, of that final food can present a potentially lethal hazard to susceptible consumers and therefore all due precautions must be taken to prevent this from happening during manufacture.[1,2] The FDA GMP Guidance[2] provides examples of how cross-contamination can occur:

"Failure to schedule the production of two different products appropriately, resulting in an allergen-containing product contaminating a product without food allergens.

Failure to adequately clean between two different formulations of a product that do and do not contain allergens, results in an allergen-containing product contaminating a product without the allergen.

Failure to store allergen-containing ingredients separately from ingredients that do not contain allergens, where leakage of allergen-containing materials results in contamination of the non-allergen-containing product.

Failure to handle powdered allergens in a way that prevents particles from blowing onto foods or food contact surfaces for foods that do not contain that allergen."

Of course, all ingredients which are known to cause allergenic or intolerance reactions must be labeled following regulations extant in the country of sale, and of course, the correct labeled packaging must be used for the correct food.

3. Thermal processing contaminants

   Thermal processing may also generate potential chemical hazards such as polycyclic hydrocarbons (PAH) during smoking of foods, furans, acrylamide, nitrosamines, monochloropropane diols (MCPDs) heterocyclic amines, and urethanes and these are discussed in Chapter 13; hazard analysis and if necessary preventative controls must be undertaken for such thermally produced compounds some of which are putative human carcinogens.

4. Addition of chemicals for fraudulent purposes (for economic gain)

   Fraudulent Adulteration unfortunately is not a rare event and could be "food fraud" or "food crime"[1]: recent examples are the substitution of horsemeat for beef in Europe which although not itself a chemical hazard, evaluations were carried out to determine if any equine veterinary drug residues constituted a public health risk. Careful hazard analysis determined they did not pose such a risk. Others are melamine in milk, lead chromate in turmeric lead oxide in paprika, and Sudan 1 in chili powder. In such cases, the hazard analysis should also consider the country of origin.[2] Chapters 16 and 23 deal with this illegal practice for economic gain in more detail and Chapter 70, the role GFSI plays to minimize and/or identify its occurrence.

5. Process water

   Water used in food manufacturing facilities and which comes into direct or indirect contact with food during production must comply with potable water regulations. Water that is recycled from other uses in the facility, in general, should not be used in situations where it can become incorporated into the foodstuff, for example, if used for cleaning materials that come into contact with food or its components during manufacture. See also paragraph 1a) above regarding naturally occurring radionuclides in water.

   More recently the presence of micro- and nanoplastic particles should be determined; see Chapter 40.

6. Facility-related chemicals and physical hazards

   Contact with the surfaces of food equipment can lead to the transfer of material to the food, such as heavy metals or residues of food from a previous batch if inadequate cleaning has not taken place.

   Contamination by the ingredients of cleaning and sanitation agents is a possibility and quality assurance and food control systems must be in place as a fundamentals basis for GMP.

   Storage of ingredients and semifinished products in a factory may require the use of fumigants and/or rodenticides and it's, therefore essential to ensure that any residues present are within acceptable limits.

   Although physical hazards do not strictly fall within the scope of "chemical changes" being discussed in this chapter they also fall within the scope of this paragraph and are of course "chemical" and fall within GMP. Metal fragments can break off during operations and be deposited in the food as can glass fragments. Both are common occurrences as are buttons and jewelry from workers. Appropriate automatic foreign body detectors are recommended but none can detect all such foreign bodies so the emphasis must be on the prevention of such occurrences.

7. Packaging and distribution

   Almost all products of food manufacturers have to be packaged for distribution and therefore the potential for interaction of the food with the packaging material with consequent contamination is a possibility. Examples have been the transfer of heavy metals from bulk tanks (and manufacturing equipment) or cans for domestic use, for example, through failures in the can coating application. More commonly the transfer of chemicals from plastics, including from labels and can lacquers, to foods has been the subject of much research and regulation, and Chapter 14 describes this in detail. The concerns about plastic waste have led to the development of various recycling methods for plastic beverage bottles and concomitant risks are addressed in chapter 15. Alongside this refilling systems for plastic beverage bottles have been used, which have an additional safety concern, for example, have they been used for storing any nonfood items, such as fabric softener? Various types of detectors are used to identify marker chemicals for misuse and again this is discussed in the second part of chapter 15.

8. Summary of actions required under GMP for effective control of chemical hazards

   Many of the chemicals in the above categories are subject to statutory limits either in the ingredients used in the formulation of the final food or in the food itself and it's the responsibility of management[1,2] to ensure that appropriate food control procedures are in place to check regulatory compliance at CCPs. However many environmental contaminants are not regulated and therefore it is incumbent upon the manufacturer in consultation with suppliers, as mentioned earlier, to ascertain if any such contamination could have occurred as part of the general information provided by suppliers on ingredient identification and provenance[4] and composition concerning regulated substances. The management should ensure adequate audit procedures are in place for both suppliers and the final product.[5]

It is therefore apparent that to fulfill the basic requirements of hazard analysis and preventive control, information on the chemical composition of ingredients is required be it regulated, natural or environmental. This will certainly require the cooperation of suppliers and traceability of ingredients to their source to ascertain likely contaminants. Further, the likelihood of process – especially heat-generated–contaminants should be known or predictable and facility/equipment contamination identified as part of GMP.

10.5 Research gaps and future directions

The information in the cited Chapters in this Book and their references provide a substantial resource for use in identifying potential sources of the deliberate and adventitious occurrence of chemicals in food raw materials and manufactured food for which subsequent hazard analysis must be undertaken as part of GMP. In addition, the European Food Safety Authority (EFSA) has published a review of chemicals in food, as previously mentioned. EFSA has also initiated annual requests to the EU Member States to submit information on continuous collection of chemical contaminants occurrence data in food and feed.[5] As an example the list of chemicals requested in 2021 is:

'Process contaminants

- Furan, 2-methylfuran, 3-methylfuran, 2,5-dimethylfuran, 2-ethylfuran and 2-pentyfuran
- Acrylamide
- PAHs
- 3-MCPD, 3-MCPD esters, 2-MCPD esters, and glycidyl esters
- Ethyl Carbamate.

Organic contaminants

- Dioxins and PCBs
- Non-dioxin-like PCBs
- Brominated Flame Retardants
- PFAS
- Chlorinated Paraffins
- Melamine and analogs
- Benzene
- Perchlorate.

Inorganic

- Cadmium
- Lead
- Arsenic (inorganic and total)
- Mercury (methyl mercury and total mercury)
- Fluorine in feed
- Nitrates and Nitrites
- Inorganic tin
- Aluminum
- Nickel.

Mycotoxins

- Aflatoxins (B1 in feed, B1, B2, G1 and G2 and Total in food, M1 in dairy)
- Ochratoxin A
- Deoxynivalenol (and acetylated derivatives and DON-3-glucoside)
- Zearalenone and modified forms
- Fumonisins and modified forms
- Alternaria toxins (alternariol, alternariol monomethyl ether, tenuazonic acid, tentoxin)
- Patulin
- T-2 and HT-2 and modified forms
- Nivalenol and modified forms
- Ergot sclerotia
- Ergot alkaloids
- Enniatins
- Sterigmatocystin
- Beauvericin
- Citrinin
- Moniliformin
- Diacetoxyscirpenol
- Phomopsins.

Plant toxins

- Opium alkaloids
- Quinolizidine alkaloids
- Pyrrolizidine alkaloids
- Glucosinolates
- Glycoalkaloids
- Tropane alkaloids
- Hydrocyanic acid
- Erucic acid
- Tetrahydrocannabinol
- Specific for feed
    - Free Gossypol
    - Theobromine
    - Ricin
    - Abrin
    - Crotin I

Organochlorine compounds specific for feed

- Aldrin
- Dieldrin
- Camphechlor
- Chlordane
- DDT
- Endosulfan
- Endrin
- Heptachlor

- Hexachlorobenzene (HCB)
- Hexachlorocyclohexane (HCH-alpha, beta, and gamma isomers)'

Collectively these "lists" provide alerts as to what might be present in food ingredients in Europe but may occur in other geographies and which need to be part of the discussion with suppliers and subject to hazard analysis as appropriate.

A further resource is the EFSA publication "Compendium of botanicals reported to contain naturally occurring substances of possible concern for human health when used in food and food supplements"[4] as mentioned earlier in 1a).

As the data accumulates on the occurrence in food/ingredients of all the above naturally occurring chemicals, pesticide residues, veterinary drug residues, mycotoxins, process-related and environmental contaminants, along with all the other groups of chemicals which collectively make up the final chemical composition of food post-manufacture and distribution, prior to home preparation and consumption, the use of AI / ML is increasingly being used to predict future levels and help risk evaluation. The use of this tool is discussed in Chapter 67 .

Another rapidly developing technology that is being used in food safety and antifraud contexts in the agrifood industry is "block chain", which allows for the tracking of data and its modification over time, as discussed in Chapter 68.

The previous discussion demonstrates the complex and dynamic nature of the agri-food business, but now is being further exacerbated by climate change as well as being impacted by other industries and household waste as environmental contaminants, so methodologies for identifying emerging contaminants in food are being published. As an example, EFSA published a paper on "A systematic procedure for the identification of emerging chemical risks in the food and feed chain" in 2014.[6] Additional discussions of emerging contaminants are also reviewed in Chapters 17–24 and Chapter 72—climate change.

To conclude, management of the changes to the chemical composition of food through its manufacturing and distribution stages to ensure its safety and integrity requires a wide variety of hazard analyses and risk evaluations and controls, based on reliable data, as discussed above, and undertaken by responsible management and qualified staff within comprehensive GMP Guidelines, such as those referred to in this chapter.

References

1. Manning L. *Food & Drink –Good Manufacturing Practice: A Guide To It's Responsible Management*. 7th ed. Institute of Food Science and Technology (IFST) (UK), Wiley; 2018.
2. US Department of Health and Human Services, Food Safety Modernisation Act (FSMA), Final Rule for Preventative Controls for Human Food, Good Manufacturing Practice, Hazard Analysis and Risk-Based Preventative Controls for Human Food, 2020.
3. Available at <https://www.efsa.europa.eu/en/topics/topic/chemicals-food>.
4. Available at <https://efsa.onlinelibrary.wiley.com/doi/pdf/10.2903/j.efsa.2009.281>.
5. Available at <https://www.efsa.europa.eu/en/call/call-continuous-collection-chemical-contaminants-occurrence-data-0>
6. EFSA Supporting Publication EN-547, A systematic procedure for the identification of emerging chemical risks in the food and feed chain, 2014.

Chapter 11

Global regulations for the use of food additives and processing aids

Youngjoo Kwon[1], Rebeca López-García[2], Susana Socolovsky[3] and Bernadene Magnuson[4]

[1]Department of Food Science and Biotechnology, Ewha Womans University, Seoul, South Korea, [2]Logre International Food Science Consulting, Mexico City, Mexico, [3]Pentachem Consulting Group, Buenos Aires, Argentina, [4]Health Science Consultants Inc, Collingwood, Canada

Abstract

Direct food additives can be broadly defined as substances that are intentionally added to food or beverages during preparation or storage to achieve a particular technical effect within the food. In contrast, processing aids are used to facilitate food processing only and are not intended to alter the characteristics of the food itself. In this chapter, the regulations, definitions, and approval processes for food additives and processing aids are reviewed for the following specific countries/jurisdictions: Argentina, Australia, Brazil, Canada, China, the European Union, Japan, New Zealand, and the United States. Although there are some differences, all have regulations that require an evaluation before market approval to ensure that the food containing the additives is safe for the entire population. A positive list of approved food additives is publicly available in all jurisdictions, with some exceptions for the United States. The safety assessment principles applied during evaluation are based on principles developed by the Joint FAO/WHO Expert Committee on Food Additives, which are described. Future challenges include developing an understanding of the appropriate application of non-animal toxicology testing alternatives into safety assessments, addressing emerging concerns such as potential effects on the microbiome, continued efforts to harmonize global regulations, and addressing consumer concerns to promote optimal use of limited food supplies for a growing global population.

Keywords: Additives; processing aid; regulations; JECFA; CODEX; safety assessment; harmonization

Chapter Points

- History of food additive regulation
- Overview of global food regulatory agencies
- Country specific regulations, definitions, and approval processes for food additives and processing aids for: Argentina, Australia, Brazil, Canada, China, the European Union, Japan, New Zealand, and the United States
- Summary of food additive and processing aid regulations
- Research gaps and future directions

11.1 Introduction

The history of food additives, broadly defined as a substance added intentionally to foods to achieve a particular effect such as changing color, flavor, or texture or to preserve the food, began in ancient times.[1] Examples include the production of salt from seaweed and use as both a flavoring and preservative. Cookbooks from the 1700s describe the use of food coloring derived from cochineal and other sources. Concern about the safety of food additives also has a long history, beginning with the practice of using additives for food adulteration, which became increasingly common in the early 1800s. Such practices resulted in the development of food safety regulations, methods for food analyses, and safety testing of food additives in the early 1900s.

As discussed below, by the 1950s, international agencies were established to develop globally accepted methods for toxicology testing and safety assessment of the use of food additives. Methods and regulations have continued to evolve with advances in science; however, the controversies and concerns regarding the safety of food additives continue, fueled by consumer chemophobia and marketing scare campaigns. A greater understanding of the scrutiny of the use of food additives and the rigor of safety assessment by global food regulatory agencies may alleviate unwarranted consumer fear. A comparison of requirements for premarket approvals in various jurisdictions illustrates the adoption of similar approaches and

Present Knowledge in Food Safety. DOI: https://doi.org/10.1016/B978-0-12-819470-6.00067-6

principles, promoting regulatory harmonization and facilitating global trade. As the human population expands along with the loss of agricultural land, efficient use of all food resources, which often requires the use of food additives to maintain or improve safety, freshness, taste, and appearance, thereby reducing food loss and waste will be needed.

11.1.1 International scientific and advisory committees

11.1.1.1 Food and Agricultural Organization and the World Health Organization

Protecting the wholesomeness of the global food supply has been the function of national governments for centuries. However, with communication, global trade, and technological development, the food supply can no longer be considered local. Food control and protection of public health is most certainly a global task that is addressed by the Food and Agricultural Organization (FAO)[2] and the World Health Organization (WHO) Codex Alimentarius Commission (CAC)[3]. This Commission is one of the best-known and most successful cooperative projects between two United Nations agencies. The First FAO Regional Conference for Europe, meeting in Rome in October 1960[2], stated: "The desirability of international agreement on minimum food standards and related questions (including labeling requirements, methods of analysis, etc.) was recognized as an important means of protecting consumer's health, ensuring quality, and reducing trade barriers, particularly in the rapidly integrating market of Europe."[2] In November 1961 the CAC was established as a joint FAO/WHO organization to address the safety and nutritional quality of foods to promote trade.[4] Since its inception, the Codex Alimentarius (CA), or food code, has become the global reference point for consumers, food producers and processors, national food control agencies, and the international food trade.[5] The CA has extensive influence in the protection of public health, and fair practices in the food trade.[3]

11.1.1.2 Joint FAO/WHO Expert Committee on Food Additives

The main FAO/WHO expert body responsible for food additive safety assessment is the Joint FAO/WHO Expert Committee on Food Additives (JECFA)[6], which was established in 1955 to consider chemical, toxicological, and other aspects of contaminants, and residues of veterinary drugs in food for human consumption. The JECFA is an independent scientific expert committee charged with performing risk assessments and advice to FAO, WHO, the member countries of both organizations, and the Codex Alimentarius Commission. This committee provides:

1. Risk assessments/safety evaluations of food additives, processing aids, residues of veterinary products, contaminants, and natural toxins
2. Exposure assessment to chemicals
3. Specifications and analytical methods, residue definition, and Maximum Residue Limits proposals
4. Guidelines for the safety assessment of chemicals in foods are consistent with current thinking on risk assessment in toxicology and other relevant sciences.

The initial steps of this committee were to establish general principles regarding the technical purpose of food additives as well as principles of evaluation to protect public health. The Committee has established that the use of food additives should be technologically justified to:

1. Maintain the nutritional quality of food,
2. Enhance quality or stability to prevent food waste,
3. Make food attractive to consumers, and
4. Provide essential aids to processing.

The Committee established that the use of food additives must have a technological justification and established that food additives should not be used to:

1. Deceive the consumer,
2. Result in a substantial reduction of the nutritional value of food,
3. Achieve an effect that can be obtained by Good Manufacturing Practices,
4. Disguise the use of faulty processing or handling techniques.

For the safety evaluation of food additives, the Committee established solid general principles that included:

1. It is impossible to establish absolute proof of non-toxicity for all members of the human population.
2. Critically designed animal studies to provide a reasonable basis for evaluating the safety of food additives are needed.
3. The decision for a safe level for a food additive is based on knowledge of the minimum dietary level that produces no unfavorable response in test animals.
4. Decisions on the use of food additives must be based on the considered judgment of properly qualified scientists that the intake of the additive will be below any level that could be harmful to consumers.
5. The fate of the additive during food processing and preparation should be considered because of the possible formation of toxic substances and the interaction of the food additive with components of food or other food additives.
6. Consideration should be given to groups within the population who for medical reasons may be especially vulnerable to certain food additives.

As will be discussed below, although animal testing was a central component of the JECFA principles for safety assessment and remains to be used today, the scientific and regulatory communities have long recognized the need to find alternatives to reliance on animal toxicity testing methods and derivation of acceptable dietary levels of exposure. Further understanding of how predictive assays of biological activity of compounds can be integrated into safety assessments is needed to achieve the reduction of the use of animal testing methods.

The Committee also established that positive lists are better for food additives because the use of prohibited lists could entail exposure to potentially harmful compounds before sufficient evidence was accumulated to place the additive on the list. Also, consumers should be aware of the permitted lists of additives.

11.1.1.3 JECFA general principles of food additive safety evaluation

The Committee decided that it was only possible to formulate general recommendations on testing procedures since additives are a diverse group of chemical compounds with different structures, physicochemical properties, and conditions of human exposure. Thus using a rigid set of mandatory tests is not considered desirable and may not fully address specific concerns of individual additives. General principles of food additive evaluation include:

1. The selection of animal species for testing indicated that background information on species/strain, natural disease rates, tumor incidence, and duration of life was essential for the proper interpretation of experimental results.
2. The importance of animal housing, diets, control groups, and statistical procedures for the design of studies, and their interpretation.
3. The importance of dose selection emphasizes the need to magnify the dose in experimental animals to overcome statistical limitations of the test design and to provide a means of studying dose-response relationships.
4. The need for biochemical mechanistic investigations to detect subtle physiological changes and to assist in data interpretation.
5. The need to examine the potential for food additives to induce carcinogenesis, stating that no proven carcinogen should be considered suitable for use as a food additive in any amount.[6]
6. The results of the toxicological evaluations are the basis for the allocation of an acceptable daily intake (ADI) for food additives, or in the case of contaminants the Committee considered unavoidable, a tolerable intake.

Codex standards[7] for food additives are based on the principle that lifetime exposure daily to any of the chemicals approved for food use should result in no appreciable health risk. This is commonly known as the ADI approach and is used for the approval of food additive applications. As the safety evaluation of food additives involves testing using animal models, the Committee considered the issues associated with the extrapolation of animal studies to humans and determined that a safety margin of 100 applied at doses identified to cause no adverse effect in animals provided an adequate margin of safety for most substances proposed as food additives. More recently, the use of the benchmark dose approach instead of the traditionally used no-observed-adverse-effect level approach, has been recommended in some jurisdictions[8] since it makes more extended use of dose-response data and it allows for a quantification of the uncertainties in the dose-response data.

The toxicological assessment of food additives is used to identify any potential hazard of consumption of the food additive at different exposure levels. Risk assessment involves determining the expected population exposure levels to the food additive from foods in which it will be used and comparing that to the ADI to assess the potential risk of harm to consumers.[9] Further discussion of the process of risk analysis of components in foods, including risk management and risk communication, is outside the scope of this review. In countries with limited risk assessment capabilities, the JECFA scientific opinion is used by local authorities to make risk management decisions, such as establishing the maximum use levels and approved food categories for the food additive. Other countries have decided to directly adopt Codex Standards into their national system.

The principles of JECFA are still quite relevant and have been pivotal in the development of national food control systems. The early work done by the Committee and the level of expertise of the original Committee members resulted in a solid reference tool that has guided many governments and organizations.

11.1.1.4 International Programme on Chemical Safety

The International Programme on Chemical Safety (IPCS) is a joint venture of the United Nations Environment Programme, the International Labour Organisation, and the World Health Organization. In 1987, in response to numerous recommendations by JECFA, the IPCS convened a Task Force to review current knowledge and advances in toxicological science and to develop criteria for testing and evaluating the safety of food additives and contaminants. Thus in 1987 the Environmental Health Criteria 70 (EHC70) entitled Principles for the Safety

Assessment of Food Additives and Contaminants in Food was published. This document was subsequently updated by the IPCS in 2009, with the publication of EHC240, entitled Principles, and Methods for the Risk Assessment of Chemicals in Food.[10] These guidelines address the considerable changes that have taken place in the procedures and complexity of assessments of chemicals in food since the preparation of the original guidance documents for the work of JECFA. Since its publication in 2009 the practices have evolved further. Thus in 2020 FAO and WHO updated sections on genotoxicity, dose-response assessment, and derivation of health-based guidance values, dietary exposure assessment of chemicals in food, and enzymes. These updated sections are currently available in the online version of the Environmental Health Criteria 240.[10]

11.2 Regulations in different jurisdictions

A summary of the regulation of food additives and processing aids (where not included in the regulation for food additives), and laws about their safety are tabulated below. The countries that were chosen included: Argentina, Australia, Brazil, Canada, China, the EU, Japan, New Zealand, and the United States. These countries include both those with well-established regulatory systems (i.e., Australia, Canada, Japan, New Zealand, and the EU and the USA) and several that are currently in the process of changing and/or modernizing their food regulatory systems (i.e., Argentina, Brazil, and China). For each target country, the following information was sought and is summarized in table format (Tables 11.1–11.8):

- A brief historical overview of the main regulatory body/scientific advisory body and their roles and responsibilities concerning the regulation of chemicals added to food.
- A discussion of the regulatory framework.
- Pertinent regulations.
- A brief summary of submission requirements and the process for the approval of food additives.

11.3 Global regulation and safety assessment of food additives and processing aids

In general, each of the target countries has a regulatory system in place for the scientific evaluation and approval of food additives; however, several are undergoing change, refinement, and working towards harmonization with other countries. The EU adopted regulations to establish a common authorization procedure for food additives to move away from authorization at the national level for each member state.[21]

Other efforts to harmonize food standards among countries include Australia and New Zealand with joint labeling and compositional standards under the Australia NZ Food Standard Code.[12] In South America, the South American Common Market, known as Mercosur,[24] represents Brazil, Argentina, Uruguay, Paraguay, and Venezuela. While having their regulatory systems in place, many of the country's food standards are gradually being replaced by official Mercosur standards as they are developed.

11.4 Food additive regulations

Although the precise definition of a food additive differs among different countries, in general, a food additive is defined as a substance added to foods intentionally to achieve a technological function in the final product. In most jurisdictions, a permitted list of food additives is published and available to the public. The exception to this is the USA, which will be discussed further below. The permitted list contains food additives, which are deemed safe for human consumption under the specified conditions of use. If a food additive is not on the permitted list or its use is not permitted in a particular food and an applicant wants to use the food additive, the applicant must apply to the regulatory agency to approve its use in the respective country, following the conditions and requirements laid out by the respective authoritative body.

One point to be emphasized is that there is no distinction between naturally occurring compounds and synthetically generated compounds with respect to global food additive regulations and requirements for safety assessment. Although there is a wide held belief that a natural source of a compound imparts safety, there is no toxicological scientific evidence to support this misconception. Many of the most toxic compounds identified are naturally occurring, such as ricin from the seeds of the castor oil plant. Naturally occurring toxins in foods represent significant food safety issues for both humans and livestock.[23] Thus novel food additives derived from natural sources must undergo safety assessment to the same degree as a synthetic compound.

In Argentina and Brazil, food additives are regulated under Mercosur standards (GMC 11/06, 34/10, and 35/10).[22] For new food additives, applicants must submit to the Comisión Nacional de Alimentos (CONAL)[12] or Agência Nacional de Vigilância Sanitária[14] (for Argentina and Brazil, respectively), which will subsequently forward the application to Mercosur's Sub Work Group #3. In Canada, all new food additives or changes to the permitted uses of already approved food additives under Division 16 of the Food and Drug Regulations must undergo a premarket assessment focused on safety.[16] Similarly, in Japan[19] and China,[17] a safety assessment was conducted on all currently permitted food additives. In order to increase consistency in

TABLE 11.1 Regulatory framework on food additives and processing aids in Argentina.

Argentina Regulatory authority	*Name:* **Ministry of Health (Ministerio de Salud) and The National Administration of Drugs, Foods, and Medical Technology (Administración Nacional de Medicamentos, Alimentos y Tecnología Médica (ANMAT)[11]**
	Website: https://www.argentina.gob.ar/salud https://www.argentina.gob.ar/anmat
	Historical overview: ANMAT was created by Presidential Decree 1490/92 http://www.anmat.gov.ar/webanmat/Legislacion/NormasGenerales/Decreto_1490-1992.pdf
	Role/responsibility: ANMAT is a decentralized body of the National Public Administration, established by Decree 1490/92. It assists in the protection of human health, ensuring the quality of products within its jurisdiction: medicines, food, medical products, diagnostic reagents, cosmetics, dietary supplements, and household products. Its jurisdiction covers the entire country. Since its creation in 1992, a body of professionals and technicians work with modern technology effectively to implement the processes of authorization, registration, regulation, monitoring, and control of products used in medicine, human food, and cosmetics. It depends both technically and scientifically on the norms and directives set forth by the Secretary for Policies, Regulations, and Institutions of the Ministry of Health, with a system of economic and financial autarchy. In this context, ANMAT's main objective is "to ensure that medicines, food and medical devices available to the population, have proven effectiveness (achieving the therapeutic, diagnostic or nutrition targets), safety (high ratio benefit/risk) and quality (responding to the needs and expectations of citizenship) . . ."
Advisory Scientific body	National Committee of Food (CONAL)[12] http://www.conal.gob.ar/ Historical overview: Created by Presidential Decree 815/99 http://www.conal.gob.ar/decretos/Decreto_815/815-99.htm Role/responsibility: CONAL functions as an advisory body that provides support and monitoring to the National Food Inspection System (Sistema Nacional de Control de Alimentos—SNCA), which enforces the Argentine Food Code (also known as Código Alimentario Argentino—CAA). CONAL reviews all the petitions for incorporation to the CAA (new ingredients, food additives and processing aids, materials in contact with foods, etc.) When pertinent because of harmonization requirements with Mercosur, CONAL requests treatment of the matter at the Mercosur level.
Framework regulation	Argentine Food Code (CAA) https://www.argentina.gob.ar/anmat/codigoalimentario The CAA regulates local food production; however, as harmonized Mercosur regulations become available, the CAA incorporates those regulations into the CAA through *Resoluciones Conjuntas* issued by the Ministry of Health and the Ministry of Agriculture, Livestock, and Fisheries. The CAA is a set of sanitary provisions, analytical standards, and rules for the commercial identification of products. It has more than 1400 articles divided into 22 chapters that include general provisions related to food factories and food trade, conservation and food processing, use of utensils, containers, packaging, standards for labeling and advertising of food, technical specifications of the different types of foods and beverages, processing aids, and food additives. *Historical overview:* The Argentine Food Code came into effect by Law 18,284, regulated by Decree 2126/71, of which Annex I is the text of the CAA
Part of an overarching international organization	Member of the World Trade Organization since 1995. Member of the Codex Alimentarius Commission. Mercosur (which was established in 1991 and encompasses Argentina, Brazil, Uruguay, Paraguay, and as of 2006, Venezuela) Mercosur standards are influenced by the European Union, the Codex Alimentarius Commission, and the USFDA
Regulatory overview of specific food chemical groups	
Direct food additives	*Definition*: It is an ingredient added to food intentionally, without the purpose of nourishing, to modify the physical, chemical, biological or sensory characteristics, during manufacturing, processing, preparation, treatment, packaging, conditioning, storage, transportation, or handling of food. This will result, or can reasonably be expected to result (directly or indirectly), that the additive itself or its products become a component of that food. This term does not include contaminants or nutritional substances that are incorporated into a portion of food to maintain or improve its nutritional properties.

(*Continued*)

TABLE 11.1 (Continued)

Argentina Regulatory authority	*Name:* **Ministry of Health (Ministerio de Salud) and The National Administration of Drugs, Foods, and Medical Technology (Administración Nacional de Medicamentos, Alimentos y Tecnología Médica (ANMAT)[11]** *Regulations:* Argentina has incorporated Mercosur regulations: • Mercosur GMC 11/06—MERCOSUR Technical Regulation on the harmonized general list of food additives and their functional classes. (Currently under revision) • Mercosur GMC 34/10—Provisions for food additives authorized for use according to Good Manufacturing Practices (GMP) • Mercosur GMC 35/10—Technical Regulation on maximum limits for additives excluded from the list of food additives authorized for use according to Good Manufacturing Practices (GMP) Argentina has adopted Mercosur regulations that establish food additives permitted in 12 harmonized food categories and conditions. These are called "Mercosur Technical Regulation on Allocation of Additives and Their Maximum Concentrations for Food Category 21: Industrial Cooking Preparations," for example. Harmonized food categories are: dairy products, edible ices, confectionery, cereals, and cereal products, bakery ware, meat, and meat products, soups and broths, sauces, dressings and condiments, non-alcoholic beverages, savory snack foods, desserts, and powdered desserts, culinary industrial products Provisions for food additives are outlined in Chapter XVIII of the Argentine Food Code https://www.argentina.gob.ar/sites/default/files/capitulo_xviii_aditivosactualiz_2020-01.pdf Low and no-calorie sweeteners: Chapter XVII of the Argentine Food Code provides outdated information on LNCS. *Guidance document*: http://www.conal.gob.ar/Documentos/INSTRUCTIVO_Presentacion_ante_CONAL_17_10.pdf *The approval process for new substances*: • An application to modify the Code is required to approve the use of a new food additive or to modify the approval for use in a different food category, change usage levels, etc. Information required as specified in the Guideline document includes: • Product Identification: description, scientific name, common name, denomination of sale, manufacturing process • Characteristics: qualitative and quantitative composition, bioavailability, technological function, proposed use and levels of use, technical specifications (identity, quality, purity, stability), conditions of use, manufacturing methods, instructions for storage and handling, preparation and consumption, analytical method for detection • Use of food additives in other countries and international regulations (EU, FDA, CODEX) national regulations (C.A.A.), regional regulations (MERCOSUR), Publications of official bodies, and proof of approval in other countries. • Safety of the food additive: metabolism studies, toxicity studies, allergenicity studies.
Processing aid	*Definition*: A processing aid is any substance, excluding equipment and utensils, that is not consumed by itself as a food ingredient and which is intentionally used in the processing of raw materials, foods, or ingredients, for a technological purpose during treatment or processing. It must be removed from the food or inactivated; the presence of traces of the substances or their derivatives may be admitted in the final product. Definition as per Mercosur regulation GMC 26/03 which is currently under review. It is expected to be gazetted by the end of 2021 *Regulation*: Chapter XVI of the CAA "CORRECTIVOS Y ADJUVANTES", defines the functions of processing aids, following the provisions of Mercosur Resolution GMC No. 084/93. It does not provide a list of authorized processing aids and/or enzymes in the MERCOSUR, thus authorization and use are done following the regulations of each member country. Enzymes: To enable the Sanitary Authorization of new enzymes to be used as processing aids, article 1263 of the Argentine Food Code (CAA Chapter XVI) was modified in 2019, introducing a

(Continued)

TABLE 11.1 (Continued)

Argentina Regulatory authority	*Name:* **Ministry of Health (Ministerio de Salud) and The National Administration of Drugs, Foods, and Medical Technology (Administración Nacional de Medicamentos, Alimentos y Tecnología Médica (ANMAT)[11]**
	positive list of enzymes. Likewise, article 1263 bis, "Protocol for the Evaluation of an Enzyme as a processing aid", was included in the aforementioned Code, to evaluate whether other enzymes that are not included in the list of article 1263 could be admitted.
	Guidance document: https://www.argentina.gob.ar/sites/default/files/capitulo_xvi_correctivosactualiz_2020-01.pdf https://www.argentina.gob.ar/sites/default/files/anmat_instructivo_enzimas_02.pdf
	Approval process for a new substances: A detailed dossier on the new enzyme should be submitted following guidance set forth in article 1263 bis Chapter XVI of the CAA.

TABLE 11.2 Regulatory framework on food additives and processing aids in Australia and New Zealand.

Australia and New Zealand Regulatory authority	*Name:* **Food Standards Australia New Zealand[13]**
	Website: www.foodstandards.gov.au
	Historical overview:
	• In 1991 the National Food Authority (NFA) was created. The role of the NFA was to prepare and recommend standards to the National Foods Standards Council (NFSC), consisting of Commonwealth, state and territory health ministers. • Australia and New Zealand established Joint Food Standards in December, 1995, which aimed to harmonize food standards, reduce compliance costs and remove regulatory barriers to trade in food. FSANZ, as we now know it, was established on 1 July 2002.
	Role/responsibility:
	• FSANZ is a Government agency that develops and administers the Australia New Zealand Food Standards Code (the Code). • The Code regulates the use of ingredients, processing aids, colorings, additives, vitamins, and minerals. The code also covers the composition of some foods e.g., dairy, meat, and beverages as well as standards developed by new technologies such as genetically modified foods. • FSANZ is also responsible for labeling both packaged and unpackaged food, including specific mandatory warnings or advisory labels. • In Australia, FSANZ has a broader coverage and prepares standards across the food supply chain. FSANZ develops standards for primary production and processing and food hygiene. FSANZ also set residue limits for agricultural and veterinary products. In New Zealand, these activities are undertaken by the New Zealand Ministry for Primary Industries. • FSANZ develops standards in consultation with other government agencies and stakeholders, the Australia and New Zealand Ministerial Forum on Food Regulation sets policy guidelines for the development of food standards by FSANZ. • FSANZ also has many other functions in Australia including coordinating food surveillance and food recall systems, conducting research, and supporting the Department of Agriculture in its duty to inspect imported foods. • FSANZ's ultimate goal is to ensure Australia and New Zealand have a safe food supply and well-informed consumers. • FSANZ is not responsible for the following: (1) decide overarching food policy, (2) enforce the Code, (3) provide advice on food compliance issues, (4) regulate therapeutic goods e.g., medicines and complementary medicines, (5) regulate industrial chemicals, and (6) inspect and sample imported food.

(Continued)

TABLE 11.2 (Continued)

Australia and New Zealand Regulatory authority	*Name:* **Food Standards Australia New Zealand**[13]
Advisory Scientific body	*Internal body*: FSANZ Board • 12 members, must include qualified people from all walks of life. Members are drawn from relevant specialist areas such as public health, nutrition, food science, consumer affairs, medical science, food safety, veterinary science, food production, the food industry, food retailing, international trade, food regulation, and government. *External body:* FSANZ Fellows • Developed to create a network of experts who can provide FSANZ with objective expert advice and critical review. Also helps to develop academic links and networks.
Framework regulation	Australia New Zealand Standards Code (the Code): The Code regulates all aspects of food including labeling and other information requirements, foods requiring premarket clearance (novel foods, food produced using gene technology, irradiation of food), substances added to or present in food (processing aids, vitamins, and minerals, food additives), microbiological limits and processing requirements, and contaminants and residues. In addition, applied in Australia only, food safety standards and primary production standards are also included. (https://www.foodstandards.gov.au/code/Pages/default.aspx)
Part of an overarching international organization	• FSANZ supports the work of the WHO and FAO by participating in expert consultations and meetings, including the JECFA. • Australia (FSANZ) and China are co-chairs of the Asia-Pacific Economic Cooperation (APEC) Food Safety Cooperation Forum.
Regulatory overview of specific food chemical groups	
Direct food additives	*Definition*: • Section 1.1.2-11: A substance is used as a food additive concerning a food if it is added to the food and: performs one or more of the technological purposes listed in Schedule 14; and is a substance (identified in subsection 1.1.2-11(2)): o any of the following: (1) a substance that is identified in Schedule 15, an additive permitted at GMP (listed in section S16-2), (2) a coloring permitted at GMP (listed in section S16-3), (3) a coloring permitted to a maximum level (listed in section S16-4) o any substance that is: (1) a non-traditional food and (2) has been concentrated or refined, or synthesized, to perform one or more of the technological purposes listed in Schedule 14. *Regulation*: • Standard 1.3.1—Food Additives • Foods by category type are set out in: o Schedule 15: Substances that may be used as food additives o Schedule 16: Types of substances that may be used as food additives • 1.3.1—3 describes "when food additives may be used as ingredients in foods" • 1.3.1—4 describes "maximum permitted levels of food additives in foods" • 1.3.1—5 describes "limitation on use of intense sweeteners" • 1.3.1—6 describes "food additives performing the same purpose" *Guidance document*: • Application Handbook (https://www.foodstandards.gov.au/code/changes/pages/applicationshandbook.aspx *The approval process for new substances*: • An application to vary the Code is required to approve the use of a new food additive in the food supply or to change the permissions for a currently used food additive. • Information required as specified in Guideline 3.1.1 includes: • Technical information on the food additive: o Nature and technological purpose o Information and specification to enable identification and purity o Chemical and physical properties of the additive

(*Continued*)

TABLE 11.2 (Continued)

Australia and New Zealand Regulatory authority	*Name:* **Food Standards Australia New Zealand**[13]
	o Manufacturing process and impurities o Information for food labeling o Analytical method for detection • Safety of the food additive o Toxicokinetics and metabolism o Toxicity, and, if necessary, its degradation products and major metabolites o Safety assessment reports prepared by international agencies or other national government agencies, if available • Dietary exposure to the food additive o Food groups or foods proposed to contain the food additive or changes to currently permitted foods o Maximum proposed levels of the food additive for each food group or food. o The percentage of the food group in which the food additive is proposed to be used o Use of the food additive in other countries, if applicable
Processing aid	*Definition*: • Section 1.1.2-13: a substance that is used to preform a technological purpose during the course of food processing; and does not perform a technological purpose in a food for sale. *Regulation*: • Food Standard Code 1.3.3—processing aids o A substance may be used if: (1) permitted to be used as a processing aid for that food by the Standard; and (2) the proportion used is no more than the maximum level necessary to achieve the technological purpose under conditions of GMP. *Guidance document*: (https://www.foodstandards.gov.au/code/changes/pages/applicationshandbook.aspx) *Approval process for a new substances*: • An application is required to approve the use of a new processing aid or to change the permissions for a currently used processing aid specified in Schedule 18—Processing aids. • The following information is required in addition, to that specified in Guideline 3.1.1 – • Technical information (type and identity) • Chemical and physical properties • Manufacturing process, Specifications and purity • Analytical method for detection • Use of the chemical as a food processing aid in other countries • Safety including: toxicokinetics and metabolism, toxicity of processing aid and, if necessary, its major metabolites, potential allergenicity. • Dietary exposure • Additional information related to the safety of processing aid derived from a microorganism o Source, pathogenicity and toxicity, and genetic stability of microorganism • Additional information related to the safety of an enzyme processing aid derived from a genetically-modified microorganism o Methods used in the genetic modification

common areas of the procedural aspects of food additives' approval in the EU, guidelines for evaluation by EFSA and decision-making by the Commission, are provided in Regulation (EC) No. 1331/2008 (adopted December 16, 2010) which establishes a common authorization procedure for food additives, food enzymes and food flavorings.[24]

In the USA, substances to be added to food are subject to a premarket approval requirement unless they are exempt as outlined below. Rulis and Levitt[25] provide an excellent detailed description of the food additive approval process in the US. The 1958 Food Additive Amendments of the Federal Food, Drug and Cosmetic Act (FFDCA) required demonstration of the safety of food additives, but also included two clauses to exempt food additives currently in use from safety assessments by making them "grandfathered" ingredients. This included food additives that had been previously sanctioned for use in foods and food additives that were "generally recognized as safe" (GRAS) for

TABLE 11.3 Regulatory framework on food additives and processing aids in Brazil.

Brazil Regulatory authority	***Name:*** **Ministry of Health (Ministério da Saude) through its regulatory agency Agencia Nacional de Vigilancia Sanitária (ANVISA[14]—National Agency of Sanitary Surveillance)** *Website:* • Ministry of Health: https://www.gov.br/saude/pt-br (Ministerio da Saude 2021) • ANVISA: https://www.gov.br/anvisa/pt-br • Mercosur: http://www.mercosul.gov.br/[15] *Historical overview*: ANVISA was established by Law 9.782, as of 26 January 1999 *Role/responsibility*: The institutional purpose of the agency is to foster the protection of the health of the population by exercising sanitary control over the production and marketing of products and services subject to sanitary surveillance. The latter embraces premises and manufacturing processes, as well as the range of inputs and technologies concerned with the same. In addition, the agency exercises control over ports, airports, and borders and also liaises with the Brazilian Ministry of Foreign Affairs and foreign institutions over matters concerning international aspects of sanitary surveillance
Advisory Scientific body	Name: ANVISA is designated an autonomous agency operating under a special regime. This means that it is an independently administered, financially autonomous regulatory agency with the security of tenure for its directors during the period of their mandates. It is managed by a Collegiate Board of Directors, comprised of five members Website: http://portal.anvisa.gov.br/wps/portal/anvisa/home Historical overview: No authoritative statement was found Role/responsibility: ANVISA's function is to evaluate the safety of the use of food additives and ingredients in foods. There are specific workgroups, comprised of university professors who give technical support if needed. These groups work mainly in the approval of novel foods and novel food ingredients with functional health claims.
Framework regulation	No authoritative statement found
Part of an overarching international organization	Member of the World Trade Organization since 1995 Member of the Codex Alimentarius Commission. Mercosur (which was established in 1991 and includes Argentina, Brazil, Uruguay, Paraguay, and as of 2006, Venezuela). Mercosur standards are influenced by the European Union, the Codex Alimentarius Commission, and the USFDA
Regulatory overview of specific food chemical groups	
Direct food additives	*Definition*: It is an ingredient added to food intentionally, without the purpose of nourishing, to modify the physical, chemical, biological or sensory characteristics, during manufacturing, processing, preparation, treatment, packaging, conditioning, storage, transportation, or handling of food. This will result, or can reasonably be expected to result (directly or indirectly), that the additive itself or its products become a component of that food. This term does not include contaminants or nutritional substances that are incorporated into a food to maintain or improve its nutritional properties. *Regulations:* Brazil has adopted Mercosur regulations that establish food additives permitted in 12 harmonized food categories and conditions. These are called "Mercosur Technical Regulation on Allocation of Additives and Their Maximum Concentrations for Food Category 21: Industrial Cooking Preparations," for example. Harmonized food categories are dairy products, edible ices, confectionery, cereals and cereal products, bakery ware, meat, and meat products, soups and broths, sauces, dressings and condiments, non-alcoholic beverages, savory snack foods, desserts, and powdered desserts, culinary industrial products. Brazil has produced additional regulations for non-harmonized categories such as: RESOLUTION OF THE COLLEGIATE BOARD—RDC No. 7, OF 6 MARCH 2013—Provides for the approval of the use of processing aids for the manufacture of fruit and vegetable products (including edible mushrooms).

(Continued)

TABLE 11.3 (Continued)

Brazil Regulatory authority	*Name:* **Ministry of Health (Ministério da Saude) through its regulatory agency Agencia Nacional de Vigilancia Sanitária (ANVISA[14]—National Agency of Sanitary Surveillance)**
	RESOLUTION—RDC No. 329, DECEMBER 19, 2019—Establishes food additives and processing aids authorized for use in fish and fish products. Brazil has incorporated Mercosur regulations: • Mercosur GMC 34/10—Provisions for food additives authorized for use according to Good Manufacturing Practices (GMP) (internalized in Brazil by means of Resolução RDC 45 dated 3 November 2010) • Mercosur GMC 35/10—Technical Regulation on maximum limits for additives excluded from the list of food additives authorized for use according to Good Manufacturing Practices (GMP) (internalized in Brazil by means of Resolução RDC 46 dated 3 November 2010). Brazil has not incorporated Mercosur GMC 11/06—List of permitted food additives ANVISA published in 2008 a regulation for low and no calorie sweeteners: Resolução RDC 18/08
	Guidance document: Guia de procedimentos para pedidos de inclusão e extensão de uso de aditivos alimentares e coadjuvantes de tecnologia de fabricação na legislação Brasileira—Gerência de Avaliação de Risco e Eficácia para Alegações—GEARE/Gerência Geral de Alimentos—GGALI Guide for Applications for Inclusion and Extension of Use of Food Additives and Processing Aids in the Brazilian Legislation. Risk And Effectiveness Evaluation Management For Claims—GEARE/ General Food Management—GGALI.
	Approval process for a new substances: The regulatory process includes the case-by-case assessment of new substances, at the request of the interested party, who must submit: proof of safety of use, the technological need, the proposed usage level, the estimated intake for the additive and internationally recognized references. For a food additive or a processing aid to be approved in Brazil, internationally recognized references are considered, such as Codex Alimentarius, the European Union and additionally the U.S. Food and Drug Administration—FDA. These criteria are established by Brazilian legislation—Ordinance SVS/MS No. 540/1997 and MERCOSUR GMC/RES. No. 52/98.
Processing aid	*Definition:* A processing aid is any substance that is not consumed by itself as a food ingredient and that is used intentionally in the preparation of raw materials, foods or their ingredients, to obtain a technological purpose during treatment or manufacturing. It must be eliminated from the food or inactivated, and the presence of traces of substances or their derivatives may be admitted in the final product.
	Regulations Same regulations apply for processing aids as for food additives
	Guidance document: Guia de procedimentos para pedidos de inclusão e extensão de uso de aditivos alimentares e coadjuvantes de tecnologia de fabricação na legislação Brasileira—Gerência de Avaliação de Risco e Eficácia para Alegações—GEARE/Gerência Geral de Alimentos—GGALI Guide for Applications for Inclusion and Extension of Use of Food Additives and Processing Aids in the Brazilian Legislation. Risk And Effectiveness Evaluation Management For Claims—GEARE/ General Food Management—GGALI.
	Approval process for a new substances: *Refer to food additives* Enzymes or enzyme preparations used as processing aids are regulated by Resolutions-RDC No 53/2014 and No 54/2014. RDC No 53/2014 provides for the list of enzymes, food additives and vehicles authorized in enzymatic preparations for use in food production in general. RDC No 54/2014 provides for the Technical Regulation on enzymes and enzymatic preparations for use in food production. Its Annex provides the information required in the technical-scientific report for enzyme safety assessment. https://www.legisweb.com.br/legislacao/?id = 275613

use as food. Thus a food additive premarket approval is not required for use of a new food additive if the user is determined to be GRAS.[21] This can be done by experts qualified by scientific training and experience to evaluate its safety under the conditions of intended use, through scientific procedures, or through experience based on common use in food before 1958. The requirement for "general recognition" of safety is often met through peer-reviewed publications of

TABLE 11.4 Regulatory framework on food additives and processing aids in Canada.

Canada Regulatory authority	*Name:* **Health Canada (HC) Food Directorate**[16] *Website*: https://www.canada.ca/en/health-canada/corporate/about-health-canada/branches-agencies/health-products-food-branch/food-directorate.htm *Historical overview:* The Food and Drugs Act was introduced in 1920, with ongoing revisions. • *Role/responsibility:* • Establishing policies, setting standards, and providing advice and information on the safety and nutritional value of food, and promoting the nutritional health and well-being of Canadians. • Administering the provisions of the Food and Drugs Act that relate to public health, safety, and nutrition.
Regulatory enforcement	• *Name:* Canadian Food Inspection Agency (CFIA) • *Website:* https://www.inspection.gc.ca/eng/1297964599443/1297965645317
Framework regulation	Food and Drug Regulations: https://laws-lois.justice.gc.ca/eng/regulations/c.r.c._c._870/index.html
Part of an overarching international organization	• Member of the Codex Alimentarius Commission since it was established in 1963 • Member of the World Trade Organization since 1995
Regulatory overview of specific food chemical groups	
Direct food additives	• *Definition:* According to the Food and Drugs Regulations B.01.001, "a food additive means any substance the use of which results, or may reasonably be expected to result, in it or its by-products becoming a part of or affecting the characteristics of a food, but does not include: • Any nutritive material that is used, recognized or commonly sold as an article or ingredient of food; • Vitamins, mineral nutrients and amino acids, other than those listed in the tables to Division 16 • Spices, seasonings, flavoring preparations, essential oils, oleoresins and natural extractives; • Agricultural chemicals, other than those listed in the tables to Division 16, • Food packaging materials and components thereof; and • Drugs recommended for administration to animals that may be consumed as food". • It should be noted that a substance not present in the final food but which has affected the characteristics of that food would be regulated as a food additive. The official food additive provisions are listed in the tables of B.16.100 of the Food and Drug Regulations. Listings of permitted food additives include the common name of the food additive, a list of the foods in which the additive may be used, and the maximum level of use. Table III lists food additives that may be used as coloring agents; Table IX lists sweeteners permitted for use as a food additive. *Regulation*: Division B.16 https://laws.justice.gc.ca/eng/regulations/C.R.C._c._870/ *Guidance document:* https://www.canada.ca/en/health-canada/services/food-nutrition/reports-publications/guide-preparation-submissions-food-additives.html • *Approval process for new substances:* A submission for a food additive is required if a petitioner is seeking approval for use in Canada of a new food additive not currently regulated in the Food and Drug Regulations, and for an extension of the use of an existing food additive, e.g., the use of an existing food additive in a different food or the use of a food additive at a higher maximum level of use. General requirements include: • Identity and purpose/function of the food additive • Method of manufacture • Chemical and physical properties • Specifications and residue data • Efficacy data demonstrating the technical effect and Proposed maximum level of use • Safety data including toxicological and pharmacokinetic studies • Food intake data • Nutritional safety considerations • Labeling information • A sample of the food additive • Other non-statutory requirements for submissions on food additives: • Consumer benefits and food quality considerations • Information on evaluations, approvals, and authorizations of other national/international • Environmental assessment of new food additives

(Continued)

TABLE 11.4 (Continued)

Canada Regulatory authority	*Name:* **Health Canada (HC) Food Directorate**[16]
Processing aids	*Definition*: According to the Food Directorate, "a food processing aid is a substance that is used for a technical effect in food processing or manufacture, the use of which does not affect the intrinsic characteristics of the food and results in no or negligible residues of the substance or its by-products in or on the finished food". This definition implies the absence of residues of any given chemical and its by-product in the final food product, which is different from Australia's definition of a processing aid (in which the absence of by-products is not mentioned). Also, the characteristics of the final food must not be affected by the use of any given chemical classified as a processing aid. The definition of processing aid in Canada differs from the definition used by the Codex Alimentarius Commission. The CAC definition does not have a limitation on residue levels and does not refer to affecting the characteristics of the food. These restrictions must be included in the Directorate's definition because a substance is considered to be a food additive, under the Canadian regulatory definition of food additive, if use of the substance results in residues in the food or affects the characteristics of the food
	Approval process for a new substances: The use of a processing aid does not require a submission like a food additive but a petitioner may seek a so-called "Letter of Opinion" from the Bureau of Chemical Safety of HC's Food Directorate, confirming that, under its conditions of use, the substance in question is considered to be a processing aid and is acceptable for use.

TABLE 11.5 Regulatory framework on food additives and processing aids in China.

China Regulatory authority	*Name*: **Ministry of Health of the People's Republic of China, 2021**[17]
	Website: http://english.gov.cn/2005-10/09/content_75326.htm
	Historical overview: Established November 1949
	Role/responsibility:
	• To draft health laws, regulations and policies; to propose health development programs and strategic goals; to formulate technical protocols, health standards, supervise their enforcement and coordinate nationwide allocation of health resources • To supervise communicable disease prevention and treatment, food health, occupational, environmental, radiological and school health. To formulate food and cosmetics quality control protocols and be responsible for their accreditation. • To organize and guide multilateral and bilateral governmental and non-governmental health and medical cooperation and exchanges and medical aid to other countries, to participate in major health events initiated by international organizations • To coordinate medical and health exchanges and collaborations between China and the World Health Organization and other international organizations • To undertake other work as designated by the State Council
Advisory scientific body	Same as Regulatory authority (above)
Framework regulation	Food Safety Law of the People's Republic of China (adopted February 2009)
Part of an overarching international origination	• Member of the World Trade Organization since 2001. • Member of the Codex Alimentarius Commission.
Regulatory overview of specific food chemical group	
Direct food additives	*Definition*: "An artificially chemosynthetic or natural substance to be added to foods in order to improve food quality, color, fragrance and taste, and for the purpose of preservation and processing technology. Nutrition enhancers, gum-based substances in chewing gum, flavoring agents, and processing aids in the food industry are also included."

(Continued)

TABLE 11.5 (Continued)

China Regulatory authority	*Name*: **Ministry of Health of the People's Republic of China, 2021**[17] *Regulation*: • National Standard GB-2760-2007—Hygienic Standards for the Use of Food Additives • National Food Safety Standard—Standards for uses of food additives GB-2760-xxxx • Administrative Licensing Regulation for New Varieties of Food Additive *Guidance document*: Order No. 73: Measures for Administration of New Food Additives (English translation) (http://gain.fas.usda.gov/Recent%20GAIN%20Publications/Food%20Additive%20Registration_Beijing_China%20-%20Peoples%20Republic%20of_5-12-2010.pdf) *Premarket approval process* for a new substances: The application shall include: • Generic name, functions, dosage and scope of use of additives • Documents demonstrating technical necessity and efficiency of additives • Quality requirements, manufacturing process and testing methods of food additives, and testing methods of such additives or relevant explanations • Safety assessment data, including raw materials or sources, chemical constitution and physical properties, manufacturing process, and toxicological safety assessment data. • Label, specifications, and sample of food additives • Data on permission of manufacture and use granted by other countries or regions.
Enzymes	*Definition*: "Biological products directly extracted from edible or non-edible parts of a plant or animal or fermented and extracted from traditional or genetically modified microorganisms (including but not limited to bacteria, actinomycetes, and fungi) that are used in food processing and have a special catalytic function." A list of allowable food enzyme preparations is available (https://apps.fas.usda.gov/newgainapi/api/report/downloadreportbyfilename?filename = Standard%20for%20Food%20Additive%20Use%20-%20GB2760-2015_Beijing_China%20-%20Peoples%20Republic%20of_4-28-2015.pdf) *Regulation*: Hygienic Standard for Enzyme Preparations Used in Food Processing (Notified to the WTO as G/SPS/N/CHN/112 on 5 January 2009) *Guidance document*: See "Direct food additives" (above)
Processing aids	• *Definition:* A substance or material (not including apparatus or utensils), and not consumed as a food ingredient by itself, and only used to fulfill a certain technological purpose during processing or treatment. • *Regulation:* See "Direct food additives" (above)

TABLE 11.6 Regulatory framework on food additives and processing aids in the European Union.

European Union Regulatory authority	*Name*: **European Commission (EC)—Directorate General for Health and Food Safety**[18]
	Website: https://ec.europa.eu/food/safety_en *Historical overview:* • The predecessor of the EU was created in the aftermath of the Second World War. The first steps were to foster economic cooperation: the idea being that countries that trade with one another become economically interdependent and so more likely to avoid conflict. • The result was the European Economic Community (EEC), created in 1958, and initially increasing economic cooperation between six countries: Belgium, Germany, France, Italy, Luxembourg and the Netherlands. Since then, 22 other members joined and a huge single market (also known as the 'internal' market) has been created and continues to develop towards its full potential. • On 31 January 2020 the United Kingdom left the European Union. • What began as a purely economic union has evolved into an organization spanning policy areas, from climate, environment and health to external relations and security, justice and migration. A name change from the European Economic Community (EEC) to the European Union (EU) in 1993 reflected this.

(Continued)

TABLE 11.6 (Continued)

European Union Regulatory authority	*Name*: **European Commission (EC)—Directorate General for Health and Food Safety**[18]
Advisory scientific body	*Name*: European Food Safety Authority (EFSA)
	Website: https://www.efsa.europa.eu/
	Historical overview:
	• EFSA is a European agency funded by the EU that operates independently of the European legislative and executive institutions (Commission, Council, Parliament) and EU Member States. • Set up in 2002 following a series of food crises in the late 1990s to be a source of scientific advice and communication on risks associated with the food chain. The agency was legally established by the EU under the General Food Law- Regulation 178/2002. • The General Food Law created a European food safety system in which responsibility for risk assessment (science) and for risk management (policy) are kept separate. EFSA is responsible for the former area, and also has a duty to communicate its scientific findings to the public. • Regulation (EC) No 178/2002 of the European Parliament and Council (January 2002) laying down the general principles and requirements of food law, establishing the ESFA and procedures of food safety • Commission Regulation (EC) No 1304/2003 (July 2003) on the procedure applied by the European Food Safety Authority to request for scientific opinions referred to it • Commission Regulation (EC) No 2230/2004 (December 2004) detailed rules for the implementation of European Parliament and Council Regulation (EC) No 178/2002 with regard to the network of organizations operating in the fields within EFSA's mission
	Role/responsibility:
	• The Authority shall provide scientific advice and scientific and technical support for the Community's legislation and policies in all fields which have a direct or indirect impact on food and feed safety. It shall provide independent information on all matters within these fields and communicate risks (178/2002/EC, Article 22) • As the risk assessor, EFSA produces scientific opinions and advice that form the basis for European policies and legislation. Includes: o Food and feed safety o Nutrition o Animal health and welfare o Plant protection o Plant health. • Communicating on risks associated with the food chain is another key part. Scientific results cannot always be easily converted into simple guidelines and advice that non-scientists can understand. One of EFSA's tasks, therefore is to communicate clearly not only to its principal partners and stakeholders but also to the public at large, to help bridge the gap between science and the consumer.
Framework regulations	Regulation (EC) No 178/2002 the general principles and requirements of food law, establishing the ESFA and procedures in matters of food safety
Part of an overarching international organization	• Member of the World Trade Organization since 1995 • Member of the Codex Alimentarius Commission
Recent and/or pending changes	• Regulation (EU) 2019/1381 on the transparency and sustainability of the EU risk assessment in the food chain amends mainly Regulation (EC) No 178/2002. It seeks to do the following: o Ensure more transparency: o Increase the independence and robustness of submitted scientific studies: o Strengthen governance and scientific cooperation: o Develop comprehensive risk communication: • It also amend Regulations (EC) No 1829/2003, (EC) No 1831/2003, (EC) No 2065/2003, (EC) No 1935/2004, (EC) No 1331/2008, (EC) No 1107/2009, (EU) 2015/2283 and Directive 2001/18/EC.

(Continued)

TABLE 11.6 (Continued)

European Union Regulatory authority	*Name*: **European Commission (EC)—Directorate General for Health and Food Safety**[18]
Regulatory overview of specific food chemical groups	
	Definition:
Direct food additives	• Regulation (EC) No 1333/2008: "Food additives shall mean any substance not normally consumed as a food in itself and not normally used as a characteristic ingredient of food, whether or not it has nutritive value, the intentional addition of which to food for a technological purpose in the manufacture, processing, preparation, treatment, packaging, transport or storage of such food results, or may be reasonably expected to result, in it or its by-products becoming directly or indirectly a component of such foods". o The following are not considered to be food additives: i) monosaccharides, disaccharides or oligosaccharides and foods containing these substances used for their sweetening properties; ii) foods, whether dried or in concentrated form, including flavorings incorporated during the manufacturing of compound foods, because of their aromatic, sapid or nutritive properties together with a secondary coloring effect; iii) substances used in covering or coating materials, which do not form part of foods and are not intended to be consumed together with those foods; iv) products containing pectin and derived from dried apple pomace or peel of citrus fruits or quinces, or from a mixture of them, by the action of dilute acid followed by partial neutralization with sodium or potassium salts (liquid pectin); v) chewing gum bases; vi) white or yellow dextrin, roasted or dextrinated starch, starch modified by acid or alkali treatment, bleached starch, physically modified starch and starch treated by amylolitic enzymes; vii) ammonium chloride; viii) blood plasma, edible gelatin, protein hydrolysates and their salts, milk protein and gluten; ix) amino acids and their salts other than glutamic acid, glycine, cysteine and cystine and their salts having no technological function; x) caseinates and casein; xi) inulin;
	Regulation:
	• All additives in the EU must be authorized and listed with conditions of use in the EU's positive list based on: a safety assessment, technological need, ensuring that use of the additive will not mislead consumers • Regulation EC 1333/2008 sets the rules on food additives: definitions, conditions of use, labeling and procedures. • It contains: o Annex I: Technological functions of food additives o Annex II: Union list of food additives approved for use in food additives and conditions of use o Annex III: Union list of food additives approved for use in food additives, food enzymes and food flavorings, and their conditions of use o Annex IV: Traditional foods for which certain EU countries may continue to prohibit the use of certain categories of food additives o Annex V: Additives labeling information for certain food colors • The list of authorized food additives approved for use in food additives, enzymes and flavorings can be found in the Annex of Commission Regulation (EU) No 1130/2011 which amends Annex III to Regulation (EC) No 1333/2008. The additives approved for use in flavorings can be found in part 4 of this Annex. • Food additives must comply with specifications which should include information to adequately identify the food additive, including origin, and to describe the acceptable criteria of purity. • Regulation (EU) No 231/2012 laid down specifications for food additives listed in Annexes II and III to Regulation (EC) No 1333/2008. • Commission Regulation (EU) No 257/2010 set up a program for the re-evaluation of approved food additives in accordance with Regulation (EC) No 1333/2008.

(*Continued*)

TABLE 11.6 (Continued)

European Union Regulatory authority	*Name*: **European Commission (EC)—Directorate General for Health and Food Safety**[18]
	Guidance document: • Guidance notes on the classification of food extracts with coloring properties—The guidance document is currently being reviewed by the Commission services. • Guidance document describing the food categories in Part E of Annex II to Regulation (EC) No 1333/2008 on Food Additives—The guidance document describing the food categories was elaborated by Commission services after consultation with the EU countries' experts on food additives and the relevant stakeholders. The descriptions of the categories can be useful for an EU country's control authorities and food industry to assure correct implementation of the food additives legislation. • The practical guidance for applicants on food additives, food enzymes and food flavorings—This guidance is to provide applicants with practical information which aims at facilitating the preparation and submission of application for establishing or updating the Union lists.
	Approval process for a new substance: • The Commission, an EU country or an interested party can start the procedure through an application for updating the EU lists of authorized food additives, food enzymes and flavorings. o Applicants send their applications to the Commission. If the requested use is liable to have an effect on human health, the Commission will ask the European Food Safety Authority (EFSA) for an opinion. o EFSA must give an opinion within 9 months of receipt of a valid application. o The Commission submits a draft regulation to the Standing Committee o The proposed regulation can be adopted with regulatory procedure with scrutiny (Art. 5a of Decision 1999/468/EC) • Requirements for the application includes data of risk assessment and risk management of food additives, food enzymes and flavorings • based on the Requirements set in Regulation EU 234/2011 as amended by Commission Implementing Regulation (EU) No 562/2012
Enzymes	*Definition*: • Regulation (EC) No 1332/2008 (Article 3): A food enzyme means a product obtained from plants, animals or microorganisms or products thereof including a product obtained by a fermented process using microorganisms: i) containing one or more enzymes capable of catalyzing a specific biochemical reaction; and ii) added to food for a technological purpose at any stage of the manufacturing, processing, preparation, treatment, packaging, transport or storage of foods.
	Regulation: • Regulation (EC) No 1332/2008 only covers food enzymes added to food for a technological purpose in the manufacture, processing, preparation, treatment, packaging, transport or storage of food, including enzymes used as processing aids. Does not include food enzymes intended for human consumption e.g., for nutritional or digestive purposes. • All food enzymes are subject to safety evaluation by the EFSA and subsequently approved by the EC by means of their inclusion into the Union list of food enzymes. A food enzyme will be included in the EU list only if: o Does not pose a health concern to the consumer o There is a technological need o Its use does not mislead the consumer.
	Guidance document: Refer to direct food additives
Food processing aid	*Definition*: Processing aid shall mean any substance which:
	o is not consumed as a food by itself; o is intentionally used in the processing of raw materials, foods or their ingredients, to fulfill a certain technological purpose during treatment or processing; and o may result in the unintentional but technically unavoidable presence in the final product of residues of the food processing aid or its derivatives provided they do not present any health risk and do not have any technological effect on the final product
	Regulation: No specific regulations

TABLE 11.7 Regulatory framework on food additives and processing aids in Japan.

Japan Regulatory authority	***Name*: Ministry of Health Labour and Welfare (MHLW)[19]** *Website:* https://www.mhlw.go.jp/english/ *Historical overview*: • In 1947, then Ministry of Health and Welfare (the present Ministry of Health, Labour and Welfare (MHLW)) enacted the Food Sanitation Act (FSA) as the first comprehensive Act for food safety/hygiene, and introduced a positive list system for food additives. The, designation system had been applied only to chemically synthesized additives until 1995 when the FSA was amended. • Currently, all types of additives are equally subject to the designation system, synthetic and natural origin, with some exceptions (JETRO[20]). *Role/responsibility*: • MHLW formulates and implements various food safety policies based on scientific principles in collaboration with many relevant bodies including consumers, food business operators and other stakeholders from various fields. • Under the Food Sanitation Act and other related acts, the MHLW establishes food safety standards and other regulations for foods, food additives and food utensils, containers/packaging based on scientific evidence to protect the health of Japan's people.
Advisory scientific body	*Name*: Food Safety Commission (FSC) *Website*: http://www.fsc.go.jp/english/index.html *Role/responsibility*: • Undertakes risk assessment, and is independent from risk management organizations such as the Ministry of Agriculture, Forestry and Fisheries, the Ministry of Health, Labour and Welfare, and the Consumer Affairs Agency. • Primary goals: o Conducting risk assessment on food in a scientific, independent, and fair manner, and making recommendations to relevant ministries based upon the results. o Implementing risk communication among stakeholders such as consumers and food-related business operators. o Responding to food-borne accidents and emergencies.
Framework regulation	• Japan carries out food safety work under the Food Safety Basic Law and related laws. • Covers a wide range of responsibilities from regulating the manufacture, import, and sale of food, food additives, and food apparatus and containers/packages to provide necessary information to consumers and businesses.
Part of an overarching international organization	Member of the World Trade Organization since 1995 Member of the Codex Alimentarius Commission
Recent and/or pending changes	Since the last amendment of the Food Sanitation Act in 2003, the circumstance of food safety has been changing and globalization of food has developed. Taking into account the present conditions and issues regarding food safety, the amendment of the Food Sanitation Act was promulgated on June 2018.
Regulatory overview of specific food chemical group	
	Definition: "food additives" are:
Direct food additives	o substances used in or on food in the process of manufacturing food, or o substances used for the purpose of processing or preserving food. • Consequently, "food additive" includes both substances remaining in the final products, such as food colors and preservatives, and substances not remaining in the final products, such as processing aids. Food additives are classified into four categories: o Designated Additives o Existing Food Additives o Natural Flavoring Agents o Ordinary food used as a food additive

(Continued)

TABLE 11.7 (Continued)

Japan Regulatory authority	*Name*: **Ministry of Health Labour and Welfare (MHLW)[19]**
	Regulation:
	• Food additives that are permitted for use in food are limited to those listed at the following URLs, excluding natural flavorings and ordinary foods used as food additives. *Designated additives*: designated by MHLW as substances that are unlikely to harm human health based on Article 10 of FSA. http://www.ffcr.or.jp/zaidan/FFCRHOME.nsf/pages/list-desin.add-x • *Existing food additives*: Other than the designated additives, certain substances are permitted for use and distribution in Japan, as exception, for the reason that they are widely used in Japan and have a long history of consumption by humans. This additive status was created in 1995 when the FSA was revised and all additives (not only chemically synthesized substances but also natural origin) came to be subject to the designation system. http://www.ffcr.or.jp/zaidan/FFCRHOME.nsf/pages/list-exst.add o *Natural flavoring agents*: are obtained from animals and plants and used for flavoring food. http://www.ffcr.or.jp/zaidan/FFCRHOME.nsf/pages/list-nat.flavors o *Ordinary foods used as food additives*: generally provided for eating or drinking as food and also used as food additives (e.g., strawberry juice and agar). • http://www.ffcr.or.jp/zaidan/FFCRHOME.nsf/pages/list-general.provd.add Standards for use of Food additives: o Food additives with use standards (i.e., target foods and maximum use limits/residue limits) shall meet these standards, when these substances are used. http://www.ffcr.or.jp/zaidan/FFCRHOME.nsf/pages/stanrd.use
	Establishment of specifications and standards:
	• The Food Sanitation Law requires the MHLW to prepare an official compilation of food additive specifications and standards. The compilation contains compositional specifications and standards for manufacturing and use of additives. The compilation is updated every several years to introduce new and improved test methods commensurate with the progress in science and technology, and to achieve international harmonization of standards. • Japan's Specifications and Standards for Food Additives is the English translation of the official compilation of food additives. Current publication (9th edition) was revised according to the errata published by November 30, 2018 (the latest update was on March 3, 2019). • Japan External Trade Organization (JETRO) provides publications (the latest update was on April 2011) to present an outline of specification and standards for foods, milk and milk products, food additives, apparatus and container/packages, which are regulated under the Food Sanitation Act and relevant legislations.
	Guidance document:
	Guidelines for the Designation of Food Additives and Revision of Standards for Use of Food Additives: https://www.mhlw.go.jp/english/topics/foodsafety/foodadditives/dl/tenkabutu-shiteikijunkaiseishishin-english.pdf
	Approval process for a new substance:
	• Requires both risk assessment by the Food Safety Commission of Japan (FSCJ) and review by the MHLW. • Information required includes: ◦ Documents on origin or development, and use status in other countries ◦ Physicochemical properties and specifications ◦ Manufacturing methods, Identification tests, Purity, Residues, Stability ◦ Effectiveness and comparison with other similar food additives, Stability and Effects on nutritional components in food. ◦ Safety: Metabolism and pharmacological studies, various toxicity studies, ◦ Daily intake of the food additive ◦ Standards for use
Enzymes	*Definition*: No authoritative statement found
	Regulation: Enzymes listed as a permitted food additive can be used in food under the conditions indicated; however, for enzymes produced by genetically modified microorganisms, a safety

(Continued)

TABLE 11.7 (Continued)

Japan Regulatory authority	*Name*: Ministry of Health Labour and Welfare (MHLW)[19]
	assessment would be required under Standards for the Safety Assessment of Food (additives) Produced Using Genetically Modified Microorganisms (only available in Japanese)
	Guidance document: No authoritative guidance document found
	Approval process for a new substance: No authoritative statement found
Processing aids	• The scope of food additives referred to by the FSA is different from that defined by the CAC. • Processing aids (e.g., infiltration-supporting agents), which are not defined by the CAC as food additives, are categorized as food additives in Japan.
	Regulation: Refer to direct food additives (above)
	Guidance document: Refer to direct food additives (above)
	Approval process for a new substance: Refer to direct food additives (above)

the pivotal safety data, although other approaches can be used. It is important to emphasize that the GRAS determination of a compound is based on the intended use(s) and levels of use in specific foods, which will determine the anticipated consumer exposure and thus safety. Therefore the specified use, and not the substance in general, is determined to be GRAS. Other uses are not GRAS.

The reason that the US does not have a comprehensive positive food additive list is that FDA notification of the GRAS determination is voluntary. There is no publicly available list of the uses of substances that have been "self-determined" to be GRAS without FDA notification. It is unknown how many food additives have been introduced into the US food supply through the self-determined GRAS process, but estimates suggest that the majority of GRAS determinations are not notified.[26] Recommendations to address this issue were published in 2010,[27] but as recently reviewed by,[28] these recommendations have not been fully implemented resulting in continued gaps in the US FDA oversight of food additive safety and a lack of a complete positive list of food additives used in this jurisdiction.

11.5 Processing aids regulations

The definition of processing aids varies across the target countries; however, in general, processing aids are substances not consumed as food ingredients by themselves and are used intentionally in processing or in the production of raw materials, ingredients, or foods to achieve a technological purpose. As illustrated in the Codex inventory of processing aids, except for enzymes and solvents, most processing aids have not been evaluated by JECFA. Furthermore, this inventory is not considered to be complete. The development of a comprehensive Codex database of processing aids is under discussion.

In Canada, processing aids are permitted for use without premarket notification providing they meet the specific criteria for the definition of a processing aid (i.e. results in no or negligible residues in the food). If they do not meet these criteria, the processing aid is considered to be a food additive and the approval process for direct food additives would be applicable. Similarly in the EU, no regulations pertain to processing aids specifically; however, if a processing aid does not meet the criteria for the definition of a processing aid, it is classified as a food additive. Processing aids are regulated as food additives in China and Japan. In Argentina and Brazil, processing aids are not harmonized in Mercosur. The only harmonized regulation is 84/93, which establishes the definitions of the functions of processing aids. In Australia/New Zealand, processing aids are regulated under Food Standard 1.3.3, a general standard for processing aids. In the US, processing aids would be known as "secondary direct food additives" and regulated as either direct food additives or food contact substances.

11.6 Research gaps and future directions

A long history of safe use of food additives in the global food supply demonstrates the robustness and highly conservative process of the food additive safety assessment methods used, which evolved from the principles and guidelines established by JECFA.[6] Although the definitions, regulations, and approval processes may vary among all different jurisdictions, in general, there are many similarities in terms of the data requirements and considerations for assessment of the safety of use of substances added to food, including the use of positive lists of approved substances, premarket approval, and separation between science and policy decisions.

TABLE 11.8 Regulatory framework on food additives and processing aids in the United States.

United States Regulatory authority	*Name*: **US Food and Drug Administration**[21]
	https://www.fda.gov/food/food-ingredients-packaging/
	Historical overview: (June 29, 2018)
	• Since 1848 the federal government has used chemical analysis to monitor the safety of agricultural products. Although it was not known by its present name until 1930, FDA's modern regulatory functions began with the passage of the 1906 Pure Food and Drugs Act. Since then, the FDA has changed along with social, economic, political and legal changes in the United States.
	Role/responsibility related to food: (March 28, 2018)
	• FDA is responsible for protecting the public health by ensuring the safety of nation's food supply.
Advisory scientific body	*Name*: USFDA Science Board and USFDA Food Advisory Committee
	Websites:
	USFDA Science Board: https://www.fda.gov/advisory-committees/committees-and-meeting-materials/science-board-food-and-drug-administration USFDA Food Advisory Committee: https://www.fda.gov/advisory-committees/committees-and-meeting-materials/food-advisory-committee
	Role/responsibility:
	• The Science Board shall provide advice to the Commissioner and other appropriate officials on specific complex scientific and technical issues important to FDA and its mission, including emerging issues within the scientific community. • FDA's advisory committees are established to provide functions, which support the agency's mission of protecting and promoting the public health, while meeting the requirements set forth in the Federal Advisory Committee Act.
Framework regulations	Code of Federal Regulations https://www.ecfr.gov/cgi-bin/text-idx?SID = 6ba0a6620c258cee683e814692be783d&mc = true&node = pt21.3.170&rgn = div5
Part of an overarching international organization	Member of the World Trade Organization (WTO) Participates and exercises leadership in the Codex Alimentarius Commission (https://www.fda.gov/food/international-interagency-coordination/international-cooperation-food-safety)
Regulatory overview of specific food chemical groups	
Direct food additives	*Definition*:
	• A substance added directly to food can fall into one of several categories: food additive, prior sanctioned substance, color additive, or the use of the substances is considered GRAS (Generally Recognized as Safe), depending on its intended use and the mechanism through which approval is sought. • o The term "food additive" means any substance the intended use of which results or may reasonably be expected to result, directly or indirectly, in its becoming a component or otherwise affecting the characteristics of any food (including any substance intended for use in producing, manufacturing, packing, processing, preparing, treating, packaging, transporting, or holding food; and including any source of radiation intended for any such use); if such substance is not GRAS or sanctioned prior to 1958 or otherwise excluded from the definition of food additives. • *Direct food additives* are substances intentionally added to foods whose use has been approved usually in response to a food additive petition by the manufacturer. • *Color additives* are substances that are capable (alone or through reaction with other substances) of imparting color when added or applied to food. Substances intended to be used solely for purposes other than coloring, that may also impart color, do not fall within this category.

(*Continued*)

TABLE 11.8 (Continued)

United States Regulatory authority	*Name*: **US Food and Drug Administration**[21]
	• *Prior-sanctioned substances* are chemicals that were government-approved for use in food prior to 1958 • *GRAS substances* are substances "generally recognized among experts qualified by scientific training and experience to evaluate their safety, as having been adequately shown through scientific procedures (or, in the case of a substance used in food prior to 1 January 1958, through either scientific procedures or experience based on common use in food) to be safe under the conditions of its intended use".
	Regulation:
	21 CFR §§70-82 and §§170-189 https://www.accessdata.fda.gov/scripts/cdrh/cfdocs/cfCFR/CFRSearch.cfm • Under sections 201(s) and 409 of the Act, and FDA's implementing regulations in 21 CFR 170.3 and 21 CFR 170.30, the use of a food substance may be GRAS either through scientific procedures or, for a substance used in food before 1958, through experience based on common use in food. Under 21 CFR 170.30(b), general recognition of safety through scientific procedures requires the same quantity and quality of scientific evidence as is required to obtain approval of the substance as a food additive. https://www.fda.gov/food/food-ingredients-packaging/generally-recognized-safe-gras
	Guidance document: https://www.fda.gov/food/food-ingredients-packaging/food-additives-petitions
	Approval process for new substances:
	• Same as described for food ingredients above. In this case, the petitions submitted would be food additive or color additive petitions. o 21 CFR Part 71--Color Additive Petitions o 21 CFR Parts 171--Food Additive Petitions • Voluntary GRAS notifications submitted by a manufacturer are reviewed by the agency, and if the agency's review of this notification raises no concerns, the USFDA would send a letter stating that it has "no questions" regarding the manufacturer's conclusion. An inventory of notifications and agency responses is available. https://www.fda.gov/food/generally-recognized-safe-gras/gras-notice-inventory
Enzymes	*Definition*: There is no specific regulation governing enzymes. They would be regulated as direct or indirect additives, or GRAS substances depending on their intended use and the method used to allow the substances in food.
	Regulation: See "Direct food additives" (above)
	Guidance document: See "Direct food additives" (above)
	Approval process for new substances: See "Direct food additives" (above)
Food processing aids	*Definition*:
	• A subcategory of direct food additives, known as "secondary direct additives". These have a technical effect in food during processing but not in the finished food (e.g., processing aid). Some food processing aids also meet the definition of a food contact substance. • In general, food contact substances are substances that may come into contact with food as part of packaging or processing equipment but are not intended to be added directly to food. Additional "indirect" additives that are effective as part of the food contact substance notification program or that are exempted from regulation as food additives in accordance with 21 CFR 170.39. Threshold of Regulation Exemptions for substances used in food-contact articles are listed in separate inventories.
	Regulation: See "Direct food additives" (above) and food contact substances (indirect food additives) as follow; Indirect food additives mentioned in Title 21 of the U.S. Code of Federal Regulations (21CFR) used in food-contact articles, include adhesives and components of coatings (Part 175), paper and paperboard components (Part 176), polymers (Part 177), and adjuvants and production aids (Part 178). Currently, additional indirect food additives are authorized through the

(*Continued*)

TABLE 11.8 (Continued)

United States Regulatory authority	*Name*: US Food and Drug Administration[21]
	food contact notification program. In addition, indirect food additives may be authorized through 21 CFR 170.39. A substance used in a food contact article may be exempted from the requirement of a food additive listing regulation if the use in question has been shown to meet the requirements in 21 CFR 170.39.
	Guidance document: See "Direct food additives" (above)
	Approval process for a new substance: See "Direct food additives" (above)

There is recognition that the use and development of food additives will need to continue as the global population expands concurrently with limitations on the expansion of food production, requiring efficient use and preservation of the quality of food. However, food additive safety continues to be a topic both of consumer concern, and scientific research and debate. Efforts to refine the process of assessment of the biological activity of food additives, and of consumer exposure levels as dietary patterns and food choices change, therefore need to continue to improve confidence in the overall risk assessment and use of food additives. In addition, there is a need to improve risk communications strategies to address consumer, nutrition, and other health professionals' concerns that are not familiar with the risk assessment processes conducted before any compound makes it to the market.

Future directions and research gaps include strategies for integration of novel non-animal toxicology methodologies into risk assessment and tolerance settings; determination of the toxicological significance of observed alterations in the gut microbiome; evaluation of the toxicological impact of exposure to mixtures of food additives, and development of effective communication strategies to combat misinformation on food safety in general.

The development of non-animal methods to investigate biological activity and toxicity of chemicals has been a subject of research for many years, to reduce the use of animals, and to reduce the cost and time required for safety assessment. Models include human stem cell cultures, 3-D cell cultures, organs-on-chips, microarrays, adverse outcome pathway development, models to study digestion, bioavailability, kinetics, and biotransformation, and quantitative structure-activity relationship (QSAR) models. These methods are widely used for toxicity screening in product development and in establishing priority compounds for evaluation. However, except for QSAR models, there is little use of these methods in regulatory approval approaches for food ingredients.[29] Greater understanding of how these methods can be used to establish reference values such as the ADI is needed.

Although consideration of the potential impact on the gut microbiota has long been a part of the safety assessment of non-absorbed food ingredients such as novel dietary fiber, the gut microbiome has emerged as an important potential target for many other compounds in foods. One group of food additives that have received considerable attention based on reports of alteration of the gut microbiome is non-caloric sweeteners.[15] The difficulty is in the interpretation of the significance of the various microbiome alterations reported in studies, which are not consistent in direction or phyla from study to study,[30] and are not associated with a toxicology endpoint. As discussed in a recent review[31] the criteria for diagnosis or confirmation of gut microbiome toxicity have not been established with specific and effective biomarkers. Standardization of experimental design, the inclusion of appropriate negative controls, and strict control of other dietary factors are critical as

"The gut microbiome and its functions will change under various environmental pressure at almost all times, however, not all changes are necessarily adverse and lead to adverse outcomes. Therefore it is imperative to develop strategies identifying alterations that adversely influence human health".[31]

Different methods for sampling and evaluation of changes in the microbiome are often not comparable. Also, as animal models for human microbiota are not well established, it is difficult to predict the relevance of outcomes observed in animals to human health with complex host-microbiota interaction.

Although the approach for safety assessments of individual food additives is well established, there is a need for improvement in the safety assessment of mixtures of compounds, which may be used as food ingredients. Work towards this goal by EFSA has resulted in the development of the MixTox framework for risk assessment of mixtures. This framework has been used in the risk assessment of combined exposure to multiple chemicals in essential oils.[32] This approach may be a useful new tool in the risk assessment of mixtures of compounds to be used as food additives.

Lastly, ongoing efforts to harmonize food regulations as illustrated by Australia and New Zealand, Mercosur, and by the EU, are needed globally to reduce the burden on regulatory agencies for food additive review and approvals, and to free up resources to address other pressing food safety and food security issues. Harmonization of global food regulations is envisioned to promote the use of all available foods through free trade, support farmers, and reduce food loss, food waste, and ultimately reduce hunger and poverty globally.

References

1. Trager J. *The Food Chronology*. New York: Henry Holt; 1995.
2. FAO. Report of the Conference for Europe. Rome; 10–15 October 1960.
3. FAO. Resolution No. 12/61. Report of the eleventh session of the Conference. Rome; 4–24 November 1962.
4. Codex Alimentarius Commission. *Understanding the Codex Alimentarius*. 3rd ed. Rome, Italy: Food and Agriculture Organization of the United Nations (FAO) and World Health Organization (WHO); 2006. Joint FAO/WHO Food Standards Programme.
5. Codex Alimentarius Commission. *Procedural Manual in Joint FAO/WHO Food Standards Programme*. Rome, Italy: Food and Agricultural Organization of the United Nations; 2005.
6. JECFA. Procedures for the Testing of Intentional Food Additives to Establish Their Safety for Use. Second Report of the Joint FAO/WHO Expert Committee on Food Additives (JECFA), in World Health Organization Technical Reort Series No. 144. Geneva, Switzerland; 1958.
7. Codex Alimentarius. *Codex Alimentarius International Food Standards*. [Internet], Rome, Italy: Codex Alimentarius Commission. <http://www.fao.org/fao-who-codexalimentarius/codex-texts/list-standards/en/> Accessed January 2021.
8. EFSA Scientific Committee, et al. Update: use of the benchmark dose approach in risk assessment. *EFSA J*. 2017;15(1):4658.
9. Randal AW. *Scientific Basis for Setting Food Standards Through Codex Alimentarius*. Rome: Food, Nutrition and Agriculture; 2002:7–14.
10. WHO. *Principles and methods for the risk assessment of chemicals in food. Environmental Health Criteria 240*. Geneva, Switzerland: World Health Organization; 2009.
11. ANMAT. Ministry of Health (Ministerio de Salud) and The National Administration of Drugs, Foods, and Medical Technology (Administración Nacional de Medicamentos, Alimentos y Tecnología Médica). VISTO el Decreto N-1269/92y el expediente Nº 2020–16.628/92-1 del registro de la Secretaria de Salud del Ministerio de Salud y Accion Social, y [History], Buenos Aires: República Argentina. <http://www.anmat.gov.ar/webanmat/Legislacion/NormasGenerales/Decreto_1490-1992.pdf>; 1992 Accessed January 2021.
12. Punt A, et al. Non-animal approaches for toxicokinetics in risk evaluations of food chemicals. *ALTEX*. 2017;34(4):501–514.
13. [CONAL] La Comisión Nacional de Alimentos (National Committee of Food). Reglamento go to Guia. [Internet]. Buenos Aires: República Argentina; 2011. <www.conal.gov.ar>.
14. FSANZ, Food Standards Australia New Zealand. Canberra, Australia: Foods Standards Australia New Zealand. <https://www.foodstandards.gov.au/Pages/default.aspx>; 2019 Accessed November 2020.
15. ANVISA. Ministry of Health (Ministério da Saude) through its regulatory agency Agencia Nacional de Vigilancia Sanitária (ANVISA—National Agency of Sanitary Surveillance) [Internet], Brasilia: Agência Nacional de Vigilância Sanitária. <https://www.gov.br/anvisa/pt-br> Accessed January 2021.
16. Lobach AR, Roberts A, Rowland IR. Assessing the in vivo data on low/no-calorie sweeteners and the gut microbiota. *Food Chem Toxicol*. 2019;124:385–399.
17. Health Canada (HC) Food Directorate. Ottawa, ON: Health Canada. <https://www.canada.ca/en/health-canada/corporate/about-health-canada/branches-agencies/health-products-food-branch/food-directorate.htm> Accessed January 2021.
18. Ministry of Health of the People's Republic of China. Beijing, China; 2021. <http://english.gov.cn/2005-10/09/content_75326.htm> Accessed January 2021.
19. European Commission (EC) Directorate General for Health and Food Safety [Internet], Brussels, Belgium: European Commission. <https://ec.europa.eu/food/safety_en> Accessed December 2020.
20. MHLW. *Ministry of Health, Labor and Welfare, Japan*. [Internet]. Tokyo, Japan: Ministry of Health, Labor and Welfare, Japan. <https://www.mhlw.go.jp/english/> Accessed December 2020.
21. JETRO. Specifications, and Standards for Foods, Food Additives, etc. Under the Food Sanitation Act 2011. Tokyo, Japan: Japan External Trade Organization (JETRO). <https://www.jetro.go.jp/ext_images/en/reports/regulations/pdf/foodext2010e.pdf> Accessed January 2021.
22. US Food and Drug Administration. Silver Spring, MD: US Food and Drug Administration. <https://www.fda.gov/food/food-ingredients-packaging/>; 2020 Accessed December 2020.
23. EFSA Panel on Food Additives and Nutrient Sources added to Food (ANS). Guidance for submission for food additive evaluations. *EFSA J*. 2012;10(7):2760.
24. Mercosur. [Internet], Braslia: Mercosur. <http://www.mercosul.gov.br/> Accessed January 2021.
25. WHO. *Natural Toxins in Food (Factsheet)*. Geneva, Switzerland: World Health Organization; 2018. <https://www.who.int/news-room/fact-sheets/detail/natural-toxins-in-food> Accessed 10.02.20.
26. Rulis AM, Levitt JA. FDA'S food ingredient approval process: safety assurance based on scientific assessment. *Regul Toxicol Pharmacol*. 2009;53(1):20–31.
27. Neltner TG, Kulkarni NR, Alger HM, et al. Navigating the U.S. food additive regulatory program. *Comp Rev Food Sci Food Saf*. 2011;10:342–368.
28. U.S. Government Accountability Office. FDA should strengthen its oversight of food ingredients determined to be generally recognized as safe (GRAS). <https://www.gao.gov/products/A88948>; 2010 Accessed January 2021.
29. Faustman C, et al. Ten years post-GAO assessment, FDA remains uninformed of potentially harmful GRAS substances in foods. *Crit Rev Food Sci Nutr*. 2021;61(8):1260–1268.
30. Serrano J, et al. High-dose saccharin supplementation does not induce gut microbiota changes or glucose intolerance in healthy humans and mice. *Microbiome*. 2021;9(1):11.
31. Tu PC, et al. Gut microbiome toxicity: connecting the environment and gut microbiome-associated diseases. *Toxics*. 2020;8(1):19.
32. EFSA, et al., Animal Health Risk Assessment of Multiple Chemicals in Essential Oils for Farm Animals. EFSA Supporting publication (EN-1760); 2020:1760.

Chapter 12

Direct addition of flavors, including taste and flavor modifiers

Ivonne M.C.M. Rietjens[1], Samuel M. Cohen[2], Gerhard Eisenbrand[3], Shoji Fukushima[4], Nigel J. Gooderham[5], F. Peter Guengerich[6], Stephen S. Hecht[7], Thomas J. Rosol[8], Matthew J. Linman[9], Christie L. Harman[9] and Sean V. Taylor[9]

[1]*Division of Toxicology, Wageningen University, Wageningen, The Netherlands,* [2]*Department of Pathology and Microbiology, University of Nebraska Medical Center, Omaha, NE, United States,* [3]*Food Chemistry and Toxicology, University of Kaiserslautern, Heidelberg, Germany,* [4]*Japan Bioassay Research Center, Hadano, Kanagawa, Japan,* [5]*Department of Metabolism, Digestion and Reproduction, Imperial College London, London, United Kingdom,* [6]*Department of Biochemistry, Vanderbilt University School of Medicine, Nashville, TN, United States,* [7]*Masonic Cancer Center and Department of Laboratory Medicine and Pathology, University of Minnesota, Minneapolis, MN, United States,* [8]*Department of Biomedical Sciences, Heritage College of Osteopathic Medicine, Ohio University, Athens, OH, United States,* [9]*Flavor and Extract Manufacturers Association, Washington, DC, United States*

Abstract

The addition of flavorings to food and beverages provides practically unlimited opportunities for innovation, for maintaining and enhancing palatability, and is one essential element of a stable supply of nutritious consumer products. A safety evaluation by the Flavor and Extract Manufacturers Association (FEMA) Expert Panel provides a pathway for flavor producers and users to achieve regulatory authority to use for substances under the conditions of intended use as a flavoring. This chapter describes the factors that contribute to the safety assessment process that is conducted by the Expert Panel, and provides examples of specific flavorings and types of flavorings that are considered. The chapter also describes future issues and opportunities likely to be encountered within the context of the FEMA generally recognized as safe assessment of flavorings.

Keywords: Flavor; food flavorings; risk assessment; safety evaluation; exposure; toxicity; natural flavoring complexes

12.1 Introduction

Since ancient times herbs, spices, and other flavoring materials have been used to flavor foods to make them more alluring or improve their palatability. Over time and with the advent of a flavor-producing industry, flavors added to foods now also include, for example, natural extracts, mixtures distilled from natural sources, and single chemical substances with flavoring properties (whether isolated from a natural source or synthesized in a laboratory setting). Additionally, advances in chemical synthesis and the identification and cloning of taste receptors have resulted in the introduction of flavorings that are not found in nature and that have been created to exert specific flavor effects, such as modifying the impact of other flavorings within foods.

Given that all these flavorings are intentionally added to our food, there is a need for their premarket safety evaluation and postmarket vigilance. The safety evaluation of flavors in the United States started within the framework of the 1958 Food Additives Amendment to the United States Federal Food, Drug, and Cosmetics Act. The origins and early work of the Flavor and Extract Manufacturers Association (FEMA) Expert Panel have been reviewed.[1] This initial work resulted in a 1965 publication that provided the first list of 1124 flavorings that the FEMA Expert Panel considered generally recognized as safe (GRAS).[2] Since 1965 the FEMA Expert Panel has continued to publish its findings related to the GRAS evaluations of flavors.[3–5]

Within Europe, the formal safety evaluation and regulation of food flavors started in 1970 with a Council of Europe Expert Committee. This work resulted in the 1973 publication of the "Blue Book," which presented a list of permitted flavoring substances,[a] while it is only since 2012 that regulation European Union (EU) 872/2012 came into force containing a list of flavoring substances that can be used in food in the EU,[6] based on safety

Present Knowledge in Food Safety. DOI: https://doi.org/10.1016/B978-0-12-819470-6.00074-3

evaluations by the European Food Safety Authority (EFSA). This list is commonly referred to as the "Union List." The food industry can only use chemically defined flavoring substances in the EU that are on the Union List as outlined in Regulation EU 872/2012. Transitional measures for other flavorings such as those made from non-food sources to be evaluated and authorized later were established in Regulation EU 873/2012, which was amended by Regulation EU 2018/1259. In addition, other expert scientific bodies, for example, the Joint Food and Agriculture Organization of the United Nations (FAO)/WHO Expert Committee on Food Additives (JECFA), and national regulatory agencies, including the Japanese Food Safety Commission (JFSC) and the UK Food Standards Agency, among others, have established programs for the safety evaluation of food flavors.

The present chapter provides an overview of the type of flavors used in food and the procedures generally used for their safety evaluation. It also presents some examples illustrating these principles.

12.2 Types of flavors

Based on the definition provided by the Codex Alimentarius Guidelines for the Use of Flavorings (CAC/GL 66-2008), food flavorings are "products that are added to food to impart, modify, or enhance the flavor of food with the exception of flavor enhancers considered as food additives under the Codex Class Names and the International Numbering System for Food Additives—CAC/GL 36-1989. Flavorings do not include substances that have an exclusively sweet, sour, or salty taste (e.g., sugar, vinegar, and table salt). Flavorings may consist of flavoring substances, natural flavoring complexes, thermal process flavorings, or smoke flavorings and mixtures of them and may contain non-flavoring food ingredients within defined conditions such as carriers, solvents, etc. Flavorings are not intended to be consumed as such."

This implies that the universe of flavorings can consist of individual compounds (referred to as chemically defined flavorings) found within and isolated from natural sources, chemically defined flavorings that are identical to those found in nature but created using nonnatural methods, chemically defined flavorings not found in nature, complex mixtures used as flavoring ingredients (commonly referred to as natural flavoring complexes, or NFCs), process flavorings or smoke flavorings. Examples of chemically defined flavorings that have been identified from natural sources include benzaldehyde (almond flavor), isoamyl acetate (banana), limonene (citrus), methyl anthranilate (grape), and allyl hexanoate (pineapple). While found in nature, many of these are now synthesized using simple chemical building blocks, as this is typically a more efficient method to prepare flavorings of suitable purity and identity. This group of flavorings consists of about 1700 substances. It also provides the chemical starting point for about 350 chemically defined substances that are not found in nature but are structurally related to naturally occurring flavoring substances. One such flavoring is cinnamyl propionate which is structurally related to cinnamyl acetate and cinnamyl butyrate; all provide a cinnamon tone with different intensity, for example, from a mild cinnamon undertone and mostly fruity and/or floral aroma, to strong cinnamon aroma with mild fruit or floral tones.

The second group of flavorings consists of NFCs which are complex mixtures obtained from plants or other natural sources via various extraction methods. This group includes commonly known essential oils, such as citrus oils (lemon, lime, orange), mint oils (peppermint, spearmint), and oils derived from culinary spices (cloves, cinnamon, ginger, allspice, black pepper). Another group are extracts derived from botanicals, such as vanilla extract obtained from vanilla pods. Essential oils are NFCs produced by distillation and hence are composed of volatile compounds with only trace amounts of nonvolatile constituents, if at all detectable. In contrast, NFCs produced by extraction contain both volatile and nonvolatile constituents (vanilla extract). About 300 NFCs have been defined that are used as food flavorings in almost all food categories. Most NFCs contain hundreds of chemically identified volatile constituents, only a few of which generally being responsible for the flavor effect of the NFC.

Process flavorings are produced by heating precursor substances in a carefully controlled reaction/process to create a complex mixture of flavoring substances. These flavoring mixtures are generated mainly via the Maillard reaction, which normally occurs when food is heated. Smoke flavorings are extracted from smoke and produce flavors that mimic the flavor experience from consuming foods that are smoked using traditional methods. In the safety assessment all categories of food flavorings present their own challenges, although the applied procedures share common considerations. In the following sections, these aspects will be discussed in more detail.

12.3 Levels of use and uses

The GRAS concept establishes the safety of flavors at their intended use and use levels. Thus procedures for their safety assessment require information on uses and intended levels of use. Each safety dossier that is evaluated must contain detailed information on the food categories in which a flavor is intended to be used and the anticipated average usual and maximum usual use levels. These data can be used for the exposure assessment that forms an integral part of the safety assessment and can be performed as outlined in the next section. Within the safety evaluation the actual proposed maximum levels of use are often limited because of palatability issues (i.e., use at higher levels in the final food product would result in intolerable taste perception). In addition, maximum use levels may have to be limited for flavorings that possess modifying properties to comply with the requirement that they should not have inherent sweetness or saltiness under conditions of intended use in the finished food product. This requirement originates from the fact that the Codex Alimentarius definition of flavorings excludes compounds with exclusively sweet, sour or salty taste.[7] In the United States, a substance that would impart sweetness at the intended levels of use is excluded from the definition of flavoring substances as evaluated within the FEMA GRAS process.[8] A substance that has, for example, inherent sweetness (or as other examples, imparts an exclusively salty or sour effect) at intended levels of use would instead be considered a non-flavoring food ingredient that would be subject to a different approval process.[b] Evaluation of the proposed intended use and use levels of flavorings with modifying properties, also called flavor modifiers, generally requires sensory testing, including a test to demonstrate that the compound does not have inherent sweetness or saltiness under the conditions of intended use. This test includes sensory testing of the compound in water or a suitable substitute matrix, against the threshold of sweetness (1.5% sucrose in a water base) or saltiness (0.25% sodium chloride in a water base) to establish if the proposed use levels are less sweet or salty than these thresholds.[8] For other matrices, specific threshold levels for sucrose and/or sodium chloride can be established to perform the test to confirm the lack of inherent sweetness/saltiness up to the maximum intended level of use as a flavoring. For flavorings with modifying properties the maximum use level in a food category can be set at the highest level at which the substance to be evaluated is inherently less sweet than 1.5% sucrose and/or less salty than 0.25% sodium chloride references in the relevant matrix.

12.4 Exposure assessment

The exposure assessment is an essential element of the safety evaluation process for food flavorings. It is also the part of a safety evaluation where the most significant degree of uncertainty is often found. This is reflected by the many procedures available for exposure assessment of food flavors and the ongoing debate about the method of choice for estimating flavor exposure. This is in part caused by the fact that although suggested typical and possible maximum use levels for all food categories are part of the dossier submitted for safety evaluation, these levels are generally estimates by flavorists as to what concentrations would ultimately be found in a final food product. This uncertainty results from the fact that approved flavorings are not applied as such but rather are formulated into compounded flavors, combinations of flavors designed to imitate a natural flavor or heighten a flavor experience. Compounded flavors are then incorporated into final food products by food manufacturers. Notably final food products could in some cases include multiple compounded flavor formulations. Additional challenges are presented by the fact that there are over 20,000 different food products available to consumers, almost 3000 flavor ingredients that have been approved for use in food, and food (and thus flavor consumption) is nonhomogeneous across consumer populations. As a result of these complexities, obtaining accurate intake estimates from dietary analysis for diverse eater populations has proven difficult.[9]

Several methods have been defined and used over the years to estimate daily exposure to flavorings and have been extensively covered in a recent review.[10] These methods can generally be divided into two categories: volume-based methods and use level–based methods.

12.4.1 Volume-based methods for exposure assessment

The volume-based method used by the FEMA Expert Panel calculates the so-called *per capita* intake (PCI) based on the annual volume of production (poundage) of the flavoring of interest in the United States. For new flavorings under evaluation for GRAS status in the United States, the annual volume is estimated by the industry member submitting the GRAS application for the potential flavoring under review. For substances for which GRAS status has already been attained, industry surveys that provide annual volume of use data for flavorings are performed on a regular basis.[10–13] This industry-wide data can be used to provide helpful postmarket monitoring of flavoring usage and exposure. The FEMA Expert Panel regularly reevaluates flavorings with uses in food determined as FEMA GRAS based on increases in use as determined from industry surveys.

Based on the annual volume of use for a flavor, whether it is anticipated in a premarket setting or based on the reported volume of use, the PCI in μg/person/day is calculated as follows:

$$\text{PCI} = \frac{\text{Annual volume (United States)} \times 10^9}{\text{CF} \times \text{population (United States)} \times \text{days}}$$

where: PCI, μg/person/day; annual volume (United States), kg/year; 10^9, unit conversion, μg/kg; CF, correction factor, unitless (see below); population, number of persons; days, 365 days/year.

A correction factor (CF) of 0.6 or 0.8 has been applied when calculating exposure based on anticipated volume or reported volume, respectively. In general, this CF accounts for the fact that while industry surveys gather data from the majority of the industry, some fraction of the industry does not provide data. In a typical volume of use survey, flavor manufacturers comprising more than 90% of the flavor industry respond to the survey, but a CF of 0.8 (assuming that companies covering 80% of the market have responded) has been applied to ensure a conservative approach.[14] For those new flavorings undergoing evaluation by the FEMA Expert Panel, a more conservative CF of 0.6 is used.[14]

The PCI provides an intake estimate based on the assumption that the consumption of the flavor is spread among the entire population. The FEMA Expert Panel has concluded that this assumption is likely valid for flavors with a high reported volume of use (greater than 22,700 kg/year). For flavors with a reported volume of use less than 22,700 kg (50,000 lb) it is assumed that consumption will be distributed among only 10% of the entire population.[14] For these lower-volume flavorings the PCI is multiplied by 10 to account for the fact that a 10% "eaters only" population is consuming the flavoring, and the exposure value is referred to as the PCI × 10.[15,16] JECFA applies the same "eaters only" assumption in its volume-based approach to estimate exposure and refers to it as the maximized survey-derived daily intake (MSDI).[17] In Europe, from 2000 onward,[18] the MSDI was also used for volume-based flavoring exposure estimates. In the EU the MSDI is calculated as follows:

$$\text{MSDI} = \frac{\text{Annual volume (EU)} \times 10^9}{\text{CF} \times \text{population (EU)} \times 0.1 \times \text{days}}$$

where: MSDI, μg/person/day; annual volume (based on volumes from EU volume of use surveys), kg/year; 10^9, unit conversion, μg/kg; CF, correction factor, unitless, and based on the response rate from the national and/or regional volume of use survey; population, number of persons; 0.1, 10% of the population; days, 365 days/year.

This formula is comparable to the PCI × 10 as it uses the number of consumers estimated to be 10% of the total population, regardless of the scale of the annual volume. The applied CF depends on the response rate for the surveyed region and considers that industry survey data on poundage may be incomplete.

12.4.2 Use level–based methods for exposure assessment

In addition to volume-based methods, several use level–based methods for flavor exposure assessment have also been developed, each with advantages and disadvantages. One use level–based approach is the so-called "possible average daily intake" (PADI) method.[19] The PADI is based on the intended mean use level of the flavor ingredient for 34 defined food categories, combined with the amounts of those foods consumed. Another method, the theoretical added maximum daily intake (TAMDI),[20] which was used in Europe, is based on the same approach as the PADI method but uses 18 food categories (that are then summed over seven food groupings) instead of 34 different food and beverage categories as well as maximum use levels. TAMDI utilizes the intake data from the 1988 Dietary and Nutritional Survey of British adults and maximum instead of mean intended use levels.[21] Analysis of the accuracy of these methods, when compared to actual intake data, indicates that the PADI and TAMDI approaches dramatically overestimate daily consumer exposures.[9,22] The overestimates are primarily because these methods estimate the consumer intake by multiplying the average or maximum intended use level for the flavoring in all 33 food categories or seven food groups with the average amount consumed of that food category/group on a daily basis, subsequently adding up the intake over all the food categories.[4,9] These approaches assume that all food categories are consumed daily and that all foods in a food category always contain the flavoring under evaluation at the proposed use levels.[19,22,23] This is usually not the case; proposed use levels are often not the actual levels consumed. For instance, due to the volatile loss of flavors during food processing, such as by heating or baking, application levels may be significantly higher than the levels of flavorings present in the final food product.[22] Additionally, even within the same food category, use levels vary significantly depending upon the specific food matrix in which the flavoring is used and whether the flavoring provides a dominant or supporting flavor note. Additionally, flavorings are used to impart a specific flavor to the food to which it is added and would not be used in all food products in a given food category (e.g., a blueberry yogurt would not contain a flavoring that imparts a chocolate flavor). The exaggeration of intake by the PADI and TAMDI methods is supported by the fact that these intake estimates, for the vast majority of flavors, would require annual production volumes that exceed the actual yearly production volumes of the flavors by up to four orders of magnitude, especially for the flavors with low reported annual poundage.[9,22,24,25]

Studies of actual flavor intake based on detailed dietary analysis of large groups of consumers confirmed that actual intakes are likely closer to the values obtained using volume-based methods than to values obtained by the PADI or TAMDI methods [9,23,26] Comparison of PADI or TAMDI values to those obtained by the PCI × 10 method revealed that the PADI and TAMDI approaches overestimate the intake by three orders of magnitude, especially for low volume flavoring substances.[9,24,25]

Only for high volume flavoring substances (e.g., with volume > 22,700 kg/year) was the PADI comparable to the PCI × 10.[9]

To account for this overestimation of daily intake by the PADI and TAMDI use level–based methods, other use level–based methods have been developed, including the modified TAMDI (mTAMDI) approach that EFSA introduced in 2004,[27] the single-portion exposure technique (SPET) developed by JECFA in its 2006 and 2007 meetings[24,28] and the added portion exposure technique (APET),[29] that was included in the joint EFSA-FAO 2011 guidance.[30] The mTAMDI differs from the TAMDI in that it uses average intended use levels instead of the maximum intended use levels.[27,31] The mTAMDI still presents a very conservative intake estimate since it (1) aggregates exposure from 18 food categories into seven larger food groups, (2) assumes that the flavoring is present in all foods within a food category, and (3) that all food categories are consumed every day. The SPET method, which JECFA now employs alongside the MSDI approach, does not sum all exposures per food category but instead considers only the food subcategory among 83 subcategories (under 16 primary food categories) that results in the highest potential dietary exposure calculated from the intended average ("usual") use levels of a flavor reported (using the food categorization system of the Codex General Standard on Food Additives).[24,28,29] Similar to SPET, the APET method that EFSA now uses for exposure estimates within the Common Authorization Procedure (CAP) submissions,[32] adds the highest potential dietary consumption within the "Beverages" and the "Solid foods" groups. The SPET and APET methods were developed to estimate exposure for a regular consumer loyal to a specific food and/or specific beverage, which are both assumed to contain the flavoring under consideration, which is quite conservative given the likelihood of addition for low volume flavorings is quite low.

12.5 Safety evaluation

When the estimated daily exposure to a food flavoring has been quantified, the corresponding risk assessment compares these exposure data to a relevant point of departure that results from the hazard assessment of the flavor of interest. This risk, or safety assessment of flavorings, differs from that of most food additives in that it uses a group-based/read-across approach based on structure-activity relationships. The group-based approach utilizes the structural similarities between various flavorings, allowing flavorings to be grouped based on chemical/structural relations. Read-across of relevant biological data (e.g., toxicological study results, metabolic outcomes) between the flavorings within a group avoids the extensive animal-based testing that would otherwise be required for all individual flavorings. Both JECFA and EFSA have evaluated the safety of flavoring substances within groups of structurally and metabolically related substances. JECFA assigns flavoring substances into 58 groups.[33] New flavoring substance evaluations by JECFA are published as addenda to existing group evaluations. EFSA reorganized JECFA's groups into 34 groups of flavorings in the EU market according to their chemical structure and denoted their safety evaluations as "Flavor Group Evaluations".[18] This grouping and the accompanying chemical group designation (EC-CG 1-34) has been included in the European Commission Regulation (EC) No 1565/2000, Annex 1.[18] The safety evaluation of flavoring substances belonging to the same chemical group has been based on data for substances determined to represent the whole group or subgroups of higher structural similarity within larger groups. With the advent of the Common Authorization Procedure (CAP), EFSA still uses the read-across concept to provide supporting data for flavorings under review. Still, each flavoring is typically considered within the results of its own evaluation.

Other safety assessment bodies have adopted similar approaches to the use of "read-across," including for example the JFSC. In all cases the use of read-across relies primarily upon an expert judgment of the above considerations (structure, likely metabolic outcomes, and toxic potential), but there is increasing interest in identifying additional support for read-across via in silico methods.[34]

Another general characteristic in which safety evaluation of flavors differs from that of food additives is that the generally low levels of use and the correspondingly low exposure levels enable the use of the threshold of toxicological concern (TTC) concept. This concept assumes that a certain level of exposure is insignificant from a toxicological point of view. A low level of exposure with a negligible risk can be defined based on knowledge of only the chemical structure of the compound under consideration. If the estimated daily exposure is below the TTC, further safety testing would not be required. The FEMA Expert Panel as well as JECFA and EFSA utilize the TTC concept in their flavor safety evaluations. Use of chemical grouping, read-across, and the TTC approach are essential characteristics of the safety evaluation of all types of flavoring substances, including individual compounds, NFCs, process flavorings, or smoke flavorings. In the following sections some further details on the safety evaluation of these groups of flavorings are provided.

12.5.1 Safety evaluation of individual flavor compounds

The safety assessment of individual flavor compounds includes thorough evaluation of all the available data on the candidate flavor ingredient and structurally related substances in the same chemical group. This includes information on chemical specifications, metabolism, toxicity, and genotoxicity of the substance and its structural relatives. The safety evaluation uses the TTC to evaluate if estimated daily exposure resulting from intended uses exceeds the TTC relevant for the Cramer Class into which the compound under consideration has been assigned.[35] Three TTC values have been defined for compounds that do not raise a concern for genotoxicity and belong to one of the three Cramer classes: Cramer Class I, II, or III. The Cramer class for a compound can be determined by answering a series of questions on its structural characteristics embedded within a so-called "decision tree."[35] In recent years computer programs to assign a compound to a Cramer Class based on its chemical structure have been developed. They include, for example, ToxTree (http://toxtree.sourceforge.net/),[36] which has been adopted for use in Europe by the European Commission Joint Research Center (https://ec.europa.eu/jrc/en/scientific-tool/toxtree-tool). The TTC for Cramer Class I compounds, including flavorings for which the chemical structure suggests low toxicity and an initial presumption of safety, amounts to 1800 μg/person/day. For flavorings in Cramer Class II which are of expected intermediate toxicity a TTC of 540 μg/person/day applies, and for Cramer Class III which contains compounds with no initial presumption on safety because they contain structural alerts for toxicity a TTC of 90 μg/person/day has been defined.[37–39] These TTC values are based on a bodyweight of 60 kg and the 5th percentiles of the distribution of no observed adverse effect level (NOAEL) values of substances in each class with an additional 100-fold safety factor, resulting in a highly conservative threshold for each class.[37–39]

Additional toxicity data would not be required when the estimated daily intake of a flavoring substance resulting from its intended use and use levels remains below the relevant TTC. A prerequisite for this approach is that the substance does not raise concerns for genotoxicity. However, for compounds with a structural alert for genotoxicity based on tumor data for a large set of genotoxic carcinogens, a TTC of 0.15 μg/person/day has been established.[38] This TTC can be applied to compounds that do not belong to one of the TTC-excluded classes including high potency carcinogens such as aflatoxin-like, azoxy- or *N*-nitroso-compounds and benzidines, certain inorganic substances, metals and organometallics, certain proteins, steroids, known or predicted bio-accumulators, nanomaterials, and radioactive materials.[38,40] When individual flavor compounds raise concern for genotoxicity that could ultimately manifest as adverse human health effects (e.g., carcinogenicity) and exceed the relevant TTC, they are generally not considered suitable for flavor use. However, a positive in vitro genotoxicity result has to be evaluated within the framework of all available data especially because several factors—including negative results in subsequent in vivo genotoxicity assays for either the compound itself or for its structural analogs, inconsistent data, additional negative in vitro results, considerations on the underlying mode of action, and/or arguments pointing at possible false positives resulting from cytotoxicity—may overrule these initial concerns.[41–44]

When the estimated daily intake of a proposed flavor ingredient exceeds the TTC of its relevant Cramer Class the safety evaluation must be based on experimental data from toxicity studies conducted on the substance and/or its structural analogs. In these subsequent considerations it is evaluated whether an adequate margin of safety exists between the NOAELs or, if NOAELs are absent, the lowest observed adverse effect levels (LOAELs) available for the compound under consideration or its structural analogs and the estimated consumer intake. Determining whether a margin of safety is adequate to conclude on the safe use of a flavor at its intended uses and use levels depends on expert judgment. Given the self-limiting nature of most flavorings the estimated daily intake under the intended conditions of use of a food flavoring is generally low enough to either be below the relevant TTC and, if not, to result in margins of safety that amount to several orders of magnitude. For example, ethyl vanillin had a reported poundage of 435,000 kg in the 2015 FEMA Poundage and Technical Effect Survey,[10] resulting in an intake based on PCI of 77 μg/kg bw/day. Based on a good laboratory practice (GLP), 90-day repeated dose oral toxicity study of ethyl vanillin in rats,[45] a NOAEL was assigned at 500 mg/kg bw/day, thus resulting in a margin of safety of >6000. Thus, even for a large volume flavor the margin of safety is often substantial.

When considering individual flavor compounds their assumed or known metabolic fate is also taken into account, evaluating whether the chemical may be expected to be converted to innocuous products and readily excreted. This group-based approach using the TTC is common to the safety evaluations performed by the different regulatory bodies when evaluating individual flavor compounds. Subtle differences exist in evaluating all available data as a whole using a weight-of-evidence approach or evaluating the different aspects in a stepwise approach in which further evaluation of the compound may be postponed until additional data become available. This subtle difference becomes most evident in the review of genotoxicity data, for example, the FEMA Expert Panel, JECFA, and EFSA may all conclude that evidence for in vivo genotoxicity raises a concern, but the EFSA stepwise approach may prevent further evaluation of the flavoring while JECFA and the FEMA Expert Panel would evaluate the genotoxicity data within the framework of all other data before concluding on the safety in use.[44,46,47] Despite this, all the safety evaluations use a weight-of-evidence approach integrating all data relevant for a particular endpoint of interest, for example genotoxicity, including considerations on the mode of action, the relevance of an observation for the human situation, data quality, and sources of uncertainty and their impact on the assessment outcome.[44]

It is of interest to note that a recent evaluation of the available data on genotoxicity of individual flavor ingredients revealed that the majority of flavor ingredients have given negative results in all in vitro and/or in vivo genotoxicity/mutagenicity tests conducted on them.[44] Of the limited positive responses reported for flavor ingredients most were obtained from older, often obsolete genotoxicity assays that fall short of current testing guidelines or are no longer in use due to inherent limitations.[44] It has also been argued that the statistical probability of 5% false-positive outcomes at the 95% confidence level typically used in statistical analysis of test results is likely to result in a higher chance for positive responses with a larger number of in vitro genotoxicity tests conducted on a substance.[42,43] This may also be one reason why positive results for a flavor ingredient in an in vitro assay are most often not confirmed in a subsequent in vivo study.[33,44]

12.5.2 Safety evaluation of natural flavoring complexes

The safety evaluation of NFCs essentially uses the same concepts as outlined above for the safety evaluation of individual flavoring substances. However, the complex nature of the NFCs, their many constituents, and the potential presence of unidentified constituents require additional considerations. The procedure for the safety evaluation for NFCs has been described in detail in publications of the FEMA Expert Panel[25,48] with a recent update.[14] The procedure is based on a thorough identification of the chemical composition of the NFC and evaluation of the chemical and biological properties of the constituents (Fig. 12.1).

The updated approach[14] includes a more detailed assessment of unidentified constituents. In this updated procedure the NFC passes through a 14-step process. In Step 1 data are gathered and the consumption of the NFC as a flavor relative to intake from the natural source when consumed as food is assessed. For example, based on the percent volatile oil in the cassia/cinnamon spice, an estimated 348,000 kg of cassia/cinnamon oil would be expected to be consumed in the United States per year by

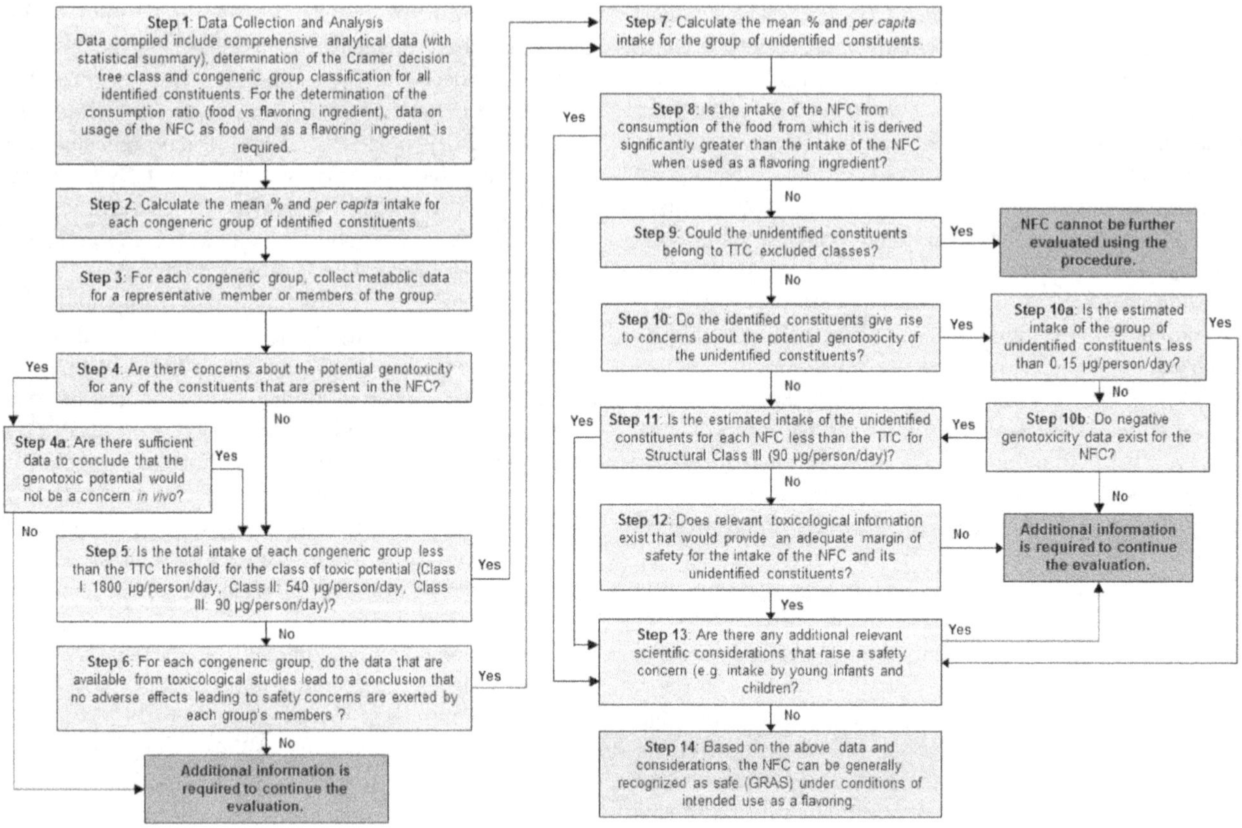

FIGURE 12.1 Revised procedure for the safety evaluation of natural flavoring complexes. *Reproduced from Cohen SM, Eisenbrand G, Fukushima S, et al. Updated procedure for the safety evaluation of natural flavor complexes used as ingredients in food. Food Chem Toxicol. 2018;113:171–178. https://doi.org/10.1016/j.fct.2018.01.021.*

consuming the cinnamon spice, which is significantly higher than the most recent volume for cassia bark oil as a flavor ingredient (26,200 kg).[49]

In this first step of the NFC safety evaluation the identified constituents are ordered into congeneric groups containing constituents with similar structural characteristics expected to share similar kinetic and toxicological properties. Given that the metabolic pathways in plants and other natural sources from which NFCs are obtained are limited, the 36 congeneric groups appear to be sufficient to sort the NFC constituents.[14] In the subsequent steps the safety assessment of the NFC is based on evaluation of the daily estimated exposure from each congeneric group, summing up the exposure of its constituents and assigning to the group the Cramer Class of the constituent in the group with the Cramer Class of most significant concern. In Steps 2 through 6 the exposure and potential toxicity of the identified constituents sorted in their congeneric groups are evaluated using the TTC concept and scientific data on metabolism and toxicity for each congeneric group. This includes the evaluation of potential genotoxicity. For most congeneric groups sufficient data from in vitro and in vivo genotoxicity testing on relevant constituents are available to exclude concerns over genotoxicity for the whole group.[50] However, given that NFCs are extracts from plants and other natural sources the presence of compounds of concern with respect to genotoxicity and/or carcinogenicity can sometimes not be avoided. This holds for example for NFCs derived from plants like basil (*Ocimum basilicum*), fennel (*Foeniculum vulgare*), and nutmeg (*Myristica fragrans*) that may contain a substantial amount of hydroxyallylbenzene and hydroxypropenylbenzene derivatives, including compounds like safrole, estragole, and/or methyl eugenol.[51–53] These natural constituents may raise concern because they have been shown to yield DNA adduct formation and induce liver tumors at high dose levels in experimental animals.[53–59] To assess the safety of NFCs containing these constituents, in the first instance the TTC approach can still be applied to the respective congeneric group, where a TTC of 0.15 μg/person/day has been established for compounds with a structural alert for genotoxicity as covered earlier.[38]

Since these hydroxyallylbenzene and hydroxypropenylbenzene constituents do not belong to a TTC-excluded class, the exposure resulting from the use of the NFC at intended use and use levels can be compared to the TTC of 0.15 μg/person/day. When exposure to the respective congeneric group in the NFC is below this TTC, the presence of these constituents does not raise a safety concern. In cases where exposure exceeds the TTC the exposure can be evaluated using the margin of exposure (MOE) approach developed for compounds that are both genotoxic and carcinogenic.[60,61] In this approach the MOE is defined as the ratio between the lower confidence limit of the benchmark dose associated with a 10% increase in tumor incidence above background level ($BMDL_{10}$), a value that can be derived from available tumor data, and the estimated daily intake. When the MOE for intake of the compound and/or congeneric group of concern is above 10,000, the respective exposure would not raise a safety concern.[61] An example is clove bud oil, which contains methyl eugenol. Based on the estimated intake of methyl eugenol resulting from use of clove bud as a flavor and a previously published $BMDL_{10}$ of 22.2 mg/kg bw/day for methyl eugenol,[62,63] the MOE for this intake of methyl eugenol from use of clove bud oil is >1,400,000.[64] It should be noted that at the time of this publication, the FEMA Expert Panel was conducting a GRAS re-evaluation of the group of NFCs containing the hydroxyallylbenzene and hydroxypropenylbenzene constituents and will apply a new $BMDL_{10}$ value derived from updated BMD calculation approaches.

After evaluating the safety of all the groups of identified constituents present in an NFC, Steps 7–12 of the procedure address the potential toxicity and genotoxicity, of the group of unidentified constituents. Formally, the TTC for general toxicity cannot be applied to unidentified constituents because the TTC approach is based on the chemical structure of the constituent under consideration. However, similar to the proposal for the use of the TTC for the safety evaluation of unidentified constituents in nonintentionally added substances (NIAS) migrating from food contact materials into food,[65] the updated procedure for the safety evaluation of NFCs [14] considers the application of the TTC to the group of unidentified constituents present in NFCs provided they do not belong to a TTC excluded class. In line with what was proposed for unidentified NIAS,[65] it is evaluated whether the unidentified constituents in an NFC belong to a TTC excluded class based on (1) expert judgment on the product, contaminants, production process, packaging, transport, and storage; (2) basic analytical chemistry knowledge; (3) analytical chemistry approaches; and/or (4) bioassays.[14] Bioassays may be used to overcome concerns over genotoxicity, detect mixture effects, and/or ascertain that unidentified constituents do not belong to a TTC excluded class since they may detect compounds like aflatoxins using enzyme-linked immunosorbent assay (ELISA) or steroids, for instance by using reporter gene assays. For NFCs, the expert judgment reveals that their identified constituents provide information on the relevant biosynthetic pathways active in the botanical from which the NFC is derived. The constituents of an NFC are generally derived from the photosynthesis-driven pathways that generate primary and secondary plant constituents, such as the shikimic acid pathway and carbohydrate, lipid and protein biosynthesis, turnover, and storage, resulting in chemical profiles with predictable structural variation [66] and generally lacking structural alerts for genotoxicity. However, if the identified constituents of an NFC have a biologically relevant structural alert for genotoxicity, such as the presence of identified hydroxyallylbenzenes and hydroxypropenylbenzene derivatives, evaluation of the group of unknowns may be based on the TTC of 0.15 μg/person/day for compounds with a structural alert for genotoxicity, and/or applying the MOE approach with the value of 10,000 to evaluate potential concerns over the intake of the group of unidentified constituents and the $BMDL_{10}$ for the most active congener.[60,61] When a concern over genotoxicity for the group of unidentified constituents can be excluded, the TTC of Cramer Class III of 90 μg/person/day can be applied to evaluate the estimated daily exposure to the fraction of unknowns as a result of the use of the NFC under evaluation.

In the final Steps 13 and 14 of the procedure for safety evaluation of NFCs, the overall safety is evaluated along with considerations of potential biologically relevant interactions among constituents.[14] Children's exposure is also considered in this step, taking their lower body weight into account (see also section on future directions).

Although EFSA does not assess the safety of flavoring substances obtained from botanical sources, the evaluation of botanical materials for use in food supplements by EFSA depends on whether intake from these applications exceeds intake levels from historical use. If estimated intake exceeds historical use, existing information of adverse effects and additional data are required, including data for metabolism, toxicokinetic profile, and toxicological studies including genotoxicity.[67] When intake is comparable to historical human intake, the safety evaluation includes comparison with health-based guidance values, such as the acceptable daily intake (ADI) or tolerable daily intake (TDI) or application of the TTC. At the same time, the MOE approach is adopted for constituents with genotoxicity concerns, taking into account intake from all sources.[67] JECFA evaluates the safety of natural extracts in the context of their use as food additives but does not currently conduct safety assessments for NFCs. JECFA has carried out a pilot program to consider the safety evaluation of NFCs (JECFA, 2004) but has not yet finalized an NFC evaluation procedure (JECFA, 2004).

12.5.3 Safety evaluation of process flavors

As noted above, process flavorings are the product of heating starting materials under well-defined reaction conditions to produce a complex mixture of flavoring substances that are designed to mimic the flavor and aroma of cooked foods. Like home cooking, the heating/reaction process produces several types of chemicals mainly from Maillard reactions. The goal of process flavor manufacturers is to prepare such products safely and with high consistency from batch-to-batch and ensure that such products are safe for humans.

As with all flavors, the safety considerations for process flavors involve estimating the human exposure, appropriately characterizing the product (including the product consistency) and considering the metabolic impact and relevant toxicological information. Given the especially broad range of process flavors that are in use by the flavor and food industries, it was concluded that conducting FEMA GRAS on a one-by-one basis would not provide a timely and appropriate approach for the safety evaluation. As an alternative, the flavor industry undertook a program to provide relevant data to consider the safety of process flavors and then presented those data in a report to the FEMA Expert Panel.[68] This analytical testing program evaluated 102 process flavors commonly added to food in the United States for the presence of polycyclic heteroaromatic amines (PHAs).[68] No PHAs were detected in 90 out of 102 process flavor samples while only two samples detected the presence of a single PHA above the limit of detection. As a result of that work and considerations of all data that would be considered relevant for review within that context, The Expert Panel concluded that "process flavors do not present a safety concern under current conditions of use."[69]

12.5.4 Safety evaluation of smoke flavorings

Smoke flavorings are generally produced by thermal degradation of wood and extraction of the resulting smoke. They are added to foods to confer a smoked flavor. They may replace traditional smoking or be added to foods that would traditionally not be smoked. Since 2008 smoke flavors intended for use on the EU market have to be evaluated for their safety by the EFSA. The original guidance, and the more recently published, updated guidance for submitting a dossier on a smoke flavoring primary product for evaluation by EFSA outlines the details of the data required for the safety evaluation, including the toxicological tests required.[31,70] Given that the smoke flavors are complex mixtures, detailed chemical identification and quantification is needed, including quantification of the volatile fraction and the fraction of unidentified constituents as well as quantification of a series of 16 polycyclic aromatic hydrocarbons (PAHs), including the eight carcinogenic and genotoxic PAHs (PAH8) proposed by EFSA to be used for risk assessment of PAHs.[31] The toxicological data required for safety evaluation of smoke flavors consist in the first instance of a battery of tests to exclude concerns over genotoxicity and a 90-day feeding study in rats, according to OECD 408.[31] Provided concerns over genotoxicity can be excluded, this 90-day study should give the NOAEL (or LOAEL) to establish the margin of safety for the estimated human exposure resulting from the proposed uses and use levels. An exposure assessment is required to obtain these safety margins, preferably performed using a method specifically designed to assess the dietary exposure to smoke flavors.[31] Upon evaluating the suitability of the MSDI, SPET, and TAMDI/mTAMDI methods for exposure assessment outlined above, in the original guidance EFSA developed two methods for exposure assessment specifically for smoke flavors. This appeared necessary to evaluate the consequences of authorizing the smoke flavors in only traditionally smoked products. These methods are the so-called Smoke Flavoring Theoretical Added Maximum Daily Intake (SMK-TAMDI) and the Smoke Flavoring European Prospective Investigation into Cancer and Nutrition (EPIC) model (SMK-EPIC).[31] These two methods are both use level–based approaches. In the updated smoke flavoring guidance, EFSA has indicated that a new exposure estimation tool should be used, DietEx, to estimate chronic dietary exposure to substances present in food (e.g., intentionally added or naturally present chemicals, contaminants, proteins, novel food ingredients).[70]

In the SMK-TAMDI, dietary exposure is estimated using the intended upper use levels in 18 food categories combined with standard portion sizes. For the exposure assessment for each out of three food categories ("Beverages," "Traditionally smoked solid foods," and "Other solid foods not traditionally smoked") only the food category from the group resulting in the highest potential dietary exposure is considered for further evaluation. The SMK-TAMDI is calculated by summing these highest potential dietary exposures for the food category of each of the three food groups.

The SMK-EPIC method was developed because most food consumption surveys do not discriminate between smoked and nonsmoked foods and beverages, hampering the definition of portion sizes in the use level–based exposure assessments for smoke flavors. The SMK-EPIC method uses the food consumption data from the EPIC where consumption of smoked meat and several other food categories possibly being smoked were quantified.

Dietary exposure assessment by all five methods, including the two newly defined methods, provided exposure estimates in the same order of magnitude.[31] In subsequent risk assessments, EFSA used the SMK-TAMDI and SMK-EPIC methods to calculate the margins of exposure and conclusions on the safety in use of the respective smoke flavors. It remains to be seen how the exposure assessment tool for smoke flavors that has been referenced in the updated guidance will compare to either SMK-TAMDI or SMK-EPIC.

In the United States, in contrast to the EU, only two specific smoke flavors have gone through a safety evaluation conducted by the FEMA Expert Panel and have been granted FEMA GRAS status under conditions of use as a flavoring.

12.6 Examples

The following sections provide some examples to illustrate the principles underlying the safety assessment of the direct addition of flavors, including taste and flavor modifiers to food. These examples also illustrate the differences in the regulatory framework across international jurisdictions.

12.6.1 Diacetyl: generally recognized as safe implies safe at proposed uses and use levels

Diacetyl is used as a food flavor in the United States, Europe, and the rest of the world. It provides a "buttery flavor" to a wide range of foods including snack foods, candies, baked goods, flavored coffees, and popcorn. In 2000 the National Institute of Occupational Safety and Health recommended respiratory protection for all workers in microwave popcorn production because it was recognized that factory workers in popcorn processing factories could develop bronchiolitis obliterans, a rare type of lung disease.[71–74] For this reason, bronchiolitis obliterans is sometimes also referred to as "popcorn lung" or "popcorn workers lung." When in 2007 a consumer of relatively large amounts of microwaved popcorn presented the first known case of a consumer diagnosed with bronchiolitis obliterans this initiated a discussion on the GRAS status of diacetyl butter flavor, since evidence suggested that inhaling diacetyl fumes would be a potential cause of the disease.[71] Use as a flavor includes oral consumption but would not include inhaling the flavor from freshly microwaved popcorn bags. As a result, the GRAS status of diacetyl as a food flavoring was continued. While popcorn producers have announced their intention to replace diacetyl butter flavor with another flavoring, diacetyl is still considered safe for all approved uses and use levels in food, including the flavoring of microwave popcorn.

This example is a good illustration that conclusions on the safety of a food flavor relate to its intended use and use levels in food and its estimated daily exposure via oral consumption.

12.6.2 Coumarin: carcinogenicity threshold, remarkable species differences, and differences in regulation between the European Union and United States

Coumarin is a naturally occurring flavoring substance and a notable ingredient within some NFCs, including cassia cinnamon and lavender.[75] Long-term studies in mice and rats at high oral dose levels resulted in induction of liver and lung tumors associated with hepatic and pulmonary toxicity. Because of these adverse effects in rodents, the use of coumarin was banned in the United States in 1954 and coumarin is currently listed among the "Substances Generally Prohibited from Direct Addition or Use as Human Food," by the Food and Drug Administration (FDA).[c] In contrast use of coumarin in food is allowed in Europe, where both the German Federal Institute for Risk Assessment (BfR)[76,77] and EFSA[78] established a TDI of 0.1 mg/kg bw/day while also maximum use limits for specific food categories are established.[79] BfR and EFSA both also concluded that moderate exceedance of the TDI for short periods, specified by EFSA as intakes three times higher than the TDI for one or two weeks, would not be of safety concern.[76,77,80] This difference in the regulatory status of coumarin in the United States and Europe relates to differences in the regulatory framework across these jurisdictions. While the prohibition of coumarin in the United States preceded it by four years, incorporating the Delaney Clause[d] within the 1958 Food Additives Amendment to the Federal Food, Drug and Cosmetic Act has effectively prevented any attempts to reintroduce coumarin as a food additive in the United States. This decision ignores whether the mode of action underlying the carcinogenicity includes genotoxicity or rather a mechanism for which a safe level of exposure can be established, or even if the mode of action is irrelevant to humans. EFSA concluded that a study on possible DNA adduct formation in the kidney and liver of exposed experimental animals revealed that coumarin does not bind to DNA, supporting a nongenotoxic mode of action for tumor induction and enabling the establishment of a TDI. This TDI was based on a NOAEL of 10 mg coumarin/kg bw/day for liver toxicity in dogs, considered the most sensitive species, and a default uncertainty factor of 100 to take intraspecies and interspecies differences into account.[78] In a later opinion EFSA also evaluated studies showing a substantial interspecies difference in the bioactivation of coumarin in rats and humans, with humans mainly detoxicating coumarin by 7-hydroxylation catalyzed by cytochrome P450 (CYP)2A6 while rats predominantly catalyze bioactivation of coumarin via 3,4-coumarin epoxide formation leading to generation of the proposed toxic intermediate *o*-hydroxyphenyl acetaldehyde (oHPA) (Fig. 12.2). This remarkable species difference in the bioactivation of coumarin could in theory be used to derive a compound-specific assessment factor, reducing the default uncertainty factor of 10 for interspecies differences to eliminate the factor 4.0 for interspecies differences in kinetics. This would result in an overall uncertainty factor of 25 instead of the default value of 100 now used to establish the TDI. Physiologically based pharmacokinetic modeling studies on oHPA formation and bioactivation of coumarin in humans as compared to rats, also including

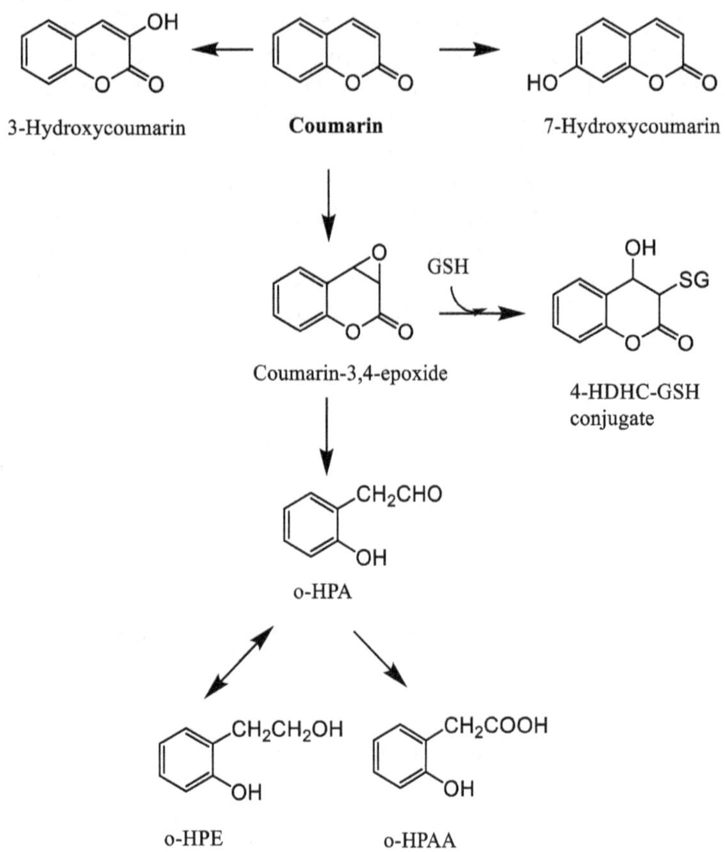

FIGURE 12.2 Metabolic pathways for coumarin, presenting detoxification via 7-hydroxylation and bioactivation via coumarin-3,4-epoxide formation leading to *o*-hydroxyphenyl acetaldehyde (oHPA).

individuals with homozygous CYP2A6 deficiency resulting in reduced possibilities for 7-hydroxylation of coumarin, indicated the level of oHPA formation to be lower in humans than in rats even for the CYP2A6-deficient individuals.[81] However, EFSA indicated that these physiologically-based kinetic (PBK) model–based predictions remained unsubstantiated and in vivo metabolic data on coumarin in CYP2A6-deficient individuals would be necessary to elucidate what pathways replace inefficient or even wholly absent 7-hydroxylation.[80] The example of coumarin clearly illustrates the need for evaluation of toxicity data in the context of insight on the underlying mode of action and presents an important difference in the regulatory framework between the United States and Europe.

12.6.3 Alkenylbenzenes versus naturals containing them: different approach in European Union and United States

Another example where differences in regulatory approaches become apparent is the regulation of plant-derived NFCs. While in the United States botanically sourced NFCs have regulatory authority to be used in food based on GRAS determinations or (in principle) review by the FDA within the context of food additive petitions, in the EU botanicals and botanical extracts are not subject to premarket safety evaluation and approval. This can be illustrated by considering the NFCs containing group 21 constituents (hydroxyallylbenzene and hydroxypropenylbenzene derivatives), including compounds like safrole, estragole, and/or methyl eugenol. Some of these compounds are also evaluated for flavor use as individual substances. In the United States both the individual substances and the related NFCs are subject to premarket safety evaluation within the framework of the GRAS concept. These safety evaluations are performed as outlined above. As noted previously, at the time of this publication the FEMA Expert Panel was in the process of conducting GRAS re-assessments for the NFCs that contain these constituents.

In Europe evaluation of the safety of these individual natural flavorings would be performed by EFSA, which provides the basis for the EU decision to include the compound on the positive list under Regulation EU 872/2012.[6] In 2001 the Scientific Committee on Food, the predecessor of EFSA, concluded that methyl eugenol, estragole, and safrole are genotoxic and carcinogenic and indicated the need for a reduction in exposure and restrictions in the levels of use.[82–84] This resulted in regulatory restrictions for the use of safrole, estragole, and methyl eugenol in Europe.[79]

In contrast, botanicals and botanical extracts, and thus also herbs and spices, essential oils, and other extracts containing safrole, estragole, and/or methyl eugenol are not subject to a safety evaluation by EFSA. This implies that in Europe the addition of methyl eugenol to food is regulated,[79] while basil extracts containing estragole and/or methyl eugenol are not. The lack of a regulatory framework in the EU on botanicals and botanical preparations has raised attention, including from national food safety authorities in Europe and EFSA. As a result, EFSA's Scientific Committee provided guidance on the data needed to conduct safety assessments of a botanical or a botanical preparation.[67] They also issued a Compendium of Botanicals (https://www.efsa.europa.eu/en/microstrategy/botanical-summary-report) which presents a database of botanicals that are reported to contain naturally occurring substances of possible concern for human health when present in food. For example, regarding basil (*O. basilicum*) the Compendium lists estragole as a substantial constituent (20%–50%) of the essential oil. Currently these actions did not result in a framework for premarket safety evaluations of botanicals or botanical preparations. EFSA indicates that the presence of a substance of concern in a botanical does not necessarily imply that the substance will be present at a level that would raise a health concern. Thus the Compendium may support possible hazard identification at the present state of the art but does not provide a risk or safety assessment.

12.7 Discussion and conclusions

This chapter on the direct addition of flavors, including taste and flavor modifiers, to food illustrates that food flavors often are of no concern because of their long history of safe use, the available safety data from toxicity and other studies, and their low use levels resulting in low levels of estimated daily exposure. These characteristics explain why safety evaluations of other food-borne constituents, including food additives and pesticides, received a higher priority and that safety evaluation of food flavors in some jurisdictions started only in the last several decades. While the FEMA Expert Panel began to perform safety evaluations of food flavoring in the 1960s to establish GRAS status, safety evaluation of food flavors by EFSA and other regulatory authorities started in the 21st century. This may be one of the reasons underlying the notable differences in the procedures applied. Some intake methods are still under development that acknowledge previously applied use level–based methods, like the PADI and TAMDI, while trying to improve upon them, since these older methods result in exceedingly high estimated exposure levels that are orders of magnitude higher than exposure estimates based on anticipated or reported annual production volumes.

There are also remarkable differences between different jurisdictions in the regulatory framework regarding flavor use. As a result, flavors considered safe and allowed for use in some parts of the world can be excluded from food use in others. In the United States, this can be due to the so-called "Delaney Clause," which prevents the use of a flavor even when mode of action–based considerations support the definition of a safe level of exposure to a carcinogenic compound that does not act via a genotoxic mode of action as illustrated by coumarin. It can also be due to different regulatory frameworks as illustrated for plant-based NFCs. On the other hand, the use of a group-based approach and read-across methods may result in differences in expert judgments and resulting differences in conclusions regarding safety of use of a flavor ingredient. For example, the FEMA Expert Panel evaluation of perillaldehyde (*p*-mentha-1,8-dien-7-al) differed from that of EFSA, as detailed in a recent review.[44] Briefly, the FEMA Expert Panel considered results from an in vivo comet assay to be not biologically relevant. It noted that the %tail DNA did not extend beyond the historical control range and the increase was only observed in animals with liver toxicity. Based on the weight of evidence, it did not consider perillaldehyde to raise a genotoxic concern.[44,85] By contrast, EFSA interpreted the comet assay results differently and thus still had a concern for genotoxicity for perillaldehyde.[86] More recently, published data from a study in transgenic rodents has confirmed the lack of in vivo mutagenic potential of perillaldehyde.

Despite these differences the overall conclusion is that flavorings generally do not raise safety concerns because of their low levels of use resulting in estimated exposure levels below the relevant TTC values and/or resulting in margins of exposure that amount to several orders of magnitude. A recent overview of their genotoxicity revealed that most flavor ingredients have given negative results in all in vitro or in vivo genotoxicity/mutagenicity tests conducted on them.[44]

However, some research areas of interest that provide future directions may also be defined and are summarized in the next section.

12.8 Future directions

12.8.1 Intake by children

One issue to consider when addressing current research gaps and future directions relates to estimates of intake by children and the impact of those estimates on safety evaluations. TTC values are currently considered for a 60 kg person, and the corresponding margins of safety or exposure are generally calculated based on intake estimates for adults. To evaluate children's exposure, one could convert TTC values, expressed on a per-person basis, to TTC values expressed per kg bodyweight using a relevant typical child's body weight (e.g., 20 kg). In addition, one could consider that food and beverage intake, including portion sizes, by children would also be lower on a per person basis and calculate children's specific levels of intake using modifications to the standard approaches described above. Recent procedures on flavor safety evaluation and/or use of the TTC discuss this topic and provide guidance on dealing with this issue.[14,32] In its updated procedure for the safety evaluation of NFCs, for instance, the FEMA Expert Panel considers that intake by older infants and young children should particularly be considered when estimated exposures for adults (of a congeneric group) approaches the TTC, since the margins of safety could in theory not be sufficient to cover the potentially higher intake by children when considered on a bodyweight basis. A comprehensive evaluation of children's diets, and corresponding consideration of how intake estimates could be modified, could possibly be addressed with data available from dietary recall surveys from national nutrition surveys, but thus far the scholarship on this is limited, and the potential impact of modifying intake estimates for children has not been effectively explored for flavorings. The Expert Panel also notes that childhood exposure occurs over a small percentage of the total typical lifetime, while the consideration of toxicity within the context of a safety evaluation is based on chronic (i.e., lifetime) exposure.

12.8.2 Use of threshold of toxicological concern for unidentified constituents

Since the TTC cannot be applied to compounds of unknown chemical structure, the use of the TTC in the evaluation of the group of unidentified constituents within an NFC also requires further attention. Within the current state-of-the-art approach it is assumed that the TTC can be applied for unidentified constituents of complex mixtures provided that these unidentified constituents are reasonably unlikely to belong to a TTC-excluded class.[14] Tools to provide helpful information regarding this include instrumental analytical methods and the use of bioassays. For example, bioassays may be used to overcome concerns over genotoxic potential, detect mixture effects, and/or ascertain that the unidentified constituents do not belong to a TTC-excluded class, since they may detect compounds like aflatoxins or steroids. It would be helpful to extend research defining the limits of detection of genotoxic or endocrine active constituents in a complex mixture by such bioassays. Recent evaluations have concluded that currently available bioassays could detect endocrine-active compounds that migrated from various food contact materials into food during production, packaging, preparation, serving, transport, processing, and storage with sufficient detection limits.[87–89]

In contrast, a study investigating the suitability of the Ames test to characterize the mutagenicity of individual compounds present in complex food contact material migrates, concluded that only 4 out of 40 genotoxic chemicals potentially associated with food contact materials on which data were available could be detected at the pragmatic threshold of 0.01 mg/kg of the complex mixture.[89] This would imply that the Ames test cannot be used as the only test to evaluate the genotoxicity of complex mixtures but would have to be combined with data from analytical chemistry, knowledge of the manufacturing process, and expert judgment. Performing similar analyses for compounds expected to occur in NFCs would be useful.

12.8.2.1 Reanalysis of the threshold of toxicological concern of 0.15 μg/person/day for compounds with a structural alert for genotoxicity

The TTC of 0.15 μg/person/day for compounds with a structural alert for genotoxicity, used in the evaluation of constituents in NFCs that may raise a concern for genotoxicity, is derived based on linear extrapolation of available TD_{50} values, representing dose levels that induce 50% tumor incidence to virtual safe dose levels inducing an extra tumor incidence above background levels of one in a million upon lifetime exposure. However, the current state-of-the-art the MOE approach is the preferred method of choice for evaluating compounds that are genotoxic and carcinogenic.[60,61] It could also be claimed that the TTC value for these compounds should be redefined based on the MOE value of 10,000 and $BMDL_{10}$ values derived from the tumor data that originally provided the TD_{50} values. An effort to redefine the TTC for genotoxicity, taking this preferred state-of-the-art methodology for risk assessment of both genotoxic and carcinogenic compounds into account, would have practical value for the safety evaluation of all chemicals, including flavorings, that are not members of TTC-excluded classes.

12.8.2.2 Exposure assessments

As described above, several methods have been used to carry out an exposure assessment of flavorings, and the alignment of approaches within the safety evaluation community would be desirable. Given that safety evaluations conclude on the safety in use of the flavorings *at the intended use and use levels*, it would be preferable to rely upon use levels–based estimation methods in an ideal scenario. However, the available use level–based methodologies overestimate actual exposure levels by orders of magnitude due to assumptions that flavorings would be present in every food in a food category. Further work to refine approaches for exposure assessment of flavors would be valuable.

12.8.2.3 Extending the database of available studies for read-across

As described above, read-across of data between flavorings is a shared practice in the safety evaluations conducted by JECFA, EFSA, and the FEMA Expert Panel. Continual research and development by flavoring producers has contributed to the expansion of the palette of flavorings with uses that are considered FEMA GRAS. To ensure that appropriate data—data from studies in line with current guidelines and focusing on materials of significant use—continue to be available, it is helpful for additional data to be collected to ensure that the underlying dataset for read-across remains robust and up-to-date. Given these considerations it is of interest to take note of recent studies conducted on some flavorings, sometimes conducted at the request of EFSA, the data of which have been applied for read-across to new flavorings. As the database of available safety studies for flavorings continues to increase, it also allows for more detailed analysis into safety trends for this large group of chemicals.

Endnotes

[a]"Flavoring Substances and Natural Sources of Flavorings, Council of Europe," 1973.

[b]FDA, 2014. High intensity sweeteners, available at: https://www.fda.gov/food/food-additives-petitions/high-intensity-sweeteners.

[c]21CFR189.30(b). Food containing any added coumarin as such or as a constituent of tonka beans or tonka extract is deemed to be adulterated under the act, based upon an order published in the Federal Register of March 5, 1954 (19 FR 1239).

[d]The Delaney Clause prohibits the FDA from approving the use in food of any substance found to cause cancer in animals or humans.

References

1. Oser BL, Ford RA. FEMA expert panel: 30 years of safety evaluation for the flavor industry. *Food Technol.* 1991;46(11):84–97.
2. Hall RL, Oser BL. Recent progress in the consideration of flavoring ingredients under the Food Additives Amendment. 3. GRAS substances. *Food Technol.* 1965;19(2). Suppl.
3. Hallagan JB, Hall RL. FEMA GRAS – a GRAS assessment program for flavor ingredients. *Regul Toxicol Pharmacol.* 1995;21(3):422–430. Available from: https://doi.org/10.1006/rtph.1995.1057.
4. Hallagan JB, Hall RL. Under the conditions of intended use – new developments in the FEMA GRAS program and the safety assessment of flavor ingredients. *Food Chem Toxicol.* 2009;47(2):267–278. Available from: https://doi.org/10.1016/j.fct.2008.11.011.
5. Hallagan JB, Hall RL, Drake J. The GRAS provision – the FEMA GRAS program and the safety and regulation of flavors in the United States. *Food Chem Toxicol.* 2020;138:111236. Available from: https://doi.org/10.1016/j.fct.2020.111236.
6. Commission Implementing Regulation (EU) No 872/2012 of 1 October 2012 adopting the list of flavouring substances provided for by Regulation (EC) No 2232/96 of the European Parliament and of the Council, introducing it in Annex I to Regulation (EC) No 1334/2008 of

the European Parliament and of the Council and repealing Commission Regulation (EC) No 1565/2000 and Commission Decision 1999/217/EC Text with EEA relevance 1-161; 2012.

7. Codex Alimentarius Commission. *Guidelines for the Use of Flavourings*. CAC/GL 66-2008. In: (CCFA) CCoFA, Ed.; 2008.
8. Harman CL, Hallagan JB. Sensory testing for flavorings with modifying properties. *Food Technol*. 2013;67(11):44–47.
9. Smith RL, Cohen SM, Doull J, et al. Criteria for the safety evaluation of flavoring substances. *Food Chem Toxicol*. 2005;43(8):1141–1177. Available from: https://doi.org/10.1016/j.fct.2004.11.012.
10. Harman CL, Bastaki M, Aubanel M, et al. *Methodologies employed for estimating flavoring substance intake. Reference Module in Food Science*. Elsevier; 2018.
11. Gavin CL, Williams MC, Hallagan JB. *2005 Poundage and Technical Effects Survey*. Washington, DC: Flavor and Extract Manufacturers Association of the United States (FEMA); 2008.
12. Harman CL, Lipman MD, Hallagan JB. *2010 Poundage and Technical Effects Survey*. Washington, DC: Flavor and Extract Manufacturers Association; 2013.
13. Lucas CD, Putnam JM, Hallagan JB. *Poundage and Technical Effects Update Survey*. Washington, DC: Flavor and Extract Manufacturers Association of the United States; 1995:1999.
14. Cohen SM, Eisenbrand G, Fukushima S, et al. Updated procedure for the safety evaluation of natural flavor complexes used as ingredients in food. *Food Chem Toxicol*. 2018;113:171–178. Available from: https://doi.org/10.1016/j.fct.2018.01.021.
15. Rulis AM, Hattan DG, Morgenroth 3rd VH. FDA's priority-based assessment of food additives. I. Preliminary results. *Regul Toxicol Pharmacol*. 1984;4(1):37–56. Available from: https://doi.org/10.1016/02732300(84)90005-9.
16. Woods LA, Doull J. GRAS evaluation of flavoring substances by the Expert Panel of FEMA. *Regul Toxicol Pharmacol*. 1991;14(1):48–58. Available from: https://doi.org/10.1016/0273-2300(91)90051-v.
17. JECFA. *Evaluation of Certain Food Additives and Contaminants (Forty-Sixth Report of the Joint FAO/WHO Expert Committee on Food Additives). WHO Technical Report Series*. 868. World Health Organization; 1997.
18. European Commission. Regulation (EC) No 1565/2000 of 18 July 2000 laying down the measures necessary for the adoption of an evaluation programme in application of Regulation (EC) No. 2232/96. *Official Journal of the European Communities*. 2000; L 84:8–16.
19. Oser BL, Hall RL. Criteria employed by the expert panel of FEMA for the GRAS evaluation of flavouring substances. *Food Cosmet Toxicol*. 1977;15(5):457–466. Available from: https://doi.org/10.1016/s0015-6264(77)80014-x.
20. Arcella D, Leclercq C. Assessment of dietary intake of flavouring substances within the procedure for their safety evaluation: advantages and limitations of estimates obtained by means of a per capita method. *Food Chem Toxicol*. 2005;43(1):105–116. Available from: https://doi.org/10.1016/j.fct.2004.08.017.
21. Cadby P. Estimating intakes of flavouring substances. *Food Addit Contam*. 1996;13(4):453–460. Available from: https://doi.org/10.1080/02652039609374430.
22. Young KWH, Danielewska-Nikiel B, Munro IC. An evaluation of the maximized survey-derived daily intake (MSDI) as a practical method to estimate intake of flavouring substances. *Food Chem Toxicol*. 2006;44(11):1849–1867. Available from: https://doi.org/10.1016/j.fct.2006.06.004.
23. Lambe J, Cadby P, Gibney M. Comparison of stochastic modelling of the intakes of intentionally added flavouring substances with theoretical added maximum daily intakes (TAMDI) and maximized survey-derived daily intakes (MSDI). *Food Addit Contam*. 2002;19(1):2–14. Available from: https://doi.org/10.1080/02652030110071327.
24. JECFA. *Sixty-Seventh Meeting of the Joint FAO/WHO Expert Committee on Food Additives. Summary and Conclusions. WHO Technical Report Series*. Rome, 20–29 June 2006; 2006:940.
25. Smith RL, Cohen SM, Doull J, et al. A procedure for the safety evaluation of natural flavor complexes used as ingredients in food: essential oils. *Food Chem Toxicol*. 2005;43(3):345–363. Available from: https://doi.org/10.1016/j.fct.2004.11.007.
26. Hall RL, Ford RA. Comparison of two methods to assess the intake of flavouring substances. *Food Addit Contam*. 1999;16(11):481–495. Available from: https://doi.org/10.1080/026520399283777.
27. EFSA. *7th Plenary Meeting of the Scientific Panel on Food Additives, Flavourings, Processing Aids and Materials in Contact with Food (AFC)*. Brussels, 12–13 July 2004; 2004.
28. JECFA. *Evaluation of Certain Food Additives and Contaminants (Sixty-eighth Report of the Joint FAO/WHO Expert Committee on Food Additives). WHO Technical Report Series*; 2007:No. 947(68).
29. JECFA. *Safety Evaluation of Certain Food Additives and Contaminants (Sixty-Ninth Meeting of Committee on Food Additives). WHO Food Additive Series*; 2009:No. 60.
30. European Food Safety Authority (EFSA), Food and Agriculture Organization of the United Nations (FAO). Towards a harmonised Total Diet Study approach: a guidance document. *EFSA J*. 2011;9(11):2450. Available from: https://doi.org/10.2903/j.efsa.2011.2450.
31. EFSA. Scientific Opinion on Dietary exposure assessment methods for smoke flavouring primary products. *EFSA J*. 2009;RN-284:1–30.
32. EFSA. Guidance on the data required for the risk assessment of flavourings to be used in or on foods. *EFSA J*. 2010;8(6):1623–1676.
33. JECFA. *Food Safety – JECFA Monographs*. JECFA; 2018:2022. <http://www.who.int/foodsafety/publications/monographs/en/>.
34. Benfenati E, Chaudhry Q, Gini G, Dorne JL. Integrating in silico models and read-across methods for predicting toxicity of chemicals: a step-wise strategy. *Environ Int*. 2019;131:105060. Available from: https://doi.org/10.1016/j.envint.2019.105060.
35. Cramer GM, Ford RA, Hall RL. Estimation of toxic hazard—a decision tree approach. *Food Cosmet Toxicol*. 1978;16(3):255–276. Available from: https://doi.org/10.1016/s0015-6264(76)80522-6.
36. Patlewicz G, Jeliazkova N, Safford RJ, Worth AP, Aleksiev B. An evaluation of the implementation of the Cramer classification scheme in the Toxtree software. *SAR QSAR Environ Res*. 2008;19(5–6):495–524. Available from: https://doi.org/10.1080/10629360802083871.
37. Kroes R, Galli C, Munro I, et al. Threshold of Toxicological Concern for chemical substances present in the diet: a practical tool for assessing the need for toxicity testing. *Food Chem Toxicol*. 2000;38(2–3):255–312.
38. Kroes R, Renwick AG, Cheeseman M, et al. Structure-based thresholds of toxicological concern (TTC): guidance for application to substances present at low levels in the diet. *Food Chem Toxicol*. 2004;42(1):65–83. Available from: https://doi.org/10.1016/j.fct.2003.08.006.
39. Munro IC, Ford RA, Kennepohl E, Sprenger JG. Correlation of structural class with no-observed-effect levels: a proposal for

establishing a threshold of concern. *Food Chem Toxicol.* 1996;34 (9):829–867. Available from: https://doi.org/10.1016/s0278-6915 (96)00049-x.
40. EFSA. Review of the Threshold of Toxicological Concern (TTC) approach and development of new TTC decision tree. *EFSA Suppor Publ.* 2016;13(3):1–50. Available from: https://doi.org/ 10.2903/sp.efsa.2016.EN-1006. 1006e.
41. Kirkland D. Improvements in the reliability of in vitro genotoxicity testing. *Expert Opin Drug Metab Toxicol.* 2011;7(12):1513–1520. Available from: https://doi.org/10.1517/17425255.2011.627855.
42. Kirkland D, Aardema M, Henderson L, Müller L. Evaluation of the ability of a battery of three in vitro genotoxicity tests to discriminate rodent carcinogens and non-carcinogens: I. Sensitivity, specificity and relative predictivity. *Mutat Res.* 2005;584(1–2):1–256. Available from: https://doi.org/10.1016/j.mrgentox.2005.02.004.
43. Kirkland D, Pfuhler S, Tweats D, et al. How to reduce false positive results when undertaking in vitro genotoxicity testing and thus avoid unnecessary follow-up animal tests: report of an ECVAM Workshop. *Mutat Res.* 2007;628(1):31–55. Available from: https://doi.org/10.1016/ j.mrgentox.2006.11.008.
44. Gooderham NJ, Cohen SM, Eisenbrand G, et al. The safety evaluation of food flavoring substances: the role of genotoxicity studies. *Crit Rev Toxicol.* 2020;50(1):1–27.
45. Hooks WN, Kirk SJ, Smith HL, et al. Ethyl vanillin toxicity to rats by repeated dietary administration for 13 weeks. Unpublished report No EVT 2/920067 of Huntingdon Research Centre Ltd Submitted to WHO by Ethyl Vanillin Task Force, International Food Additives Council (IFAC) Atlanta, Georgia, USA; 1992.
46. EFSA. Scientific opinion on genotoxicity testing strategies applicable to food and feed safety assessment. *EFSA J.* 2011;9(9):2379. Available from: https://doi.org/10.2903/j.efsa.2011.2379.
47. JECFA. *Guidance Document for WHO Monographers and Reviewers Evaluating Flavouring Agents. Geneva: World Health Organization*; 2017. Version 1.
48. Smith RL, Adams TB, Cohen SM, et al. Safety evaluation of natural flavour complexes. *Toxicol Lett.* 2004;149(1–3):197–207. Available from: https://doi.org/10.1016/j.toxlet.2003.12.031.
49. Rietjens IMCM, Cohen SM, Eisenbrand G, et al. FEMA GRAS assessment of natural flavor complexes: cinnamomum and myroxylon-derived flavoring ingredients. *Food Chem Toxicol.* 2020;135:110949. Available from: https://doi.org/10.1016/j.fct.2019.110949.
50. Cohen SM, Eisenbrand G, Fukushima S, et al. FEMA GRAS assessment of natural flavor complexes: citrus-derived flavoring ingredients. *Food Chem Toxicol.* 2019;124:192–218. Available from: https://doi.org/10.1016/j.fct.2018.11.052.
51. Alajlouni AM, Al-Malahmeh AJ, Isnaeni FN, Wesseling S, Vervoort J, Rietjens IMCM. Level of alkenylbenzenes in parsley and dill based teas and associated risk assessment using the margin of exposure approach. *J Agric Food Chem.* 2016;64(45):8640. Available from: https://doi.org/10.1021/acs.jafc.6b03650.
52. van den Berg SJPL, Alhusainy W, Restani P, Rietjens IMCM. Chemical analysis of estragole in fennel based teas and associated safety assessment using the Margin of Exposure (MOE) approach. *Food Chem Toxicol.* 2014;65:147–154. Available from: https://doi. org/10.1016/j.fct.2013.12.035.
53. Rietjens IMCM, Boersma MG, Woude H, Jeurissen SM, Schutte ME, Alink GM. Flavonoids and alkenylbenzenes: mechanisms of mutagenic action and carcinogenic risk. *Mutat Res.* 2005;574. Available from: https://doi.org/10.1016/j.mrfmmm.2005.01.028.
54. Paini A, Scholz G, Marin-Kuan M, et al. Quantitative comparison between in vivo DNA adduct formation from exposure to selected DNA-reactive carcinogens, natural background levels of DNA adduct formation and tumour incidence in rodent bioassays. *Mutagenesis.* 2011;26(5):605–618. Available from: https://doi.org/ 10.1093/mutage/ger022.
55. Rietjens IMCM, Cohen SM, Fukushima S, et al. Impact of structural and metabolic variations on the toxicity and carcinogenicity of hydroxy- and alkoxy-substituted allyl- and propenylbenzenes. *Chem Res Toxicol.* 2014;27(7):1092–1103. Available from: https:// doi.org/10.1021/tx500109s.
56. Miller EC, Swanson AB, Phillips DH, Fletcher TL, Liem A, Miller JA. Structure-activity studies of the carcinogenicities in the mouse and rat of some naturally occurring and synthetic alkenylbenzene derivatives related to safrole and estragole. *Cancer Res.* 1983;43 (3):1124–1134.
57. Phillips DH, Reddy MV, Randerath K. 32P-post-labelling analysis of DNA adducts formed in the livers of animals treated with safrole, estragole and other naturally-occurring alkenylbenzenes. II. Newborn male B6C3F1 mice. *Carcinogenesis.* 1984;5 (12):1623–1628. Available from: https://doi.org/10.1093/carcin/ 5.12.1623.
58. Randerath K, Haglund RE, Phillips DH, Reddy MV. 32P-post-labelling analysis of DNA adducts formed in the livers of animals treated with safrole, estragole and other naturally-occurring alkenylbenzenes. I. Adult female CD-1 mice. *Carcinogenesis.* 1984;5 (12):1613–1622. Available from: https://doi.org/10.1093/carcin/ 5.12.1613.
59. NTP. NTP toxicology and carcinogenesis studies of methyleugenol (CAS NO. 93-15-2) in F344/N rats and B6C3F1 mice (gavage studies). *Natl Toxicol Progr Tech Rep Ser.* 2000;491:1–412.
60. Benford D, Bolger PM, Carthew P, et al. Application of the margin of exposure (MOE) approach to substances in food that are genotoxic and carcinogenic. *Food Chem Toxicol.* 2010;48:S2–S24.
61. EFSA. Opinion of the Scientific Committee on a request from EFSA related to a harmonised approach for risk assessment of substances which are both genotoxic and carcinogenic. *EFSA J.* 2005;282:1–31.
62. van den Berg S, Restani P, Boersma M, Delmulle L, Rietjens IMCM. Levels of genotoxic and carcinogenic compounds in plant food supplements and associated risk assessment. *Food Nutr Sci.* 2011;2:989–1010. Available from: https://doi.org/10.4236/ fns.2011.29134.
63. Suparmi S, Ginting AJ, Mariyam S, Wesseling S, Rietjens IMCM. Levels of methyleugenol and eugenol in instant herbal beverages available on the Indonesian market and related risk assessment. *Food Chem Toxicol.* 2019;125:467–478. Available from: https:// doi.org/10.1016/j.fct.2019.02.001.
64. Gooderham NJ, Cohen SM, Eisenbrand G, et al. FEMA GRAS assessment of natural flavor complexes: clove, cinnamon leaf and West Indian bay leaf-derived flavoring ingredients. *Food Chem Toxicol.* 2020;145:111585. Available from: https://doi.org/10.1016/ j.fct.2020.111585.
65. Koster S, Boobis AR, Cubberley R, et al. Application of the TTC concept to unknown substances found in analysis of foods. *Food*

Chem Toxicol. 2011;49(8):1643–1660. Available from: https://doi.org/10.1016/j.fct.2011.03.049.

66. Schwab W, Davidovich-Rikanati R, Lewinsohn E. Biosynthesis of plant-derived flavor compounds. *Plant J.* 2008;54(4):712–732. Available from: https://doi.org/10.1111/j.1365-313X.2008.03446.x.
67. EFSA, EFSA Scientific Committee. Guidance on safety assessment of botanicals and botanical preparations intended for use as ingredients in food supplements, on request of EFSA. *EFSA J.* 2009;7(9):1249–1267. Available from: https://doi.org/10.2093/j.efsa.2009.1249.
68. Hallagan JB. The safety assessment of process flavors. Process and reaction flavors. In: ACS Symposium Series. 905. American Chemical Society; 2005:26–40.
69. Newberne P, Smith RL, Doull J, et al. GRAS flavoring substances 19. *Food Technol.* 2000;54(6):66–68. 70, 72–74, 76–84.
70. EFSA. Scientific guidance for the preparation of applications on smoke flavouring primary products. *EFSA J.* 2021;19(3):e06435. Available from: https://doi.org/10.2903/j.efsa.2021.6435.
71. Rigler MW, Longo WE. Emission of diacetyl (2,3 butanedione) from natural butter, microwave popcorn butter flavor powder, paste, and liquid products. *Int J Occup Environ Health.* 2010;16(3):291–302. Available from: https://doi.org/10.1179/107735210799160237.
72. Hallagan JB. The use of diacetyl (2,3-butanedione) and related flavoring substances as flavorings added to foods—workplace safety issues. *Toxicology.* 2017;388:1–6. Available from: https://doi.org/10.1016/j.tox.2017.05.010.
73. Kreiss K. Recognizing occupational effects of diacetyl: what can we learn from this history? *Toxicology.* 2017;388:48–54. Available from: https://doi.org/10.1016/j.tox.2016.06.009.
74. Anders MW. Diacetyl and related flavorant α-diketones: biotransformation, cellular interactions, and respiratory-tract toxicity. *Toxicology.* 2017;388:21–29. Available from: https://doi.org/10.1016/j.tox.2017.02.002.
75. Abraham K, Wöhrlin F, Lindtner O, Heinemeyer G, Lampen A. Toxicology and risk assessment of coumarin: focus on human data. *Mol Nutr Food Res.* 2010;54(2):228–239. Available from: https://doi.org/10.1002/mnfr.200900281.
76. Federal Institute of Risk Assessment (BfR). Consumers, who eat a lot of cinnamon, currently have an overly high exposure to coumarin. BfR Health Assessment; 16 June 2006. <https://mobil.bfr.bund.de/cm/349/consumers_who_eat_a_lot_of_cinnamon_currently_have_an_overly_high_exposure_to_coumarin.pdf>.
77. Federal Institute of Risk Assessment (BfR). High daily intakes of cinnamon: health risk cannot be ruled out. BfR Health Assessment; 18 August 2006. <https://mobil.bfr.bund.de/cm/349/high_daily_intakes_of_cinnamon_health_risk_cannot_be_ruled_out.pdf>.
78. EFSA. Opinion of the Scientific Panel on food additives, flavourings, processing aids and materials in contacts with Food (AFC) on a request from the commission related to coumarin. *EFSA J.* 2004;104:1–36.
79. European Commission. Regulation (EC) No 1334/2008 of the European Parliament and of the Council of 16 December 2008 on flavourings and certain food ingredients with flavouring properties for use in and on foods and amending Council Regulation (EEC) No 1601/91, Regulations (EC) No 2232/96 and (EC) No 110/2008 and Directive 2000/13/EC. *Official Journal of the European Union.* 2008;354:34–50.
80. EFSA. Coumarin in flavourings and other food ingredients with flavouring properties – Scientific Opinion of the Panel on food additives, flavourings, processing aids and materials in contact with food (AFC). *EFSA J.* 2008;6(10):793. Available from: https://doi.org/10.2903/j.efsa.2008.793.
81. Rietjens IMCM, Boersma MG, Zaleska M, Punt A. Differences in simulated liver concentrations of toxic coumarin metabolites in rats and different human populations evaluated through physiologically based biokinetic (PBBK) modeling. *Toxicol In Vitro.* 2008;22(8):1890–1901. Available from: https://doi.org/10.1016/j.tiv.2008.09.004.
82. Opinion of the Scientific Committee on Food on estragole (1-Allyl-4-methoxybenzene). European Commission Health & Consumer Protection Directorate-General; 2001.
83. Opinion of the Scientific Committee on Food on methyleugenol (1-allyl-1,2-dimethoxybenzene. European Commission Health & Consumer Protection Directorate-General; 2001.
84. Opinion of the Scientific Committee on Food on the safety of the presence of safrole (1-allyl-3,4-methylene dioxybenzene) in flavorings and other food ingredients with flavoring properties. European Commission Health & Consumer Protection Directorate-General; 2002.
85. Cohen SM, Fukushima S, Gooderham NJ, et al. FEMA Expert Panel review of p-mentha-1,8-dien-7-al genotoxicity testing results. *Food Chem Toxicol.* 2016;98(Pt B):201–209. Available from: https://doi.org/10.1016/j.fct.2016.10.020.
86. EFSA. Scientific Opinion on Flavouring Group Evaluation 208 Revision 2 (FGE0.208Rev2): consideration of genotoxicity data on alicyclic aldehydes with α,β-unsaturation in ring/side-chain and precursors from chemical subgroup 2.2 of FGE.19. *EFSA J.* 2017;15(5):e04766. Available from: https://doi.org/10.2903/j.efsa.2017.4766.
87. Severin I, Souton E, Dahbi L, Chagnon MC. Use of bioassays to assess hazard of food contact material extracts: state of the art. *Food Chem Toxicol.* 2017;105:429–447. Available from: https://doi.org/10.1016/j.fct.2017.04.046.
88. Groh KJ, Geueke B, Muncke J. Food contact materials and gut health: implications for toxicity assessment and relevance of high molecular weight migrants. *Food Chem Toxicol.* 2017;109(Pt 1):1–18. Available from: https://doi.org/10.1016/j.fct.2017.08.023.
89. Rainer B, Pinter E, Czerny T, et al. Suitability of the Ames test to characterise genotoxicity of food contact material migrates. *Food Addit Contam Part A Chem Anal Control Expo Risk Assess.* 2018;35(11):2230–2243. Available from: https://doi.org/10.1080/19440049.2018.1519259.

Chapter 13

Production of contaminants during thermal processing in both industrial and home preparation of foods

Franco Pedreschi[1] and María Salomé Mariotti[2]

[1]*Departamento de Ingeniería Química y Bioprocesos, Pontificia Universidad Católica de Chile, Santiago, Chile,* [2]*Escuela de Nutrición y Dietética, Facultad de Medicina, Universidad Finis Terrae, Santiago, Chile*

Abstract

The problem of processing contaminants is now one of the most challenging issues the food industry needs to address. Heat processing contaminants may be defined as substances that are produced in a food when it is cooked or processed, and they are not present or present at much lower concentrations in the raw, unprocessed food. These heat toxic compounds and undesirable either because they have an adverse effect on product quality or because they are potentially harmful.

It is important to highlight that Maillard Reaction (Mr) is the most important chemical reaction occurring during food processing at high temperature unit operations since it is crucial for the development of attractive sensory food attributes of the final products, improving their digestibility, ensuring microbial safety, and developing flavor and taste to name just three. On the other hand, Mr has shown that heating of starchy and protein food matrixes can generate various kinds of potentially toxic compounds (PTCs). Consequently, PTCs could be mitigated by favoring the processing conditions under which Mr is inhibited and/or reducing the PTC crucial precursors in raw food materials before being heated at high temperature unit operations such as frying, extrusion, roasting, grilling, baking, and among others. Mr also plays a crucial role in the heat formation of some PCTs such as acrylamide (AA), furan, 5-hydroxymethylfurfural (HMF), and heterocyclic amines (HAs) either in starchy and/or protein food matrixes processed by excessive heating.

In this chapter, we will present some of the most important PTCs in foods such as AA, furan, HMF, and HAs. We will show you some mitigation strategies for PTCs considering the following issues: (1) raw materials and precursor contents specific for the formation of one or more PCTs, (2) heating processing conditions, and (3) mecanism(s) of PTC formation under specific conditions. This information will help you to generate foods heated at high processing temperatures while minimizing PCT formation and preserving the quality attributes of the desired food product. In this way, we will contribute in reducing the exposure of consumers to dietary PCTs.

Keywords: Heating; acrylamide; Maillard Reaction; furan; 5-hydroxymethylfurfural; heterocyclic amines

13.1 Introduction

Heat treatment of foods is a key operation not only in the industry but also at home resulting in the development of a large range of flavors and tastes through the Maillard Reaction (Mr).[1] At the same time, potential toxic compound (PTC) generation during processing has become an interesting area of research because of the hazardous potential of these compounds. It has been postulated that specific PCTs formed depend not only in the original raw material composition but also on the high temperature profile.[2]

Mitigation of PCTs could be achieved by diminishing the food precursors in the raw materials and/or inhibiting the processing conditions which favored the reactions that led to the formation of PCTs.[2] Since PTC formation reactions are usually also responsible for the attractive color, flavor, and texture of the final product, the challenge is how to mitigate the formation of these compounds without affecting negatively the final attractive sensory attributes of foods and thus preserving consumer acceptance.[3,4] PCT formation could be mitigated by removing precursors in raw materials (asparagine, reducing sugars, ascorbic acid, reducing sugars, creatinine, free amino acids, and among others) or by favoring conditions under which critical PCT formation reactions such as Mr are inhibited (thermal load reduction, formulation change, addition of amino acids,

Present Knowledge in Food Safety. DOI: https://doi.org/10.1016/B978-0-12-819470-6.00036-6

addition of antioxidants, treatment with asparaginase, and among others).[5,6]

PCTs are formed naturally during thermal processing of foods through the complex Mr taking place and exhibit possible harmful human effects.[7] Among the several PCTs described in the literature, acrylamide (AA), 5-hydroxymethylfurfural (HMF), furan, and heterocyclic amines (Has) have attracted the attention of the scientific community in the recent years. In Mr, the interaction between food with an specific composition and the heat process applied results in the development of complex oxidation and glycation reactions, which give rise to a mixture of flavored compounds and PTCs.[8] Interestingly, most of the PCTs have not been precisely evaluated regarding to their potential health effects. However, epidemiological studies have identified possible relations between some health parameters and the ingestion of foods processed at high temperatures, such as for instance an association between the consumption of meat rich in mutagenic HAs and cancer.

For instance, specifically for AA mitigation in the new EU regulation leaves the food industry with the challenge of maintaining product brands while meeting the new restrictions. PCT mitigation strategies must be designed specifically to face the manufacturing heating process and the chemical composition of the raw materials for each processed matrix. In this chapter, we will focus on some relevant PCTs such as AA, furan, HMF, and HAs during processing at high temperature unit operations in starchy and protein (meat) food matrixes.

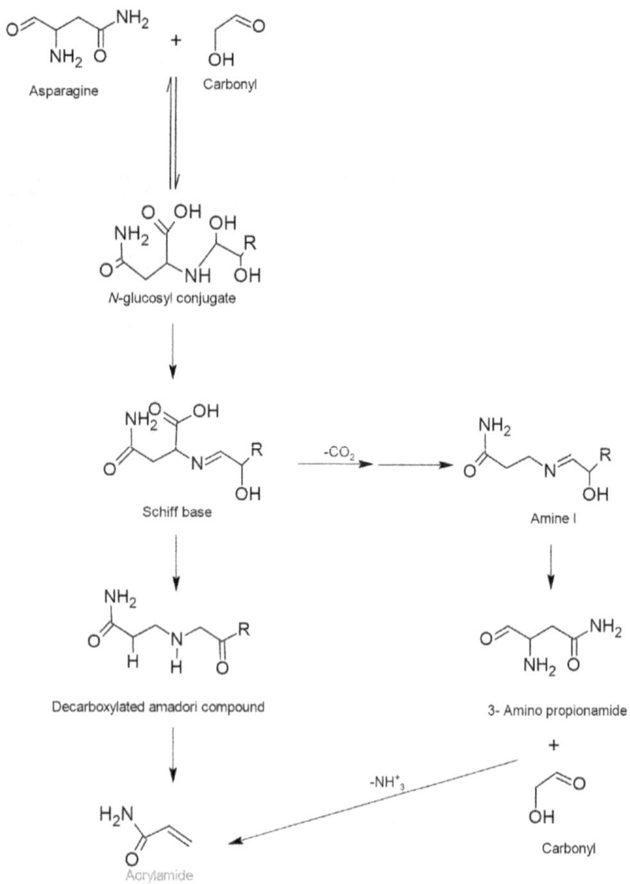

FIGURE 13.1 Acrylamide formation through the Maillard Reaction. *Adapted from Pedreschi F, Mariotti M, Granby K. Current issues in dietary acrylamide: formation, mitigation and risk assessment.* J Sci Food Agric. *2014;94:9–20.*

13.2 Potential heat toxic compounds

13.2.1 Acrylamide

AA is produced as byproduct of the Mr in starchy foods such as potato and cereal products processed at high temperatures (>120°C).[9–11] Acrylamide is formed in foods mainly by Mr during heat treatment and it is predominantly formed from asparagine in the presence of reducing sugars in certain foods when exposed to temperatures higher than 120°C at low-moisture conditions[1] (Fig. 13.1). Raw materials which contain the above-mentioned precursors in significant levels are cereals, potatoes, green coffee, and various kinds of vegetables and fruits. It is worth to mention that reducing sugars such as glucose and fructose are the major contributors to AA in potato-based products.[12] On the other hand, the limiting substrate of AA formation in cereals and coffee is the free amino acid asparagine.[13] Foodstuffs prepared from these raw materials by thermal processing are suspicious of high AA content, independent commercial, or home preparation.

AA is known as a neurotoxin in humans and it is classified as a probable human carcinogen by the International Agency of Research on Cancer.[14] AA induces tumors in several organs in mice and rats and exerts reproductive and neurotoxic damage.[15,16] Currently, according to the World Health Organization, AA belongs to the group of carcinogenic and genotoxic compounds; it is considered that there is not a reliable threshold exposure limit for its reaction. In 2015 the European Food Safety Authority (EFSA) confirmed that AA in food potentially increases the risk of developing cancer for consumers of all age.[17]

The main sources of human dietary exposure to AA are those of fried potatoes (272–570 μg/kg), bakery products (75–1044 μg/kg), breakfast cereals (149 μg/kg), and coffee (229–890 μg/kg).[18] The distribution of AA levels in particular food categories is summarized in the scientific opinion of the EFSA.

Current policy is that practical measures should be taken voluntarily to reduce AA formation in vulnerable foods and so lessen human exposure to this chemical.[3] A new EU regulation set a benchmark level for AA in potato chips at 750 μg/kg.[19] In this sense, heat processed products must have AA levels lower than the benchmark levels and "as low as reasonable achievable" principle. Among the most relevant intervention for AA mitigation, we have storage and selection of raw material with low level of precursors, adjustment of heat transfer, application of additives preventing AA formation, and enzymatic treatment with asparaginase to eliminate asparagine.[1]

Acrylamide is metabolized in the body to glycidamide. Both are conjugated with urinary mercapturic acid, forming adducts with hemoglobin as well as DNA. They can be used as biomarkers for measuring the exposure to AA. In epidemiological studies, AA intake was not associated with an increased risk of most common cancers but the evidence is limited and inconsistent.[1]

13.2.2 Furan

Furan (C_4H_4O) is a small organic compound (M_w: 68 g/mol) with high volatility (boiling point: 31°C) and lipophilicity used in various chemical-manufacturing industries.[20] The broad number of foods that have been shown to contain furan suggest that multiple pathways are involved in furan formation in foods.[20,21] The thermal degradation and rearrangement of sugars and amino acids,[22] as well as the thermooxidation of polyunsaturated fatty acids (PUFAs)[22] and ascorbic acid,[4] have been proposed as the mechanisms responsible for its generation in foods[20,23] (Fig. 13.2).

Carbohydrates, amino acids, carbohydrate–amino acid mixtures, vitamins, PUFAs, and carotenoids have been reported as precursors for furan formation. In this respect, some factors such as heating temperature, pH, and moisture content have been shown to have a considerable effect on furan generation, most of the mechanistic insights into the formation of furan depend on them.[22,24] Despite its high volatility, furan has also been found in low-moisture foods processed in open containers such as potato chips, salty crackers, crisp breads, and toasted breads.[5,25] Furan levels in food are reported to range from a few μg/kg to 7000 μg/kg. Finally, the presence of furan in a broad range of heat processed foods (0–6000 μg/kg) has received considerable attention due to the fact that this heat-induced contaminant is considered as a "possible carcinogenic compound to humans."[5] The highest furan concentrations were found in roasted and instant coffee, followed by baby foods and soups.

The study of this contaminant really became a potential concern in the mid-1990s when based on research made in laboratories with animals exposed to high furan doses, this contaminant was considered as a possible carcinogen to humans (2B) by the International Agency for Research on Cancer.[14] The mechanism of furan-induced carcinogenicity in rodents as well as the level and effect of fura nonhumans has not yet been clarified. The liver is the target organ of furan-induced toxicity in rats and mice with a clear dose-dependency and probably acting by a genotoxic mechanism. Due to the limited relevant experience with regard to furan toxic effects associated with neither human exposure nor epidemiology, a final conclusion concerning genotoxic or mutagenic activity of this molecules has not been drawn yet.[1]

13.3 5-Hydroxymethylfurfural

HMF is a furanic compound formed as an intermediate in Mr when carbohydrates are heated in the presence of amino acids or proteins or, alternatively, by the thermal dehydration

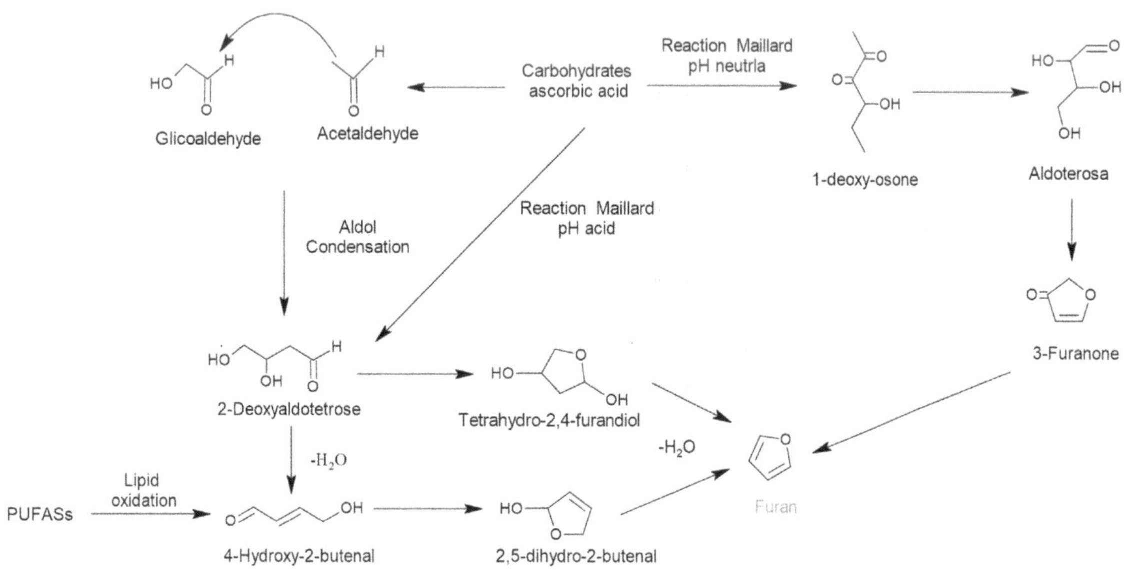

FIGURE 13.2 Mechanisms of furan formation. *Adapted from Mariotti M, Granby K, Rozowski J, Pedreschi F. Furan: a critical heat induced dietary contaminant.* Food Funct. *2013;4:1001–1105.*

of a sugar under acidic conditions[7] (Fig. 13.3).[26] HMF has been identified in a wide variety of foods processed at high temperatures (110°C–121°C) including dairy products, fruit juices, alcoholic beverages, honey, and among others.[27,28]

HMF is considered potentially carcinogenic to humans or might be metabolized by humans to potentially carcinogenic compounds and it is mainly formed through Mr and can be regarded as one of the most important heat-induced contaminants occurring in bread bakery products.[7] To date, studies could not confirm the potential human health risks of HMF but available in vitro and in vivo data give rise to concern about its genotoxicity. HMF has been recently shown to be converted in vivo to which is a genotoxic compound.[29]

The effect of HMF on human health has long been subject of research. It is still unclear whether dietary exposure to HMF is a health risk to humans.[30] However, some findings indicate that HMF exhibits potential genotoxic and mutagenic activity upon metabolic activation to 5-sulfoxymethylfurfural.[7]

Pedreschi et al.[6] significantly mitigated the formation of HMF in Chilean bread by incorporating polyphenols extracted from Tara (*Caesalpinia spinosa*) pods. These authors highlight the potential of using polyphenolic extracts to reduce the exposure of consumers to dietary NFCs. In addition, Barrios-Rodríguez et al.[30] assessed the effect of formulation and heat treatment on the formation of HMF, nonenzymatic browning and rheology of dulce de leche (DL). HMF in DL was mitigated in 35% in a

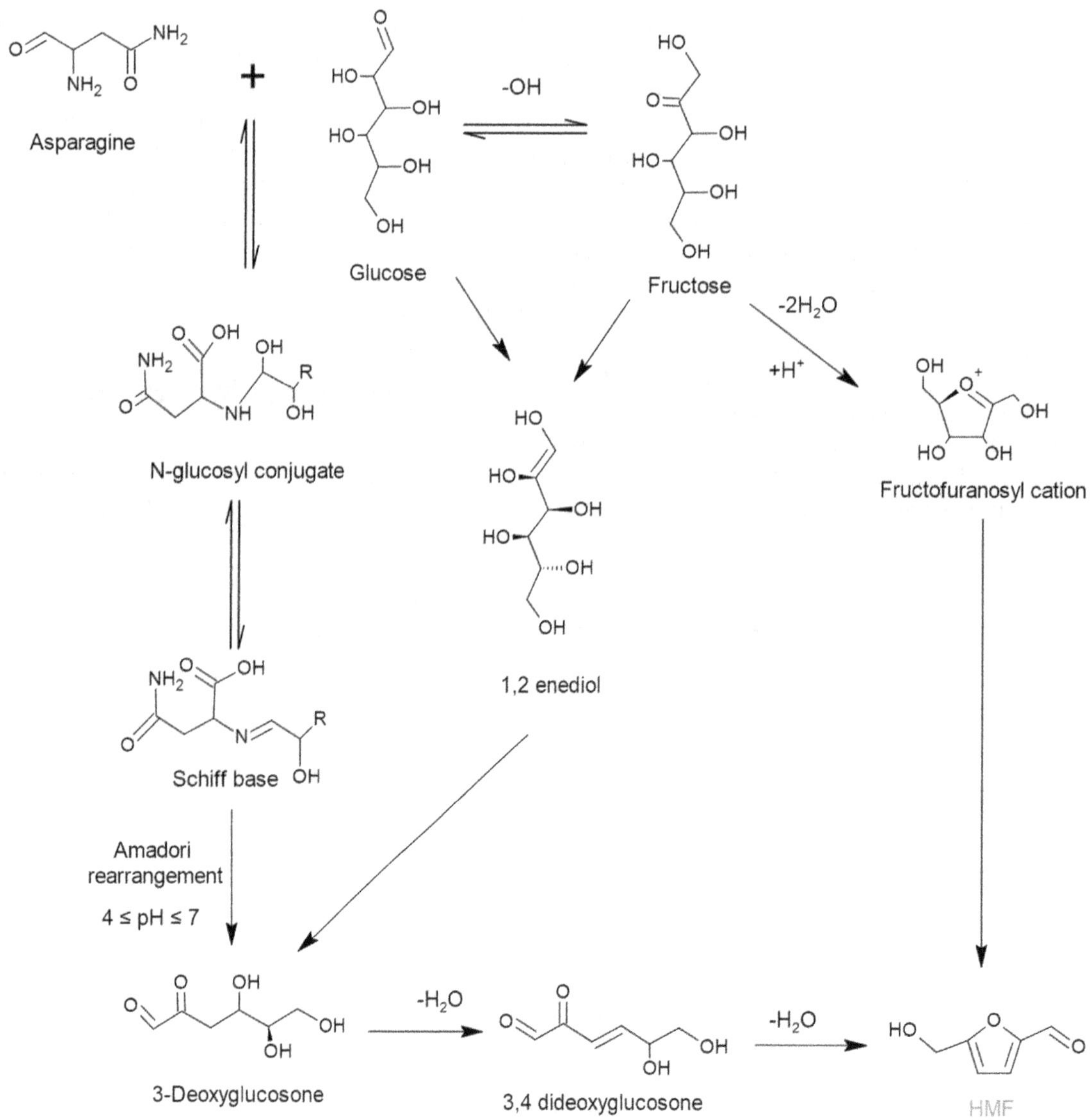

FIGURE 13.3 Mechanisms of HMF formation. *Adapted from Lee C, Chen K, Lin J, et al. Recent advances in processing technology to reduce 5-hydroxymethylfurfural in foods.* Trends Food Sci Technol. *2019;93:271–280.*

lactose-free formulation by lowering the process temperature. Moreover, HMF formation was reduced up to 80% replacing sucrose by tagatose without affect the quality parameters.

13.3.1 Heterocyclic amines

HAs are formed during intensive heating of protein-rich foods as pyrolysates from amino acids or as a part of the Mr from carbohydrates, amino acids, and creatine. Of the 30 compounds described up to date, only 10 are known to be carcinogenic in rodents.[1] The concentrations found in heated meat or fish are in the low ppb range (0–10 ng/g) of HAs. Intensive heat treatments result in significantly higher concentrations. Normally, 2-amino-1-methyl-6-phenylimidazol[4,5-b]pyridine is the compound occurring at higher concentrations with values of up to 480 ng/g, for example, barbecued chicken meat.

Mechanisms of HAs formation are seen in Fig. 13.4. For the formation of HAs during cooking of meat foods, some precursors are necessary which comprise mainly carbohydrates, amino acids, and in some cases creatine[31] (Fig. 13.4). Complex and to a great extent not yet characterized reaction pathways result in the formation of HAs. Some of these compounds contain an imidazole group, which is derived directly from the creatine. The other parts of the molecules are formed from the carbohydrates and amino acids. The complex reaction pathways need high temperature above 150°C to proceed significantly.[32]

HAs comprise c.20 compounds, of which 10 have been demonstrated to be carcinogenic. On the other hand, the "nonpolar" HAs are formed from direct degradation of amino acids. The epidemiological evidence suggests that consumption of well done or grilled meat may link with increased cancer risk in humans.[33] HAs are well known for their mutagenicity and the carcinogenicity in laboratory rodents. Although the results from the animal and tissue culture studies are unambiguous, it is difficult to derive these results from epidemiological studies. The epidemiological evidence suggests that consumption of well done or grilled

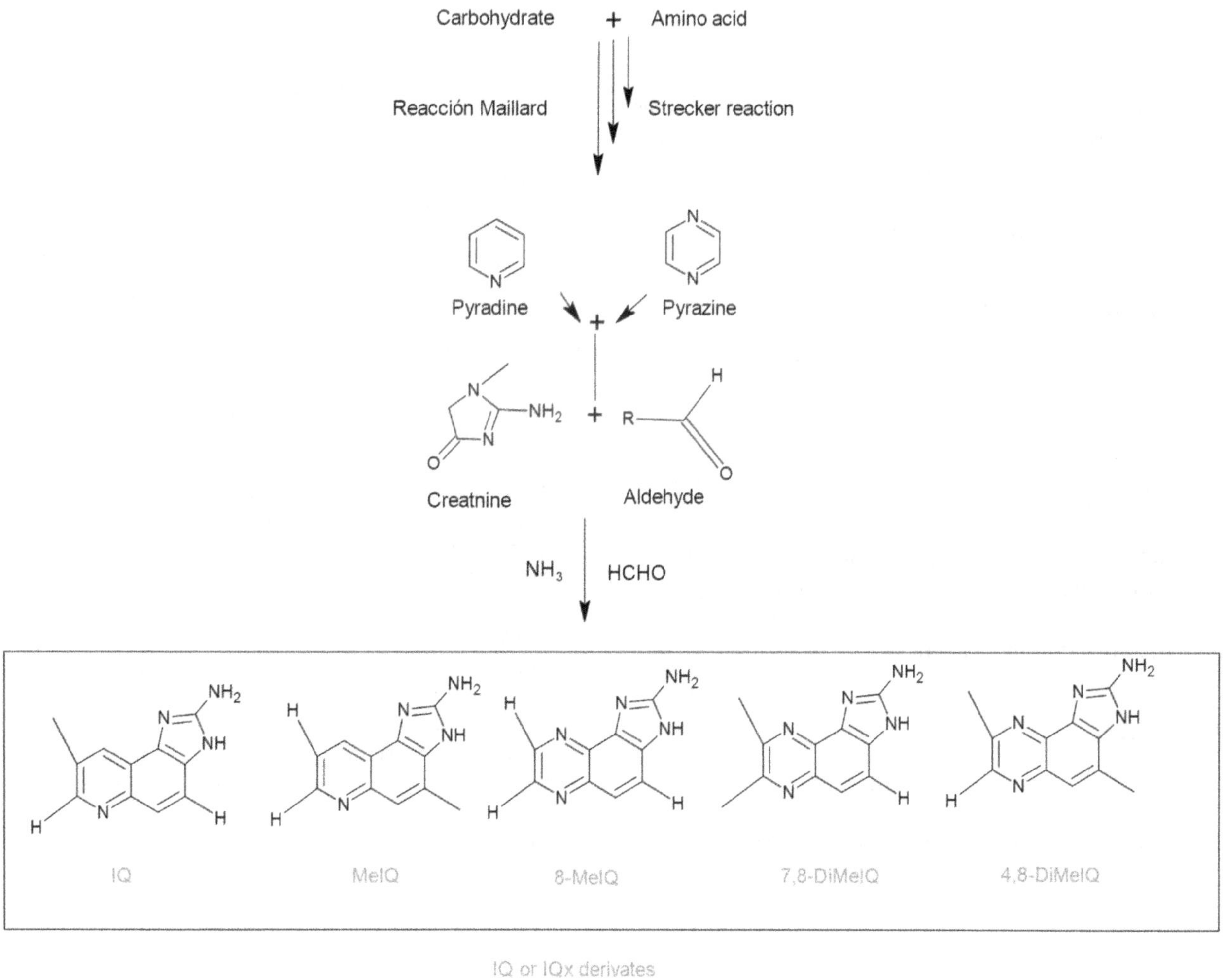

FIGURE 13.4 Mechanisms of HAAs formation. *Adapted from Rosario et al. (2020).*

meat may be associated with increased cancer risk in humans.[31] Furthermore, the carcinogenic effects of these HAs may be inhibited or enhanced by many factors, including interaction of HA mixtures. It is, therefore, difficult for human epidemiological studies to establish associations between cancer risk and specific HAs.[33]

There are several ways to reduce the exposure to HAs. The simplest way is to reduce the consumption of red meat, especially when it is over done. During cooking, too high temperatures for much time should be avoided. Many controversial results have been obtained for the use of, for example, antioxidant spices or a variety of other food additives or ingredients. On the other hand, reduce temperature cooking could avoid the formation of HAs.[31]

13.4 Future prospects

"Tailor-made" PCT mitigation strategies must be designed specifically to face the manufacturing heating process and the chemical composition and microstructure for each processed food matrix. Besides, rapid methods to identify and quantify PCTs should be developed by using some important physical surface properties of heated foods such as color intensity, darkness, lightness, degree of heterogeneity in core surface distribution, and among others. Finally, the PCTs presented here are naturally occurring constituents of our daily diet. Avoiding them will be a difficult task but reducing their intake will be possible by responsible cooking and/or by changing our eating habits.

Acknowlegdments

This study was financially supported by FONDECYT Project No 1190080, Fondo Nacional de Desarrollo Científico y Tecnológico, ANID, Chile.

Conflicts of interest

The authors declare that they have no conflict of interest. The authors have no affiliation with any organization with a direct or indirect financial interest in the subject matter discussed in the manuscript.

References

1. Murkovic M, Pedreschi F, Ciesarová Z. Process contaminants: a reviewIn: *Reference Module in Food Science*. 2018;.
2. Pedreschi F, Murkovic M. Potentially toxic components by excessive heat processing. In: Urribari J, ed. *Dietary AGES and Their Role in Health Disease*. New York: CRC Press; 2017.
3. Pedreschi F, Mariotti M, Granby K. Current issues in dietary acrylamide: formation, mitigation and risk assessment. *J Sci Food Agric*. 2014;94:9–20.
4. Mariotti M, Granby K, Fromberg A, Risum J, Agosin E, Pedreschi F. Furan occurrence in starchy food model systems processed at high temperatures: effect of ascorbic acid and heating conditions. *J Agric Food Chem*. 2012;60:10162–10169.
5. Mariotti M, Granby K, Rozowski J, Pedreschi F. Furan: a critical heat induced dietary contaminant. *Food Funct*. 2013;4:1001–1105.
6. Pedreschi F, Saavedra I, Bunger A, et al. Tara pod (*Caesalpinia spinosa*) extract mitigates neo-contaminant formation in Chilean bread preserving their sensory attributes. *LWT-Food Sci Technol*. 2018;95:119–122.
7. Capuano E, Fogliano V. Acrylamide and 5-hydroxymethylfurfural (HMF): a review on metabolism, toxicity, occurrence in food and mitigation strategies. *LWT-Food Sci Technol*. 2011;44 (4):793–810.
8. Birlouez-Aragon I, Morales F, Fogliano V, Pain JP. The health and technological implications of a better control of neoformed contaminants by the industry. *Pathol Biol*. 2010;58:232–238.
9. Mottram D, Wedzicha A, Dodson A. Acrylamide is formed in the Maillard reaction. *Nature*. 2002;419:448–449.
10. Yalayan V, Wnorowski A, Perez Locas C. Why asparagine needs carbohydrated to generate acrylamide. *J Agric Food Chem*. 2003;51:1753–1757.
11. Zyzak D, Sanders R, Stojanovic M, Tallmadge D, Ebehart H. Acrylamide formation mechanism in heated foods. *J Agric Food Chem*. 2003;51:4782–4787.
12. Brathen E, Kita A, Knutsen S, Wicklund T. Addition of glycine reduces the content of acrylamide in cereal and potato products. *J Agric Food Chem*. 2005;48:2271–2275.
13. Halford N, Curtis T, Muttucumaru N, Postles J, Elmore S, Mottram D. The acrylamide problem: a plant and agronomic science issue. *J Exp Botany*. 2012;63(8):2841–2851.
14. IARC. Dry cleaning, some chlorinated solvents and other industrial chemicals. In *Monographs on the Evaluation of Carcinogenic Risks to Humans*. Lyon, France, Chapter 63, 1995:394–407.
15. LoPachin R. The changing view of acrylamide neurotoxicity. *NeuroToxicology*. 2004;25:617–630.
16. Rosén J, Hellenas K. Analysis of acrylamide in cooked foods by liquid chromatography tandem mass spectrometry. *Analyst*. 2002;127:880–882.
17. EFSA (European Food Safety Authority). Scientific opinion on acrylamide on food EFSA panel on contaminants in the food chain. *EFSA J*. 2015;13(6):4104.
18. EFSA (European Food Safety Authority). Update on acrylamide levels in food from monitoring years 2007 to 2010. *EFSA J*. 2012;10:2938–2976.
19. Powders G, Mottram D, Curtis A, Halford N. Acrylamide levels in potato crisps in Europe from 2002 to 2016. *Food Addit Contam A*. 2017;34(12):2085–2100.
20. Crews C, Castle L. A review of the occurrence, formation and analysis of furan in heat-processed foods. *Trends Food Sci Biotechnol*. 2007;18:365–372.

21. Perez Locas C, Yaylayan V. Origin and mechanistic pathways of formation of the parent furan. A food toxicant. *J Agric Food Chem.* 2004;52:6830–6836.
22. Owczarek-Fendor A, De Meulanaer B, Scholl G, et al. Importance of fat oxidation in starch based emulsions in the generation of the process contaminant furan. *J Agric Food Chem.* 2010;58:9579–9586.
23. Hasnip S, Crews C, Castle L. Some factors affecting the formation of furan in heated foods. *Food Addit Contam.* 2006;23:219–227.
24. Fan X, Huang L, Sokoral K. Factors affecting thermally induced furan formation. *J Agric Food Chem.* 2008;56:9490–9494.
25. Anese M, Suman M. Mitigation strategies of furan and 5-hydroxymethylfurfural in food. *Food Res Int.* 2013;51:257–264.
26. Lee C, Chen K, Lin J, et al. Recent advances in processing technology to reduce 5-hydroxymethylfurfural in foods. *Trends Food Sci Technol.* 2019;93:271–280.
27. Husoy T, Haugen M, Murkovic M, et al. Dietary exposure of 5-hydroxymethylfurfural from Norwegian food and correlations with urine metabolites of short-time exposure. *Food Chem Toxicol.* 2008;46(12):3697–3702.
28. Ramirez A, García-Villanova B, Guerra-Hernandez E. Hydroxymethylfurfural and methylfurfural content of selected bakery products. *Food Res Int.* 2000;33(10):833–838.
29. Abraham K, Gurtler R, Berg K, Heinemeyer G, Lampen A, Appel K. Toxicology and risk assessment of 5-hydroxymethylfurfural in food. *Mol Nutr Food Res.* 2011;55(5):667–678.
30. Barrios-Rodríguez Y, Barrera J, Zuñiga R, Pedreschi F, Mariotti MS. Effect of formulation and heat treatment on 5-hydroxymethylfurfural formation and quality parameters in dulce de leche. *Food Addit Contam A.* 2021;. Available from: https://doi.org/10.1080/19440049.2021.1905187.
31. Murkovic M, Pichel N. Analysis of 5-hydroxymethylfurfural in coffee, dried fruits and urine. *Mol Nutr Food Res.* 2006;50:842–846.
32. Murkovic M, Weber H, Geiszler S, Frohlich K, Pfannhauser W. Formation of the food associated carcinogen 2-amino-1-methyl-6-phenylimidazol [4,5-b]pyridine (PhIP) in model systems. *Food Chem.* 1999;65:233–237.
33. NTP (National Toxicology Program). *Reporto n carcinogens.* 13th ed. Research Triangle Park, NC: U.S. Department of Health and Human Services, Public health Service; 2014.

Chapter 14

Migration of packaging and labeling components and advances in analytical methodology supporting exposure assessment

Cristina Nerín, Elena Canellas and Paula Vera
University of Zaragoza, Campus Rio Ebro, Zaragoza, Spain

Abstract

Nowadays, food industries offer products of nutritional and sensory quality to the consumers in which the packaging plays a fundamental role for the achievement of this objective. However, it can also become a serious problem if some aspects are not controlled, such as the mass transfer through it, known as migration. Migration has a great toxicological interest, as it implies the contamination of food from the packaging material. In this process, not only the material but everything applied on it, such as varnishes, printing inks, or adhesives, contribute as source of chemicals. Migration also affects the quality of packaged food, sometimes providing strange smells or tastes to the packaged food.

There are different types of packaging, which can be classified according to their functions or their materials, being the plastics and specifically the polyolefins the most commonly used as food packaging materials. They are normally found combined with other materials forming complex laminates. Nowadays, there is a search to reduce the environmental problems associated with the plastics due to nonbiodegradability. And then, new compostable and biodegradable materials have been developed for this purpose.

As any material requires additives and components other than the pure macromolecule to have the right functionality, there is a wide spectrum of chemical substances that may be transferred as migrants. The migrants can be grouped as intentionally added substances (IAS), like monomers and additives, and non-IAS, like impurities, degradation products, or reaction by-products (neoformed). To guaranty the food safety of packaged food, advanced analytical techniques are required to determine these migrant compounds at high sensitivity and selectivity for volatile, nonvolatile compounds and metals.

Keywords: Packaging; migration; NIAS; IAS; food contact materials; adhesives; printing inks; varnishes; labels; analytical techniques

14.1 Introduction

14.1.1 Types of food packaging and labeling

Packaging is an indispensable element in the food industry; its main function is to protect the food preserving its nutritional, sensorial, and health quality, minimizing any external incidence or contamination.

This protection can be passive or active: the first one avoids the food's physical deterioration and/or prevents its chemical or microbiological contamination. It provides a barrier against different parameters such as oxygen, humidity, microorganisms, light, temperature, aromas, flavors, and so on, which may reduce the quality of the food-producing microbiological alterations, lipid oxidations, vitamin destructions, or browning. Active protection helps to maintain a favorable atmosphere for food, preventing chemical and/or microbiological deterioration, and ultimately extending its shelf life. This is possible through components which can be added either as a label or be incorporated directly in the material of the container. This type of packaging is known as active packaging. Some good examples are moisture scavengers, antimicrobial or antioxidant packaging.

A secondary function of food packaging, of increasing importance, is to provide nutritional information, ingredients, traceability, manufacturer, and other important information to consumers. These details are found in the labeling, which in addition to providing information, have a clear objective of influencing consumers' choices, who have a critical interest in healthy and safe consumption.[1] The European Regulation No 1169/2011[2,3] establishes the requirements that labeling of food has to fulfill.

Other important functions of increasing demand of the packaging are convenience, tamper indications, and

Present Knowledge in Food Safety. DOI: https://doi.org/10.1016/B978-0-12-819470-6.00005-6

antifraud devices. Convenience concerns ease of access, re-sealing, handling, disposal, and microwave heating or cooking options using directly the same packaging, to minimize the time and effort to prepare the food. The packaging has facilitated the possibility of shopping in one-stop shop and the availability of food from around the world. Tamper and antifraud indications concern the use of special features designed to reduce or eliminate the risk of adulteration or tampering.[3] Some examples are special printing or holograms on bottle and cans such as graphics or text that irreversibly change upon opening.[4]

Perhaps one of the last innovations deals with intelligent packaging, that provides an informative response as result of a change produced either in the packaged food or in its headspace or outside in the environment. Some examples are the response against the presence of bacteria, microorganisms, or molds and also, the response against the change of gases concentration in the headspace or the cold chain breaking.[5–7]

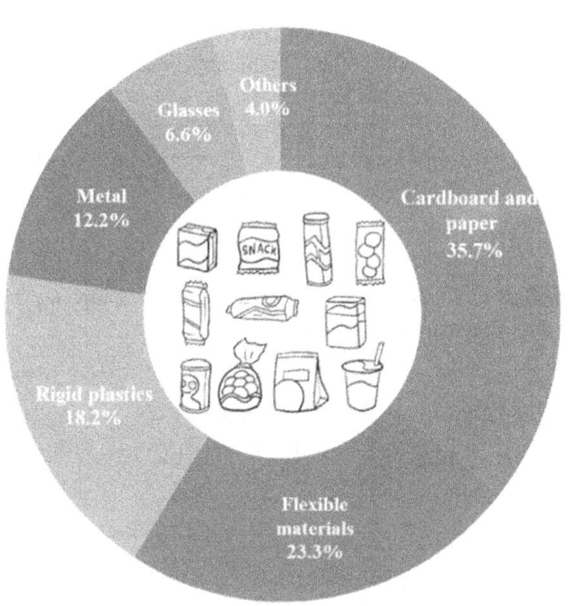

FIGURE 14.1 Materials used in food packaging. *World Packaging Organisation (WPO), 2017.*

14.1.2 Types of food packaging materials and labels

The packaging can be classified according to their functions in three categories: primary packaging, which contains the food packaged in direct contact. Some examples of this type are individual wrappers, films, bottles, trays, cans, jars, and so on; Secondary packaging assembles the primary packaging, and it consists of outer wrapping that assists in displaying, storing, shipping, and protecting products, as shrink-wrap around groups of individual bottles or canned of water soft drinks, and so on; and finally, tertiary packaging is used to protect and transport the packaging mentioned above, like corrugated boxes of cardboard or wooden boxes, pallets, plastic film to transport pallets, and so on.

Another way to classify the food packaging is based on the materials used to manufacture them. These materials include different types of plastics, papers, cardboards, metals, glasses, or woods. They can be used individually or combining different types of materials forming multilayers or laminates. Fig. 14.1 shows the percentage of world packaging market by material.

As can be seen, plastics, paper, and board are the most abundant materials used for food packaging, either alone or in combination with other materials. Under the frame of plastics, only conventional polymers are included, as biopolymers, which recently burst onto the market and will probably increase in the near future, can be included under the term "others." There have been numerous advancements in improving the performance of food packaging system, more especially, on the technology involved in film formation. It includes polymer composites (formed from a combination of different materials processed together, at least one is a polymer), blends of polymeric materials (mixture of polymers), and the formation of multilayers (several layers coextruded or laminated), or coatings (applied on the surface). Multilayer materials consist of several polymers joined to improve the characteristics of packaging and can have between 2 and 12 layers. It can be classified as flexible packages (such as films), semirigid packages (such as beverage cartons, trays, and multilayer bottles), or rigid ones. Within the group of flexible packaging are (1) flexible polymer composites without barrier layer, (2) flexible polymer composites with barrier layer, (3) flexible polymer composites with metal oxide coatings, (4) thermoformed plastic composites, and (5) plastic composites with aluminum foil.[8]

The selection of the material mainly depends on the necessary requirements to comply with the functions to protect and preserve the food, minimizing the external factors. Therefore this choice is completely related to the characteristics of the food packaged (pH, fat content, if it is solid or liquid), as well as with the technical requirements throughout the supply chain, such as mechanical resistance, barrier to gases, solvents, odors, humidity, microbes, thermal resistance, and inertness. Marketing needs are also crucial for this choice, as consumer attraction and identification of content (labeling, printing, etc.), and of course, the cost of the material used, play an important role.[4,9]

Labels can be made of either plastic or paper, virgin or recycled, and attached to the packaging material by thermosealing, which stretches plastic to cover the full container as a sleeve in a bottle, or by using adhesive. Electronic tags for radiofrequency identification can be printed on different materials and used as labels as well.

Table 14.1 shows a brief description of these materials found in the market, their main applications, as well as their advantages and disadvantages.

As Fig. 14.1 shows, the major percentage of food packaging contains plastics (43%, combining the amount of flexible materials and rigid plastics).

Polyolefins such as polypropylene and polyethylene (PP and PE) are the most common synthetic plastics used, with 63% of the global production as shown in Fig. 14.2. It displays the different types of plastics and their percentages produced worldwide for food packaging. However, it is expected that this figure will change over the coming years.

TABLE 14.1 Types of packaging classified according to the materials, their manufacture, their main uses, and some advantages and disadvantages.

Materials	Manufacture	Uses	Advantages	Disadvantages
Plastic	Polycondensation, the polymer chain grows by condensation reactions between molecules and formation of low molecular weight by-products such as water and methanol Polyaddition, monomers with at least 2 functional groups such as alcohol, amine, or carboxylic groups are combined to form a larger molecule	• Bottles of water, fruit juices, soft drinks, and oils • Trays of meat, fish, and fruits • Bags of frozen products • Cans for fresh cheese, yogurt, precooked food, and so on	Versatility: different forms and the most diverse designs (easy to print) Chemical resistant Inexpensive and lightweight Heat sealable[4,10]	Variable permeability to light, gases, vapors, and low molecular weight molecules. Variable recyclability Possible migration of components
Paper	Interlaced network of cellulose fibers derived from wood by using sulfate and sulfite Pulped and bleached are treated with chemicals such as slimicides and strengthening agents to improve its properties like barrier, strength, oil resistance, smooth and glossy finish	• Sacks for sugar, biscuits, and confectionary • Bags for dried fruits and vegetables • Wrapping of flour, snack foods, cookies, candy bars, oily foods, fast foods, and baked goods • Laminated with plastic or aluminum for soups, herbs, and spices	Cheap It is a resource that can be 100% recyclable	Not thermosealable Not oil resistance Low wet Poor barrier properties, need to laminate with other materials like aluminum or plastics as PE to improve their properties Possible migration of components
Cardboard	Is thicker than paper with a higher weight per unit area and often made in multiple layers	• Corrugated boxes for fruits and vegetables • Tubes for salt and other condiments • Coated with wax or laminated with PE for direct food contact, take-out food • Laminated with PE for fruit juices • soft drinks and milk • Outer layers of cartons for foods such as tea and cereals • Laminated with plastics or aluminum as coffee and milk powder	Resistance to impact abrasion and crushing damage Cheap It is a resource that can be 100% recyclable	Not thermosealable Not oil resistance Low wet Poor barrier properties, need to laminate with other materials like aluminum or plastics as polyethylene to improve their properties Possible migration of components

(Continued)

TABLE 14.1 (Continued)

Materials	Manufacture	Uses	Advantages	Disadvantages
Aluminum	Metal combined with oxygen as alumina. Magnesium and manganese added to improve its strength properties	• Cans of soft drink, pet food, seafood, and prethreaded closures • Aluminum foil to wrap food and thicker foils to store precooked meals trays or ready-to-eat foods • Lamination binding with paper or plastic film for dried soups, herbs, and spices	Excellent physical protection Barrier to moisture, air, odors, light, and microorganisms Not acceptable for acidic food Other protection is not required Good flexibility Excellent malleability Decorative potential Recyclability	Very expensive Requires a huge amount of bauxite (scarce) Low mechanic resistance No transparency Migration of the aluminum to acidic foods
Steel	Tinplate Coating both sides of low-carbon steel by dipping sheets of steel in molten tin or by the electro-deposition of tin on the steel sheet	• Cans for drinks, processed foods, and aerosols • Containers for powdered foods and sugar- or flour-based confections • Package closures • Package for sterile products	Common and high velocities of manufacture Excellent barrier properties to gases, water vapor, light, and odors Can be heat-treated Sealed hermetically Outstanding graphical decoration Relatively low weight and high strength Easily recycled many times without loss of quality	Expensive (lower than aluminum) Chemical and electrochemical reactivity Susceptible Corrosion and oxidation
	Tin-free steel Electrolytic chromium or chrome oxide–coated steel	• Food cans • Trays • Bottles caps and closures • Large containers for bulk sale and storage of ingredients	Excellent adhesion of coatings such as paints, lacquers, and inks Formability and strength Sulfur compounds-resistant Heat resistant	Expensive (less than tinplate) Humidity and acid reactivity
Glasses	Mixture of silica (the glass former), sodium carbonate (the melting agent), and limestone/calcium carbonate and alumina (stabilizers) to high temperatures until the materials melt into a thick liquid	• Jars of jams, sauces, and pickles • Bottles of beer, water, and wine	Odorless and chemically inert Impermeable to gases and vapors Ability to withstand high processing temperatures Rigid and transparent Reusable and recyclable	Heavy weight adding to transportation costs Brittleness and susceptibility to breakage
Wood	Pulp from polar or pine	• Barrels for liquids like wine, beer, liqueurs, or oil • Boxes for fruits, vegetables, fish, and seafood	Cheap High resistance to impact and compression Recyclable and reusable materials	Used only for packaging of huge amount of food or drinks

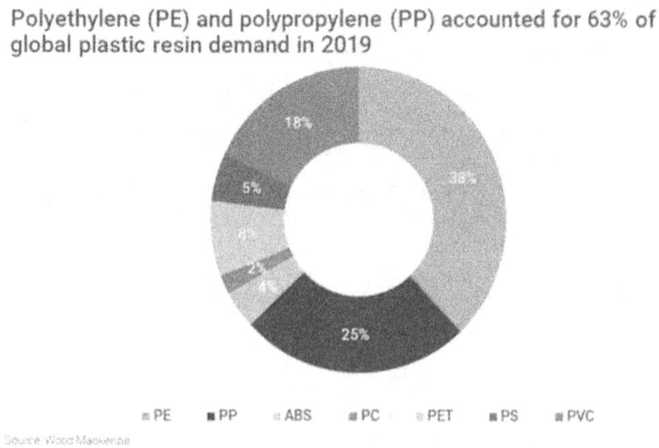

FIGURE 14.2 Different types of plastics used in the packaging industry worldwide. *Wood Mackenzie (2019).*

The environmental pressure, not only from the authorities, but also from eco-organizations and consumers, has increased the development of recycling technologies and production of compostable and biodegradable biopolymers at industrial scale. The abuse of plastics and the overpackaging will be reduced, and thus a rational and more balanced use of plastic packaging will remain.

As it has already mentioned above, there is a search to reduce the environmental problems associated with these nonbiodegradable materials. Research studies have been focused on developing new biopolymeric materials as raw materials for food packaging, mainly based on materials from renewable sources that are abundant in nature. In general, these materials are cheap and many of them are considered as waste or by-products reducing environmental problems. Therefore they are an alternative in several applications such as cutlery, plates, drinking cups, lids, straws, stirrers, overwrap and lamination films, containers for food dispensed at gourmet food stores, and fast-food establishments due to their capabilities to prevent moisture loss, aromas loss, solute transport, water absorption in the food matrix, or oxygen penetration.[11,12]

Table 14.2 describes these different types of synthetic and bioplastics used in the packaging market, with their main applications and characteristics.

14.1.2.1 Legislation

To guarantee the safety of the packaging, the materials must fulfill the European Regulation No 1935/2004 about materials and articles into contact with food, which provides a harmonized legal EU framework. It sets out the general principles of safety and inertness for all food contact materials (FCM).[19,20]

In addition, the European Regulation No 10/2011/EU[20,21] offers a positive list of compounds as monomers, starting substances and partial list of additives authorized as well as their specific migration limits (SML). These limits must not be exceeded by the migration value of each migrant compound obtained in the specific migration assays described earlier.

For those nonlisted compounds, their migration should not be higher than 0.01 mg/kg (ratio 6:1).[21] If the migrants found are not authorized, their toxicity should be confirmed, either by experimental data of toxicity, if any, or through a theoretical approach based on their chemical structure. The theoretical toxicity and the classification of analytes can be provided by the threshold of toxicological concern (TTC) and Cramer classes. Cramer classifies the compounds according to their chemical structure into three categories (class I, class II, and class III that correspond to low, medium, and high toxicity, respectively) and sets the maximum migration recommended for each class I, II, and III as 1.8, 0.54, and 0.09 mg/kg, respectively. TTC approach has been recommended by the European Food Safety Authority (EFSA).[22,23]

It must be highlighted that this legislation is only related to plastic materials intended to come into contact with food. But due to the lack of other legislations for other FCM, it can be applied to all packaging materials.

The case of paper and board is a little different. The document approved by the Council of Europe recommends, in addition, to carry out the migration tests. As was mentioned earlier, these tests are usually done with MPPO as solid simulant. A list of migrants with SML also appears in the RESAP (Resolution approved by the Council of Europe) and limits a series of substances, including metals such as Cd, Hg, and Pb. There are also restrictions on specific pollutants in the paper and board intended to be in contact with food.

Besides the main materials described above, such as the different types of plastics, papers, cardboards, metals, glasses, or woods used as FCM, there are other types of materials such as adhesives, printing inks, varnishes, and lacquers that are part of the packaging, and therefore their migrations must be considered.

14.2 Migration sources (materials, adhesives, printing inks, varnishes, etc.)

14.2.1 Direct migration

14.2.1.1 Definition of migration and its mechanism

After having described the complexity of food packaging, in which not only monolayers of one material, but also multilayer and multimaterial packaging with adhesives, varnishes, and printing inks applied on them, are very common, it is clear that the food packaging as a whole contains a wide spectrum of chemical substances that may be transferred to the food in contact with them. This

TABLE 14.2 Types of plastic and bioplastics used as food packaging materials, their main applications and characteristics.

Types of plastic	Applications	Characteristics
PP Polypropylene	Yoghurt containers, straws, margarine tubs	Low cost Good mechanic properties as flexibility, strength, lightness Moisture and chemical resistance Easy processability[9,13,14]
HDPE High-density polyethylene	Brick for milk, juice, cereal box liners, margarine tubs, trash, and retail bags	Stiff, strong, and tough resistant to chemicals and moisture Permeable to gas Easy to process, and easy to form[4,15,16]
LDPE Low-density polyethylene	Food wrap, bread bags, grocery bags. Film applications where heat sealing is necessary. Bread and frozen food bags, flexible lids, and squeezable bottles	Flexible, strong, and tough Easy to seal Resistant to moisture Relatively transparent[4]
PET Reaction of terephthalic acid with ethylene glycol	Beverages and mineral waters bottles Semirigid sheets for thermoforming (trays and blisters) Thin-oriented films (bags and snack food wrappers).	Good barrier to gases and moisture Good resistance to heat, mineral oils, solvents, and acids, but not to bases Glass-like transparency and light weight
Polyethylene naphthenate (PEN) Condensation polymer of dimethyl naphthalene dicarboxylate and ethylene glycol	Bottles for beer Carbonated beverages	Very expensive Barrier protection against transfer of flavors and odors Properties for carbon dioxide, oxygen, and water vapor are superior to PET Better performance at high temperatures
Polyvinylchloride (PVC) Addition polymer of vinyl chloride	Oil bottles Films for meat	Protection against transfer of gases, flavors, and odors Excellent resistance to chemicals (acids and bases) and oil Easily thermoformed Migration of plasticizers (phthalates) Environmental problem because of its chlorine content[9]
Polyvinylidene chloride (PVDC) Addition polymer of vinylidene chloride	Packaging of poultry, cured meats, cheese, snack foods, tea, coffee, and confectionary Hot filling, retorting, low-temperature storage, and modified atmosphere packaging	Thermosealable Excellent barrier to water vapor, gases, and fatty and oily products Migration of plasticizers and problems with chlorine[9]
Polystyrene (PS) Addition polymer of styrene	Hot beverage cups, plates, and bottles Take-home boxes, egg cartons, meat trays	Clear, hard, and brittle with a relatively low melting point Can be recycled or incinerated
Polyamide (PA) (Nylon) Condensation reaction between diamine and acid polyamide	Boil in bag Films	Good chemical resistance (oil, fats, acid foods) Good barrier (oxygen, odors, and flavors) Resistance at very high and low temperatures

(Continued)

TABLE 14.2 (Continued)

Types of plastic	Applications	Characteristics
EVOH Copolymer of ethylene and vinyl alcohol	Multilayered coextruded films, not in direct contact with liquids	Good barrier of gases, flavors, and odors Excellent barrier to oil and fat Very moisture sensitive[8]
Polylactic acid (PLA) Copolymerization of poly(D-lactic acid) and poly(L-lactic acid)	Short-term food packaging applications (take away) Cutlery, covered jars, windows of the boxes, trays, and bottles Combined with other materials for enhancing the properties: • PLA/cellulose/Ag nanoparticles → Increased strength for plastic shelf life. • PLA/polyurethane softening → flexibility agent[17]	High transparency Mechanical properties are assimilated to PET and PS Heat sealing at temperatures lower than those of polyolefins Biodegradable[8]
Polyhydroxylalkanoates (PHAs) Obtained from bacterial fermentation There are more than a hundred different monomers, hydroxyvalerate, butyrate, and so on	Short-term food packaging applications Combined materials for enhancing the properties: • PHA/zein increase storage time • PHA/nanokeratin increase shelf life and barrier properties[17]	Completely biodegradable Good mechanical properties comparable with polyolefins High crystallinity, melting temperature, and good resistance to organic solvents
Polyhydroxybutyrate (PHB) Produced by certain microorganisms as a carbon assimilation product (from glucose or starch)	Films for cheese Combined materials for enhancing the properties: • PHB/ZnO improved mechanical properties • PHB/PLA stabilized the film produced • PHB/presence of chlorinated agent increased storage[18]	Biocompatibility, biodegradability Optical properties and ultraviolet-resistivity[17] Poor mechanical strength and thermal
Polycaprolactone (PCL) Ring-opening polymerization	• PCL/nanocomposite shelf life of the packed material. • PCL/chitosan film improved barrier properties	Flexible, biodegradable, and nontoxic, Easy to process and hydrophobic fossil-based polymer[17]
Starch Composed of two isomers, amylose (linear structure) and amylopectin (highly branched structure) Different origins; corn, potato, or pea	• Starch/basil/green tea; smart packaging biodegradable plastic material. Where polyphenolic helped in the preservation of the food by retarding the oxidative reactions. Chlorophyll and carotenoids allowed pH sensitive.[17] • Corn starch/Chitosan: films, good pH sensitivity	Cheap, abundant, and biodegradable Susceptible to moisture attacks Easily modified with surface additives Good sealability and printability properties without surface treatment[11]
Cellulose Polysaccharide-containing many linked glucose units. From wood, cotton, hemp, and plant materials or synthesized by tunicates and microorganisms	Film for fresh fruit, meat, and cheese • Cellulose/polyvinyl alcohol/ carboxymethylcellulose; films for enhanced mechanical thermal properties to some extent[17]	Renewability and low cost Biodegradability and biocompatibility Chemical stability[11]

process is usually called "migration." Thus migration is a submicroscopic process of mass transfer of components present in food packaging to food, as a consequence of the tendency toward equilibrium of all chemical systems. Their consequences are the alteration of physicochemical and mechanical characteristics of the packaging material together with changes in the composition of the food that can significantly affect its quality, sensory characteristics, or may be toxic to the human body.

Volatile, semivolatile, and nonvolatile compounds, as well as metals in different chemical forms can migrate from the packaging materials in their final format, that means, once manufactured, printed, and so on. Among the potential migrants, monomers and additives as intentionally added substances (IAS) are found. However, as result of polymerization and manufacturing processes, impurities from raw materials and interaction between ingredients, either in the production process or in the packaging, non-IAS (NIAS) can appear.[23]

Migration is controlled by two mechanisms: partition and diffusion. The partition expresses the distribution of the migrant between two phases when the thermodynamic equilibrium is established. The partition coefficient (K) [Eq. (14.1)] is defined as the relationship between the equilibrium concentration of the migrant in both phases in (mol/m^3):

$$K_{1,2} = Ceq(1)/Ceq(2) \quad (14.1)$$

where $K_{1,2}$ is the partition coefficient, Ceq (1) is the concentration of the migrant in phase 1 (package), and Ceq (2) is the concentration in phase 2 (food).

When the constant $K_{1,2}$ has a value $K > 1$, the element has a great tendency to remain in phase 1 (packaging); on the contrary, if the value is <1, it has a tendency to migrate to the phase 2 (food). The partition constant largely depends on the solubility, that is, the affinity of the migrant with the packaging materials or with the food. It also depends on the temperature, chemical structure and size of the migrant compound, fat content and crystallinity of the food.[24–26]

The diffusion (D) of a molecule in a matrix is a kinetic parameter that is related to the mobility of the molecules in the material. It is represented by a flow magnitude (J) that crosses perpendicularly through an area of different sections in a homogeneous phase, with a concentration gradient of migrants. It is based on a steady-state dimensional process, which can be described according to Fick's first law:

$$J = -D(C)dC/dx \quad (14.2)$$

where J is the migrant flow (mol/m^2/s), D (C) is the diffusion coefficient (m^2/s), C is the migration concentration compound (mol/m^3), and x is the thickness of the material (m). This equation gets more complex depending on the number of layers in multilayer or laminated materials.

The diffusion coefficient depends on the size, molecular weight, shape, and flexibility of the migrant compound, as well as the characteristics of the packaging material, such as the type of material (paper, polymer, etc.), its crystallinity, glassy or gummy state, porosity, plasticization, and formulation.[24–26] Very big molecules, such as those heavier than 1500 Da, cannot diffuse through the packaging and consequently, they cannot migrate.

Fig. 14.3 shows an example of migration of a multilayer complex, showing the parameters that would depend on its hypothetical migration, such as the partition coefficients (K) between different materials and the diffusion coefficients (D) in these materials.

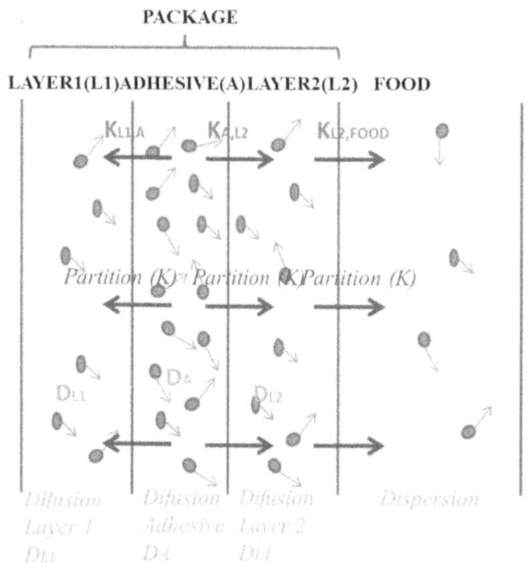

FIGURE 14.3 Migration of a multilayer package and the parameters that depend on this migration.

14.2.1.2 Migration analysis

The migration can be determined by conventional approach of direct experimental migration tests using analytical methods to identify and quantify the migrants[16,21,27–29] or using mathematical models as predicting tools to provide insights for the design and evaluation of the packaging material.[8,30,31] The first one is time-consuming but it is the basic assay which allows determination of accurate and nonpredictive migration values, as well as identification and quantification of migrants, including NIAS. Therefore this kind of assay provides a complete overview of all compounds that could migrate from the package.

In practice, the migration tests consist of two different kinds of assays: overall migration and specific migration. Overall migration refers to the total mass that is transferred from the container to the food, and the total mass must not exceed 60 mg of total constituents released per kilogram of food simulant.[20,21] On the other hand, the specific migration represents the amount of each specific substance that is transferred to 1 kg food.

All these assays are carried out with different simulants according to Commission Regulation 10/2011/EU[20,21] where the contact conditions, both time and temperature, as well as the simulants, are established. The simulants tested mimic the behavior of food and are chosen depending on their final uses according to the intended food: for example, ethanol 10% (simulant A), acetic acid 3% (simulant B), and ethanol 20% (simulant C) are selected when the material is intended for hydrophilic food character. Ethanol 50% (simulant D1) shall be used for alcoholic foods with an alcohol content of above 20% and for oil in water emulsion. Any vegetable oil (simulant D2) containing less than 1% unsaponifiable matter, that can be replaced by 95% ethanol and/or isooctane, were selected for fatty foods. Finally, poly(2,6-diphenyl-*p*-phenylenoxide) (MPPO, simulant E) is used for dry foods.

Migration from paper and board is described by the Council of Europe (ref.: RESAP 2005, etc.), where recommendations for testing and migration limits are established. For this purpose, the simulant should be MPPO, as liquid simulants destroy the paper packaging. When paper or board is covered by a plastic layer, then liquid simulants can be used. In these cases, the same simulants used for plastics migration testing are also used. One key point in this frame is the amount of MPPO used in the test, to completely cover the material during the test. In order to have reliable results from any laboratory involved in the tests, a norm has been launched[32] in which 4 g of MPPO per dm^2 of paper surface is established.

14.2.1.2.1 Adhesives

Adhesives are widely used in flexible laminates structures to join the different layers materials. Around 80% of FCM contain various kinds of adhesives in their structures. In some cases, tie layers are used to glue different materials in a laminate, as it is the case of polyethylenterephthalate (PET) and PE. However, the composition can be similar to that of some adhesives. Despite the abundance of chemical formulas and the number of chemicals involved in this sector, there is no specific legislation for these kinds of materials.

The most common adhesive studied in migration is that based on polyurethane (PU). It is widely used, due to its excellent adhesion properties, chemical and temperature resistance, and its ease of application at fast roll-to-roll lamination speeds, especially to join plastic-plastic materials.[33] The most common migrant compounds found in this type of adhesives are the cyclic oligomers as by-products of polyester synthesis[34,35] in the adhesive production and the primary aromatic amines (PAAs)[36–38] generated as NIAS when the residual isocyanates, one of the main monomers of PU, enter in contact with humidity and degrade into PAAs. This degradation takes place when the curing process is not complete, and thus residual isocyanates still remain in the system. Some producers add small amounts of epoxy resins to PU adhesives to increase the resistance of the final multilayer. This practice is not recommended in FCM, as migrants of concern such as bisphenol A (BPA), bisphenol A diglycidyl ethers (BADGE), and their derivatives amount others, migrate to the packaged product.[39–42]

Other type of adhesives are the acrylic ones, commonly used to join laminates formed by cardboard or paper with plastic films or to stick label directly attached to the food.[43,44] Several surfactants based on 2,4,7,9-tetramethyl-5-decyne-4,7-diol (TMDD) 2-butoxyethanol and 2,4,7,9-tetramethyl-5-decyne-4,7-diol 10 and ethoxylated compounds were found as migrants that should be removed from the formula.[25,45] Acrylic adhesives are usually water-based and can be seen as environmentally friendly and efficient alternative to solvent-based adhesives, avoiding their low-volatile organic compounds. They have adjustable permeability and economic practicality.[46] However, isothiazolinones are added as biocides, providing the protection against microorganisms that is prone to occur in aqueous media, and their migrations have to be studied.[47] Hot-melt adhesives are used to glue cardboard boxes but also in other applications such as to seal paper or aluminum closures on the edge of plastic boxes. They are based on paraffinic waxes, hydrocarbon resins, and polyolefins. The most common migrants found from them were aromatic hydrocarbons as 9,10-dihydroanthracene and dehydroabietin derivatives.[24,48,49]

Other types of adhesives such as rubber and vinylic used in special applications in FCM, have been also studied.[26,50] Natural adhesives based on gelatin or polysaccharides, commonly used in the paper sector, are rarely employed in food packaging materials.

14.2.1.2.2 Varnishes and lacquers

Varnishes or coatings play an important role in FCM, as they are used not only for decoration and better appearance, but also for supplying additional functionalities such as higher barrier properties, antislip, thermosealing properties, or additional protection of ink. In this way, they can be classified into interior and exterior coatings. Protective interior coatings, also called lacquers, are designed to avoid possible interaction between the food and the metal packaging (cans). One of the most effective coatings is phenolic epoxy, which combines properties such as chemical resistance, excellent adhesion to the substrate, good flexibility, and high resistance to high-temperature sterilization. However, the migration of Bisphenol A, a common monomer used in epoxy resins, as a synthetic endocrine-disrupting chemical, and its derivative BADGE must be considered.[51] Also, acrylic coatings are used for generating white films resistant to wear or abrasion, with good pigmentation properties. Other types of coatings are polyesters and alkyds based on natural unsaturated oils (soy, flax seed) and/or fatty acids.

14.2.1.2.3 Wax

Wax is used as treatment, coating, laminate, and impregnation of materials such as board, paper, and aluminum.

Furthermore, it may be used as a direct coating on fruit and cheese. It is also used as a lubricant to reduce friction in the manufacturing process and as a good moisture barrier to protect dry foods from environmental moisture or to reduce moisture lost. It is based on petroleum such as paraffin waxes or made of natural material such as beeswax, soy wax, or candelilla wax.[48,52]

The waxes and their components may migrate into food, including antioxidants, plasticizers, water proofing agents, and mineral oils.[53,54] Due to the fact that the waxes also have small amounts of polymeric material, they are regulated under No 10/2011/EU.[20,21]

14.2.1.2.4 Printing inks

Printing inks on FCM are used for consumer information as well as for marketing purposes. Inks are used with many different packaging materials such as plastics, paper, board, glass, and cork. They consist of coloring matters (pigments or dyes), vehicles (resins), solvents (depending on the printing process), and a large number of additives.

Even though they are applied on the outside of the packaging, their migration through the different material layers can occur. This migration depends on the material properties; for example, carton and board have a high permeability, whereas glass has no permeability. Besides, other transfer of matter can be carried out based on set-off phenomena, discussed in detail in the next subsection.[48,52]

Several studies have found components of printing inks in foodstuffs, such as plasticizers, ultraviolet (UV) initiators, and benzophenones.[29,55–57]

No specific EU harmonized legislation on printing inks for food contact has been issued; but in Europe, Switzerland, in 2005, was the first country that included arrangements for printing inks in its national regulation on FCM.[58]

14.2.2 Set-off phenomena

The set-off phenomena is a special case of migration, where compounds from the outer layer of a food packaging material migrate to the inner and consequently migrate to food. It occurs in the manufacturing process, when both layers come into direct contact between them. This migration can occur, for example, from printing inks when beverage cartons or multilayer plastics are stored in rolls,[2,57,59] or when paper cups are stacked one inside the other.[56] It is also produced from varnishes in contact from its exterior coating.[29]

Fig. 14.4 shows two examples of this phenomena as migration of printing inks from paper cups stacked and from multilayer plastics rolled.

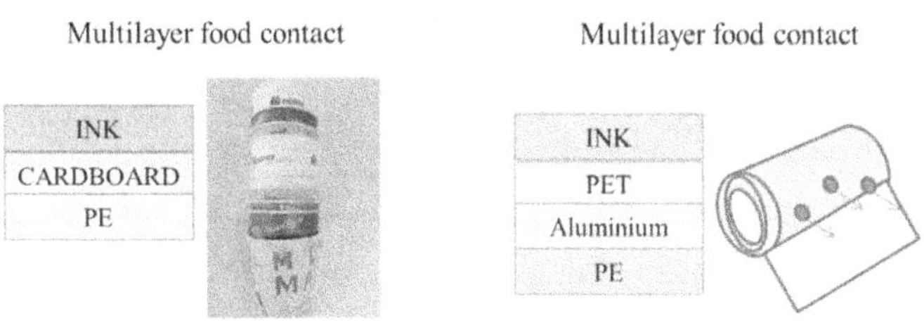

FIGURE 14.4 Examples of set-off phenomena.

14.3 Components

Migrants can be classified in two large groups of substances according to their origin: IAS and NIAS.

14.3.1 Intentionally added substances

IAS are the compounds added in purpose in the manufacture of a food contact material and involve monomers, additives to provide specific functions, and so on. There are different categories depending on their use. Table 14.3 shows the classification of IAS, the packaging materials where they are added, and the migration studies recently published about it.

A monomer is a molecule that can react together with other monomer molecules to form a larger polymer chain. The monomer used in each kind of polymer has a different chemical nature. Therefore it will have a different migration tendency and a different toxicity. Theoretically, the monomers used should be absent in the polymer, as they should react and disappear. However, some traces of residual monomers can be trapped into the polymer and later migrate. Almost all monomers involved in the polymeric FCM have SMLs and should be carefully controlled.

Bisphenol A is an important monomer in the production of polycarbonate. It has been a target with respect to food safety, since it is an endocrine disruptor. Nowadays, there are safer alternatives but its migration is still under study.[60] Moreover, epoxy resins of bisphenol A type contain oligomers such as BADGE usually applied as starting materials for cold-cured epoxy resins. Migration of BADGE and its derivatives have been studied in both simulants and food.[61–63] Migration of all residual monomers has been studied in depth, and the main references are shown in Table 14.3.

Other IAS used as plasticizers such as phthalates,[69] which are endocrine disruptors, have been intensively

TABLE 14.3 Classification of the intentionally added substances, the packaging materials where they are added, and the migration studies about these compounds.

Family	Migrants	Material	References about migration of the compounds
Monomers	Bisphenol A	Polycarbonate	60
	BADGE	Epoxy resin	61–63
	Styrene	Polystyrene	64
	Monoethylene glycol and terephthalic acid	PET	65
	Caprolactam and oligomers from PA	Polyamide	66–68
Plasticizers	Phthalates	PVC, PVA, PE, PP	61–63,69–73
	Adipates	PET, PVC, PE	15,74
	Citrates	PVC	75,76
	ESBO	PVC	77,78
	Sebacates	PVC	79,80
Antioxidants	Synthetics: Tinuvin P, Tinuvin 326, Tinuvin 776 DF, Tinuvin 234, Chimassorb 81, Irganox 1076, Irganox 1330, Irganox 1010, Irganox168 and Irganox P-EPQ, butylated hydroxyanisole, butylated hydroxytoluene, propyl gallate, and tertiary butylhydroquinone	PE, PP, adhesive, hot melt, PET	11–14,16
	Natural: α-tocopherol, essential oils, selenium	Adhesive	81–84
Photoinitiators	Benzophenone and derivatives: 1-hydroxycyclohexyl-1-phenyl ketone, 2,2′-dimethoxy-2-phenylacetophenone, 2-ethylhexyl 4-dimethylaminobenzoate, 2-methyl-4′-(methylthio)-2-morpholinopropiophenone, 2-isopropylthioxanthone	Varnishes, inks, and paper	81–83,85
Slip additives	Fatty acid amines	Polyolefins, PS, and PVC	86,87
Light stabilizers	Chimassorb 944 and Tinuvin 770	Polyolefins	88,89
Mineral oils	MOSH MOAH	Paper and board, adhesives, inks	48,90–93
Metals	Iron and lead	Cans	94
	Antimony	PET	95
	Lead (Pb), cadmium, zinc, and arsenic (As)	Paper and board	96,97
	Cadmium	Cork	98
Nanoparticles	Silver nanoparticles	Plastic materials	99
	Zinc oxide nanoparticles	Plastic materials, alginate film	100
	Selenium nanoparticles	Adhesive/ multilayer	101

BADGE, Bisphenol A diglycidyl ethers; *ESBO*, epoxidized soybean oil; *MOAH*, mineral oil aromatic hydrocarbons; *MOSH*, mineral oil saturated hydrocarbons; *PE*, polyethylene; *PP*, polypropylene; *PS*, polystyrene; *PVA*, polyvinyl acetate.

studied in many samples, even in bottled water made from PET[70] and in edible oils and fatty foods,[71–73] where they are more soluble. Adipates from PVC films to food,[15,74] tributyl acetyl citrate (ATBC),[75,76] epoxidized soybean oil (ESBO) from gaskets for glass jar lids, and film wraps and sebacates from PVC were also studied.[77–79]

Antioxidants are added to the plastics and labels, mainly to polyolefins, to reduce the rate of oxidation caused from UV light and air. Tinuvin P, Tinuvin 326, Tinuvin 776 DF, Tinuvin 234, Chimassorb 81, Irganox 1076, Irganox 1330, Irganox 1010, Irganox 168, and Irganox P-EPQ, butylated hydroxyanisole, butylated hydroxytoluene, propyl gallate, and tertiary butylhydroquinone are the most widely known chemical antioxidant substances. Their migration has been broadly studied.[11–14,16] Moreover, some natural antioxidants such as tocopherols and tocotrienols (vitamin E), ascorbate (vitamin C), vitamin A and carotenoids (β-carotene, lycopene, lutein, etc.) are also added to FCM.[81] Migration from essential oils used as antioxidants in food packaging has been broadly studied.[82,83,85] There are also other antioxidants to protect and extend the shelf life of the packaged food instead of protecting the polymer, what is called active packaging. One example is nanoselenium, which acts as antioxidant for food,[84] when added to a multilayer without being in direct contact with food, or essential oils and their major components.[102–106]

Photoinitiators are compounds that produce free radicals when exposed to UV light and initiate the polymer chain growth. They are essential ingredients of all UV-curable adhesives, inks, and coatings. These compounds have a high tendency to migrate to food and their migration has been deeply studied. Benzophenone,1-hydroxycyclohexyl-1-phenyl ketone, 2,2′-dimethoxy-2-phenylacetophenone, 2-Ethylhexyl 4-dimethylaminobenzoate, 2-methyl-4′-(methylthio)-2-morpholinopropiophenone, and 2-isopropylthioxanthone, among others have been reported from varnishes, inks, and paper.[81–83,85]

Fatty acid amides are applied as lubricants in a wide range of plastics such as polyolefins, polystyrene (PS), and PVC. These compounds and other substances used to lubricate have been reported to migrate from packaging polymers and cans.[86,87]

Light stabilizers prevent the damage to plastics caused by exposure to the environmental parameters of light, heat, and air. Polymeric hindered amines such as Chimassorb 944 and Tinuvin 770 are applied in polyolefins as light stabilizers.[88,89]

Mineral oil hydrocarbons are derived from crude oil and include mineral oil saturated hydrocarbons and mineral oil aromatic hydrocarbons (MOAH). They are used as lubricants, defoaming, cleaning, and nonstick agents. MOAH represent the most toxic fraction due to its mutagenic and carcinogenic properties. The migration of these compounds has been studied by many researchers and mainly found from paper and board,[90–92] adhesives,[48] and also added to inks for packaging.[93] Different polymers are now under study to act as efficient barriers for mineral oils in food packaging, mainly applied to paper and board packaging.[107]

Metals such as iron and lead migration from cans has been studied,[94] and antimony has been reported to migrate from PET.[95] Paper is another important source of heavy metals, lead (Pb), cadmium, zinc, and arsenic (As) migrated from paper or recycled paper,[96] in some cases coming from colorants,[97] and cadmium has been reported to migrate from cork stoppers.[98]

Silver has been used in food packaging in the nanoform state, to provide antimicrobial, antifungal, antiyeasts, and antiviral activity. Morais et al. did a review about 26 food contact articles and showed that only two showed no evidence of migration. However, these results are questionable, because all studies present conflicting, contradictory, or questionable results[99] mainly due to the difficulties in demonstrating the migration of nanoparticles (NPs)[108,109] or the dissolved metal as an ion. Zinc oxide NPs have also antimicrobial properties, Aristizabal-Gil et al. recorded that depending on the percentage of NPs the maximum migration limit was exceeded.[100] In contrast, no-migrating selenium NPs inserted in multilayer materials has been demonstrated.[101]

14.3.2 Nonintentionally added substances

NIAS can be impurities, reaction products, breakdown products, degradation products, and so on. The term NIAS was introduced for FCM made from plastics in Europe in the legal context of regulation 10/2011/EU. Nevertheless, NIAS are not limited to plastics as they can also migrate from nonplastic materials, since impurities and reaction by-products can be produced in all materials that form a food contact material. Table 14.4 shows some examples of NIAS, the packaging materials where they come from, and the migration studies done about it.

Toxic PAAs are reaction products from residual isocyanates in PU adhesives and have been broadly studied as they are the most common NIAS in the packaging industry.[37,38]

NIAS coming from polyolefins have been studied recently. Methyl and ethyl 3-(3,5-di-tert-butyl-4-hydroxyphenyl) propanoate were found to be degradation products of either Irganox 1010 or Irganox 1076 detected in migration from PE and PP.[14,16] Moreover, breakdown products including hexa-heptadecanamide, *N,N′*-1,2-ethanediylbis- and 11-eicosenamide were identified together with impurity reaction products, for example, dibutyl amine or compounds of unknown origin like phosphine oxide and tributyl-.[16] Moreover, other by-product of the antioxidant

Irganox 1010, tert-butyl-1-oxaspiro(4,5)deca-6-9-diene-2,8-dione was identified in PP and in multilayer samples of PE/PET, PP/PP, PE/PA, low-density polyethylene/PP, and PE/PVDC.[110,111]

NIAS have been also found migrating from paper and board. Dialkyl diketene dimers are used as sizing agents in the manufacture of paper and board for food contact applications to increase wetting stability. Unbound residues can hydrolyze and decarboxylate into dialkylketones which are NIAS that can migrate to fatty foods.[112]

Other source of NIAS are cans. Bis(2-hydroxy-3-tert-butyl-5-methylphenyl)dicyclopentane,1-tetradecanesulfonic acid, 1-pentadecanesulfonic acid, 1-hexadecanesulfonic acid, and naphthalene-2-sulfonic acid were identified as

TABLE 14.4 Examples of nonintentionally added substances, the packaging materials where they were found, and the migration studies recently conducted.

Nonintentionally added substances	Source	Material	References
Primary aromatic amines	Diisocyanates	Polyurethane	37,38
Methyl and ethyl 3-(3,5-di-tert-butyl-4-hydroxyphenyl)propanoate	Degradation products of either Irganox 1010 or Irganox 1076	Polyolefin	14,16
Hexa-heptadecanamide, *N,N′*-1,2-ethanediylbis- and 11-eicosenamide	Alkylamide breakdowns	Polyolefin	16
Dibutyl amine or compounds of unknown origin like phosphine oxide and tributyl-	Impurities	Polyolefin	16
Tert-butyl-1-oxaspiro (4,5) deca-6–9-diene-2,8-dione	By-product of the antioxidant Irganox 1010	PE/PET, PP/PP, PE/PA, LDPE/PP, and PE/PVDC	110,111
Dialkylketones	Dialkyl diketene dimers that hydrolyze and decarboxylate	Paper and board	112
Bis(2-hydroxy-3-tert-butyl-5-methylphenyl) dicyclopentane,1-tetradecanesulfonic acid, 1-pentadecanesulfonic acid, 1-hexadecanesulfonic acid, and naphthalene-2-sulfonic acid	Fragments of polymeric anionic surfactants based on sodium C14–17 sec-Alkyl sulfonate	Sealants can	29
2-Propenoic acid,1,1′-[2-[[3-[2,2-bis[[(1-oxo-2-propen-1-yl)oxy]methyl]butoxy]-1-oxopropoxy]methyl-2-ethyl-1,3-propanediyl] ester, 5, 11-diethyl-7-oxo-4,6,10,12-tetraoxopentadecane-3,13-diyl diacrylate and 2-{2-[2-(acryloyloxy)-1-methylethoxy]-1-methylethoxy}-1-methylethyl acrylate	Reaction product with monomer and impurities	Ultraviolet varnishes	29
2-(12-(Methacryloyloxy) dodecyl)malonic acid	Methyl methacrylate derivative	Acrylic adhesive	50
Methyl-3-(3,5-di-tert-butyl-4-hydroxyphenyl) propanoate	Degradation product from Irganox 1076	Hot-melt adhesive for labels	43
Tripropylene glycol diacrylate, 10-heneicosene and α-tocopherol acetate, *N,N*-diethyldodecanamide, *N*-[(9Z)-9-octadecen-1-yl]acetamide, 1-palmitoylglycerol, and glycerol stearate		Nanocomposites prepared with PLA/PL and ZnO nanoparticles	113
Oligomer	Either present in the polymer or produced during the degradation of polymers	PET, polyester, polystyrene, polybutylene terephthalate, and polyethylene naphthenate, PLA, bioadhesives	28,114–118

LDPE, Low-density polyethylene; *PE*, polyethylene; *PLA*, polylactic acid; *PP*, polypropylene.

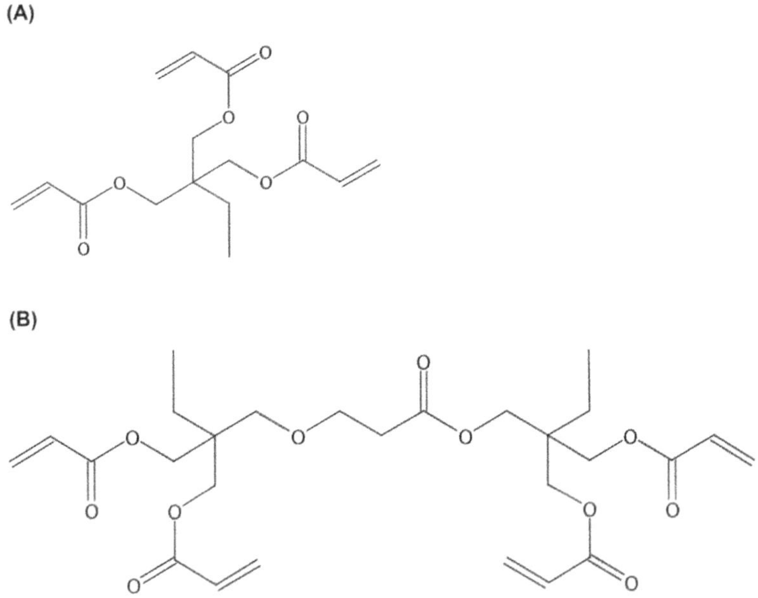

FIGURE 14.5 Molecular structure of the (A) monomer 2-Propenoic acid, 1,1′-[2-ethyl-2-[[(1-oxo-2-propen-1-yl) oxy]methyl]-1,3-propanediyl] ester (TMPTA) and (B) the NIAS found: 2-propenoic acid,1,1′-[2-[[3-[2,2-bis[[(1-oxo-2-propen-1-yl)oxy]methyl]butoxy]-1-oxopropoxy] methyl]-2-ethyl-1,3-propanediyl] ester from varnishes.[29]

NIAS, since they are fragments of polymeric anionic surfactants based on sodium C14−17 sec-Alkyl sulfonate. They came from the sealing used in food cans.[29]

The compounds 2-propenoic acid,1,1′-[2-[[3-[2,2-bis [[(1-oxo-2-propen-1-yl)oxy]methyl]butoxy]-1-oxopropoxy]methyl-2-ethyl-1,3-propanediyl] ester, 5, 11-diethyl-7-oxo-4,6,10,12-tetraoxopentadecane-3,13-diyl diacrylate, and 2-{2-[2-(acryloyloxy)-1-methylethoxy]-1-methylethoxy}-1-methylethyl acrylate, which were reaction products from monomers and impurities, were identified as NIAS from UV varnishes and migrated to food simulants. Fig. 14.5 shows the molecular structure of the original monomer and the NIAS found.[29]

NIAS coming from several types of adhesives have been studied. The compound 2-(12-(methacryloyloxy) dodecyl)malonic acid was a NIAS, which could be a methyl methacrylate derivative from acrylic adhesive.[45] Moreover, the compound methyl-3-(3,5-di-tert-butyl-4-hydroxyphenyl)propanoate, a degradation product from Irganox 1076, was identified in the migration of a shelf-adhesive label used for direct contact on food.[44]

Other NIAS such as tripropylene glycol diacrylate, 10-heneicosene, α-tocopherol acetate, *N,N*-diethyldodecanamide, *N*-[(9Z)-9-octadecen-1-yl]acetamide, 1-palmitoylglycerol, and glycerol stearate were identified from nanocomposites prepared with polylactic acid (PLA)/PL and ZnO NPs.[113]

Oligomers are considered within the broad group NIAS. Oligomers migrating from PET, polyester, PS, polybutylene terephthalate, and polyethylene naphthenate have been described in the literature.[114−117] Additionally, migration of oligomers from biopolymers such as PLA[118] and from bioadhesives[28] have been recently studied.

14.4 Analytical techniques

Fig. 14.6 shows a scheme of the main analytical techniques used for the analysis of migrants coming from food packaging. The analytical techniques have been classified according to the chemical nature of the migrant, volatiles, nonvolatiles, and metals. Nevertheless, the selected technique inside each chemical classification depends on the sensitivity and selectivity required.

14.4.1 Volatile compounds

For volatile compounds, the technique gas chromatography coupled to mass spectrometry (GC-Ms) is capable of detecting analytes at trace levels.[119] This technique is generally used after an extraction technique. The most recent and useful extraction techniques are solid-phase microextraction (SPME), stir bar sorptive extraction (SBSE), hollow-fiber liquid-phase microextraction (HFLPME), and fabric phase sorptive extraction (FPSE).[43,56,120−125]

SPME is based on the absorption of the volatile compounds in a microfiber, SBSE is based on magnetic stirring rod coated by a sorbent, HFLPME is based on the extraction, concentration and separation using a semipermeable membrane, and finally FPSE is based on natural or synthetic fabric covered by ultrathin coating sorbent used as substrate.

The most common GC-Ms instruments use electron impact ionization, where analytes ionization is induced by 70 electron volt (eV) electrons. Due to the fact that the same conditions are used in all the instruments, databases are available. Therefore the identification of compounds according to their fragmentation pattern is easier.

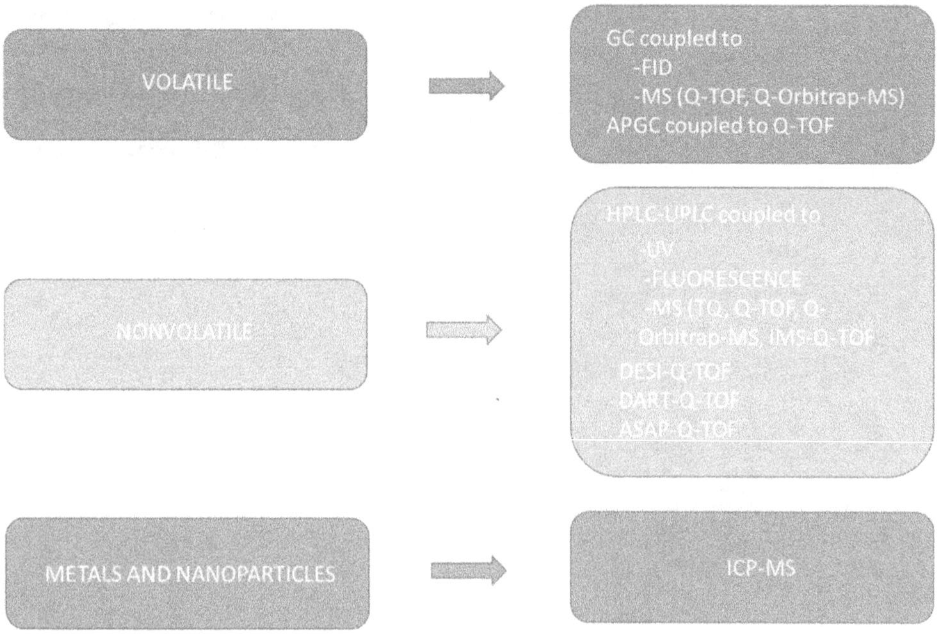

FIGURE 14.6 Scheme of the main analytical techniques used for the analysis of migrants coming from food packaging.

However, databases are incomplete and NIAS are not included, since sometimes they are from decomposition of molecules or neoformed compounds.

For the analysis of NIAS, high resolution techniques are required to obtain the exact mass for the identification of unknowns. The analysis of NIAS is a very challenging work, since complex and expensive analytical techniques are required and very highly experienced analysts are necessary to interpret the mass spectra.

GC-MS can be coupled to a quadrupole time-of-flight analyzer mass spectrometer (APGC-MS-Q-TOF). This technique consists of a soft mass spectrometry, where the sample ions with different masses are accelerated to the same kinetic energy and the time taken for each ion to reach the detector at a known distance is measured. This technology has been recently used for the analysis of NIAS in food packaging migration, to identify NIAS coming from plastics and adhesives used in food packaging.[27,44,126,127] Fig. 14.7 shows an example of the identification done through APGC-MS-Q-TOF.[44] Spectra of each chromatographic peak are studied in order to elucidate the chemical structure of the compounds. In the first place, the low energy spectra are studied in order to obtain a molecular formula. Taking the accurate mass of the molecular ion in each spectrum, different possibilities for the molecular formula were established. Once the molecular formula of each accurate mass is known, it is then necessary to use a database of chemicals to obtain a list of candidates for the identification. Then, using the high energy function the fragmentation spectra are obtained. The accurate masses of the fragments are considered in order to find out if they could be generated from the candidates in the databases in order to confirm their identification.

Orbitrap uses another technology to obtain high-resolution mass spectra. In an Orbitrap, ions are tangentially injected into an electrical field between the electrodes and become trapped, because their electrostatic attraction to the inner electrode is counteracted by centrifugal force, then the ions go around the central electrode. Additionally, the ions also move in front and behind through the axis of the central electrode. Ions with a specific mass–charge relationship move in rings that oscillate around the central spindle and finally high mass accuracy is obtained. GC-Q-Orbitrap-Ms have been used recently for the analysis of NIAS,[113] where three volatile NIAS were detected (tripropylene glycol diacrylate, 10-heneicosene and α-tocopherol acetate).

14.4.2 Nonvolatile compounds

For the study of nonvolatile compounds the most common sensitive technique used to analyze a target compound is liquid chromatography coupled to mass spectrometry (LC-Ms-MS), and it has been widely used in migration studies.[128] There are not databases for LC-Ms spectra, since the ionization and fragmentation depend on many experimental factors. Therefore for the analysis of NIAS high resolution techniques are required. Both Orbitrap and Q-TOF mass spectrometers are also coupled to liquid chromatography and both have been widely used for the detection and identification of NIAS.[23,80,113]

Nevertheless, sometimes even using high resolution techniques such as those mentioned above, it is not

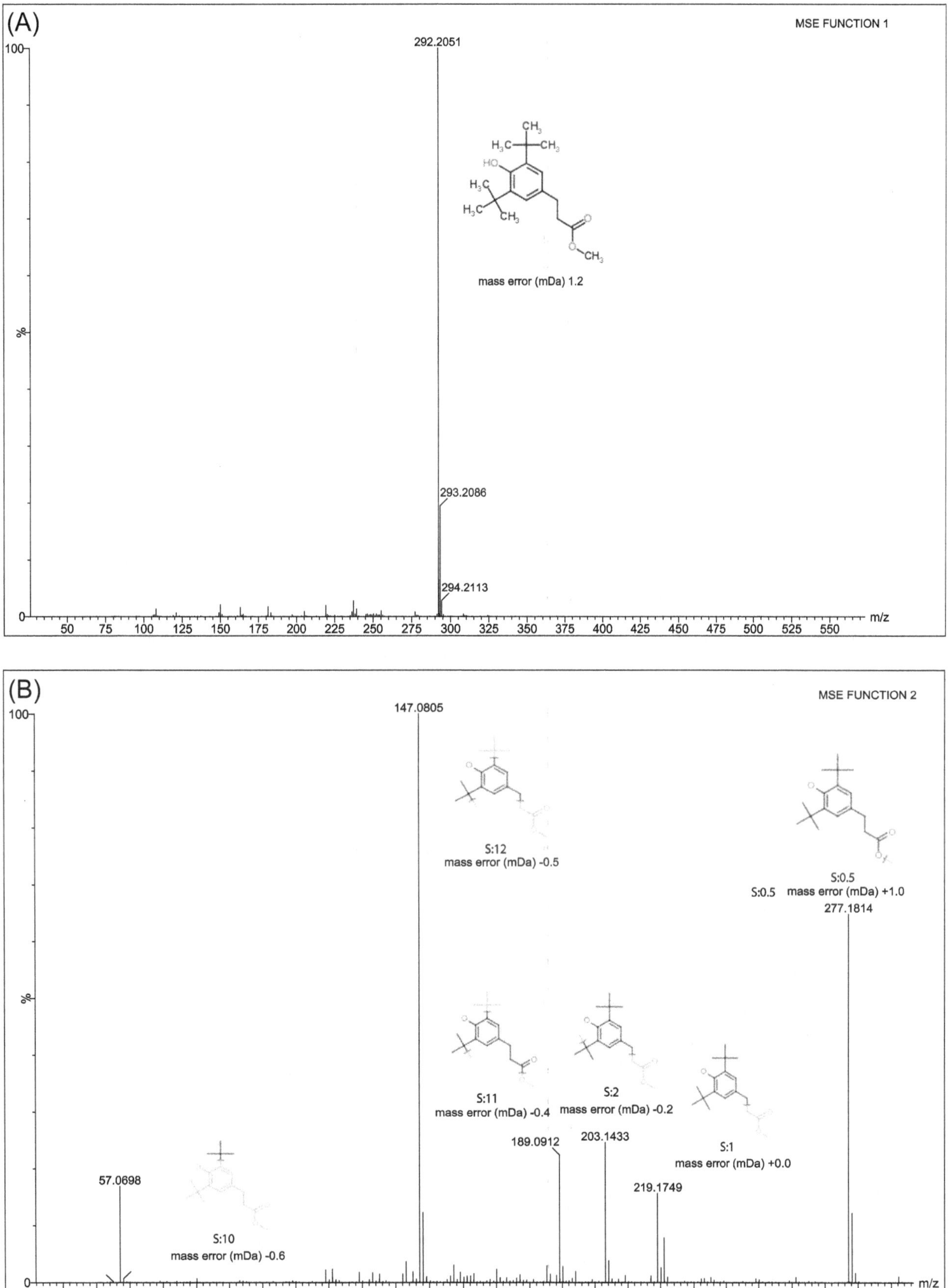

FIGURE 14.7 Function 1 (A) and function 2 (B) of the compound methyl-3-(3,5-di-tert-butyl 4-hydroxyphenyl)propanoate obtained by APGC-MS-Q-TOF at a cone voltage of 30 V .[44]

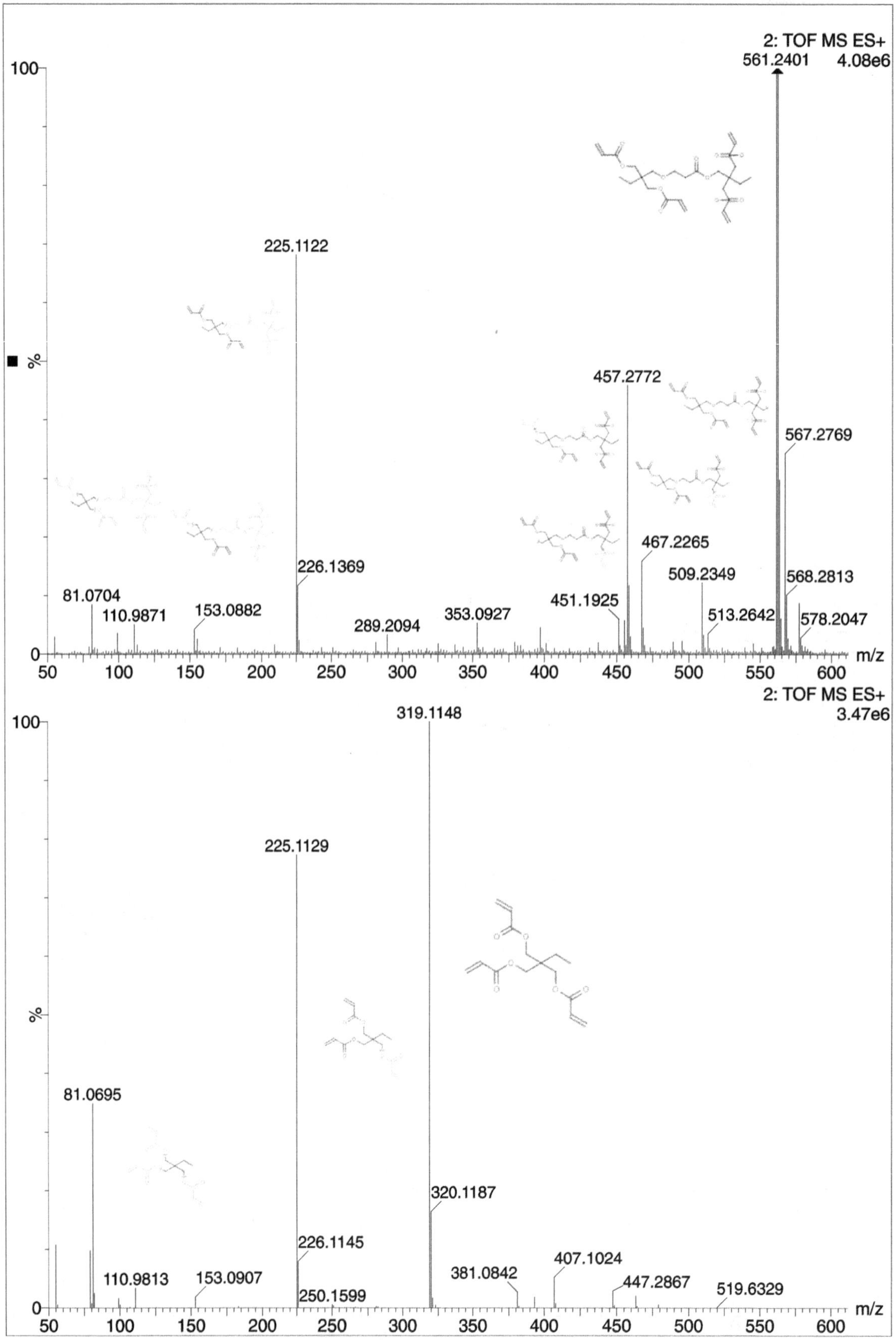

FIGURE 14.8 Spectra of 2-propenoic acid,1,1′-[2-ethyl-2-[[(1-oxo-2-propen-1-yl)oxy]methyl]-1,3-propanediyl] ester (TMPTA) and 2-propenoic acid,1,1′-[2-[[3-[2,2-bis[[(1-oxo-2-propen-1-yl)oxy]methyl]butoxy]-1-oxopropoxy]methyl]-2-ethyl-1,3-propanediyl] ester. Molecular structure of the compounds and the fragments of the molecules in high-energy spectra.[29]

possible to identify all NIAS present in a sample, due to the complexity related to the mass spectra interpretation, the presence of adducts, and sometimes the lack of additional fragmentation. Software tools and technologies such as mass spectrometry at elevated energy (MS^E) are of great help to identify the chemical structure of unknowns and NIAS. In addition, the new technique ion mobility quadrupole time-of-flight mass spectrometry (IMS-Q-TOF) coupled to the ultrahigh pressure liquid chromatography contribute to obtain cleaner spectra. Drift tube ion mobility spectrometry is a rapid gas phase separation technique, that is easily combined with Ms for high-throughput multidimensional separations. Ions are subjected to a constant electric field while traveling through a buffer gas and separate quickly based on ion shape and size, where compact species drift faster than those with extended structures. The ions are characterized based on their collision cross-section (a parameter related to the ion's rotationally averaged size, shape, total charge, and charge distribution). This technique has been recently used for the identification of NIAS from food packaging.[16,29]

Fig. 14.8 shows the identification of some NIAS from its high-energy spectra obtained by IMS-Q-ToF.[29]

14.4.3 Metals and nanoparticles

For the analysis of metals and NPs, the most used technique is inductively coupled plasma mass spectrometry (ICP-Ms). NPs require the use of single-particle mode technique (sp-ICP-Ms), where distinction of dissolved metal and the NP-form can be unequivocally analyzed. ICP-Ms has been used for the migration analysis of heavy metals coming from food packaging[95,129,130] and sp-ICP-Ms for migration of NPs from food packaging.[109,131–133] Moreover, an important application of this technique is the analysis of NP migrants in food, since they have recently been incorporated in food packaging materials.

14.5 Research gaps and future directions

Food packaging and labeling play an important role in food safety. Migration from them is a reality and should be seriously considered. Food packaging materials are in continuous development, trying to find better and safer materials as well as environmentally friendly solutions. Conventional materials, and mainly the plastics, are now the target of criticisms because of their persistence in the environment and the migration of their components. However, biopolymers are not free of substances of concern and also require thorough studies to guaranty their safety in use.

Fortunately, together with the development of packaging materials, analytical technology is also advancing very fast and can provide the high sensitivity required to detect traces and ultratraces of migrants in both simulants and food. However, there are still many unidentified migrants from packaging, since these are difficult to detect and characterize, and this requires the improvement of analytical techniques. There is also an important lack of pure standards for confirming the identification and quantification of many migration products, which requires new scientific developments applicable to food packaging materials. For example, more effort is needed in building the databases of migrants, especially those of nonvolatile compounds. Criteria for quantifying NIAS, especially for those that do not have pure standards, are needed for establishing the risk assessment of packaging materials and labels.

It is true that food packaging materials and labeling require a continuous effort to develop better formula, decrease the migration, eliminate the potential toxic compounds, and improve the performance. This is an important feature, where the research institutes or universities and the industrial sector can work together under the frame of "safety by design." This means that packaging materials, adhesives, printing inks, varnishes, coatings, and so on can be designed in a safer way, where potential migrating compounds would be removed and substituted by others of no concern.

References

1. Seyedhamzeh S, Nedjat S, Hosseini H, Shakibazedeh E, Viera AJ, Motlagh AD. Potential effect of different nutritional labels on food choices among mothers: a study protocol. *BMC Public Health.* 2020;20(1).
2. Clemente I, Aznar M, Nerin C, Bosetti O. Migration from printing inks in multilayer food packaging materials by GC-MS analysis and pattern recognition with chemometrics. *Food Addit Contam Part A Chem.* 2016;33(4):703–714.
3. Spink J, Ortega DL, Chen C, Wu F. Food fraud prevention shifts the food risk focus to vulnerability. *Trends Food Sci Technol.* 2017;62:215–220.
4. Marsh K, Bugusu B. Food packaging – roles, materials, and environmental issues. *J Food Sci.* 2007;72(3):R39–R55.
5. Nerin C, Vera P, Canellas E, Active and intelligent food packaging, in: V. Ravishankar Rai, A. Jamuna Bai (Ed.), Food safety and protection 2017, CRC Press.
6. de Abreu DAP, Cruz JM, Losada PP. Active and intelligent packaging for the food industry. *Food Rev Int.* 2012;28(2):146–187.
7. Fang ZX, Zhao YY, Warner RD, Johnson SK. Active and intelligent packaging in meat industry. *Trends Food Sci Technol.* 2017;61:60–71.
8. Anukiruthika T, Sethupathy P, Wilson A, Kashampur K, Moses JA, Anandharamakrishnan C. Multilayer packaging: advances in preparation techniques and emerging food applications. *Compr Rev Food Sci Food Saf.* 2020;19:1156–1186.

9. Raheem D. Application of plastics and paper as food packaging materials – an overview. *Emir J Food Agric.* 2013;25(3):177–188.
10. Lara W. *Food science and quality control.* Edtech Press; 2019.
11. Cazon P, Velazquez G, Ramirez JA, Vazquez M. Polysaccharide-based films and coatings for food packaging: a review. *Food Hydrocoll.* 2017;68:136–148.
12. Byun Y, Kim YT. *Utilization of bioplastics for food packaging industry.* London: Academic Press Ltd, Elsevier Science Ltd; 2014.
13. Vera P, Canellas E, Nerin C. Compounds responsible for off-odors in several samples composed by polypropylene, polyethylene, paper and cardboard used as food packaging materials. *Food Chem.* 2020;309.
14. Vera P, Canellas E, Nerin C. Identification of non volatile migrant compounds and NIAS in polypropylene films used as food packaging characterized by UPLC-MS/QTOF. *Talanta.* 2018;188:750–762.
15. Cao XL, Zhao W, Churchill R, Hilts C. Occurrence of di-(2-ethylhexyl) adipate and phthalate plasticizers in samples of meat, fish, and cheese and their packaging films. *J Food Prot.* 2014;77(4):610–620.
16. Vera P, Canellas E, Barknowitz G, Goshawk J, Nerin C. Ion-mobility quadrupole time-of-flight mass spectrometry: a novel technique applied to migration of nonintentionally added substances from polyethylene films intended for use as food packaging. *Anal Chem.* 2019;91(20):12741–12751.
17. Din MI, Ghaffar T, Najeeb J, Hussain Z, Khalid R, Zahid H. Potential perspectives of biodegradable plastics for food packaging application – review of properties and recent developments. *Food Addit Contam Part A Chem.* 2020;37(4):665–680.
18. Yeo JCC, Muiruri JK, Thitsartarn W, Li ZB, He CB. Recent advances in the development of biodegradable PHB-based toughening materials: approaches, advantages and applications. *Mater Sci Eng C Mater Biol Appl.* 2018;92:1092–1116.
19. Regulation (EC) No 1935/2004 of the European Parliament and of the Council of 27 October 2004 on materials and articles intended to come into contact with food. 2004.
20. Commission Regulation (EU) No 10/2011 of 14 January 2011 on plastic materials and articles intended to come into contact with food. 2011.
21. Wrona M, Nerin C. Analytical approaches for analysis of safety of modern food packaging: a review. *Molecules.* 2020;25(3).
22. EFSA Scientific Committee. Scientific opinion on exploring options for providing advice about possible human health risks based on the concept of threshold of toxicological concern (TTC). *EFSA J.* 2012;10:2750.
23. Nerin C, Alfaro P, Aznar M, Domeno C. The challenge of identifying non-intentionally added substances from food packaging materials: a review. *Anal Chim Acta.* 2013;775:14–24.
24. Vera P, Aznar M, Mercea P, Nerin C. Study of hotmelt adhesives used in food packaging multilayer laminates. Evaluation of the main factors affecting migration to food. *J Mater Chem.* 2011;21(2):420–431.
25. Canellas E, Aznar M, Nerin C, Mercea P. Partition and diffusion of volatile compounds from acrylic adhesives used for food packaging multilayers manufacturing. *J Mater Chem.* 2010;20(24):5100–5109.
26. Nerin C, Gaspar J, Vera P, Canellas E, Aznar M, Mercea P. Determination of partition and diffusion coefficients of components of two rubber adhesives in different multilayer materials. *Int J Adhes Adhes.* 2013;40:56–63.
27. Canellas E, Vera P, Domeno C, Alfaro AP, Nerin C. Atmospheric pressure gas chromatography coupled to quadrupole-time of flight mass spectrometry as a powerful tool for identification of non intentionally added substances in acrylic adhesives used in food packaging materials. *J Chromatogr A.* 2012;1235:141–148.
28. Canellas E, Vera P, Nerin C. UPLC-ESI-Q-TOF-MSE and GC-MS identification and quantification of non-intentionally added substances coming from biodegradable food packaging. *Anal Bioanal Chem.* 2015;407(22):6781–6790.
29. Canellas E, Vera P, Nerin C. Ion mobility quadrupole time-of-flight mass spectrometry for the identification of non-intentionally added substances in UV varnishes applied on food contact materials. A safety by design study. *Talanta.* 2019;205:120103.
30. Brandsch J, Mercea P, Ruter M, Tosa V, Piringer O. Migration modelling as a tool for quality assurance of food packaging. *Food Addit Contam.* 2002;19:29–41.
31. Gavriil G, Kanavouras A, Coutelieris FA. Food-packaging migration models: a critical discussion. *Crit Rev Food Sci Nutr.* 2018;58(13):2262–2272.
32. AENOR. UNE-EN-14338:2004. Papel y cartón para contacto alimentario. Condiciones para la determinación de la migración desde el papel y cartón utilizando óxido de polifenileno modificado (MPPO) como simulante. 2004.
33. Zhang N, Kenion G, Bankmann D, Mezouari S, Hartman TG. Migration studies and chemical characterization of low molecular weight cyclic polyester oligomers from food packaging lamination adhesives. *Packag Technol Sci.* 2018;31(4):197–211.
34. Ramos MJG, Lozano A, Fernandez-Alba AR. High-resolution mass spectrometry with data independent acquisition for the comprehensive non-targeted analysis of migrating chemicals coming from multilayer plastic packaging materials used for fruit puree and juice. *Talanta.* 2019;191:180–192.
35. Ubeda S, Aznar M, Vera P, et al. Overall and specific migration from multilayer high barrier food contact materials - kinetic study of cyclic polyester oligomers migration. *Food Addit Contam Part A Chem.* 2017;34(10):1784–1794.
36. Campanella G, Ghaani M, Quetti G, Farris S. On the origin of primary aromatic amines in food packaging materials. *Trends Food Sci Technol.* 2015;46(1):137–143.
37. Pezo D, Fedeli M, Bosetti O, Nerin C. Aromatic amines from polyurethane adhesives in food packaging: the challenge of identification and pattern recognition using Quadrupole-Time of Flight-Mass Spectrometry(E). *Anal Chim Acta.* 2012;756:49–59.
38. Aznar M, Canellas E, Nerin C. Quantitative determination of 22 primary aromatic amines by cation-exchange solid-phase extraction and liquid chromatography-mass spectrometry. *J Chromatogr A.* 2009;1216(27):5176–5181.
39. Perez-Lamela C, Paseiro-Losada P, Cortizas-Castro D, Rodriguez-Hergueta A, Simal-Lozano J. Isolation and characterization of BADGE hydrolysis products. *Int J Environ Anal Chem.* 2002;82(3):123–132.
40. Salafranca J, Batlle R, Nerin C. Use of solid-phase microextraction for the analysis of bisphenol A and bisphenol A diglycidyl ether in food simulants. *J Chromatogr A.* 1999;864(1):137–144.
41. Nerin C, Ubeda JL, Alfaro P, et al. Compounds from multilayer plastic bags cause reproductive failures in artificial insemination. *Sci Rep.* 2014;4.
42. Nerin C, Philo MR, Salafranca J, Castle L. Determination of bisphenol-type contaminants from food packaging materials in

aqueous foods by solid-phase microextraction-high-performance liquid chromatography. *J Chromatogr A*. 2002;963(1–2):375–380.
43. Canellas E, Vera P, Nerin C. Multiple headspace-solid phase microextraction for the determination of migrants coming from a self-stick label in fresh sausage. *Food Chem*. 2016;197:24–29.
44. Canellas E, Vera P, Nerin C. Atmospheric pressure gas chromatography coupled to quadrupole-time of flight mass spectrometry as a tool for identification of volatile migrants from autoadhesive labels used for direct food contact. *J Mass Spectrom*. 2014;49(11):1181–1190.
45. Canellas E, Vera P, Nerin C. Migration assessment and the 'threshold of toxicological concern' applied to the safe design of an acrylic adhesive for food-contact laminates. *Food Addit Contam Part A Chem Anal Control Expo Risk Assess*. 2017;34(10):1721–1729.
46. Rosero-Moreano M, Canellas E, Nerin C. Three-phase hollow-fiber liquid-phase microextraction combined with HPLC-UV for the determination of isothiazolinone biocides in adhesives used for food packaging materials. *J Sep Sci*. 2014;37(3):272–280.
47. Zhong HN, Li ZC, Chen S, Zeng Y, Zheng JG, Li D. Simultaneous quantitative analysis of six isothiazolinones in water-based adhesive used for food contact materials by high-performance liquid chromatography-tandem mass spectrometry (HPLC-MS/MS). *Molecules*. 2019;24(21).
48. Lommatzscha M, Biedermann M, Grob K, Simat TJ. Analysis of saturated and aromatic hydrocarbons migrating from a polyolefin-based hot-melt adhesive into food. *Food Addit Contam Part A Chem*. 2016;33(3):473–488.
49. Vera P, Canellas E, Nerin C. Identification of non-volatile compounds and their migration from hot melt adhesives used in food packaging materials characterized by ultra-performance liquid chromatography coupled to quadrupole time-of-flight mass spectrometry. *Anal Bioanal Chem*. 2013;405(14):4747–4754.
50. Canellas E, Vera P, Nerin C. Risk assessment derived from migrants identified in several adhesives commonly used in food contact materials. *Food Chem Toxicol*. 2015;75:79–87.
51. Guo MM, He MF, Zhong JJ, et al. High-performance liquid chromatography (HPLC)-fluorescence method for determination of bisphenol A diglycidyl ether (BADGE) and its derivatives in canned foods. *Sci Total Environ*. 2020;710:134975.
52. Food Packaging Forum, October 10, 2012.
53. Nowacka M, Rybak K, Wiktor A, et al. The quality and safety of food contact materials - paper and cardboard coated with paraffin emulsion. *Food Control*. 2018;93:183–190.
54. Biedermann M, Ingenhoff JE, Zurfluh M, et al. Migration of mineral oil, photoinitiators and plasticisers from recycled paperboard into dry foods: a study under controlled conditions. *Food Addit Contam Part A Chem*. 2013;30(5):885–898.
55. Aznar M, Alfaro P, Nerin C, Jones E, Riches E. Progress in mass spectrometry for the analysis of set-off phenomena in plastic food packaging materials. *J Chromatogr A*. 2016;1453:124–133.
56. Asensio E, Peiro T, Nerin C. Determination the set-off migration of ink in cardboard-cups used in coffee vending machines. *Food Chem Toxicol*. 2019;130:61–67.
57. Aznar M, Domeno C, Nerin C, Bosetti O. Set-off of non volatile compounds from printing inks in food packaging materials and the role of lacquers to avoid migration. *Dye Pigment*. 2015;114: 85–92.
58. Domeno C, Aznar M, Nerin C, Isella F, Fedeli M, Bosetti O. Safety by design of printed multilayer materials intended for food packaging. *Food Addit Contam Part A Chem*. 2017;34 (7):1239–1250.
59. Scarsella JB, Zhang N, Hartman TG. Identification and migration studies of photolytic decomposition products of UV-photoinitiators in food packaging. *Molecules*. 2019;24(19).
60. Ye SJ, Ye RH, Shi YD, et al. Highly sensitive aptamer based on electrochemiluminescence biosensor for label-free detection of bisphenol A. *Anal Bioanal Chem*. 2017;409(30):7145–7151.
61. Cardama AL, Sendon R, Bustos J, Santillana MI, Losada PP, de Quiros ARB. GC-MS screening for the identification of potential migrants present in polymeric coatings of food cans. *Polymers*. 2019;11(12).
62. Kudlak B, Jatkowska N, Kubica P, Yotova G, Tsakovski S. Influence of storage time and temperature on the toxicity, endocrine potential, and migration of epoxy resin precursors in extracts of food packaging materials. *Molecules*. 2019;24(23).
63. Kudlak B, Szczepanska N, Nedyalkova M, Simeonov V, Namiesnik J. Chemometric assessment and best-fit function modelling of the toxic potential of selected food packaging extracts. *Molecules*. 2018;23(11).
64. Pilevar Z, Bahrami A, Beikzadeh S, Hosseini H, Jafari SM. Migration of styrene monomer from polystyrene packaging materials into foods: characterization and safety evaluation. *Trends Food Sci Technol*. 2019;91:248–261.
65. Brenz F, Linke S, Simat T. Qualitative and quantitative analysis of monomers in polyesters for food contact materials. *Food Addit Contam Part A Chem*. 2017;34(2):307–319.
66. Borzi F, Torrieri E, Wrona M, Nerin C. Polyamide modified with green tea extract for fresh minced meat active packaging applications. *Food Chem*. 2019;300.
67. Kappenstein O, Ebner I, Forster C, et al. Validation and application of an LC-MS/MS method for the determination of cyclic oligomers originating from polyamide 6 and polyamide 66 in food simulant. *Food Addit Contam Part A Chem*. 2018;35(7):1410–1420.
68. Felix JS, Monteiro M, Manzoli JE, et al. Identification and migration of degradation compounds from irradiation of multilayer polyamide 6 films for meat foodstuffs and cheese. *Anal Bioanal Chem*. 2008;391(3):847–857.
69. Mariana M, Feiteiro J, Verde I, Cairrao E. The effects of phthalates in the cardiovascular and reproductive systems: a review. *Environ Int*. 2016;94:758–776.
70. Khaustov A, Redina M, Goryainov S. Migration of PAHs and phthalates from package materials during water storage: glass or plastic? *Polycycl. Aromat. Compd*. 2022;42(2):358–370. Available from: https://doi.org/10.1080/10406638.2020.1734033.
71. Luo Q, Liu ZH, Yin H, et al. Global review of phthalates in edible oil: an emerging and nonnegligible exposure source to human. *Sci Total Environ*. 2020;704:135369.
72. Yang JL, Song WZ, Wang XJ, et al. Migration of phthalates from plastic packages to convenience foods and its cumulative health risk assessments. *Food Addit Contam Part B Surveill*. 2019;12 (3):151–158.
73. Bogdanovicova S, Jarosova A, Mihok M, Jandasek J. The migration of phthalates from packaging into food depending on the heat processing and fat content of meat products. 2015.
74. Bhunia K, Sablani SS, Tang J, Rasco B. Migration of chemical compounds from packaging polymers during microwave, conventional heat treatment, and storage. *Compr Rev Food Sci Food Saf*. 2013;12(5):523–545.

75. Ibarra VG, Sendon R, Garcia-Fonte XX, Losada PP, de Quiros ARB. Migration studies of butylated hydroxytoluene, tributyl acetylcitrate and dibutyl phthalate into food simulants. *J Sci Food Agric.* 2019;99(4):1586–1595.
76. Kim H, Kim GB, Choi MS, Kim IS, Gye MC, Yoo HH. Liquid chromatography-tandem mass spectrometric analysis of acetyl tributyl citrate for migration testing of food contact materials. *Microchem J.* 2018;139:475–479.
77. Bandele OJ, Cureton LT, Bailey AB, Ogungbesan A. A review of dietary exposure and toxicological information on epoxidised soybean oil (ESBO) in food-contact applications. *Food Addit Contam Part A Chem.* 2018;35(11):2204–2219.
78. Choi MS, Rehman SU, Kim H, et al. Migration of epoxidized soybean oil from polyvinyl chloride/polyvinylidene chloride food packaging wraps into food simulants. *Environ Sci Pollut Res.* 2018;25(5):5033–5039.
79. Ezerskis Z, Morkunas V, Suman M, Simoneau C. Analytical screening of polyadipates and other plasticisers in poly(vinyl chloride) gasket seals and in fatty food by gas chromatography-mass spectrometry. *Anal Chim Acta.* 2007;604(1):29–38.
80. Vaclavikova M, Paseiro-Cerrato R, Vaclavik L, Noonan GO, DeVries J, Begley TH. Target and non-target analysis of migrants from PVC-coated cans using UHPLC-Q-Orbitrap MS: evaluation of long-term migration testing. *Food Addit Contam Part A Chem.* 2016;33(2):352–363.
81. Blanco-Zubiaguirre L, Zabaleta I, Usobiaga A, et al. Target and suspect screening of substances liable to migrate from food contact paper and cardboard materials using liquid chromatography-high resolution tandem mass spectrometry. *Talanta.* 2020;208:11.
82. Lago MA, Rodriguez-Bernaldo de Quiros A, Sendon R, Bustos J, Nieto MT, Paseiro P. Photoinitiators: a food safety review. *Food Addit Contam Part A Chem.* 2015;32(5):779–798.
83. Luis Aparicio J, Elizalde M. Migration of photoinitiators in food packaging: a review. *Packag Technol Sci.* 2015;28(3):181–203.
84. Kim YT, Min B, Kim KW. *General characteristics of packaging materials for food system.* London: Academic Press Ltd, Elsevier Science Ltd; 2014.
85. Lago MA, Sendon R, Bustos J, Nieto MT, Losada PP, de Quiros ARB. Migration studies of two common components of UV-curing inks into food simulants. *Molecules.* 2019;24(19):11.
86. Schaefer A, Kuchler T, Simat TJ, Steinhart H. Migration of lubricants from food packagings – screening for lipid classes and quantitative estimation using normal-phase liquid chromatographic separation with evaporative light scattering detection. *J Chromatogr A.* 2003;1017(1–2):107–116.
87. Cooper I, Tice PA. Migration studies on fatty-acid amide slip additives from plastics into food simulants. *Food Addit Contam.* 1995;12(2):235–244.
88. Noguerol-Cal R, Lopez-Vilarino JM, Fernandez-Martinez G, Gonzalez-Rodriguez MV, Barral-Losada LF. Liquid chromatographic methods to analyze hindered amines light stabilizers (HALS) levels to improve safety in polyolefins. *J Sep Sci.* 2010;33(17–18):2698–2706.
89. Wang CY, Li CF, Lin JF, Xie TT, Chu NQ. Simultaneous determination of the specific migration amounts of light stabilizers and antioxidants in plastic materials in contact with foodstuffs by ultra-high performance liquid chromatography/orbitrap high resolution mass spectrometry. *Chin J Chromatogr.* 2017;35(5):509–519.
90. Fengler R, Gruber L. Mineral oil migration from paper-based packaging into food, investigated by means of food simulants and model substances. *Food Addit Contam Part A Chem.* 2020;37:845–857.
91. Pack EC, Jang DY, Cha MG, et al. Potential for short-term migration of mineral oil hydrocarbons from coated and uncoated food contact paper and board into a fatty food simulant. *Food Addit Contam Part A Chem.* 2020;37:858–868.
92. Wagner M, Oellig C. Screening for mineral oil saturated and aromatic hydrocarbons in paper and cardboard directly by planar solid phase extraction and by its coupling to gas chromatography. *J Chromatogr A.* 2019;1588:48–57.
93. Tarnow P, Hutzler C, Grabiger S, Schoen K, Tralau T, Luch A. Estrogenic activity of mineral oil aromatic hydrocarbons used in printing inks. *PLoS One.* 2016;11(1):e0147239.
94. Kassouf A, Chebib H, Lebbos N, Ouaini R. Migration of iron, lead, cadmium and tin from tinplate-coated cans into chickpeas. *Food Addit Contam Part A Chem.* 2013;30(11):1987–1992.
95. Welle F, Franz R. Migration of antimony from PET bottles into beverages: determination of the activation energy of diffusion and migration modelling compared with literature data. *Food Addit Contam Part A Chem.* 2011;28(1):115–126.
96. Mohammadpour I, Ahmadkhaniha R, Jeddi MZ, Rastkari N. Heavy metals in recycled pastry packages and pastries. *Acta Aliment.* 2016;45(4):509–514.
97. Mertoglu-Elmas G. The effect of colorants on the content of heavy metals in recycled corrugated board papers. *BioResources.* 2017;12(2):2690–2698.
98. Corona T, Iglesias M, Antico E, eds. Migration of components from cork stoppers to food: challenges in determining inorganic elements in food simulants. *J Agric Food Chem.* 2014;62(24):5690–5698.
99. Morais LD, Macedo EV, Granjeiro JM, Delgado IF. Critical evaluation of migration studies of silver nanoparticles present in food packaging: a systematic review. *Crit Rev Food Sci Nutr.* 2020;60:3083–3102.
100. Aristizabal-Gil MV, Santian-Toro S, Sanchez LT, Pinzon MI, Gutierrez JA, Villa CC. ZnO and ZnO/CaO nanoparticles in alginate films. Synthesis, mechanical characterization, barrier properties and release kinetics. *LWT Food Sci Technol.* 2019;112:108217.
101. Vera P, Echegoyen Y, Canellas E, et al. Nano selenium as antioxidant agent in a multilayer food packaging material. *Anal Bioanal Chem.* 2016;408(24):6659–6670.
102. Clemente I, Aznar M, Nerin C. Synergistic properties of mustard and cinnamon essential oils for the inactivation of foodborne moulds in vitro and on Spanish bread. *Int J Food Microbiol.* 2019;298:44–50.
103. Gavril GL, Wrona M, Bertella A, et al. Influence of medicinal and aromatic plants into risk assessment of a new bioactive packaging based on polylactic acid (PLA). *Food Chem Toxicol.* 2019;132:110662.
104. Silva F, Caldera F, Trotta F, Nerin C, Domingues FC. Encapsulation of coriander essential oil in cyclodextrin nanosponges: a new strategy to promote its use in controlled-release active packaging. *Innov Food Sci Emerg Technol.* 2019;56:102177.

105. Simionato I, Domingues FC, Nerin C, Silva F. Encapsulation of cinnamon oil in cyclodextrin nanosponges and their potential use for antimicrobial food packaging. *Food Chem Toxicol*. 2019;132:110647.
106. Wrona M, Silva F, Salafranca J, Nerin C, Alfonso MJ, Caballero MA. Design of new natural antioxidant active packaging: screening flowsheet from pure essential oils and vegetable oils to ex vivo testing in meat samples. *Food Control*. 2021;120:107536.
107. Diehl H, Welle F. How to determine functional barrier performance towards mineral oil contaminants from recycled cardboard. *Food Packag Shelf Life*. 2015;5:41–49.
108. Echegoyen Y, Nerin C. Nanoparticle release from nano-silver antimicrobial food containers. *Food Chem Toxicol*. 2013;62:16–22.
109. Echegoyen Y, Rodriguez S, Nerin C. Nanoclay migration from food packaging materials. *Food Addit Contam Part A Chem*. 2016;33(3):530–539.
110. Ibarra VG, de Quiros ARB, Losada PP, Sendon R. Identification of intentionally and non-intentionally added substances in plastic packaging materials and their migration into food products. *Anal Bioanal Chem*. 2018;410(16):3789–3803.
111. Ibarra VG, de Quiros ARB, Losada PP, Sendon R. Non-target analysis of intentionally and non intentionally added substances from plastic packaging materials and their migration into food simulants. *Food Packag Shelf Life*. 2019;21:100325.
112. Lestido-Cardama A, Stormer A, Franz R. Dialkylketones in paperboard food contact materials-method of analysis in fatty foods and comparative migration into liquid simulants vs foodstuffs. *Molecules*. 2020;25(4):915.
113. Martinez-Bueno MJ, Hernando MD, Ucles S, Rajski L, Cimmino S, Fernandez-Alba AR. Identification of non-intentionally added substances in food packaging nano films by gas and liquid chromatography coupled to orbitrap mass spectrometry. *Talanta*. 2017;172:68–77.
114. Bauer A, Jesus F, Ramos MJG, Lozano A, Fernandez-Alba AR. Identification of unexpected chemical contaminants in baby food coming from plastic packaging migration by high resolution accurate mass spectrometry. *Food Chem*. 2019;295:274–288.
115. Maria H, Pim DV, Roland F. Oligomers in polyethylene naphthalate and polybutylene terephthalate – identification and exploring migration. *Food Packag Shelf Life*. 2018;17:171–178.
116. Gelbke HP, Banton M, Block C, et al. Risk assessment for migration of styrene oligomers into food from polystyrene food containers. *Food Chem Toxicol*. 2019;124:151–167.
117. Pietropaolo E, Albenga R, Gosetti F, et al. Synthesis, identification and quantification of oligomers from polyester coatings for metal packaging. *J Chromatogr A*. 2018;1578:15–27.
118. Ubeda S, Aznar M, Alfaro P, Nerin C. Migration of oligomers from a food contact biopolymer based on polylactic acid (PLA) and polyester. *Anal Bioanal Chem*. 2019;411(16):3521–3532.
119. Sung JH, Park HJ. Derivatization GC-MS techniques on plastic food contact materials. 2009.
120. David F, Ochiai N, Sandra P. Two decades of stir bar sorptive extraction: a retrospective and future outlook. *TRAC Trends Anal Chem*. 2019;112:102–111.
121. Oliveira EC, Echegoyen Y, Cruz SA, Nerin C. Comparison between solid phase microextraction (SPME) and hollow fiber liquid phase microextraction (HFLPME) for determination of extractables from post-consumer recycled PET into food simulants. *Talanta*. 2014;127:59–67.
122. Liu PY, Zhao CX, Zhang YJ, Chen YJ. Simultaneous determination of 10 photoinitiators in milk by solid-phase microextraction coupled with gas chromatography/mass spectrometry. *J Food Sci*. 2016;81(5):T1336–T1341.
123. Su QZ, Vera P, Nerin C. Direct immersion-solid-phase microextraction coupled to gas chromatography-mass spectrometry and response surface methodology for nontarget screening of (semi-) volatile migrants from food contact materials. *Anal Chem*. 2020;92(7):5577–5584.
124. Aznar M, Alfaro P, Nerin C, Kabir A, Furton KG. Fabric phase sorptive extraction: an innovative sample preparation approach applied to the analysis of specific migration from food packaging. *Anal Chim Acta*. 2016;936:97–107.
125. Otoukesh M, Nerin C, Aznar M, Kabir A, Furton KG, Es'haghi Z. Determination of adhesive acrylates in recycled polyethylene terephthalate by fabric phase sorptive extraction coupled to ultra performance liquid chromatography-mass spectrometry. *J Chromatogr A*. 2019;1602:56–63.
126. Osorio J, Dreolin N, Aznar M, Nerin C, Hancock P. Determination of volatile non intentionally added substances coming from a starch-based biopolymer intended for food contact by different gas chromatography-mass spectrometry approaches. *J Chromatogr A*. 2019;1599:215–222.
127. Su QZ, Vera P, Van de Wiele C, Nerin C, Lin QB, Zhong HN. Non-target screening of (semi-)volatiles in food-grade polymers by comparison of atmospheric pressure gas chromatography quadrupole time-of-flight and electron ionization mass spectrometry. *Talanta*. 2019;202:285–296.
128. Simal-Gandara J, Damant AP, Castle L. The use of LC-MS in studies of migration from food contact materials: a review of present applications and future possibilities. *Crit Rev Anal Chem*. 2002;32(1):47–78.
129. Lee JG, Hwang JY, Lee HE, Kim TH, Choi JD, Gang GJ. Effects of food processing methods on migration of heavy metals to food. *Appl Biol Chem*. 2019;62(1).
130. Xue MG, Wang SF, Huang CX. Determination of heavy metals (Pb, Cr, Cd and Hg) in printing inks and their effect on the recovery of waste paper and board. 2010.
131. Hetzer B, Burcza A, Graf V, Walz E, Greiner R. Online-coupling of AF(4) and single particle-ICP-MS as an analytical approach for the selective detection of nanosilver release from model food packaging films into food simulants. *Food Control*. 2017;80:113–124.
132. Metak AM, Nabhani F, Connolly SN. Migration of engineered nanoparticles from packaging into food products. *LWT Food Sci Technol*. 2015;64(2):781–787.
133. Tsagkaris AS, Tzegkas SG, Danezis GP. Nanomaterials in food packaging: state of the art and analysis. *J Food Sci Technol*. 2018;55(8):2862–2870.

Chapter 15

Safety assessment of refillable and recycled plastics packaging for food use

Forrest L. Bayer[1] and Jan Jetten[2]

[1]*Bayer Consulting and UW Imaging, LLC, Atlanta, GA, United States,* [2]*Ex-TNO, Zeist, The Netherlands*

Abstract

This chapter will discuss the various toxicological criteria/concepts and safety considerations that have evolved to ensure that refillable and recycled plastics can safely be used in direct food contact applications. In addition it will summarize the scientific literature that has been developed over a number of years covering detailed investigations by many researchers to validate the concepts and regulations, approvals, and authorization processes employed. The strict criteria developed by governments and these investigations insure the safety of both refillable and recycled plastics used in direct food contact applications.

Keywords: Recycled and refillable plastics; safety in food contact articles; reuse; returnable; PET; sniffer; legislation; guidelines

Part A Recycled plastics in food contact applications

15.1 History

The discovery, development, and evolution of plastics have been at a historical pace. The use of plastics has permeated throughout societies' lifestyles. A key area of this evolution has been in the food packaging area. The predominant plastics that have achieved a significant footing in the food packaging area are polyethylene terephthalate, polyolefins, styrene, and polycarbonate (PC). This expansion has occurred due to a variety of factors such as, cost, lightweight, suitable barrier properties, and a resistance to breakage. This has resulted in a significant decrease in the use of various metals and glass in the various packaging applications.

Bakelite discovered in 1907 is considered to be the first modern synthetic plastic. The early development of polymers centered in fiber industry applications. The first of these polymers was rayon followed by polyethylene (PE) in 1933 (Imperial Chemicals Industries, LLC) and the discovery of polyester by John Rex Winfield in the late 1930s. This discovery was patented in 1941 but was not made public until 1946 due to wartime restrictions. As a result of this early research, the fundamental dynamics of polymerization expanded widely. This resulted in creating many new plastics and a multitude use of applications. In 1950 1.5 million metric tons of plastics were produced worldwide. This figure has grown to the global production of 359 million metric tons of plastics in 2018.

The use of plastics has permeated throughout our society in a multitude of applications. These include but are not limited to fabrics, construction, packaging, electronics, automotive, and medicine.

The unique properties of plastics have created these multitude of uses. One of the prime properties of plastics is their durability. This in and of itself has also created the side issue with regards to their life expectancy. This durability and man's inability to properly manage end of life use has created major problems with regards to litter, waste disposal (landfill) and improper discharge into our rivers and oceans.

The volume of plastics produced, as can be seen in Fig. 15.1, dictates a need for responsible waste management. The challenge to manage plastics end of life use was recognized in the early 1980s when refillable plastic PET bottles entered the marketplace in the early 80s. These bottles are one approach to social responsibility in that they extended the life expectancy for the use of plastic bottles in food contact applications. However, eventually these bottles need to find a way to be dealt with. The predominant approach is through recycling. Discussion of the refillable plastics will be given in detail in part B of this chapter.

The volume of resin used is typically predominated by the use in plastics packaging. The bulk of those applications are in single serve or single use (one-way) packages.

Present Knowledge in Food Safety. DOI: https://doi.org/10.1016/B978-0-12-819470-6.00021-4

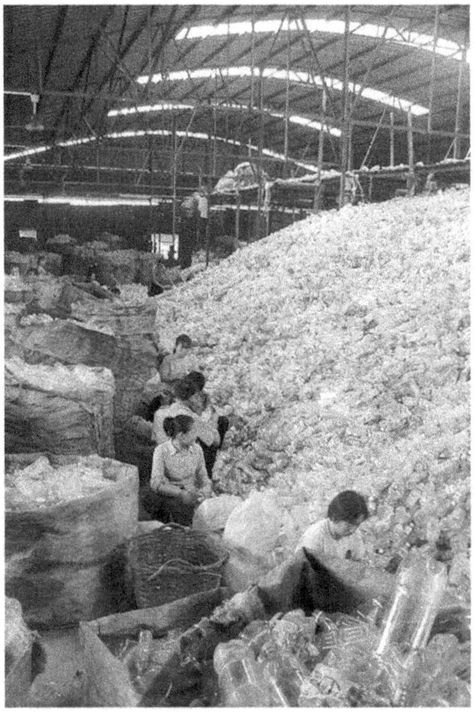

FIGURE 15.1 Polyethylene terephthalate bottle sortation plant in China.

Consumer desire has continued to increase conversion of metals and glass packaging to plastics has created both a need and a business opportunity for the recycling of plastics for various uses. These include, but are not limited to the use of recycled plastics in food contact applications.

15.2 Regulations—Authorization and approvals for recycled plastics and food contact applications

The predominant factor that inhibited the use and expansion of recycled plastics in the food contact applications was based on the lack of a regulatory framework to allow such applications and knowledge how to safely use postconsumer materials for food and thus to allow such applications. The situation existed because most established regulations governing the safe use of materials in food contact applications were developed decades before there was a need or desire for the use of recycled materials back into direct food contact applications. In general, most regulations neither specifically allowed nor prohibited the use of recycled plastics in food contact applications, although the safe use was dictated by all regulations. There were, however, also regulations that existed in about a half a dozen countries that strictly prohibited the use of recycled materials in food contact applications. Today, these regulations have been rescinded.

15.3 North America

15.3.1 United States

Recycled plastics presently are predominantly used in fibers, sheet and film, strapping, food and beverage bottles and nonfood containers. However, use in food and beverage bottles did not originally exist. The major thrust for use of postconsumer plastics in food contact applications occurred in the late 1980s. This was due to the fact that the consumer goods companies and resin companies saw a growing need to manage for sustainability reduce litter and divert material from landfill. Therefore in the late 80s a group of industry representatives met with the US Food and Drug Administration (FDA) to discuss how the use of recycled plastics in food contact applications might be achieved. Both parties had a common goal in mind; ensure consumer safety. The predominant concern that the FDA had was that after the original use of the container the consumer might mix or store some deleterious/toxic substance in the container and that after use this container would enter the plastics recycle feed stream. Typical substances of concern were pesticides/herbicides, petrochemicals or other household chemicals.

The regulators were faced with a dilemma. Traditionally, in reviewing a potential substance for use in food or food contact applications, the identity, chemistry and toxicology are clearly defined. In this instance, regulators had no way of knowing what potential hazardous chemical might enter as part of the plastics recycling stream. This created a challenge for assessing the safety of the recycled plastics material for use in food contact applications.

15.4 Safety criteria

Fortunately, the US FDA had been investigating alternative approaches for safety assessment without compromising the safety of the consumer. Their work was based on a concept put forth by Frawley,[1] who worked on packaging for the US based company Hercules. He proposed that there might be a human no effect level that could be used to establish the safety of chemicals that have not gone through traditional testing for toxicological scrutiny. The US FDA picked up his original concept. Their work resulted in a concept known as the Threshold of Regulation (TOR). The FDA had considered this concept for a number of years. They believed that the potential risk from a toxin was related to dietary intake rather than on the level migrating Rulis et al.[2] The toxic endpoint that was chosen was carcinogenesis. It was believed that this end point would act as a conservative measure for protection for all types of toxic effects.[3–7] This TOR concept became part of the US Code of Federal Regulations in July 1995 US FDA.[8,9] The use of the TOR criteria for safety considerations of recycled plastics has been described in detail by Thorsheim and Armstrong,[10] Bayer et al.,[11] Kuznesof and van der Veer,[12] Sadler,[13] Bayer.[14] Acceptance by other regulatory bodies of new concepts such as the TOR, takes time. The European Commission's Scientific Committee on Foods (SCF)[15] in their review indicated the concept gave reasonable assurance but wanted to see data on further endpoints.[16] The WHO Joint Expert Committee on Food Additives adopted the concept for the safety evaluation of flavors.[17] Cheeseman et al.[18] reviewed short-term toxicity data, genotoxicity and structure–activity relationships in support of a potentially higher threshold, finding that for many substances a higher threshold than proposed for the TOR would be appropriate and that the carcinogenic endpoint is the most conservative. Kroes et al.[19] under the auspices of the International Life Science Institute (ILSI) reviewed toxicological endpoints not only suggested by the SCF but additional endpoints and found that in fact, carcinogenicity was the most sensitive endpoint. This TOR concept used for food packaging in the United States is more commonly recognized in other countries as the threshold of toxicological concern (TTC). The principals of the TOR are based on the same principles as the TTC. Considerable work has continued to expand and validate the safety of the concept in assuring consumer safety. Additionally, Kroes et al.[20] expanded the work to look at low levels of substances of concern at low levels in the diet. Barlow[21] and Boobis et al.[22] have published a comprehensive review on the use of the TTC and on the endpoints for use of chemicals of high levels of concern.

The TTC Concept has been accepted by a variety of authorities: (1) European Medicines Agency (EMEA) to assess genotoxic impurities in pharmaceutical preparations, (2) the former EC SCF and is now used by the European Food Safety Authority (EFSA) to evaluate flavoring substances, (3) has been endorsed by the WHO International Program on Chemical Safety for the Risk Assessment of Chemicals, and (4) also by the EU Scientific Committee on Toxicology, Ecotoxicology and the Environment.

15.4.1 US FDA guidance criteria

The US FDA did not formally adopt the TOR until 1995. However, from the beginning, they employed this concept as a key criterion for the use of recycled plastics approved for food contact applications. The discussions between the industry and US FDA eventually allowed the US FDA to create a guidance document for use of recycled plastics and food contact applications. The FDA chose not to establish a formal regulation, but to create a process for industry to voluntarily submit data to the FDA for review based on meeting criteria established in the guidance document. If all criteria were met, the FDA would issue a "Letter of No Objection" (LNO).

The first publication of the guidance document was issued (May 1992) and titled "Points to Consider for the Use of Recycled Plastics in Food Packaging: Chemistry Considerations." This document was updated in August 2006. Key criteria outlined in the guidance documents are as follows:

1. Each recycling technology is different and must individually meet the recommendations.
2. Only food grade plastics are allowed—sorting efficiency of 99% is required.
3. Food grade plastics used in nonfood applications may be used as a feed stream source, but require different test approaches.
4. Challenge test must be performed to demonstrate capability of technology to decontaminate.
5. Challenge surrogates: would be defined to cover the four basic physical and chemical properties of compounds such as polar volatile, polar non volatile, nonpolar volatile, non polar non volatile and an organo metallic compounds.
6. Surrogate concentrations and exposure times are defined.
7. Any changes to the process which could reduce decontamination, would require a repeat of surrogate challenge test.
8. Establish potential for contamination of food products ensuring the TOR concept is achieved;
   a. Assume 100% migration to the food
   b. Determine level in plastic and use recognized models to predict migration to food[23]
   c. Do migration test with actual food under actual use conditions
   d. Do migration test in accordance with regulatory guidelines
   e. Migration must be nondetectable at detection limits of analytical methodology or based on a suitable criteria such as the TOR.
9. The finished recycled material must comply with all virgin resin specifications
10. The US FDA adopted recycling definitions previously defined by the[24]:
    a. Preconsumer scrap: Primary recycling
    b. Physical reprocessing: Secondary recycling
    c. Chemical reprocessing: Tertiary recycling.

Currently the US FDA has listed on their website as of November 12, 2019 a total of 222 LNOs. The breakdown of the LNOs relative to types of plastics are as follows: polyethylene terephthalate (PET) 163, polyolefins; linear low density polyethylene (LLDPE), high-density polyethylene (HDPE) and polypropylene (PP) 28; polystyrene

(PS) 23, acrylics (3), PC (1), silicon and carbon coatings (2) and 1 listed as miscellaneous. The predominance of aqueous compatible food contact applications has been for PET and in a few instances polyolefins. The first LNO was issued on February 21, 1990 for recycled PS used in egg cartons, the second on June 1990 for grocery bags and the third LNO was issued on January 9, 1991 for the use of recycled PET in soft drink containers. This third LNO resulted in the first field trials of recycled PET soft drink containers in April 1991, followed by a major roll-out in September 1991. Since that pivotal date, billions of recycled PET content containers have been placed in the marketplace with no reported issues of health and safety to the consumer.

The primary reason that there have been no issues of health and safety with the use of recycled plastics in direct food contact applications is because of the ultra conservative approach taken by regulators to ensure consumer safety. The US FDA in their development of the points to consider document requires or assumes the following conservatism's[14]:

1. No data existed on the frequency of contamination in the recycle feed stream, therefore they required a worst-case scenario of contaminating 100% of the test material being subjected to the proposed recycling technology. In reality, there are many operational factors in plants supplying recycled plastics for food contact operations that would preclude this from happening. First, many operators have specific requirements for bales with feedstock input quality assurance checks looking for bottles or material not meeting the specific requirements. Secondly, all bottles or material will initially be separated and inspected by one or a combination of the following:
   a. The feedstock material may be individually manually inspected on the line for rejecting material that may be suspect due to discoloration or the deformation of the material
   b. The material then may pass through a series of sophisticated mechanical sorters for selecting or rejecting material not meeting specified criteria
   c. After mechanical sortation, it is a fairly common practice to subject bottles to a final manual inspection in order to reduce any potential troublesome material entering into the next phase of operation.

   That step is generally grinding the material to a specified size. Many operations now employ highly sophisticated flake sorters using lasers scanning multiple wave length at a rate of one million scans per second to accept or reject specified material. A very comprehensive study undertaken in Europe showed a contamination level in the order of one in 3000–4000 bottles.[25] In the original guidance document (May 1992) 100% concentrations or user strengths were proposed for the surrogate contaminants. Thus using a representative surrogate such as toluene for gasoline resulted in exceedingly high levels of contamination for this representative surrogate that would never be achieved in real life. This was modified in the US FDA's August 2006 Guidance Document to lower calculated values based on values derived from theoretical calculations and some actual comparisons of absorb levels of compounds by Begley et al.[26] and Demertzis et al.[27]
2. Nevertheless, these concentrations are still so high that they actually change the material properties and will affect diffusion.
3. Calculation of the migratable level of a contaminant was based on using a 100% consumption factor for the recycled resin. In essence this means that there would be recycled plastic in every food contact application where plastic was being used. This is a highly unlikely scenario.
4. The recycled article is assumed to contain 100% recycled resin. There is no way that all food contact applications of plastics would all contain 100% content resin simply due to availability for all applications.
5. Any contaminant absorbed into the plastic is assumed to migrate at a 100% level into the food source. Based on simple diffusion theory data in the literature it is well known that compounds with high absorptivity for the plastic will readily permeate the plastic but will also be easily removed. Conversely, compounds with low absorptivity in the plastic will not readily absorb into the plastic but if absorbed, also will be difficult to remove.
6. Certainly the potential exists for the consumer to misuse or contaminate a potential plastic that might enter in the feed stream used in recycling for food contact applications. Each recycling system used in food contact applications has fairly sophisticated sortation systems encompassing one or both mechanical and or manual sortation systems to remove highly discolored or suspicious plastic materials. Given that this frequency of contamination has been shown to be on the order of one bottle in 3000–4000,[25,28–30] one can easily calculate that there is a tremendous dilution of the original contaminant in the feed stream material by simply mixing in with the other feed stream material. As an example, if a bottle was contaminated at a 1000 mg/kg level and this bottle was one in 4000, dilution takes place in many steps involved in the recycling process such as grinding, elutriation, sink float, and washing. These result in a homogeneous mix and therefore simple dilution of the individual

contaminate to a level of 250 μg/kg prior to the effects of further decontamination. Thus before the further decontamination process, the dilution reduced level is only slightly above the target of 220 μg/kg for PET.[31] Therefore the US FDA assumptions and calculations used in the assessment are ultra conservative, thus assuring consumer safety.

15.4.2 Canada/Mexico

Canada developed a set of guidelines for using recycled plastics in food contact applications. The criteria listed in their guidance document were based on the US FDA criteria. Canada also chose not to formalize an official regulation but to review technologies on a case-by-case basis and issues a LNO as in the United States.

Mexico does not have formal regulations for food contact packaging. However, they have reviewed the concept of recycled material being used into contact applications and have indicated that as long as the technologies meet the US FDA criteria, they would allow the technologies to be used. The first plant in Mexico became operational in 2005. As of 2016, the National Standardization and Certification Organismo issued a voluntary standard NMX-E-263-CNCP regarding post consumer recycled PET for food packaging. The standard follows the US FDA guidance document.

15.5 Europe

Until 2008, European wide regulations for packaging only existed for virgin plastics. There were no regulations or directives allowing for the use of recycled material in food contact applications. Five European countries had specific regulations prohibiting the use of recycled material in these types of applications. Therefore, it was necessary for interested parties desiring to use recycled plastics materials back into food contact applications to meet with the individual national governments. The desire was to have the individual national governments adopt the same scientific principles established by the US FDA. During the 90s, success was achieved in the number of countries: Austria, Belgium, The Czech Republic, Finland, Germany, Hungary, The Netherlands, Norway, Slovakia, Slovenia, Sweden, Switzerland and the United Kingdom agreed to this approach. Both Germany and Switzerland went on to establish their own specific criteria also based on the FDA criteria. The EU Commission funded a project (AIR2-CT93−104) in 1993 to establish criteria to ensure the safe use of recycle and refillable plastics in food packaging. Unfortunately, upon completion of the project very little was done with the data established for recycled plastics. Subsequently, the ILSI packaging-working group took upon themselves to draft a guidance document ILSI.[32] What they developed was based predominantly on the US FDA guidelines and data from the Air2 −CT93−104 project. Due to continued pressure from many parties, a second European study, FAIR-CT98−4318 was funded and initiated. This project involved over 30 different entities encompassing recycle plastics commercial operations and Government and private research institutes. The focus was to fill in existing gaps in information related to the average contamination levels of postconsumer recycle plastics. A second objective was to investigate the potential variation between different types of collection systems and how consumer behavior might vary in various EU countries.

A similar study had been conducted in the United States.[33] That study had focused on demonstrating that recycled plastics could be used from either deposit collection systems which focus predominantly on food contact plastics or nonfood plastic containers available in other collections systems to varying degrees. This project focused specifically on PET. This was due to the fact that the polymer industry had clearly stated that all commercial PET was food grade. Material was obtained from five different types of commercial feed streams covering materials that were 100% from deposit systems to 100% nonfood containers. Approximately 500 kg on each of these five different types of feeds streams were processed at a commercial operation that had obtained a LNO from the US FDA for processing recycle plastics for food contact applications. The five resultant feed stream materials were then analyzed by a variety of analytical techniques to ascertain that the 5 types of resulting material streams all met US FDA criteria for food contact applications. The final conclusion drawn was that even using 100% feed streams containing food grade PET with nonfood items in them could be rendered equivalent to a 100% deposit stream and still meet all of the US FDA criteria for food use. These and other data caused FDA changing their position and allowing for the use of nonfood containers made from food grade plastics.

The EU FAIR project collected and analyzed 944 samples from 12 European countries (689 PET flakes samples from commercial washing plants), (38 Pelletized samples) and (217 "Super Clean" pellets). "Super Clean" pellets were from the plants utilizing decontamination technologies that were authorized in specific EU countries on a similar basis as the US FDA criteria. The analysis of the data showed PET related substances such as acetaldehyde (average concentration of 2.9 mg/kg) and food related substances, like limonene (average concentration 18.6 mg/kg). Limonene is represented by far the most dominant post consumer contaminant. This compound was in general accompanied by other nontoxic flavors or aromas in a proportion of 15% or lower compared to limonene. These results are in-line with other studies.[33−37]

Just 3 washed PET flake samples were found that were potentially related to misused PET bottles, most likely by storage of household chemicals such as pesticides and herbicides or other aggressive solvent cocktails used in their formulations (toluene and possibly xylenes). Statistical evaluation of the samples revealed postconsumer PET feed streams might have a potentially contaminated bottle at a rate of 1 to 3000–4000 bottles. These contaminants were only found in the washed PET flake. Further subjecting the washed PET flake to a "Super Cleaning" process would reduce the level of contamination below the limit of 10 μg/kg migration for limonene and far lower for all other compounds. The final conclusion of the study was that postconsumer PET articles produced by these modern "super cleaning" technologies are as safe as food contact articles from virgin PET. The FAIR project resulted in a guidance document being developed.[25]

At the completion of the project, a symposium was held in the Versa, Italy (February 2002). The data from the FAIR project and numerous other studies were presented and reviewed. At the completion of the symposium, a decision was made in DG SANCO to initiate the development of regulations allowing for the use of recycled plastics in food contact applications. The EFSA produced a final document in 2008 resulting in the Commission issuing (Commission Regulation (EC) No 282/2008 of March 27, 2008). The regulation stipulated that the resultant material must meet criteria as noted in Commission Regulation (EC) No 2002/72; (EC) No 2023/2006; and (EC) No 1935/2004.

A full guidance document as how to meet these criteria was published only in 2011.[38]

The key criteria required were very similar in scope to the US FDA criteria:

1. A complete description of the process
2. Characterization of the input material
3. Determination of the decontamination efficiency of the process via a surrogate challenge test after washing
4. Characterization of the recycled plastic
5. Description of the intended application
6. Evidence of compliance with regulations
7. Identification of critical process steps
8. Description of quality assurance systems.

A number of governments in Europe, Latin America, and Asia had adopted the same basic criteria for safety (carcinogenicity) as had been developed and put forth by the US FDA. This end point resulted in a dietary intake of 1.5 μg per kilogram per day. The EFSA, however, chose the far more conservative endpoint of genotoxicity. Based on the Threshold of Toxological Concern using genotoxicity as the end point, EFSA established it's dietary intake on calculating values for infants and toddlers and adults. This resulted in the dietary intakes of 0.0025 μg/kg bw/day (infants), 0.03 μg/kg bw/day (toddlers), and 0.15 bw/day (adults). Using the body weight of an infant of 5 kg results in the final concentration of 0.1 μg/kg being established based on a threshold for structural alerts raising concern for potential mutagenicity. EFSA, based on a review of the FAIR project and other data, established a standard value of 3 mg/kg of a contaminant in the recycle stream. They realized that this level was far too low as a target value in the surrogate challenge test, based on the high efficiency previously demonstrated by the various "supercycle" processes. They recommended target contamination levels between 200 and 1000 mg/kg for the input surrogates. The evaluation process is essentially based on the overall cleaning efficiency demonstrated by the cleaning process. The artificially contaminated material after washing is analyzed to differentiate between the initial contamination and the residual contamination in the full process output, monitoring the decrease at each critical step. This yields a cleaning efficiency for the recycling process. These Challenge Test's higher contamination values are then normalized to the standardized initial concentration of 3 mg/kg using a factor for the respective modeled substance. Likewise, the final concentrations also have to be corrected by the same factor. Using the approved Fickian based migration-modeling equation, EFSA calculated a modeled concentration (Cmod) that could be in the PET bottle that couldn't exceed the adjusted target value for genotoxicity. Infant calculated values (being the standard), for toluene, chlorobenzene, methyl salicylate, phenylcyclohexane, benzophenone, lindane, and methyl stearate respectively were 0.09, 0.09, 0.13, 0.14, 0.16, 0.31, and 0.32 mg/kg. Thus the residual concentration (Cres) needs to be less than Cmod. EFSA[38,39] is well aware that factors used in calculating migration over-estimate migration are by a minimum factor of fivefold for low molecular weight compounds and upto 100 fold for higher molecular weight compounds. EFSA therefore increased dietary intakes for genotoxicity by a factor of five. The resulting values calculated for infants, toddlers and adults were respectively 0.1, 0.15, and 0.75 μg/kg. For conservatism only the 0.1 μg/kg applies.

This requires the technology provider to determine the cleaning efficiency of the decontamination process and then calculate the residual concentration using the following equations:

1. Percent cleaning efficiency = 1− (Conc. final/Conc. initial) × 100
2. Cres = 3 mg/kg × (1% cleaning efficiency)
3. Cres < Cmod for each surrogate.

If the concentration (C) residual is less than concentration (C) modeled for each surrogate compound, then the technology meets the necessary criteria for decontamination.

To date, it has been shown that technologies that have met the US FDA guidance document criteria have also met the criteria as established for Europe by EFSA. Therefore the extensive analytical migration data developed for specific technologies submitted to the US FDA could also be used in Europe.

EFSA, through October 2019 has listed the review of 116 plastics recycling process for food contact applications (97 PET and 9 for either HDPE or PP).

15.6 South America

A number of countries in South America were interested in pursuing the use of recycled plastics in food contact applications. Symposiums and conferences were held a number of times in the 1990s covering the science and safety that had been developed in the United States and Europe. In 2002 a concerted effort was initiated in the Mercosur countries, Argentina, Brazil, Paraguay, Uruguay, and Venezuela to review all existing data on recycling technologies for the use of postconsumer plastics in food contact applications. They sought advice from both US FDA and European officials. In 2007 they enacted legislation for postconsumer PET for the Mercosur countries under resolution GMC 30/07. This resolution follows a combination of both US FDA and EFSA guidelines. The member countries are supposed to incorporate the resolution into their own National laws within a 6-month period. Paraguay transposed the Mercosur resolution into their National legislation under a decree 1319/2018.

Key elements of the Mercosur resolution encompass the following:

1. Processed postconsumer PET material must meet all compliance requirements for Virgin PET for food contact
2. Authorized processes must be registered by the respective national governments
3. Responsibilities:
   a. Proposed recycle technologies must have successfully completed a surrogate challenge test for validation
   b. Tests for conditions of use
   c. Plants must be authorized by the appropriate sanitary authority
   d. The package processor must be a registered entity and maintain all appropriate documentation and have full ability for package traceability
   e. The food processor is only allowed to use authorized material/packages and demonstrate full traceability.

Bolivia: issued Supreme Decree 0559/2010 making it mandatory for the Bolivian Institute of Standardization and Quality standard 716002:2009 on postconsumer PET. The standard follows US FDA and or EU. In 2016 Supreme Decree 2887/2016 complemented the previous decrees and established a minimum of 30% postconsumer PET to be used in the manufacture of PET bottles. A multi–ministerial resolution 1/2017 established that the National Service of Agriculture and Livestock Health and Food Safety (SENASAG) must implement the 2016 Supreme Decree. SENASAG issued a resolution 47/2018 requiring regulation and registration of companies that manufacture or import postconsumer PET.

Columbia: established regulations in 2012 based on the Mercosur criteria.

Ecuador: Resolution 16003/*2016* of the Under-Secretariat of Quality, Ministry of Industries and Productivity, makes mandatory Ecuador standard RTE INEN 291–*2016* on PCR-PET (it follows US-FDA and/or EU).

Peru: Supreme Decree 7/1998 was modified by Supreme Decree 038/2014 allowing for the use of postconsumer PET for food packaging. Under the 2014 decree, a certificate of conformity may be issued by a body accredited by any one of three Peruvian authorities: National Institute for the Competence Defense and the Intellectual Property, International Laboratory Accreditation Corporation, and Inter-American Accreditation Cooperation.

Chili: In the mid to late 1990s the Chilean government had convened an expert group to review the potential of using postconsumer PET from a select source in multilayer bottles. This use was authorized and implemented for a number of years; however, this application has been abandoned due to economics.

15.7 Central America

Costa Rica: In 2017 Costa Rica enacted decree 40393/2017. This degree made it mandatory the Costa Rican Standard RTCR 480–2016 for the use of postconsumer PET in food contact. The standard was based on US FDA criteria.

El Salvador/Guatemala: Reportedly draft guidelines have been prepared in both countries. However, at this time these drafts do not appear to have been enacted.

15.8 Asia-Pacific

Australia/New Zealand: Australian and New Zealand align a number of their food and packaging regulations along the lines of those of the US FDA. After careful review of the US FDA guidance document, Australia issued a letter of no objection in1993 for the use of postconsumer recycled PET in multilayer PET packages for food use. In 1999, Australia authorized the first plant to use postconsumer recycled PET in direct food contact applications. These authorizations seem to be out of step with the Australian Standard AS 2070–1999 that expressly forbids the use of recycled plastics in direct food contact. However, this standard was meant to harmonize Australian regulations with other international bodies such as the US FDA and Europe both of which have had provisions and or regulations for the use of recycled plastics in food contact applications. The Australian Packaging Covenant states that in communication with Food Standards Australia and New Zealand representatives have indicated that the food standards code is currently under revision and a reference to AS 2070–1999 will most likely be removed in the revision.

Philippines: based on a careful review of the US FDA criteria in their guidance document, the Filipino FDA issued a LNO for the first postconsumer PET recycling plant for food contact applications in 2007.

China: Industry began working in 2004 with the governing factions of the Chinese authorities to establish a process for the use of recycled plastics and food contact applications. After a 2.5-year review of the US FDA criteria and relevant scientific information, a letter of authorization was issued in 2007 for a postconsumer PET recycling plant in Beijing producing material for food contact applications. China has not progressed any further to establish specific regulations or guidelines for this use. The Chinese National Health and Family Planning Commission has been instructed by the government to undertake a total review and rewrite of existing packaging regulations and other food additive regulations. The new revised packaging regulations have been completed but it may be sometime before new food additive regulations can be finalized. It is not expected of that recycling regulations for food contact will be developed until the completion of the food additive regulations.

Japan: The Japanese Health Ministry authorized the use of chemical depolymerization processes in producing food grade PET from postconsumer plastics as far back as 1995. This was in line with the US, in several European countries, and in Canada. Japan's National Institute of Health Sciences undertook a diligent review of scientific literature and the US FDA guidelines and drafted a proposed guidance document. The Ministry of Health, Labor and Welfare authorized the guidance document 0427 NO 2 April 27, 2012.

15.9 Africa

South Africa: presently, it is the only country on the continent of Africa that has looked at the use of postconsumer plastics in food contact applications. South Africa does not have formalized packaging regulations and relies on the legal aspects of producer responsibility. Following requests from industry, a joint group with officials from the South African Bureau of Standards was established which developed a guidance document based on the US FDA criteria.

15.10 Conclusion

At present, national regulations, guidance criteria, authorization processes or approvals for the use of recycle plastics in the food contact applications only exist in about 45 countries globally. To date, those processes are based on sound science and extreme safety conditions such as the TOR (carcinogenicity) in the United States and the TTC (genotoxicity) in Europe to ensure consumer health and safety. The added requirements to demonstrate compliance also create the additional factors ensuring safety. These include but are not limited to the following:

1. Worst case scenario of contamination requires 100% of material to be contaminated for testing technologies
2. High levels of surrogate contaminants are used to demonstrate capabilities of proposed technologies
3. Practicality dictates that ground flake be contaminated which directly results in increased surrogate absorption by a factor of 5–100 times
4. Consumption factors assume 100% of the food contact application will use recycled plastic
5. The recycled content in the article is assumed to be 100%
6. If there is a contaminant in the material, it will be assumed to migrate 100% to the food product.

Numerous scientific studies have been conducted over the past 30 years. These studies have helped to substantiate the overall safety of using recycled plastics in food contact applications as well as demonstrating the over conservatisms of the regulations and guidelines that have been established.

1. Barrier layer inhibition of minimum of 25 μ between potential contaminant (United States)
2. Efficiency of contaminant removal via washing
3. Efficiency of contaminant removal via extrusion
4. Efficiency of contaminant removal via "super cleaning"
5. Contaminant absorption in flakes versus whole bottles
6. Typical absorb compounds in postconsumer PET recycle streams in Europe, the United States, Japan, and Australia
7. Establishment of general level of incidental contamination in European postconsumer PET recycle streams
8. Establishment of over estimation of migration in currently accepted mathematical models of migration.

There will be a need for collection volumes of recycled plastics to significantly increase. Whether it is from industry making sustainability commitments or governmental mandated requirements, PET in the United States alone would require collection and processing an additional 1.7 million metric tons by 2025 and 2.7 million metric tons by 2030.[40] This would also increase the need for an additional capacity for processing the material estimated to be 3 billion dollars capitol costs by 2030. It is estimated that this would require a 78% recycling rate in the United States by 2030. Similar scenarios can be constructed for Europe and other countries. It is clear that to meet either sustainability or governmental mandates that many additional countries will have to establish regulations, guidance documents or approval/authorization processes to allow the expansion for use of recycled plastics in food contact applications. Consumer safety must be insured without overburdening and creating insurmountable cost economics. It is imperative to establish those new regulations and procedures based on the strong safety criteria developed by the US FDA and EFSA Europe in order to avoid a patchwork of regulations requiring vastly different criteria, which could result in international trade issues and additional cost barriers.

The safety of using recycled plastics in food contact applications has been assured based on exceedingly stringent safety and test procedures. Government and scientific studies have validated all aspects of these criteria. Finally, billions of food packages utilizing postconsumer recycled plastics based on these criteria have been used in and around the globe for the past three decades without any incidents of safety concerns.

Part B Refillable plastic food contact materials

15.11 History and perspective of returnable refillable plastic food containers

Used Food contact materials (FCM) are reused in either recycling processes, as feedstock for new FCM or can be returned to a filling/bottling company. But, according to EU Packaging Waste Directive 94/62/EC "*reuse*" *shall mean any operation by which packaging, which has been conceived and designed to accomplish within its life cycle a minimum number of trips or rotations, is refilled or used for the same purpose for which it was conceived, with or without the support of auxiliary products present on the market enabling the packaging to be refilled; such reused packaging will become packaging waste when no longer subject to reuse*."

Refillable FCM reused at home are not covered by this definition. In this chapter, the quality and safety aspects of articles returned to for example, a bottler for refilling are described. Fig. 15.2 shows that refillable bottle systems create the shortest loop in a circular bottle economy.

Glass packaging has been used for more than 2000 years as reusable packaging but only in the 20th century returnable refillable glass containers became rather common in many countries all over the world. These refillable containers are locally collected, returned to the bottler and there inspected for damage, visual contaminants, cleaned, sanitized, and refilled. This initially required, for safety reasons, rather heavy bottles and costly transport. In the late 1960s, many containers were designed for single-use. This often allowed for thinner, lightweight one-way glass bottles and eliminated the cost of collection, inspection and cleaning. Refillable glass packaging can be reused up to ca 30 times, depending on the market requirements while for refillable PET (RefPET) a trippage rate of $\geq 12-14$ is mentioned.

15.12 Refillable plastic containers for consumer market

Refillable plastic containers have a relative short history. As recently as 1960, 95% of all soft drinks and 53% of all packaged beer was sold in refillable glass deposit bottles that were reused 20 or more times (Environmental Encyclopedia, 2020). The first plastic refillables made of HDPE plastic were introduced in the mid-1960s in the United States and from 1974 for 8 years in Ontario, Canada.[41]

At that time the US FDA was confronted with reuse of lightweight, unbreakable refillable PE dairy containers as an alternative for heavy glass.

In the early 1970s, PET was produced by using stretch blow molding technology, resulting in the first oriented three-dimensional structures.[42] The development of lightweight, clear, transparent, tough, unbreakable PET bottles with good gas barrier properties led to a fast expanding use for (soft) drinks and many other applications. Today, depending on the monomers, treatment and thus obtained physical properties, refillable polyester containers can be used for hot [crystalline PET (CPET), heat-set PET or polyethylene naphthalate (PEN)] or cold fill applications.

In 1978 in the United States, polycarbonate (PC) replaced refillable PE containers in some dairy markets.[43] The rigid and very clear returnable LEXAN PC dairy container, developed in the early 1970, offered the advantages of both glass and HDPE plastic without the disadvantages.[44] After the early use of refillable PE dairy bottles in the United States, there was no significant follow up for refillable plastics due in part to widespread use and recycling of one-way PET bottles. Refillable plastic containers never became popular in the United States, although during the 1980s and 1990s, many US dairies

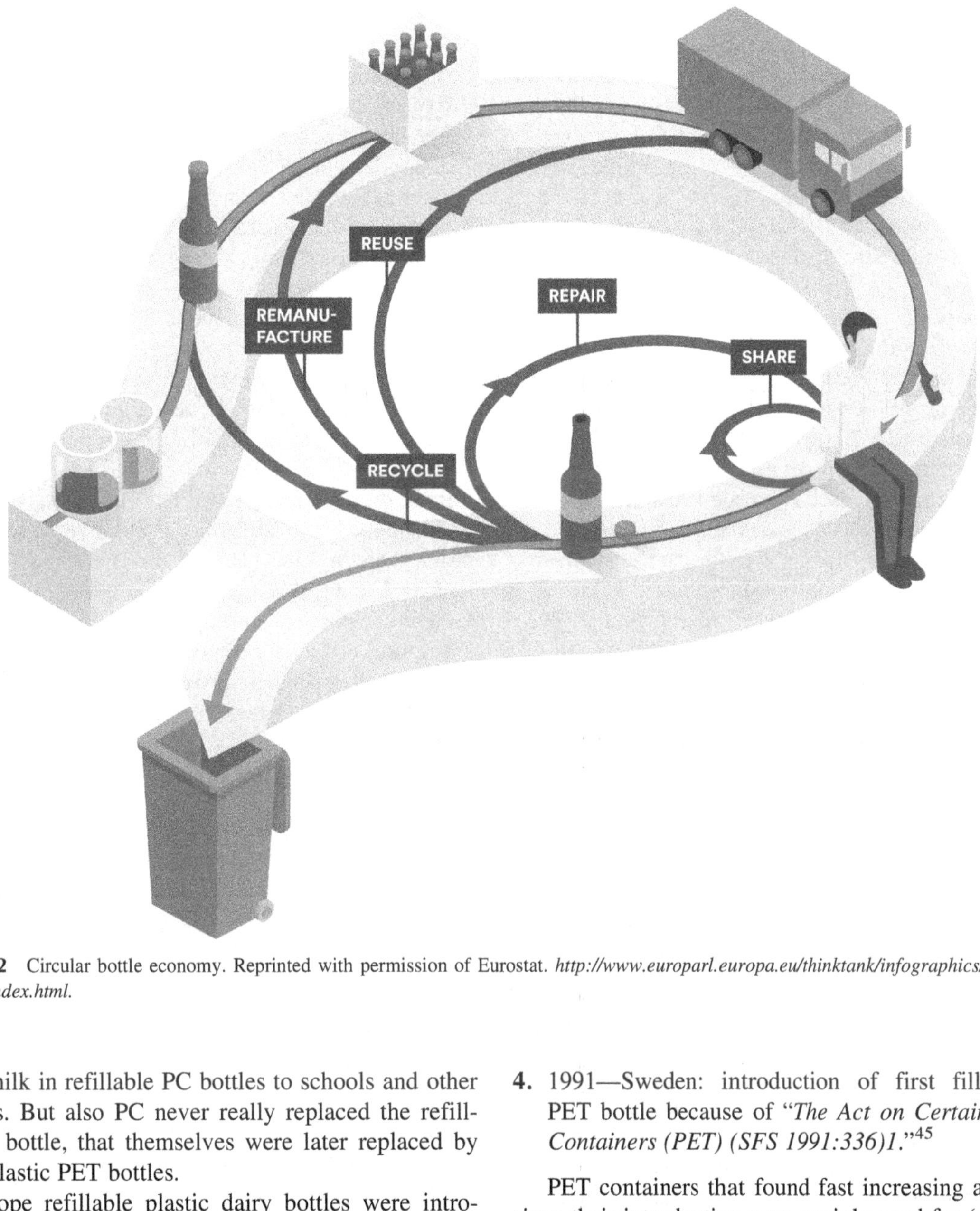

FIGURE 15.2 Circular bottle economy. Reprinted with permission of Eurostat. *http://www.europarl.europa.eu/thinktank/infographics/circulareconomy/public/index.html.*

supplied milk in refillable PC bottles to schools and other institutions. But also PC never really replaced the refillable glass bottle, that themselves were later replaced by one-way plastic PET bottles.

In Europe refillable plastic dairy bottles were introduced for the first time in Switzerland in 1981. As the result of growing environmental awareness and the resulting introduction of National and European, for example, packaging waste legislations many other countries followed are:

1. 1977—Denmark: ban on one-way packaging for carbonated soft drinks. Only reusable packaging for carbonated beverages allowed, while all other beverages could be sold in one-way packaging.
2. 1983—Germany: introduction of refillable 3-L PC dairy bottle.[41]
3. 1986—Germany: first trials of RefPET in Cologne, Germany.
4. 1991—Sweden: introduction of first fillable 1.5 L PET bottle because of "*The Act on Certain Beverage Containers (PET) (SFS 1991:336)1*."[45]

PET containers that found fast increasing applications since their introduction were mainly used for (carbonated) beverages while, for example, PC and HDPE, and low-density polyethylene (LDPE) were mainly used for dairy.

15.13 Shift away from refillable plastic

Especially during the 1970–90s, refillable plastic bottles (mainly polyesters) were increasingly used all over the world but especially in the European Community.[46] By the introduction of the regulations and guidelines for the closed loop recycling concept "*threshold of regulation*" in the United States[47,48] and later in the EU recycling regulation 282/2008, it became possible to close the material loop completely by (mainly) mechanical recycling processes.

From that time, it was no longer necessary to collect, inspect, and wash relative heavy refillable plastic bottles that were increasingly replaced, first, in the United States and later also in Europe, by light weight one-way plastic bottles. Yet, the share of refillable lightweight refillable glass bottles and PET bottles decreased all over the World[45,49,50,50] (Rehkopf, 2019). In Asia, South America, that is, in Brazil (Lemons Junior et al., 2019)[91] refPET bottles are still used in significant numbers. According to EU report "A European Strategy for Plastics in a Circular Economy"[51] "*reuse of consumer plastic packaging is not very common. Use of refillable plastic containers (e.g., some PET bottles, some hygiene and detergent bottles) happens only when this is mandated (e.g., in Germany), but has declined to very low levels in general in Europe.*" On 6 March 2020, 15 European countries and 66 companies have entered into a partnership (European Plastic Pact) committed to making all plastic packaging recyclable and suitable for reuse. A large beverage company like PepsiCo is following recent environmental based regulations and announced in 2019 that it can avoid the use of 67 billion plastic bottles through 2025, thanks to the expansion of its SodaStream system that allows consumers to create customized beverages at home with reusable bottles.[52] By 2025, all their packaging needs to be recyclable, compostable or biodegradable."

15.14 Safety and quality of refillable containers

Both refillable glass and plastic bottles are collected, transported to bottlers, inspected, washed and refilled. RefPET bottles and standard one-way PET bottles have a similar chemical composition but refillables contain approximately twice as much resin for increased wall thickness. This provides the sturdiness, thermal stability and other attributes needed to handle reusable packages. To ensure the refillable plastic bottles are not distorted, the cleaning conditions are often milder than for glass or during other forms of recycling. The maximum washing temperatures range from 58°C–60°C (amorphous PET) to ca 95°C (heat-set PET and PEN). This is more than enough to allow hot filling and pasteurization of many food products[53] (Packaging Europe, 2017).

Glass however is generally considered inert, while plastics are not. Absorption of chemicals by plastics from previous use or misuse and subsequent release into new fillings might cause a safety or quality risk. Although, metals like lead and cadmium can also migrate from glass into food, Glassallianceeurope.eu.[54] and Gasaway[55] reported that pesticide ingredients were shown to be removed from commercially caustic washed glass returnable containers previously exposed to pesticide formulations.

The quality, safety, and material properties of refillable plastic packaging have been investigated thoroughly. The majority of the published scientific papers on the safety of refillables originate from the 1970s and especially from the 1990s. From around 2000, the published studies focus on quality issues like flavor carry-over, and on-methods to determine plastics absorbed and desorbed by chemicals adequately. The degree of absorption and desorption of substances depends from the inertness of a plastic that is determined by its physical and chemical composition, the technique used to produce containers and the properties of the interacting chemicals stored in them. For example, PP and PE are among the most used materials in plastic food packaging.[56] Their inertness is generally considered much lower than that of PET. Recycling of polyolefin packaging for food contact applications requires more advanced cleaning and assessment protocols, because diffusion of most substances is much faster than in PET. This results in strongly increasing migration rates, and thus of sorption of substances from food and misuse. According to van Willige[57] the extent of absorption of flavor compounds by LLDPE is influenced by food components in the order:

Oil or fat >> polysaccharides and proteins > disaccharides

PC is rather inert but also very vulnerable for many contaminants. Gasaway[44] reports that 30% of the 85 pesticides investigated were incompatible with Lexan PC. Similar results of contact with solvents and other substances such as anise flavor at high concentrations, Dettol (chloroxylenol) and other chemicals, were reported.[58–60] They report stress cracking, hazing and other damage to the bottles (often after washing) so that they could be detected by pre- and postwashing inspection systems.

PET is relative inert compared to other plastics but is also not compatible with certain contaminants. Feron et al.[61] reported that 12 test substances used in a misuse study were incompatible with PET and clearly damaged the bottles. PET is a glassy polymer at room temperature and in the vast majority of conditions of use, while polyolefins are rubbery and have poor barrier properties. The diffusion coefficient of a given substance is much lower in PET than in polyolefins so that the possible migration of absorbed contaminants is much lower for PET. The high absorption of polyolefins is also one of the reasons why refilling of plastics is mainly limited to polyesters.

Inertness testing can be done in many ways. The voluntary Industrial Code of Practices for PET and PC[62–64] included procedures for testing of the chemical resistance of bottles.

In EU project AIR2-CT93–1014[65] a quick predictive absorption test[60] with PET and PC bottle strips, exposed to surrogate contaminant cocktails with different chemical properties, showed a good correlation with the results of whole bottles. Quick rinsing (20 s) of contaminated PET bottles with 95% ethanol seemed to be as effective in removing surrogate contaminants as commercial washing of bottles. In 2004, Franz and Palzer et al.,[27] issued an official European procedure "Certification of a refillable PET bottle material with respect to chemical Inertness behavior according to a PR-CEN standard method, BCR-712." This method gave enforcement laboratories *"for the first time a systematic control possibility to check the food safety of refilled PET bottles taken from the market."* This test considers the effects of mechanical stress influences on the inertness of PET material and, in case of complaint, allows the enforcement authorities to determine the cause (bottle manufacture process/wash/refill system/too many trips). The inertness of common packaging polymers decreases as follows:

PEN > PET > rigid PVC > PS > HDPE, PP > LDPE.

Van Lune et al.,[66] Widén and Hall,[67] and van Willige et al. (2002) reported the relative high inertness of PEN compared with standard PET and other materials. Jetten[68] reported similar results for high and low copolymer NDC (naphthalenedicarboxylic acid) containing polyester bottles for beer. Carbonyl compounds from beer (major flavor substances) showed that high-NDC (naphthalenedicarboxylic acid) bottles are much more inert than standard PET and better than low-NDC and heat-set PET bottles. Depending on temperature, the total absorption of flavor compounds by polyolefins (LLDPE and PP) was upto 2400 times higher than by PET, PEN, and PC. Their low absorption and better cleanability, but also that of for example, ethylene vinyl alcohol (EVOH) and rigid polyvinylchloride (PVC), makes them more suitable for use as a refillable food packaging than PS and HDPE.[69,70,71,72]

Jetten et al.[60] and Jetten and de Kruijf[73] developed "a set of quality criteria and methods for sensory evaluation, chemical and microbiological safety-in-use of refillable PET, PC and vending PP cups (premarket) for industry and regulatory authorities." Flavor carry-over was observed for all products tested while lipstick could not be removed from cups. Most misuse and flavor chemicals caused an off-flavor to water stored in PET and PC bottles but repeated washing (PET and PC) did not affect:

1. Overall migration into standard EU food simulants, including 95% ethanol
2. (Specific) migration levels of monomers and oligomers (of PET)
3. Odor and taste of bottled water exposed to the contaminants and mixed fruit and anise sirup
4. Intrinsic properties (oxygen, carbon dioxide and water barrier, degradation and surface characteristics).

The hydrophobicity of 15 times washed PC bottles (contact angle goniometry) was affected. According to Tawfik et al.[74], the impact strength and modulus of elasticity properties of PET strips was significantly ($P < .05$) affected by the level of d-limonene absorbed. The elongation was not influenced. Van Willige et al. (2002) also showed that oxygen permeability in PET was not significantly affected by absorption of flavor compounds.

Between 1994 and 2011 several studies were done with (heat-set) PET, PC, PVC, HDPE and PP refillable containers to investigate the effect of (repeated) washing conditions on flavor carry-over and inertness of container[58,69] Franz et al. 1998,[60,75] van Willige et al.[76,77] Caustic and additive concentrations but also carbonation level and pH of beverages had little effect on decontamination and absorption. Repeated washing did affect inertness of standard PET while for other materials and heat-set PET no effect was reported. It was concluded that all plastic containers contain residues of test substances but polyolefins (PP, HDPE) and PVC appear to retain significantly more contaminants compared with the more polar polymer types (PC and PET) and of course glass.

15.15 Flavor carry-over and effects of repeated use on materials

Absorption of essential flavor constituents from food by plastics is called flavor scalping. It changes (minimizes) the flavor of packed foods. Absorbed flavor compounds from previous uses belong to common contaminants in postconsumer plastic packaging as they may remigrate into new filled beverages, affecting the quality. This is called flavor carry-over. Flavors can also permeate through a packaging causing flavor loss. This is less likely to occur in case of thick-walled refillable bottles. Off-flavors may originate from intended applications but also from misuse of the packaging by consumers. For example, chemicals present in personal hygiene products, cleaning agents and foods and beverages like sirups used at home, could also migrate into plastic. Not only do such components pose a health risk, they could also influence the organoleptic properties of the re-filled foodstuffs.

Several authors used the flavor component d-limonene (major citrus compound, present in most soft drinks) to develop optimal washing processes or analytical methods to determine the inertness of plastic containers. According to Franz et al.[25–28] and Welle[76] limonene is present as a contaminant at μg/kg level in almost any (98%) postconsumer PET recyclate and can even be used to recognize or identify postconsumer recyclates. They report an average limonene level of 2.9 mg/kg (range 0.1–20 mg/kg) in conventional recycled PET flake (rinsed, flaked, washed, and surface dried). After deep cleansing it was never detected. Remigration into water never reached the taste threshold level of 35 μg/L water.

15.16 Contaminants from misuse

In the second half of the 1970s, researchers published research on the migration and retention of pesticides and household chemicals stored into HDPE and PC (Lexan) returnable milk bottles.[44,55,78,79] Ca. 31% of the pesticides were incompatible with PC. Misuse of containers was investigated by sniffer detector, sensory evaluation and extraction. Their results showed implications for PC, HDPE as well as glass, while the majority of the test substances were not detected by the sniffer. Bodyfelt reported that 11 out of 16 common substances, including pesticides, stored in HDPE bottles passed undetected. Milk stored in 5 of these 11 "detector-accepted" washed bottles contained either pesticide residues in excess of legal tolerance limits or had objectionable off-flavors. Pesticide ingredients were however also extracted from commercially caustic washed glass returnable containers previously exposed to pesticide formulations. Landsberg tested 29 common household contaminants. The in-line contamination detector allowed nine washed treated PE containers and five treated PC containers to pass undetected. Each retained sufficient contaminant to produce an off-odor in milk.

Gasaway[55] showed that sensory testing of washed containers was more effective in detection of off-odors than the contaminant detector. All three types of washed containers exposed to pesticides exhibited off-odors. Pesticides could be detected in milk stored in the washed containers (PC: 6 out of 85 and PE: 22 out of 85).

In 1993 European project[65] "*Programme to establish criteria to ensure the safety-in-use of recycled and re-used plastics for food packaging*" was launched by major EU research organizations. The United Kingdom, Spain, France, The Netherlands, Germany, and Sweden were involved. The objective for refillables was "*to define the boundaries were use and re-use in food applications is acceptable or unacceptable*." Safety (chemical and microbiological) and quality (odor/flavor carry-over) using repeatedly washed refillable PET and PC was investigated. This required development of new analytical methods for plastics. Jetten et al.[60] described new methods to test the quality (sensory) and safety (microbial and chemical) of refillable PET, PC, and PP containers.

In 1994, Feron et al. published the results of large studies on the health and safety aspects of refPET bottles, including and extending the results of the safety studies of the 1970s. As part of a multiclient project in which the entire refillables chain participated (producers of resin, detergents, blow molders and bottlers), the potential public health risks of the reuse of possible misused refPET bottles was investigated extensively. Project partners also provided research data on 1.5 L PET containers and their safety from previous studies conducted on their behalf by independent contract laboratories. The results of five of these studies, along with the project results of a complementary study carried out at by R&D organization TNO, were compiled and published. RefPET bottles were exposed to 62 contaminants, (pesticides but also substances like a cyanide and aflatoxins), commercially or simulated, washed, filled with a simulated beverage, and stored for various lengths of time.

The hazard assessment of the contaminant residue remigrations involved comparing the Acceptable Daily Intakes (ADIs), set by the Joint FAO/WHO Committee on Pesticide Residues, with the "maximum potential exposure" (MPE) calculated from the amount migrated per bottle. Comparisons of the MPEs with the estimated non-toxic doses (ENTDs) were also made during the hazard assessment. The estimated chance of a consumer contacting more than two bottles in a year ranged from approximately 1/100,000 to less than 1/1000,000, depending on the exposure assumptions used. Gasaway[44,55] and Jonker et al.[80] reported that the probability of contaminated milk being purchased in a returnable PC or HDPE bottle once in a person's lifetime was calculated to be 1 in 20,000,000. The evaluation of Feron et al. showed that even under exaggerated exposure conditions, there is no public health concern. The low risk of exposure to toxic contaminants was also shown by Bayer.[33] Evaluation of five different postconsumer PET feed-streams (deposit and curbside) showed that citrus compound limonene, present at 18 ppm, was the predominant contaminant in the "deposit" feed-stream (100% beverage bottles). Methyl salicylate, present at 15.3 ppm, was the predominant contaminant in "food-grade" PET used in nonfood applications (100% nonfood containers such as mouthwash, detergents, and cleaners). The concentrations in caustic hot washed material ranged from 28–39 mg/kg and it was concluded that this PET, regardless of the source of the feed-stream, could be mechanical recycled for new food contact applications.

15.17 Contamination rate

According to the ILSI Task Force (1994), the number of consumer complaint for refillables were comparable with those for other packages. For the number of PET bottles contaminated by previous use or consumer misuse different figures are reported that range from 1:3000[26] to 1:10,000 (ILSI Task Force). According to Konkol[71] contaminants in washed PET and HDPE obtained from curbside collection are rather similar and the relationship between these contaminants and the original ingredients of the bottle gives support of the assumption that most contaminants arise from the "normal" use of plastic bottles and not consumer misuse. According to Widén et al.[50] the frequency of off-odor products (consumer complaints) due to the reuse of contaminated water and soft drink PET bottles can be estimated to 9 in 1,000,000.

15.18 Food contact material regulations

Since the introduction of PET bottles many countries approved this material for use as FCM.[81] FCM like PET, but also other materials, are made of known substances for which the safety is controlled by legislation. This is necessary because substances like monomers and additives can migrate into packed foods. The rate and amounts depend on time, temperature, contact medium, physical- and chemical properties of the food contact material. Therefore, in 1976, the EU introduced Council Directive 76/893/EEC, including chapter number 13, comprising a positive list of allowed monomers and additives that may be used for the production of FCM, and their migration limits into food.

The US Federal FDA Food Drugs and Cosmetics Act (FFDCA) has no positive list but all FCMs including resins and colorants must comply with the act. But, substances and their migration limits also must ensure the safety of FCM. PET, for example, as a new material was judged safe and approved for food contact in the late 1970s under FDA food additive regulation 21 CFR 177.1630 and 21 CFR 177.1315 as a container for soft drinks.

The two major FCM regulations in the world are those of the EU and the US FDA. They served as a basis for many other national regulations.

In 1990, the EU introduced Directive 90/128/EEC on plastic FCM. At present (2021), the safety of FCM is oulined in plastics regulation (EU) 1935/2004 and plastics regulation (EU) No. 10/2011. FCM other than plastic do not have specific rules at EU level.[51] Both EU and FDA specify use conditions such as hot fill and require material allowance test conditions that meet the type of use (such as refill).

15.19 Refillable food contact materials regulations

Refillables require further assurance of packaging quality and safety as they may absorb chemicals from previous use or even consumer misuse and thus may contain unknown substances. Specific regulations for plastic refillables are however lacking in most countries, although safety is always a requirement. Besides they are subject to good manufacturing practices (GMP) requirements like (EC) No 2023/2006 and FDA 21 CFR Section 174.5. Upon introduction, the safety of returnable refillable plastic containers was tested all over the world (see Section 16.2). Dedicated legislation was most often considered unnecessary because test results of safety studies on (simulated) misused containers, evaluated by the authorities, demonstrated their safety. Controlled sanitation and inspection as required by FDA was considered sufficient. The ILSI Task Force on Refillable PET packaging[82] describes the global legal requirements and the results of safety testing upto 1994. Their overall conclusion is that refillable PET, the most used plastic, is allowed by most countries without specific, dedicated legal requirements. In 1994 Plastic refillable bottles were already permitted in many countries including The Netherlands, Brazil, Germany, Denmark, Sweden, Mexico, Chile, Argentina, and Thailand. Development of major legal and governmental safety requirements are described below.

15.20 United States and Canada

In 1965 the US Public Health Service (USPHS) allowed the unlimited use of refillable polyethylene (HDPE) dairy containers, provided certain provisions of the Grade "A" Pasteurized Milk Ordinance 1965 which were met. One of the seven safeguards required for use of a returnable plastic containers drew attention everywhere. It concerned the new condition that a "sniffer" detector should be installed in the process to identify and remove containers that were contaminated with volatile substances after consumer use.[44]

In the 1970s, the US FDA placed no restrictions on reuse and/or refilling of plastic bottles (with no recycling) provided were:

1. Properly sanitized
2. Made in accordance with GMP, as required by 21 CFR 174.5.

In 1992 the FDA made some recommendations in their "Points to consider for the use of recycled plastic in food packaging: Chemistry consideration, May 1992"[47,82]:

1. Educate the consumer (considered most important) to avoid storing household chemicals, such as pesticides and automotive fluids, in reusable containers;
2. Label the bottles "*for food use only*";
3. Require a deposit on the bottles to minimize the possibility of consumers contaminating the bottle;
4. Hydrocarbon sniffer or color scanners could be part of the screening process for chemical contaminants;
5. Reusable containers, unlike those intended for recycling, would be returned directly to the store by the consumer or collected at the home by the distributor.

In their guidance on the use of recycled plastic FCM for Industry[48] the FDA declares that "*EPA considers recycling to be the processing of waste to make new articles.*" Because bottles intended for reuse are not made to be discarded and become waste, reuse is not considered recycling by EPA. Reuse is regarded as one way to minimize the amount of material entering the environment. "*In simple reuse, the package remains intact and is reused in its original form.*"

Canada has, like the United States no specific regulations for plastic refillables as industry has refused to formally consider refillable plastic container options and governments have generally avoided examining these technologies as part of 3Rs policy-making processes.[83]

15.21 European Union

Non-intentionally added substances such as misuse chemicals and residues of previous fillings as occurring with refillable, reusable plastic FCM are not (yet) specifically addressed in EU regulations and directives. The safety is however covered by article 3 of framework regulation (EC) No 1935/2004 that requires that materials and articles, including active and intelligent materials and articles, shall be manufactured in compliance with GMP so that, under normal or foreseeable conditions of use, they do not transfer their constituents to food in quantities which could:

1. endanger human health or;
2. bring about an unacceptable change in the composition of the food or;
3. bring about a deterioration in the organoleptic characteristics thereof.

However, upon introduction, several countries evaluated the safety of refillable PET bottles. The Norwegian Government Industry Quality Control concluded that "*there are no microbiological or toxicological reasons to impede the use of REFPET for use with nonalcoholic carbonated beverages.*"[82] Other European countries like Italy and Denmark allowed the use of REFPET beginning in the 1990s, while referring to applicable FCM regulations after evaluation of safety studies. In 1993 European project AIR2-CT93–1014[65] was launched to develop quality and safety criteria (chemical, microbial, and flavor) for refillables. But it did not result in legislation.

15.22 MERCOSUR and South America

In South America, the MERCOSUR trade organization including Argentina, Brazil, Paraguay, Uruguay, Venezuela (currently suspended) and associated states, Bolivia (in the process of accession), Chile, Colombia, Ecuador have regulations. Guyana, Peru, and Surinam have regulations that are also harmonized with food packaging requirements in the EU, the United States, and the German BfR as well as other countries around the world.[84]

GMC Resolution 56/92 "*General provisions on food contact plastics*" applies to all plastic containing FCMs and established positive lists. In addition, "due to the phenomena of sorption and desorption, food contact plastics must be manufactured only with virgin materials, and reuse of plastic packaging is forbidden in general, with the exceptions established by the MERCOSUR legislation (i.e., PET refillable bottles and PCR-PET packages). Nonalcoholic carbonated soft drinks in returnable packaging of PET are regulated in MERCOSUR Ordinance n.105/99–Annex IX under GMC no. 16/93.[84,85] This regulation applies mainly to PET refillable (i.e., returnable) bottles, which have been in the MERCOSUR Ms markets since that year (for instance, in Argentina and Brazil). It states that carbonated, nonalcohol containing beverages that are sold in returnable plastic containers between the states must comply with the demands given in the annex to the resolution. "*This is not necessarily applicable to export outside the member states.*" Apart from general food safety, GMP and use requirements comparable with those of the FDA: the returnable plastic packages must:

1. Be registered at the Authorities and get formal approval,
2. Be resistant to all processes to which they are submitted during their return cycles,
3. Be labeled for explicit exclusive product use,
4. For QA control have sampling procedures and analytical methods as determined by the American Public Health Association,
5. Have instruments that can be used to inspect 100% of the containers for the presence of foreign contaminants,
6. Have adequate equipment for cleaning returnable containers a control system as well as
7. Have dedicated adequately trained staff that uses the equipment.
   a. Have periodic microbiological controls. Microbiological requirements on washed plastic bottles for this application are:
      i. Absence of coliforms and
      ii. Mesophilic aerobic bacteria: maximum 1 colony forming unit mL1 (of internal package volume).

In 1993, sections 196 and 196 bis were also included in the **Argentine** Food Code where reuse is specified in detail.

Chile, Decree No. 977/1996 and its amendments, Sanitary Food Regulation (Reglamentos Sanitario de los Alimentos) Title II–Foods (Título II–De los Alimentos), Paragraph III–Packages and Articles (Parrafo III–De los Envases y utensilios) contains a paragraph specific for reuse. Article 128 permits the use of returnable packages provided they allow adequate cleaning and sanitation.

Article 129 establishes that packages that have been in contact with nonfood products or which are incompatible with foods must not be used to hold foodstuffs.[86]

15.23 Code of practices

The ILSI provided draft guidelines in 1994 for the safe use of PRB's while in 1993 and 1995 voluntary Code of Practices for refillable PET and PC bottles, for soft drinks, mineral waters and dairy were introduced.[62,63] They were produced under supervision of the Dutch contract R&D organization TNO and incorporate the combined expertise of 20–26 leading companies representing the entire involved chain of reuse. In particular, producers of: bottles, raw materials, washing systems and equipment were involved. To protect quality and consumer safety they provide guidelines and specifications for proper production and handling of plastic refillable bottles (incl. pre- and postwash inspection). The COPs for soft drinks and mineral water were endorsed by Union of European Soft Drink Associations (UNESDA) and Confederation of European Soft Drink Associations and were recognized as authoritative for all parties involved. The COP for refillable PC dairy containers[63] was endorsed by the German Milchwerke Westfalen, for example, a second edition of the COP for polyester bottles with an extended scope was published in 2000 (TNO). It also covered other polyester-based materials like heat-set PET and PEN and described quality and safety requirements for the chain involved with soft drinks and mineral waters. It was endorsed by branch organizations for soft drinks (UNESDA/CISDA), natural mineral waters' Union European and International Grouping of Natural Mineral Water Industries and Spring Waters (UNESEM) and by the ILSI whose contribution were also incorporated.

15.24 Microbial safety

Microbiological safety of refillables was investigated extensively by the Health and Environmental Science Institute of ILSI. Data were collected from bottlers in The Netherlands, Argentina, Germany, and Norway.[82] These data indicated that bottles, as well as returnable glass with and without rough interiour defects, were cleaned and sanitized. Given the nature of soft drink products (e.g., acidity), processes and raw materials, the risk of transmission of pathogenic bacteria or viruses was considered extremely low. In the United States, a soil test (cleanability) was developed by the US Society of Soft Drink Technologist that included dirt and microbes. Jetten et al.[60] and Jetten and de Kruijf[73] also developed a challenge test to verify microbial safety of PET, PC bottles and PP vending cups with sporeformers.

Devlieghere and Huyghebaert[87] investigated anherence and removal of microorganims with glass, HDPE, PP, PC, PET, and PVC bottles. The influence of temperature, caustic concentration and additive on the remaining microorganisms was limited but strongly depends on the type of material. Optimization of process parameters resulted in much better cleaning and the following classification in decreasing order of microbial rinsibility could be made:

$$Glass > PET > PC > PP = PVC > HDPE.$$

15.25 Sniffer detection technology

It is generally recognized that GMP procedures, including visual and electronic inspection systems, are required to eliminate abused bottles and maintain quality. It became clear rather early that existing sniffers did not suffice. Bodyfelt et al.[78] and Landsberg et al.[79] used in-line contamination detectors to detect residues of household chemicals (pesticides, herbicides, beverages and other substances) in multiuse PC, PE, and glass containers. These detectors did not give adequate consumer protection to the refillable PE or PC milk container systems as they allowed many containers to pass undetected. The detectors were not capable of detecting, for example, those test containers, which had held water based, nonhydrocarbon substances of low volatility. Neither the PE nor the PC containers appeared to comply with the Grade Pasteurized Milk Ordinance 1965 recommendations of the United States Public Health Service (USPHS). Glass showed no absorption problems.

Initially, the volatile content of bottles was measured everywhere by simple photoionization detectors (PIDs). Investigations above, performed during the 1970s and 80s resulted by the end of the 1980s in the development and use of more sophisticated empty bottle inspectors (EBI). These were based on gas chromatography detection like FID, ECD, and MSD (relative slow), as well as infrared (relative fast for hydrocarbons) and extensive visual inspection.[46]

Soon it became clear that with these systems, the detection of a common contaminant, like urea/ammonia, was not sufficient.[88,89] To that end, two new systems were introduced: Chemical Luminescence (indirectly after burning a gas probe) and directly, and more sensitive by a microwave-process analyzer (MIPAN) that detects ammonia compounds, such as liquids containing ammonia, decayed organic compounds, cigarettes or urine. In the next phase it was realized that nonvolatile substances (e.g., flavor residues from detergents) but also mineral water (no masking flavor), required other detection systems.[89,90] Therefore in 1995, the so-called USM residual liquid analyzer (widely applicable to detergents and nonvolatile hydrocarbons) was developed.

Re-use also requires prior to washing and sanitizing visual substance screening of the postconsumer containers with color scanners.[71]

According to Bayer[41] a refillable PET line requires:

1. Either a manual or electronic (visual camera) system to insure that each bottle on the line has had the closure removed
2. Electronic contaminant detection systems periodically calibrated with appropriate standards fully operational at all times
3. Filling operations to stop in case of failure of operation of either criterion at any time.
4. Modern contaminant detectors (Sniffers) developed are based on the following detection technologies:
   a. Pulsed fluorescence (polycyclic aromatic compounds at ppb level)
   b. Electrolytic chemiluminescence
   c. Mass spectrometry
   d. Infrared spectrophotometry (e.g., hydrocarbons)
   e. Microwave emission
   f. Charge-coupled device camera systems
5. The conditions for operation, such as the fact that contaminant detectors must be designed for operation in a bottling line front-end environment with unwashed returned bottles, are well defined by Bayer.
6. The detectors must be capable of inline detecting:
   a. Low volatility compounds (softeners, cleaners, shampoos, etc.).
   b. Petroleum derivatives (gasoline, kerosene, paints thinner, etc.).
   c. $(NH_2)_2CO$—Urea
   d. Alcohols (beverage and nonbeverage)
   e. Aromatic compounds (anisole, toluene, etc.)
   f. Turbid liquids
   g. Decomposed organic material
   h. Local commercial products (softeners, cleaners, herbicides, fungicides, etc.).

Detection limits for such detectors are reported by Lemos Junior et al.[91] (Table 15.1).

The ILSI Task Force[82] mentions incidence data for two studies where quality control hydrocarbon sniffers caused rejects in the range of 0.3%−1%. The majority of these rejects were due to flavor components from previous fillings and not from contaminants. As shown above such a detector is not sufficient to detect all (mis)-used containers.

A hazard analysis critical control point (HACCP) approach and the use of GMP for the entire refillable process (including sniffers) are required to ensure the safety and quality.[92] The TNO COPs for refillable PET and PC bottles (1993, 1995, 2000) and the ILSI whitepaper 1994 provide detailed test protocols and requirements for inline contaminant inspection system.

Lemos Junior et al.[91] demonstrated that the number of rejected contaminated bottles is not only dependent on the detection system but also from the QA system and staff training. They developed a HACCP plan for a soft drink production line for 2 L returnable PET packaging by A.O. analysis of consumer complaints on bottles from Rio de Janeiro market during August 2013 to July 2015. The line was equipped with an All Surface Empty Bottle Inspector (ASEBI), encapsulation and metal detector and a high-end sniffer equipped with 4 sensors (Infrared pulse, Fluorescence, Radiation and Spectrometer). The results showed that the most significant complaint observed was a change of flavor, "which is commonly associated with a failure in the sniffer." However, the implementation and control of identified CCP led to the reduction of altered flavor complaint from 52% (October 2013) to 14% (July 2015).

TABLE 15.1 Detection limits of in-line contaminant detection system for refillable bottles.

Substance concentration detection system	Detection limits of sniffer	Substance concentration detection system	Detection limits of sniffer
Gasoline	0.5 μL Infrared[a]	Isopropanol	1 μL Infrared[a]
Gasoline	1 μL Fluorescent pulse	Turpentine	1 μL Infrared[a]
Diesel	2 μL Infrared[a]	*Thinner*	1 μL Infrared[a]
Diesel	1 μL Fluorescent pulse	Petroleum	2 μL Infrared[a]
Exxon 150	2 μL Infrared[a]	Methanol	1.5 μL Infrared[a]
Exxon 150	0.1 μL Fluorescent pulse	Isooctane	1 μL Infrared[a]
Toluene	1.5 μL Fluorescent pulse	Ethanol	15% 1 mL Infrared[a]
Kerosene	2 μL Infrared[a]	Ammonia (25%)	1 μL (9 ppm) MIPAN

[a]*Infrared USPL: Ultra short pulse laser.*

Widén et al.[50] also reported failure of sniffers for refPET bottles in the soft drink and mineral water industry. The "sniffer" devices used at the three plants all had different operating principles. They analyzed consumer complaint bottles, collected during 9 months, with GC-Ms. In some cases, the origins of the off-odors clearly seemed to originate from consumer misuse with food products (liquorish flavored alcohol, home-made alcohol containing fusel oil) or nonfood products (e.g., cleaning products, petroleum products). No real conclusions could be drawn concerning the performance of the different sniffers, except that the sniffer systems in use had passed the bottles and failed to detect and reject them.

15.26 Conclusions

All plastic refillable bottles can absorb chemicals from previous use or misuse. The degree depends from the type of polymer and the physical and chemical properties of the produced containers.

Investigations performed since the introduction of refillable systems showed that:

1. Safety is not an issue but quality problems (flavor carry-over) might occur
2. There are no countries that forbid or restrict the use but suitable EBIs are a must
3. The use of detection systems requires skilled staff, GMP and HACCP management

Anno 2020 in many countries there is a shift away from refillable to one-way bottles.

References

1. Frawley JP. Scientific evidence in common sense as a basis for food-packaging regulation. *Food Cosmet Toxicol.* 1967;5:293–308.
2. Rulis AM, Finley JW, Robinson, Armstrong DJ. Threshold of regulation, Options for handling minimal risk situations. In: Finley JW, Robinson SF, Armstrong DJ, eds. *Food Safety Assessment.* Washington, DC: American Chemical Society; 1992:380–388. ACS Symposium Series, No. 484.
3. Flamm WG, Lake RL, Lorentzen RJ, et al. *De Minimis Risk. Carcinogenic Potencies and Establishment of a Threshold of Regulation for Food– Contact Substances.* New York and London: Plenum Publishing Corporation.; 1987:87–92.
4. Rulis AM, Felix CM. De Minimis and the threshold of regulation. In: Felix CM, ed. *Food Protection Technology.* Chelsia, Michigan: Lewis Publishers Inc; 1987:29–37.
5. Rulis AM, Bonin JJ, Stevenson DE. Threshold of regulation. In: Bonin JJ, Stevenson D, eds. *Risk Assessment in Setting National Priorities.* New York and London: Plenum Publishing Corp; 1989:271–278.
6. Monroe IC. Safety assessment procedures for indirect food additives: an overview. *Regulatory Toxicol Pharmacol.* 1990;2–12.
7. Machuga EJ, Polli GH, Rulis AM. A threshold of regulation policy for food contact particles. *Food Control.* 1992;3:180–182.
8. US Food and Drug Administration. Federal register. 1993:1950, 52719–52729; vol. 58.
9. US Food and Drug Administration. Food additives: threshold of regulation of substances used in food-contact articles; Final Rule. *Fed Register.* 1995;60(36):36582–36596.
10. Thorsheim HR, Armstrong DJ. Recycled plastics for food packaging. *ChemTech.* 1993;23:55–58.
11. Bayer FL, Myers DV, Gage MJ. Considerations of pet recycling for food use. In: Rader CP, Baldwin SD, Cornell DD, Sadler GD, Stockel RF, eds. *Plastic, Rubber and Paper, Recycling: A Pragmatic Approach.* Washington, DC: American Chemical Society; 1995:152–160. Symposium Series, 609.
12. Kuznesof PM, van de Veer MC. Recycle plastics for food– contact applications: science, policy and regulations. In: Rader CP, Baldwin SD, Cornell DD, Sadler GD, Stockel RF, eds. *Plastic, Rubber and Paper, Recycling: A Pragmatic Approach.* Washington, DC: American Chemical Society; 1995:389–403. Symposium Series, 609.
13. Sadler G. Recycling of polymers for food use: a current perspective. In: Rader CP, Baldwin SD, Cornell DD, Sadler GD, Stockel RF, eds. *Plastic, Rubber and Paper, Recycling: A Pragmatic Approach.* Washington, DC: American Chemical Society; 1995:380–388. Symposium Series, 609.
14. Bayer FL. The threshold of regulation and its application to indirect food additive contaminants in recycle plastics. *Food Addit Contam.* 1997;14:661–670.
15. Scientific Committee on Foods (SCF). Opinion on response to requests from the commission for SCF opinion on the scientific basis of the concept of threshold of regulation in relation to food contact materials. Annex VII to document III/ 5557/96. Brussels: EC; 1996.
16. European Commission. Directorate–General III Industry, Industry, Scientific Committee for Foods, Request for the opinion of the Scientific Committee for Foods on the scientific basis of the concept of a Threshold of Regulation. C S/P M/ 2636. Brussels: EC; 1995.
17. Joint F AO/WHO Expert Committee on Certain Food Additives, Evaluation of certain food additives and contaminants. 49th Report of the Joint FAO/WHO Expert Committee on Food Additives, vol. 884. Geneva: WHO; 1–84; 1997:1–89. 1 – 89. WHO Technical Reports Series.
18. Cheeseman MA, Machuga EJ, Bailey AB. A Tiered approach to threshold of regulation. *Food Chem Toxicol.* 1999;37:287–412.
19. Kroes R, Galli C, Munro I, et al. Threshold of toxicological concern for chemical substance present in the diet: a practical tool for assessing the need for toxicity testing. *Food Chem Toxicol.* 2000;38:255–312.
20. Kroes R, Renwick AG, Cheeseman M, et al. Structure–based thresholds of toxicological concern (T TC): guidance for application to substances present at low levels in the diet. *Food Chem Toxicol.* 2004;42:65–83.
21. Barlow S. Threshold of toxicological concern (TTC). A tool for assessing substances of unknown toxicity present at low levels in the diet. ILSI Europe Concise Monograph Series; 2005.
22. Boobis A, Brown P, Cronan MTD, et al. Origin of the TTC values for compounds that are genotoxic and/or carcinogenic and an approach for their re- evaluation. *Crit Rev Toxicol.* 2017;47 (8):710–732.

23. Simoneau C, ed. Applicability of generally recognized diffusion models for the estimation of specific migration in support of EU Directive 2002/72/EC. 2. EU report 24514 EN. ISBN 978-92-79-16586-3; 2010.
24. US Environmental Protection Agency (EPA), Characterization of Municipal Solid Waste in the United States: 1994 Update, EPA/530-S-94-042, Washington, DC 20460, Table 7; 1994.
25. Franz R, Mauer A, Welle F. European survey on post-consumer polyethylene terephthalate (PET) materials to determine contamination levels and maximum consumer exposure from food packages made from recycled PET. *Food Addit Contam.* 2004b;21 (3):265–286.
26. Begley TH, McNeal TP, Biles JE, Paquette KE. Evaluating the potential for recycling all PET bottles into new food packaging. *Food Addit Contam.* 2002;19(1):135–143. Supp. 1.
27. Demertzis PG, Johansson F, Lievens C, Franz R. Development of a quick inertness test procedure for multi-use PET containers—sorption behavior of bottle wall strips. *Packaging Technol Sci.* 1997;10:45–58.
28. Franz R, Bayer F, Welle F. Guidance and criteria for safe recycling of post-consumer polyethylene terephthalate (PET) into new food packaging applications. Report EUR 2155. ISBN 92-894-6776-2; 2004a:1–37.
29. Franz R, Palzer G, Gawlik BM, Bernreuther A, Lamberty A, Bennink D. Certification of a refillable PET bottle material with respect to chemical inertness behaviour to a pr-CEN standard method. Report EUR 21075, ISBN 92-894-7220; 2004c, 1–68.
30. Franz R. Progamme on the recyclability of food–packaging materials with respect to food safety considerations: polyethylene terephthalate (PET), paper and board, and plastics covered by functional barriers. *Food Addit Contam.* 2002;19:93–100.
31. US Food and Drug Administration. Office of Food Additive Safety Division of Food Contact Notifications HFS-275, Guidance for industry: use of recycled plastics in food packaging (chemistry considerations). College Park, MD: Center for Food Safety and Applied Nutrition, Food and Drug Administration; 2006:20740.
32. ILSI. *Recycling of Plastics for Food Contact Use, Guidelines Prepared Under the Responsibility of the International Life Sciences Institute (ILSI) European Packaging Material Task Force.* Brussels: International Life Science Institute; 1998.
33. Bayer FL. Polyethylene terephthalate recycling for food-contact applications: testing, safety and technologies: a global perspective. *Food Addit Contam.* 2002;19(Suppl)):111–134.
34. Blanchard F, Christael A, Gorski G, Welle F. Drinks from the detergent bottle. *Kunstoffe.* 2003;9:145–148.
35. Franz R, Welle F. Analytical screening and assessment of commercial available post–consumer PET recyclers for reuse and food packaging. *Dtsch Lebensmittel-Rundschau.* 1999;95:94–100.
36. Pierce DE, King DB, Sadler G. Analysis of contaminants in recycling polyethylene terephthalate by thermal extraction gas chromatography–mass spectrometry. In: Rader CP, Baldwin SD, Cornell DD, Sadler GD, Stockel RF, eds. *Plastic, Rubber and Paper, Recycling: A Pragmatic Approach.* Washington, DC: American Chemical Society; 1995:458–471. Symposium Series, 609.
37. Triantafyllou VI, Karmani AG, Akrida-Demertzi K, Demertziz PG. Studies on the usability of recycle pet for food packaging applications. *Eur Food Res Technol.* 2002;215:243–248.
38. EFSA Journal. Scientific Opinion on the criteria to be used for safety evaluation of a mechanical recycling process to produce recycled PET intended to be used or manufacture of materials and articles in contact with food. *EFSA J.* 2011;9(7):2184.
39. Welle F. Is PET bottle-to-bottle recycling is safe? Evaluation of post – consumer recycling processes according to the EFSA guidelines. *Res Convers Recycling.* 2013;73:41–45.
40. Bermish M. J Soc Chem Ind UK, 40, 2020.
41. Bayer FL. Refillable PET Bottles REFPET. Coca Cola presentation; 2013:1–43.
42. Petcore -Europe, <https://www.petcore-europe.org/what-is-pet.html>; 2020.
43. Platt B, Rowe D. Reduce, reuse, refill! Washington, DC: Institute for Local Self-Reliance), produced under a joint project with the GrassRoots Recycling Network; 2002.
44. Gasaway JM. Significance of abuse chemical contamination of returnable dairy containers: pesticide storage and detector evaluation. *J Food Prot.* 1978;41(11):851–862.
45. Amano M. PET bottle system in Sweden and Japan: an integrated analysis from a life-cycle perspective. Masters' Thesis for LUMES—Lund University International Master's Programme. In: Environmental Science 2003–2004; 2004:147.
46. Komolprasert V, Lawson A. Considerations for reuse of poly(ethylene terephthalate) bottles in food packaging: migration study. *J Agric Food Chem.* 1997;45(2):444–448.
47. US Food and Drug Administration. Center for food safety and applied nutrition, points to consider for the use of recycled plastics in food packaging: chemistry considerations, (HFS–245). Washington, DC; 1992:20204.
48. Golding A. Reuse of primary packaging. Final report. Part I—main report. <http://ec.europa.eu/environment/waste/studies/packaging/reuse_main.pdf>; 1999:1–107.
49. Widén H, Leufven A, Nielsen T. Identification of chemicals, possibly originating from misuse of refillable PET bottles, responsible for consumer complaints about off-odours in water and soft drinks. *Food Addit Contam.* 2005;22(7):681–692.
50. Rehkopf L. 2019, Container Deposit Legislation; https://www.encyclopedia.com/environment/encyclopedias-almanacs-transcripts-and-maps/container-deposit-legislation.
51. European Commission. FIP scientific network for the cooperation and harmonisation of risk assessment of FCM. In: The 'EFSA FCM Network' Meeting. Environmental Encyclopedia, 2020. <https://www.encyclopedia.com/environment/encyclopedias-almanacs-transcripts-and-maps/container-deposit-legislation>; 2018.
52. PepsiCo. <https://www.beveragedaily.com/Article/2019/09/24/PepsiCo-We-re-radically-reinventing-how-we-think-about-packaging>; 2019.
53. Packaging Europe (2017, 27, July), https://packagingeurope.com/molding-options-for-heat-setting-pet/.
54. Glassallianceeurope.eu. Guidelines on lead leaching from glass tableware into foodstuffs, 2003; <https://www.glassallianceeurope.eu>; 2017.
55. Gasaway JM. Significance of abuse chemical contamination of returnable dairy containers: sensory and extraction studies. *J Food Prot.* 1978;41(11):863–877.
56. Garcia PS, Cruz SA, Nerín C. Comparison of different extrusion processes for cleaning the recycled polypropylene removing volatile and non-volatile contaminants. *Prog Rubber, Plast Recycling Technol.* 2014;30(1):1–18.
57. van Willige RWG. Effects of flavour absorption on foods and their packaging materials. Thesis. ISBN: 90-5808-640-2. Wageningen Universiteit; 2002:1–152.

58. Devlieghere F, De Meulenaer B, Sekitoleko P, Garcia AAE, Huyghebaert A. Evaluation, modeling and optimization of the cleaning process of contaminated plastic food refillables. *Food Addit Contam.* 1997;14(6–7):671–683.
59. Jetten J, van den Berg F, Feron VJ. Quality monitoring of synthetic refillable packagings. Progress report IV. Analytical and sensory study on absorption and desorption properties of refillable polycarbonate bottles. TNO-report V94.335. Zeist: TNO; 1994.
60. Jetten J, de Kruijf N, Castle L. Quality and safety aspects of reusable plastic food packaging materials: a European study to underpin future legislation. *Food Addit Contam.* 1999;16(1):25–36.
61. Feron VJ, Jetten J, De Kruijf N, van den Berg F. Polyethylene terephthalate bottles: a health & safety assessment. *Food Addit Contam.* 1994;11(5):571–594.
62. TNO. Guidelines for an industrial code of practice for refillable PET bottles, 1st ed., TNO Nutrition and Food Research, Jetten et al., ed. ISBN 90-6743-294-6; 1993–1994.
63. TNO. Guidelines for an industrial code of practice for refillable polycarbonate bottles, 1st ed. TNO Nutrition and Food Research, Jetten et al., ed.; 1995.
64. TNO. Guidelines for an industrial code of practice for refillable PET bottles, 2nd ed. TNO Nutrition and Food Research, Jetten et al., ed; 2001.
65. AIR2-CT93-1014. Final report of EU funded AIR project AIR2-CT93–1014, Programme to establish criteria to ensure the quality and safety of recycled and re-used plastics for food packaging. Brussels; 1997.
66. Van Lune FS, Nijssen LM, Linssen JPH. Absorption of methanol and toluene by polyester-based bottles. *Packag Technol Sci.* 1997;10:221–227.
67. Widén H, Hall G. Sensory characterization of polyester-based bottle material inertness using threshold odour number determination. *LWT–Food Sci Technol.* 2007;40:1–7.
68. Jetten J. Evaluation of beer packaging. In: EBC Symposium, Beer in plastic bottles. Oslo. In: EBC monograph 30. ISBN 3-41-00784-8; 2000:15–27.
69. Nielsen TJ. Limonene and myrcene sorption into refillable polyethylene terephthalate bottles, and washing effects on removal of sorbed compounds. *J Food Sci.* 1994;59(1):227–230.
70. ILSI Europe Packaging Material Task Force. ILSI Europe report series: recycling of plastics for food contact use: GUIDELINES. ISBN 1-57881-035-3; 1998:1–24.
71. Konkol L. Contaminant levels in recycled PET plastics. PhD Dissertation. Victoria University, Australia; 2004:1–319.
72. Welle F. Develop a food grade HDPE recycling process. ISBN 1-84405-225-7. The Waste & Resources Action Programme; 2004, 2005:1–137.
73. Jetten J, de Kruijf N. Quality and safety aspects of reusable plastic food packaging materials: influence of reuse on intrinsic properties. *Food Addit Contam.* 2002;19(1):76–88.
74. Tawfik MS, Devlieghere F, Huyghebaert A. Influence of D-limonene absorption on the physical properties of refillable PET. *Food Chem.* 1998;61(1–2):157–162.
75. Franz R, Huber M, Welle F. Recycling of Post-Consumer (Polyethylene terephthalate) for diret food contact- a Feasibility Study using a Simplified Challange Test. *Deutsch Lebensmittle Rundschau.* 1998;94:303–308.
76. Welle F. Maximum concentrations of limonene in mineral water bottles containing postconsumer PET recyclates without organoleptic deteriorations. FHIV factsheet. 2009:1.
77. Hayashi E, Imai T, Niimi H. Safety verification for reuse of pet and glass bottles. *J Food Hyg Soc Jpn.* 2011;52(2):112–116.
78. Bodyfelt FW, Morgan ME, Scanlan RA, Bills DD. Critical study of the multiuse polyethylene plastic milk container system. *J Milk Food Technol.* 1976;39(7):481–485.
79. Landsberg JD, Bodyfelt FW, Morgan ME. Retention of chemical contaminants by glass, polyethylene, and polycarbonate multiuse milk containers. *j Food Prot.* 1977;40(11):772–777.
80. Jonker D, Woutersen RA, Jetten J, Volmuth TA, Feron VJ. Safety aspects of returnable polyethylene terephthalate (PET) bottles. Europak 96. In: *The Eighth International Conference on Plastics for Packaging Food and Beverage Industry*; 1996: 410–421.
81. De Cort S, Godts F, Moreau A. Packaging materials 1. Polyethylene terephthalate (PET) for food packaging applications. Updated version. ISBN 9789078637431. ILSI Europe; 2017:1–27.
82. ILSI Task Force on refillable PET packaging. White paper on refillable plastic packaging made from PET (polyethylene terephthalate). International Life Sciences Institute (ILSI), North America; 1994:1–114.
83. Ontario Blue Box system. Ontario's blue box system: a case study of government's role in the technological change process, 1970–1991: <http://www.envstudiesyork.ca/public/law/bluebox.htm>; 1994, envstudiesyork.ca.
84. TUV-Sud. <https://www.tuvsud.com/en/e-ssentials-newsletter/food-and-health-essentials/e-ssentials-2-2017/food-packaging-requirements-in-brazil>; 2017.
85. Ariosti A. MERCOSUR legislation on food contact materials. *Encyclopaedia (Ref Module Food Sci).* 2018;1–19. Available from: https://doi.org/10.1016/b978-0-08-100596-5.21879-9.
86. Rijk R, Veraart R, eds. *Global Legislation for Food Contact Materials.* Weinheim: WILEY-VCH Verlag GmbH & Co. KGaA; 2010:1–389. ISBN: 978-3-527-31912-1.
87. Devlieghere F, Huyghebaert A. Removal of microorganisms from polymer bottles by caustic washing. *Lebensm-Wiss u-Technol.* 1997;30:62–69.
88. Drinktec UNISENSOR Sensorsysteme GmbH <https://exhibitors.drinktec.com/en/exhibitor-details/product-presentation/product-presentation-detail/objId/282/actionproDrink/detail/controllerpro/Products/>; 2017.
89. Unkrig G, Pschichholz M. Fremdstoffen auf der Spur. Neue Verpackung; 2003:66–69.
90. Castle L. Recycled and re-used plastics for food packaging? *Packaging Technol Sci.* 1994;7:291–297.
91. Lemos Junior WJF, do Amaral dos Reis LP, de Oliveira VS, Lopes LO, Pereira KS. Reuse of refillable PET packaging: approaches to safety and quality in soft drink processing. *Food Control.* 2019;100:329–334.
92. Bovee EHG, De Kruijf N, Jetten J, Barendsz AW. HACCP approach to ensure the safety and quality of food packaging. *Food Addit Contam.* 1997;14(6–7):721–735.

Chapter 16

Preventing food fraud

Steven M. Gendel
Gendel Food Safety LLC, Silver Spring, MD, United States

Abstract
Food fraud is an international problem that causes economic harm and threatens food safety. Individual facilities are responsible for assessing the food fraud risk for each incoming ingredient and for implementing mitigation programs to reducing this risk. While there are several guidance documents available to help facilities meet this responsibility, all of them recognize the importance of supply chain controls and ingredient testing in an effective fraud mitigation program. Because food fraud mitigation plays a critical role in food safety and quality assurance systems, facilities must be able to create an integrated system that addresses all three needs synergistically. In the future, the food industry and regulatory authorities will need to recognize that effective fraud mitigation will require taking a systems-based approach rather than the current approach focused on individual facilities.

Keywords: Food fraud; food authenticity; food safety; fraud mitigation

16.1 Introduction

Food fraud occurs in many forms (Table 16.1). All forms of fraud cause economic harm to consumers who do not receive the product they pay for. Further, fraud can harm consumer health by the addition of toxic adulterants or the removal of essential nutrients. Harm can also occur because fraud seldom happens under sanitary or food-safe conditions. Fraud threatens public confidence in the overall integrity of the food supply, the industry, and regulatory authorities.

There is a great deal of evidence that fraud is an important and continuing problem. A 2010 report from the (then) Grocery Manufacturing Association estimated that the food fraud represents a \$10–\$15 billion burden on industry and consumers each year.[3] As of December 2020 the Decernis Food Fraud Database (which tracks all types of food fraud) included 1670 incident records involving 2248 adulterants, of which 44% were considered as potentially hazardous (according to the scheme described in Ref. [4]).

The most disconcerting indicator of the persistence and scale of food fraud comes from the reports of Operation OPSON, which is coordinated by Europol and Interpol. Each year, over about 3–4 months, multiple national and international enforcement agencies carry out targeted actions aimed at finding and removing fake and substandard foods and beverages. Summary data on product seizures from most of the OPSON operations are shown in Table 16.2. Also, each year several hundred people were arrested or referred to authorities for further legal action. These data and other news reports show that fraud continues to be "big business" even when significant efforts are being made to stop it. A detailed analysis of the results and information from national authorities suggest that, even though OPSON is nominally an international effort, some countries show little commitment to finding and responding to food fraud.

16.2 Overview of food fraud mitigation

The only way to avoid the economic and health consequences of fraud is to interrupt the flow of fraudulent ingredients and information. Because fraud can occur at any step in a supply chain, the primary responsibility for control generally rests with individual facilities and companies. GFSI (Global Food Safety Initative) benchmarking requirements for certification programs include a requirement for a certified facility to have a food fraud vulnerability assessment and a mitigation plan.[5] In the United States, Food and Drug Administration food safety regulations require that covered facilities consider hazards "intentionally introduced for purposes of economic gain" in their Food Safety Plan.[6] Similar requirements exist for facilities in other countries.

Because the food industry is familiar with HACCP-type (Hazard Analysis and Critical Control Points) food safety systems, they often try to address fraud using a

Present Knowledge in Food Safety. DOI: https://doi.org/10.1016/B978-0-12-819470-6.00013-5

TABLE 16.1 Some major forms of food fraud.[a]

Type of fraud	Description
Dilution/adulteration	Increasing volume or weight by addition, usually by adding a less valuable or undesirable substance
Enhancement	Concealing quality or identity such as by adding undeclared colors or flavors
Removal	Removing a valuable constituent and selling the remainder as if it were intact
Mislabeling/ misidentification	Providing inaccurate label information about properties such as nutritional content, geographic origin, expiration date, or production method
Illegal ingredients	Use of ingredients that are not approved or that are not fit for food use
Counterfeit documentation	Providing false information about the composition, properties, safety, regulatory status, or commercial status of an ingredient
Species substitution	Use of a different plant or animal species than claimed

[a]*Based on Refs.* [1,2].

TABLE 16.2 Summary of OPSON results.[a]

Operation number	Start date	Duration (months)	Product seizures (tons)	Product seizures (Liters)
1[b]	12/2011	0.25	2654	>13,000
2[b]	12/2012	1	262	35,702
3	12/2013	2	5661	739,816
4	12/2014	2	11,592	814,563
5	11/2015	4	11,131	1,449,056
6	12/2016	4	13,407	26,336,305
7[b]	12/2017	4	3620	9,700,000
8[b]	12/2018	5	16,000	33,000,000
9[b]	12/2019	7	5000	(>2000 tons)

[a]*Results of OPSON operations are available at https://www.europol.europa.eu/operations/opson.*
[b]*Information on OPSON 1 and 2 were obtained from the OPSON 3 report. Information on OPSON operations 7, 8, and 9 was obtained from agency press releases; no formal report has been published for these operations.*

similar approach.[7–10] This approach can obscure the important differences between fraud and safety:

1. The universe of problems encompassed under the rubric of fraud is much larger than for food safety. Importantly, this universe includes deception through forgery and mislabeling that are actions rather than material hazards (i.e., physical, chemical, or biological hazards).
2. Because fraud is the result of deliberate and changeable human action, it is more appropriate to apply the concepts of vulnerabilities and mitigations rather than hazards and controls.
3. The fact that fraud can occur at any point in a supply chain, possibly several times in the same supply chain, and in multiple forms means that fraud cannot always be "controlled" at "critical control points." It needs to be addressed by every participant in the supply chain.
4. The lack of a systems-based approach, in contrast to a facilities-based approach, to fraud can make it difficult for individual companies and facilities to appreciate the importance of the problem or the need to implement mitigation strategies.

16.3 Developing food fraud mitigation plans

Until the food industry, national food regulators, and other stakeholders can develop a systems-based approach to food fraud, individual companies and facilities will continue to bear primary responsibility for creating and implementing fraud mitigation plans. The most effective approach to this is based on the broad concepts that underlay most risk mitigation systems. These are to:

1. Identify and evaluate vulnerabilities,
2. Identify actions that can be taken to decrease vulnerability,
3. Implement and monitor these actions, and
4. Evaluate the effectiveness of the actions.

Because threats, vulnerabilities, and resources change, this process needs to be repeated regularly.

To date the focus for vulnerability identification and evaluation has been on the biochemical properties of incoming ingredients and materials because these considerations are similar to, and overlapping with, those addressed in food safety systems. However, it is important to also consider vulnerabilities associated with potential documentation fraud, particularly for credence claims such as "organic," "sustainable," or geographic origin.

Several resources describe the factors to be considered when evaluating vulnerability. These resources include both general and sector-specific guidance (Table 16.3). These resources generally recommend considering historical data along with information on current conditions such as price fluctuations, weather events that affect primary production, and geopolitical pressures. Vulnerability evaluation will, for facilities with many ingredients, also need to consider prioritization to identify those ingredients that carry the highest risk.

Most assessment guides place significant emphasis on the role of supplier relationships. For example, the Food Chemicals Codex (FCC) Food Fraud Mitigation Guide says that the "...the closer the relationship between buyer and supplier, the more knowledge and confidence each party will have in [the] other." The level of knowledge and confidence needed to have the needed confidence can be very difficult to achieve in an industry where ingredient uses change frequently as new products are developed and the industry responds to consumer fads. The recent experience with pandemic-related supply chain disruptions shows that relying on supplier relationships for risk mitigation is not feasible when it is difficult or impossible to track rapidly evolving supply chains.[11] It is also difficult to have knowledge and confidence without a mechanism to evaluate whether the vulnerability assessments and mitigation efforts at one facility are concordant with those of other facilities along an entire supply chain.

TABLE 16.3 Examples of food fraud guidance.

Source	Title	Web address	Last update
Food Chemicals Codex (FCC)	Food Fraud Mitigation Guidance	https://www.usp.org/food-safety-integrity	2020
FSSC22000	Guidance on Food Fraud Mitigation	https://www.fssc22000.com/wp-content/uploads/fssc-22000-guidance-on-food-fraud-final-100418.pdf	2018
PwC	Food Fraud Vulnerability Assessment and Mitigation	https://www.pwc.com/vn/en/publications/2017/pwc-food-fraud-vulnerability-assessment-and-mitigation-november.pdf	2016
SSafe	Excel spreadsheet that facilitates assessment and identifies the most significant vulnerabilities for each ingredient	https://www.ssafe-food.org/our-projects/	2018
Food and Drink Federation	Food Authenticity	http://www.fdf.org.uk/corporate_pubs/Food-Authenticity-guide-2014.pdf	2014
Food and Drink Federation	Guidance on Authenticity of Herbs and Spices	http://www.fdf.org.uk/herbs-spices-guidance.aspx	2016
American Spice Trade Association	Identification and Prevention of Adulteration	https://www.astaspice.org/food-safety-technical-guidance/best-practices-and-guidance/identification-prevention-adulteration-guidance-document/	2016
Nestle	Food Fraud Prevention	https://www.nestle.com/sites/default/files/asset-library/documents/library/documents/suppliers/food-fraud-prevention.pdf	2016

Once vulnerabilities have been identified, it is possible to determine what actions are needed to mitigate these vulnerabilities. This determination can be unexpectedly complex. For example, in a facility with many inputs, the most significant vulnerabilities are likely to be different for different ingredients. For example, one ingredient might be vulnerable to adulteration by dilution, while another might be vulnerable to substitution with nonfood-grade material. This diversity can lead to the need for a fraud mitigation program requiring many different types of mitigations.

One of the complexities of developing a fraud mitigation plan for multiple ingredients is that a facility needs to have an appropriate way to characterize each ingredient. That is, facilities need to know what to expect before they can determine if those expectations are being met. Many facilities do not have the expertise to do this for multiple ingredients. For example, a company making a product based on a particular plant protein is likely to have the expertise to create specifications that define the expected biochemical characteristics of that protein but is less likely to be able to draft equally sophisticated specifications for the spices, binders, flavors, colors, and preservatives that are part of the final product. One efficient way to address this need is to rely on specifications developed by an independent Standard Development Organization such as the Food Chemicals Codex, the Joint Expert Committee on Food Additives, and the Codex Alimentarius.

Because fraud and adulteration can happen at any point in a supply chain, including during transport, testing of incoming ingredients will be a crucial component of most fraud mitigation programs. Many facilities carry out ingredient testing as part of their QA program and these tests can be useful for fraud mitigation either as they are currently used or with only minor enhancements. For example, a facility that evaluates the presence of peaks at a few wavelengths in a spectral scan of an ingredient could use the entire scan for product fingerprinting. Integrating fraud mitigation with an existing quality assurance program will reduce the overall complexity of the mitigation effort and is likely to improve the utility of the quality assurance system as well.[12] This also supports the importance of considering safety, integrity, and food defense together as part of the overall food safety culture of an organization.[13]

Facilities need to use appropriate and informative testing methods. This means that the test methods used must be capable of differentiating questionable or unusual material from authentic or normal material. As with ingredient specifications, it is unlikely that most facilities will have the expertise needed to choose the best method(s) for all the ingredients that they use. In many cases, facilities can rely on methods contained in standards such as those from the Food Chemicals Codex.[14] Methods that are part of an FCC ingredient standard have been validated for suitability for identity and purity testing of that ingredient. These standards are more robust for use in fraud mitigation than nonspecific methods such as the Kjeldahl technique for protein determination in dairy products, or Brix measurement of sugar content in juice.[14]

Because many of the newer methods used in fraud mitigation systems require somewhat complex equipment (nuclear magnetic resonance or mass spectrometry) many facilities rely on contract laboratories to carry out these analyses.[15] In general, laboratories that are certified to meet appropriate standards (such as ISO 17025) will provide accurate and reliable results.[16] However, as with assessing an ingredient supplier, there are important precautions that should be exercised when assessing a contract laboratory. The first is to ensure that the scope of certification for the laboratory covers the tests that will be carried out. The second is to check that the laboratory participates in a proficiency testing program that includes those tests if such a program is available. Regardless of whether there is an appropriate proficiency program, the laboratory should have a documented process for demonstrating analyst proficiency and for ensuring that each test is carried out only by an analyst with documented skills. Third, the contracting facility should review the methods that will be used by the laboratory. This means that the contracting facility needs more than a statement that a particular test will be carried out according to an in-house SOP (Standard Operating Procedure); it is the content of that SOP that is important. The contracting facility should determine whether the methods being used are those in a recognized standard and that the performance of the assays has been fully validated in-house. This is particularly important if the laboratory has modified the standard method.

Facilities and contract laboratories doing fraud-related testing need to consider whether the tests need to be highly sensitive. The appropriate level of sensitivity will depend on the ingredient and the type of fraud that is of concern. For example, if historical data or economic considerations show that an ingredient is prone to adulteration at high levels (e.g., 25% replacement), a relatively insensitive and rapid assay would be sufficient. Also, high precision will not be needed in this case. For example, if the facility is concerned about adulteration at the 25% level, an assay with a precision of 5% may be adequate.

Facilities will also need to consider whether to use targeted or nontargeted testing. The difference between them, and the factors to be considered in developing a nontargeted testing program have been described in Gao et al.[17] Nontargeted testing, sometimes referred to as fingerprinting, is a versatile approach that is particularly suitable for ingredients with a history of different problems. Detailed guidance on how to implement a nontargeted testing scheme is available in the Food Chemicals Codex.[18]

Using testing as part of a fraud mitigation program will be effective only if the testing is coupled to an appropriate sampling scheme.[19] This means that a facility will need to decide how often to sample and test each incoming ingredient and will need to ensure that the tested samples are representative of the batch or lot being evaluated. Because fraud can occur at any step in the supply chain, including during transport between facilities, ideally each shipment of incoming ingredients should be sampled and tested by each facility. In many cases, as discussed above, this lot-by-lot testing can be integrated with existing quality assurance testing. Further, the frequency of fraud testing can be adjusted as facilities gain experience in fraud mitigation and in response to external factors that change patterns of vulnerability. Facilities that only store or reship sealed products will need to consider the potential for documentation fraud, but it should not be necessary for these facilities to open and test batches of ingredients.

In the past, testing was only effective in detecting the types of fraud that altered the chemical composition of an ingredient. This includes activities such as dilution, removal, adulteration, and substitution. Recently methods have been developed that can be used to detect fraud related to claims such as organic or country of origin.[15,20] Unfortunately, many of these methods require the use of advanced technology such as mass spectrometry or nuclear magnetic resonance. While the cost of these methods is decreasing, they are likely to be impractical for many small and medium food manufacturers and facilities in many parts of the world. This suggests that food scientists and analysts who are developing and improving fraud detection methods should concentrate on those, such as spectrophotometric fingerprinting or antibody-based lateral flow devices, that can be applied easily and at a low cost. Methods that provide rapid pass/fail determinations when applied "at the loading dock" are likely to be widely used. When a rapid pass/fail system is used, batches that do not pass can be further evaluated using more advanced laboratory techniques.

It is worth noting that widespread availability of effective rapid methods would be useful for on-site use by government inspectors, auditors, and purchasers evaluating suppliers. By allowing more frequent testing at low cost, these technologies could make it more difficult for fraud to go undetected.

The third step in the fraud mitigation process is to implement and monitor the identified actions. This means that each facility should frequently review actions and records to demonstrate that the mitigation plan is being applied as designed. This review is also necessary to ensure that any process failures can be identified and corrected before they impact the integrity of food products.

The last step in the fraud mitigation process, evaluating effectiveness, is likely to be difficult. One tool that may be useful is to conduct mock (or tabletop) exercises such as is done with recall processes. Further, a detailed review of the fraud assessment and mitigation plan by an outside source will be useful. This review should go beyond simply verifying that a plan exists but should also evaluate the quality of the planning and implementation processes.

The use of contract manufacturing or copacking creates additional layers of complexity for a food fraud mitigation program. In many cases, the partners in the contract arrangement will have different degrees of experience with, and understanding of, vulnerability assessment and fraud mitigation. It is important that fraud, as well as safety, is addressed collaboratively in a contract arrangement.

16.4 Research gaps and future directions

Fraud remains a critical problem for the food industry, consumers, and regulators. As seen here, mitigating the risk of fraud can be difficult. This difficulty is compounded by the evolution of fraud beyond physical product risk to include information and labeling risks. Unfortunately, many fraud risk mitigation strategies have been adapted from food safety systems that deal with physical/chemical risks that are amenable to statistical description, and that can be controlled or eliminated by processing. On the other hand, integrating fraud mitigation with safety and food defense efforts will strengthen the response to all three threats.

The increased use of electronic record-keeping and networked information systems create new opportunities for fraud. The food industry will need to remain cognizant of the fact that they produce a physical product and that it will continue to be important to focus on protecting ingredients and materials, not just business records. That reflects the fact that the chain of physical custody is not necessarily the same as the chain of commerce, particularly in a multinational food system.

Increasing fraud vulnerability is a consequence of the increasing complexity of the food supply system. While the steps described here are important for risk mitigation at the facility or corporate level, it is clear that industry and regulators need to begin transitioning to a systems-based approach that leverages visibility and data sharing. An example of a successful systems approach to food safety is that of the Voluntary Control System (VCS) of SGF International that was developed by the fruit juice industry.[21] This system includes controls at every step in the manufacturing process, auditing, an analytical scheme, and checks on traceability. The VCS also includes the collection of retain samples at both receipt and shipping by all participants, sampling during all facility audits, and retail sampling. Because this program covers a large proportion of the European fruit juice industry, the effectiveness of the program can be evaluated using information such as from the Rapid Alert System for Food and Feed (RASFF) and national regulatory authorities. In the United States, the National Organic Program (NOP) of the U.S. Department of Agriculture (USDA) Agricultural Marketing Service is also taking a systems approach to protecting the integrity of the USDA Organic label. The NOP is working to implement a process that starts with soil on the farm and includes all steps and inputs through to the final consumer packaging.

The success of the fruit juice VCS suggests that system-based approaches to fraud assessment and mitigation could be successful in other industry segments. The current fragmented response to fraud improves the odds that fraudulent activity will not be detected. Moving to systems thinking for products such as olive oil, honey, meat, or spices would allow the industry to efficiently use resources in a way that provides an advantage not available to those who engage in food fraud.

References

1. Global Food Safety Initiative. Tackling food fraud through food safety management systems. <https://mygfsi.com/wp-content/uploads/2019/09/Food-Fraud-GFSI-Technical-Document.pdf>; Published 2018 Accessed 30.12.20.
2. Spink, J. Food fraud and adulteration: where we stand today. In: Melton, L, Shahidi, F, Varelis, P, (eds.) Encyclopedia of food chemistry. New York: Elsevier; 2019: 657–662.
3. Grocery Manufacturers Association. *Consumer Product Fraud: Deterrence and Detection*. Washington, DC: Grocery Manufacturers Association; 2010.
4. Everstine K, Abt E, McColl D, et al. Development of a hazard classification scheme for substances used in the fraudulent adulteration of foods. *J Food Prot*. 2018;81:31–36.
5. Global Food Safety Initiative. Benchmarking requirements 2020. <https://mygfsi.com/news-and-resources/?type = publications>; Published February 2020 Accessed 30.12.020.
6. US Food and Drug Administration. Electronic Code of Federal Regulations: Title 21 –Food and Drugs, Part 117 – Current Good Manufacturing Practice, Hazard Analysis, Risk-Based Preventive Controls for Human Food. <https://www.ecfr.gov/cgi-bin/text-idx?SID = 404a42953dbdf255c7ad63aa9555c825&mc = true&node = -pt21.2.117&rgn = div5>; 2015.
7. Codex Alimentarius. *General Principles of Food Hygiene*. Codex Stan CXC 1-1969; 2011.
8. Cook J, Marsh K, Spink J. VACCP: HACCP for vulnerability assessments. Food Engineering. <https://www.foodengineeringmag.com/articles/95205-vaccp-haccp-for-vulnerability-assessments>; Published February 17, 2016 Accessed 30.12.20.
9. Wareing P, Hines T. Knowing your HACCP from your TACCP and VACCP. Leatherhead Food Research. <https://www.leatherheadfood.com/files/2016/08/White-Paper-Knowing-your-HACCP-from-your-TACCP-and-VACCP-FINAL1.0.pdf>; Published 2016 Accessed 31.12.20.
10. Lupo L. Employing TACCP and VACCP for food safety and quality. Quality Assurance and Food Safety. <https://www.qualityassurancemag.com/article/employing-taccp-and-vaccp-for-food-safety-and-quality/>; Published March 2019 Accessed 30.12.20.
11. Whitworth J. Food fraud rise 'inevitable' because of COVID-19. Food Safety News. < https://www.foodsafetynews.com/2020/05/food-fraud-rise-inevitable-because-of-covid-19/>; Accessed 31.12.20.
12. Ali I. *Food quality assurance: principles and practices*. Boca Raton, FL: CRC Press; 2003.
13. Yiannis F. *Food safety culture: creating a behavior-based food safety management system*. New York: Springer-Verlag; 2008.
14. Food Chemicals Codex. Rockville, MD: US Pharmacopeia. <https://www.foodchemicalscodex.org/>; Published 2020 Accessed 30.12.20.
15. Hellberg R, Everstine K, Sklare S. *Food fraud: a global threat with public health and economic consequences*. Cambridge, MA: Academic Press; 2020.
16. International Organization for Standardization. ISO/IEC 17025 – Testing and calibration laboratories. <https://www.iso.org/ISO-IEC-17025-testing-and-calibration-laboratories.html>; Published 2017 Accessed 30.12.20.
17. Gao B, Holroyd S, Moore J, Laurvick K, Gendel S, Xie Z. Opportunities and challenges using non-targeted methods for food fraud detection. *J Agric Food Chem*. 2019;67:8425–8430.
18. Food Chemicals Codex. *Food Fraud Mitigation Guide*. Rockville, MD: US Pharmacopeia; 2020.
19. Codex Alimentarius. *General Guidelines on Sampling*. Codex Stan CAC/GL 50-2004; 2004.
20. Morin J, Lees M. *Food integrity handbook: a guide to food authenticity issues and analytical solutions*. Nantes: The Food Integrity Project/Eurofins Analytics; 2018.
21. Rinke P. Best practice example of sector specific food fraud mitigation by SGF International e.V. In: Morin J, Lees M, eds. *Food integrity handbook*. Nantes: The Food Integrity Project/Eurofins Analytics; 2018:411–418.

Section V

Changes in the chemical composition of food throughout the various stages of the food chain: identification of emerging chemical risks

Chapter 17

Emerging contaminants

Eleonora Dupouy[1] and Bert Popping[2]

[1]*Food Systems and Food Safety Division (ESF), Food and Agriculture Organization of the United Nations (FAO), Rome, Italy,*
[2]*FOCOS GmbH – Food Consulting Strategically, Alzenau, Germany*

Abstract

The rapid growth of population and urbanization, increase in food demand, intensification of food production, increasingly globalized food supply, environmental degradation, and climatic changes are associated with more complex and emerging health threats from unintended and undesired contaminants in the environment and in the agrifood chains. This chapter serves as an editorial introduction for chapters 18–24 that jointly aim to contribute to better knowing and addressing the emerging contaminants by risk managers, risk assessors, and risk communicators within competent authorities in a broad range of areas of expertise and jurisdictions, including food safety, public health, food and agriculture, and environmental health. Knowing the new threats is an essential precondition for effectively handling the emerging problems and preparing to cope with related challenges through leveraging available information, taking advantage, and making use of new knowledge and new opportunities, such as new methodologies, technologies, and innovative regulatory approaches to tackle the emerging contaminants issue.

Emerging contaminants that are discussed in the following chapters (18–24) refer to a selected set of issues for which health risk is progressively increasing due to the enhancing human exposure that may result from practices applied in food chain and changes in environmental conditions. Highlights refer to increasing risks to food safety and public health from the presence in the environment of microplastics, endocrine-disrupting compounds, antimicrobial resistance genes, and climate-induced emerging contaminants including foodborne pathogens, harmful algal bloom, heavy metals, and mycotoxins (known hazards yet regaining prominence in climate changing context). The chapter 23 features emerging contaminants related to fraudulent food practices and chapter 24 is devoted to traditional and emerging trends in chemical risk assessment. Research gaps and future directions are outlined for considered themes.

Chapters 18–24 address separate themes and are therefore presented as standalone chapters in this book.

Keywords: Emerging contaminants; endocrine disruptors; antimicrobial residues; climate change; mycotoxins; food fraud; chemical risk assessment

17.1 Editorial introduction to Chapters 18–24

The origin of chemicals in foods are very different, and vary from inherent natural food constituents, through certain being purposefully added in foods formulation for their specific functions as food additives, or being residues that remain in the food, such as pesticides and veterinary drug residues after the application of adopted good practices in horticulture, livestock, and aquaculture. The intentional use of food additives, agro-chemicals, and veterinary drugs is regulated and subject to control and monitoring of their presence in food. Chemicals in food may come also as substances that migrate into foods from packaging materials or residues from applied cleaning agents. Some foods may contain toxins as naturally occurring substances formed on crops and foods under certain environmental or preservation conditions, as is the case of mycotoxins. Chemical contaminants are unintentional toxicants that may enter the food from the polluted environment (air, soil, water), as is the case of dioxins, heavy metals, and radionuclides. They may also form in food during processing at high temperatures, like acrylamide, heterocyclic aromatic hydrocarbons or heterocyclic amines. The presence of emerging chemical contaminants in food, including environmental contaminants, process contaminants, and the residues of toxicological concern is undesired. Their levels in food and the human dietary exposure through food consumption need to be subject of research, regulation, and monitoring. Avoiding or reducing consumer exposure to emerging contaminants below the levels of concern is possible through food regulation, awareness-raising, risk communication, information, and education. The body of available knowledge on contaminants and their effects on living organisms, systems, or groups of populations is critical for setting maximal limits for the level of inadvertent chemical substances in commonly consumed foods. Of critical relevance to protecting human health is risk communication about emerging

Present Knowledge in Food Safety. DOI: https://doi.org/10.1016/B978-0-12-819470-6.00047-0

contaminants and proper information of food producers, food processors, and all other relevant actors along the food chain who have an instrumental role in applying food safety standards and mitigation procedures to keep within the safe limits those contaminants that are specific for the given food chain segment or process and may end up in the produced or manufactured food.

The rapid growth of population and urbanization, increase in food demand, intensification of food production, increasingly globalized food supply, environmental degradation, and climatic changes are associated with more complex and emerging health threats from unintended and undesired contaminants in the environment and agrifood chains. The aim of this chapter is to contribute to better knowing and addressing the emerging contaminants by risk managers, risk assessors, and risk communicators within competent authorities in a broad range of areas of expertise and jurisdictions, including food safety, public health, food and agriculture, and environmental health. Knowing the new threats is an essential precondition for effectively handling the emerging problems and preparing to cope with related challenges through leveraging available information, taking advantage and making use of new knowledge and new opportunities, such as new methodologies, technologies, and innovative regulatory approaches to tackle the emerging contaminants issue.

Contaminants are defined as emerging if they are either of the following: (1) newly discovered; (2) linked for the first time to an adverse health effect in humans or to a particular food; (3) the adverse health effect increases in incidence or geographical coverage; (4) or have been around and widespread for a long time but recently have been identified through new or increased knowledge, or methods of identification and analysis of the human disease agents. Emerging contaminants in this chapter refer to a selected set of issues for which health risk is progressively increasing due to the enhancing human exposure that may result from practices applied in the food chain and changes in environmental conditions. Highlights brought in this chapter refer to increasing risks to food safety and public health from the presence in the environment of microplastics, endocrine-disrupting compounds, antimicrobial resistance (AMR) genes, and climate-induced emerging contaminants including foodborne pathogens, harmful algal bloom, heavy metals, and mycotoxins (known hazards yet regaining prominence in climate-changing context). The chapter features as well emerging contaminants related to fraudulent food practices and a section devoted to traditional and emerging trends in chemical risk assessment. Research gaps and future directions are outlined for considered themes. A brief outline of the chapters related to emerging contaminants is presented below.

Chapter 18 presents an emerging contaminant and hazard for human health and animal health related to the increasing presence of microplastics in the environment. Contaminating features of microplastics are presented from a triple perspective, as a physical hazard, chemical hazard, and vehicle for microbiological hazards.

Chapter 19 provides a comprehensive toxicological and regulatory overview of endocrine-disrupting compounds, a broad group of substances of emerging concern under research since the 1990s, highlighting their diversity, dietary sources and exposure, and approaches to regulation looking into different risk assessment paradigms used by competent authorities. The issue of endocrine disruptors is also closely linked to other emerging risks described in this chapter as microplastics (through the migration of endocrine active substances/endocrine-disrupting compounds from plastics to foods), climate change (through the need for use of new plant protection products due to migration of pests to new territories), AMR (through endocrine activity of antimicrobial growth promoters), and food fraud (due to the use of some endocrine active substances/endocrine-disrupting compounds in raw materials of components otherwise banned for use on food).

Chapter 20 highlights the emerging contaminant represented by the spread of antimicrobial residues and related AMR through the food chain, which is qualified as an emerging public health crisis, a pandemic with high risk for humanity that is projected to cause some 10 million death per year by 2050. Key actions to counteract the spread of AMR include raising awareness, data, and evidence collection through monitoring and surveillance, good practices in use of alternative practices and reduced use of antimicrobials, and intersectoral collaboration and governance. Control of AMR in foods calls for a coordinated, multidisciplinary, One Health approach, including the increased adoption of practices to keep animals and plants healthy that will reduce and eliminate the need of antimicrobials use.

Chapter 21 unfolds the scientific evidence on the impacts of climate change on food safety, highlighting the most up-to-date information on the effects of climate change on various food safety hazards, with quantification of these impacts provided where possible. The paper touches upon fostering preparedness for future challenges in keeping safe food supply and reducing health impact on future generations through foresight-based approaches.

Chapter 22 reviews the most current information related to the effect of climate change on mycotoxins. These are naturally occurring contaminants, which affect staple crops and foods at various concentrations, from very low to high. With some of them having proven carcinogenic effects. Considering the ubiquitous and unavoidable nature of human exposure to mycotoxins, the section intends to support policy-makers, decision-makers, and researchers in this area on managing the emerging risks from mycotoxins in climate change context.

Chapter 23 draws attention to food fraud as a potent entry point for contaminants in the food supply. While the motivation for food adulteration is financial gain, the limited knowledge of food composition, inappropriate handling, and lack of control may lead to food safety incidents posing a significant public health risk.

Chapter 24 provides an overview of the main concepts, conventional and emerging approaches in chemical risk assessment that allow to face the challenges related to the potential coincidental co-exposure to foodborne and nondietary chemicals and cope with data scarcity paving practical ways for addressing the emerging contaminants in the context of food safety regulation.

Chapters 18–24 address separate themes and are presented as standalone chapters in this book.

Disclaimer

The views expressed in this chapter are those of the authors and do not necessarily reflect the views or policies of their organizations.

Chapter 18

Emerging contaminants related to plastic and microplastic pollution

Ndaindila N.K. Haindongo, Christopher J. Breen and Lev Neretin
Food and Agriculture Organization of the United Nations (FAO), Office of Climate Change, Biodiversity, and the Environment (OCB), Rome, Italy

Abstract
The presence of plastic particles in food systems, which are a critical pathway for human exposure to these particles, represents a potentially dangerous, yet unclear threat to both food safety and food security. This section provides an overview of the food safety hazards related to microplastic pollution in food and agricultural systems. This includes the potential for human exposure to micro/nanoplastics pollution via food systems, the potential adverse chemical, physical, and other effects that this exposure may induce, as well as the current research gaps that constrain knowledge in this field. Future research directions are subsequently proffered. Addressing these knowledge gaps is critical, given the current magnitude of plastic pollution, as well as its projected increase, and will be crucial for ensuring global food safety and security in the long term and meeting societal goals such as the SDGs.

Keywords: Plastics pollution; microplastics; nanoplastics; emerging contaminants; plastics in agrifood systems; agricultural plastics; food safety; human health; plastic additives

18.1 Introduction

Today, the widespread utilization of plastics is driven by their valuable inherent characteristics. Plastics are typically durable, affordable, corrosion-resistant, strong, and lightweight. Consequently, they have become omnipresent in many facets of our everyday lives with a global production increasing each year by about 9% since 1950.[1] Plastics are utilized in many sectors, including as constituents in medical devices, clothing, technology, and a host of other applications[2,3].

Plastics are also ubiquitous throughout much of modern agriculture and food systems. Since the 1950s, packaging has accounted for approximately 40% of all plastics produced, and around 41% of these are used specifically for food or beverages.[4] While this figure mainly concerns the later stages of food value chains, in which feed, timber, fiber, and other products are processed, packaged, and delivered to the final consumers, plastics are also used during production, aggregation, and distribution. For example, plastics are used in agricultural mulch films, solarization and silage films, plastic tunnels and greenhouses, nets, shading, plastic reservoir and irrigation systems, and packaging containers.[5] These materials provide a variety of benefits, including increased yields, earlier harvests, frost protection, and water conservation, increased land-use efficiency, and the potential to reduce the use of pesticides and fertilizers.[5,6]

Plastic packaging also allows for the containment and preservation of food products, offering protection from external environmental perturbations such as moisture, gases, odors, dust, microorganism contamination, and physical shocks.[7] It can therefore be argued that plastics play a key role in food security by reducing food loss and waste and ensuring food safety.

Plastic consumption in agriculture is estimated at over 6.5 million tonnes annually worldwide, accounting for approximately 2% to 3% of the global production of plastic resins.[8,9] However, these figures are uncertain as they are based on a limited number of studies in selected regions.

The same characteristics that grant plastics their versatility and functionality also contribute to their persistence in the environment. Only 9% of plastics that have ever been produced have been recycled, while the remainder is either incinerated (12%) or accumulated in landfills and the natural environment (79%).[10] In a business-as-usual scenario, 12,000 billion tons of plastic are expected to accumulate in landfills (where mismanaged plastics can leak into the surrounding environment) or the natural environment by mid-century.[10] Without action, the annual flow of plastics into the ocean will nearly triple by 2040,

Present Knowledge in Food Safety. DOI: https://doi.org/10.1016/B978-0-12-819470-6.00050-0

to between 23 to 37 million tons, equivalent to 50 kg of plastic per meter of coastline worldwide.[11]

The management of increasing amounts of plastics represents a monumental and systemic economic, environmental, and social challenge: plastics pollution is proving to be an insidious and pervasive global concern. Plastics and microplastics have been found in every environmental compartment, including the deepest parts of the ocean,[12] freshwater systems,[13] polar regions of Arctic and the Antarctic,[14,15] soils (including agricultural soils),[16] the atmosphere,[17] isolated mountain areas,[18] food,[19,20] drinking water,[21] biota,[22] and even in the human placenta.[23]

18.2 Food safety risks of microplastic pollution

This section provides a brief overview of the chemical, biological, and physical pathways and impacts of microplastics on food safety. This includes indications of how microplastics are introduced into edible food through direct and indirect vectors and why this may represent potential threats to human health.

Plastics are complex chemical mixtures that, once released, can become complex stressors to human and ecosystem health. Many contain persistent, bioaccumulative, toxic, and endocrine-disrupting chemicals. Plastics can also provide an adsorption surface for ambient contaminants, allowing them to concentrate and thereby increasing their potential toxicity.

During the production process, multiple chemical constituents are added to give plastics their properties such as long shelf life, color, durability, transparency, etc. The exact chemicals used depend on the type of plastic product being produced. Typical additives include chemical compounds such as stabilizers, flame retardants, plasticizers, antioxidants, colorants, lubricants, and dyes. Many of these substances or their components (e.g., heavy metals) are classified as hazardous according to EU regulations, such as REACH (EC 1907/2006). For instance, plastic additives and constituents such as bisphenol A (BPA), heavy metals, phthalates, and some brominated flame retardants, are documented as endocrine disruptors, with the potential to damage human and/or animal health.[24–26] Attesting to this potential danger, in May 2020, the Swiss Government submitted a proposal to the Stockholm Convention on Persistent Organic Pollutants (POPs) to list the ultra-violet (UV) stabilizer, plastic additive UV-328, under the Stockholm Convention. To highlight, this is the first time that a plastics-related chemical would be considered a POP.

The ability of plastic particles to augment the potential toxicity of other contaminants in the environment is dependent on their size and shape. Larger plastic items can undergo transformation into smaller microplastic particles (0.1–5 mm), and potentially even nanoplastics (1–100 nm). These microplastics can be described as either primary or secondary, according to their source. Primary microplastics include engineered plastic microbeads, pellets, and powders used in cosmetic formulations, cleaning products, and industrial abrasives as well as microplastics resulting from vehicle tire abrasion, while secondary microplastics originate from the degradation of larger plastic items into smaller fragments.[27]

In marine environments, primary microplastics reach the ocean via road runoff, wastewater treatment systems, and wind transfer.[28–31] According to Boucher and Friot,[28] almost 1.5 million tonnes of primary microplastics are leaking into the world's oceans annually, 98% of which are from land-based sources.

Sources of secondary microplastics are often associated with maritime activities including shipping, fishing and aquaculture, recreation, and offshore activities. However, most sources are also terrestrial in origin, for example, discarded plastic bags.[32] In 2010 alone, the plastic flux to the oceans was estimated at 4.8 to 12.7 million tonnes from land-based sources. This flux is predicted to increase by an order of magnitude over the next decade.[33] However, the number of plastics measured in seawater is thought to be a mere fraction (less than 1%) of the total quantity that has been released into the oceans, estimated as at least 150 million tonnes.[31] While the relative importance of primary versus secondary sources of microplastics has yet to be determined,[28] most microplastics in the marine environment are thought to be secondary in nature.[31]

Irregular-shaped microplastics provide a greater surface area for the adsorption and concentration of hydrophobic, persistent, and bioaccumulating toxins such as dichlorodiphenyltrichloroethane (DDT), polychlorinated biphenyls (PCBs), antibiotics, and heavy metals.[24,31] Microplastic particles in the marine environment, could also potentially harbor pathogens that pose a threat to human health.[34] The level of concentration of these toxins determines the potential for deleterious effects following ingestion or inhalation by humans or animals, especially if surface electrical charges develop, which can magnify particle-cell interactions.[35] The damage to organisms that ingest microplastics at different trophic levels can cause physical damage to the gastrointestinal tract, adverse chemical reactions induced by plastic additives, or toxicity associated with chemical contaminants.[36]

While much of the attention concerning microplastic pollution has focused on marine environments, most of the microplastics that arrive in marine environments originate from terrestrial sources, with significant heterogeneity in abundance between regions. Therefore it has been estimated that microplastic pollution in terrestrial environments can be 4 to 23 times greater than in the ocean, with agricultural soils alone storing potentially more microplastics than ocean basins.[37] While plastic products used on agricultural soils are associated with yield increases, the constant accumulation of plastics in these soils has adverse impacts on soil physicochemical properties and plants, which could subsequently threaten food production systems in the long term.[38]

Microplastics can be introduced to soils via mismanagement of plastic products used in agricultural processes, or through other sources, such as atmospheric aerosols, effluents from urban and industrial centers, improper waste management and landfill leakage, and sewages and sludges.[37] Studies have demonstrated that microplastic accumulation in soils may induce negative changes in plant biomass, root characteristics, tissue elemental composition, and soil microbial activities, which could potentially have a deleterious impact on agro-ecosystems in general and terrestrial biodiversity.[39]

While there are concerns that plastics may transfer to humans via bioaccumulation in food webs, this pathway has not yet been demonstrated conclusively in research studies. Many authors have, however, noted at least the potential of this pathway to impact negatively on food webs and food safety.[40–43] Among the numerous modes of introduction of plastics into the human body is, for example, direct ingestion of microplastics via drinking water. Microplastics were detected in 92% of drinking water samples taken in the United States and 72% of those sampled in Europe.[31] However, the severity of this risk to human health is difficult to ascertain. Microplastics may also be introduced into the human body via inhalation, absorption via the skin, ingestion, and/or via their atmospheric deposition onto food products. Small plastic particles have been found in both food products and human lung tissues.[19]

Given the magnitude of plastic pollution, its projected increase, and the increasing evidence of toxic contaminants associated with microplastic polymers, scientific evidence of their risks to human health and wellbeing is also increasing.

18.3 Effects of microplastic ingestion on humans and living organisms

The potential impacts of the ingestion of microparticles by humans and other living organisms have been studied for decades. These effects include physical blockage and perforation of the gastrointestinal tract, altered growth, and tissue damage.[46] Research into the impacts of plastics is largely concentrated in Australia, Europe, and North America, leaving substantial data gaps in Africa, Oceania, and Asia.

Microplastic absorption has been detected in many fish species, even those used for human consumption from the Atlantic, Indian, and Pacific Oceans.[27] For instance, in 2016 the Food and Agriculture Organization of the United Nations (FAO) reported that microplastics have been detected in the gastrointestinal tracts of more than 50% of fish species that are important to world marine catches.[45] Considering that these particles are widely found in the gastrointestinal tract of fish, which is gutted before consumption, this therefore reduces direct human exposure. Nevertheless, small marine pelagic species such as anchovies and sardines are sometimes consumed whole.

The introduction and interaction of microplastics within the digestive process of aquatic animals may lead to complications such as intestinal blockage and reductions in animal feeding and energy assimilation.[46] Lee et al. (2013)[47] demonstrated that a high intake of microplastics might decrease food uptake which may result in reduced energy and fertility in marine copepods. On the contrary, the impacts of microplastic ingestion in marine fisheries have only been reported within laboratory settings, mostly at higher exposure levels than environmental concentrations.[45] Hence, there are limited evidence-based results on the implications associated with the uptake of microplastics by wild and farmed aquatic organisms.

Microplastics can be introduced into the human body through the consumption of fluids and food products (Appendix A). Other than marine seafood products, microplastics have also been detected in table salts,[48,49] sugar and honey,[50–52] beer,[53] wine,[54], and bottled water.[55] More recently, micro and nanoplastics were isolated from edible fruits and vegetables.[56]

According to UNEP, humans ingest about 52,000 microplastic particles per year.[57] Research has shown that the ingestion of approximately 4000 particles of microplastics by humans may lead to an inflammatory response, tissue abrasion, and reduced intestinal mucus secretion.[58,59] This may cause damage to the intestinal walls' function, increasing the permeability of the gut mucosa, triggering an imbalance of gut microbiota, and changes to nutrient uptake, such as lipogenesis triglyceride synthesis.[58] Following their absorption through the gastric mucosa, these particles may induce pro-inflammatory responses, alter gene expression, inhibit cell viability, and access the bloodstream.[60] For example, several microplastic fragments were detected in human placenta samples collected from pregnant patients.[23] It was suggested that microplastics may have entered the bloodstream and reached the placenta from the maternal respiratory system and the gastrointestinal tract.

18.4 Effects of persistent, bioaccumulative compounds associated with microplastics on humans and living organisms

The majority of the toxic substances listed by the United States Environmental Protection Agency and the

European Union have been associated with plastic debris.[61,62] A wide range of common plastic additives used during plastic manufacturing is recognized as very toxic to humans and animals when ingested. For instance, hexabromocyclododecane (HBCD), a flame retardant in some polystyrene consumer products, can be released during their production, use, and following disposal.[63] Other toxic chemicals such as phthalates, BPA, and BPS have been reported as carcinogens. They have been associated with reproductive and developmental disorders including breast cancer, neurodevelopmental disorders, metabolic disorders, blood infection, early onset of puberty, and genital defects in humans and other mammals.[64,65]

Many of these chemicals pose a serious threat to human health because they can cause a variety of impacts.[66] Phthalates are known endocrine disruptors and, as such, pregnant women are especially vulnerable to their exposure. Exposure to phthalates during pregnancy may affect thyroid function, which is essential to healthy brain development.[67] Studies from Harvard University revealed that these hormone-disrupting chemicals may increase the risk of a miscarriage.[68] Several human health studies have linked phthalate exposure to genital deformities in baby boys associated with an increased risk of reproductive health problems, and to learning and behavioral problems in older children.

According to Angelo and Meccariello (2021)[69] and Sharpe (2012),[70] exposure to chemical contamination from plastics may reduce the sperm count of young men. These findings were supported by investigations conducted on laboratory rats, revealing that some phthalates may be the reason for disorders in male offspring and fertility risks.[71] Although this is an emerging area of research and studies are still very limited, the endocrine disruptors associated with plastics have also been reported as an emerging threat to male fertility.[72,73]

Phthalates and flame retardants, usually used during plastic production, may also have toxicological impacts on terrestrial and aquatic organisms.[74] In addition, toxic, bioaccumulative, and persistent substances, including POPs and metals, present in the ambient seawater could be selectively magnified up to a million times in plastic fragments.[61,75] Because of their risks, POPs are subjected to restrictions and bans under the Stockholm Convention on POPs. Once ingested, these particles have the potential to accumulate in living organisms, including humans, and are found at higher concentrations at higher trophic levels. POPs have also been linked to cancer, reproductive issues, and other diseases in humans and wildlife.[66]

18.5 Effects of pathogenic microbes carried by microplastics on humans and living organisms

It has been documented that plastic debris can act as a substrate for diverse microbial communities[79,80,78]. Microorganisms, including plastic decomposing pathogens, have been shown to colonize microplastics. Furthermore, in the ocean, such communities are distinct from microbial communities in the surrounding surface water.[79] However, the relevance to food and the consequences to human health remain unknown.

An emerging risk is the potential of microplastics to act as vectors of pathogenic microorganisms. The attachment of harmful microbial communities to marine plastics debris was first described as the 'plastisphere' by Zettler, Mincer, and Amaral-Zettler (2013),[79] raising concerns about the spread of exotic invasive species and pathogens. It has then been widely documented that, in marine water, plastic surfaces develop a conditioning film, which subsequently leads to the formation of biofilms by various microbes, including plastic decomposing organisms and human pathogens.[79–79]

The increasing reports on the incidence of microorganisms on plastic surfaces in multiple marine regions have raised food safety threats to human health and wellbeing.[80] Some of these have been found to include potentially pathogenic organisms such as *Escherichia coli*, *Bacillus cereus*[81], and *Vibrio* spp.[86] *Vibrio* species are ubiquitous and abundant in aquatic environments.[87] They exist as part of the microflora of various marine animals, such as oysters, clams, and crabs. Among more than 70 different *Vibrio* species inhabiting marine ecosystems, at least 12 species including, *V. cholerae*, *V. parahaemolyticus*, and *V. vulnificus*, are pathogenic for humans and important to the public health.[88] These microorganisms have been reported to be agents of seafood-borne or wound infections, and they are capable of causing a potentially fatal disease known as "Vibriosis". The Center for Disease Control and Prevention estimates that Vibriosis causes 80,000 illnesses each year in the United States.[85]

Numerous researchers have reported on the alarming numbers of *Vibrios* in the plastisphere.[79,79] The ever-decreasing size of microplastics creates large surface areas where microbial "plastisphere" communities and biofilms may develop.[57] Experts have raised important questions concerning if the rising amount of plastic waste in global oceans presents opportunities for pathogenic microorganisms, including *Vibrios*, to be carried and transmitted to potential hosts. Appendix B summarizes the potential interactions of *Vibrios* with microplastics in marine ecosystems and how these might differ from interactions with natural particles, all of which might present risks to human consumers.[80]

Appendix B shows the role of different polymer surfaces (e.g., microplastics) in influencing microbial attachments, survival, and their interactions (1). The colonized pathogens are transported by ocean currents (2) and eventually ingested by marine organisms (3). Their uptake by marine organisms may increase the likelihood of disease transfers (4) from edible marine organisms to humans through direct ingestion. Microplastic surfaces have been suggested to create a niche ecosystem for the growth and spread of antimicrobial resistance (AMR). An investigation conducted by Yang et al. [86] found that microplastic surfaces contained significantly greater microbiota with ARGs and MRGs than ambient bacterial communities. In support, in-vitro studies demonstrated that these particles may play a significant role during their evolution and exchange of genes, including ARGs.[80] Considering that microplastics serve as vectors for microbes and create a favorable environment for biofilm formation, they could potentially spread AMR across aquatic and marine environments. Research has shown that bacterial communities present in biofilms are very effective at spreading and sharing ARGs.[87]

18.6 Research gaps and future directions

Understanding the impacts of microplastics on food safety at the individual level and food security at the societal level is an active area of research. While the presence of micro- and nanoplastics and synthetic polymers are increasingly documented in marine food chains, food products, and the air we breathe, more research is required to understand the effects of plastics and microplastics' exposure on human and environmental health. While there is ample attention given to the effects of microplastics on marine systems, the relative paucity of data on the effects of microplastics in terrestrial systems, including soils, needs to be addressed.

Food safety and food security are two inter-related and interdependent concepts. Food security denotes all individuals in a population having access to sufficient food to lead productive and healthy lives. However, this necessarily entails that the available food is safe, and of a suitable quality from a chemical, physical and biological standpoint. It is therefore imperative that the potential risks associated with plastics and microplastic pollution on agricultural soils and terrestrial food systems be considered, to gain a holistic overview of their impacts on entire food systems.

While there is strong evidence showing that microplastic particles act as accumulating agents for PBTs, it is still unknown whether they are more significant vectors of contamination and concentration up trophic levels compared to other pollutants. Field and laboratory exposure studies are typically limited to a small number of organisms and are therefore not able to explain the effects of microplastic exposure at a population level and the subsequent ramifications for the entire food web. Furthermore, they are unable to determine the exact mechanisms at work due to the abundant factors determining adsorption processes, such as hydrophobic and electrostatic forces, as well as physical environmental conditions, which make the environmental fate of particles highly varied and unpredictable.[88] There is also a need for research to focus on understanding the compounding effects of multiple stressors in food webs. For example, Barboza et al. (2018)[89] found that fish exposed to both mercury and microplastics suffered increased bioaccumulation of the mercury. Moreover, the adsorption of multiple deleterious contaminants, including heavy metals, antibiotics, and organic pollutants on microplastics has also been shown.[90]

Future studies should also focus on investigating the assimilation of a broader range of microplastic sizes and compositions, necessitating the development of techniques capable of identifying a range of microplastic sizes and compositions. The development of these methods will be able to exploit the increasing knowledge of the fate, bioavailability, and biological impacts of plastic contaminants.[88] Given the potential for the heightened toxicity of nanoplastics due to their higher surface area, these size fractions also require more studies. There is currently little available information on nanoplastics, even though they display a heightened potential to cross biological barriers, including the blood-brain barrier.[91]

There is a need to define the health and toxicological criteria and testing needed to establish the exposure of humans and wildlife to microplastics in aquatic environments. Thus, future studies should focus on the establishment of a common methodological approach, as currently there is a wide array of alternative reference units, sampling, and analytical and evaluation methods.[92] Moreover, the experimental design of many current studies assumes a constant plastic exposure throughout the experiment and utilizes homogenous, spherical-shaped, commercial plastics. Microplastics occurring in the environment are highly heterogenous in occurrence, size, and shape, meaning that experimental design should not consider plastic materials as homogenous when determining bioavailability.[88]

Global plastic and microplastic pollution are also influenced by global climate change, including the effects that temperature and precipitation changes might have on the distribution of microplastics in various environments. For example, as climate change induces the melting of glaciers and alters ocean currents, it could potentially magnify the delivery of microplastics to environmental compartments where they might enter food webs.[93]

In summary, microplastics in food and agricultural systems pose serious threats to human health. Given the potential adverse effects of plastic and microplastic pollution on human health and the effects of the associated harmful chemicals found in food products, it is of paramount importance to broaden the study of microplastic pollution in various food types. This includes the fate of micro- and nanoplastics and their harm to the gastrointestinal tract of humans and living organisms.[94] As plastic pollution continues to increase, it is important to assess dietary exposure, particularly for the nanoplastic size fraction.[95,96] Only by closing these research gaps can we truly determine the magnitude and scope of the impacts of plastics and microplastic pollution in the food system, and subsequently work to mitigate and reduce any potential adverse impacts. Finding solutions to the impacts of microplastics on food safety requires greater engagement by research institutions and academia, civil society, policymakers, and industry players to bring about necessary changes in policies, attitudes, and practices. Policies will play an important role in supporting research and development initiatives to address the emerging food safety risks and concerns associated with microplastics in food systems.

Appendix A

Potential risks of microplastics for human health via the food chain and dietary exposure Source[97]:

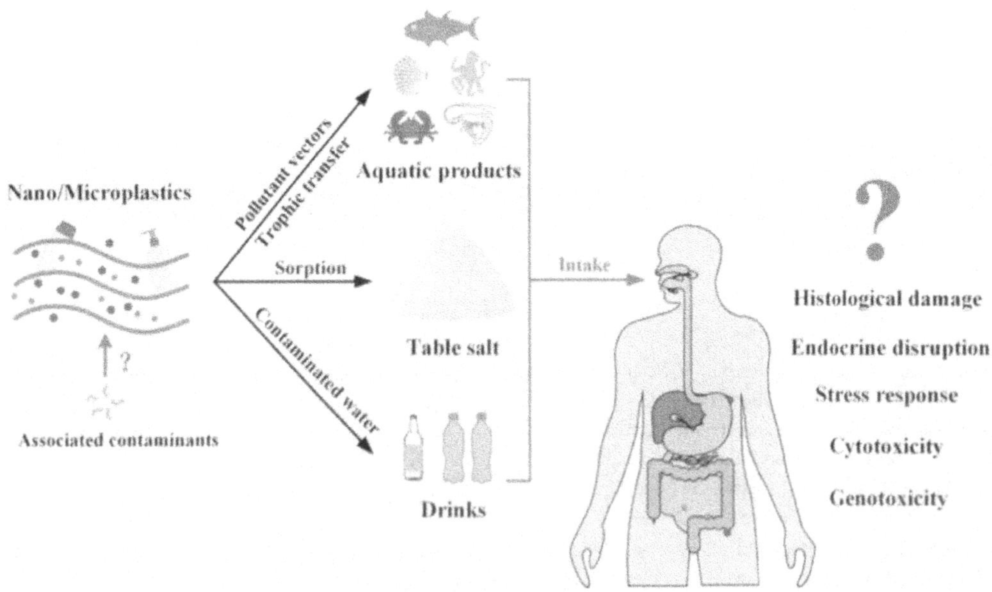

Appendix B

Summary of the potential interactions of *Vibrios* with microplastics in marine ecosystems and how these might differ from interactions with natural particles Source[80]:

Disclaimer

The views expressed in this publication are those of the author(s) and do not necessarily reflect the views or policies of the Food and Agriculture Organization of the United Nations.

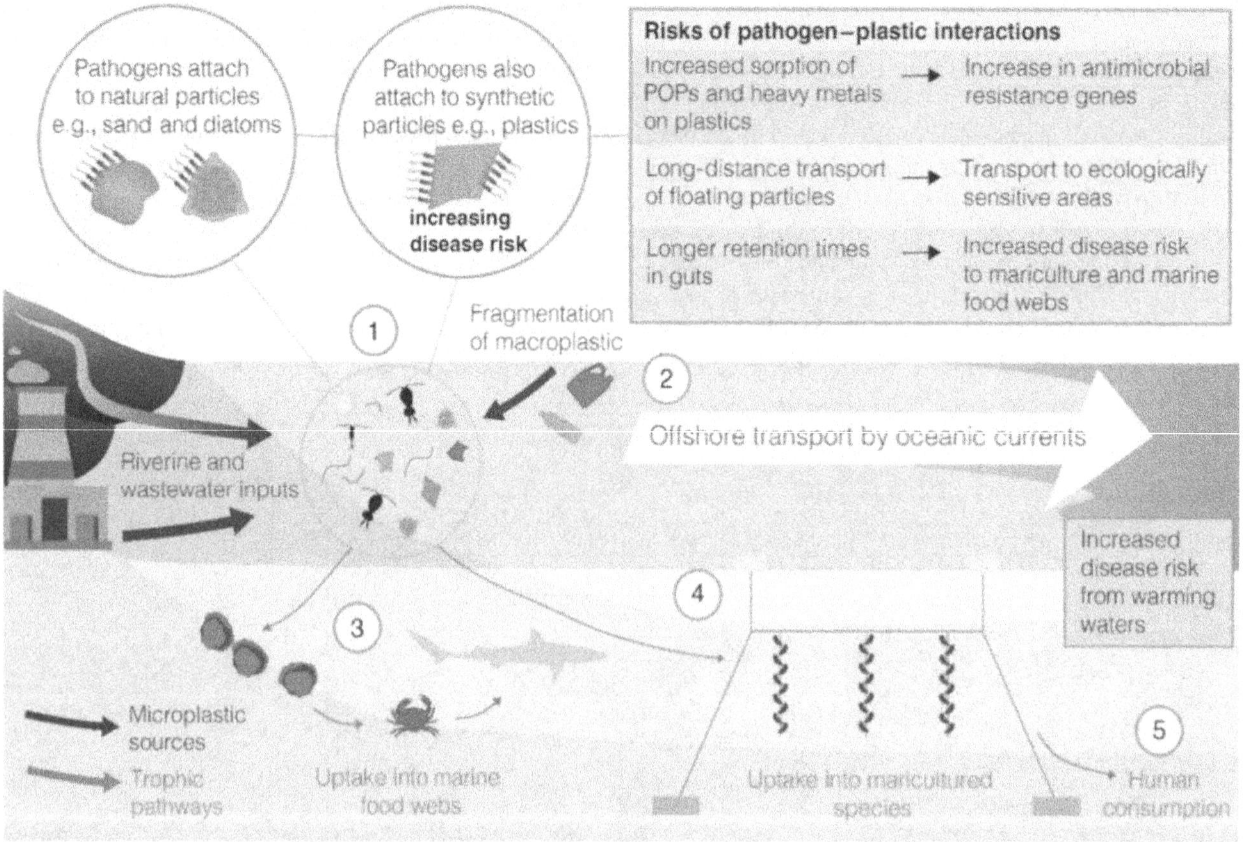

References

1. UN Environment. *Mapping of Global Plastics Value Chain and Plastics Losses to the Environment (with a Particular Focus on Marine Environment).* Ryberg, M., Laurent, A., Hauschild, M. United Nations Environment Programme. Nairobi, Kenya, 2018.
2. Andrady A, Neal M. Applications and societal benefits of plastics. *Philos Trans R Soc B Biol Sci.* 2009;364(1526):1977–1984.
3. Proshad R, Kormoker T, Islam M, Haque M, Rahman M, Mithu M. Toxic effects of plastic on human health and environment : A consequences of health risk assessment in Bangladesh. *International Journal Of Health.* 2017;10.14419/ijh.v6i1.8655.
4. Schweitzer, J., Gionfra, S., Pantzar, M., et al., Unwrapped how throw-away plastic is failing to solve europe's food waste problem (and what we need to do instead). A study by Zero Waste Europe and Friends of the Earth Europe for the Rethink Plastic Alliance. [online] Brussels: Institute for European Environmental Policy (IEEP). 2018. Available at: <http://zerowasteeurope.eu/wp-content/uploads/2018/04/Unwrapped_How-throwaway-plastic-is-failing-to-solve-Europes-food-waste-problem_and-what-we-need-to-do-instead_FoEE-ZWE-April-2018_final.pdf> Accessed 08.02.21.
5. De Lucia C, Pazienza P. Market-based tools for a plastic waste reduction policy in agriculture: a case study in the south of Italy. *J Environ Manage.* 2019;250:109468.
6. Scarascia-Mugnozza G, Sica C, Russo G. Plastic materials in European agriculture: actual use and perspectives. *J Agric Eng.* 2011;42(3):15.
7. Matthews C, Moran F, Jaiswal A. A review on European Union's strategy for plastics in a circular economy and its impact on food safety. *J Clean Prod.* 2021;283:125263.
8. Vox G, Loisi R, Blanco I, Mugnozza G, Schettini E. Mapping of agriculture plastic waste. *Agric Agric Sci Proc.* 2016;8:583–591.
9. Jansen, L., Henskens, M. and Hiemstra, F., Report on Use of Plastics in Agriculture. [online] Wageningen: Schuttelaar & Partners B.V. 2019. Available at: <https://saiplatform.org/wp-content/uploads/2019/06/190528-report_use-of-plastics-in-agriculture.pdf> Accessed 18.01.21.
10. Geyer R, Jambeck J, Law K. Production, use, and fate of all plastics ever made. *Sci Adv.* 2017;3(7):e1700782.
11. The Pew Charitable Trusts and SYSTEMIQ, Breaking the Plastic Wave: A Comprehensive Assessment of Pathways Towards Stopping Ocean Plastic Pollution. 2020 <https://www.pewtrusts.org/-/media/assets/2020/07/breakingtheplasticwave_report.pdf>.
12. Beaumont N, Aanesen M, Austen M, et al. Global ecological, social and economic impacts of marine plastic. *Mar Pollut Bull.* 2019;142:189–195.
13. Bellasi A, Binda G, Pozzi A, Galafassi S, Volta P, Bettinetti R. Microplastic contamination in freshwater environments: a review, focusing on interactions with sediments and benthic organisms. *Environments.* 2020;7(4):30.
14. Bergami E, Rota E, Caruso T, Birarda G, Vaccari L, Corsi I. Plastics everywhere: first evidence of polystyrene fragments inside the common Antarctic collembolan *Cryptopygus antarcticus. Biol Lett.* 2020;16(6):20200093. Available from: https://doi.org/10.1098/rsbl.2020.0093.

15. Obbard R. Microplastics in polar regions: the role of long range transport. *Curr Opin Environ Sci Health*. 2018;1:24–29.
16. Guo J, Huang X, Xiang L, et al. Source, migration and toxicology of microplastics in soil. *Environment International*. 2020;137:105263.
17. Prata J. Airborne microplastics: consequences to human health? *Environ Pollut*. 2018;234:115–126.
18. Scheurer M, Bigalke M. Microplastics in swiss floodplain soils. *Environ Sci Technol*. 2018;52(6):3591–3598.
19. Toussaint B, Raffael B, Angers-Loustau A, et al. Review of micro- and nanoplastic contamination in the food chain. *Food Addit Contam Part A Chem Anal Control Expo Risk Assess*. 2019;36 (5):639–673.
20. Waring R, Harris R, Mitchell S. Plastic contamination of the food chain: a threat to human health? *Maturitas*. 2018;115:64–68.
21. Pivokonsky M, Cermakova L, Novotna K, Peer P, Cajthaml T, Janda V. Occurrence of microplastics in raw and treated drinking water. *Sci Total Environ*. 2018;643:1644–1651.
22. Anbumani S, Kakkar P. Ecotoxicological effects of microplastics on biota: a review. *Environ Sci Pollut Res*. 2018;25(15): 14373–14396.
23. Ragusa A, Svelato A, Santacroce C, et al. Plasticenta: first evidence of microplastics in human placenta. *Environ Int*. 2021;146: 106274.
24. Campanale C, Massarelli C, Savino I, Locaputo V, Uricchio V. A detailed review study on potential effects of microplastics and additives of concern on human health. *Int J Environ Res Public Health*. 2020;17(4):1212.
25. The Endocrine Society and IPEN, Plastics, EDCs and Health: A Guide for public interest organizations and policy-makers on endocrine disrupting chemicals and plastics. 2020. Available at: <https://www.endocrine.org/-/media/endocrine/files/topics/edc_guide_2020_v1_6chqennew-version.pdf>.
26. Hahladakis JN, Velis CA, Weber R, Iacovidou E, Purnell P. An overview of chemical additives present in plastics: migration, release, fate and environmental impact during their use, disposal and recycling. *J Hazard Mater*. 2018;15(344):179–199. Available from: https://doi.org/10.1016/j.jhazmat.2017.10.014.
27. GESAMP, Sources, fate and effects of microplastics in the marine environment: part two of a global assessment (Kershaw, P.J., and Rochman, C.M., eds). (IMO/FAO/UNESCO-IOC/UNIDO/WMO/IAEA/UN/UNEP/UNDP Joint Group of Experts on the Scientific Aspects of Marine Environmental Protection). Rep. Stud. GESAMP No. 93, 220, 2016.
28. Boucher J, Friot D. *Primary Microplastics in the Oceans: a Global Evaluation of Sources*. Gland: IUCN; 2017.
29. Boyle K, Örmeci B. Microplastics and nanoplastics in the freshwater and terrestrial environment: a review. *Water*. 2020;12(9):2633.
30. Auta H, Emenike C, Fauziah S. Distribution and importance of microplastics in the marine environment: a review of the sources, fate, effects, and potential solutions. *Environ Int*. 2017;102: 165–176.
31. Rhodes C. Plastic pollution and potential solutions. *Sci Prog*. 2018;101(3):207–260.
32. Browne M. Sources and pathways of microplastics to habitats. In: Bergmann M, Gutow L, Klages M, eds. *Marine Anthropogenic Litter*. Cham: Springer; 2015:229–244.
33. Jambeck J, Geyer R, Wilcox C, et al. Plastic waste inputs from land into the ocean. *Science*. 2015;347(6223):768–771.
34. Keswani ADM, Gutierrez T, Quilliam RS. Microbial hitchhikers on marine plastic debris: human exposure risks at bathing waters and beach environments. *Mar Environ Res*. 2016;118:10–19, ISSN 0141-1136. Available from: https://doi.org/10.1016/j.marenvres.2016.04.006.
35. Galloway T. Micro- and nano-plastics and human health. In: Bergmann M, Gutow L, Klages M, eds. *Marine Anthropogenic Litter*. Cham: Springer; 2015:343–366.
36. Yang L, Zhang Y, Kang S, Wang Z, Wu C. Microplastics in freshwater sediment: a review on methods, occurrence, and sources. *Sci Total Environ*. 2021;754:141948.
37. de Souza Machado A, Kloas W, Zarfl C, Hempel S, Rillig M. Microplastics as an emerging threat to terrestrial ecosystems. *Global Change Biol*. 2018;24(4):1405–1416.
38. Zhang D, Ng E, Hu W, et al. Plastic pollution in croplands threatens long-term food security. *Global Change Biol*. 2020;26 (6):3356–3367.
39. de Souza Machado A, Lau C, Kloas W, et al. Microplastics can change soil properties and affect plant performance. *Environ Sci Technol*. 2019;53(10):6044–6052.
40. Carbery M, O'Connor W, Palanisami T. Trophic transfer of microplastics and mixed contaminants in the marine food web and implications for human health. *Environ Int*. 2018;115:400–409.
41. Diepens N, Koelmans A. Accumulation of plastic debris and associated contaminants in aquatic food webs. *Environ Sci Technol*. 2018;52(15):8510–8520.
42. Huerta Lwanga E, Mendoza Vega J, Ku Quej V, et al. Field evidence for transfer of plastic debris along a terrestrial food chain. *Sci Rep*. 2017;7(1).
43. Miller M, Hamann M, Kroon F. Bioaccumulation and biomagnification of microplastics in marine organisms: a review and meta-analysis of current data. *PLoS One*. 2020;15(10):e0240792.
44. Puskic PS, Lavers JL, Bond AL. A critical review of harm associated with plastic ingestion on vertebrates. *Sci Total Environ*. 2020;743. Available from: https://doi.org/10.1016/j.scitotenv.2020.140666.
45. FAO. *The State of World Fisheries and Aquaculture Meeting the Sustainable Development Goals*. Rome: Food and Agriculture Organization of the United Nations; 2018. Available from: https://doi.org/10.1364/OE.17.003331.
46. Besseling E, Wegner A, Foekema EM, Van Den Heuvel-Greve MJ, Koelmans AA. Effects of microplastic on fitness and PCB bioaccumulation by the lugworm *Arenicola marina* (L.). *Environ Sci Technol*. 2013;47(1):593–600. Available from: https://doi.org/10.1021/es302763x.
47. Lee KW, Shim WJ, Kwon OY, Kang JH. Size-dependent effects of micro polystyrene particles in the marine copepod tigriopus japonicus. *Environ Sci Technol*. 2013;47(19):11278–11283. Available from: https://doi.org/10.1021/es401932b.
48. Fadare OO, Okoffo ED, Olasehinde EF. Microparticles and microplastics contamination in African table salts. *Mar Pollut Bull*. 2021;164:112006. Available from: https://doi.org/10.1016/j.marpolbul.2021.112006.
49. Peixoto D, Pinheiro C, Amorim J, Oliva-Teles L, Guilhermino L, Vieira MN. Microplastic pollution in commercial salt for human consumption: a review. *Estuar Coast Shelf Sci*. 2019;219:161–168. Available from: https://doi.org/10.1016/j.ecss.2019.02.018.
50. Liebezeit G, Liebezeit E. Non-pollen particulates in honey and sugar. *Food Addit Contam Part A Chem Anal Control Expo Risk*

Assess. 2013;30(12):2136–2140. Available from: https://doi.org/10.1080/19440049.2013.843025.

51. Liebezeit G, Liebezeit E. Origin of synthetic particles in honeys. *Polish J Food Nutr Sci.* 2015;65(2):143–147. Available from: https://doi.org/10.1515/pjfns-2015-0025.
52. Mühlschlegel P, Hauk A, Walter U, Sieber R. Lack of evidence for microplastic contamination in honey. *Food Addit Contam Part A Chem Anal Control Expo Risk Assess.* 2017;34(11):1982–1989. Available from: https://doi.org/10.1080/19440049.2017.1347281.
53. Kosuth M, Mason SA, Wattenberg EV. Anthropogenic contamination of tap water, beer, and sea salt. *PLoS One.* 2018;13(4): e0194970. Available from: https://doi.org/10.1371/journal.pone.0194970.
54. Prata JC, Paço A, Reis V, et al. Identification of microplastics in white wines capped with polyethylene stoppers using micro-Raman spectroscopy. *Food Chem.* 2020;331:127323. Available from: https://doi.org/10.1016/j.foodchem.2020.127323.
55. Schymanski D, Goldbeck C, Humpf HU, Fürst P. Analysis of microplastics in water by micro-Raman spectroscopy: release of plastic particles from different packaging into mineral water. *Water Res.* 2018;129:154–162. Available from: https://doi.org/10.1016/j.watres.2017.11.011.
56. Oliveri Conti G, Ferrante M, Banni M, et al. Micro- and nano-plastics in edible fruit and vegetables. The first diet risks assessment for the general population. *Environ Res.* 2020;187:109677. Available from: https://doi.org/10.1016/j.envres.2020.109677.
57. UNEP. *From Pollution to Solution – A Global Assessment of Marine Litter and Plastic Pollution.* Nairobi: United Nations Environment Programme (UNEP); 2021.
58. Lu L, Wan Z, Luo T, Fu Z, Jin Y. Polystyrene microplastics induce gut microbiota dysbiosis and hepatic lipid metabolism disorder in mice. *Science of the Total Environment.* 2018;631–632:449–458. Available from: https://doi.org/10.1016/j.scitotenv.2018.03.051.
59. Revel M, Châtel A, Mouneyrac C. Micro(nano)plastics: a threat to human health? *Curr Opin Environ Sci Health.* 2018;1:17–23. Available from: https://doi.org/10.1016/j.coesh.2017.10.003.
60. Forte M, Iachettaa G, Tussellino M, et al. Polystyrene nanoparticles internalization in human gastric adenocarcinoma cells. *Toxicol In Vitro.* 2016;31:126–136. Available from: https://doi.org/10.1016/j.tiv.2015.11.006.
61. Rochman C. Classify plastic waste as hazardous. *Nature.* 2013;169–171. Available from: https://doi.org/10.1021/es303700s.
62. Secretariat of the Convention on Biological Diversity. *Marine Debris: Understanding, Preventing and Mitigating the Significant Adverse Impacts on Marine and Coastal Biodiversity.* 2016, Available from <https://www.cbd.int/doc/publications/cbd-ts-83-en.pdf>.
63. Rani M, Shim WJ, Han GM, Jang M, Song YK, Hong SH. Hexabromocyclododecane in polystyrene based consumer products: an evidence of unregulated use. *Chemosphere.* 2013;110:111–119. Available from: https://doi.org/10.1016/j.chemosphere.2014.02.022.
64. Wright SL, Thompson RC, Galloway TS. The physical impacts of microplastics on marine organisms: a review. *Environ Pollut.* 2013;178:483–492. Available from: https://doi.org/10.1016/j.envpol.2013.02.031.
65. Mishra S, Rath CC, Das AP. *Marine Microfiber Pollution: A Review on Present Status and Future Challenges.* Elsevier Ltd; 2019.
66. Azoulay, D., Villa, P., Arellano, Y., Miller, K., Thompson, K. *Plastic and Health: The Hidden Costs of Plastic Planet.* 2019. (also available at www.ciel.org/plasticandhealth).
67. Rodríguez-Carmona Y, Cantoral A, Trejo-Valdivia B, et al. Phthalate exposure during pregnancy and long-term weight gain in women. *Environ Res.* 2019;169:26–32. Available from: https://doi.org/10.1016/j.envres.2018.10.014.
68. Feldscher, K. Exposure to phthalates may raise risk of pregnancy loss, gestational diabetes. In: *University of Harvard* [online]. [Cited 11 March 2021]. 2016. <https://www.hsph.harvard.edu/news/features/phthalates-exposure-pregnancy-loss-gestational-diabetes/>.
69. Angelo SD, Meccariello R. Microplastics: a threat for male fertility. *J Environ Res PublicHealth.* 2021;. Available from: https://doi.org/10.3390/ijerph18052392.
70. Sharpe RM. Sperm counts and fertility in men: a rocky road ahead. *EMBO Rep.* 2012;13:398–403. Available from: https://doi.org/10.1038/embor.2012.50.
71. Sharpe, R. M. Are plastics making men infertile? 2015. Available from <https://theconversation.com/are-plastics-making-men-infertile-43751>. Accessed 10.03.21.
72. Carr, T. Sperm counts are on the decline – could plastics be to blame? Reproduction, 2019.
73. Sumner, R. N., Tomlinson, M., Craigon, J., England, G. C. W., Lea, R. G. Independent and combined effects of diethylhexyl phthalate and polychlorinated biphenyl 153 on sperm quality in the human and dog.2019, https://doi.org/10.1038/s41598-019-39913-9
74. Secretariat of the Convention on Biological Diversity. Impacts of Marine Debris on Biodiversity: Current Status and Potential Solutions. Montreal, 2012.
75. Mato Y, Isobe T, Takada H, Kanehiro H, Ohtake C, Kaminuma T. Plastic resin pellets as a transport medium for toxic chemicals in the marine environment. *Environ Sci Technol.* 2001;35 (2):318–324.
76. Zettler ER, Mincer TJ, Amaral-Zettler LA. Life in the "plastisphere": microbial communities on plastic marine debris. *Environ Sci Technol.* 2013;47(13):7137–7146. Available from: https://doi.org/10.1021/es401288x.
77. Harrison JP, Schratzberger M, Sapp M, Osborn AM. Rapid bacterial colonization of low-density polyethylene microplastics in coastal sediment microcosms. *BMC Microbiol.* 2014;14(1):1–15. Available from: https://doi.org/10.1186/s12866-014-0232-4.
78. McCormick A, Hoellein, T, Mason S, Schluep J, Kelly J. Microplastic is an Abundant and Distinct Microbial Habitat in an Urban River. *Environmental Science and Technology.* 2014;48 (20):11863–11871. doi:10.1021/es503610r.
79. Oberbeckmann S, Kreikemeyer B, Labrenz M. Environmental factors support the formation of specific bacterial assemblages on microplastics. *Front Microbiol.* 2018;8:2709.
80. Bowley J, Baker-Austin C, Porter A, Hartnell R, Lewis C. Oceanic hitchhikers – assessing pathogen risks from marine microplastic. *Trend Microbiol.* 2021;29(2):107–116. Available from: https://doi.org/10.1016/j.tim.2020.06.011.
81. van der Meulen, M.D., Devriese, L., Lee, J., et al. Socio-economic Impact of Microplastics in the 2 Seas, Channel and France Manche Region: An Initial Risk Assessment. MICRO Interreg project Iva. 2014.
82. Kirstein IV, Kirmizi S, Wichels A, et al. Dangerous hitchhikers? Evidence for potentially pathogenic *Vibrio* spp. on microplastic particles. *Mar Environ Res.* 2016;120:1–8.
83. Kokashvili T, Whitehouse CA, Tskhvediani A, et al. Occurrence and diversity of clinically important *Vibrio* species in the aquatic environment of Georgia. *Front Public Health.* 2015;3. Available from: https://doi.org/10.3389/fpubh.2015.00232.

84. Johnson CN, Bowers JC, Griffitt KJ, et al. Ecology of *Vibrio* parahaemolyticus and *Vibrio* vulnificus in the coastal and estuarine waters of Louisiana, Maryland, Mississippi, and Washington (United States). *Appl Environ Microbiol.* 2012;78(20):7249–7257. Available from: https://doi.org/10.1128/AEM.01296-12.
85. CDC. (2019). *Vibrio Species Causing Vibriosis.* Centers for Disease Control and Prevention. https://www.cdc.gov/vibrio/index.html please confirm
86. Yang, Y., Liu, G., Song, W., et al. Plastics in the marine environment are reservoirs for antibiotic and metal resistance genes. 2019.
87. Rodney MD. Role of biofilms in antimicrobial resistance. *ASAIO J.* 2000;47–52.
88. Pinto da Costa J, Rocha-Santos T, Duarte A. *The Environmental Impacts of Plastics and Micro-Plastics Use, Waste and Pollution: EU and National Measures.* Brussels: European Parliament; 2020. PE 658.279.
89. Barboza L, Vieira L, Branco V, et al. Microplastics cause neurotoxicity, oxidative damage and energy-related changes and interact with the bioaccumulation of mercury in the European seabass, Dicentrarchus labrax (Linnaeus, 1758). *Aquat Toxicol.* 2018;195:49–57.
90. Li J, Yang D, Li L, Jabeen K, Shi H. Microplastics in commercial bivalves from China. *Environ Pollut.* 2015;207:190–195. Available from: https://doi.org/10.1016/j.envpol.2015.09.018.
91. Prüst M, Meijer J, Westerink R. The plastic brain: neurotoxicity of micro- and nanoplastics. *Part Fibre Toxicol.* 2020;17(1).
92. Rehse S, Kloas W, Zarfl C. Microplastics reduce short-term effects of environmental contaminants. part I: effects of bisphenol A on freshwater zooplankton are lower in presence of polyamide particles. *Int J Environ Res Public Health.* 2018;15(2):280.
93. FAO, *Climate Change: Unpacking the Burden on Food Safety.* Food safety and quality series No. 8. Rome: FAO, 2020. https://doi.org/10.4060/ca8185en.
94. EFSA. Presence of microplastics and nanoplastics in food, with particular focus on seafood. *EFSA J.* 2016;14(6). Available from: https://doi.org/10.2903/j.efsa.2016.4501.
95. Gallo F, Fossi C, Weber R, et al. Marine litter plastics and microplastics and their toxic chemicals components: the need for urgent preventive measures. *Environ Sci Europe.* 2018;30(1).
96. Barboza LGA, Dick Vethaak A, Lavorante BRBO, Lundebye AK, Guilhermino L. Marine microplastic debris: an emerging issue for food security, food safety and human health. *Mar Pollut Bull.* 2018;133:336–348. Available from: https://doi.org/10.1016/j.marpolbul.2018.05.047.
97. Huang W, Song B, Liang J, et al. Microplastics and associated contaminants in the aquatic environment: a review on their ecotoxicological effects, trophic transfer, and potential impacts to human health. *Journal of Hazardous Materials.* 2020;405:124187. Available from: https://doi.org/10.1016/j.jhazmat.2020.124187.

Further reading

Barboza LGA, Lopes C, Oliveira P, et al. Microplastics in wild fish from North East Atlantic Ocean and its potential for causing neurotoxic effects, lipid oxidative damage, and human health risks associated with ingestion exposure. *Sci Total Environ.* 2020;717:134625. Available from: https://doi.org/10.1016/j.scitotenv.2019.134625.

Collard F, Gasperi J, Gabrielsen GW, Tassin B. Plastic particle ingestion by wild freshwater fish: a critical review. *Environ Sci Technol.* 2019;. Available from: https://doi.org/10.1021/acs.est.9b03083.

Daniel DB, Ashraf PM, Thomas SN, Thomson KT. Microplastics in the edible tissues of shellfishes sold for human consumption. *Chemosphere.* 2021;264:128554. Available from: https://doi.org/10.1016/j.chemosphere.2020.128554.

de Sá LC, Oliveira M, Ribeiro F, Rocha TL, Futter MN. Studies of the effects of microplastics on aquatic organisms: What do we know and where should we focus our efforts in the future? *Sci Total Environ.* 2018;645:1029–1039. Available from: https://doi.org/10.1016/j.scitotenv.2018.07.207.

FAO. Microplastics in Fisheries and Aquaculture: Status of Knowledge on Their Occurrence and Implications for Aquatic Organisms and Food Safety. Rome. 2017.

He P, et al. Municipal solid waste (MSW)landfill: a source of microplastics? Evidence of microplastics in landfill leachate. *Water Res.* 2019;159:38–45. Available from: https://doi.org/10.1016/j.watres.2019.04.060. Elsevier Ltd.

Karami A, Golieskardi A, Choo CK, Larat V, Karbalaei S, Salamatinia B. Microplastic and mesoplastic contamination in canned sardines and sprats. *Sci Total Environ.* 2018;612:1380–1386. Available from: https://doi.org/10.1016/j.scitotenv.2017.09.005.

Mazhandu Z, Muzenda E, Mamvura T, Belaid M, Nhubu T. Integrated and consolidated review of plastic waste management and bio-based biodegradable plastics: challenges and opportunities. *Sustainability.* 2020;12(20):8360.

Neves D, Sobral P, Ferreira JL, Pereira T. Ingestion of microplastics by commercial fish off the Portuguese coast. *Mar Pollut Bull.* 2015;101(1):119–126. Available from: https://doi.org/10.1016/j.marpolbul.2015.11.008.

Rahman A, Sarkar A, Yadav OP, Achari G, Slobodnik J. Potential human health risks due to environmental exposure to nano- and microplastics and knowledge gaps: a scoping review. *Sci Total Environ.* 2021;757:143872. Available from: https://doi.org/10.1016/j.scitotenv.2020.143872.

Renzi M, Blašković A, Bernardi G, Russo GF. Plastic litter transfer from sediments towards marine trophic webs: a case study on holothurians. *Mar Pollut Bull.* 2018;135:376–385. Available from: https://doi.org/10.1016/j.marpolbul.2018.07.038.

Rillig MC. Microplastic in terrestrial ecosystems and the soil? *Environ Sci Technol.* 2012;46(12):6453–6454. Available from: https://doi.org/10.1021/es302011r. *American Chemical Society.*

Senathirajah K, Attwood S, Bhagwat G, Carbery M, Wilson S, Palanisami T. Estimation of the mass of microplastics ingested – a pivotal first step towards human health risk assessment. *J Hazardous Mater.* 2021;404(PB):124004. Available from: https://doi.org/10.1016/j.jhazmat.2020.124004.

Tang Y, Liu Y, Chen Y, et al. A review: research progress on microplastic pollutants in aquatic environments. *Sci Total Environ.* 2020;142572. Available from: https://doi.org/10.1016/j.scitotenv.2020.142572.

Teng J, Wang Q, Ran W, et al. Microplastic in cultured oysters from different coastal areas of China. *Sci Total Environ.* 2019;653:1282–1292. Available from: https://doi.org/10.1016/j.scitotenv.2018.11.057.

The Guardian. 2019. <https://www.theguardian.com/us-news/2019/may/24/toxic-america-sperm-counts-plastics-research>.

Thomas, H. S. 'Software Disease' – The Hazards of Plastic, Net Wrap and Twines Plastic: net wrap and twines may be the silent killers on your operation, 2016.

Trestrail C, Nugegoda D, Shimeta J. Invertebrate responses to microplastic ingestion: Reviewing the role of the antioxidant system. *Sci Total Environ*. 2020;734:138559. Available from: https://doi.org/10.1016/j.scitotenv.2020.138559.

UNEP. *Biodegradable Plastics and Marine Litter. Misconceptions, Concerns and Impacts on Marine Environments*. Nairobi: United Nations Environment Programme (UNEP); 2015.

Wang Z, Lin T, Chen W. Occurrence and removal of microplastics in an advanced drinking water treatment plant (ADWTP). *Sci Total Environ*. 2020;700:134520. Available from: https://doi.org/10.1016/j.scitotenv.2019.134520.

WHO. Persistent Organic Pollutants: Impact on Child Health. Geneva, 2010.

Zhang Y. Microplastics and associated contaminants in the aquatic environment: a review on their ecotoxicological effects, trophic transfer, and potential impacts to human health. *J Hazardous Mater*. 2020;405:124187. Available from: https://doi.org/10.1016/j.jhazmat.2020.124187.

Chapter 19

Endocrine disruptors

Serhii Kolesnyk[1,2] and Mykola Prodanchuk[1]

[1]*L.I. Medved's Research Center of Preventive Toxicology, Food and Chemical Safety, Ministry of Health, Kyiv, Ukraine,* [2]*University of Basel, Department of Pharmaceutical Sciences, Division of Molecular and Systems Toxicology, Basel, Switzerland*

Abstract

Endocrine disruptors (EDs) are ubiquitously present substances of emerging concern. Despite different definitions of ED, the WHO definition is widely accepted. Key elements of the WHO definition are endocrine mode of action (MoA), adverse effect in an intact organism, and a causal link between MoA and adversity. This paper provides an overview of ED mechanisms of action and their impact on human health, current approaches for toxicological testing of ED, advances in analytical methodologies, and the most common dietary sources and exposure to ED are presented. Approaches to regulation looking into different (risk or hazard-based) paradigms used by competent authorities, research gaps, and future directions of research in the field of ED are discussed.

Keywords: Endocrine disruptors; emerging contaminants; chemical risk assessment; toxic endpoints

19.1 Introduction

In recent times endocrine active substances (EASs) and endocrine-disrupting chemicals (EDCs), including ones that may be present in the food, received much attention from scientists, regulators as well as society. Despite many chemicals, claimed now to have endocrine-disrupting properties, being known for a long time, more data and knowledge acquired during the last few decades made them recognized as serious and urgent threats to public health by part of the scientific community.[1–4] Meanwhile, another part of the research criticize such a special and precautionary approach to EAS, including, but not limited to (1) selective approach in some reviews to data by giving preference to studies revealing harmful effect and not considering opposite evidence; (2) lack of causality, but just inference, between exposure to some chemicals and postulated adverse effects in some studies and reviews (3) lack of objective evidence of the need for a specific approach to EDC risk/hazard assessment compared to any other chemical agents.[5–9] Therefore here the reference is made not only to new chemicals having endocrine disrupting properties but also to some old ones as emerging public health and environmental risks in terms of understanding of their health effects and approaches to their assessment. Furthermore, in this chapter, we will discuss mainly public health aspects of EDC, and their impact on environment and wildlife is mainly out of the scope of this chapter.

As with any other scientific issue before understanding more complex things it is worth looking at the history of the issue and existing terminology and definitions.

One of the most important early collaborative scientific efforts related to endocrine disruption was Wingspread Conference entitled "Chemically-induced alterations in sexual development: the wildlife/human connection" held in 1991 in the United States. The first use of the term "endocrine disruptor (ED)" is attributed to the mentioned conference.[10,11] Held in the United States later, Environmental Protection Agency (EPA) sponsored workshop on EDs defined the environmental ED as "an exogenous agent that interferes with the production, release, transport, metabolism, binding, action or elimination of natural hormones in the body responsible for the maintenance of homeostasis and the regulation of developmental processes."[12]

One of the important results of the European Workshop on "The Impact of Endocrine Disrupters on Human Health and Wildlife" held in 1996 in Weybridge, United Kingdom was agreement on a definition of an ED: "An ED is an exogenous substance that causes adverse health effects in an intact organism, or its progeny, secondary to changes in endocrine function."[13]

In the highly cited, published in 2002 under International Programme on Chemical Safety, global assessment of the current then state-of-the-science related to environmental endocrine disruption the following definition of the EDCs was provided: "An ED is an exogenous substance or mixture

Present Knowledge in Food Safety. DOI: https://doi.org/10.1016/B978-0-12-819470-6.00051-2

TABLE 19.1 Definitions of the term endocrine disruptor.

Definition	Agency	Year
An exogenous agent that interferes with the production, release, transport, metabolism, binding, action, or elimination of natural hormones in the body responsible for the maintenance of homeostasis and the regulation of developmental processes.	US EPA	1996
An exogenous substance that causes adverse health effects in an intact organism, or its progeny, secondary to changes in endocrine function. A potential ED is a substance that possesses properties that might be expected to lead to endocrine disruption in an intact organism.	EU	1996
An ED is an exogenous substance that causes adverse health effects in an organism, or its progeny, consequent to endocrine function.	The Environment Agency	1998
The term hormonally active agents (HAAs) is used to describe substances that possess hormone-like activity regardless of mechanism. Convincing evidence that an HAA can affect the endocrine system would be its ability to bind to classic hormone receptors and promote measurable responses such as the induction of hormone-responsive genes or gene products. However, chemicals can disrupt hormonal processes by a variety of other mechanisms.	National Academy of Science	1999
EDCs are substances that may interfere with the normal function of the endocrine (hormone) system of humans and animals since many of them mimic the structure of natural hormones produced in the body.	The Royal Society	2000
Substances were able to disrupt endocrine processes with the potential for impairing development and reproduction or increasing the risk of cancer.	German Consultative Study	2000
An exogenous substance or mixture that alters function(s) of the endocrine system and consequently causes adverse effects in an intact organism, or its progeny, or (sub)populations. A potential ED is an exogenous substance or mixture that possesses properties that might be expected to lead to endocrine disruption in an intact organism, its progeny, or (sub) populations.	WHO/IPCS	2002
An exogenous chemical, or a mixture of chemicals, interferes with any aspect of hormone action.	Endocrine Society	2012

that alters function(s) of the endocrine system and consequently causes adverse health effects in an intact organism, or its progeny, or (sub)populations."[1]

Mentioned above and some other definitions of EDs are presented in Table 19.1.

Despite some differences in the definitions and still open discussion around it, in the last years WHO definition becomes mostly accepted by many regulators around the world. In this definition, we may notice it consists of a few elements, including endocrine mode of action (MoA), adverse effect in an intact organism, and a causal link between MoA and adversity. This makes endocrine disruption, not a typical toxicological endpoint, where only adversity is considered.

The problem of EDs is closely linked to other emerging risks described in Section V as microplastics (through migration of EAS/EDC from plastics to foods), climate change (e.g., through the need to use new plant protection products due to migration of pests to new territories), antimicrobial resistance (through the endocrine activity of antimicrobial growth promotors) and food fraud (due to using of some EAS/EDC in raw materials or components otherwise banned for use on food).

19.2 Mechanism of action and impact of endocrine disruptors on humane health

As mentioned above, the definition of ED implies the simultaneous presence of endocrine mechanism of action and adverse effects. EDCs may exhibit their effect through a different mechanism. They may interact with hormone receptors leading to their activation or block (agonistic or antagonistic action), interfere with natural hormone synthesis, transport or metabolism (see Fig. 19.1).

Although individual susceptibility variations are pertinent for any chemical, some studies claim that EDs may be considered the best example of such variation as the mechanisms of hormone or EDCs action at the cellular and tissue levels are dependent not only on the dose/concentration but also on circadian rhythms, seasonal changes, life stage, and sex.[15]

An adverse effect related to exposure to EDCs may include both alterations in endocrine organs themselves and changes in any other organs or systems due to the integrative and regulatory role of the endocrine system and its importance during the development. There are many studies linking exposure to chemicals interfering with the endocrine system and, as a consequence, causing

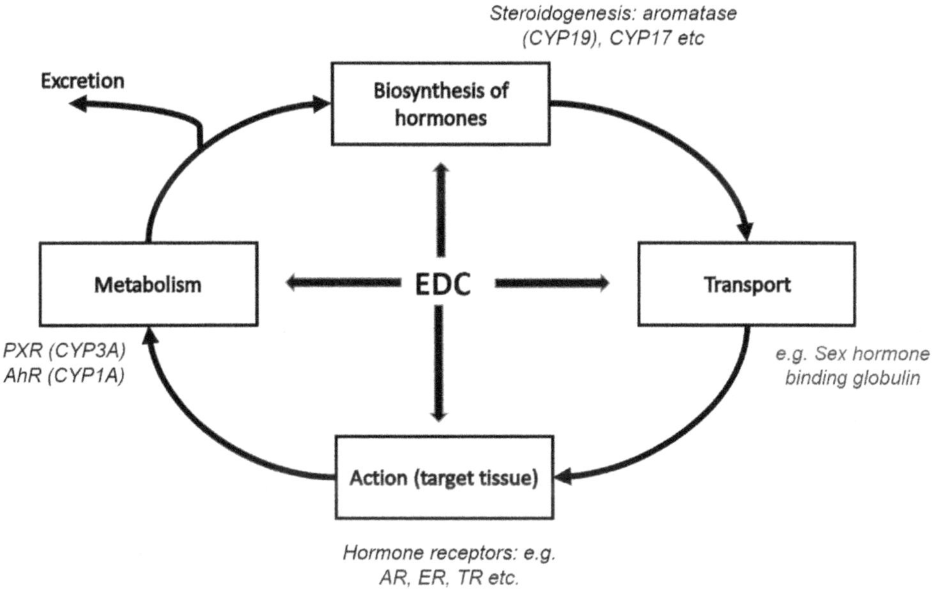

FIGURE 19.1 Different mechanisms of action of endocrine-disrupting chemical.[14] *Modified from Devillers, J., 2009. Endocrine disruption modeling, Endocr Disrupt Model. https://doi.org/10.1201/9781420076363*

various adverse effects. Among these adverse effects on human health, often mentioned are reduced fertility of men and women, impairment of brain development, cancer, metabolic disorders, etc. Impact on wildlife includes altered growth, decreased reproductive success, delayed or altered development, and population decline.[1–4]

Adverse effects of EDC on female reproductive health were revealed in the experimental and epidemiological studies.[16–20] Among adverse effects related to female reproductive health published articles mention abnormal sexual development, changed sexual behavior, irregular cyclicity, reduced fertility and infertility, polycystic ovarian syndrome endometriosis, fibrosis, preterm birth, developmental defects, mammary gland changes, and hormone-related cancers (endometrial, mammary).

Adverse effects of EDC on male reproductive health were revealed in the experimental and epidemiological studies.[21–23] These effects include failure of spermatogenesis and decreased sperm count, impairment of embryonic development, association with testicular cancer, and long-term metabolic effects.

The role of chemicals acting as EDs in metabolic disorders is also studied experimentally in vitro and in vivo[24–30] and revealed in epidemiological studies.[31–36] Mentioned studies provide a link between exposure to some chemicals with type 2 diabetes mellitus, obesity, metabolic syndrome, and, cardiovascular diseases.

It is hard to overestimate the role of the endocrine system in development, including neurodevelopment. Therefore data exist on links between exposure to EDC and neurodevelopment, such as memory, cognition, and social behavior (e.g., IQ loss, attention-deficit hyperactivity disorder).[3,37–41]

Last but not least to mention is the role of EDC in cancer development, first of all as classic tumor promotors.[3,20,42–45]

Above mentioned the nonexhaustive list of possible adverse effects should be considered with caution and just as an example since quite often adverse effects revealed in one study are not reproduced in others. Furthermore, not all studies postulating the presence of adverse effects can be given the same weight. For example, epidemiological studies with weak research design or small sample sizes are not so evident as randomized controlled trials; nonguideline studies have less weight in comparison with fully validated and regulatory accepted guideline studies conducted in the GLP environment.

19.3 Current approaches for testing and assessment of chemicals for their endocrine activity and consequent adverse effects

Due to the complex nature of the endocrine disruption (adversity, MoA, and the link between the two), it looks obvious that identification and characterization of the chemical as an ED are not possible based on any single test. Different testing strategies exist. OECD, a leading international organization in the field of development of guidelines on chemical testing, offered a conceptual tiered framework for testing and assessment of endocrine disrupters consisting of five levels[46]. Level 1 represents the assessment of existing data and the use of nontesting methods. Further levels provide conducting of various in vitro and in vivo assays to obtain data on selected endocrine mechanisms of action (Levels 2 and 3) and in vivo assays for identification of adverse effects (Levels 4 and 5). Current edition of OECD approach is available on OECD website https://www.oecd.org/chemicalsafety/testing/oecd-workrelatedtoendocrinedisrupters.htm.

In the United States the Endocrine Disruptor Screening Program (EDSP) is managed and implemented by EPA. EDSP uses a two-tiered approach to screen pesticides, chemicals, and environmental contaminants for their potential effect on estrogen, androgen, and thyroid hormone systems.[47]

The Tier 1 battery of tests consists of in vitro and in vivo screening assays. In vitro assays in the EDSP Tier 1 include the following: estrogen receptor (ER) binding—rat uterine cytosol; estrogen receptor—(hERα) transcriptional activation—Human cell line (HeLa-9903); androgen receptor (AR) binding—rat prostate cytosol; steroidogenesis—Human cell line (H295R); Aromatase—Human recombinant microsomes. In vivo assays in the EDSP Tier 1 are the following: Uterotrophic (rat), Hershberger (rat), Pubertal female (rat), Pubertal male (rat), Amphibian metamorphosis (frog), Fish short-term reproduction.

For Tier 2 testing in EDSP three testing guidelines are available now: Avian Two-Generation Toxicity Test in the Japanese Quail (890.2100); Medaka Extended One Generation Reproduction Test (890.2200); Larval Amphibian Growth and Development Assay (LAGDA) (890.2300).[48]

A comprehensive review of regulatory test methods for endocrine adverse health effects is provided by Manibusan and Touart.[49] In the mentioned review authors not only analyze currently available testing guidelines but also provide suggestions for further improvement of testing guidelines to better address endocrine-related mechanisms and endpoints.

19.4 Regulation of endocrine disrupting chemicals risk vs hazard based approach dilemma in assessment of endocrine-disrupting chemical

Currently, risk assessment is a classical approach for the regulation of chemicals in food.[50] The Procedural Manual of the FAO/WHO Codex Alimentarius Commission provides an internationally accepted definition of the relevant terms concerning risk analysis related to food safety and defines risk assessment as a scientifically based process comprising the following four steps: (1) hazard identification, (2) hazard characterization, (3) exposure assessment, and (4) risk characterization.[51] In some cases, a hazard-based approach is used, for example, for classification.[52] Such an approach skips exposure assessment and risk characterization steps and allows to make risk management decisions based on hazard identification/characterization only, often without dose-response assessment. Graphical representation of the risk assessment process and possible options of hazard and risk-based decision-making are provided in Fig. 19.2.

In some jurisdictions, a hazard-based approach was adopted for situations where the severity of consequences triggers more precautionary decision-making, for example, cut-off criteria for ingredients in plant protection products and biocides in the EU.[54,55] Substances identified as endocrine-disruptors are an example of such cut-off criteria in the EU, along with reproductive toxicants, mutagens, and carcinogens.

Discussions within the EU and internationally regarding such a precautionary approach have been going on already for more than 10 years. Cited above regulations were amended by European Commission in 2016 by scientific criteria for identification of EDs, followed by detailed EFSA/ECHA guidance for the identification of EDs published in 2018.[56] Mentioned documents (criteria and guidance) brought a better understanding of the approach to be used for the identification of the substances as EDs and as a consequence their ban from the EU market. However, the main aspect of the discussion, the hazard-based approach, was not removed, and discussions on the international level are ongoing.

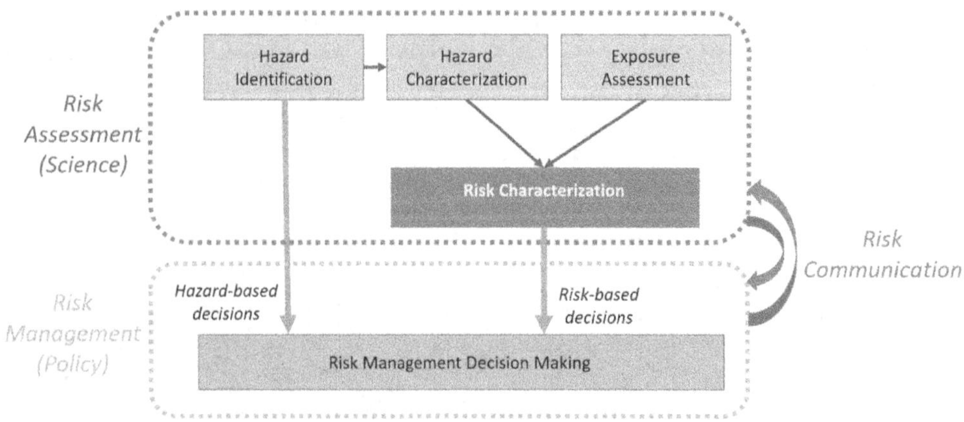

FIGURE 19.2 Scheme of the risk assessment framework and illustration of further decision making based on hazard or risk.[53] *Adapted from Slama, R., Bourguignon, J.P., Demeneix, B., et al., 2016. Scientific issues relevant to setting regulatory criteria to identify endocrine-disrupting substances in the european union. Environ Health Perspect 124, 1497–1503. https://doi.org/10.1289/EHP217.*

In the review on the role of hazard- and risk-based approaches in ensuring food safety[57] authors provide advantages and disadvantages of hazard and risk-based approaches in the food safety field together with relevant examples. Among the advantages of the hazard-based approach the authors call it is easier to implement (e.g., fewer data and expertise required) and its better understanding and perception by the public. Among the disadvantages of the hazard-based approach, the authors indicate that it cannot accommodate any flexibility being yes/no decision, drawing false conclusions about risk, loss of valuable resources due to unnecessary precaution, undermining confidence in innovation, etc. The main advantages and disadvantages of a risk-based approach, therefore mirror the disadvantages and advantages of a hazard-based approach, respectively.

Opening discussion and making conclusions related to what approach is more robust or effective is not within the scope of this section. The aim is just to present information on concerns and challenges in risk assessment of EDs which could lead regulators to take such a precautionary measure,[58–63] along with information about criticism of such an approach by its opponents.[5,64–69]

Among factors driving special attention and a more precautionary approach to EDC, including a hazard-based approach in the EU to the regulation of the plant protection products and biocides exerting endocrine-disrupting properties, often cited are the following: nonmonotonic dose-response (NMDR) curves, low-dose effects, long-term and transgenerational effects, variability of effect depending on the time of exposure (e.g., during critical periods of the organism development), the possible synergistic action of mixtures.[3,4,66,70]

The term "low dose" is used differently in different studies. In most cases it may be used to describe: (1) doses below the ones traditionally used in toxicological studies, that is, doses below the no or low adverse effect level (NOAEL or LOAEL); (2) doses in the range of typical human exposures; or (3) doses in animals that replicate the circulating concentrations of a substance in humans.[71] Closely related to the concept of a low dose is NMDR which is characterized by a dose-response relationship curve whose slope changes direction within the range of tested doses, usually "U" or inverted "U"-shaped.[72] Low dose effects and NMDR are revealed in many experimental studies, summarized, and analyzed in many reviews and reports.

Probably the biggest overview of low-dose effects and NMDR related to EDC is provided by Vandenberg and coauthors.[63] This article has received critical commentary[67] and rebuttal.[73]

Low dose effect or NMDR in the low dose end of the curve, will challenge the hazard characterization step of risk assessment, can make calculated safe or reference doses incorrect and as consequence lead to adverse effects on the levels of exposure estimated as safe.

Recently, the European Food Safety Authority (EFSA), released for public comments their draft scientific opinion on the biological plausibility of nonmonotonic dose responses and their impact on the risk assessment,[74] which follows up its previous work on the topic.[75,76] Among other, mentioned document states that "in evaluating a substance for which information on NMDR relations for one or more outcomes is obtained, the current risk assessment approach based on evaluating adverse outcomes seen in standard animal tests (as well as other observations) remains valid." Furthermore, where nonmonotonicity is taking place, the specific process is recommended to be followed considering the region of the dose-response curve where NMDR is observed, does the effect observed is apical or early/intermediate, evidence and biological relevance of the effect.[74]

The mixture effects of EDCs attracted high attention from researchers.[77–81] Concerning the mixture effects of the EDC in The Endocrine Society's Second Scientific Statement on EDCs, it is stated that there is a need for "testing mixtures of EDCs based on their structural or activity homology" in relation to the hormone-sensitive cancers in females and "expand research to mixtures of low-dose EDCs."[3] Work concerning mixtures is conducted by EFSA in the framework of establishment and evaluation of cumulative assessment groups (CAGs) of pesticides as required by EU legislation.[54] In relation to the CAG of pesticides that have chronic effects on the thyroid, it is concluded: "with varying degrees of certainty that cumulative exposure to relevant pesticides not exceeds the threshold for regulatory consideration established by risk managers."[82]

19.5 Advances in analytical methodology for detection and quantification of endocrine-disrupting chemical in food

EDC present in environmental, food, and biological samples and to which humans are exposed belong to a wide variety of chemical classes that differ greatly in their physical-chemical properties. Moreover, these substances are usually present at very low levels and in complex matrices. Therefore highly selective and sensitive methods are needed to detect and quantify these substances in the samples for checking compliance with legal limits and even more important for exposure assessment.[4]

In recent years advances in sample preparation techniques and analytical instrumentation led to tremendous improvements in the selectivity and sensitivity of the methods used to detect various classes of ED.

In the 2013 review of the analytical methodologies for the determination of EDC in biological and environmental samples information on advances in sample preparation and instrumentation was provided.[83]

19.5.1 Advances in instrumentation

The most common analytical technique employed for the detection and quantification of EDC is high-performance liquid chromatography (HPLC). In the last years, improvements achieved in the analysis are mostly achieved by coupling HPLC with different mass spectrometry detection techniques and enhancements in the development of new sorbent materials and HPLC columns. Among mentioned mass spectrometry detection techniques advances in EDC analysis were made using triple quadrupole (QqQ), time of flight (TOF), linear ion trap (LIT), and Orbitrap mass spectrometry.[83–86]

19.5.2 Sample preparation

Sample preparation (e.g., extraction and clean-up steps) is a practically inevitable step in the analysis of food matrices to obtain higher recovery and sensitivity. This step usually foresees the removal of interferences affecting the determination of the analyte, enrichment of the target compounds to detectable concentrations, and switching of solvent to the appropriate solvent for instrumental detection. Traditional methods used to extract organic compounds from the sample are liquid-liquid extraction (LLE) and solid-phase extraction (SPE). In recent years sample preparation trends existed towards automation through a coupling of sample preparation units and detection systems; the application of advanced sorbents and the application of more environmentally friendly approaches, such as reduced solvent techniques. Microextraction techniques achieving mentioned goals together with enhancement of recovery and specificity include solid-phase microextraction (SPME), stir-bar sorptive extraction (SBSE), and liquid-phase microextraction (LPME) approaches.[83]

19.6 Endocrine disruptors in food

Food is one of the major sources of exposure to EDCs. Many endocrine active or EDCs may be present in food. In Fig. 19.3 examples of the different types of endocrine active or disrupting chemicals in food are presented.

In the work of Mantovani[87] overview of EDCs, their modes of action, and the food chains more liable to contamination were made and presented here in Table 19.2. In a recently published editorial authors conclude that human exposure to synthetic EDCs is generally negligible as compared to natural compounds with higher or comparable endocrine activity.[88]

Below available data regarding main food sources and dietary exposure to some of the mentioned EAS/EDC is presented.

19.6.1 Dibenzo-p-dioxins and dibenzofurans (PCDD/F) and dioxin-like polychlorinated biphenyls (DL-PCBs)

Comprehensive data on exposure (relevant mostly to EU) and risk assessment of PCDD/F and DL-PCBs are provided in a recent EFSA publication.[89] According to the data provided the main contributors to the mean dietary exposure for the age group Infants were 'Butter and butter oil' (contributing from 6.1% to 19.6%) and 'Fatty fish' (contributing from 5.8% to 26.3%). The food categories 'Fatty fish' (contributing from 5.9% to 13.9%), 'Cheese' (contributing from 5.9% to 21.8%), and 'Livestock meat' (contributing from 7.7% to

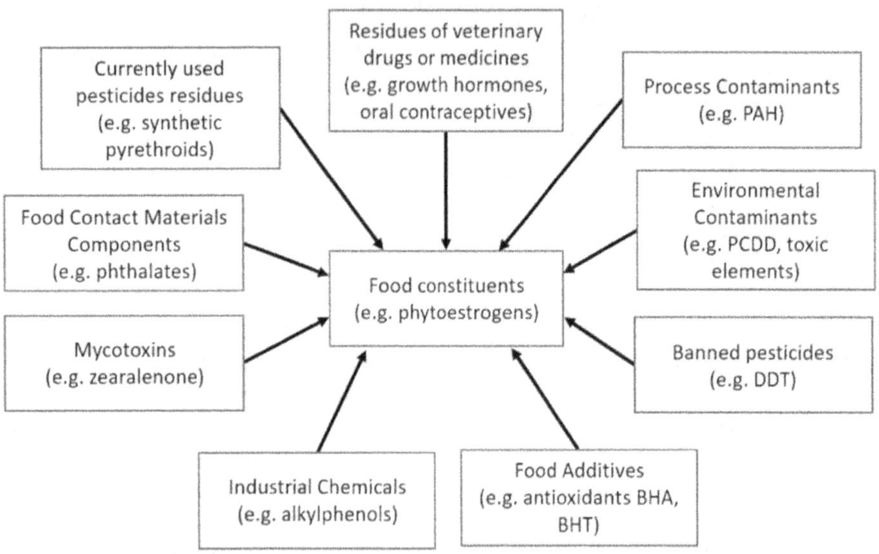

FIGURE 19.3 Possible endocrine active/disrupting chemicals in food. PAH, polycyclic aromatic hydrocarbons; PCDD, polychlorinated dibenzo-p-dioxins, DDT, dichlorodiphenyltrichloroethane; BHA, butylated hydroxyanisole; BHT, butylated hydroxytoluene.

TABLE 19.2 Overview of the main Endocrine disruptor considered, their modes of action, and the food chains more liable to contamination.[87]

Chemical(s) (Ref.)	Mode(s) of action	Food commodities
Dioxins (including dioxin-like PCB)	Act through the AhR; effects depend on sex and life stage, mainly antiestrogenic and immunotoxic actions	Bioaccumulation in lipid-rich foods, mainly of animal origin: milk, fat, and offal of grazing animals, fatty fishes; breastfeeding as well
Nondioxin-like PCB	Groups of congeners have different modes of action; estrogenicity, steroid metabolism, and thyroid as the main targets	Bioaccumulation in lipid-rich foods, mainly of animal origin: milk, fat, and offal of grazing animals, fatty fishes; breastfeeding as well
Polybrominated diphenyl ethers—PBDE	Thyroid appears as the main target, but also sex steroid balance	Bioaccumulation in lipid-rich foods, mainly fatty fishes; breastfeeding as well
Perfluorinated chemicals:PFOS and PFOA	Thyroid appears as the main target, but also sex steroid balance	Persistent but not fat-soluble: fishes, mollusks, offal
Hormone-active growth promoters	Potent steroid-like chemicals mimicking estrogens, androgens, or glucocorticoids	Prohibited in EU: possible residues in beef meat and edible organs
Ethylene bis-dithiocarbamate fungicides	A shared metabolite and environmental by-product, ethylene thiourea, is a thyrostatic agent	Treated edible crops; crops and pastures contaminated by runoff water, etc.
Chlorpyrifos and related organophosphorus insecticides	Act as ED only upon developmental exposure; neuroendocrine balance is the main target	Treated edible crops; crops and pastures contaminated by runoff water, etc.; also used as mass insecticides in farm animals
Bisphenol A (BPA)	Agonist of both estrogen receptors as well as other nuclear receptors (e.g., androgen); developmental effects on breast, reproductive, adipose, and immune tissues and the brain; highly controversial chemical	Nonpersistent but widespread in the environment (plastics, thermal paper, etc.); in foods mainly from food contact materials
Di-2-ethylhexyl phthalate and similarly acting phthalates	Interact with nuclear receptors (PPAR, etc.) impinging on early steps of steroid metabolism; effects on reproductive and metabolic development	Nonpersistent but widespread in the environment (plastics, personal care products, etc.); in foods mainly from food contact materials
Phytoestrogens	A very diverse group of chemicals including isoflavones; interact to a different extent with estrogen and androgen receptors; potential adverse effects depend on bioavailability, dose, gender, and age; soy phytoestrogens are also thyroid inhibitors	Some fruits and vegetables (soy in particular) are rich sources; high levels can be provided by soy-based foods or vegetable 'supplements'
Zearalenone	Estrogen agonist	Mycotoxin contaminating mainly cereals (corn, wheat) and derived foods
Cadmium	Endocrine actions include estrogenicity and inhibition of erythropoietin production	Widespread heavy metal: grains and seeds are the main dietary sources

Source: Adapted from Mantovani, A., 2016. Endocrine disrupters and the safety of food chains. Horm Res Paediatr 86, 279–288. https://doi.org/10.1159/000441496.

16.2%) were the main sources of exposure for toddlers. The food categories 'Fatty fish' (up to 56% contribution), 'Unspecified fish meat' (up to 53.4% contribution), 'Cheese' (up to 21.8% contribution), and 'Livestock meat' (up to 33.8% contribution) were the main sources of PCDD for the age groups of Other Children, Adolescents, Adults and Elderly. The mean upper-bond exposure for the sum of PCDD/Fs and DL-PCBs (29 congeners) ranged from 0.4 to 2.6 pg WHO2005-TEQ/kg bw per day, and the 95th percentile exposure, the UB estimates ranged from 0.9 to 6.6 pg WHO2005-TEQ/kg bw per day.

19.6.2 Polybrominated diphenyl ethers

The main dietary contributors to the PBDE exposure are "Fish and other seafood," "Meat and meat products,"

"Animal and vegetable fats and oils," "Milk and dairy products," "Eggs and egg products," "Products for special nutritional use," "Food for infants and small children" and highest dietary PBDE exposure is due to BDE-47 and \209, while the range of estimated exposure for average consumers across European countries and surveys for BDE-47 is 0.29 and 1.91 ng/kg bw per day, and for BDE-209 is 0.35 and 2.82 ng/kg bw, for minimum lower bound and maximum upper bound, respectively.[90]

19.6.3 Perfluorooctanesulfonic acid

Exposure to perfluorooctanesulfonic acid (PFOS) through food was estimated by EFSA at the level of 60 ng/kg b/w/ per day contributing mainly to fish and fishery products.[91]

19.6.4 Hormonal active growth promoters used in veterinary

Due to the EU ban on all hormonal active growth promoters, available data on the concentration of such substances in food from the EU market is limited.[92] Data on the concentrations of relevant substances and exposure assessment related to hormonal active growth promoters offered for use in productive animals can be found in the publications of the FAO/WHO Joint Expert Committee on Food Additives and Contaminants.[93] An interesting representation of the possible consumption of hormones with meat compared to daily production in the body of these hormones is provided in the article of Jeong et al.[94] According to the authors expected ingested amount of estradiol, progesterone and testosterone via consumption muscle meat from treated animals is from few hundred to few dozen thousands of times less than total daily production in the body of mentioned hormones. Nevertheless, it is worth keeping in mind that mentioned substances are highly potent in terms of their hormonal action and the endocrine system itself is extremely fine-tuned, where small fluctuations of hormone concentration may lead to big changes. Therefore such exposure data should always be assessed together with information on hazard characterization as provided in the classical risk assessment approach.

19.6.5 Pesticides

The main contributor to exposure to pesticides in the general population is residues in/on foods derived from treated crops. Therefore data on exposure to mentioned above in the Table 19.2, ethylene bis-dithiocarbamate fungicides and organophosphorus insecticides may vary considerably from region to region depending not only on the variety of the diet but also on differences in applied agricultural practice in the region. For example, using the probabilistic approach authors conclude that for the Brazilian population daily intake at the highest percentiles was a maximum of 2.0 μg carbon disulfide/kg body weight per day (upper band of the 95% confidence interval at P99.99). Tomato, rice, apple, and lettuce were the commodities that contributed most to the intake.[95] In the Danish study, the chronic exposures for adults and children were 0.35 and 0.76 μg/kg body weight day at the 99.9 percentile, representing 0.7% and 1.5%, respectively, of the acceptable daily intake for mancozeb and maneb at 50 μg/kg body weight.[96] The mean measured chlorpyrifos intake from food in the US study was assessed at the level of 0.46 μg/day.[96] In the study comparing health risks from dietary exposure (food and water) to chlorpyrifos between Danish and Chinese populations was concluded that the chronic health risk for chlorpyrifos in Denmark is 6–7-fold lower than in China, due to lower levels of exposure, which suggests that a better pesticide management policy can reduce risk levels for pesticide exposure.[97]

19.6.6 Bisphenol A

According to the EFSA risk assessment of BPA[98] diet is the main source in all population groups of external exposure to BPA. The main dietary sources of external BPA exposure were canned food and noncanned meat and meat products. In all age groups (including the most exposed groups, that is, 6–12 months infants and toddlers with levels of BPA 0.857 μg/kg bw per day) dietary exposure was more than 4-fold below the *t*-TDI (4 μg/kg bw per day), indicating no health concern from dietary exposure alone. The additional contribution from other oral sources, like dust and toy mouthing (high exposure up to 0.015 μg/kg bw per day), did not change this conclusion.[98]

19.6.7 Phtalates

In recent EFSA update of risk assessment f dibutylphthalate (DBP),butyl-benzyl-phthalate (BBP), bis(2-ethylhexyl)phthalate(DEHP), di-isononylphthalate (DINP) and di-isodecylphthala te (DIDP) for use in food contact materials exposure to individual phthalates and group exposures were estimated.[99] Thus the main contributors to group phthalates exposure of infants were 'Infant formulae, liquid' and 'Vegetable oil' and Vegetable Oil' and 'Cheese' for toddlers and adults. Estimates of dietary exposure were obtained by combining occurrence data from the literature with the consumption data from the EFSA Comprehensive Database and were as follows:

1. DBP mean of (0.042–0.769) and P95 of (0.099–1.503), lg/kg bw per day
2. BBP mean of (0.009–0.207) and P95 of (0.021–0.442), lg/kg bw per day

3. DEHP mean of (0.446–3.459) and P95 of (0.902–6.148), lg/kg bw per day
4. DINP mean of (0.232–4.270) and P95 of (0.446–7.071), lg/kg bw per day
5. DIDP mean of (0.001–0.057) and P95 of (0.008–0.095), lg/kg bw per day.

19.6.8 Phytoestrogens

Phytoestrogens are compounds present in various plants and subsequently foods that are structurally and/or functionally similar to mammalian estrogens and their active metabolites.

Most phytoestrogens are phenolic compounds, which may be grouped to polyphenols, flavonoids, and isoflavonoids.

These substances are claimed in different studies to have as beneficial health effects, but also potential to cause adverse health effects and, therefore to be EDs. Among the most often claimed beneficial health effects of phytoestrogens (mainly isoflavones) are lowered risk of osteoporosis, heart disease, breast cancer, and menopausal symptoms. Reported clinical cases or animal studies on adverse effects related to phytoestrogens are disruption of endogenous hormone levels and the ovulatory cycle; behavior changes and decreased sexual motivation, and ER-dependent gene expression in the brain. There is also evidence from animal studies of endocrine disruption during development, for example, disruption of brain sexual differentiation, and abnormal development of the female and male reproductive tract.[100]

Isoflavones and coumestans are the most widely researched groups. Information on isoflavones content in different foods may be obtained from different databases, for example, the USDA Database on the Isoflavone Content of Selected Foods.[101]

19.6.9 Zearalenone

Grains and grain-based foods, in particular grains and grain milling products, bread, and fine bakery wares, made the largest contribution to the zearalenone dietary exposure in all age classes. The estimated chronic total dietary exposures to zearalenone of adults across 19 European countries, using lower bound and upper bound concentrations, ranging from 2.4 to 29 ng/kg body weight (b.w.) per day for average consumers, and 4.7 to 54 ng/kg b.w. for 95th percentile consumers.[102]

19.6.10 Cadmium

Food is the dominating source of human exposure to cadmium in the non-smoking population. High levels of cadmium were found in algal formulations, cocoa-based products, crustaceans, edible offal, fungi, oilseeds, seaweeds, and water mollusks. Foods mostly contributing to cadmium dietary exposure across age groups are potatoes (13.2%), bread and rolls (11.7%), fine bakery wares (5.1%), chocolate products (4.3%), and leafy vegetables (3.9%) and water mollusks (3.2%). Lifetime cadmium dietary exposure, a middle bound overall weekly average was estimated at 2.04 μg/kg body weight and a potential 95th percentile at 3.66 μg/kg body weight.[103]

19.7 Research gaps and future directions of research in the field of EDC

In the already mentioned State-of-the-science of EDCs, 2012[4] the following two main areas of knowledge gaps were identified:

1. gaps in available test methods for identification and assessment of chemical's endocrine-disrupting effects and understanding of their MoA (e.g., some endocrine-related pathways are not covered, exposure periods do not cover critical developmental windows, delayed effects are not included);
2. gaps in understanding associations between exposures to EDCs and some endocrine diseases (e.g., EDC exposure and adverse pregnancy outcomes, early onset of breast development, obesity, diabetes; fetal EDC exposures and adult measures of semen quality and the risk of testicular cancer).

In the Endocrine Society's Second Scientific Statement on EDC[3] the following research gaps were identified:

1. Mechanisms of action of EDCs.
2. Translating research from animals to humans
3. The importance of life stage at evaluation and the need for longitudinal and multigenerational studies
4. Tissue- and organ-specific effects of EDCs
5. New EDCs and mixtures

A more recent overview of current gaps and needs in test methods for evaluation of EDC is provided in JRC report.[104] The mentioned report was based on the results of a survey where experts ($n = 40$) from 15 countries answered the questions about gaps in existing testing methods for identification and assessment of EDC and criteria for setting priorities for test method development and enhancement. According to mentioned report existing test, methods are not so good in predicting the development of the following endocrine-related diseases/disorders: metabolic disorders, immune-related disorders in wildlife and humans, adrenal disorders in wildlife and humans, adrenal disorders in humans, thyroid-related disorders / neurodevelopmental disorders in children.

In 2015 Endocrine Society[3] formulated the following recommendations for further research:

1. Mechanistic studies of EDC actions on nuclear hormone receptors need to be extended beyond ERs, AR, PR, GR, ThR, and PPARs to other nuclear hormone superfamily members and membrane steroid hormone receptors.
2. Investigate EDC effects on enzymes involved in steroidogenesis, hormone metabolism, and protein processing in humans and animal models.
3. Consider tissue-specific effects of EDCs.
4. Translate research from rodents into nonhuman primates, sheep, and other species; and take advantage of transgenic (especially humanized) animals, keeping in mind the need for a better understanding of hormones and early-life development in humans.
5. Test additional critical periods beyond prenatal and early postnatal—for example, adolescence as an additional sensitive developmental window.
6. Evaluate EDC outcomes at different life stages—not just adulthood.
7. Design studies to consider sex and gender differences in response to EDCs.
8. Perform longitudinal and multigenerational analyses in animals and humans.
9. Evaluate and implement emerging and sensitive testing systems, including high-throughput systems, for hazard assessment, screening, and prioritization.
10. In humans, consider genetic diversity and population differences in exposures and outcomes. This should include racial, ethnic, socioeconomic, and geographic variables.
11. Expand research to emerging "EDCs of interest" and to mixtures of low-dose EDCs.
12. The team science approach, including teams of basic, translational, and clinical scientists; epidemiologists; health care providers; and public health professionals, needs to be a priority for future research and funding.

Meanwhile, knowledge gaps exist, research related to all aspects of EDs, including new methods for chemicals assessment, analytical methodologies, and assessment approaches has been developing tremendously during the last years. As a relatively new field of research in toxicology, the issue of EDs has received much attention from both the scientific community and society in general and is one of the most dynamically developing areas. All trends that were currently seen in toxicology, including the establishment of adverse outcome pathways, development of relevant alternative testing and computational methods based on the established key events, and integrated approaches for these methods' results assessment, are fully reflected in the field of EDs' research. Despite non-testing methods are not ready yet to become the full replacement for animal testing, they already give an excellent opportunity for chemicals prioritization and more data-driven testing.[105,106]

An example of activities aimed at developing a methodology to improve the identification of EDCs is a cluster of eight EU-funded projects EURION (2019–24). Projects are focused on thyroid disruption (ATHENA, ERGO, SCREENED), metabolic disruption (OBERON, GOLIATH, and EDCMET), ED induced developmental neurotoxicity (ENDPoinTs), and female reproductive toxicity (FREIA).[107]

The US EPA is actively working to include high throughput and computational methods into its EDSP.[108]

Another important direction of further actions to enhance research and knowledge about EDCs is in addition to existing regulatory accepted guidelines relevant measurements to address endocrine-related pathways and endpoints. In the already cited above overview, Manibusan and Touart provide several suggestions to improve such methods[49] (see Table 19.3 and 19.4).

More flexibility in the use of nonguideline studies data together with a robust, fast, and efficient approach for validation of additional endpoints in the guideline studies will help us in a more comprehensive understanding of the possible effects of studied chemicals.

Therefore in the nearest future we are going to see:

1. development of new adverse outcome pathways, based on data-rich studies;
2. development and validation of new, including high throughput, in vitro assays for detection of ED MoA and screening of substances;
3. development, validation, and probably regulatory acceptance of the computational tools to address endocrine MoA and endocrine-related adverse effects;
4. addition of the new definitive ED endpoints to existing OECD testing guidelines;
5. development of more sensitive, specific, predictive, and data-rich methods/endpoints to address estrogenic, androgenic, thyroidal, and steroidogenic (EATS) modalities;
6. development of methods/endpoints specifically covering non-EATS modalities;
7. development of integrated testing and assessment strategies which will include new approach methods as its integral part;
8. a better understanding of the mixture effects of chemicals, including EDC, and methods for testing and assessment of such effects;
9. new more effective analytical and data gathering methods, including the application of emerging IT tools, for refined exposure assessment of already identified and emerging EDCs covering different sources, routes, and regimes of exposure;

TABLE 19.3 Summary of recommended test methods enhancements to address endocrine-related biological pathways.

Endocrine-related biological pathways	Test method enhancement	Added measurement(s)
Hypothalamus pituitary-gonadal axis	Repeated dose mammalian studies (e.g., OECD Test Guidelines (TG) 407–413, 422)	Additional observations on behavior could be beneficial in corroborating androgen signaling perturbationsAdded hormonal measurements (e.g., progesterone, etc.)
	Fish short-term reproductive assay (OECD TG 229) and/or Medaka extended one-generation reproduction toxicity test (OECD TG 240)	New endpoint for assessing GnRH neuron development in the brain but some logistical disadvantages with minimal added value Assess oocytes and sperm quality or a new ex vivo method for assessing oocytes and sperm derived from these fish assays.
Hypothalamus pituitary thyroid axis	Early precursor key events upstream of adverse outcomes	In vitro assays to address diagnostic, early precursor key events (e.g., thyroid transactivation reporter assays, cell proliferation assays, TPO inhibition assay, HPT regulated gene expression assays)
Hypothalamus pituitary-adrenal axis	Enhancements to existing repeated-dose mammalian studies (e.g., OECD TG 407–413, 422)	Addition of stress response relevant endpoints, glucocorticoids and corticotropin (ACTH)
	New assays for consideration of earlier key events in AOP	GhR transactivation assay (in vitro)
	Enhancement to the existing steroidogenesis assay (OCSPP 890.1550 or OECD TG 456)	Adrenal steroid synthesis assay (in vitro)
Somatotropic axis	Enhancements to existing repeated dose studies (e.g., OECD TG 407–413, 422)	Add measurements of IGF-1 serum levels or IGF-1 mRNA levels
Vitamin D signaling pathway	Vitamin D transactivation assay and AhR transactivation assay	Research on identifying biomarker endpoints that can be diagnostic of vitamin D disruption
	Enhancements to existing repeated dose studies (e.g., OECD TG 407–413, 422)	Vitamin D hydroxylase and EROD activity
Retinoid signaling pathway	Enhancements to existing repeated dose studies (e.g., OECD TG 407–413, 422)	Serum retinoid levels, EROD induction activity, CYP1A1 mRNA or protein quantification in in vivo assays
Peroxisome proliferator-activated receptor signaling pathway	PPAR transactivation reporter assays and gene microarray library as early precursor key events to supplement apical endpoints	Peroxisome proliferation measurements at different time courses and lipid accumulation measurements may be added to repeat dose toxicity studies

Source: Adapted from Manibusan, M.K., Touart, L.W., 2017. A comprehensive review of regulatory test methods for endocrine adverse health effects. Crit Rev Toxicol 47, 433–481. https://doi.org/10.1080/10408444.2016.1272095.

10. based on the above-mentioned advances, new epidemiological evidence for the number of exposure—disease associations.

19.8 Conclusions

There are many publications that chemicals identified as EDs may constitute a threat to public health and wildlife, especially taking into account their widespread presence in the environment. Therefore the great attention of academia, regulators and the general public to the issue led to the advancement of research in the field of EDC. At the same time, public concerns, and even outrage, led to a very precautionary approach to the regulation of chemicals that may be identified as EDC in some countries. The process of regulatory approach development for EDC appears to be a two-way street, where more understanding of the mechanisms, pathways, and their links to adverse outcomes will contribute to a more pragmatic and precise approach to regulation. With this in mind, it may be expected risk assessment process will be adapted to address problems and concerns related to EDC assessment. Regardless of the approach used for chemical assessment (i.e., hazard

TABLE 19.4 Summary of recommended test methods enhancements to address endocrine-related disease/disorder.

Endocrine-related disease/disorder	Test method enhancement	Added measurement(s)
Male and female reproductive health: precocious puberty	Repeated dose toxicity studies (e.g., 28/ 90-day study) (e.g., OECD TG 407–413, 422)	Hormonal measurements (e.g., LH, FSH, testosterone, estradiol, progesterone, prolactin, DHEA)
Female reproductive health: fecundityFemale reproductive health: polycystic ovaries syndromeFemale reproductive health: adverse pregnancy outcomeFemale reproductive health: endometriosis and uterine fibroidsMale reproductive health: testicular dysgenesis syndrome	No enhancements are needed at this time	No enhancements are needed at this time
Hormonal cancers: breast cancer	Adapt existing assays and diagnostic techniques	A study to address in utero to end of life duration of exposure, or from conception through a lifetime.Genetically engineered mouse models (GEMMS) or transfected organism models have been developed to study factors related to the pathogenesis of experimental prostate, ovarian, and other cancer subtypes and using more sensitive rodent strains for endocrine-related cancer
Hormonal cancers: prostate cancer and testicular cancer	Adapt existing assays and diagnostic techniques	
Hormonal cancers: thyroid	In vitro assays to establish earlier key events	TR reporter assays, TPO assay, and HTP thyroid-specific assays (NIS)
Neurodevelopment disorders	Additional research to elucidate the MoA and key events confirming the primary role of endocrine activity in the manifestations of neurodevelopmental, obesity, and diabetes multifactorial health outcomes.	
Metabolic syndrome—obesity and diabetesHuman adrenal disorders: adrenocortical hyperplasia	Repeated dose toxicity studies (e.g., 28/ 90-day study) (e.g., OECD TG 407–413, 422)	Measurements of cortisol (hydrocortisol), corticosterone, aldosterone, adrenocorticotropic hormone levels
Immune-related disorders: inflammatory, immune cancer, childhood respiratory disease	Repeated dose toxicity studies (e.g., 28/ 90-day study) (e.g., OECD TG 407–413, 422)	Functional immune tests and evaluations included in the immunotoxicity study
Vitamin D-related disorders	Repeated dose toxicity studies (e.g., 28/ 90-day study) (e.g., OECD TG 407–413, 422)	25-hydroxylase measurements, vitamin D and magnesium, biochemical markers of bone metabolism (bone-specific ALP, serum osteocalcin, serum C-telopeptide, and urinary N-telopeptide)

Source: Adapted from Manibusan, M.K., Touart, L.W., 2017. A comprehensive review of regulatory test methods for endocrine adverse health effects. Crit Rev Toxicol 47, 433–481. https://doi.org/10.1080/10408444.2016.1272095.

or risk-based) concerning their endocrine-disrupting properties, studies, or models used to generate data for such an assessment got to be well described, scientifically valid, and regulatory accepted. This ensures not only reliable but also adequate results for further assessment.

References

1. World Health Organization (WHO), International Programme on Chemical Safety. *Global Assessment of the State-of-the-Science of Endocrine Disruptors*. 2002.
2. Diamanti-Kandarakis, E., 2009. Endocrine-disrupting chemicals: an Endocrine Society scientific statement. Endocr.
3. Gore AC, Chappell VA, Fenton SE, et al. EDC-2: the endocrine society's second scientific statement on endocrine-disrupting chemicals. *Endocr Rev*. 2015;36:E1–E150. Available from: https://doi.org/10.1210/er.2015-1010.
4. Bergman Å, Heindel J, Jobling S, Kidd K, Zoeller RT. State-of-the-science of endocrine disrupting chemicals. *Toxicol Lett*. 2012;. Available from: https://doi.org/10.1016/j.toxlet.2012.03.020.
5. Dietrich DR, Aulock S, von, Marquardt H, et al. Scientifically unfounded precaution drives European Commission's recommendations on EDC regulation, while defying common sense, well-established science and risk assessment principles. *Toxicol Vitr*. 2013;27:2110–2114. Available from: https://doi.org/10.1016/j.tiv.2013.07.001.
6. Autrup H, Barile FA, Blaauboer BJ, et al. Principles of pharmacology and toxicology also govern effects of chemicals on the endocrine system. *Toxicol Sci*. 2015;146:11–15. Available from: https://doi.org/10.1093/toxsci/kfv082.
7. Lamb JC, Boffetta P, Foster WG, et al. Comments on the opinions published by Bergman et al. (2015) on critical comments on the WHO-UNEP state of the science of endocrine disrupting chemicals (Lamb et al., 2014). *Regul Toxicol Pharmacol*. 2015;73:754–757. Available from: https://doi.org/10.1016/j.yrtph.2015.10.029.
8. Lamb JC, Boffetta P, Foster WG, et al. Critical comments on the WHO-UNEP state of the science of endocrine disrupting chemicals – 2012. *Regul Toxicol Pharmacol*. 2014;69:22–40. Available from: https://doi.org/10.1016/j.yrtph.2014.02.002.
9. Rhomberg LR, Goodman JE, Foster WG, Borgert CJ, Van Der Kraak G. A critique of the European commission document, "state of the art assessment of endocrine disrupters. *Crit Rev Toxicol*. 2012;42:465–473. Available from: https://doi.org/10.3109/10408444.2012.690367.
10. Darbre PD. The history of endocrine-disrupting chemicals. *Curr Opin Endocr Metab Res*. 2019;7:26–33. Available from: https://doi.org/10.1016/j.coemr.2019.06.007.
11. Soto AM, Schaeberle CM, Sonnenschein C. From Wingspread to CLARITY: a personal trajectory. *Nat Rev Endocrinol*. 2021;. Available from: https://doi.org/10.1038/s41574-020-00460-3.
12. Kavlock RJ, Daston GP, DeRosa C, et al. Research needs for the risk assessment of health and environmental effects of endocrine disrupters: a report of the U.S. EPA-sponsored workshop. *Env Health Perspect*. 1996;104:715–740. Available from: https://doi.org/10.1289/ehp.96104s4715.
13. Bergman, A., Brandt, I., Brouwer, A., et al., European Workshop on the Impact of Endocrine Disrupters on Human Health and Wildlife, 2-4 December 1996, Weybridge, UK: Report of Proceedings, 1997.
14. Devillers J. Endocrine disruption modeling. *Endocr Disrupt Model*. 2009;. Available from: https://doi.org/10.1201/9781420076363.
15. La Merrill MA, Vandenberg LN, Smith MT, et al. Consensus on the key characteristics of endocrine-disrupting chemicals as a basis for hazard identification. *Nat Rev Endocrinol*. 2020;16:45–57. Available from: https://doi.org/10.1038/s41574-019-0273-8.
16. Canipari R, De Santis L, Cecconi S. Female fertility and environmental pollution. *Int J Env Res Public Health*. 2020;17. Available from: https://doi.org/10.3390/ijerph17238802.
17. Hipwell AE, Kahn LG, Factor-Litvak P, et al. Exposure to non-persistent chemicals in consumer products and fecundability: a systematic review. *Hum Reprod Update*. 2019;25:51–71. Available from: https://doi.org/10.1093/humupd/dmy032.
18. Karwacka A, Zamkowska D, Radwan M, Jurewicz J. Exposure to modern, widespread environmental endocrine disrupting chemicals and their effect on the reproductive potential of women: an overview of current epidemiological evidence. *Hum Fertil (Camb)*. 2019;22:2–25. Available from: https://doi.org/10.1080/14647273.2017.1358828.
19. Rattan S, Zhou C, Chiang C, Mahalingam S, Brehm E, Flaws JA. Exposure to endocrine disruptors during adulthood: consequences for female fertility. *J Endocrinol*. 2017;233:R109–R129. Available from: https://doi.org/10.1530/JOE-17-0023.
20. Scsukova S, Rollerova E, Bujnakova Mlynarcikova A. Impact of endocrine disrupting chemicals on onset and development of female reproductive disorders and hormone-related cancer. *Reprod Biol*. 2016;16:243–254. Available from: https://doi.org/10.1016/j.repbio.2016.09.001.
21. Bonde JP, Flachs EM, Rimborg S, et al. The epidemiologic evidence linking prenatal and postnatal exposure to endocrine disrupting chemicals with male reproductive disorders: a systematic review and meta-analysis. *Hum Reprod Update*. 2016;23:104–125. Available from: https://doi.org/10.1093/humupd/dmw036.
22. Sharma A, Mollier J, Brocklesby RWK, Caves C, Jayasena CN, Minhas S. Endocrine-disrupting chemicals and male reproductive health. *Reprod Med Biol*. 2020;19:243–253. Available from: https://doi.org/10.1002/rmb2.12326.
23. Sidorkiewicz I, Zaręba K, Wołczyński S, Czerniecki J. Endocrine-disrupting chemicals-mechanisms of action on male reproductive system. *Toxicol Ind Health*. 2017;33:601–609. Available from: https://doi.org/10.1177/0748233717695160.
24. Wang J, Sun B, Hou M, Pan X, Li X. The environmental obesogen bisphenol A promotes adipogenesis by increasing the amount of 11β-hydroxysteroid dehydrogenase type 1 in the adipose tissue of children. *Int J Obes*. 2013;37:999–1005.
25. Zhang H, Xue W, Li Y, et al. Perinatal exposure to 4-nonylphenol affects adipogenesis in first and second generation rats offspring. *Toxicol Lett*. 2014;225:325–332.
26. Bo E, Farinetti A, Marraudino M, et al. Adult exposure to tributyltin affects hypothalamic neuropeptide Y, Y1 receptor distribution, and circulating leptin in mice. *Andrology*. 2016;4:723–734.
27. Drobná Z, Henriksen AD, Wolstenholme JT, et al. Transgenerational effects of bisphenol A on gene expression and DNA methylation of imprinted genes in brain. *Endocrinology*. 2018;159:132–144.
28. Mimoto MS, Nadal A, Sargis RM. Polluted pathways: mechanisms of metabolic disruption by endocrine disrupting chemicals. *Curr Environ Heal Rep*. 2017;4:208–222.
29. Regnier SM, Kirkley AG, Ye H, et al. Dietary exposure to the endocrine disruptor tolylfluanid promotes global metabolic dysfunction in male mice. *Endocrinology*. 2015;156:896–910.
30. Sargis RM, Johnson DN, Choudhury RA, Brady MJ. Environmental endocrine disruptors promote adipogenesis in the 3t3-l1 cell line through glucocorticoid receptor activation. *Obesity*. 2010;18:1283–1288.

31. Bubalo NM, Balan GM, Zhminko PG, et al. Leptin as a biomarker of metabolic disorders and obesity in patients with acute herbicide poisoning based on 2,4-dichlorophenoxyacetic acid. *Bull Probl Biol Med.* 2019;3:84. Available from: https://doi.org/10.29254/2077-4214-2019-3-152-84-88.
32. Chang SC, Li WC, Huang KY, et al. Efficacy of alcohols and alcohol-based hand disinfectants against human enterovirus 71. *J Hosp Infect.* 2013;83:288–293. Available from: https://doi.org/10.1016/j.jhin.2012.12.010.
33. Ribeiro CM, Beserra BTS, Silva NG, et al. Exposure to endocrine-disrupting chemicals and anthropometric measures of obesity: a systematic review and meta-analysis. *BMJ Open.* 2020;10:e033509. Available from: https://doi.org/10.1136/bmjopen-2019-033509.
34. Tahir E, Cordier S, Courtemanche Y, et al. Effects of polychlorinated biphenyls exposure on physical growth from birth to childhood and adolescence: a prospective cohort study. *Environ Res.* 2020;189:109924. Available from: https://doi.org/10.1016/j.envres.2020.109924.
35. Tang-Péronard JL, Heitmann BL, Andersen HR, et al. Association between prenatal polychlorinated biphenyl exposure and obesity development at ages 5 and 7 y: a prospective cohort study of 656 children from the Faroe Islands. *Am J Clin Nutr.* 2014;99:5–13. Available from: https://doi.org/10.3945/ajcn.113.066720.
36. Vafeiadi M, Georgiou V, Chalkiadaki G, et al. Association of prenatal exposure to persistent organic pollutants with obesity and cardiometabolic traits in early childhood: the rhea mother-child cohort (Crete, Greece). *Environ Health Perspect.* 2015;123:1015–1021. Available from: https://doi.org/10.1289/ehp.1409062.
37. Nesan D, Kurrasch DM. Gestational exposure to common endocrine disrupting chemicals and their impact on neurodevelopment and behavior. *Annu Rev Physiol.* 2020;82:177–202.
38. Pinson A, Bourguignon J-P, Parent A-S. Exposure to endocrine disrupting chemicals and neurodevelopmental alterations. *Andrology.* 2016;4:706–722.
39. Ramhøj L, Hass U, Gilbert ME, et al. Evaluating thyroid hormone disruption: investigations of long-term neurodevelopmental effects in rats after perinatal exposure to perfluorohexane sulfonate (PFHxS). *Sci Rep.* 2020;10:1–13.
40. Repouskou A, Papadopoulou A-K, Panagiotidou E, et al. Long term transcriptional and behavioral effects in mice developmentally exposed to a mixture of endocrine disruptors associated with delayed human neurodevelopment. *Sci Rep.* 2020;10:1–16.
41. Schug TT, Blawas AM, Gray K, Heindel JJ, Lawler CP. Elucidating the links between endocrine disruptors and neurodevelopment. *Endocrinology.* 2015;156:1941–1951.
42. Alsen M, Sinclair C, Cooke P, Ziadkhanpour K, Genden E, van Gerwen M. Endocrine disrupting chemicals and thyroid cancer: an overview. *Toxics.* 2021;9:14.
43. Diamanti-Kandarakis E, Bourguignon J-P, Giudice LC, et al. Endocrine-disrupting chemicals: an endocrine society scientific statement. *Endocr Rev.* 2009;30:293–342. Available from: https://doi.org/10.1210/er.2009-0002.
44. Morgan M, Deoraj A, Felty Q, Roy D. Environmental estrogen-like endocrine disrupting chemicals and breast cancer. *Mol Cell Endocrinol.* 2017;457:89–102.
45. Rutkowska AZ, Szybiak A, Serkies K, Rachon D. Endocrine disrupting chemicals as potential risk factor for estrogen-dependent cancers. *Pol Arch Med Wewn.* 2016;126:562–570.
46. OECD. Revised Guidance Document 150 on Standardised Test Guidelines for Evaluating Chemicals for Endocrine Disruption. *OECD Series on Testing and Assessment, No. 150.* OECD; 2018:20–21. Available from: https://www.oecd-ilibrary.org/environment/guidance-document-on-standardised-test-guidelines-for-evaluating-chemicals-for-endocrine-disruption-2nd-edition_9789264304741-en. Accessed 30.03.22.
47. US EPA, Endocrine Disruptor Screening Program (EDSP) Overview [WWW Document]. 2021. URL <https://www.epa.gov/endocrine-disruption/endocrine-disruptor-screening-program-edsp-overview>.
48. US EPA. Series 890 – Endocrine Disruptor Screening Program Test Guidelines [WWW Document]. 2021. <https://www.epa.gov/test-guidelines-pesticides-and-toxic-substances/series-890-endocrine-disruptor-screening-program>.
49. Manibusan MK, Touart LW. A comprehensive review of regulatory test methods for endocrine adverse health effects. *Crit Rev Toxicol.* 2017;47:433–481. Available from: https://doi.org/10.1080/10408444.2016.1272095.
50. WTO. Agreement on the application of sanitary and phytosanitary measures. 1995..
51. FAO/WHO. Codex Alimentarius Commission – Procedural Manual twenty-seventh edition, 27th ed. Rome, 2019.
52. GHS. Globally Harmonized System of Classification and Labelling of Chemicals (GHS). United Nations, 2019.
53. Slama R, Bourguignon JP, Demeneix B, et al. Scientific issues relevant to setting regulatory criteria to identify endocrine-disrupting substances in the european union. *Environ Health Perspect.* 2016;124:1497–1503. Available from: https://doi.org/10.1289/EHP217.
54. European Parliament and the Council. Regulation (EC) No 1107/2009 of the European Parliament and of the council of 21 October 2009 concerning the placing of plant protection products on the market and repealing council directives 79/117/EEC and 91/414/EEC. *J Eur Union.* 2009;50.
55. European Parliament and the Council. Regulation (EU) No 528/2012 of the European Parliament and of the council of 22 May 2012 concerning the making available on the market and use of biocidal products. *J Eur Union.* 2012;1–123.
56. ECHA/EFSA JRC, Andersson N, Arena M, et al. Guidance for the identification of endocrine disruptors in the context of regulations (EU) No 528/2012 and (EC) No 1107/2009. *EFSA J.* 2018;16:e05311. Available from: https://doi.org/10.2903/j.efsa.2018.5311.
57. Barlow SM, Boobis AR, Bridges J, et al. The role of hazard- and risk-based approaches in ensuring food safety. *Trends Food Sci Technol.* 2015;46:176–188. Available from: https://doi.org/10.1016/j.tifs.2015.10.007.
58. Vandenberg LN, Maffini MV, Sonnenschein C, Rubin BS, Soto AM. Bisphenol-A and the great divide: a review of controversies in the field of endocrine disruption. *Endocr Rev.* 2009;30:75–95. Available from: https://doi.org/10.1210/er.2008-0021.
59. Zoeller RT, Brown TR, Doan LL, et al. Endocrine-disrupting chemicals and public health protection: a statement of principles from the endocrine society. *Endocrinology.* 2012;153:4097–4110. Available from: https://doi.org/10.1210/en.2012-1422.
60. Ashby J. Endocrine disruption occurring at doses lower than those predicted by classical chemical toxicity evaluations: the case bisphenol A. *Pure Appl Chem.* 2003;75:2167–2179. Available from: https://doi.org/10.1351/pac200375112167.

61. Phillips KP, Foster WG, Leiss W, et al. Assessing and managing risks arising from exposure to endocrine-active chemicals. *J Toxicol Environ Heal – Part B Crit Rev.* 2008;11:351–372. Available from: https://doi.org/10.1080/10937400701876657.
62. Welshons WV, Thayer KA, Judy BM, Taylor JA, Curran EM, vom Saal FS. Large effects from small exposures. I. Mechanisms for endocrine-disrupting chemicals with estrogenic activity. *Environ Health Perspect.* 2003;111:994–1006. Available from: https://doi.org/10.1289/ehp.5494.
63. Vandenberg LN, Colborn T, Hayes TB, et al. Hormones and endocrine-disrupting chemicals: low-dose effects and nonmonotonic dose responses. *Endocr Rev.* 2012;33:378–455. Available from: https://doi.org/10.1210/er.2011-1050.
64. vom Saal FS, Akingbemi BT, Belcher SM, et al. Flawed experimental design reveals the need for guidelines requiring appropriate positive controls in endocrine disruption research. *Toxicol Sci.* 2010;115:612–613. Available from: https://doi.org/10.1093/toxsci/kfq048.
65. Coady, K., Matthiessen, P., Zahner, H., et al., Endocrine disruption: where are we with hazard and risk assessment? 2016. <https://doi.org/10.7287/PEERJ.PREPRINTS.2580V1>.
66. Futran Fuhrman V, Tal A, Arnon S. Why endocrine disrupting chemicals (EDCs) challenge traditional risk assessment and how to respond. *J Hazard Mater.* 2015;286:589–611. Available from: https://doi.org/10.1016/j.jhazmat.2014.12.012.
67. Rhomberg LR, Goodman JE. Low-dose effects and nonmonotonic dose–responses of endocrine disrupting chemicals: has the case been made? *Regul Toxicol Pharmacol.* 2012;64:130–133. Available from: https://doi.org/10.1016/j.yrtph.2012.06.015.
68. Sharpe RM. Is it time to end concerns over the estrogenic effects of Bisphenol A? *Toxicol Sci.* 2010;114:1–4. Available from: https://doi.org/10.1093/toxsci/kfp299.
69. Testai E, Galli CL, Dekant W, Marinovich M, Piersma AH, Sharpe RM. A plea for risk assessment of endocrine disrupting chemicals. *Toxicology.* 2013;314:51–59. Available from: https://doi.org/10.1016/j.tox.2013.07.018.
70. Damstra, T., Barlow, S., Bergman, A., Kavlock, R., Van Der Kraak, G., Global assessment of the state-of-the-science of endocrine disruptors. WHOpublication no. WHO/PCS/EDC/02.2 180. 2002.
71. Zoeller TR, Bergman A, Becher G, et al. A path forward in the debate over health impacts of endocrine disrupting chemicals. *Environ Health A Glob Access Sci Source.* 2014;13:1–11. Available from: https://doi.org/10.1186/1476-069X-13-118.
72. Lagarde F, Beausoleil C, Belcher SM, et al. Non-monotonic dose-response relationships and endocrine disruptors: a qualitative method of assessment. *Environ Health.* 2015;14:13. Available from: https://doi.org/10.1186/1476-069X-14-13.
73. Vandenberg LN, Colborn T, Hayes TB, et al. Regulatory decisions on endocrine disrupting chemicals should be based on the principles of endocrinology. *Reprod Toxicol.* 2013;38:1–15. Available from: https://doi.org/10.1016/j.reprotox.2013.02.002.
74. EFSA. Draft EFSA Scientific Committee Opinion on biological plausibility of non-monotonic dose responses and their impact on the risk assessment, 2021.
75. EFSA. EFSA's 17th Scientific Colloquium on low dose response in toxicology and risk assessment. *EFSA Support Publ.* 2012;9:353E. Available from: https://doi.org/10.2903/sp.efsa.2012.EN-353.
76. Beausoleil C, Beronius A, Bodin L, et al. Review of non-monotonic dose-responses of substances for human risk assessment. *EFSA Support. Publ.* 2016;13. Available from: https://doi.org/10.2903/sp.efsa.2016.EN-1027.
77. Isling LK, Boberg J, Jacobsen PR, et al. Late-life effects on rat reproductive system after developmental exposure to mixtures of endocrine disrupters. *Reproduction.* 2014;147:465–476.
78. Axelstad M, Christiansen S, Boberg J, et al. Mixtures of endocrine-disrupting contaminants induce adverse developmental effects in preweaning rats. *Reproduction.* 2014;147:489–501.
79. Kolesnyk S, Riabukha O, Prodanchuk M, Zhminko P, Vasetska O. Acute mixture toxicity of pesticide formulations and perspective of use in silico methods to complement risk assessment of plant protection products. *Toxicol Lett.* 2018;295:S238. Available from: https://doi.org/10.1016/j.toxlet.2018.06.990.
80. Kortenkamp A. Low dose mixture effects of endocrine disrupters and their implications for regulatory thresholds in chemical risk assessment. *Curr Opin Pharmacol.* 2014;19:105–111.
81. Park C, Song H, Choi J, et al. The mixture effects of bisphenol derivatives on estrogen receptor and androgen receptor. *Environ Pollut.* 2020;260:114036.
82. EFSA. Cumulative dietary risk characterisation of pesticides that have chronic effects on the thyroid. *EFSA J.* 2020;18:e06088. Available from: https://doi.org/10.2903/j.efsa.2020.6088.
83. Sosa-Ferrera Z, Mahugo-Santana C, Santana-Rodríguez JJ. Analytical methodologies for the determination of endocrine disrupting compounds in biological and environmental samples. *Biomed Res Int.* 2013;2013.
84. Chiesa LM, Pavlovic R, Panseri S, Arioli F. Evaluation of parabens and their metabolites in fish and fish products: a comprehensive analytical approach using LC-HRMS. *Food Addit Contam Part A Chem Anal Control Expo Risk Assess.* 2018;35:2400–2413. Available from: https://doi.org/10.1080/19440049.2018.1544721.
85. Huysman S, Van Meulebroek L, Vanryckeghem F, Van Langenhove H, Demeestere K, Vanhaecke L. Development and validation of an ultra-high performance liquid chromatographic high resolution Q-Orbitrap mass spectrometric method for the simultaneous determination of steroidal endocrine disrupting compounds in aquatic matrices. *Anal Chim Acta.* 2017;984:140–150. Available from: https://doi.org/10.1016/j.aca.2017.07.001.
86. Lee, H.-J., Kim, C., Ryu, H.-D., Chung, E.G., Shin, D., Lee, J.K.. Simultaneous determination of pesticides and veterinary pharmaceuticals in environmental water samples by UHPLC–Quadrupole-Orbitrap HRMS Combined with On-Line Solid-Phase Extraction. Sep. 2020. <https://doi.org/10.3390/separations7010014>.
87. Mantovani A. Endocrine disrupters and the safety of food chains. *Horm Res Paediatr.* 2016;86:279–288. Available from: https://doi.org/10.1159/000441496.
88. Autrup H, Barile FA, Berry SC, et al. Human exposure to synthetic endocrine disrupting chemicals (S-EDCs) is generally negligible as compared to natural compounds with higher or comparable endocrine activity: how to evaluate the risk of the S-EDCs? *Arch Toxicol.* 2020;94:2549–2557. Available from: https://doi.org/10.1007/s00204-020-02800-8.
89. EFSA CONTAM Panel. Risk for animal and human health related to the presence of dioxins and dioxin-like PCBs in feed and food. *EFSA J.* 2018;16:e05333. Available from: https://doi.org/10.2903/j.efsa.2018.5333.

90. EFSA CONTAM Panel. Scientific opinion on polybrominated diphenyl ethers (PBDEs) in food. *EFSA J.* 2011;9:2156. Available from: https://doi.org/10.2903/j.efsa.2011.2156.
91. EFSA. Perfluorooctane sulfonate (PFOS), perfluorooctanoic acid (PFOA) and their salts. Scientific opinion of the panel on contaminants in the food chain. *EFSA J.* 2008;6:653. Available from: https://doi.org/10.2903/j.efsa.2008.653.
92. EFSA. Opinion of the scientific panel on contaminants in the food chain (CONTAM) related to hormone residues in bovine meat and meat products. *EFSA J.* 2007;5:510. Available from: https://doi.org/10.2903/j.efsa.2007.510.
93. FAO/WHO JECFA. Evaluation of certain veterinary drug residues in food. *World Health Organ Tech Rep Ser.* 2000;893 (i–viii):1–102.
94. Jeong S-H, Kang D, Lim M-W, Kang CS, Sung HJ. Risk assessment of growth hormones and antimicrobial residues in meat. *Toxicol Res.* 2010;26:301–313. Available from: https://doi.org/10.5487/TR.2010.26.4.301.
95. Caldas ED, Tressou J, Boon PE. Dietary exposure of Brazilian consumers to dithiocarbamate pesticides—a probabilistic approach. *Food Chem Toxicol.* 2006;44:1562–1571. Available from: https://doi.org/10.1016/j.fct.2006.04.014.
96. Jensen BH, Andersen JH, Petersen A, Christensen T. Dietary exposure assessment of Danish consumers to dithiocarbamate residues in food: a comparison of the deterministic and probabilistic approach. *Food Addit Contam Part A Chem Anal Control Expo Risk Assess.* 2008;25:714–721. Available from: https://doi.org/10.1080/02652030701858262.
97. Sang C, Sørensen PB, An W, Andersen JH, Yang M. Chronic health risk comparison between China and Denmark on dietary exposure to chlorpyrifos. *Environ Pollut.* 2020;257:113590. Available from: https://doi.org/10.1016/j.envpol.2019.113590.
98. EFSA CEF Panel. Scientific opinion on the risks to public health related to the presence of bisphenol A (BPA) in foodstuffs. *EFSA J.* 2015;13:3978. Available from: https://doi.org/10.2903/j.efsa.2015.3978.
99. EFSA CEP Panel, Silano V, Barat Baviera JM, et al. Update of the risk assessment of di-butylphthalate (DBP), butyl-benzyl-phthalate (BBP), bis(2-ethylhexyl)phthalate (DEHP), di-isononylphthalate (DINP) and di-isodecylphthalate (DIDP) for use in food contact materials. *EFSA J.* 2019;17:e05838. Available from: https://doi.org/10.2903/j.efsa.2019.5838.
100. Patisaul HB, Jefferson W. The pros and cons of phytoestrogens. *Front Neuroendocrinol.* 2010;31:400–419. Available from: https://doi.org/10.1016/j.yfrne.2010.03.003.
101. Bhagwat, S., Haytowitz, D.B., Holden, J.M., USDA database for the flavonoid content of selected foods, release 3. US Dep. Agric. Beltsville, MD, USA 159, 2011.
102. EFSA CONTAM Panel. Scientific opinion on the risks for public health related to the presence of zearalenone in food. *EFSA J.* 2011;9:2197. Available from: https://doi.org/10.2903/j.efsa.2011.2197.
103. EFSA. Cadmium dietary exposure in the European population. *EFSA J.* 2012;10:2551. Available from: https://doi.org/10.2903/j.efsa.2012.2551.
104. JRC, Bopp, Nepelska S, Halder M, Munn, S. M. Expert survey on identification of gaps in available test methods for evaluation of endocrine disruptors. *Publ Office Eur Union.* 2017;. Available from: https://doi.org/10.2760/844100.
105. Kolesnyk S. Risk assessment of chemicals in food and in silico toxicology. Short overview. *Inter Collegas.* 2017;4.
106. Schneider M, Pons J-L, Labesse G, Bourguet W. In silico predictions of endocrine disruptors properties. *Endocrinology.* 2019;160:2709–2716. Available from: https://doi.org/10.1210/en.2019-00382.
107. Zuang, V., Dura, A., David, et al., 2021. Non-animal methods in science and regulation – EURL ECVAM Status Report 2020-EUR 30553 EN. Publications Office of the European Union. <https://doi.org/10.2760/719755>.
108. US EPA. Use of high throughput assays and computational tools in the endocrine disruptor screening program. *Fed Regist.* 2015;80:35350–35355.

Chapter 20

Antimicrobial resistance and antimicrobial residues in the food chain

Jeffrey T. LeJeune[1,2], Alejandro Dorado Garcia[1,3] and Francesca Latronico[1,4]

[1]*Food and Agriculture Organization of the United Nations (FAO), Rome, Italy,* [2]*Food Systems and Food Safety Division (ESF), Rome, Italy,* [3]*Animal Production and Health Unit (NSA), Rome, Italy,* [4]*Joint Centre for Codex Standards and Zoonotic Diseases (CJW), Rome, Italy*

Abstract

The presence of antimicrobial-resistant microorganisms and antimicrobial residues in food are biological and chemical hazards leading to public health and food safety risks. The continued use, misuse, or abuse of antimicrobials in animals and plants, is one of the main drivers of the increased detection of antimicrobial resistance (AMR) in the food and agriculture sectors. Changes in agri-food production systems such as improved hygiene, biosecurity, and management practices are essential in minimizing the need to use antimicrobials, preventing further emergence and spread of AMR. Given the complex nature of the AMR problem, a multidisciplinary and collaborative One Health approach is needed, enabling the adoption of good practices by all actors across the food chain.

Keywords: Emerging contaminants; foodborne antimicrobial resistance; antimicrobial-resistant microorganisms; antimicrobial residues in food; biosecurity; One Health approach

20.1 Introduction

Antimicrobials, those pharmaceutical agents used to kill or inhibit the growth of microorganisms, have contributed to the treatment and control of infectious diseases in humans, animals, and plants. However, bacteria can become no longer susceptible to the effects of these drugs, a process known as antimicrobial resistance (AMR). In his acceptance speech for the Noble Prize in 1945 Alexander Fleming, the scientist credited with the discovery of the first antimicrobial (penicillin) to achieve widespread clinical use in humans, warned against the development of AMR.[1] Today we know that AMR is a result of mutations and exchange of genetic material, a process that occurs naturally, but it is exacerbated when the bacteria are under the selective pressure of the presence of antimicrobials, whether it is in a human or animal host, or in the environment.

The threat of AMR has reached pandemic proportions. The current global estimate of 700,000 annual deaths due to AMR is expected to explode to over 10 million per year by 2050 if action is not taken.[2] The primary drivers for AMR emergence include antimicrobial use in humans and animals, and potentially the contamination of the environment with antimicrobial residues. The problem of AMR is further exacerbated by the ease and speed with that resistant organisms can spread as a result of anthropological and socioeconomic factors.[3]

The One Health concept that the health of humans, animals, and the environment are inextricably interconnected is most relevant for the problem and solutions of AMR. There are multiple routes by which people can become infected with antimicrobial-resistant microorganisms or get exposed to antimicrobial residues, but under this One Health paradigm, food and water play a critical role in pathogen transmission from animals and plants because it presents a route of inoculation from these sources directly into the mouths of people.

20.2 The lifecycle of antimicrobials in food production

Antimicrobials are a key tool to maintain animal and plant health and ensure food security. They are used in agriculture to treat, control and prevent diseases in terrestrial and aquatic animals and also in plants. In the 1940s, during a nutrition feeding experiment in chickens it was discovered purely by accident, that birds consuming antimicrobials grew faster,[4] yielding an economic advantage. This finding was rapidly adopted and the use of antimicrobial growth promoters was widely incorporated throughout agriculture production systems. Some of the antimicrobials used to enhance animal growth and improve feed efficiency are considered drugs important

Present Knowledge in Food Safety. DOI: https://doi.org/10.1016/B978-0-12-819470-6.00045-7

for human medicine (e.g., tetracyclines, aminoglycosides),[5] and in some cases are even the same antimicrobials considered as a last resort in the treatment of complicated/multidrug-resistant bacterial infections in humans (e.g., colistin).[6] Antimicrobials are also used for the treatment of diseases of bees and bacterial and fungal infections in plants.[7,8]

Because of the absence of record-keeping, the exact amount of antimicrobials used on the global scale for agricultural and veterinary purposes, including aquaculture, is not precisely known. Current models estimate that, globally, by 2030, antimicrobial use for livestock and poultry production purposes will increase an additional 10% over 2017 baseline estimates, while use in aquaculture will increase by 33% during this same timeframe.[9,10] This increase in demand is driven by an increasing need for more food to meet the needs of the growing population's demand for animal-based protein sources. Parallel to this increase in use is a predicted increase in the development and spread of AMR with concatenated losses in animal production due to treatment failures and continued food contamination with antimicrobial-resistant bacteria, and impacts on food exports and international trade.[11] This pathway of increasing risk to the food chain is not unexpected: In 1969 a committee established by the UK concerning the development of AMR attributed much of the problem to the widespread use of antimicrobials for the sole purpose of growth promotion.[12]

Changes in agricultural production systems that further prevent the emergence and spread of infectious diseases—such as enhanced hygiene, biosecurity, and nutrition and management practices—can result in improved animal health, minimizing the need for antimicrobials. With optimal health and management, it is possible to achieve, without the routine use of antimicrobials for disease prevention, control, or growth promotion purposes, comparable levels of production as observed with the routine use of these medicines, but without the negative impacts associated with antimicrobial use.[13] However, antimicrobials are still used for growth promotion in many countries, despite continued calls for a prohibition of their use for this purpose by civil society, some national governments, and several international organizations.[6] The continued, and increasing, use of antimicrobials in food production means that antimicrobial residues and antimicrobial-resistant organisms—two distinctly different hazards—will continue to present as potential hazards in food.

20.3 Antimicrobial residues in foods

Following antimicrobial administration to animals, either via the feed or water, or through other routes (e.g., intravenous, intramuscular, intra-mammary, and topical), the distribution and metabolism of the drug are dependent upon a number of factors including the drug, the route of administration, the dose, the species and health status of the animal, and particularly for fish, the environmental temperature. Antimicrobials may concentrate in specific tissues such as the site of injection, in fat, in the liver, or in the kidneys. Antimicrobials and their metabolites are then, over time, excreted in the urine, feces, and milk. They may also be incorporated into eggs of chickens fed antimicrobials. Antimicrobials, notable antibiotics, have also been directly applied to meats, produce and milk post-harvest in attempts to limit food spoilage and increase shelf life, an application that is now illegal in many countries but may continue to occur [14–16]

Many regulatory authorities have adopted maximum residue limits that are permissible for antimicrobials in various tissues in different tissue types or foods. Ideally, these limits are informed by formal risk assessments and in alignment with international food standards (Codex Alimentarius) supported by recommendations of the FAO/WHO Joint Expert Committee on Food Additives. Following manufacturers' label instructions regarding the withdrawal period should result in compliance with these standards. At the end of the withdrawal period, significant amounts of antimicrobials should not remain in the animal. Therefore if in compliance with regulatory guidelines at the time of harvest, no food should contain antimicrobial residues at levels considered hazardous. Thus if regulations are followed, even previously treated animals should be virtually "antibiotic-free," yet consumers remain confused about label claims.[17] However, an unacceptable level of residues in meat, milk, and eggs can occur when the withdrawal time is not enforced, if the drugs are used other than indicated (off label use), the metabolic state of the animal, or unintentional or accidental exposure to the drug, such as feeding error or contamination carry-over in feed processing.

Foods of plant origin can become contaminated with antimicrobials because of direct application or unintentional exposure from the soil, soil amendments such as manure, or water used for irrigation, albeit at low concentrations.[18] Likewise, contamination of honey can be a result of the treatment of bees, bees feeding on contaminated food, or potentially from environmental contamination.[19] The primary mechanism to control the presence of residue of veterinary antimicrobials in foods is for producers to follow label instructions, notably adhering to preslaughter withdrawal periods.

The consumption of foods contaminated with antimicrobial residues in food can have multiple deleterious consequences on human health. First, acute or chronic toxicity could be a problem. Certain antimicrobials, such as chloramphenicol and nitrofurantoin, have been banned from use in food-producing animals because of known fetal and carcinogenic effects, for the two drugs respectively, even at very low levels.[20,21] More well-known, and potentially more prevalent, are allergic or hypersensitivity reactions among sensitive individuals who consume products contaminated with trace amounts of antimicrobials. Penicillin in milk is the classic example, being first reported in 1956.[22] More recently, there is increasing concern that very low levels of antimicrobials, levels below toxic thresholds for humans and below those known to be inhibitory to bacteria, can, if consumed, lead to disruption of the normal intestinal microbial ecology and drive AMR in the intestines.[23] The antimicrobial residues causing the greatest concern, the levels of residues causing concern, and the clinical implications, if any, of such intestinal microbial dysbiosis are not yet fully understood.

20.4 Antimicrobial resistance along the food chain

Antimicrobial-resistant organisms can enter the food chain anywhere from production to the point of consumption. These organisms include not only zoonotic pathogens responsible for foodborne diseases in humans (nontyphoidal *Salmonella* spp. and *Campylobacter* spp.) but also include pathogens not typically harbored by food-producing animals which enter the food chain from contamination with human fecal material (*Shigella* spp. and *Salmonella typhi*). In addition, it is also possible that nonpathogenic organisms such as commensal flora of animals and humans, spoilage organisms, or environmental bacterial contaminants of food harbor AMR genes on mobile genetic elements. These organisms may serve as a reservoir of these genes in food and, subsequently, a source from which these genes can be exchanged with other gut microflora, including enteric pathogens, a process that may be enhanced when humans are treated with antimicrobials. The detection of previously undescribed AMR mechanisms, such as the plasmid-mediated colistin resistance first detected in *Escherichia coli* in pigs in 2015[24] is a public health concern as it could lead to the global expansion of resistance to last-resort antimicrobials in animals and humans.

The fraction of the number of deaths and illnesses caused by antimicrobial-resistant organisms each year that are a result of foodborne transmission has not been precisely defined. Clearly, food-producing animals carry antimicrobial-resistant pathogens, foods are contaminated with antimicrobial-resistant microorganisms, and there have been foodborne illnesses caused by antimicrobial-resistant bacteria.[25–29] There is a paucity of data on food contamination with antimicrobial-resistant organisms and foodborne illnesses they cause in low- and middle-income countries (LMICs). However, is likely that the prevalence of food contamination and incidence of foodborne illnesses caused by antimicrobial-resistant microorganisms is highly variable from region to region depending upon the standards of food safety, the prevalence of AMR in the population of food-producing animals, and their environment, as well as control measures in place for infection control and antimicrobial use in human populations.[30] In one recent molecular study, approximately 20% of carriage of resistance genes among specific bacteria (i.e., genes responsible for extended-spectrum beta-lactamases in *E. coli*) among individuals in the community could be attributed to foodborne sources.[31]

20.5 Mitigation of antimicrobial resistance risks in food

By all accounts, the contamination of foods with antimicrobial residues and antimicrobial-resistant organisms, and the bigger public health threat posed by AMR in general, can be classified from a policy perspective as a "super wicked problem," a complex social problem that cannot be solved using previous linear thinking approaches because the problem itself is caused or exacerbated by interdependencies of other problems.[32] Moreover, the broader impacts and consequences of the problem are frequently dismissed to the point where resolution requires urgent action. Understanding and addressing the contributing factors and drivers of the problem are key to solving it. Super wicked problems often involve multiple diverse stakeholders with different opinions and priorities, who themselves contribute to the problem and at the same time are called to resolve it, without a central authority responsible for oversight.

Because of the complex nature and the multiple diverse drivers of AMR, the solutions to mitigate and reverse its impacts on the health of humans, animals, plants and the environment are unlikely to be resolved by the actions of any single group or organization working alone. Instead, the application of a One Health approach and express effort for all stakeholders in various disciplines (medicine, veterinary medicine, agriculture, environmental sciences, behavioral science, economics, etc.) and sectors (government, academia, private sector, civil society, etc.) to engage, communicate, coordinate and collaborate is essential to assess the costs and benefits of potential solutions, accounting for diverse priorities and perspectives of all stakeholders.[33] Moreover, enhancing diversity and leveraging the knowledge and experiences from multiple disciplines has the potential to better understand the problem and result in innovative, adaptive, and resilient approaches to arrive at holistic and sustainable solutions.

Control strategies to reduce the contamination of foods with antimicrobial-resistant organisms can be applied either during primary production, or during downstream stages of harvest, processing, packaging, transportation, storage, and preparation. Post-harvest interventions, although effective, are generally not specifically targeted toward antimicrobial-resistant organisms; however, the application of the basic principles of food hygiene and environmental sanitation, when applied correctly and consistently, will reduce contamination and cross-contamination of foods with all microbial hazards, including those that harbor AMR genetic elements. Slaughter hygiene, coupled with environmental hygiene, temperature control, and personal hygiene across all stages of the value chain from harvest to consumption requires attention by all actors in the value chain, from production to consumption. The likelihood that foods become contaminated at or after harvest with microbes resistant to antimicrobials depends upon both the prevalence and numbers of resistant microorganisms in the contamination source-on or in the live animal or food products, or in the environment where the food is processed. Proper environmental and personal hygiene among food workers can reduce cross-contamination, while live animals, either from their feathers, hide, hooves, or digestive tracts are considered the primary route of entry of pathogens into the food chain and a source of contamination of the food production environment. Thus measures specifically targeting the control of antimicrobial-resistant organisms during primary production are considered critical.

The frequency, diversity, and magnitude of contamination of live animals and plants with antimicrobial-resistant microorganisms are a reflection of their exposure to these contaminants and the selection pressure exerted by the use of antimicrobials. Thus control measures logically involve lowering exposure, achieved by adoption of best agricultural practices, and reducing selective pressure, through improved antimicrobial stewardship in agriculture.

Reaching these goals requires widespread and sweeping management transformations in the way food is produced though, in other words, behavior change. These changes involve increased emphasis and adoption of disease prevention strategies so that the need for antimicrobials to treat infections in animals is reduced and when antimicrobials are essential, they are used judiciously to minimize the selective pressure for AMR development. Interventions aimed at direct control of the use of antimicrobials in food-producing terrestrial and aquatic animals have been shown to reduce the presence of antibiotic-resistant bacteria in these animals.[34,35]

Multiple health promotion theories have been proposed to change behavior and many of these approaches have been applied to address the problem that AMR poses.[36] Effective, audience-targeted educational campaigns are important to raise awareness of the problem among individual and organizational stakeholders by providing information for those contemplating change and expanding societal support for an idea. But, unfortunately, with increased knowledge in itself, it is often inadequate to promote behavior change to alter antimicrobial use patterns.[37] Generally speaking, sustainable change occurs when stakeholders' attitudes and beliefs about the subject align more closely with a desired public health goal, and individuals are motivated to change because they perceive the change as important and beneficial, empowered with the skills to make the suggested changes, feel that their action can make a difference, and the environment is enabling for them to do so. Changing farm management practices and improving antimicrobial stewardship in agriculture production, may involve, changes to policies, regulations, and government oversight of the issue, such as ratification of guidelines limiting the use of antimicrobials for the sole use as growth promotion; and providing training on tools and adoption of best practices for disease preventions such as increased biosecurity, use of vaccination, improved nutrition, and other, non-antimicrobial, alternatives to enhance animal and plant health promotion.

Improved surveillance of antimicrobial residues and resistant organisms in foods provides evidence of the extent of the problem, allows for prioritization of risks, and, with systematic and longitudinal sampling, allows for measurement of progress towards the end goal of reducing AMR. Improved surveillance, especially in programs that integrate data from human, animal, plant, and environmental sectors in LMICs will advance the fight against AMR.[38] A major challenge facing widespread behavior change related to the control of AMR is infrastructure and economic barriers may limit opportunities to adopt changes, especially in LMICs. Therefore investments in incentives, training, laboratory capacity, surveillance, opportunities for observational learning, examples of economic feasibility, and other resources under various conditions can all provide an environment more enabling for the adoption of behavior changes to tackle AMR.

Antimicrobials are valuable tools to treat diseases in animals and plants. Their efficacy needs to be maintained for sustainable food production. Inappropriate use of antimicrobials in agriculture threatens the continued value as infections resistant to antimicrobials emerge. Moreover, the presence of veterinary drug residues and the increased pressure for the selection of antimicrobial-resistant microorganisms in food-producing animals, caused by inappropriate antimicrobial use, presents a food safety hazard. This challenge is best addressed by a coordinated and collaborative One Health approach involving multiple disciplines and multiple sectors. Due to global trade in food products and the proclivity of microbes to not respect geopolitical borders, action must be taken on a global scale to reduce this threat to the safety of the food supply and public health.

Disclaimer

The views expressed in this publication are those of the authors and do not necessarily reflect the views or policies of the Food and Agriculture Organization of the United Nations.

References

1. Fleming A. *Penicillin*. Stockholm: Nobel Lecture; 1945.
2. Review on Antimicrobial Resistance. Antimicrobial Resistance: Tackling a Crisis for the Health and Wealth of Nations. 2014. Available at https://amr-review.org/sites/default/files/AMR%20Review%20Paper%20-%20Tackling%20a%20crisis%20for%20the%20health%20and%20wealth%20of%20nations_1.pdf.
3. Collignon P, Beggs JJ, Walsh TR, Gandra S, Laxminarayan R. Anthropological and socioeconomic factors contributing to global antimicrobial resistance: a univariate and multivariable analysis. *Lancet Planet Health*. 2018;2(9):e398–e405.
4. Stokstad E, Jukes TH, Pierce J, Page Jr A, Franklin AL. The multiple nature of the animal protein factor. *J Biol Chem*. 1949;180:647–654.
5. WHO. *WHO List of Critically Important Antimicrobials for Human Medicine (WHO CIA List)*. World Health Organization; 2019.
6. Góchez D, Raicek M, Pinto Ferreira J, Jeannin M, Moulin G, Erlacher-Vindel E. OIE annual report on antimicrobial agents intended for use in animals: methods used. *Front Vet Sci*. 2019;6:317.
7. Reybroeck W, Daeseleire E, De Brabander HF, Herman L. Antimicrobials in beekeeping. *Vet Microbiol*. 2012;158(1):1–11.
8. Taylor P, Reeder R. Antibiotic use on crops in low and middle-income countries based on recommendations made by agricultural advisors. *CABI Agric Biosci*. 2020;1(1):1–14.
9. Schar D, Klein EY, Laxminarayan R, Gilbert M, Van Boeckel TP. Global trends in antimicrobial use in aquaculture. *Sci Rep*. 2020;10(1):21878.
10. Tiseo K, Huber L, Gilbert M, Robinson TP, Van Boeckel TP. Global trends in antimicrobial use in food animals from 2017 to 2030. *Antibiotics (Basel)*. 2020;9(12).
11. World Bank W. *Drug-Resistant Infections: A Threat to Our Economic Future*. World Bank; 2017.
12. Swann M.M., Joint Committee on the use of Antibiotics in Animal Husbandry and Veterinary Medicine. Report of the joint committee on the use of antibiotics in animal husbandry and veterinary medicine. 1969.
13. Jul P, et al. *Tackling antimicrobial use and resistance in pig production. Lessons learned in Denmark*. Rome: FAO and Denmark Ministry of Environment and Food; 2019:52.
14. Hassabo A, Eisa M, Ishag I, Osman S, Bushara I. Usage of antibiotic as milk preservative in the slums of Khartoum state. *J Anim Prod Adv*. 2012;2(2):138–141.
15. Vaughn RH, Stewart GF. Antibiotics as food preservatives. *JAMA*. 1960;174(10):1308–1310.
16. Eckert JW. *Control of postharvest diseases with antimicrobial agents. Post-Harvest Physiol Crop Preserv*. Springer; 1983:265–285.
17. Bowman M, Marshall KK, Kuchler F, Lynch L. Raised without antibiotics: lessons from voluntary labeling of antibiotic use practices in the broiler industry. *Am J Agric Econ*. 2016;98(2):622–642.
18. Pan M, Chu LM. Fate of antibiotics in soil and their uptake by edible crops. *Sci Total Environ*. 2017;599-600:500–512.
19. Kaufmann A, Kaenzig A. Contamination of honey by the herbicide asulam and its antibacterial active metabolite sulfanilamide. *Food Addit Contam*. 2004;21(6):564–571.
20. Settepani JA. The hazard of using chloramphenicol in food animals. *J Am Vet Med Assoc*. 1984;184(8):930–931.
21. Chain EPo Ci t F. Scientific opinion on nitrofurans and their metabolites in food. *EFSA J*. 2015;13(6):4140.
22. Bierlein K. Repeated anaphylactic reactions in a patient highly sensitized to penicillin; a case report. *Ann Allergy*. 1956;14(1):35–40.
23. Subirats J, Domingues A, Topp E. Does dietary consumption of antibiotics by humans promote antibiotic resistance in the gut microbiome? *J Food Prot*. 2019;82(10):1636–1642.
24. Liu YY, Wang Y, Walsh TR, et al. Emergence of plasmid-mediated colistin resistance mechanism MCR-1 in animals and human beings in China: a microbiological and molecular biological study. *Lancet Infect Dis*. 2016;16(2):161–168.
25. Hölzel CS, Tetens JL, Schwaiger K. Unraveling the role of vegetables in spreading antimicrobial-resistant bacteria: a need for quantitative risk assessment. *Foodborne Pathog Dis*. 2018;15(11):671–688.
26. Kimera ZI, Mshana SE, Rweyemamu MM, Mboera LEG, Matee MIN. Antimicrobial use and resistance in food-producing animals and the environment: an African perspective. *Antimicrobial Resist Infect Control*. 2020;9(1):37.
27. Singh AS, Nayak BB, Kumar SH. High prevalence of multiple antibiotic-resistant, extended-spectrum β-lactamase (esbl)-producing *Escherichia coli* in fresh seafood sold in retail markets of Mumbai, India. *Vet Sci*. 2020;7(2):46.
28. Brown AC, Grass JE, Richardson LC, Nisler AL, Bicknese AS, Gould LH. Antimicrobial resistance in Salmonella that caused foodborne disease outbreaks: United States, 2003–2012. *Epidemiol Infect*. 2017;145(4):766–774.
29. EFSA and ECDC. The European Union summary report on antimicrobial resistance in zoonotic and indicator bacteria from humans, animals and food in 2018/2019. *EFSA J*. 2021;18:6490.
30. Duarte ASR, Röder T, Van Gompel L, et al. Metagenomics-based approach to source-attribution of antimicrobial resistance determinants – identification of reservoir resistome signatures. *Front Microbiol*. 2021;11(3447).
31. Mughini-Gras L, Dorado-García A, van Duijkeren E, et al. Attributable sources of community-acquired carriage of *Escherichia coli* containing β-lactam antibiotic resistance genes: a population-based modelling study. *Lancet Planet Health*. 2019;3(8):e357–e369.
32. Littman J, Viens A, Silva DS. *The super-wicked problem of antimicrobial resistance. Ethics and Drug Resistance: Collective Responsibility for Global Public Health*. Cham: Springer; 2020.

33. WHO. *Taking A Multisectoral One Health Approach: A Tripartite Guide to Addressing Zoonotic Diseases in Countries.* Food & Agriculture Org; 2019.
34. Tang KL, Caffrey NP, Nóbrega DB, et al. Restricting the use of antibiotics in food-producing animals and its associations with antibiotic resistance in food-producing animals and human beings: a systematic review and meta-analysis. *Lancet Planet Health.* 2017;1 (8):e316–e327.
35. Wang Y, Xu C, Zhang R, et al. Changes in colistin resistance and mcr-1 abundance in *Escherichia coli* of animal and human origins following the ban of colistin-positive additives in China: an epidemiological comparative study. *Lancet Infect Dis.* 2020;20 (10):1161–1171.
36. Nutbeam D, Harris E, Wise W. *Theory in a Nutshell: A Practical Guide to Health Promotion Theories.* McGraw-Hill; 2010.
37. Pearson M, Chandler C. Knowing antimicrobial resistance in practice: a multi-country qualitative study with human and animal healthcare professionals. *Glob Health Action.* 2019;12(sup1):1599560.
38. WHO. *Integrated Surveillance of Antimicrobial Resistance in Foodborne Bacteria: Application of a One Health Approach: Guidance From the WHO Advisory Group on Integrated Surveillance of Antimicrobial Resistance (AGISAR)*; 2017.

Chapter 21

Climate change as a driving factor for emerging contaminants

Keya Mukherjee
Food Systems and Food Safety Division (ESF), Food and Agriculture Organization of the United Nations (FAO), Rome, Italy

Abstract

Climate change has multifaceted impacts on various biological and chemical contaminants found in both food and water, thereby increasing the risk of exposure to such hazards through our diets. Expansion of the global agrifood system and increased globalization of the food supply chains can amplify foodborne hazards along the way. This enhances the possibility of unsafe food produced on one side of the world having implications for public health and economic growth on the other side. A number of climate-vulnerable regions that are facing these food safety challenges lack adequate capacity to detect and manage foodborne illness outbreaks, making it difficult to mitigate damage to local economies and public health. This chapter illustrates how climate change affects some of the key food- and waterborne hazards and lays down some approaches that can be taken across the food and agricultural sector to tackle the global issue.

Keywords: Climate change; emerging contaminants; foodborne pathogens and parasites; algal blooms; heavy metals; mycotoxins; One Health

21.1 Introduction

Food links human health to our environment. To sustain a growing global population, enormous gains in food production have been made, but it has come at a tremendous cost to the environment. It is estimated that 34% of the total greenhouse gas emissions in 2015 (or 18 Gt CO_2 equivalent per year) came from our food systems.[1] Such emissions from agriculture are on the rise, propelled by increased global food demand and changes in food consumption patterns due to rising incomes in different regions. In addition, agriculture is increasingly putting pressure on our finite land and water resources. According to estimates,[2] nearly half of all cultivated land on the planet is devoted to growing staple crops (wheat, rice, maize, etc.) and 70% of freshwater worldwide is used by agriculture.[3]

In the coming decades, sustaining agricultural productivity to meet the growing demand for food that is safe for consumption will be more challenging due to climate change. Various environmental conditions induced by climate change have an impact on food availability,[4] as well as food safety,[5] all along the entire food chain starting from production through processing, storage, and distribution, right until the food is consumed. Unsafe food is unfit for consumption. With sufficient, affordable, nutritious, and safe food being key components of food security, climate change impacts on food safety are closely linked to food security.

Elevated temperatures, changes in water availability, deteriorating soil quality, extreme weather events, rising sea levels, and ocean acidification, among other factors, have serious implications for both biological and chemical contaminants in food by altering their occurrence and virulence. This increases the risk of human exposure to foodborne hazards.

21.1.1 Climate change increases the risk of exposure to foodborne contaminants

While global food chains, such as for sugar, cocoa, tea, and spices, have existed for centuries, today's supply chain landscape is more complex. It involves moving much larger quantities of commodities and at a greater speed between regions that are geographically very distant. Food distribution networks are vulnerable to extreme weather events, some of the obvious ones are floods, droughts, or fires. While it is arguably true that weather and natural disasters have always been unpredictable to some degree, climate change makes them even more difficult to predict. This impedes preparing in advance, causing economic losses as well as public health concerns by

Present Knowledge in Food Safety. DOI: https://doi.org/10.1016/B978-0-12-819470-6.00048-2

increasing the risks of human exposure to foodborne hazards. Moreover, increased globalization of food supply chains facilitates the amplification of foodborne hazards along the way, enhancing the chances that unsafe food produced in one country can affect consumers on the other side of the world. This is a major issue for populations living in countries that tend to import a majority of their food, for instance, small island developing states (SIDS).[6] Other vulnerable populations at risk of exposure to food safety hazards under climate change are the poor, especially from regions where malnutrition and food insecurity remain critical issues. Such areas also tend to have fewer resources for putting in place adequate climate change adaptation and mitigation measures. In addition to conflicts, prolonged droughts and hurricanes can make areas inhabitable for people, leading to migrations. Such displaced populations are also at a higher risk of not having enough access to safe food and water. Additionally, competition for limited resources, under climate change conditions and propelled by population growth, is leading to greater intrusion of humans into wildlife habitats increasing the risk of zoonotic diseases.

The effects of climate change on some key foodborne hazards are described below.

21.1.1.1 Foodborne pathogens and parasites

Rising temperatures and altered precipitation patterns, due to climate change, are expected to affect the geographic distribution and persistence of both foodborne pathogens and parasites. Higher incidences of infections by several foodborne pathogens, like *Salmonella* spp. and *Campylobacter* spp., in different parts of the world are linked to increasing temperatures.[7,8] Higher temperatures also favor greater pest growth and activity and therefore, influence contact between food and pathogen-carrying insects, like flies.[9]

Increased frequency and severity of extreme weather events, like hurricanes, cause recurring, widespread flooding which increases the risk of human exposure to waterborne diseases such as cholera. This is especially acute in areas where basic public infrastructure for hygiene and sanitation is inadequate.[9] Between 2000 and 2014, the number of cholera cases in East Africa increased by 50,000 and this was attributed to El Niño events. Strong El Niño events can cause severe droughts in areas with dry climates, bring intense flooding in wetter regions, and cause more hurricanes to form in the Pacific. Under rising global temperatures, El Niño events are expected to be more intense leading to major socioeconomic and health consequences.[10,11] An onset of El Niño conditions is suggested to play a role in the epidemiology of *Vibrio parahaemolyticus*, a marine pathogenic bacteria that cause foodborne illnesses through consumption of contaminated raw or insufficiently cooked seafood (crustaceans and mollusks). Geographic expansion of *V. parahaemolyticus* is leading to cases being reported from areas with few previous incidents, like Northern Europe and South America.[12] In addition, widespread marine pollutants like microplastics can contain waterborne pathogens, including *V. cholerae* and *V. parahaemolyticus*, as part of their "plastisphere".[13,14] With climate change altering ocean circulation patterns, the effects of this on the distribution of microplastics in the marine environment, and potentially on the spread of pathogenic bacteria, have yet to be investigated.[15]

Many foodborne parasites have complicated life cycles that transpire through multiple hosts. Climate change may affect the survival and transmission rates of parasites as well as the abundance and migration of reservoir hosts.[16] In addition, the dynamic relationships between parasites, hosts, and their environments are likely to either increase or decrease based on the sensitivity of both hosts and parasites to climate change. For instance, temperature influences the survival of viable *Giardia* cysts.[17] Warming temperatures are also predicted to alter the geographical distribution of waterborne *Schistosoma* sp., with the risk of infections expected to increase by 20% in most of East Africa.[18]

Excessive rainfall and flooding can overwhelm storm tanks in wastewater treatment plants allowing untreated wastewater overflows into waterways, affecting freshwater quality. Prolonged droughts, on the other hand, can put stress on the availability and usage of water in a given area. This can affect businesses, such as food processing plants, where sanitation measures may be reduced or restricted to compensate for the lack of sufficient water, thereby compromising food safety. Power outages, common during extreme weather events, affect the storage conditions of food in homes and retail stores.

Flooding in areas with animal farms where antibiotics are used also facilitates the spread of antibiotic-resistant bacteria into the surrounding environment. Recent evidence points to a potential association between rising temperatures and increased rates of antimicrobial resistance in human pathogens (*Escherichia coli*, *Klebsiella pneumonia*, and *Staphylococcus aureus*).[19,20] Various food- and waterborne pathogens are increasingly showing resistance to clinically important antibiotics, which is worrisome. These pathogens include *V. cholerae*, *Campylobacter* spp., *Listeria monocytogenes*, *Salmonella* spp., *E. coli*, and *Arcobacter* spp.[21–28]

21.1.1.2 Algal blooms

Algae are essential components of the aquatic ecosystem and produce more than half of the oxygen in the earth's atmosphere. Uncontrolled growth of algal species is termed as an algal bloom and this happens due to various environmental and anthropogenic conditions, occurring in both freshwater and marine ecosystems. An overabundance of nitrogen and phosphorus-rich fertilizer applications combined with more frequent and intense precipitation are among the factors leading to increased eutrophication and algal blooms in water bodies. When algal blooms die and decompose, they deplete the surrounding area of oxygen creating "dead" zones or hypoxic areas that cannot support marine life. This results in severe ramifications to the ecosystem in the area and massive economic losses to coastal communities. Today a large number of these "dead" zones are in major fishing areas.

Certain algal species produce marine toxins (phycotoxins) that can bioaccumulate in fish and shellfish. Consumption of such contaminated seafood constitutes the primary route for exposure to phycotoxins in humans. Exposure to marine toxins causes toxic syndromes with symptoms ranging from skin, eye or ear irritations to more severe reactions such as liver and kidney damage as well as gastrointestinal, cardiovascular, respiratory, and neurological conditions.[29] Blooms by both toxic and nontoxic algal species can also affect the availability of potable drinking water in an area.[30,31]

Ciguatera poisoning is a major foodborne illness that affects the tropical and sub-tropical regions of the Pacific Ocean, Indian Ocean, and the Caribbean Sea. Extreme weather events, like hurricanes, can impact reef ecosystems that can lead to an increased abundance of *Gambierdiscus* spp. responsible for ciguatera poisoning.[32] Climate change is not only affecting the frequency of storms and hurricanes but also causing the sea surface temperatures to rise. Both of these factors affect the distribution and proliferation of ciguatoxin and make the occurrence of ciguatera poisoning less predictable, underscoring the need for monitoring and surveillance in affected regions.[32] There are also increased incidences of ciguatera poisoning in places with no prior history of such illnesses. This is concerning as some of the affected regions have no risk management measures in place to manage the outbreak putting public health at risk.[5,32]

21.1.1.3 Heavy metals

While metals like cadmium, lead, mercury, and arsenic[1] occur naturally in the environment (soil, air, and water), they can be found in food either due to their presence in the environment or as a result of anthropogenic activities and contamination of food during production and storage. On land, climate change can cause heavy precipitation events and flooding[33,34] in mining areas that can lead to overflows from toxic waste sites, altering the distribution of contaminants in the area, and compromising food and water quality. Rising soil temperatures and flooding events are expected to facilitate the uptake of heavy metals (like arsenic) by staple crops such as rice, which is known to accumulate heavy metals in the plant as well as the grain.[35,36] This threatens the health of millions of people, mainly in low- to middle-income countries (LMIC).

The bioaccumulation of methylmercury in the aquatic food chain is a major concern, as ocean and freshwater fish are generally the largest source of foodborne mercury exposure in humans. Methylmercury has toxic impacts on the nervous, immune, and digestive systems of humans and also poses a threat to the development of a child *in utero* as well as in early life. Thawing of permafrost regions due to rising temperatures can release large quantities of historically trapped mercury into our aquatic ecosystems where the inorganic form of mercury gets methylated. According to Schuster et al.,[37] the Arctic permafrost contains 1,656 $\pm$ 962 Gg of mercury, which is approximately ten times the total amount of mercury released by anthropogenic sources to date. Warmer ocean temperatures are linked to the methylation of inorganic mercury[38] and increased bioaccumulation of methylmercury in commercial fish species, such as the European seabass (*Dicentrarchus labrax*).[39] One of the reasons for this accumulation can be attributed to the higher metabolism of predatory fish species in warmer waters which can lead to greater consumption of prey.[40]

21.1.1.4 Mycotoxins

Mycotoxins are toxic metabolites produced by various fungi that contaminate staple and cash crops (maize, nuts, rice, and spices). Therefore, contamination by mycotoxins can pose a barrier to international trade and cause economic losses. Dietary exposure to mycotoxins can occur either directly through the consumption of contaminated food, or indirectly via the consumption of products derived from animals raised on contaminated feed. Aflatoxin, ochratoxin A, fumonisin, deoxynivalenol, and zearalenone are the five most significant mycotoxins in agriculture.[41] These toxins exert toxic effects on the kidneys, as well as on the reproductive, immune, and gastrointestinal systems.[42,43] Exposure to mycotoxins increases the risk for liver cancer.[44] There is growing evidence that exposure to fumonisins and aflatoxins or a combination of both can cause stunting in children.[45–49] Children suffering from high exposure to aflatoxins can also suffer from micronutrient deficiencies, making this a dual food safety and malnutrition concern.[50] In addition, these toxins are generally not eliminated by food processing, compounding the seriousness of the issue.[51] Due to the serious health effects of such toxins, their presence in crops is limited by regulatory limits in most countries.

Some of the important factors that influence mycotoxin production—temperature, relative humidity, and crop damage by pests—are all affected by climate change. With global warming making cooler temperate zones conducive to agriculture, agricultural pests and fungal species can spread to new habitats. Increased growth and geographic niche expansion of insects, as seen more recently with desert locusts from the Horn of Africa, can be attributed to conditions created by climate change.[52] When insects feed on plants, fungal spores carried by the insects can be introduced inside plants. Moreover, damage from insects can cause stress in plants, making them more susceptible to fungal infections.

There are reports of migration of mycotoxins into areas with no history of prior contamination.[53–55] Some of these regions lack the capacity for outbreak management making it difficult to curtail damage to the local economies and public health. In addition, increases in temperatures are expected to cause a shift in the types of mycotoxins produced by any given fungal species in a certain area, that is, from those that are currently dominant to other related compounds. For instance, while zearalenone was once the more common mycotoxin found in infected maize in the United States of America, deoxynivalenol has emerged as the dominant mycotoxin recently. *Fusarium graminearum* is the causal species for the formation of both mycotoxins.[54] Poor post-harvest conditions for drying, storage, and transportation facilities under climate change conditions are also increasing the risk of exposure to aflatoxins and ochratoxin A.

21.2 Conclusion

The complexity of our food system combined with the varied impacts climate change has on the different foodborne hazards shows that this is a multidisciplinary issue that requires the engagement of stakeholders from all sectors of the "farm-to-fork" continuum, including the public health sector — a One Health approach. Stronger collaboration among the relevant stakeholders will bring about holistic solutions to issues as well as help to focus expertise and resources in a way that prevents duplication of efforts. This is especially useful in countries where financial and human resources are scarce. Foodborne illnesses are usually under-reported and this makes it difficult to estimate the foodborne disease burden and conduct timely detection of outbreaks. Systematic monitoring of food and environmental contaminants, and surveillance of foodborne diseases in conjunction with transparent data sharing with all relevant partners are important to quickly identify potential foodborne risks in food chains. Combining all this with technology-driven traceability in the food chain will facilitate tracking and removing of contaminated food products before it becomes a public health issue.

Disclaimer

The views expressed in this publication are those of the author(s) and do not necessarily reflect the views or policies of the Food and Agriculture Organization of the United Nations.

Endnotes

[a]Arsenic, though a metalloid, is often considered collectively under heavy metals.

References

1. Crippa M, Solazzo E, Guizzardi D, Monforti-Ferrario F, Tubiello FN, Leip A. Food systems are responsible for a third of global anthropogenic GHG emissions. *Nat Food.* 2021;2:198–201. Available from: https://doi.org/10.1038/s43016-021-00225-9.
2. Ritchie, H. Half of the world's habitable land is used for agriculture. Our World in Data. 2019. Accessed May 22 2022. Available from: https://ourworldindata.org/global-land-for-agriculture.
3. Food and Agriculture Organization of the United Nations (FAO). *Water for Sustainable Food and Agriculture A Report Produced for the G20 Presidency of Germany.* Rome: FAO; 2017. Available from: https://www.fao.org/3/i7959e/i7959e.pdf.
4. Wang R, Rejesus RM, Tack JB, Balagtas JV, Nelson AD. Quantifying the yield sensitivity of modern rice varieties to warming temperatures: evidence from the Philippines. *Am J Agric Econ.* 2021;1–22. Available from: https://doi.org/10.1111/ajae.12210.
5. FAO. *Climate change: unpacking the burden on food safety. Food Safety and Quality Series No. 8.* Rome: FAO; 2020. Available from: https://doi.org/10.4060/ca8185en.
6. FAO. The future of food safety. First FAO/WHO/AU International Food Safety Conference Addis, 12–13 February 2019. Available from: http://www.fao.org/3/ca4289en/CA4289EN.pdf.
7. Kuhn KG, Nygård KM, Guzman-Herrador B, et al. *Campylobacter* infections expected to increase due to climate change in northern Europe. *Sci Rep.* 2020;10:13874. Available from: https://doi.org/10.1038/s41598-020-70593-y.
8. Lake IR. Food-borne disease and climate change in the United Kingdom. *Environ Health.* 2017;16:117. Available from: https://doi.org/10.1186/s12940-017-0327-0.
9. Intergovernmental Panel on Climate Change (IPCC). Climate change 2007: impacts, adaptation and vulnerability. In: Parry ML, Canziani OF, Palutikof JP, van der Linden PJ, Hanson CE, eds. *Contribution of Working Group II to the Fourth Assessment Report of the Intergovernmental Panel on Climate Change.* Cambridge, United Kingdom of Great Britain and Northern Ireland and New York: Cambridge University Press; 2007. Available from: https://www.ipcc.ch/report/ar4/wg2/.
10. Moore SM, Azman AS, Zaitchik BF, et al. El Niño and the shifting geography of cholera in Africa. *Proc Natl Acad Sci USA.* 2017;114(17):4436–4441. Available from: https://doi.org/10.1073/pnas.1617218114.
11. Wang B, Luo X, Yang Y-M, et al. Historical change of El Niño properties sheds light on future changes of extreme El Niño. *Proc*

Natl Acad Sci USA. 2019;116(45):22512–22517. Available from: https://doi.org/10.1073/pnas.1911130116.

12. Abanto M, Gavilan RG, Baker-Austin C, Gonzalez-Escalona N, Martinez-Urtaza J. Global expansion of Pacific Northwest *Vibrio parahaemolyticus* sequence type 36. *Emerg Infect Dis*. 2020;26(2):323–326. Available from: https://doi.org/10.3201/eid2602.190362.
13. Kirstein IV, Kirmizi S, Wichels A, et al. Dangerous hitchhikers? Evidence for potentially pathogenic *Vibrio* spp. on microplastic particles. *Mar Environ Res*. 2016;120:1–8. Available from: https://doi.org/10.1016/j.marenvres.2016.07.004.
14. Zettler ER, Mincer TJ, Amaral-Zettler LA. Life in the "plastisphere": microbial communities on plastic marine debris. *Environ Sci Technol*. 2013;47(13):7137–7146. Available from: https://doi.org/10.1021/es401288x.
15. Welden NA, Lusher AL. Impacts of changing ocean circulation on the distribution of marine microplastic litter. *Integr Environ Assess Manag*. 2017;13(3):483–487. Available from: https://doi.org/10.1002/ieam.1911.
16. Short EE, Caminade C, Thomas BN. Climate change contribution to the emergence or re-emergence of parasitic diseases. *Infect Diseases Res Treat*. 2017;. Available from: https://doi.org/10.1177/1178633617732296.
17. Brunn A, Fisman DN, Sargeant JM, Greer AL. The influence of climate and livestock reservoirs on human cases of Giardiasis. *EcoHealth*. 2019;16:116–127. Available from: https://doi.org/10.1007/s10393-018-1385-7.
18. McCreesh N, Nikulin G, Booth M. Predicting the effects of climate change on *Schistosoma mansoni* transmission in eastern Africa. *Parasites Vectors*. 2015;8:4. Available from: https://doi.org/10.1186/s13071-014-0617-0.
19. MacFadden DR, McGough SF, Fisman D, Santillana M, Brownstein JS. Antibiotic resistance increases with local temperature. *Nat Clim Change*. 2018;8(6):510–514. Available from: https://doi.org/10.1038/s41558-018-0161-6.
20. McGough SF, MacFadden DR, Hattab MW, Molbak K, Santillana M. Rates of increase of antibiotic resistance and ambient temperature in Europe: a cross-national analysis of 28 countries between 2000–2016. *bioRxiv*. 2018;. Available from: https://doi.org/10.1101/414920.
21. Dengo-Baloi LC, Sema-Baltazar CA, Manhique LV, Chitio JE, Inguane DL, Langa JP. Antibiotics resistance in El Tor *Vibrio cholerae* 01 isolated during cholera outbreaks in Mozambique from 2012 to 2015. *PLoS One*. 2017;12(8):e0181496. Available from: https://doi.org/10.1371/journal.pone.0181496.
22. Elmali M, Can HY. Occurrence and antimicrobial resistance of *Arcobacter* species in food and slaughterhouse samples. *Food Sci Technol*. 2017;37(2):280–285. Available from: https://doi.org/10.1590/1678-457x.19516.
23. Henderson JC, Herrera CM, Trent MS. AlmG, responsible for polymyxin resistance in pandemic *Vibrio cholerae*, is a glycyltransferase distantly related to lipid a late acyltransferases. *J Biol Chem*. 2017;292(51):21205–21215. Available from: https://doi.org/10.1074/jbc.RA117.000131.
24. Olaimat AN, Al-Holy MA, Shahbaz HM, et al. Emergence of antibiotic resistance in *Listeria monocytogenes* isolated from food products: a comprehensive review. *Compr Rev Food Sci Food Saf*. 2018;17(5):1277–1292. Available from: https://doi.org/10.1111/1541-4337.12387.
25. Poirel L, Madec JY, Lupo A, et al. Antimicrobial resistance in *Escherichia coli*. *Microbiology Spectr*. 2018;6(4). Available from: https://doi.org/10.1128/microbiolspec.ARBA-0026-2017.
26. Van Puyvelde S, Pickard D, Vandelannoote K, et al. An African *Salmonella typhimurium* ST313 sublineage with extensive drug-resistance and signatures of host adaptation. *Nat Commun*. 2019;10(1):4280. Available from: https://doi.org/10.1038/s41467-019-11844-z.
27. Wang X, Biswas S, Paudyal N, et al. Aniktibiotic resistance in *Salmonella typhimurium* isolates recovered from the food chain through national antimicrobial resistance monitoring system between 1996 and 2016. *Front Microbiol*. 2019;10:985. Available from: https://doi.org/10.3389/fmicb.2019.00985.
28. Wang Z, Zhang M, Deng F, et al. Emergence of multidrug-resistant *Campylobacter* species isolates with a horizontally acquired rRNA methylase. *Antimicrob Agents Chemother*. 2014;58(9):5405–5412. Available from: https://doi.org/10.1128/AAC.03039-14.
29. Grattan LM, Holobaugh S, Morris JG. Harmful algal blooms and public health. *Harmful Algae*. 2016;57:2–8. Available from: https://doi.org/10.1016/j.hal.2016.05.003.
30. Lee, J.J. Driven by climate change, algae blooms behind Ohio water scare are new normal. *National Geographic*. 6 August 2014. https://www.nationalgeographic.com/news/2014/8/140804-harmful-algal-bloom-lake-erie-climate-change-science/.
31. Villacorte LO, Tabatabai SAA, Anderson DM, Amy GL, Schippers JC, Kennedy MD. Seawater reverse osmosis desalination and (harmful) algal blooms. *Desalination*. 2015;360:61–80. Available from: https://doi.org/10.1016/j.desal.2015.01.007.
32. FAO and World Health Organization (WHO). Report of the Expert Meeting on Ciguatera Poisoning. Rome, 19–23 November 2018. *Food Safety and Quality*. 2020;9. Available from: https://doi.org/10.4060/ca8817en.
33. Knutson T, Camargo SJ, Chan JCL, et al. Tropical cyclones and climate change assessment: part I: detection and attribution. *Bull Am Meteorol Soc*. 2019;100(10):1987–2007. Available from: https://doi.org/10.1175/BAMS-D-18-0189.1.
34. Knutson T, Camargo SJ, Chan JCL, et al. Tropical cyclones and climate change assessment: part II. Projected response to anthropogenic warming. *Bull Am Meteorol Soc*. 2019;. Available from: https://doi.org/10.1175/BAMS-D-18-0194.1.
35. Muehe EM, Wang T, Kerl CF, Planer-Friedrich B, Fendorf S. Rice production threatened by coupled stresses of climate and soil arsenic. *Nat Commun*. 2019;10(1):4985. Available from: https://doi.org/10.1038/s41467-019-12946-4.
36. Neumann RB, Seyfferth AL, Teshera-Levye J, Ellingson J. Soil warming increases arsenic availability in the rice rhizosphere. *Agric Environ Lett*. 2017;2(1):170006. Available from: https://doi.org/10.2134/ael2017.02.0006.
37. Schuster PF, Schaefer KM, Aiken GR, et al. Permafrost stores a globally significant amount of mercury. *Geophys Res Lett*. 2018;45(3):1463–1471. Available from: https://doi.org/10.1002/2017GL075571.
38. Dijkstra JA, Buckman KL, Ward D, Evans DW, Dionne M, Chen CY. Experimental and natural warming elevates mercury concentrations in estuarine fish. *PLoS One*. 2013;8(3):e58401. Available from: https://doi.org/10.1371/journal.pone.0058401.
39. Maulvault AM, Custodio A, Anacleto P, et al. Bioaccumulation and elimination of mercury in juvenile seabass (*Dicentrarchus*

labrax) in a warmer environment. *Environ Res*. 2016;149:77–85. Available from: https://doi.org/10.1016/j.envres.2016.04.035.

40. Schartup AT, Thackray CP, Qureshi A, et al. Climate change and overfishing increase neurotoxicant in marine predators. *Nature*. 2019;572(7771):648–650. Available from: https://doi.org/10.1038/s41586-019-1468-9.
41. Lee HJ, Ryu D. Worldwide occurrence of mycotoxins in cereals and cereal-derived food products: public health perspectives of their co-occurrence. *J Agric Food Chem*. 2017;65(33):7034–7051. Available from: https://doi.org/10.1021/acs.jafc.6b04847.
42. International Agency for Research on Cancer (IARC). Improving public health through mycotoxin control. In: *IARC Scientific Publication No. 158*. Lyon, France; 2012. https://publications.iarc.fr/Book-And-Report-Series/Iarc-Scientific-Publications/Improving-Public-Health-Through-Mycotoxin-Control-2012.
43. Alshannaq A, Yu JH. Occurrence, toxicity, and analysis of major mycotoxins in food. *Int J Environ Res Public Health*. 2017;14(6). Available from: https://doi.org/10.3390/ijerph14060632.
44. Liu Y, Wu F. Global burden of aflatoxin-induced hepatocellular carcinoma: a risk assessment. *Environ Health Perspect*. 2010; 118(6):818–824. Available from: https://doi.org/10.1289/ehp.0901388.
45. IARC. Mycotoxin control in low- and middle- income countries. In: *IARC Working Group Report No. 9*. Lyon, France; 2015. https://publications.iarc.fr/Book-And-Report-Series/Iarc-Working-Group Reports/Mycotoxin-Control-In-Low--And-Middle-income-Countries-2015
46. Watson S, Moore SE, Darboe MK, et al. Impaired growth in rural Gambian infants exposed to aflatoxin: a prospective cohort study. *BMC Public Health*. 2018;18(1):1247. Available from: https://doi.org/10.1186/s12889-018-6164-4.
47. Chen C, Mitchell NJ, Gratz J, et al. Exposure to aflatoxin and fumonisin in children at risk for growth impairment in rural Tanzania. *Environ Int*. 2018;115:29–37. Available from: https://doi.org/10.1016/j.envint.2018.03.001.
48. Chen C, Riley RT, Wu F. Dietary fumonisin and growth impairment in children and animals: a review. *Compr Rev Food Sci Food Saf*. 2018;17(6):1448–1464. Available from: https://doi.org/10.1111/1541-4337.12392.
49. FAO and WHO. *Evaluation of certain contaminants in food. Eighty-Third Report of the Joint FAO/WHO Expert Committee on Food Additives*. Rome: FAO; 2016. Available from: https://apps.who.int/iris/handle/10665/254893.
50. Watson S, Chen G, Sylla A, Routledge MN, Gong YY. Dietary exposure to aflatoxin and micronutrient status among young children from Guinea. *Mol Nutr Food Res*. 2016; 60(3):511518. Available from: https://doi.org/10.1002/mnfr.201500382.
51. Bullerman LB, Bianchini A. Stability of mycotoxins during food processing. *Int J Food Microbiol*. 2007;119(1-2):140–146. Available from: https://doi.org/10.1016/j.ijfoodmicro.2007.07.035.
52. Salih AAM, Baraibar M, Mwangi KK, Artan G. Climate change and locust outbreak in east Africa. *Nat Clim Change*. 2020;10:584–585. Available from: https://doi.org/10.1038/s41558-020-0835-8.
53. Balbus JM, Boxall AB, Fenske RA, McKone TE, Zeise L. Implications of global climate change for the assessment and management of human health risks of chemicals in the natural environment. *Environ Toxicol Chem*. 2013;32(1):62–78. Available from: https://doi.org/10.1002/etc.2046.
54. Miller JD. Changing patterns of fungal toxins in crops: challenges for analysts. *J AOAC Int*. 2016;99(4):837–841. Available from: https://doi.org/10.5740/jaoacint.16-0110.
55. Miller JD. Mycotoxins in food and feed: a challenge for the twenty-first century. In: Li D-W, ed. *Biology of Microfungi*. Cham, Switzerland: Springer International; 2016:469–493.

Chapter 22

Emerging mycotoxin risks due to climate change. What to expect in the coming decade?

Angel Medina
Environment and Agrifood Theme, Cranfield University, Cranfield, United Kingdom

Abstract
Mycotoxins are toxic secondary metabolites produced by fungi that are commonly found in the environment. They can cause disease and death in humans and other animals through the ingestion of contaminated products. Environmental conditions are the most important factors affecting the production of these mycotoxins and thus climate change (CC) is becoming a paramount force shaping mycotoxins contamination worldwide and mycotoxicological research. In this chapter, we review the latest literature regarding the most important toxins, the most important effects of environmental condition in the production of such toxins by several fungal species, and the current science on the changes driven by CC. Moreover, we discuss on the need for analytical techniques that can help us to cope with these changes forecasted for the coming years.

Keywords: Climate change; analysis; mycotoxins; legislation; fungi; forecast

22.1 Important mycotoxins in food

Mycotoxins are a diverse group of toxic secondary metabolites produced by fungi that are commonly found in the environment. They are commonly synthesized as secondary metabolites by certain filamentous fungi that colonize crops throughout the food chain and are capable of causing disease and death in humans and in animals through the ingestion of contaminated products. Six major classes of mycotoxins have been defined: aflatoxins, trichothecenes, fumonisins, zearalenone, ochratoxins, and ergot alkaloids. They are produced by different species of fungi, with many of these species being able to produce more than one mycotoxin simultaneously. The more important mycotoxins are produced by fungus from *Aspergillus*, *Fusarium*, and *Penicillium* species, commonly associated with foods commodities (see Table 22.1).

22.2 Factors affecting the production of mycotoxins

When it comes to the most important factors affecting the production of these mycotoxins, a paramount role is played by environmental conditions. Indeed, it is their major adaptability to different environments, very harsh for other microorganisms, what allow these fungal species to grow and thrive in food products containing low amounts of water, very acidic pH values, or high concentrations of NaCl, among others.

A major force transforming the environmental conditions that these fungal species will suffer in the field, and other steps of different food chains worldwide, is climate change (CC). The last report of the Intergovernmental Panel on Climate Change (IPCC) revealed that warming of the climate system is unequivocal, with many of the observed changes over the last few decades being unprecedented.[1] Indeed, more recent forecasts of CC prediction are suggesting different scenarios of temperature and CO_2 changes depending on socio-economic behavior, which could lead to increases from +3.5°C to 7.5°C and from 500 to 1200 ppm.[2] Such CCs could have significant impacts on the life cycles of toxigenic fungi and modify host–resistance and host–pathogen interactions.

On the one side, it has been described that plant pathogens are predicted to move globally and change the diversity of diseases and pests invading staple crops with both

Present Knowledge in Food Safety. DOI: https://doi.org/10.1016/B978-0-12-819470-6.00053-6

TABLE 22.1 Important food commodities for which EU legislative limits exist in relation with the contamination by different fungal species.

	Aflatoxins	Ochratoxin A	Fusarium mycotoxins[a]	Patulin	Ergot alkaloids
Main producing fungal species					
	Aspergillus flavus, A. parasiticus	*Penicillium verrucosum, P. nordicum, Aspergillus steynii, A. westerdijkiae, A. niger, A. carbonarius*	*Fusarium graminearum, F. culmorum, F. avenaceum, F. verticillioides, F. temperatum, F. proliferatum*	*Penicillium expansum*	*Claviceps purpurea*
Food commodities					
Cereals	+	+	+		+
Maize	+	+	+		
Baby foods	+	+	+	+	
Groundnuts	+	+			
Nuts	+	+			
Spices	+	+			
Dried fruit		+		+	
Coffee		+			
Cocoa		+			
Grape juice		+			
Fruit	+	+		+ (Apple)	
Milk, egg	+				
Wine		+			

[a]*Includes: trichothecenes, fumonisins, and zearalenone.*

economic and social costs.[3,4] Recent predictions by Bebber et al.[5] suggest that pests and diseases are migrating to the poles at the rate of 3–5 km/year, with the diversity of pest populations becoming significantly changed.[6] Pest damage of ripening crops, especially cereals, can predispose them to infection/colonization by mycotoxigenic fungal pathogens leading to increased mycotoxin contamination.

Second, this could have significant impacts on the resilience of different toxigenic species and their ability to produce mycotoxins. Most importantly could modify the current pattern of mycotoxins produced by these species leading to the prevalence of different toxins in the coming years.[7] Environmental stress has been shown to have significant consequences for secondary metabolite production, especially mycotoxins.[8,9] Therefore it is very important to know the biodiversity of species that can contaminate a crop and the changes in environmental conditions that can occur in a CC scenario.

22.3 Predicted climate changes and their potential effects on future mycotoxins contamination

Based on the present available data, atmospheric concentrations of CO_2 are expected to double or triple (from 350–400 to 800–1200 ppb) in the next 25–50 years. Thus different regions worldwide will be impacted by the increases in temperature of 2°C–5°C. It is important to highlight that these changes will not be homogeneous around the globe. On the contrary, some regions will be specific hotspots where these changes can be more dramatic, and in others, the changes will be mild. This is coupled with elevated CO_2 (800–1200 ppm) and more frequent drought episodes, which in turn might have a profound effect on mycotoxigenic fungi and mycotoxin production.[2]

Under such scenario, there is a real possibility of new and emerging combinations of mycotoxins getting into the food/feed chains.[7]

In the last 5 years, evidence is accumulated to show the potential effect of these environmental changes on several fungal species. The information points out to some positive impacts for particular fungus-crop systems. A good example is the potential reduction of *Penicillium expansum* because of the increased temperature and hence the reduced threat from patulin in pome fruits.[10]

However, most literature points out to potential increase in mycotoxins problems in the coming decades.

It has been predicted that in Europe in the next 50–100 years due to the forecasted environmental changes leading to hotter and dryer weather, *Aspergillus flavus* may outcompete *Aspergillus carbonarius*, with aflatoxins (AFs) becoming a greater risk than ochratoxin A (OTA). This shift is toxicologically important as aflatoxins exhibit a much greater toxicity and are considered a carcinogen for humans.

The growth patterns of *Fusarium* species such as *F. graminearum* and *F. verticillioides* have been shown to change under interacting CC-related conditions in vitro.[7]

Other studies on ochratoxigenic species such as *A. carbonarius*, *Aspergillus westerdijkiae*, *Aspergillus steynii*, and *Penicillium verrucosum* on different matrices have also examined effects of CC-related abiotic factors on growth and toxin contamination.[11–14] Overall, the growth rates of the *Aspergillus* section *Circumdati* and *Nigri* species were not affected by CC-related interacting abiotic factors. However, in vitro experiments, both on coffee-based media and on stored coffee beans, suggested that there was a stimulation of OTA production (e.g., *A. westerdijkiae*), while for other species (e.g., *A. carbonarius*) there was a reduction in toxin contamination.[13]

In addition, Cervini et al. studied strains of *A. carbonarius* isolated from grapes and showed that while growth was relatively unaffected on grape-based media by CC-related interacting factors (+4°C, 400 vs 1000 ppm CO_2, water stress), toxin production was stimulated for some strains, and this was confirmed with an increase in relative gene expression of cluster genes involved in toxin biosynthesis.[14]

Furthermore, the effect of increases in temperature and CO_2 concentration was recently studied in *Alternaria alternata* strains by Siciliano et al.[15] They used four different strains, three different host plants, and six different combinations of increased temperature range (day/night) and CO_2. The results showed that mycotoxin production was very variable and influenced by strain and host plant factors. In particular, tenuazonic acid was the most frequent mycotoxin produced among the four toxins quantified.

Among all mycotoxigenic species, *A. flavus* is the one that has received more attention with regard to the impacts of existing and forecasted CC-related abiotic factors on aflatoxin contamination of maize. Studies in vitro and on harvested maize grain have shown that growth is relatively unaffected, while AFB_1 is significantly stimulated when exposed to CC-related abiotic factors compared to existing conditions (30 vs 37°C; 400 vs 1000 ppm CO_2; 0.995 vs 0.93 water activity). This was supported by the increased relative expression of biosynthetic genes involved in toxin production.[16] Further transcriptomic data analyses showed changes in secondary metabolite gene clusters (aflatoxins, cyclopiazonic acid), universal regulators, sugar transporters, and other stress-related pathways. Garcia-Cela et al.[17] has recently described that there are not only changes in the amounts of toxins produced but also a shift in production under elevated CO_2 conditions making the toxins appear earlier. This compendium of information about *A. flavus* suggests that there are changes in amounts produced, changes in the time that the fungus needs to produce the toxin but also suggest switches in secondary metabolite production patterns under CC conditions.[17–19]

Overall, the available information suggests that positive and deleterious effects might happen due to the effects of CC-interacting abiotic factors. The data suggest that the effects are more important on specific individual mycotoxigenic species.

For some species, survival under the forecasted conditions will be more difficult and we might find a geographical shift. Others might remain in the same geographical location or even expand their presence to new areas with related implication in monitoring programs and legislative limits or adaptation. Other potential scenario will be for those species that need to produce new or a different battery of secondary metabolites to cope with the new environment thus changing those molecules that are currently toxicologically important for human health and hence prompting for a need of new regulations or analysis for such emerging mycotoxins.

22.4 Current analytical techniques and future analytic challenges

Since their discovery, many different analytical techniques have been used to analyze mycotoxins, such as thin-layer chromatography, high-performance liquid chromatography in combination with different detectors (e.g., fluorescence, diode array, ultraviolet), gas chromatography (GC) in combination with electron capture detectors, liquid chromatography coupled with mass spectrometry (LC–MS), liquid chromatography-tandem mass spectrometry (LC–MS/MS), and gas chromatography-tandem mass spectrometry (GC–MS/MS) for mycotoxin analysis, with chromatographic techniques being dominant.[20]

However, because of their high price per sample and the need of expensive equipment and trained personnel, the usage of these techniques has normally been restricted to research environments or to big corporations.

In most key places along the food chain, other techniques that, although are not as precise and sensitive, offer good results in terms of identifying the levels of a toxin or sometimes mixtures of toxins are used as they allow for a quick evaluation without the need of extra investment. In this category, the mayor techniques are enzyme-linked immunosorbent assay, lateral-flow devices, and biosensors based upon biological binding elements, such as antibodies (immunosensors and immunoassays) and also aptamers (aptasensors) that have proved to be useful tools for mycotoxins identification.[20,21] A recent interesting development that could be also adapted in industrial setups is the use of hyperspectral imaging.

22.5 Emerging mycotoxins threats under climate change conditions

Although in the last decade different definitions have been used,[22] defined them as mycotoxins neither routinely determined, nor legislatively regulated; however, the evidence of their incidence is rapidly increasing. As described earlier, the forecasted climatic conditions will differentially affect the growth of different fungi (and the formation of different toxins) in different parts of the world, and hence some populations will be more affected than others, but mycotoxins will certainly remain a global challenge.

There have been important advances in LC-MS and LC-MS/MS analytical techniques to study small molecules in food commodities. Currently some methods can measure and quantify more than 500 different molecules in a single run.[23] Thus the information that we have now about the contamination of certain commodities in not only restricted to the legislated toxins as it was years ago.

Thus these new comprehensive datasets point out the importance on some other fungal metabolites, which although exhibit lower toxicity that the current legislated toxins are constantly present in some food commodities of their incidence has been increasing during the recent years. In this group of metabolites, we could mention some fungal metabolites as enniatins, beauvericin, moniliformin, fusaproliferin, fusaric acid, culmorin, butenolide, sterigmatocystin, emodin, mycophenolic acid, alternariol, alternariol monomethyl ether, and tenuazonic acid (see Ref.[24] for an extended review).

Similarly, analytical advances led to the discovery of the so-called "masked mycotoxins." This term refers to the plant phase-II conjugated metabolites of mycotoxins that are normally produced in the natural detoxification process in plants (see Ref.[25] for an extensive review). They pose serious safety concerns as they can accumulate in the edible parts of contaminated crops and thus could be a relevant part of the total mycotoxins load since they can be reverted to the original free-mycotoxin molecule due to the digestive and intestinal processed in humans and animals.

Hence, a further potential effect of environmental changes will be the potential effects on the plant metabolism and thus the way they detoxify mycotoxins and also the susceptibility of the plants to be colonized by the mycotoxigenic fungal pathogenes (viz. drought makes maize more susceptible to *Aspergillus* colonization).

Unfortunately, there are no studies looking to the effects that environmental changes might have to the detoxification of mycotoxins by different plant species.

22.6 Research gaps and future directions

As highlighted previously, inevitably, under the forecasted climatic conditions, food safety will be jeopardized in different ways.

Taking the current knowledge in consideration can be found that there are several research gaps and areas that require future developments (Fig. 22.1).

More work needs to be developed to fully understand the potential changes in the production of current mycotoxins and other emerging toxic compounds that might happen in the coming years under CC conditions. Are the ratios of secondary metabolites going to change? Which mycotoxins will be toxicologically important for humans and animals in the future?

Another research gap is the effect that CC will have on free versus plant-bound (masked) mycotoxins. Will CC modify the plant metabolism and hence increase or

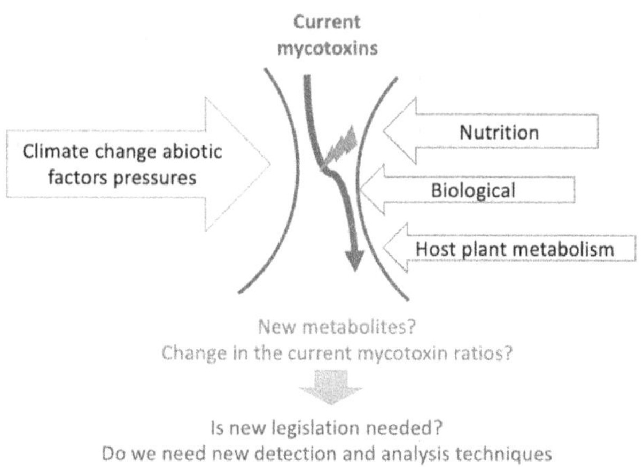

FIGURE 22.1 Pictorial representation of the effects that different factors will have on mycotoxins contamination under the forecasted environmental conditions.

reduce the proportion of these molecules accumulated in the edible parts of the crops?

Some recent data indicate that there are certain mechanisms of fungal adaptation to the new environmental conditions, that sometimes make fungal strains to acclimatize to the new conditions modifying their ability to produce different secondary metabolites. In some cases, this results in increases in toxin production. However, only few papers have been published in this area and thus work needs to be done so we can fully understand the risks to come.

Taking into consideration all the above, an important question arises about whether all these changes will make existing legislation out of step with potential problems for consumers around the globe. How can we get prepared for this? This is an area that needs much more work in the coming years.

Will the current analytical methods be able to cope with the rapid changes in years to come? While chromatographic methods with spectrophotometric detector can be easily adjusted to detect different molecules, the rapid test used by industry and producers might not be able to cope with such rapid changes. Both immunoassays and aptasensors technologies relay in extensive research to redevelop the assays for different molecules. This will be even more challenging when the new molecules that we need to detect are very closely related with previous toxins. Thus the ability of farmers, small industries, and other actors in the food chain to develop reliable and accurate mycotoxin tests to protect the final consumers will depend on multiple factors for which answers are not clear yet, including: the ability of our current legislation to adapt to these potential molecule shifts (not only kind of toxin also geographical location), our ability to predict these changes and the development of extensive research in the detection area to adapt the tests to the new requirements. Surely a big challenge that as a society we will need to tackle in the near future.

References

1. Intergovernmental Panel on Climate Change (IPCC). Climate Change 2014: Synthesis Report. Contribution of Working Group I, II, III to the IPCC's Fifth Assessment Report of the Intergovernmental Panel on Climate Change. Geneva, Switzerland, Intergovernmental Panel on Climate Change (IPCC). Available online: <https://www.ipcc.ch/report/ar5/syr/>; 2020 Accessed 27.09.20.
2. Gidden MJ, Riahi K, Smith SJ, et al. Global emissions pathways under different socioeconomic scenarios for use in CMIP6: a dataset of harmonized emissions trajectories through the end of the century. *Geosci Model Dev Discuss (GMDD)*. 2018;1–42. Available from: https://doi.org/10.5194/gmd-2018-266.
3. Medina A, Rodriguez A, Sultan Y, Magan N. Climate change factors and *A. flavus*: effects on gene expression, growth and aflatoxin production. *World Mycotoxin J*. 2015;8:171–179.
4. Bebber DP, Gurr SJ. Crop-destroying fungal and oomycete pathogens challenge food security. *Fungal Gen Biol*. 2015;74:62e64.
5. Bebber DP, Ramotowski MAT, Gurr SJ. Crop pests and pathogens move poleward in a warming world. *Nat Clim Change*. 2013;3:985e988.
6. Crespo-Perez V, Regniere J, Chuine I, Rebaudo F, Dangles O. Changes in the distribution of multispecies pest asemblages affect levels of crop damage in warming tropical Andes. *Glob Change Biol*. 2015;21:82e96.
7. Medina A, Gilbert MK, Mack BM, et al. Interactions between water activity and temperature on the *Aspergillus flavus* transcriptome and aflatoxin B1 production. *Int J Food Microbiol*. 2017;256:36–44.
8. Medina, A., Rodriguez, A., Magan, N.. Changes in environmental factors driven by climate change: effects on the ecophysiology of mycotoxigenic fungi. In: Botana, L.M., Sainz, M.J. (Eds.), Climate Change and Mycotoxins. Walter De Gruyter, Berlin, 2015.
9. Schmidt-Heydt M, Parra R, Geisen R, Magan N. Modelling the relationship between environmental factors, transcriptional genes and deoxynivalenol mycotoxin production by two *Fusarium* species. *J R Soc Interface*. 2011;8:117e120.
10. Paterson RRM, Lima N. Further mycotoxin effects from climate change. *Food Res Int*. 2011;44:2555–2566.
11. Abdelmohsen S, Verheecke-Vaessen C, Garcia-Cela E, Medina A, Magan N. Solute and matric potential stress on *Penicillium verrucosum*: impact on growth, gene expression and ochratoxin A production. *World Mycotoxin J*. 2020;13:345–353.
12. Akbar A, Medina A, Magan N. Resilience of *Aspergillus westerdijkiae* strains to interacting climate-related abiotic factors: effects on growth and ochratoxin A production on coffee-based medium and in stored coffee. *Microorganisms*. 2020;8:1268.
13. Akbar A, Medina A, Magan N. Impact of interacting climate change factors on growth and ochratoxin A production by *Aspergillus* section *Circumdati* and *Nigri* species on coffee. *World Mycotoxin J*. 2016;9:863–874.
14. Cervini C, Gallo A, Piemontese L, et al. Effects of temperature and water activity change on ecophysiology of ochratoxigenic *Aspergillus carbonarius* in field-simulating conditions. *Int J Food Microbiol*. 2020;315:108420.
15. Siciliano I, Berta F, Bosio P, Gullino ML, Garibaldi A. Effect of different temperatures and CO_2 levels on Alternaria toxins produced on cultivated rocket, cabbage and cauliflower. *World Mycotoxin J*. 2017;10:63–71.
16. Medina A, Gonzalez-Jartin JM, Sainz MJ. Impact of global warming on mycotoxins. *Curr Opin Food Sci*. 2017;18:76–81.
17. Garcia-Cela E, Verheecke-Vaessen C, Gutierrez-Pozo M, et al. Unveiling the effect of interacting forecasted abiotic factors on growth and aflatoxin B1 production kinetics by *Aspergillus flavus*. *Fungal Biol*. 2021;125(2):89–94.
18. Medina A, Akbar A, Baazeem A, Rodriguez A, Magan N. Climate change, food security and mycotoxins: do we know enough? *Fungal Biol Rev*. 2017;31:143–154.
19. Perrone G, Ferrara M, Medina A, Pascale M, Magan N. Toxigenic fungi and mycotoxins in a climate change scenario: ecology,

genomics, distribution, prediction and prevention of the risk. *Microorganisms*. 2020;8(10):1496.

20. Tittlemier SA, Brunkhorst J, Cramer B, et al. Developments in mycotoxin analysis: an update for 2019–2020. *World Mycotoxin J.* 2021;14(1):3–26.
21. Tittlemier SA, Cramer B, Dall'Asta C, et al. Developments in mycotoxin analysis: an update for 2017–2018. *World Mycotoxin J.* 2019;12(1):3–29.
22. Vaclavikova M, Malachova A, Veprikova Z, Dzuman Z, Zachariasova M, Hajslova J. 'Emerging' mycotoxins in cereals processing chains: changes of enniatins during beer and bread making. *Food Chem.* 2013;136:750–757.
23. Sulyok M, Stadler D, Steiner D, Krska R. Validation of an LC-MS/MS-based dilute-and-shoot approach for the quantification of> 500 mycotoxins and other secondary metabolites in food crops: challenges and solutions. *Anal Bioanal Chem.* 2020;1–14.
24. Gruber-Dorninger C, Novak B, Nagl V, Berthiller F. Emerging mycotoxins: beyond traditionally determined food contaminants. *J Agric Food Chem.* 2017;65(33):7052–7070.
25. Berthiller, F., Maragos, C.M. and Dall'Asta, C. Chapter 1: Introduction to masked mycotoxins, in Masked Mycotoxins in Food: Formation, Occurrence and Toxicological Relevance, pp. 1–13. RSC Publishing. 2015 doi:10.1039/9781782622574-00001.

Chapter 23

Emerging contaminants in the context of food fraud

Simon Douglas Kelly

Food Safety and Control Laboratory, Joint FAO/IAEA Centre of Nuclear Techniques in Food and Agriculture, Department of Nuclear Sciences and Applications, International Atomic Energy Agency, Vienna International Centre, Vienna, Austria

Abstract

Food fraud may be defined as intentionally causing a mismatch between food product claims and food product characteristics. This deception is intentional and usually motivated by the economic gain on the part of the perpetrator. Obvious examples are substituting inferior products for foods with added-value quality claims, such as organic, free-range, wild-caught, natural, Protected Designation of Origin, and so on. In addition, rather than completely substituting a food product it may be extended or fortified with an adulterant, or mixture of adulterants, that ostensibly maintains or enhance its characteristics whilst reducing production costs. It is at this point that the interface between food fraud and food safety is often breached. The unintended (side) effects of food fraud may result in significant harm to human health, or at worst death if toxic or contaminated adulterants are unwittingly added to foods and beverages.

Keywords: Food fraud; food adulteration; emerging contaminants; food safety; food authenticity; food integrity

23.1 Introduction

Food fraud may be defined as intentionally causing a mismatch between food product claims and food product characteristics.[1] This deception is usually motivated by an economic gain on the part of the perpetrator. Obvious examples are substituting food products, which have added-value claims, for example organic, free-range, wild-caught, natural, Protected Designation of Origin,[2] etc., with similar but physically indiscernible products from a relatively inexpensive source for example conventional, barn-fed, farmed, nature-identical, non-appellation, etc, respectively. Rather than completely substituting a food product it may also be extended or fortified with an adulterant, or mixture of adulterants, that ostensibly maintains or artificially enhance its favored characteristics, whilst reducing production costs. It is predominantly at this point that the interface between food fraud and food safety may be breached with potentially disastrous consequences. The unintended side-effects of food fraud may result in significant harm to human health or at worst fatalities. The most notorious, and often cited, example in recent history was the ill-fated addition of melamine to milk powder to increase its apparent protein concentration and increase its trade value, which came to light in 2008. This adulteration caused renal failure in adults, and[3] infant mortality and subsequently led to widespread global recalls along milk powder supply chains affecting many different sectors of the food industry. It also had a significant financial impact and caused long-lasting damage to the reputation of the Chinese dairy and infant formula industries.[4] Food Fraud is a hidden activity and the sheer breadth and scale of unscrupulous activity, from individual market traders to international organized crime groups, makes it incredibly difficult to predict when food adulterants will manifest themselves as food contaminants. On the face of it, those carrying out food adulteration want to make a significant profit but wish to go undetected, and so it is not in their interests to produce unsafe adulterated foods that result in chronic illness or death. Nevertheless, insufficient knowledge and consideration of potential toxicity, human error, and/or human nature inevitably will result in cases where adulterants or substituents impact food safety, and this may be viewed through the lens of emerging contaminants in the context of food fraud.

23.2 Veterinary drugs residues in food

One aspect of food fraud that is often overlooked is its cyclical nature. Some events which grow into scandals

Present Knowledge in Food Safety. DOI: https://doi.org/10.1016/B978-0-12-819470-6.00052-4

may seem extraordinarily unique at the time. However, "There is nothing new in the world except the history you do not know" . This statement by Harry S. Truman certainly applies to food authenticity and fraud. For example, the Horsemeat scandal was identified by the routine meat speciation surveillance conducted by the Food Safety Authority of Ireland in January 2013. This increasingly rare activity of proactively monitoring retail food authenticity identified horsemeat in beef meat products sold in food outlets in the United Kingdom and the Republic of Ireland.[5] What is less well known, is that in 1948 there was a widespread undeclared substitution of horsemeat for beef in the United Kingdom.[6] At that time, it was claimed that up to 3 million people per week were buying horsemeat, but only 50% of those were knowingly buying it from licensed butchers at the post-war controlled price of one shilling per pound. The other 50% was being illegally sold fraudulently as 'black-market' beef steaks or veal through restaurants and non-licensed food outlets. This situation arose due to shortages of beef meat in post-war Britain and the significant price differences between bovine and equine carcasses. In the context of chemical contaminants, the 2013 horsemeat scandal revealed both the shortcomings in management and the hidden complexity of meat supply chains. The anti-inflammatory drug phenylbutazone was known to be present in horse carcasses illegally entering the food chain.[7] Once again, a fraudulent practice, which on the face of it appeared to only affect consumers by preventing them from making informed choices about the type of meat they were eating and with economic inconvenience associated with the substitution, became an unintended food safety issue due to the risks of ingesting medicated horsemeat not destined for food production. This prompted The European Commission to request the European Food Safety Authority and the European Medicines Agency to jointly assess the risk to consumers of residues of phenylbutazone in horse meat in the context of fraudulent practices.[8] It concluded that the likelihood of a consumer being both exposed to phenylbutazone residues and being susceptible to developing aplastic anemia was insignificant. Furthermore, the risks associated with eating residues of phenylbutazone on organ toxicity and carcinogenicity were considered to be very low due to infrequent exposure directly from horse meat or adulterated beef-based products. Nevertheless, the ramifications of the horsemeat scandal sent shockwaves through the food industry and led to the Elliott Review into the integrity and assurance of food supply networks.[9] Looking forward, the possibility of contaminants associated with horses with an unknown veterinary medicine history entering the human food chain uncontrolled remains a real risk. In all likelihood, this will still be due to inadequate animal welfare and traceability systems in some equine exporting countries, despite official controls and audits from importing countries. Figures from animal welfare advocacy groups claim that approximately 17,000 tons of horsemeat are imported into the EU and Switzerland on an annual basis.[10] Another intentionally deceptive action designed to provide the perpetrators with a competitive advantage was the undeclared use of the pesticide fipronil in the treatment of parasitic red mites on egg-laying chickens in 2017. The mite can lead to reduced egg-laying capacity and increased susceptibility to disease in hens. Critically fipronil is licensed for use as veterinary medicine to treat parasitic mites in dogs but not for use in animals or animal products intended for human consumption, such as chickens' eggs. The detection of fipronil residues in eggs in July 2017 led to millions of them being withdrawn from sale and destroyed across the European Union.[11] The illegal use of fipronil and the consequent contamination of eggs showed how rapid action can have a significant effect on outcomes when contaminants are detected in food. However, the scandal highlighted limitations in the risk assessments used by regulators to estimate prolonged exposure to consumers, which led to arguably unnecessary destruction of eggs.

23.3 Food adulteration with extraneous additives

The authenticity of dairy products is an age-old problem. The dilution and adulteration of liquid milk with water and other 'ingredients' has a long history. In some villages in the United Kingdom, the water pump in the market square is affectionately known as the "iron cow" referencing the alleged practice of diluting milk by market traders in the late 18th and early 19th centuries. This was often accompanied by a recipe to extend milk and fool the lactometer (a traditional instrument used to check the density and indicate the 'richness' and purity of milk). Common exogenous additives to hide the dilution and maintain the density and color of milk were sugar, salt, and caramel. Although this may seem rather trivial from a food safety perspective, these rather crude adulteration practices are still a daily fact of life in many developing countries and they pose a significant and potentially dangerous problem. This is reflected in milk as probably the second most adulterated food product globally, after olive oil.[12] For example, in 2014, Aziz and Khan reported on a survey of milk adulteration from retail outlets in Islamabad, Pakistan, that included 280 milk samples gathered throughout 1-year.[13] They found a range of chemical adulterants, but the most prevalent was carbonate (27%), followed, in order of decreasing incidence, by hydrogen peroxide (7%) and starch (5%). Added water, as an adulterant, was found in almost all samples (99% of buffalo milk and 88% of cows' milk). The average of added/extraneous water was found to be 36% and 25%, for buffalo and cows' milk respectively. This kind of activity does not go unnoticed and this was demonstrated through recent enforcement activity in Pakistan where 4000 L of adulterated milk was destroyed because detergents are often used to form emulsions with cheap vegetable oils and nitrogenous compounds, such as urea, added to increase the apparent protein content.[14] Extended bovine milk not only poses an immediate acute toxic threat due to the possible use of chemical preservatives such as formaldehyde but there is also a potential long-term chronic risk for lower concentrations or less harmful contaminants. Indeed, even if adulterants pose no short or long-term toxic effects on human health, diluted milk will potentially have a long-term negative impact on nutrition, especially among vulnerable groups such as infants and young children.[15]

23.4 Illegally produced or counterfeit alcohol

One of the most pervasive and potentially dangerous areas of fraud is the illicit trade in alcohol in which it has been estimated that nearly 26% of all alcohol consumed globally is counterfeit or from illegal production.[16] The problem of illicit alcohol is ubiquitous and exists in both developing and developed countries alike. It is often linked to organized crime and often has the worst attributes of counterfeiting due to the impact on human health caused by the use of cheap sources of inadequately distilled spirits, or industrial or denatured ethanol. Formulations, of denatured alcohol, which should be used as a solvent or fuel, intentionally contain 'contaminants' such as pyridine and/or methanol to prevent its recreational use. At the same time, these additives make denatured alcohol toxic and potentially fatal if consumed in large quantities.[17] Denatonium benzoate is often added as an aversive agent (bitterant known as Bittrex) to dissuade human consumption of even the smallest quantities. In addition, these additives are designed to be difficult to remove, however sodium hypochlorite, in the form of household bleach, is used to remove the Bittrex.[18] This process does not remove methanol, which is acutely toxic and has led to many serious neurological defects, kidney failure, blindness, and fatalities. The World Health Organization has tracked methanol poisonings involving illicit alcohol in Cambodia, the Czech Republic, Ecuador, Estonia, India, Indonesia, Kenya, Libya, Nicaragua, Norway, Pakistan, Turkey, and Uganda. Each of those instances involved 20–800 victims.[19]

23.5 Definitions and databases

In the many examples of food adulteration and fraud described above, some features represent the height of sophisticated adulteration to crude attempts or gross adulteration. However, the unintended side-effects resulting from the associated chemical contaminants can be a common feature that has an immediate and disastrous effect on human health, a longer-term chronic effect, or a cumulative deleterious effect on nutrition. Perhaps, surprisingly, there have been very few attempts to characterize the hazards associated with the fraudulent adulteration of foods. In 2018 a panel of experts in food safety and toxicology from the food industry, academia, and the US Food and Drug Administration developed a classification system for food adulterants based on their associated health hazards and applied it to 2970 records in the US Pharmacopeial Convention's food fraud database.[20] The main group of potentially hazardous adulterants was subdivided into four further groups including those that were likely to cause fatalities in "1a" through to "1d", which included adulterants that lacked sufficient safety information or regulatory authorization. The categorization aimed to provide a framework within which food fraud mitigation strategies could be developed predominantly by the food industry, where increasingly the responsibility lies to understand vulnerabilities and protect consumers and honest traders from fraud. Another interesting development in the characterization of adulterants is the FADB-CHINA, which is "A Molecular Level Food Adulteration Database in China Based on Molecular Fingerprint and Structural Similarity Prediction Expansion".[21] The open-access database permits the user to search for structural similarities between known adulterants and contaminants and potential analogs that can be used to a similar effect. The developers included significant amounts of information based on previously published research on pharmaceuticals, pesticides, veterinary drugs, industrial dyes, and industrial chemicals that had been added to food in violation of regulations because of their properties and relatively low cost. This constituted 26 related compound databases and lists, which were managed by authoritative international organizations or published in peer-reviewed journals. The database may be searched through specific adulterants or food types to obtain relevant information on potential contaminants. Database resources of this type highlight the plethora of ingredients and/or chemicals that may be added to food and are described as economically motivated adulteration. Consequently, this emphasizes the challenge in trying to identify emerging contaminants that may result from food fraud either directly or indirectly as we have seen above.

23.6 Early warning systems

Because food fraud can impact human health, and damage consumer trust and sectors or entire industries, it is essential that it is detected at an early stage. The development of food fraud early warning systems linked to trade data or other safety systems is a relatively recent concept that potentially could save lives and livelihoods. One such system was reported in 2016 and was based on a Bayesian Network (BN) algorithm linked to adulteration and fraud notifications reported in the European Union's "Rapid Alert System for Food and Feed (RASFF)" for the period between 2000 and 2013.[22] The BN algorithm was then used to 'predict' 88 food fraud notifications reported in RASFF in 2014. These validation steps correctly predicted 80% of food fraud types when similar events had been reported previously in RASFF. This success rate fell to 52% when the country of origin or the product-country combination had not been recorded before in the RASFF database. It was concluded that the model could assist risk managers and border control officers to decide which fraud type to check when importing products.

23.7 Research gaps and future directions

As shown in these fraud examples that lead to harmful contaminants in food, understanding the complexity of supply chains and points of vulnerability are paramount. Examination of the ease with which raw materials or ingredients can be substituted or extended will give some insight into the possibilities to adulterate and possible unintended contamination events. Unfortunately, the capacity for humans to make gross errors of judgment are infinite in terms of harmful compounds which may be unintentionally added to food. However, it is also clear that the practice of food adulteration has a long and repetitive history and as a consequence, it is worthwhile taking the time to perform an in-depth assessment of the major factors influencing a food product's inherent vulnerabilities. The importance of proactively screening foods in the retail marketplace for contaminants and adulterants cannot be overstated. One area of analytical research that is emerging as a powerful tool to screen for emerging chemical contaminants resulting from food fraud is non-targeted analysis (NTA). In this approach a range of low resolution spectroscopic and high resolution mass spectrometric techniques are being applied, often in conjunction with chemometrics, without any prior knowledge of target adulterants that may unintentionally impact food safety. However, there are many challenges associated with the use of NTA by both industry and regulatory stakeholders. These include; an incomplete set of definitions of terms; the perennial problem of obtaining authentic foods, that contain all the inherent variability due to permissible industrial processing, to construct reference databases; consistent and widely accepted multivariate models that can also be used in a court of law for enforcement activities; and the legislative framework within which to set NTA.[23] Steps are being taken to address some of these challenges by standard-setting organizations, such as the US Pharmacopeia.[24] Suffice to say that non-targeted methods will not completely replace targeted methods on specific adulterants. Rather, non-targeted approaches will be used to rapidly screen foods, especially at points of entry in supply chains, where significant decisions about the passage of food at sea and airports are taken. Targeted testing for specific contaminants identified by NTA can often be confirmed by the same techniques for example, high-resolution mass spectrometry. However, when the point of use techniques such as hand-held vibrational spectroscopy is used, additional orthogonal testing with targeted chemical and or analytical confirmatory analysis will be required.[25] Ultimately, combining both NTA and targeted methods will facilitate rapid testing and save money. Undoubtedly there will be an increase in the use of rapid screening at ports of entry using NTA. Because food fraud is by definition a hidden activity its true extent and prevalence can only be the subject of speculation. It is to the detriment of any domestic food supply chain to ignore the potential hazards of food fraud, which can manifest itself as unintended unsafe food effects associated with existing or emerging contaminants. Ultimately, food fraud, illicit trade, and counterfeit agrochemicals undermine sustainable farming practices and threaten the delivery of safe and sustainable food supplies, which undermines progress toward the sustainable development goal of zero hunger.[26] Greater effort is needed to understand that food fraud and food safety are inherently linked and should not necessarily be separated and should be addressed together through the concept of 'Food Integrity'.

Disclaimer

The views expressed in this publication are those of the author and do not necessarily reflect the views or policies of the International Atomic Energy Agency

References

1. CWA17369. Cen workshop agreement: Authenticity and fraud in the feed and food chain -Concepts, terms, and definitions; 2019.
2. Kelblová H. The new community regulation on quality schemes for agricultural products and foodstuffs–obligations and opportunities for producers. *Procedia Econ Financ.* 2014;12:296–301.
3. Hau AKC, Kwan TH, Li PKT. Melamine toxicity and the kidney. *J Am Soc Nephrol.* 2009;20(2):245–250.

4. Maitiniyazi S, Canavari M. Understanding Chinese consumers' safety perceptions of dairy products: A qualitative study. *Br Food J.* 2021;123(5):1837–1852.
5. Brooks S, Elliott CT, Spence M, Walsh C, Dean M. Four years post-horsegate: An update of measures and actions put in place following the horsemeat incident of 2013. *NPJ Sci Food.* 2017;1(1):1–7.
6. British Pathe News. The British horsemeat scandal. <https://www.britishpathe.com/video/the-horsemeat-scandal>; 1948 Accessed 10.04.21.
7. Dodman N, Blondeau N, Marini AM. Association of phenylbutazone usage with horses bought for slaughter: A public health risk. *Food Chem Toxicol.* 2010;48(5):1270–1274.
8. Anon. Joint statement of EFSA and EMA on the presence of residues of phenylbutazone in horse meat. *EFSA J.* 2013;11(4):3190.
9. Elliott C. *Elliott Review into the Integrity and Assurance of Food Supply Networks-Final Report: A National Food Crime Prevention Framework.* London, UK: Department for Environment, Food & Rural Affairs Food Standards Agency; 2014.
10. Whitworth J. EU rejects call to stop Argentinian horsemeat imports. *Food Safety News.* 2021;. April 8.
11. Van der Merwe D, Jordaan A, Van den Berg M. *Case report: fipronil contamination of chickens in the Netherlands and surrounding countries. Chemical Hazards in Foods of Animal Origin.* Wageningen Academic Publishers; 2019:363–373.
12. Moore JC, Spink J, Lipp M. Development and application of a database of food ingredient fraud and economically motivated adulteration from 1980 to 2010. *J Food Sci.* 2012;77(4):R118–R126.
13. Aziz T, Khan H. A survey on milk adulteration at retail outlets of Islamabad, Pakistan. *Carpathian J Food Sci Technol.* 2014;6 (2):44–52.
14. Urdu Point. PFA disposes off 4000 liters adulterated milk. <https://www.urdupoint.com/en/pakistan/pfa-disposes-off-4000-liters-adulterated-milk-1165396.html>; 2021 Accessed 10.04.21.
15. Handford CE, Campbell K, Elliott CT. Impacts of milk fraud on food safety and nutrition with special emphasis on developing countries. *Compr Rev Food Sci Food Saf.* 2016;15(1):130–142.
16. Euromonitor International. *Size and Shape of the Global Illicit Alcohol Market.* London: Euromonitor International; 2018. Available from: https://www.tracit.org/uploads/1/0/2/2/102238034/illicit_alcohol__-_white_paper.pdf. Accessed 10.04.21.
17. World Health Organization. *Global Status Report on Alcohol and Health.* 2011. ISBN 978 92 4 156415 1.
18. Kwiatkowski A, Czerwicka M, Smulko J, Stepnowski P. Detection of denatonium benzoate (Bitrex) remnants in noncommercial alcoholic beverages by Raman spectroscopy. *J Forensic Sci.* 2014;59 (5):1358–1363.
19. Food Safety News. Methanol deaths in Costa Rica are likely due to alcohol fraud. <https://www.foodsafetynews.com/2019/07/methanol-deaths-in-costa-rica-are-likely-due-to-alcohol-fraud/>; 2019 Accessed 10.04.21.
20. Everstine K, Abt E, McColl D, et al. Development of a hazard classification scheme for substances used in the fraudulent adulteration of foods. *J Food Prot.* 2018;81(1):31–36.
21. FADB-CHINA. A molecular level food adulteration database in China based on molecular fingerprint and structural similarity prediction expansion. <http://www.rxnfinder.org/FADB-China/>; 2016 Accessed 10.04.21.
22. Bouzembrak Y, Marvin HJ. Prediction of food fraud type using data from rapid alert system for food and feed (RASFF) and bayesian network modelling. *Food Control.* 2016;61:180–187.
23. McGrath TF, Haughey SA, Patterson J, et al. What are the scientific challenges in moving from targeted to non-targeted methods for food fraud testing and how can they be addressed?–spectroscopy case study. *Trends Food Sci Technol.* 2018;76:38–55.
24. United States Pharmacopeia. *Appendix XVIII: Guidance on Developing and Validating Non-Targeted Methods for Adulteration Detection. Food Chemicals Codex.* 3rd supplement to 11th edition Rockville, MD: USP; 2019.
25. Gao B, Holroyd SE, Moore JC, Laurvick K, Gendel SM, Xie Z. Opportunities and challenges using non-targeted methods for food fraud detection. *J Agric Food Chem.* 2019;67(31):8425–8430.
26. TACIT. Transnational alliance to combat illicit trade: mapping the impact of illicit trade on the sustainable development goals, Chapter 1. <www.tracit.org/publications.html>; 2019 Accessed 10.04.21.

Chapter 24

Trends in risk assessment of chemical contaminants in food

Eleonora Dupouy

Food Systems and Food Safety Division (ESF), Food and Agriculture Organization of the United Nations (FAO), Rome, Italy

Abstract

A plethora of chemicals are used in agrifood production and exist in the environment that potentially may end up as contaminants in food. At low levels, humans are usually exposed to many synthetic chemicals in addition to those naturally occurring. This paper provides a brief overview of the main concepts, conventional and emerging approaches in chemical risk assessment that allow to face the challenges related to the potential exposure to foodborne chemicals and cope with data scarcity paving practical ways for addressing the emerging contaminants in the context of food safety regulation. It highlights also the research gaps and future directions. Understanding the principles and approaches of toxicological risk assessment is important for the policy-makers and regulatory competent authorities, and also for key actors in the food supply chain, such as food producers, food manufacturers, and food processors.

Keywords: Emerging contaminants; chemical risk assessment; risk perception; food safety regulation

24.1 Introduction

A plethora of chemicals are used in agri-food production and exist in the environment that potentially may end up as contaminants in foods. Contaminants can enter the food at any point along the food chain: during production, harvesting, manufacturing, packaging, distribution and may originate from a variety of sources, such as environment (water, soil, air), processing under certain conditions, migration from packaging materials, etc. At low levels, humans are exposed usually to many synthetic chemicals in addition to those naturally occurring for which there would be no expectations for any appreciable negative health outcomes. The purpose of risk assessment is to understand the risks associated with a particular food safety hazard, including the nature of adverse health effects (known and potential), such as hepatotoxicity, neurotoxicity, carcinogenesis, etc., estimate the risk in terms of the probability of occurrence and severity of health effects, identify the population at risk (general, children, pregnant women, etc.), and clarify uncertainties in the available data (limited toxicological data, exposure estimates, etc.).

Regardless of good practices applied by food business operators, complete avoidance of contaminants in food is not feasible due to their occurrence in the environment (soil, water). Dietary exposure to low levels of undesired non-intended chemicals in food is unavoidable. There is always some risk of toxic effects either due to the unintended chemical contamination, overconsumption of food, displaying an allergy, or other unpredictable individual sensitivity following the food ingestion. However, although foods may contain contaminants or naturally occurring toxins, the incidence of chemical foodborne adverse health effects is rather low and rare which may be explained by the levels of exposure well below the safety threshold and by the natural protective processes and repair mechanisms acting in the body. Potential adverse health effects caused by chemicals may include genotoxic effects that may lead to either mutagenicity, teratogenicity, or carcinogenicity, and non-genotoxic effects that may include functional or morphological changes, allergy, immunotoxicity, neurotoxicity, cytotoxicity, nephrotoxicity, hepatotoxicity, reproductive and developmental toxicity, etc. A substance usually displays more than one adverse effect, among which one is most significant and critical. Unless high dietary exposure of humans to certain chemicals is identified and quantified, a challenge remains linking the adverse health effects and a specific chemical.

The purpose of risk assessment is to understand the risks associated with a particular food safety hazard, including the nature of adverse health effects (known and

Present Knowledge in Food Safety. DOI: https://doi.org/10.1016/B978-0-12-819470-6.00046-9

potential), estimate the risk in terms of probability of occurrence and severity of adverse health effects, identify the population at risk (general, children, pregnant women, etc.), and uncertainties related to the available data, such as limited toxicological data, food consumption, exposure estimates, etc. Current regulatory practice is based on a hazard-based approach to quantify chemicals' risk combined with risk-based management to limit the exposure of humans and of the environment to acceptable levels. The use of chemical risk assessment provides a scientific basis for the tolerable levels of contaminants and acceptable levels of residues and food additives in foods which in combination with systematic regulatory control prove to be an effective approach for consumer health protection through risk-based paradigm and risk management measures.

Risk assessment is the scientific component and integral part of a broader food safety risk analysis framework along with other two interlinked components - risk management and risk communication. Risk assessment consists of characterization or quantification of the hazard for potential adverse effects to life and health resulting from the occurrence of a chemical and exposure to it through all possible routes. Risk analysis is widely used as a central methodology in food safety standards-setting and in food control regulation to ensure an appropriate level of consumer protection through sound scientific and risk-based management options. FAO and WHO provided definitions of the key terms related to the food safety risk analysis framework, as well as methodology and guidance to national governments on working principles for risk assessment, risk communication, and risk management with regard to food safety hazards for humans health.[1] One of the important challenges in chemical risk assessment consists of multiple and various types of chemicals that may be present in food for which quantitative hazard data for risk assessment is incomplete, limited, or absent to characterize the associated risk for human health following the exposure to those chemicals through food consumption.[2] In real life the exposure is occurring not only to one substance in one food at a time, but to complex mixtures from a variety of foods compounded with the exposure to non-dietary chemicals of different application areas through various pathways, and rarely with only one critical effect.

This paper provides a brief overview of the main concepts, conventional and emerging approaches in chemical risk assessment that allow to face the challenges related to the potential exposure to foodborne chemicals and cope with data scarcity paving practical ways for addressing the emerging contaminants in the context of food safety regulation. Understanding the principles and approaches of toxicological risk assessment is important for the policymakers and regulatory competent authorities, and also for key actors in the food supply chain, such as food producers, food manufacturers, and food processors.

24.2 Fundamentals of chemical risk assessment: concepts, principles, methods

Chemical risk assessment serves to establish whether the presence of certain chemicals in food and in what quantities may pose a risk to human health. The approach based on the relativity concept regarding food safety of chemical substances has been intuited in the 16th century by Paracelsus' reflection that the dose makes the poison, meaning that consumers can be adequately protected by limiting their exposure to hazards. The relative nature of chemical food safety is expressed through dose-response data and knowledge as a basis for concluding on a safety level. It took time for the insight of Paracelsus for chemical risk assessment to develop through 1970s, the 1980s and get accepted in the early 1990s as a scientific comparative evaluation method. Food safety risk assessment became a systematic discipline with remarkable progress in quantitative risk assessment methods and a better understanding of foodborne chemicals' health effects that required establishing competent authorities' control on human exposure to chemicals for their health protection.[3,4] The introduction of the risk concept, understanding, and applying it has particular importance for consumer health protection in the context of the need to ensure food security and reduce food losses. Risk-based approaches help food safety risk managers decide on suitable and feasible risk management measures to ensure safe levels of chemicals in foods and reach an acceptable risk.

The fundamentals of chemical risk assessment, including definitions, principles, and methods are described by FAO and WHO.[12] Risk assessment as a scientific discipline is realized through a structured process for organizing data, information, and knowledge for a better understanding of the interaction between hazards, food, and human illness. Four steps of risk assessment are common both for chemical and microbiological hazards[5,6] (Fig. 24.1).

Defining a compound's safety benchmark is based on comparing the dose-dependent response differences in the test and control samples in various settings, such as animal experiments, field trials, or epidemiological studies. The risk assessment process takes into account all relevant scientific data available at the time it is undertaken (chemical, toxicological, epidemiological, occurrence of the compound in food, food consumption, level of exposure, etc.), including appropriate analysis and consideration of related uncertainties. Risk assessment has to be

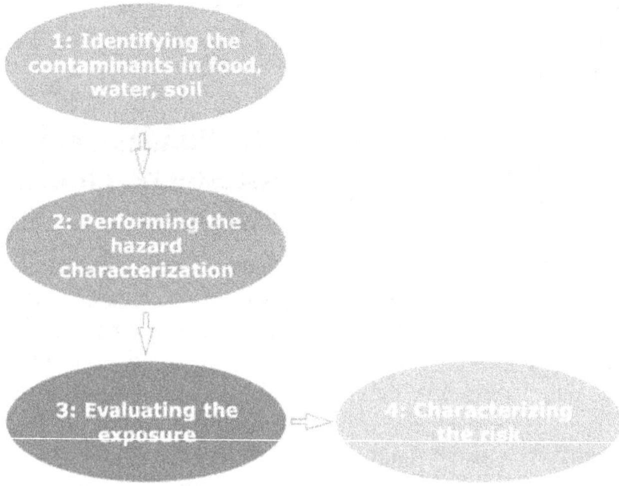

FIGURE 24.1 Four steps of risk assessment.

functionally separated from risk management to ensure objectivity and scientific independence of the process, to ensure that the results are unbiased and free of political or socio-economic considerations.[7,8]. While functionally separated, regular communication between risk assessors and risk managers is recommended on an interactive and iterative basis, as and when may be needed or required. Effective communication is important for the benefit of proper identification of the problem and formulation of the risk assessment's scope. Risk assessment questions formulated by risk managers guide the assessors in identifying possible hazards, health impact, vulnerable (sub) populations, the likelihood of causing harm, and finally identifying risk in quantitative or qualitative terms while recognizing and paying due attention to uncertainties.

24.2.1 Hazard identification

Hazard identification consists in the determination of substances capable of causing adverse health effects under certain conditions of exposure to a given organism, system, or (sub)population and which may be present in a particular food or group of foods. Hazard identification aims to identify potential critical toxicological endpoints of chemicals that may be of relevance to human health. At this step are described and documented the chemical structure of the contaminant and its physicochemical properties. Furthermore, "there should be documented and discussed the pathways of formation or synthesis and the recommended methods for the quantitative analysis of the compound."[9] Identifying the relationships between the structure of a compound and its toxicological activity is one of the fundamental tools in toxicological research and risk assessment. Structure-activity-relationships (SAR) informs the structural classification and may be indicative of some specific types of effect in chemicals with similar structure. This SAR approach is useful to support the initial screening and suggest the toxicity studies that are of greatest importance to focus further for risk assessment purposes.

24.2.2 Hazard characterization

Hazard characterization refers to a qualitative and/or quantitative evaluation of the nature of adverse health effects associated with the presence in food of a certain toxic substance. Hazard characterization includes toxicokinetics and toxicodynamics studies that investigate the absorption, distribution of the substance in the target tissues and storage sites, its metabolization, and excretion of the toxicant or its metabolites. For risk assessment, a detailed consideration of the mode of action, mechanism of action, and sensitivity of various endpoints is needed.[9] The mode of action for a toxicological effect is represented by a "biologically plausible sequence of key events, starting with the interaction of an agent with a cell, through functional and anatomical changes, leading to an observed effect supported by robust experimental observations and mechanistic data."[10,11] Toxicological data needed for chemical risk assessment include detailed information for understanding the mechanistic aspects, including mechanism of action at the molecular level, the mode of action of the toxic substance at the cellular level, and the sensitivity to the adverse effect (from dose-response studies). Usually, the mechanisms of action are determined in the in vitro studies using biological units, such as organs, cells, and subcellular entities, or separate substances, such as enzymes. In case when substances display more than one mode of action, affecting several target organs, the most sensitive adverse effect is considered the critical endpoint. In vitro studies are largely used to define the mode of action of a compound and often follow and build on findings from in vivo experiments on mice or rats (the most frequently used animals).

The dose-response assessment is a process that determines the relationship between the level of exposure (dose) to the scrutinized compound and the severity and/or frequency of associated adverse health effects (response). The purpose of dose-response assessment is to derive **health-based guidance values** (HBGV). The setting of health-based guidance values provides quantitative risk assessment information for risk managers, enabling them to make decisions on appropriate protection measures for human health. HBGV for substances found in food, including drinking water, is the quantitative expression of the range of dietary exposure (either acute or chronic) that would be expected to be without appreciable health risk.[12] For most unavoidable chemical contaminants the HBGV used is the **tolerable daily intake value (TDI)** expressed on a body-weight basis (mg/kg bw/day), that can be ingested daily over a lifetime without appreciable health risk. A different term is used for HBGV for substances purposely added to food, such as food additives, or used in food production, such as residues of pesticides and veterinary drugs, for which the determined HBGV is **acceptable daily intake (ADI)**. While the methodology for setting the TDI and ADI is similar, different terms bear different connotations with reference to the unavoidability and "permissibility" for the intake of contaminants associated with food consumption. In the case of contaminants which can display acute toxicity, the **acute reference dose** (ARfD) is determined which is defined as "an estimate of the amount of a substance in the food and/or drinking-water, normally expressed on a body-weight basis, that can be ingested in a period of 24 h or less, without appreciable health risk to the consumer, based on all the known facts at the time of the evaluation."[12] In a food safety risk assessment all available data from in vivo studies, as well as in vitro studies, will be considered, as applicable and available. The values of ADI, TDI, and ARfD are derived based on the lowest relevant **no-observable-adverse-effect-level (NOAEL)** dose from the dose-response curves in the most sensitive animal species reduced quantitatively by 100 uncertainty factor (UF). The UF 100 consists of factor 10 for animal-to-human extrapolation and related interspecies differences and another 10 factor takes into account different sensitivity of humans for the adverse effect, i.e. inter-individual variation as individuals generally vary in terms of the dose that can cause harm to them. The uncertainty/safe factor ensures that both sensitive individuals and average persons are sufficiently protected. Additional factors may apply to consider higher uncertainty in cases of important data gaps, such as limitations of toxicological and exposure data, and the absence of animal studies/NOAEL. Lower UFs may be used if the HBGVs are derived from epidemiological human data.[7] In such cases, there is no use of the uncertainty factor 10x for the interspecies difference. Determining toxicity HBGVs from studies conducted in laboratory animals is the most reliable source of toxicological data along with observational epidemiological studies in humans where available. However, the tests on animals are both resource- and time-intensive and increasingly raise ethical issues. To address this matter, the HBGVs available from earlier toxicological studies are used in various computational models that serve to derive pragmatic tools used to define health-based reference values, for screening to prioritize testing, and for other practical purposes.

24.2.2.1 Benchmark dose modeling

An alternative technique for the evaluation of dose-response data is the Benchmark Dose (BMD) dose-response computational modeling approach that is increasingly used to derive HBGVs. The BMD allows deriving more information from available dose-response datasets and with higher statistical precision for the point of departure/reference point with subsequent deriving more precise exposure limits. Applying targeted theoretical levels for adverse effects, the BMDL (BMDL stands for BMD lower confidence bound), allows for a more explicit definition of exposure limits. The BMD approach can apply to combined similar datasets for the same chemical in a single analysis, which further increases precision and also allows for combining a dose-response dataset with historical data for other similar chemicals that increases significantly the utility of this technique.[13–15] BMD software allows as well the selection of valid datasets for the identification of potential critical endpoints that should be further analyzed. The BMD modeling is "a considerable step forward from the perspective of the reduction, replacement, and refinement of in vivo testing methods since more information is obtained from the same number of animals, or, similar information may be obtained from fewer animals.[14]

24.2.2. 2 Approach to identifying the genotoxic and carcinogenic potential of chemicals

A range of endpoints is used in regulatory chemical risk assessment, such as genotoxicity, carcinogenicity, immunotoxicity, reproductive and developmental toxicity, etc. Among them, the genotoxic and carcinogenic potential is the most alarming and major endpoints the assessment of which is a basic requirement. Regulatory genotoxicity assessment aims to identify chemicals of genotoxic and carcinogenic concern for excluding their approval for purposeful use in food or the other uses in the food chain or for the reduction of their levels in foods to as low as reasonable achievable (ALARA) by technically and financially feasible risk management measures.[16] Carcinogenesis is a complex biological process that develops usually over a long time and requires certain key changes to accumulate in the body. Some chemicals are both genotoxic and carcinogenic. Genotoxic and carcinogenic are those compounds that induce cancer through a genotoxic mode of action. Due to linkages between cancer and accumulation of genetic damage in cells, test strategies for cancer hazard identification focus primarily on identifying genotoxicity through a tiered approach starting with a set of well-established and standardized in vitro genotoxicity tests. A positive in vitro finding requires subsequent in vivo testing to confirm the positive in vitro result. The high frequency of false-positive in vitro genotoxicity results is a problem as it requires unnecessary in vivo confirmation studies.[10] The strategic orientation in the regulatory genotoxic hazard assessment is to enhance the performance of in vitro testing batteries to reduce the need for in vivo follow-up tests. The available at present in vitro tests are not considered sufficient to fully replace animal tests needed to evaluate chemicals' safety and efforts are oriented at improving the accuracy of the core in vitro testing battery, considering the most suitable combinations of in vitro tests, developing novel tests, optimizing the use of animals for in vivo testing (e.g. integrating different endpoints into a single study, including genotoxicity endpoints into a short-term repeated dose toxicity studies.[17]

Various tools are used in risk assessment, including the classification of contaminants as genotoxic, or non-genotoxic. However, some non-genotoxic chemicals can induce cancer as well and while the mechanisms through which non-genotoxic carcinogens induce cancer are increasingly elucidated, test strategies to provide the mode of action are lacking at present. New test methods for the detection of non-genotoxic carcinogens are in strong demand. Using genotoxicity assays to predict carcinogenic potential has the significant drawback that risks from non-genotoxic carcinogens remain largely undetected unless carcinogenicity studies are performed. Compiled genotoxicity and carcinogenicity databases from different sources (regulatory authorities, research, industry) are useful tools and important references to support food safety chemical risk assessment. For a comprehensive review of test methods for cancer hazard identification that have been adopted by the regulatory authorities, the reader is referred to Luijten et al., 2016.[10] The authors highlight as well alternative testing methods thought capable of detecting both genotoxic as well as non-genotoxic carcinogens and improving understanding of the related mode of action.

To fill the toxicological data gap for a large number of various chemicals in alignment with the strong emphasis on reducing, minimizing, and replacing animal testing methods in toxicological studies, alternative non-testing methods, are rapidly developing. One of the fundamental non-testing methods to assess genotoxic or carcinogen hazards is the (quantitative) structure-activity relationships ((Q)SAR) which are based on the linkage between the structure and the toxicity of a compound. Chemicals are grouped and classified according to their structure as a basis to predict their adverse health effect. Also for identifying the genotoxic feature of a chemical, various computational modeling has been developed and are available, some free of charge, and others on a commercial basis. However, generally, there is significant commonality between the available computational models as most of them operate with the same sets of experimental data.[10]

24.2.2.3 Practical approaches to mixture risk assessment

The current practice of chemical risk assessment is principally based on characterizing the risk following the exposure to individual contaminants or single chemicals deliberately used during food production or in other applications. Meanwhile in real life consumers may be exposed to low levels of more than one chemical substance at a time. Within the context of human health, animal health, and environmental health, the is a growing recognition of the need to consider in the risk assessment the combined exposure to mixtures of chemicals and the aggregate exposure to single same chemicals from various sources, pathways, and routes of exposure. The combined effect in chemical mixtures would depend on the type of chemicals' interactions that may include dose addition, synergism, and potentiation (meaning more than the additive effect of single components), antagonism, inhibition, masking (less than an additive effect). Where interactions are known to exist, mixture risk assessments are routinely conducted, and good practice that builds on various regulatory frameworks exists at international, regional, and national levels. For example, JECFA and JMPR have considered the combined effect in the evaluation of some food additives, pesticides, and veterinary drugs, that were formulated as mixtures, as well as have considered some co-occurring contaminants in the mixtures.[12] FAO and WHO provide continuous support to the development of practical approaches, guidance, and recommendations for the implementation of risk assessment of combined dietary exposures to multiple chemicals.[5] The importance to address the complex task of chemical mixtures in risk assessment is gaining momentum. Competent public authorities across the world and dedicated thematic research groups have developed pragmatic step-wise frameworks that are fit for purpose to address the combined exposure to multiple chemicals for risk assessment that integrate chemical and toxicological data while using the opportunities of digitalization and availability of big data.

The efforts to consider chemical mixtures risk assessment for regulatory purposes are increasingly conducing to innovative research which materialize in alternative to single chemicals-centered approaches and tools, some with public access and others available on a commercial basis. New mechanism-based practical tools for multiple chemical risk assessments continue to be conceptualized and developed.[11,18–22]

24.2.3 Exposure assessment

Exposure assessment refers to the quantitative evaluation of the likely intake of a certain substance with food as well as via other routes of exposure if relevant (inhalation through the lungs, penetration through the skin).[12] Quantitative assessment of the exposure requires food consumption data by the exposed groups of the population, as well as the occurrence and level of a scrutinized substance in the consumed food. In case of exposure from various pathways and several sources, aggregate exposure has to be taken into account.

Humans are potentially exposed to many different chemicals. These may include foodborne chemicals, and non-dietary substances, such as anthropogenic chemicals, manufactured, by-products, metabolites, and abiotically formed transformation products.[21] Therefore, there is an increasing need for strategies and practical tools to mainstream exposure assessment to multiple chemicals and their combined effects. As the body of knowledge is continuously evolving, the approaches to the assessment of safe exposure are continuously revisited for alignment with the latest scientific developments and achieved insights in the overall risk assessment framework at any given time to ensure their robustness and reliability.[23]

24.2.3.1 Threshold of Toxicological Concern

Considering that a high number of chemicals in the environment and food that may be ingested in very low doses and for which little or no toxicity data exists, a pragmatic principle of the Threshold of Toxicological Concern (TTC) is used to prioritize targeted chemical testing.

The TTC is a scientific risk-based approach that consists of the establishment of a human exposure threshold value for a chemical or groups of chemicals below which there would be no expectation for any appreciable risk to human health. The establishment of a TTC is based on the analysis of available toxicological data considering the chemical structures of a wide range of substances, both genotoxic and non-genotoxic. Thus, the TTC allows for an estimate of the probability of no adverse effects from a substance of unknown toxicity for which the daily intake exposure is known as being very low. The derived TTC values are a practical substitute for substance-specific hazard information that is used to manage the risk for a broad range of substances to which the human exposure is so low that performing toxicity studies appears as not justified. The TTC concept does not apply to chemicals that are regulated and for which specific requirements exist regarding their risk assessment, including "no threshold" substances that have the potential of displaying adverse health effects unless the exposure level is completely absent (none). Major historical data sets obtained from various toxicity studies (acute, sub-chronic, and chronic) that are continuously completed and updated, as well as knowledge are used for setting the TTCs values, such as (i) databases for carcinogens, (ii) non-cancer toxicological endpoints databases, and (iii) knowledge regarding the distribution of potencies of relevant classes of chemicals for which sufficient toxicity data are available. Two ways of setting the TTC value are used are based on (i) a predicted tumor risk of *one in a million*, derived through the analysis of genotoxic chemicals data, or (ii) on frequency distributions (5th percentile) of NOAELs of non-genotoxic chemicals.[2] The first application of the TTC concept refers to the adoption in 1995 by the FDA of a TTC value of 0.025 microgram/body weight/day for food contact materials. Further practical application of the TTC approach extended to set the safe threshold for food flavoring substances (EFSA & JECFA), pesticide metabolites in groundwater (EU), genotoxic impurities in pharmaceuticals (EMEA), genotoxic constituents in herbal substances and preparations (EMEA), micro-pollutants and impurities in drinking water (AUS).[24] The TTC approach is considered not applicable to the following chemical groups/endpoints for the following reasons[25]

- "heavy metals and polyhalogenated dibenzo-p-dioxins, polyhalogenated dibenzofurans and polyhalogenated biphenyls, or any other substances with a potential for bioaccumulation in the body, e.g. ochratoxin A, are excluded from the TTC approach, because the safety factors used may not be high enough to account for differences between species in their elimination from the body, or they were not included in the original databases used to develop the TTC principle, or toxicological data sufficient to perform a full chemical-specific evaluation is available.
- endocrine-disrupting chemicals, including steroids, due to little and inconsistent data at lower doses;
- high molecular weight chemicals, such as polymers, are excluded because their toxicity data were not in the databases used to develop TTC.
- proteins are excluded from the TTC approach because of the potential for allergenicity or other biological activities, and because they were not included in the original database used to develop the TTC principle.

- allergy, hypersensitivity, and intolerance should at present not be evaluated using the TTC principle, due to too uncertain dose-response data, whereas other immunotoxic effects are included."

Other chemicals excluded from the application of the TTC principle are radioactive substances and mixtures of substances containing unknown chemical structures.

For non-genotoxic substances, maximum exposure levels (TTCs) can be considered safe.

24.2.3.2 Margin-of-Exposure

Margin-of-Exposure (MOE) is a tool that helps to estimate the level of concern with particular reference to substances that are genotoxic and carcinogenic. The 64th JECFA meeting recommended that advice on substances that are both genotoxic and carcinogenic should be based on estimated MOEs.[15] MOE reflects the "margins of safety between carcinogenic doses in experimental animals and exposure levels in humans."[26] Margin-of-Exposure is calculated as the ratio of a toxicological reference dose (NOAEL) obtained from animal toxicity studies to the theoretical, estimated, or predicted human exposure level or dose (MOE = NOAEL/Exposure).[12] For the MOE calculation the $BMDL_{10}$ value is usually used as Reference Point for a carcinogenic effect in animal experiments. This value is compared with the exposure dose of an average consumer or high consumers groups. The MOE is a dimensionless value. The Margin-of-Exposure for genotoxic and carcinogenic contaminants is "of concern" for MOE values less than 10,000, "of low concern" for MOE values between 10,000 and 1,000,000, and "of no concern" for MOE values over 1,000,000.[15,27] For substances with Margin-of Exposure values over one million, risk managers may decide if a low priority for risk management actions would apply or on applying risk management measures that further reduce consumer exposure to the scrutinized substances.

24.2.4 Risk characterization

Risk characterization consists of a qualitative estimate in terms of low, moderate, high, and/or quantitative/numerical estimation of the probability of occurrence and the severity of an adverse effect (known or potential) in a certain population. Risk characterization is the final step of risk assessment that derives from the analysis of data and evidence collected in previous steps of chemical risk assessment (1-2-3), assessors' reflections, and conclusions. Risk characterization takes into account and acknowledges the overall uncertainties in the interpretation related to data limitation, time limitation, related to sampling and extrapolation, etc. When characterizing risk, the assessors may use also probability expressions, such as "likely"/"unlikely." Science- and evidence-based risk characterization are key for effective risk communication and decisions on risk management options.

24.3 Risk perception in food safety risk assessment

Risk assessment, as the scientific component of risk analysis methodology that quantifies objectively food safety risk, the involved experts basing their judgment on scientific and statistical estimates. Meanwhile, as scientific data are not always complete, safety decisions imply as well some uncertainty related to extrapolation from limited evidence, and subjective perception of risk, which "can only be minimized but never eliminated."[23] Safety assessment is a multidisciplinary science in continuous development as knowledge and experience accumulate with the outcome depending on the available data and tools, knowledge, and a certain subjectivity of risk perception. It is thought that some degree of subjective judgment possibly exists at every step of risk assessment that may translate into vulnerability to bias. Jenkins et al (2020)[28] suggest that the psychological construct of risk needs to be acknowledged within the risk assessment. A review of relevant research performed by this research group has identified 12 non-technical factors that could affect risk assessment and risk management decisions along with psychological perspectives on possible sources of bias that may arise at any step of risk assessment. Authors bring recommendations on the ways to overcome the psychological aspects of a standardized risk assessment. An important factor that is essential both for new knowledge development and related risk perception is time. A logical framework that recognizes time as the factor shaping the interaction between scientific evidence and risk perception and ensures that the pace of food safety standards development and the pace of innovations are synchronized is proposed by Fernandez & Paoletti.[23]

24.4 Research gaps and future directions

Current needs for improvements refer especially to the gaps in hazard characterization and exposure assessment. Data gaps for individual chemicals and especially for emerging contaminants, limited toxicity studies, and exposure data are the major bottlenecks in chemical risk assessment. While the additive effects of simultaneous exposure to a group of related substances are well understood and routinely addressed in food safety risk assessments, questions with regard to possible non-linear interactions are less well understood and remain the subject of intense research efforts at a global level. Scientific and regulatory communities converge on the necessity for advancements toward a more integrated, harmonized, and systematic assessment of the risk from the exposure to coincidental multiple chemicals that may derive from various sources, pathways, routes, and areas of application. Addressing the multiple exposures to chemicals through multiple pathways relies on both strengthening the generation of data relevant for toxicological risk assessment, and on strengthening the transdisciplinary coordination and cooperation for data sharing from the research community, regulators, and industry with associated involvement in the policy dialog of a broad range of stakeholders. Areas of further research intensification include identifying and prioritizing emerging contaminants and chemical mixtures, strengthening predictive modeling of exposure to a variety of typical mixtures of chemicals, and applying new approach methodologies for chemical testing, risk assessment procedures, and modern epidemiological studies. Opportunities for prospective mixture risk assessment and evaluation of possible combined exposures to (real-life) chemical mixtures to human health, animal health, and ecological risk are to be grasped and unfolded. The newly accumulated knowledge may reveal that what was unsafe in the past may be safe and vice versa. Systematic reviews are key to identifying the chemicals that would need a re-evaluation of their safety through risk assessment updates using next-generation approaches.[2,23,29] A more precise risk assessment would benefit from research and scientific advancement in developing the understanding of mechanistic aspects, applying the next generation of techniques for identifying the points of departure, developing harmonized and effective strategies for BMD and other modeling techniques.[30] Research efforts are needed as well to address regulatory and policy alignment for a collaborative chemical safety governance at all levels.[11,17]

Disclaimer

The views expressed in this publication are those of the author and do not necessarily reflect the views or policies of the Food and Agriculture Organization of the United Nations.

References

1. FAO and WHO. Working Principles for Risk Analysis for Food Safety for Application by Governments. Rome, Italy; 2007. http://www.fao.org/documents/card/fr/c/fdaaa09d-8a3f-50c6-b801-945ffcac73a2/.
2. Pham LL, Borghoff SJ, Thompson CM. Comparison of threshold of toxicological concern (TTC) values to oral reference dose (RfD) values. *Regul Toxicol Pharmacol.* 2020;113:104651. Available from: https://doi.org/10.1016/j.yrtph.2020.104651. Epub 2020 Mar 27. PMID: 32229245.
3. Rodricks JV. When risk assessment came to washington: a look back. *Dose Response.* 2019;17(1). Available from: https://doi.org/10.1177/1559325818824934. PMID: 30783394; PMCID: PMC6366000.
4. Wu F, Rodricks JV. Forty years of food safety risk assessment: a history and analysis. *Risk Anal.* 2020;40:S1. Available from: https://doi.org/10.1111/risa.13624.
5. FAO and WHO. *FAO/WHO Expert Consultation on Dietary Risk Assessment of Chemical Mixtures (Risk Assessment of Combined Exposure to Multiple Chemicals).* Geneva: WHO; 2019, 16-18 April 2019. Available from: https://www.who.int/foodsafety/areas_work/chemical-risks/Euromix_Report.pdf.
6. FAO. Food Safety Risk Analysis. A Guide for National Food Safety Authorities. Rome, Italy; 2006. http://www.fao.org/3/a0822e/a0822e.pdf.
7. Benford DJ. *Risk Assessment of Chemical Contaminants and Residues in Food. In: Chemical Contaminants and Residues in Food.* Elsevier Ltd.; 2017:3–13. Available from: https://dx.doi.org/10.1016/B978-0-08-100674-0.00001-1.
8. FAO/WHO. Working Principles for Risk Analysis for Food Safety for Application by Governments. Rome, Italy; 2007. http://www.fao.org/3/a1550t/a1550t.pdf.
9. Cartus A, Schrenk D. Current methods in risk assessment of genotoxic chemicals. *Food Chem Toxicol.* 2017;106(B):574–582. Available from: https://doi.org/10.1016/j.fct.2016.09.012.
10. Luijten M, Olthof ED, Hakkert BC, et al. An integrative test strategy for cancer hazard identification. *Crit Rev Toxicol.* 2016;46(7):615–639. Available from: https://doi.org/10.3109/10408444.2016.1171294. Epub 2016 May 3. PMID: 27142259.
11. Boberg J, Dybdahl M, Petersen A, Hass U, Svingen T, Vinggaard AM. A pragmatic approach for human risk assessment of chemical mixtures. *Curr Opin Toxicol.* 2019;15:1–7. Available from: https://doi.org/10.1016/j.cotox.2018.11.004.
12. FAO/WHO/IPCS. Environmental Health Criteria 240. Principles and methods for the risk assessment of chemicals in food. <https://apps.who.int/iris/bitstream/handle/10665/44065/WHO_EHC_240_eng.pdf>; 2009.
13. EFSA Scientific CommitteeHardy A, Benford D, Halldorsson T, et al. Update: use of the benchmark dose approach in risk assessment. *EFSA J.* 2017;15(1):41. Available from: https://doi.org/10.2903/j.efsa.2017.4658. 4658.
14. Wout Slob. Benchmark dose and the three Rs. Part I. Getting more information from the same number of animals. *Crit Rev Toxicol.* 2014;44(7):557–567. Available from: https://doi.org/10.3109/10408444.2014.925423.
15. FAO and WHO, JECFA (Joint FAO (Food and Agriculture Organization of the United Nations) and WHO (World Health Organization)), 2006. Expert Committee on Food Additives – JECFA. Sixty-Fourth Meeting, WHO/IPCS Safety Evaluation of Certain Contaminants in Food. In: *WHO Food Additives Series 55.*
16. Barlow SM, Boobis AR, Bridges J, et al. The role of hazard- and risk-based approaches in ensuring food safety. *Trends Food Sci Technol.* 2015;46:176–188. Available from: https://doi.org/10.1016/j.tifs.2015.10.007.
17. Corvi R, Madia F. In vitro genotoxicity testing - Can the performance be enhanced? *Food Chem Toxicol.* 2017 August;106 (Pt B):600–608, Epub 2016 Aug 21. Available from: https://doi.org/10.1016/j.fct.2016.08.024.
18. Rotter S, Beronius A, Boobis AR, et al. Overview on legislation and scientific approaches for risk assessment of combined exposure

to multiple chemicals: the potential EuroMix contribution. *Crit Rev Toxicol.* 2018;48(9):796–814. Available from: https://doi.org/10.1080/10408444.2018.1541964. Epub 2019 Jan 10. PMID: 30632445.

19. Bopp SK, Kienzler A, Richarz AN, et al. Regulatory assessment and risk management of chemical mixtures: challenges and ways forward. *Crit Rev Toxicol.* 2019;49(2):174–189. Available from: https://doi.org/10.1080/10408444.2019.1579169. Epub 2019 Apr 1. PMID: 30931677.
20. Cheng F, Li H, Brooks BW, You J. Retrospective risk assessment of chemical mixtures in the big data era: an alternative classification strategy to integrate chemical and toxicological data. *Environ Sci Technol.* 2020;54:5925–5927.
21. Drakvik E, Altenburger R, Aoki Y, et al. Statement on advancing the assessment of chemical mixtures and their risks for human health and the environment. *Environ Int.* 2020;134:105267. Available from: https://doi.org/10.1016/j.envint.2019.105267. Epub 2019 Nov 6. PMID: 31704565; PMCID: PMC6979318.
22. Teuschler LK. Deciding which chemical mixtures risk assessment methods work best for what mixtures. *Toxicol Appl Pharmacol.* 2007;223(2):139–147. Available from: https://doi.org/10.1016/j.taap.2006.07.010. PMID: 16997340.
23. Fernandez A, Paoletti C. What is unsafe food? Change of perspective. *Trends Food Sci Technol.* 2021;109:725–728. Available from: https://doi.org/10.1016/j.tifs.2021.01.041.
24. Patlewicz G. March *Threshold of Toxicological Concern Approach in Regulatory DecisionMaking: The Past, Present, and Future.* SOT FDA Colloquia on Emerging Toxicological Science Challenges in Food and Ingredient Safety; 2016.
25. SCHER/SCCP/SCENIHR. *scientific opinion on the use of the Threshold of Toxicological Concern (TTC) approach for the safety assessment of chemical substances.* 2008;SCCP/1171/08,:19.11.08. Available from: https://ec.europa.eu/health/ph_risk/committees/documents/sc_o_001.pdf.
26. Schrenk D. Modern concepts in chemical risk assessment. *Encycl Food Chem.* 2019;1:685–689. Available from: https://doi.org/10.1016/B978-0-08-100596-5.21791-5. ISBN 9780128140451.
27. EFSA Scientific CommitteeBoris A, Sue B, Andrew C, et al. Statement on the applicability of the Margin of Exposure approach for the safety assessment of impurities which are both genotoxic and carcinogenic in substances added to food/feed. *EFSA J.* 2012;10(3):2578. 5 pp.
28. Jenkins SC, Harris AJL, Osman M. Influence of psychological factors in food risk assessment – a review. *Trends Food Sci Technol.* 2020;103:282–292. Available from: https://doi.org/10.1016/j.tifs.2020.07.010.
29. Whaley P, Halsall C, Ågerstrand M, et al. Implementing systematic review techniques in chemical risk assessment: challenges, opportunities and recommendations. *Environ Int.* 2016;92-93:556–564. Available from: https://doi.org/10.1016/j.envint.2015.11.002. Epub 2015 Dec 11. PMID: 26687863; PMCID: PMC4881816.
30. Levorato S, Rietjens IMCM, Carmichael PL, Hepburn PA. Novel approaches to derive points of departure for food chemical risk assessment. *Curr Opin Food Sci.* 2019;27:139–144. Available from: https://doi.org/10.1016/j.cofs.2019.02.016.

Section VI

Changes in pathogenic microbiological contamination of food pre- and post-farm gate/fishing

Chapter 25

Common and natural occurrence of pathogens, including fungi, leading to primary and secondary product contamination

Maristela S. Nascimento[1] and Marta H. Taniwaki[2]

[1]*University of Campinas, Campinas, Brazil,* [2]*Institute of Food Technology, Campinas, Brazil*

Abstract

This chapter summarizes some characteristics of the main pathogenic bacteria found in foods (*Staphylococcus aureus, Clostridium, Bacillus cereus, Listeria monocytogenes, Escherichia coli, Salmonella, Campylobacter, Shigella, Yersinia, Brucella, Cronobacter*), and the three most important fungal genera producing mycotoxins: *Aspergillus, Fusarium,* and *Penicillium.* The ecology and factors governing the growth of these microorganisms are described, as well as some foodborne outbreaks that have resulted, associated with different types of foods. In addition, the potential routes of contamination of these microorganisms in primary and secondary production steps are discussed, with the exception of water, will be addressed in this chapter.

Keywords: Bacteria; fungi; mycotoxins; foodborne outbreak; food production chain; food safety

25.1 Introduction

The World Health Organization (WHO) estimates that 600 million cases of foodborne illnesses occur annually around the world, with 420,000 deaths.[1] In 2018 EU authorities reported 5146 foodborne outbreaks resulting in 48,365 illnesses.[2] Meanwhile, in the United States in 2017, 841 outbreaks with 14,481 cases and 20 deaths were reported.[3] On the other hand, according to the WHO, Africa has the highest proportional burden of foodborne diseases in the world with 91 million falling ill each year and 137,000 dying of the same cause, representing one-third of the global death toll for foodborne diseases.[1] In addition, an economic impact study done by the World Bank (WB) in 2019 estimated that unsafe foods cost low- and middle-income economies mainly in Sub-Saharan Africa and Southeast Asia, about $110 billion in lost productivity and medical expenses alone each year.[4]

Vegetables and animal products can become contaminated with foodborne pathogens during preharvest, harvest, and postharvest stages. Cross-contamination and poor agricultural practices are frequently implicated contributors. Contamination may originate directly or indirectly from soil, feces, water, manure, biosolids, dust, insects, animals, equipment, transport containers, and food handlers.[5–7] Furthermore, fungal spores commonly occur in air, dust, soil, and water. Consequently, foods become contaminated with mixed spores of fungal species from these sources. Under favorable conditions, fungi can grow in food and cause deterioration. However, not all fungal species that are present are capable of causing spoilage and the most undesirable consequence is the production of mycotoxins in food and feed. The presence of mycotoxins in a food indicates that, at some stage in production or processing, conditions became favorable for growth of a toxigenic fungus and mycotoxin production. Therefore a better understanding of these routes of contamination is essential for the production of good quality and safe food.

25.2 Foodborne pathogenic bacteria

25.2.1 Staphylococcus aureus

Staphylococcus aureus is a Gram-positive coccus arranged in a format of clusters of grapes. It is a facultative anaerobe, nonspore-forming, catalase, thermonuclease, and

Present Knowledge in Food Safety. DOI: https://doi.org/10.1016/B978-0-12-819470-6.00018-4

coagulase positive organism. Some strains are able to produce staphylococcal enterotoxins (SEs, SEA to SEE, SEG to SEI, SER to SET) with emetic activity.[8] Usually, they are produced when the bacterial population achieves 10^5 CFU/g and at temperatures of between 10°C and 46°C, with optimum production at 34°C–40°C. On the other hand, bacterial growth occurs between 7°C and 47.8°C, with optimum growth between 30°C and 40°C.[9] The pH for growth ranges from 4.2 to 9.3, with an optimum around 7.0. *S. aureus* is able to grow at a water activity (a_w) of 0.83 and tolerates high concentrations of NaCl (up to 15%).[10] The production of enterotoxins could occur in a wide variety of foods, such as milk products, mixed foods, meat and meat products, egg and egg products, cakes, and ice cream.[11] The SEs are heat-stable and the thermal resistance varies according to the type of enterotoxin, reaching up to 121°C for 28 min.[12] In the EU, the prevalence of the bacterium in animals is in the region of 19% and in food, 8.4%, whereas the enterotoxins were detected in 1.2% of the food samples analyzed in 2018.[2] In China, the prevalence of *S. aureus* in raw milk ranged from 22.0% to 46.2%.[13,14] Regarding raw meat, *S. aureus* was recovered from 67.9% of raw poultry, 54.5% of raw beef, and 50.4% of raw pork samples collected between 2011 and 2016 in China.[15] In the United States in 2010–11, 27.9% of retail meat was positive for this pathogen.[16] In Brazil from 2008 to 2014, *S. aureus* was responsible for 23% of foodborne outbreaks linked to fruit and vegetables.[17] Food handlers are the main source of food contamination via direct contact. According to the Food and Drug Administration (FDA) of the United States,[9] the species can occur naturally in the nose, throat, or skin of at least 50% of healthy people. A recent public health concern involving this species is the spread of antibiotic-resistant strains such as methicillin-resistant *S. aureus* (MRSA). In swine farms in Denmark, the prevalence of livestock-associated MRSA (LA-MRSA) has increased from 16% in 2010 to 88% in 2016.[18]

25.2.2 Clostridium

Clostridium is an anaerobic, Gram-positive, spore-forming, immotile rod-shaped bacterium, which is also catalase negative. *C. perfringens* and *C. botulinum* are the foremost foodborne pathogens of this *genus*.

25.2.2.1 *Clostridium botulinum*

Strains of *C. botulinum* are grouped into proteolytic and nonproteolytic strains due to their ability to produce proteases and are also grouped according to the production of one of eight antigenically distinct toxins (A, B, C, D, E, F, G, and H).[19] Group I (proteolytic strains) produces the neurotoxins A, B, F, and H. Their spores are highly heat resistant ($D_{100°C}$ 25 min) and germinate in a_w greater than 0.94 (10% NaCl) and a pH higher than 4.6.[20,21] Growth is inhibited at temperatures below 10°C.[22,23] Group II (nonproteolytic strains) produces neurotoxins B, E, and F and ferments a range of carbohydrates. Their spores are moderately thermally resistant ($D_{100°C} < 0.1$ min) and can germinate in a_w above 0.97 (5% NaCl) and at a pH greater than 5.0.[20,24] The strains of this group are psychrotrophic and are capable of growing and producing toxins at temperatures above 3°C.[22,23] The toxins are heat labile and can be destroyed if heated at 80°C for 30 min or longer. The spores are widely dispersed in nature, including soil, sediments, and manure.[9] Foodborne botulism cases are very rare and are usually associated with consumption of inadequately home-canned or home-prepared foods.[24] In 2018 an outbreak of type A botulism with seven cases was linked to a homemade savory jelly in Denmark.[25] In the same year in the United States, three cases of botulism were associated with home-canned peas.[26] In addition, in 2017, 19 foodborne botulism cases and 3 deaths were reported; for 16 of these cases the foods involved were identified as nacho cheese, herbal deer antler tea, seal blubber with seal oil, and dried herring in seal oil.[27] Honey is an important vehicle of infant botulism. Austin[28] reported that the incidence of *C. botulinum* spores in honey ranges from 2% to 26% depending upon the production region. In Poland and the United States, spores were isolated from 8.5% and 10% of the honey samples tested.[29,30]

25.2.2.2 *Clostridium perfringens*

C. perfringens is classified into seven toxin types (A, B, C, D, E, F, and G) based on the production of six major toxins (CPA, CPB, ETX, ITX, CPE, and NetB). *C. perfringens* type F formerly classified as type A produces CPA and CPE, and is linked to foodborne diseases, with an infectious dose $\geq 10^5$ CFU/g.[31] *C. perfringens* spores are resistant to radiation, desiccation, freezing, refrigeration, and heat (100°C for up to 60 min).[9] The optimum growth temperature is between 37°C and 45°C. Furthermore, the species grows well at a pH of 6.0–7.0 and is inhibited at pH <5, NaCl >6%, 10,000 ppm $NaNO_3$, or 400 ppm $NaNO_2$.[32] *C. perfringens* is widely spread in the environment,[9] mainly in the soil and dust, but it is also part of the intestinal microbiota of humans and animals, making feces an important route of contamination.[9] According to the Centers for Disease Control and Prevention (CDC),[3] *C. perfringens* was the third most common bacteria responsible for 5% of foodborne disease outbreaks in the United States in 2017. Meat and poultry were reported as frequent food vehicles for *C. perfringens* type A.[33] In 2012 in Michigan, United States, an investigation of a large outbreak involving 108 cases identified chicken taco meat mixture as the source of *C. perfringens*.[34] Furthermore, an outbreak with 58 cases was associated with the consumption of minced beef during a Handball Championship for children in Greece.[35] Outbreaks involving cooked meat-based foods are most commonly implicated, while outbreaks involving plant foods are not commonly reported, even though the organism may be present. In Poland 7.7% of vegetables and fruit tested positive for the presence of this species.[29]

25.2.3 Bacillus cereus

The *Bacillus cereus* group comprises nine *species*: *B. anthracis, B. cereus, B. mycoides, B. pseudomycoides, B. thuringiensis, B. weihenstephanensis, B. cytotoxicus, B. bombysepticus, B. toyonensis*.[36] *B. cereus* species is a Gram−positive, rod-shaped, facultative anaerobic, catalase positive, oxidase negative, and spore-forming bacterium. Motility is variable, with Logan and DeVos[37] reporting more than 85% of strains showing motility, whereas Tallent et al.[38] and Bennett et al.[39] reported 50% and between 50 and 90% motility, respectively. The optimum growth temperature is around 35°C, and the minimum is 4°C for some psychrotolerant strains.[9] The pH values for growth range from 4.9 to 9.3 and the minimum a_w is 0.93.[9] This pathogen produces six types of toxins, including nonhemolytic enterotoxin and cytotoxin K linked to the diarrheal syndrome, and the emetic toxin cereulide responsible for the emetic syndrome.[37,40] The infectious dose of *B. cereus* ranges between 10^5 and 10^8 cells or spores per gram.[40] Spores and vegetative cells of *B. cereus* are widespread in nature and have often been recovered from soil, dust, and raw materials.[41] The most commonly associated foods with outbreaks are rice, pasta, vegetables, meat, milk, and dairy products.[42] According to the European Food Safety Authority (EFSA),[43] from 2007 to 2014, 6657 cases and 413 outbreaks caused by *B. cereus* were reported in the EU. In China, the prevalence of *B. cereus* in raw milk was reported as 34.4%.[44] In Wisconsin (United States), *B. cereus* was found in 9%, 35%, 14%, and 48% of raw milk, pasteurized milk, Cheddar cheese, and ice cream samples, respectively.[45] The pathogen was also isolated from vegetable samples at a rate of 50% in China,[46] 20%−48% in South Korea,[47,48] and 57% in Mexico.[49] In meat and meat products, the prevalence was reported as 22.4% in Turkey[50] and 30%−40% in Serbia.[51]

25.2.4 Listeria monocytogenes

The genus *Listeria* embraces 26 species, five of them identified for the first time in 2021.[52] It is characterized as a Gram-positive, rod-shaped or coccoid, facultative anaerobic, and catalase positive bacterium. The organism is immotile at 35°C, but motile at 25°C. It is able to hydrolyze esculin and ferment glucose without gas production.[53] It is a psychrotrophic bacterium, growing from −2°C to 45°C, with an optimum of between 30°C and 37°C.[54] The organism is not heat resistant and is therefore killed by pasteurization temperatures. Postprocessing contamination is often the cause of foodborne listeriosis outbreaks. The pH for growth ranges from 4.1 to 9.6, with an optimum of between 6 and 8. In addition, it survives in salinity up to 20% NaCl and grows well at a salt concentration of between 10% and 12%. The minimum a_w required for growth is 0.90,[55] but it may survive for long periods at values around 0.83.[56] *L. monocytogenes* is the species that currently causes the greatest concern in public health, with a high hospitalization rate (94%) and a mortality rate of between 20% and 25%. It is a ubiquitous microorganism, widespread in the environment, and able to persist in the food-processing environment for extended periods of time.[56] A great variety of food categories have been linked to listeriosis incidents and the biggest concern lies with ready-to-eat (RTE) foods,[9] which do not undergo a further listericidal treatment before consumption. A survey carried out from 2010 to 2017 indicated that the most frequently implicated food vehicles in the EU were mixed food, followed by fish and fish products, vegetables, and seafood.[2] *L. monocytogenes* is frequently found in raw meat, for example, 3.5% of commercial ground beef tested positive for *L. monocytogenes* in the United States,[57] while 2.5% beef and 26.7% pork tested positive in Argentina whereas the prevalence rate in Uruguay was 28.6% for beef, 30% for pork, and 50% for chicken.[58] However, presence in raw meat is expected, considering that the organism is present in environments where food animals are farmed; therefore it is not surprising that raw meat and poultry would frequently contain low levels of *L. monocytogenes*. Furthermore, cattle can be a reservoir of *Listeria* and may shed the organism in their feces.[59,60] According to Lee et al.,[61] the prevalence rate of *L. monocytogenes* in raw milk varies throughout the world; in the United States it ranges from 0% to 19.7%, in South America from 0% to 3.7% whereas in Europe it reaches values up to 28.6%. Vegetables can also be contaminated via several environmental sources. The prevalence of the pathogen in fresh vegetables varies worldwide, with 2.22% in Brazil,[62] 10.2% in Chile,[63] 4.18% in Spain,[64] 13.6% in Turkey,[65] and 5.0% in the Czech Republic.[66] In the United States, five outbreaks with 50 cases and five deaths were described during 2018−19.[67] Meanwhile, in 2018, 14 outbreaks involving 158 cases were reported in the EU.[2] Whole cantaloupe was the vehicle of an outbreak that occurred in 2011 in the United States with 147 cases and 33 deaths.[68] Other outbreaks have occurred due to contaminated ice cream, fresh cheeses made from unpasteurized milk, caramel apples, smoked fish, a variety of processed meats, and certain salads. The biggest listeriosis outbreak reported so far occurred in South Africa (SA) in 2017–18 and resulted in 937 cases and at least 193 deaths. A RTE processed meat was identified as the source of the ST6 strain that was identified through the use of Whole Genome Sequencing. One of the more important differences between this outbreak in SA and others is the high percentage of neonates affected.[69]

25.2.5 Escherichia coli

The species is a Gram-negative, facultative anaerobic, motile, nonspore-forming, rod-shaped bacterium.[70] *E. coli* is a coliform and commonly used as a fecal indicator in microbiological testing of food.[71] It can grow between 7°C and 46°C, with an optimum of around 37°C; it requires a pH value >5.4 for growth and survives a salt concentration of 6%.[72] *E. coli* serotypes are characterized by combinations of somatic (O), flagellar (H), and capsular (K) surface antigens, which can be detected through various molecular techniques including serology.[9] The strains mainly responsible for enteric disorders are classified into six pathotypes: enterotoxigenic *E. coli* (ETEC), enteropathogenic *E. coli* (EPEC), enteroaggregative *E. coli* (EAEC), enteroinvasive *E. coli* (EIEC), Shiga toxin-producing *E. coli* (STEC) that includes enterohemorrhagic *E. coli* (EHEC), and diffuse adherence *E. coli* (DAEC). The most lethal is EHEC; the members of this pathotype are Shiga-toxin (Stx) producers (STEC). Although *E. coli* O157:H7 is responsible for most outbreaks worldwide, other non-O157 EHEC serotypes referred to as the "big 6" (O111, O26, O121, O103, O145, and O45) are a focus of concern.[73] It is estimated that STEC causes 265,000 illnesses each year in the United States with at least 30 deaths.[74] Ruminants, in particular, cattle and sheep, are the main animal reservoirs. *E. coli* O157:H7 was detected in 53% of cattle herds in Sweden.[75] In 2018 the frequency of EHEC in herds of the EU was cattle (5.1%), pigs (10%), and goats and sheep (10.5%).[2] Although meat and their products are the main sources of EHEC, in the last few decades, the number of outbreaks linked to fresh produce, particularly leafy greens and sprouts, has increased[2,3] and is a growing cause for concern. *E. coli* O157:H7 can be transferred from manure-amended soil or manure compost–amended soil to leafy greens and root vegetables where it can persist for long periods of time. Zhang et al.[76] found that *E. coli* O157:H7 could survive for at least 25 days on lettuce leaf surfaces. The largest reported EHEC outbreak occurred in 2011 in the EU, with the majority of cases in Germany. The outbreak was caused by the serotype O104:H4. It resulted in 3842 cases, 855 with bloody diarrhea and hemolytic uremic syndrome (HUS), while 53 deaths were reported. The implicated food vehicle was sprouts of fenugreek seeds originating from Egypt. The serotype O104:H4 combined virulence characteristics of EHEC and EAEC, which had not been previously described in any EHEC strain.[77] This demonstrates the constant evolvement of foodborne pathogens.

25.2.6 Salmonella

Salmonella is a Gram-negative, rod-shaped bacterium, which is nonspore-forming, facultative anaerobic and oxidase negative.[78] The *genus* contains two *species—S. bongori* and *S. enterica*—the latter is divided into six *subspecies*: *enterica, salamae, arizonae, diarizonae, houtenae, indica*.[79] Another form of classification widely used is by serotype; there are over 2500 *Salmonella* serotypes. The classification is based on the antigenic composition of cellular structures (capsule, cell wall, and flagella), according to the Kauffman–White typing scheme.[80] In the EU, the five most commonly recovered serovars are *S.* Enteritidis, *S.* Typhimurium, monophasic *S.* Typhimurium, *S.* Infantis, and *S.* Derby.[2] *Salmonella* can grow at a temperature range of 5°C–47°C, with an optimum of 35°C–37°C. The pH for growth varies between 4.0 and 9.0, and the minimum a_w for growth is 0.94.[9] This bacterium is widely dispersed in the environment and the primary reservoir is the intestinal tract of vertebrates, including livestock, wildlife, birds, domestic pets, and humans.[9] In the EU, the prevalence in breeding flocks of *Gallus gallus* and of turkey in 2018 was 2% and 3.9%, respectively.[2] *Salmonella* was the most frequent bacterium involved in foodborne outbreaks in the United States in 2017 with 3007 illnesses. The most common vehicles were chicken and fruit.[3] In the EU, salmonellosis is the second most common foodborne illness, accounting for 1581 outbreaks and 91,857 cases reported in 2018, and the main vehicle identified was eggs and egg products (46%).[2] A multicountry outbreak of *Salmonella* Enteritidis, involving eggs occurred in the EU from 2016 to 2020 totaling 1041 cases.[81] Uniquely, *S.* Enteritidis can contaminate eggs by trans-ovarian or trans-shell infection. Elsewhere, *Salmonella* was detected in 26.3% of poultry and 6.7% of pork meat in Argentina,[58] and in 41% of retail ground poultry in Tulsa (OK, United States).[82] Demirci et al.[83] found that the prevalence of *Salmonella* in raw milk varies according to species; in cow milk it was 4.2%, in sheep milk 3.1%, and in goat milk 1.5%. Although animal foods are the most common linked to salmonellosis outbreaks, in the last few decades the reporting of outbreaks due to consumption of vegetables and low moisture food has increased.[84] In the United States between 2010 and 2017, *Salmonella* was linked to 56 multistate outbreaks associated with fresh produce with a total of 3778 cases and 16 deaths.[85] In addition, the pathogen was responsible for 30% of the outbreaks in fruit and vegetables in Brazil from 2008 to

2014.[17] Furthermore, *Salmonella* was found on 77% of waterleaf and 53% of pumpkin samples in Nigeria.[86] In the Philippines, the prevalence in fresh vegetables, fruit, and sprouted seeds was 24.7%.[87] Regarding low-moisture foods, several outbreaks have been reported. Although *Salmonella* cannot grow in water activity lower than 0.94, it can remain viable for a long time. The pathogen was recovered after 240 and 330 days of storage at 28°C in raw in-shell peanuts and unblanched peanut kernels, respectively.[88] Importantly, the common thread in outbreaks linked to low-moisture foods is the very low levels of *Salmonella* present in those products. Furthermore, a low water activity has a synergistic effect on its heat resistance. Nascimento et al.[89] reported that 8.86 min at 110°C was needed to reduce 1 log of *Salmonella* during the dry roasting of cocoa nibs. In 2018 two multistate outbreaks involving dried coconut and cereal were reported in the United States[90,91] with one of the largest outbreaks linked to peanut butter in the United States between 2008 and 2009. The latter outbreak resulted in 714 illnesses and 9 deaths.[92] Other outbreaks associated with low-moisture foods are listed in Table 25.1.[93–101]

25.2.7 Campylobacter

The genus *Campylobacter* is characterized as a Gram-negative rod with a curved- to S-shaped morphology. It is nonspore-forming, microaerophilic (prefers 3%–6% oxygen), oxidase, and catalase positive.[102] The majority of species are motile, showing motility characteristic of movements in a "corkscrew" fashion. The optimum growth temperature varies according to species, but ranges between 30°C and 43°C; however, most of them do not grow below 25°C–30°C. The optimum pH is 6.5–7.5, with a maximum of 9.5, and they cannot grow at 2% NaCl.[102] *Campylobacter* spp. associated with foodborne illness are thermotolerant and these are *C. jejuni*, *C. coli*, *C. lari*, and *C. upsaliensis*.[103] Food-producing animals, such as chickens, cattle, sheep, and pigs, can be a reservoir of this bacterium. In the EU, *Campylobacter* was found in 72% of turkeys, 26% in broilers, 2% in pigs, and 3% in bovine.[2] In Greece, *Campylobacter* spp. were detected on 47%–67% of goat carcasses and 62%–86% of sheep carcasses.[104] Inadequate processing and cross contamination, for example, in the consumer's kitchen seem to be the most common causes of outbreaks.[105] *Campylobacter* is regarded as one of the most important causes of foodborne disease in the EU and the United States. In 2018, 246,571 cases were reported in the EU and the main foods involved were milk and broiler meat.[2] Meanwhile, in the United States, 17 outbreaks with 117 campylobacteriosis cases were reported in 2017.[3] In the United Kingdom, 79.2% of the broiler batches collected from 37 abattoirs were contaminated with *Campylobacter*.[106] *Campylobacter* was also found on fresh produce due to cross-contamination in the field, especially by poultry manure. Karikari et al.[107] reported that 42% of market vegetables and 24% of vegetables collected from farms in Ghana had *Campylobacter*. In another study, beans and sprouts were the vegetable group with the greatest prevalence (11.1%).[108]

25.2.8 Shigella

The genus *Shigella* embraces four *species*: *S. dysenteriae*, *S. sonnei*, *S. flexneri*, *S. boydii*.[109] They are characterized as rod-shaped bacteria, Gram-negative, nonmotile,

TABLE 25.1 Salmonellosis outbreaks associated with low moisture foods.

Food	Year	Country	Cases	References
Brazil nuts	2019	United Kingdom, France, Luxembourg, Netherlands, Canada	123	EFSA and ECDC[93]
Powdered infant formula (PIF)	2017–18	France, Spain, Greece	39	Jourdan-da Silva et al.[94]
Pistachios	2016	United States	11	CDC[95]
Nut butter spread	2015	United States	13	CDC[96]
Tahini sesame paste	2013	United States	16	CDC[97]
Chocolate	2001–02	Europe, Canada	439	Werber et al.[98]
Snack	1994–95	United States, United Kingdom, Israel	>2200	Shohat et al.[99]; Killalea et al.[100]
Potato chips	1993	Germany	1000	Lehmacher et al.[101]

nonspore-forming, oxidase negative, and H_2S-negative.[110] The temperature for growth ranges from 7°C to 46°C. *Shigella* grows between pH values of 4.8 and 9.3, and tolerates 5%–6% NaCl.[111] The only host and main reservoir are humans, and transmission usually occurs from person to person. However, it can also be transmitted by contaminated water and food, and the foremost contamination routes are feces and food handlers.[9] According to the CDC, *Shigella* is estimated to cause 80–165 million cases and 600,000 deaths annually worldwide, with 99% of the illnesses in developing countries.[112] In Nigeria, *Shigella* was found in 57% of waterleaf, 33% of pumpkin,[86] 2.1% of bovine raw milk, and 1.5% of sheep's raw milk.[83]

25.2.9 Yersinia

Yersinia is characterized as a rod-shaped or coccobacillus bacterium. It is Gram-negative, facultative anaerobic, oxidase negative, catalase and urease positive, and motile at temperatures below 30°C. The optimum growth temperature is 28°C–29°C, but some *species* are psychrotrophic and can grow between −2°C and 45°C.[113] *Yersinia* tolerates up to 5% NaCl, and proliferates between pH 4.6 and 9.6.[114] The main foodborne pathogenic *species* are *Y. enterocolitica* and *Y. pseudotuberculosis*. *Yersinia* has been isolated from the intestinal tract of many domestic and wild animals.[115] In the EU in 2018, the prevalence of *Y. enterocolitica* in pork and beef was 5% and 30%, respectively.[2] Furthermore, between 2005 and 2018, pig meat and products thereof were the food categories most reported to cause yersiniosis. In the EU in 2018, *Y. enterocolitica* was responsible for 12 outbreaks with 58 cases.[2] Although pigs have been identified as a major reservoir for *Y. enterocolitica*, outbreaks have also been traced to milk. An outbreak of yersiniosis associated with improperly pasteurized milk was reported in the United States in 2011 with 22 cases.[116] Ahmed et al.[117] isolated *Y. enterocolitica* from 22% of raw milk and 4% of pasteurized milk samples, and Drake et al.[118] from 7.5% raw milk samples. *Y. enterocolitica* is heat labile, being eliminated by pasteurization, therefore its presence in pasteurized milk could be related to failure of the heat process or to postprocess contamination.[119] In addition, contamination of fruits and vegetables by this pathogen can occur at any step of the production chain, especially during preharvesting through soil or water contaminated with animal feces or manure. *Y. enterocolitica* was isolated from 5.8% of fruits, vegetables, and sprouts in the EU.[120] In Finland, *Yersinia* spp. was recovered from 33% of fresh leafy vegetables.[121] A higher contamination rate was reported in India, with 67.9% of carrot samples testing positive.[122]

25.2.10 Brucella

The genus *Brucella* embraces Gram-negative, nonspore-forming, small coccobacilli, which are catalase negative and oxidase positive. Growth temperature varies between 6°C and 42°C, and they grow at a pH of between 4.5 and 8.7. Brucellosis is considered an occupational disease that affects veterinarians and farm workers, who can be infected by contaminated secretions, tissues, and fetuses, when handling such materials.[123] However, the bacterium can also be transmitted by food and the main vehicles are unpasteurized milk and soft cheeses made from unpasteurized milk.[9] The habit of consuming unpasteurized milk and dairy products from informal markets plus poor sanitary control of the dairy herd contribute to making *Brucella* an endemic problem in developing countries. The average incidence rate of *B. abortus* varied from 0.03 to 33.93/100,000 cattle in Brazil from 2014 to 2018.[124] In Pakistan, the prevalence in small ruminants ranged from 13.5% to 42.6%,[125,126] and in large ruminants from 3.84% to 47.19%.[127,128] According to McDermott et al.,[129] in 2013 the prevalence of *Brucella* in Africa and Asia ranged between 0% and 88.8% in sheep and goats and 0% and 68.8% in cattle. Moreover, the authors reported a prevalence of 11% in veterinarians, livestock handlers, and abattoir workers. Between 2005 and 2017, 16 foodborne outbreaks of brucellosis were reported in the EU with 153 cases and 1 death; 4 of them were associated with cheeses.[2] In 2018 in Italy, the prevalence of *Brucella* in this food category was 3%. At the same time, a low number of cattle herds were reported positive (0.18%) for *Brucella* in nonofficially brucellosis-free regions in the EU.[2] The presence of *Brucella* in cheeses made with pasteurized milk can be due to cross-contamination and poor food hygiene, since this bacterium is unable to survive to pasteurization.[72]

25.2.11 Cronobacter

Cronobacter, previously named *Enterobacter sakazakii*, was accepted as a new *genus* in 2007.[130] At present, the *genus* contains seven *species*: *C. sakazakii*, *C. malonaticus*, *C. turicensis*, *C. muytjensii*, *C. dublinensis*, *C. universalis*, and *C. condimenti*.[131] It is a Gram-negative, rod-shaped, nonsporulating, and motile bacterium.[131] *Cronobacter* spp. particularly affect neonates and young infants and are classified as a severe hazard, with a high-mortality rate up to 80%.[132] Between 1961 and 2018, 183 cases of *Cronobacter* infant infections were reported worldwide; most cases were in the United States (79), followed by the United Kingdom (35).[133] This pathogen is widely spread in the environment and has a great resistance to osmotic stress. *Cronobacter* has been isolated from powdered infant formula (PIF), rehydrated infant formula, and utensils used to prepare infant formula.[134] Its survival in PIF for up to 2 years has been reported.[9] In a survey conducted in the EU, 1.5% samples including PIF and dairy products were positive for *C. sakazakii*.[2] PIF can become contaminated by cross-contamination due to poor hygiene practices. *Cronobacter* can also affect adults, especially elderly and immunocompromised and most cases are nosocomial.[135,136]

25.3 Toxigenic fungi

The three fungal genera of most importance in the spoilage of foodstuffs and in the production of mycotoxins are *Aspergillus*, *Fusarium*, and *Penicillium*. Mycotoxins are toxic metabolites, produced by some fungal species during their growth, with mutagenic, teratogenic, and carcinogenic effects on humans and animals.[137,138] Production occurs only as a result of fungal growth: the presence of spores of a particular fungus on a foodstuff does not mean that mycotoxin was necessarily produced. However, if environmental conditions, especially temperature and water activity (a_W), are favorable for fungal growth, toxin production may occur at any period during growing, harvesting, drying, or storage of food commodities. Mycotoxins may occur in processed foods, but are less frequent than in commodities such as grains or nuts, since during processing most fungi are killed. However, mycotoxins are typically chemically stable once formed and persist in food even after the destruction of the fungi that produced them.[138] According to a Food and Agriculture Organization (FAO) study, approximately 25% of the global food and feed output is contaminated by mycotoxins.[139]

25.3.1 Aspergillus

The genus *Aspergillus* is among the most abundant and widely distributed organisms on earth and at the moment comprises 339 known species.[140] This genus has a great impact on several areas of research. On the positive side, it is being used in biotechnology for the production of metabolites such as antibiotics, organic acids, medicines, enzymes, or as agents in food fermentations. On the negative side, some species can be pathogens in animals and humans, food spoilage agents causing changes in the sensorial, nutritional, and quality aspects such as: pigmentation, discoloration, rot, unpleasant flavors, and odors. However, the most undesirable consequence is the production of mycotoxins in food and feed.[141]

Aspergillus species are widespread geographically and can be either beneficial or harmful microorganisms; however, they have mainly a saprophytic lifestyle and predominantly grow on plant decaying materials. Aspergilli are one of the major causes of degradation of agricultural products, as they can contaminate food and feed at different stages, including pre- and postharvest, processing, and handling.[142] *Aspergillus* species are well adapted to growth in the tropics and subtropical countries, as common species rarely grow below 10°C and most grow strongly at 37°C or above. Most species that occur commonly in foods are xerophilic, able to grow down to, or near to, 0.80 water activity. Some are strictly saprophytic, growing only after harvest, while some are commensals, able to grow in some plant crops and developing nuts or kernels before harvest without causing damage to the crop.[143]

Some *Aspergillus* species are opportunistic pathogens without host specialization, and are frequently isolated as food contaminants. *A. niger, A. flavus*, and *A. fumigatus* cause animal and human diseases, like mycotoxicoses, noninvasive, and invasive infections in immune-compromised patients, and hypersensitive reactions (e.g., asthma, allergic alveolitis) due to exposure to fungal fragments.[142]

The groups of toxigenic *Aspergillus* most commonly found in food are: *Aspergillus* section *Flavi* (aflatoxins B_1, B_2, G_1, G_2, cyclopiazonic acid), *Aspergillus* section *Circumdati* [ochratoxin A (OTA)], and *Aspergillus* section *Nigri* (OTA and fumonisins B_2 and B_4) that will be described below.

25.3.1.1 *Aspergillus* section *Flavi*

Aspergillus section *Flavi* are producers of aflatoxins and other mycotoxins. Currently, 16 species of this group are recognized as aflatoxin producers: *A. flavus, A. parasiticus, A. nomius, A. pseudonomius, A. novoparasiticus, A. pseudotamarii, A. togoensis, A. pseudocaelatus, A. luteovirescens, A. minisclerotigenes, A. arachidicola, A. sergii, A. transmontanensis, A. aflatoxiformans, A. austwickii*, and *A. cerealis*.[144]

Aflatoxins are the most relevant mycotoxins in food because they are the most toxic and carcinogenic to humans and animals. Due to their extreme hepatocarcinogenicity, extensive research has been conducted on the natural occurrence, identification, characterization, biosynthesis, and control of production.[137] According to the International Agency for Research on Cancer (IARC),[145] aflatoxin B1 is the most potent of aflatoxins and was classified as a Group 1 carcinogen.

Several species of *Aspergillus* section *Flavi* producing aflatoxins have been described, but the most common in food are: *A. flavus, A. parasiticus, A. nomius*, and related species. These species are commensal with peanuts and maize and grow in these plants under unfavorable growth conditions, such as drought stress, which permits infection of developing nuts or grains, and hence the production of aflatoxins before harvest.[146]

A. flavus isolates produce B aflatoxins and some also produce cyclopiazonic acid. On a worldwide basis, about 40% of *A. flavus* isolates produce aflatoxins, though percentages of toxin producing isolates may vary with land use.[147] Isolates of *A. parasiticus* produce both B and G aflatoxins but not cyclopiazonic acid, and almost all isolates are toxigenic.[147]

A. flavus and *A. parasiticus* have similar growth patterns. Both grow at temperatures ranging from 10°C−12°C to 42°C−43°C, with an optimum from 30°C−33°C,[143] with aflatoxins being produced from 12°C−40°C. The optimum a_w for growth is near 0.996, with minima reported as 0.80 to 0.82−0.83. Aflatoxins are generally produced in greater quantity at higher a_w values (0.98−0.99) with toxin production apparently ceasing at or near a_w 0.85. Although growth can take place over the pH range of just above 2.0 up to 10.5 (*A. parasiticus*) or 11.2 (*A. flavus*), aflatoxin production has been reported for *A. parasiticus* only between pH 3.0 and 8.0, with an optimum near pH 6.0.[143]

25.3.1.2 *Aspergillus* section *Circumdati*

Aspergillus section *Circumdati* comprises 27 accepted species; 13 species are able to produce OTA: *A. affinis, A. cretenses, A. flocculosus, A. fresenii, A. muricatus, A. occultus, A. ochraceus, A. pseudoelegans, A. pulvericola, A. roseoglobulosus, A. sclerotiorum, A. steynii*, and *A. westerdijkiae*. In addition, seven species produce OTA inconsistently and/or in trace amounts: *A. melleus, A. ostianus, A. persii, A. salwaensis, A. sesamicola, A. subramanianii*, and *A. westlandensis*.[148]

The species belonging to the *Aspergillus* section *Circumdati* are important because of the production of several mycotoxins including OTA,[149] penicillic acid,[150] xanthomegnin, viomelein, and vioxantin.[150−152] Among these, OTA is the most potent, exhibiting carcinogenic, teratogenic, and immunotoxic properties in rats. The IARC has classified this compound as a possible human carcinogen (Group 2B), based on sufficient evidence of carcinogenicity in experimental animal studies but inadequate evidence in humans.[153] The target organ of toxicity in all mammalian species tested is the kidneys, in which lesions can be produced by both acute and chronic exposure.

The main OTA producer species in *Aspergillus* section *Circumdati* are *A. ochraceus, A. westerdijkiae*, and *A. steynii*.[154] These three species have similar growth requirements apart from the difference in maximum growth temperature, 40°C for *A. ochraceus* and about 5°C lower for the other species *A. westerdijkiae* and *A. steynii*. These latter two species are distinguished from *A. ochraceus* by their inability to grow on Czapek Yeast Autolysate agar at 37°C. These three species are xerophilic, growing down to a_w of 0.8 or below, and as such can be isolated from stored dry foods.

25.3.1.3 *Aspergillus* section *Nigri*

At present, *Aspergillus* section *Nigri* comprises 27 accepted species; five of these produce OTA: *A. carbonarius, A. lacticoffeatus, A. niger, A. sclerotioniger*, and *A. welwitschiae*.[140,155,156]

Aspergillus niger is the representative species of the section and it is the most frequently reported in food, together with *A. carbonarius, A. japonicus*, and *A. aculeatus*. Recently, *A. tubingensis, A. uvarum*, and *A. welwitschiae* have also been found as food contaminating species.[142]

A. niger has usually been regarded as a benign fungus and has been widely used in enzyme production and ingredients for food processing. It holds GRAS (generally recognized as safe) status from the USA/FDA. Usually only a low percentage of *A. niger* isolates are able to produce OTA. Although *A. niger* is very frequently isolated, it is not a significant source of OTA as a rule.

A. carbonarius is the largest OTA producer within the *Aspergillus* section *Nigri*. The percentage of ochratoxigenic strains in *A. carbonarius* varies from 70% to 100%[155,157,158] whereas for *A. niger* it has been restricted to only 3%−10% of isolates.[155,157]

Frisvad et al.[159] reported the production of fumonisin B_2 (FB_2) by *A. niger* for the first time, after the genome of *A. niger* had been fully sequenced. Until then, the production of fumonisin had been reported only in *Fusarium* species. Later on, *A. welwitschiae* was dismembered from the *A. niger* taxon.[160] OTA, FB_2, and FB_4 were produced by some isolates of both species.[161,162] The cooccurrence of OTA, FB_2, and FB_4 in foods is of concern since these species are commonly found.

A. niger grows at a minimum of 6°C−8°C and a maximum of 45°C−47°C, while *A. carbonarius* grows from 10°C to 41°C. The a_w for *A. niger* germination was reported at 0.77 at 35°C. For *A. carbonarius*, the optimum a_w for growth is 0.96−0.98, with a minimum near to a_w 0.85 at 25°C−30°C.[143] The black spores of this group apparently protect the fungus from sunlight and ultraviolet rays, providing a competitive advantage in habitats such as drying yards and vineyards.[143] As a result, species in *Aspergillus* section *Nigri* are the source of OTA in products such as grapes,[163,164] dried fruits,[165,166] coffee,[157,167] and cocoa.[158] *A. welwitschiae* has been found in dried fruits, grapes, coffee beans, and cocoa.[168,169] Gherbawy et al.[170] and Silva et al.[156] reported *A. welwitschiae* as the prevalent species in onion samples. Logrieco et al.[171] showed that black aspergilli, and in particular strains belonging to *A. niger* and *A. welwitschiae*, could contribute to some extent to the contamination of maize by fumonisins in association with *Fusarium verticillioides*. This fact is of great concern since maize is consumed as a staple food in several Latin American and African countries.

25.3.2 Penicillium

Penicillium is the more diverse genus, in terms of numbers of species and range of habitats. It produces a very wide range of compounds, some of these are known as pharmaceuticals, such as penicillin (antibiotic, *Penicillium rubens*), griseofulvin (antifungal, *Penicillium griseofulvum*), and mycophenolic acid (immunosuppressant, *Penicillium brevicompactum*), among others. Other industrial applications include the production of organic acids and enzymes.[172]

In general, *Penicillium* species are strictly aerobic, able to grow in a wide range of physicochemical environments.[173] Some of them are fruit pathogens (*P. expansum* on apples, *P. digitatum* and *P. italicum* on citrus fruits). Some species grow in low-water content feeds (*P. brevicompactum, P. chrysogenum*, and *P. implicatum*), and others at low oxygen tension (*P. roqueforti*).

The range of mycotoxin classes produced by *Penicillium* is broader than for any other fungal genus. OTA is undoubtedly the most important toxin produced by a *Penicillium* species. Some minor mycotoxins (non-regulated) produced include: citreoviridin, citrinin, cyclopiazonic acid, penicillic acid, and roquefortine C.[173]

Most of the *Penicillium* foodborne species are psychrophilic, some are hardly able to grow at 37°C, but they are mainly mesophilic with optimum temperatures around 25°C. *P. verrucosum* and *P. nordicum* are OTA producers in cool temperate climates, ranging across Northern and Central Europe, Canada, and Northern Asia. The physiology of these two species is very similar. Both grow from about 0°C–31°C, with optimum at 20°C. The minimum a_w for germination and growth is 0.80.[143] Maximum OTA production occurs at about 20°C, and is possible down to about a_w of 0.85.[72]

P. verrucosum is the major OTA producer in cereal products, especially bread and flour-based foods, and is found in the meat of animals that eat contaminated cereals as a major dietary component.[138] *P. verrucosum* is not found in warmer climates, so small grains from the tropics and warm temperate zones do not contain OTA.[143] *P. nordicum* is closely related to *P. verrucosum* but does not occur in cereals. However, it has been found in manufactured meat products such as salami and ham, and can produce OTA there.

Patulin, a genotoxic mycotoxin, is produced by a large number of species belonging to *Penicillium, Aspergillus, Paecilomyces*, and *Byssochlamys* genera. It has been found frequently in apples decayed by *Penicillium expansum*, especially those that have fallen on the soil surface. Use of poor quality apples can lead to contamination of apple juice by patulin.[174] *P. expansum* with the potential of producing patulin was isolated from a variety of fruits including apples, apricots, black mulberries, cherries, kiwis, lingon berries, nectarines, plums, strawberries, and white mulberries.[173,175] The presence of patulin has been found in several fruit juices of pear (64.1%), peach (6.7%), apricot (25.9%), and mixed juices (31.0%) with an average of 0.3–5.1 μg/kg.[176]

25.3.3 Fusarium

Many *Fusarium* species are plant pathogens, while others are saprophytic; most can be found in the soil. In terms of foods, *Fusarium* species are most often encountered as contaminants of cereal grains, seeds, beans, and milled cereal products such as flour and corn meal, barley malt, animal feeds, and necrotic plant tissue.

Some *Fusarium* species produce several toxic or biologically active metabolites. The trichothecenes are a group of closely related compounds that are esters of sesquiterpene alcohols that possess a basic trichothecene skeleton and an epoxide group. The trichothecenes are divided into three groups: the type A trichothecenes (diacetoxyscirpenol, T-2 toxin, HT-2 toxin, and neosolaniol); the type B trichothecenes [deoxynivalenol (DON), 3-acetydeoxynivalenol, 15-acetyldeoxnyivalenol, nivalenol, and fusarenon-X]; and the type C (macrocyclic trichothecenes known as satratoxins). Of these, the toxin most commonly found in cereal grains or most often associated with human illness is DON. Other *Fusarium* toxins associated with diseases are zearalenone and the fumonisins.

The most important general observation to be made about the production of mycotoxins by *Fusarium* species is that they all grow at high a_w (>0.9), so that toxin production in crops occurs before harvest as a result of growth of the causal fungus in the living plant and seed or during early stages of drying. Production of mycotoxins ceases long before the crops are fully dried, but can occur during storage under flooding or other catastrophic conditions.[138]

Wheat and maize are the crops in which *Fusarium* mycotoxins have the most frequent occurrence and greatest impact. However, toxigenic *Fusarium* species can occur in all small grain crops, as well as many other crops such as asparagus, figs, forage grasses, soybean and other legumes, spice plants, medicinal plants, and some nut crops such as pistachio. *Fusarium* toxins also can occur in spoiled food products made from plants that are not necessarily hosts for pathogenic infections. As a consequence of crop contamination, *Fusarium* toxins occur in prepared animal feeds and human food products, including fermented products such as beer,[177] since these toxins are heat stable.

25.3.3.1 *Fusarium species producing fumonisins*

Fumonisins are produced by *F. verticillioides* (known in older literature as *F. moniliforme)* and some closely related species, in particular, *F. proliferatum*. These species are systemic in maize worldwide, being always present in the plants, and even in healthy kernels.

F. verticillioides grows at a maximum temperature of 32°C–37°C, a minimum of 2.5°C–5°C, and at an optimum near 25°C. The minimum a_w for growth has been reported as 0.87 at 25°C.[143] FB_1 and FB_2 were produced at a_w as low as 0.92 but were not detected at a_w 0.89–0.91.[178,179]

Fumonisins are found primarily in maize and sorghum, as are *F. verticillioides* and *F. proliferatum* and rarely infect other crops. Although these two species are found in all maize growing regions, these fungi are most prolific in humid tropical and subtropical regions.[180] In general, fumonisin levels are influenced by insect damage, moisture content of the soil, high daytime maximum temperatures, and nutrient-deficient soils.[181,182] Although fumonisin formation is believed to occur predominantly in maize at preharvest, there are some reports that the toxin forms postharvest, mainly when maize is inadequately stored at high temperatures and high relative humidity (RH).[178,181,183]

25.3.3.2 *Fusarium species producing deoxynivalenol*

DON is produced by *Fusarium graminearum* (often listed as *Gibberella zeae*, its sexual stage), *F. culmorum*, and less commonly some related species. *F. graminearum* occurs in maize, and both *F. graminearum* and *F. culmorum* occur in small grains, especially wheat and barley. These species are pathogens, invading plants and grains by causing diseases, known as *Gibberella* ear rot in maize and *Fusarium* head blight in wheat, barley, and triticale. Epidemics of *Gibberella* ear rot require the congruence of three factors: airborne or insect-borne spores, inoculation at the susceptible time, and appropriate moisture and temperature. This disease is prevalent in north temperate climates especially in wet years and much less commonly in the tropics.[138]

F. graminearum grows at 15°C–37°C, with optimal temperatures between 24°C and 26°C. The minimum a_w for growth is close to 0.90 at 15°C–25°C.[143] The range of a_w for DON production is 0.95–0.995 at temperatures of 25°C–30°C.[184]

DON is the most common trichothecene found in grains; therefore the greatest potential exists for it to occur in finished foods and food ingredients such as wheat flour bread, pasta, corn, cornmeal, breakfast cereals, corn chips, snack foods, popcorn, and beer.[143,185] Cereal grains and nuts are often used as ingredients in commercial pet food as well. Cereal by-products, furthermore, may be diverted to animal feed even though they may contain concentrated levels of mycotoxins. Commonly found mycotoxins in pet food include *Fusarium* toxins, aflatoxins, and ochratoxins, among others.[186,187]

25.3.3.3 *Fusarium species producing zearalenone*

Several species of the genus *Fusarium* produce zearalenone including *F. culmorum, F. equiseti*, and *F. graminearum*, the same *Fusarium* species that produce DON and nivalenol, and generally under the same conditions. Different members of the genus *Fusarium* capable of producing zearalenone may survive in the temperate and/or tropical zones.[188]

Although zearalenone is probably most common in maize, it can also be found in barley, oats, wheat, rice, and sorghum, together with their related products. Production of zearalenone in maize appears to occur later during kernel development, which differs from DON that occurs relatively early in kernel development in both wheat and maize.[188]

25.4 Routes of contamination

25.4.1 Feces and manure

Livestock is an important reservoir for a number of foodborne pathogens. Consequently, their feces often used as biological soil amendments are considered one of the main root causes of microbial contamination, especially in primary production.[189] This contamination can occur through direct or indirect contact with feces or raw manure or inadequately treated manure. According to the *Codex Alimentarius Commission*, manure is defined as animal excrement, which may be mixed with litter or other material and may be fermented or otherwise treated.[190]

Foodborne outbreaks due to the application of contaminated animal waste have been widely reported. Manure, feral swine feces, and compost were suspected to be the contamination source of three *E. coli* O157:H7 outbreaks associated with the consumption of leafy vegetables in 2005 in Sweden, in 2006 in the United States and Canada, and in 2019 in the United States, respectively.[3,191,192] Furthermore, a listeriosis outbreak was linked to the consumption of coleslaw, which was made from cabbage fertilized with sheep manure.[193] Feces can also contaminate milk during milking and meat during slaughtering. *Salmonella* was detected on 17.1% and *E. coli* O157 on 1.5% of small-ruminant hide surfaces.[194] The prevalence of some foodborne pathogens in feces and manure is shown in Table 25.2.[194–213]

The survival and fate of pathogens in feces, manure, slurry, or composting depend on multiple factors such as

TABLE 25.2 Prevalence of foodborne pathogens in feces and manure.

Microorganism	Sample	Animal	Prevalence (%)	Country	Reference
Listeria monocytogenes	Feces	Various	13.5	ND	Lyautey et al.[195]
L. monocytogenes	Manure	Pig	18.2	ND	Pourcher et al.[196]
L. monocytogenes	Manure	ND	25	ND	Orzi et al.[197]
L. monocytogenes	Manure	ND	40		Le Maréchal et al.[198]
L. monocytogenes	Manure	ND	8.0	Iran	Gholipour[199]
Clostridium botulinum type D, and E	Manure	Cows	8.3, and 12.5	ND	Neuhaus et al.[200]
C. botulinum	Manure	ND	60	ND	Le Maréchal et al.[198]
C. botulinum	Manure	Poultry	56.5	ND	Souillard et al.[201]
Bacillus cereus	Feces, liquid manure		78.9, 100	China	Cui et al.[202]
Salmonella	Feces	Sheep	7.0	United States	Edrington et al.[203]
Salmonella	Feces	Goats and lambs	10.3 and 11.4	ND	Hanlon et al.[194]
Salmonella	Feces	Poultry	52.4	ND	Kagambèga et al.[204]
Salmonella	Manure	Pig	50	ND	Pourcher et al.[196]
Salmonella	Manure	Pig	1.6	Germany	
Salmonella	Manure	Swine	38.5	United States	Pornsukarom and Thakur[205]
Salmonella	Manure	ND	100		Le Maréchal et al.[198]
Arcobacter butzleri	Feces	Cow	4–40	ND	Golla et al.[206]; Grove-White et al.[207]; Vilar et al.[208]
Brucella spp.	Manure	Cows and goats	33	ND	Morales-Estrada et al.[209]
Campylobacter	Feces	Goats	35.1	Congo	Mpalang et al.[210]
Campylobacter spp.	Feces	Goats and lambs	71.0 and 75.0	United States, Mexico, and Bahamas	Hanlon et al.[194]
Campylobacter spp.	Feces	Poultry	68	ND	Kagambèga et al.[204]
Campylobacter	Manure	Pig	36.5	ND	Farzan et al.[211]
Campylobacter spp.	Manure	ND	100	ND	Le Maréchal et al.[198]
E. coli O157:H7	Feces	Lambs	9.0	United States	Edrington et al.[203]
E. coli O157:H7	Feces	Goats and sheep	3.3 and 5.4	Ethiopia	Mersha et al.[212]
E. coli O157:H7	Feces	Goats and lambs	19.7 and 9.8	United States, Mexico, and Bahamas	Hanlon et al.[194]
Yersinia enterocolitica	Manure and feces	ND	5.8	Canada	Farzan et al.[211]
Y. enterocolitica	Stool and manure	Pig	7.2	ND	Bozcal et al.[213]

ND, Not declared.

environmental conditions (temperature, pH, UV, moisture), aeration, soil type, dry matter content, holding time, species, concentration, and interaction of microorganisms and compost-type treatment.[214,215] According to Nicholson et al.,[216] the survival of *Campylobacter, E. coli* O157:H7, *L. monocytogenes*, and *Salmonella* in solid manure varied from 2 to 32 days, the most resistant bacterium was *E. coli* O157:H7 and the least was *Campylobacter*. However, a long-term survival of *E. coli* O157:H7 has been reported. In dairy cow compost, this pathogen survived for 154 days and up to 168 days at 22°C and 5°C, respectively.[217] In high moisture content bovine manure, it survived for over 70 days at 5°C and for 49 days at 30°C.[218] In addition, non-O157 STEC persisted for over 125 days in dairy compost stored at 4°C and 22°C.[219] A study from sub-Saharan Africa recovered *S.* Typhimurium after 14 weeks in high-density inoculated manure.[220] In poultry compost, *Salmonella* remained viable for 77 days at 22°C and up to 168 days at 5°C.[217] *Campylobacter* survived in goose feces for up to 7 days in winter compared with less than 2 days in summer.[221] Smith et al.[222] reported that *C. jejuni* survived for 72 h at 20°C, 25°C, and 30°C under aerobic and low-RH conditions. *Brucella* spp. survived for up to 122 days at room temperature in cow feces[223] and *L. monocytogenes* for up to 6 months in dairy slurry[216] and up to 40 days in digestates.[224]

To reduce the initial microbial load in manure, slurry, and other natural fertilizers, proper physical, chemical, or biological treatment methods (composting, pasteurization, natural and artificial drying, UV irradiation, alkaline digestion, or combinations of these) should be adopted.[190] However, few studies have been conducted to validate whether the processes inactivate foodborne pathogens. Based on that, Canadian authorities specify 3, 15, and 12 months for tree fruits and grapes, small fruits, and vegetables, respectively, as the minimum holding time delay between manure application and harvesting of these crops.[225] In the United States, a 90- or 120-day interval between application of untreated manure and harvesting of crops is recommended.[226] Furthermore, the FDA Food Safety Modernization Act (FSMA) establishes as microbiological standards for soil amendments of animal origin: <3 MPN *Salmonella* spp. per 4 g of total solids (dry weight basis) and <1000 MPN fecal coliforms per gram of total solids (dry weight basis).[227]

25.4.1.1 Compost

Composting is a biological aerobic or anaerobic process in which microorganisms convert organic wastes into a product that can be used as fertilizer.[190] Compost is widely used in the production of food crops in both developing and developed countries. The process needs to be carried out under controlled conditions aiming to reduce initial pathogen load and at the same time stabilize and convert the organic wastes into products that can be easily handled.[228] The microbial activity generates heat ($\geq$55°C) to kill enteric bacterial pathogens originally present in the feedstocks.[229] According to Qian et al.,[230] thermophilic composting resulted in reductions of the pathogenic bacteria population from 77% to 97%. Heat treatment (55°C) resulted in 3 and 4 log reductions of *E. coli* O157:H7 in dairy cattle manure after 30 and 100 min, respectively.[231] The presence of niches with different temperatures during the composting process can lead to the survival of pathogens.[232] *E. coli* and *Salmonella* could persist on the heap surface of poultry compost during the first composting phase.[233] However, composting at 64°C caused a reduction of 7 log CFU of *Salmonella* after 20 days.[234]

25.4.2 Seeds

Seeds are an agricultural input that play a relevant role in microbial contamination in the field, especially for sprouts. In the United States, seed sprouts were linked to 38% of foodborne outbreaks reported from 2006 to 2014.[235] In 2009 contaminated seeds were responsible for an outbreak of *Salmonella* in alfalfa sprouts involving 235 cases.[236] In addition, in 2011 a large outbreak of *E. coli* O104:H4 occurred in Germany and other countries resulting in 3911 cases, 47 deaths, and 777 patients with HUS. Fenugreek sprouts germinated locally from contaminated seeds imported from Egypt 2 years earlier were identified as the primary source of the outbreak.[237] In 2014 in the United States, an outbreak of *E. coli* O121 was associated with clover sprouts likely produced from contaminated seeds.[238] In case of fungi, infection by *Fusarium* species may sometimes occur in developing seeds, especially in cereals, which may be a potential for toxin production.[137]

The use of manure-amended soil when germinating seeds can be an important route for transfer of pathogens to fresh produce. Semenov et al.[239] reported that *S.* Typhimurium and *E. coli* O157:H7 colonized the rhizosphere and phyllosphere of cress and oat seedlings after seeds had been germinated in soil mixed with manure previously contaminated with either pathogen. According to the ICMSF,[132] cultivating seeds using Good Agricultural Practices (GAP) and preinspecting batches are useful tools to prevent microbial contamination of fresh produce, especially, sprouts.

25.4.3 Soil

Soil is a natural source of a large variety of spore-forming and nonspore-forming microorganisms, including foodborne pathogens[240] and fungi.[137] Some of them are ubiquitous in soil and others can be introduced by amendments, water, or animals.[241] The microbial diversity and concentration are very high in the top 10 cm of the soil and decrease with depth.[242] The prevalence of some foodborne pathogens in soil is shown in Table 25.3.[205,243–255]

Survival of microorganisms in soil depends on several factors, including temperature, soil moisture, RH, rate of ultraviolet radiation, presence of plants, nutrient availability, agronomic practices, microbial competition, and soil type.[256,257] The long-term persistence of foodborne pathogens in soil is of particular concern especially in fresh produce crops that undergo minimal processing prior to consumption. Moist and organic soils permit longer survival than dry and low-organic soils.[258] *Salmonella* survival was enhanced in clay loam compared to sand, at lower temperatures, and in manure-amended soils compared to unamended soils.[259] This was attributed to higher organic matter and nutrient content, as well as more alkaline pH.[260] In addition, according to some studies, *Salmonella* persistence in soil ranges from 21 to 332 days.[205,261–263] Another relevant pathogen that is carried by soil is *E. coli* O157:H7; it can persist in soil between 12 and 217 days.[264–266] Poultry litter amended soils significantly supported *E. coli* O157:H7 survival compared to horse manure amended soils.[267] This pathogen population declined 1 log CFU/g after 29 and 37 days, in sandy and clay soils, respectively.[263] In a study using a soil system held at 25°C, both *E. coli* O157:H7 and *Salmonella* were affected by moisture content with greater losses in soils adjusted to 40% water-holding capacity (WHC) compared to soils adjusted to 20% WHC.[268] In addition to these two bacteria, there are data in the literature on the survival of other foodborne pathogens. *B. abortus* and *B. suis* survived for more than 60 days and up to 28 days in soil, respectively.[269,270] *C. botulinum* type D persisted in amended soils for over 939 days[271] and *C. jejuni* for at least 28 days in clay loam.[272] Furthermore, Huang, Flint, and Palmer[273] reported 1 g of soil containing 50–380,000 CFU of *B. cereus* spores.

Uncultivated soils contain very low numbers of *A. flavus*, but soils in peanut fields usually contain 100–1000 propagules/g. Under drought stress conditions, this number may rise to 10^4–10^5 CFU/g.[274] Direct entry to developing peanuts through the shell by *A. flavus* in the soil appears to be the main method for nut infection.[275] The major causes of preharvest infection are high spore numbers in soil and plant stress induced by drought and/or high soil temperatures.

As is the case with peanuts, the soil in which maize is grown is often highly contaminated with *A. flavus* sclerotia (resting bodies) and conidia, as a result of colonization of unharvested grains or kernels. These particles provide a ready source of inoculation of future crops, entering developing cobs either during silking or by insect damage, providing access to ripening kernels. Colonization of the silks also allows invasion of the cobs directly.[276] Maize is particularly sensitive to drought stress, which increases *A. flavus* density in soil and reduces the plant defense mechanisms.

TABLE 25.3 Prevalence of foodborne pathogens in soil.

Microorganism	Prevalence (%)	Country	Reference
Bacillus cereus	27.5	Nigeria	Mgbakogu and Eledo[243]
B. cereus	72	Ghana	Owusu-Kwarteng et al.[244]
Listeria monocytogenes	17	–	Locatelli et al.[245]
L. monocytogenes	2	India	Kulesh et al.[246]
Clostridium perfringens	41	–	Nayel et al.[247]
C. perfringens	25.5	Greece	Stefanis et al.[248]
C. botulinum, C. perfringens	1, 38	Costa Rica	del Mar Gamboa et al.[249]
C. botulinum, C. perfringens	10, 10	Nigeria	Makut et al.[250]
Salmonella	10.7	United States	Pornsukarom and Thakur[205]
Cronobacter sakazakii	33.33	–	Singh et al.[251]
Brucella abortus, B. melitensis	1.8, 0.31	Pakistan	Ahmed et al.[252]
Campylobacter	10	–	Schets et al.[253]
Escherichia coli	54	Bangladesh	Pickering et al.[254]
EPEC, *Shigella*, STEC, *E. coli* O157	30, 25, 15, 7.5	India	Shrivastava et al.[255]

Brazil nuts are harvested from the ground, beneath trees growing naturally in Amazonian forests. Harvesting is intermittent, up to a month apart, providing time for the ever-present aflatoxigenic species to infect the nuts.[277] In the case of pistachio nuts, entry of *A. flavus* into the nuts depends on the time of splitting of hulls. Nuts in which hull splitting occurs early are much more susceptible to *A. flavus* invasion on the tree.[278] However, it is known that some cultivars are more prone to early splitting than others, and this is especially important where nuts are harvested from the ground, after contact with the soil.[278]

In some countries, figs are harvested from the ground. Immature figs are not colonized by *A. flavus*, but once they are ripe, infection occurs readily and fungal growth continues during drying.[279,280]

Coffee samples collected from the ground showed high levels of OTA, indicating that infection mostly occurred after harvest, and fungal sources were likely to be the soil.[157]

25.4.4 Dust

Dust is a vehicle for spreading contamination through the air in both field and manufacturing environments. This may occur by emission of bioaerosols from the farms or indirectly by contamination of tools, farming implements, clothing, etc., which are brought inside the farm buildings.[281,282] An example of the spreading potential is the study conducted by Berry et al.,[283] who detected *E. coli* O157:H7 in leafy green samples planted up to 180 m away from a cattle feedlot. Moreover, *Salmonella* was isolated from 40.3% of dust samples collected in the surrounding environment of layer farms in Korea.[284] Several factors may influence the survival of bacteria in aerosols and in settled dust, such as composition and structure of dust particles, microbial species, RH, and temperature.[285–287] LA-MRSA was recovered even after 66–72 days in swine farm dust.[288] In turkey manure dust, the microbial survival was influenced by the moisture content. *Salmonella* was recovered after 68, 88, and 291 days in 15%, 10%, and 5% moisture content, respectively.[289]

The principal mechanisms of *Fusarium* species infection include splash dispersal of infective material from the soil by rain during anthesis (wheat and barley) or silking (maize), together with transfer of infective material by wind.

25.4.5 Insects and wildlife

Insects act as mechanical and biological vectors that can spread foodborne pathogens throughout the food production chain.[290,291] Some species that feed on plants can also provide a direct route for internalizing pathogens into fresh produce.[292] They are equally attracted to excrements and human food sources and are commonly found in manure piles and feedlots.[293,294] According to Martínez-Vaz et al.[295] farms practicing mixed farming represents a more significant contamination risk. Studies verified the ability of flies to transfer *E. coli* O157:H7 from manure to spinach leaves[292,296] and apples.[297] *C. sakazakii*, *B. cereus*, *E. coli* 0157:H7, and *S. dysenteriae* were detected in house flies in Florida.[298] *E. coli* was found in 54% of flies[254] and *E. coli* O157:H7 was isolated in 5.2% of flies sampled from cattle and swine farms.[299] In addition, *Campylobacter* was recovered from 5% of flies in poultry farms[300] and from 25% of flies in cattle farms.[301] In Serbia, 1.6% of honey bees had *C. botulinum* spores,[302] and in India, *L. monocytogenes* was recovered from 3.9% of invertebrates on goat farms.[246]

High levels of aflatoxins in early split pistachio nuts were associated with navel orange worm (*Amyelois transitella*) infestation.[278] It appears probable that the most important route for entry of *A. flavus* to maize is through insect damage.[303,304] For fumonisin, studies from natural occurrence and experimental infections clearly demonstrate the importance of drought stress and insect damage at the same time as temperatures that are favorable. Factors that control insects confer resistance to other ear diseases (*Fusarium* ear rot, *Gibberella* ear rot), and adaptations, including drought and temperature tolerance, are important in reducing the risk of fumonisin accumulations in maize.[137] Insects play an important role in the infection of maize since they act as wounding agents or as the vector spreading the fungus to the maize plant.[305] Higher levels of fungal infection in crops infested with the western corn rootworm beetle (*Diabrotica virgifera*) than in those which were not demonstrated that the beetle was a vector for *F. moniliforme* (*F. verticillioides*) and *F. subglutinans* infection.[306]

Just like insects, wildlife, especially small mammals and birds, are considered an important reservoir of foodborne pathogens, shedding them into the environment through feces.[307] *L. monocytogenes* was detected in 3.2% of the intestinal tracts of wild rodents in China[219] and in 36% of wild birds in Japan.[308] A survey carried out from 2012 to 2015 in Germany, France and the Czech Republic noted *S. aureus* in 15.3% of wild rodents and shrews.[309] In Finland, *Yersinia* spp. were isolated from 8% of wild small mammals,[310] and in China, the prevalence of *Y. enterocolitica* in rodents was 3.4%.[311] A large outbreak of *E. coli* O157:H7 associated with spinach in the United States had feces of feral swine as the primary contamination source.[192] Physical damage to the developing maize crop has also been shown to promote fungal infection. Transmission of *F. graminearum* in maize can be increased as a consequence of physical damage, mediated by either birds or insects. Sutton et al.[312] showed a positive correlation between the amount of bird damage and the level of zearalenone contamination. Thus these data emphasize the relevance of proper pest control in different steps of the food production chain.

25.4.6 Food handlers

Some bacteria are commonly found on human skin, in nasal cavities, oral secretions, and feces. Consequently, humans are a potential contamination source of food during the manual harvest of fresh produce, egg collection, milking, and in intensive production systems.[313] In the United States during the 2000s, 647 foodborne outbreaks were attributed to food worker transmissions.[314] The main factors that support this transmission are poor personal hygiene habits due to improper food safety training, working while sick or the presence of asymptomatic carriers. It is estimated that between 1% and 10% of the population are healthy carriers of *L. monocytogenes*.[315] In addition, between 25% and 40% of the population carries *S. aureus* on their skin or in nasal passages.[316] In Egypt, the prevalence of *S. aureus* in hand and nasal swabs of retail handlers was 76% and 64%, respectively.[317] In Iran, the same species was recovered from 65.4% of food handler nostrils and 46% of fingernails, while 0.9% had *Shigella boydii* in their stool samples.[318] Ivbule et al.[319] reported that 21.1% of workers of pig slaughterhouses were carriers of MRSA. Bogdanovicova et al.[320] isolated *E. coli* from 11% of staff hands, *B. cereus* from 30.2%, and *S. aureus* from 18.9%. Furthermore, *Salmonella* and *Shigella* prevalence rates in food handlers ranged from 1% to 42.3% and 0% to 15.5% in sub-Saharan African countries, respectively.[321–324] A study carried out in China from 2012 to 2017 isolated *Salmonella* from 193 out of 214,542 food handlers' fecal samples, of which 73.4% of the isolates were multidrug-resistant.[325] Brar and Danyluk[326] reported that *S. enterica* was transmitted from gloves to tomatoes during harvesting. In a bell pepper farm, 17.3% and 15.3% of workers had *Salmonella* and *E. coli*, respectively, on their washed hands before starting work.[327] On British chicken farms, 39% and 18% of the workers' shoes and hands tested positive for *Campylobacter*.[328] Jimenez et al.[329] observed that the bidirectional transfer of *S.* Typhimurium between bare and gloved hands was reduced on hands by using a combination of hand-washing and application of alcohol-based hand gel. It emphasizes the importance of maintaining a training program that focuses on the need for and relevance of a high degree of personal cleanliness and proper personal behavior.

25.4.7 Facilities, equipment, and utensils

Microorganisms can contaminate facilities such as green houses, packinghouses, and animal houses as transient or permanent residents. Poor conditions of equipment and facilities and ineffective hygiene can favor this contamination.[330] The shared use of facilities and tools for handling animals and vegetables on a farm increases the risk of cross-contamination. Foodborne pathogens may enter the food processing environment from raw materials or the movement of workers or equipment.[331] *E. coli* was detected in 33% of the samples of a conveyor system at a melon farm in Texas.[332] Two studies verified that coring knives were able to transfer *E. coli* O157:H7 to lettuce.[333,334] In Finland, *L. monocytogenes* was detected in 39% of the milk filter socks in milk facilities.[335] Furthermore, Fox et al.[331] detected *L. monocytogenes* in 13.1% of the milk processing environment and 12.3% of samples external to the milk processing environment. The pulsed field gel electrophoresis analysis indicated the external farm environment may be the source of contamination. In packinghouses *L. monocytogenes* was isolated from 0.8% to 5.8% of environmental samples and in fresh-cut facilities from <0.4% to 1.6%.[336] *Cronobacter* was detected in 16.7% of the milking machine samples in one farm and in 55.6% of the floor of livestock building samples on another farm in Ukraine.[337] *Salmonella* was detected in 2.6% of samples among harvest, field containers, unloading ramps, packing bins, and sorting on a bell pepper farm.[327]

Mechanical harvesting machines, including combine harvesters, are potential spreaders of contamination.[338] A survey conducted in Brazil throughout the peanut production chain identified mechanized threshing as the main contamination source of *Salmonella*, corresponding to 55% of positive samples.[339] An aggravating factor during mechanized harvesting and transportation is the physical injury of plant tissue that can expose internal surfaces to microbial contamination.[340] In chicken farms in the United Kingdom, 41% and 38% of vehicles were contaminated by *Campylobacter* on the exterior and interior, respectively.[328]

The long-term persistence of pathogens in the environment is directly related to the capacity of biofilm formation by the contaminating microorganism. Fox et al.[331] isolated the same *L. monocytogenes* strain from the same milk facility over 10 years later. *S. aureus* can persist from 7 days to 7 months on surfaces.[341] A trace back investigation of an outbreak caused by *Y. pseudotuberculosis* O:1 in Finland identified the carrot-peeling line in the fresh-food processing plant as one of the contamination sources of the grated carrots.[342] Egg water wash in a packing facility was the likely source of *Salmonella* in a multistate outbreak associated with shell eggs, which resulted in 3578 cases in 2010 in the United States.[343] In 2010 a listeriosis outbreak in the United States associated with precut celery had as its primary contamination source the machine blades.[344] In 2011 another listeriosis outbreak in the United States linked to cantaloupes, resulted in 147 cases and 33 deaths. In the latter case, improper sanitation and improper processing equipment were identified as the likely cause of contamination.[345] In 2012, 261 illnesses and 3 deaths occurred in the United States in another salmonellosis outbreak related to cantaloupes. The contamination of the cantaloupes started in the production fields and was spread by operations and practices within the packinghouse.[346] The FDA identified the apple packing facility as the contamination source of *L. monocytogenes* in an outbreak involving 35 cases associated with caramel apples.[347]

25.4.8 Drying and storage

Drying of crops is a critical process in reducing development of mycotoxins. Grains and nuts are often dried in the field, with consequent poor control over conditions. In subtropical and temperate regions, the weather is usually drier at harvest time and field drying is effective. In tropical countries, groundnuts are frequently harvested and left to dry in stacks in the field, or are separated from plants at harvest and dried on the ground, on some form of matting, or on plastic sheets.

Storage practices in developed countries normally prevent development of mycotoxins after drying. However, less than ideal storage conditions in developing countries are sometimes inadequate, permitting increases in moisture content, leading to spoilage or production of mycotoxins.

Crops susceptible to aflatoxin formation are mostly nuts and oilseeds, where soluble solids (sugars) in the dried commodity are low, and oil content is high. Sorption isotherms of these commodities are similar.[348] *A. flavus* and *A. parasiticus* cannot grow below a a_w of about 0.80, equivalent to about 10% moisture content in these commodities. However, storage above 8% moisture content (about 0.7 a_w) can lead to fungal spoilage. Fungal growth may result in a moisture increase, creating conditions under which *A. flavus* can grow, so 8% moisture must be considered the safe moisture content for these commodities. However, such a low moisture content can be difficult to maintain in practice.[137]

Fungal growth in grain is also closely associated with a_w. Researchers have shown that the recommended a_w to avoid fungal growth is generally less than 0.70. In general, the moisture content of grains during storage should not be higher than 15%. Appropriate level of moisture content of grain should be determined based on cereal variety, kernel size, grain quality, storage period, and storage condition (e.g., temperature). In addition, safe storage guidance may be provided to reflect the environmental situation in each region.[349]

25.5 Research gaps and future directions

Mitigating risk of contamination is challenging during primary production, especially due to poor agricultural practices and because of the ubiquitous behavior of microorganisms. Moreover, in most investigations, the route of contamination, the primary source, and the specific vehicle involved in foodborne outbreaks are lacking. In fact, nowadays with the globalization of the food production chain, it is an even greater challenge. Therefore further studies are needed to obtain data on the behavior and prevalence of pathogens and toxigenic fungi in the early stages of the food production chain so that effective control measures for microbial contamination of food can be implemented.

References

1. World Health Organization. WHO Estimates of the Global Burden of Foodborne Diseases: Foodborne Disease Burden Epidemiology Reference Group 2007–2015. Switzerland, WHO Press, World Health Organization. 2015. <https://apps.who.int/iris/bitstream/handle/10665/199350/9789241565165_eng.pdf> Accessed 02.02.21.
2. European Food Safety Authority and European Centre for Disease Prevention and Control. The European Union One Health 2018 Zoonoses Report. *EFSA J.* 2019;17(12):5926. Accessed October 1, 2020.
3. Centers for Disease Control and Prevention. Surveillance for Foodborne Disease Outbreaks, United States, 2017, Annual Report. <https://www.cdc.gov/fdoss/pdf/2017_FoodBorneOutbreaks_508.pdf>; 2019 Accessed 01.10.20.
4. Jaffee S, Henson S, Unnevehr L, Grace D, Cassou E. The safe food imperative. International Bank for Reconstruction and Development/The World Bank: Washington, DC. 2019. <https://openknowledge.worldbank.org/bitstream/handle/10986/30568/9781464813450.pdf?sequence = 6&isAllowed = > Accessed 02.02.21.
5. Tournas VH. Spoilage of vegetable crops by bacteria and fungi and related health hazards. *Crit Rev Microbiol.* 2005;31:33–44.
6. Beuchat LR. Vectors and conditions for preharvest contamination of fruits and vegetables with pathogens capable of causing enteric diseases. *Br Food J.* 2006;108:38–53.
7. Matthews KR. Sources of enteric pathogen contamination of fruits and vegetables: future directions of research. *Stewart Postharvest Rev.* 2013;9:1–5.
8. Argudín MÁ, Mendoza MC, Rodicio MR. Food poisoning and *Staphylococcus aureus* enterotoxins. *Toxins.* 2010;2:1751–1773.
9. Food and Drug Administration. Bad Bug Book Handbook of Foodborne Pathogenic Microorganisms and Natural Toxins. 2nd (ed.) <https://www.fda.gov/media/83271/download>; 2012 Accessed 01.10.20.
10. Le Loir Y, Baron F, Gautier M. *Staphylococcus aureus* and food poisoning. *Genet Mol Res.* 2003;2:63–76.

11. Adams MR, Moss MO. *Food Microbiology*. 3rd ed. Cambridge: Royal Society of Chemistry; 2008.
12. Rall VL, Vieira FP, Rall R, et al. PCR detection of staphylococcal enterotoxin genes in *Staphylococcus aureus* strains isolated from raw and pasteurized milk. *Vet Microbiol*. 2008;132:408–413.
13. Liu H, Li S, Meng L, et al. Prevalence, antimicrobial susceptibility, and molecular characterization of *Staphylococcus aureus* isolated from dairy herds in northern China. *J Dairy Sci*. 2017;100: 8796–8803.
14. Wang W, Lin X, Jiang T, et al. Prevalence and characterization of *Staphylococcus aureus* cultured from raw milk taken from dairy cows with mastitis in Beijing, China. *Front Microbiol*. 2018;9:1–16.
15. Wu S, Huang J, Wu Q, et al. *Staphylococcus aureus* isolated from retail meat and meat products in China: incidence, antibiotic resistance and genetic diversity. *Front Microbiol*. 2018;9:1–14.
16. Ge B, Mukherjee S, Hsu CH, et al. MRSA and multidrug-resistant *Staphylococcus aureus* in U.S. retail meats, 2010–2011. *Food Microbiol*. 2017;62:289–297.
17. Elias SO, Decol LT, Tondo EC. Foodborne outbreaks in Brazil associated with fruits and vegetables: 2008 through 2014. *Food Qual Saf*. 2018;2:173–181.
18. Ministry of Environment and Food in Denmark. About the Danish Smiley Scheme. <http://www.findsmiley.dk/english/Pages/About.aspx>; 2017. Accessed 01.10.20.
19. Bhunia Mechanisms AK. *Food Science Text Series Foodborne Microbial Pathogens*. Indiana: Springer; 2018.
20. Hauschild AHW. Clostridium botulinum. In: Doyle MP, ed. *Foodborne Bacterial Pathogens*. New York, NY: Marcel Dekker; 1989:111–189.
21. Talon R, Leroy S, Vermassen A, et al. Réduction des nitrates, nitrites dans les produits carnés: quelles conséquences? Quelles solutions? *Innov Agron*. 2015;44:25–34.
22. Johnson EA. Clostridium botulinum. In: Doyle MP, Buchanan RL, (eds.) Food Microbiology: Fundamentals and Frontiers. 4th ed. Washington, DC: ASM Press; 2013:288-304.
23. Lund BM, Peck MW. Clostridium botulinum. In: Lund BM, Baird-Parker AC, Gould GW, eds. *The Microbiological Safety and Quality of Food*. Gaithersburg, MD: Aspen; 2000:1057–1109.
24. Carter AT, Peck MW. Genomes, neurotoxins and biology of *Clostridium botulinum* group I and group II. *Res Microbiol*. 2015;166:303–317.
25. Technical University of Denmark. Annual Report on Zoonoses in Denmark 2018. <https://www.food.dtu.dk>; 2019. Accessed 01.09.20.
26. Bergeron G, Latash J, Da Costa-Carter CA, et al. Notes from the field: botulism outbreak associated with home-canned peas - New York City, 2018. *Morb Mortal Wkly Rep*. 2019;68:251–252.
27. Centers for Disease Control and Prevention. National Botulism Surveillance Summary. <https://www.cdc.gov/botulism/surv/2017/index.html>; 2017. Accessed 01.10.20.
28. Austin JW. *Clostridium*: occurrence and detection of *Clostridium botulinum* and botulinum neurotoxin. *Encycl Food Heal*. 2016;2016:155–159.
29. Grenda T, Grabczak M, Kwiatek K, et al. Prevalence of *C. botulinum* and *C. perfringens* spores in food products available on Polish market. *J Vet Res*. 2017;61:287–291.
30. Midura TF, Snowden S, Wood RM, et al. Isolation of *Clostridium botulinum* from honey. *J Clin Microbiol*. 1979;9:282–283.
31. Rood JI, Adams V, Lacey J, et al. Expansion of the *Clostridium perfringens* toxin-based typing scheme. *Anaerobe*. 2018;53:5–10.
32. Rainey HG. *Understanding and managing public organizations*. 5th ed. San Francisco, CA: Jossey-Bass, Inc.; 2009.
33. Lindström M, Heikinheimo A, Lahti P, et al. Novel insights into the epidemiology of *Clostridium perfringens* type A food poisoning. *Food Microbiol*. 2011;28:192–198.
34. London AE, Payne JA, Hartl B. Outbreak caused by *Clostridium perfringens* infection and intoxication at a county correctional facility. *J Environ Health*. 2017;80:8–13.
35. Mellou K, Kyritsi M, Chrysostomou A, et al. *Clostridium perfringens* foodborne outbreak during an athletic event in Northern Greece, June 2019. *Int J Environ Res Public Health*. 2019;16 (20):3967. Available from: https://doi.org/10.3390/ijerph16203967.
36. Stenfors Arnesen LP, Fagerlund A, Granum PE. From soil to gut: *Bacillus cereus* and its food poisoning toxins. *FEMS Microbiol Rev*. 2008;32:579–606.
37. Logan NA, DeVos P. Genus *Bacillus*. In: DeVos P, Garrity GM, Jones D, et al., eds. *Bergey's Manual of Systematic Bacteriology*. 2nd ed. New York, NY: Springer; 2009:21–128.
38. Tallent SM, Kotewicz KM, Strain EA, et al. Efficient isolation and identification of *Bacillus cereus* group. *J AOAC Int*. 2012;95:446–451.
39. Bennett RW, Tallent SM, Hait JM. *Bacillus cereus* and *Bacillus cereus* toxins. In: Salfinger Y, Tortorello ML, eds. *Compendium of Methods for the Microbiological Examination of Foods*. 5th ed. Washington, DC: American Public Health Association (APHA); 2015:375–390.
40. Lindbäck T, Granum PE. Bacillus cereus. In: Doyle M, Diez-Gonzalez F, Hill C, eds. *Food Microbiology: Fundamentals and Frontiers*. 5th ed. Washington, DC: ASM Press; 2019:541–554.
41. European Food Safety Authority. Opinion of the scientific panel on biological hazards on *Bacillus cereus* and other *Bacillus* spp in foodstuffs. *EFSA J*. 2005;175:1–48. Accessed October 1, 2020.
42. Ryu JH, Beuchat LR. Biofilm formation and sporulation by *Bacillus cereus* on a stainless-steel surface and subsequent resistance of vegetative cells and spores to chlorine, chlorine dioxide, and a peroxyacetic acid-based sanitizer. *J Food Prot*. 2005;68:2614–2622.
43. European Food Safety Authority, EFSA Panel on Biological Hazards. Scientific opinion on the risks for public health related to the presence of *Bacillus cereus* and other *Bacillus* spp. including *Bacillus thuringiensis* in foodstuffs. *EFSA J*. 2016;14(7):4524. Accessed October 1, 2020.
44. Lan X, Wang J, Zheng N, et al. Prevalence and risk factors for *Bacillus cereus* in raw milk in Inner Mongolia, Northern China. *Int J Dairy Technol*. 2018;71:269–273.
45. Tewari A, Abdullah S. *Bacillus cereus* food poisoning: international and Indian perspective. *J Food Sci Technol*. 2015;52:2500–2511.
46. Yu P, Yu S, Wang J, et al. *Bacillus cereus* isolated from vegetables in China: incidence, genetic diversity, virulence genes, and antimicrobial resistance. *Front Microbiol*. 2019;10:1–10.
47. Kim YJ, Kim HS, Kim KY, et al. High occurrence rate and contamination level of *Bacillus cereus* in organic vegetables on sale in retail markets. *Foodborne Pathog Dis*. 2016;13:656–660.
48. Park KMIN, Jeong M, Park KEEJAI, et al. Prevalence, enterotoxin genes, and antibiotic resistance of *Bacillus cereus* isolated from raw vegetables in Korea. *J Food Prot*. 2018;81:1590–1597.

49. Flores-Urbán KA, Natividad-Bonifacio I, Zquez-Quiñones CRVÁ, et al. Detection of toxigenic *Bacillus cereus* strains isolated from vegetables in Mexico City. *J Food Prot*. 2014;77:2144–2147.
50. Güven K, Mutlu MB, Avci Ö. Incidence and characterization of *Bacillus cereus*. *J Food Saf*. 2005;26:30–40.
51. Milojevic L, Velebit B, Djordjevic V, et al. Screening of *Bacillus cereus* presence in minced meat and meat products originating from Serbian retail facilities. *IOP Conf Ser Earth Environ Sci*. 2019;333:1–6.
52. Carlin CR, Liao J, Weller D, et al. *Listeria cossartiae* sp. nov., *Listeria immobilis* sp. nov., *Listeria portnoyi* sp. nov. and *Listeria rustica* sp. nov., isolated from agricultural water and natural environments. *Int J Syst Evol Microbiol*. 2021;71:004795. Available from: https://doi.org/10.1099/ijsem.0.00479.
53. McLauchlin J, Rees CED, Genus I. *Listeria* Pirie 1940. In: DeVos P, Garrity GM, Jones D, et al., eds. *Bergey's Manual of Systematic Bacteriology*. New York: Springer; 2009:244–257.
54. Liu D, Lawrence ML, Ainsworth AJ, et al. Comparative assessment of acid, alkali and salt tolerance in *Listeria monocytogenes* virulent and avirulent strains. *FEMS Microbiol Lett*. 2005;243:373–378.
55. Donnelly CW, Diez-Gonzalez F. Listeria monocytogenes. In: Labbé RG, Garcia S, eds. *Guide to Foodborne Pathogens*. Chichester: Wiley; 2013:45–74.
56. Ly V, Parreira VR, Farber JM. Current understanding and perspectives on *Listeria monocytogenes* in low-moisture foods. *Curr Opin Food Sci*. 2019;26:18–24.
57. Samadpour M, Barbour MW, Nguyen T, et al. Incidence of enterohemorrhagic *Escherichia coli*, *Escherichia coli* O157, *Salmonella*, and *Listeria monocytogenes* in retail fresh ground beef, sprouts, and mushrooms. *J Food Prot*. 2006;69:441–443.
58. Pereira JG, Soares VM, Tadielo LE, et al. Foods introduced into Brazil through the border with Argentina and Uruguay: pathogen detection and evaluation of hygienic-sanitary quality. *Int J Food Microbiol*. 2018;283:22–27.
59. Haley BJ, Sonnier J, Schukken YH, et al. Diversity of *Listeria monocytogenes* within a U.S. Dairy Herd, 2004-2010. *Foodborne Pathog Dis*. 2015;12:844–850.
60. Rocha PRDA, Lomonaco S, Bottero MT, et al. Ruminant rhombencephalitis-associated *Listeria monocytogenes* strains constitute a genetically homogeneous group related to human outbreak strains. *Appl Environ Microbiol*. 2013;79:3059–3066.
61. Lee SHI, Cappato LP, Guimarães JT, et al. *Listeria monocytogenes* in milk: occurrence and recent advances in methods for inactivation. *Beverages*. 2019;5:14.
62. Byrne V, de V, Hofer E, Vallim DC, et al. Occurrence and antimicrobial resistance patterns of *listeria monocytogenes* isolated from vegetables. *Braz J Microbiol*. 2016;47:438–443.
63. Cordano AM, Jacquet C. Listeria monocytogenes *isolated from vegetable salads sold at supermarkets in Santiago, Chile: Prevalence and strain characterization. Int J Food Microbiol*. 132. 2009176–179.
64. Moreno Y, Sánchez-Contreras J, Montes RM, et al. Detection and enumeration of viable *Listeria monocytogenes* cells from ready-to-eat and processed vegetable foods by culture and DVC-FISH. *Food Control*. 2012;27:374–379.
65. Cetinkaya F, Elal Mus T, Yibar A, et al. Prevalence, serotype identification by multiplex polymerase chain reaction and antimicrobial resistance patterns of *Listeria monocytogenes* isolated from retail foods. *J Food Saf*. 2014;34:42–49.
66. Vojkovská H, Myšková P, Gelbíčová T, Skočková A, Koláčková I, Karpíšková R. Occurrence and characterization of food-borne pathogens isolated from fruit, vegetables and sprouts retailed in the Czech Republic. *Food Microbiol*. 2017;63:147–152.
67. Centers for Disease Control and Prevention. Listeria outbreaks. <https://www.cdc.gov/listeria/outbreaks/index.html>; 2020. Accessed 01.10.20.
68. McCollum JT, Cronquist AB, Silk BJ, et al. Multistate outbreak of listeriosis associated with cantaloupe. *N Engl J Med*. 2013;369:944–953.
69. Thomas J, Govender N, McCarthy KM, et al. Outbreak of listeriosis in South Africa associated with processed meat. *N Engl J Med*. 2020;382:632–643.
70. Croxen MA, Law RJ, Scholz R, et al. Recent advances in understanding enteric pathogenic *Escherichia coli*. *Clin Microbiol Rev*. 2013;26:822–880.
71. van Elsas JD, Semenov AV, Costa R, et al. Survival of *Escherichia coli* in the environment: fundamental and public health aspects. *ISME J*. 2011;5:173–183.
72. International Commission on Microbiological Specifications for Foods. *Microorganisms in Foods 5. Microbiological Specifications of Food Pathogens*. London: Chapman and Hall; 1996.
73. Karmali MA, Gannon V, Sargeant JM. Verocytotoxin-producing *Escherichia coli* (VTEC). *Vet Microbiol*. 2010;140:360–370.
74. Scallan E, Hoekstra RM, Angulo FJ, et al. Foodborne illness acquired in the United States—major pathogens. *Emerg Infect Dis*. 2011;17:7–15.
75. Widgren S, Söderlund R, Eriksson E, et al. Longitudinal observational study over 38 months of verotoxigenic *Escherichia coli* O157: H7 status in 126 cattle herds. *Prev Vet Med*. 2015;121:343–352.
76. Zhang G, Ma L, Phelan VH, et al. Efficacy of antimicrobial agents in lettuce leaf processing water for control of *Escherichia coli* O157.H7. *J Food Prot*. 2009;72:1392–1397.
77. Buchholz U, Bernard H, Werber D, et al. German outbreak of *Escherichia coli* O104:H4 associated with sprouts. *N Engl J Med*. 2011;365:1763–1770.
78. Brenner DJ, Farmer III JJ. Family I. Enterobacteriaceae. In: Brenner DJ, Krieg NR, Staley JT, eds. *Bergey's Manual of Systematic Bacteriology*. New York, NY: Springer; 2005:587–607.
79. Euzéby JP. List of prokaryotic names with standing in nomenclature – Genus *Salmonella* website. <http://www.bacterio.cict.fr/s/salmonella.html>; 2012. Accessed 01.10.20.
80. Grimont PAD, Weill FX. *Antigenic Formulae of the Salmonella Serovars*. 9th ed. Paris: Institute Pasteur; 2007.
81. European Food Safety Authority and European Centre for Disease Prevention and Control. Rapid outbreak assessment: multi-country outbreak of *Salmonella enteritidis* infections linked to eggs - Third update. <https://www.ecdc.europa.eu/en/publications-data/multi-country-outbreak-salmonella-enteritidis-infections-linked-egg>; 2020. Accessed 30.10.20.
82. Gad AH, Abo-Shama UH, Harclerode KK, et al. Prevalence, serotyping, molecular typing, and antimicrobial resistance of *Salmonella* isolated from conventional and organic retail ground poultry. *Front Microbiol*. 2018;9:1–10.
83. Demirci M, Yiğin A, Altun S, et al. *Salmonella* Spp. and *Shigella* Spp. detection via multiplex real-time PCR and discrimination via MALDI-TOF MS in different animal raw milk samples. *Niger J Clin Pract*. 2019;22:1083–1090.

84. Beuchat LR, Komitopoulou E, Beckers H, et al. Low–water activity foods: increased concern as vehicles of foodborne pathogens. *J Food Prot.* 2013;76:150–172.
85. Carstens CK, Salazar JK, Darkoh C. Multistate outbreaks of foodborne illness in the United States associated with fresh produce from 2010 to 2017. *Front Microbiol.* 2019;10:1–15.
86. Lennox JA, Eja M, Edeghor U, et al. Incidence of *Salmonella* and *Shigella* species on some selected fruits and vegetables obtained from open area markets in calabar metropolis. *Int J Curr Microbiol App Sci.* 2015;4:262–268.
87. Vital PG, Dimasuay KGB, Widmer KW, et al. Microbiological quality of fresh produce from open air markets and supermarkets in the Philippines. *Sci World J.* 2014;1–7.
88. Nascimento MS, Carminati JA, Morishita KN, et al. Long-term kinetics of *Salmonella* Typhimurium ATCC 14028 survival on peanuts and peanut confectionery products. *PLoS One.* 2018;13: e0192457. Available from: https://doi.org/10.1371/journal.pone.0192457.
89. Nascimento MS, Brum DM, Pena PO, et al. Inactivation of *Salmonella* during cocoa roasting and chocolate conching. *Int J Food Microbiol.* 2012;159:225–229.
90. Centers for Disease Control and Prevention. Multistate outbreak of Salmonella Typhimurium infections linked to dried coconut (final update). <https://www.cdc.gov/salmonella/typhimurium-03-18/index.html>; 2018. Accessed 01.10.20.
91. Centers for Disease Control and Prevention. Multistate outbreak of Salmonella Mbandaka infections linked to Kellogg's honey smacks cereal (final update). <https://www.cdc.gov/salmonella/mbandaka-06-18/index.html>; 2018. Accessed 01.10.20.
92. Centers for Disease Control and Prevention. Multistate outbreak of Salmonella Typhimurium infections linked to peanut butter, Minnesota, USA; 2008-2009. 2009. Morb Mortal Wkly Rep 58:85-90.
93. European Food Safety Authority and European Centre for Disease Prevention and Control. Multi-country outbreak of *Salmonella* Typhimurium and *S.* Anatum infections linked to Brazil nuts – 21 October 2020. Available from: <https://www.efsa.europa.eu/en/supporting/pub/en-1944>; 2020. Accessed 30.10.20.
94. Jourdan-da Silva N, Fabre L, Robinson E, et al. Ongoing nationwide outbreak of *Salmonella* Agona associated with internationally distributed infant milk products, France, December 2017. *Euro Surveill.* 2018;23:17–00852. Available from: https://doi.org/10.2807/1560-7917.ES.2018.23.2.17-00852.
95. Centers for Disease Control and Prevention. Multistate outbreak of Salmonella montevideo and Salmonella Senftenberg infections linked to wonderful pistachios (final update). <https://www.cdc.gov/salmonella/montevideo-03-16/index.html>; 2016. Accessed 01.10.20.
96. Centers for Disease Control and Prevention. Multistate outbreak of Salmonella Paratyphi B variant L(+) tartrate(+) infections linked to JEM raw brand sprouted nut butter spreads (final update). <https://www.cdc.gov/salmonella/paratyphi-b-12-15/index.html>; 2015. Accessed 01.10.20.
97. Centers for Disease Control and Prevention. Multistate outbreak of Salmonella Montevideo and Salmonella Mbandaka infections linked to tahini sesame paste (final update). <https://www.cdc.gov/salmonella/montevideo-tahini-05-13/>; 2013. Accessed 01.10.20.
98. Werber D, Dreesman J, Feil F, et al. International outbreak of *Salmonella* Oranienburg due to German chocolate. *BMC Infect Dis.* 2005;5:7–17.
99. Shoha T, Green MS, Merom D, Gill ON, et al. International epidemiological and microbiological study of outbreak of *Salmonella agona* infection from ready to eat savoury snack—II: Israel. *Br Med J.* 1996;313:1107–1109.
100. Killalea DLR, Ward D, Roberts Jde Louvois, et al. International epidemiological and microbiological study of outbreak of *Salmonella agona* infection from ready to eat savoury snack—I: England and Wales and the United States. *Br Med J.* 1996;313:1105–1107.
101. Lehmacher AJ, Bockemühl J, Aleksic S. Nationwide outbreak of human salmonellosis in Germany due to contaminated paprika and paprika-powdered potato chips. *Epidemiol Infect.* 1995;115:501–511.
102. Vandamme P, Dewhirst FE, Paster BJ, et al. Genus I. Campylobacter. In: Brenner DJ, Krieg NR, Staley JT, (eds.) Bergey's Manual of Systematic Bacteriology. New York, NY: Springer; 2005:1147–1160.
103. Euzéby JP. List of prokaryotic names with standing in nomenclature website. Genus *Campylobacter*. <http://www.bacterio.net/campylobacter.html>; 2010 Accessed 01.10. 20.
104. Lazou T, Dovas C, Houf K, et al. Diversity of *Campylobacter* in retail meat and liver of lambs and goat kids. *Foodborne Pathog Dis.* 2014;11:320–328.
105. Brown LG, Khargonekar S, Bushnell L. Frequency of inadequate chicken cross-contamination prevention and cooking practices in restaurants. *J Food Prot.* 2013;76:2141–2145.
106. Lawes JR, Vidal A, Clifton-Hadley FA, et al. Investigation of prevalence and risk factors for *Campylobacter* in broiler flocks at slaughter: results from a UK survey. *Epidemiol Infect.* 2012;140:1725–1727.
107. Karikari AB, Obiri-Danso K, Frimpong EH, et al. Antibiotic resistance of *Campylobacter* recovered from faeces and carcasses of healthy livestock. *Biomed Res Int.* 2017;4091856. Available from: https://doi.org/10.1155/2017/4091856.
108. Mohammadpour H, Berizi E, Hosseinzadeh S, et al. The prevalence of *Campylobacter* spp. in vegetables, fruits, and fresh produce: a systematic review and *meta*-analysis. *Gut Pathog.* 2018;10:1–12.
109. Strockbine NA, Maurelli AT. Family I. Enterobacteriaceae. Genus XXXV. Shigella Castellani and Chalmers 1919, 936. In: Brenner DJ, Krieg NR, Staley JT, (eds.) Bergey's Manual of Systematic Bacteriology. New York, NY: Springer; 2005:811–823.
110. Lampel KA. Shigella species. In: Labbé RG, Garcia S, (eds.) Guide to Foodborne Pathogens. Chichester: Wiley; 2013:138–147.
111. Binet R, Lampel K. Shigella species. In: Doyle M, Buchanan R, (eds.) Food Microbiology: Fundamentals and Frontiers. 4th ed. Washington, DC: ASM Press; 2013:339–376.
112. Watkins LKF, Appiah GD. Shigellosis. In: Centers for Disease Control and Prevention. CDC Yellow Book. <https://wwwnc.cdc.gov/travel/yellowbook/2020/travel-related-infectious-diseases/shigellosis>; 2020. Accessed 01.10.20.
113. Robins-Browne RM. Yersinia enterocolitica. In: Doyle M, Buchanan R, (eds.) Food Microbiology: Fundamentals and Frontiers. 4th ed. Washington, DC: ASM Press; 2013:400–440.

114. Stern NJ, Pierson MD, Kotula AW. Effects of pH and sodium chloride on *Yersinia enterocolitica* growth at room and refrigeration temperatures. *J Food Sci.* 1980;45:64–67.
115. Schaake J, Drees A, Grüning P, et al. Essential role of invasin for colonization and persistence of *Yersinia enterocolitica* in its natural reservoir host, the pig. *Infect Immun.* 2014;82:960–969.
116. Longenberger AH, Gronostaj MP, Yee GY, et al. Yersinia enterocolitica infections associated with improperly pasteurized milk products: Southwest Pennsylvania, March-August, 2011. Epidemiol Infect 2014;142:1640–1650.
117. Ahmed HA, Tahoun ABMB, Abou Elez RMM, et al. Prevalence of *Yersinia enterocolitica* in milk and dairy products and the effects of storage temperatures on survival and virulence gene expression. *Int Dairy J.* 2019;94:16–21.
118. Drake FN, Davis S, Khatiwada J, et al. Identification and antimicrobial susceptibility of *Yersinia enterocolitica* found in chitterlings, raw milk and swine fecal samples. *Adv Microbiol.* 2018;08:804–820.
119. Bernardino-Varo L, Quinones-Ramírez EI, Fernandez FJ, et al. Prevalence of *Yersinia enterocolitica* in raw cow's milk collected from stables of Mexico City. *J Food Prot.* 2013;76:694e698.
120. Verbikova V, Borilova G, Babak V, et al. Prevalence, characterization and antimicrobial susceptibility of *Yersinia enterocolitica* and other *Yersinia* species found in fruits and vegetables from the European Union. *Food Control.* 2018;85:161–167.
121. Nousiainen LL, Joutsen S, Lunden J, et al. Bacterial quality and safety of packaged fresh leafy vegetables at the retail level in Finland. *Int J Food Microbiol.* 2016;232:73–79.
122. Sabbithi A, Naveen Kumar R, Kashinath L, et al. Microbiological quality of salads served along with street foods of Hyderabad, India. *Int J Microbiol.* 2014;1–6.
123. Corbel MJ. Food and Agriculture Organization of the United Nations, World Health Organization & World Organization for Animal Health. Brucellosis in humans and animals. World Health Organization. <https://apps.who.int/iris/handle/10665/43597>; 2006. Accessed 01.10.20.
124. Ribeiro CM, De Carvalho JLB, De Santis Bastos PA, et al. Spatial and temporal trend analysis of bovine brucellosis in Brazil, 2014 to 2018. *Semin Agrar.* 2020;41:1279–1290.
125. Iqbal Z, Jamil H, Qureshi ZI, et al. Seroprevalence of ovine brucellosis by modified rose bengal test and ELISA in Southern Punjab, Pakistan. *Pak Vet J.* 2013;33:455–457.
126. Mirza MA, Jalvi MA, Razzak A. Screening of goat flocks for Brucellosis using Rose Bengal Plate Test. *Pak Vet J.* 1998;18:146–149.
127. Soomro AH, Kamboh AA, Rind R, et al. Study on prevalence and risk factors of brucellosis in cattle and buffaloes in district Hyderabad, Pakistan. *J Anim Health Product.* 2014;2:33–37.
128. Nasir A, Shah M, Rashid M. Current status of Brucellosis in cattle in various government livestock farms in Panjab. *Int J Agric Biol.* 1999;1:337–338.
129. McDermott J, Grace D, Zinsstag J. Economics of brucellosis impact and control in low-income countries. *Rev Sci Tech.* 2013;32:249–261.
130. Iversen C, Lehner A, Mullane N, et al. The taxonomy of *Enterobacter sakazakii*: proposal of a new genus *Cronobacter* gen. nov. and descriptions of *Cronobacter sakazakii* comb. nov. *Cronobacter sakazakii* subsp. *sakazakii*, comb. nov., *Cronobacter sakazakii* subsp. *malonaticus* subsp. nov., *Cronobacter turicensis* sp. nov., *Cronobacter muytjensii* sp. nov., *Cronobacter dublinensis* sp. nov. and *Cronobacter genomospecies* 1. *BMC Evol Biol.* 2007;7:1–11.
131. Iversen C, Mullane N, McCardell B, et al. *Cronobacter* gen. nov., a new genus to accommodate the biogroups of *Enterobacter sakazakii*, and proposal of *Cronobacter sakazakii* gen. nov., comb. nov., *Cronobacter malonaticus* sp. nov., *Cronobacter turicensis* sp. nov., *Cronobacter* muytjensii sp. nov., *Cronobacter dublinensis* sp. nov., *Cronobacter genomospecies* 1, and of three subspecies, *Cronobacter dublinensis* subsp. *dublinensis* subsp. nov., *Cronobacter dublinensis* subsp. *lausannensis* subsp. nov. and *Cronobacter dublinensis* subsp. *lactaridi* subsp. nov. *Int J Syst Evol Microbiol.* 2008;58:1442–1447.
132. International Commission on Microbiological Specifications for Food. *Microorganisms in Foods 8. Use of data for assessing process control and product acceptance.* New York: Springer; 2011.
133. Strysko J, Cope JR, Martin H, et al. Food safety and invasive *Cronobacter* infections during early infancy, 1961–2018. *Emerg Infect Dis.* 2020;26:857–865.
134. Codex Alimentarius. *Code of Hygienic Practice for Powdered Formulae for Infants and Young Children. (CAC/RCP 66-2008 Revision 1: 2009).* Rome: Joint FAO/WHO Food Standards Program; 2009.
135. Holý O, Forsythe S. *Cronobacter* spp. as emerging causes of healthcare-associated infection. *J Hosp Infect.* 2014;86:169–177. Available from: https://doi.org/10.1016/j.jhin.2013.09.011.
136. Patrick ME, Mahon BE, Greene SA, et al. Incidence of *Cronobacter* spp. infections, United States, 2003-2009. *Emerg Infect Dis.* 2014;20:1520–1523. Available from: https://doi.org/10.3201/eid2009.140545.
137. Pitt JI, Wild CP, Baan RA, et al. *Improving Public Health Through Mycotoxin Control.* Lyon: IARC (International Agency for Research on Cancer № 158); 2012.
138. Taniwaki MH, Pitt JI. Mycotoxins. In: Doyle MP, Diez-Gonzalez F, Hill C, eds. *Food Microbiology: Fundamentals and Frontiers.* 5th ed. Washington, DC: ASM Press; 2019:585–608.
139. Food and Agriculture Organization. *Worldwide Regulations for Mycotoxins in Foods and Feeds in 2003.* Rome: FAO Food and Nutrition; 2004.
140. Samson RA, Visagie CM, Houbraken J, et al. Phylogeny, identification and nomenclature of the genus *Aspergillus. Stud Mycol.* 2014;78:141–173.
141. Perrone G, Susca A, Cozzi G, et al. Biodiversity of *Aspergillus* species in some important agricultural products. *Stud Mycol.* 2007;59:53–66.
142. Perrone G, Gallo A. *Aspergillus* species and their associated mycotoxins. In: Moretti A, Susca A, eds. *Mycotoxigenic Fungi: Methods and Protocols, Methods in Molecular Biology.* Totowa, NJ: Humana Press; 2017:33–50.
143. Pitt JI, Hocking AD. *Fungi and Food Spoilage.* 3rd ed. New York, NY: Springer; 2009.
144. Frisvad JC, Hubka V, Ezekiel CN, et al. Taxonomy of *Aspergillus* section *Flavi* and their production of aflatoxins, ochratoxins and other mycotoxins. *Stud Mycol.* 2019;93:01–63.
145. International Agency for Research on Cancer. *Some naturally occurring substances: food items and constituents, heterocyclic aromatic amines and mycotoxins. IARC Monographs on the*

Evaluation of Carcinogenic Risks to Humans. Vol. 56. Lyon: International Agency for Research on Cancer; 1993.

146. Taniwaki MH, Pitt JI, Magan N. *Aspergillus* species and mycotoxins: occurrence and importance in major food commodities. *Curr Opin Food Sci*. 2018;23:38–43.
147. Frisvad JC, Thrane U, Samson RA, et al. Important mycotoxins and the fungi which produce them. In: Hocking AD, Pitt JI, Samson RA, et al., (eds.) Advances in Food Mycology. New York, NY: Springer; 2006:3-31
148. Visagie CM, Houbraken J, Frisvad JC, et al. Identification and nomenclature of the genus *Penicillium*. *Stud Mycol*. 2014;78:343–371.
149. Van der Merwe KJ, Steyn PS, Fourie L, et al. Ochratoxin A, a toxic metabolite produced by *Aspergillus ochraceus* Wilh. *Nature*. 1965;205:1112–1113.
150. Ciegler A. Bioproduction of ochratoxin A and penicillic acid by members of the *Aspergillus ochraceus* group. *Can J Microbiol*. 1972;18:631–639.
151. Robbers JE, Hong S, Tuite J, et al. Production of xanthomegnin and viomellein by species of *Aspergillus* correlated with mycotoxicosis produced in mice. *Appl Environ Microbiol*. 1978;36:819–823.
152. Frisvad JC, Frank JM, Houbraken JAMP, et al. New ochratoxin A producing species of *Aspergillus* section *Circumdati*. *Stud Mycol*. 2004;50:23–43.
153. International Agency for Research on Cancer. *Ochratoxin A. IARC Monographs on the Evaluation of Carcinogenic Risks to Humans, v.56. Some Naturally Occurring Substances: Food Items and Constituents, Heterocyclic Aromatic Amines and Mycotoxins*. Lyon: International Agency for Research on Cancer; 1994:489–521.
154. Visagie CM, Varga J, Houbraken J, et al. Ochratoxin production and taxonomy of the yellow aspergilli (*Aspergillus* section *Circumdati*). *Stud Mycol*. 2014;78:1–6.
155. Samson RA, Houbraken JAMP, Kuijpers AFA, et al. New ochratoxin or sclerotium producing species in *Aspergillus* section *Nigri*. *Stud Mycol*. 2004;50:45–61.
156. Silva JJ, Iamanaka BT, Ferranti LS, et al. Diversity within *Aspergillus niger* clade and description of a new species: *Aspergillus vinaceus* sp. nov. *J Fungi*. 2020;6:371.
157. Taniwaki MH, Pitt JI, Teixeira AA, et al. The source of ochratoxin A in Brazilian coffee and its formation in relation to processing methods. *Int J Food Microbiol*. 2003;82:73–179.
158. Copetti MV, Pereira JL, Iamanaka BT, et al. Ochratoxigenic fungi and ochratoxin A in cocoa during farm processing. *Int J Food Microbiol*. 2010;143:67–70.
159. Frisvad JC, Smedsgaard J, Samson RA, et al. Fumonisin B_2 production by *Aspergillus niger*. *J Agric Food Chem*. 2007;55:9727–9732.
160. Perrone G, Stea G, Epifani F, et al. *Aspergillus niger* contains the cryptic phylogenetic species *A. awamori*. *Fungal Biol*. 2011;115:1138–1150.
161. Mogensen JM, Frisvad JC, Thrane U, et al. Production of fumonisin B2 and B4 by *Aspergillus niger* on grapes and raisins. *J Agric Food Chem*. 2010;58:954–958.
162. Frisvad JC, Larsen TO, Thrane U, et al. Fumonisin and ochratoxin production in industrial *Aspergillus niger* strains. *PLoS One*. 2011;6:e23496. Available from: https://doi.org/10.1371/journal.pone.0023496.
163. Da Rocha Rosa CA, Palacios V, Combinas M, et al. Potential ochratoxin A from wines grapes in Argentina and Brazil. *Food Addit Contam*. 2002;19:408–414.
164. Battilani P, Pietri A, Bertuzzi T, et al. Occurrence of ochratoxin A-producing fungi in grapes grown in Italy. *J Food Prot*. 2003;66:633–636.
165. Iamanaka BT, Taniwaki MH, Menezes HC, et al. Incidence of toxigenic fungi and ochratoxin A in dried fruits sold in Brazil. *Food Addit Cont*. 2005;22:1258–1263.
166. Abarca ML, Accensi F, Bragulat MR, et al. *Aspergillus carbonarius* as the main source of ochratoxin A contamination in dried vine fruits from the Spanish market. *J Food Prot*. 2003;66:504–506.
167. Joosten HMLJ, Goetz J, Pittet A, et al. Production of ochratoxin A by *Aspergillus carbonarius* on coffee cherries. *Int J Food Microbiol*. 2001;65:39–44.
168. Massi FP, Sartori D, Ferranti LS, et al. Prospecting for the incidence of genes involved in ochratoxin and fumonisin biosynthesis in Brazilian strains of *Aspergillus niger* and *Aspergillus welwitschiae*. *Int J Food Microbiol*. 2016;221:19–28.
169. Ferranti LS, Fungaro MHP, Massi FP, et al. Diversity of *Aspergillus* section *Nigri* on the surface of *Vitis labrusca* and its hybrid grapes. *Int J Food Microbiol*. 2018;268:53–60.
170. Gherbawy Y, Elhariry H, Kocsubé S, et al. Molecular characterization of black *Aspergillus* species from onion and their potential for ochratoxin A and fumonisin B_2 production. *Foodborne Pathog Dis*. 2015;12:414–423.
171. Logrieco AF, Haidukowski M, Susca A, et al. *Aspergillus* section *Nigri* as contributor of fumonisin B2 contamination in maize. *Food Addit Contam Part A*. 2014;31:149–155.
172. Houbraken J, de Vries RP, Samson RA. Modern taxonomy of biotechnologically important *Aspergillus* and *Penicillium* species. *Adv Appl Microbiol*. 2014;86:199–249.
173. Perrone G, Susca A. *Penicillium* species and their associated mycotoxins. In: Moretti A, Susca A, eds. *Mycotoxigenic Fungi: Methods and Protocols, Methods in Molecular Biology*. Totowa, NJ: Humana Press; 2017:107–121.
174. Sanchis V, Magan N. Environmental conditions affecting mycotoxin. In: Magan N, Olsen M, eds. *Mycotoxins in Food Detection and Control*. Cambridge: Woodhead Publishing Limited; 2004:174–189.
175. Reddy KRN, Spadaro D, Lore A, et al. Potential of patulin production by *Penicillium expansum* strains on various fruits. *Mycotox Res*. 2010;26:257–265.
176. Spadaro D, Garibaldi A, Gullino ML. Occurrence of patulin and its dietary intake through pear, peach, and apricot juices in Italy. *Food Addit Contam Part B*. 2008;1:134–139.
177. Munkvold GP. *Fusarium* species and their associated mycotoxins. In: Moretti A, Susca A, eds. *Mycotoxigenic Fungi: Methods and Protocols, Methods in Molecular Biology*. Totowa, NJ: Humana Press; 2017:51–106.
178. Marin S, Sanchis V, Vinas I, et al. Effect of water activity and temperature on growth and fumonisin B1 and B2 production of *Fusarium proliferatum* and *F. moniliforme* on maize grain. *Lett Appl Microbiol*. 1995;21:298–301.
179. Marin S, Magan N, Belli N, et al. Two dimensional profiles of fumonisin B sub(1) production by *Fusarium moniliforme* and *Fusarium proliferatum* in relation to environmental factors and

potential for modelling toxin formation in maize grain. *Int J Food Microbiol.* 1999;51:159–167.

180. Bakan B, Melcion D, Richard-Molard D, et al. Fungal growth and *Fusarium mycotoxin* content in isogenic traditional maize and genetically modified maize grown in France and Spain. *J Agric Food Chem.* 2002;50:728–731.
181. Le Bars J, Le Bars P, Dupuy J, et al. Biotic and abiotic factors in fumonisin B1 production and stability. *J Assoc Anal Chem.* 1994;77:517–521.
182. Miller JD. Factors that affect the occurrence of fumonisin. *Environ Health Perspect.* 2001;109:321–324.
183. Cahagnier B, Melcion D, Richard-Moulard D. Growth of *Fusarium moniliforme* and its biosynthesis of fumonisin B1 on maize grain as a function of different water activities. *Lett Appl Microbiol.* 1995;20:247–251.
184. Ramirez ML, Chulze S, Magan N. Temperature and water activity effects on growth and temporal deoxynivalenol production by two Argentinean strains of *Fusarium graminearum* on irradiated wheat grain. *Int J Food Microbiol.* 2006;106:291–296.
185. Scott PM, Kanhere SR, Weber D. Analysis of Canadian and imported beers for *Fusarium* mycotoxins by gas chromatography-mass spectrometry. *Food Addit Contam.* 1993;10:381–389.
186. Leung MCK, Dıaz-Llano G, Trevor K, et al. Mycotoxins in pet food: a review on worldwide prevalence and preventative strategies. *J Agric Food Chem.* 2006;54:9623–9635.
187. Atungulu GG, Mohammadi-Shad Z, Wilson S. Mycotoxin issues in pet food. In: Ricke SC, Atungulu GG, Rainwater CE, et al., (eds.) *Food and Feed Safety Systems and Analysis.* Cambridge: Academic Press; 2017:25-44.
188. Alldrick AJ, Hajšelová M. Zearalenone. In: Magan N, Olsen M, (eds.) Mycotoxins in Food Detection and *Controled.* Cambridge: Woodhead Publishing Limited; 2004:353-366.
189. Stein RA, Katz DE. *Escherichia coli*, cattle and the propagation of disease. *FEMS Microbiol Lett.* 2017;364:1–11.
190. Codex Alimentarius. *Code of Hygienic Practice for Fresh Fruits and Vegetables CXC 53-2003.* Rome: Joint FAO/WHO Food Standards Program; 2017.
191. Söderström A, Österberg P, Lindqvist A, et al. A large *Escherichia coli* O157 outbreak in sweden associated with locally produced lettuce. *Foodborne Pathog Dis.* 2008;5:339–349.
192. Jay MT, Cooley M, Carychao D, et al. *Escherichia coli* O157: H7 in feral swine near spinach fields and cattle, central California coast. *Emerg Infect Dis.* 2007;13:1908–1911.
193. Newell DG, Koopmans M, Verhoef L, et al. Food-borne diseases—the challenges of 20 years ago still persist while new ones continue to emerge. *Int J Food Microbiol.* 2010;139:S3–S15.
194. Hanlon KE, Miller MF, Guillen LM, et al. Presence of *Salmonella* and *Escherichia coli* O157 on the hide, and presence of *Salmonella, Escherichia coli* O157 and *Campylobacter* in feces from small-ruminant (goat and lamb) samples collected in the United States, Bahamas and Mexico. *Meat Sci.* 2018;135:1–5.
195. Lyautey E, Hartmann A, Pagotto F, et al. Characteristics and frequency of detection of fecal *Listeria monocytogenes* shed by livestock, wildlife, and humans. *Can J Microbiol.* 2007;53:1158–1167.
196. Pourcher AM, Ziebal C, Kervarrec M, et al. Sanitary status of 44 hog manures in Brittany: comparison of the effectiveness of manure treatments based on the levels of indicator bacteria and two pathogenic bacteria. *J Agric Sci Technol.* 2012;2:303–313.
197. Orzi V, Scaglia B, Lonati S, et al. The role of biological processes in reducing both odor impact and pathogen content during mesophilic anaerobic digestion. *Scie Total Environ.* 2015;526: 116–126.
198. Le Maréchal C, Druilhe C, Repérant E, et al. Evaluation of the occurrence of sporulating and nonsporulating pathogenic bacteria in manure and in digestate of five agricultural biogas plants. *MicrobiologyOpen.* 2019;8:1–10.
199. Gholipour S, Nikaeen M, Farhadkhani M, et al. Survey of *Listeria monocytogenes* contamination of various environmental samples and associated health risks. *Food Control.* 2020;108:1–6.
200. Neuhaus J, Schrödl W, Shehata AA, et al. Detection of *Clostridium botulinum* in liquid manure and biogas plant wastes. *Folia Microbiol.* 2015;60:451–456.
201. Souillard R, Le Marechal C, Balaine L, et al. Manure contamination with *Clostridium botulinum* after avian botulism outbreaks: management and potential risk of dissemination. *Vet Rec.* 2020;187:233–238.
202. Cui Y, Liu X, Dietrich R, et al. Caracterização de isolados de *Bacillus cereus* de fazendas leiteiras locais na China. *FEMS Microbiol Lett.* 2016;363:1–6.
203. Edrington TS, Long M, Ross TT, et al. Prevalence and antimicrobial resistance profiles of *Escherichia coli* O157: H7 and *Salmonella* isolated from feedlot lambs. *J Food Prot.* 2009;72:1713–1717.
204. Kagambèga A, Thibodeau A, Trinetta V, et al. *Salmonella* spp. and *Campylobacter* spp. in poultry feces and carcasses in Ouagadougou. *Burkina Faso Food Scie Nutr.* 2018;6: 1601–1606.
205. Pornsukarom S, Thakur S. Assessing the impact of manure application in commercial swine farms on the transmission of antimicrobial resistant *Salmonella* in the environment. *PLoS One.* 2016;11:1–17.
206. Golla SC, Murano EA, Johnson LG, Tipton NC, et al. Determination of the occurrence of *Arcobacter butzleri* in beef and dairy cattle from Texas by various isolation methods. *J Food Prot.* 2002;65:1849–1853.
207. Grove-White DH, Leatherbarrow AJH, Cripps PJ, et al. Temporal and farm-management-associated variation in faecal pat prevalence of *Arcobacter* spp. in ruminants. *Epidemiol Infect.* 2014;142:861–870.
208. Vilar MJ, Pena FJ, Perez I, et al. Presence of *Listeria, Arcobacter*, and *Campylobacter* spp. in dairy farms in Spain. *Berl Münch Tierärztl Wochenschr.* 2010;123:58–62.
209. Morales-Estrada AI, Hernández-Castro R, López-Merino A, et al. Isolation, identification, and antimicrobial susceptibility of *Brucella* spp. cultured from cow and goat manure in Mexico. *Arch Med Vet.* 2016;48:231–235.
210. Mpalang RK, Boreux R, Melin P, et al. Prevalence of *Campylobacter* among goats and retail goat meat in Congo. *J Infect Dev Ctries.* 2014;8:168–175.
211. Farzan A, Friendship RM, Cook A, et al. Occurrence of *Salmonella, Campylobacter, Yersinia enterocolitica, Escherichia coli* O157 and *Listeria monocytogenes* in swine. *Zoonoses Public Health.* 2010;57:388–396.
212. Mersha G, Asrat D, Zewde BM, et al. Occurrence of *Escherichia coli* O157: H7 in faeces, skin and carcasses from sheep and goats in Ethiopia. *Lett Appl Microbiol.* 2010;50:71–76.

213. Bozcal E, Uzel A, Aydemir S, Skurnik M. Isolation of pathogenic *Yersinia enterocolitica* strains from different sources in Izmir region, Turkey. *Folia Microbiol (Praha)*. 2015;60:523–529.
214. Ingram DT, Millner PD. Factors affecting compost tea as a potential source of *Escherichia coli* and *Salmonella* on fresh produce. *J Food Prot*. 2007;70:828–834.
215. Kim J, Jiang X. The growth potential of *Escherichia coli* O157: H7, *Salmonella* spp. and *Listeria monocytogenes* in dairy manure-based compost in a greenhouse setting under different seasons. *J Appl Microbiol*. 2010;109:2095–2104.
216. Nicholson FA, Groves SJ, Chambers BJ. Pathogen survival during livestock manure storage and following land application. *Bioresour Technol*. 2005;96:135–143.
217. Chen Z, Kim J, Jiang X. Survival of *Escherichia coli* O157: H7 and *Salmonella enterica* in animal waste-based composts as influenced by compost type, storage condition and inoculum level. *J Appl Microbiol*. 2018;124:1311–1323.
218. Semenov AV, Van Bruggen AH, Van Overbeek L, et al. Influence of temperature fluctuations on *Escherichia coli* O157: H7 and *Salmonella enterica* serovar Typhimurium in cow manure. *FEMS Microbiol Ecol*. 2007;60:419–428.
219. Wang H, Dharmasena M, Chen Z, et al. Persistence of non-O157 Shiga toxin–producing *Escherichia coli* in dairy compost during storage. *J Food Prot*. 2017;80:1999–2005.
220. Ongeng D, Muyanja C, Geeraerd AH, et al. Survival of *Escherichia coli* O157:H7 and *Salmonella enterica* serovar *Typhimurium* in manure and manure-amended soil under tropical climatic conditions in Sub-Saharan Africa. *J Appl Microbiol*. 2011;110:1007–1022.
221. Moriarty EM, Weaver L, Sinton LW, et al. Survival of *Escherichia coli*, *Enterococci* and *Campylobacter jejuni* in Canada goose faeces on pasture. *Zoonoses Public Health*. 2012;59:490–497.
222. Smith S, Meade J, Gibbons J, et al. The impact of environmental conditions on *Campylobacter jejuni* survival in broiler faeces and litter. *Infect Ecol Epidemiol*. 2016;6:1–7.
223. Mitscherlich E, Marth EH. *Microbial Survival in the Environment: Bacteria and Rickettsiae Important in Human and Animal Health*. Madison, WI: Springer Science & Business Media; 2012.
224. Maynaud G, Pourcher AM, Ziebal C, et al. Persistence and potential viable but non-culturable state of pathogenic bacteria during storage of digestates from agricultural biogas plants. *Front Microbiol*. 2016;7:1469.
225. Olaimat AN, Holley RA. Factors influencing the microbial safety of fresh produce: a review. *Food Microbiol*. 2012;32:1–19.
226. U.S. Department of Agriculture. Electronic Code of Federal Regulations: National Organic Program. T CFR part 205:203. <http://www.law.cornell.edu/cfr/text/7/205.203>, 2000.
227. Food and Drug Administration. FSMA Final Rule on Produce Safety: Standards for the Growing, Harvesting, Packing, and Holding of Produce for Human Consumption.<https://www.fda.gov/food/food-safety-modernization-act-fsma/fsma-final-rule-produce-safety#:~:text = About%20the%20Final%20Rule &text = The%20Produce%20Safety%20rule%20establishes,FDA%20Food%20Safety%20Modernization%20Act.>; 2015. Accessed 20.10. 20.
228. Warriner K, Huber A, Namvar A, et al. Recent advances in the microbial safety of fresh fruits and vegetables. *Adv Food Nutr Res*. 2009;57:155–208.
229. Berry ED, Millner PD, Wells JE, et al. Fate of naturally occurring *Escherichia coli* O157:H7 and other zoonotic pathogens during minimally managed bovine feedlot manure composting processes. *J Food Prot*. 2013;76:1308–1321.
230. Qian X, Sun W, Gu J, et al. Reducing antibiotic resistance genes, integrons, and pathogens in dairy manure by continuous thermophilic composting. *Bioresour Technol*. 2016;220:425–432.
231. Singh R, Jiang X, Luo F. Thermal inactivation of heat-shocked *Escherichia coli* O157:H7, *Salmonella*, and *Listeria monocytogenes* in dairy compost. *J Food Prot*. 2010;73:1633–1640.
232. Agostini F, Sundberg C, Navia R. Is biodegradable waste a porous environment? A review. *Waste Manag Res*. 2012;30:1001–1015.
233. Shepherd Jr MW, Liang P, Jiang X, et al. Microbiological analysis of composts produced on South Carolina poultry farms. *J Appl Microbiol*. 2010;108:2067–2076.
234. Sunar NM, Stentiford EI, Fletcher LA, et al. *Survival of* Salmonella *spp. in composting using vial and direct inoculums technique*. *Proceedings of the ORBIT International Conference of Organic Resources in Carbon Economy*. Greece: Crete; 2010:886–892.
235. Centers for Disease Control and Prevention. Multistate Outbreak of Shiga Toxin-Producing *Escherichia coli* O121 Infections Linked to Raw Clover Sprouts (Final Update). 2. <https://www.cdc.gov/ecoli/2014/o121-05-14/index.html>; 2014. Accessed 01.10.20.
236. Jung Y, Jang H, Matthews KR. Effect of the food production chain from farm practices to vegetable processing on outbreak incidence. *Microb Biotechnol*. 2014;7:517–527.
237. European Food Safety Authority. Shiga toxin-producing *E. coli* (STEC) O104:H4 2011 outbreaks in Europe: taking stock. *EFSA J*. 2011;9(10):2390. Accessed October 1, 2020.
238. Centers for Disease Control and Prevention. Multistate outbreak of Shiga toxin-producing *Escherichia coli* O121 infections linked to raw clover sprouts. Available from: <https://www.cdc.gov/ecoli/2014/o121-05-14/index.html>; 2014. Accessed 01.10.20.
239. Semenov AV, Franz E, van Bruggen AH. COLIWAVE a simulation model for survival of *E. coli* O157: H7 in dairy manure and manure-amended soil. *Ecol Model*. 2010;221:599–609.
240. Whipps J, Hand P, Pink D, et al. Phyllosphere microbiology with special reference to diversity and plant genotype. *J Appl Microbiol*. 2008;105:1744–1755.
241. Santamaría J, Toranzos GA. Enteric pathogens and soil: a short review. *Int Microbiol*. 2003;6:5–9.
242. Eilers KG, Debenport S, Anderson S, et al. Digging deeper to find unique microbial communities: the strong effect of depth on the structure of bacterial and archaeal communities in soil. *Soil Biol Biochem*. 2012;50:58–65.
243. Mgbakogu RA, Eledo BO. Incidence, characterization and pathological features of *Bacillus cereus* in soil, raw cereals and meat in Anambra State, Eastern Nigeria. *J Nat Sci Res*. 2015;5:67–76.
244. Owusu-Kwarteng J, Wuni A, Akabanda F, et al. Prevalence, virulence factor genes and antibiotic resistance of *Bacillus cereus* sensu lato isolated from dairy farms and traditional dairy products. *BMC Microbiol*. 2017;17:1–8.

245. Locatelli A, Spor A, Jolivet C, et al. Biotic and abiotic soil properties influence survival of *Listeria monocytogenes* in soil. *PLoS One*. 2013;8:1–8.
246. Kulesh R, Shinde SV, Khan WA, et al. The occurrence of *Listeria monocytogenes* in goats, farm environment and invertebrates. *Biol Rhythm Res*. 2019;1–10. Available from: https://doi.org/10.1080/09291016.2019.1660836.
247. Nayel M, El-Sify A, Akram S, et al. Molecular typing of *Clostridium perfringens* isolates from soil, healthy, and diseased sheep in Egypt by multiplex PCR. *J Vet Med Res*. 2013;22:53–57.
248. Stefanis C, Alexopoulos A, Voidarou C, et al. Prevalence of *C. perfringens* in agricultural fields with different vegetation types. *Folia Microbiol*. 2014;59:1–4.
249. del Mar Gamboa M, Rodríguez E, Vargas P. Diversity of mesophilic clostridia in Costa Rican soils. *Anaerobe*. 2005;11:322–326.
250. Makut MD, Obiekezie SO, Owuna G. Isolation and screening for biobutanol producing *Clostridium* species from the soil environment of Keffi Metropolis. *South Asian J Res Microbiol*. 2018;1:1–6.
251. Singh N, Goel G, Raghav M. Prevalence and characterization of *Cronobacter* spp. from various foods, medicinal plants, and environmental samples. *Curr Microbiol*. 2015;71:31–38.
252. Ahmed R, Muhammad K, Rabbani M, et al. Spatial distribution of soil borne *Brucella* species specific DNA in Punjab. *Pak Pak J Zoo*. 2017;49:1739–1748.
253. Schets FM, Jacobs-Reitsma WF, van der Plaats RQ, et al. Prevalence and types of *Campylobacter* on poultry farms and in their direct environment. *J Water Health*. 2017;15:849–862.
254. Pickering AJ, Ercumen A, Arnold BF, et al. Fecal indicator bacteria along multiple environmental transmission pathways (water, hands, food, soil, flies) and subsequent child diarrhea in rural Bangladesh. *Environ Sci Technol*. 2018;52:7928–7936.
255. Shrivastava AK, Mohakud NK, Panda S, et al. Major enteropathogens in humans, domestic animals, and environmental soil samples from the same locality: prevalence and transmission considerations in coastal Odisha, India. *Epidemiol Health*. 2020;42:1–9.
256. Alegbeleye OO, Singleton I, Sant'Ana AS. Sources and contamination routes of microbial pathogens to fresh produce during field cultivation: a review. *Food Microbiol*. 2018;73:177–208.
257. Ryser ET, Marth EH. *Listeria, listeriosis, and food safety*. 3rd ed. Boca Raton, FL: CRC Press; 2007.
258. Buchanan RL, Gorris LG, Hayman MM, et al. A review of *Listeria monocytogenes:* an update on outbreaks, virulence, dose-response, ecology, and risk assessments. *Food Control*. 2017;75:1–13.
259. Phan-Thien K, Metaferia MH, Bell TL, et al. Effect of soil type and temperature on survival of *Salmonella enterica* in poultry manure-amended soils. *Lett Appl Microbiol*. 2020;71:210–217.
260. Fongaro G, García-González MC, Hernández M, et al. Different behavior of enteric bacteria and viruses in clay and sandy soils after biofertilization with swine digestate. *Front Microbiol*. 2017;8:1–9.
261. Jacobsen CS, Bech TB. Soil survival of *Salmonella* and transfer to freshwater and fresh produce. *Food Res Int*. 2012;45:557–566.
262. Islam M, Morgan J, Doyle MP, et al. Fate of *Salmonella enterica* serovar Typhimurium on carrots and radishes grown in fields treated with contaminated manure composts or irrigation water. *Appl Environ Microbiol*. 2004;70:2497–2502.
263. Nyberg KA, Ottoson JR, Vinnerås B, et al. Fate and survival of *Salmonella* Typhimurium and *Escherichia coli* O157:H7 in repacked soil lysimeters after application of cattle slurry and human urine. *J Sci Food Agric*. 2014;94:2541–2546.
264. Islam M, Doyle MP, Phatak SC, et al. Persistence of enterohemorrhagic *Escherichia coli* O157:H7 in soil and on leaf lettuce and parsley grown in fields treated with contaminated manure composts or irrigation water. *J Food Prot*. 2004;67:1365–1370.
265. Sharma M, Millner PD, Hashem F, et al. *E. coli* survival duration in manure-amended soils is affected by spatiotemporal, agricultural, and weather factors: a multi-season, multi-site field study in the Mid-Atlantic US. *Appl Environ Microbiol*. 2018;85:1–23.
266. Baker CA, Lee S, De J, et al. Survival of *Escherichia coli* O157 in autoclaved and natural sandy soil mesocosms. *PLoS One*. 2020;15:1–16.
267. Sharma M, Millner PD, Hashem F, et al. Survival and persistence of nonpathogenic *Escherichia coli* and attenuated *Escherichia coli* O157:H7 in soils amended with animal manure in a greenhouse environment. *J Food Prot*. 2016;79:913–921.
268. Erickson MC, Habteselassie MY, Liao J, et al. Examination of factors for use as potential predictors of human enteric pathogen survival in soil. *J Appl Microbiol*. 2014;116:335–349.
269. Aune K, Rhyan JC, Russell R, et al. Environmental persistence of *Brucella abortus* in the Greater Yellowstone Area. *J Wildl Manage*. 2012;76:253–261.
270. Worth Calfee M, Wendling M. The effects of environmental conditions on persistence and inactivation of *Brucella* suis on building material surfaces. *Lett Appl Microbiol*. 2012;54:504–510.
271. Gessler F, Böhnel H. Persistence and mobility of a *Clostridium botulinum* spore population introduced to soil with spiked compost. *FEMS Microbiol Ecol*. 2006;58:384–393.
272. Jäderlund L, Sessitsch A, Arthurson V. Persistence of two *Campylobacter jejuni* strains in soil and on spinach plants. *Appl Environ Soil Sci*. 2011;1–7.
273. Huang Y, Flint SH, Palmer JS. *Bacillus cereus* spores and toxins—the potential role of biofilms. *Food Microbiol*. 2020;90:103493. Available from: https://doi.org/10.1016/j.fm.2020.103493.
274. Horn BW, Greene RL, Dorner JW. Effect of corn and peanut cultivation on soil populations of *Aspergillus flavus* and *A. parasiticus* in southwestern Georgia. *Appl Environ Microbiol*. 1995;61:2472–2475.
275. Diener UL, Cole RJ, Sanders TH, et al. Epidemiology of aflatoxin formation by *Aspergillus flavus*. *Annu Rev Phytopathol*. 1987;25:249–270.
276. Giorni P, Camardo Legierri M, Magan N, et al. Comparison of ecological needs for sporulation of *Aspergillus flavus* sclerotia on natural and artificial substrates. *Fungal Biol*. 2012;116:637–642.
277. Johnsson P, Lindblad M, Thim AM, et al. Growth of aflatoxigenic moulds and aflatoxin formation in Brazil nuts. *World Mycotoxin J*. 2008;1:127–137.
278. Doster MA, Michailides TJ. *Aspergillus* molds and aflatoxins in pistachio nuts in Calfornia. *Phytopathology*. 1994;84:583–590.

279. Buchanan JR, Sommer NF, Fortlage RJ. Aspergillus flavus infection and aflatoxin production in fig fruits. *Appl Microbiol.* 1975;30:238–241.
280. Le Bars J. Contribution to a practical strategy for preventing aflatoxin contamination of dried figs. *Microbiol Aliment Nutr.* 1990;8:265–270.
281. Bos ME, Verstappen KM, Van Cleef BA, et al. Transmission through air as a possible route of exposure for MRSA. *J Expo Sci Environ Epidemiol.* 2016;26:263–269.
282. Dahms C, Hübner NO, Cuny C, et al. Occurrence of methicillin-resistant *Staphylococcus aureus* in farm workers and the livestock environment in Mecklenburg-Western Pomerania, Germany. *Acta Vet Scand.* 2014;56:1–8.
283. Berry ED, Wells JE, Bono JL, et al. Effect of proximity to a cattle feedlot on *Escherichia coli* O157:H7 contamination of leafy greens and evaluation of the potential for airborne transmission. *Appl Environ Microbiol.* 2015;81:1101–1110.
284. Im MC, Jeong SJ, Kwon YK, et al. Prevalence and characteristics of *Salmonella* spp. isolated from commercial layer farms in Korea. *Poult Sci J.* 2015;94:1691–1698.
285. Madsen AM, Schlünssen V, Olsen TT, et al. Airborne fungal and bacterial components in PM1 dust from biofuel plants. *Ann Occup Hyg.* 2009;53:749–757.
286. Tang JW. The effect of environmental parameters on the survival of airborne infectious agents. *J R Soc Interface.* 2009;6: S737–S746.
287. Zhao Y, Aarnink AJ, De Jong MC, et al. Airborne microorganisms from livestock production systems and their relation to dust. *Crit Rev Environ Sci Technol.* 2014;44:1071–1128.
288. Feld L, Bay H, Angen Ø, et al. Survival of LA-MRSA in dust from swine farms. *Ann Work Expo Health.* 2018;62:147–156.
289. Oni RA, Sharma M, Buchanan RL. Survival of *Salmonella enterica* in dried turkey manure and persistence on spinach leaves. *J Food Prot.* 2015;78:1791–1799.
290. Humphrey T, O'Brien S, Madsen M. *Campylobacters* as zoonotic pathogens: a food production perspective. *Int J Food Microbiol.* 2007;117:237–257.
291. Lim JA, Lee DH, Heu S. The interaction of human enteric pathogens with plants. *Plant Pathol J.* 2014;30:109–116.
292. Talley JL, Wayadande AC, Wasala LP, et al. Association of *Escherichia coli* O157: H7 with filth flies (Muscidae and Calliphoridae) captured in leafy greens fields and experimental transmission of *E. coli* O157: H7 to spinach leaves by house flies (Diptera: Muscidae). *J Food Prot.* 2009;72:1547–1552.
293. Zurek L, Gorham JR. Insects as vectors of foodborne pathogens. In: Voeller, J.G. (eds.) Wiley Handbook of Science and Technology for Homeland Security. Hoboken, NJ: Wiley; 2008:1-16.
294. Khamesipour F, Lankarani KB, Honarvar B, et al. A systematic review of human pathogens carried by the housefly (*Musca domestica* L.). *BMC Public Health.* 2018;18:1–15.
295. Martínez-Vaz BM, Fink RC, Diez-Gonzalez F, et al. Enteric pathogen-plant interactions: molecular connections leading to colonization and growth and implications for food safety. *Microbes Environ.* 2014;29(2):123–135. Available from: https://doi.org/10.1264/jsme2.me13139.
296. Wasala L, Talley JL, DeSilva U, et al. Transfer of *Escherichia coli* O157: H7 to spinach by house flies, *Musca domestica* (Diptera: Muscidae). *Phytopathology.* 2013;103:373–380.
297. Janisiewicz WJ, Conway WS, Brown MW, et al. Fate of *Escherichia coli* O157: H7 on fresh-cut apple tissue and its potential for transmission by fruit flies. *Appl Environ Microbiol.* 1999;65:1–5.
298. Butler JF, Garcia-Maruniak A, Meek F, et al. Wild Florida house flies (*Musca domestica*) as carriers of pathogenic bacteria. *Florida Entomol.* 2010;93:218–223.
299. Keen JE, Wittum TE, Dunn JR, et al. Shiga-toxigenic *Escherichia coli* O157 in agricultural fair livestock, United States. *Emerg Infect Dis.* 2006;12:780.
300. Choo LC, Saleha AA, Wai SS, et al. Isolation of *Campylobacter* and *Salmonella* from houseflies (*Musca domestica*) in a university campus and a poultry farm in Selangor, Malaysia. *Trop Biomed.* 2011;28:16–20.
301. Aung WW. Occurrence of *Campylobacter* spp. and their antibiotic resistance profiles in cattle and farm environment. (Doctoral thesis). Universiti Putra Malaysia, Malaysia, 2014.
302. Matović K, Mišić D, Karabasil N, et al. *Clostridium botulinum* spores in European honey bees from Serbia. *J Apic Res.* 2019;58:420–426.
303. Lillehoj EB, Kwolek WF, Guthrie WD, et al. Aflatoxin accumulation in preharvest maize kernels: interaction of three fungal species, European corn borer and two hybrids. *Plant Soil.* 1982;65:95–102.
304. Bilgrami KS, Ranjan KS, Sinha AK. Impact of crop damage on occurrence of *Aspergillus flavus* and aflatoxin in rainy-season maize (*Zea mays*). *Indian J Agric Sci.* 1992;62:704–709.
305. Fandohan P, Hell K, Marasas WFO, et al. Infection of maize by *Fusarium* species and contamination with fumonisin in Africa. *Afr J Biotechnol.* 2003;2:570–579.
306. Abramson D. Mycotoxin formation and environmental factors. In: Sinha KK, Bhatnagar D, eds. *Mycotoxins in Agriculture and Food Safety.* New York, NY: Marcel Dekker, Inc.; 1998:255–277.
307. Cernicchiaro N, Pearl DL, McEwen SA, et al. Association of wild bird density and farm management factors with the prevalence of *E. coli* O157 in dairy herds in Ohio (2007–2009). *Zoonoses Public Health.* 2012;59:320–329.
308. Hellström S, Kiviniemi K, Autio T, et al. *Listeria monocytogenes* is common in wild birds in Helsinki region and genotypes are frequently similar with those found along the food chain. *J Appl Microbiol.* 2008;104:883–888.
309. Mrochen DM, Schulz D, Fischer S, et al. Wild rodents and shrews are natural hosts of *Staphylococcus aureus. Int J Med Microbiol.* 2018;308:590–597.
310. Joutsen S, Laukkanen-Ninios R, Henttonen H, et al. *Yersinia* spp. in wild rodents and shrews in Finland. *Vector-Borne Zoonotic Dis.* 2017;17:303–311.
311. Liang J, Duan R, Xia S, et al. Ecology and geographic distribution of *Yersinia enterocolitica* among livestock and wildlife in China. *Vet Microbiol.* 2015;178:125–131.
312. Sutton JC, Baliko W, Funnell HS. Relation of weather variables to incidence of zearalenone in corn in Southern Ontario. *Can J Plant Sci.* 1980;60:149–155.
313. Gil MI, Selma MV, Suslow T, et al. Pre-and postharvest preventive measures and intervention strategies to control microbial food safety hazards of fresh leafy vegetables. *Crit Rev Food Sci Nutr.* 2015;55:453–468.

314. Greig JD, Todd EC, Bartleson CA, et al. Outbreaks where food workers have been implicated in the spread of foodborne disease. Part 1. Description of the problem, methods, and agents involved. *J Food Prot.* 2007;70:1752–1761.
315. Hernandez-Milian A, Payeras-Cifre A. What is new in listeriosis? *Biomed Res Int.* 2014;2014:358051. Available from: https://doi.org/10.1155/2014/358051.
316. Francois P, Huyghe A, Charbonnier Y, et al. Use of an automated multiple-locus, variable number tandem repeat-based method for rapid and high-throughput genotyping of *Staphylococcus aureus* isolates. *J Clin Microbiol.* 2005;43: 3346–3355.
317. Nossair MA, Ibrahim HA, Khalifa E, et al. *Staphylococcus aureus* isolated from raw meat products and food handlers: prevalence, antimicrobial susceptibility and molecular characterization. *Life Sci J.* 2018;15:14–21.
318. Nasrolahei M, Mirshafiee S, Kholdi S, et al. Bacterial assessment of food handlers in Sari City, Mazandaran Province, north of Iran. *J Infect Public Health.* 2017;10:171–176.
319. Ivbule M, Miklaševičs E, Čupāne L, et al. Presence of methicillin-resistant *Staphylococcus aureus* in slaughterhouse environment, pigs, carcasses, and workers. *J Vet Res.* 2017;61:267–277.
320. Bogdanovicova K, Kamenik J, Dorotikova K, et al. Occurrence of foodborne agents at food service facilities in the Czech Republic. *J Food Prot.* 2019;82:1096–1103.
321. Mobolaji OA, Olubunmi OF. Assessment of the hygienic practices and the incidence of enteric bacteria in food handlers in small businesses in an urban area in Abeokuta. *Int J Microbiol Res.* 2014;5:41–49.
322. Nigusse D, Kumie A. Food hygiene practices and prevalence of intestinal parasites among food handlers working in Mekelle university student's cafeteria, Mekelle. *Global Adv Res J Soc Sci.* 2012;1:65–71.
323. Ifeadike CO, Ironkwe OC, Adogu POU, et al. Prevalence and pattern of bacteria and intestinal parasites among food handlers in the Federal Capital Territory of Nigeria. *Niger Med J.* 2012;53:166–171.
324. Mama M, Alemu G. Prevalence, antimicrobial susceptibility patterns and associated risk factors of *Shigella* and *Salmonella* among food handlers in Arba Minch University, South Ethiopia. *BMC Infect Dis.* 2016;16:1–7.
325. Xu H, Zhang W, Guo C, et al. Prevalence, serotypes, and antimicrobial resistance profiles among *Salmonella* isolated from food catering workers in Nantong, China. *Foodborne Pathog Dis.* 2019;16:346–351.
326. Brar PK, Danyluk MD. *Salmonella* transfer potential during hand harvesting of tomatoes under laboratory conditions. *J Food Prot.* 2013;76:1342–1349.
327. Beltran M, Gerba CP, Porto Fett A, et al. Prevalence and characterization of *Listeria monocytogenes, Salmonella* and Shiga toxin-producing *Escherichia coli* isolated from small Mexican retail markets of queso fresco. *Int J Environ Health Res.* 2015;25:140–148.
328. Ridley A, Morris V, Gittins J, et al. Potential sources of *Campylobacter* infection on chicken farms: contamination and control of broiler-harvesting equipment, vehicles and personnel. *J Appl Microbiol.* 2011;111:233–244.
329. Jimenez M, Siller JH, Valdez JB, et al. Bidirectional *Salmonella enterica* serovar *Typhimurium* transfer between bare/glove hands and green bell pepper and its interruption. *Int J Environ Health Res.* 2007;17:381–388.
330. Buchholz AL, Davidson GR, Marks BP, et al. Quantitative transfer of *Escherichia coli* O157: H7 to equipment during small-scale production of fresh-cut leafy greens. *J Food Prot.* 2012;75:1184–1197.
331. Fox EM, Leonard N, Jordan K. Physiological and transcriptional characterization of persistent and nonpersistent *Listeria monocytogenes* isolates. *Appl Environ Microbiol.* 2011;77:6559–6569.
332. Castillo A, Mercado I, Lucia LM, et al. *Salmonella* contamination during production of cantaloupe: a binational study. *J Food Prot.* 2004;67:713–720.
333. McEvoy JL, Luo Y, Conway W, et al. Potential of *Escherichia coli* O157: H7 to grow on field-cored lettuce as impacted by postharvest storage time and temperature. *Int J Food Microbiol.* 2009;128:506–509.
334. Taormina PJ, Beuchat LR, Erickson MC, et al. Transfer of *Escherichia coli* O157: H7 to iceberg lettuce via simulated field coring. *J Food Prot.* 2009;72:465–472.
335. Castro H, Ruusunen M, Lindström M. Occurrence and growth of *Listeria monocytogenes* in packaged raw milk. *Int J Food Microbiol.* 2017;261:1–10.
336. Sullivan G, Wiedmann M. Detection and prevalence of *Listeria* in US produce packinghouses and fresh-cut facilities. *J Food Prot.* 2020;83:1656–1666.
337. Berhilevych O, Kasianchuk V. Identification of *Cronobacter* spp (*Enterobacter sakazakii*) from raw milk and environmental samples of dairy farms. *Eastern-European J Enterp Technol.* 2017;6 (11):4–10.
338. Yang Y, Wan C, Xu H, et al. Development of a multiplexed PCR assay combined with propidium monoazide treatment for rapid and accurate detection and identification of three viable *Salmonella enterica* serovars. *Food Control.* 2012;28:456–462.
339. Nascimento MS, Carminati JA. Silva ICRN, et al. *Salmonella, Escherichia coli* and *Enterobacteriaceae* in the peanut supply chain: from farm to table. *Food Res Int.* 2018;105–930-935.
340. Bartz JA, Spiceland D, Teplitski M, et al. Factors affecting proliferation of *Salmonella enterica* in tomato fruit tissues (abstr). *Phytopathology.* 2013;103:12–23.
341. Kramer A, Guggenbichler P, Heldt P, et al. Hygienic relevance and risk assessment of antimicrobial-impregnated textiles. *Biofunct Text Skin.* 2006;33:78–109.
342. Kangas S, Takkinen J, Hakkinen M, et al. *Yersinia pseudotuberculosis* O:1 traced to raw carrots, Finland. *Emerg Infect Dis.* 2008;14:1959–1961.
343. Centers for Disease Control and Prevention. Multistate outbreak of human *Salmonella* enteritidis infections associated with shell eggs. <https://www.cdc.gov/salmonella/2010/shell-eggs-12-2-10.html>; 2010. Accessed 01.10.20.
344. Gaul LK, Farag NH, Shim T, et al. Hospital-acquired listeriosis outbreak caused by contaminated diced celery—Texas, 2010. *Clin Infect Dis.* 2013;56:20–26.

345. Centers for Disease Control and Prevention. Multistate outbreak of listeriosis linked to whole cantaloupes from Jensen Farms, Colorado. <https://www.cdc.gov/listeria/outbreaks/cantaloupes-jensen-farms/index.html>; 2012. Accessed 01.10.20.

346. Centers for Disease Control and Prevention. Multistate outbreak of *Salmonella* Typhimurium and *Salmonella* Newport infections linked to cantaloupe. <https://www.cdc.gov/salmonella/typhimurium-cantaloupe-08-12/index.html#:~:text = to%20Chamberlain%20farms.-,Among%2021%20people%20in%20the%20Salmonella%20Newport%20outbreak%20for%20whom,and%20tested%20samples%20of%20cantaloupe>; 2012. Accessed 01.10.20.

347. Centers for Disease Control and Prevention. Multistate outbreak of listeriosis linked to commercially produced, prepackaged caramel apples made from Bidart Bros. apples (final update). <https://www.cdc.gov/listeria/outbreaks/caramel-apples-12-14/index.html>; 2015. Accessed 01.10.20.

348. Iglesias HH, Chirife J. *Handbook of Food Isotherms*. New York, NY: Academic Press; 1982.

349. Codex Alimentarius. *Code of Practice for the Prevention and Reduction of Mycotoxin Contamination in Cereals. (CXC 51-2003 Adopted in 2003. Amended in 2014, 2017. Revised in 2016)*. Rome: Joint FAO/ WHO Food Standards Program; 2017.

Chapter 26

Contributions of pathogens from agricultural water to fresh produce

Zeynal Topalcengiz[1], Matt Krug[2], Joyjit Saha[3], Katelynn Stull[3] and Michelle Danyluk[4]

[1]*Department of Food Engineering, Faculty of Engineering and Architecture, Muş Alparslan University, Muş, Turkey,* [2]*Southwest Florida Research and Education Center, Institute of Food and Agricultural Sciences, University of Florida, Immokalee, FL, United States,* [3]*Citrus Research and Education Center, Institute of Food and Agricultural Sciences, University of Florida, Lake Alfred, FL, United States,* [4]*Department of Food Science and Human Nutrition, Citrus Research and Education Center, Institute of Food and Agricultural Sciences, University of Florida, Lake Alfred, FL, United States*

Abstract

Water used during the production, harvest, and postharvest handling of fresh fruits and vegetables is known to contribute to their microbiological quality and is often identified as the source of foodborne pathogens during outbreak investigations. Often, the focus of preharvest agricultural waters is on irrigation water, but other water uses such as spray application, frost protection, washing, and hydrocooling where water touches the harvested portion of the crop should be treated equally. This chapter builds upon previous and recent research as well as reviews on microbiological contamination of produce from agricultural water. It includes evaluations on the role agricultural waters play in produce safety, what is known about the prevalence of foodborne pathogens and microbiological indicators in agricultural waters; the fate of foodborne pathogens in agricultural waters and mitigation options to manage risks from agricultural waters.

Keywords: Water; agricultural water; irrigation water; produce; produce safety; fruits; vegetables

26.1 Introduction

Worldwide consumption of fresh produce has shown a considerable increase in the past two decades[1,2] with a notable rise in global distribution.[3] In 2017, the United States alone produced about 11.7 billion pounds of fresh produce valued at $18.9 billion.[4] However, with the increased consumption, the incidence of produce associated illness outbreaks have also risen sharply. There is increasing evidence that consumption of raw fresh produce is a major factor contributing to human illness, due to the potential for contamination with pathogenic microorganisms. In the United States, fresh produce-related outbreaks have accounted for a large portion of all reported foodborne illness outbreaks over the last several decades.[5,6] According to the Centers for Disease Control and Prevention (CDC), between 1998 and 2018, fresh produce was responsible for 355 foodborne illness outbreaks with 10,324 cases, 624 hospitalizations, and 14 deaths.[7–10,11] Not limited to the US, there has also been an increasing number of produce associated outbreaks in the European Union (EU) and some of them have revealed unique and unexplained links between the implicated food and etiological agents such as *Shigella* and imported baby corn,[12] *Yersinia pseudotuberculosis* and lettuces,[13] and Noroviruses and raspberries.[14,15] In Australia, from 2001 to 2005, fresh produce accounted for 4% of all the reported foodborne illness outbreaks.[16]

Investigation of fresh produce linked to foodborne illness outbreaks provided some of the best insights into the microbial etiology and the types of process failures leading to these outbreaks. Most of these outbreaks were associated with the contamination of enterohemorrhagic *Escherichia coli* (e.g., *E. coli* O157:H7), *Salmonella* spp., or Norovirus[7,11,17–20] either during the production, processing, or packing stage.[2,21] Contamination of produce can occur via a number of routes, including contact with soil or improperly composted manure, the use of contaminated agricultural or postharvest washing water or transmission from infected food handlers.[22,23] Although the use of poor quality water during produce production has been correlated with increased incidence of outbreaks,[24] direct evidence of irrigation water causing foodborne diseases is relatively rare.[25] It is important to remember that agricultural water is used in many ways while growing, harvesting, and packing fresh fruits and vegetables and that agricultural water can come from many sources with varying degrees of inherent

Present Knowledge in Food Safety. DOI: https://doi.org/10.1016/B978-0-12-819470-6.00075-5

risk. When assessing the risk associated with different agricultural waters, it is critical to evaluate the source of the water including the hazards likely present (i.e., surface water vs groundwater), the way the water is applied to the crop (i.e., onto the harvested portion or not), and the time of the water application (i.e., close to harvest or not).

Role of agricultural water during pre- and postharvest activities such as irrigation, spray application of pesticides, frost protection, washing, and hydrocooling in foodborne outbreaks is of great interest to this chapter and will be discussed in detail, with a focus on water that touches the harvested portion of the crop before it is harvested. The chapter builds upon previous and recent research as well as reviews on microbiological contamination of produce from agricultural water.

26.2 Agricultural water's role in produce safety

26.2.1 Outbreaks linked to agricultural water

A comprehensive list of trace-back investigation findings for foodborne illness outbreaks linked to agricultural water use is presented for different parts of the world in Table 26.1.

The majority of these foodborne illness outbreaks results from crop contamination in the field and suggests contamination due to poor quality of irrigation water. There are three outbreaks specifically linked to wash water during postharvest handling. Importantly, a source for most of these outbreaks associated with irrigation

TABLE 26.1 Trace back investigations of foodborne outbreaks associated with produce linked to contaminated agricultural water.

Year	Country	Implicated food	Pathogen	Cases	Source of contamination (confirmation status)	Reference
1999	United States	Mangoes	*Salmonella* Newport	79	Wash water (confirmed)	Sivapalasingam et al.[26]
2000	Germany	Herbs	*Cyclospora cayetanensis*	34	Irrigation water (not confirmed)	Döller et al.[27]
2001	United States	Mangoes	*Salmonella* Newport	26	Wash water (confirmed)	Gibbs et al.[28]
2002	United States	Tomatoes	*Salmonella* Newport	510	Irrigation water (confirmed)	Greene et al.[29]
2004	Norway	Lettuce	*Salmonella* Thompson	21	Irrigation water (not confirmed)	Nygård et al.[30]
2005	Denmark	Raspberries	Norovirus	1000	Irrigation water (not confirmed)	Sarvikivi et al.[31]
2005	Sweden	Lettuce	*Escherichia coli* O157	135	Irrigation water (not confirmed)	Uyttendaele et al.[2]
2005	United States	Tomatoes	*Salmonella* Newport	72	Irrigation water (not confirmed)	Gurtler et al.[32]
2006	United States	Spinach	*E. coli* O157	205	Irrigation water (confirmed)	Gelting et al.[33]
2006	Australia	Papaya	*Salmonella* Litchfield	26	Wash water (confirmed)	Gibbs et al.[28]
2008	United States	Peppers	*Salmonella* Saintpaul	1500	Irrigation water (not confirmed)	Barton Behravesh et al.[34]
2011	Canada	Basil	*C. cayetanensis*	17	Irrigation water (Not confirmed)	Hoang et al.[35]
2013	Sweden	Salad	*E. coli* O157	19	Irrigation water (not confirmed)	Uyttendaele et al.[2]
2013	United Kingdom	Watercress	STEC	19	Irrigation water (not confirmed)	Uyttendaele et al.[2]
2016	United States	Alfalfa Sprouts	*Salmonella* Cubana	25	Irrigation water (confirmed)	Centers for Disease Control and Prevention CDC[36]
2018	United States	Lettuce	*E. coli* O157:H7	210	Irrigation water (not confirmed)	Centers for Disease Control and Prevention CDC,[8,9]
2018	United States	Lettuce	*E. coli* O157:H7	62	Irrigation water (confirmed)	Centers for Disease Control and Prevention CDC[37]

water quality could not be confirmed with direct evidence. In only 4 of the 14 outbreaks, agricultural water was confirmed as the source; the evidence was circumstantial at most.

In many traceback investigations a suggestive link between irrigation water and contaminated produce is assumed with no real evidence (i.e., no direct match with the outbreak strains). Since most of these outbreaks undergo an epidemiological investigation based on questions and answers from the affected individuals, the real source of contamination is often never ascertained.[16,26,27,29,32,34] For instance, the organism involved in an outbreak associated with iceberg lettuce in Sweden was isolated from cattle upstream but not directly from the water.[2] Similarly, outbreak strains obtained from the nationwide 2008 US outbreak of *Salmonella* SaintPaul in peppers could not be traced back to the irrigation water.[34] Cooley et al.[38] reported the results of the extensive sampling of a farm associated with three separate outbreaks between 2002 and 2003 that could not be matched with the clinical strains associated with the three outbreaks. Studies by Lynch et al.[39] have shown that once a particular transmission pathway is identified, repeated outbreaks and investigations lead to a bias in causation. Investigators may either speculate or assume a source of contamination due to the lack of sufficient data.

Agricultural waters have been implicated as a preharvest contamination source for major produce-related outbreaks. Two multistate outbreaks of *Salmonella* serotype Newport originated from tomatoes grown on the eastern shore of Virginia in 2002 and 2005 in the United States. Both *S.* Newport strains had the same pulsed-field gel electrophoresis (PFGE) pattern.[29,40] In 2006, potential water issues were related to fresh spinach during the multistate *E. coli* O157:H7 outbreak in the United States with circumstantial evidence. During the investigation, outbreak strains of *E. coli* were obtained from the surrounding river water and sediment. Analysis of the available data suggested that there was no definitive determination about how the spinach was contaminated with the outbreak strain. However, transmission of the pathogen to the shallow aquifer supplying irrigation well water during the recharge of the irrigation well by contaminated river water was identified as the possible reason for the source of the outbreak. This was likely due to the water table level in the well dropping during the late growing season due to increased water use during the harvest season.[33] In 2008, the *E. coli* O157:H7 outbreak in the US was associated with the consumption of contaminated shredded lettuce, and the outbreak was linked to the accidental mixing of irrigation well water and a dairy manure lagoon.[41] In 2016, the *Salmonella* outbreak associated with the consumption of alfalfa sprouts in the United States and was attributed to the irrigation water. The outbreak strain of *Salmonella* Cubana from an alfalfa sprout lot had the same DNA fingerprint as the strains isolated in the irrigation water.[36] A recent multistate outbreak of *E. coli* O157:H7 in the United States, in 2018, linked to romaine lettuce was confirmed of their source of contamination as irrigation water.[37]

Contrary to preharvest water use, most of the outbreaks associated with postharvest water were confirmed. In the United States, the first *Salmonella* outbreak associated with postharvest water use was traced back to imported mangoes from Brazil in 1999. Hot water treatment of mangoes in the packinghouse, a process to prevent importation of the Mediterranean fruit fly, led to contamination by *Salmonella*.[26] The detection of outbreak strains in the river water used for processing mangoes confirmed the source of contamination.[26] Another *Salmonella* outbreak associated with mangoes occurred in 2001 as part of the same program, where growers in Peru were dipping fruit in untreated water from the river.[28] Later in 2006, an outbreak associated with *Salmonella* in papaya in Australia occurred due to a similar reason, that is, untreated river water used to wash the fruits before packaging.[28]

In some countries, including Senegal, South Africa, Mexico, and India, the quality of agricultural water has been documented to influence microbial quality in fresh produce.[2,42–44] Poor microbiological quality of irrigation water, often having a waste origin, has frequently been associated with the incidence of human pathogens in leafy vegetables in some of these countries. The incidence of foodborne and waterborne diseases such as shigellosis, salmonellosis, typhoid fever, and infectious hepatitis is higher in communities practicing wastewater irrigation. In Mexico, a study revealed that rates of diarrhea are significantly higher in households irrigating with untreated wastewater than in households irrigating with rainfall. In Morocco, untreated wastewater usage for irrigation significantly increased the rate of salmonellosis among children.[45] The lack of surveillance and reporting infrastructure systems in many countries and challenging traceback to flowing water sources often makes it challenging to locate a specific source.

26.2.2 Microbial water quality standards

The microbiological quality of water touching the harvested portion of produce is commonly believed to relate directly to the safety of produce. Agricultural water quality is usually monitored by the presence or population of indicator organisms. Indicator organisms, not pathogenic themselves, are assumed to show the presence of fecal contamination and possible pathogen contamination from feces. Indicator microorganisms indicate general fecal contamination and should not be used interchangeably with the Index microorganism. Indicator microorganisms exceeding specific limits do not represent the presence of pathogen; the index microorganism shows the possible occurrence of ecologically similar pathogens.[46,47] The intention for the use of an index microorganism is to predict the presence of a specific pathogen, whereas the intention of the use of an indicator microorganism is indirect prediction of pathogen presence due to fecal contamination.[46]

Some of the primary reasons for using indicator organisms to establish microbial water quality rather than actual pathogen are driven by the complex procedures for enumeration of pathogen populations, high cost, and the length of time required to obtain results. Populations of indicator organisms are typically enumerated with easy detection methods using inexpensive and simple techniques. Indicator organisms for irrigation water testing can include counts of total coliforms, fecal coliforms, *E. coli*, fecal streptococci, and nematode eggs.[48] The US Environmental Protection Agency (EPA), in 1973, stated "total coliforms" are considered the indicator organism; however, later it was changed to "fecal coliforms" since fecal contamination was found to be the only possible source of pathogen contamination in waters.[49] Because total coliform and fecal coliform counts can enumerate bacteria of nonfecal origin, the indicators of choice have been changed to generic *E. coli* and, in some cases, fecal *Streptococci*. In some countries, additional standards have been adopted to include nematode and helminth egg counts or virus counts.[50] Nematode eggs are used to estimate the risk of infection from *Ascaris* spp., *Trichuris* spp., and hookworms from treated wastewater in regions where these organisms are endemic.[23] In the United States, Arizona has a virus standard of 1 plaque-forming unit (PFU)/40 L and *Giardia* cysts of 1 per 40 L in addition to a fecal coliform standard of 25/100 mL.[50] As indicator microorganisms are accepted as increasing evidence of a likelihood of potential contamination of food or water, it is predicted that their presence would ideally correlate with ecologically closely related pathogens or other enteric organisms.

The monitoring of fecal indicator organisms has been used as a mitigation to ensure produce safety; however, there are questions about their accuracy to assess potential pathogen presence in agricultural water sources. The correlation between indicator microorganisms and pathogens has been reported as present, weak, or temporal, especially in water sources sampled for both generic *E. coli* and *Salmonella* spp.[49,51] Required standards for agricultural water quality cannot guarantee the safety of produce. For example, generic *E. coli* populations in six agricultural ponds from Central Florida were in compliance with metrics required by the Produce Safety Rule (PSR) under the Food Safety Modernization Act (FSMA) in the United States, despite the presence of pathogenic genes associated with Shiga toxin-producing *E. coli* (STEC) and pathogenic *Salmonella* spp.[52] For the same agricultural surface water sources in Florida, metrics required by FSMA (a minimum of 20 initial samples collected over 2–4 years followed by rolling recent 15 samples with a minimum of five annual samples) are determined insufficient for certain characterization of microbiological water quality.[53] In another study, a rigorous sampling program is concluded as essential for effective monitoring of microbial water quality due to high spatiotemporal variabilities in generic *E. coli* populations.[54] These discrepancies between generic *E. coli* populations and pathogen presence have led to some researchers proposing alternative fecal indicator organisms or methodologies for more successful predictions.

Predictions of indicator microorganisms and pathogens in agricultural water sources have been suggested as a more economic and faster alternatives compared to conventional methods. However, numerous studies with statistical and computer-based approaches have attempted to predict or link pathogen presence or microbial quality of surface water to various types of microbiological indicators, chemical, physical, meteorological, or landscape predictors with moderate, little or no agreement.[53,55–68] Despite encouraging and promising results of statistical models and machine learning algorithms, the success of prediction models is limited by factors including the use of datasets, obtained from a specific area, unstable environmental conditions in sampling areas, the lack of animal activity measurement in and around the water source, and terrestrial variables.

The United States selected generic *E. coli* as the indicator organism for water testing requirements for PSR under FSMA as mentioned above. This metric originated from the recreational water requirements of the US EPA. Sweden also bases irrigation water quality standards on those for recreational water.[69] The use of recreational water standards is questioned by some, as they are established by considering the exposure of full-body exposure and do not take into account the rapid die-off during postirrigation intervals and exposure to environmental stresses associated with crop production.[70] To meet realistic expectations by taking into account economic considerations and other geological factors, guidelines governing the microbial quality of irrigation water vary considerably between countries and between sources such as groundwater, surface water, and human wastewater. Guidelines for the microbial quality of surface water tend to be more lenient than those for wastewater since it is less likely to contain human pathogens and enteric viruses.[23] Potable water or rainwater, groundwater from deep wells, and groundwater from shallow wells have lower tendencies to contaminate produce than surface water and inadequately treated wastewater.[71] A guideline by the US EPA for surface water for irrigation of crops recommends a range from <100 to <1000 fecal coliforms per 100 mL.[23] In the United States, the groundwater is often considered a microbiologically safe source for irrigation water.[50] Similar to the US EPA guidelines, most irrigation water is withdrawn from surface water or groundwater sources in Canada.[72] Canadian Water Quality Guidelines for the Protection of Agricultural Water Uses recommends a maximum of 1000 coliforms per 100 mL and 100 fecal coliforms per 100 mL of irrigation water.[23,73] Among all the sources, guidelines for reclaimed wastewater for irrigational use are the strictest due to possible high numbers of human pathogens present in untreated wastewater.

Guidelines can also be based on an essential distinction between crops likely to be eaten uncooked (restricted) and crops that will be cooked (unrestricted).[49,74] The quality of water recommended for irrigation of crops likely to be consumed raw is often higher than that for processed or fodder crops. For example, water quality requirements in the PSR under FSMA do not apply to agricultural waters that do not directly contact the harvestable portion of the produce as drip irrigation of tree crops, or for crops that undergo commercial processing.[75] The US EPA guidelines for reclaimed wastewater recommends zero and <200 fecal coliforms per 100 mL for produce that would be eaten raw and processed, respectively.[49] The World Health Organization (WHO) allows up to 1000 fecal coliforms per 100 mL of reclaimed wastewater, one viable intestinal nematode egg per liter of water for raw consumed produce and up to 100,000 fecal coliforms per 100 mL of water for processed produce before consumption.[74]

The wastewater irrigation standards recommended by the US EPA are based on a zero-risk approach where a single pathogenic microorganism poses a potential public health risk, whereas the WHO guidelines are based on the model-generated risk assessment predicted from epidemiological data obtained from outbreaks.[74] Based on the model, WHO calculates the level of water treatment required to keep the level of increased infections up to 10^{-4} infections per person per year.[74] Although high-quality irrigation water is always desirable, in some countries, the economic costs associated with treating wastewater to achieve this high level of water quality is not feasible.[23] Therefore the development of guidelines and regulations dealing with microbial standards based upon prior experience is necessary, rather than an empirical method, and what is achievable under good practices.[2,74] The fit for purpose standard for the microbiological quality of surface water emphasizes site-specific analysis for specific crop, pathogen, irrigation system, water sources, and management. One of the ways to achieve this expectation is to use quantitative microbial risk assessment (QMRA) to establish irrigation water standards.

26.2.3 Quantitative microbial risk assessment

QMRA can help producers and regulatory agencies to conduct meaningful exposure assessments despite the variability of different production practices, water sources, and uses of water associated with produce production.[76] QMRA has made it possible to perform a dynamic risk assessment dealing realistically with the factors that may influence the level of a foodborne pathogen in foods consumed by the population.[76] Risk assessment[77] has a specific framework and starts with identification of the hazard followed by exposure assessment, hazard characterization, and risk characterization. QMRA for irrigation waters establishes a relationship between the concentrations of pathogenic microorganisms in irrigation water and the probability of illness due to ingestion of pathogens with the contaminated produce.[78]

Using QMRA, WHO revised the guidelines for wastewater use in agriculture by replacing the fecal coliform standards with more health-based targets such as fecal coliforms. Using this approach, O'Toole et al.[79] showed how to translate every step in water treatment, irrigation and farming practices based on health outcome. They also proposed how QMRA could be used in a regulatory framework to guide farm managers to the interventions in the farm-to-fork chain in produce. In another study using QMRA to improve irrigation water quality, Ottoson et al.[80] showed how a reduction of 2 $\log_{10}$ CFU *E. coli*/100 mL in the irrigation water would reduce STEC illnesses through the consumption of iceberg lettuce by five times. Ottoson et al.[80] also recommended to increase the time between irrigation and harvest besides controlling the microbial quality of the irrigation water source. Stine et al.[50] reported that *Salmonella* concentrations on furrow-irrigated lettuce could range between 1.5×10^2 and 7.2×10^6 CFU/100 mL based on the last irrigation event. Another study by Stine et al.,[50] utilizing QMRA, estimated that less than one hepatitis A virus per 10 L of irrigation water could result in a risk exceeding 1:10,000 per year considering the exposure and the survival of the virus from crop till harvest time. More recently, pathogen-specific irrigation QMRA were also developed, notably for viruses on lettuce,[81] enteric virus infection on cucumber, broccoli, cabbage, or lettuce, *Cryptosporidium* and *Giardia* on irrigated tomatoes, bell peppers, cucumbers, and lettuce, and norovirus (NoV) and *Ascaris* infection helping risk managers and regulators to be more specific.[49]

QMRA models are based upon the premise that the response of microbial populations to different environmental factors are reproducible. This allows, based on past observations, the prediction of the microbial population response to changing environmental conditions.[82] However, the behavior of microorganisms in response to environmental factors could change. Therefore "predictive models are never perfect, due to intrinsic inaccuracies, extrapolations, and unexpected biological behavior."[83] Although it could lead us to estimate the trends, it is essential to know the reliability of predictions or recommendations derived from these models.[84] Furthermore, development and validation of QMRA models are data-intensive which might be costly at the beginning.[85] However, once the model has been built, the effect of new parameters such as changes in exposure conditions could be evaluated by using equations to reduce cost over time. Over the last decade, the exponential growth of QMRA in various domains indicates its success and acceptability, and its role in establishing agricultural water quality standards.

26.3 Foodborne pathogens and microbial indicators in agricultural waters

The previous section described the increasing numbers of produce-associated foodborne illness outbreaks and some of the foodborne pathogens attributed to these outbreaks. Domesticated and wild animal feces can serve as the main sources for pathogen contamination of agricultural water sources.[86,87] The following section discusses what is known about the prevalence and concentration of different types of bacteria, viruses, and parasites in agricultural waters. The interplay of pathogen presence and environmental aspects of both the location of water sources and the surrounding water environment on pathogen levels is also examined. Differences in the sampled volume of water, and testing methodologies, make direct comparisons between reported pathogen prevalence challenging.

26.3.1 Prevalence of foodborne pathogens in agricultural waters

26.3.1.1 Bacterial pathogen prevalence

Indicator organism and pathogen presence have been characterized for different agricultural water sources and regions. Many of the studies referenced samples for a small selection of the types of pathogens that can be found in particular regions. Particularly, indicator organisms such as generic *E. coli* are typically sampled for in studies. A limitation in comparing prevalences in different studies is the differing volumes of water sampled; as a larger volume of water is sampled, the limit of detection decreases, and the likelihood of finding something increases. In Ontario, Canada, at the South Nation River basin, samples were collected that tested positive for *Listeria monocytogenes* (74/321; 23%), *E. coli* O157:H7 (5/423; 1%), *Salmonella* spp. (72/751; 10%), and *Campylobacter* spp. (181/628; 29%).[88] In South Alberta, Canada, *E. coli* O157:H7 was detected in 1.3% and 2% of 90 mL surface water samples in the Oldman River Basin for each year over 2 years of sampling.[89] In the same study, *Salmonella* was isolated at 5.5% in the first year and 14.9% in the second year of sampling in 90 mL of samples.[89] In another survey conducted in Canada, Johnson et al.[90] reported that the prevalence of *E. coli* O157:H7 and *Salmonella* spp. was 0.9% and 6.25% in 90 mL water samples in more than 1,400 samples, respectively. In the United States, in Pennsylvanian surface waters used for irrigation, no *E. coli* O157:H7 was detected in 100 mL samples, while 5/153 (3%) samples were positive for *Salmonella* spp. from 90 mL samples.[91] Two L surface water samples from drainage ditches, canals, and water reservoirs used for crop irrigation in the southeast area of Spain were sampled; the authors noted that these sources of water can be mixed with reclaimed water from wastewater treatment plants. Of these samples, *Salmonella* spp. was confirmed in 49/113 samples (43%), *E. coli* O157:H7 was confirmed in 14/113 (12%) of samples, and non-O157:H7 STEC was confirmed in 12/113 samples (11%).[63] These researchers noted that of their water sources, samples with the most positives were from drainage ditches, followed by canals, and then water reservoirs. Researchers in New York, United States, sampled surface water used for irrigation of spinach fields and noted 33/62 (52%) of 250 mL samples were positive for *L. monocytogenes*.[92] While these studies all differ in terms of pathogen tested for, water source, sampling scheme, and methods and volume used, it is important to note that pathogens are consistently found in agricultural waters in a wide variety of regions.

26.3.1.2 Virus prevalence

Researchers in South Korea sampled 300 L of groundwater sources for NoVs, adenoviruses (AdVs), enteroviruses (EVs), and rotaviruses (RVs). Five of the 29 samples tested positive for EV, 2 samples were positive for AdVs, and 1 sample was positive for NoVs. While groundwater does not have the same level of risk as surface water, these researchers note that viruses are still found in groundwater sources, as contamination from surrounding aquifers can occur.[93,94] Expanding on this, in Italy NoVs were found in 4/26 (15.38%) groundwater samples.[95] A research group in Europe took irrigation water samples from berry farms in Finland, the Czech Republic, Serbia and Poland with samples tested for hepatitis A virus (HAV) and NoVs.[94] Of these samples, no HAV was detected while 2/36 samples were positive for NoVs.[94] In Italy, 20 L groundwater well samples were tested for NoVs, RVs, EVs, and HAV; 23/147 samples in wells with suitable water (defined as no microorganism of fecal origin exceeding Italian Ministerial Decree DM 185/03 where water is acceptable when *E. coli* < 100 CFU/100 mL and *Salmonella* spp. absent from 1000 mL of water in one of two samples) were positive for viruses, with no HAV being detected.[96] Similar to bacteria, the amount and types of viruses detected differed, but researchers detected them in various locations and sources of water.

26.3.1.3 Parasitic pathogen prevalence

Spanish researchers detected parasitic pathogens *Giardia intestinalis*, *Acanthamoeba castellanii*, *Toxoplasma gondii*, and *Entamoeba histolytica*, in surface irrigation water samples.[97] For these samples, 1.5 L was used for DNA detection with an additional 500 mL used to detect *Cryptosporidium* oocysts and *Giardia* cysts. These researchers note the difficulty of detecting parasites in water samples, especially as molecular techniques for confirmation are not widely used.[97] In Mexico, *Cryptosporidium* oocysts and *Giardia* cysts were detected in surface water used for irrigation. Forty-nine samples were taken from an irrigation canal, four were taken from an agricultural wastewater canal, and five taken from a river; 48% of samples were positive for *Cryptosporidium* oocysts and 50% were positive for *Giardia* cysts.[98] Surface water samples between 100 and 400 L were taken from sources used for irrigation in Costa Rica, Mexico, Panama, and the US and were tested for *Giardia* cysts and *Cryptosporidium* oocysts. Out of 25 total samples, 60% tested positive for *Giardia* cysts with a geometric mean of 369 cysts per 100 L and 36% of samples tested positive for *Cryptosporidium* oocysts with a geometric mean of 227 oocysts per 100 L. The US had less than 1% of samples testing positive for *Cryptosporidium* oocysts.[99] Similar to bacteria and viruses, parasitic pathogens are consistently found in agricultural waters in a wide variety of regions.

26.3.2 Regional differences on the presence of foodborne pathogens

As noted in the previous section, different types of pathogens are typically present when sampled in various locations. While seasonal variations and weather will be discussed in section 26.3.3 on environmental impacts, other regional variables can impact pathogen type and distribution. Surrounding land use, soil type, and types of water used can all vary by region. Evaluating surrounding land use is an important part of risk assessment as activities can serve as a source of contamination. Regions where animal husbandry is geographically close to agricultural water sources can contribute to contamination, notably when runoff occurs. Of importance for the microbial quality of groundwater is soil type, as it serves as a natural filtration of bacteria.[100] Regions that have loose soil experience a greater pathogen filtration effect than those regions where stony soil is found.[49] Clay soils and others susceptible to shrinking or cracking are not as effective at limiting bacterial transport as the bacteria can pass through these spaces.[101] The makeup of soil and its ability to retain moisture and nutrients impact bacterial presence as they can utilize these resources for survival.[101] When raw, untreated wastewater is used for agricultural water purposes, there are higher numbers of pathogens present; this occurs more in some countries than others, especially in those where population growth outpaces sanitation and wastewater management practices.[49,102] Many growers in these countries, especially those in urban and peri-urban areas, often have no realistic alternative to irrigation water than wastewater.[102] This is an ongoing challenge for the safety of crops due to the negative impact untreated wastewater has on human health.

26.3.3 Environmental impacts on the presence of foodborne pathogens

26.3.3.1 Seasonal differences

Seasonal shifts are not only associated with changes in weather but also changes in bacteria prevalence. The changes in temperature and precipitation amounts associated with seasonal shifts are accompanied by changes in pathogen populations. Changes in human and animal reservoir shedding may contribute to a seasonal effect.[51] Belgian researchers reported that a seasonal effect was noted for detection of enterohemorrhagic *E. coli*, *Salmonella* spp., *Campylobacter* spp., and three indicator organisms: total coliforms, enterococci, and *E. coli* with summer months showing elevated numbers of organisms.[103] However, there have been studies where seasons did not have a statistically significant impact on pathogen populations in agricultural water, but other environmental factors did.[51]

Seasonality can be broken into two major variables: temperature and precipitation. Higher temperatures have shown a correlation with pathogen presence.[51,63,104] In a study that took place in Southern Georgia in the United States, rainfall, dissolved oxygen concentration, and temperature were noted with the collection of irrigation water samples for bacterial quantification. Of the environmental variables recorded, higher temperatures were associated with the presence of *Salmonella* spp. and generic *E. coli*.[51] Higher water temperatures in correlation with weather temperatures provide a growing environment that is beneficial to not just *Salmonella* spp. and *E. coli*, but many foodborne bacterial pathogens. The researchers in

Spain who sampled water from drainage ditches, canals, and water reservoirs noted a temperature effect with *E. coli* where higher water temperatures were moderately, but statistically significantly associated with *E. coli* presence. This was seen with the samples from drainage ditches and water reservoirs, yet not canals; researchers hypothesized that this was due to discharge from a nearby wastewater treatment plant where contamination occurred regularly and was independent of temperature.[63] The severity of climate change and the associated rising air and water temperatures and weather changes, including severe weather events, may have an impact on microbial water quality in the future.[105]

Precipitation has also shown an association with increased levels of bacteria.[38,49,52] It is recommended to growers sampling their production water to wait after rain events for a more accurate representation of their water. Rain can result in runoff, that may contain pathogens, into production water systems while also recirculating what has settled on the bottom of production water systems; this exemplifies the importance of knowing the surrounding environment and land use to agricultural water sources. A study in Ohio in the United States characterized that precipitation had an impact on generic *E. coli* and total coliforms from two locations; in one irrigation canal and four water reservoirs.[106] Researchers determined that samples from the canals had higher *E. coli* and total coliforms counts after 20 mm of rain. However, the counts of total coliforms and *E. coli* from the water reservoirs were not associated with precipitation in the previous 24 h.[106] The difference between the canal and water reservoirs in the precipitation's impact on the bacteria was hypothesized to be from the increased opportunity for runoff into the canals after rain and the depth of water being low enough for the sediment suspension to have a greater impact.[106] Alternatively, large rain amounts can increase the volume of water in a system leading to dilution of pathogens, which also contributes to an inaccurate representation of water quality when sampling.[49] In a study in Central Florida, US, six agricultural ponds were sampled for indicator organisms: total coliforms, enterococci, and generic *E. coli*, while also noting environmental factors including precipitation. Researchers did note an increased amount (4.3 MPN/100 mL) of total coliforms after rain; this did not amount to a statistically significant correlation between precipitation and bacterial population.[52] While precipitation has shown increases in bacterial populations, this cannot be assumed for all types of pathogens and water sources.

Giardia lamblia cysts and *Cryptosporidium* oocysts were sampled from the Delaware River in Trenton, New Jersey, United States; researchers were sampling within the scope of drinking water. However, this water source is used for agricultural water purposes.[107] Researchers noted a strong correlation between rainfall and the presence of *Giardia* cysts and *Cryptosporidium* oocysts. It is important to note during the sampling period that rainfall for this location was above average.[108] As for bacteria, these researchers suggest that the increased surface runoff resuspension within the water system leads to increased numbers of parasites during sampling.[108] In a Norwegian study researchers sampled surface water sources and groundwater for *E. coli*, *Giardia* cysts, and *Cryptosporidium* oocysts. Concentrations of *E. coli* increased in surface water after rainfall while there was no detection of *Giardia* cysts or *Cryptosporidium* oocysts when in dry seasons, but they detected oocysts and cysts after rainfall.[105] There was no detection of *E. coli*, *Giardia* cysts, or *Cryptosporidium* oocysts in the groundwater sources. The dry season during the sampling period included the driest May in a century. This study illustrates the difference between the presence of pathogens or indicators in water sources and the importance of risk evaluation.

The South Korean researchers who detected viruses in groundwater noted that there was no temperature effect on the presence of enteric viruses; yet there was a significance between temperature and detection of bacterial indicator organisms.[93] A temperature effect was seen when researchers in Spain sampled surface water, reclaimed water subjected to secondary treatment, and reclaimed water subjected to tertiary treatment for NoV genogroup I (GI), NoV genogroup II (GII), and HAV. Higher temperature was associated with higher prevalence of NoV GI and NoV GII, although the NoV GII viruses experienced this effect when the temperature was between 7°C and 8°C or 9°C and 10°C compared to 11°C–12°C. There were not enough samples with HAV detected for a temperature effect to be determined.[109]

26.3.3.2 Temporal variations

Temporal variations in pathogen prevalence in water samples depending on the time of day of sampling have been described. Some studies have indicated that within their sampling scheme, there is a diurnal effect. The inactivation rate of indicator microorganisms was reported greater under sunlight exposure than in the darkness in estuary and irrigation pond water.[110,111] In the Southwestern United States, researchers took 802 samples of irrigation canal water at the same location at four different times throughout the day: before 0900, between 0900 and 1200, between 1200 and 1300, and after 1300 h. *E. coli* and total coliforms were enumerated from these samples. There was a statistically significant difference between morning sampling times and afternoon sampling times leading researchers to suggest water samples be taken before 1200 h. This was demonstrated by a statistically significant difference between *E. coli* collected between 0700 and 1200 h compared to those collected between

1200 and 1600 h with geometric means of 24.8 ± 164 MPN/100 mL for the morning compared to the afternoon of 15.4 ± 117 MPN/100 mL; however, there was no relationship between sampling time and total coliform populations. Researchers also noted that their region had high levels of UV which could contribute to bacterial death as the day went on.[104] In Canada, samples were taken every 15 min over 24 h from three streams; *E. coli* was enumerated from these samples. Researchers noted that there was variability in population numbers throughout the day but did not suggest sampling at any specific times.[112]

26.3.3.3 Spatial variations

The spatial distribution of pathogens within a system is varied dependent upon the type of system and the surrounding environment. A higher occurrence of pathogens would exist at the point of contamination, for example near a location in a pond where runoff occurred.[49] For researchers who were determined to find the best location to sample from an irrigation canal in Arizona, United States, they found that *E. coli* was distributed evenly in the various locations they sampled. They noted that in other studies point-source contamination could occur, but that bacteria distributed themselves similarly to what they found.[104] The impact of water source elevation on fecal coliform populations was characterized by Maeys and others in British Columbia, Canada, in rivers. They demonstrated that higher elevation sites contained lower amounts of fecal coliforms, with mid-range elevation sites containing the highest levels of fecal coliforms.[113] The surrounding land use at these locations was noted as an important factor; these authors also noted that sampling could be influenced by the flow and geographic location of pool sites where bacteria may flow out of the system before sampling can occur.[112]

The relationship between indicator organisms, agricultural water, and the environment is not a one-size-fits-all situation as seen by some of the differing results presented. Correlation with microbiological indicator and environmental factors can vary depending on sampling frequency, sites, and time.[60,114,115] It is important to note that pathogens have been detected in agricultural water systems in various regions and that there are a multitude of factors contributing to their presence and persistence.

26.4 Fate of foodborne pathogens in agricultural waters

There are several potential risks associated with using microbiologically compromised water for produce irrigation. The capability of pathogens to survive in the environment and on produce is an essential determinant for the risk of human illness. After introduction to water sources, pathogens can survive for prolonged times in agricultural water sources and may result in contaminated product.[86,116] Data on the fate, survival, and transport of pathogenic and indicator microorganisms is highly relevant for areas where the microbial quality of irrigation water is critical. The contamination of agricultural surface water sources may be affected due to runoff water, weather events, time of day (solar radiation), precipitation, animal activities, turbidity, and other environmental factors.[52,53] Examples can be expanded as direct fecal matter from domesticated animals or wildlife, runoff from lands that have manure applied or stored, overflow from drainage fields, or discharge from faulty sewer lines. The interaction of water with bottom sediment and bank soils, periphyton, and algae can affect the microbial concentration of water during storage and transport through canals or irrigation ditches. Irrigation water distribution systems can also impact the microbial quality of water. For example, biofilm formation within irrigation pipes and subsequent interaction with water during transport will lead to the degradation of microbial quality of the irrigation water used in the field. It is important to consider all inputs and variables of irrigation water sources and distribution systems to better understand the potential risks of transporting contamination (Fig. 26.1).

26.4.1 Foodborne pathogens survival in water

The ability of bacteria, viruses, and parasites to survive in irrigation water sources is dependent on several factors such as temperature, sunlight (UV radiation), available nutrients, pH, or indigenous biota. Inactivation patterns differ between surface water and groundwater and between pathogen types, serotypes, and strains. The general rate of decay of microbial populations in the environment is demonstrated in the following equation (derived from Cho and coworkers[117,118]):

$$N_t/N_0 = 10^{-kt} \tag{26.1}$$

N_t = number of bacteria at time t
N_0 = number of bacteria at time 0 (initial)
t = time in days
k = die-off rate constant (day)

Eq. (26.1) illustrates microbial decay following first-order kinetics as initially suggested by Chick[119]; however, it does not account for the effects of temperature and other parameters on the decay constant (k). To account for temperature, an Arrhenius-type equation [Eq. (26.2)] is used (derived from Pachepsky and coworkers[49,118,120]).

$$k = k_{20}\Theta^{T-20} \tag{26.2}$$

k = die-off rate constant (day)
k_{20} = die-off rate at 20°C

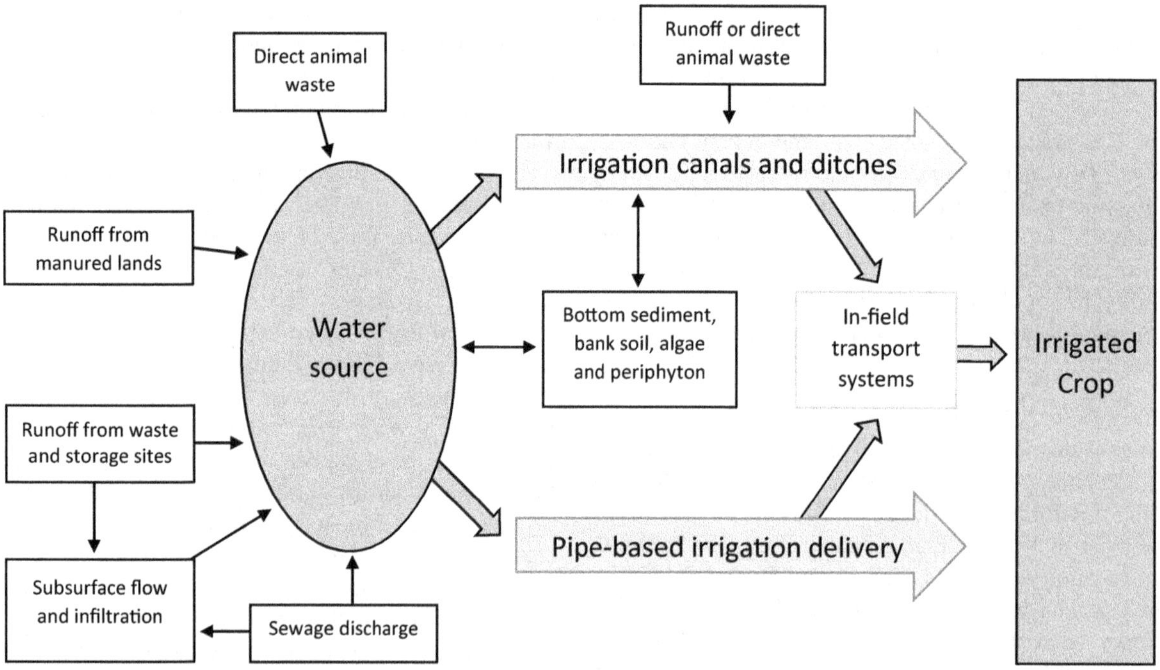

FIGURE 26.1 Overview of processes and factors affecting the microbial quality of irrigation water (modified from Pachepsky and coworkers[49]).

T = temperature (°C)
Θ = Temperature correction factor

Using Eqs. (26.1) and (26.2) or other derivatives, researchers have estimated the inactivation rates for indicator and pathogenic microorganisms in different environmental conditions. Although Eqs. (26.1) and (26.2) suggest die-off rates following first-order kinetics, this should not always be assumed.[120,121] Commonly, the decay rate of fecal microorganisms will shift during the process indicating biphasic decay.[120,122,123] Several inactivation curves have been observed for various fecal-derived microorganisms with created uncertainty in fate and transport models in watersheds.[121] Recent legislative activity in the United States, PSR under FSMA, has encouraged modeling as part of water management programs.[75] Further development of fate and transport models for watersheds that incorporate environmental parameters and scenarios may potentially help determine if these standards can be met in different management and environmental conditions.[117] An overview of current fate and transport models for watersheds is found in Cho et al.[117]

While there are common factors that contribute to the die-off and survival of indicator and pathogenic microorganisms, the effect of these factors may vary considerably depending on the type of microorganism or other environmental conditions.[121] It is important to note that both viruses and parasites are unable to replicate outside of a host, but bacteria are capable of growth and replication outside of a host given the right conditions. However, viruses and parasites are known to be more tolerant to environmental extremes and therefore have a generally lower die-off rate and increased survival expectancy in the environment compared to bacteria.[124,125]

In relation to the microbial quality of irrigation sources, certain types of microorganisms are more prevalent and are the focal point of related research. *E. coli* O157:H7 is frequently associated with water-related outbreaks. The presence of total coliforms in water has long been used to infer fecal contamination.[126] Within the coliform group, *E. coli* has shown to be an even more specific indicator of fecal contamination.[127] Generic *E. coli* and coliforms are used to set microbial quality testing thresholds for food safety irrigation water standards and regulations around the world.[2] Common viruses that can be transmitted through water include, but are not limited to, NoV, RVs, poliovirus, and Hepatitis A.[128] Several parasites including *Cryptosporidium* and *Giardia*[129] are often transmitted through water, causing waterborne and foodborne outbreaks. An extended list of bacteria, viruses, and parasites that can be transmitted by water is found in Yates.[130]

26.4.1.1 Temperature

Temperature is an important environmental factor that can influence survival of bacteria, viruses, and parasites. Generally, the survival of microorganisms increases as the temperature decreases, although the extent may depend on microorganism type or other environmental variables. Studies have demonstrated an increased microbial decay constant, k (day^{-1}), at higher temperatures (23°C–30°C) compared to lower temperatures (4°C–9°C) in various surface waters for coliforms,[131] generic *E. coli*,[116,131,132] *E. coli* O157:H7,[116,131,133,134] *Salmonella*,[132,133,135] and *Enterococcus*.[131,132] Conversely, Cho et al.[136] observed a positive correlation of coliform and *E. coli* survival and increased temperatures (25°C–30°C) in surface water which suggests seasonal variability and potential bacterial regrowth under warmer conditions.[136] Increased decay rates at higher temperatures have also been observed in surface and groundwaters for viruses[121,133,137] and parasites.[138]

26.4.1.2 Sunlight (UV radiation)

The full effect of sunlight (UV radiation) on microbial populations in water sources is difficult to determine as direct sunlight is often associated with higher temperatures. However, Whitman et al.[139] observed increased generic *E. coli* levels in freshwater as cloud cover increased, thereby decreasing sunlight. Nguyen et al.[140] observed higher inactivation rates of *E. coli* and *Enterococcus* in open-water wetlands compared to the vegetative wetlands, thought to be because of higher exposure to sunlight. This effect has also been observed for virus and parasite inactivation in marine water and freshwater.[141,142]

26.4.1.3 Nutrients

Although adding nutrients to water may aid microorganism survival, it has not always shown to be a strong predictor of occurrence in surface water.[143] Surface water samples exposed to liquid discharges in cattle feedlots tend to have more STEC positive in runoff from corrals' nonexposed surface waters.[144] Tanaro et al.[145] observed that the addition of dairy cattle manure containing carbon, nitrogen, and phosphorus to water lead to an initial spike in the concentration of coliforms; however, the die-off rates measured prenutrient addition, were restored after the initial growth occurred. *E. coli* O157:H7 has been shown to die out over time in carbon-limited environments,[146] but is also known to survive in low nutrient environments as it exhibits a high degree of catabolic flexibility.[147] In groundwater, both *E. coli* and viruses have been shown to have a decreased decay rate in the absence of protein- or carbon-based nutrients.[148]

26.4.1.4 pH

The pH level of water may also influence microorganism survival, as the die-off rate of fecal indicator organisms in surface water has been shown to decrease significantly when below pH 6 or above pH 8.[117] Similarly, McFeters and Stuart[149] observed a greatly reduced *E. coli* survival when water pH was below 5.5 or above 8. Overall, the idea that pH effect on bacterial inactivation is lowest at pH levels between 6 and 8 is supported.[49,121,150]

26.4.1.5 Water source

The source of water often plays a key role in initial microbial quality and variability in decay rate. Since surface water is exposed to the environment, it is more likely exposed to UV radiation, temperature, and other environmental conditions when compared to groundwater. Surface water is also more susceptible to direct contact with contaminants (e.g., manure). This infers that groundwater should be of better microbial quality than surface water, however, groundwater can still become contaminated if located close to a contamination source or due to inadequate well quality.[56] An overview of research related to different water sources, including groundwater, lakes, and rivers is found in Pandey et al.[151]

26.4.1.6 Environmental reservoirs—bottom sediments and bank soils

Different microorganism reservoirs such as bottom sediments, bank soils, or aquatic biota are often present in irrigation water sources and affect microbial water quality. Sediments have increasingly been recognized as reservoirs of indicator and pathogenic microorganisms in freshwater[49,144] and *E. coli* O157:H7 has been isolated from sediment during the investigation of recent produce outbreaks.[152] The United States Food and Drug Administration (USFDA)[153] demonstrated the ability of *E. coli* to survive and grow in streambed sediments. Rainfall or other events can cause sediment movement and resuspension and increase microorganism levels in the water. The concentration of *E. coli* in stream water was shown to increase by two orders of magnitude after artificial flooding events.[154] Spatial variability of *E. coli* concentrations is known to be high in sediments[49] and areas of high concentrations (hot spots) can affect nearby or downstream zones during sediment resuspension.[155] These hot spots increase the unpredictability of *E. coli* concentrations during sampling and present a challenge for fate and transport models.[155] Viruses can also be found in sediments, however, they may be more prevalent in water and top sediments rather than bottom sediments.[156]

Bank soils are another microorganism reservoir that can affect microbial quality of water. Populations of *E. coli* in soils usually decrease as the distance from the water's edge increases.[157,158] Although this suggests that a higher water content of soils could help the survival of *E. coli*, studies have shown that upon soil drying, *E. coli* can survive and even multiply.[158,159] Furthermore, *E. coli* populations in soils have been shown to move downslope towards rivers due to erosion or runoff events.[160] Soils and sediments are likely to directly impact the microbial quality of irrigation water transported via canals and ditches and can potentially affect other water sources depending on storage conditions.

26.4.1.7 Aquatic biota

Naturally occurring biota (e.g., algae, amoebae) found in aquatic ecosystems can also be beneficial to the survival and growth of pathogens and indicator organisms as they can act as a reservoir for these microorganisms. Bacterial pathogens such as STEC, *Salmonella*, *Shigella*, and *Campylobacter* have been found to be associated with green algae growing in lake water.[161] Thomas et al.[162] also suggest that free-living amoebae benefit the growth of bacteria such as *L. monocytogenes* and *Vibrio cholerae* and also certain viruses. Although these aquatic biota have been shown to facilitate pathogen survival, little is known in regard to their role as a reservoir in irrigation systems.[49]

26.4.2 Foodborne pathogen survival in water distribution systems

26.4.2.1 Biofilms

The formation of biofilms in water distribution systems is a well-known phenomenon. Biofilms are a complex mixture of microbes, organic, and inorganic matter that accumulate amidst a microbially produced organic polymer matrix attached to the inner surface of these distribution systems.[163] Biofilms act as microbial reservoir which may significantly impact the microbial quality of water during transport through water distribution systems. Microorganisms that accumulate in biofilms may be shed into the water column as water passes through.

Biofilms are known to form on a variety of surfaces such as metal, glass, rubber, plastic, and wood. The adhesion of biofilms to surfaces is also dependent on other physicochemical properties such as texture (smooth or rough), surface charge, hydrophobicity, temperature, pH, or composition of preconditioning solution.[164,165] Generally, surfaces that are rough, porous, or absorbent present a suitable environment for biofilm formation as they may entrap organic material and microorganisms. Biofilms have also been shown to form on a wide variety of produce surfaces.[166]

Any pathogen or indicator organism present in water may attach or become enmeshed in a biofilm. Survival time within a biofilm will vary depending on the organism and environmental conditions. Although certain pathogens may not be suited to grow in an irrigation water distribution system environment, they may accumulate in a biofilm and have extended survival.[163] Once biofilms have formed on a surface, they are difficult to remove and are much more resistant to cleaning, sanitizing, and environmental stressors than single-cell organisms.[166,167]

26.4.2.2 Effect of biofilms in pipe-based irrigation systems

Although biofilm formation in drinking water distribution systems has been widely studied, research on the role of biofilms in irrigation water distribution systems has been limited.[168] These systems all share common basic features, but they may differ by the initial water source (i.e., surface water, groundwater) and the various irrigation methods (i.e., sprinkler, drip, micro jet, subirrigation). Furthermore, the length and complexity of the piping systems that connect source water to irrigation point will vary extensively between different systems. Irrigation water distribution systems are also more exposed and susceptible to environmental factors. All of these components make it difficult to fully understand the role of biofilms in these systems and extent to which downstream water used for fresh produce application may be affected (i.e., inadequate microbial quality).

Some recent research has studied biofilms within irrigation water distribution systems. Pachepsky et al.[169] evaluated the effect of biofilms formed in irrigation pipes on microbial quality of irrigation water by measuring *E. coli* levels at the source (creek water) and at the end (sprinklers) over a 4-week period. Results indicated significant differences in *E. coli* levels of incoming water and sprinkler water; however, the dynamics were different for each irrigation event (four total) and over time during the 2-h irrigation events. Initially, *E. coli* levels of incoming water were measured much higher than sprinkler water and this difference increased over time whereas later events measured higher in the sprinkler water compared to incoming water, and this difference decreased over time. These results suggest that initially *E. coli* was being released from the water to the pipe surface and in later irrigation events *E. coli* was released from biofilms into the water passing through.[169] Other research[170] investigated the genetic make-up of biofilms formed over time in drip irrigation systems using reclaimed water and treated wastewater. The results suggest that microbial communities able to grow at high temperatures (i.e., thermophilic bacteria) were more likely to be sourced from the incoming water into the biofilms forming.[170]

Further research on biofilms in irrigation water distribution systems is warranted but does present challenges. These complex systems are close-ended which can make it difficult to obtain relevant samples. Sampling may often require the removal and disruption of the distribution system infrastructure, which is difficult if the system is still actively in use. Also, since biofilms are composed of several different organisms, it is sometimes difficult to quantify the level of embedded pathogens and measure their impact on downstream water. However, this research is vital to better help the produce industry understand biofilm management and reduce the risk of fresh produce being contaminated from this source. Yuan and Oliver[168] provide a further overview of current research and offer potential considerations for future research related to this topic.

26.4.3 Foodborne pathogen fate during and after application to produce crops

Pathogens that survive transport through a distribution system present a contamination risk during and after the application of irrigation water that contacts fresh produce. It is important to understand the potential of postirrigation pathogen survival so that appropriate and adequate mitigation techniques may be implemented into the process.

Several studies have investigated the survival of *E. coli* O157,[171–174] *Salmonella*,[174] *L. monocytogenes*,[175] nonpathogenic *E. coli*,[176] or *Listeria innocua*[123,177] on the surface of lettuce or spinach as a result of contaminated irrigation water. Overall, it is evident that these microorgansims can survive on the surface of leafy greens for an extended period postirrigation treatment; however, the extent of the contamination and length of survival vary significantly depending on environmental conditions and irrigation method.[23] As mentioned above, the decay rate of fecal microorganisms shifts during their time on the surface of produce crops to a biphasic decay. Other studies evaluated the ability of *E. coli* O157:H7 to internalize into the leaf of the plant after treatment with contaminated irrigation water at the root[178] or the leaves directly.[171] There is evidence that this phenomenon can occur, however, this was only observed when the contaminated irrigation water was inoculated at very high levels (≥7 log CFU/mL) and not under field conditions.

Other commodities besides leafy greens may also become contaminated from irrigation water.[23] Islam et al.[179] demonstrated that *E. coli* O157:H7 applied through irrigation water could survive for an extended period on onions (74 days) and carrots (168 days). Regardless of the commodity, anytime irrigation water is applied to fresh produce in a manner likely to have direct contact with the edible portion of the crop, the microbial quality of the water is very important.

26.5 Agricultural water management and mitigations

Agricultural water has been implicated as the source of pathogen contamination causing foodborne outbreaks. Transfer of pathogens to the harvested portion of produce is unavoidable in case of direct contact with contaminated water. Various standards, control and management strategies, and corrective measures are recommended for agricultural water sources to enhance produce safety with legal regulations.

26.5.1 Management and testing

Monitoring of microbiological water quality is considered an essential measure for the assessment of potential contamination risk of produce in the preharvest farming environment. Various standards are required by different local and international organizations, guidelines, and agencies, as discussed above. The absence of universally accepted water quality management practices is not surprising due to lack of scientific consensus around the parameters. In general, different criteria on the population of generic *E. coli* in 100 mL water sample are set to assess the risk of pathogen contamination.[75,180–182] For agricultural water sources, some recommended microbiological water quality standards and criteria have been adopted from guidelines for drinking, environmental and recreational waters. Besides general agreement about the use of generic *E. coli* as indicator in waters, recommended maximum concentration of indicator microorganisms is not standardized. Parameters including number of samples, time of sampling, and accepted test methodologies, are not standardized and vary significantly. Insufficient standards and metrics by authorities and the absence of a rigorous sampling program may limit the success of effective monitoring.[53,54] The economic burden of frequent water sampling is not acceptable for growers due to high costs.

Appropriate risk management measures may vary according to type of crop. Limited agreement about the fate, presence, transfer, and survival of pathogens in agricultural water and on produce after irrigation makes it difficult to have conclusive recommendations to enhance agricultural water quality.[182] Recent guidelines for management of agricultural water quality require various standards for waters touching the edible part of produce, fruits, and vegetables. For example, "no detectable generic *E. coli* in 100 mL of agricultural water" is applied to sprouts by the USFDA.[75] Surface waters applied by sprinkle and overhead irrigation to crops represents an important and largely uncontrolled risk to fresh produce food safety. The use of agricultural water for diverse foliar applications increases the risk of contamination. Unfortunately, management techniques must be site specific if they are to be effective at all. Relying more on mitigation through the application of controls or water treatments, when there is an inherent risk of a water supply or product, is deemed unacceptable otherwise.

Preharvest and postharvest water quality management practices are early in their development and continue to evolve.

26.5.2 Control and water treatment

Understanding the characteristics of the individual water source is important to implement water quality intervention strategies for produce safety. In general, the availability of natural water sources and the presence of distribution canals are the primary reason for the choice of water sources by growers for agricultural purposes. Unless it is contaminated with runoff or wastewater, groundwater typically maintains good quality. The microbiological quality of groundwater is generally expected to be high and meet any microbiological requirements for agricultural water, however, pathogens can be introduced directly to the groundwater via the well opening. More than 50% of the waterborne illnesses in the United States are caused by the consumption of contaminated groundwater via septic tanks, landfills and artificial recharge of groundwater, and treated sewage effluent from irrigated crops.[183] Conversely, reclaimed waters may contain high salts, heavy metals, and pathogens and other high-risk chemicals for health and may negatively impact the safety of produce.[184] To reduce the risk of pathogen transmission to produce, preventative strategies and mitigation measures can be used for agricultural water sources.[185] These strategies and measures aim to prevent contamination of water sources and to treat contaminated water for minimization of pathogen transfer to produce.

To minimize contamination of produce, the possibility of pathogen transfer into water sources should be considered in the first place. The most effective approach to minimize produce contamination in the field is the prevention of agricultural water sources from potential contamination sources. Several preventive strategies can be applied depending on water source, type of crop, and type of irrigation. Agricultural water sources should be conserved from potential sources of contamination with preventive methods such as fencing, sediment basins, hedgerows, runoff protection, grass waterways, and filter strips.[186] The type of irrigation can affect the transfer of pathogens onto produce sourced from agricultural water. Enhanced risk of *E. coli* contamination of produce has been reported for sprinkle and furrow irrigation compared to subsurface drip irrigation.[176,187] It is important that growers use irrigation methods that minimize contact between produce and contaminated agricultural waters. There are other preventive strategies for agricultural water including concurrent use of irrigation and break time between final irrigation and harvesting.[49] The risk of contamination due to increased microbiological populations in agricultural water sources after rain can be reduced by changing time of irrigation and/or having a gap between harvest and last irrigation.[185] Several waiting periods between last irrigation and harvest have been suggested for different microorganisms and field conditions however, no conclusive and certain time interval has been reached.

Pathogens can be transferred to agricultural waters from contamination sources developed in irrigation systems. Maintenance of irrigation systems should be performed regularly to reduce the formation of biofilms in water distribution systems. Animals should be deterred from water sources as much as possible since they are natural reservoirs of pathogens. As the USFDA pointed out in a report on a 2019 outbreak investigation linked to leafy greens in the Western United States, water source can be protected from contamination adjacent to cattle grazing lands by increasing the buffer zone, and adding physical barriers such as berms, diversion ditches, and vegetative strips.[188]

The risk of produce contamination with pathogens can be reduced in agricultural waters through several mitigation measures. Treatment of water is another alternative strategy to reduce pathogen populations. Removal of suspended material, filtration of water, waste stabilization ponds, oxidation reduction, electrolysis, UV treatment and solar-driven disinfection, chlorination, ozonation, ultrasound, and heat treatment are some potential techniques.[49,185,189] All these mitigation strategies have advantages and drawbacks in applying water from different water sources with various microbial loads and characteristics and cannot be realistically applied to all water used during produce production worldwide.

26.5.3 Corrective actions and measures (before and after using water)

Despite the inevitable spatial and temporal fluctuations of indicator microorganism populations, especially in surface waters that are open to unstable environmental factors affecting agricultural water quality, a risk-based approach can be used to minimize risks associated with agricultural water use. Depending on microbiological limits defined in guidelines or regulations, different options are proposed to ensure produce safety while supplying enough fresh fruits and vegetables to markets. For example, in the US FDA PSR, growers can still continue using their water sources even if water quality requirements are not met as per the required quality standards. If growers cannot find alternative water sources within required water quality standards, there are options for the water exceeding these numbers in the PSR[75]:

1. Preharvest interval: Application of time interval as days between last irrigation and harvest to reduce the generic *E. coli* populations to meet the required

microbiological quality requirements by assuming a die-off rate of 0.5 log per day. The final rule allows a maximum interval of four days preharvest (2 log reduction).
2. Harvest and storage interval: Application of time interval as days between harvest and storage or microbial removal rates during treatments (i.e., commercial washing) to reduce generic *E. coli* populations to meet the required microbiological quality requirements with supported data as a peer-reviewed paper.
3. Re-inspect the water system, identify problems, make necessary changes, and confirm effectiveness.
4. Treatment of water.

Defining corrective actions that give produce growers an option to continue using the water but still reducing risk is necessary in cases where agricultural water quality may change, but sustainability and food security must be maintained.

Development of an ultimate decision tree to ensure the use of safe agricultural water for growers from all regions and countries is not possible due to lack of universal water quality standards and limited knowledge of possible contamination risks for specific sites.[182] Risk assessment should be done based on parameters including type of crop, type of irrigation, foliar or nonfoliar use. Fig. 26.2 shows a generalized scheme for growers to use agricultural water that is safe. If water quality does not meet the standards, preventive strategies, and valid intervention measures, such as chemical treatments can be performed with a supportive risk assessment. Corrective actions should be taken after preventive measures to decrease risk of contamination.

26.6 Conclusions/future needs

The quality of agricultural waters used during produce production is known to play a role in the safety of fresh fruits and vegetables. Microbiological hazards, including foodborne bacterial, parasitic, and viral pathogens, are regularly found in agricultural waters in a wide variety of regions when surveys are performed. Differences between volume of sampled water and testing methodologies make direct comparisons challenging between reported pathogen prevalences. The interplay of pathogen presence and environmental aspects of both the location of water sources and the surrounding water environment on pathogen levels should be explored further. The presence of microbiological hazards in agricultural water does not necessarily indicate a risk with its use during produce production. Agricultural water is used in many ways while growing, harvesting, and packing fresh fruits and vegetables. When assessing the risk associated with agricultural waters, the way the water is applied to the crop and the time of the water application are critical variables; however, much remains to be discovered about the impact of each variable in different production environments. No "one single fit for purpose standard" for the microbiological quality of water to assure produce safety is currently agreed upon. Instead, site-specific analysis for specific crop, pathogen, irrigation system, water source, and management are used; there is potential for QMRA in this area.

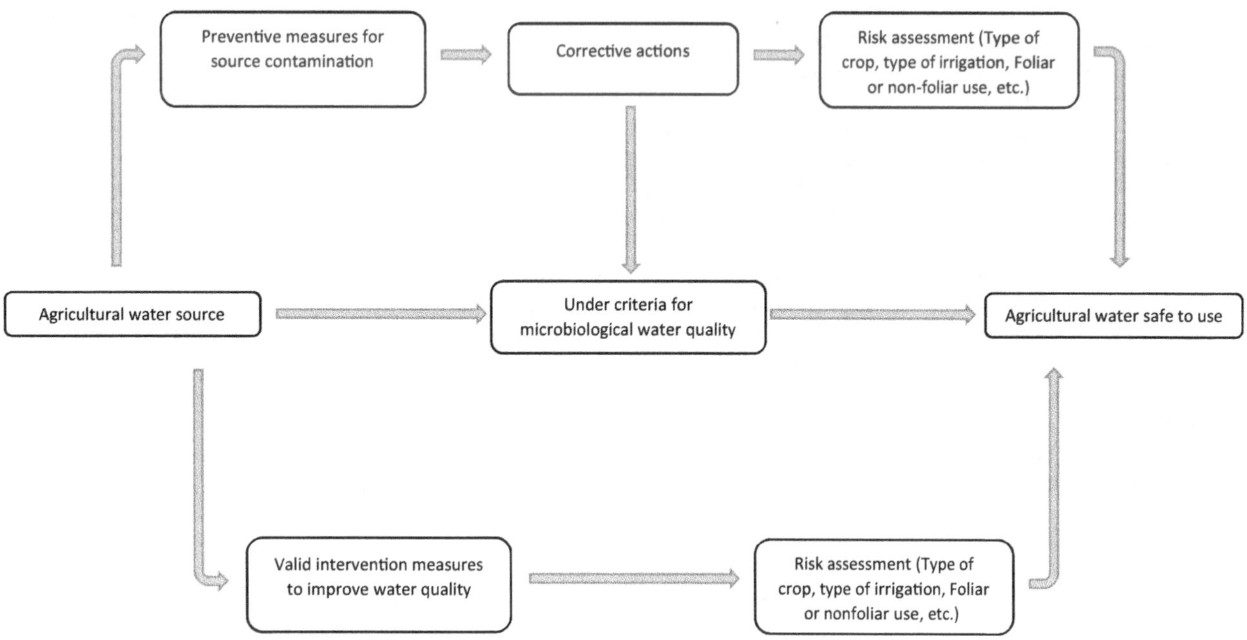

FIGURE 26.2 A generalized scheme for growers to use agricultural water that is safe to use.

References

1. León JS, Jaykus LA, Moe CL. Food safety issues and the microbiology of fruits and vegetables. *Microbiol Safe Foods*. 2009;255–281.
2. Uyttendaele M, Jaykus LA, Amoah P, et al. microbial hazards in irrigation water: standards, norms, and testing to manage use of water in fresh produce primary production. *Compr Rev Food Sci Food Saf*. 2015;14:336–356.
3. Johnson R. *The US Trade Situation for Fruit and Vegetable Products*:7–5700. 2014 <https://fas.org/sgp/crs/misc/RL34468.pdf> Accessed 10.10.18.
4. Parr B, Bond JK, Minor T. *U.S. Department of Agriculture, Economic Research Service: Falling Exports More Than Offset Production Declines to Raise Per Capita Availability*; 2018. <https://www.ers.usda.gov/webdocs/publications/88712/vgs-360.pdf?v = 0>.
5. DeWaal CS, Glassman M. *Outbreak Alert 2001–2010*; 2013. <https://cspinet.org/sites/default/files/attachment/outbreak_alert_2013_final.pdf>.
6. Fischer N, Bourne A, Plunkett D. *Outbreak Alert! 2015*; 2015. <https://cspinet.org/sites/default/files/attachment/outbreak-alert-2015.pdf>.
7. Callejon RM, Rodriguez-Naranjo MI, Ubeda C, Hornedo-Ortega R, Garcia-Parrilla MC, Troncoso AM. Reported foodborne outbreaks due to fresh produce in the United States and European Union: trends and causes. *Foodborne Pathog Dis*. 2015;12:32–38.
8. Centers for Disease Control and Prevention (CDC). Multistate outbreak of *E. coli* O157:H7 infections linked to romaine lettuce. 2018 <https://www.cdc.gov/ecoli/2018/o157h7-04-18/index.html>.
9. Centers for Disease Control and Prevention (CDC). Multistate outbreak of Shiga toxin-producing *Escherichia coli* O157:H7 infections linked to leafy greens. 2018. <https://www.cdc.gov/ecoli/2017/o157h7-12-17/index.html>.
10. Centers for Disease Control and Prevention (CDC). Multistate state outbreak by *E. coli* O157:H7 was linked to lettuce that was grown in the Yuma, Arizona region in 2018. 2018. <https://www.cdc.gov/ecoli/2018/o157h7-04-18/index.html>.
11. Centers for Disease Control and Prevention (CDC). National outbreak reporting system. 2018e. <https://wwwn.cdc.gov/norsdashboard/>.
12. Lewis HC, Kirk M, Ethelberg S, et al. Outbreaks of shigellosis in Denmark and Australia associated with imported baby corn, August 2007–final summary. *Euro Surveill*. 2007;12:E071004.2.
13. Jalava K, Hallanvuo S, Nakari UM, et al. Multiple outbreaks of *Yersinia pseudotuberculosis* infections in Finland. *J Clin Microbiol*. 2004;42:2789–2791.
14. Hjertqvist M, Johansson A, Svensson N, et al. Four outbreaks of norovirus gastroenteritis after consuming raspberries, Sweden, June-August 2006. *Eurosurveillance*. 2006;11:3038.
15. Le Guyader FS, Mittelholzer C, Haugarreau L, et al. Detection of noroviruses in raspberries associated with a gastroenteritis outbreak. *Int J Food Microbiol*. 2004;97:179–186.
16. Kirk M, Fullerton K, Gregory J. Fresh produce outbreaks in Australia 2001–2006. Board 21. In: *2008 International Conference on Emerging Infectious Diseases Program and Abstracts Book*. Atlanta, GA: Centers for Disease Control and Prevention; 2008:49–50.
17. Bennett SD, Sodha SV, Ayers TL, Lynch MF, Gould LH, Tauxe RV. Produce-associated foodborne disease outbreaks, USA, 1998-2013. *Epidemiol Infect*. 2018;146:1397–1406.
18. Beuchat LR. Pathogenic microorganisms associated with fresh produce. *J Food Prot*. 1996;59:204–216.
19. Hanning IB, Nutt J, Ricke SC. Salmonellosis outbreaks in the United States due to fresh produce: sources and potential intervention measures. *Foodborne Pathog Dis*. 2009;6:635–648.
20. Sivapalasingam S, Friedman CR, Cohen L, Tauxe RV. Fresh produce: a growing cause of outbreaks of foodborne illness in the United States, 1973 through 1997. *J Food Prot*. 2004;67:2342–2353.
21. Esseili MA, Gao X, Tegtmeier S, Saif LJ, Wang Q. Abiotic stress and phyllosphere bacteria influence the survival of human norovirus and its surrogates on preharvest leafy greens. *Appl Env Microbiol*. 2016;82:352–363.
22. Beuchat LR, Ryu JH. Produce handling and processing practices. *Emerg Infect Dis*. 1997;3:459–465.
23. Steele M, Odumeru J. Irrigation water as source of foodborne pathogens on fruit and vegetables. *J Food Prot*. 2004;67:2839–2849.
24. United States Food and Drug Administration (USFDA). Guide to minimize microbial food safety hazards for fresh fruits and vegetables. 1998 <https://www.fda.gov/media/117408/download> Accessed 10.05.21.
25. Centers for Disease Control and Prevention. Outbreaks of *Shigella sonnei* infection associated with eating fresh parsley–United States and Canada, July-August 1998. *MMWR Morb Mortal Wkly Rep*. 1999;48:285.
26. Sivapalasingam S, Barrett E, Kimura A, et al. A multistate outbreak of *Salmonella enterica* Serotype Newport infection linked to mango consumption: impact of water-dip disinfestation technology. *Clin Infect Dis*. 2003;37:1585–1590.
27. Döller PC, Dietrich K, Filipp N, et al. Cyclosporiasis outbreak in Germany associated with the consumption of salad. *Emerg Infect Dis*. 2002;8:992.
28. Gibbs R, Pingault N, Mazzucchelli T, et al. An outbreak of *Salmonella enterica* serotype Litchfield infection in Australia linked to consumption of contaminated papaya. *J Food Prot*. 2009;72:1094–1098.
29. Greene S, Daly E, Talbot E, et al. Recurrent multistate outbreak of *Salmonella* Newport associated with tomatoes from contaminated fields, 2005. *Epidemiol Infect*. 2008;136:157–165.
30. Nygård K, Lassen J, Vold L, et al. Outbreak of *Salmonella* Thompson infections linked to imported rucola lettuce. *Foodborne Pathog Dis*. 2008;5:165–173.
31. Sarvikivi E, Roivainen M, Maunula L, et al. Multiple norovirus outbreaks linked to imported frozen raspberries. *Epidemiol Infect*. 2012;140:260–267.
32. Gurtler JB, Harlee NA, Smelser AM, Schneider KR. *Salmonella enterica* contamination of market fresh tomatoes: a review. *J Food Prot*. 2018;81:1193–1213.
33. Gelting RJ, Baloch MA, Zarate-Bermudez MA, Selman C. Irrigation water issues potentially related to the 2006 multistate *E. coli* O157: H7 outbreak associated with spinach. *Agric Water Manag*. 2011;98:1395–1402.
34. Barton Behravesh C, Mody RK, Jungk J, et al. 2008 outbreak of *Salmonella* Saintpaul infections associated with raw produce. *N Engl J Med*. 2011;364:918–927.
35. Hoang L, Fyfe M, Ong C, et al. Outbreak of cyclosporiasis in British Columbia associated with imported Thai basil. *Epidemiol & Infect*. 2005;133:23–27.

36. Centers for Disease Control and Prevention (CDC). Multistate outbreak of *Salmonella* infections linked to Alfalfa sprouts from one contaminated seed lot (final update). 2016. <https://www.cdc.gov/salmonella/muenchen-02-16/index.html>.
37. Centers for Disease Control and Prevention (CDC). Outbreak of *E. coli* infections linked to romaine lettuce. 2018. <https://www.cdc.gov/ecoli/2018/o157h7-11-18/index.html>.
38. Cooley M, Carychao D, Crawford-Miksza L, et al. Incidence and tracking of *Escherichia coli* O157:H7 in a major produce production region in California. *PLoS One*. 2007;2:e1159.
39. Lynch MF, Tauxe RV, Hedberg CW. The growing burden of foodborne outbreaks due to contaminated fresh produce: risks and opportunities. *Epidemiol Infect*. 2009;137:307–315.
40. Centers for Disease Control and Prevention (CDC). Multistate outbreaks of *Salmonella* infections associated with raw tomatoes eaten in restaurants – United States, 2005–2006. *MMWR Morbidity Mortal Wkly Rep*. 2007;56(35):909–911.
41. Turner K, Moua CN, Hajmeer M, Barnes A, Needham M. Overview of Leafy Greens–Related Food Safety Incidents with a California Link: 1996 to 2016. *J Food Prot*. 2019;82:405–414.
42. Ibenyassine K, Mhand RA, Karamoko Y, Anajjar B, Chouibani M, Ennaji M. Bacterial pathogens recovered from vegetables irrigated by wastewater in Morocco. *J Environ Health*. 2007;69:47–51.
43. Minhas P, Sharma N, Yadav R, Joshi P. Prevalence and control of pathogenic contamination in some sewage irrigated vegetable, forage and cereal grain crops. *Bioresour Technol*. 2006;97:1174–1178.
44. Ndiaye ML, Niang S, Pfeifer HR, Peduzzi R, Tonolla M, Dieng Y. Effect of irrigation water and processing on the microbial quality of lettuces produced and sold on markets in Dakar (Senegal). *Irrig Drain*. 2011;60:509–517.
45. Melloul AA, Hassani L. *Salmonella* infection in children from the wastewater-spreading zone of Marrakesh city (Morocco). *J Appl Microbiol*. 1999;87:536–539.
46. Cordier JL. Microbiological criteria and indicator microorganisms. In: *Food Microbiology; Fundamentals and Frontiers*. 4th ed. 2012.
47. Mossel DA, Struijk CB. *Escherichia coli*, other *Enterobacteriaceae* and additional indicators as markers of microbiologic quality of food: advantages and limitations. *Microbiologia*. 1995;11(1):75–90.
48. Ashbolt NJ, Grabow WO, Snozzi M. 13 Indicators of microbial water quality; 2001. <https://www.who.int/water_sanitation_health/dwq/iwachap13.pdf>.
49. Pachepsky Y, Shelton DR, McLain JE, Patel J, Mandrell RE. Irrigation waters as a source of pathogenic microorganisms in produce: a review. *Advances in agronomy*. 113. Elsevier; 2011:75–141.
50. Stine SW, Song I, Choi CY, Gerba CP. Application of microbial risk assessment to the development of standards for enteric pathogens in water used to irrigate fresh produce. *J Food Prot*. 2005;68:913–918.
51. Antaki EM, Vellidis G, Harris C, Aminabadi P, Levy K, Jay-Russell MT. Low concentration of *Salmonella enterica* and generic *Escherichia coli* in farm ponds and irrigation distribution systems used for mixed produce production in Southern Georgia. *Foodborne Pathog Dis*. 2016;13:551–558.
52. Topalcengiz Z, Strawn LK, Danyluk MD. Microbial quality of agricultural water in Central Florida. *PLoS One*. 2017;12:1–18.
53. Havelaar AH, Vazquez KM, Topalcengiz Z, Muñoz-Carpena R, Danyluk MD. Evaluating the U.S. food safety modernization act produce safety rule standard for microbial quality of agricultural water for growing produce. *J Food Prot*. 2017;80:1832–1841.
54. Pachepsky Y, Kierzewski R, Stocker M, et al. Temporal stability of *Escherichia coli* concentrations in waters of two irrigation ponds in Maryland. *Appl Env Microbiol*. 2018;84(3):e01876–17.
55. Abimbola OP, Mittelstet AR, Messer TL, Berry ED, Bartelt-Hunt SL, Hansen SP. Predicting *Escherichia coli* loads in cascading dams with machine learning: an integration of hydrometeorology, animal density and grazing pattern. *Sci Total Env*. 2020;722:137894.
56. Benjamin L, Atwill ER, Jay-Russell M, et al. Occurrence of generic *Escherichia coli*, *E. coli* O157 and *Salmonella* spp. in water and sediment from leafy green produce farms and streams on the Central California coast. *Int J Food Microbiol*. 2013;165(1):65–76.
57. Bradshaw JK, Snyder BJ, Oladeinde A, et al. Characterizing relationships among fecal indicator bacteria, microbial source tracking markers, and associated waterborne pathogen occurrence in stream water and sediments in a mixed land use watershed. *Water Res*. 2016;101:498–509.
58. Buyrukoğlu G, Buyrukoğlu S, Topalcengiz Z. Comparing regression models with count data to artificial neural network and ensemble models for prediction of generic *Escherichia coli* population in agricultural ponds based on weather station measurements. *Microb risk Anal*. 2021;19:100171.
59. Buyrukoğlu S. New hybrid data mining model for prediction of *Salmonella* presence in agricultural waters based on ensemble feature selection and machine learning algorithms. *J Food Saf*. 2021;2021:e12903.
60. McEgan R, Mootian G, Goodridge LD, Schaffner DW, Danyluk MD. Predicting *Salmonella* populations from biological, chemical, and physical indicators in Florida surface waters. *Appl Env Microbiol*. 2013;79:4094–4105.
61. Park Y, Kim M, Pachepsky Y, et al. Development of a nowcasting system using machine learning approaches to predict fecal contamination levels at recreational beaches in Korea. *J Env Qual*. 2018;47(5):1094–1102.
62. Polat H, Topalcengiz Z, Danyluk MD. Prediction of *Salmonella* presence and absence in agricultural surface waters by artificial intelligence approaches. *J Food Saf*. 2020;40:e12733.
63. Truchado P, Hernandez N, Gil MI, Ivanek R, Allende A. Correlation between *E. coli* levels and the presence of foodborne pathogens in surface irrigation water: establishment of a sampling program. *Water Res*. 2018;128:226–233.
64. Truitt LN, Vazquez KM, Pfuntner RC, Rideout SL, Havelaar AH, Strawn LK. Microbial quality of agricultural water used in produce preharvest production on the eastern shore of Virginia. *J Food Prot*. 2018;81(1):1661–1672.
65. Vereen Jr. E, Lowrance RR, Jenkins MB, Adams P, Rajeev S, Lipp EK. Landscape and seasonal factors influence *Salmonella* and *Campylobacter* prevalence in a rural mixed use watershed. *Water Res*. 2013;47(16):6075–6085.
66. Weller D, Brassill N, Rock C, et al. Complex interactions between weather, and microbial and physicochemical water quality impact the likelihood of detecting foodborne pathogens in agricultural water. *Front Microbiol*. 2020;11:134.

67. Weller DL, Love TMT, Belias A, Wiedmann M. Predictive models may complement or provide an alternative to existing strategies for managing enteric pathogen contamination of Northeastern streams used for produce production. *Front Sustain Food Syst.* 2020;4:561517.
68. Wu J, Long SC, Das D, Dorner SM. Are microbial indicators and pathogens correlated? A statistical analysis of 40 years of research. *J Water Health.* 2011;9(2):265–278.
69. Söderström A, Österberg P, Lindqvist A, et al. A large *Escherichia coli* O157 outbreak in Sweden associated with locally produced lettuce. *Foodborne Pathog Dis.* 2008;5:339–349.
70. Suslow T, Oria M, Beuchat L, et al. Production practices as risk factors in microbial food safety of fresh and fresh-cut produce. *Compr Rev Food Sci Food Saf.* 2003;2:38–77.
71. Leifert C, Ball K, Volakakis N, Cooper J. Control of enteric pathogens in ready-to-eat vegetable crops in organic and 'low input' production systems: a HACCP-based approach. *J Appl Microbiology.* 2008;105:931–950.
72. Martin F, Bootsma A, Coote D, et al. Canada's rural water resources. In: Coote DR, Gregorich LJ, eds. 2000.
73. Williamson DA. *Manitoba Water Quality Standards, Objectives, and Guidelines.* Water Quality Management Section, Manitoba Conservation; 2000.
74. Blumenthal UJ, Mara DD, Peasey A, Ruiz-Palacios G, Stott R. Guidelines for the microbiological quality of treated wastewater used in agriculture: recommendations for revising WHO guidelines. *Bull World Health Organ.* 2000;78:1104–1116.
75. United States Food and Drug Administration (USFDA). Federal register notice: standards for the growing, harvesting, packing, and holding of produce for human consumption; final rule. 2015 <https://www.gpo.gov/fdsys/pkg/FR-2015-11-27/pdf/2015-28159.pdf> Accessed 17.12.18.
76. Buchanan RL, Whiting RC. Concepts in predictive microbiology. In: Proceedings of the *Fiftieth Annual Reciprocal Meat Conference*, Champaign, IL; 1997.
77. Codex-Alimentarius-Commission. *Principles and Guidelines for the Conduct of Microbiological Risk Assessment. CAC/GL-30*; 1999.
78. Haas CN, Rose JB, Gerba CP. *Quantitative Microbial Risk Assessment.* John Wiley & Sons; 1999.
79. O'Toole J, Sinclair M, Leder K. Quantitative microbial risk assessment and Australian Guidelines for Water Recycling: two case studies. *Food Aust.* 2010;62:408–412.
80. Ottoson JR, Nyberg K, Lindqvist R, Albihn A. Quantitative microbial risk assessment for *Escherichia coli* O157 on lettuce, based on survival data from controlled studies in a climate chamber. *J Food Prot.* 2011;74:2000–2007.
81. Petterson SR, Teunis PF, Ashbolt NJ. Modeling virus inactivation on salad crops using microbial count data. *Risk Anal.* 2001;21:1097–1108.
82. Ross T, McMeekin T. Predictive microbiology. *Intl J Food Microbiol.* 1994;23:241–264.
83. Zwietering MH, den Besten HM. Modelling: one word for many activities and uses. *Food Microbiol.* 2011;28:818–822.
84. Guillier L. Predictive microbiology models and operational readiness. *Proc Food Sci.* 2016;7:133–136.
85. Mejlholm O, Dalgaard P. Microbial challenge tests and predictive modelling software for evaluating and improving food safety – a case study with *Listeria monocytogenes* and ready-to-eat foods. In: *XV National Congress SI Di. LV.* 2013.
86. Topalcengiz Z, Spanninger PM, Jeamsripong S, et al. Survival of *Salmonella* in various wild animal feces that may contaminate produce. *J Food Prot.* 2020;83:651–660.
87. Topalcengiz Z, Jeamsripong S, Spanninger PM, et al. Survival of Shiga toxin-producing *Escherichia coli* (STEC) in various wild animal feces that may contaminate produce. J Food Prot. 2020b;83:1420–1429.
88. Wilkes G, Edge T, Gannon V, et al. Seasonal relationships among indicator bacteria, pathogenic bacteria, *Cryptosporidium* oocysts, Giardia cysts, and hydrological indices for surface waters within an agricultural landscape. *Water Res.* 2009;43:2209–2223.
89. Gannon VPJ, Graham TA, Read S, et al. Bacterial Pathogens in Rural Water Supplies in Southern Alberta. *Can J Toxicol Env Health A.* 2004;67:1643–1653.
90. Johnson JYM, Thomas JE, Graham TA, et al. Prevalence of *Escherichia coli* O157:H7 and *Salmonella* spp. in surface waters of southern Alberta and its relation to manure sources. *Can J Microbiol.* 2003;48(5):326–335.
91. Draper AD, Doores S, Gourama H, LaBorde LF. Microbial survey of pennsylvania surface water used for irrigating produce crops. *J Food Prot.* 2016;79(6):902–912.
92. Weller D, Wiedmann M, Strawn LK. Spatial and temporal factors associated with an increased prevalence of *Listeria monocytogenes* in spinach fields in New York State. *Appl Env Microbiol.* 2015;81:6059–6069.
93. Cheong S, Lee C, Song SW, Choi WC, Lee CH, Kim SJ. Enteric viruses in raw vegetables and groundwater used for irrigation in South Korea. *Appl Env Microbiol.* 2009;75:7745–7751.
94. Kokkinos P, Kozyra I, Lazic S, et al. Virological quality of irrigation water in leafy green vegetables and berry fruits production chains. *Food Env Virol.* 2017;9:72–78.
95. Gabrieli R, Maccari F, Ruta A, Panà A, Divizia M. Norovirus detection in groundwater. *Food Env Virol.* 2009;1:92–96.
96. De Giglio O, Caggiano G, Bagordo F, et al. Enteric viruses and fecal bacteria indicators to assess groundwater quality and suitability for irrigation. *Int J Env Res Public Health.* 2017;14.
97. Moreno Y, Moreno-Mesonero L, Amorós I, Pérez R, Morillo JA, Alonso JL. Multiple identification of most important waterborne protozoa in surface water used for irrigation purposes by 18S rRNA amplicon-based metagenomics. *Int J Hyg Env Health.* 2018;221:102–111.
98. Chaidez C, Soto M, Gortares P, Mena K. Occurrence of *Cryptosporidium* and *Giardia* in irrigation water and its impact on the fresh produce industry. *Int J Env Health Res.* 2005;15: 339–345.
99. Thurston-Enriquez JA, Watt P, Dowd SE, Enriquez R, Pepper IL, Gerba CP. Detection of protozoan parasites and microsporidia in irrigation waters used for crop production. *J Food Prot.* 2002;65 (2):378–382.
100. Liu H, Whitehouse CA, Li B. Presence and persistence of *Salmonella* in water: the impact on microbial quality of water and food safety. *Front Public Heal.* 2018;6:1–13.
101. Jamieson RC, Gordon RJ, Sharples KE, Stratton GW, Madani A. Movement and persistence of fecal bacteria in agricultural soils and subsurface drainage water: a review. *Can Biosyst Eng / Le Genie des Biosyst au Can.* 2002;44:1–9.

102. Qadir M, Wichelns D, Raschid-Sally L, et al. The challenges of wastewater irrigation in developing countries. *Agric Water Manag*. 2010;97:561–568.
103. Holvoet K, Sampers I, Seynnaeve M, Uyttendaele M. Relationships among hygiene indicators and enteric pathogens in irrigation water, soil and lettuce and the impact of climatic conditions on contamination in the lettuce primary production. *Int J Food Microbiol*. 2014;171:21–31.
104. Lothrop N, Bright KR, Sexton J, Pearce-Walker J, Reynolds KA, Verhougstraete MP. Optimal strategies for monitoring irrigation water quality. *Agric Water Manag*. 2018;199:86–92.
105. Paruch AM, Mæhlum T, Robertson L. Changes in microbial quality of irrigation water under different weather conditions in southeast Norway. *Env Process*. 2015;2:115–124.
106. Won G, Kline TR, LeJeune JT. Spatial-temporal variations of microbial water quality in surface reservoirs and canals used for irrigation. *Agric Water Manag*. 2013;116:73–78.
107. United State Department of the Interior. Agency specific procedures for implementing the council on environmental quality's principles, requirements, and guidelines for water and land related resources implementation studies. 2015 <https://www.doi.gov/sites/doi.gov/files/elips/documents/707_dm_.pdf> Accessed 10.05.21.
108. Atherholt TB, LeChevallier MW, Norton WD, Rosen JS. Effect of rainfall on *Giardia* and crypto. *J Am Water Work Assoc*. 1998;90:66–80.
109. López-Gálvez F, Truchado P, Sánchez G, Aznar R, Gil MI, Allende A. Occurrence of enteric viruses in reclaimed and surface irrigation water: relationship with microbiological and physicochemical indicators. *J Appl Microbiol*. 2016;121:1180–1188.
110. Chandran A, Hatha MAA. Relative survival of *Escherichia coli* and *Salmonella* Typhimurium in a tropical estuary. *Water Res*. 2005;39:1397–1403.
111. Maıga Y, Wethe J, Denyigba K, Ouattara AS. The impact of pond depth and environmental conditions on sunlight inactivation of *Escherichia coli* and enterococci in wastewater in a warm climate. *Can J Microbiol*. 2009;55:1364–1374.
112. Meays CL, Broersma K, Nordin R, Mazumder A, Samadpour M. Diurnal variability in concentrations and sources of *Escherichia coli* in three streams. *Can J Microbiol*. 2006;52.
113. Meays CL, Broersma K, Nordin R, Mazumder A, Samadpour M. Spatial and annual variability in concentrations and sources of *Escherichia coli* in multiple watersheds. *Env Sci Technol*. 2006;40:5289–5296.
114. Santiago-Rodriguez TM, Tremblay RL, Toledo-Hernandez C, Gonzalez-Nieves JE, Ryu H, Santo Domingo JW. Microbial quality of tropical inland waters and effects of rainfall events. *Appl Env Microbiol*. 2012;78:5160–5169.
115. Won G, Schlegel PJ, Schrock JM, LeJeune JT. Absence of direct association between coliforms and *Escherichia coli* in irrigation water and on produce. *J Food Prot*. 2013;76(6):959–966.
116. Topalcengiz Z, Danyluk MD. Fate of generic and Shiga toxin-producing *Escherichia coli* (STEC) in Central Florida surface waters and evaluation of EPA Worst Case water as standard medium. *Food Res Int*. 2019;120:322–329.
117. Cho KH, Pachepsky YA, Oliver DM, et al. Modeling fate and transport of fecally-derived microorganisms at the watershed scale: state of the science and future opportunities. *Water Res*. 2016;100:38–56.
118. Pachepsky YA, Sadeghi AM, Bradford SA, Shelton DR, Guber AK, Dao T. Transport and fate of manure-borne pathogens: modeling perspective. *Agr Water Manage*. 2006;86:81–92.
119. Chick H. An investigation of the laws of disinfection. *J Hyg*. 1908;8:92–158.
120. Blaustein RA, Pachepsky Y, Hill RL, Shelton DR, Whelan G. *Escherichia coli* survival in waters: temperature dependence. *Water Res*. 2013;47:569–578.
121. Bradford SA, Morales VL, Zhang W, et al. Transport and fate of microbial pathogens in agricultural settings. *Crit Rev Env Sci Tec*. 2013;43:775–893.
122. Hellweger FL, Bucci V, Litman MR, Gu AZ, Onnis-Hayden A. Biphasic decay kinetics of fecal bacteria in surface water not a density effect. *J Environ Eng*. 2009;135(5):372–376.
123. Oliver JD, Page T, Heathwaite AL, Haygarth PM. Re-shaping models of *E. coli* population dynamics in livestock feces: increased bacterial risk to humans? *Env Int*. 2010;36:1–7.
124. Ferguson C, de Roda Husman AM, Altavilla N, Deere D, Ashbolt N. Fate an transport of surface water pathogens in watersheds. *Crit Rev Env Sci Tec*. 2003;33(3):299–361.
125. Payment P, Locus A. Pathogens in water: value and limits of correlation with microbial indicators. *Ground Water*. 2011;49(1):4–11.
126. Santiago-Rodriguez TM, Toranzos GA, Arce-Nazario JA. Assessing the microbial quality of a tropical watershed with and urbanization gradient using traditional and alternate fecal indicators. *J Water Health*. 2016;14(5):796–807.
127. Toranzos GA, McFeters GA, Borrego JJ, Savill M. Detection of microorganisms in environmental freshwaters and drinking waters. In: Hurst C, Crawford R, Garland J, Lipson D, Mills A, Stetzenbach L, eds. *Manual of Environmental Microbiology, 3rd ed*. Washington, DC: ASM Press; 2007:249–264.
128. Abbaszadegan M, Alum A. Waterborne enteric viruses: diversity, distribution, and detection. In: Yates MV, Nakatsu CH, Miller RV, Pillai SD, eds. *Manual of Environmental Microbiology, 4th ed*. Washington, DC: ASM Press; 2016:1–13.
129. Alum A, Villegas EN, Keely SP, Bright KR, Sifuentes LY, Abbaszadegan M. Detection of protozoa in surface and finished waters, 4th ed. In: Yates MV, Nakatsu CH, Miller RV, Pillai SD, eds. *Manual of Environmental Microbiology*. Washington, DC: ASM Press; 2016:1–25.
130. Yates MV. Drinking water microbiology, p. 83–89. In T. Schmidt (ed.), Encyclopedia of Microbiology, 4th ed. Elsevier. 2019.
131. Easton JH, Gauthier JJ, Lalor MM, Pitt RE. Die-off of pathogenic *E. coli* O157:H7 in sewage contaminated waters. *Am Wat Res*. 2005;41(5):1187–1193.
132. Pachepsky YA, Blaustein RA, Whelan G, Shelton DR. Comparing temperature effects on *Escherichia coli, Salmonella*, and *Enterococcus* survival in surface waters. *Lett Appl Microbiol*. 2014;59:278–283.
133. Ibraham EME, El-Liethy MA, Abia ALK, Hemdan BA, Shaheen MN. Survival of *E. coli* O157:H7, *Salmonella* Typhimurium, HAdV2, and MNV-1 in river water under dark conditions and varying storage temperatures. *Sci Total Env*. 2019;648:1297–1304.
134. Wang G, Doyle MP. Survival of enterohemorrhagic *Escherichia coli* O157:H7 in Water. *J Food Prot*. 1998;61(6):662–667.
135. Topalcengiz Z, McEgan R, Danyluk MD. Fate of *Salmonella* in Central Florida surface waters and evaluation of EPA worst case water as a standard medium. *J Food Prot*. 2019;82:916–925.

136. Cho KH, Pachepsky YA, Kim M, et al. Modeling seasonal variability of fecal coliform in natural surface waters using the modified SWAT. *J Hydrol*. 2016;535:377–385.
137. de Roda Husman AM, Lodder WL, Rutjes SA, Schijven JF, Teunis PFM. Long-term inactivation study of three enteroviruses in artificial surface and groundwaters, using PCR and cell culture. *Appl Env Microb*. 2009;75(4):1050–1057.
138. Walker MJ, Montemagno CD, Jenkins MB. Source water assessment and nonpoint sources of acutely toxic contaminants: a review of research related to survival and transport of *Cryptosporidium parvum*. *Water Resour Res*. 1998;34(12):3382–3392.
139. Whitman RL, Nevers MB, Korinek GC, Byappanahalli MN. Solar and temporal effects on *Escherichia coli* concentration at a Lake Michigan swimming beach. *Appl Env Microbiol*. 2004;70 (7):4276–4285.
140. Nguyen MT, Jasper JT, Boehm AB, Nelson KL. Sunlight inactivation of fecal indicator bacteria in open-water unit process treatment wetlands: modeling endogenous and exogenous inactivation rates. *Water Res*. 2015;83:282–292.
141. Johnson DC, Enriquez CE, Pepper IL, Davis TL, Gerba CP, Rose JB. Survival of *Giardia*, *Cryptosporidium*, poliovirus, and *Salmonella* in marine waters. *Water Sci Tec*. 1997;35(11–12):261–268.
142. Sattar SA. *Giardia Cyst and Cryptosporidium Oocyst Survival in Watersheds and Factors Affecting Inactivation*. AWWA Research Foundation, Ontario; 1999.
143. Wilkes G, Edge TA, Gannon VPJ, et al. Associations among pathogenic bacteria, parasites, and environmental and land use factors in multiple mixed-use watersheds. *Water Res*. 2011;45:5807–5825.
144. Shelton DR, Pachepsky YA, Kiefer LA, Blaustein RA, McCarty GW, Dao TH. Response of coliform populations in streambed sediment and water column to changes in nutrient concentrations in water. *Water Res*. 2014;59:316–324.
145. Tanaro JD, Piaggio MC, Galli L, et al. Prevalence of *Escherichia coli* O157:H7 in surface water near cattle feedlots. *Food Pathog Dis*. 2014;11:960–965.
146. Vital M, Hammes F, Egli T. *Escherichia coli* O157 can grow in natural freshwater at low carbon concentrations. *Env Microbiol*. 2008;10(9):2387–2396.
147. Van Elsas JD, Semonov AV, Costa R, Trevors JT. Survivial of *Escherchia coli* in the environment: fundamental and public health aspects. *ISME J*. 2010;5:173–183.
148. Gordon C, Toze S. Influence of groundwater characteristics on the survival of enteric. *Viruses J Appl Micro*. 2003;95 (3):536–544.
149. McFeters G, Stuart D. Survival of coliform bacteria in natural waters: field and laboratory studies with membrane-filter chambers. *Appl Microbiol*. 1972;24(5):805–811.
150. Foppen JW, Schijven J. Transport of *E-coli* in columns of geochemically heterogeneous sediment. *Water Res*. 2006;39 (13):3082–3088.
151. Pandey PK, Kass PH, Soupir ML, Biswas S, Singh VP. Contamination of water resources by pathogenic bacteria. *AMB Express*. 2014;4:51.
152. Pachepsky YA, Shelton DR. *Escherichia coli*. And fecal coliforms in freshwater and estuarine sediments. *Crit Rev Env Sci Tec*. 2011;41(12):1067–1110.
153. United States Food and Drug Administration (USFDA). *Investigation report: factors potentially contributing to the contamination of leafy greens implicated in the fall 2020 outbreak of E. coli O157:H7*. 2021. <https://www.fda.gov/media/147349/download>; Accessed 01.06.21.
154. Muirhead RW, Davies-Colley RJ, Donnison AM, Nagels JW. Faecal bacteria yields in artificial flood events: quantifying in-stream stores. *Water Res*. 2004;38(5):1215–1224.
155. Cho KH, Pachepsky YA, Kim JH, Guber AK, Shelton DR, Rowland R. Release of *Escherichia coli* from bottom sediment in a first-order creek: experiment and reach-specific modeling. *J Hydrol*. 2010;391:322–332.
156. Ferguson CM, Coote BG, Ashbolt NJ, Stevenson IM. Relationships between indicators, pathogens and water quality in an estuarine system. *Water Res*. 1996;30:2045–2054.
157. Byanppanahalli M, Fowler M, Shively D, Whitman R. Ubiquity and persistence of *Escherichia coli* in a Midwestern coastal stream. *Appl Env Microbiol*. 2003;69(8):4549–4555.
158. Desmarais TR, Solo-Gabriele HM, Palmer CJ. Influence of soil on fecal indicator organisms in a tidally influenced subtropical environment. *Appl Env Microbiol*. 2002;68(3):1165–1172.
159. Solo-Gabriele HM, Wolfert MA, Desmarais TR, Palmer CJ. Sources of *Escherichia coli* in a coastal subtropical environment. *Appl Env Microbiol*. 2000;66(1):230–237.
160. Ishii S, Yan T, Shively DA, Byappanahalli MN, Whitman RL, Sadowsky MJ. Cladophora (Chlorophyta) spp. harbor human bacterial pathogens in nearshore water of Lake Michigan. *Appl Env Microbiol*. 2006;72(7):4545–4553.
161. Byappanahalli MN, Sawdey R, Ishii S, et al. Seasonal stability of Cladophora-associated *Salmonella* in Lake Michigan watersheds. *Water Res*. 2009;43:806–814.
162. Thomas V, McDonnell G, Denyer SP, Maillard JY. Free-living amoebae and their intracellular pathogenic microorganisms: risks for water quality. *Fems Microbiol Rev*. 2010;34(3):231–259.
163. United States Environmental Protection Agency (USEPA). *Health risks from microbial growth and biofilms in drinking water distribution systems*. 2002 <https://www.epa.gov/sites/production/files/2015-09/documents/2007_05_18_disinfection_tcr_whitepaper_tcr_biofilms.pdf>; Accessed 01.06.21.
164. Fechner LC, Gourlay-France C, Tusseau-Vuillemin MH. Linking community tolerance and structure with low metallic contamination: a field study on 13 biofilms sampled across the Seine river basin. *Water Res*. 2014;52:152–162.
165. Srey S, Jahid IK, Ha SD. Biofilm formation in food industries: a food safety concern. *Food Control*. 2013;31:572–585.
166. Jahid IK, Ha SD. A review of microbial biofilms of produce: future challenge to food safety. *Food Sci Biotechnol*. 2012;21:299–316.
167. Lajhar SA, Brownlie J, Barlow R. Characterization of biofilm-forming capacity and resistance to sanitizers of a range of *E. coli* pathotypes from clinical cases and cattle in Australia. *BMC Microbiol*. 2018;18:41.
168. Yuan Y, Olivier H. Biofilm research within irrigation water distribution systems: trends, knowledge gaps and future perspectives. *Sci Total Env*. 2019;673:254–265.
169. Pachepsky Y, Morrow J, Guber A, Shelton D, Rowland R, Davies G. Effect of biofilm in irrigation pipes on microbial quality of irrigation water. *Lett Appl Microbiol*. 2011;54:217–224.

170. Sanchez O, Ferrera I, Garrido L, Gomez-Ramos MDM, Fernandez-Alba AR, Mas J. Prevalence of potentially thermophilic microorganisms in biofilms from greenhouse-enclosed drip irrigation systems. *Arch Microbiol*. 2014;196:219–226.
171. Erickson MC, Webb CC, Diaz-Perez JC, et al. Surface and internalized *Escherichia coli* O157:H7 on field-grown spinach and lettuce treated with spray-contaminated irrigation water. *J Food Prot*. 2010;73(6):1023–1029.
172. Markland SM, Shortlidge KL, Hoover DG, et al. Survival of Pathogenic *Escherichia coli* on basil, lettuce, and spinach. *Zoonoses Public Health*. 2013;60:563–571.
173. Van der linden I, Cotty B, Uttendaele M, Vlaemynch G, Maes M, Heyndrickx M. Long-term survival of *Escherichia coli* O157:H7 and *Salmonella enterica* on butterhead lettuce seeds, and their subsequent survival and growth on the seedlings. *Int J Food Microbiol*. 2013;161(3):214–219.
174. Van der Linden I, Cottyn B, Uyttendaele M, et al. Enteric pathogen survival varies substantially in irrigation water from Belgian lettuce producers. *Int J Env Res Public Health*. 2014;11:10105–10124.
175. Olmez H, Temur SD. Effects of different sanitizing treatments on biofilms and attachment of *Escherchia coli* and *Listeria monocytogenes* on green leaf lettuce. *LWT – Food Sci Technol*. 2010;43:964–970.
176. Fonseca JM, Fallon SD, Sanchez CA, Nolte KD. *Escherichia coli* survival in lettuce fields following its introduction through different irrigation systems. *J Appl Microbiol*. 2011;110 (4):893–902.
177. Oliviera M, Usall J, Vinas I, Solsana C, Abadias M. Transfer of *Listeria innocua* from contaminated compost and irrigation water to lettuce leaves. *Food Microbiol*. 2010;28:590–596.
178. Chitarra W, Decastelli L, Garibaldi A, Gullino ML. Potential uptake of *Escherichia coli* O157:H7 and *Listeria monocytogenes* from growth substrate into leaves of salad plants and basil grown in soil irrigated with contaminated water. *Int J Food Microbiol*. 2014;189:139–145.
179. Islam M, Doyle MP, Phatak SC, Millner P, Jiang X. Survival of *Escherichia coli* O157:H7 in soil and on carrots and onions grown in fields treated with contaminated manure composts or irrigation water. *Food Microbiol*. 2005;22:63–70.
180. European Commission. Council directive 98/83/EC of 3 November 1998 on the quality of water intended for human consumption. *J Eur Communities*. 1998;41:32–54.
181. The California leafy green marketing agreement. *Commodity specific food safety guidelines for the production and harvest of lettuce and leafy greens*, 2019 *[Online]*. <https://lgma-assets.sfo2.digitaloceanspaces.com/downloads/190419-CA-LGMA-Metrics_Accessible_0605.pdf>; Accessed 30.06. 20.
182. World Health Organization (WHO). *Safety and quality of water used in food production and processing: meeting report*. 2019. <https://www.who.int/foodsafety/publications/mra_33/en/>.
183. Yates MV, Gerba CP, Kelley LM. Virus persistence in groundwater. *Appl Environ Microbiol*. 1985;49:778–781.
184. Chen W, Lu S, Jiao W, Wang M, Chang AC. Reclaimed water: a safe irrigation water source? *Environ Dev*. 2013;8:74–83.
185. Banach JL, van der Fels-Klerx HJ. Microbiological reduction strategies of irrigation water for fresh produce. *J Food Prot*. 2020;83(6):1072–1087.
186. Robins P, *Co-management of water quality and food safety*. 2012. Available from: <http://www.vineyardteam.org/files/resources/Robins,%20Paul.pdf>; Accessed 02.06.21.
187. Song I, Stine SW, Choi CY, Gerba CP. Comparison of crop contamination by microorganisms during subsurface drip and furrow irrigation. *J Environ Eng*. 2006;132:1243–1248.
188. United States Food and Drug Administration (USFDA). *Factors potentially contributing to the contamination of Romaine lettuce implicated in the three outbreaks of E. Coli O157:H7 during the fall of 2019*. 2019 <https://www.fda.gov/food/outbreaks-foodborne-illness/factors-potentially-contributing-contamination-romaine-lettuce-implicated-three-outbreaks-e-coli>; Accessed 10.05.21.
189. Allende A, Monaghan J. Irrigation water quality for leafy crops: a perspective of risks and potential solutions. *Int J Environ Res Public Health*. 2015;12(7):7457–7477.

Chapter 27

Microbial pathogen contamination of animal feed

Elena G. Olson[1], Tomasz Grenda[2], Anuradha Ghosh[3] and Steven C. Ricke[1]

[1]*Department of Animal and Dairy Sciences, University of Wisconsin-Madison, Madison, WI, United States,* [2]*Department of Hygiene of Animal Feedingstuffs, National Veterinary Research Institute, Pulawy, Poland,* [3]*Biology Department, Pittsburg State University, Pittsburg, KS, United States*

Abstract

Animal feed production is a complex process involving several steps during feed milling. In feed manufacturing, there are numerous opportunities to introduce microorganisms from various environmental and other sources. While most of these microorganisms are likely nonpathogenic, pathogens can also be members of feed microbial populations. In addition to fungi, several bacterial pathogens have been identified. They are believed to be associated with animal feed and include *Listeria*, Clostridia, pathogenic *Escherichia coli*, and *Salmonella*, as well as others that are less well characterized. Of the pathogens known to contaminate animal feeds, *Salmonella* has probably been the most extensively characterized. Much of the focus has been on designing intervention strategies to reduce *Salmonella* population levels on feeds. In this chapter, a survey of some of the pathogens found in feeds will be discussed, along with sources of feed microbial contamination, and finally future directions for applying molecular technologies such as microbiome sequencing to characterize feed microbial communities.

Keywords: Animal feed; cross-contamination; rendering; pathogens; *Salmonella*; *Clostridia*; *Listeria monocytogenes*; pathogenic *Escherichia coli*; antibiotic resistance

Chapter points

1. Animal feed microorganisms may cause epidemiological risk for animals, economic losses to feed manufacturers and farmers, and some of them potential risk for consumers.
2. The origins and sources for microbial feed contamination are considerable and potentially variable by being somewhat dependent on a combination of environmental and manufacturing operational differences.
3. *Salmonella* species are one of the more extensively characterized pathogens in all animal feeds.
4. *Listeria monocytogenes*, pathogenic *Escherichia coli*, and *Clostridium* spp. have also been associated with animal feeds.
5. Although the prevalence of *Salmonella*, *E. coli*, and *Enterococcus* is common in animal feed ingredients, antimicrobial resistance is not typically observed at high frequencies.

27.1 Introduction

Microbial contamination of animal feeds can originate from a wide range of sources during production and harvesting of the cereal grain, such as soil from which the cereal crop grows, airborne transmission, water sources, animals grazing on adjoining pastures along with exposure of feeds during harvesting, processing, and storage.[1] Given the variety of environmental sources, it is not surprising that the microorganisms contaminating animal feeds are likely to be quite diverse. Some of these organisms can cause deterioration of feed during storage, reducing feed quality. Ultimately, the microorganisms that contaminate the grain being processed for feed may impact the performance of the food animal consuming the feed and/or contribute to animal disease. In addition, animal feed can serve as a vector for microorganisms that cause foodborne illness in humans. Therefore animal feed microorganisms may represent epidemiological risk for animals, economic losses to feed manufacturers and farmers, and some of them, because of their zoonotic character, also a potential risk for consumers.

There are other concerns for microbial contamination of animal feeds. For example, fecal sources and slurry can be contamination routes in pastures and, depending on proximity, eventually contaminate the grain sources that comprise animal feeds. The resulting

Present Knowledge in Food Safety. DOI: https://doi.org/10.1016/B978-0-12-819470-6.00023-8

contaminated feeds could potentially impact the animal host, leading to colonization of the host animal by foodborne pathogens. Frequently, animal excreta can become a source of environmental contamination and an epidemiological risk for other animals that contact these environments. Given the variety of pathogens and their genetic variants, a wide range of microbiological methods are needed as analytical tools to detect pathogens, design strategies for controlling their dissemination, and animal feed safety.[2–4] Control measures may vary depending on the type of microorganism. For example, spore formers represent a different intervention challenge versus a pathogen that may only exist as a vegetative cell on the animal feed. Therefore it is critical to understand the likelihood of pathogens contaminating animal feeds, their potential sources, and the inherent risk of exposure for food animals consuming these feeds. Once these factors have been identified, appropriate control strategies can be devised to lower the risk.

Microbial contamination of animal feeds has been reviewed over the years, emphasizing different aspects of microbial contamination, such as focusing on specific pathogens or surveys of feed treatments to limit pathogen contamination.[1,5,6] More specifically, there has been extensive research on *Salmonella* and poultry feeds, given the concern over the relationship between poultry and foodborne *Salmonella* species.[7,8] However, feeds for other food animals represent potential microbial contamination problems as well. The type of microbial contamination can undoubtedly vary depending on the type of feed, for example, silage versus cereal grain. Likewise, the food animal's susceptibility can vary both as a function of species such as ruminant versus nonruminant and the level of environmental stress that the animal may be encountering.

Similarly, the age of an animal is a factor. A young calf with a developing rumen may be more susceptible to foodborne pathogen colonization than an adult ruminant animal with a fully functional rumen containing a diverse set of fermentative microorganisms. This would be true of other animal species in a similar context, such as young chickens being much more likely to be colonized by *Salmonella*. However, adult animals can also be susceptible to pathogen colonization in the gastrointestinal tract under certain circumstances, such as nutritional stress.[9] Exposure to microbially contaminated feed can thus serve as a source of pathogens to susceptible animals. Consequently, microbial feed contamination remains an ongoing concern during all phases of animal production. The current review's objective is to discuss the potential sources of microbial contamination in animal feeds and the pathogenic microorganisms likely to occur on feeds.

27.2 Animal feed and microbial contamination—general concepts

In the United States, the feed industry is a major commercial enterprise, and as animal production increases, it is likely to continue to expand.[10] In 2016 over 236 million tons of animal feed were distributed to nine animal species, including the top three food animal commodities: cattle (74.7 million tons), broilers (56.3 million tons), and pigs (46.3 million tons), which contributed to $297.1 billion in sales.[11] Also, there is a total of approximately 8000 feed mills and 264 protein renderers in the United States [US Food and Drug Administration's (FDA)]. This growth in the US feed industry has been influenced by the vertical integration in some animal commodity groups, such as the broiler industry.[12] The operational aspects of animal feed milling have also evolved over the years.

Meeting the specific nutritional needs of such a wide range of food animal species adds to feed milling and manufacturing complexity. This becomes further complicated when the age of the animal and growth nutrient requirements associated with specific growth phases are factored into feed formulation. Consequently, the vast array of specialized feed additives and other nutrient supplements has continued to expand. This, in turn, has multiplied the number of potential opportunities for microbial contamination of feeds as they are being mixed and distributed. Consequently, not only does the introduction of ingredients during feed milling provide more sources for contamination but the potential for microbial cross-contamination is also more likely.

Microbial feed contamination can arise at any production step, such as raw ingredients, transportation, warehousing, manufacturing, and animal housing.[1,13] Thus there is a significant probability of contamination of animal feed and animal feed ingredients between manufacturing facilities, resulting in pathogen exposure to animals and eventually meat products for human consumption.[14] Microbial contamination of animal feed pre- and postfarmgate affects colonization and potentially disease incidence in food animals. Thus food animals can be a principal reservoir for several bacterial pathogens, such as *Campylobacter*, nontyphoidal *Salmonella*, and Shiga toxin–producing *Escherichia coli* (STEC).[14–17] While the animal host harboring these pathogens may be asymptomatic, they remain carriers of the foodborne pathogens potentially on extended periods of their growth cycle. When the respective food animals are harvested and processed for meat, the presence of pathogens in the gastrointestinal tract can also influence the carcass's potential level of pathogen contamination during processing. However, the range of factors that impact this transmission is complex and subject to numerous mitigating circumstances.

European Union (EU) legislation is not very prescriptive concerning microbiological contaminants in feed. Only a general approach in Directive 2003/99/EC obligates the Member States to monitor different zoonoses and salmonellosis for all food chain links, including feedstuffs. Member states are obliged to implement a control program against *Salmonella* according to Regulation (EC) 2160/2003. Based on these two regulations, each Member State must form national monitoring programs for feedstuff control of these biological agents. Specific microbiological criteria for every feedstuff and feedstuff ingredient are not described in detail. Only a general notice is expressed in Regulation (EC) 183/2005 art. 5, p. 3, according to which: "feed business operators must comply with specific microbiological criteria and implement measures to meet targets." The mentioned "target" has not been entirely specified until now. However, the most thoroughly determined microbiological criteria refer to processed animal proteins (PAP) derived from animal by-products classified as category 3 material according to Regulation (EC) 1069/2009. Based on the implementation of Regulation (EU) 142/2011 of Regulation (EC) 1069/2009, microbiological criteria are dependent on processing methods.

Regarding the regulation mentioned above, insects could be submitted to processing methods one to five and seven. Samples of the final products taken during or on-withdrawal from storage at the processing plant must comply with standards limited to Enterobacteriaceae enumerated from 1 g and *Salmonella* absence in 25 g. Moreover, according to the Regulation, requirements regarding processing method number seven are also described. In this method, the final product sampling is conducted daily for 30 production days in compliance with the microbiological standards, including requirements limited to Enterobacteriaceae number in 1 g, *Salmonella* spp. absence in 25 g, and *Clostridium perfringens* absence in 1 g.

In the United States, the Feed Contaminants Program (7371.003) is one of several food safety-related compliance programs controlled by the FDA.[18] During assessment, the Center for Veterinary Medicine (CVM) suggests that investigators perform activities on more than one program, such as collecting feed for microbial samples [Feed Manufacturing Compliance Program (7371.004)], collecting milk samples for aflatoxin analysis [Milk Safety Program (7318.003)], and executing a bovine spongiform encephalopathy (BSE)-related inspection [BSE/Ruminant Feed Ban Inspections (7371.009)].[18] Under sample collection guidelines, CVM states a preference for only two pathogens, *Salmonella* and *E. coli* O157:H7.[18] In addition, Program 7371.003 states that discrete prudence and inspectional conclusions should guide sampling, and priority should be held for animal feed and feed constituents associated with food-producing animals, laying hens, and milking cows over nonfood-producing animals.[18] Additionally, whether the feed or its components should be submitted to further heat treatments must be determined, especially during microbial sampling.[18] Investigational samples should be gathered to acquire surveillance data or to examine contaminated samples.[18]

Interestingly, dioxin and bacterial contaminants are the only directed assignments to survey sections of production that CVM issues, and their application is currently based on inactive PAC codes 71003H and 71003I.[18] To further analyze feed samples for *Salmonella* and *E. coli* O157:H7, Program 7371.003 suggests applying methodology described in Bacteriological Analytical Manual (BAM) Online, Chapters 4A and 5. Analysis of 10 subsamples combined into a total of 375 grams for *Salmonella* is advised. For *E. coli* O157:H7, testing individual subsamples using 25 g from each subsample is instructed in Program 7371.003.

Establishing regulations regarding animal feed manufacturing and limiting pathogens in feeds is a challenge from both a sampling and detection standpoint. Given the potential for microbial contamination of animal feed and the wide range of pathogens that can come in contact with feed, developing strategies for assessing microbial contamination levels and applying the appropriate control measures remain difficult. The origins and sources for microbial feed contamination are considerable and potentially variable, being somewhat dependent on a combination of environmental and manufacturing operational differences. In the following sections, some of the potential sources for microbial contamination of feeds will be discussed, and the respective impact on overall feed contamination.

27.3 Potential sources of microbial contamination in feed manufacturing

27.3.1 Feed manufacturing steps as a source of cross-contamination

Besides the individual feed manufacturing steps, general feed mill and farm methods can affect finished feed products' biological safety.[1] Factors outside of manufacturing processes include sanitation practices, quality of raw feed constituents, and other biosecurity procedures within the feed mill.[1] Furthermore, the surrounding environment in the rendering facilities can contribute to bacterial contamination of the final rendered product. Gong and Jiang[19] detected the highest concentrations of *Salmonella*'s in areas of the rendering plant where the raw constituents were received. *Salmonella* was present in biofilms in rendered constituents before grinding procedure, and finished meal-loading out spaces, potentially appearing in the final meal product. The machinery, plant environment, and employees can all serve as potential sources of contamination. While not fully documented in the feed mill, some lessons can be learned from the food industry and manufacturing facilities. For example, foodborne pathogens, such as *E. coli* O157:H7, *Listeria monocytogenes*, *Yersinia enterocolitica*, and *Campylobacter jejuni* form biofilms on food surfaces and food contact equipment.[20–22] Some bacteria can generate biofilms on processing machinery, conveyor belts, storage containers, and the floor of the manufacturing plant. In feed mills, additional recontamination risks exist during bulk storage and the transportation of raw materials to the feed facility, specifically liquids (Kinley et al.).[1]

Contaminated feed constituents can contaminate manufacturing equipment, resulting in cross-contamination of other products. More so, while the use of chemicals may eliminate *Salmonella* in feed, Muckey et al.[23] detected viable *Salmonella* cells on the surface of the sampling locations. Gebhardt et al.[24] and Huss et al.[25] concluded that dust gathered from animal feed contact surfaces can carry biological pathogens and, thus represents one of the highest risks for cross-contamination in feed manufacturing facilities. In an artificially inoculated feed with *E. faecium* study on the manufacturing process, Huss et al.[25] observed that most animal and nonanimal feed contact surfaces were positive for the indicator bacteria. These experiments indicate how the magnitude of biological material in dust particles can be particularly challenging for minimizing microbial contamination during animal feed processing. Furthermore, Huss et al.[25] suggested that extremely persistent interventions, such as heat and chemical agents, may be essential to more thoroughly decontaminate animal feed processing surfaces.

Besides bacterial risks correlated with certain feed ingredients, accidental batch-to-batch cross-contamination can occur when feed is made for more than one animal species in the same facility. For instance, Okuma and Hellberg[26] found that numerous animal species were not identified on pet food labels. Their findings suggest that the amount of raw ingredients cross-contamination led to increased recalls due to the ambiguity of consequential ongoing production processes or lack of appropriate clean-outs between product manufacturing steps. Also, mammalian animal proteins are banned in ruminant feed due to a potential risk of transmission of BSE to humans. This fact provides a reason for another concern for cross-contamination during feed formulation processes. If such ingredients are formulated in the same facilities, the cross-contamination between the feeds can occur and thus potentially lead to dissemination of disease.

27.3.2 Rendering

Animal feed is formulated to optimize animal performance to maximize efficient animal product harvests for human consumption. More than 900 safe agricultural constituents are approved for animal feed use in the United States.[27] Although mammalian animal protein is banned in ruminant feeds in the United States and Canada, fats and proteins manufactured by rendering are still the major nutritional contributors to the livestock industries.[1,28] Since consumers in the United States consider less than 50% of the animal edible, the process of rendering recycles over 50% of the left-over meat and other body parts into a value-added product, which in turn improves the sustainability of animal production.[1,29] Annually, the United States produces 11.2×10^9 pounds of protein and 10.0×10^9 pounds of fat.[30] Nearly 85% of these products are used to manufacture animal feed components and are considered primary feed ingredients in poultry and aquaculture.[30–32] Rendering sources include meat processing plants, dead animals from various places, such as animal shelters, restaurants, and retail grocery store wastes.[33] Other animal tissues can occur in feeds as well. For example, when comparing 16S rRNA gene sequences of mitochondrial DNA in feeds, Yang et al.[34] identified dog, cat, and rat or mouse tissues in the animal feed samples.

While adding rendered animal proteins to feed delivers many fundamental nutrients and minerals essential for animal growth and development, animal feed is also a source of foodborne pathogens that can contribute to human foodborne illnesses.[14] Although the rendering process consists of applying high heat and removing moisture while separating the fat, the finished meal can still become recontaminated with bacteria postrendering.[1] When such contaminated products are used in animal feed, pathogen inoculation of animals in the food chain occurs and leads to possible human exposure. Because animal proteins used for feed mixing are potential natural reservoirs of human pathogens, such as *Salmonella*, *L. monocytogenes*, *C. jejuni*, and *C. perfringens*, there is a microbiological safety concern.[1] Hofacre et al.[35] determined that poultry meal contained bacterial populations ranging from 1.6 to 4.02 $\log_{10}$ colony forming units/g. While *Salmonella* was isolated from 14% of the meat and bone samples, *Acinetobacter colcoaceticus*, *Citrobacter freundii*, and *Enterobacter cloacae* were the other most commonly isolated bacteria from poultry meal.[35] In some studies, *Enterococci* spp. were detected in rendered animal meals[36,37]. In a 2003 national survey conducted by the FDA on 122 rendered meal samples, 84% were contaminated with *Enterococcus* spp. that were further identified as *E. faecium* (86.5%), *Enterococcus faecalis* (7.5%), *Enterococcus gallinarum* (2%), *Enterococcus hirae* (1.5%), and *Enterococcus avium* (0.5%). *Enterococci* contamination within the animal feed is not as surprising, as *Enterococcus* species can be heat tolerant.[38]

Raw rendered materials have been notorious for being one of the most commonly contaminated animal feed ingredients.[39] Over 40 years later, Kinley et al.[30] obtained similar results after isolating *Enterococcus* species in 81.3% of the samples and *Salmonella* from 8.7% of the samples containing rendered animal products. In addition, Troutt et al.[40] detected 71.4% *C. perfringens*, 8.3% *L. monocytogenes*, 76.2% *Listeria* spp., 20% *C. jejuni*, and 29.8% *Campylobacter* spp. in raw materials used for rendered by-product manufacturing. Moisture is one of the main control points for averting microbial growth of the rendered product. Kinley et al.[30] concluded that when protein meals were not adequately dried, microbial contamination increased in blood and feather meals. More so, although moisture levels in animal feeds can remain low for most bacterial growth, *Salmonella*, if present, can persist for extended periods during storage.[41]

27.3.3 Animal versus plant-derived bacterial contamination in feeds

Ingredients used to formulate animal feed rations are derived primarily from the processing of plants, mainly grains and oilseed meals, along with animal by-products, such as rendered products and fish meal, in addition to purified vitamins, minerals, and other feed supplements.[42,43] From 2007 to 2009 surveillance data, it was reported that 41.3% of the animal-derived and 10.6% of the plant-based ingredients were contaminated with *Salmonella*.[1,44] Ge et al.[45] observed that none of the 201 feed ingredient samples from rendering plants yielded detectable *Campylobacter* or *E. coli* O157:H7, while 22.9% of samples were contaminated with *Salmonella*, 39.3% with *E. coli*, and 86.6% with *Enterococcus*. Furthermore, while animal by-products had a considerably higher contamination rate of *Salmonella*, plant feed sources were more often contaminated with *E. coli* and *Enterococcus*.[45] The incidence of *Salmonella* within animal by-products ranged from 10% in feather meal, 38.9% in meat and bone meal, to 80% in a fish meal.[45] Other studies described fish meal as being particularly problematic.[46,47]

The incidence of *Salmonella*, *E. coli*, or *Enterococcus* did not vary considerably between the meat and bone meal, poultry meal, or blood meal.[45] In contrast, amongst plant by-products, only soybean meal (9.7%) and cottonseed meal (12.5%) tested positive for *Salmonella*; while the incidence of *E. coli* and *Enterococcus* between alfalfa meal and oilseed by-products was considerably higher than that in corn by-products.[45] The much higher incidence of *Salmonella* among animal versus plant by-products also validated two FDA/CVM surveys.[44,48] Based on an extensive Great Britain survey between 1987 and 2006, rapeseed meal, soybean meal, and fish meal were reported to be the top three feed sources with detectable *Salmonella* contamination.[46]

Fecal contamination of feeds is prevalent on farms and represents a potentially important route of cattle exposure to *E. coli* and other pathogens.[49] Lynn et al.[50] found that 30% of cattle feed samples in the United States contained *E. coli*. Replication of fecal *E. coli* was demonstrated by D'Mello[49] in various animal feeds held under conditions mimicking summer months occurring on cattle farms in the United States. The probability for microbial exposure also occurs when poultry litter materials are fed to cattle.[49] For instance, in California, two such poultry waste products were made commercially accessible as cattle feed.[49] Although appropriate heat-processing before distribution significantly decreased the risk of contamination by *E. coli*, *Salmonella* spp., and *Campylobacter* spp.; contamination with *Salmonella enterica* generally ranged up to 19% in cattle feeds in United States, Europe, and South Africa.[49,51]

Cereal grains and animal-based feeds are not the only potential source of pathogens. The term "feed" is commonly used in its broadest context to incorporate cereal grain-based feed mixtures of traditional ingredients as well as forage-based feed sources such as silages.[49] *L. monocytogenes* tends to occur in poor-quality forages.[49] Grass must remain under anaerobic conditions with a low pH to ensure *Listeria*'s exclusion during ensiling.[49] Nevertheless, in big-bale silage, aerobic processes may occur, increasing pH, thus providing essential components for *Listeria* growth that can persist through low temperatures and excessive levels of dry matter.[49] Contamination of cattle feed with *Listeria* is critical as exposure can lead to abortion and life-threatening diseases in animals and humans.[49] Previously, *E. coli* O157, but not *Campylobacter*, has been detected in cattle feed.[52,53] Ge et al.[45] did not recover any *Campylobacter* or *E. coli* O157:H7 from 201 feed ingredients, corroborating that feed component is a far less significant source for these particular foodborne pathogens at least for these specific feed ingredients.

27.4 Microbial pathogen contamination of feeds—general concepts

While animal feeds harbor a wide range of microorganisms, feed is undoubtedly a potential vector for foodborne pathogen transmission as well. However, the role of animal feed and foodborne pathogen occurrence in animal production is complicated. For example, several *Salmonella* infections in animals have been traced to contaminated animal feed.[54–57,58]Moreover, evidence exists that bacteria pathogenic to humans are not always pathogenic to animals and can be readily transmitted to food animals via contaminated feed, ultimately appearing on animal carcasses intended for human ingestion.[14,59]

Humans can become infected after ingesting a contaminated meat product, and raw produce or other foods contaminated with animal feces or cross-contaminated by contact with uncooked meat.[14,60–64]

Salmonella species are one of the most characterized pathogens associated with animal feeds.[1] Since 1958, several *Salmonella* outbreaks have been traced back to animal feed.[65–70] Furthermore, several experimental studies demonstrated that animals fed artificially contaminated feed containing *Salmonella* experienced colonization by the microorganism and disease resulting from exposure to that organism.[71,72] However, pathogens, such as *E. coli*, *C. perfringens*, and *Campylobacter*, can remain relatively asymptomatic in the animal, making it hard to assess as a preventative strategy. This can also be true of *Salmonella*. For instance, Harris et al.[73] isolated 13 *Salmonella* species serotypes from swine feed across 30 farms, where the history of salmonellosis was not previously observed.

Although many foodborne outbreaks have been linked to contaminated meat, there is a lack of investigations that trace the source of contamination through the food supply chain to the farm of origin.[14] More so, these investigations lack the in-depth microbiological assessment of animal feed.[14] Therefore surveillance of animal feed, food-producing animals, and human illness for bacterial contamination is not adequately integrated to distinguish outbreaks that may be specifically linked to contaminated animal feed.[14] However, bacterial contamination of animal feed is still considered a possible critical route for the entry of pathogens into human food products. Thus safeguarding pathogen-free animal feed can potentially lead to significant reduction in the occurrence of associated foodborne diseases. According to the European Food Safety Authority (EFSA) opinion from 2008, *Salmonella* spp. was recognized as a significant feed microbiological contaminant. However, besides *Salmonella* spp., other potential hazards have been reported and/or suggested, namely *Campylobacter* spp., *L. monocytogenes*, *E. coli* O157:H7, and *Clostridium* spp. The following sections describe some of the more extensively examined foodborne pathogens that have been consistently associated with animal feeds or in some cases feed has at least been suggested as a potential source for the corresponding pathogen.

27.4.1 Salmonella

Salmonella infection of food animals remains a persistent problem for animal production. It is worth noting that out of the more than 2500 various *Salmonella* serotypes, only a few are pathogenic to a particular animal but can remain asymptomatic with other animal species.[1] Thus the specific strain is considered an adulterant only when feed is intended for poultry, livestock, and equine farms and is pathogenic to the animal consuming the feed.[1,74] Conversely, due to a high chance of human contact, there is a zero *Salmonella* tolerance in pet food.[1,74] Some serovars of *Salmonella* are considered to be adapted to particular livestock species causing characteristic disease symptoms in that respective animal species. *S.* Gallinarum and *S.* Pullorum cause fowl typhoid and pullorum disease in poultry, respectively.[3] *S.* Choleraesuis is responsible for enteritis and septicemia in pigs.[3] *S.* Dublin is a cause of septicemia, abortion, or enteritis in cattle; and *S.* Abortusovis usually causes abortion in sheep.[3]

However, *Salmonella* infection of animals is not limited to host-specific disease-causing serovars but can originate from nonhost adapted serovars, several of which are responsible for human foodborne salmonellosis. Colonization in the gastrointestinal tract by these serovars is a challenge for control measures as detectable disease symptoms may only occasionally appear, with the majority of colonization that occurs only resulting in an asymptomatic carriage in the *Salmonella* colonized animal. While animals are frequently infected by other *Salmonella*-positive animals or various environmental routes and vectors such as insects, the infection can also originate via contaminated feed.[75]

Transfer of *Salmonella* strains can occur from consumption of contaminated feedstuffs by animals. Still, *Salmonella*'s animal feed contamination can vary depending on the type of feed, feed mill operations, antimicrobial agents added to the feed, and storage conditions before feeding, just to name a few.[1] Even if it is difficult to evaluate the exact source of contamination (feed, environmental sources, milling operations, among others), there always exists a possible transmission of *Salmonella* through feed.[4] The overall prevalence of *Salmonella*-positive units in animal- and vegetable-derived feed supplies in 2018 in the EU was 0.93% of 28,680 reported units. The *Salmonella* contamination of compound feeds (or the finished feed for animals), according to EFSA Report from 2018, was relatively low for all animal populations: 0.52% of 10,497 tested samples for poultry, 0.45% of 7259 tested samples for cattle, and 0.33% of 4251 tested samples for pigs.[76]

The four essential feeding groups for livestock in the EU are industrially compounded feeds, home-grown cereals, forages, and purchased feedstuffs.[77] Among feed constituents, oilseeds and PAP are considered high-risk feed materials that can introduce *Salmonella* to the food chain.[46] According to literature reports, nonprocessed cereals are generally characterized by a low prevalence of *Salmonella*, while nonprocessed soybeans can be frequently contaminated with this pathogen.[77] Limited information is available on *Salmonella* occurrence in forages and for on farm-mixing of feeds. The EFSA Panel of Biological Hazards has recommended collecting more data on feed proportions.

Annual culture-confirmed human infection surveys regarding *Salmonella* indicate that the five most prevalent serovars in decreasing order are Enteritidis, Newport, Typhimurium, Javiana, and monophasic Typhimurium in the United States (Centers for Disease Control and Prevention, 2016) and Enteritidis, Typhimurium, monophasic Typhimurium, Infantis, and Newport in the European Union.[78] Regular monitoring of *Salmonella* prevalence in feed indicated five serovars that could be considered critical: *S.* Enteritidis, *S.* Typhimurium, *S.* Infantis, *S.* Virchow, and *S.* Hadar.[68] Rendered animal products are often contaminated with *Salmonella*. In a 1993 survey, the USFDA CVM identified *Salmonella* in nearly a 50% of 151 feed ingredients sampled.[48] Epidemiological findings have linked human disease-causing *Salmonella* spp. to contaminated animal feed.[14] For instance, *S.* Heidelberg outbreak in 1963 led to 77 infections from drinking milk and was linked to bovine mastitis caused by the same *Salmonella* serotype, which was found in the meat and bone meal fed to the cows.[70] *Salmonella* was detected in 84.2% of the broiler premix over four months, 81% of the meat meal, and 40% of the feather meal produced in Ontario feed mills.[79] The Animal Protein Producers Industry weekly examined samples from rendered animal products at the end of the processing line for *Salmonella* for at least 52 tests a year. Typically, 25% of the samples tested positive for *Salmonella*.[80] Results from 197 *Salmonella*-positive samples during a particular year insinuated that the average most probable number (MPN) per gram was 16.3, with a range of 0.278 MPN/g.[80] Out of all *Salmonella* serovars found in the previously discussed study, four were associated with foodborne disease, namely, *S.* Typhimurium, *S.* Agona, *S.* Enteritidis, and *S.* Infantis. In addition, samples that tested positive for *Salmonella* were poultry or feather meal.[80]

A potential rationalization for this type of outcome is that the raw poultry products might consist of more significant *Salmonella* numbers upon entering the rendering plants. It would therefore necessitate additional heat exposure compared to the other meal types. Heat processing is a common practice in feed manufacturing, providing for improved antimicrobial and nutritional value of animal feed.[49] Thus the initial bacterial load of raw constituents should result in microbiologically safe meal products following proper heat processing. However, this assumption may not always be the case. Troutt et al.[40] detected over 84.5% *Salmonella*-positive samples from raw rendered materials and 26.1% *Salmonella*-positive samples from the final rendered product. In addition, numerous other studies, such as Kinley et al.,[30] Sapkota et al.,[42] Franco,[80] and Laban et al.,[81] detected the presence of *Salmonella* in the final rendered products, such as animal feed.

Cross-contamination may be one of the primary reasons for the presence of *Salmonella* in the finished products. Kinley et al.[30] hypothesized that the likely source of contamination of the rendered constituents was the raw animal by-product. In addition, Kinley et al.[30] presented baseline data on bacterial contamination levels in newly rendered meals. Kinley et al.[30] demonstrated that the heat used by rendering process is sufficient in eliminating bacterial contamination, indicating that contamination with *Salmonella* occurred during postprocessing. As a part of this study, heat-tolerant enterococci served as a marker for the bacterial load to help determine whether the meal products had been heated sufficiently or had become contaminated by raw ingredients or the manufacturing environment.[30] Liu et al.[82] also demonstrated the successful application of *E. faecium* as a *Salmonella* surrogate in thermal processing for low-moisture foods over a wide range of water activities.

Historically, a wide range of antimicrobial chemicals and other control measures using external agents have been explored over the years to decrease *Salmonella* contamination in animal feeds and potentially in animals consuming the treated feeds. These interventions have been extensively discussed in a series of comprehensive reviews and will not be discussed in detail in the current study.[1,5,8,83–85] More recently, other control measures have been examined. Novel feed machinery such as hygienizers has been recommended to decrease *Salmonella* associated with mash feed due to the ability to sustain conditioned feed temperatures for a prolonged period of time.[86] By utilizing a hygienizer, Boltz et al.[86] examined feed processing and the variation in reduction of the *Salmonella* surrogate (*E. faecium*) among feeds subjected to standard pelleting and more thermally aggressive pelleting. Boltz et al.[86] observed a 3-log reduction of *E. faecium* in typical pelleting and a 4-log reduction in more thermally aggressive pelleting. In addition, the more thermally aggressive pelleting reduced pellet mill motor load and increased hot pellet temperature and stability[86]. Boltz et al. (2019) concluded that utilization of more thermally aggressive pelleting may enhance manufacture effectiveness, pellet attributes, and reduce *Salmonella* concentration. Such technologies appear promising for decreasing *Salmonella* contamination, but follow-up studies with different *Salmonella* serovars will be critical given the variability in thermal tolerances among different serovars.[87,88] In addition, nutritional studies will need to be conducted to determine whether any decrease in nutritional quality results from the extended heat treatment of the feed mixtures.

While animal feed and *Salmonella* contamination have a long history of research and attempts to limit contamination, challenges remain. Given that there are over 2500 *Salmonella* distinct serotypes,[89] identifying individual serovars in the laboratory can be labor-intensive. This becomes critical since some of these serovars have been identified as primary causative agents for foodborne disease and/or have been identified with recent outbreaks, including *S. enterica* serovar Enteritidis, Typhimurium, Heidelberg, Reading, and Infantis, among others. Over the years, several serovars have been consistently detected in animal feeds, but sporadic appearances of other serovars also occur. Given a large number of serovars that potentially could contaminate feeds, isolation and identification of *Salmonella* from feeds have not been amendable to comprehensive survey analytics for in-depth tracking and interpretation. However, advances in detection methods and whole-genome sequencing have vastly improved both initial identification and tracking capabilities for identifying the culprit serovars and their respective strain variants responsible for specific salmonellosis outbreaks.[90] Some of these advanced methods have been recently employed for the identification of *Salmonella* from animal feeds. For example, based on clustered regularly interspaced short palindromic repeats (CRISPR) to molecular serotype *Salmonella* isolates from over 100 US feed mills, Shariat et al.[91] identified serovars *S.* Infantis and *S.* Tennessee as being the most commonly isolated serovars in the feed samples collected from these feed mills. These improved diagnostic tools offer the potential to better understand the role that *Salmonella* contaminated feed may play in the dissemination of specific serovars and strains in animal feed mill operations and feed distribution systems throughout animal production.

27.4.2 Campylobacter

According to the EFSA opinion from 2008,[2] *Campylobacter* is considered as one of the more common causes of foodborne diseases. This Gram-negative, thermophilic bacterium colonizes the intestinal mucosa of most warm-blooded hosts, including livestock and humans. It is commonly found in avian intestines.[92] Generally, in birds, *Campylobacter* spp. exist in a relatively asymptomatic type of relationship. Animal feed is not generally considered a primary vehicle for *Campylobacter* transmission since this microorganism survives poorly under dry environmental conditions such as the low water activity characteristic of dry feedstuffs.[1] In addition, its minimal resistance to disinfectants and heat would suggest a limited capability to survive under conditions associated with feed processing.[1,93] Therefore this pathogen has not been considered epidemiologically significant concerning feed production, storage, and distribution.[94,95]

However, the ability of *Campylobacter* to exist in a viable nonculturable state has been suggested as one avenue that *Campylobacter* could still be present in animal feed.[1,93] In accordance with this suggestion, *C. jejuni* has been shown to survive and sometimes grow when introduced into poultry feed matrices after storage of the feed for a few days.[83,96] In short, the lack of discovery of *Campylobacter* in routine feed sampling surveys may be a combination of it being viable but nonculturable under these conditions and lack of sufficiently sensitive detection technologies to detect low numbers of this pathogen. When detection and quantitation methodologies improve in their sensitivity for identifying viable *Campylobacter*, the role of animal feed in *Campylobacter* dissemination may need to be re-assessed and interpretations modified accordingly.

27.4.3 Listeria monocytogenes

L. monocytogenes is a ubiquitous microorganism that can be isolated from soil, water, sewage, and forage and can grow over a wide range of temperatures from $-1.5°C$ to $45°C$.[97] Occasionally, this pathogen has also been detected in different food animal species, resulting in contaminated meat products. Most animals are asymptomatic intestinal carriers.[98,99] However, listeriosis's clinical symptoms have been described sporadically in various ruminant species.[1,100,101] *L. monocytogenes* prevalence in animal feed generally occurs relatively infrequently in low water activity animal feeds such as hay and cereal grains.[102] However, *Listeria* spp. have been detected in poultry feeds before and after heat treatment.[52,103,104] Whyte et al. (2003)[52] observed that much of the feed mill's environment was contaminated with *Listeria* spp., which could suggest that recontamination of pelleted feed may also occur.

Listeria have been isolated from silages fed to ruminants, and there are several factors such as pH and silage quality that may contribute to its prevalence.[1] The occurrence of *L. monocytogenes* in silages has been linked to listeriosis in cattle, sheep, and goats.[1,105–107] There is also evidence of an association between spoiled silage and listeriosis in livestock.[108] For example, the higher risk of *L. monocytogenes* in raw milk was noted when cattle were fed with silage held at pH 4 and above.[108] It would be of interest to further characterize silage management and the likelihood of *Listeria* becoming established in the silage matrix. Factors that may need to be considered include sources that could potentially introduce *Listeria* to silage during the ensiling process and conditions that encourage its proliferation during the fermentation. It would also be of interest to determine if certain silage microbial community members are potentially inhibitory to *Listeria* and if management strategies could be developed to support these antagonistic microorganisms.

27.5 Pathogenic Escherichia coli

E. coli O157:H7 is also considered by EFSA as a critical zoonotic agent which is rarely detected in feed.[78] STEC strains can be harbored in cattle and represent a high potential for transmission to humans in beef products such as ground beef.[15] The serotype *E. coli* O157:H7 is one of the leading causes of hemorrhagic colitis and hemolytic-uremic syndrome in humans.[109] It has been suggested that *E. coli* O157 could be transmitted through feed and thus be a potential source of this pathogen in cattle.[110–112] According to Hancock et al.[113] 0.5% of purchased feed stored at the farm was positive for *E. coli* O157:H7 that was able to multiply in the presence of sufficient humidity.[50,102] Also, some reports have indicated that the time and temperatures used in commercial pelleting processes are insufficient to inactivate *E. coli* O157:H7.[114] It would be of interest to screen animal feeds for other pathogenic *E. coli* serovars besides *E. coli* O157:H7 since several pathogenic *E. coli* serovars are known to be associated with ruminants.[15] It is conceivable that other *E. coli* serovars may possess properties that would allow them to survive in animal feed consumed by ruminant animals.

27.5.1 Clostridia

Clostridium spp. are comprised of anaerobic Gram-positive bacteria producing highly resistant spores that are difficult to eliminate during animal feed production. Spores are particularly a problem for animal feeds that are thermally processed and likely to resist other antimicrobial treatments such as acids.[1] Clostridia are ubiquitous in the environment and mainly present in the top layers of soils and dust, water, and digestive tracts of humans and animals.[115] Also, radical inactivation methods of processing such as soybean extraction with hexane, toasting soybean meal, or thermal treatment of meat in the oven are not sufficient to inactivate all spores.[116] Many clostridial strains can survive temperatures up to 80°C; therefore an optimal temperature of 83°C for pelleting of feed should be sufficient to destroy spores,[117] but would likely depend on time of exposure and other potential factors. According to Prió et al.,[118] little or no correlation has been observed between clostridial contamination levels in feed materials and animal feeds prepared from them (in the form of a meal or pellet).

Conventional pelleting may not be sufficient to effectively control the contamination level of clostridia and would likely depend on temperature and other factors. Moreover, additional contamination may occur during further processing. Most clostridial strains are saprophytes; however, some of them could be pathogenic to humans and animals.[119] *C. perfringens* and *Clostridium botulinum* strains are of the most significant concern regarding feed hygiene and epidemiological significance.[120] Ricke[93] suggested that preventing spore formation initially and minimizing numbers of the spore formers represents a practical overall management strategy. To avoid formation spores, antimicrobial interventions that target vegetative cells could be potentially administered.[93] It would be presumed that some (or at least a few) of the antimicrobial agents already being used during feed processing and manufacture could be potential candidates. However, concentrations and timing of application for limiting *Clostridia* spp. specifically would need to be determined to optimize efficacy against these microorganisms.

C. perfringens can be isolated from the environment, feed, and water.[121] Frequently it is transmitted to feed in the form of vegetative cells or thermoresistant spores and is particularly prevalent in soil-contaminated feed materials, for example, root crops.[122] This species is capable of producing up to 30 toxins, and its strains are classified into seven categories (A–G) according to the combination of the significant toxins α, β, ι, ϵ, *C. perfringens* enterotoxin, and necrotic enteritis B-like (NetB) they produce.[123] Besides the listed major toxins, numerous minor ones can be produced by this microorganism as well.

Among feed materials, animal proteins and compound feeds usually are more likely to be contaminated frequently with *C. perfringens*,[122] and higher contamination levels have been observed.[124] *C. perfringens* commonly occurs in the intestinal tracts of livestock (75%–95% of broilers chickens).[121] This bacterium is considered an opportunistic pathogen, and its occurrence is not obviously associated with disease occurrence; therefore expression of pathogenicity of these microorganisms remains unclear.[121,125,126] However, feed contamination by *C. perfringens* has been associated with fowl necrotic enteritis outbreaks.[127,128] One study included four pig farms with higher mortality for necrotic enteritis observed in piglets.[129] *C. perfringens* type A has also been considered an indigenous microorganism in the digestive tract of cattle.[130]

It should be noted that *C. perfringens* type A pathogenesis may depend on physiological predisposing factors during host exposure.[130] This may include predisposing factors such as intestinal damage caused by coccidial pathogens in poultry.[121] Type A has been associated with several cattle diseases, such as clostridial enteritis in neonates, where calves afflicted with hemorrhagic abomasitis or abomasal ulceration are frequently observed.[130] Hemorrhagic enteritis in adult cattle and calves can also occur, while in some cases type A hemorrhagic enteritis and sudden death in veal calves occurred during specific feeding times.[130] Some *C. perfringens* type A isolates that possess the ability to produce β2-toxin can develop (along with α-toxin) hemorrhagic lesions in the small intestine such as those that occur in bovine enterotoxemia. Isolates of *C. perfringens* type A have also been suggested to cause jejunal hemorrhage syndrome (JHS) in beef and dairy cattle. However, further experiments on reproducing JHS from this microorganism were not sufficiently convincing, suggesting that the possibility exists of other contributing or predisposing factors being present in the etiology of this disease. The recently described toxin type G can produce NetB toxin and may play an essential role in necrotic enteritis in broiler chickens.[130]

C. botulinum is a pathogen that is able to produce one of the most potent toxins (BoNTs) known to occur in the environment. Botulism occurs among various animal species; however, it has been frequently observed in cattle and is caused by BoNT/C and D or its mosaic variants. According to Moeller et al.,[131] the median toxic dose (MTD50) of BoNT/C for cattle is 0.388 ng/kg (3.88 mouse lethal doses/kg). This indicates that cattle are 12.88 times more sensitive to BoNT/C than mice on a per-kilogram weight basis. Botulism cases in cattle are generally sporadic, but when they do occur they can be economically severe.[132] They are primarily associated with feeding haylage or silage contaminated by this microorganism or BoNT/C, D or its mosaic variants.[132] Botulism cases have been linked to feeding with insufficiently acidified silage contaminated with *C. botulinum* from the soil or ingestion of silage made from contaminated brewers' grain. Spreading of contaminated poultry litter on pasture can also be a source of cattle botulism as well as contamination of inside layers of silage bales via contact with bird or small ruminant carcasses.[124] Large outbreaks of botulism have also been observed in fur animals resulting from *C. botulinum* multiplication in the slaughterhouse by-products that are used for feeding these animals.[133].

C. botulinum as a species is characterized by considerable genetic diversity, especially in strains classified in group III that are responsible for most of the cattle botulism outbreaks.[134] In the past few decades, an increasing number of botulism D and mosaic D/C linked outbreaks associated with direct contact with poultry litter have been reported involving spores of type D, D/C (which possesses a gene encoding for two-thirds of the type D toxin and gene encoding for one-third of the type C toxin).[135]. It has been hypothesized that *C. botulinum* group III could have originally been in poultry litter because of its known asymptomatic carriage in animals.[135] Litter material containing the spores or the BoNTs could, in turn, be dispersed in the silage pasture via wind, runoff water, or scavengers. It appears that poultry are less susceptible than cattle to type D botulism[135] and the mosaic D/C form. Asymptomatic carriage of type D and its mosaic variant is still hypothetical and remains the focus of ongoing investigations and further interpretation. It would appear reasonable to advise from a farm management standpoint that safe storage and proper disposal of poultry and ruminant litter be practiced in order to prevent cattle botulism outbreaks.[136]

27.6 Fungi

In addition to bacteria, fungi in the feed are also of considerable concern for feed quality and potential animal health related to mycotoxin production and development of strategies for detoxifying animal feeds.[1,137] Several distinct taxonomic groups of fungi can be associated with animal feeds. Feedstuff contamination with fungi and their spores has been the subject of several literature reports.[138–141] According to a report by Hegazy et al.,[141] primary molds observed in ruminant feeds are *Penicillium* spp., *Aspergillus flavus*, *Cladosporium* spp., *Mucor* spp., *Trichoderma* spp., *Aspergillus niger*, *Alternaria* spp., *Rhizopus* spp., *Fusarium* spp., *Aspergillus fumigatus*, and *Aspergillus terreus*. Cegielska-Radziejewska et al.[139] reported that the most common genera of fungi detected in poultry feed included *Aspergillus*, *Rhizopus*, and *Mucor*.

Fungi are widely distributed in soil, air, plant material, and the mycotoxins produced by them cause serious hygienic risk for livestock consuming commercial animal feeds that are contaminated with these toxins.[138,140] In addition, fungal spores from feed and feed material such as moldy hay, silage, brewers' grain, and sugar-beets if inhaled and consumed, could cause various mycoses such as ringworm and mycotic abortion (in cattle).[138–140] However, some fungi have been utilized as probiotics and exhibit a beneficial impact on animal health, for example, *Saccharomyces cerevisiae*, *Aspergillus oryzae*, *Pleurotus* spp., *Antrodia cinnamomea*, and *Cordyceps militaris*.[142] These fungi are rich in functional components such as glucans, polysaccharides, polyphenols, triterpenes, ergosterol, adenosine, and laccases, which play an essential role immune system regulation.[142]

27.7 Antibiotic-resistant bacteria in feed

The prevalence and antimicrobial sensitivity of foodborne pathogens and indicator microorganisms in animal feed is not well understood.[45] Hofacre et al.[35] observed that 85% of the poultry and meat and bone meal samples contained bacteria resistant to amoxicillin, ampicillin, clavulanic acid, and cephalothin. Ge et al.[45] reported that 201 feed ingredient samples from animal and plant by-products of the 74 recovered *Salmonella* isolates were pan-susceptible to 17 tested antimicrobials. In addition, *E. coli* and *Enterococcus* isolates exhibited antimicrobial resistance to five tested antimicrobials. Furthermore, resistance rates were higher among isolates recovered from by-products of animal origin than of plant. These facts suggest that although the prevalence of *Salmonella*, *E. coli*, and *Enterococcus* is common in animal feed ingredients, antimicrobial resistance is not typically observed at high frequencies.[45]

Where antibiotic resistance may originate remains unclear. Likewise, whether feed plays a role remains unknown as well or if medicated feeds serve as a potential selective agent for antibiotic-resistant bacteria. Animal studies involving unmedicated feeds may offer some insight.

For example, in a pasture flock surveillance study, Melendez et al.[143] characterized 59 *Salmonella* isolates from various farm places, such as animal feed and water, and from retail carcasses attained from a resident natural foods store and a manufacturing plant. The majority of the isolated *Salmonella* serotypes were *S.* Kentucky (53%), *S.* Enteritidis (24%), *S.* Barely (10%), *S.* Mbandaka (7%), *S.* Montevideo (5%), and *S.* Newport (2%). However, although originating from antibiotic-free production systems, all isolates were resistant to sulfixasole and novobiocin, a few were additionally resistant to other antibiotics, and most isolates contained class I integrons. Based on this, it is difficult to conclude where the antibiotic resistance occurring in these isolates from antibiotic free husbandry practices may have originated and if feed had any impact. Comparative additional studies need to be conducted using medicated versus unmedicated feeds and comparing the antibiotic-resistant microbial profiles from the respective feed microbial populations.

Salmonella in feeds may not be the only organism possessing antibiotic resistance. Other microorganisms present in animal feeds could also present antibiotic resistance issues that may be a concern as well. For example, *Enterococcus* spp. have also been isolated and characterized from poultry feeds.[104,144] *Enterococci* have commonly been used as probiotics in food production but also account for over 10% of nosocomial infection in the United States, causing bacteremia, endocarditis, and other diseases with *E. faecalis* and *E. faecium* being responsible for the majority of these infections.[145,146] Notably, in the last 10 years, *E. faecium* has become more conspicuous in part due to its acquired drug resistance.[147]

Generally, *Enterocci* attain drug resistance by horizontal gene transfer of plasmids or transposons or via point mutation.[147] In addition, *Enterococci* are resistant to various stresses, including mild heat and a wide variety of antibiotics, specifically vancomycin, which is a significant concern.[148,149] Thus it is essential to identify plausible reservoirs of enterococci to control potential contamination with these bacteria. The incidence and significance of particular plasmids in *Enterococci* and their function in propagating antibacterial resistance among *Enterococci* in animals and feed has not been established.[147] Moreover, the research remains at a disadvantage because of the lack of a standardized categorization system applied in surveys and epidemiological studies.[147]

27.8 Conclusions and future directions

The ecology of microbial feed contamination remains a highly complex and still largely uncharacterized microbial ecosystem. Given the wide range of potential environmental sources for microbial contaminants that can come in contact with animal feed both from the multitude of ingredients, cross-contamination at the feed mill, and during transportation to the farm, it would be anticipated that a fairly wide range of different microorganisms could be present in the feed matrices. Many animal feed microbial communities are relatively benign and would have minimal impact on the animal consuming the feed. However, some of these microorganisms would be considered pathogenic and could colonize the animal consuming the feed. In some cases, this could lead to systemic infection and result in infectious diseases occurring in the animal.

Animal feeds have been identified as sources for several pathogens, including *Listeria*, Clostridia, pathogenic *E. coli*, and *Salmonella*. Probably the best-documented and most common pathogen associated with animal feeds is *Salmonella*. *Salmonella* spp. have been repeatedly isolated and identified from a wide range of animal feeds and feed ingredients. Numerous *Salmonella* serovars have been found in animal feeds, and specific serovars appear to occur more commonly as feed contaminants. Foodborne *Salmonella*'s presence in animal and poultry feed has been a public health concern from a food safety standpoint since food animals are known to be a reservoir for foodborne illness in humans. Consequently, numerous attempts have been made over the years to devise and implement antimicrobials that limit and reduce the level of *Salmonella* contamination in feed. Along with chemical-based interventions, heat treatment application during animal feed processing has been promoted to reduce *Salmonella* levels in feeds. However, more research is needed as *Salmonella* can elicit antimicrobial and thermal resistance responses, which can vary among serovars.

Historically, characterization of microorganisms in animal feeds has been primarily culture-based, resulting in limited ability to fully catalog animal feed microbial community taxonomies. This, in part, is no doubt due to the emphasis on just a few of the feed microorganisms present that are of primary concern, such as the foodborne pathogen *Salmonella*. However, the sampling logistics for acquiring sufficient samples from large batches of commercial feed prohibit retrieving representative numbers of samples that can capture the relatively infrequent occurrence of *Salmonella* in these massive volumes of animal feeds generated at the feed mill.[1] As a result, *Salmonella* spp. may very well be at too low a population level to base antimicrobial efficacy only on their detection and quantitation, and this in turn becomes a challenge for designing the practical implementation of feed interventions. Consequently, other microbial methods and strategies are needed to assess the potential impact of interventions on pathogens such as *Salmonella*. Therefore the identification of nonpathogenic indicator microorganisms that mimic the pathogen's behavior, but can occur at much higher and more consistent levels represents an alternative approach that should provide sufficient baseline data for evaluation of antimicrobial efficacy.

Traditionally, the choice of an indicator microorganism in feeds would be based on other nonfeed microbial ecosystems. However, these indicator microorganisms would not necessarily represent microorganisms that are likely present on a feed. Therefore different approaches are needed to identify optimal indicator microorganisms that are more reflective of the feed microbial community and parallel *Salmonella* and other pathogens of interest as they would potentially exist in feeds. The emergence and adoption of 16S rDNA microbiome sequencing has provided a means to conduct a comprehensive survey of microbial communities in complex microbial ecosystems such as the gastrointestinal tract of animals, food production, and humans.[150] While only limited studies have used microbiome characterization in animal feeds,[1,83,84] there is an opportunity to profile shifts in microbial populations in response to the application of various interventions and compare those responses to the impact on *Salmonella* and other pathogens in these same feed matrices. Such an approach would seem to offer a more precise means to predict the efficacy of a particular antimicrobial or other feed processing steps during feed manufacturing. Before this can become a standard approach, more microbiome characterization of a wide range of animal feeds must be conducted to establish core or signature microbial populations that might be characteristic of different feed types and feed ingredients. Once such data baselines are assembled, the compiled information can be used to standardize microbial quality expectations for individual feeds and feed mill operations.

References

1. Ricke SC. Chapter 8. Feed hygiene. In: Dewulf J, Van Immerseel F, eds. *Biosecurity in Animal Production and Veterinary Medicine – From Principles to Practice*. Leuven: ACCO (Academische Coöperative Vennootschap cvba); 2018: 177–209.
2. EFSA. European Commission on Microbiological Risk Assessment in feeding stuffs for food-producing animals – Scientific Opinion of the Panel on Biological Hazards on a request from the Health and Consumer Protection Directorate General. *EFSA J*. 2008;720:1–84.
3. EFSA. The community summary report on trends and sources of zoonoses, zoonotic agents, antimicrobial resistance and foodborne outbreaks in the European Union in 2007. *EFSA J*. 2009;223. Accessed 04.02.21.
4. EFSA. The community summary report on foodborne outbreaks in the European Union in 2007. *EFSA J*. 2009;271. Accessed 04.02.21.
5. Wales AD, Allen VM, Davies RH. Chemical treatment of animal feed and water for the control of *Salmonella*. *Foodborne Path Dis*. 2010;7:1–15.
6. Maciorowski KG, Herrera P, Jones FT, et al. Effects of poultry and livestock feed with bacteria and fungi. *Anim Feed Sci Technol*. 2007;133:109–136.
7. Williams JE. Salmonellas in poultry feeds – a worldwide review. Part I. Introduction. *World's Poult Sci J*. 1981;37:6–19.
8. Maciorowski KG, Jones FT, Pillai SD, et al. Incidence and control of food-borne *Salmonella* spp. in poultry feeds – a review. *World's Poult Sci J*. 2004;60:446–457.
9. Ricke SC. Insights and challenges of *Salmonella* infections in laying hens. *Curr Opin Food Sci*. 2017;18:43–49.
10. Einstein-Curtis A. USDA: US feed use, animal production is expected to grow. <https://www.feednavigator.com/Article/2020/01/22/USDA-US-feed-use-animal-production-expected-to-grow>; Published 2020 Accessed 01.02.21.
11. Koeleman E. Insight into the US animal feed market. <https://www.allaboutfeed.net/animal-feed/feed-processing/insight-into-the-us-animal-feed-market/>; Published 2018 Accessed 29.03.21.
12. Dittoe DK, Ricke SC, Kiess AS. Chapter 1. Commercial poultry production and gut function – historical perspective. pp. 3–30. In S.C. Ricke (Ed.) *Improving Gut Function in Poultry*. Burleigh Dodd Publishing, Cambridge; 2006.
13. Van Houte G. Reducing the risk of Salmonella re-contamination feed. <https://www.poultryworld.net/Health/Articles/2020/4/Reducing-the-risk-of-salmonella-re-contamination-in-feed-566977E/>; Published 2020 Accessed 02.02.21.
14. Crump JA, Griffin PM, Angulo FJ. Bacterial contamination of animal feed and its relationship to human foodborne illness. *Clin Infect Dis*. 2002;35(7):859–865. Available from: https://doi.org/10.1086/342885.
15. Baker CA, Rubinelli PM, Park SH, et al. Shiga toxin-producing *Escherichia coli* in food: incidence, ecology, and detection strategies. *Food Control*. 2016;59:407–419.
16. Magwedere K, Rauff D, De Klerk G, et al. Incidence of nontyphoidal *Salmonella* in food-producing animals, animal feed, and the associated environment in South Africa, 2012–2014. *Clin Infect Dis*. 2015;61(4):S283–S289. Available from: https://doi.org/10.1093/cid/civ663.
17. Mead PS, Slutsker L, Dietz V, et al. Food-related illness and death in the United States. *Emerg Infect Dis*. 1999;15:607–625.
18. Food and Drug Administration (FDA). Compliance program guidance manual. <https://www.fda.gov/media/74766/download>; Published 2010 Accessed 24.03.21.
19. Gong C, Jiang X. Characterizing *Salmonella* contamination in two rendering processing plants. *J Food Prot*. 2017;80(2):265–270. Available from: https://doi.org/10.4315/0362-028X.JFP-16-210.
20. Chae MS, Schraft H. Comparative evaluation of adhesion and biofilm formation of different *Listeria monocytogenes* strains. *Int J Food Microbiol*. 2000;62(1–2):103111.

21. Doyle MP, Beuchat LR, Montville TJ. *Food microbiology: fundamentals and frontiers*. 2nd ed. Washington, DC: ASM Press; 2001.
22. Kumar CG, Anand SK. Significance of microbial biofilms in food industry: a review. *Int J Food Microbiol*. 1998;42(1–2):927.
23. Muckey M, Huss AR, Yoder A, et al. Research note: evaluating the roles of surface sanitation and feed sequencing on mitigating *Salmonella* Enteritidis contamination on animal food manufacturing equipment. *Poult Sci*. 2020;99(8):3841–3845. Available from: https://doi.org/10.1016/j.psj.2020.04.016.
24. Gebhardt JT, Woodworth JC, Jones CK, et al. Evaluating the impact of VevoVitall and/or CRINA as potential porcine epidemic diarrhea virus mitigation strategies as determined by polymerase chain reaction analysis and bioassay. 2016 Kansas State University Swine Day. *KS Agric Exp Stn Res Rep*. 2016;2:8.
25. Huss AR, Cochrane RA, Deliephan A, et al. Evaluation of a biological pathogen decontamination protocol for animal feed mills. *J Food Prot*. 2015;78:1682–1688.
26. Okuma TA, Hellberg RS. Identification of meat species in pet foods using a real-time polymerase chain reaction (PCR) assay. *Food Control*. 2015;50:9–17.
27. American Feed Industry Association. (AFIA). How feed is made. <https://www.afia.org/feedfacts/how-feed-is-made/>; Published 2021 Accessed 04.02.21.
28. WATTPoultry.com. Even safer feed: validating cross-contamination control. <https://www.wattagnet.com/articles/186-even-safer-feed-validating-cross-contamination-control>; Published 2021 Accessed 04.02.21.
29. North American Renderers Association (NARA). Sustainability. <https://nara.org/sustainability/>; Published 2020 Accessed 02.02.20.
30. Kinley B, Rieck J, Dawson P, et al. Analysis of *Salmonella* and enterococci isolated from rendered animal products. *Can J Microbiol*. 2010;56:65–73.
31. Swisher K. The global market for rendered products. In *Essential Rendering: All About Animals By-products Industry*. Edited by D. L. Meeker. Kirby Lithographic Company Inc., Arlington, VA. 2006;pp. 213229.
32. Meeker DL, Hamilton CR. An overview of the rendering industry. In *Essential Rendering: All About the Animal By-products Industry*. Edited by D.L. Meeker. Kirby Lithographic Company Inc., Arlington, VA. 2006; pp.117.
33. CRS Report for Congress. Animal rendering: economics and policy. <https://www.everycrsreport.com/files/20040317_RS21771_99c9bda76377d8e94144ca033cb5f43b57f1dde7.pdf>; Published 2004 Accessed 13.03.21.
34. Yang L, Tan Z, Wang D, et al. Species identification through mitochondrial rRNA genetic analysis. *Sci Rep*. 2014;4:4089. Available from: https://doi.org/10.1038/srep04089.
35. Hofacre CL, White DG, Maurer JJ, et al. Characterization of antibiotic-resistant bacteria in rendered animal products. *Avian Dis*. 2001;45(4):953961.
36. Schwalbe RS, McIntosh AC, Qaiyumi S, et al. Isolation of vancomycin-resistant enterococci from animal feed in USA. *Lancet*. 1999;353(9154):722.
37. Cullen, P., Mcdermott, S.D., Carter, P.J., Paige, J.C., and Wagner, D.D. 2003. Prevalence and antibiotic susceptibility profiles of Enterococcus spp. recovered from rendered animal feed commodities: results of a national survey [online]. 2003 FDA Science Forum Poster Abstract Board H-01. 24–25 April 2003. Washington, D.C. Available from http://www.accessdata.fda.gov/scienceforums/forum03/H-01.htm
38. McAuley C.M., Gobius K.S., Britz M.L., Craven H.M., Heat resistance of thermoduric enterococci isolated from milk. Int J Food Microbiol. 2012;154(3):162-8. Available from: https://doi.org/10.1016/j.ijfoodmicro.2011.12.033. Epub 2012 Jan 3. PMID: 22260926.
39. Loken KI, Culbert KH, Solee RE, Pomeroy BS. Microbiological quality of protein feed supplements produced by rendering plants. *Appl Microbiol*. 1968;1:1002–1005.
40. Troutt HF, Schaeffer D, Kakoma I, et al. Director's Digest #312 *Prevalence of Selected Foodborne Pathogens in Final Rendered Products: Pilot Study*. Fats and Proteins Research Foundation, Inc.; 2001.
41. Meat Research Corporation. *Prevention of Post-processing Contamination of Stock Meal with Salmonella and Other Pathogens*. Sydney, NSW: Australian Meat Corporation; 1997.
42. Sapkota AR, Lefferts LY, McKinzie S, et al. What do we feed food-production animals? A review of animal feed ingredients and their potential impacts on human health. *Environ Health Perspect*. 2007;115(5):663–670.
43. Li J, Wang T, Shao B, et al. Plasmid-mediated quinolone resistance genes and antibiotic residues in wastewater and soil adjacent to swine feedlots: potential transfer to agricultural lands. *Environ Health Perspect*. 2012;120(8):1144–1149. Available from: http://doi.org/10.1289/ehp.1104776.
44. Li X, Bethune LA, Jia Y, et al. Surveillance of *Salmonella* prevalence in animal feeds and characterization of the *Salmonella* isolates by serotyping and antimicrobial susceptibility. *Foodborne Pathog Dis*. 2012;9(8):692–698. Available from: https://doi.org/10.1089/fpd.2011.1083.
45. Ge B, LaFon PC, Peggy J, Carter SD, et al. Retrospective analysis of *Salmonella, Campylobacter, Escherichia coli*, and *Enterococcus* in animal feed ingredients. *Foodborne Pathog Dis*. 2013;10(8):684–691.
46. Papadopoulou C, Carrique-Mas JJ, Davies RH, et al. Retrospective analysis of *Salmonella* isolates recovered from animal feed in Great Britain. *Vet Rec*. 2009;165:681–688.
47. Veldman A, Vahl HA, Borggreve GJ, et al. A survey of the incidence of *Salmonella* species and Enterobacteriaceae in poultry feeds and feed components. *Vet Rec*. 1995;136:169–172.
48. McChesney D.G., FDA survey results: *Salmonella* contamination of finished feed and primary meal ingredients. Presented at Feed Safety Committee of the United States Animal HealthAssociation, 99th Annual Meeting, Reno, Nevada, 1995
49. D'Mello JPF. Assessing quality and safety of animal feeds [Contaminants and toxins in animal feed]. Scottish Agricultural College (SAC) in Edinburgh, United Kingdom. http://www.fao.org/tempref/docrep/fao/007/y5159e/y5159e04.pdf>; Published 2007 Accessed 04.03.21.
50. Lynn TV, Hancock DD, Besser TE, et al. The occurrence and replication of *Escherichia coli* in cattle feeds. *J Dairy Sci*. 1998;81:1102–1108.
51. Jeffrey JS, Kirk JH, Atwill ER, et al. Research notes: prevalence of selected microbial pathogens in processed poultry waster used as dairy cattle feed. *Poult Sci*. 1988;77(6):808–811.
52. Whyte P, McGill K, Collins JD. A survey of the prevalence of *Salmonella* and other enteric pathogens in a commercial poultry feed mill. *J Food Saf*. 2003;23:13–24.

53. Davis MA, Hancock DD, Rice DH, et al. Feedstuffs as a vehicle of cattle exposure to *Escherichia coli* O157:H7 and *Salmonella enterica*. *Vet Microbiol.* 2003;95:199–210.
54. Anderson RJ, Walker RL, Hird DW, Blanchard PC. Case-control study of an outbreak of clinical disease attributable to *Salmonella* Menhaden infection in eight dairy herds. *J Am Vet Med Assoc.* 1997;210:528–530.
55. Glickman LT, McDonough PL, Shin SJ, et al. Bovine salmonellosis attributed to *Salmonella* Anatum-contaminated haylage and dietary stress. *J Am Vet Med Assoc.* 1981;1981(17):1268–1272.
56. Boyer CI, Bruner DW, Brown JA. *Salmonella* organisms isolated from poultry feed. *Avian Dis.* 1958;2:396–401.
57. Zecha BC, McCapes RH, Dungan WH, et al. The Dillon Beach Project: a five-year epidemiological study of naturally occurring *Salmonella* infection in turkeys and their environment. *Avian Dis.* 1977;21:141–159.
58. Boyer CI, Narotsky S, Bruner DW. Salmonellosis in turkeys and chickens associated with contaminated feed. *Avian. Dis.* 1962;6:43–50.
59. Wigley P. *Salmonella enterica* in the chicken: how it has helped our understanding of immunology in a non-biomedical model species. *Front Immunol.* 2014;5:482. Available from: https://doi.org/10.3389/fimmu.2014.00482.
60. Breuer T, Benkel DH, Shapiro RL, et al. A multistate outbreak of *Escherichia coli* O157:H7 infections linked to alfalfa sprouts grown from contaminated seeds. *Emerg Infect Dis.* 2001;7:977–982.
61. Shiferaw B, Yang S, Cieslak P, et al. Prevalence of high-risk food consumption and food-handling practices among adults: a multistate survey, 1996 to 1997. *J Food Prot.* 2000;63:1538–1543.
62. Food Safety News (FSN). Nearly half of people risk illness from undercooked burgers. <https://www.foodsafetynews.com/2020/07/nearly-half-of-people-risk-illness-from-undercooked-burgers/>; Published 2020 Accessed 01.02.21.
63. Food Safety News (FSN). CDC shares data on *E. coli* and *Salmonella* in beef. <https://www.foodsafetynews.com/2014/10/cdc-shares-mass-of-data-on-e-coli-and-salmonella-in-beef/>; Published 2014 Accessed 01.02.21.
64. Mead PS, Griffin PM. *Escherichia coli* O157:H7. *Lancet.* 1998;352:1207–1212.
65. Pennington JH, Brooksbank NH, Pool PM, et al. *Salmonella* Virchow in a chicken-packing station and associated rearing units. *Br Med J.* 1968;4:804–806.
66. Semple AB, Turner GC, Lowry DM. Outbreak of food poisoning caused by *Salmonella virchow* in spit-roasted chicken. *Br Med J.* 1968;4:801–803.
67. Clark GM, Kaufmann AF, Gangarosa EJ, et al. Epidemiology of an international outbreak of *Salmonella* Agona. *Lancet.* 1973;2:490–493.
68. Ferrari RG, Rosario DKA, Cunha-Neto A, et al. Worldwide epidemiology of *Salmonella* serovars in animal-based foods: a meta-analysis. *Appl Environ Microbiol.* 2019;85(14). Available from: https://doi.org/10.1128/AEM.00591-1. e00591-19.
69. Hirsch W, Sapiro-Hirsch R. The role of certain animal feeding stuffs, especially bone meal, in the epidemiology of salmonellosis. *Bull Hyg.* 1958;33:647.
70. Knox WA, Galbraith NC, Lewis MJ, et al. A milkborne outbreak of food poisoning due to *Salmonella heidelberg*. *J Hyg.* 1963;61:175–185.
71. Gordon RF, Tucker JF. The epizootiology of *Salmonella menston* infection of fowls and the effect of feeding poultry food artificially infected with *Salmonella*. *Br Poult Sci.* 1965;6(3):251–264. Available from: https://doi.org/10.1080/00071666508415581.
72. Hinton M. *Salmonella* infection in chicks following the consumption of artificially contaminated feed. *Epidemiol Infect.* 1988;100(2):247–256. Available from: https://doi.org/10.1017/S0950268800067388.
73. Harris IT, Fedorka-Cray PJ, Gray JT, et al. Prevalence of *Salmonella* organisms in swine feed. *J Am Vet Med Assoc.* 1977;210(3):382–385.
74. Food and Drug Administration (FDA). Guidance for FDA staff. Compliance policy guide Sec. 690.800 Salmonella in food for animals. <https://www.fda.gov/media/86240/download#:~:text=FDA%20considers%20an%20animal%20feed,the%20FD%26C%20Act%20(21%20U.S.C.&text=Cases%20of%20contamination%20involving%20other,case%2Dby%2Dcase%20basis>; Published 2013 Accessed 29.03.21.
75. Park SY, Woodward CL, Kubena LF, et al. Environmental dissemination of foodborne *Salmonella* in preharvest poultry production: reservoirs, critical factors and research strategies. *Crit Rev Environ Sci Technol.* 2008;38:73–111.
76. European Food Safety Authority and European Centre for Disease Prevention and Control (EFSA and ECDC). The European Union One Health 2018 Zoonoses Report. *EFSA J.* 2019;17(12): e05926. Accessed 04.02.21.
77. Wierup M, Widell S. Estimation of costs for control of *Salmonella* in high-risk feed materials and compound feed. *Infect Ecol Epidemiol.* 2014;4. Available from: https://doi.org/10.3402/iee.v4.23496.
78. European Food Safety Authority (EFSA). . The European Union summary report on trends and sources of zoonoses, zoonotic agents and food-borne outbreaks in 2017. *EFSA J.* 2018;16(12):e05500. Available from: https://doi.org/10.2903/j.efsa.2018.5500.
79. Hacking WC, Mitchell WR, Carlson HC. *Salmonella* investigation in an Ontario feed mill. *Can J Comp Med.* 1977;42:400406.
80. Franco DA. A survey of *Salmonella* serovars and most probable number (MPN) in rendered animal protein meals: inferences for animal and human health. *J Environ Health.* 2005;67(6):18–22.
81. Laban SE, Moustafa GZ, Anwer W, et al. Microbial load of poultry by-products following rendering process. *Glob Vet.* 2014;12(6):756–759.
82. Liu S, Tang J, Tadapaneni RK, et al. Exponentially increased thermal resistance of *Salmonella* spp. and *Enterococcus faecium* at reduced water activity. *Appl Environ Microbiol.* 2018;84(8). Available from: https://doi.org/10.1128/AEM.02742-17.
83. Ricke SC, Dittoe DK, Richardson KE. Formic acid as an antimicrobial for poultry production: a review. *Front Vet Sci.* 2020;7:563. Available from: https://doi.org/10.3389/fvets.2020.00563.
84. Ricke SC, Richardson K, Dittoe DK. Formaldehydes in feeds and interaction with the poultry gastrointestinal tract microbial community. *Front Vet Sci.* 2019;6:188. Available from: https://doi.org/10.3389/fvets.2019.00188.
85. Dittoe DK, Ricke SC, Kiess AS. Organic acids and potential for modifying the avian gastrointestinal tract and reducing pathogens and disease. *Front Vet Sci.* 2018;5:216. Available from: https://doi.org/10.3389/fvets.2018.00216.

86. Boltz TP, Boney JW, Shen C, et al. The effect of standard pelleting and more thermally aggressive pelleting utilizing a hygieniser on feed manufacture and reduction of *Enterococcus faecium*, a *Salmonella* surrogate. *J Appl Poult Res.*. 2019;28:1226–1233. Available from: http://doi.org/10.3382/japr/pfz088.
87. Dawoud TM, Davis ML, Park SH, et al. *Salmonella* thermal resistance – molecular responses. *Front Vet Sci.* 2017;4:93. Available from: https://doi.org/10.33889/fvets.2017.00093.
88. Jarvis NA, O'Bryan CA, Dawoud TM, et al. An overview of *Salmonella* thermal destruction during food processing and preparation. *Food Control.* 2016;68:280–290.
89. Foley SL, Johnson TJ, Ricke SC, et al. *Salmonella* pathogenicity and host adaptation in chicken-associated serovars. *Microbiol Mol Biol Rev.* 2013;77:582–607.
90. Ricke SC, Kim SA, Park SH. Molecular-based identification and detection of *Salmonella* in food production systems: current perspectives. *J Appl Microbiol.* 2018;125:313–327.
91. Shariat NW, Feye KM, Richards AK, et al. Incidence of *Salmonella* serovars isolated from commercial animal feed mills in the United States and serovar identification using CRISPR analysis. *J Appl Microbiol.* 2020;. Available from: https://doi.org/10.1111/jam.14933.
92. Horrocks SM, Anderson RC, Nisbet DJ, et al. Incidence and ecology of *Campylobacter* in animals. *Anaerobe.* 2009;15:18–25.
93. Ricke SC. Chapter 7. Ensuring the safety of poultry feed. In: Mead GC, ed. *Food Safety Control in Poultry Industry.* Cambridge: Woodhead Publishing Limited; 2005:174–194.
94. Sörqvist S. Heat resistance in liquids of *Enterococcus* spp., *Listeria* spp., *Escherichia coli, Yersinia enterocolitica, Salmonella* spp. and *Campylobacter* spp. *Acta Vet Scand.* 2003;44(1):1–19.
95. Newell DG, Fearnley C. Sources of *Campylobacter* colonization in broiler chickens. *Appl Environ Microbiol.* 2003;69(8):4343–4351.
96. Alves MBR, Fonseca BB, Melo RT, Mendonça EP, et al. Feed can be a source of *Campylobacter jejuni* infection in broilers. *Br Poult Sci.* 2017;58:46–49. Available from: http://doi.org/10.1080/00071668.2016.1258691.
97. Lado BH, Yousef AE. Characteristics of *Listeria monocytogenes* important to food processors (Chapter 6) In: Ryser ET, Marth EH (eds) *Listeria, Listeriosis and Food Safety.* 3rd ed., CRC Press Taylor & Francis Group, Boca Raton, FL; 2007, 157–213.
98. CFSPH. Technical fact sheet. Listeriosis. The Center for Food Security& Public Health, Iowa State University. <https://www.cfsph.iastate.edu/FastFacts/pdfs/listeriosis_F.PDF>; Published 2006 Accessed 29.03.21.
99. Food and Drug Administration (FDA). Get the facts about Listeria. <https://www.fda.gov/animal-veterinary/animal-health-literacy/get-facts-about-listeria>; Published 2020 Accessed 29.03.21.
100. Anon. Enter-net annual report 2004; surveillance of enteric pathogens in Europe and beyond. Enter-Net <http://ecdc.europa.eu/documents/ENTER_NET/annual_report2004.pdf>; 2006.
101. Anon. *Salmonella* in livestock production in GB: 2005 report. Veterinary Laboratories Agency. <http://www.defra.gov.uk/corporate/vla/science/science-salm-rep05.htm>; 2006.
102. Fenlon DR, Wilson J. Growth of *Escherichia coli* O157 in poorly fermented laboratory silage: a possible environmental dimension in the epidemiology of *E. coli* O157. *Lett Appl Microbiol.* 2000;30:118–121.
103. Blank G, Savoie S, Campbell LD. . Microbiological decontamination of poultry feed-evaluation of steam conditioners. *J Sci Food Agric.* 1996;72:299–305.
104. Olson E, Micciche A, Sevigny J, et al. Draft genome sequences of 11 bacterial strains isolated from commercial corn-based poultry feed. *Microbiol Resour Announc.* 2020;9, e00170-20. Available from: https://doi.org/10.1128/MRA.00170-20.
105. Skovgaard N, Morgen CA. Detection of *Listeria* spp. in faeces from animals, in feeds, and in raw foods of animal origin. *Int J Food Microbiol.* 1988;6:229–242.
106. Wagner M, Melzner D, Bagò Z, et al. Outbreak of clinical listeriosis in sheep: evaluation from possible contamination routes from feed to raw produce and humans. *J Vet Med B.* 2005;52 (6):278–283. Available from: https://doi.org/10.1111/j.1439-0450.2005.00866.x.
107. Nightingale KK, Schukken YH, Nightingale CR, et al. Ecology and transmission of *Listeria monocytogenes* infecting ruminants and in the farm environment. *Appl Environ Microbiol.* 2004;70: 4458–4467.
108. El Marnissi B, Bennani L, Cohen N, et al. Presence of *Listeria monocytogenes* in raw milk and traditional dairy products marketed in the north-central region of Morocco. *Afr J Food Sci.* 2013;7(5):87–91.
109. Kutkowska J, Michalska-Szymaszek M, Matuszewska R, et al. Cell-surface antigens and virulence factors of *Escherichia coli* O157. *Adv Microbiol.* 2015;54(1):53–64.
110. Sargeant JM, Gillespie JR, Oberst RD, et al. Results of a longitudinal study of the prevalence of *Escherichia coli* O157:H7 on cow-calf farms. *Am J Vet Res.* 2000;61:1375–1379.
111. Dargatz DA, Wells SJ, Thomas LA, et al. Factors associated with the presence of *Escherichia coli* O157 in feces of feedlot cattle. *J Food Prot.* 1997;60:466–470.
112. Dodd CC, Sanderson MW, Sargeant JM, et al. Prevalence of *Escherichia coli* O157 in cattle feeds in midwestern feedlots. *Appl Environ Microbiol.* 2003;69(9):5243–5247. Available from: https://doi.org/10.3390/antibiotics8020059.
113. Hancock D, Besser T, Lejeune J, et al. The control of VTEC in the animal reservoir. *Int J Food Microbiol.* 2001;66:71–78.
114. Hutchison ML, Thomas DJI, Avery SM. Thermal death of *Escherichia coli* O157:H7 in cattle feeds. *Lett Appl Microbiol.* 2007;44:357–363.
115. Bintsis T. Foodborne pathogens. *AIMS Microbiol.* 2017;3 (3):529–563. Available from: https://doi.org/10.3934/microbiol.2017.3.529.
116. Frazier WC, Westhoff DC. *Food Microbiology.* 4th ed. New York: McGraw-Hill; 1988.
117. Furuta K, Oku I, Morimoto S. Effect of steam temperature in the pelleting process of chicken food on the viability of contaminating bacteria. *Lab Anim.* 1980;14:293–296.
118. Prió P, Gasol R, Soriano RC, et al. Effect of raw material microbial contamination over microbiological profile of ground and pelleted feeds. In: Brufan J, *Feed Manufacturing in the Mediterranean Region. Improving Safety: From Feed to Food,* CIHEAM, Zaragoza. 2001;197- 199.
119. Wells CL, Wilkins TD. Chapter 18 – *Clostridia*: sporeforming anaerobic bacilli. In: Baron S, ed. *Medical Microbiology.* 4th ed. Galveston, TX: University of Texas Medical Branch at Galveston; 1996. https://www.ncbi.nlm.nih.gov/books/NBK8219/.

120. Grenda T, Grabczak M, Kwiatek K, et al. Prevalence of *C. botulinum* and *C. perfringens* spores in food products available on Polish Market. *J Vet Res*. 2017;61(3):287–291. Available from: https://doi.org/10.1515/jvetres-2017-0038.
121. Van Immerseel F, De Buck J, Pasmans F, et al. *Clostridium perfringens* in poultry: an emerging threat for animal and public health. *Avian Pathol*. 2004;33(6):537–549.
122. Xylouri E, Papadopoulou C, Antoniadis G, et al. Rapid identification of *Clostridium perfringens* in animal feedstuffs. *Anaerobe*. 1997;3:191–193.
123. Kiu R, Hall LJ. An update on the human and animal enteric pathogen *Clostridium perfringens*. *Emerg Microbes Infect*. 2018;7:1–15. Available from: https://doi.org/10.1038/s41426-018-0144-8.
124. Relun A, Dorso L, Douart A, Chartier C, Guatteo R, Mazuet C, Popoff MR, Assié S. A large outbreak of bovine botulism possibly linked to a massive contamination of grass silage by type D/C Clostridium botulinum spores on a farm with dairy and poultry operations. Epidemiol Infect. 2017 Dec;145(16):3477–3485. https://doi.org/10.1017/S0950268817002382. Epub 2017 Nov 2. PMID: 29094676; PMCID: PMC9148736.
125. Songer JG. *Clostridial* enteric diseases of domestic animals. *Clin Microbiol Rev*. 1996;9(2):216–234.
126. Craven SE. Colonization of the intestinal tract by *Clostridium perfringens* and fecal shedding in diet-stressed and unstressed broiler chickens. *Poult Sci*. 2000;79(6):843–849. Available from: https://doi.org/10.1093/ps/79.6.843.
127. Dosoky RM. The role of environment in the occurrence of clostridial infection among fowl. *Assiut Vet Med J*. 1990;24 (47):165–171.
128. Frame DD, Bickford AA. An outbreak of coccidiosis and necrotic enteritis in 16-week-old cage-reared layer replacement pullets. *Avian Dis*. 1986;30(3):601–602.
129. Udovičić I. Necrotic enteritis in pigs: contamination of feed for sows with Clostridium perfringens. In: Proceedings of the *Thirteenth International Pig Veterinary Society Congress*. Bangkok, Thailand. June 1994; 26–30.
130. Goossens E, Valgaeren BR, Pardon B, et al. Rethinking the role of alpha toxin in *Clostridium perfringens*-associated enteric diseases: a review on bovine necro-haemorrhagic enteritis. *Vet Res*. 2017;48(9). Available from: https://doi.org/10.1186/s13567-017-0413-x.
131. Moeller Jr RB, Puschner B, Walker RL, et al. Determination of the median toxic dose of type *C. botulinum* toxin in lactating dairy cows. *J Vet Diagn Invest*. 2003;15:523–526.
132. Nakamura K, Kohda T, Umeda K, et al. Characterization of the D/C mosaic neurotoxin produced by *Clostridium botulinum* associated with bovine botulism in Japan. *Vet Microbiol*. 2010;140:147–154.
133. Lindström M, Nevas M, Kurki J, et al. Type C botulism due to toxic feed affecting 52,000 farmed foxes and minks in Finland. *J Clin Microbiol*. 2004;42(10):4718–4725.
134. Skarin H, Håfström T, Westerberg J, et al. *Clostridium botulinum* group III: a group with dual identity shaped by plasmids, phages and mobile elements. *BMC Genomics*. 2011;12:185. Available from: https://doi.org/10.1186/1471-2164-12-185.
135. Le Maréchal C, Woudstra C, Fach P. Botulism. In: Uzal FA, Songer JG, Prescott JF, Popoff MR, eds. *Clostridial Diseases of Animals*. Ames, IA: Blackwell Publishing; 2016:303–330.
136. Otter A, Livesey C, Hogg R, Gray D. Risk of botulism in cattle and sheep arising from contact with broiler litter. *Vet Rec*. 2006;159(6):186–187.
137. Oguz H. A review from experimental trials on detoxification of aflatoxin in poultry feed. *Eurasian J Vet Sci*. 2011;27:1–12.
138. Queiroz B, Pereyra CM, Keller KM, et al. Fungal contamination and determination of fumonisins and aflatoxins in commercial feeds intended for ornamental birds in Rio de Janeiro, Brazil. *Lett Appl Microbiol*. 2013;57(5):405–411. Available from: https://doi.org/10.1111/lam.12127.
139. Cegielska-Radziejewska R, Stuper K, Szablewski T. Microflora and mycotoxin contamination in poultry feed mixtures from western Poland. *Ann Agric Environ Med*. 2013;1:30–35.
140. Variane ACF, dos Santos FC, Fernandes de Castro F, et al. The occurrence of aflatoxigenic *Aspergillus* spp. in dairy cattle feed in Southern Brazil. *Braz J Microbiol*. 2018;49 (4):919–928.
141. Hegazy SMS, Hassan WH, Shawki HM, et al. Study on toxigenic fungi in ruminant feeds under desert conditions with special references to its biological control. *Beni-Suef Univ J Basic Appl Sci*. 2015;4:167–173.
142. Chuang WY, Hsieh YC, Lee TT. The effects of fungal feed additives in animals: a review. *Animals (Basel)*. 2020;10(5):805. Available from: https://doi.org/10.3390/ani10050805.
143. Melendez SN, Hanning I, Han J, et al. *Salmonella enterica* isolates from pasture-raised poultry exhibit antimicrobial resistance and class I integrons. *J Appl Microbiol*. 2010;109:1957–1966. Available from: https://doi.org/10.1111/j.1365-2672.2010.04825.x.
144. Olson EG, Dittoe DK, Micciche AC, et al. Identification of bacterial isolates from commercial poultry feed via 16S rDNA. *J Environ Sci Health B*. 2021;56:272–281. Available from: https://doi.org/10.1080/03601234.2020.1868236.
145. Franz CMAP, Stiles ME, Schleifer KH, et al. Enterococci in foods a conundrum for food safety. *Int J Food Microbiol*. 2003;88 (2–3):105122.
146. Bhonchal Bhardwaj S. Enterococci: an important nosocomial pathogen. In: Kırmusaoğlu S, Bhonchal Bhardwaj S, eds. *Pathogenic Bacteria*. IntechOpen; 2019. Available from: https://doi.org/10.5772/intechopen.90550. Available from: <https://www.intechopen.com/books/pathogenic-bacteria/enterococci-an-important-nosocomial-pathogen>.
147. Jensen LB, Garcia-Migura L, Valenzuela AJS, et al. A classification system for plasmids from enterococci and other Gram-positive bacteria. *J Microbiol Methods*. 2010;80(1):25–43. Available from: https://doi.org/10.1016/j.mimet.2009.10.012.
148. Wegener HC. Antibiotics in animal feed and their role in resistance development. *Curr Opin Microbiol*. 2003;6(5):439–445.
149. Manero A, Vilanova X, Cerd-Cullar M, et al. Vancomycin- and erythromycin-resistant enterococci in a pig farm and its environment. *Environ Microbiol*. 2006;8(4):667–674.
150. Ricke SC, Hacker J, Yearkey K, et al. Chapter 19. Unravelling food production microbiomes: concepts and future directions. In: Ricke SC, Atungulu GG, Park SH, Rainwater CE, eds. *Food and Feed Safety Systems and Analysis*. San Diego, CA: Elsevier Inc; 2017:347–374.

Chapter 28

Zoonoses from animal meat and milk

Abani K. Pradhan[1,2] and Shraddha Karanth[1]

[1]*Department of Nutrition and Food Science, University of Maryland, College Park, MD, United States,* [2]*Center for Food Safety and Security Systems, University of Maryland, College Park, MD, United States*

Abstract

Cases of foodborne zoonoses are on the rise, impacted by a number of intrinsic (food, animal, environment) and extrinsic (effect of intensive meat farming, world trade, population expansion) factors. In this chapter, we focus primarily on pathogens that can infect humans via their bovine (cattle, buffalo, etc.), porcine (pigs and wild boar), ovine (sheep and goats), and/or avian (chicken, turkey, geese, ducks, etc.) reservoirs, particularly through the consumption of meat and milk. Additionally, we discuss some major factors impacting the proliferation and persistence of major zoonotic agents in these food vehicles and their overall public health impact. Finally, we discuss routes to take to control and reduce the incidence of these agents.

Keywords: Foodborne zoonoses; microbial zoonotic agents; bacteria; domestic ruminants; milk; meat microbiology

Chapter points

- Changing global landscapes, human interference, and environmental fluctuations have encouraged a number of dangerous microbial agents to diversify their host range, by making the jump across the animal–human interface.
- A number of these pathogens affect humans almost exclusively via the consumption of the meat and milk of infected animals or contaminated food items.
- Prominent bacterial, viral, and parasitic foodborne zoonotic agents include *Escherichia coli*, *Salmonella*, *Listeria*, Hepevirus, and *Toxoplasma gondii*.
- A number of intrinsic and extrinsic factors impact the incidence and persistence of these agents worldwide.
- There is a critical need for improvement in detection methods and consumer education to reduce the public health burden of these zoonoses.

28.1 Introduction

Foodborne pathogens are a major concern for food safety. Historically, humans are exposed to these pathogens via the consumption of contaminated animal products, such as their meat or milk. A majority of these pathogens have zoonotic importance, exerting a significant impact on public health. Zoonotic diseases or zoonoses (singular: zoonosis), as suggested by their name [from the *Greek*: nosos = disease; zoos = living (animal)], are infectious diseases that are transmitted between vertebrate species such as from animals to humans (or vice versa) under natural conditions.[1] The name was coined by Rudolf Virchow during his study of trichinellosis in 1885.[2] As described by Lloyd-Smith et al.,[3] a majority of pathogens (approximately 75%) that infect humans tend to originate in nonhuman hosts, or also circulate in animal reservoirs. In fact, an estimated 816 out of 1407 human pathogens (58%) reviewed by Woolhouse and Gowtage-Sequeria[4] have been broadly classified as zoonotic. Influenza, the Ebola virus, mad cow disease, and the plague are just some of the examples of pathogens that have transcended the animal–human divide to infect humans and cause global outbreaks that significantly impact worldwide health and commerce. Foodborne pathogens with zoonotic potential are of particular concern since they do not solely depend on human hosts for their proliferation and survival.[5] Moreover, foodborne zoonoses have proven to be difficult to eliminate as they have at least one ever-present nonhuman reservoir, such as a domesticated animal, food animal, or a wild animal.[6] In this chapter, we focus on foodborne zoonoses and zoonotic agents (bacterial, viral, parasitic, fungal, and others) that cause disease in humans, particularly as a result of the consumption of animal meat and milk: what they are, what drives their incidence, and how they spread. We also focus on some major animal meat and milk-driven zoonotic agents and their impact on animal and human health, including their

Present Knowledge in Food Safety. DOI: https://doi.org/10.1016/B978-0-12-819470-6.00029-9

modes of transmission, diagnosis, and potential treatment strategies (Box 28.1).

The overall incidence of foodborne zoonoses is a sum total of the incidence of foodborne illness, or illness caused by the consumption of contaminated animal, fowl, and fish products (meat and milk) and nonfood transmission via some form of contact with animals that are traditionally raised for their meat or food by-products such as milk or eggs. The latter type could be transmitted when humans come in contact with infected animals, via occupational exposure (by farm workers, veterinarians, etc.), as well as through vectors (such as mosquitos, ticks, rodents, etc.).[7] Based on this definition, foodborne zoonoses can be divided into those caused by zoonotic agents that transcend the human–animal interface either directly or indirectly. Direct transmission constitutes disease caused by direct handling of infected animals, via inhalation, or by the oral route (i.e., consumption of infected meat or milk), whereas indirect transmission, also known as vector-based transmission, is usually caused by hematophagous arthropods[2,8] or pests such as rodents (Table 28.1).

BOX 28.1

A more popular way to classify zoonotic agents of human disease would be based on their taxonomic classification (i.e., bacteria, virus, fungus, parasite, etc.). In this chapter, this is retained as a subclassification, in order to differentiate between zoonotic diseases caused by consumption of infected meat, milk, and eggs and those caused by mere contact with meat animals. While the primary focus of this chapter is the former, we have also described some nonalimentary (i.e., nonmeat-/milk-/egg-related) zoonotic agents in some detail, in accordance with the definition of a foodborne zoonosis by Scallan et al.[7]

In recent years, there has been an uptick in the incidence of infections caused by foodborne pathogens, such as *Campylobacter*, *Escherichia coli*, and *Vibrio* spp. A 2020 study,[9] which analyzed the results of routine monitoring conducted by the US Centers for Disease Control and Prevention's (CDC) Foodborne Diseases Active Surveillance Network, of the incidence of laboratory-diagnosed infections caused by major foodborne pathogens, determined a sharp increase in the incidence of these pathogens in 2019 compared to the previous three years. They also observed a sharp shift in the pathogenic species responsible for more recent outbreaks compared to previous years from, for example, *Salmonella* and *E. coli*, to *Shigella*, *Listeria*, and *Campylobacter*.[9] This is especially concerning, given the widespread implementation of initiatives keyed toward controlling or reducing the incidence of such pathogens in our food sources. Studies have speculated that a combination of factors drive this increase and change, including the rapid growth in worldwide population and wealth demographics and the resultant changes in nutritional, agricultural, and trade practices, globalization, changes in land use, rapid urbanization (especially in developing countries or countries that have seen rapid economic growth in the past few decades), deforestation, encroachment on wildlife, and climate change.[10]

28.2 Factors impacting increase in zoonotic incidences worldwide

Zoonoses affecting humans due to contact with, or consumption of, major food animals and their products are on the rise. The environment in which livestock and poultry

TABLE 28.1 Modes of zoonotic transmission.

Mode of transmission	Specifications	Select examples
Direct contact		
Oral/alimentary	Consumption of infected animal meat/milk; food contaminated with pathogens	*Salmonella, Listeria, Escherichia coli, Trichinella*
Cutaneous/percutaneous	Contact with infected lesions or wounds, bites from infected animals	*Erysipelothrix*
Aerogenic	Inhalation of aerosolized pathogens	*Chlamydia, Coxiella burnetii*
Occupational	Veterinarian, farm worker, slaughterhouse worker, and so on	*Burkholderia, Corynebacterium*
Recreational	Petting zoos, domestic contact	
Indirect contact		
Vector-based	Via bites from ticks, mosquitoes	*Francisella*, Nairovirus

are raised constitutes a number of risk factors for pathogen growth, persistence, and transfer. Moreover, animals tend to shed a number of pathogenic agents in their feces, with subsequent human infection occurring additionally as a result of direct contact with the feces of an infected animal, aerogenically, or passed on by common animal vectors such as ticks, flies, and mosquitos. Subsequent infection is dependent on a number of factors—farming practices (industrial vs small scale), animal housing conditions (closed quarters vs free range), climate, and diet, among others. In this section, we deal with factors that have impacted this rise in, and persistence of, foodborne zoonoses.

28.2.1 Population expansion, urbanization, and international trade

The last century has been characterized by unprecedented changes in our world. There has been a sharp increase in worldwide population estimates, drastic changes in world demographics, and greater connectivity and the globalization of economic networks. These numbers are only projected to increase. The world is also shifting to an urban setting, with over half the world's ($\sim$57%) population living in urbanized areas compared to 1950 ($\sim$30%). Combined with increasing life expectancy and accessibility, this has led to a drastic increase in the demand for nutritious, safe, and diverse foods. Countries have had to ramp up food production in order to feed this growing population, using the finite resources, such as arable land, pasture land, animal food and feed, and freshwater, that the world has to offer. This situation is exacerbated by the increase in international travel and trade, brought about by globalization-supported accessibility.

These developments have led to major changes in global dietary habits. In fact, the Food and Agriculture Organization of the United Nations (FAO) estimates a global increase in per capita consumption of livestock milk and meat of 1.3% and 1.5% per annum, respectively.[11] Additionally, given current knowledge of the nutritional benefits of animal-based products, most humans would include some livestock products in their diet, given a choice.[12] This is because, in order to obtain all essential nutrients from a completely plant-based diet, one would need to consume a diverse complement of grains, fruits, vegetables, nuts, and seeds. Compared to plant-based food sources, meat is an energy-dense source of high-quality protein, containing high levels of important micronutrients such as thiamin, niacin, vitamin B12, calcium, iron, zinc, potassium, and phosphorous.[12,13] Similarly, animal milk is another important source of protein, fats, and carbohydrates, and micronutrients such as calcium, phosphorous, iron, vitamin A, and riboflavin.[12,14] Therefore, as concluded by Salter,[12] people in countries with greater economic stability tend toward a diet high in animal meat and milk.

28.2.2 Plant-based to animal-based and small-scale to industrialized food production practices

Clearly, the world food economy is driven by the increase in population, income growth, and trends in diets and food consumption patterns. Global meat consumption increased by 58% in the 50 years between 1968 and 2018.[15] Studies conducted in 2018 estimate that livestock accounts for 60% of all mammal biomass, far surpassing that of all wild mammals combined (4%).[16,17] This is particularly visible in developing countries, which account for 85% of the increase in global meat consumption. This increasing trend toward an animal-based diet could be attributed directly to rapid population growth and upward economic mobility in these areas. The FAO, in fact, reports a 5%–6% increase in meat consumption and 3.4%–3.8% increase in milk and dairy product consumption per capita in developing countries over the past few decades.[11] As a result, the past few decades have seen a rapid increase in global production of food animals and their products. This is particularly true in countries previously considered to be poorer, such as Brazil and China, relative to the static levels seen in the top producers from the 1990s—North America, Europe, and Australasia.[11] For reference, compared to the 9.05 million tons of meat animals produced in 1961, Asian countries were estimated to have produced 143.71 million tons of the same in 2018, a 1489% increase. In contrast, North American production of meat animals saw just a 187% jump in the same time period.[18] However, this increase in production does not equate to a proportional increase in land mass being used for grazing purposes, indicating the use of cost- and space-cutting operations in meat production.

Since the 1940s, agricultural and food animal production has become increasingly industrialized worldwide (so-called livestock farming) compared to traditional entrepreneurial small-scale farms and businesses. In the case of food animals, this involves high-throughput animal husbandry, wherein a very large number of animals and/or birds (in the thousands) are bred under mostly crowded, controlled conditions, with access to specially formulated diets and large-scale antibiotic treatment to ensure animal health and growth.[19] These methods are viewed as being necessary to ensure a uniform end-product (be it animal meat or animal product, such as eggs or milk).[16] However, in recent times, questions have been raised about the negative impacts of employing such methods and the escalating numbers of livestock and its resultant radical ecological change on animal health and welfare, consumer health, and the environment. A particular matter of concern is that the closed-in surroundings of such farms result in a "blurring of the lines" in the human–animal–environment interface—in essence, the close contact between confined animals in overcrowded farms allows for easier transmission of dangerous pathogenic and disease-causing entities among the confined food animals, wild animals, humans, and the environment via direct and indirect transmission,[16] posing a significant risk to public health. For reference, current agricultural practices have resulted in the creation of conditions that are responsible for >50% of all zoonotic infectious diseases in humans, numbers that will likely increase as agriculture intensifies to meet current demand.[20]

28.2.3 Blurring of the animal–human–environment interface

Many studies have speculated on the interplay between pathogens, hosts, and the environment being a primary driver of the emergence and persistence of zoonoses.[4,10,21,22] For example, changes in the environment and consequently, host characteristics, have been identified as important links to the creation of novel transmission patterns and persistence of pathogens in the environment.[10] These transmission patterns could be driven by closer contact with novel host types (such as humans) due to deforestation, game hunting, and increased interspecies contact; redistribution of pathogens, vectors, or hosts due to geographic redistribution. This, coupled with the rapidly growing human population, has resulted in wildlife coming into urban areas and humans living ever closer to their livestock, which narrows the animal–human divide considerably, supporting the emergence and persistence of zoonotic agents in the environment.

28.2.3.1 Human-mediated factors impacting the emergence and spread of zoonoses

Anthropogenic activities have resulted in substantial modifications that have, in turn, accelerated the evolution of a large number of pathogens. As a result, recent decades have seen an increase in the burden of infectious diseases in both high- and low-income countries because of the emergence of new pathogens and re-emergence of old pathogens with newfound resistance to current pathogen control measures.[4] Some of these activities include pollution, habitat encroachment, urbanization, trade practices leading to introduction of nonnative species in certain areas, and extensive usage of antibiotics and vaccines in the meat and milk industry (Box 28.2).

BOX 28.2

Globalization has resulted in a myriad of activities that contribute to blurring the lines between the human–animal interface. Urbanization impacts land-use patterns, leading to a decrease in worldwide "green cover," bringing about major changes in the natural habitats (environmental, animal, and human) of pathogens, promoting their proliferation. Deforestation leads to a disturbance in cross-species transmission rates in multihost disease systems. This also eventually leads to habitat encroachment, which increases the exposure of pathogens to a rich pool of novel hosts and vectors.[23,24] This is evidenced by, for example the increase in incidences of the Crimean Congo hemorrhagic fever in Turkey, which is associated with excessive usage of agricultural land, creating optimal habitat conditions for the growth of *Hyalomma marginatum* ticks, primary vectors, and reservoirs of its causative Nairovirus.[2] Another example is the direct correlation found between incidences of avian influenza H5N1 and the development of peri-urban lands.[25] A more pressing problem contributing to the rise of these diseases is increasing consumer demand for meat-based foods. This has led to a drastic increase in livestock production, particularly in poorer and developing countries, which have relatively weaker veterinary and public health infrastructure, lack of knowledge of prevalent and emerging infectious diseases, and poor living and sanitation conditions.[26] The combination of traditional animal rearing, and intensive livestock farming, with increased usage of antibiotics and hormones, could help existing animal-specific pathogens to jump the animal–human barrier, as well as support the re-emergence of previously eradicated zoonoses. Finally, increasing travel to "exotic locations," resulting in nonimmune travelers being exposed to pathogens and vectors endemic to these areas, and the global food trade, leading to novel vectors and pathogens moving across international borders, round out some of the most common anthropogenic factors contributing to zoonotic disease emergence and re-emergence.

28.2.3.2 Climate change

Climate change is one of the many factors with implications on the incidence of foodborne diseases and zoonoses. However, the exact connections between climate change and food safety are unclear, due to the attendant uncertainties governing them both. Climactic factors that could directly affect the occurrence and transmission of zoonotic pathogens include fluctuations in temperature and precipitation patterns, occurrence of extreme weather events, and changes in the transport pathways of complex contaminants.[27] Climate change–related indirect drivers of foodborne zoonoses incidence and intensity include variations in agriculture and animal husbandry practices, food and feed manufacturing and processing, transport and handling practices, and evolving consumer behavior towards food and food animals.[28]

In terms of the food industry and the microbial agents governing it, climate has been reported to have both direct and indirect impacts. The direct impact of climate change includes changes in host immunity, likely increasing their susceptibility to disease. Animal hosts of foodborne pathogens are also impacted by the increased physiological stress and altered geographic ranges and seasonality. Indirectly, climate change causes changes in contact between vectors, pathogens, and hosts (potentially leading to increased dissemination of disease agents), and/or increased pathogen persistence in a livestock environment.[29] Climate change has also resulted in the formation of conditions that are extremely favorable for the growth of both the pathogens themselves, as well as vectors that can transmit these pathogens among host species. Environmental variables in any given place, such as temperature and amount of vegetation, are important contributors determining the distribution of many arthropod species, with their presence or absence defined by these variables, as well as subtle changes in the seasonality of the variables.[19] For example, climate change is considered an important contributor to the increase in incidence of mosquitos responsible for the dissemination of West Nile Virus, which is fatal to both food animals and humans, via changes in range and distribution of vector movement and rate and seasonality of vector growth.[30,31] Moreover, the behavior of foodborne parasites has been definitively linked to climate change—foodborne parasites pass through a range of external environments and hosts during their life cycle, which in turn exposes them to the direct and indirect effects of climate change.[32]

In summary, rapid scientific and medical advancements have provided us with the means to immediately reduce the burden of microbial diseases—recent years have seen a substantial increase in the use of technologies such as antibiotics and other drugs against pathogenic infection, organ transplantation, immune therapy against debilitating diseases, and a significant increase in the number of immunological disorders. This has a serious effect on the susceptibility of human hosts to diseases. This, combined with the natural adaptability of pathogens of animal origin, leads to an interesting, potentially fatal interplay between new and old zoonoses of food animal origin and human hosts.

28.3 Common foodborne zoonotic agents

A large number of foodborne zoonotic agents are ubiquitous by nature—they are naturally found in the soil, water, in animals, plants, and in some cases, in humans. Pathogens can also be introduced to the food product during harvesting, slaughter, processing, transport, and storage of finished products. Moreover, many zoonotic agents are shed in animal feces, which tends to persist in the environment and water sources for extended periods of time, paving the way for further contamination and cross-contamination (in the form of contaminated produce, for example). Consumer impact and activities cannot be discounted—foods are subject to improper consumer handling, temperature abuse, and cross-contamination on a regular basis, accounting for a large percentage of recent foodborne outbreaks. Overall, these factors contribute to the occurrence and persistence of zoonotic outbreaks in both animal and human hosts (Table 28.2).

Included herein is a list of common zoonotic agents, primarily bacteria, viruses, and protozoa of public health importance (i.e., that cause disease in humans due to) via *the consumption of infected or contaminated animal meat and milk.* It is important to note that the complete list of zoonotic agents is exhaustive, and includes agents that cause disease due to nonfood-related exposure to disease agents, including exposure to nonfood animal–related zoonotic agents, inhalation of airborne zoonotic particles, contact with contaminated offal or excreta or droppings of infected animals and birds, or occupational exposure to zoonotic agents (veterinarians, animal care workers, slaughterhouse workers, etc.).

In this chapter, we focus on zoonotic agents spread due to the consumption of the meat and/or milk of (1) ruminants, including cattle, bison, sheep, and goats; (2) swine, including domestic pigs and wild boars; and (3) poultry (chicken, turkey, geese, ducks, and swans) and their eggs.

28.3.1 Bacteria

Bacteria are the most common agents of foodborne illness worldwide. Single-celled, ubiquitous organisms, most bacteria are nonpathogenic and tend to be host-specific. In fact, the human gastrointestinal tract is host to over 300 species of bacteria. However, some bacterial species have made the shift across the animal–environment–human divide, developing zoonotic potential. Accordingly, most bacterial foodborne diseases were initially attributed to contact with, or consumption of, animal meat, milk, or eggs (Box 28.3).

In this section, we cover bacterial zoonoses that specifically infect human hosts via the consumption of animal meat, milk, and eggs. Herein, we focus on their mode of transmission, host range, illness symptoms, treatment, and prevention strategies. Other zoonotic bacteria that are transmitted to humans via nonfoodborne contact, such as exposure to food animals (including the causative agents

TABLE 28.2 General features of most foodborne zoonotic agents.

Pathogen	General intrinsic factors impacting persistence, infection	Control strategies	References
Bacteria	Bacterial numbers (generally high numbers required, with exceptions)	Reducing water content (water activity, $a_w < 0.91$)	33
	Oxygen (facultative anaerobes, with exceptions)	Temperature <4°C and >60°C (<40°F and >140°F)	
	High-fat, high-protein content in host environment	Reducing pH (<7)	
Virus	Host cell for replication	High temperature treatment at 100°C (212°F)	34
	Viral shedding by hosts	Ultra-high temperature pasteurization	
	Generally host-specific	Pasteurization of solid foods (meat) at 70°C for 2 min and milk using HTST (71°C for 15 s)	
		Treatment with 10% sodium chlorite	
Parasites	Capable of colonizing multiple matrices	Freezing at −21°C for 1−7 days	35,36
		Gamma irradiation	
		Cooking meat to a core temperature of 60°C−75°C for 15−30 min or pasteurizing milk at 71°C for 15 s (HTST)	

HTST, High temperature short time.

BOX 28.3

Pathogenic bacteria cannot be detected by human senses (looks, smell, and taste)—thus it is hard to know if contaminated food should not be eaten. They cause foodborne illness in one, or a combination of three ways—infection, intoxication, and toxico-infection. Infection occurs from consuming food contaminated with live pathogenic bacteria, which attack the intestinal cells directly (e.g., *Salmonella*). Intoxication is caused by consuming food contaminated with dangerous toxins produced by bacteria, not the bacteria itself—thus the bacteria could have been killed by various food processing methods, but can still cause disease if it has had enough time to produce the toxin (e.g., *Staphylococcus aureus*). Finally, toxico-infection occurs when bacterial agents enter the intestines live, after surviving the acidic environment of the stomach, and produce harmful toxins inside the digestive system [e.g., *Clostridium perfringens*, Shiga-toxigenic *E. coli* (STEC)]—this is very common too in cases of infant botulism, where *Clostridium botulinum* is the causative agent.

of Q fever, dermatophilosis, tularemia, pasteurellosis, among others), are outside the scope of this chapter.

28.3.1.1 Bacillus anthracis

Bacillus anthracis, the causative organism of anthrax, is a zoonotic organism with major public health and bioterrorism implications. Known since ancient times, with references in the ancient texts of the Greeks, Romans, Hindus, and Chinese, it is a highly contagious and fatal disease. Mainly associated with and found in herbivores and domesticated animals, in recent times, anthrax is a common occurrence in countries where widespread vaccination of animals is not practiced.

First isolated and described by Robert Koch in 1876, *B. anthracis* is an aerobic, Gram-positive spore-forming bacillus.[37] The spores are highly resistant to inactivation and can persist in soil or the environment for long durations, thereby infecting grazing animals such as goats, sheep, and cattle.[38] Disease occurs when anthrax spores enter the body, germinate, multiply, and release toxins.[39] Infected animals exhibit a per-acute septic infection with a rapidly fatal course and sudden death. In cattle and sheep, specifically, the course of illness may last 1−2 h, with clinical signs, including a fever up to 41.7°C (107°F), muscle tremors, respiratory distress, and convulsions, mostly going unnoticed. Additionally, *postmortem*, a bloody discharge may be observed from the natural openings of the body, along with rapid bloating, a lack of rigor mortis, and the presence of unclotted blood (due to a toxin released by *B. anthracis*).[39]

Human infections, on the other hand, while uncommon, can take the form of a cutaneous (via contact with infected animal parts during slaughter), gastrointestinal (via ingestion of raw, undercooked infected meat), or pulmonary (via inhalation of airborne spores) infection, based on the mode of transmission.[2,38] The most common and mass outbreaks of anthrax have been via the cutaneous and pulmonary routes, with recent gastrointestinal outbreaks seen in Volgograd in 2000,[2] Bangladesh in 2010,[6] and in India in 2014.[40] The mortality rates of the different types of anthrax also vary, with cutaneous, gastrointestinal, and pulmonary anthrax having mortality rates of 20%, 25%–75%, and 67%–88%, respectively. Symptoms of intestinal anthrax tend to appear between 1 and 7 days, and may include severe abdominal pain, nausea, vomiting, severe diarrhea, and bleeding from the gastrointestinal tract (stomach and intestines). Untreated symptoms could lead to septicemia, meningitis, and/or pneumonia.[41]

Anthrax cannot be diagnosed based on disease symptoms alone, however, as symptoms can mimic those seen in pneumonia in humans,[42] and must be confirmed by bacterial culture or polymerase chain reaction (PCR). Although the most effective means to control the spread of anthrax is by mass vaccination, routine preexposure vaccination is only recommended for people who are regularly in direct contact with cattle or other reservoirs of the bacterium. Currently, penicillin and doxycycline curative is the preferred mode of treatment against *B. anthracis* in humans, as approved by the US FDA.

28.3.1.2 Brucella spp

The genus *Brucella* is a group of nonmotile Gram-negative coccobacilli comprising several different species, including *Brucella abortus*, *Brucella melitensis*, *Brucella suis*, and *Brucella canis*, which are collectively responsible for brucellosis. This bacterium has a wide natural host range based on the species and the biotype within each species, including domestic ruminants such as cows and bison (*B. abortus*), pigs and wild boar (*B. suis* biotypes 1–3), and sheep and goats (*B. melitensis*).[2,6]

Brucella spp. can survive for extended periods of time in meat, milk, eggs, skin, and excreta, although not in the environment. Humans are primarily introduced to these bacteria through the consumption of the meat and unpasteurized milk and milk products of infected animals, although cases of occupational exposure are not unheard of. Humans afflicted with brucellosis can exhibit undulant fever, and other serious, debilitating, and potentially chronic symptoms such as hyperhidrosis, headaches, myalgia, formation of granulomas, edema, endocarditis, as well as damage to the kidneys and other organs, among others. Acute forms of brucellosis in humans are rare (fatality rate in untreated cases is 2%–5%). Most patients exhibit symptoms between 2 and 4 weeks, followed by spontaneous recovery, while others develop intermittent fever and other persistent symptoms that wax and wane at 2- to 14-day intervals. A majority of people with undulant fever recover completely in 3–12 months. However, some patients become chronically ill.[2,6]

Brucella is diagnosed primarily by bacterial culture. Although this is time-consuming due to *Brucella* spp. being fastidious, it remains the gold standard recommended by the US CDC, over *Brucella* standard agglutination and PCR tests.[43,44] Since a vaccination is not available, the most effective preventative strategies against this bacteria are to eradicate the bacteria in their natural hosts, as well as to educate the masses about the importance of dairy pasteurization.[2,44]

28.3.1.3 Campylobacter spp

Campylobacter spp., comprising *Campylobacter jejuni* and *Campylobacter coli* among others (which form a very small percentage of *Campylobacter*-related human infections, and are therefore not the focus of this section), is a Gram-negative, motile, bacillus, long recognized as a responsible agent of enteritis, gastroenteritis, and campylobacterosis in humans. The many species of *Campylobacter* normally colonize the gastrointestinal tracts of domestic or wild animals and are increasingly being found in many foods of animal origin.[45] While usually asymptomatic in its poultry hosts (which are reservoirs for this bacterium), it can manifest as a number of symptoms ranging from moderate to severe in its animal (cattle and pigs) and human hosts.[2]

Campylobacter's main environmental niche is the intestinal tract of poultry and other avian species. It is transmitted to humans via the fecal-oral route, through the consumption and handling of contaminated, undercooked poultry meat and water, although raw milk, raw red meat and fruit and vegetable-related cases are not unheard of.[46–48] Although a majority of the cases of *Campylobacter* infection are self-limiting, some may lead to severe complications including rare cases of bloodstream infections, even death, and life-threatening postinfection sequelae.[49] One of the most prominent sequelae of *Campylobacter*-related gastroenteritis is Guillain–Barré Syndrome, an acute peripheral demyelinating polyneuropathy causing weakness in the extremities, and, in severe cases, paralysis.[50] *Campylobacter* infections have also been linked with other sequelae such as reactive arthritis, bursitis, postinfectious bowel syndrome, pregnancy loss,[51] occasional cases of meningitis in infants,[52] and myocarditis.[53] Thus *Campylobacter* infections are a notifiable disease in a number of developed countries including the United States and Canada. Bacterial culture remains the gold standard for detecting these bacteria, although molecular detection methods such as immunological assays and PCR have also been used in certain cases.

28.3.1.4 Clostridium spp

Clostridia (*C. botulinum*, *C. perfringens*, and *C. difficile*) are a group of highly virulent anaerobic Gram-positive rod-shaped spore-forming bacteria with significant public health impact. *Clostridium* species are endemic to the soil, and are commonly seen in the digestive tract of vertebrates such as pigs, cattle, sheep, goats, horses, and poultry, with spores surviving in vegetables, fruits, and grains such as rice, as well as the soil. The spores produced are very hardy—these function as a form of survival mode for bacteria, allowing them to withstand the unfavorable conditions brought on by food processing (such as high cooking temperatures), proliferating at a faster rate when conditions become favorable again (e.g., slow cooling of the food— it is recommended to reduce the cooling time by refrigeration).[54] This is why commercial canning for low-acid canned foods (or foods with a pH > 4.6) must be subjected to a 12-D log reduction heating step to ensure there are no surviving spores that could germinate, grow, and flourish in an anaerobic environment. Typically, foods must be heated to 121°C for 15 min (which is the temperature–time combination required to completely inactivate spores). While not a contagious disease, *Clostridium* (especially *C. botulinum*) is of special concern to the food industry and consumers alike due to its ability to produce enterotoxins, which are responsible for food poisoning, and, depending on the species, exposure time, and severity, paralysis, and death.[6]

C. botulinum is the causative agent of botulism in both animals (mammals and birds) and humans. Botulism is an alimentary intoxication caused by the released enterotoxin. The most effective among the various subtypes of neurotoxins that can be released by *C. botulinum* can cause irreversible neuromotoric (or flaccid) paralysis (with a fatality rate of 15%–75%) after an incubation period ranging from 12 h to several days, resulting in loss of motility, diplopia,[a] strabism,[b] and paralysis of the respiratory muscles. Botulism is diagnosed by detecting botulotoxin in the stool and vomit of infected individuals, and can only be treated with stomach and intestinal lavage or administering the poly- or monovalent botulinum antitoxin. Humans with occupational exposure to *C. botulinum* are also vaccinated with the toxoid.[2]

C. perfringens is estimated to be the second leading bacterial cause of foodborne illness in the United States. Foodborne illness caused by this bacterium can take one of two forms—gastroenteritis, which in severe cases can result in damage to the small intestine and possibly death, and pig-bel disease (aka enteritis necroticans), a fatal symptom characterized by swelling of the gut. Most cases of death are due to severe dehydration brought on by fluid imbalance, and mostly occur in children and infants (*C. perfringens* is a recognized cause of sudden infant death syndrome, or SIDS), the elderly, and the immunocompromised.[54] The mode of action of foodborne *C. perfringens* is via infection, wherein live cells are ingested in food and proliferate in the alimentary canal—*C. perfringens* multiply within the host body, form endospores under the harsh environment caused by stomach acids within the host, with toxins being released upon cell lysis. Symptoms include pronounced diarrhea and abdominal cramp appearing within 8–16 h, with most cases resolving within 12–24 h.[54,55]

Clostridium difficile, like most other clostridia, is a Gram-positive spore-forming, rod-shaped bacteria. However, unlike other species, *C. difficile* requires a strictly anaerobic environment to proliferate, making it difficult to isolate and grow. While mostly a nosocomial (hospital-acquired) infection associated with antimicrobial therapy (which disrupts the colonic microbiota, leaving it susceptible to infections), the past two decades have seen a sharp rise in the isolation of *C. difficile* ribotypes from uncooked, ready-to-eat retail meats which are also associated with human cases of *Clostridium*-associated colitis.[56]

28.3.1.5 Pathogenic *Escherichia coli* group

E. coli is a genus of Gram-negative, aerobic rod–shaped bacteria, which are the main enteric bacteria colonizing the human gut. Some nonpathogenic variants even form a part of normal intestinal flora. The organism is used extensively as a model organism to study bacterial physiology, metabolism, genetic regulation, signal transduction, and cell wall structure and function. However, a few variants of *E. coli* have been shown to be pathogenic to humans. Among the six recognized pathogenic *E. coli* pathotypes, enterotoxigenic *E. coli*, enteropathogenic *E. coli*, enterohemorrhagic *E. coli* (EHEC), and enteroaggregative *E. coli* are well-known foodborne pathogens. Among these, EHEC is the most common pathogen, being implicated in foodborne outbreaks worldwide (with an estimated >63,000 cases in the United States annually), and is also directly related to animal meat and milk.[7,54,57] Foodborne outbreaks attributed to the other pathogenic variants are generally as a result of cross-contamination or fecal contamination of food sources by infected animals or humans, and are not specifically considered to be zoonotic; thus the remainder of this section will focus on EHEC.

EHEC, a subset of the Shiga-like toxin (Stx)-producing STEC, are some of the major causative agents of bloody diarrhea and hemolytic uremic syndrome (HUS). The pathogenic mechanism of EHEC is by binding strongly to host epithelial cells, producing attachment lesions, and producing toxins that result in cell death.

Serotype O157:H7 is the prototypic strain among the many serotypes associated with EHEC. However, a number of other serotypes, chief among them O111, O26, O121, O103, O145, O45, O113, and O91, have been isolated from human cases of infection. EHEC colonizes the intestine of several food animals, particularly cattle (which function as a reservoir for these bacteria), and has also been isolated from the feces of sheep, goats, pigs, and chickens. In fact, beef and ground beef remain two major food vehicles implicated in human outbreaks in several developed countries.

EHEC is primarily transmitted via the consumption of contaminated meat, milk, and eggs, and produce irrigated with contaminated water and manure, and water; however, outbreaks have also been linked to direct contact with infected animals and humans. The minimum infectious dose of EHEC is believed to be low; the dose for O157:H7 is suspected to be among the lowest, with a range of 10–100 colony forming units (CFU). Infections from EHEC range from asymptomatic to severe. The primary symptom is nonspecific gastrointestinal disease, including diarrhea, vomiting, and nausea. Hemorrhagic colitis is an acute symptom, manifesting as abdominal cramps and bloody diarrhea; this can be fatal if it progresses to HUS, which is characterized by acute renal failure, hemolytic anemia, and thrombocytopenia. The most effective treatment strategy is rehydration; antibiotic treatment is generally not recommended for EHEC infections, as it has been shown to aggravate HUS symptoms in some patients. EHEC infections are diagnosed by culture, antibody tests, and PCR.[7,54,57]

28.3.1.6 Listeria spp

Listeria spp. is a genus of Gram-positive, facultative anaerobic, motile, rod-shaped bacteria, which is among the leading causes of death from foodborne illness. Among the five species belonging to this genus, only *Listeria monocytogenes* is considered to be pathogenic to humans. *L. monocytogenes* can tolerate and grow under refrigeration temperatures (i.e., it is a psychro-tolerant bacterium), making it a bacterium of specific concern since it can multiply in foods that are expected to have a longer shelf life under refrigeration conditions.[58] *L. monocytogenes* is also one of the only bacteria that are transmitted exclusively through food (i.e., is exclusively foodborne).[2,54,59]

L. monocytogenes is the causative organism of listeriosis, a serious infection with an estimated human health burden of 1600 infections and 260 deaths in the United States every year.[60,61] In humans, *L. monocytogenes* is transmitted via consumption of contaminated food or ready-to-eat (RTE) meat (no further cook step) and unpasteurized dairy products.[41,61,62] Human listeriosis manifests as mild (noninvasive) to severe (invasive) gastrointestinal infections, or, in severe cases, septicemia, meningitis, encephalitis, or abortion (in infected pregnant women).[2,63] Most severe cases are seen in immunocompromised people, the elderly, the very young or pregnant women. The incubation period of *L. monocytogenes* also varies according to the observed clinical manifestations: 6–240 h for gastrointestinal forms; 1–12 days for bacteremia; 1–14 days for central nervous system cases; and 17–67 days for pregnancy-related cases.[64]

Listeriosis is diagnosed based on clinical symptoms in the infected, detection of bacteria in a blood smear, cerebrospinal fluid, meconium of newborns, from the feces, or vomit of infected individuals. Additionally, in recent years, regulatory agencies have embraced novel methods such as Pulsed Field Gel Electrophoresis (PFGE), Multilocus Sequence Typing (MLST), and Whole Genome Sequencing (WGS) to detect the foodborne sources of human outbreaks of listeriosis based on the pathogen's genomic signatures.[65] In most mild cases, infections are self-limiting.[2]

28.3.1.7 Mycobacterium spp

Tuberculosis (TB) is one of the most devastating bacterial infectious diseases worldwide. While the main cause of TB in humans is *Mycobacterium tuberculosis*, which is host-specific to humans, certain cases can be attributed to zoonotic versions of the bacteria including *Mycobacterium bovis* and *Mycobacterium avium* subsp. *paratuberculosis* (henceforth referred to as *M. paratuberculosis*). Zoonotic transmission of these agents is primarily attributed to the consumption of contaminated animal products, such as unpasteurized milk.[66]

Studies have suggested that zoonotic TB accounted for a significant proportion (3%–10% attributed to *M. bovis*) of the cases seen in the Western world in recent history, particularly in children who consumed whole, raw milk,[2,67] until the implementation of standardized milk pasteurization programs.[68] In fact, in developed countries, where standardized pasteurization programs have been running for a few decades, zoonotic cases of TB from *M. bovis* have been practically eradicated. This, compounded by the fact that *M. bovis*, like *M. tuberculosis*, appears to be best adapted to its host species (i.e., does not transmit easily between humans), has resulted in very few cases of foodborne cases of TB in developed countries (although foodborne TB is prevalent in countries where TB is endemic in cattle and pasteurization programs are not strictly enforced, such as a few countries in the African and Indian subcontinents).

M. bovis infection manifests as a pulmonary or extrapulmonary progressive disease accompanied with fever and gastrointestinal, urogenital, meningeal, or skin-related symptoms. *M. paratuberculosis* is transmitted aerogenically among infected animals such as cattle[2] and galliforms,[69] or via ingestion of contaminated water, feed or exposure to contaminated feces of infected animals. In humans, *M. paratuberculosis* manifests as avian TB (transmitted via contact with infected poultry) or as paratuberculosis (via consumption of contaminated milk, and less frequently, meat).[2] Some studies also suggest that zoonotic *M. paratuberculosis* is responsible for Crohn's disease in humans, although the scientific consensus is not fixed on this point.[70–73]

Disease is diagnosed by X-ray tomography, microscopy, or by 8-week cultivation of sputum, cerebrospinal fluid, urine, or pus in Löwenstein–Jensen medium. Multiplex PCR is also used in some cases. Unless *M. bovis* is treated sufficiently with a range of antibiotics including rifampicin and pyrazinamide and other tuberculostatics, it could be lethal, particularly in young children and immunocompromised individuals. The same treatment strategy is utilized for *M. paratuberculosis* infections; however, this treatment is rarely long-term, with relapses common. A more effective strategy is to prevent the occurrence of disease with the *M. bovis*-attenuated BCG (Bacillus Calmette-Guérin) vaccine, or by implementing domestic eradication programs.[2]

28.3.1.8 *Salmonella* spp

Salmonella enterica subsp. *enterica* is a major foodborne pathogen; as of 2015, *Salmonella* was ranked among the top four global causes of diarrheal disease in the world.[74] *Salmonella* is one of the top causes of foodborne gastroenteritis worldwide; in 2011 Scallan et al.[7] reported that an estimated >1 million nontyphoidal *Salmonella* infections occurred in the United States every year. In developed and high-income countries, foodborne *Salmonella* is primarily acquired by consuming infected animal meat or animal products (or food products contaminated during farming or processing). Infected or contaminated poultry meat and eggs are top causes of *Salmonella* infections in humans, primarily because *Salmonella* is commensal in chicken guts, and improper handling during slaughter and processing could lead to cross-contamination.[75] However, recent outbreak data have also identified products from other animal sources—cattle, pigs, sheep, and goats, as well as nonanimal sources such as nuts, fruits, and vegetables—as novel routes for human infection.[65,76,77]

S. enterica subsp. *enterica* is a Gram-negative facultative anaerobic, rod-shaped bacterium with a highly diverse sero-profile. As of 2020, this subspecies of bacteria comprises over 50 serogroups and >2600 serovars based on the O (somatic/surface) and H (flagellar) antigens that each bacterial type presents. What sets *Salmonella* apart from most other bacterial zoonoses is that many of these serovars have demonstrated pathogenic potential, and have been implicated in a number of outbreaks worldwide. In fact, between 1998 and 2017, over 250 *Salmonella* serovars have been implicated in food-related outbreaks.[77] *Salmonella* has a high minimum infectious dose of 10^6 cells, although highly virulent strains could infect humans with just 10 cells. However, since *Salmonella* is ubiquitous, sources of contamination and cross-contamination are manifold, including farm environments, at slaughter, in produce irrigation water, during food transportation, and in consumer homes. Moreover, *Salmonella* replicates easily in food (under nutrient availability conditions) at room temperature. This allows for easy infection with *Salmonella*.

Salmonella is transmitted from infected to uninfected hosts primarily via the fecal-oral contamination route or via direct contact with infected animals or individuals. In humans, *Salmonella* causes salmonellosis (all serovars except *S.* Typhi and *S.* Paratyphi, also known as nontyphoidal serovars) or typhoid fever (*S.* Typhi and *S.* Paratyphi only, which are only found in humans), depending on the serovars. Nontyphoidal salmonellosis (NTS) is primarily characterized by nonspecific gastrointestinal illness. However, acute symptoms (dehydration due to fluid loss) and chronic (reactive arthritis, septicemia, and bacteremia, among others) sequelae can also be observed in severe cases. NTS has a relatively low mortality rate, at $\sim 1\%$, but the rate is higher in immunocompromised individuals.[2,54] Culturing fecal samples remains the gold standard for *Salmonella* identification, although PCR and novel sequencing technologies, including WGS, are being used increasingly to identify specific serovars and epidemiologically connect human cases of infection with the causative food sources (Karanth et al., unpublished data). In most cases of infection, antibiotic treatment is not recommended, as it has been shown to prolong the infectious course of the illness; instead, most infected individuals are provided with supportive care (mostly rehydration) as the illness is mainly self-limiting.

28.3.1.9 *Staphylococcus* spp

S. aureus are nonmotile, Gram positive, facultative anaerobic, nonspore-forming bacteria that can be found on the skin of most mammals and birds, as well as in the mouth, blood, mammary glands, and intestinal, genitourinary, and upper respiratory tracts of infected hosts. This bacteria is among the most resistant nonspore-forming bacteria, surviving in a dry state for long periods of time; in fact, its resistant capacity is demonstrated by its frequent isolation from the air, water, sewage, and dust.[78] Kloos[79] proposed that *Staphylococcus* is host-specific, due to coevolving with its specific host—studies have shown *S. aureus* strains living in different habitats acquire unique phenotypic traits that do not allow for existing outside of that specific host system. Accordingly, a majority of human-associated cases of *S. aureus* are attributed to contact with infected humans (nosocomial infections) or to food contaminated due to handling by infected humans. However, human infections with certain strains of *S. aureus* (such as strain ST398) specific for animal hosts have been recently identified, raising considerable speculation about the zoonotic potential of these animal-associated clones.[80]

28.3.1.10 *Yersinia spp*

Yersinia is a genus of bacteria comprising 11 species, four of which are pathogenic. Among these, *Yersinia enterocolitica* and *Yersinia pseudotuberculosis* are foodborne pathogens that cause yersiniosis in humans. *Yersinia* spp. is widespread in the environment, and is isolated from cattle, pigs, birds, small mammals, and domestic or companion animals, introducing multiple potential sources of infection to humans. Domestic and wild pigs are the main reservoir of *Y. enterocolitica*, and pork, especially medium-rare or underdone pork products are the most important sources of human infection. Although this bacterium is one of the rarer causes of gastroenteritis, it is of importance as it is primarily associated with improper food processing practices. *Y. enterocolitica* is a psychrotroph, and can survive at temperatures as low as 4°C. In fact, at this temperature, the bacterium may produce a heat-stable enterotoxin which is resistant to 121°C for 30 min. It can also survive in pH conditions ranging from 4 to 10, with an optimal pH at 7.6. This bacterium can also persist longer in cooked food such as vacuum-packed meat, pasteurized liquid eggs, boiled eggs, pasteurized whole milk, and cheese, because of increased nutrient availability.[54,81,82]

In the United States, *Y. enterocolitica* infections were believed to have accounted for approximately 3% (~97,000 cases, ~530 hospitalizations, and ~30 deaths) of all foodborne infections, accounting for underreporting and potentially undiagnosed cases.[7] In Europe, ~7000 cases of yersiniosis were reported in 2011, a 3.5% jump from those reported in 2010. As of 2012, although no foodborne cases of *Y. pseudotuberculosis* were reported in the United States, multiple outbreaks from consumption of contaminated water and food were reported from Japan. Although fatalities due to *Yersinia* are rare, infections can result in significant economic and public health burden. *Y. enterocolitica* and *Y. pseudotuberculosis* infections can clinically manifest as self-limiting, nonspecific gastroenteritis; however, chronic sequelae include autoimmune complications, such as reactive arthritis, hyperthyroidism, Graves' disease, Hashimoto's thyroiditis, and (in the case of *Y. pseudotuberculosis*) Kawasaki disease.[2,54]

Yersiniosis is diagnosed by isolating the organism from the stool, blood, or vomit of infected human hosts, and subsequently confirmed by serological identification or PCR. Since infection with *Yersinia* can sometimes be confused with Crohn's disease, it is important to accurately diagnose infections in order for the right treatment strategy to be employed.[2,83]

28.3.2 Viruses

A number of viral outbreaks, such as influenza, have been recorded since the early 1990s. These were of particular concern to the general public due to the large number of cases involved in each outbreak. A majority of these outbreaks originated from animals; however, the actual outbreaks were due to direct contact with viral particles, aerogenic transmission, or by person-to-person contact. However, since viruses tend to mutate at a rapid pace, concerns have arisen regarding the potential of a mutated virus being transmitted through food.[6]

Viruses are very small microorganisms; yet, they represent the pinnacle of adaptation and survivalism. Each group of virus affects a specific host range and cell type. Therefore foodborne viruses are of particular concern for their zoonotic and pandemic potential, as they would have undergone several generations of genetic recombination and pass through highly selective evolutionary bottlenecks in order to infect a nonspecific host (such as a human).[84] Recent years have seen the emergence of a number of zoonotic diseases of viral origin. Although a majority of these are related to environmental cross-contamination (and are therefore nonspecific to a food source) or transmission due to proximity to infected animals, a few viruses have been associated specifically with the consumption of meat and other products from infected animals. The ongoing coronavirus (COVID-19) pandemic is one such example of a zoonosis that has transcended the animal (bats)—human barrier. However, currently, there is no evidence that it is transmitted via food.[85]

Herein, a zoonotic viral species that has been definitively associated with animal meat/milk/egg consumption are discussed; additional viruses that infect humans via exposure to food animals and have zoonotic potential, such as the causative agents of West Nile fever, rabies, cowpox, Crimean Congo hemorrhagic fever, Newcastle disease, Rift Valley fever, and vesicular stomatitis, as well as the Orthomyxoviridae family of viruses, but are transmitted aerogenically or via direct contact with infected animals, are not included in this chapter.

28.3.2.1 Hepevirus

Hepevirus (Hepatitis E virus; HEV) is the causative agent behind Hepatitis E,[34,86] a major viral foodborne zoonosis. Hepatitis E is an important disease in developing countries in Asia and Africa, and is also responsible for large outbreaks in some developed countries (which are primarily associated with travel to endemic areas). Of the four genera in the Hepeviridae family, genotypes 3 and 4 have been associated with sporadic and cluster cases of Hepatitis E.[86] The host range of zoonotic HEV includes humans, pigs,[87,88] chicken, small mammals, and fish.

The main modes of transmission of this virus to humans are via direct contact with infected animals, and consumption of animal meat and meat products contaminated with the virus, unlike the Hepatitis A virus, which follows a food contact–based transmission pattern. Studies have shown that HEV remains fully active in contaminated pig liver. Moreover, medium-to-rare cooking conditions, approximating a cooking temperature of 56°C, are ineffective in inactivating the virus.[89] Alternative routes of transmission of the virus to humans include the consumption of fish and shellfish contaminated with infected swine bodily waste,[90] as well as water contaminated with infected animal and human wastes.[91] HEV is dangerous to pregnant women, and can be transmitted from mother to child. HEV can also be transmitted from person to person within the household of an infected individual.

HEV manifests as viral hepatitis in humans, which is characterized by increased levels of bile in the blood, causing infected individuals to have a yellow pallor, similar to the symptoms seen in patients afflicted with Hepatitis A. However, compared to Hepatitis A, HEV has a significantly higher mortality rate in high-risk groups, such as pregnant women in their third trimester, immunocompromised individuals, and individuals with preexisting liver conditions.[92] Infected individuals are diagnosed by enzyme-linked immunosorbent assay (ELISA) and supportive care is offered to the infected (i.e., no set treatment strategy). Preventative measures include the use of good hygiene practices, especially among handlers of domestic pigs and boars, and avoiding drinking untreated water or consumption of undercooked meat.[87]

28.3.3 Parasites

Over the decades, a number of parasites potentially associated with meat and animal food products have been identified and characterized. However, attributing a parasitic outbreak exclusively to a food source has been a challenge, as these microorganisms have shown an uncanny ability to colonize and thrive in multiple matrices, including the animal itself, water bodies, and the environment, making it difficult to identify the exact point of contact with the human host. Excluding enteric protozoa, foodborne parasitic agents were reported to be responsible for approximately 48% of the 91.1 million cases of human disease worldwide as of 2010, with a majority of cases concentrated in low-income countries.[93] Many of these parasites are associated with multiple meat animals, such as pigs, cows, and other domestic ruminants (including goats and sheep). This chapter focuses on the most prominent zoonotic parasites associated with the consumption of animal meat and milk, with those associated with nonfoodborne exposure to meat animals (e.g., *Giardia* spp., *Trypanosoma cruzi*), not included.

28.3.3.1 Cryptosporidium parvum

Cryptosporidium spp. is a eukaryotic enteric alveolate parasite that has a life cycle that supports both waterborne and foodborne transmission, and consequently, is frequently isolated from humans and ruminants, primarily in low-income countries. *Cryptosporidium parvum*, the major zoonotic species, is transmitted primarily in contaminated water, although studies have shown zoonotic transmission via milk from infected ruminants.[94] A lesser known species, *Cryptosporidium meleagridis*, mainly colonizes turkeys (and subsequently humans). Infected hosts excrete oocysts of *C. parvum*, which is eventually ingested by other animals and humans via contaminated water and food. However, *Cryptospridium* spp. is chiefly considered to be a waterborne zoonotic agent, since it is widely spread in infective environments, and is believed to be resistant to disinfection treatment that drinking water is normally subjected to (e.g., chlorine treatment).[2,95,96] Moreover, waterborne outbreaks of *Cryptosporidium* spp. are generally clustered together and can be traced definitively back to water distribution networks, whereas foodborne outbreaks tend to be more widely spread, allowing for potential misclassification of suspected outbreaks as sporadic cases (as opposed to outbreak cases).

In humans, *Cryptosporidium* spp. causes cryptosporidiosis, an enteric disease, with symptoms including fever, headache, abdominal pain, diarrhea, and vomiting. The minimum infective dose of *C. parvum* for humans is just 30 oocysts, and since infected hosts tend to shed thousands of oocycts into the environment, this is a parasite of high importance to food safety.[97] Moreover, its potential for causing multiple relapses in infected humans, as well as capacity for human-to-human transmission, typifies its significant impact on public health. However, since the heat treatments used to decontaminate beef carcasses have been proven to be effective in inactivating the infective oocysts, proper cooking (of meat) and pasteurization (of milk) are believed to be sufficient to reduce the risk of transmission of this parasite.[95–97] *C. parvum* infection is diagnosed in humans by microscopy of stool samples,

ELISA, or specialized real-time polymerase chain reaction (RT-PCR).

28.3.3.2 Sarcocystis spp

Protozoan parasites of the genus *Sarcocystis*, belonging to the same Sarcocystidae family as *T. gondii*, have a slightly different transmission cycle compared to most other parasites in this list—they require two hosts to complete their life cycle, and are dependent on the prey-predator host network, with sexual reproduction occurring primarily in the predator host (such as wild animals and humans), and asexual reproduction occurring in the prey host (such as cattle and pigs). Definitive hosts such as humans and other carnivores are infected by intermediate hosts such as cattle and ruminants by the alimentary route (i.e., consumption of muscle tissues infected with cysts containing bradyzoites), while intermediate hosts are infected by coming into contact with resistant oocysts shed by definitive hosts in their feces/stool. However, in some cases, humans can also serve as the intermediate host, with significantly different clinical manifestations of the infection. Two species of *Sarcocystis* have been identified with foodborne zoonotic potential—*Sarcocystis bovihominis* (cattle → humans) and *Sarcocystis suihominis* (pigs → humans).[35,98]

Humans infected with this parasite present with sarcosporidiosis, with intestinal symptoms observed in humans serving as definitive hosts, and musculoskeletal symptoms and development of sarcocysts in humans serving as intermediate hosts.[2] Humans are primarily infected by consuming raw or undercooked beef or pork infected with mature cysts of *S. suihominis* or *bovihominis*. *Sarcocystis* infection is diagnosed by identification of oocysts or sporocysts in the feces/stool of infected hosts, and in humans, the cyst stages are identified by histological examination of biopsied muscle tissue. The best means to deal with infections is by preventing them in the first place, by heat treatment at 60°C for 20 min (or 70°C for 15 min), or freezing at −4°C for at least 48 h (which is sufficient to render bradyzoites noninfectious) prior to preparing and consuming meat.[98,99]

28.3.3.3 Taenia spp

Taenia spp. is a genus comprising many intestinal zoonotic cestodes (tapeworms) that infect cattle (*Taenia saginata*) and pigs (*Taenia solium*), among others. *T. solium* is the causative agent of cysticercosis, a disease with serious public health impact, as well as taeniasis. Humans are definitive hosts of these cestodes, with the metacestode larval stage colonizing intermediate hosts (cattle, pigs). Although both *T. saginata* and *T. solium* are distributed widely across the globe, the actual number of foodborne illnesses attributable to each is hard to quantify as it is difficult to differentiate the various species, and due to the asymptomatic nature of most infections.[100] Like most other parasites on this list, *Taenia* spp. is transmitted across animals and humans via the fecal-oral route. In fact, humans living in close proximity to infected humans are at high risk of getting infected themselves. Although this genus is found nearly worldwide, it is endemic to low-income and developing countries and areas with poor access to basic sanitation services. However, it is important to note that, since human-to-human transmission is a certainty via the fecal-oral route, it is possible to contract this parasite in regions that have no known proximity to any of the animal carriers, as long as a human carrier is present close by.

T. saginata shed by a definitive host in the form of eggs is consumed by cattle during grazing, subsequently colonizing their intestines. After hatching in the intestine, oncospheres are liberated from the eggs, and cross the intestinal barrier to the blood stream, eventually forming cysts, also known as cysticerci, in various parts of the body. The muscle and other meat of such an infected animal, when consumed raw or undercooked by humans, are responsible for human cysticercosis from *T. saginata*.[98] There are, however, two modes of transmission of *T. solium* to humans—direct contact with the eggs, resulting in cysticercosis (in both pigs and humans), and consumption of the mature tapeworm in undercooked pork meat, causing taeniasis. The foodborne route does not directly result in cysticercosis in humans, although the colonizing mature *T. solium* can lay eggs within the intestinal epithelium, eventually resulting in cysticercosis.[35,101]

Human infection with *T. solium* can result in the development of cysticerci in the muscles, eyes, brain, or spinal cord. Development of these cysts in the neural system results in a dangerous form of cysticercosis known as neurocysticercosis, which can cause strokes, paralysis, and eventually death. Muscular cysticercosis is a less serious version of the disease, which can manifest as mostly asymptomatic tender lesions under the skin on the muscles.[35,102] On the other hand, cysticercosis caused by *T. saginata* can be either asymptomatic, or manifest as nonspecific abdominal disorders such as nausea, vomiting, and so on. Taeniasis can result in digestive issues, including abdominal pain, loss of appetite, weight loss, and an upset stomach. Taeniasis caused by *T. saginata* tends to be more severe than that caused by *T. solium*, as the former is much larger in size (up to 10 m) than *T. solium* (up to 3 m). A primary symptom of taeniasis is the active passing of tapeworm segments, also known as proglottids, through the anus and in the stool.[35,102]

Infections are usually confirmed by magnetic resonance imaging (MRI) or a computed tomography (CT) scan, with blood tests also being effective in diagnosing heavy infections. While most people with cysticercosis need not receive any specific form of treatment, some cases may require surgical intervention.[101]

28.3.3.4 *Toxoplasma gondii*

T. gondii, which belongs to the protozoan family Sarcocystidae, is a foodborne parasite of major public health importance. Scallan et al.[7] estimated that toxoplasmosis (infection with *T. gondii*) is the most prevalent parasitic infection with an estimated ~80,000 annual cases in the United States. It has been speculated that *T. gondii* is capable of infecting all warm-blooded animals, including humans. Although a parasite of specific concern in the mid- to late-1900s, the overall number of foodborne outbreaks of *T. gondii* has reduced over the decades due to the implementation of stringent processing standards. Moreover, recent studies have shown low prevalence of *T. gondii* in naturally infected meats in the United States. However, *T gondii* has proven to be difficult to completely control or eradicate, especially due to the vast number of potential sources of infection and its close association with domestic cats, which are both a reservoir (and only host that supports oocyst formation) and disseminator of the infectious cysts of the parasite. *T. gondii* is transmitted to humans through two primary foodborne routes: via tissue cysts in infected animal meat, or via oocyst contamination of various food vehicles, including produce. Moreover, it can be transmitted transplacentally from a pregnant woman to her fetus, which would result in central nervous system abnormalities, ocular disease, or death of the fetus.[2,35,54]

Pigs and sheep act as major intermediate hosts of *T. gondii* (most warm-blooded animals, however, act as intermediate hosts); as a result, foodborne toxoplasmosis is primarily associated with infected pork, lamb, mutton, and pig offal. Proper cooking (with the appropriate time-temperature combination), commercial freezing, and irradiation have proven to be effective in controlling *T. gondii* in meat.[103] On the other hand, vacuum packing and chilling have not shown any efficacy against *T. gondii* viability. Therefore, it is extremely important to educate consumers, especially those in the high-risk categories about the best measures to deal with this parasite; in fact, it is suggested that pregnant women stay away from cats and undercooked meat products.[104,105]

Human symptoms of *T. gondii* infection range from mild to moderate to severe, with abortions and congenital defects being the most prominent acute effects. Chronic sequelae include ocular disease, and chronic mental, behavioral, and neurological issues, including meningoencephalitis and chorioretinitis.[106] Pregnant women and immunocompromised individuals are especially at risk from this parasite. *T. gondii* infection is diagnosed by serological assay (like ELISA; which remains the gold standard testing methodology), although studies have shown the efficacy of molecular methods such as PCR.[107]

28.3.3.5 *Trichinella spiralis*

Trichinella spiralis, also known as roundworm, is a historically relevant parasite belonging to the phylum Nematoda. *T. spiralis* is the causative agent of trichinellosis, and is primarily transmitted to humans via the consumption of undercooked meat. This is a parasite of concern, particularly in the pork industry, since it is endemic to pig breeding operations.[108] The encysted larval stage of the parasitic life cycle is primarily associated with human cases of disease; larvae reside in animal skeletal muscles, thereby infecting animals and humans that consume them.[6,54] Therefore, stringent testing and inspection of pork and meat facilities play a significant role in reducing the public health impact of this parasite. As a result, in recent years, *Trichinella* has been controlled to a great degree in most developed and high-income countries. However, the same cannot be said of lower income and developing countries, and literature regarding the prevalence of *T. spiralis* in meats in these countries is sparse.[107]

The consumption of undercooked, infected pork is one of the primary sources of *T. spiralis* infection. Game meats and leafy greens irrigated with larvae-contaminated water are additional sources of *T. spiralis*. In leafy greens, the preharvest intervention strategies that were developed decades earlier to control the risk posed by this parasite to human consumers remain the industry gold standard even today. This parasite can also be inactivated by proper cooking of meat (recently reduced by the United States Department of Agriculture to at least 62°C from the earlier Information and Communications Technology (ICT) in Agriculture recommended 71°C) by consumers, as well as commercial freezing, and irradiation.[6]

Trichinellosis manifests as nonspecific gastrointestinal symptoms (including diarrhea, abdominal pain, and vomiting), followed by facial edema, conjunctivitis, fever, and myalgia. Severe forms of this infection affect the circulatory (myocarditis) and central nervous systems.[6] Chronic sequelae include chronic muscle pain. Trichinellosis is primarily diagnosed by antibody testing, as well as muscle biopsy.[108]

28.4 Research gaps and future directions

The food industry must, by law, develop and implement effective control measures to ensure food safety and quality. In the animal meat and milk industry, this means having a thorough understanding of the zoonoses relevant to specific food products. Such an understanding must consider both known pathways and mechanisms employed by pathogens, as well as those that could potentially arise because of pathogen genetic recombination and adaptation to new environments. Moreover, since new pathogens are constantly being discovered, it is important to study and track them in order to develop and retain a diverse profile of pathogens and their food sources.[109] For example, although *E. coli* O157:H7 was first associated with insufficiently cooked hamburgers in 1982, more recent outbreaks have been associated with both animal products, such as unpasteurized milk and cheeses, as well as nonanimal food sources, such as unpasteurized fruit juices, sprouts, and more recently, leafy greens such as spinach (Box 28.4).[110]

28.4.1 Consumer awareness and education

Previous epidemiological surveillance has indicated that consumer behavior is a hidden, but very important, contributor to foodborne disease outbreaks. Obviously, consumers are not given sufficient, easy-to-understand information about habits that can lead to foodborne disease outbreaks, and how to prevent them. Consumers, as a rule, are aware of the need for food safety, but their knowledge about food safety practices remains asymmetric. For example, prior studies have shown that only a third of the participating consumers follow cold chain transport principles for perishable foods.[113] Thus, it is important to educate consumers about the real risks associated with incorrect handling of meat, milk, and egg products, in order to reduce the risk of zoonotic disease emergence. Combining such education with knowledge about, and skills for, effective food handling, transport, and storage practices can serve the purpose of potentially changing the consumer's perceived risk of foodborne diseases, and thereby their habits related to food safety practices. Such education can come in the form of leaflets and flyers from federal regulatory agencies, posters, newsletters, signs, videos, television and radio advertisements, internet advertisements, and more.[114]

BOX 28.4

Previously a matter of concern only for individuals afflicted with bacterial disease, antimicrobial resistance has become a matter of serious concern over the past three decades. The development of antimicrobial resistance in pathogens of concern for both humans and animals can be directly attributed to the use (or misuse) of antibiotics in clinical and veterinary practice—to promote growth and as a prophylaxis to prevent disease in animals. However, based on the delivery system, animals can end up being administered sublethal doses of antibiotics, which in turn can sensitize the pathogenic agent against it. Transfer of the resistance gene via mobile genetic elements through the microbial population, in turn, results in the selection and proliferation of the resistant phenotype. When these infect humans, antimicrobial therapy would not work against them, causing serious disease.[111] In recent times, studies have shown the efficacy of natural antimicrobials, such as lactic acid bacteria, in controlling pathogen numbers in milk and meat-based food items.[112]

28.4.2 Detection methods—scope for improvement

As seen for a majority of the included foodborne zoonoses, traditional culture methods remain the gold standard method for detection. However, in addition to being time-consuming, these methods are inefficient in determining the various subtypes and serovars of pathogens, especially bacteria. Studies have shown that not all subtypes of bacteria are made equal—some (like EHEC O157:H7) have the capability of causing severe disease, while others may be relatively harmless.[54] This highlights the need for the widespread acceptance and utilization of molecular subtyping methods such as whole genome sequencing in the identification of zoonotic agents, which, in addition to being rapid, remove the need for a multitude of confirmatory tests, and are highly specific. Alternatively, current research is severely lacking in knowledge regarding the interplay between "healthy" and "dangerous" microbes within a host environment. Such information can be gleaned by specific analyses of the microbiome and microbial ecology, which in turn would help in the development of microbiome-based intervention strategies in the animal host and food processing environment.[115]

Endnotes

[a]Double vision

[b]Disorder wherein eyes are misaligned (do not line up in the same direction)

References

1. Mantovani A. Notes on the development of the concept of zoonoses. WHO Mediterranean Zoonoses Control Centre Information Circular; 2001: 51 pp.
2. Hubálek Z, Rudolf I. *Microbial Zoonoses Sapronoses*. Springer Science Business Media; 2011. Available from: http://doi.org/10.1007/978-90-481-9657-9_2.
3. Lloyd-Smith JO, George D, Pepin KM, et al. Epidemic dynamics at the human-animal interface. *Science*. 2009;326(5958):1362–1367.
4. Woolhouse ME, Gowtage-Sequeria S. Host range and emerging and reemerging pathogens. *Emerg Infect Dis*. 2005;11:1842–1847.
5. Karesh WB, Cook RA. The human-animal link. *Foreign Aff.* 2005;84(4):38–50.
6. Todd E. Foodborne diseases: overview of biological hazards and foodborne diseases. *Encycl Food Saf.* 2014;221–242.
7. Scallan E, Hoekstra RM, Angulo FJ, et al. Foodborne illness acquired in the United States – major pathogens. *Emerg Infect Dis*. 2011;17(1):7–15.

8. Animal and Plant Health Inspection Service – United States Department of Agriculture (USDA APHIS). Zoonotic diseases of sheep and goats. <https://www.aphis.usda.gov/aphis/ourfocus/animalhealth/sa_animal_disease_information/sheep-goat/zoonotic>; 2020 Accessed 10.01.21.
9. Tack DM, Ray L, Griffin PM, et al. Preliminary incidence and trends of infections with pathogens transmitted commonly through food—foodborne diseases active surveillance network, 10 U.S. sites, 2016–2019. *MMWR Morb Mortal Week Rep*. 2020;69(17):509–514.
10. Engering A, Hogerwerf L, Slingenbergh J. Pathogen–host–environment interplay and disease emergence. *Emerg Microb Infect*. 2012;2. Available from: https://doi.org/10.1038/emi.2013.5.
11. Food and Agricultural Organization of the United Nations. Livestock commodities. In: Bruinsma J, ed. *World Agriculture – Towards 2015/2030. An FAO Perspective*. 2003;XII: 432.
12. Salter AM. Improving the sustainability of global milk and meat production. *Proc Nutr Soc*. 2016;76(1):22–27.
13. Wyness L, Weichselbaum E, O'Connor A, et al. Red meat in the diet: an update. *Nutr Bull*. 2011;36:34–77.
14. Kliem KE, Givens DI. Dairy products in the food chain: their impact on health. *Annu Rev Food Sci*. 2011;2:21–36.
15. Whitnall T, Pitts N. Meat consumption. Meat consumption – <Agricultural Commodities March 2019 (awe.gov.au)> Department of Agriculture; 2020 Accessed 01.05.21.
16. Burkart MR. Diffuse pollution from intensive agriculture: sustainability, challenges, and opportunities. *Water Sci Technol*. 2007;55 (3):17–23.
17. Bar-On YM, Phillips R, Milo R. The biomass distribution on Earth. *Proc Natl Acad Sci U S A*. 2018;115:6506–6511.
18. Ritchie H, Roser M. Meat and dairy production. OurWorldInData. org. <https://ourworldindata.org/meat-production>; 2017 Accessed 17.05.21.
19. Graham JP, Leibler JH, Price LB, et al. The animal-human interface and infectious disease in industrial food animal production: rethinking biosecurity and biocontainment. *Public Health Rep*. 2008;123(3):282–299.
20. Espinosa R, Tago D, Treich N. Infectious diseases and meat production. *Environ Resour Econ*. 2020;76:1019–1044.
21. Schrag SJ, Wiener P. Emerging infectious disease: what are the relative roles of ecology and evolution? *Trends Ecol Evol*. 1995;10:319–324.
22. Plowright RK, Sokolow SH, Gorman ME, Daszak P, Foley JE. Causal inference in disease ecology: investigating ecological drivers of disease emergence. *Front Ecol Environ*. 2008;6:420–429.
23. Vora N. Impact of anthropogenic environmental alterations on vector-borne diseases. *Medscape J Med*. 2008;10(10):238.
24. Murray KA, Daszak P. Human ecology in pathogenic landscapes: two hypotheses on how land use change drives viral emergence. *Curr Opin Virol*. 2013;3(1):79–83.
25. Loth L, Gilbert M, Osmani MG, Kalam AM, Xiao X. Risk factors and clusters of Highly Pathogenic Avian Influenza H5N1 outbreaks in Bangladesh. *Prev Vet Med*. 2010;96(1–2):104–113.
26. Bett B, Kiunga P, Gachohi J, et al. Effects of climate change on the occurrence and distribution of livestock diseases. *Prev Vet Med*. 2017;137(Pt B):119–129.
27. Food and Agricultural Organization of the United Nations (FAO). Food safety and climate change. In: *FAO Conference on Food Security and the Challenges of Climate Change and Bioenergy*. <http://www.fao.org/ag/agn/agns/files/HLC1_Climate_Change_and_Food_Safety.pdf>; 2008 Accessed 06.05.21.
28. Tirado MC, Clarke R, Jaykus LA, McQuatters-Gollop A, Frank JM. Climate change and food safety: a review. *Food Saf Int*. 2010;43:1745–1765.
29. McMichael AJ, Woodruff RE, Hales S. Climate change and human health: present and future risks. *Lancet*. 2006;367:859–869.
30. Ebi KL, Lindgren E, Suk JE, Semenza JC. Adaptation to the infectious disease impacts of climate change. *Clim Change*. 2013;118:355–365.
31. Paz S. Climate change impacts on West Nile virus transmission in a global context. *Philos Trans R Soc B*. 2015;370:20130561.
32. Polley LR. Foodborne parasites and climate change. In: Gajadhar A, ed. *Foodborne Parasites in the Food Supply Web*. 1st ed. Cambridge: Woodhead Publishing; 2015:482.
33. Roberts CA. *The Food Safety Information Handbook*. Greenwood Publishing Group; 2001.
34. Hollinger FB, Ticehurst JR. Hepatitis A virus. In: Fields BN, Knipe DM, Howley PM, eds. *Fields Virology*. 3rd ed. Philadelphia, PA: Lippincott-Raven; 1996:735–782.
35. World Health Organization. Multicriteria-based ranking for risk management of food-born parasites. Microbiological Risk Assessment Series (MRA) 23. 2014.
36. Franssen F, Gerard C, Cozma-Petruţ A, et al. Inactivation of parasite transmission stages: efficacy of treatments on food of animal origin. *Trends Food Sci Technol*. 2019;83:114–128.
37. Goel AK. Anthrax: a disease of biowarfare and public health importance. *World J Clin Cases*. 2015;3(1):20–33.
38. U.S. Food and Drug Administration. Anthrax. <Anthrax | FDA>; 2018 Accessed 06.05.21.
39. United States Department of Agriculture – Animal and Plant Health Inspection Service (USDA APHIS). Anthrax factsheet. <anthraxpdf (fdlp.gov)>; 2001 Accessed 07.05.21.
40. Rastogi A. Anthrax; Anthrax | National Health Portal Of India (nhp.gov.in)>; 2015 Accessed 08.05.21.
41. McLauchlin J, Mitchell RT, Smerdon WJ, Jewell K. *Listeria monocytogenes* and listeriosis: a review of hazard characterisation for use in microbiological risk assessment of foods. *Int J Food Microbiol*. 2004;92:15–33.
42. U.S. Centers for Disease Control and Prevention. Florida retiree gets – and survives – anthrax. <Florida Retiree Gets—and Survives—Anthrax | CDC>; 2020 Accessed 08.05.21.
43. U.S. Centers for Disease Control and Prevention. Brucellosis. <CDC - Home - Brucellosis>; 2021 Accessed 08.05.21.
44. U.S. Centers for Disease Control and Prevention. Brucellosis reference guide: Exposures, testing and prevention. <Brucellosis Reference Guide: Exposures, Testing and Prevention (cdc.gov)>; 2017 Accessed 08.05.21.
45. Man SM. The clinical importance of emerging *Campylobacter* species. *Nat Rev Gastroenterol Hepatol*. 2011;8(12):669–685.
46. Inglis GD, Kalischuk LD, Busz HW. Chronic shedding of *Campylobacter* species in beef cattle. *J Appl Microbiol*. 2004;97:410–420.
47. Stafford RJ, Schluter PJ, Wilson AJ, et al. Population-attributable risk estimates for risk factors associated with *Campylobacter* infection, Australia. *Emerg Infect Dis*. 2008;14:895–901.
48. Meldrum RJ, Griffiths JK, Smith RMM, Evans MR. The seasonality of human *Campylobacter* infection and *Campylobacter* isolates

from fresh, retail chicken in Wales. *Epidemiol Infect.* 2005;133:49–52.

49. Huang H, Brooks BW, Lowman R, Carrillo CD. *Campylobacter* species in animal, food, and environmental sources, and relevant testing programs in Canada. *Can J Microbiol.* 2015;61(10):701–721.
50. Rees JH, Soudain SE, Gregson NA, Hughes RA. *Campylobacter jejuni* infection and Guillain–Barré Syndrome. *N Engl J Med.* 1995;333:1374–1379.
51. Blaser MJ, Engberg J. Clinical aspects of *Campylobacter jejuni* and *Campylobacter coli* infections. In: Nachamkin I, Szymanski CM, Blaser MJ, eds. *Campylobacter.* 3rd ed. Washington, DC: ASM Press; 2008:99–121.
52. Goossens H, Henocque G, Kremp L, et al. Nosocomial outbreak of *Campylobacter jejuni* meningitis in newborn infants. *Lancet.* 1986;328:146–149.
53. Pena LA, Fishbein MC. Fatal myocarditis related to *Campylobacter jejuni* infection: a case report. *Cardiovasc Pathol.* 2007;16:119–121.
54. U.S. Food and Drug Administration. *Bad Bug Book, Foodborne Pathogenic Microorganisms and Natural Toxins*, 2nd ed. <Bad Bug Book (fda.gov)>; 2012 Accessed 12.05.21.
55. Bhunia AK. *Foodborne Microbial Pathogens: Mechanisms and Pathogenesis*. Berlin: Springer Science & Business Media; 2018.
56. Songer JG. Clostridia as agents of zoonotic disease. *Vet Microbiol.* 2010;140(3–4):339–404.
57. European Food Safety Authority (EFSA). The European Union summary report on trends and sources of zoonoses, zoonotic agents and food-borne outbreaks in 2014. *EFSA J.* 2015;13(12):4329. Available from: https://doi.org/10.2903/j.efsa.2015.4329.
58. Swaminathan B, Gerner-Smidt P. The epidemiology of human listeriosis. *Microbes Infect.* 2007;9:1236–1243.
59. Drevets DA, Bronze MS. *Listeria monocytogenes*: epidemiology, human disease, and mechanisms of brain invasion. *FEMS Immunol Med Microbiol.* 2008;53(2):151–165.
60. U.S. Centers for Disease Control and Prevention. Listeria (listeriosis). <Listeria (Listeriosis) | Listeria | CDC>; 2021 Accessed 12.05.21.
61. World Health Organization. Listeriosis. <Listeriosis (who.int)>; 2021 Accessed 12.05.21.
62. Jordan K, McAuliffe O. *Listeria monocytogenes* in foods. *Adv Food Nutr Res.* 2018;86:181–213.
63. Ferreira V, Wiedmann M, Teixeira P, Satsiewicz MJ. *Listeria monocytogenes* persistence in food-associated environments: epidemiology, strain characteristics, and implications for public health. *J Food Prot.* 2014;77(1):150–170.
64. Goulet G, King LA, Vaillant V, De Valk H. What is the incubation period for listeriosis? *BMC Infect Dis.* 2013;13:11.
65. Chen J, Karanth S, Pradhan AK. Quantitative microbial risk assessment for *Salmonella*: inclusion of whole genome sequencing and genomic epidemiological studies, and advances in the bioinformatics pipeline. *J Agric Food Res.* 2020;2:100045.
66. Müller B, Dürr S, Alonso S, et al. Zoonotic *Mycobacterium bovis*-induced tuberculosis in humans. *Emerg Infect Dis.* 2013;19(6):899–908.
67. Grange JM. *Mycobacterium bovis* infection in human beings. *Tuberculosis (Edinb).* 2001;81(1–2):71–77.
68. Torgerson PR, Torgerson DJ. Public health and bovine tuberculosis: what's all the fuss about? *Trends Microbiol.* 2010;18(2):67–72.
69. Morishita TY. *Chapter 18 – Galliformes. Fowler's Zoo and Wild Animal Medicine*. 8. 2015143–155.
70. Collins MT. *Mycobacterium paratuberculosis*: a potential foodborne pathogen? *J Dairy Sci.* 1997;80(12):3445–3448.
71. Nacy C, Buckley M. *Mycobacterium Avium Paratuberculosis: Infrequent Human Pathogen or Public Health Threat?* Washington DC: American Society of Microbiology; 2008.
72. Naser SA, Sagramsingh SR, Naser AS, Thanigachalam S. *Mycobacterium avium* subspecies *paratuberculosis* causes Crohn's disease in some inflammatory bowel disease patients. *World J Gastroenterol.* 2014;20:7403–7415.
73. Pal M, Rahman MT. *Mycobacterium avium* subspecies *paratuberculosis*: an emerging bacterial disease of global public health significance. *Microbes Health.* 2015;4(1):4–13.
74. Kirk MD, Pires SM, Black RE, et al. World Health Organization estimates of the global and regional disease burden of 22 foodborne bacterial, protozoal, and viral diseases, 2010: a data synthesis. *PLoS Med.* 2015;12:e1001921.
75. Gharieb RM, Tartor YH, Khedr MH. Non-typhoidal *Salmonella* in poultry meat and diarrhoeic patients: prevalence, antibiogram, virulotyping, molecular detection and sequencing of class I integrons in multidrug resistant strains. *Gut Pathol.* 2015;7:1–11.
76. U. S. Centers for Disease Control and Prevention. Reports of selected Salmonella outbreak investigations. Salmonella homepage. <Outbreaks Involving Salmonella | CDC>; 2021 Accessed 22.05.21.
77. U. S. Centers for Disease Control and Prevention. National Outbreak Reporting System (NORS). <National Outbreak Reporting System (NORS) | CDC>; 2021 Accessed 22.05.21.
78. Bacon RT, Sofos JN. Characteristics of biological hazards in foods. In: Schmidt RH, Rodrick GE, eds. *Food Safety Handbook.* New Jersey: John Wiley & Sons; 2003:157–195.
79. Kloos WE. Natural populations of the genus *Staphylococcus. Annu Rev Microbiol.* 1980;559–592.
80. Wulf M, Voss A. MRSA in livestock animals – an epidemic waiting to happen? *Clin Microbiol Infect.* 2008;14:519–521.
81. European Food Safety Authority. The European Union summary report on trends and sources of zoonoses, zoonotic agents and food-borne outbreaks in 2011. *EFSA J.* 2013;11:3129–3379.
82. Sabina Y, Rahman A, Ramesh CHR, Montet D. *Yersinia enterocolitica*: mode of transmission, molecular insights of virulence, and pathogenesis of infection. *J Pathol.* 2011;. Available from: https://doi.org/10.4061/2011/429069.
83. Baumgartner A, Küffer M, Suter D, Jemmi T, Rohner P. Antimicrobial resistance of *Yersinia enterocolitica* strains from human patients, pigs and retail pork in Switzerland. *Int J Food Microbiol.* 2007;115:110–114.
84. Walker JW, Han BA, Ott IM, Drake JM. Transmissibility of emerging viral zoonoses. *PLoS One.* 2018;. Available from: https://doi.org/10.1371/journal.pone.0206926.
85. International Commission on Microbiological Specifications for Foods. ICMSF opinion on SARS-CoV-2 and its relationship to food safety. <https://www.icmsf.org/in-the-news/announcements/>; 2020 Accessed 14.08.21.
86. Hoofnagle JH, Nelson KE, Purcell RH, Hepatitis E. *N Engl J Med.* 2012;367(13):1237–1244. Available from: https://doi.org/10.1056/NEJMra1204512.

87. Meng XJ. From barnyard to food table: the omnipresence of hepatitis E virus and risk for zoonotic infection and food safety. *Virus Res*. 2011;161(1):23–30.

88. Drobeniuc J, Favorov MO, Shapiro CN, et al. Hepatitis E virus antibody prevalence among persons who work with swine. *J Infect Dis*. 2001;184(12):1594–1597.

89. Feagins AR, Opriessnig T, Guenette DK, Halbur PG, Meng XJ. Inactivation of infectious hepatitis E virus present in commercial pig livers sold in local grocery stores in the United States. *Int J Food Microbiol*. 2008;123(1–2):32–37.

90. Song YJ, Jeong HJ, Kim YJ, et al. Analysis of complete genome sequences of swine hepatitis E virus and possible risk factors for transmission of HEV to humans in Korea. *J Med Virol*. 2010;82 (4):583–591.

91. Said B, Ijaz S, Kafatos G, et al.Hepatitis E Incident Investigation Team Hepatitis E outbreak on cruise ship. *Emerg Infect Dis*. 2009;15(11):1738–1744.

92. Anelich L. Foodborne disease: prevalence of foodborne diseases in Africa. In: Motarjami Y, Moy G, Todd E, eds. *Encyclopedia of Food Safety*. 1. 2014:262–275.

93. Torgerson PR, Devleesschauwer B, Praet N, et al. World Health Organization estimates of the global and regional disease burden of 11 foodborne parasitic diseases, 2010: a data synthesis. *PLoS Med*. 2015;. Available from: https://doi.org/10.1371/journal.pmed.1001920.

94. Harper CM, Cowell NA, Adams BC, Langley AJ, Wohlsen TD. Outbreak of *Cryptosporidium* linked to drinking unpasteurised milk. *Commun Dis Intell*. 2002;26:449–500.

95. Karanis P, Kourenti K, Smith HV. Waterborne transmission of protozoan parasites: a worldwide review of outbreaks and lessons learnt. *J Water Health*. 2007;5:1–38.

96. Smith HV, Caccio SM, Cook N, Nichols RAB, Tait A. *Cryptosporidium* and *Giardia* as foodborne zoonoses. *Vet Parasitol*. 2007;149(1–2):29–40.

97. Moriarty EM, Duffy G, McEvoy JM, et al. The effect of thermal treatments on the viability and infectivity of *Cryptosporidium parvum* on beef surfaces. *J Appl Microbiol*. 2005;98:618–623.

98. Tzipori S, Jaskiewicz JJ. *Protozoan diseases: cryptosporidiosis, giardiasis, and other intestinal protozoan diseases. International Encyclopedia of Public Health*. 2nd ed. Academic Press; 2017.

99. Saleque A, Juyal PD, Bhatia BB. Effect of temperature on the infectivity of *Sarcocystis miescheriana* cysts in pork. *Vet Parasitol*. 1990;36(3–4):343–346.

100. Craig P, Ito A. Intestinal parasites. *Curr Opin Infect Dis*. 2007;20:524–532.

101. Murrell KD, Dorny P, Flisser A, et al., eds. *WHO/FAO/OIE Guidelines for the surveillance, prevention and control of taeniosis/cysticercosis* (139 pp.). Paris: OIE. <http://www.oie.int/doc/ged/d11245.pdf>; 2005 Accessed 24.08.13.

102. U.S. Centers for Disease Control and Prevention. Parasites – cysticercosis: epidemiology & risk factors. <CDC - Cysticercosis - Epidemiology & Risk Factors>; 2021 Accessed 21.05.21.

103. Rani S, Pradhan AK. Evaluating uncertainty and variability associated with *Toxoplasma gondii* survival during cooking and low temperature storage of fresh cut meats. *Int J Food Microbiol*. 2021;341:109031.

104. Dubey JP, Hill DE, Fournet V, et al. Low prevalence of viable *Toxoplasma gondii* in fresh, unfrozen, American pasture-raised pork and lamb from retail meat stores in the United States. *Food Control*. 2020;109:106961.

105. Rani S, Cerqueira-Cézar CK, Murata FHA, et al. Distribution of *Toxoplasma gondii* tissue cysts in shoulder muscles of naturally infected goats and lambs. *J Food Prot*. 2020;83(8):1396–1401.

106. Flegr J. Effects of *Toxoplasma* on human behaviour. *Schizophr Bull*. 2007;33(3):757–776.

107. Rani S, Pradhan AK. Evaluation and meta-analysis of test accuracy of direct PCR and bioassay methods for detecting *Toxoplasma gondii* in meat samples. *LWT*. 2020;131:109666.

108. U. S. Centers for Disease Control and Prevention. Parasites – Trichinellosis: Resources for health professionals. <CDC - Trichinellosis - Resources for Health Professionals>; 2021 Accessed 01.06.21.

109. Jevšnik M, Hlebec V, Raspor P. Consumers' awareness of food safety from shopping to eating. *Food Control*. 2008;19 (8):737–745.

110. Smoot L, Cordier JL. *Emerging foodborne pathogens and the food industry. Foodborne Pathogens*. Woodhead Publishing; 2009:154–181.

111. Cork S, Hall D, Liljebjelke K. *One Health Case Studies: Addressing Complex Problems in a Changing World*. 5m Books Ltd.; 2016.

112. Abdelhamid AG, El-Dougdoug NK. Controlling foodborne pathogens with natural antimicrobials by biological control and antivirulence strategies. *Heliyon*. 2020;6(9):e05020.

113. Patil SR, Morales R, Cates S, Anderson D, Kendall D. An application of *meta*-analysis in food safety consumer research to evaluate consumer behaviors and practices. *J Food Prot*. 2004;67 (11):2587–2595.

114. Yiannas F. *Communicating food safety effectively. Food Safety Culture*. New York: Springer; 2009:1–7.

115. Kovac J. Precision food safety: a paradigm shift in detection and control of foodborne pathogens. *mSystems*. 2019;4(3). Available from: https://doi.org/10.1128/mSystems.00164-19.

Chapter 29

Abattoir hygiene

Ivan Nastasijevic[1], Marija Boskovic[2] and Milica Glisic[2]

[1]*Institute of Meat Hygiene and Technology, Belgrade, Serbia,* [2]*Faculty of Veterinary Medicine, University of Belgrade, Belgrade, Serbia*

Abstract

Abattoirs have important role in surveillance, control, and eradication of diseases of animal health importance, as well as control, reduction, and prevention of foodborne hazards of public health importance. To achieve control and prevention of cross-contamination of carcasses and meat with foodborne hazards, the abattoir hygiene should be applied throughout the slaughter and dressing, up to the chilling of carcasses. This is based on strict adherence to good hygiene practices and the overall hygiene requirements at abattoir, named prerequisite programs (layout and design of production facility, equipment, tools, ventilation, trained workers), supplemented with risk-based food safety management system (hazard analysis and critical control point) and chilled carcass safety assurance system in the farm-abattoir continuum. Therefore abattoir hygiene has an important impact on final microbiological status of chilled carcass, as well as prevention and minimization of consumers exposure to foodborne hazards associated with meat consumption.

Keywords: Abattoir hygiene; foodborne; hazard; chilled carcass; food safety

29.1 Introduction

29.1.1 The role of abattoirs—past and current status

Animal slaughter to provide meat for consumption is one of humanity's most ancient activities. The first attempt to recognize the public health impact associated with animal slaughter and meat consumption was done by the early Roman Empire, which regulated this activity by setting up public spaces called *macella*. Such places represented a space where animals could be slaughtered and meat can be sold.

Throughout the middle ages and up to the beginning of the 19th century most animals, in Europe and United States, were slaughtered in the open air, usually in yards at the back of small, private butcher's shops.[1] For example, the predecessors of public abattoirs can be found in Spain with municipal slaughter points traced back to 11th century (1020) in Leon, 13th century (1202) in Madrid, 14th century (1398) in Toledo and up to establishing a first centralized abattoir in Barcelona in 15th century (1456).

The transformation of thousand years' old agrarian to an industrial economy, increased urban population, and growing awareness over hygiene have led to the first public abattoirs at the beginning of the 19th century. In France, in 1807, Napoleon issued an order that public abattoirs should be built to provide the meat supply for the city of Paris and other French cities, as well. The idea was to centralize the slaughter of animals in establishment where stricter hygiene measures can be applied and where carcasses/meat could be routinely inspected. Many other European countries and United States throughout the second half of 19th century and beginning of 20th century followed that example and developed regulations for construction and operation of public abattoirs, including meat marketing. In the United States the development of "Chicago Union Stockyards" in the 19th century forever transformed the production of meat and the physical landscape.

Abattoirs are, therefore, institutions and locations from which many economic and geographical changes in the production of food, cultural attitudes toward slaughter of animals, social changes, sensibilities, and relations between humans and meat-producing animals can be followed and understood.

The first legislation regulating public abattoirs and meat marketing (distribution, retail) in the beginning of 20th century differed in some European countries. The "French model" recommended that, due to difficulty in preserving meat, mainly because of the lack of refrigerated transport, public abattoirs should be constructed close to centers of consumption and close to livestock market to which animals were brought from the farm. Contrary to this, in the United States, Netherlands, and Denmark the decision was to locate public abattoirs with cold storage close to centers of production, from where carcasses would be transported to centers

Present Knowledge in Food Safety. DOI: https://doi.org/10.1016/B978-0-12-819470-6.00002-0

of consumption.[2] In both approaches, meat preservation depended on the microbial status of carcass, which leads back to the abattoir hygiene level.

However, increased size of meat production due to industrialization of animal slaughter and increased demand also brought other challenges related to transmission of zoonoses and zoonotic foodborne diseases to consumers.

Zoonoses can be defined as: "any disease or infection caused by all types of agents (bacteria, parasites, fungi, viruses and unconventional agents) transmissible from vertebrate animals to humans and *vice versa*."[3] They are recognized as important public health problems also causing economic disruption and decreased productivity in animal populations and increased morbidity and mortality in humans.

Increased food trade at local and international level is attracting additional attention to biosecurity on farm and control measures related to abattoir hygiene to decrease the potential for transmission of zoonoses and zoonotic foodborne diseases from food-producing animals via food chain (Fig. 29.1).[4]

Meat-producing animals are usually coming from different sources to abattoir. They may come not only from farms with high-level biosecurity measures, where prevalence of hazards of public health importance is very low or negligible, but also from farms with poor biosecurity level, where the prevalence of hazards is high, including less-controlled livestock markets. Different batches of animals may carry in their gastrointestinal tract and fecally shed different level of hazards of public health importance (*Salmonella*, *Campylobacter*, Shiga toxin-producing *E. coli* (STEC), *Listeria monocytogenes*, *Yersinia*, *Clostridium perfringens*). It may lead to cross-contamination of animal hides, skins, or feathers during transportation and in abattoir lairage, and subsequent transfer to carcasses/meat during slaughter and dressing. Therefore abattoirs present a "central place" where application of effective and efficient control measures has a crucial public health role in control and prevention of zoonotic foodborne hazards and their transmission to consumers via meat consumption. The major roles of abattoirs are achieved through some veterinary public health (VPH) functions.

29.2 Veterinary public health

VPH was defined for a first time in 1975 as "the component of public" health activities devoted to the application of veterinary skills, knowledge, and resources to the protection and improvement of human health.[5] VPH definition expanded further in 1999 and included "the sum of all contributions to the physical, mental, and social well-being of humans through an understanding and application of veterinary science."[6] In most countries, VPH activities encompass the surveillance, prevention, and control of zoonoses, food hygiene, and animal-related aspects of the protection of the environment.[5] Some VPH functions applied in abattoirs related to meat hygiene and environmental protection are as follows: prevention and control of zoonoses and other diseases transmitted by meat, including antimicrobial resistance; supervision of abattoir hygiene and prevention of carcass/meat cross-contamination with microbiological hazards of public health importance; audit of abattoirs, their operations and products, including slaughter, dressing, chilling, storage, and distribution; antemortem and postmortem meat inspection; safe collection and disposal of dead animals, condemned meat, inedible animal by-products and of other animal wastes; control of environmental pollution by wastewaters treatment; supervision of export and import of meat from the hygienic viewpoint.

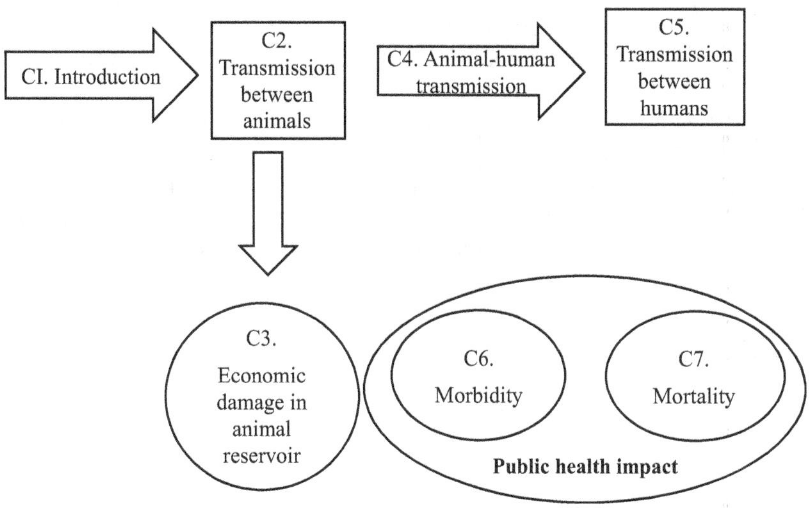

FIGURE 29.1 The pathway from introduction of a zoonotic pathogen to public health impact, represented by seven criteria, C1–C7.[4]

29.2.1 Prevention and control of zoonoses and other meat-borne diseases

Abattoir hygiene is closely related to prevention and control of zoonoses and meat-borne diseases. Q-fever, brucellosis, and tularemia are major zoonotic diseases for slaughterhouse workers (occupational diseases).

From recently, new zoonotic public health risks emerged due to spreading of previously unknown pathogens originated from animal reservoirs such as bats (Severe Acute Respiratory Syndrome associated with coronavirus, SARS-CoV, SARS-CoV-2/COVID-19), camels (Middle East Respiratory Syndrome coronavirus, MERS-CoV), birds/poultry (Avian Flu/H5N1), and pigs (Swine Flu, H1N1). These events that caused epidemics and pandemics showed that certain habits in some regions of world associated with poor slaughter hygiene, such as butchering of wild animals in "wet markets," as well as poor animal breeding activities, can pose a significant public health risk. For example, the outbreak of COVID-19, provoked by SARS-CoV-2, was most probably linked with butchering of wild animals (e.g., pangolin) with potential origin from wildlife farm, as intermediary hosts to whom the virus was spread from a primary reservoir (horseshoe bats).[7,8] It is believed (although still without firm scientific evidence and confirmation) that the disease subsequently spread to humans working at or visiting this wet market triggering multiple chains of transmission that enabled further sustained transmission in the human population,[9,10] first in China and subsequently on a global level.

Other reemerged zoonoses of bacterial and viral origin are, for example, *Mycobacterium bovis*, *Brucella* spp., and Hepatitis E.[11] These zoonoses should be considered as emerging risks in animal breeding and meat production and should be addressed by specific preventive measures, for example, farm biosecurity and abattoir hygiene, respectively.

Zoonotic diseases that are regularly surveyed in abattoirs are as follows: trichinellosis (*Trichinella* spp.), echinococcosis (*Echinococcus granulosus*, *Echinococcus multilocularis*), cysticercosis (*Cysticercus cellulosae*, *Cysticercus bovis*, *Cysticercus ovis*), sarcocystosis (*Sarcocystis* spp.), brucellosis (*Brucella melitensis*, *Brucella abortus*), leptospirosis (*Leptospira interrogans*), listeriosis (*L. monocytogenes*), tuberculosis (*Mycobacterium bovis*), tularemia (Francisella tularensis), anthracosis (*Bacillus anthracis*), Q-fever (*Coxiella burnetii*), leishmaniosis (*Leishmania donovani*), and Rift Valley fever (*Phlebovirus*).

Zoonotic meat-borne pathogens that are regularly surveyed in abattoirs are as follows: *Salmonella* spp., *Campylobacter* spp., STEC, and *L. monocytogenes*. Epidemiological studies provide essential knowledge of zoonoses and help to determine the most suitable method of control.[12] To achieve a defined level of public health protection, animal health and public health activities should be integrated as fully as possible. Special emphasis should be put on biosecurity measures applied on farm and, good hygiene practices (GHP) and risk-based food safety management system applied in abattoirs, that is, hazard analysis and critical control point (HACCP).

29.2.2 Antemortem and postmortem meat inspection

Abattoir is the place where the meat inspection is carried out, both antemortem (meat-producing animals' health status) and postmortem (carcasses/offal' wholesomeness for consumption). Traditional practices of meat inspection are not always suitable for detecting the main zoonotic foodborne hazards such as *Campylobacter* and *Salmonella* or contamination by chemical substances such as persistent organic pollutants or prohibited substances.[13] This is due to substantial changes over the recent decades in modern animal- and meat-production systems that have led to a significant change in meat-borne threats to public health.[14] For example, traditional zoonoses, such as tuberculosis, brucellosis, anthrax infection, trichinellosis, and cysticercosis became much less important,[15] while bacterial agents carried and excreted (primarily via feces) by healthy food-producing animals, showing no symptoms, have emerged as the most relevant (*Campylobacter*, *Salmonella*, Shiga toxin-producing *E. coli* (STEC)). It has to be understood that abattoir hygiene is of crucial importance for prevention and reduction of cross-contamination of carcasses/meat. Further, public concern regarding the presence of harmful chemical in meat, in particular industrial contaminants and antibiotics, has also increased.[16]

All those "new" agents are macroscopically invisible, as they cause no lesions in organs/tissues and so cannot be detected by traditional meat inspection which includes visual observation, palpation, and incision. For this reason, the European Commission decided that meat inspection practices in the European Union (EU) should be modernized.[14,16–20] The similar approach has been taken in the United States where regulation on "Modernization of Swine Slaughter Inspection" has been introduced.[21] In the EU, the European Food Safety Authority (EFSA) identified foodborne biological and chemical hazards for all types of meat-producing animals and meat thereof, considered, and ranked them according to their risk for public health (Table 29.1).[4,13,16–19]

29.3 Prerequisite programs for abattoirs

Prerequisite programs (PRPs) represent basic conditions and activities that are necessary within the abattoirs for production of safe meat.[22,23] Well-established, fully operational, and verified PRPs, that are designed according to

TABLE 29.1 Ranking of main biological and chemical hazards identified for each animal species.[4,13,16–19]

Species	Biological hazards				Chemical hazards
	High	**Medium**	**Low**	**Undetermined**	
Cattle			*Campylobacter* spp. *(thermophilic)*		Dioxins, dioxin-like polychlorinated biphenyls (DL-PCBs)
	STEC	N/A	*Yersinia enterocolitica/ pseudotuberculosis*	*Toxoplasma gondii*	
	Salmonella enterica		*ESBL/AmpC Escherichia coli*	*Trichinella* spp.	
			Cysticercus (Taenia saginata)		
			Mycobacterium bovis		
Sheep and goats			*Campylobacter* spp. *(thermophilic)*		Dioxins, DL-PCBs
	STEC		*S. enterica*		
	T. gondii	N/A	*Y. enterocolitica/ pseudotuberculosis*	*Trichinella* spp.	
			ESBL/AmpC E. coli		
Porcines	*S. enterica*	*Y. enterocolitica/ pseudotuberculosis*	*Campylobacter* spp. *(thermophilic)*	N/A	Dioxins, DL-PCBs
		T. gondii	STEC		
		Trichinella spp.	*ESBL/AmpC E. coli*		
			Cysticercus (Taenia solium)		
			Mycobacterium avium (hominissuis)		
Solipeds	*Trichinella*	N/A	*Campylobacter* spp. *(thermophilic)*	*T. gondii*	Phenylbutazone,[a] chemical elements *(cadmium)*
			S. enterica		
			Y. enterocolitica/ pseudotuberculosis		
			STEC		
			ESBL/AmpC E. coli		
Poultry (broilers)	*Campylobacter* spp. *(thermophilic)*	*ESBL/AmpC E. coli*	N/A	*E. coli (process hygiene)*	Dioxins, DL-PCBs, chloramphenicol, nitrofurans, nitroimidazoles
	S. enterica				
Farmed game (deer)	*T. gondii*	N/A	N/A	N/A	N/A
Farmed game (wild boar)	*S. enterica*	N/A	N/A	N/A	N/A
	T. gondii				
Farmed game (reindeer, ostriches, rabbits)		N/A			N/A

N/A, Not applicable; *STEC*, Shiga toxin-producing *E. coli*.
[a]*EFSA recommended that phenylbutazone, which is not allowed in the food chain, be specifically included in the National Residue Control Plans for solipeds.*

principles of GHP and good manufacturing practice (GMP), enable implementation of safety and quality management systems during slaughter and processing.[24] It is food business operators' (FBO) responsibility to ensure that abattoir's location, construction, and operating procedures are in accordance with all applicable regulations, standards, codes of practice, and guidelines.[23] PRPs in abattoirs are the foundation for building a risk-based food safety management system (HACCP) and may include as follows: establishment design and facilities (location, premises and rooms, equipment, facilities), establishment maintenance and sanitation (maintenance and cleaning, cleaning programs, pest control systems, waste management), establishment personal hygiene (health status, illness and injuries, personal cleanliness, personal behavior, visitors), including traceability (lot identification, labeling), and product recall system.[22,25,26]

29.3.1 Layout

Premises of PRPs for abattoirs refer to the location, layout of buildings and associated utilities, materials used, and the equipment installed. Proper location choice means a well-connected area (surrounded by roadways) that is protected from external contaminants that may compromise the safety of meat (flooding, airborne contaminants, pests). Also, supplies of air, water, energy, and other utilities must be ensured.[23,24] The layout of entire abattoir should be in accordance with forwarding flow principle and consider: Reception; Lairage; Slaughter hall with the stunning place, bleeding area, hoisting area, flaying section, evisceration area, carcass splitting and carcass washing area; Chills and frozen storage; Auxiliary facilities—offal rooms, dry goods store, and sanitary facilities (changing rooms, toilets, hygiene lobby with hot and cold potable running water, hands-free handwashing stations, hand sanitizers, and hand-drying equipment or supplies); Inspection facilities.[26] Considering the operations that are performed in the abattoirs (sticking/bleeding, scalding, dehiding/dehairing/defeathering, evisceration, carcass splitting, trimming, washing, chilling), these facilities should be designed so there is the physical separation between dirty (live animals, inedible by-products) and clean areas (edible meat), with a progressive processing line that disables cross-contamination. Additional measures for the prevention of cross-contamination, cleaning and disinfecting, and personal hygiene must be applied. All facilities, workrooms and equipment should be constructed to allow effective cleaning and monitoring of hygiene status, while for different chemicals (cleaning materials, lubricants, branding ink) safe storage must be ensured,[24,27] including "food grade" certification.

29.3.2 Equipment

The equipment in abattoirs, used for slaughter procedures, heat treatment, storage, chilling and freezing, control and monitoring of humidity and airflow, should be located, designed, and installed to permit adequate cleaning, disinfection, and maintenance.[25,28] Material used for equipment and containers construction must be resistant, impervious, and easy-to-clean (e.g., wood is not permitted), while the functions of equipment should be continuously monitored and controlled. Preventive maintenance and calibration of equipment should be specifically defined (list of equipment, detailed procedures, schedules and frequencies of maintenance and calibration activities).[23,24] The elements of equipment and containers that come into contact with meat are particularly important since they affect food safety.[24]

The spreading of bacteria in abattoir environment, and consequently the cross-contamination of the carcasses by potentially pathogenic bacteria, highly depends on hygienic conditions of the walls, floors, ceilings, and hard-to-clean equipment.[29] For example, the highest percentage of *Salmonella* spp. and *L. monocytogenes*-positive samples originates from the tray used to collect viscera, dehairing conveyor, splitting machine, and a cutting room table, besides lairage and ground floor.[30] In addition, of all equipment sites examined that included hooks, worktables, chopping blocks, knives, cleavers, dehairing devices, and cold room hooks, *Salmonella* and *Yersinia*-positive samples were from worktables, *Listeria* was isolated from chopping blocks swabs, while *Salmonella* was detected in cleavers swabs.[31] *L. monocytogenes* is usually isolated from poultry plucker, *Staphylococcus aureus* from rubber fingers, *Yersinia enterocolitica* from trolleys and wheels, *S. enteritidis* from gutters and drains, and *S. Typhimurium* from work surfaces and conveyor belts swabs in abattoirs.[32] Further, after cleaning and disinfection procedures *Salmonella* spp. was found on the splitting machine and dehairing conveyor, and *L. monocytogenes* on the table in the cutting room.[30] The presence of various microorganisms in scraper/swab samples in raw meat facilities was reported after standard cleaning/disinfection procedures had been applied.[33] Although progress has been made in machine design in effort to improve hygiene, improper cleaning and disinfection protocols and inadequate equipment maintenance still may represent a major problem regarding abattoir hygiene.

An additional and more complex problem in the abattoirs are biofilms, which are protective reservoirs for pathogens harbored in abattoir environment.[34] The equipment itself could also be the vector to move the contamination from one biofilm hotspot to another. This usually includes fixed pieces of equipment with moving parts or pieces of equipment (e.g., chains) which are a mile long and travel through the slaughterhouse. Standard hygiene regimes and monitoring of cleanliness via swabbing are not efficient enough in the detection of biofilms and Viable-But Nonculturable bacteria. Therefore different biofilm eradication strategies are developed and include the use of physical methods (sonication/activated water with low frequencies sound waves and brushing); chemicals (biocides: Cl_2, H_2O_2, QAC); and new techniques with enzymes, plasma ion, and electrolyzed water.[32,33,35] Recently, the use of antimicrobial materials in the production of food contact equipment has been proposed, such as copper alloys in food processing, copper alloy conveyor belts, and so on.[32,34]

29.3.3 Ventilation

The ventilation system in the abattoirs should provide adequate means of natural or mechanical airflow so the condensation and airborne contamination of meat and meat products be minimized. Also, it should be able to control the ambient temperatures, humidity, and odors that might affect the meat suitability. Ventilation systems with integrated collectors for control of air pollutants are of great importance for a suitable work environment, reduced smell nuisance, and environmental pollution, so the health and welfare of workers and neighboring residents of such facilities do not be disturbed.[24] Dust dissemination in indoor air and inhalation of bio-aerosols are known to cause various health effects: infections, hypersensitivity, toxic reactions, irritations, and inflammatory responses.[36] Dust particles are carriers for gases, microorganisms, and endotoxins, while the main sources of airborne microbiota in these facilities include feed, litter material, animals and their feces.[37] Crowded and cooled conditions for workers in abattoirs and meat processing facilities make these workplaces high risk for the exposure to potential biological hazards.[38] Namely, the enclosed spaces in abattoirs can help to confine aerosols and allow them to build up to potentially infectious levels. This gains special attention due to the problems that the COVID-19 pandemic and SARS-CoV-2 transmission causes for the food industry.[39] The higher generation rate and accumulation potential of airborne microbiota with lower clearance by ventilation routs lead to the increased concentration of Gram-positive bacteria.[40] It is also found that bacteria and yeast isolated from bio-aerosol environment of abattoirs have an important role in carcass contamination.[41] Customized, properly designed airflow distribution systems, with adequate capacity, air-exchange rate, and the additional installations that increase ventilation effectiveness are necessary in slaughterhouses.

29.3.4 Veterinary-sanitary requirements

Veterinary-sanitary issues encompass antemortem and postmortem inspection which are connected with food safety management activities related to GHPs and HACCP.[42] Official veterinary meat inspection targets hazards that cause clinical signs and/or detectable lesions in animals at slaughter, and have an important role in both animal and public health protection.[24]

To enable efficient inspection and maintenance of sanitary conditions, FBO should provide suitable and properly located offices so the authorized veterinary inspectors could control all activities in the slaughterhouse. There should be appropriate facilities for inspection of animals before slaughter, while offices for postslaughter inspection should be free from vapors and steam, equipped with abundant artificial light, hot and cold water, and with disinfectant solutions, racks, and watertight metal containers for veterinary confiscations, a sterilizer for instruments, a microscope, and a compressorium.[27]

Traditional meat safety system in abattoirs achieved through GHP/HACCP meat inspection, and monitoring of slaughter process hygiene supported with swab sampling and laboratory analyses, have numerous deficiencies and do not provide enough protection in relation to the current priority meat-borne biological and chemical hazards.[43] That is why the new meat safety assurance system (MSAS) that is risk-based and longitudinally integrated into the whole meat chain is developed with intention of its implementation in the EU Member States.[44] In this way, the intensity of meat inspection procedures is adjusted according to the Food Chain Information (FCI) and Harmonized Epidemiological Indicators (HEI) analyses, in farm-to-abattoir continuum; farm and abattoir risk categorization defines if the visual-only inspection (VOI) will be carried out in low-risk animals or more stringent inspection procedures or additional carcass treatments will be performed in high-risk animals.[44]

29.4 Animal welfare in abattoir hygiene context

29.4.1 Transport of animals from farm/livestock market to abattoir

Although slaughter at a stationary plant at the farm can reduce stress related to transport and minimize exposure to unfamiliar environments and contact with other animals,[45] the majority of farms do not have conditions for on-farm slaughter. The transport of animals from farm to the slaughterhouse, including their lay-over in lairage, is an integral part of today's livestock industry.[46,47] Animals may be exposed to numerous stressogenic factors including high stocking densities, mixing with unknown animals, long transport duration, abnormal temperatures, noise, vibrations, pollution, hunger and thirst, rough handling that compromise animal welfare, and have an adverse effect on meat quality and safety.[47–49] Animals exposed to one or multiple factors mentioned above may experience stress, injury, fatigue, dehydration, core body temperature, mortality, and morbidity. In addition, poor conditions in animal transport may lead to increased dirtiness of animal hides/skins and increased risk for subsequent cross-contamination during slaughter and dressing.

Some animals when stressed are more prone to shed pathogenic bacteria including *Escherichia coli* O157: H7 and *Salmonella* spp.[50,51] Thus increased shedding of pathogenic bacteria and compromised immunity increase the probability of contaminating healthy animals especially in high-density situations like the transport truck. The vehicles that have not been properly cleaned and disinfected can be also sources of cattle contamination.[48]

Moreover, stress during transport and lairage may cause shrink loss, increase incidence of dark firm dry or pale soft exudative meat, and increased carcass trim due to bruising.[46,47]

In all, animal transport to the slaughterhouse has become a cause for concern because of animal welfare considerations, consequentially impact on meat safety and quality, and associated economic losses.[47]

During animal transport loading and unloading are the most stressful processes.[52,53] Steep loading ramps present animals with a difficult obstacle to negotiate and are commonly associated with injuries and prolapses.[54] For cattle, pigs, and sheep the maximum recommended angle for adjustable ramps is 25 and 20 degrees for nonadjustable ramps.[55,56] Grandin[57] suggested that loading ramps should have a slope of 11 degrees, but if other factors, like nonslip floors and cleats, were optimized, slopes of no more than 20–25 degrees could be climbed without significant problems.[53] The welfare of animals depends greatly on the training of stock persons. Quiet handling by well-trained people, who know how to take advantage of animal flight zone to move an animal from place to place without using stick or electric goads, is crucial.[49] Also, mixing unfamiliar animals from different social and age groups during loading or transport should be avoided because of fighting and aggressive behavior.[47,53,54] During transport, all animals should be able to stand and lie down and have access to water. Optimal stocking density for pigs should be 0.42 m^2 per 100 kg.[58] Optimal stocking density for cattle depends on the animal size and weight but also on their physiological condition, on the weather conditions, and on the duration of transport itself. For heavy cattle (550 kg) the specified space is 1.3–1.6 m^2.[53,58] Although the duration of the transport has a negative impact on animal' welfare, it is reported that short (15 min) transport showed an intense stress response and suggested that pigs submitted to short transport could need longer lairage time, while transport of 3 h could allow the animals to adapt to transport conditions and then could act as a resting period like a lairage time.[59] For transport longer than 8 h, the animals should be given a rest period and if necessary, feed.[58] Furthermore, due variation of weather condition, ventilation systems are essential during transport. For cattle, the minimum airflow rate should not be lower than 60 m^3/h per 100 kg live weight.[58]

Along with behavioral measures, some physiological measures that can be used to assess animal welfare and stress during transport are as follows: temperature, heart rate, breathing rate, adrenal medullary hormones, adrenal cortical hormones (e.g., cortisol), acute phase proteins (e.g., haptoglobin), pituitary hormones (e.g., oxytocin), enzymes (e.g., creatine kinase, lactate dehydrogenase), hematocrit, and so on.[60]

29.4.2 Lairage

Cross-contamination during lairage affects the process hygiene at slaughter and increase the public health risk for consumers.[61] From the perspective of abattoir hygiene, lairage can be considered as a reservoir for pathogenic bacteria.

Lairage allows animals to recover from the stresses of handling and transport and is also a point for antemortem inspection.[62,63] On the other hand, lairage has been identified as a major contributor of animal, and subsequently carcass, contamination with different pathogens, for example, *Salmonella* spp., *Campylobacter* spp., *E. coli* O157, and *L. monocytogenes*.[64] In order to ensure animal welfare, pens should meet number of requirements.[63] The lairage should be designed to allow a one-way flow of animals from unloading from transporting vehicles and placement to holding pens, to the point of slaughter, with a minimum number of abrupt corners. In red meat abattoirs, pens, passageways, and races should be arranged in such a way as to permit inspection of animals at any time, and to permit the removal of sick or injured animals when appropriate, for which separate accommodation should be provided.[65] In poultry abattoirs, the unloading space should be available, where containers with perforated or flexible bottoms, in which birds are transported, should be unloaded with particular care in order to avoid injury of animals.[65]

Cattle lairage pens may be constructed of solid rendered block wall or tubular galvanized steel at least 1.80 m high, while pig pens are preferably constructed with solid walls. The pens should be long and narrow to allow more pigs to rest along the walls[66] or to prevent bulls' aggressions allowing each bull to "defend" a line of fence, compared to squarer pens of the same area.[63] Mixing unfamiliar animals especially pigs and overcrowding in lairage should be avoided because it inevitably causes fighting, which results in skin bruises, stress, and poor pork quality.[67] Also, this practice cause dissemination of pathogens from infected to noninfected animals. Holding pen floors, entrance gates of stun boxes, and stun box floors are the most frequently contaminated sites in cattle lairages.[64] Hygienic interventions of pens are recommended as GHPs. The cleaning and disinfection of lairage pen environment may potentially reduce the bacterial contamination in beef products.[68] Presence of *Salmonella* spp. in trucks and lairage (18.75%) after cleaning and disinfection, points out that among the other measures the intensification of the cleaning and disinfection in the lairage is required to decrease or eliminate the risk of *Salmonella* spp. infection or recontamination from the environment in pork from organic or eco-friendly systems.[69] However, no pathogen elimination was achieved by these preharvest measures. The difficulty in cleaning and disinfection is also result of the lairage construction.[70] Uneven floor and wall surfaces contain different size holes in which disinfection solutions penetrate badly. Disinfection is especially important when it comes to hide contamination.[71] Hides contaminated with pathogens in the lairage environment present big challenges for the beef industry since this could negate preharvest intervention efforts[72,73] and subsequently contaminate carcasses.[72] Thus even the absence of pathogens on cattle hides when the animals arrive at a processing plant does not ensure that carcasses will remain free of pathogens.[72] This is why an effective hide intervention, apart from cleaning and disinfection, such as hide-on carcass washing, is needed to reduce contamination.[72,73]

According to the UK Farm Animal Welfare Committee, animals are required to have sufficient space to stand up, lie down, and turn around without difficulty when penned. Recommended minimum stocking rates for cattle, pigs and heavy pigs, calves, and sheep are 2.3–2.8, 0.6, and 0.75 m^2/head, respectively.[66] This space allows animal to lie down simultaneously in the holding pens overnight. Moreover, during lairage and fasting times the water amount should be calculated to minimize the potential loss of carcass yield and at same time reduce the volume of gastrointestinal contents in order to reduce the risk of carcass contamination during slaughter.[62] Apart from space requirements, ventilation and temperature in the lairage should be of an adequate standard, while the environment should be reasonably quiet.[63] To avoid heat stress during warm weather and calm animals after transport, water misting/showers are used.[67,74] This practice is considered beneficial since it removes fecal matter on the animal before slaughter.[62]

Although numerous studies suggested lairage to be a hotspot for animal contamination it should be mentioned that some studies reported opposite findings on the effect of lairage on increase prevalence of pathogen microorganism in slaughter animals; a model has been developed suggesting that transport and lairage stages are unlikely to be responsible for a large increase in average prevalence of foodborne pathogenic microorganisms at the EU Member States level.[75] It is also confirmed transport and lairage do not cause an increase in the prevalence of *E. coli* O157 fecal shedding in cattle.[76,77]

29.4.3 Stunning

The stunning process has aim to minimize the pain and suffering associated with slaughter (fear and distress) and should produce a rapid onset of stress-free insensibility of sufficient duration to keep the animal unconscious until harvested.[78] Different stunning methods, their descriptions, and indicators used to assess animal unconscious are presented in Table 29.2.[79–84] Although there are many articles and official reports that cover the stunning in animals and its relation to animal welfare, the focus will be put mainly on aspects of stunning and food safety.

In cattle, small ruminants, and horses captive bolt is used for stunning. During this process, penetration of skin and scull may pose risk of internal and/or external microbial contamination of edible tissues and organs and has an impact on the hygienic status of carcasses/meat.

For example, it is reported that the marker organisms (nalidixic acid–resistant *E. coli* K12 or *Pseudomonas fluorescens*) previously inoculated into the sheep brain through the stun wound immediately after stunning by a penetrative captive bolt pistol, were found after slaughtering and dressing on average, in blood and liver of 90% animals, lungs and spleen of 80%, lymph nodes of 30%, in deep muscle of 20% and on carcass surface of 50% of brain-inoculated animals.[85] Furthermore, when the pistol which had been used to stun one brain-inoculated lamb was used to stun consecutive, noninoculated lambs, the marker organisms were found, on average, in stun wounds of 100%, in blood of 30%, and on the carcass surface of 40% consecutively stunned animals, showing that this stunning method may pose a risk for cross-contamination. During stunning process, penetration can cause brain tissue and cerebrospinal fluid leakage from the bolt hole in the head for at least 55 min, and consequently contributes to contamination of the surrounding area of the hide as well as the bleeding area and equipment in the abattoir.[86] Therefore edible carcasses can be contaminated with pathogens and bovine spongiform encephalopathy–causing agent (prion) during the physical movement associated with hide pulling and head removal.[86] Thus, from meat safety point of view, penetrative stunning may carry

TABLE 29.2 Most common stunning methods in pig, cattle, and poultry.[79–84]

Animal species	Type of stunning	Max. stun/stick interval	Properties	Stage	Indicators	Additional indicators	References
Pig	Electrical stunning	20 s	≥ 1.25 A	End of stunning and shackling	Tonic–clonic seizures, breathing, corneal/palpebral reflex	Spontaneous blinking, posture, vocalizations	EFSA[79] OIE[80]
				Sticking	Breathing, tonic/clonic seizures, muscle tone	Spontaneous blinking, corneal/palpebral reflex, vocalizations	EFSA[79] OIE[80]
				Bleeding	Breathing muscle tone	Spontaneous blinking, corneal/palpebral reflex, vocalizations	EFSA[79] OIE[80]
	Carbon dioxide stunning	60 s	≥ 80% Preferably 90% ideally 3 min	End of stunning and shackling	Muscle tone, breathing corneal/palpebral reflex	Response to nose prick or ear pinch, vocalizations	EFSA[79] OIE[80]
				Sticking	Muscle tone, breathing, vocalizations	Corneal/palpebral reflex, response to nose prick or ear pinch	EFSA[79] OIE[80]
				Bleeding	Muscle tone, breathing	Corneal/palpebral reflex, vocalizations	EFSA[79] OIE[80]
Cattle	Electrical stunning	23 s (adult) 12 s (calves)	≥ 1.5 A (adult cattle) ≥ 1.0 A (calves-less than six months of age) at least 10 s on the head and 45 s on the heart		Posture, breathing, tonic–clonic seizures	Nystagmus, response to nose prick or pinch, vocalizations, spontaneous blinking	OIE[80] Grandin[81] Verhoeven et al.[82] EFSA[83]
	Captive bolt stunning		The captive bolt must be fired at the cross-over point of imaginary lines drawn between the base of the horns and the contralateral eyes	After stunning until shackling	Posture, breathing, tonic seizure, corneal/palpebral reflex	Muscle tone, eye movements, vocalization	EFSA[79]
				Neck cutting or sticking	Body movements, muscle tone, breathing	Eye movements, corneal/palpebral reflex, spontaneous blinking	EFSA[83]
				Bleeding	Muscle tone, breathing, spontaneous blinking		

Poultry	Electrical stunning	20 s	Chickens: 50–200 Hz,100 mA	Between exit from the waterbath and neck cutting	Tonic seizures, breathing, spontaneous blinking	corneal/palpebral reflex, vocalizations	OIE[80] EFSA[84]
			200–400 Hz, 150 mA				
			400–1500 Hz, 200 mA				
			Turkeys: 50–200 Hz, 250 mA	Bleeding	Wing flapping, breathing	Corneal/palpebral reflex, spontaneous swallowing, head shaking	
			200–400 Hz, 400 mA				
			400–1500 Hz, 400 mA				
	Stunning with gas mixtures		$\geq$2 min 40% CO_2, 30% O_2 30% N, followed by $\geq$1 min 80% CO_2	Shackling	Breathing, muscle tone, wing flapping, spontaneous blinking	Corneal/palpebral reflex, vocalizations	OIE[80]
			$\geq$1 min 30% CO_2, followed by $\geq$1 min $\geq$60% CO_2				
			$\geq$2 min $\geq$55% CO_2				
			$\geq$2 min Ar, N, or other inert gases or their mixture, $\leq$2% O_2 in final mixture				
			$\geq$2 min CO_2, Ar, N, or other inert gases, $\leq$30% CO_2, $\leq$2% O_2 in final mixture				EFSA[84]

a risk. However, nowadays animal stunning has been primarily viewed from an animal welfare perspective. From this point of view, some concerns exist about using alternative stunning method in cattle. Namely, electrical stunning provokes short duration of unconsciousness and this method can be ineffective due to technical shortcomings.[87]

However, in pigs most of the stunning failures occurred when CO_2 stunning were applied due to insufficient dwell time, followed by head-only stunning, while most effective method was electrical stunning where the two-cycle method (head/heart current) was applied.[88] Furthermore, it is supposed that gas stunning method increases the risk of *Salmonella* spp. contamination in pigs. Unlike electrical stunning, treatment with CO_2 relaxes muscles and may lead to increased *Salmonella* spp. shedding.[79] This phase of slaughter process and its link with contamination of pig carcasses need further investigation.[89]

In broilers, it has been suggested that stunning bath, along with plucking machine and chiller, is one of the areas of major cross-contamination of carcasses.[90] The risk factor for *Campylobacter* spp. carcasses contamination during electrical stunning has been also observed.[91] It has been found that *Campylobacter* counts on broilers stunned by gas where 2.8 and 2.7 log colony forming unit (CFU)/g after plucking and washing, respectively, while on broilers stunned with electricity, *Campylobacter* loads were 3.3 and 3.2 log CFU/g, respectively. Electrical stunning may induce defecation and the fecal material can be spread on the carcass during processes where significant amounts of water are applied.[91,92] Thus it is suggested that gas stunning technique is better method since the induction of unconsciousness is rapid and requires less exposure time for broilers, and result in improved product quality and yield by eliminating the risk of broken bones, bruising, and hemorrhaging that may occur during electrical water bath.[93]

29.5 Slaughter and dressing in abattoir hygiene context

Abattoirs should have slaughter lines designed to work at adequate speeds to allow constant progress of hygienic slaughter and dressing processes to prevent and/or decrease cross-contamination between carcasses, equipment, tools, and workers. In cases when more than one slaughter line is operational and working at the same time (e.g., bovine and pig slaughter lines working simultaneously), the adequate separation of the lines should be enabled. When the same slaughter line is used for slaughter of different animal species (e.g., bovine and sheep or bovine and pigs) the lines should be used alternatively, at different time/shifts, with thorough cleaning and sanitation between two shifts.

At all times during slaughter and dressing, GHP and standard operating procedures (SOPs) should be applied to maintain the abattoir hygiene level and prevent cross-contamination of carcasses.

29.5.1 Stunning, sticking, and bleeding of slaughter animals

Animals should be stunned in a manner to be unconscious prior to sticking and bleeding. Exceptions are made only in case of religious purposes (Halal or Kosher slaughter) when ritual slaughter is practiced provided that the slaughter method is humane. The animal should be unconscious long enough to allow sticking to be carried out and for brain death due to the lack of blood supply (cerebral anoxia). Sticking is intended to cut the major blood vessels (brachiocephalic trunk) in neck area, to provoke intensive bleeding and to allow blood to drain from the carcass (cattle, pigs).[94]

The bleeding knife should be always sharpened. Bleeding should be carried out by an incision made with a knife in the jugular furrow at the base of the neck, the knife being directed toward the entrance of the chest to sever all the major blood vessels arising from the heart. For the purposes of good hygiene "two knives system" should be used (e.g., operator must work with the clean knife, while other knife is placed in a "sterilizer" box at minimum temperature of 82°C; after several moves are done with one knife, the operator should wash the knife with water, at working station and place it in a sterilizer box; the second, clean knife must be taken from the sterilizer box and the work should be continued with this knife; the procedure must be repeated at all times during sticking/bleeding), the first to open the skin ("skin preparation") and the second to sever the blood vessels. In poultry, sheep, goats, and ostriches, the throat is cut behind the jaw.

Cattle bleeding is carried out with opening of the skin at the neck, between brisket and jaw through a 30 cm longitudinal cut. A clean and sharp knife should be used and inserted at a 45-degree angle to cut the jugular and carotid vessels.[94]

In sheep and goats, bleeding can be carried out in a similar way as for cattle. The trachea and esophagus of animals intended for human consumption must remain intact during bleeding, except in the case of slaughter according to a religious custom.

Certain delay is needed between stunning and sticking/bleeding, but it should be definitely short period of time (e.g., less than one minute); in poultry it should be within 15 s of stunning. This is because a prolonged delay in bleeding may result in a level of consciousness being regained, in particular where animals have been stunned electrically.[94]

There are five major control points to be monitored during stunning, sticking, and bleeding within risk-based food safety management system: (1) stunning efficacy, (2) bleed rail insensibility, (3) vocalization, (4) slipping and falling, and (5) electric prods.

29.5.2 Dehiding of cattle and small ruminants

GHP should be always followed in a manner that the outer side of the hide must never touch the skinned carcass/meat. Operators must not touch the skinned surface with the hand that was in contact with the skin. "Two knives" system should be always applied.[94]

29.5.2.1 Legs

Dehiding and removal of legs are done at hindleg (tarsal) and foreleg (carpal). The removal of forelegs should be done when carcass is in vertical position, before dehiding.

29.5.2.2 Head

After bleeding, while the animal is still hanging from the shackling chain, the horns are removed and the head is skinned. The head is detached by cutting through the neck muscles and the occipital joint. The head should be hanged on a hook and washed, prepared for the meat inspection.

High-throughput plants with conveyer system and overhead rails convey the carcass from the sticking/bleeding point to the chilling room. In cattle, conveyer system allows hide removal to be carried out on the hanging carcass. A single operator may work with a hydraulic platform which is raised and lowered as required.

In small ruminants, dehiding procedure should be carried out with strict adherence to GHP since sheep fleeces may be heavily contaminated with excessive amount of dirt and feces. To prevent cross-contamination of carcasses, the meat handler should take care that the fleece or hair must never touch skinned carcass, neither operator should touch carcass with the hand that previously was in contact with the fleece.

29.5.3 Scalding, dehairing, singeing, and polishing of pigs

Operational steps in slaughtering of pigs include scalding and dehairing, followed by singeing and polishing, before evisceration. Scalding is carried out in water at around 60°C (58°C–62°C) for about 6 min (5–10 min) which loosens the hair in the follicle. Pigs are placed in scalding tank in a horizontal (water-based scalding) or a vertical position (vertical condensation scalding). Scalding and dehairing may be combined in one operation in the simple scalding tank. Inside the tank there are rotating rubber-tipped paddles which are started after closing the lid. As the hair is loosened by the scalding water it is removed by the rubbing effect of the paddles against the skin.[94] From the point of hygiene, the vertical condensation scalding is more beneficial, as pig carcasses are not mixed together in a scalding tank, but conveyer system is transporting pig carcasses through the specially designed condensation chamber, so that carcasses are not directly immersed in water (except frontal part of head), but exposed to the condensed steam. Such closed scalding system is operating by injecting steam and water into a circulating air stream, air is heated and humidified. Suspended by one of the hind legs, the pigs are scalded with hot, water-saturated (close to 100%) air, which condenses on the carcasses' surfaces.[94] Scalding temperature should be carefully monitored as by too low temperature the hair will not be loosened, while at too high temperature the skin will be cooked, reddish and the hair difficult to remove.

The singeing and polishing of pig carcasses are applied immediately after scalding and dehairing to reduce and/or eliminate microbiological load on surface of the skin of scalded and dehaired pigs. Carcasses are singed (manually or in singeing chamber with sensors) using a gas flame for around 25 s. Polishing is done in a chamber with a cold-water spray and rubber flails rotating and moving in opposing directions. Afterward, carcasses are transported into the "clean" dressing area and prepared for bunging (tying off), to prevent leakage of the intestinal content, and evisceration.

29.5.4 Evisceration

Evisceration is the step which should be always carried out, in all species, with care and strict adherence to GHP to prevent the rupture of viscera and spillage of intestinal content to the surface of carcass. The clean, sterilized knife should be always used for the cut at brisket and abdominal wall. A "two knives" system should be always applied. A full traceability must be provided so that all viscera are identified with associated carcass until the postmortem veterinary inspection has been performed.[94]

29.5.4.1 Cattle

The first step is to saw down the brisket at middle line. In slaughterhouses with a conveyer system, the brisket saw is regularly used. Furthermore, the cut is carried out along the abdominal cavity middle line. The viscera are separated into thoracic viscera (lungs, heart), paunch (liver, abdominal fat), and intestines, for postmortem inspection and washing/cleaning.

It is important that, before the evisceration, ties are made at the esophagus/stomach, stomach/duodenum boundaries, so that the esophagus and rectum are properly tied off during hide removal. This will prevent cross-contamination of carcass with intestinal content.

29.5.4.2 Small ruminants

A small cut is made in the abdominal cavity wall, at middle line just above the brisket, and the fingers of the other hand are inserted to lift the body wall away from the viscera. The cut is than continued to within about 5 cm of the cod fat or udder.[94] The omentum is withdrawn, the rectum loosened, and the viscera freed and taken out. The esophagus is pulled up through the diaphragm. The breastbone is split down the middle line with precaution not to puncture the thoracic organs which are then removed.

29.5.4.3 Pigs

The rectum is loosened and tied off. The cut is done along the body wall (abdominal and thoracic middle line), from the crotch to the neck through the skin. The cut is done through the pelvis to remove the bladder and sexual organs (in males, the foreskin must not be punctured as its content is a serious source of carcass contamination). The removal of abdominal and thoracic viscera is carried out. The kidneys are removed after the splitting of carcass. At all times, the contact with the floor or standing platform should be avoided during evisceration.

29.5.5 Splitting, washing, and dressing of carcasses

GHP should be practiced during splitting, washing, and dressing of carcasses in order to prevent cross-contamination with bone fragments or pathogenic microorganisms. Splitting saw or cleaver should be always sterilized in hot water (≥82°C) between carcasses.[94]

29.5.5.1 Cattle

The splitting operation is carried out facing the back of the carcass. In slaughterhouses with conveyer system the carcass saw is regularly used to split the carcass, while in some small-scale slaughterhouses the cleaver can be used. The carcass is split down the backbone from the pelvis to the neck. The use of carcass saw gives better result, but the attention should be made to bone dust which should be removed. In case when a cleaver is used, it is necessary to saw through the rump and loin, in particular in older animals.

29.5.5.2 Sheep

Since sheep and lamb carcasses are generally sold entire, there is a rare occasion to split their carcasses. If necessary, their carcasses can be split by saw or cleaver (the saw is better choice for older animals).

29.5.5.3 Pigs

The pig carcass should be split down the backbone (as for cattle), but the head is generally left intact (or split into two halves).

29.5.5.4 Carcass dressing

The goal of carcass dressing or trimming is to remove all damaged or visually contaminated parts (fecal or intestinal content, dirt, bone fragments, blood stains, abscesses) to standardize the presentation of carcasses prior to weighing and to decrease the probability for bacterial growth originated from cross-contamination with bacteria.[94] The dressing should be done always with the clean knife, previously sterilized in hot water (≥82°C).[94]

In cattle and other ruminants, the Specified Risk Materials (SRMs) (certain tissues which are associated with the pathogenesis of transmissible spongiform encephalopathies/TSEs) should be removed from the carcass (Table 29.3). SRM is recognized as responsible for acquiring transmissible spongiform encephalopathies (TSEs), including bovine spongiform encephalopathy (BSE) first recognized in bovine animals in 1986. In the following years, TSEs were also recognized in other animal species (e.g. scrapie in sheep and goats; chronic wasting disease (CWD) in deer). TSEs/BSE were recognized as important public health issue since a new variant of Creutzfeldt-Jakob Disease (nvCJD) was identified and described in 1996. After this finding, the increasing evidence was obtained to support the similarity between the BSE agent and nvCJD in humans. Therefore, SRMs is considered as inedible and cannot be used for human consumption.[95–98]

29.5.5.5 Carcass washing

The primary goal of carcass washing is to remove visible dirt and blood stains and to improve the overall appearance of carcass after chilling. Washing is done with water satisfying requirements for drinking water. Washing is no substitute for GHP during slaughter and dressing, because it helps additional spread of bacteria throughout the carcass rather than reduce total numbers. Washing should be always carried outgoing vertically down from rump and hind legs to the brisket, head, and forelegs, applying simultaneously horizontal movements.[94] Stains and gut contents must be cut off. Attention should be given to the internal surface of carcass in order to cut off the sticking

TABLE 29.3 Specified Risk Materials (SRMs) in cattle.[165–168]

All ages	Tonsils, distal ileum (80 inches or 203 cm of unstretched small intestine or the last four meters of the small intestine), the caecum and the mesentery (which cannot be dissociated from the mesenteric nerves, the celiac and mesenteric ganglion complex and the mesenteric fat); *Note: The remaining parts of the bovine intestines, e.g. duodenum, the colon and the small intestine except for the last four meters should be excluded*
12 months or older*[166]	Skull, brain, eyes, spinal cord, vertebral column
30 months or older	Skull, brain, eyes, spinal cord, vertebral column

**Undetermined BSE risk - The cattle population of a country, zone or compartment poses an undetermined BSE risk if it cannot be demonstrated that it meets the requirements of another category.*

wound and remove stains and dirt from the pelvic region. It is not allowed to use wiping cloths.

Since wet surface of carcass may favor the bacterial growth the chilling should start immediately after carcass washing. In the chilling room, if designed and operating efficiently, the carcass surface will quickly dry out, thus inhibiting bacterial growth.

29.5.6 Chilling procedures (carcasses and offal)

Microbial contamination of carcasses is easy to occur during meat production and, while most of the microorganisms transferred to carcasses are saprophytic or spoilage microorganisms there is a possibility that pathogens are present.[99,100] In order to prevent this microbial growth and extend the meat shelf life, in abattoirs the primary chilling is performed, that include rapid carcasses cooling so that the temperature at the carcass warmest point reaches <7°C for beef, pig, and lamb, and <4°C for poultry carcasses, while for edible offal the temperature <3°C must be ensured. These temperatures are usually achieved within 16–24 h in small carcasses (lamb), in less than 48 h in large carcasses (beef, pork), and less than 2 h in poultry carcasses (internal deep breast).[27,101]

Contamination during the chilling process may occur through contact of the carcass with contaminated surfaces or workers' hands, through water splashes, direct contact between carcasses (where the fecal contamination is present on the surface of one carcass), and from the air. However, under proper hygiene conditions, the major concern during chilling is survival and growth of existing microorganism rather than new contamination.[100] Contrarily, contamination that occurs during evisceration process is likely to be reduced by chilling. Since the complete elimination of pathogens is not possible, chilling, as the last step in meat production, has the objective to reduce microorganisms on carcass surfaces or prevent their growth.[102] The microbiological safety of chilled foods depends on numerous factors such as type of pathogens present, their loads, presence of other microbiota, the conditions of storage (temperature, the relative humidity, atmosphere), as well as food characteristics.[103,104] Although the relative humidity, carcass surface pH, and a_w may limit bacterial growth on carcasses during chilling, temperature remains a critical factor for meat safety.[103–105] Chilling extends the lag phase of bacteria.[99] Different chilling regimes are used for different animal species. Chilling processes must consider meat safety, shelf-life, and quality, but also the impact on palatability traits and economic concerns.[106]

In general, beef carcasses are chilled by a flow of refrigerated air (dry chilling) or by intermittently spraying with chilled water or antimicrobials (spray chilling).[107] In United States and Canada spray chilling is usually used in large-scale meat-packing plants, while in smaller packing plants in North America, as well as in the EU, Australia, and New Zealand dry chilling is the prevalent method of beef carcasses chilling.[108–110] STEC and *Salmonella* spp. continue to be a major food safety concern for the beef industry.[111] For example, a decrease in *S. Typhimurium* and *E. coli* O157 counts on beef during conventional chilling has been reported.[112] The inhibitory effect of low temperatures was confirmed when after 1 h of carcasses chilling *E. coli* counts decreased from 3.30 to 2.04 log CFU/cm^2, while no *E. coli* was recovered after 67 h of chilling.[113] Results from several studies suggest that spraying with antimicrobials greatly increases the antibacterial effect of chilling. It has been found that chlorine dioxide caused approximately 3 log CFU/cm^2 reduction in *E. coli* numbers when applied during spray chilling, while after application immediately prior to regular spray chilling the reduction was approximately 1 log CFU/cm.[2,111] In addition, both chlorine dioxide and peroxyacetic acid (at ≥20 and ≥200 ppm, respectively) applied during spray chilling decreased the number of both, *E. coli* and *S. enterica*, by more than 4 log CFU/cm^2.

Thus an oxidant-based application during spray chilling could be effective to reduce the enteric pathogen contamination on beef meat.

The two most widely employed practices by poultry establishments for primary chilling of carcasses are water immersion chilling and air chilling, with and without incorporation of water sprays.[114] In the EU, most plants use an air-chill method, while ice-water immersion is a predominant way of poultry carcass chilling in the United States.[115] *Campylobacter* spp. and *Salmonella* spp. are the bacteria most associated with a foodborne illness caused by the consummation of contaminated poultry, which is why the primary objective of chilling poultry is to reduce the number of these pathogens. Significant reduction of *Campylobacter* spp., *E. coli*, and *Salmonella* spp. can be obtained during both chilling procedures.[115,116]

The effect of chilling in the water and chilling in the air on different bacterial groups on broiler carcasses has been studied. It was observed that the numbers of psychrotrophs, pseudomonads, Lactic Acid Bacteria (LAB), and *Brochothrix thermosphacta* recovered from water-chilled carcasses were all 0.4 or more log lower than the numbers recovered from air-chilled carcasses.[117] The incidence of *Salmonella* spp. and *Campylobacter* spp. tends to be significantly lower in air-chilled broilers, suggesting that cross-contamination may be more prevalent for immersion-chilled broilers.[118]

Carcass chilling is a routine aspect of pork production. The pork industry currently uses either blast chilling or conventional chilling.[99] Literature data on the effects of blast chilling on the microbiological quality of pork are inconclusive. For example, it is reported that blast chilling was significantly more effective in reducing populations of *L. monocytogenes*, *S.* *Typhimurium*, and *Campylobacter coli* than conventional chilling.[99] The better effect of blast chilling was attributed to the high air velocity. Blast chilling lowers the temperature at a rapid rate and may provoke cold shock, especially in particularly sensitive Gram-negative microorganisms including *E. coli* and Enterobacteriaceae. Contrarily, with conventional chilling, microorganisms may adapt to the low temperatures more slowly, thereby preventing cold shock.[99] Blast chilling is proved to be effective against *Campylobacter* spp.[119] The prevalence of this bacteria decreased from 56.7% to 1.7% on pig carcasses. In addition, a significant decrease of coliform bacteria, thermotolerant coliform bacteria, and *E. coli* counts was reported. However, this type of chilling did not have an effect on pathogenic *Y. enterocolitica* O:3/biovar 4 (8.3% prevalence before and after blast chilling), nor on the number of aerobic microorganisms. Conventional chilling of pork carcasses also reduces levels of Campylobacter *jejuni*.[120] Interestingly, both the conventional method and blast chilling were equally effective at decreasing the prevalence of *Campylobacter* spp. on pig carcasses from 7.4% to 0%.[99] Similarly, it was reported that the type of chilling (fast or conventional chilling) had no impact on the recovery of four strains of *Salmonella* from pork skin.[121] In addition, overnight chilling decreased the prevalence of *Campylobacter* spp. on pork carcasses from 7% (immediately before chilling) to 0%.[122] It was confirmed that the chilling operation has a significant effect on the reduction of pathogenic *Salmonella* occurrence in pig carcasses.[123] Different findings among studies and abattoirs are attributed to differences in sampling sites, method of swabbing, chilling equipment, cross-contamination of carcasses, level of *Salmonella* infection at slaughterhouses, differences in the microbiological protocol, season, year and country, and so on.[123] Overall, an effective and well-designed chilling regime should be considered as an integral part of abattoir hygiene providing "farm-to-chilled carcass continuum."[19]

29.5.7 Animal by-product utilization

Industrial processing of livestock and poultry generates significant amounts of by-products.[124] The amount of waste range between ~33% to ~43% of the live animal weight.[125] The final destination of animal by-products is determined based on the risks they pose to the food and feed chain. The abattoir hygiene also encompasses the proper collection and disposal of animal by-products. Animal by-products are divided into three categories:

- Category 1 is a high-risk material (among the other carcasses and all body parts of animals suspected of being infected with transmissible spongiform encephalopathy, carcasses of wild animals suspected of being infected with a disease that humans or animals could contract, etc.);
- Category 2 (animal by-products not included in definitions for Category 1 or 3, products containing residues of authorized veterinary drugs and contaminants exceeding the permitted levels, animals and parts of animals that die other than by being slaughtered for human consumption and fetuses, products of animal origin that have been declared unfit for human consumption due to the presence of foreign bodies in those products, manure and digestive tract contents, blood from any animal which has not passed antemortem inspection);
- Category 3 is a low-risk material (including among the others animal meat not intended for human consumption from healthy animals, fat or lard, pig incised offal, pig spleens, stomachs, and intestines from mammals or ratites empty of digestive material—except the last 4 m of bovine small intestine and cecum and ovine and caprine ileum which are Category 1, blood, hides,

skins, hooves, feathers, wool, horns, and hair from animals that had no signs of infectious disease at death).[126]

All mixture containing Categories 1, 2, and 3 are treated as Category 1 material.[126] Use of animal by-products is restricted and they are mainly used in animal feed, as fertilizers, or are disposed according to regulations.[124] The burden of animal by-products is not only related to abattoir hygiene or biosecurity, but also to the fact that nonutilization or underutilization of animal by-products leads to loss of potential revenues and increasing cost of disposal of these products.

29.5.8 Wastewater management

Slaughtering and cleaning of slaughterhouse facilities result in the generation of a high quantity of slaughterhouse wastewater (SWW).[127] For each cow and pig processed, approximately 700 and 330 L of wastewater are generated, respectively.[128] Wastewater contains large amounts of fats, proteins, and fibers, microorganisms, detergents, and disinfectants used for cleaning.[127] Frequently heavy metals and veterinary drugs are also present.[127,129]

SWW contains coliforms and *Streptococcus* spp. However, since the major part of the organic contaminants came from blood, stomach, and intestinal content.[129] SWW may contain different pathogens of enteric origin including *Salmonella* spp., *E. coli*, and *C. jejuni*, gastrointestinal parasites such as *Ascaris* spp., *Giardia lamblia*, *Cryptosporidium parvum*, and enteric viruses.[130] SWW are considered to be one of the most important hotspots for antibiotic-resistant bacteria, due to high cell densities in a nutrient-rich environment like wastewater horizontal gene transfer occurs between bacteria.[131,132] Inadequate discharge of wastewater causes harborage sites for pests (rodents) nearby abattoir, as well as environmental pollution, and poses a serious health threat for human and animals which is why SWW needs to be treated in a wastewater treatment plant before being released into the environment.[133,134]

SWW processing is usually performed in several steps, including preliminary, primary, secondary, and even tertiary treatment.[133] Numerous methods can be applied after preliminary treatment and they can be divided into following subgroups: land application, physicochemical treatment, biological treatment, advanced oxidation processes, and combined processes.[135] Some of the common methods used for SWW treatment are described in Table 29.4.[133,136–139] Taking into consideration that SWW are reach in organic content the predominant treatment methods are biological.[135] Usually, anaerobic treatment followed by aerobic treatment is used. SWW may contain some toxic and/or nonbiodegradable organic substances which is why after anaerobic–aerobic processes and some other methods like advanced oxidation processes or combined processes should be used.[133]

29.6 Food safety management system in the context of abattoir hygiene

In recent years, meat industry and regulatory authorities have attempted to limit the presence of pathogens on carcasses or reduce it to acceptable levels by the application of risk-based meat safety system within slaughterhouses and meat processing plants.[140] The Hazard Analysis and Critical Control Points (HACCP) system is the most widely used internationally accepted food safety management system in the world. The HACCP plans for slaughter and dressing are designed to assist in the management and control of the mainly biological hazards in slaughtering process founded on adherence to Good Hygiene Practice (GHP)/Standard Operating Procedures (SOPs) at each operational step along the slaughter line. Meat operators are required to apply the seven principles of HACCP defined by Codex Alimentarius[25] which are also incorporated to legislation at international level (EU, United States, Euroasian Customs Federation, United Kingdom, Australia, New Zealand, etc.): (1) hazard analysis, (2) identification of critical control points (CCPs), (3) establishing critical limits at each CCP, (4) monitoring of each CCP, (5) corrective actions at each CCP, (6) HACCP verification/validation, and (7) HACCP documentation.[25,141] This ensures the prevention or minimization of microbial contamination of final carcasses from feces, hide, intestinal contents, lymph nodes, processing equipment, water, air, and workers.[142,143]

There are two main HACCP types: the so-called "nonintervention" HACCP (GHP-based) and "intervention" HACCP (hazard-based).[144] It was reported that microbiological safety of meat improved after intervention HACCP implementation in cattle, pig, and poultry abattoirs in the United States.[145] Similar effect of nonintervention HACCP system was found in cattle and pig abattoirs.[144]

29.6.1 Nonintervention hazard analysis and critical control point

The nonintervention HACCP system is GHP-based and relies only on the use of abattoir hygiene, namely strict preventive hygiene measures and procedures during slaughter and dressing, that is, does not include carcass decontamination treatment.[144] The EU countries are more inclined to this system and the EU legislation made HACCP mandatory in the meat industry since January 1,

TABLE 29.4 Some slaughterhouse wastewater (SWW) treatment options.[133,136–139]

Treatment		Methods	Description	Source
Physicochemical treatment methods		Dissolved air flotation	Air bubbles injected at the bottom of the flotation tank, transport light solids, and other material (fat and grease) to the surface where the scum is consistently skimmed off	Mittal[136]
		Coagulation and flocculation	Chemical treatment applied prior to sedimentation and filtration to enhance the ability of a treatment process to remove particles by adding different coagulants	Mittal[136]
		Electrocoagulation	Generating coagulant species in situ by electrolytic oxidation of sacrificial anode materials triggered by electric current applied through the electrodes	Hakizimana et al.[137]
		Membrane technology	During this process microfiltration, ultrafiltration, nanofiltration, and reverse osmosis are used to remove articulates, colloids, macromolecules, organic matter, and pathogens	Bustillo-Lecompte and Mehrvar[133]
Biological treatment	Anaerobic treatment	Anaerobic filter	Fixed-bed biological reactors with filtration chambers	Bustillo-Lecompte and Mehrvar[133]
		Anaerobic baffled reactor	Series of compartments and baffles under which the SWW flows under and over from the inlet to the outlet	Bustillo-Lecompte and Mehrvar[133]
		Anaerobic lagoon	Basins—3–5 m deep with a retention time of 5–10 days. Influent WW flow is near the bottom of the lagoon and it is not mechanically mixed, although some gas mixing can occur	Mittal[136]
		Upflow anaerobic sludge blanket reactor	Process consist from three phases—liquid, solid (the sludge or biomass), and gas (gases formed during the digestion process, mainly CO_2 and CH_4)	Mittal[136]
	Aerobic treatment	Rotary biological contactor	WW come in contact with a biological medium to absorb and metabolize the organic content and remove other pollutants	Mittal[136]
		Activated sludge process	The sludge is maintained by continually recycling a fraction of the settleable solids (contain an active microbial population) separated after aeration back to the aeration basin	Mittal[136]
		Aerobic sequencing batch reactor	Process consists of five stages: filling, reaction, settling, decanting/drawing, and idle	Bustillo-Lecompte and Mehrvar[133]
		Aerobic lagoons	Earthen basins that use algae in combination with other microorganisms for WW treatment. O_2 is supplied naturally by the wind, through photosynthesis and by mechanical means	Mittal[136]
Advanced oxidation processes		Gamma radiation	Using ionizing radiation to remove toxic organic chemicals and biological contaminants	Melo et al.[138]
		Ozonation	Using different (usually low) concentrations of ozone for the removal of organics	Bustillo-Lecompte and Mehrvar[133]
		Ultraviolet (UV)/ H_2O_2	The degradation and detoxification of pollutants in the UV/ H_2O_2 process rely on highly reactive species, hydroxyl radicals (OH)	Cao and Mehrvar[139]

2006.[27] Generally, optimal hygienic practices in abattoir and effective process hygiene management are crucial for successful working of the nonintervention HACCP system and overcoming the threat posed by various foodborne safety hazards.[146] In cattle slaughterhouses this HACCP system usually includes some GHP-based measures: lairage (animal handling, logistic slaughter, hide/fleece cleanliness assessment, hide/fleece clipping/shearing, hide/fleece washing) and four CCPs: (1) dehiding, (2) evisceration, (3) removal of the spinal cord (SRM), and (4) chilling. From the carcass hygiene point of view, dehiding and evisceration are two operational steps that determine if the fecal or rumen material will get onto the carcass, while not completely removed spinal cord may pose a risk to consumer health (variant Creutzfeldt–Jakob disease).[146] In pig slaughterhouses, GHP-based measures include as follows: lairage (animal handling, logistic slaughter, washing) and three CCPs: scalding/singeing, evisceration, and chilling.[140]

SOPs of GMP that prevent cross-contamination associated with these CCPs are numerous and include as follows: sterilization of all the equipment used in water at 82°C, rodding with the crocodile clip/plastic ring or the use of an applicator with potato starch cone, bagging and tying of the rectum, and controlled condition in the cold room (temperature, relative humidity, airflow, carcass grade and spacing).[146]

This HACCP system applied in abattoirs considers close and constant monitoring of the CCPs by visual inspection performed by trained personnel. In addition to this purpose, online monitoring systems, few microbiological systems and some new imaging technologies have been developed which enables lesions and fecal contamination detection, data recording, collection, and processing that pointed out where the problem occurs during the process (specific operation) and suggest corrective measures that should be taken.[44,146,147] The corrective actions involve immediate trimming of feces, ingesta, spinal cord tissue using a sterilized knife (zero tolerance), replacing/retraining the operating person, replacement of knives ("two knives" system), steels and scabbards, checking the sterilizers, and so on.[140,146] Also, some additional measures are proposed, such as dividing into two categories based on the physiological state and cleanliness score and slaughtering under specific conditions for high-risk animals (very dirty animals or animals that have bad hide, skin or fleece).[148]

Unlike the intervention system that achieves a consistent reduction in microbial load with less personnel involved and larger investments, no-intervention system is relatively inexpensive, easy to implement, and is more preventive since it identifies the exact cause of carcass contamination. However, this system relies more on human effort so the possibility for error is considerably higher than for the intervention system and its effectiveness highly depends on personnel training and commitment.[140,146]

29.6.2 Intervention hazard analysis and critical control point

This type of HACCP system is hazard-based and is designed to reduce pathogenic bacteria from the carcass by introducing CCPs where the specific control measures/interventions are applied. The US legislation permits and regulates decontamination techniques of intervention HACCP system that include different procedures applied after slaughter designed to remove bone dust, blood clots, and to reduce bacterial contamination on the carcasses. These specific interventions in beef processing plants usually involve: spraying/washing of carcasses—cold (10°C–15°C), warm (15°C–40°C), or hot (75°C–85°C) potable water in a cabinet system or hand sprayed at different pressures; steam vacuuming of small areas on the carcasses; steam pasteurization at 100°C; organic acid washes (lactic or acetic), hot (50°C–55°C) or cold; spray chilling with antimicrobials.[111,146,149] For these interventions adequate critical limits are determined, processes are continuously monitored, equipment is regularly calibrated, and the corrective actions that can be taken are established.[146]

In contrast to the cattle or sheep, pig slaughter operations involve scalding, mechanical dehairing, singeing, and polishing, so the skin is commonly not removed from the carcasses.[150] As a result of the mentioned stages, pig carcass surfaces are visibly clean and free of hair, but might be highly contaminated with bacteria.[151] Since the skin of pig carcasses is an important contamination source, of particular importance are decontamination interventions that basically comprise physical, chemical, and biological treatments.[152] Physical decontamination treatments for pig carcasses include phases of the normal pig slaughter process, such as scalding and singeing, and other methods that are additionally applied with the specific objective of pig carcass decontamination: chilling,[107] water spraying (cold and warmwater preslaughter, preevisceration, final carcass washing; hot water—after polishing, before- and after-carcass splitting),[151,153] steam treatment (commercial steam unit (82°C–85°C, 60 s); strong jet of steam (90°C–95°C, 0.013 s, 4–6 bar) at the end of slaughter process,[154,155] and irradiation (γ rays or electron beams, 1 kGy dose).[140] Chemical decontamination treatments comprise the spraying of pig carcasses before evisceration or at the end of slaughter with organic acids (1%, 2%, 4% lactic acid, 1.5% acetic and citric acid) or different chlorine-based or phosphate-based treatments.[156] Biological interventions such as decontamination treatments consider the use of bacteriophages and bacteriocins.[152]

Similarly, the poultry carcass decontamination techniques also include water-based treatments (hot water, steam, electrolyzed water), irradiation, ultrasound, air chilling or freezing, and chemical interventions (organic acids, acidified sodium chlorite, trisodium phosphate).[157]

However, in a number of investigations is shown that interventions have no, or a little effect, (only at specific carcass sites) on reduction of carcasses bacterial numbers. Also, in many cases bacteria are simply redistributed from one area to another, implying that interventions, like washing, is more related to improving carcass appearance and not food safety.[146,152,158] Furthermore, reduced efficacy of different treatments can be caused by covering a small carcass area, not reaching optimal heating or cooling temperature in all areas of the carcass, insufficient time to achieve pasteurizing effect, and not enough time for operatives online to finish the job.[146]

29.7 Discussions and future directions

The changes that recently happened in meat chain production encompassed new technologies, including increased automation and robotization, artificial intelligence and nanotechnologies (sensing systems), production of alternative meat using precision fermentation technology (cultured meat), and three-dimensional printing of meat. These novel approaches to meat production should decrease the labor-dependent process (of critical importance in emergency situations and crises such as the COVID-19 pandemic), while also providing climate change resilience and environmental sustainability.

Apart from the abundant changes mentioned above, meat safety remains at the forefront of public health and social-economic concerns.[159] Abattoir hygiene is strongly associated with major meat safety challenges. Namely, poor hygiene in slaughter and dressing may lead to cross-contamination of carcasses with food safety hazards that can be considered as traditional, new, or emerging. These hazards enter the meat chain in multiple points along the farm – abattoir – meat processing – distribution – retail – consumer continuum. Other challenges include the need for development of rapid testing and pathogen detection methodologies with sufficient sensitivity and specificity (e.g. Whole Genome Sequencing – WGS[160]), traceability systems (block chain technology), agreement and allocation of responsibilities between veterinary and public health authorities regarding monitoring and surveillance systems for zoonotic diseases (including food borne), establishment of government policy regarding maximum allowed contamination level-appropriate level of protection (MACL-ALOP) for food which should reach the consumer,[161] as well as establishment of risk-based food safety objectives in meat production/processing, together with complete and routine implementation of risk-based food safety management system (HACCP).[162,163]

29.7.1 Farm-to-chilled carcass approach

In 2005 Codex Alimentarius Commission issued a Code of Hygienic Practice for Meat[22] and recommended integrated and risk-based approach to achieving meat safety. In this document, it is suggested that "hygiene measures should be applied at those points in the meat chain where they will be of greatest value in reducing foodborne risks to consumers." The abattoir hygiene is of utmost importance for reduction of these foodborne risks by preventing and minimizing cross-contamination of carcasses/meat during operational steps in slaughter and dressing.

From recently, the EFSA adopted several scientific opinions related to public health hazards to be covered by inspection of meat.[13,16–19] The farm-to-chilled carcass approach to ensure meat safety and safeguard public health has been recommended. Two key elements of such MSAS were suggested, as follows: (1) risk categorization of slaughter animals (on farm) for high-priority biological hazards based on improved FCI, and (2) risk categorization of abattoirs according to their capability to control those hazards. In addition, VOI has been recommended whenever it is feasible, based on a risk categorization of slaughter animals on farm and risk categorization of abattoirs.[13,16–19] This is because the omission of palpation and incision during post-mortem inspection of slaughter animals, intended for routine slaughter, may decrease spreading and cross-contamination with the high-priority biological hazards.[14,164]

MSAS should be based on FCI from farm to abattoir (bottom-up) and *vice versa* (top-down), as well as harmonized epidemiological indicators (HEI) related to major meat-borne pathogens and chemical contaminants. FCI should include data on prevalence/concentration of major foodborne hazards of public health importance at farm, transport/lairage, and abattoir. These data should be result from targeted sampling (pooled feces on farm or carcass swabs at abattoir), microbiological detection (and serotyping), and auditing (animal welfare and biosecurity on farm; GHP/HACCP at abattoir). HEI can be used to consider improvement and modernization of meat inspection methods and to carry out risk analysis to support such decisions (Fig. 29.2). It is foreseen that the indicators will be used in the bovine/pig/poultry carcass MSAS to help categorize farms/herds and abattoirs according to the risk related to the hazards, as well as setting appropriate specific hazard-based targets in/on bovine/pig/poultry carcasses and, when appropriate, in bovine/pig/poultry farms.

Risk managers will have the possibility to operate within the MSAS, taking into consideration FCI and HEI and making decisions based on the situation related to the

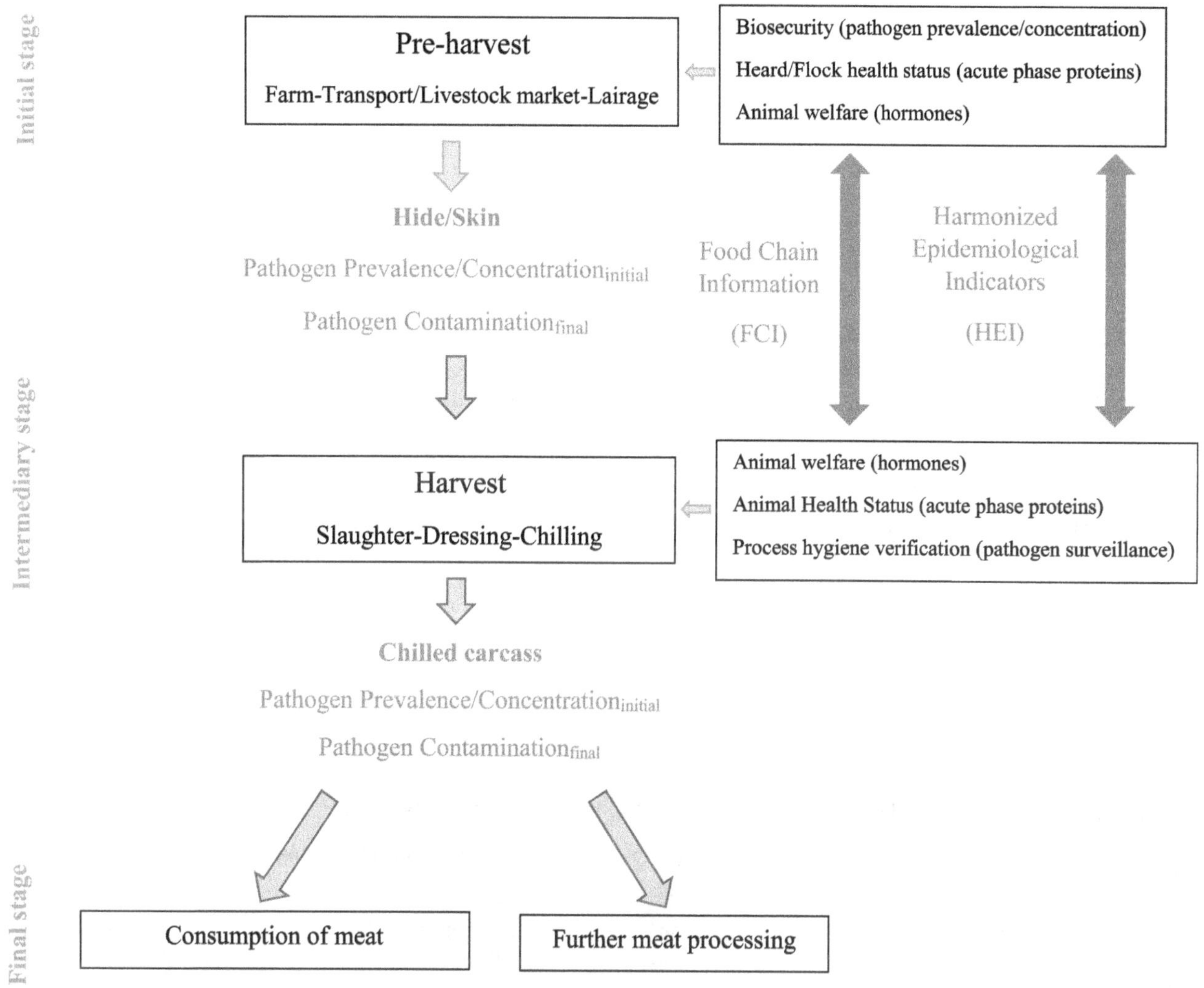

FIGURE 29.2 A model to set up harmonized epidemiological indicators for meat safety assurance system based on prevalence and/or level of hazard in the farm-to-chilled carcass continuum.

level/type of meat inspection that should be applied, for example, classical antemortem and postmortem inspection or VOI.

Some HEIs for bovine, pig, and poultry carcasses are given in Table 29.5–29.7.[16,17,19]

29.7.2 Automation and robotics in abattoir

Automation and robotization have led to significant increases in slaughter line speed for beef, pork, sheep, poultry, and fish operations and have begun to take over the meat processing business. The meat industry is changing slaughter methods from conventional manual handling to an automated and robot-driven process. For example, the fastest line currently observed in broiler slaughter line enables speed at 13,500/h.[162] The automated pig slaughter/dressing lines include separation of the pelvic bone, carcass opening, breastbone splitting, and neck clipping, and run with capacities varying from 300 to1280 pigs per hour. The automation and robotization in beef slaughter have certain limitations regarding development of technology for the slaughter process; this has been quite limited partly due to the biological variation in animals and the cost/benefit of applying complex technology.[162] Mostly, development was recorded in the area of manually operated tools. For example, in the United States there is a development allowing a high line speed in beef slaughter of 300 head/per hour; it is achieved by dividing slaughter and dressing processes across more meat handlers and by ensuring the animals slaughtered are relatively homogenous in size, as slaughter lines are usually specialized for steers or heifers. These plants run in several shifts.[163]

In the EU, most of large-scale abattoirs run in single shifts at line speeds from 30–75 head/per hour and these plants are seldom specialised, which means they operate

TABLE 29.5 Harmonised epidemiological indicators for human pathogenic Shiga toxin-producing *E. coli* (STEC) in the bovine carcass safety assurance system (adapted from EFSA, 2013b).[19]

Indicator(animal/food category)	Meat chain phase	Analytical/diagnostic method	Sample
HEI 1: Practices which increase the risk of introducing pathogenic STEC into the farm (purchase policy, mixing with other herds, access to pasture, access to surface water)	Farm	Auditing	N/A*
HEI 2: On-farm practices and conditions	Farm	Auditing	N/A
HEI 3: Pathogenic STEC status of the group(s) of bovine animals containing animals to be slaughtered within one month	Farm	Microbiology	Pooled (composite) faeces or floor samples
HEI 4: Transport and lairage conditions	Transport and lairage	Auditing	N/A
HEI 5: Visual inspection of hide conditions of animals at lairage (clean animal scoring system)	Abattoir	Visual inspection	N/A
HEI 6: Pathogenic STEC on incoming animals (after bleeding and before dehiding)	Abattoir	Microbiology	Hide swabs
HEI 7: Pathogenic STEC on carcases pre-chilling	Abattoir	Microbiology	Carcass swabs
HEI 8: Pathogenic STEC on carcases post-chilling	Abattoir	Microbiology	Carcass swabs

Not applicable.

TABLE 29.6 Harmonized epidemiological indicators (HEIs) for *Salmonella* in the pig carcass safety assurance system.

Indicator (animal/food category)	Meat chain phase	Analytical/diagnostic method	Sample
HEI 1: *Salmonella* in breeding pigs	Farm	Microbiology (detection and serotyping)	Pooled (composite) feces sample
HEI 2: *Salmonella* in fattening pigs prior to slaughter	Farm	Microbiology (detection and serotyping)	Pooled (composite) feces sample
HEI 3: Controlled housing conditions at farm	Farm	Auditing	N/A
HEI 4: Transport and lairage conditions	Transport and lairage	Auditing of time, mixing of batches, and reuse of pens in lairage	N/A
HEI 5: *Salmonella* in fattening pigs—evisceration stage	Abattoir	Microbiology (detection and serotyping)	Ileal content
HEI 6: *Salmonella* in fattening pigs—carcasses after slaughter process before chilling	Abattoir	Microbiology (detection and serotyping)	Carcass swabs
HEI 7: *Salmonella* in fattening pigs—carcasses after slaughter process and after chilling	Abattoir	Microbiology (detection and serotyping)	Carcass swabs

N/A, not applicable.
Source: Adapted from European Food Safety Authority. Technical specifications on harmonised epidemiological indicators for public health hazards to be covered by meat inspection of swine. *EFSA J*. 2011;9:2371. https://doi.org/10.2903/j.efsa.2011.2371 (Accessed 27.10.20).

with all types of cattle.[163] This implies the new, automated technology, must be flexible and should match the large biological variation of carcass dimensions.

Modern technologies are also common in pork and poultry meat harvest (slaughter/dressing, chilling). Shorter time is allowed for deboning; robots are designed to cut meat and they are replacing traditional manual operations. However, this can also be a challenge regarding meat safety because high speed equipment is not always equipped to respond to frequent variations in carcass size/

TABLE 29.7 Harmonized epidemiological indicators (HEIs) for the poultry carcass safety assurance system.

Indicator (animal/food category)	Meat chain phase	Analytical/diagnostic method	Sample
HEI 1: *Salmonella* and *ESBL/AmpC E. coli* in parent flock	Farm	Microbiology (detection and serotyping)	Pooled (composite) feces sample
HEI 2: *Salmonella, Campylobacter*, and *ESBL/AmpC E. coli* in production flock	Farm	Microbiology (detection and serotyping)	Pooled (composite) feces sample
HEI 3:*Campylobacter* and *ESBL/AmpC E. coli* in incoming batches intended for slaughter	Abattoir	Microbiology (detection)	Ileal content
HEI 4: *Salmonella, Campylobacter*, and *ESBL/AmpC E. coli* in carcasses after chilling	Abattoir	Microbiology (detection and serotyping)	Neck skin samples or carcass swabs

Source: Adapted from European Food Safety Authority. Technical specifications on harmonised epidemiological indicators for biological hazards to be covered by meat inspection of poultry. *EFSA J*. 2012;10:2764. https://doi.org/10.2903/j.efsa.2012.2764 (Accessed 27.10.20).

conformation and, therefore, requires development and installation of tailor-made sensors and IT control systems. Automation and robotization requires progress in breeding and genetics to provide greater carcass uniformity, which would help in operating automated equipment.[163] Some alternative approaches have been also recently suggested, like the meat factory cell (MFC).[164] The MFC concept is different from the conventional slaughter and dressing approach that uses the conveyer system with workers' positions along the slaughter line at numerous operational stations. MFC is based on individual cell stations instead of a conveyer; the slaughter and meat primal cutting is carried out in a way that carcass is disassembled from "outside-in", where limbs, neck, back and loin are removed before internal organs, so that primal cuts' cross-contamination is minimised.[164] However, this concept and its advantages related to improvement of hygiene, food safety, and cost benefit are under development and consideration.

29.7.3 Future perspectives—looking ahead

In all, the meat industry has undergone substantial changes over the previous several decades due to development of new technologies in primary production and meat processing. In terms of "traditional" meat production, abattoirs still have very important role in surveillance, control, and eradication of specific diseases of animal health importance, as well as control, reduction, and prevention of hazards of public health importance. Therefore application of GHP and the overall hygiene requirements at abattoir during slaughter and dressing of animals still remain of utmost importance for microbiological status of chilled carcass, as this may have public health consequences associated with presence of foodborne hazards on/in meat. Parallel to that, it has been observed that current, traditional meat inspection protocols (antemortem and postmortem), based on visual inspection, palpation, and incision, had not been changed since the end of the 19th century, and is not fully efficient in terms of the current needs for consumer protection. Namely, public health hazards associated with meat are, nowadays, the zoonotic food (meat) borne pathogens that are responsible for the majority of human illnesses attributed to meat consumption. Traditional meat inspection cannot respond effectively to detection of such foodborne hazards but can even increase cross-contamination due to palpation and/or incision procedures. Therefore abattoir hygiene should be an essential issue within the modern MSAS or carcass safety assurance system, based on farm-to-chilled carcass continuum. The risk managers who are responsible for decision-making within MSAS, should decide on the level and type of antemortem and postmortem inspection in abattoir, based on information available from farm of origin (farm biosecurity, animal health, and animal welfare) and the level of abattoir hygiene and its public health hazards' risk-reduction capacity. Therefore abattoir hygiene in slaughter and dressing of animals supported with GHP/HACCP in abattoirs and FCI/HEI in farm-abattoir continuum should be a foundation of farm-to-chilled carcass assurance system.

References

1. Fuentes JM, Lopez-Sanchez M, Garcia AI, et al. Public abattoirs in Spain: History, construction characteristics and the possibility of their reuse. *J Cult Herit*. 2015;16:632–639.
2. Briz J. Anotaciones a los mercados y flujos ganaderos enei vacuno para carne. *Rev Estud Agrosoc*. 1979;106:71–99.
3. World Health Organization. Zoonoses. https://www.who.int/topics/zoonoses/en/. (Accessed on June 1, 2020).

4. European Food Safety Authority. Scientific opinion on the development of a risk ranking framework on biological hazards. EFSA Panel on Biological Hazards (BIOHAZ). *EFSA J.* 2012;10:2724. Available from: https://doi.org/10.2903/j.efsa.2012.2724 (Accessed on June 15, 2020).
5. Food and Agriculture Organization, World Health Organization. The veterinary contribution to public health practice. Joint FAO/WHO expert committee on veterinary public health. World Health, https://apps.who.int/iris/bitstream/handle/10665/38156/WHO_TRS_573_eng.pdf?sequence = 1&isAllowed = y Published 1975. (Accessed on May 25, 2020).
6. World Health Organization. Future trends in veterinary public health. https://apps.who.int/iris/bitstream/handle/10665/42460/WHO_TRS_907.pdf?sequence = 1. Published 2002. (Accessed on May 25, 2020).
7. Zhang T, Wu Q, Zhang Z. Probable pangolin origin of SARS-CoV-2 associated with the COVID-19 outbreak. *Curr Biol.* 2020;30:1346–1351.
8. Touati R, Haddad-Boubaker S, Ferchichi I, et al. Comparative genomic signature representations of the emerging COVID-19 coronavirus and other coronaviruses: High identity and possible recombination between bat and pangolin coronaviruses. *Genomics.* 2020;112:4189–4202.
9. Liu Z, Bing X, Zhi XZ. Novel Coronavirus Pneumonia Emergency Response Epidemiology Team (NCPERET). The epidemiological characteristics of an outbreak of 2019 novel coronavirus diseases (COVID-19) in China. 2020;41:145–151. https://doi.org/10.3760/cma.j.issn.0254-6450.2020.02.003 (Accessed on February 10, 2021).
10. Mizumoto K, Kagaya K, Zarebski A, et al. Estimating the asymptomatic proportion of coronavirus disease 2019 (COVID-19) cases on board the Diamond Princess cruise ship, Yokohama, Japan, 2020. *Euro Surveill.* 2020;25:2000180. Available from: https://doi.org/10.2807/1560-7917.ES.2020.25.10.2000180 (Accessed on February 10, 2021).
11. Rabozzi G, Bonizzi L, Crespi E, et al. Emerging zoonoses: the "One Health Approach". *Saf Health Work.* 2012;3:77–83.
12. Mantovani A. Zoonoses control and veterinary public health. *Rev Sci Tech Off Int Epiz.* 1992;11:205–218.
13. European Food Safety Authority. Meat inspection: EFSA completes review of practices and recommends improvements. https://www.efsa.europa.eu/en/press/news/130627-0. Published 2013. (Accessed on May 28, 2020).
14. Buncic S, Alban L, Blagojevic B. From traditional meat inspection to development of meat safety assurance programs in pig abattoirs – The European situation. *Food Control.* 2019;106:106705. Available from: https://doi.org/10.1016/j.foodcont.2019.06.031 (Accessed on September 23, 2020).
15. Edwards DS, Johnston AM, Mead GC. Meat inspection: An overview of present practices and future trends. *Vet J.* 1997;154:135–147.
16. European Food Safety Authority. Technical specifications on harmonised epidemiological indicators for public health hazards to be covered by meat inspection of swine. *EFSA J.* 2011;9:2371. Available from: https://doi.org/10.2903/j.efsa.2011.2371 (Accessed on October 27, 2020).
17. European Food Safety Authority. Technical specifications on harmonised epidemiological indicators for biological hazards to be covered by meat inspection of poultry. *EFSA J.* 2012;10:2764. Available from: https://doi.org/10.2903/j.efsa.2012.2764 (Accessed on October 27, 2020).
18. European Food Safety Authority. Scientific Opinion on the public health hazards to be covered by inspection of meat (solipeds). *EFSA J.* 2013;11:3263. Available from: https://doi.org/10.2903/j.efsa.2013.3263 (Accessed on October 27, 2020).
19. European Food Safety Authority. Technical specifications on harmonised epidemiological indicators for biological hazards to be covered by meat inspection of bovine animals. *EFSA J.* 2013;11:3276. Available from: https://doi.org/10.2903/j.efsa.2013.3276 (Accessed on October 27, 2020).
20. Blagojevic B, Nesbakken T, Alvseike O, Vågsholm I, Antic D, Johler S, Houf K, Meemken D, Nastasijevic I, Vieira Pinto M, Antunovic B, Georgiev M, Alban L. Drivers, opportunities, and challenges of the European risk-based meat safety assurance system. *Food Control.* 2021;124:107870.
21. Food Safety and Inspection Service/USDA. Modernization of swine slaughter inspection. https://www.federalregister.gov/documents/2019/10/01/2019-20245/modernization-of-swine-slaughter-inspection. Published 2019. (Accessed on May 28, 2020).
22. Codex Alimentarius Commission. Code of hygienic practice for meat. CAC/RCP 58-2005; 2005.
23. International Organization for Standardisation. ISO 22000:2018. Food safety management systems. Requirements for any organization in the food chain; 2018.
24. Food and Agriculture Organization. Technical guidance principles of risk-based meat inspection and their application. Rome, Italy; 2019.
25. Codex Alimentarius Commission. General principles of food hygiene. CAC/RCP 1-1969, Rev. 4-2003; 2003.
26. Howlett B, Bolton DJ, O'Sullivan C. *Development of pre-requisite programmes and HACCP principles for Irish beef slaughterhouses.* Dublin, Ashtown: Teagasc-The National Food Centre; 2005.
27. European Commission. Regulation (EC) 853/2004 of the European Parliament and of the Council of 29 April 2004 laying down specific hygiene rules for on the hygiene of foodstuffs. OJEU, 2004;139:55-205. https://eur-lex.europa.eu/legal-content/EN/ALL/?uri = celex%3A32004R0853. (Accessed on October 27, 2020).
28. European Hygiene Engineering Design Group. Hygienic Design Principles – Doc. 8. 3rd edition. download.PDF.EHEDG.DOC_08_E_2018. Published 2018. (Accessed on February 1, 2021).
29. Rivas T, Vizcaino JA, Herrera FJ. Microbial contamination of carcasses and equipment from an Iberian pig slaughterhouse. *J Food Prot.* 2020;63:1670–1675.
30. Conter M, Zanardi E, Ghidini S, et al. Microbiological condition of carcasses and equipment in a pig slaughterhouse and evaluation of a steam decontamination system. *Ital J Food Sci.* 2006;18:387–396.
31. Sammarco ML, Ripabelli G, Ruberto A, et al. Prevalence of Salmonellae, Listeriae, and Yersiniae in the slaughterhouse environment and on work surfaces, equipment, and workers. *J Food Prot.* 1997;60:367–371.
32. Keevil CW. Biofilms in the food industry, VBNC and resistance; requiring new means of detection and control. Paper presented at: Barcelona Biofilm Summit; 7th October, 2020; Barselona, Spain.
33. Limburn R. Breacking cover: Species diversity in bacteria biofilms and cleaning for removal. Paper presented at: Barcelona Biofilm Summit; 7th October, 2020; Barselona, Spain.

34. Warnes SL, Highmore CJ, Keevil CW. Horizontal transfer of antibiotic resistance genes on abiotic touch surfaces: implications for public health. *Mbio.* 2012;3. Available from: https://doi.org/10.1128/mBio.00489-12. e00489-12.
35. Nahar S, Mizan MFR, Ha AJW, et al. Advances and future prospects of enzyme-based biofilm prevention approaches in the food industry. *Compr Rev Food Sci F.* 2018;17:1484–1502.
36. Adeeb F, Shooter D. Emission and evolution of air-borne microflora in slaughter houses. *Indoor Built Environ.* 2003;12:179–184.
37. Donham KJ. Relationships of air quality and productivity in intensive swine housing. *Agri-Practice.* 1990;10:15–26.
38. Husman T. Health effects of indoor-air microorganisms. *Scand J Work Environ Health.* 1996;5–13.
39. Zuber S, Brüssow H. COVID 19: challenges for virologists in the food industry. *Microb Biotechnol.* 2020;1–13. Available from: https://doi.org/10.1111/1751-7915.13638.
40. Whyte RT. Aerial pollutants and the health of poultry farmers. *Worlds Poult Sci J.* 1993;49:139–156.
41. Rahkio TM, Korkeala HJ. Airborne bacteria and carcass contamination in slaughterhouses. *J Food Prot.* 1997;60:38–42.
42. Nastasijevic I, Tomasevic I, Smigic N, et al. Hygiene assessment of Serbian meat establishments using different scoring systems. *Food Control.* 2016;62:193–200.
43. Blagojevic B, Antic D. Assessment of potential contribution of official meat inspection and abattoir process hygiene to biological safety assurance of final beef and pork carcasses. *Food Control.* 2014;36:174–182.
44. Blagojevic B. A path towards modernisation of meat safety assurance in European abattoirs. *IOP Conf Ser Earth Environ Sci.* 2019;333:012013. Available from: https://doi.org/10.1088/1755-1315/333/1/012013.
45. Hultgren J. Is livestock transport a necessary practice? Mobile slaughter and on-farm stunning and killing before transport to slaughter. *CAB Reviews.* 2018;13:1–15.
46. Speer NC, Slack G, Troyer E. Economic factors associated with livestock transportation. *J Anim Sci.* 2001;79:E166–E170.
47. Schwartzkopf-Genswein KS, Faucitano L, Dadgar S, et al. Road transport of cattle, swine and poultry in North America and its impact on animal welfare, carcass and meat quality: A review. *Meat Sci.* 2012;92:227–243.
48. Niyonzima E, Ongol MP, Kimonyo A. Risk factors and control measures for bacterial contamination in the bovine meat chain: A review on *Salmonella* and pathogenic *E. coli*. *J. Food Res.* 2015;4:98–121.
49. Grandin T. *Livestock handling and transport.* Oxfordshire, UK: CABI; 2019.
50. Gopinath S, Carden S, Monack D. Shedding light on *Salmonella* carriers. *Trends Microbiol.* 2012;20:320–327.
51. Pfeiffer CS, King DA, Lucia LM, et al. Influence of transportation stress and animal temperament on fecal shedding of *Escherichia coli* O157: H7 in feedlot cattle. *Meat Sci.* 2009;81:300–306.
52. Warriss PD. The welfare of slaughter pigs during transport. *Anim Welf.* 1998;7:365–381.
53. Villa PD, Marahrens M, Calvo AV, et al. Project to develop animal welfare risk assessment guidelines on transport. EFSA Supporting Publications, 2009;6:21E. https://doi.org/10.2903/sp.efsa.2009.EN-21 (Accessed on December 8, 2020).
54. Warriss PD, Brown SN, Adams SJM, et al. Relationships between subjective and objective assessments of stress at slaughter and meat quality in pigs. *Meat Sci.* 1994;38:329–340.
55. Grandin T. Design of loading facilities and holding pens. *Appl Anim Behav Sci.* 1990;28:187–201.
56. Garcia A, McGlone JJ. Loading and unloading finishing pigs: effects of bedding types, ramp angle, and bedding moisture. *Animals.* 2015;5:13–26.
57. Grandin T. Effect of animal welfare audits of slaughter plants by a major fast food company on cattle handling and stunning practices. *J Am Vet Med Assoc.* 2000;216:848–851.
58. European Commission. Regulation (EC). No 1/2005 of 22 December 2004 on the protection of animals during transport and related operations and amending Directives 64/432/EEC and 93/119/EC and Regulation (EC) No 1255/97. OJEU. 2005;3:1-44. https://eur-lex.europa.eu/legal-content/en/ALL/?uri = CELEX%3A32005R0001.
59. Pérez MP, Palacio J, Santolaria MP, et al. Influence of lairage time on some welfare and meat quality parameters in pigs. *Vet Res.* 2002;33:239–250.
60. Broom DM. Animal welfare complementing or conflicting with other sustainability issues. *Appl Anim Behav Sci.* 2019;219:104829.
61. Nastasijevic I, Lakicevic B, Raseta M, et al. Evaluation of pig welfare in lairage and process hygiene in a single abattoir. *Meat Technology.* 2018;59:8–22.
62. Warriss PD. Optimal lairage times and conditions for slaughter pigs: a review. *Vet Rec.* 2003;153:170–176.
63. Weeks CA. A review of welfare in cattle, sheep and pig lairages, with emphasis on stocking rates, ventilation and noise. *Anim Welf.* 2008;17:275–284.
64. Small A, Reid CA, Avery SM, et al. Potential for the spread of *Escherichia coli* O157, *Salmonella*, and *Campylobacter* in the lairage environment at abattoirs. *J Food Prot.* 2002;65:931–936.
65. World Organisation for Animal Health. Terrestrial Animal Health Code Slaughter of animals, Chapter 7.5, Lairage design and construction. https://www.oie.int/doc/ged/D10905.PDF. Published 2018. (Accessed on March 1, 2020).
66. Collins DS, Huey RJ. *Gracey's meat hygiene.* Hoboken, NJ: John Wiley & Sons; 2014.
67. Faucitano L. Invited review: Effects of lairage and slaughter conditions on animal welfare and pork quality. *Can J Anim Sci.* 2010;90:461–469.
68. Bulut E. Controlling public health risks posed by zoonotic pathogens in beef cattle production through consumption of meat products and exposure to environmental pathways. Doctoral dissertation. Lincoln: University of Nebraska; 2019.
69. Hernández M, Gómez-Laguna J, Luque I, et al. *Salmonella* prevalence and characterization in a free-range pig processing plant: tracking in trucks, lairage, slaughter line and quartering. *Int. J. Food Microbiol.* 2013;162:48–54.
70. Swanenburg M, Berends BR, Urlings HAP, et al. Epidemiological investigations into the sources of *Salmonella* contamination of pork. Proceedings of the 4th International symposium on the epidemiology and control of *Salmonella* and other food borne pathogens in pork. Iowa State University;2001:301-303.
71. Small A, James C, James S, et al. Presence of *Salmonella* in the red meat abattoir lairage after routine cleansing and disinfection and on carcasses. *J. Food Prot.* 2006;69:2342–2351.

72. Arthur TM, Bosilevac JM, Brichta-Harhay DM, et al. Source tracking of *Escherichia* coli O157: H7 and *Salmonella* contamination in the lairage environment at commercial US beef processing plants and identification of an effective intervention. *J Food Prot.* 2008;71:1752–1760.
73. Wheeler TL, Kalchayanand N, Bosilevac JM. Pre-and post-harvest interventions to reduce pathogen contamination in the US beef industry. *Meat Sci.* 2014;98:372–382.
74. Walia K, Argüello H, Lynch H, et al. The efficacy of different cleaning and disinfection procedures to reduce *Salmonella* and *Enterobacteriaceae* in the lairage environment of a pig abattoir. *Int J Food Microbiol.* 2017;246:64–71.
75. Hill AA, Simons RL, Swart AN, et al. Assessing the effectiveness of on-farm and abattoir interventions in reducing pig meat–borne Salmonellosis within EU Member States. *Risk Anal.* 2016;36:546–560.
76. Minihan D, O'Mahony M, Whyte P, et al. *J Vet Med B.* 2003;50:378–382.
77. Jaros P, Cookson AL, Reynolds A, et al. The effect of transportation and lairage on faecal shedding and carcass contamination with *Escherichia coli* O157 and O26 in very young calves in New Zealand. *Epidemiol Infect.* 2018;146:1089–1100.
78. Craig EW, Fletcher DL, Papinaho PA. The effects of antemortem electrical stunning and postmortem electrical stimulation on biochemical and textural properties of broiler breast meat. *Poult Sci.* 1999;78:490–494.
79. European Food Safety Authority Panel on Animal Health and Welfare (AHAW). Guidance on the assessment criteria for studies evaluating the effectiveness of stunning interventions regarding animal protection at the time of killing. *EFSA J.* 2013;11:3486. Available from: https://doi.org/10.2903/j.efsa.2013.3486 (Accessed on October 27, 2020).
80. World Organisation for Animal Health. Terrestrial Animal Health Code – 28/06/2019. Slaughter of animals, Chapter 7.5. https://www.oie.int/fileadmin/Home/eng/Health_standards/tahc/current/chapitre_aw_slaughter.pdf; 2019. (Accessed on September 27, 2020).
81. Grandin T. *Improving animal welfare: a practical approach.* 3rd edition Oxfordshire, UK: CABI; 2021.
82. Verhoeven MTW, Gerritzen MA, Hellebrekers LJ, et al. Indicators used in livestock to assess unconsciousness after stunning: a review. *Animal.* 2015;9:320–330.
83. European Food Safety Authority. Opinion of the scientific panel for animal health and welfare on a request from the Commission related to welfare of animals during transport. *EFSA J.* 2004;44:1–36. Available from: https://doi.org/10.2903/j.efsa.2004.44 (Accessed on October 27, 2020).
84. European Food Safety Authority Panel on Animal Health and Welfare (AHAW). Scientific Opinion on monitoring procedures at slaughterhouses for poultry. *EFSA J.* 2013;11:3521. Available from: https://doi.org/10.2903/j.efsa.2013.3521. Accessed on October 27, 2020.
85. Buncic S, McKinstry J, Reid CA, et al. Spread of microbial contamination associated with penetrative captive bolt stunning of food animals. *Food control.* 2002;13:425–430.
86. Prendergast DM, Sheridan JJ, Daly DJ, et al. Dissemination of central nervous system tissue from the brain and spinal cord of cattle after captive bolt stunning and carcass splitting. *Meat Sci.* 2003;65:1201–1209.
87. Von Holleben KV, Von Wenzlawowicz M, Gregory N, et al. Report on good and adverse practices-Animal welfare concerns in relation to slaughter practices from the viewpoint of veterinary sciences. *Dialrel Deliverable.* 2010;1:3. Available from: https://www.vetjournal.it/archivio_pdf/2010/4069.pdf.
88. Von Wenzlawowicz M, Von Holleben K, Eser E. Identifying reasons for stun failures in slaughterhouses for cattle and pigs: a field study. *Anim Welf.* 2012;21:51–60.
89. Swart AN, Evers EG, Simons RLL, et al. Modeling of *Salmonella* contamination in the pig slaughterhouse. *Risk Anal.* 2016;36:498–515.
90. Fluckey WM, Sanchez MX, McKee SR, et al. Establishment of a microbiological profile for an air-chilling poultry operation in the United States. *J Food Prot.* 2003;66:272–279.
91. Seliwiorstow T, Baré J, Berkvens D, et al. Identification of risk factors for *Campylobacter* contamination levels on broiler carcasses during the slaughter process. *Int J Food Microbiol.* 2016;226:26–32.
92. Warriss PD, Wilkins LJ, Brown SN, et al. Defaecation and weight of the gastrointestinal tract contents after feed and water withdrawal in broilers. *Br Poult Sci.* 2004;45:61–66.
93. Battula V, Schilling MW, Vizzier-Thaxton Y, et al. The effects of low-atmosphere stunning and deboning time on broiler breast meat quality. *Poult Sci.* 2008;87:1202–1210.
94. Humane Slaughter Association. On-farm killing for disease control purposes. www.hsa.org.uk/downloads/killing-for-disease-control.pdf; 2017. (Accessed on October 27, 2020).
95. FAO (2001) Guidelines for Humane Handling, Transport and Slaughter of Livestock. Chapter 7: Slaughter of livestock. Published 2001. https://www.fao.org/3/x6909e/x6909e.pdf (accessed on February 1, 2021).
96. Chang VP, Mills EW, Cutter CN. Reduction of bacteria on pork carcasses associated with chilling method. *J Food Prot.* 2003;66:1019–1024.
97. Koutsoumanis K, Sofos JN. Microbial contamination of carcasses and cuts. *Enc of Meat Sci.* 2004;67:1624–1629.
98. Nastasijević I, Lakićević B, Petrović Z. Cold chain management in meat storage, distribution and retail: A review. *IOP Conf Ser Earth Environ Sci.* 2017;85:012022. Available from: https://doi.org/10.1088/1755-1315/85/1/012022.
99. Lenahan M, Crowley H, O'Brien SB, et al. The potential use of chilling to control the growth of *Enterobacteriaceae* on porcine carcasses and the incidence of *E. coli* O157: H7 in pigs. *J Appl Microbiol.* 2009;106:1512–1520.
100. Lebert I, Baucour P, Lebert A, et al. Assessment of bacterial growth on the surface of meat under common processing conditions by combining biological and physical models. *J Food Eng.* 2005;68:89–98.
101. James SJ, James C. Chilling and freezing. In: Motarjemi J, Lelieveld H, eds. *Food safety management.* Amsterdam, The Netherlands: Elsevier; 2014:481–510.
102. Sukted N, Tuitemwong P, Erickson LE, et al. Reducing risk of campylobacteriosis from poultry: a mini review. *Int J Food Process Technol.* 2017;4:41–52.
103. Zhang Y, Mao Y, Li K, et al. Effect of carcass chilling on the palatability traits and safety of fresh red meat. *Compr Rev Food Sci Food Saf.* 2019;18:1676–1704.
104. Savell JW, Mueller SL, Baird BE. The chilling of carcasses. *Meat Sci.* 2005;70:449–459.

105. European Food Safety Authority. Revision of the joint AFC/BIOHAZ guidance document on the submission of data for the evaluation of the safety and efficacy of substances for the removal of microbial surface contamination of foods of animal origin intended for human consumption. *EFSA J*. 2010;8:1544. Available from: https://doi.org/10.2903/j.efsa.2010.1544 (Accessed on October 27, 2020).
106. Algino RJ, Ingham SC, Zhu J. Survey of antimicrobial effects of beef carcass intervention treatments in very small state-inspected slaughter plants. *J Food Sci*. 2007;72:173–179.
107. Visvalingam J, Liu Y, Yang X. Impact of dry chilling on the genetic diversity of *Escherichia coli* on beef carcasses and on the survival of *E. coli* and *E. coli* O157. *Int J Food Microbiol*. 2017;244:62–66.
108. Kocharunchitt C, Mellefont L, Bowman JP, et al. Application of chlorine dioxide and peroxyacetic acid during spray chilling as a potential antimicrobial intervention for beef carcasses. *Food Microbiol*. 2020;87:103355. Available from: https://doi.org/10.1016/j.fm.2019.103355. Accessed on July 15, 2020.
109. Reid R, Fanning S, Whyte P, et al. The fate of *Salmonella Typhimurium* and *Escherichia coli* O157 on hot boned versus conventionally chilled beef. *Meat Sci*. 2017;126:50–54.
110. Liu Y, Youssef MK, Yang X. Effects of dry chilling on the microflora on beef carcasses at a Canadian beef packing plant. *J Food Prot*. 2016;79:538–543.
111. Nagyová A, Korim P, Mellen M, et al. The efficacy of air spray chilling and its impact on microbial quality of broiler carcasses. *Ital J Anim Sci*. 2015;14:3740. Available from: https://doi.org/10.4081/ijas.2015.3740. Accessed on July 15, 2020.
112. Berrang ME, Meinersmann RJ, Smith DP, et al. The effect of chilling in cold air or ice water on the microbiological quality of broiler carcasses and the population of *Campylobacter*. *Poult Sci*. 2008;87:992–998.
113. Smith DP, Cason JA, Berrang ME. Effect of fecal contamination and cross-contamination on numbers of coliform, *Escherichia coli*, *Campylobacter*, and *Salmonella* on immersion-chilled broiler carcasses. *J Food Prot*. 2005;68:1340–1345.
114. Barbut S, Moza LF, Nattress F, et al. The microbiological conditions of air-or water-chilled carcasses produced at the same poultry packing plant. *J Appl Poult Res*. 2009;18:501–507.
115. Sanchez MX, Fluckey WM, Brashears MM, et al. Microbial profile and antibiotic susceptibility of *Campylobacter* spp. and *Salmonella* spp. in broilers processed in air-chilled and immersion-chilled environments. *J Food Prot*. 2002;65:948–956.
116. Nesbakken T, Eckner K, Røtterud OJ. The effect of blast chilling on occurrence of human pathogenic *Yersinia enterocolitica* compared to *Campylobacter* spp. and numbers of hygienic indicators on pig carcasses. *Int J Food Microbiol*. 2008;123:130–133.
117. Bracewell AJ, Reagan JO, Carpenter JA, et al. Comparison of sampling methods for isolation of *Campylobacter jejuni coli* from pork skin. *J Food Prot*. 1986;49:532–533.
118. Vanantwerpen G, De Zutter L, Berkvens D, et al. Impact of the sampling method and chilling on the *Salmonella* recovery from pig carcasses. *Int J Food Microbiol*. 2016;232:22–25.
119. Pearce RA, Wallace FM, Call JE, et al. Prevalence of *Campylobacter* within a swine slaughter and processing facility. *J Food Prot*. 2003;66:1550–1556.
120. Gonzales-Barron U, Cadavez V, Sheridan JJ, et al. Modelling the effect of chilling on the occurrence of *Salmonella* on pig carcasses at study, abattoir and batch levels by meta-analysis. *Int J Food Microbiol*. 2013;163:101–113.
121. Martínez-Alvarez O, Chamorro S, Brenes A. Protein hydrolysates from animal processing by-products as a source of bioactive molecules with interest in animal feeding: A review. *Food Res. Int*. 2015;73:204–212.
122. Hamilton CR. *Real and perceived issues involving animal proteins. Protein sources for the animal feed industry*. Bangkok, Thailand: FAO Expert Consultation and Workshop; 2002:255–276.
123. European Commission. Regulation (EC) No 1069/2009 of the European Parliament and of the Council of 21 October 2009 laying down health rules as regards animal by-products and derived products not intended for human consumption and repealing Regulation (EC) No 1774/2002 (Animal by-products Regulation). OJEU. 2009;300:1-33.
124. Bustillo-Lecompte CF, Mehrvar M. Treatment of actual slaughterhouse wastewater by combined anaerobic–aerobic processes for biogas generation and removal of organics and nutrients: An optimization study towards a cleaner production in the meat processing industry. *J Clean Prod*. 2017;141:278–289.
125. López-López A, Barrera-Fraire J, Vallejo-Rodriguez R, et al. Estudio comparativo entre un proceso fisicoquímico y uno biológico para tratar agua residual de rastro. *Interciencia*. 2008;33:490–496.
126. Tritt WP, Schuchardt F. Materials flow and possibilities of treating liquid and solid wastes from slaughterhouses in Germany. A review. *Bioresour Technol*. 1992;41:235–245.
127. Mittal GS. Characterization of the effluent wastewater from abattoirs for land application. *Food Rev Int*. 2004;20:229–256.
128. Van Elsas JD, Bailey MJ. The ecology of transfer of mobile genetic elements. *FEMS Microbiol Ecol*. 2002;42:187–197.
129. Savin M, Bierbaum G, Hammerl JA, et al. ESKAPE bacteria and extended-spectrum-β-lactamase-producing *Escherichia coli* isolated from wastewater and process water from German poultry slaughterhouses. *Appl Environ Microbiol*. 2020;86. Available from: https://doi.org/10.1128/AEM.02748-19. Accessed on July 15, 2020.
130. Bustillo-Lecompte CF, Mehrvar M. Slaughterhouse wastewater characteristics, treatment, and management in the meat processing industry: A review on trends and advances. *J Environ Manage*. 2015;161:287–302.
131. Bibbal D, Um MM, Diallo AA, et al. Mixing of Shiga toxin-producing and enteropathogenic *Escherichia coli* in a wastewater treatment plant receiving city and slaughterhouse wastewater. *Int J Hyg Environ Health*. 2018;221:355–363.
132. Valta K, Kosanovic T, Malamis D, et al. Overview of water usage and wastewater management in the food and beverage industry. *Desalination Water Treat*. 2015;53:3335–3347.
133. Mittal GS. Treatment of wastewater from abattoirs before land application—a review. *Bioresour Technol*. 2006;97:1119–1135.
134. Hakizimana JN, Gourich B, Chafi M, et al. Electrocoagulation process in water treatment: A review of electrocoagulation modeling approaches. *Desalination*. 2017;404:1–21.
135. Melo R, Verde SC, Branco J, et al. Gamma radiation induced effects on slaughterhouse wastewater treatment. *Radiat Phy Chem*. 2008;77:98–100.

136. Cao W, Mehrvar M. Slaughterhouse wastewater treatment by combined anaerobic baffled reactor and UV/H_2O_2 processes. *Chem Eng Res Des*. 2011;89:1136–1143.
137. Milios KDEZP, Drosinos EH, Zoiopoulos PE. Carcass decontamination methods in slaughterhouses: a review. *J Hell Vet Medical Soc*. 2014;65:65–78.
138. Bolton DJ, Pearce R, Tergny A, et al. *Hazard analysis and critical control point (HACCP) and hygiene control auditing in Irish beef abattoirs*. Teagasc, Ashtown, Dublin: Food Research Centre; 2007.
139. Tergney A, Bolton DJ. Validation studies on an online monitoring system for reducing faecal and microbial contamination on beef carcasses. *Food Control*. 2006;17:378–382.
140. Nørrung B, Buncic S. Microbial safety of meat in the European Union. *Meat Sci*. 2008;78:14–24.
141. Nastasijevic I, Mitrovic R, Popovic K, et al. The effects of a non-intervention HACCP implementation on process hygiene indicators on bovine and porcine carcasses. *Meso*. 2009;11:232–239.
142. Rose BE, Hill WE, Umholtz R, et al. Testing for *Salmonella* in raw meat and poultry products collected at federally inspected establishments in the United States, 1998 through 2000. *J Food Prot*. 2002;65:937–947.
143. Bolton DJ, Doherty AM, Sheridan JJ. Beef HACCP: intervention and non-intervention systems. *Int J Food Microbiol*. 2001;66:119–129.
144. Sheridan JJ. Monitoring CCPs in HACCP systems. In: Brown M, ed. *HACCP in the meat industry*. Sawston, Cambridge: Woodhead Publishing; 2000:203–230.
145. Byrne B, Dunne G, Lyng J, et al. The development of a 'clean sheep policy'in compliance with the new Hygiene Regulation (EC) 853/2004 (Hygiene 2). *Food Microbiol*. 2007;24:301–304.
146. Bosilevac JM, Nou X, Osborn MS, et al. Development and evaluation of an on-line hide decontamination procedure for use in commercial beef processing plant. *J Food Prot*. 2005;68:265–272.
147. Borch E, Nesbakken T, Christensen H. Hazard identification in swine slaughter with respect to foodborne bacteria. *Int J Food Microbiol*. 1996;30:9–25.
148. Gill CO, Bedard D, Jones T. The decontaminating performance of a commercial apparatus for pasteurizing polished pig carcasses. *Food Microbiol*. 1997;14:71–79.
149. Loretz M, Stephan R, Zweifel C. Antibacterial activity of decontamination treatments for cattle hides and beef carcasses. *Food Control*. 2011;22:347–359.
150. Bolton DJ, Pearce RA, Sheridan JJ, et al. Washing and chilling as critical control points in pork slaughter hazard analysis and critical control point (HACCP) systems. *J Appl Microbiol*. 2002;92:893–902.
151. Trivedi S, Reynolds AE, Chen J. Use of a commercial household steam cleaning system to decontaminate beef and hog carcasses processed by four small or very small meat processing plants in Georgia. *J Food Prot*. 2007;70:635–640.
152. Pipek P, Houška M, Hoke K, et al. Decontamination of pork carcasses by steam and lactic acid. *J Food Eng*. 2006;74:224–231.
153. Prasai RK, Acuff GR, Lucia LM, et al. Microbiological effects of acid decontamination of beef carcasses at various locations in processing. *J Food Prot*. 1991;54:868–872.
154. Loretz M, Stephan R, Zweifel C. Antimicrobial activity of decontamination treatments for poultry carcasses: a literature survey. *Food Control*. 2010;21:791–804.
155. Bell RG. Distribution and sources of microbial contamination on beef carcasses. *J Appl Microbiol*. 1997;82:292–300.
156. Sofos J. Challenges to meat safety in the 21st century. *Meat Sci*. 2008;78:3–13.
157. Nastasijevic I, Milanov D, Velebit B, Djordjevic V, Swift C, Painset A, Lakicevic B. Tracking of *Listeria monocytogenes* in meat establishment using Whole Genome Sequencing as a food safety management tool: A proof of concept. *International Journal of Food Microbiology*. 2017;257:157–164.
158. Nastasijevic I, Proscia F, Boskovic M, et al. The European Union control strategy for *Campylobacter* spp. in the broiler meat chain. *J Food Saf*. 2020;40:e12819.
159. Nastasijevic I, Schmidt JW, Boskovic M, et al. Seasonal prevalence and characterization of Shiga toxin-producing Escherichia coli on pork carcasses at three steps of the harvest process at two commercial processing plants in the US. *Appl. Environ. Microbiol*. 2020;87:e01711–20. Available from: https://doi.org/10.1128/AEM.01711-20.
160. Nastasijevic I, Mitrovic R, Buncic S. The occurence of *Escherichia coli* O157 in/on faeces, carcasses and fresh meats from cattle. *Meat Science*. 2009;82:101–105.
161. Alban L, Petersen JV, Bækbo AK, et al. Modernising meat inspection of pigs – A review of the Danish process from 2006-2020. *Food Control*. 2021;119:107450.
162. Barbut S. Review: Automation and meat quality-global challenges. *Meat Sci*. 2014;96:335–345.
163. Madsen NT, Nielsen JU, Mønsted JK. Automation – The meat factory of the future. 52nd International Congress of Meat Science and Technology, 13-18 August, Dublin, Ireland. 2006:35-42.
164. Alvseike O, Prieto M, Torkveen K, et al. Meat inspection and hygiene in a Meat Factory Cell - An alternative concept. *Food Control*. 2018;90:32–39.
165. Regulation (EC) 999/2001 of the European Parliament and of the Council laying down rules for the prevention, control and eradication of certain transmissible spongiform encephalopathies. https://eur-lex.europa.eu/legal-content/en/TXT/PDF/?uri = CELEX:02001R0999-20130701&from = en (accessed on 23 March 2021).
166. EFSA. Scientific Opinion on BSE risk in bovine intestines and mesentery. *EFSA Journal*. 2014;12(2):3554.
167. Commission Regulation (EU) 2015/728 amending the definition of specified risk material set out in Annex V to Regulation (EC) No 999/2001 of the European Parliament and of the Council laying down rules for the prevention, control and eradication of certain transmissible spongiform encephalopathies. https://eur-lex.europa.eu/legal-content/EN/TXT/PDF/?uri = CELEX:32015R0728&from = EN (accessed on 23 March 2021).
168. OIE Terrestrial Animal Health Code (2021) CHAPTER 11.4. BOVINE SPONGIFORM ENCEPHALOPATHY. Article 11.4.14. https://www.oie.int/fileadmin/Home/eng/Health_standards/tahc/current/chapitre_bse.pdf (accessed on 23 march 2021).

Chapter 30

Dairy production: microbial safety of raw milk and processed milk products

Victor Ntuli[1], Thulani Sibanda[2,3], James A. Elegbeleye[2], Desmond T. Mugadza[4], Eyassu Seifu[5] and Elna M. Buys[2]

[1]*Department of Biology, National University of Lesotho, Maseru, Lesotho,* [2]*Department of Consumer and Food Sciences, University of Pretoria, Hatfield, South Africa,* [3]*Department of Applied Biology and Biochemistry, National University of Science and Technology, Bulawayo, Zimbabwe,* [4]*Department of Food Science and Nutrition, Midlands State University, Gweru, Zimbabwe,* [5]*Department of Food Science and Technology, Botswana University of Agriculture and Natural Resources, Gaborone, Botswana*

Abstract

Dairy production is important for the survival of billions of people across the globe who consume milk and dairy products every day. Milk and its products are a source of essential nutrients, such as proteins, fats, vitamins, and minerals necessary for human health. The production and consumption of dairy products are increasing worldwide. As the single most important raw material in dairy production, the quality of raw milk is central to the quality and safety of all dairy products. Owing to its highly nutritious nature, milk serves as an excellent growth medium for a wide range of microbes. Microbial contamination of milk and dairy products along the value chain remains a daunting task for the dairy industry. Notwithstanding the different process technologies (both conventional and novel) that have been adopted by the dairy industry, microbial spoilage of milk and its products still causes major losses in the industry. Furthermore, several foodborne disease outbreaks have been implicated in milk and dairy products around the world. Enteric pathogens such as *Salmonella* serovars, *Campylobacter* spp., Shiga toxin-producing *Escherichia coli*, *Listeria monocytogenes*, and enterotoxin producing *Staphylococcus aureus* are the most commonly implicated organisms in dairy-borne disease outbreaks. In order to manage food safety in the dairy industry, any approach to food safety reform must be proactive and risk-based. However, this approach is still posing a challenge in developing countries where the dairy sector is predominated by the informal value chains. Irrespective of the scales of production (large or small scale) and sector (formal or informal), the dairy industry should apply principles of good hygiene practices and good manufacturing practices, coupled with identification and management of possible sources of contamination, in order to curb the challenges of quality and safety.

Keywords: Dairy value chain; microbial contamination; food safety; hygiene; risk-based approach

30.1 Introduction

Milk is an essential component of the human diet consumed by approximately 80% of the world's population.[1] It is a source of essential nutrients, such as proteins, fats, vitamins, and minerals necessary for human health.[2] Milk is one of the most produced and valuable agricultural commodities accounting for 27% of the global added value of livestock and 10% of the global added value to agriculture.[3] Globally, about 881 billion liters of milk are produced annually, most of it (81%) coming from cattle, and the remainder coming from other dairy species such as buffaloes, goats, camels, and sheep.[1]

As the single most important raw material in dairy production, the quality of raw milk is central to the quality and safety of all dairy products. The highly nutritious nature of milk makes it an attractive medium for microbial growth. Several contamination sources and risk factors expose raw milk to microbial hazards at the farm level and along the dairy value chain.[4] At the farm, contamination of raw milk can emanate from within the udder (in the case of infected animals suffering from mastitis), the milking environment and from milk handling and storage equipment. Bioaerosols and dust in milking parlour environments can be sources of contamination with soilborne organisms, fecal and animal skin microflora. In addition, bacterial biofilms in milking machines, and milk pipelines can be another source of raw milk contamination. With so many sources of contamination, the microflora of raw milk is very diverse. It includes soilborne and waterborne microorganisms such as *Curtobacterium* spp., *Bacillus* spp., *Corynebacterium* spp., *Aerococcus* spp., *Staphylococcus* spp. and *Pseudomonas* spp. The microflora also include

Present Knowledge in Food Safety. DOI: https://doi.org/10.1016/B978-0-12-819470-6.00076-7

animal-derived commensal bacteria such as lactic acid bacteria (LABs) and pathogenic bacteria such as Shiga toxin-producing *Escherichia coli*, *Salmonella* serovars, *Campylobacter* spp., *Listeria monocytogenes*, *Staphylococcus aureus*, and *Yersinia enterocolitica*.[5]

The presence of microorganisms in milk has two main consequences. The growth of spoilage organisms that secrete hydrolytic enzymes can cause spoilage and quality defects in milk. Microbial spoilage of milk is a major cause of losses in the dairy industry. The deterioration in quality is exacerbated by inadequate cooling conditions in the storage of raw milk and inadequate cold chain post-milking. The second consequence of microbial presence in milk is the health risk to consumers arising from the growth of foodborne pathogens. Enteric pathogens such as *Salmonella enterica*, *Campylobacter* spp., Shiga toxin-producing *E. coli* (STEC), and *L. monocytogenes* are common fecal contaminants of raw milk.[5] Other zoonotic pathogens such as *Mycobacterium* spp., *Brucella* spp., *Coxiella burnetii*, *S. aureus*, and *Streptococcus* spp. can also be transferred into raw milk from infected animals.[6,7] Unlike spoilage organisms that cause noticeable quality deterioration in milk, the growth of pathogenic organisms may not produce any discernible effects on quality. Thus, contaminated milk poses a great public health risk as it can be consumed without any objectionable quality defects.

Microbial growth in milk is a major risk factor limiting the shelf life of raw milk. Hence, milk is frequently processed into fresh dairy products such as pasteurized milk, ultra-high temperature (UHT) milk, and extended shelf life (ESL) milk. Of these processes, pasteurization (heat treatment at 72°C for 15 s) is considered the most fundamental step in milk processing. It is a process designed to keep the microbial load of milk low, before further processing into other value-added dairy products such as cheeses and yogurt, butter, and sour cream.[8] Although pasteurization has been effective as a primary step in controlling the microbial load in milk, the spoilage and safety of pasteurized milk are still a major issue in the dairy industry.[9] Moreover, some heat-resistant (thermoduric vegetative) bacterial species and spore-formers can survive the pasteurization processing and cause spoilage of the pasteurized milk.[9] Because of the low-temperature storage of pasteurized milk, the spoilage is often a result of psychrotolerant spore-formers such as *Bacillus* spp. and *Paenibacillus* spp. that survive the thermal processing conditions.[10] Besides the psychrotolerant spore-formers, heat-labile psychrotolerant Gram-negative bacterial species introduced into the product through post-pasteurization contamination are also a significant factor in the spoilage of pasteurized milk.[9] Among the psychrotolerant post-pasteurization contaminants, *Pseudomonas* species are typically the most common causes of spoilage of pasteurized milk. Their adaptation and rapid growth rate under low-temperatures favors their growth in refrigerated pasteurized milk.[9]

As most pathogens associated with milk and dairy products are susceptible to pasteurization, most dairy-borne disease outbreaks are often due to consumption of raw milk or raw-milk-derived products.[11] Notwithstanding the bactericidal effectiveness of pasteurization, incidents of illnesses and outbreaks linked to the consumption of pasteurized milk and its products are still common.[12] Hence, the control and management of microbial hazards in dairy foods is a matter that must incorporate all stages of the value chain. These include farm-level good hygiene practices (GHP) involving animal hygiene, hygiene of the milking environment, the milking equipment and cow health- as well as hazard analysis critical control point (HACCP) systems during processing.[13] In addition to the implementation of GHP and HACCP, risk-based approaches can provide a way of limiting the risk of illnesses associated with pathogens in dairy foods. Using risk-based approaches, processes and operations where a higher probability of contamination, cross-contamination and pathogen growth exists, are given more attention.

30.2 Dairy value chain

The microbial quality and safety of dairy products are a cumulative function of the contamination risks and the growth or inactivation probabilities of the contaminating microorganisms and pathogens from the point of milking up to the consumer. The contamination risks and growth probabilities of the contaminant microflora are influenced by hygiene practices and the handling of milk at the farm level, storage and transportation of raw milk to processing facilities, processing conditions, handling and storage of processed products at the wholesale, retail, and consumer stages. The main stages of the dairy value chain and their associated microbial quality and safety risk factors are shown in Fig. 30.1.

In developed countries (and some developing countries), dairy value chains are formal and are characterized by large commercial farms with modern production technology implementing global standards on good agricultural practices. Although the implementation of food safety standards at different stages of the formal value chains aims to reduce the risk of microbial hazards, many cases of dairy-based foodborne diseases continue to be reported worldwide.[12,14] Several risk factors are associated with every stage of the value chain (summarized in Fig. 30.1). Hence, food safety failures at any stage of the value chain can result in a magnified risk along the chain.

Unlike the situation in developed countries, dairy value chains in most developing countries are predominantly informal. For instance, more than 80% of the milk

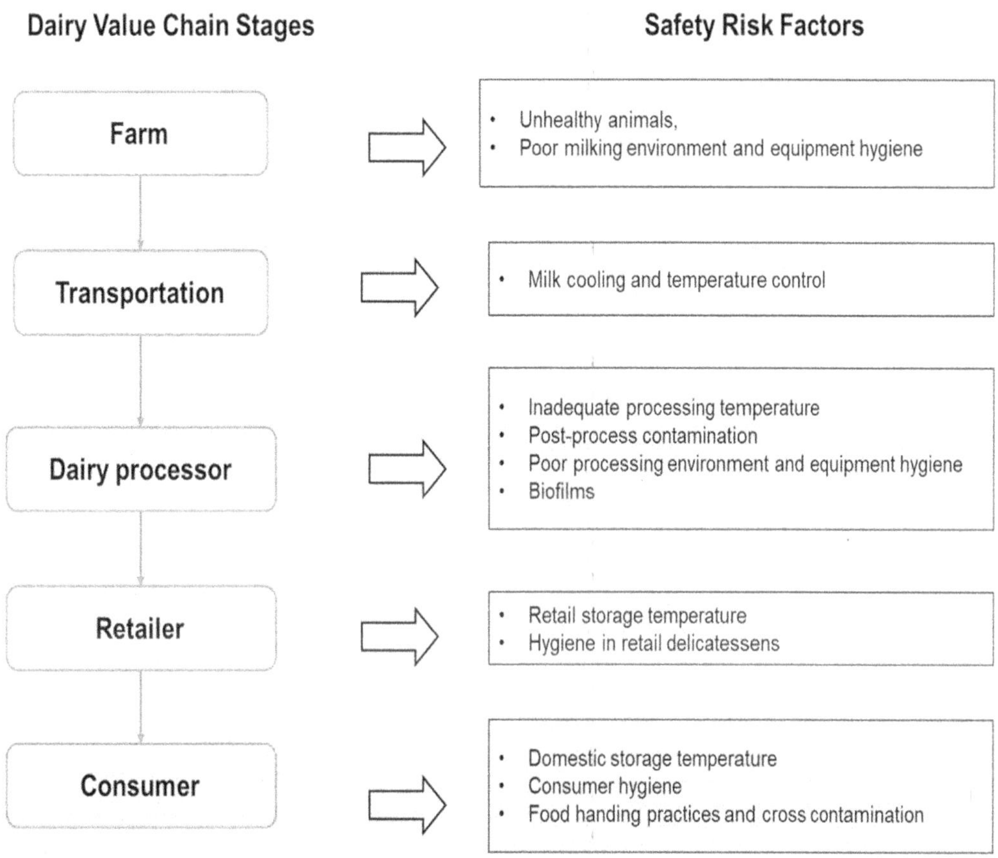

FIGURE 30.1 Dairy value chain and associated risk factors of microbial contamination and growth.

supply in Zambia and Kenya is from informal milk producers and is supplied through informal value chains.[15,16] The informal milk supply chains depend on traditional rural farmers (usually producing milk from indigenous non-dairy breeds for subsistence and family income) and small-holder dairy farms that keep small (3–15) herds of dairy cows and informal milk traders as a supply line to the consumers.[16] In countries where informal rural and smallholder farmers are the predominant raw milk suppliers, the milk can also be channeled to formal processing plants through milk collection centers and dairy cooperatives.[15] Milk collection centers provide facilities for cooling and further distribution to commercial processors. The several nodes of such informal milk value chains and their cross intersection with formal value chains make such supply chains a major safety risk even for products produced through formal commercial processors.

Depending on regulations in each county, milk collection in formal systems is usually done by certified collectors who sample the milk for quick testing to check for compliance with standards such as antibiotic residues. If the milk complies with the required standards, it is pumped from the bulk tanks at farms into the milk trucks.[17] A truckload may contain milk from several farms when it is delivered to the processing plant. Before unloading at the processing plant, the milk passes through a series of preliminary analytical tests such as acidity, antibiotic residuals, added water, fat, and protein content. Compliance failures especially with antibiotic testing would normally result in rejection of the entire truckload. However, failure to comply with other tests would normally result in the classification of the milk load as low-grade which can be used for the processing of low-value dairy products.[18] In some instances, raw milk can be pasteurized at the farm before transportation to processing plants, and in some cases, milk processing can also be conducted on-site.

30.3 Microbiology of raw milk

Milk is a sterile fluid as it is secreted into the alveoli of the udder of healthy animals. However, depending on the level of milking hygiene, milk is almost immediately contaminated at the point of milking. Because of its high nutrient content and nearly neutral pH, it is a good medium for microbial growth. The immediate sources of milk contamination include the exterior of the udder, and the milking and storage equipment. The microflora of raw milk is very diverse; it consists of organisms that are part of the natural flora of healthy animals (skin and gastrointestinal tract commensals), and organisms that cause systemic and gastrointestinal tract infections in dairy animals.[5,19] The microflora also includes soilborne and waterborne organisms as well as organisms from animal feed and vegetation. Animal feed and feed ingredients have been implicated as an important source of microbial contamination of milk at farm level.

30.3.1 Pathogenic organisms

Most milk-borne pathogens are either zoonotic organisms that infect dairy cows or commensal organisms that are part of the natural flora of healthy animals. In some instances, milk-borne pathogens can be environmental saprophytes introduced into the milk from the milking environment while some can be introduced into the milk by personnel during milking. Among the systemic infections, mastitis has the greatest influence on the microbiology of raw milk. Mastitis is an inflammation of the mammary gland primarily caused by bacterial intramammary infections. Based on the extent of inflammation, mastitis can be clinical (with visible signs such as a swollen udder and watery milk with clots) or subclinical which is asymptomatic. Because of its asymptomatic nature, subclinical mastitis is a major risk factor in the transmission of milk-borne pathogens as infected animals shed the pathogens into the milk together with somatic cells. The most identified causes of subclinical mastitis are *S. aureus* and *Streptococcus agalactiae*.[20] These bacterial species are part of the natural flora of the cow's udder and teat skin that can colonize and grow into the teat canal. Other pathogens include *E. coli*, *Klebsiella* spp., *Enterobacter* spp., *Pseudomonas* spp., *Streptococcus uberis*, and *Bacillus* spp.[21] Thus, milk from infected animals is considered to be a main source of milk-borne pathogens with enterotoxigenic *S. aureus* as the leading risk in raw milk and raw milk-derived products.[21]

In addition to mastitis, raw milk consumption has for a long time been known to be a risk factor for the transmission of other zoonotic pathogens that cause systemic infections in dairy animals. These include *Mycobacterium bovis* and *Mycobacterium avium* subspecies *paratuberculosis* (MAP),[22] which cause bovine tuberculosis (TB) and Johne's disease respectively. Due to the universal implementation of pasteurization, zoonotic TB outbreaks are now rare in developed countries. However, sporadic cases still occur due to on-farm consumption of raw milk. Notwithstanding the well known success of pasteurization in attenuating the human risk of zoonotic TB, low levels of MAP have been detected in retail pasteurized milk.[23,24] The reason for this has not been clearly understood. Intracellular MAP within the somatic cells may be protected against heat inactivation during pasteurization.[24] Several milk-borne human MAP infection outbreaks have been reported across the globe. Table 30.1 presents some of the disease outbreaks traced to the consumption of some milk and dairy products since 2000 in Europe and United States.

Like many other livestock animals, dairy animals can be asymptomatic carriers of several enteric pathogens such as *Salmonella* serovars, *Campylobacter* spp., *E. coli* O157:H7, and *L. monocytogenes*.[41] Most commonly, these organisms are harboured as commensals in the gastrointestinal tracts and are introduced into milk during milking through fecal contamination of the udder. Milking hygiene is a key factor in modulating the risk of fecal contamination. Since the udder of the dairy animals can come into direct contact with the dung, cleaning the udder before milking is one of the most important hygienic practices to reduce the transmission of pathogens through fecal contamination. A 90% reduction of teat contamination can be achieved with good udder preparation before milking.[42]

30.3.2 Spoilage organisms

While it is not a food safety risk factor, the deterioration in milk quality as a result of microbial growth is a major concern for the dairy industry. Milk spoilage is a result of microbial growth and enzyme production that result in the degradation of lipids and proteins leading to the release of metabolites that have negative effects on milk quality. If raw milk is kept unrefrigerated, the most common spoilage problem is souring due to mesophilic LABs. However, the greatest challenge is attributed to the growth of psychrotrophic organisms in raw and pasteurized milk stored at low temperatures. The low-temperature spoilage is mainly due to the growth of psychrophilic *Pseudomonas* spp. and *Acinetobacter* spp. as raw milk contaminants or as post-pasteurization contaminants.[9] Moreover, spoilage can also result from heat-stable enzymes produced by *Pseudomonas* spp. during growth of the organisms in low-temperature stored raw milk before pasteurization.[43] As a ubiquitous environmental saprophyte, contamination with *Pseudomonas* spp. can emanate from water, bulk milk tank surfaces, udder teats, and milking equipment.[44]

Apart from psychrotrophic vegetative bacterial species, psychrotolerant spore-forming bacteria also represent a major challenge in the spoilage of thermally processed dairy products. The Gram-positive psychrotolerant spore-formers include *Bacillus* spp. (*B. licheniformis*, *B. cereus*, *B. pumilus*, *B. sporothermodurans*, *B. weihenstephanensis*), and *Paenibacillus* spp. (*P. odorifer*, *P. graminis*, and *P. amylolyticus*).[10,45] In terms of ecology, the spore-formers are ubiquitously found around the dairy farm

TABLE 30.1 Disease outbreaks traced to consumption of some milk and dairy products since 2000 in Europe and United States.

Pathogen	Country	Year	Implicated dairy products	Number of cases	Reference
Salmonella serovars	France	2018	Raw goats' milk cheese	153	Robinson et al.[25]
	France	2017	Infant milk products	22	Jourdan-Da Silva et al.[26]
	France	2015–2016	Raw milk cheese	83	Ung et al.[27]
Escherichia coli (STEC)	France	2019	Soft raw cow's milk cheeses	13	Jones et al.[28]
	USA	2014	Aged raw milk Gouda cheese	41	Mccollum et al.[29]
	Canada	2013	Aged raw milk Gouda cheese	29	Currie et al.[30]
Campylobacter spp.	Italy	2018	Cheese	222	Sorgentone et al.[31]
	England	2016	Raw milk	69	Kenyon et al.[32]
	USA	2012	Unpasteurized milk	81	Longenberger et al.[33]
Listeria monocytogenes	Austria and Germany	2009–2010	Acid curd cheese "Quargel"	14	Fretz et al.[34]
	Canada	2008	Pasteurized cheese	38	Gaulin et al.[35]
	United States	2009	Mexican-style cheese	8	Jackson et al.[36]
Staphylococcus aureus	Switzerland	2014	Soft cheese made from raw milk	14	Johler et al.[37]
	Germany	2013	Ice cream	13	Fetsch et al.[38]
	Japan	2000	Powdered skim milk products	13 420	Asao et al.[39]
	Austria	2007	Pasteurized milk products	40	Schmid et al.[40]

STEC, Shiga toxin-producing *Escherichia coli.*

environment, being abundant in soil, vegetation, silage, and the gastrointestinal tracts of dairy animals. Apart from the contamination of raw milk at the farm, spore-formers present a big challenge along the dairy product processing continuum as they are hard to eliminate once such organisms colonize storage tanks, pipework, and product packaging lines.

30.4 Dairy processing and safety of processed products

Raw milk is a very perishable commodity with a short shelf life. The usable life of milk can be extended for several days through techniques such as cooling, pasteurization and fermentation. Milk is further processed into high-value dairy products with longer shelf lives. Dairy processing involves the conversion of raw milk into fluid milk products, fermented milk products like yogurt and cheese, evaporated and condensed milk, dry milk products, whey and whey products, ice cream, and butter and spreads.

Irrespective of prior pasteurization, milk arriving at the dairy processing plant should be transported at temperatures between 4°C and 6°C.[17] Having passed the preliminary analytical tests, the milk is subsequently processed into different value-added products. Although the dairy industry is still employing conventional processing technologies, different new processing techniques have evolved over time, bringing with them new and unforeseen quality and safety consequences.[46] Potential threats to human health can arise from errors in pasteurization and emergence of heat-resistant pathogens. Cross-contamination of finished products with raw material, inadequate sanitation procedures in the plant environment, or inadequately sanitized equipment has resulted in dairy products with reduced shelf life. Other critics have pointed out the lack of a system involving good laboratory methods for detecting and tracing sources of microbial contamination in the dairy plant environment as the main limitation to achieving an acceptable level of food safety with prolonged shelf life.[46]

The size or scale (large or small) of production influences the operating practices and safety of dairy products.[47] In most developing countries, dairy industries that process more than 10,000 L of milk per day are classified as large-scale.[47] Apart from scales of production, large-scale industries have fairly adopted and implemented food safety management systems (FSMS) while small-scale dairy industries generally lack such management systems.[47,48] Due to the lack of FSMS, small-scale dairy industries have been being characterized by poor dairy product quality.[48]

30.4.1 Thermal processing and quality of fresh milk products

Thermal processing of milk is arguably the principal method of eliminating pathogenic and spoilage organisms, and ensuring safety and long shelf life. The intentional heating of milk above 50°C for a sufficient time such that there is a reduction in the concentration of one or more microorganisms is considered heat treatment. Thus the heat treatment concept covers an infinite number of time–temperature combinations. Although heating has the beneficial effect of reducing microbial load, it results in some inevitable negative consequences such as the loss of nutritional value, loss of bioactive compounds (such as antioxidant, antithrombotic, antitumor, and antiinflammatory activities), and loss of the sensory qualities of milk. A range of novel thermal processing techniques have been developed to improve the quality of foods, at the same time minimizing the negative impacts associated with thermal degradation. Numerous investigations on dielectric heating (which includes microwave heating and radio-frequency heating), ohmic heating, inductive heating, and infrared heating have demonstrated their effectiveness in ensuring product safety, quality, and acceptability.[49] Although efforts have been made to improve milk processing to inactivate microorganisms, there is no ultimate technology that eliminates pathogens from the food supply chain. A combination of multiple thermal and nonthermal interventions also known as the hurdle approach, has shown some potential in improving food safety. Moreover, while novel thermal processes have been partially adopted in dairy industries, the processing of milk is still largely dependent on the conventional thermal processes such as thermization, pasteurization, and ultra-heat treatment.

30.4.1.1 Pasteurized milk

Pasteurization is the oldest and yet still the most widely used technology in dairy processing. The modern process of milk pasteurization [high-temperature, short-time (HTST) process] is based on continuous plate pasteurizers in which the milk is heated to a temperature of 72°C for 15 s in a holding tube followed by rapid cooling.

Except for spore-formers, the time-temperature conditions of HTST pasteurization are considered sufficient to eliminate most bacterial pathogens found in raw milk. With the decimal reduction times (*D*-values) for pathogens such as *E. coli* O157:H7 (16.2 s at 63°C), *L. monocytogenes* (33.3 s at 63°C), *M. bovis* (6.6 s at 64°C), *Campylobacter* spp. (0.12–0.14 min at 60°C), and *Salmonella* serovars (0.11 min at 62.8°C), the HTST process can achieve >5 log reduction of these pathogens in milk.[50]

Although the HTST pasteurization process greatly reduces the safety risks associated with milk and dairy products, infections and outbreaks resulting from consumption of contaminated products derived from pasteurized milk continue to be a challenge for the dairy sector.[51] Most of the safety challenges of pasteurized milk products are attributed to post-pasteurization contamination emanating from filling machines and bacterial biofilms on milk post-pasteurization contact surfaces.[50] Apart from post-pasteurization contamination, the presence of pathogens directly associated with raw milk such as *L. monocytogenes*, *E. coli*, and MAP, could be an indication of faulty pasteurization.[50] Besides the issues of microbial safety risks, pasteurized milk generally has a short shelf life of 2–20 days under refrigerated storage.[52] The major limiting factor to the shelf life is spoilage due to psyschrotrophs, principally *Pseudomonas* spp. These organisms are frequent post-pasteurization contaminants and can multiply at refrigeration temperatures. Moreover, the growth of psychrotrophs in refrigerated raw milk before processing has a significant impact on the quality and shelf life of pasteurized milk as heat-stable proteases and lipases secreted at this stage can cause quality deterioration post-pasteurization. Therefore, the total microbial load and the types of organisms present in the raw milk, have a substantial influence on the quality and shelf life of the pasteurized milk.[50]

30.4.1.2 Ultra-high temperature (UHT) processed milk

UHT milk is milk that has been processed at ultra-high temperatures and filled under aseptic conditions into hermetically sealed packaging, thus producing a commercially sterile product. Typically, UHT milk is processed at 125°C–154°C for 1–8 s, followed by quick cooling to ambient temperature.[53] As a commercially sterile product, UHT milk has a shelf life of 4–9 months unrefrigerated. Notwithstanding the ultra-high heat sterilization treatment, some heat-resistant spore-forming bacteria such as *B. cereus*, *B. sporothermodurans*, and *Geobacillus stearothermophilus* have been isolated from UHT milk.[54] Their presence in UHT milk has been attributed to several factors that include intrinsic high heat resistance, survival of clean in place (CIP) procedures, and post-sterilization contamination.[54,55] With respect to intrinsic heat resistance, *B. sporothermodurans* spores have been found to possess a very high thermal resistance, with *D*-values at 140°C (D_{140}) ranging from 3.4 to 7.9 s.[56] In a survey of UHT milk brands sold in South Africa, Tabit[56] found that 50% of them were positive for *B. sporothermodurans* with counts ranging from 2.25 to 4.11 $\log_{10}$ CFU/mL.

30.4.1.3 Extended shelf life (ESL) milk

ESL or ultra-pasteurized milk is produced by thermal processing using temperature conditions that are between the HTST pasteurization and the UHT sterilization processes. There is no consensus in the dairy sector on the shelf life of ESL milk, although, the product can have a refrigerated life span of 21–45 days.[57] Some manufacturers, however, claim that the product can stay up to 90 days if properly refrigerated.[58] Although ESL milk has a shorter shelf life as compared to UHT milk, it is more superior in terms of sensory properties, having less pronounced cooked or scorched flavors. The precise definition of ESL milk and its manufacturing processes varies in many national jurisdictions. Generally, the product is manufactured using two principal technologies (thermal treatment alone or a combination of heat treatment and membrane filtration). The widely used method is a thermal process in which conditions are more severe than pasteurization but less severe than UHT processing (direct or indirect heating at 123°C–127°C with a holding time of 1–5 s).[57] In the alternative method, nonthermal processes such as microfiltration through ceramic membranes with an average pore diameter of 0.8–1.4 μm and bactofugation are usually combined with a final thermal pasteurization treatment.[57] The later process is reported to achieve a spore reduction of 3–5 $\log_{10}$ CFU/mL.[57]

Given that ESL milk is usually not packaged under aseptic conditions, spoilage challenges are also reported.[45] Spoilage of ESL milk can occur as a result of spore-forming bacteria whose spores are not destroyed by the heating process or by post-pasteurization contamination due to poor hygiene practices or by process biofilms especially around the filler nozzle and other parts of the processing equipment.[45,59] Among the spore-formers, *Bacillus* spp. (in particular psychrotrophic strains) have been identified as a major challenge. The most common and problematic post-process contaminants of ESL milk are the Gram-negative psyschrotrophs, principally Pseudomonads. Studies have also shown the presence of mesophilic organisms in ESL milk stored under refrigeration.[45] These mesophiles include the *Bacillus* spp. and *Paenibacillus* spp. which harbour genes for cold adaptation and growth.[45] Other common spoilage organisms in commercial ESL milk include *Rhodococcus* spp, *Anquinibacter* spp. *Arthrobacter* spp. *Microbacterium* spp. *Enterococcus* spp. *Staphylococcus* spp. *Micrococcus spp.* and coryneforms.[57] A further consideration that can affect ESL milk is the initial bacterial load in the raw milk received for processing. The higher the bacterial count in the raw milk, the higher will be the residual count in the heated milk.[53,58] For good quality ESL milk, the total count in the raw milk should not exceed 10^5 CFU/mL.[57]

30.4.2 Quality of fermented dairy products

Preservation of food by fermentation has been practiced since time immemorial and fermented milk is one of the oldest examples of fermented foods. Until now, fermented dairy products continue to contribute to the socio-economic development and food security of people in both rural and urban communities across the globe. Fermented dairy products are produced using spontaneous fermentation or starter cultures. Spontaneous fermentation uses the natural microflora associated with raw milk. Spontaneous fermentation has occasionally been associated with pathogens, predominantly, because of poor hygiene.[60] Using certain strains of starter cultures (LAB, yeasts, and molds), a lot of commercial fermented dairy products such as cultured buttermilk, sour cream, yogurt, and cheeses are among the most common dairy products produced across the globe. Other, less known products include *kefir*, *koumiss*, acidophilus milk, and new yogurts containing *Bifidobacterium* spp. are also consumed in different parts of the world.[60]

With a rising consumer demand for additive-free and minimally processed foods, innovative food processing technologies are gaining more attention and are increasingly being adopted within the dairy industry.[61] Of interest is the application of new starter cultures (probiotics, *kombucha*), as well as quality improving ingredients like transglutaminase, milk protein fractions, and functional components of plant origin.[61] Other novel processing technologies of interest to dairy fermentations are high-pressure processing, high-pressure homogenization, and ultrasonic processing because of their potential to achieve a specific and/or novel functionality or to improve efficiency.[61] Certainly, novel trends in fermented dairy technology contribute to the creation of various products with high nutritive value. However, new food safety challenges arising from the introduction of novel processing techniques need to be recognized.

30.4.2.1 Microbial quality of cheese

Cheese is a fermented dairy product that can be made using pasteurized or raw milk. Cheese made from raw milk imparts different flavours and texture characteristics to the finished cheese. The product comes in different varieties, ranging from soft, and semi-soft to hard cheeses. In terms of macrostructure, cheese is a stabilized curd of milk solids produced by coagulation of the milk caseins. The coagulum entraps fats, proteins, vitamins, calcium, and phosphorus. Microbial contamination of the cheese is intrinsically linked to the dairy value chain, from production through handling and processing to consumption. The various sources of microbial contamination that have been implicated in cheese processing include raw materials (milk and cheese ingredients), personnel, packaging material, and the processing environment.[62] As ready-to-eat (RTE) foods, cheeses are high-risk products with respect to human listeriosis outbreaks due to their ability to support the growth of *L. monocytogenes* through a long refrigerated shelf life and the lack of further treatment before consumption.[62,63]

Soft and semi-soft cheeses have previously been associated with outbreaks of listeriosis and most of these outbreaks were from cheeses made from unpasteurized milk. However, for cheeses made from pasteurized milk, post-process contamination of the product by *L. monocytogenes* and other enteric pathogens has been reported.[62] Soft cheeses are relatively more vulnerable to post-pasteurization bacterial contamination and subsequent outgrowth than hard cheeses.[64] Bacterial contamination of soft cheeses is attributed to low acidity and high moisture content. Soft cheeses like Camembert have a moisture content $> 70\%$ and a pH range of 5.5–5.8, whereas hard cheeses like Cheddar have a moisture content $< 42\%$ and a pH < 5.45.[65] As a result, psychrotrophic pathogens like *L. monocytogenes* can readily multiply in soft cheeses during refrigerated storage. On the other hand, while several pathogens can be inactivated during storage in hard cheeses, *E. coli*, *L. monocytogenes*, *Brucella* spp., and *Salmonella* can still be detected after long ripening periods.[62]

The occurrence of pathogenic and spoilage microorganisms in fermented dairy products is influenced by a number of factors which include the health status of the dairy herd, hygiene level in the farm environment, milking and storage conditions, geographic location, season, and processing of the milk.[60] Therefore, to reduce the risk associated with fermented dairy products, there is a need for a continuous system of preventive measures beginning with the safety of animal feed, through good farming practices and on-farm controls, to good manufacturing and hygiene practices, consumers' safety awareness, and proper application of FSMS throughout the dairy chain.[60]

30.5 Hygiene in dairy processing

Contamination of the milk typically occurs when the raw milk comes into contact with contaminated teats and milking equipment, feed, water, and soil at the farm level. Due to the susceptibility of raw milk to contamination, good hygiene and sanitary conditions of the dairy environment are crucial and imperative matters as they directly impact the quality and safety of the dairy products. The challenge of ensuring the safety and quality of products necessitates the development of FSMS targeted at producers and personnel at all levels of the value chain.

30.5.1 Sources of contamination in dairy processing

Contaminated water, aerosols, and packaging materials are some of the entry points for microbial contamination of dairy products. The microbes may also form biofilms that can persist in the processing environment. This makes the need for GHP in the dairy chain a critical issue that will aid in the production of a safe and quality product. Therefore constant monitoring and improvement of hygiene and safety control measures to meet the rising demands of both regulatory standards and consumers are crucial in the dairy industry.

30.5.1.1 Bioaerosols

Air often serves as a medium for microdroplets and suspended inanimate and biological agents, including viruses, bacteria, parasites, yeasts, molds, skin particles, dust and water droplets.[66] Microbial aerosols can be free-floating bacterial or fungal spores either suspended in droplets or adhered to dust or skin particles. The quality of air inside dairy processing areas plays a vital role in the final quality of processed milk products. This is because milk products are highly susceptible to extraneous contamination by microbes, and the indoor air of the dairy processing plant is a vehicle for such biological aerosols or contaminants.[67] These bioaerosols may harbor pathogenic organisms or spoilage microbes, that affect both safety and product shelf life.[67]

A critical factor in controlling airborne microbial contamination of processing areas is the management of air quality entering processing plants through the use of clean air systems. The air entering the processing plant is usually filtered to remove suspended particulate matters such as microbes, after which it is cooled and gently pumped into processing areas. Nonetheless, factors such as personnel clothing and footwear, structures, ingredients, and food contact surfaces may initiate the release of bioaerosols into the processing environments causing product contamination if uncontrolled.[67] For example, microorganisms such as *L. monocytogenes* and *E. coli* can be dispersed in the aerosols produced by cleaning operations such as applying hoses and spray lances and condensate on the cooling fins of evaporative chillers.[68] Other factors responsible for the generation of aerosols are industry operations such as milling, weighing powdery substances, spray drying, vacuuming, and handling of dry ingredients.[69]

The concentration of microbes suspended in an aerosol is dependent on several factors which include the size of the particulate materials in suspension, location, season, weather conditions, and the level ground covering in the vicinity of processing plants.[70] Furthermore, the size of the suspended particulate matter influences the dispersion of aerosols. For instance, particulate materials of more than 15–20 μm easily fall close to the point of dispersion, while lighter particles can be airborne for an extended period and travel further to the point of dispersion in slow-moving air.[69] Thus a regular monitoring of the microbial load in air within processing environments is an essential tool in management of airborne contamination.

30.5.1.2 Contaminated water

In the dairy industry, water is used for cleaning equipment during the production cycle, steam generation and cooling systems. The dairy industry consumes vast amounts of water and generates huge volumes of wastewater. Contaminated water used for equipment cleaning can serve as a transmission vehicle for foodborne pathogens in dairy processing. Most dairy processing plants use treated municipal water for their operations. The microbial quality of water supplied from municipality treatment facilities depends on the efficiency of the treatments to remove enteric pathogenic bacteria, viruses, and parasites.[71] Although conventional water treatment facilities are designed to remove pathogens, bacteria growing in pipeline biofilms can be a source of contamination of purified water within the supply system.[71] Additionally, due to corrosion of the piping system (because of pipe aging) or other poor engineering design in municipal reticulation systems, potable water supply systems can be contaminated through leakages. Leakages arising from sewage runoff, overloaded sewage treatment systems, septic systems, and leaking sanitary sewer pipes impose the greatest risk to the contamination of purified potable water.[71] Because of this, most dairy processing plants further treat the municipal water by processes such as filtration. However, depending on the maintenance of the purifying system, it can accumulate sludge, scale, rust, algae, or slime deposits in the water distribution systems and potentially represent a temporary reservoir of undesirable microbial contaminants (some of which can be pathogenic).[72] Therefore a good water supply in dairy production is a principal starting point in controlling microbial contamination dairy products.

30.5.1.3 Personnel hygiene

Poor personnel hygiene is frequently one of the sources of contamination in dairy processing. In most cases, negligence is often cited as the cause of poor personnel hygiene. Critics believe that most foodborne illness outbreaks are caused by food workers' contact with food, particularly those that are ill or chronically infected.[73] As carriers of foodborne pathogens, infected workers can be reservoirs and vehicles for the contamination of dairy products.

Microorganisms can colonize the human external body surfaces such as the skin and hair, and mucosal surfaces such as nose, and mouth, or be excreted from the alimentary tract via faeces.[73] The most implicated microorganisms to increase the risk of cross-contamination from personnel to food products or process environments in the food industry are the microorganisms that reside on the skin. These microorganisms can be transient or resident skin microflora. Gram-negative bacteria such as *Salmonella* spp., *E. coli*, *Pseudomonas* spp., and *Klebsiella* spp. are examples of transient organisms that can be acquired from handling of raw materials, contaminated equipment, contaminated clothing, or touching other body parts or through poor toilet hygiene. In most cases, the transient organisms do not have sufficient residence time to multiply, and are easily removed by hand washing with detergents.[73] Some of the transient organisms like *S. aureus* can reside on localized skin lesions for longer periods, making them temporary residents. Resident skin microorganisms are generally not food pathogens and can live and multiply on the skin and constitute the normal microflora.[73] Although not a common threat in the dairy industry (because they do not multiply in the food), viruses can also be transferred by food handlers to the food via contaminated hands or droplets via coughing or sneezing.

The personnel who often dismantle and reassemble machinery for cleaning procedures and those who maintain the operation of machinery during production are often a source of contamination. Besides such contamination, the movement of personnel from processing areas of low-hygiene to high-hygiene areas increases the risk of product contamination. Arrangements averting the free flow of movement between low- and high-hygiene areas should be installed, such as a hygiene lobby or barriers, where a change of protective clothing should be required if the staff member moves from a low hygiene to a high hygiene area. Other considerations that can be put in place may involve compartmentalizing processing lines and preventing rotation on the job within the same processing day.[74]

30.5.1.4 Biofilms

Biofilms are surface or substratum communities of attached microorganisms surrounded by extracellular polymeric substances, often behaving differently than their planktonic counterparts.[75] Essentially, microbes exist in their natural environments as biofilms and not as single cells as obtainable on culture media in the laboratory. The biofilm structure is dispersed by detaching and reattaching to another part of the dairy processing line during the downstream process termed "sloughing off."[76] They often grow on different processing equipment parts, such as ultrafiltration membranes etc. Biofilms in the dairy processing plant present a daunting challenge as they are about 1000 times more resistant to disinfection than the planktonic cells, making their control and prevention crucial.[59] Their establishment in dairy processing lines creates a contamination reservoir. Some factors that influence the formation of biofilms include the surface roughness of the equipment, conditioning films such as remnants of milk on equipment, the composition of the processed product, electrostatic charge, and hydrophobicity of the surface.[77]

The quality of the raw milk to be processed is a strong determinant in the formation of biofilms. Some contaminating microbes, such as the spores of *Bacillus* spp., survive the pasteurization process and the cleaning in place (CIP) regimes. They later establish in the processing lines, making their control a challenge. The biofilm structure, especially the inner part, is a well-known zone for high sporulation and formation of persister cells. These spores within biofilms have been demonstrated to be capable of forming fresh biofilms post-CIP.[55]

30.5.1.5 Sanitization and cleaning in place (CIP)

The CIP system involves the automated cleaning of hard-to-reach internal parts of processing equipment and pipelines without them being dismantled. The cleaning solutions that are used are often recycled and reused. The automation of these systems allows for a safe and economic optimization of the process.[78] CIP is an integral part of the food safety systems that are put in place to eliminate potential microbial contaminants in the food industry. Most CIP regimes use various biocides, usually in combination at an appropriate flow rate and temperature. However, the effectiveness of the sanitizing strength of the CIP system is hindered by the resistance of some bacteria, due to repeated disinfectant exposure and a consequent build-up of biofilms on equipment surfaces.[78] The standard CIP regime in a dairy processing plant is given as: water rinse, 1% sodium hydroxide at 65°C for 10 min, water rinse, 1.0% nitric acid at 65°C for 10 min, water rinse. There are other alternatives, such as caustic and acid blends that have effectively removed attached bacteria.[79]

Bacteria become attached when they survive a bactofugation or microfiltration process. The bactofugation and microfiltration processes take place before the pasteurization of milk, which significantly reduces the concentration of the contaminating microbes. Nonetheless, some microbes, especially the thermophilic spore-formers, survive the process or cause post-processing contamination, thus reducing the shelf life of the products.[80] Since the traditional CIP methods may fail to remove vegetative cells, biofilms and spores of these contaminants, this challenge has generated the demand for innovative techniques in the dairy industry. An investigation by Pretorius and Buys[55] revealed that simulated CIP treatment is not very effective when applied against *B. cereus* spores isolated from the filler nozzles, nor did it prevent subsequent germination. High-pressure spray and mechanical scrubbing are highly effective in removing biofilms that develop on exposed surfaces, but not for removing biofilms in crevices within the dairy factory.

The perceived reasons for the resistance of biofilms to biocides used in CIP are multifactorial. These may include reduced penetration of the biocide within the biofilm structure due to the complexity and the production of extra polymeric substances, reduced metabolism, stress response, and changes in quorum sensing among the cells within the biofilm.[81] It is therefore important to design the most effective CIP regime for a dairy processing plant.

Another problem associated with the CIP chemicals used in the dairy industry is the transfer of chemical residues from sanitized surfaces to the milk. This has necessitated the need for safe, efficient, and environmentally compatible chemicals for the dairy industry, such as food-grade and edible surfactants. Monitoring fouling during the CIP process is vital in controlling contamination by spoilage and pathogenic microbes in the dairy processing plant.

30.5.1.6 Packaging material

Packaging material in the dairy industry is of critical importance because of its impact on the quality, safety, cost, and marketing of the commodities to consumers. Although interest has shifted towards novel applications such as smart or intelligent packaging, modified atmosphere packaging, active packaging, and sustainability, studies have shown that packaging material can be a source of contamination for various dairy products.[82]

Food packaging material has the potential to affect the quality of food as there are possible interactions between the food and the packaging material, which include permeability of gases and water vapor into or out of the package, and migration of package components into the food. This interaction has a direct bearing on the quality and shelf life of products. The dairy industry is no different; here, packaging materials can play an important role in the microbiological quality of milk and milk products. This can occur by directly influencing the microbial load due to the presence of microbes on their surfaces or indirectly due to the permeable character of the packaging material, thereby allowing the growth of microbes that may be present.[83] Proper selection of packaging material in the dairy industry is therefore essential to provide a barrier that retains the quality of the product and also allows for a reasonable shelf life, among other factors.[83]

30.6 Risk-based preventative approach to dairy food safety

The dairy industry has evolved into one of the largest and most modernized food sectors characterized by large volumes of milk and a wide variety of dairy products in the food market. Partly, the dynamics of the dairy industry are influenced by an increase in the population, changes in food regulations, and consumer demands for safe and healthy milk product selection that is supplemented with a great variety and availability in the market. Although consumer trends are global, the nature and extent of their influence are shaped by geography, cultural norms, government policy, and socio-economic status. In most developing countries, particularly in Africa, the dairy industry is predominated by the informal sector, which is characterized by unregistered milk suppliers and processors who do not apply FSMS.[48]

As the industry is expanding and operating in a globalized environment, new challenges to food safety are continuing to emerge. Globalization of the food industry exposes populations worldwide to entirely new and unique food hazards. Regrettably, the dairy industry remains one of the most implicated food sectors associated with foodborne outbreaks globally. Efforts have been made by the dairy industry to adopt different strategies for managing food safety. However, in most developing countries, the policies are more reactive rather than proactive. A reactive system is hazard-based, which uses the premise that the mere presence of a potentially harmful agent at a detectable level in food (testing food to determine safety) is justification for legislation and/or risk management action.[84] However, it is also well known that the presence of a hazard does not necessarily mean that the product is harmful to human health.

In order to manage food safety amid an expanding dairy industry, any approach to food safety reform must be proactive and risk-based.[85] A risk-based food safety management methodology allows the consideration of exposure in assessing whether there may be any unacceptable risks to human health. When considering a preventive approach to food safety management, all aspects of a food safety system, from farm-to-fork (raw material, distribution, food processing, retail, and consumer behavior), are taken into account, ensuring that the combined efforts of all actors along the food chain provide safe and suitable dairy products rather than separating responsibility for any particular component of the chain. A systematic evaluation of hazards and associated risks at each point in the supply chain is required. Additionally, a risk-based approach tries to answer the following questions: where is the risk highest?, which food safety interventions should be prioritized?, and which risk mitigation measure is the most effective?. Undoubtedly, using a risk-based system, the FSMS in the dairy industry would improve through applying more effort towards managing the greatest risks, while fully understanding the factors that contribute to the risk, and allocating resources appropriately to prevent the risks and their root causes, and truly evaluating the effects of those efforts.[86,87] Apart from benefiting the dairy industry alone, a risk-based approach to food safety is also used by regulatory bodies that monitor food safety. Risk-based resource allocation focuses government efforts on the greatest risks and the greatest opportunities to reduce the risk, wherever they may arise. To promote a risk-based approach to food safety in the dairy industry, concepts such as qualitative and quantitative risk assessments, including HACCP-based FSMS are central.

30.6.1 Microbiological risk assessment and role in dairy food safety

The objective of ensuring safe food for the consumer has been a major preoccupation of governments and international organizations. Globalization of the dairy industry has posed challenges in the management of food safety. Food safety hazards such as microorganisms may enter at various stages along a dairy supply chain. Several interventions have been implemented to control microbial hazard presence in dairy products. These include good manufacturing practices (GMP) and HACCP principles, which are applied at specific stages of the production process, acting as preventive measures, and not the entire food production chain. Foodborne outbreaks from milk and dairy products are still reported regardless of FSMS programmes in place. Food safety management in the dairy industry should be risk-based and focus on the most relevant food safety hazards. The most prominent and central approach to risk-based preventative approaches to dairy food safety is food safety risk assessment. Risk assessment offers a means of improving and managing food safety associated with pathogenic microorganisms as well as chemical hazards. Microbial risk assessment is a valuable tool used to organize and analyze scientific information to estimate the probability and severity of any adverse risk posed by a pathogen in a particular dairy commodity. Risk assessment can be defined as the measurement of risk and identification of factors that influences it. It is an independent scientific process that can be conducted qualitatively (through descriptive measures as high, medium or low probability of contamination) or quantitatively (through numerical measures such as pathogen prevalence and modeling pathogen responses in foods). The process includes four stages: (1) hazard identification, (2) exposure assessment, (3) hazard characterization, and (4) risk characterization as outlined by the Codex Alimentarius Commission.[89] Risk assessment can be used to; review the safety of new products under development; evaluate the most effective control measures to address a particular food safety hazard; and establish food safety priorities. Apart from benefiting the dairy industry and protecting the consumer from food safety hazards, outputs and decisions from risk assessments can be used to facilitate international trade.

Risk assessment studies have been carried out to quantify the risk posed by pathogenic organisms in milk at national and regional levels by different researchers across the globe.[89] To date, quantitative microbial risk assessment (QMRA) for the major milk-borne pathogens has been conducted. EFSA[90] and Giacometti et al.[91–93] conducted risk assessments for *L. monocytogenes*, *Campylobacter jejuni*, STEC O157, and *Salmonella* spp. in raw drinking milk in Europe. The risk of listeriosis associated with the consumption of milk was also evaluated in the United States.[94] However, few risk assessment studies on pathogen-contaminated foods have been carried out in developing countries such as those in Africa. Among the few studies, Grace et al.[95] and Makita et al.[96] estimated the risk of hemolytic uremic syndrome (HUS) and brucellosis incidence respectively in informally marketed milk in Africa. Ntuli et al.[97] estimated the risk of HUS associated with the consumption of bulk milk sold directly from producer to consumer in South Africa. Most risk assessment studies carried out for pathogen-contaminated raw or pasteurized milk identified that temperature and storage time are the main factors influencing the product safety risk. For preventative measures, especially in countries where the sale of raw milk is permitted (sold via vending machines or outlets), the risk assessors recommended the boiling of milk before consumption.[98] The major shortcoming outlined by researchers who conducted QMRA in developing countries was applying risk-based methods to diverse, nonlinear, shifting, and data-scarce systems in which formal and informal food supply systems coexist and overlap. The major drawback is that risk assessments are expensive and time-consuming and because of the complexity of value chains, the approach has not been widely adopted in developing countries where the informal sector predominates and resources are limited.

A review by Verraes et al.[64] indicated that microbiological hazards and risks associated with dairy products manufactured from raw milk vary with the type of the product. They reported that the main microbiological hazards associated with raw milk soft and fresh cheeses were *L. monocytogenes*, STEC, *S. aureus*, *Salmonella*, and *Campylobacter* spp., whereas the microbiological hazards associated with raw milk butter and cream included *L. monocytogenes*, STEC, and *S. aureus*. They also highlighted that raw milk dairy products may also be contaminated with *Brucella* spp., *M. bovis*, and the tick-borne encephalitis virus. To limit the exposure to pathogens due to consumption of dairy products made from raw milk, several control measures can be applied from farm to fork and these control measures can vary depending on the point/source of contamination across the dairy value chain.[64] Ramos et al.[98] reviewed risk assessment studies conducted from 2015 to 2018 on cheese produced from raw or pasteurized milk. The target organisms in the risk assessments were STEC, *L. monocytogenes*, *S. aureus*, and *Clostridium* spp. In general, the studies reviewed by Ramos et al.[98] noted that the risk of infection was influenced by the initial concentration of the pathogen in the raw material, particularly for raw milk cheeses. The studies also revealed that the storage condition of cheese also influences the risk of consuming contaminated cheeses.[98]

Microbial risk assessment has also been applied as a microbial source tracking tool in the dairy industry. Vissers et al.[99] applied QMRA to the microbial contamination of farm tank milk related to the amount of dirt transmitted to milk via the exterior of teats using spores of mesophilic aerobic bacteria as a marker for transmitted dirt. The authors found that silage was the main source of butyric acid bacteria and *Clostridium spp.* spores in milk.

30.6.2 HACCP –based food safety systems

The establishment of a HACCP system in the dairy industry is the first step towards managing the safety of milk and dairy products. HACCP and its evolution to preventive controls have been hailed as promoting a risk-based approach to food safety. Although not common, the application of HACCP programmes on dairy farms has improved the quality and safety of milk intended for processing for those dairy farms that have adopted the system.[100] On-farm HACCP does not only cover milk safety but has components that improve the welfare of dairy animals and environmental protection as demanded by consumers and retailers. On-farm HACCP is linked to both operational management and food chain quality assurance. Given that dairy animals are one of the main reservoirs of pathogenic microorganisms, the presence of pathogens in milk is because of direct contact with the contamination sources which include the infected udder and fecal contamination. On-farm HACCP systems apply cost-effective, accurate, and reproducible practices to monitor certain points which are contamination routes. However, this system is less effective for small-holder dairy farmers due to the high costs associated with testing methodologies. Other approaches to managing animal health problems and addressing pathogens have been developed specifically for the dairy industry. A joint guidance on Good Dairy Farming Practices (GDFP) was prepared and published by the International Dairy Federation (IDF) and the Food and Agriculture Organization (FAO) in an effort to improve the safety of milk at dairy farms.[100] Good agricultural practices are still applied at dairy farms. However, for the practices to be effective, they should focus on the areas such as animal health, milking hygiene, animal feeding and water safety, animal welfare, and the environment.[100]

In dairy processing, the implementation of HACCP has been primarily reported as an effective approach to improve the safety of dairy products. For effective management of safety in the dairy industry at the processing level, GHP, HACCP-based systems, and other risk management metrics should be applied. An effective HACCP-based programme requires the appropriate expertise.

Dairy manufacturers must understand and be able to document their production practices and demonstrate their understanding of the various biological and other classes of hazards that could be introduced and controlled at each step. Dairy products are susceptible to microbial hazards; therefore temperature treatment is very important for rendering the end product safe. In the dairy industry, temperature–time combinations during processing are considered a critical control point.

Notwithstanding the effectiveness of HACCP-based programmes in dairy safety, the system has not received widespread adoption except in countries where it is mandatory.[47,48] In some countries where such systems are not mandatory, industries implement the HACCP-based FSMS as a response to consumer demand. The process requires a critical multidisciplinary review of existing management systems, the establishment of limits via the identification of critical control points, the use of routine surveillance procedures, effective record keeping, and documentation of standard processes. Because of these confines, several dairy farmers and processors in the developing world have favored alternative approaches such as hurdle technology.[46]

30.7 Gaps and future directions

The dairy industry is diverse and complex. Factors affecting microbiological quality and safety of milk and milk products involve everything from production (farming), processing, distribution, trade (including multinational companies), and strict regulation. Like any other food industry, the dairy sector is battling to adjust and manage the rising global milk consumption as a result of population growth and changing socio-economic dynamics which demand diverse, convenient, safe, and high-quality milk and milk products. On the other hand, food regulations are evolving to meet quality and safety requirements. In view of this, the industry has invested in novel production and processing technologies in order to meet some of the consumer demands as well as changing food regulations. As much as the adoption of novel technologies is showing improvement in quality and the convenience and availability of dairy products, there are safety concerns that still need to be taken into consideration. More research needs to be conducted that provides information concerning source tracking of spoilage and pathogenic organisms at farms and in dairy processing environments. This also includes improvements in dairy farm management and cleaning regimes in processing environments. New technologies such as whole-genome sequencing can assist the dairy industry in surveillance and microbiological source tracking of contaminants.

Many regulatory authorities in developing countries are adopting and implementing a risk-based preventative approach to improve food safety. However, in yet other developing countries where the food supply chain is an interconnection between the formal and informal sector and is predominated by the informal sector, this approach is still in its infancy. Research is still required in order to understand the complexities of the informal sector in order to apply practical risk-based food safety measures that are appropriate for this sector. This includes source tracking of microbial contamination in milk which is produced and supplied in the informal sector. More data are required related to the informal dairy sector so that a HACCP system can be developed that is appropriate in order to improve the safety of milk and milk products in this vast and important sector.

References

1. IDF. The global impact of dairy. <https://fil-idf.org/dairys-global-impact/>; 2021.
2. Haug A, Høstmark AT, Harstad OM. Bovine milk in human nutrition – a review. *Lipids Health Dis.* 2007;6:1–16.

3. FAO. The global dairy sector: facts 2019. <http://www.dairydeclaration.org/Portals/153/Content/Documents/DDOR%20Global%20Dairy%20Facts%202019.pdf>; 2019.
4. Grace D, Wu F, Havelaar AH. MILK Symposium review: foodborne diseases from milk and milk products in developing countries—review of causes and health and economic implications. *J Dairy Sci*. 2020;103:9715–9729.
5. Idland L, Granquist EG, Aspholm M, Lindbäck T. The prevalence of *Campylobacter* spp., *Listeria monocytogenes* and Shiga toxin-producing *Escherichia coli* in Norwegian dairy cattle farms; a comparison between free stall and tie stall housing systems. *J Appl Microbiol*. 2022;132:3952–3972.
6. Collins ÁB, Floyd S, Gordon SV, More SJ. Prevalence of *Mycobacterium bovis* in milk on dairy cattle farms: an international systematic literature review and meta-analysis. *Tuberculosis*. 2022;132:102166.
7. Rabaza A, Fraga M, Corbellini LG, Turner KME, Riet-Correa F, Eisler MC. Molecular prevalence of *Coxiella burnetii* in bulk-tank milk from bovine dairy herds: systematic review and meta-analysis. *One Health*. 2021;12:100208.
8. Yu J, Mo L, Pan L, et al. Bacterial microbiota and metabolic character of traditional sour cream and butter in Buryatia, Russia. *Front Microbiol*. 2018;9:2496.
9. Martin NH, Boor KJ, Wiedmann M. Symposium review: effect of post-pasteurization contamination on fluid milk quality. *J Dairy Sci*. 2018;101:861–870.
10. Ivy RA, Ranieri ML, Martin NH, et al. Identification and characterization of psychrotolerant sporeformers associated with fluid milk production and processing. *Appl Environ Microbiol*. 2012;78:1853–1864.
11. Costard S, Espejo L, Groenendaal H, Zagmutt FJ. Outbreak-related disease burden associated with consumption of unpasteurized cow's milk and cheese, United States, 2009–2014. *Emerg Infect Dis*. 2017;23:957.
12. Hanson H, Whitfield Y, Lee C, et al. Listeria monocytogenes associated with pasteurized chocolate milk, Ontario, Canada. *Emerg Infect Dis*. 2019;25:581.
13. De Oliveira CAF, Da Cruz AG, Tavolaro P, Corassin CH. *Food safety: good manufacturing practices (GMP), sanitation standard operating procedures (SSOP), hazard analysis and critical control point (HACCP). Antimicrobial Food Packaging*. Elsevier; 2016.
14. Rietberg K, Lloyd J, Melius B, et al. Outbreak of *Listeria monocytogenes* infections linked to a pasteurized ice cream product served to hospitalized patients. *Epidemiol Infect*. 2016;144:2728–2731.
15. Kang'ethe EK, Grace D, Roesel K, Mutua F. *Food Safety Landscape Analysis: The Dairy Value Chain in Kenya. Nairobi, Kenya*: International Livestock Research Institute (ILRI); 2020.
16. Phiri BSJ, Sakumona M, Hang'ombe BM, Fetsch A, Schaarschmidt S. The traditional dairy value chain in Zambia and potential risk factors to microbiological food safety. *Food Control*. 2021;124:107885.
17. Burke N, Zacharski KA, Southern M, Hogan P, Ryan MP, Adley CC. *The dairy industry: process, monitoring, standards, and quality. Descriptive Food Science*. IntechOpen; 2018:162.
18. Murphy SC, Martin NH, Barbano DM, Wiedmann M. Influence of raw milk quality on processed dairy products: how do raw milk quality test results relate to product quality and yield? *J Dairy Sci*. 2016;99:10128–10149.
19. Artursson K, Schelin J, Lambertz ST, Hansson I, Engvall EO. Foodborne pathogens in unpasteurized milk in Sweden. *Int J Food Microbiol*. 2018;284:120–127.
20. Elhaig MM, Selim A. Molecular and bacteriological investigation of subclinical mastitis caused by *Staphylococcus aureus* and *Streptococcus agalactiae* in domestic bovids from Ismailia, Egypt. *Trop Anim Health Prod*. 2015;47:271–276.
21. Van Engelen E, Dijkstra T, Meertens NM, Van Werven T. Bacterial flora associated with udder cleft dermatitis in Dutch dairy cows. *J Dairy Sci*. 2021;104:728–735.
22. Béné C, Prager SD, Achicanoy HAE, et al. Understanding food systems drivers: a critical review of the literature. *Glob Food Security*. 2019;23:149–159.
23. De La Rua-Domenech R. Human *Mycobacterium bovis* infection in the United Kingdom: incidence, risks, control measures and review of the zoonotic aspects of bovine tuberculosis. *Tuberculosis*. 2006;86:77–109.
24. Gerrard ZE, Swift BMC, Botsaris G, et al. Survival of *Mycobacterium avium* subspecies paratuberculosis in retail pasteurised milk. *Food Microbiol*. 2018;74:57–63.
25. Robinson E, Travanut M, Fabre L, et al. Outbreak of *Salmonella* Newport associated with internationally distributed raw goats' milk cheese, France, 2018. *Epidemiol Infect*. 2020;148:e180.
26. Jourdan-Da Silva N, Fabre L, Robinson E, et al. Ongoing nationwide outbreak of *Salmonella* Agona associated with internationally distributed infant milk products, France, December 2017. *Eurosurveillance*. 2018;23:17-00852.
27. Ung A, Baidjoe AY, Van Cauteren D, et al. Disentangling a complex nationwide *Salmonella* Dublin outbreak associated with raw-milk cheese consumption, France, 2015 to 2016. *Eurosurveillance*. 2019;24:1700703.
28. Jones G, Lefèvre S, Donguy M-P, et al. Outbreak of Shiga toxin-producing *Escherichia coli* (STEC) O26 paediatric haemolytic uraemic syndrome (HUS) cases associated with the consumption of soft raw cow's milk cheeses, France, March to May 2019. *Eurosurveillance*. 2019;24:1900305.
29. Mccollum JT, Williams NJ, Beam SW, et al. Multistate outbreak of *Escherichia coli* O157: H7 infections associated with in-store sampling of an aged raw-milk Gouda cheese, 2010. *J Food Prot*. 2012;75:1759–1765.
30. Currie A, Galanis E, Chacon PA, et al. Outbreak of *Escherichia coli* O157: H7 infections linked to aged raw milk Gouda cheese, Canada, 2013. *J Food Prot*. 2017;81:325–331.
31. Sorgentone S, Busani L, Calistri P, et al. A large food-borne outbreak of campylobacteriosis in kindergartens and primary schools in Pescara, Italy, May–June 2018. *J Med Microbiol*. 2021;70:001262.
32. Kenyon J, Inns T, Aird H, et al. Campylobacter outbreak associated with raw drinking milk, North West England, 2016. *Epidemiol Infect*. 2020;148.
33. Longenberger AH, Palumbo AJ, Chu AK, Moll ME, Weltman A, Ostroff SM. *Campylobacter jejuni* infections associated with unpasteurized milk—multiple states, 2012. *Clin Infect Dis*. 2013;57:263–266.
34. Fretz R, Sagel U, Ruppitsch W, et al. Listeriosis outbreak caused by acid curd cheese 'Quargel', Austria and Germany 2009. *Eurosurveillance*. 2010;15:19477.
35. Gaulin C, Levac E, Ramsay D, et al. *Escherichia coli* O157: H7 outbreak linked to raw milk cheese in Quebec, Canada: use of exact probability calculation and case-case study approaches to foodborne outbreak investigation. *J Food Prot*. 2012;75:812–818.

36. Jackson KA, Biggerstaff M, Tobin-D'angelo M, et al. Multistate outbreak of *Listeria monocytogenes* associated with Mexican-style cheese made from pasteurized milk among pregnant, Hispanic women. *J Food Prot.* 2011;74:949–953.
37. Johler S, Weder D, Bridy C, et al. Outbreak of staphylococcal food poisoning among children and staff at a Swiss boarding school due to soft cheese made from raw milk. *J Dairy Sci.* 2015;98:2944–2948.
38. Fetsch A, Contzen M, Hartelt K, et al. *Staphylococcus aureus* food-poisoning outbreak associated with the consumption of ice-cream. *Int J Food Microbiol.* 2014;187:1–6.
39. Asao T, Kumeda Y, Kawai T, et al. An extensive outbreak of staphylococcal food poisoning due to low-fat milk in Japan: estimation of enterotoxin A in the incriminated milk and powdered skim milk. *Epidemiol Infect.* 2003;130:33.
40. Schmid D, Fretz R, Winter P, et al. Outbreak of staphylococcal food intoxication after consumption of pasteurized milk products, June 2007, Austria. *Wien Klinische Wochenschr.* 2009;121:125–131.
41. Castro H, Jaakkonen A, Hakkinen M, Korkeala H, Lindström M. Occurrence, persistence, and contamination routes of *Listeria monocytogenes* genotypes on three Finnish dairy cattle farms: a longitudinal study. *Appl Environ Microbiol.* 2018;84:e02000-17.
42. Bekuma A, Galmessa U. Review on hygienic milk products practice and occurrence of mastitis in cow's milk. *Agric Res Technol.* 2018;18:1–11.
43. Fusco V, Chieffi D, Fanelli F, et al. Microbial quality and safety of milk and milk products in the 21st century. *Compr Rev Food Sci Food Saf.* 2020;19:2013–2049.
44. Vidal A, Saran Netto A, Vaz ACN, et al. *Pseudomonas* spp.: contamination sources in bulk tanks of dairy farms. *Pesqui Vet Bras.* 2017;37:941–948.
45. Mugadza DT, Buys EM. Diversity of *Bacillus cereus* strains in extended shelf life. *Int Dairy J.* 2017;73:144–150.
46. Ruegg PL. Practical food safety interventions for dairy production. *J Dairy Sci.* 2003;86:E1–E9.
47. Opiyo BA, Wangoh J, Njage PMK. Microbiological performance of dairy processing plants is influenced by scale of production and the implemented food safety management system: a case study. *J Food Prot.* 2013;76:975–983.
48. Njage PMK, Opiyo B, Wangoh J, Wambui J. Scale of production and implementation of food safety programs influence the performance of current food safety management systems: case of dairy processors. *Food Control.* 2018;85:85–97.
49. Soni A, Samuelsson LM, Loveday SM, Gupta TB. Applications of novel processing technologies to enhance the safety and bioactivity of milk. *Compr Rev Food Sci Food Saf.* 2021;20:4652–4677.
50. Sarkar S. Microbiological considerations: pasteurized milk. *Int J Dairy Sci.* 2015;10:206–218.
51. Clough HE, Clancy D, French NP. Quantifying exposure to verocytotoxigenic *Escherichia coli* O157 in milk sold as pasteurized: a model-based approach. *Int J Food Microbiol.* 2009;131:95–105.
52. Stratakos AC, Inguglia ES, Linton M, et al. Effect of high pressure processing on the safety, shelf life and quality of raw milk. *Innov Food Sci Emerg Technol.* 2019;52:325–333.
53. Deeth H. *Improving UHT processing and UHT milk products. Improving the Safety and Quality of Milk.* Elsevier; 2010.
54. Alonso VPP, De Oliveira Morais J, Kabuki DY. Incidence of *Bacillus cereus*, *Bacillus sporothermodurans* and *Geobacillus stearothermophilus* in ultra-high temperature milk and biofilm formation capacity of isolates. *Int J Food Microbiol.* 2021;354:109318.
55. Pretorius C, Buys EM. Extended shelf life milk processing: effect of simulated cleaning in place on the germination and attachment of *Bacillus cereus* spores. *Int J Dairy Technol.* 2021;74:75–83.
56. Tabit FT. Prevalence and growth characteristics of *Bacillus sporothermodurans* in UHT milk. *Br Food J.* 2018;120:2250–2260.
57. Deeth H. Optimum thermal processing for extended shelf-life (ESL) milk. *Foods.* 2017;6:102.
58. Lorenzen PC, Clawin-Rädecker I, Einhoff K, et al. A survey of the quality of extended shelf life (ESL) milk in relation to HTST and UHT milk. *Int J Dairy Technol.* 2011;64:166–178.
59. Elegbeleye JA, Buys EM. Potential spoilage of extended shelf-life (ESL) milk by *Bacillus subtilis* and *Bacillus velezensis*. *LWT.* 2022;153:112487.
60. Owusu-Kwarteng J, Akabanda F, Agyei D, Jespersen L. Microbial safety of milk production and fermented dairy products in Africa. *Microorganisms.* 2020;8:752.
61. Carić MD, Milanović SD, Iličić MD. Novel trends in fermented dairy technology. *Zb Matice Srpske Prir Nauk.* 2019;136:9–21.
62. Pal M, Mulu S, Tekle M, Pintoo SV, Prajapati J. Bacterial contamination of dairy products. *Beverage Food World.* 2016;43:40–43.
63. Rosshaug PS, Detmer A, Ingmer H, Larsen MH. Modeling the growth of *Listeria monocytogenes* in soft blue-white cheese. *Appl Environ Microbiol.* 2012;78:8508–8514.
64. Verraes C, Vlaemynck G, Van Weyenberg S, et al. A review of the microbiological hazards of dairy products made from raw milk. *Int Dairy J.* 2015;50:32–44.
65. Mcintyre L, Wilcott L, Naus M. Listeriosis outbreaks in British Columbia, Canada, caused by soft ripened cheese contaminated from environmental sources. *BioMed Res Int.* 2015;2015:131623.
66. Oliveira M, Tiwari BK, Duffy G. Emerging technologies for aerial decontamination of food storage environments to eliminate microbial cross-contamination. *Foods.* 2020;9:1779.
67. Masotti F, Cattaneo S, Stuknytė M, De Noni I. Airborne contamination in the food industry: an update on monitoring and disinfection techniques of air. *Trends Food Sci Technol.* 2019;90:147–156.
68. Dobeic M, Kenda E, Mičunovič J, Zdovc I. Airborne *Listeria* spp. in the red meat processing industry. *Czech J Food Sci.* 2011;29:441–447.
69. Burfoot D. *Aerosols as a contamination risk. Handbook of Hygiene Control in the Food Industry.* Elsevier; 2016.
70. Zara G, Budroni M, Mannazzu I, Fancello F, Zara S. Yeast biofilm in food realms: occurrence and control. *World J Microbiol Biotechnol.* 2020;36:1–10.
71. Lechevallier MW, Au K-K. *Water Treatment and Pathogen Control.* Iwa Publishing; 2004.
72. Nriagu J, Xi C, Siddique A, Vincent A, Shomar B. Influence of household water filters on bacteria growth and trace metals in tap water of Doha, Qatar. *Sci Rep.* 2018;8:1–16.
73. Margas E, Holah JT. *Personal hygiene in the food industry. Hygiene in Food Processing.* Elsevier; 2014.
74. Aalto-Araneda M, Lundén J, Markkula A, Hakola S, Korkeala H. Processing plant and machinery sanitation and hygiene practices associate with *Listeria monocytogenes* occurrence in ready-to-eat fish products. *Food Microbiol.* 2019;82:455–464.

75. Elegbeleye JA, Buys EM. Molecular characterization and biofilm formation potential of *Bacillus subtilis* and *Bacillus velezensis* in extended shelf-life milk processing line. *J Dairy Sci.* 2020;103:4991–5002.
76. Kim S-K, Lee J-H. Biofilm dispersion in *Pseudomonas aeruginosa. J Microbiol.* 2016;54:71–85.
77. Teh KH, Flint S, Bremer P. *Raw milk quality influenced by biofilms and the effect of biofilm growth on dairy product quality. Biofilms in the Dairy Industry.* John Wiley & Sons; 2015:65–98.
78. Tang X, Flint SH, Bennett RJ, Brooks JD. The efficacy of different cleaners and sanitisers in cleaning biofilms on UF membranes used in the dairy industry. *J Membr Sci.* 2010;352:71–75.
79. Bremer PJ, Fillery S, Mcquillan AJ. Laboratory scale Clean-In-Place (CIP) studies on the effectiveness of different caustic and acid wash steps on the removal of dairy biofilms. *Int J Food Microbiol.* 2006;106:254–262.
80. Mugadza DT, Buys E. *Bacillus* and *Paenibacillus* species associated with extended shelf life milk during processing and storage. *Int J Dairy Technol.* 2018;71:301–308.
81. Otter JA, Vickery K, Walker JTD, et al. Surface-attached cells, biofilms and biocide susceptibility: implications for hospital cleaning and disinfection. *J Hosp Infect.* 2015;89:16–27.
82. Temelli S, Anar Ş, Sen C, Akyuva P. Determination of microbiological contamination sources during Turkish white cheese production. *Food Control.* 2006;17:856–861.
83. Simon M, Hansen AP. Effect of various dairy packaging materials on the shelf life and flavor of pasteurized milk. *J Dairy Sci.* 2001;84:767–773.
84. Barlow SM, Boobis AR, Bridges J, et al. The role of hazard-and risk-based approaches in ensuring food safety. *Trends Food Sci Technol.* 2015;46:176–188.
85. Koutsoumanis KP, Aspridou Z. Moving towards a risk-based food safety management. *Curr Opin Food Sci.* 2016;12:36–41.
86. Farrell D, Gebre B, Hudspeth C, Sellgren A. *Risk-Based Resource Allocation.* McKinsey Center for Government; 2013.
87. Wallace RB, Oria M, National Research C. *Adopting a risk-based decision-making approach to food safety. Enhancing Food Safety: The Role of the Food and Drug Administration.* National Academies Press (US); 2010.
88. Codex Alimentarius Commission. Principles and guidelines for the conduct of microbiological risk assessment. 1999. CAC/GL, 30.
89. Ntuli V. *Shigatoxin Producing Escherichia coli O157 and Non-O157 Serotypes in Producer-Distributor Bulk Milk* [Ph.D. thesis]. Pretoria, South Africa: University of Pretoria; 2017.
90. EFSA. Scientific opinion on the public health risks related to the consumption of raw drinking milk. *EFSA J.* 2015;13:3940.
91. Giacometti F, Bonilauri P, Albonetti S, et al. Quantitative risk assessment of human salmonellosis and listeriosis related to the consumption of raw milk in Italy. *J Food Prot.* 2015;78:13–21.
92. Giacometti F, Serraino A, Bonilauri P, et al. Quantitative risk assessment of verocytotoxin-producing *Escherichia coli* O157 and *Campylobacter jejuni* related to consumption of raw milk in a province in Northern Italy. *J Food Prot.* 2012;75:2031–2038.
93. Giacometti F, Bonilauri P, Piva S, et al. Paediatric HUS cases related to the consumption of raw milk sold by vending machines in Italy: quantitative risk assessment based on *Escherichia coli* O157 official controls over 7 years. *Zoonoses Public Health.* 2017;64:505–516.
94. Latorre AA, Pradhan AK, Van Kessel JAS, et al. Quantitative risk assessment of listeriosis due to consumption of raw milk. *J Food Prot.* 2011;74:1268–1281.
95. Grace D, Omore A, Randolph T, Kang'ethe E, Nasinyama GW, Mohammed HO. Risk assessment for *Escherichia coli* O157: H7 in marketed unpasteurized milk in selected East African countries. *J Food Prot.* 2008;71:257–263.
96. Makita K, Fèvre EM, Waiswa C, Eisler MC, Welburn SC. How human brucellosis incidence in urban Kampala can be reduced most efficiently? A stochastic risk assessment of informally-marketed milk. *PLoS One.* 2010;5:e14188.
97. Ntuli V, Njage PMK, Bonilauri P, Serraino A, Buys EM. Quantitative risk assessment of hemolytic uremic syndrome associated with consumption of bulk milk sold directly from producer to consumer in South Africa. *J Food Prot.* 2018;81:472–481.
98. Ramos GLPA, Nascimento JS, Margalho LP, et al. Quantitative microbiological risk assessment in dairy products: concepts and applications. *Trends Food Sci Technol.* 2021;111:610–616.
99. Vissers MMM, Driehuis F, Te Giffel MC, De Jong P, Lankveld JMG. Quantification of the transmission of microorganisms to milk via dirt attached to the exterior of teats. *J Dairy Sci.* 2007;90:3579–3582.
100. Papademas P, Bintsis T. Food safety management systems (FSMS) in the dairy industry: a review. *Int J Dairy Technol.* 2010;63:489–503.

Chapter 31

Reduction of risks associated with processed meats

Lynn M. McMullen
Department of Agricultural, Food and Nutritional Science, University of Alberta, Edmonton, AB Canada

Abstract

Meat processors have been challenged to reduce the microbiological risks associated with their products while meeting consumer demands for high quality, minimally processed, convenient products with "clean labels." This has led to the search for new or alternative sources of antimicrobial compounds and the development of nonthermal technologies that could reduce the microbiological risks for consumers while maintaining product quality. This chapter reviews the sources of contamination of processed meats, the application of novel or alternative sources of antimicrobial compounds and nonthermal processes, and their ability to reduce risks associated with processed meats. Some challenges from the use of either novel antimicrobials or processing technologies have been documented and warrant further investigation.

Keywords: Processed meat safety; novel antimicrobials; clean label antimicrobials; plant extracts; bacteriocins; bacteriophage; nonthermal processing; atmospheric cold plasma; ultraviolet-C radiation

Chapter points

1. The safety of processed meats is complex and depends on intrinsic and extrinsic factors to reduce risks for consumers. Contamination of meat and ingredients with pathogens can occur at multiple stages during processing.
2. Consumer demands for minimally processed products and "clean labels" with limited naming of synthetic additives have led the meat processing industry and researchers to look for alternative technologies to minimize potential food safety risks.
3. The use of antimicrobials is one strategy to reduce microbial risks and help the industry meet consumer demands. Novel antimicrobials, new sources of established antimicrobials, and mixtures of antimicrobials have been one approach to reducing risks. To overcome interactions with product and processing parameters, approaches using nanotechnology and other novel delivery systems have been researched.
4. The use of nonthermal technologies has gained attention as an approach to reducing risks without impacting the quality parameters of processed meats. High-pressure processing has been successfully commercialized to reduce risks but it is not without issues with injured cells that may grow during extended storage. Atmospheric cold plasma and ultraviolet-C radiation are two technologies that are gaining attention by the research community for application to processed meats but more research is needed before they can be applied commercially.
5. Microbial risks associated with processed meats can be best mitigated through a multihurdle approach as the use of a single approach is limited in its ability to reduce or eliminate hazards.
6. For commercial application, research on novel technologies needs to include validation that replicates industrial practice as closely as possible and needs to demonstrate efficacy without impacting quality parameters.

31.1 Introduction

The World Health Organization defines processed meats as "meat that has been transformed through salting, curing, fermentation, smoking, or other processes to enhance flavor or improve preservation."[1] This includes a wide variety of products that can include fully cooked products, partially processed products that require thermal processing by consumers, or fermented products that receive no thermal processing but can be safe for consumption. For all processed meat products, a "farm to fork" approach is needed to ensure that microbiological risks are reduced in raw meat and other ingredients that are destined for use in

Present Knowledge in Food Safety. DOI: https://doi.org/10.1016/B978-0-12-819470-6.00059-7

processed meats. The safety of processed meat products is dependent on the processing parameters (i.e., thermal and nonthermal processing, drying, curing, fermentation, and chilling) and the intrinsic and extrinsic properties of the product including water activity, pH, antimicrobials, and packaging technologies used. The safety of processed meats is dependent on the use of a combination of control measures to reduce the risks for consumers and including adequate microbial control on the inputs to the process, a bactericidal process (where possible), prevention of post-processing contamination, and if necessary, adequate refrigeration of the final product.

The raw meat used in processing can be contaminated with a variety of pathogens that must be controlled through thermal and nonthermal processing technologies, ingredient formulation, and/or environmental controls. The organisms that need to be controlled include enterohaemorrhagic *Escherichia coli* (EHEC), *Salmonella enterica*, *Campylobacter jejuni*, *Campylobacter coli*, *Yersinia enterocolitica*, *Listeria monocytogenes*, *Clostridium botulinum*, and *Clostridium perfringens*, *Bacillus cereus* and *Staphylococcus aureus*. The occurrence of these organisms on raw meat depends on a number of factors that start with the carriage in animals and hygiene during the harvest of meat. The contamination of raw meat and abattoir hygiene is covered elsewhere (see Chapter 29—Abattoir hygiene).

Salmonella, *Campylobacter* spp., *Yersinia*, *S. aureus*, and EHEC are generally controlled during meat processing by thermal processing technologies; however, *Salmonella* and EHEC can be a risk in dried fermented meats.[2] *Salmonella* has been identified as a risk in par-cooked poultry products, which are not always fully cooked by consumers prior to consumption.[3] *Salmonella* has also been associated with fully cooked meat products and salted dried meat products.[4] *Bacillus cereus* intoxications have been linked to meat products[4] but they are usually associated with starch-based food products and seldom associated with processed meats. *S. aureus* intoxications have been linked to consumption of ham[4] and cases are usually linked to postprocessing contamination and temperature abuse of products.

As many processed meats are ready-to-eat (RTE) and do not undergo any thermal treatment by the consumer, it is critical that postprocessing contamination of these products is controlled or that the growth of pathogens in these products is reduced or eliminated. One of the main concerns for RTE meats is contamination with *L. monocytogenes*, a psychrotrophic pathogen that is tolerant to salt and nitrite. There have been several large outbreaks of listeriosis associated with RTE meats, the most recent in South Africa being the largest with over 1000 cases of listeriosis and 216 deaths.[5] Prevention of postprocessing contamination through environmental controls, including good hygienic design, sanitation, or controlling the presence of the organism through thermal or nonthermal treatments postpackaging, are options for processors. Many jurisdictions have regulatory requirements that limit the number of *L. monocytogenes* that can be present on the surface of RTE meats or limit the growth to <100 CFU/g during storage. To control the growth of *L. monocytogenes* on RTE meats during refrigerated storage, processors can reformulate with a variety of antimicrobial agents.

The endospores of *Cl. botulinum* and *Cl. perfringens* survive thermal processing so the outgrowth of endospores must be controlled through postprocessing temperature control (cooling to prevent germination and refrigeration to prevent growth) and antimicrobial ingredients.

Spices added to processed meats can also be a source of pathogens and mycotoxins. Spices are notorious for contamination with *Salmonella* and have been implicated in outbreaks and recalls associated with processed meats.[6–8] Spices can also be a source of mycotoxins[9,10] but the growth of toxigenic molds on dry processed meats can also be a source of mycotoxins[11] although the presence of molds on dried, cured meats does not always mean that mycotoxins are produced in the product. Franciosa et al. detected mycotoxin-producing species of molds from casings used in the production of Salame Piemonte; however, no mycotoxins were detected in the final product.[12] The production of mycotoxins in dry fermented sausages is complex and is likely dependent on the conditions of ripening and the ingredients. The product water activity (a_w) and relative humidity (RH) in the drying chamber are critical parameters for the control of ochratoxin A production by *Penicillium nordicum*.[13] Spices were recently implicated as the source of ochratoxin A in dry-cured meats in Croatia as aflatoxin B1 was detected in samples but no toxigenic molds were detected.[11] However, oregano and rosemary can reduce the production of ochratoxin A in dry-cured fermented meats.[14] Although spices can introduce hazards to processed meat, they are also a source of strong antimicrobials that have been applied to control the growth of pathogens in processed meats.

As the meat industry is moving towards meeting consumer demands for minimally processed meat products with limited synthetic additives, the industry is challenged to ensure the safety of processed meats. The research literature available on novel antimicrobials and technologies is extensive and has been the subject of several reviews. For example, the use of emerging thermal and nonthermal processing technologies to improve the safety of meat products was recently reviewed by Singh et al.[15] Others have reviewed the use of novel antimicrobials to enhance the safety of processed meats.[16–18] This chapter will focus on the most recent advances in novel antimicrobials and nonthermal processing technologies. Novel thermal technologies will not be covered as the most recent advances are reviewed by Singh et al.[15]

31.2 Antimicrobials in processed meat formulations

There are many antimicrobials that are used to reduce the risks associated with foodborne pathogens in or on processed meats. In the age of "clean labels" and the desire to avoid chemical names, the choice of antimicrobials for use in processed meats has expanded substantially. Some of the "new" alternatives contain the same active ingredient as traditional antimicrobials while others represent new compounds that may be used as antimicrobials. Table 31.1 gives examples of the application of novel compounds or combinations of compounds and their impact on the growth of *L. monocytogenes* in processed meats. The α- and β-acids extracted from hops stop the growth of *L. monocytogenes* in a deli-style ham stored at abusive temperatures[20] while others have limited effect.

Single antimicrobials are seldom used as a hurdle to the growth of pathogens in processed meats. They are often combined or are used in combination with processing technologies for additive or synergistic effects. When combined, antimicrobials can often be used at lower concentrations, or processing technologies can be used at lower intensity without compromising their antimicrobial effects.[24] Much of the recent research has evaluated combinations of antimicrobials with processing technologies to eliminate or reduce microbial hazards in processed meats.

31.2.1 Nitrate and nitrite

Nitrate and nitrite have a long history of use to control the outgrowth of the endospores of *C. botulinum* in processed meats and other foods. The exact origin of its use

TABLE 31.1 Application of novel antimicrobials to control the growth of *Listeria monocytogenes* in processed meats.

Active compound	Product	Concentration	Source	Storage conditions	Impact	
Beta-acids	Pork bologna	800 ppm	Hops	7°C, 28 days	>4 log CFU/g reduction	19
Beta-acids	Deli style turkey	5 ppm	Hops	4°C or 7°C up to 60 days	0 growth	20
Alpha-acids	Deli style turkey	5 ppm	Hops	4°C or 7°C up to 60 days	0 growth	20
Beta-phenylethylamine	Lyoner slices	20 mg/g	–	4°C or 10°C for 11 or 7 days, respectively	2 log reduction compared to control	21
Liquid (LBV) or dry buffered vinegar (DBV)	Mortadella	Liquid: 1 or 1.5% Dry: 0.4, 0.6 or 1%	–	Vacuum packaged, 4°C or 12°C up to 120 or 28 days, respectively	LBV decreased CFU by <1 log CFU/slice after 120 days at 4°C. DBV (0.4% or 0.6%), had no antimicrobial effect, regardless of temperature. 1% DBV inhibited growth at 12°C.	22
Ethyl-N-dodecanoyl-L-arginate hydrochloride	Ham formulated with buffered vinegar, buffered vinegar/K-lactate, or K-lactate/K-acetate/Na-diacetate.	Surface treatment with 44 ppm solution	–	Vacuum packaged, sliced and stored at 4°C for 120 days or whole hams stored at −2.2°C for 3 months then 4°C for 120 days.	0.9–1.9 Log CFU reduction/slice during storage at 4°C; 4.2–5.2 log reduction per ham when product held at −2.2°C	23

is unknown but it is likely linked to unintentional addition with the addition of salt as a drying agent.[25,26] Nitrate must be converted to nitrite for biological activity. This is achieved through conversion by starter cultures that express nitrate reductases. Nitrite is reduced to nitric oxide which can react with microbial DNA, proteins, and lipids to act as an antimicrobial.[27] Nitric oxide is also the precursor of peroxynitrite which as a strong oxidant, has complex antimicrobial effects on both *Cl. botulinum* and *Cl. perfringens*.[28] For details on the antibacterial mechanism of nitrite, the reader is referred to the detailed review by Majou and Christieans.[28]

The endospores of *Cl. botulinum* and *Cl. perfringens* can be found in meat and meat products and their germination, outgrowth, and growth of viable cells are the targets for control. *Cl. botulinum* produces botulinum toxin or botulin (a potent neurotoxin) during growth thus all efforts must be made to control the growth of this organism in processed meats. *Cl. perfringens* causes a toxic infection as a result of ingestion of the organism, thus growth in foods must be controlled. Cooked meats that are held in the "danger zone" are typically associated with outbreaks of *Cl. perfringens* toxic infection. The presence of endospores in meat products can be prevented through adequate thermal processing of shelf-stable canned meats and in other meat products, storage at refrigeration temperatures (<3°C) or nitrite can be used to control the outgrowth of endospores of both of these organisms. The potential formation of nitrosamines, which have been linked to cancer, has resulted in the search for alternatives to nitrate/nitrite.

Alternatives to nitrite as a curing agent in processed meats have been the subject of years of investigation. Progress has been made on identifying alternatives to the use of nitrite when evaluating the quality parameters but there has been nothing described that can reduce the microbiological risks associated with processed meats. Alternatives such as beetroot powder,[29] prickly pear extract,[30] radish powder, and oregano essential oil,[31] and heme pigments[32] have been investigated as replacements for nitrite but the research has focused on the impact on chemical stability and sensory quality and there is little if any evidence they can inhibit the outgrowth of endospores. A reduction in a_w, a lower pH, and a competitive microbiota may be more important to the control of clostridia in RTE meats than the presence of nitrite. A combination of red wine and garlic used in the production of chouriço (a cold smoked, dried sausage with an a_w of <0.90 after 30 days drying) was suggested as a replacement for nitrite to control the outgrowth of endospores.[33] In a controlled laboratory setting, Hospital et al. found that the reduction or removal of nitrite had no impact on toxin production by *Cl. botulinum* in dry fermented sausages.[34] It is critical to note that nitrite is important to the safety of fermented sausages if other hurdles to the growth of *Cl. botulinum* fail or if product and processing conditions vary, thus the risks associated with the removal of nitrite from cured meats need to be carefully evaluated.

To meet the demand for "clean labels" and avoid naming "nitrite" or "nitrate" on labels, formulations can include alternative natural sources of nitrate or nitrite. In North America, fermented celery powder is used as a source of nitrite as it does not change the sensory properties of processed meats.[35] In Europe, Swiss chard is used as a source of natural nitrate as celery is considered to be an allergen in the EU.[36] Yong et al. reviewed the use of pre-converted nitrite in cured meats and pointed out that one of the weaknesses of natural nitrite is that the vegetable powders containing nitrite may impart off-flavors to meat products.[37] However, the use of plant-derived nitrite does not always impart off-flavors.[38] Natural sources of nitrite can produce products that have the superior sensory quality to synthetic sources of nitrite.[39] In terms of meat safety, natural sources of nitrite are able to control the growth of *Cl. perfringens*[40] and toxin production by *Cl. botulinum*[41] in deli-style turkey products when the source of nitrite provides similar nitrite "rate of addition" to that used for products formulated with synthetic nitrite.

Sodium nitrite also inhibits the growth of *L. monocytogenes* on RTE meats.[42,43] Natural source nitrite from celery was able to inhibit the growth of *L. monocytogenes* and *S. aureus* in naturally cured ham during extended cooling times.[44] Plasma activated water has been proposed as an alternative source of nitrite in processed meats. Beef jerky cured with plasma-activated brine as a nitrite source had a 1-log CFU/g of *L. innocua* as compared to controls cured with sodium nitrite.[45] However, the impact of plasma-activated water on the outgrowth of endospores of *Cl. botulinum* is unknown and will need to be evaluated before this technology can be used for enhancing the safety of cured meats.

The ability of nitrite to control the growth of pathogens in cooked processed meats will depend on the intrinsic properties of the meat product, including the addition of other ingredients that may have synergistic effects, and extrinsic properties, including the size of the product and cooling processes.

31.2.2 Acids and sodium salts of acids

Mixtures of sodium or potassium lactate with diacetates are used as antimicrobials to control the growth of *L. monocytogenes* in vacuum packaged ready-to-eat meats. Research on the use of lactates in combination with acetate has been done since the early 1990s and demonstrates that the combination can control the growth of *L. monocytogenes* on RTE meats.[46–48] Lactates have also been investigated for their ability to control the growth of *Cl. botulinum* and *Cl. perfringens* in uncured, cooked meats.[49–53] Recent work on the use of combinations of lactate/diacetate with other antimicrobials has demonstrated that combinations of lactates with nisin enhance the antimicrobial efficacy of potassium lactate/diacetate.[54]

To meet clean label requirements, processors have incorporated fruit extracts or dried powders to provide a source of acid and these are often considered to be flavorings rather than antimicrobials. The addition of low concentrations (1%–1.5%) of vinegar-based formulations with citrus extract or lemon juice powder to sous vide processed chicken breasts inhibited the growth of *Cl. perfringens* stored at abusive temperatures (16°C) for 16 days.[55] The citrus extract and lemon juice powder are a source of citric acid which can have synergistic antimicrobial activity with acetic acid.[55] Buffered vinegar can be used as a clean label ingredient to replace other antimicrobials that control the growth of *L. monocytogenes*. Dried or liquid buffered vinegar added to formulations for a "clean label" mortadella provided equivalent control as potassium lactate/sodium diacetate blend for the growth of *L. monocytogenes*.[22] A cultured sugar and vinegar blend, which is likely to contain bacteriocins, inhibit the growth of *L. monocytogenes* in uncured, deli-style turkey breast.[56]

The use of clean-label antimicrobials can help processors meet regulatory requirements for control of the growth or presence of *L. monocytogenes* in RTE meats. In the United States, clean label alternatives are important to the organic and natural processed meat producers as they cannot use traditional antimicrobials in their products due to label restrictions.[56]

31.2.3 Plant extracts and essential oils

The essential oils of plant materials have been investigated as potential antimicrobials for use in processed meats and can inhibit a wide range of microorganisms, including those of concern in processed meats. They can be added as flavoring ingredients which may have the benefit of a more "clean label" for processed meats.[18] The application of essential oils and plant extracts in meats has recently been reviewed[17,18,57] and the use of the phytochemical constituents of Mediterranean plants in meat products was reviewed by Alirezalu et al.[58] In all cases, the authors point out the limitations for direct use in processed meats as a result of their impact on flavor characteristics and the potential interaction with the components of products to reduce their antimicrobial efficacy in meats.

The antimicrobial activity of plant extracts can be attributed to a range of bioactive compounds including phenolics, terpenes, and acids. Generally, essential oils with high concentrations of phenolic compounds have greater antimicrobial activity than those with lower concentrations of phenolic compounds.[58] Essential oils from oregano, rosemary, and thyme (0.005%) inhibited the growth of *L. monocytogenes* during the drying of chouriço.[59] One of the drawbacks of the application of essential oils as antimicrobials is the potential negative impact on the sensory properties of the meat product. Combinations of essential oils with other antimicrobials to take advantage of potential synergistic effects, or encapsulation of essential oils have been proposed as strategies to mitigate this issue.[18] A combination of cinnamaldehyde and 2-hydroxycinnamic acid at low concentrations was able to inhibit the growth of *Salmonella* Enteritidis and *L. monocytogenes in vitro* but was not able to reduce these pathogens on cooked ham.[60] Although screening *in vitro* provides valuable insight into the antimicrobial efficacy of essential oils, the importance of interactions with a food matrix cannot be overlooked. Nanoemulsions of essential oils have been evaluated for their antimicrobial activity and have been used in combination with nonthermal processing technologies. Nanoemulsions of blends of 5 essential oils reduced the growth of *Cl. sporogenes* (used as a surrogate for *Cl. botulinum*) in a low-nitrite mortadella after 10 days storage at 14°C but there was little difference from the control after 20 days of storage.[61] Washing RTE chicken meat with nano emulsified linalool (25 min) reduced populations of *Salmonella* and *E. coli* O157:H7 by <2 log CFU/g on RTE chicken meat; however, when combined with cold atmospheric plasma, reductions of both organisms were increased to above 3 logs CFU/g.[62] The effects of this treatment were evaluated immediately after treatment and it is unknown if sublethally injured cells would resuscitate and grow during extended storage at abusive temperatures.

More research is needed on the antimicrobial effects of essential oils, their specific antimicrobial components, and interactions with the complex matrices of processed meats to ensure that they provide an adequate hurdle to the growth of foodborne pathogens in processed meats that can be exposed to variable environmental conditions.

31.2.4 Bacteriocins and bacteriocin-producing organisms

Bacteriocins are ribosomally-synthesized peptides with antimicrobial activity against bacterial species that are closely related to the producer organism.[63] Bacteriocins produced by lactic acid bacteria have been commercialized for use in many different food systems, including processed meats. Some of the commercially available preparations are listed in Table 31.2 and include partially

TABLE 31.2 Commercially available bacteriocin preparations.

Antimicrobial	Producer strain(s) of bacteriocins	Type of preparation	Supplier
Nisin	*Lactococcus lactis* subsp. *lactis*	Partially purified culture supernatant	Dupont nutrition and biosciences Chr Hansen
Nisin A, rosemary extract	*Lactococcus lactis* subsp. *lactis*	Partially purified culture supernatant	Dupont nutrition and biosciences
Pediocin PA-1/ACH/ sakacin A	*Pediococcus acidilactici* *Latilactobacillus curvatus*	Freeze-dried culture for use in salami and dry fermented sausages	Chr Hansen
Plantaricin/carnocin	*Lactiplantibacillus plantarum*, *Staphylococcus carnosus*	Freeze-dried cultures	Danisco DuPont nutrition and biosciences
Carnobacteriocin BM1, carnocyclin, piscicolin	*Carnobacterium maltaromaticum*	Partially purified culture supernatant with or without live culture	Griffith Foods Ltd.
Leucocin	*Leuconostoc carnosum*	Freeze-dried culture	Chr. Hansen
Sakacin	*Latilactobacillus sakei*	Freeze-dried culture	Chr. Hansen
Divercin and other undisclosed bacteriocins	*C. divergens*, *C. maltaromaticum*, *L. sakei*	Freeze-dried culture	Sacco

purified preparations, the bacteriocin-producing culture, or a combination of the two. In processed meats, the main target of research has been on inhibition of the growth of *L. monocytogenes* on RTE processed meats. Recent publications have reported inhibition of the growth of *L. monocytogenes* on cooked ham,[64,65] frankfurters,[66] fresh mutton sausage,[67] and dry-cured ham[68] by either culture supernatants of bacteriocin-producing cultures or by the live bacteriocinogenic culture.

The most effective inhibition of *L. monocytogenes* occurs when the bacteriocins or bacteriocin-producing organisms are on the surface of processed meats.[69] This has been accomplished commercially with spray systems that deliver the antimicrobial to the product at the time of packaging. A novel approach to the delivery of bacteriocins to the surface of processed meats is to treat casings with the bacteriocin before processing. Natural and artificial casings treated with sakacin G, a bacteriocin produced by *Latilactobacillus curvatus* ACU-1, were able to inhibit the growth of *L. monocytogenes* in model processed meat systems.[70] Casings would deliver the bacteriocin to the surface of processed meat without modifications to production processes. This has distinct advantages for the delivery of partially-purified bacteriocins or culture supernatants but cannot be used for delivery of live organisms to the surface of cooked processed meats as the organisms are unlikely to survive a thermal process. The use of packaging materials that deliver bacteriocins to the surface of processed meat is another approach that has some merit (see the section on antimicrobial packaging).

There is a significant body of research literature on the use of bacteriocins in conjunction with other antimicrobials and technologies. Mathur et al. reviewed the literature and pointed out that combinations of bacteriocins with other antimicrobials can have either synergistic or additive effects.[71] More recent research has demonstrated additive effects when bacteriocins are combined with high hydrostatic pressure processing (HPP). The combination of nisin,[72,] or lactocin AL705[73] with HPP can result in additive antimicrobial effects and prevents the growth of surviving cells of *L. monocytogenes* during storage.

Recent research has demonstrated fairly success in the reduction or removal of biofilms from surfaces with bacteriocins. Capidermicin, produced by *Staphylococcus capitis*, was able to remove preformed biofilms from the surface of a microtiter plate but was not able to stop biofilm formation by *L. monocytogenes*.[74] The cell-free supernatants containing bacteriocins from *Enterococcus faecium* 20, 22, or 24 reduce the viability of biofilms of *L. monocytogenes* on polystyrene[75] and a "bacteriocin-like inhibitory substance" produced by *E. faecium* DB1 was recently shown to decrease biofilm formation by *Cl. perfringens* on stainless steel.[76] The use of bacteriocins to control environmental contamination is an emerging area of application. Most of the research has been done on microtiter plates or on small stainless steel coupons in a laboratory setting. Before bacteriocins can be utilized in this manner, research needs to be done to determine efficacy under conditions that more closely represent the environment in a meat processing facility and to assess their impact on the microbiota and storage life of processed meat products. The economics of their use in the processing environment would have to compete favorably with other sanitation strategies.

One of the limitations of the use of bacteriocins in processed meats is their narrow spectrum of activity.[77] Attempts to bioengineer variants of different bacteriocins to improve activity have generally had limited success. However, recently Nyhan et al. evaluated combinations of 36 culture-free supernatants of *L. lactis* subsp. *lactis* that produce nisin derivatives and discovered a combination of two nisin derivatives that had enhanced antilisterial activity in a frankfurter homogenate stored at 4°C or 20°C.[78] The double combination of a derivative with a substitution of methionine for glutamine at position 17 with a derivative that has a substitution of asparagine for proline at position 20 was able to inhibit the growth of *L. innocua* better than combinations of other derivatives, including combinations of three derivatives or nisin A.[78] This is the first report of enhanced antilisterial efficacy of bioengineered derivatives of a bacteriocin applied in a meat matrix. Of note, an enhanced effect was not observed in chocolate milk, emphasizing the matrix-dependent activity of bacteriocins in food.

While bacteriocins hold promise for improving the safety of processed meats, their use is not without challenges. The development of resistance to bacteriocins has been identified as a potential downside to their use in foods[71,79] and some strains of *L. monocytogenes* may be inherently resistant to bacteriocins. Strains of *L. monocytogenes* that are recommended for use in challenge studies[80] are resistant to leucocin A, a Class II bacteriocin produced by *Leucontostoc gelidum* UAL187.[81] However, the presence of different carbohydrates can impact the resistance of *L. monocytogenes* to bacteriocins. *L. monocytogenes* FSLR2−499, which is resistant to leucocin A on the surface of frankfurters, became sensitive to leucocin A when it was grown in the presence of mannose *in vitro*.[82] Carbohydrates also impact the resistance of *L. monocytogenes* to carnocyclin A, a circular bacteriocin.[82] Tessema et al. also reported similar changes in resistance to sackacin P when strains of *L. monocytogenes* are grown in the presence of different carbohydrates.[83] All of the research on these changes in the resistance of *L. monocytogenes* to bacteriocins has been done *in vitro* and the potential impact of different carbohydrates in processed meats on the resistance of *L. monocytogenes* to bacteriocins still needs to be unraveled.

An emerging area of research is the combination of bacteriocins with nanoparticles for enhanced antimicrobial efficacy. Observations of enhanced activity of bacteriocins with gold[84] and silver[85,86] nanoparticles have been observed *in vitro* against foodborne pathogens of concern to processed meats, including *S. aureus* and *L. monocytogenes*. Bacteriocins have been incorporated into other nanostructures, such as cellulose nanocrystals,[87] nanoliposomes,[88] polyvinyl alcohol/polylactide particles[89], and these delivery systems have demonstrated enhanced antibacterial activity than the bacteriocin alone. However, to date, none of these nanostructures have been tested for their antimicrobial efficacy in processed meats. Assessment of the antibacterial efficacy of combinations of bacteriocins with nanoparticles in meats is essential before claims of enhanced activity for meat applications can be made.

31.2.5 Bacteriophage

Another biological approach to controlling pathogens in processed meats is the use of lytic bacteriophages that target a specific pathogen. Lytic bacteriophages infect the target host where they replicate and cause lysis of the bacterial cell as they release their progeny. Phage cocktails for controlling *L. monocytogenes* on the surface of processed meats are commercially available. These have regulatory approval in Australia, Canada, Israel, New Zealand, Switzerland, and the United States as processing aides[90] and are not declared on ingredient labels. The use of bacteriophage to control pathogens in foods has been reviewed by Polaska and Soklowska,[90] Kawacka et al.,[91] and Vikram et al.[92] Each of these reviews includes reference to commercial products that are available for control of pathogens on processed meats and reference research that has demonstrated the ability of cocktails of bacteriophage to control the growth of *L. monocytogenes* on processed RTE meats.

The combination of bacteriophage with other antimicrobials has shown promise as a means of controlling the growth of *L. monocytogenes* in RTE processed meats. Resendiz-Moctezuma et al.[54] used a model ham system to compare the efficacy of a lytic bacteriophage (P100) alone or in combination with several different antimicrobials using a response surface experimental design. A combination of P100 with nisin resulted in synergistic interactions in the control of the growth of *L. monocytogenes*.[54]

There have been reports of initial reductions of *L. monocytogenes* inoculated onto processed meats with bacteriophage and subsequent regrowth during storage[93] indicating a lack of inactivation by bacteriophage.[91] This could be a result of poor distribution of the phage on the product surface or the development of resistance to bacteriophage. Although Chibeu et al.[93] ruled out the possibility of the development of resistance to bacteriophage, strains of phage-resistant *L. monocytogenes* serotype 1/2a have been isolated from turkey processing facilities in the USA.[94] The phage-resistant strains are lacking in glycosylated teichoic acid surface receptors,[95] which serve as bacteriophage receptors and are important in biofilm formation.[96] Without glycosylated teichoic acids, the phage-resistant strains should not form structure biofilms and should easily be washed from surfaces in processing facilities.[97] Explanations for the persistence of the phage-resistant strains of *L. monocytogenes* remain to be uncovered.

31.2.6 Novel antimicrobial strategies

Chitosan, a linear polysaccharide, has been evaluated for application as an antimicrobial for processed meats. Most of the research has focused on the use of chitosan-based films on the surface of products and most of the research has incorporated other antimicrobials or films that have been used in conjunction with nonthermal processing to achieve antimicrobial effects. Films with chitosan, nisin, and rice bran extract (as a source of γ-oryzanol) and applied to dry-cured Iberian ham that was subsequently subjected to high-pressure treatment (600 MPa, 8 min) resulted in a 6-log reduction of *L. monocytogenes.*[98] Starch-based films with chitosan reduced initial cell numbers and inhibited the growth of *L. monocytogenes* on ham during 28 days storage at 4°C.[99] Biopolymer films with chitosan and other antimicrobials could be developed as alternatives to plastic packaging.

The search for novel antimicrobial strategies using biological agents other than those normally found in food has identified predatory protozoa as a novel solution to the destruction of pathogens. *Tetrahymena pyriformis*, nonpathogenic predatory protozoa, can reduce populations of *L. monocytogenes* in experimental conditions.[100] Exposure of planktonic cells and surface-attached cells of *L. monocytogenes* to *T. pyriformis* resulted in a 2-log reduction in *L. monocytogenes*. The authors envisioned that this strategy could be used to control *L. monocytogenes* in food processing environments.[100] This strategy must be validated in food products or in an environment that simulates a processing environment before conclusions can be made on its efficacy and potential application to improve the safety of RTE meats. The acceptance of this approach by the industry and consumers needs to be validated.

Strategies to reduce environmental contamination and the presence of biofilms of *L. monocytogenes* can reduce the risk of contamination of RTE meats. Stainless steel surfaces with nanotechnological coatings are bactericidal to foodborne pathogens by reducing surface adhesion and subsequent growth on stainless steel.[101] This type of approach may reduce the populations of all bacteria present in a facility. However, it may not be advantageous to remove the microbiota that is normally present in a meat processing facility as a background microbiota could provide antimicrobial effects to control the growth of *L. monocytogenes* during storage.[102]

31.3 Nonthermal processing technologies to reduce risks

Nonthermal processing technologies, such as (HPP), are used commercially to reduce the risk of pathogens in processed meat products. These technologies can assist the industry in meeting consumer demands for minimally processed, limited ingredient processed meats while ensuring the safety of the products. While each technology may have an impact on the safety of processed meats, they are often used in combination or are used in conjunction with antimicrobials to provide additional hurdles to pathogen survival and growth. Examples of research where nonthermal processes are combined with antimicrobials are summarized in Table 31.3.

31.3.1 High hydrostatic pressure processing

High hydrostatic pressure has been used as a nonthermal intervention since the early 2000s to reduce the risks associated with postprocessing contamination of ready-to-eat meats with *L. monocytogenes*. As reviewed by Li et al.,[108] HPP can reduce a target pathogen from <1 to >8 log CFU/g or cm^2, depending on the target organism and the characteristics of the product. Gram-negative organisms tend to be more susceptible to the effects of pressure than gram-positive organisms. The impact of HPP on cell constituents including membranes and cytoplasmic components was recently reviewed by Li et al. who outlined the specific impacts of HPP on cellular targets and described the impact of intrinsic and extrinsic factors on the efficacy of HPP.[108]

One of the intrinsic factors that are important to the lethality of HPP is a_w. In dry-cured ham, the lethality of HPP is less than 1 log CFU/g for Shiga-toxin producing *E. coli*, as reviewed by Li et al.[108] and can be <2 log CFU/g for *L. monocytogenes.*[109,110] Others have reported log reductions between 2 and 2.5 log CFU/g in similar dry-cured products.[111,112] This may not be sufficient to reduce the food safety risks for consumers as dry-cured ham can contain 5 log CFU/g of *L. monocytogenes.*[113] The low lethality of HPP has been linked to the low a_w in dry-cured ham. High-pressure treatment of dry-cured ham with an a_w of 0.92 resulted in a 2.5 to 2.8 log reduction after HPP whereas in ham with an a_w of 0.88, a 1 log reduction was observed.[114] As a result, research has focused on the use of multiple hurdles to achieve a greater reduction of *L. monocytogenes* in low a_w meat products.

While HPP can reduce populations of *Listeria*, it has little impact on the endospores of *Cl. perfringens* or *Cl. botulinum*, unless it is combined with temperatures close to that used in retorting (120°C). The advantage is the shorter processing time which reduces the impact on the quality parameters of the product. In nitrite-free processed

TABLE 31.3 Examples of research that has combined different antimicrobials with nonthermal processing technologies to improve the safety of processed meats.

Target organism	Antimicrobial	Processing technology	Product	Storage conditions	Impact	Reference
Listeria monocytogenes	Nisin	HHP (500 MPa; 3 min)	Cooked ham	–	HHP alone:	72
	Rosemary extract	HHP (500 MPa; 3 min)	Cooked ham		No effect	72
	Rosemary extract	Cold plasma	Cooked ham		No effect	103
	K lactate +/– Na diacetate	HHP (400 MPa, various times)	Cooked ham	No storage post HHP	Increased lactate reduced the ability of HHP to achieve 2 log reduction	104
	K lactate/Na diacetate	HHP 600 MPa, 6 min	Cooked ham	Vacuum package and stored at 8, 12, and 20°C.	Presence of antimicrobial stimulated post-HHP growth	105
Salmonella Typhimurium	Linalool nanoemulsion (surface treatment 25 min)	Cold atmospheric plasma (5 min) before 25 min nanoemulsion wash	Cooked chicken	–	>3.24 log CFU/g reduction	62
	Lactic acid	UV-C light	Dry-cured pork loin		1.3 log CFU/g reduction using 0.36 J/cm2 with 7.7% lactic acid	106
Escherichia coli O157	Linalool nanoemulsion (surface treatment 25 min)	Cold atmospheric plasma (5 min) before 25 min nanoemulsion wash	Cooked chicken	–	2.76 log CFU/g reduction	62
	Clove oil (1%)	Atmospheric cold plasma (15 min)	Beef jerky		>7 log CFU/g reduction	107

meats, the addition of 1% vinegar to the formulation and application of HPP (500 MPa, total 12 min) can inhibit the growth of *Cl. perfringens*.[115] The interest in nitrite-free or low nitrite products to meet consumer demands increases the need for alternative hurdles to the growth of spore-forming organisms.

Although HPP results in a decrease in numbers of viable cells post-treatment, there is evidence of sublethal injury and regrowth of *L. monocytogenes* during storage after pressure treatment in cooked, cured RTE ham.[116] This regrowth can be prevented by the presence of a competitive microbiota that survives HPP.[72] The ability of nonpathogenic organisms to survive HPP and their impact on pathogen growth during postprocessing storage requires further investigation to understand the mechanisms and potentially develop a microbiome-based system to provide enhanced hurdles to control *L. monocytogenes* in HPP-treated RTE meats.

31.3.2 Atmospheric cold plasma

Atmospheric cold plasma (ACP) is a novel nonthermal technology that can reduce risks associated with the presence of pathogens in processed meats. The antimicrobial efficacy of plasma technology is based on the ionization of gas to form positive and negative ions, free radicals, and other reactive species, and is influenced by product and process factors, and the target organism as reviewed by Feizollahi et al.[117]

Recent research on the application of cold plasma to control *Listeria* on the surface of processed meats found that ACP treatment was able to reduce populations by

1.75 log CFU/cm^2 on the surface of low salt (1% NaCl) ham at treatment temperatures of 4°C and 23°C; post-treatment storage resulted in further reductions of *Listeria*.[103] Different package atmospheres can influence the efficacy of ACP treatment with atmospheres containing oxygen having the greatest antimicrobial efficacy immediately after treatment and during post-treatment storage.[118] A modified atmosphere containing 20% oxygen was able to reduce populations of *L. monocytogenes* on ham by >6 log CFU/cm^2 during post-treatment storage of ham subjected to ACP after packaging.[118] The presence of oxygen during ACP treatment results in the production of reactive oxygen and nitrogen species that increase the antibacterial efficacy of ACP.

As with other processing technologies, the combination of ACP with other antimicrobials has greater antimicrobial effects but effects depend on the target organism and the antibacterial agent. For example, treatment of beef jerky with a combination of 1% clove oil and ACP was able to reduce *E. coli* O157:H7 to below detection limits (>7 log CFU/g reduction) while counts of *S. aureus* were only reduced by 1–2 log CFU/g. The authors attributed the high reductions of *E. coli* to the ability of the reactive species to cause changes in membrane structure.[107] In contrast the addition of bacteriocins or a combination of sodium lactate and sodium diacetate did not improve the antimicrobial efficacy of ACP applied to ham.[118] The additive or synergistic effects observed with additives are likely related to the mode of action of the antimicrobial and the ability of ACP to potentiate the effects.

The use of ACP is not without issues as the reactive species that are responsible for the antimicrobial effects also cause lipid oxidation in processed meats, which affects the quality of the product.[118] For the commercial application of ACP to be realized, reductions in the presence of pathogens on meats and the impacts on quality parameters have to be balanced. More research on the use of modified atmospheres and combinations of technologies to enhance the antimicrobial efficacy of ACP is needed to optimize the impacts on meat safety and to understand the underlying mechanisms of the antimicrobial effects.

31.3.3 Ultraviolet-C radiation

Ultraviolet-C radiation (UV-C; 200–280 nm) may enhance the safety of processed meats and has been investigated as a postpackaging treatment to control pathogens on the surface of RTE meats. Research in the late 2000's evaluated the efficacy of UV-C to reduce populations of *E. coli* and *L. monocytogenes*. The reduction of pathogens on the surface of RTE meats by UV-C has typically been <2 log CFU/g. UV-C treatment of frankfurters containing potassium lactate and sodium diacetate resulted in a <2 log reduction with a UV-C treatment of 4 J/cm^2; however, an additional 2.5 log reduction in *L. monocytogenes* occurred during post-treatment storage.[119] The role of potassium lactate and sodium diacetate in lethality during UV-C is unknown as the experiment did not have controls without added acids. However, others have found that acids do not enhance the efficacy of UV-C treatment. Treatment of dry-cured pork loin with 0.33 J/cm^2 UV-C light combined with 6.5% lactic acid resulted in a 1.2 log CFU/g reduction of *S.* Typhimurium, whereas the same UV-C treatment with 0.1% lactic acid resulted in a 1.0 log reduction.[106]

The exposure of the organism to the meat matrix prior to UV-C treatment can reduce the antimicrobial efficacy of UV-C treatment. Mutz et al. evaluated the impact of UV-C on the inactivation of *S.* Typhimurium on dry-fermented sausages and found that if the organisms had time to adapt to the meat matrix, the efficacy of UV-C treatment was reduced. [120] Cells that were adapted to the meat matrix prior to treatment were more resistant to the UV-C treatment. The authors suggested that the resistance was the result of adaptation to stress which in turn allowed a more efficient cellular response to the damage induced by UV-C, although the relationship between *in vivo* stress and resistance to UV-C remains unknown.[120]

There are few reports on the use of UV-C to reduce risks associated with RTE meats. The importance of adaptation to stress in the meat environment needs further study prior to the adaption of this technology. In addition, as a surface treatment, the impacts of the microbiome on meat are unknown and require further investigation. Although UV-C treatments could provide the meat processing industry with a low-cost alternative for reducing the risks associated with RTE meats, more research is needed to provide validation that it can be used to meet regulatory requirements for the presence of pathogens in RTE meats.

31.3.4 Other nonthermal processing technologies to improve the safety of processed meats

Technologies using either high pressure or supercritical carbon dioxide have promise as emerging technologies to enhance the safety of processed meats. The high-pressure carbon dioxide that is saturated with water reduces populations of *E. coli* and *Salmonella* on beef jerky by >5 log CFU/cm^2.[121] This is the only report of the use of saturated high-pressure carbon dioxide to reduce pathogens on meat products and with the level of inactivation achieved, the technology warrants further investigation for application to other processed meats. Supercritical carbon dioxide is limited in its antimicrobial efficacy on meat products but when combined with high-power ultrasound and a saline solution used during processing, *E. coli* was reduced by 3.6 log CFU/g on dry-cured ham.[122] These carbon-dioxide-based technologies are viewed as environmentally-friendly nonthermal technologies and have promise for meat safety applications in the future.

Pulsed light technology has gained attention as a potential nonthermal processing technology for processed meats. Pulsed light (8.4 J/cm^2) reduced populations of *L. innocua* on Serrano and Iberian ham by 2 and 1 log CFU/cm^2, respectively.[123] Earlier studies reported similar log reductions for *L. monocytogenes* on bologna, cooked ham, and dry-cured meats.[15]

The use of electron beam irradiation and pulsed electric fields to reduce risks associated with processed meats has been recently reviewed by Singh et al.[15] and there have been no further advancements in the application of these technologies to processed meats.

31.4 Research gaps and future directions

Regulatory agencies and the World Health Organization have suggested that processors take steps to lower the sodium concentration in RTE meats to lower the risk of hypertension in humans. Sodium chloride acts as a hurdle to the growth of pathogens in processed meats and plays an important technological role in the production of good-quality processed meat products. There is a papacy of literature on the impact of lower sodium concentrations on the growth of pathogens in processed meats. On vacuum-packaged ham formulated with 0.3 or 0.75% NaCl, *L. monocytogenes* was able to increase more than 2-logs after 15 days storage at 4°C whereas on ham formulated with 1% NaCl, the length of the lag phase was increased and *L. monocytogenes* did not increase by 2-logs until after 22 days of storage.[124] Replacement of NaCl with other salts may be an option to meet requirements for sodium reduction. Replacement of NaCl with KCl or $CaCl_2$ in the manufacture of biltong, a marinated and dried raw beef product that is similar to beef jerky, provided a 5-log reduction of *Salmonella* during processing, which produces a safe product. There are limits on the salt reduction that can be achieved in processed meats due to the loss of the functional properties required for processing and product quality. However, the impact on the potential survival and/or growth of pathogens on low salt processed meats needs to be investigated further.

Research on the interaction of technologies used to control pathogens in meat is needed as there is evidence of some antagonistic effects when combinations of antimicrobials are used [125] or when antimicrobials are used in combination with processing technologies.[126] The combination of antimicrobials and technologies needs to be validated in processed meat products to ensure that there are no antagonistic effects, including the risk of pathogen growth during post-treatment refrigerated storage. The recovery of sublethally injured cells on processed meats is an important parameter that is often overlooked in challenging studies and has not been sufficiently documented.

One aspect of the microbiology of processed meats that are often overlooked in research is the importance of a competitive microbiota. Processed meat products are typically not sterile (there are a few exceptions) and in the assessment of the efficacy of antimicrobials and processing technologies researchers seldom consider that pathogens are not in a sterile environment and that the background microbiota can impact the antimicrobial efficacy of any proposed treatment. For example, Teixeira et al.[72] demonstrated that the presence of a competitive meat microbiota prevented the recovery of sublethally injured *L. monocytogenes* after pressure treatment. Similar observations were documented by Zhao et al. in their assessment of the antilisterial properties of a starch-based antimicrobial packaging film.[99] Challenge studies should be designed to include the presence of a competitive microbiota to assess the impact of new technologies to control pathogens in meats in the presence of a background microbiota.

Processing treatments that are intended to target pathogens may also have an impact on the composition of the autochthonous microbiota, which may, in turn, impact the growth of spoilage organisms. For example, the presence of nisin provided selective pressure on a competitive microbiota that was co-inoculated with *L. monocytogenes*, selecting for the growth of *Leuconostoc gelidum*; however, high-pressure treatment selected for the growth of *Brochothrix thermosphacta*.[72] Although both of these organisms are meat spoilage bacteria, it is possible that they could provide hurdles to the growth of pathogens on RTE meats. Our ability to investigate the impact of novel processes and antimicrobials on the microbiota and safety of processed meats is enhanced by recent advancements in next-generation sequencing technologies, which to date have not been used extensively in research on processed meats.

Many of the newer approaches to improve the safety of processed meats do not result in large reductions in the numbers of the target pathogen. Further research should consider unique combinations of technologies that can optimize the inactivation of pathogens while having a limited impact on the sensory quality of the product.

The safety of processed meats is a complex and multifaceted topic that depends on the product characteristics (intrinsic factors) and processes, packaging, and storage conditions (extrinsic factors). Recent research demonstrates that novel applications of antimicrobials and processes or combinations of the two may enhance the safety of processed meats. As with any other approaches to food safety, advancements in the safety of processed meats have to be considered in the context of the impacts on the quality parameters and consumer acceptability.

References

1. World Health Organization. Cancer: Carcinogenicity of the consumption of red meat and processed meat. 2015. <https://www.who.int/news-room/q-a-detail/cancer-carcinogenicity-of-the-consumption-of-red-meat-and-processed-meat>. Accessed 03.09.21.
2. Bennett SD, Walsh KA, Gould LH. Foodborne disease outbreaks caused by *Bacillus cereus, Clostridium perfringens*, and *Staphylococcus aureus* – United States, 1998–2008. *Clin Infect Dis*. 2013;57(3):425–433. Available from: https://doi.org/10.1093/cid/cit244.
3. Trmcic A, Man S, Tamber S, Prystajecky N, McIntyre L. A survey of raw frozen breaded chicken products for *Salmonella* in British Columbia, Canada, and phylogenetically associated illnesses. *J Food Prot*. 2020;83(2):315–325. Available from: https://doi.org/10.4315/0362-028X.JFP-19-224.
4. Omer MK, Álvarez-Ordoñez A, Prieto M, Skjerve E, Asehun T, Alvseike OA. A systematic review of bacterial foodborne outbreaks related to red meat and meat products. *Foodborne Pathog Dis*. 2018;15(10):598–611. Available from: https://doi.org/10.1089/fpd.2017.2393.
5. Smith AM, Tau NP, Smouse SL, et al. Outbreak of *Listeria monocytogenes* in South Africa, 2017–2018: laboratory activities and experiences associated with whole-genome sequencing analysis of isolates. *Foodborne Pathog Dis*. 2019;16(7):524–530. Available from: https://doi.org/10.1089/fpd.2018.2586.
6. CDC. CDC - Multistate Outbreak of *Salmonella* Montevideo – May 4, 2010 – *Salmonella*. 2010. <https://www-cdc-gov.login.ezproxy.library.ualberta.ca/salmonella/2010/montevideo-5-4-2010.html>. Accessed 03.08.21.
7. Zhang G, Hu L, Pouillot R, et al. Prevalence of *Salmonella* in 11 spices offered for sale from retail establishments and in imported shipments offered for entry to the United States. *J Food Prot*. 2017;80(11):1791–1805. Available from: https://doi.org/10.4315/0362-028X.JFP-17-072.
8. Zweifel C, Stephan R. Spices and herbs as source of *Salmonella*-related foodborne diseases. *Food Res Int*. 2012;45(2):765–769. Available from: https://doi.org/10.1016/j.foodres.2011.02.024.
9. Banach JL, Stratakou I, van der Fels-Klerx HJ, de Besten HMW, Zwietering MH. European alerting and monitoring data as inputs for the risk assessment of microbiological and chemical hazards in spices and herbs. *Food Control*. 2016;69:237–249. Available from: https://doi.org/10.1016/j.foodcont.2016.04.010.
10. Aziz NH, Youssef YA, Aziz NH. Occurrence of aflatoxins and aflatoxin-producing moulds in fresh and processed meat in Egypt. *Food Addit Contam*. 1991;8(3):321–331. Available from: https://doi.org/10.1080/02652039109373981.
11. Zadravec M, Vahčić N, Brnić D, et al. A study of surface moulds and mycotoxins in Croatian traditional dry-cured meat products. *Int J Food Microbiol*. 2020;317(June 2019):108459. Available from: https://doi.org/10.1016/j.ijfoodmicro.2019.108459.
12. Franciosa I, Coton M, Ferrocino I, et al. Mycobiota dynamics and mycotoxin detection in PGI salame piemonte. *J Appl Microbiol*. 2021;. Available from: https://doi.org/10.1111/jam.15114. Published online.
13. Delgado J, Rondán JJ, Núñez F, Rodríguez A. Influence of an industrial dry-fermented sausage processing on ochratoxin A production by *Penicillium nordicum*. *Int J Food Microbiol*. 2021;339 (July 2020). Available from: https://doi.org/10.1016/j.ijfoodmicro.2020.109016.
14. Álvarez M, Rodríguez A, Núñez F, Silva A, Andrade MJ. In vitro antifungal effects of spices on ochratoxin A production and related gene expression in *Penicillium nordicum* on a dry-cured fermented sausage medium. *Food Control*. 2020;114(February):107222. Available from: https://doi.org/10.1016/j.foodcont.2020.107222.
15. Singh M, Novoa Rama E, Kataria J, Leone C, Thippareddi H. Emerging meat processing technologies for microbiological safety of meat and meat products. *Meat Muscle Biol*. 2020;4(2). Available from: https://doi.org/10.22175/mmb.11180.
16. Delgado-Pando G, Ekonomou SI, Stratakos AC, Pintado T. Clean label alternatives in meat products. *Foods*. 2021;10(7):1615. Available from: https://doi.org/10.3390/foods10071615.
17. Papadochristopoulos A, Kerry JP, Fegan N, Burgess CM, Duffy G. Natural antimicrobials for enhanced microbial safety and shelf-life of processed packaged meat. *Foods*. 2021;10(7):1–42. Available from: https://doi.org/10.3390/foods10071598.
18. Ji J, Shankar S, Royon F, Salmieri S, Lacroix M. Essential oils as natural antimicrobials applied in meat and meat products—a review. *Crit Rev Food Sci Nutr*. 2021;0(0):1–17. Available from: https://doi.org/10.1080/10408398.2021.1957766.
19. Kramer B, Mignard C, Warschat D, Gürbüz S, Aiglstorfer P, Muranyi P. Inhibition of *Listeria monocytogenes* on bologna by a beta acid rich hop extract. *Food Control*. 2021;126(February):108040. Available from: https://doi.org/10.1016/j.foodcont.2021.108040.
20. Sansawat T, Lee HC, Singh P, Ha SD, Kang I. Inhibition of *Listeria monocytogenes* in deli-style Turkey using hop acids, organic acids, and their combinations. *Poult Sci*. 2019;98 (3):1539–1544. Available from: https://doi.org/10.3382/ps/pey398.
21. Muchaamba F, Stephan R, Tasara T. Β-Phenylethylamine as a natural food additive shows antimicrobial activity against listeria monocytogenes on ready-to-eat foods. *Foods*. 2020;9(10):1–19. Available from: https://doi.org/10.3390/foods9101363.
22. Porto-Fett ACS, Campano SG, Rieker M, et al. Behavior of *Listeria monocytogenes* on mortadella formulated using a natural, clean-label antimicrobial agent during extended storage at 4 or 12°C. *J Food Prot*. 2018;81(5):769–775. Available from: https://doi.org/10.4315/0362-028X.JFP-17-400.
23. Luchansky JB, Campano SG, Shoyer BA, Porto-Fett ACS. Viability of listeria monocytogenes on boneless, water-added hams, commercially prepared with and without food-grade chemicals, during extended storage at 4 and/or −2.2 degrees C. *J Food Prot*. 2016;79(4):613–619. Available from: https://doi.org/10.4315/0362-028X.JFP-15-431.
24. Leistner L. Basic aspects of food preservation by hurdle technology. *Int J Food Microbiol*. 2000;55(1-3):181–186. Available from: https://doi.org/10.1016/S0168-1605(00)00161-6.
25. Binkerd E, Kolari O. The history and use of nitrate and nitrite in the curing of meat. *Food Cosmet Toxicol*. 1975;13(6):655–661. Available from: https://doi.org/10.1016/0015-6264(75)90157-1.

26. Pegg R, Shahidi F. *Nitrite Curing of Meat – The N-Nitrosamine Problem and Nitrite Alternatives*. Food and Nutrition Press, Inc; 2000.
27. Fang FC. Mechanisms of nitric oxide-related antimicrobial activity. *J Clin Invest*. 1997;99(12):2818–2825.
28. Majou D, Christieans S. Mechanisms of the bactericidal effects of nitrate and nitrite in cured meats. *Meat Sci*. 2018;145(July):273–284. Available from: https://doi.org/10.1016/j.meatsci.2018.06.013.
29. Aykln-Dinçer E, Güngör KK, Çağlar E, Erbaş M. The use of beetroot extract and extract powder in sausages as natural food colorant. *Int J Food Eng*. 2021;17(1):75–82. Available from: https://doi.org/10.1515/ijfe-2019-0052.
30. Kharrat N, Salem H, Mrabet A, et al. Synergistic effect of polysaccharides, betalain pigment and phenolic compounds of red prickly pear (Opuntia stricta) in the stabilization of salami. *Int J Biol Macromol*. 2018;111:561–568. Available from: https://doi.org/10.1016/j.ijbiomac.2018.01.025.
31. Ozaki MM, Santos M, dos, Ribeiro WO, et al. Radish powder and oregano essential oil as nitrite substitutes in fermented cooked sausages. *Food Res Int*. 2021;140(August 2020):109855. Available from: https://doi.org/10.1016/j.foodres.2020.109855.
32. De Maere H, Chollet S, De Brabanter J, Michiels C, Paelinck H, Fraeye I. Influence of meat source, pH and production time on zinc protoporphyrin IX formation as natural colouring agent in nitrite-free dry fermented sausages. *Meat Sci*. 2018;135(August 2017): 46–53. Available from: https://doi.org/10.1016/j.meatsci.2017.08.024.
33. Patarata L, Martins S, Silva JA, Fraqueza MJ. Red wine and garlic as a possible alternative to minimize the use of nitrite for controlling *Clostridium sporogenes* and *Salmonella* in a cured sausage: Safety and sensory implications. *Foods*. 2020;9(2). Available from: https://doi.org/10.3390/foods9020206.
34. Hospital XF, Hierro E, Stringer S, Fernández M. A study on the toxigenesis by *Clostridium botulinum* in nitrate and nitrite-reduced dry fermented sausages. *Int J Food Microbiol*. 2016;218:66–70. Available from: https://doi.org/10.1016/j.ijfoodmicro.2015.11.009.
35. Sebranek JG, Jackson-Davis AL, Myers KL, Lavieri NA. Beyond celery and starter culture: advances in natural/organic curing processes in the United States. *Meat Sci*. 2012;92(3):267–273. Available from: https://doi.org/10.1016/j.meatsci.2012.03.002.
36. Mermelstein NH. Formulating processed meats for clean labeling. *Food Technol*. 2018;72(12):59–62.
37. Yong HI, Kim TK, Choi HD, Jang HW, Jung S, Choi YS. Clean label meat technology: pre-converted nitrite as a natural curing. *Food Sci Anim Resour*. 2021;41(2):173–184. Available from: https://doi.org/10.5851/kosfa.2020.e96.
38. Shin DM, Hwang KE, Lee CW, Kim TK, Park YS, Han SG. Effect of Swiss chard (*Beta vulgaris* var. *cicla*) as nitrite replacement on color stability and shelf-life of cooked pork patties during refrigerated storage. *Korean J Food Sci Anim Resour*. 2017;37(3): 418–428. Available from: https://doi.org/10.5851/kosfa.2017.37.3.418.
39. Martínez-Zamora L, Peñalver R, Ros G, Nieto G. Substitution of synthetic nitrates and antioxidants by spices, fruits and vegetables in clean label Spanish chorizo. *Food Res Int*. 2021;139(January 2020). Available from: https://doi.org/10.1016/j.foodres.2020.109835.
40. King AM, Glass KA, Milkowski AL, Sindelar JJ. Impact of clean-label antimicrobials and nitrite derived from natural sources on the outgrowth of *Clostridium perfringens* during cooling of deli-style turkey breast. *J Food Prot*. 2015;78(5):946–953. Available from: https://doi.org/10.4315/0362-028X.JFP-14-503.
41. Golden MC, Wanless BJ, David JRD, et al. Effect of cultured celery juice, temperature, and product composition on the inhibition of proteolytic *Clostridium botulinum* toxin production. *J Food Prot*. 2017;80(8):1259–1265. Available from: https://doi.org/10.4315/0362-028X.JFP-17-011.
42. Golden MC, McDonnell LM, Sheehan V, Sindelar JJ, Glass KA. Inhibition of *Listeria monocytogenes* in deli-style turkey breast formulated with cultured celery powder and/or cultured sugar-vinegar blend during storage at 4°C. *J Food Prot*. 2014;77(10):1787–1793. Available from: https://doi.org/10.4315/0362-028X.JFP-14-059.
43. McDonnell LM, Glass KA, Sindelar JJ. Identifying ingredients that delay outgrowth of *Listeria monocytogenes* in natural, organic, and clean-label ready-to-eat meat and poultry products. *J Food Prot*. 2013;76(8):1366–1376. Available from: https://doi.org/10.4315/0362-028X.JFP-12-501.
44. Wu J, Acuff J, Waterman K, Ponder M. Evaluation of *Listeria monocytogenes* and *Staphylococcus aureus* survival and growth during cooling of hams cured with natural-source nitrite. *J Food Prot*. 2021;84 (2):286–290. Available from: https://doi.org/10.4315/JFP-20-249.
45. Inguglia ES, Oliveira M, Burgess CM, Kerry JP, Tiwari BK. Plasma-activated water as an alternative nitrite source for the curing of beef jerky: influence on quality and inactivation of *Listeria innocua*. *Innov Food Sci Emerg Technol*. 2020;59(December 2019):102276. Available from: https://doi.org/10.1016/j.ifset.2019.102276.
46. Schlyter JH, Glass KA, Loeffelholz J, Degnan AJ, Luchansky JB. The effects of diacetate with nitrite, lactate, or pediocin on the viability of *Listeria monocytegenes* in turkey slurries. *Int J Food Microbiol*. 1993;19(4):271–281. Available from: https://doi.org/10.1016/0168-1605(93)90019-D.
47. Glass KA, Granberg DA, Smith AL, et al. Inhibition of *Listeria monocytogenes* by sodium diacetate and sodium lactate on wieners and cooked bratwurst. *J Food Prot*. 2002;65(1):116–123. Available from: https://doi.org/10.4315/0362-028X-65.1.116.
48. Mbandi E, Shelef LA. Enhanced inhibition of *Listeria monocytogenes* and *Salmonella enteritidis* in meat by combinations of sodium lactate and diacetate. *J Food Prot*. 2001;64(5):640–644. Available from: https://doi.org/10.4315/0362-028X-64.5.640.
49. Meng J, Genigeorgis CA. Modeling lag phase of nonproteolytic *Clostridium botulinum* toxigenesis in cooked turkey and chicken breast as affected by temperature, sodium lactate, sodium chloride and spore inoculum. *Int J Food Microbiol*. 1993;19(2):109–122. Available from: https://doi.org/10.1016/0168-1605(93)90177-I.
50. Mass M, Glass KA, Doyle MP. Sodium lactate delays toxing production by *Clostridium botulinum* in cook-in-bag turkey products. *Appl Environ Microbiol*. 1989;55(9):2226–2229.
51. Redondo-Solano M, Valenzuela-Martinez C, Juneja VK, Burson DE, Thippareddi H. Control of *Clostridium perfringens* spore germination and outgrowth by potassium lactate and sodium diacetate in ham containing reduced sodium chloride. *LWT – Food Sci Technol*. 2021;137(September 2020):110395. Available from: https://doi.org/10.1016/j.lwt.2020.110395.
52. Juneja VK, Thippareddi H. Inhibitory effects of organic acid salts on growth of *Clostridium perfringens* from spore inocula during chilling of marinated ground turkey breast. *Int J Food Microbiol*. 2004;93(2):155–163. Available from: https://doi.org/10.1016/j.ijfoodmicro.2003.10.012.
53. Juneja VK, Thippareddi H. Control of *Clostridium perfringens* in a model roast beef by salts of organic acids during chilling. *J Food*

Saf. 2004;24(2):95–108. Available from: https://doi.org/10.1111/j.1745-4565.2004.tb00378.x.

54. Resendiz-Moctezuma C, Rezac SD, Miller MJ, Stasiewicz MJ. Enabling cost-effective screening for antimicrobials against *Listeria monocytogenes* in ham. *J Food Prot.* 2021;84(5):802–810. Available from: https://doi.org/10.4315/JFP-20-435.
55. Smith CJ, Olszewska MA, Diez-Gonzalez F. Selection and application of natural antimicrobials to control *Clostridium perfringens* in sous-vide chicken breasts. *Int J Food Microbiol.* 2021;347(March):109193. Available from: https://doi.org/10.1016/j.ijfoodmicro.2021.109193.
56. Weyker RE, Glass KA, Milkowski AL, Seman DL, Sindelar JJ. Controlling *Listeria monocytogenes* and *Leuconostoc mesenteroides* in uncured deli-style turkey breast using a clean label antimicrobial. *J Food Sci.* 2016;81(3):M672–M683. Available from: https://doi.org/10.1111/1750-3841.13232.
57. Pateiro M, Munekata PES, Sant'Ana AS, Domínguez R, Rodríguez-Lázaro D, Lorenzo JM. Application of essential oils as antimicrobial agents against spoilage and pathogenic microorganisms in meat products. *Int J Food Microbiol.* 2021;337(May 2020). Available from: https://doi.org/10.1016/j.ijfoodmicro.2020.108966.
58. Alirezalu K, Pateiro M, Yaghoubi M, Alirezalu A, Peighambardoust SH, Lorenzo JM. Phytochemical constituents, advanced extraction technologies and techno-functional properties of selected Mediterranean plants for use in meat products. A comprehensive review. *Trends Food Sci Technol.* 2020;100(April):292–306. Available from: https://doi.org/10.1016/j.tifs.2020.04.010.
59. García-Díez J, Alheiro J, Pinto AL, et al. Behaviour of food-borne pathogens on dry cured sausage manufactured with herbs and spices essential oils and their sensorial acceptability. *Food Control.* 2016;59:262–270. Available from: https://doi.org/10.1016/j.foodcont.2015.05.027.
60. Corrêa JAF, Santos JVG, dos, Evangelista AG, Pinto ACSM, de Macedo REF, Luciano FB. Combined application of phenolic acids and essential oil components against *Salmonella* Enteritidis and *Listeria monocytogenes* in vitro and in ready-to-eat cooked ham. *LWT – Food Sci Technol.* 2021;149(June). Available from: https://doi.org/10.1016/j.lwt.2021.111881.
61. Pinelli JJ, Helena de Abreu Martins H, Guimarães AS, et al. Essential oil nanoemulsions for the control of *Clostridium sporogenes* in cooked meat product: an alternative? *LWT – Food Sci Technol.* 2021;143(July 2020). Available from: https://doi.org/10.1016/j.lwt.2021.111123.
62. González-González CR, Labo-Popoola O, Delgado-Pando G, Theodoridou K, Doran O, Stratakos AC. The effect of cold atmospheric plasma and linalool nanoemulsions against *Escherichia coli* O157:H7 and *Salmonella* on ready-to-eat chicken meat. *LWT – Food Sci Technol.* 2021;149(May). Available from: https://doi.org/10.1016/j.lwt.2021.111898.
63. Cotter PD, Ross RP, Hill C. Bacteriocins-a viable alternative to antibiotics? *Nat Rev Microbiol.* 2013;11(2):95–105. Available from: https://doi.org/10.1038/nrmicro2937.
64. Iacumin L, Cappellari G, Colautti A, Comi G. *Listeria monocytogenes* survey in cubed cooked ham packaged in modified atmosphere and bioprotective effect of selected lactic acid bacteria. *Microorganisms.* 2020;8(6):1–18. Available from: https://doi.org/10.3390/microorganisms8060898.
65. de Azevedo POS, Mendonça CMN, Seibert L, et al. Bacteriocin-like inhibitory substance of *Pediococcus pentosaceus* as a biopreservative for *Listeria* sp. control in ready-to-eat pork ham. *Braz J Microbiol.* 2020;51(3):949–956. Available from: https://doi.org/10.1007/s42770-020-00245-w.
66. Vijayakumar PP, Muriana PM. Inhibition of *Listeria monocytogenes* on ready-to-eat meats using bacteriocin mixtures based on mode-of-action. *Foods.* 2017;6(3):1–13. Available from: https://doi.org/10.3390/foods6030022.
67. Junges da Costa R, Pereira da Silva A, Nobre da Fonseca R, et al. Characterization of *Enterococcus faecium* EO1 isolated from mutton and activity of bacteriocin-like substances in the control of *Listeria monocytogenes* in fresh mutton sausage. *LWT – Food Sci Technol.* 2021;141(September 2020):1–8. Available from: https://doi.org/10.1016/j.lwt.2021.110954.
68. Montiel R, Quesille-Villalobos A, Alessandria V, Medina M, Cocolin LS, Rantsiou K. Antilisterial effect and influence on *Listeria monocytogenes* gene expression of enterocin or *Enterococcus faecalis* in sliced dry-cured ham stored at 7°C. *J Food Prot.* 2019;82(9):1598–1606. Available from: https://doi.org/10.4315/0362-028X.JFP-19-024.
69. Zhou H, Xie Y, Liu H, Jin J, Duan H, Zhang H. Effects of two application methods of plantaricin BM-1 on control of *Listeria monocytogenes* and background spoilage bacteria in sliced vacuum-packaged cooked ham stored at 4°C. *J Food Prot.* 2015;78(10):1835–1841. Available from: https://doi.org/10.4315/0362-028X.JFP-14-594.
70. Rivas FP, Cayré ME, Campos CA, Castro MP. Natural and artificial casings as bacteriocin carriers for the biopreservation of meats products. *J Food Saf.* 2018;38(1). Available from: https://doi.org/10.1111/jfs.12419.
71. Mathur H, Field D, Rea MC, Cotter PD, Hill C, Ross RP. Bacteriocin-antimicrobial synergy: A medical and food perspective. *Front Microbiol.* 2017;8(JUN):1–18. Available from: https://doi.org/10.3389/fmicb.2017.01205.
72. Teixeira JS, Repková L, Gänzle MG, McMullen LM. Effect of pressure, reconstituted RTE meat microbiota, and antimicrobials on survival and post-pressure growth of *Listeria monocytogenes* on ham. *Front Microbiol.* 2018;9(AUG):1–11. Available from: https://doi.org/10.3389/fmicb.2018.01979.
73. Dallagnol AM, Barrio Y, Cap M, et al. *Listeria* inactivation by the combination of high hydrostatic pressure and lactocin AL705 on cured-cooked pork loin slices. *Food Bioprocess Technol.* 2017;10(10):1824–1833. Available from: https://doi.org/10.1007/s11947-017-1956-6.
74. Lynch D, Hill C, Field D, Begley M. Inhibition of *Listeria monocytogenes* by the *Staphylococcus capitis* - derived bacteriocin capidermicin. *Food Microbiol.* 2021;94(October 2020). Available from: https://doi.org/10.1016/j.fm.2020.103661.
75. Rocha KR, Perini HF, de Souza CM, et al. Inhibitory effect of bacteriocins from enterococci on developing and preformed biofilms of *Listeria monocytogenes, Listeria ivanovii* and *Listeria innocua. World J Microbiol Biotechnol.* 2019;35(7):1–11. Available from: https://doi.org/10.1007/s11274-019-2675-0.
76. Lee JS, Park SW, Lee HB, Kang SS. Bacteriocin-like inhibitory substance (BLIS) activity of *Enterococcus faecium* DB1 against biofilm formation by *Clostridium perfringens. Probiotics Antimicrob Proteins.* 2021;. Available from: https://doi.org/10.1007/s12602-021-09813-4 (0123456789).
77. Soltani S, Hammami R, Cotter PD, et al. Bacteriocins as a new generation of antimicrobials: toxicity aspects and regulations. *FEMS Microbiol Rev.* 2021;45(1):1–24. Available from: https://doi.org/10.1093/femsre/fuaa039.

78. Nyhan L, Field D, Hill C, Callanan M, Begley M. Investigation of combinations of rationally selected bioengineered nisin derivatives for their ability to inhibit *Listeria* in broth and model food systems. *Food Microbiol.* 2021;99(May). Available from: https://doi.org/10.1016/j.fm.2021.103835.
79. do C de F Bastos M, Coelho MLV, da S. Santos OC. Resistance to bacteriocins produced by gram-positive bacteria. *Microbiol – SGM.* 2015;161:683–700. Available from: https://doi.org/10.1099/mic.0.082289-0.
80. Fugett E, Fortes E, Nnoka C, Wiedmann M. International Life Sciences Institute North America *Listeria monocytogenes* strain collection: development of standard *Listeria monocytogenes* strain sets for research and validation studies. *J Food Prot.* 2006;69(12):2929–2938. Available from: https://doi.org/10.4315/0362-028X-69.12.2929.
81. Balay DR, Dangeti RV, Kaur K, McMullen LM. Purification of leucocin A for use on wieners to inhibit *Listeria monocytogenes* in the presence of spoilage organisms. *Int J Food Microbiol.* 2017;255:25–31. Available from: https://doi.org/10.1016/j.ijfoodmicro.2017.05.016.
82. Balay DR, Gänzle MG, McMullen LM. The effect of carbohydrates and bacteriocins on the growth kinetics and resistance of *Listeria monocytogenes. Front Microbiol.* 2018;9(MAR):347. Available from: https://doi.org/10.3389/fmicb.2018.00347.
83. Tessema GT, Møretrø T, Snipen L, Axelsson L, Naterstad K. Global transcriptional analysis of spontaneous sakacin p-resistant mutant strains of *Listeria monocytogenes* during growth on different sugars. *PLoS One.* 2011;6(1). Available from: https://doi.org/10.1371/journal.pone.0016192.
84. Singh AK, Bai X, Amalaradjou MAR, Bhunia AK. Antilisterial and antibiofilm activities of pediocin and LAP functionalized gold nanoparticles. *Front Sustain Food Syst.* 2018;2(November):1–15. Available from: https://doi.org/10.3389/fsufs.2018.00074.
85. Sidhu PK, Nehra K. Bacteriocin-capped silver nanoparticles for enhanced antimicrobial efficacy against food pathogens. *IET Nanobiotechnol.* 2020;14(3):245–252. Available from: https://doi.org/10.1049/iet-nbt.2019.0323.
86. Amer SA, Abushady HM, Refay RM, Mailam MA. Enhancement of the antibacterial potential of plantaricin by incorporation into silver nanoparticles. *J Genet Eng Biotechnol.* 2021;19(1). Available from: https://doi.org/10.1186/s43141-020-00093-z.
87. Bagde P, Vigneshwaran N. Improving the stability of bacteriocin extracted from *Enterococcus faecium* by immobilization onto cellulose nanocrystals. *Carbohydr Polym.* 2019;209(January):172–180. Available from: https://doi.org/10.1016/j.carbpol.2019.01.027.
88. Niaz T, Shabbir S, Noor T, Imran M. Antimicrobial and antibiofilm potential of bacteriocin loaded nano-vesicles functionalized with rhamnolipids against foodborne pathogens. *LWT – Food Sci Technol.* 2019;116(April):108583. Available from: https://doi.org/10.1016/j.lwt.2019.108583.
89. Holcapkova P, Hrabalikova M, Stoplova P, Sedlarik V. Core–shell PLA–PVA porous microparticles as carriers for bacteriocin nisin. *J Microencapsul.* 2017;34(3):243–249. Available from: https://doi.org/10.1080/02652048.2017.1324919.
90. Połaska M, Sokołowska B. Bacteriophages—a new hope or a huge problem in the food industry. *AIMS Microbiol.* 2019;5(4):324–347. Available from: https://doi.org/10.3934/microbiol.2019.4.324.
91. Kawacka I, Olejnik-Schmidt A, Schmidt M, Sip A. Effectiveness of phage-based inhibition of *Listeria monocytogenes* in food products and food processing environments. *Microorganisms.* 2020;8(11):1–20. Available from: https://doi.org/10.3390/microorganisms8111764.
92. Vikram A, Woolston J, Sulakvelidze A. Phage biocontrol applications in food production and processing. *Curr Issues Mol Biol.* 2020;40:267–302. Available from: https://doi.org/10.21775/cimb.040.267.
93. Chibeu A, Agius L, Gao A, Sabour PM, Kropinski AM, Balamurugan S. Efficacy of bacteriophage LISTEX™P100 combined with chemical antimicrobials in reducing *Listeria monocytogenes* in cooked turkey and roast beef. *Int J Food Microbiol.* 2013;167(2):208–214. Available from: https://doi.org/10.1016/j.ijfoodmicro.2013.08.018.
94. Kim J-W, Siletzky RM, Kathariou S. Host ranges of *Listeria*-specific bacteriophages from the turkey processing plant environment in the United States. *Appl Environ Microbiol.* 2008;74(1):6623. 2230. https://doi.org.login.ezproxy.library.ualberta.ca/10.1128/AEM.01282-08.
95. Brown P, Chen Y, Parsons C, et al. Whole genome sequence analysis of phage-resistant listeria monocytogenes serotype 1/2a strains from turkey processing plants. *Pathogens.* 2021;10(2):1–13. Available from: https://doi.org/10.3390/pathogens10020199.
96. Hsu CY, Cairns L, Hobley L, Abbott J, O'Byrne C, Stanley-Wall NR. Genomic differences between *Listeria monocytogenes* EGDe isolates reveal crucial roles for sigB and wall rhamnosylation in biofilm formation. *J Bacteriol.* 2020;202(7):1–13. Available from: https://doi.org/10.1128/JB.00692-19.
97. Brauge T, Faille C, Sadovskaya I, et al. The absence of *N*-acetylglucosamine in wall teichoic acids of *Listeria monocytogenes* modifies biofilm architecture and tolerance to rinsing and cleaning procedures. *PLoS One.* 2018;13(1):1–19. Available from: https://doi.org/10.1371/journal.pone.0190879.
98. Martillanes S, Rocha-Pimienta J, Llera-Oyola J, et al. Control of *Listeria monocytogenes* in sliced dry-cured Iberian ham by high pressure processing in combination with an eco-friendly packaging based on chitosan, nisin and phytochemicals from rice bran. *Food Control.* 2021;124(September 2020). Available from: https://doi.org/10.1016/j.foodcont.2021.107933.
99. Zhao Y, Teixeira JS, Saldaña MDA, Gänzle MG. Antimicrobial activity of bioactive starch packaging films against *Listeria monocytogenes* and reconstituted meat microbiota on ham. *Int J Food Microbiol.* 2019;305(June):108253. Available from: https://doi.org/10.1016/j.ijfoodmicro.2019.108253.
100. Meinersmann RJ, Berrang ME, Rigsby LL. Recoverability of *Listeria monocytogenes* after coculture with *Tetrahymena pyriformis. J Food Saf.* 2020;40(3):1–6. Available from: https://doi.org/10.1111/jfs.12778.
101. Di Cerbo A, Mescola A, Rosace G, et al. Antibacterial effect of stainless steel surfaces treated with a nanotechnological coating approved for food contact. *Microorganisms.* 2021;9(2):1–18. Available from: https://doi.org/10.3390/microorganisms9020248.
102. Fagerlund A, Langsrud S, Møretrø T. Microbial diversity and ecology of biofilms in food industry environments associated with *Listeria monocytogenes* persistence. *Curr Opin Food Sci.* 2021;37:171–178. Available from: https://doi.org/10.1016/j.cofs.2020.10.015.
103. Yadav B, Spinelli AC, Govindan BN, Tsui YY, McMullen LM, Roopesh MS. Cold plasma treatment of ready-to-eat ham: influence of process conditions and storage on inactivation of *Listeria innocua. Food Res Int.* 2019;123(December 2018):276–285. Available from: https://doi.org/10.1016/j.foodres.2019.04.065.
104. Serra-Castelló C, Ferrocino I, Jofré A, Cocolin L, Bover-Cid S, Rantsiou K. Unravelling the molecular mechanisms underlying

the protective effect of lactate on the high-pressure resistance of *Listeria monocytogenes*. *Biomolecules.* 2021;11(5):1–16. Available from: https://doi.org/10.3390/biom11050677.

105. Bover-Cid S, Serra-Castelló C, Dalgaard P, Garriga M, Jofré A. New insights on *Listeria monocytogenes* growth in pressurised cooked ham: a piezo-stimulation effect enhanced by organic acids during storage. *Int J Food Microbiol.* 2019;290(August 2018):150–158. Available from: https://doi.org/10.1016/j.ijfoodmicro.2018.10.008.
106. Rosario DKA, Mutz YS, Castro VS, Bernardes PC, Rajkovic A, Conte-Junior CA. Optimization of UV-C light and lactic acid combined treatment in decontamination of sliced Brazilian dry-cured loin: *Salmonella* Typhimurium inactivation and physicochemical quality. *Meat Sci.* 2021;172(January 2020):108308. Available from: https://doi.org/10.1016/j.meatsci.2020.108308.
107. Yoo JH, Baek KH, Heo YS, Yong HI, Jo C. Synergistic bactericidal effect of clove oil and encapsulated atmospheric pressure plasma against *Escherichia coli* O157:H7 and *Staphylococcus aureus* and its mechanism of action. *Food Microbiol.* 2021;93(August 2020):103611. Available from: https://doi.org/10.1016/j.fm.2020.103611.
108. Li H, Sun X, Liao X, Gänzle M. Control of pathogenic and spoilage bacteria in meat and meat products by high pressure: challenges and future perspectives. *Compr Rev Food Sci Food Saf.* 2020;19(6):3476–3500. Available from: https://doi.org/10.1111/1541-4337.12617.
109. Pérez-Baltar A, Serrano A, Medina M, Montiel R. Effect of high pressure processing on the inactivation and the relative gene transcription patterns of Listeria monocytogenes in dry-cured ham. *LWT – Food Sci Technol.* 2021;139(July 2020). Available from: https://doi.org/10.1016/j.lwt.2020.110555.
110. Montiel R, Peirotén Á, Ortiz S, et al. Inactivation of *Listeria monocytogenes* during dry-cured ham processing. *Int J Food Microbiol.* 2020;318(September 2019):108469. Available from: https://doi.org/10.1016/j.ijfoodmicro.2019.108469.
111. Cava R, Higuero N, Ladero L. High-pressure processing and storage temperature on *Listeria monocytogenes*, microbial counts and oxidative changes of two traditional dry-cured meat products. *Meat Sci.* 2021;171(August 2020):108273. Available from: https://doi.org/10.1016/j.meatsci.2020.108273.
112. Cava R, García-Parra J, Ladero L. Effect of high hydrostatic pressure processing and storage temperature on food safety, microbial counts, colour and oxidative changes of a traditional dry-cured sausage. *LWT – Food Sci Technol.* 2020;128(April):109462. Available from: https://doi.org/10.1016/j.lwt.2020.109462.
113. Hereu A, Bover-Cid S, Garriga M, Aymerich T. High hydrostatic pressure and biopreservation of dry-cured ham to meet the Food Safety Objectives for *Listeria monocytogenes*. *Int J Food Microbiol.* 2012;154(3):107–112. Available from: https://doi.org/10.1016/j.ijfoodmicro.2011.02.027.
114. Pérez-Baltar A, Alía A, Rodríguez A, Córdoba JJ, Medina M, Montiel R. Impact of water activity on the inactivation and gene expression of *Listeria monocytogenes* during refrigerated storage of pressurized dry-cured ham. *Foods.* 2020;9(8). Available from: https://doi.org/10.3390/foods9081092.
115. Lee SH, Choe J, Shin DJ, et al. Combined effect of high pressure and vinegar addition on the control of *Clostridium perfringens* and quality in nitrite-free emulsion-type sausage. *Innov Food Sci Emerg Technol.* 2019;52(July 2018):429–437. Available from: https://doi.org/10.1016/j.ifset.2019.02.006.
116. Teixeira JS, Maier MB, Miller P, Gänzle MG, McMullen LM. The effect of growth temperature, process temperature, and sodium chloride on the high-pressure inactivation of *Listeria monocytogenes* on ham. *Eur Food Res Technol.* 2016;242(12):2021–2029. Available from: https://doi.org/10.1007/s00217-016-2700-6.
117. Feizollahi E, Misra NN, Roopesh MS. Factors influencing the antimicrobial efficacy of Dielectric Barrier Discharge (DBD) Atmospheric Cold Plasma (ACP) in food processing applications. *Crit Rev Food Sci Nutr.* 2020;61(4):666–689. Available from: https://doi.org/10.1080/10408398.2020.1743967.
118. Yadav B, Spinelli AC, Misra NN, Tsui YY, McMullen LM, Roopesh MS. Effect of in-package atmospheric cold plasma discharge on microbial safety and quality of ready-to-eat ham in modified atmospheric packaging during storage. *J Food Sci.* 2020;85(4):1203–1212. Available from: https://doi.org/10.1111/1750-3841.15072.
119. Sommers CH, Cooke PH, Fan X, Sites JE. Ultraviolet light (254 nm) inactivation of *Listeria monocytogenes* on frankfurters that contain potassium lactate and sodium diacetate. *J Food Sci.* 2009;74(3):114–119. Available from: https://doi.org/10.1111/j.1750-3841.2009.01081.x.
120. Mutz YS, Rosario DKA, Bernardes PC, Paschoalin VMF, Conte-Junior CA. Modeling *Salmonella* Typhimurium inactivation in dry-fermented sausages: Previous habituation in the food matrix undermines UV-C decontamination efficacy. *Front Microbiol.* 2020;11(April). Available from: https://doi.org/10.3389/fmicb.2020.00591.
121. Schultze DM, Couto R, Temelli F, McMullen LM, Gänzle M. Lethality of high-pressure carbon dioxide on Shiga toxin-producing *Escherichia coli, Salmonella* and surrogate organisms on beef jerky. *Int J Food Microbiol.* 2020;321:1–8. Available from: https://doi.org/10.1016/j.ijfoodmicro.2020.108550.
122. Castillo-Zamudio RI, Paniagua-Martínez I, Ortuño-Cases C, García-Alvarado MA, Larrea V, Benedito J. Use of high-power ultrasound combined with supercritical fluids for microbial inactivation in dry-cured ham. *Innov Food Sci Emerg Technol.* 2021;67(June 2020). Available from: https://doi.org/10.1016/j.ifset.2020.102557.
123. Fernández M, Hospital XF, Cabellos C, Hierro E. Effect of pulsed light treatment on *Listeria* inactivation, sensory quality and oxidation in two varieties of Spanish dry-cured ham. *Food Chem.* 2020;316(January):126294. Available from: https://doi.org/10.1016/j.foodchem.2020.126294.
124. Liu X, Shand P, McMullen LM. Growth of *Listeria monocytogenes* on sodium reduced ham. In: *Proceedings of the 58th ICoMST.*; 2012:LOWSALTP-86.
125. Rúa J, Del Valle P, De Arriaga D, Fernández-Álvarez L, García-Armesto MR. Combination of carvacrol and thymol: Antimicrobial activity against *Staphylococcus aureus* and antioxidant activity. *Foodborne Pathog Dis.* 2019;16(9):622–629. Available from: https://doi.org/10.1089/fpd.2018.2594.
126. Serra-Castelló C, Jofré A, Belletti N, Garriga M, Bover-Cid S. Modelling the piezo-protection effect exerted by lactate on the high pressure resistance of *Listeria monocytogenes* in cooked ham. *Food Res Int.* 2021;140(July 2020). Available from: https://doi.org/10.1016/j.foodres.2020.110003.

Chapter 32

Pathogens and their sources in freshwater fish, sea finfish, shellfish, and algae

Foteini F. Parlapani[1], Ioannis S. Boziaris[1] and Christina A. Mireles DeWitt[2]

[1]*Lab of Marketing and Technology of Aquatic Products and Foods, Department of Ichthyology and Aquatic Environment, School of Agricultural Sciences, University of Thessaly, Volos, Greece,* [2]*Seafood Research and Education Center, Coastal Oregon Marine Experiment Station, Department of Food Science and Technology, College of Agricultural Sciences, Oregon State University, Astoria, OR, United States*

Abstract

Fish production is one of the most important solutions to tackle the great challenges of the 21st century, such as how to feed people in the context of a growing population. However, pathogens such as bacteria, including antimicrobial-resistant populations and viruses, can be present in the water column and fish (also including shellfish) threatening food security and public health. Pathogens can be transferred from human settlements, cropping systems, livestock systems, animal slaughtering and processing industries, and from other sources of human and animal activity, into the aquatic environment and contaminate fish. Fish contamination can be also continued in harvesting, handling, packaging, processing, and distribution, because of poor hygiene or sanitary practices in the post-farm gate. Such pathogens can end up in humans through the food value chain and fall ill after eating contaminated fish. Several pathogenic strains, serotypes or serovars of *Vibrio vulnificus*, *Vibrio parahaemolyticus*, *Vibrio cholerae*, *Salmonella enterica*, *Aeromonas* sp., *Listeria monocytogenes*, and *Clostridium botulinum* are responsible for thousands of cases and deaths associated with fish consumption around the globe. Of them, *Vibrio*, *Salmonella*, *Aeromonas*, and *L. monocytogenes* isolated from farmed fish, have been found to present antibiotic resistance to various antimicrobial agents. Researchers can now detect such pathogenic bacteria using cutting-edge methodologies for example, conventional PCR, Real-Time PCR, High-Resolution Melting, and technologies such as Next Generation Sequencing. Such innovations have immensely contributed to our understanding of how to solve problems of stakeholders related to seafood safety, minimize hazard related issues, and tackle food and economic losses in pre- and post- fish farm gate, thereby providing products of the highest safety in the world.

Keywords: Fish; pathogens; microbial contamination sources; microbial hazards; *Vibrio*; *Salmonella*; *Aeromonas*; *Listeria*; *Clostridium*; viruses; algae; outbreaks; antibiotic resistance; public health concerns; hazard detection; traditional PCR; real-time PCR; multiplex PCR; high-resolution melting; next generation sequencing; 16S rRNA amplicon sequencing; Shotgun metagenomics; whole-genome sequencing; microbial source tracking

32.1 Introduction

Fisheries and aquaculture are important sources of food, nutrition, income, and livelihoods for hundreds of millions of people worldwide. Nevertheless, the presence of pathogens such as bacteria, including antimicrobial-resistant populations and viruses in aquatic environments, threaten natural systems, fish production, and public health. Furthermore, their presence creates food and economic losses and present challenges for protection agencies, scientists, and stakeholders all around the world. Pathogens can be transferred from inland to the aquatic environment through various sources, reservoirs, and pathways, then to fish and ultimately the consumers' table through the food value chain. Biological contaminants such as foodborne pathogens have also emerged in oceans due to climate change and frequent outbreaks are predicted to occur in the future due to contaminated seafood consumption.[1] Microbiological methods, antibody-based methods, optical and electrochemical methods have been used to detect pathogens in seafood and the water column of harvesting or growing areas. Pathogens and their sources in fish during farming, primary processing in aquaculture, or the processing continuum in the food industry are now detected using cutting-edge methodologies and technologies. Novel research and digital approaches are being established as next-generation monitoring solutions to create a healthy aquatic environment and to protect public health in the context of climate

Present Knowledge in Food Safety. DOI: https://doi.org/10.1016/B978-0-12-819470-6.00056-1

change, thus contributing to the 'Sustainable Development Goals'[2] and the "One Health" approach.[3]

32.2 Microbial hazards associated with fish

Pathogens can be transferred from inland to aquatic environments by drainage or wastewater discharges that result from human and animal activity. In the food production, processing, and distribution continuum, poor hygiene and unsanitary practices can lead to pathogens from, for example, workers, equipment, working surfaces, vehicles, washing water, and ice. Pathogenic bacteria such as *Vibrio*, *Salmonella*, *Aeromonas*, *Listeria*, *Clostridium*, and viruses such as enteroviruses, hepatitis viruses, adenoviruses, rotavirus, and small round viruses for example, Norwalk virus, can contaminate finfish and shellfish. Therefore marine or freshwater fish can serve as vectors of foodborne, waterborne, or environmental pathogens that can cause human infections. Guidance for identification and control of microbial hazards associated with finfish and shellfish is provided by the US Food and Drug Administration Fish and Fishery Products Hazards and Controls Guidance.[4] This Controls Guidance helps seafood processors identify both species and processing microbial hazards. In addition, safety levels for pathogens are provided in Appendix 5: FDA and EPA Safety Levels in Regulations and Guidance Table A-5. In the same Controls Guidance, Appendix 4: Bacterial Pathogen Growth and Inactivation provides the limiting conditions for pathogen growth in Table A-1. Tables A-3 and A-4 provide inactivation conditions for *Listeria monocytogenes* and *Clostridium botulinum*. The Controls Guidance helps processors develop and implement a robust hazard analysis critical control point program to control the microbial hazards associated with seafood.

32.2.1 Vibrio

Vibrio vulnificus, *Vibrio parahaemolyticus*, and *Vibrio cholerae* are widely distributed bacteria in the aquatic environment (marine, estuarine) and frequently contaminate seafood. The consumption of raw or undercooked shellfish contaminated with toxigenic *Vibrio* strains usually causes serious human infections such as gastroenteritis, septicemia, or wound infection. *V. vulnificus* has been characterized as the most dangerous *Vibrio* species for consumer's health as it causes septicemia. This bacterium is responsible for more than 95% of raw and cooked seafood consumption-related deaths in the United States of America. The illnesses reported in the United States have often been related to the consumption of raw oysters.[5] From 1991 to 2010, *V. vulnificus* infections linked to the consumption of raw or cooked oysters were reported in 61 of 88 patients in California and 231 in other states. Of these confirmed cases, 39 (64%) and 106 (46%), respectively, died.[6] There were also 125 confirmed cases and 44 deaths in Florida, from 1981 to 1992. Of these cases, 88% of the patients with septicemia ate raw oysters.[7] The consumption of raw seafood, fish or mollusks particularly oysters and clams, or the exposure of the patients to contaminated seawater, were probably the main causes of 588 *V. vulnificus* infection cases and 285 deaths in Korea, from 2001 to 2010.[8] Taiwan and Japan also present a significant number of reported cases and deaths, while *V. vulnificus* infection cases and deaths are extremely low in Europe.[9] However, the true incidence of *V. vulnificus* is unknown in Europe due to the lack of data and publications in peer-reviewed literature.

V. parahaemolyticus is the most important cause of bacterial gastroenteritis associated with raw seafood consumption in the United States and Asia, but outbreaks are reported rarely in Europe.[10] The organism was first identified as a cause of foodborne outbreaks in Japan in 1950 when 20 ill persons died due to the consumption of contaminated cooked sardines.[11] From 1994 to 2008, there were thousands of seafood-related outbreaks and reported cases of *V. parahaemolyticus* infection sporadically in Japan.[12] In February 1996 an unusual increase of *V. parahaemolyticus* cases was documented in the Infectious Diseases Hospital in Calcutta, India. The *V. parahaemolyticus* serotype O3:K6, an identical type to those isolated from the patients in Calcutta, or its serovariants, had been spread into Asia, America, Africa, and Europe in the following months.[13] In the United States, the first confirmed foodborne outbreak from *V. parahaemolyticus* was documented due to the consumption of steamed crab in Maryland in August 1971 contaminated during transport and storage with live crab.[14,15] In 1997 outbreaks of *V. parahaemolyticus* (209 persons ill) due to the consumption of raw oysters from the United States (California, Oregon, and Washington) and Canada (British Columbia) were reported.[16] One year later, 416 infectious cases were recorded due to the consumption of raw oysters harvested from Galveston Bay in Texas, United States.[17] In 1998 the serotype O3:K6 also emerged as a principal cause of illness for the first time in the United States and then in Puerto Montt, Chile.[12] From 2004 to 2006, all reported cases caused by *V. parahaemolyticus* in Chile, were related to the serovar O3:K6. In 2007 the number of cases caused by the pandemic serotype O3:K6 decreased since 40% of the clinical cases concerned the serotype O3:K59.[18,19] However, in 2008 the findings changed, and the epidemiological status returned to the previous pattern. Nevertheless, in 2009 only 64% of the clinical cases were associated with the pandemic serotype, while the other 36% of cases were related to a non-pandemic *tdh*- and *trh*-negative strain which was identified for the first time in shellfish in 2006.[18] In Europe, some cases observed from Spanish hospital records, including two isolates belonging to the serotype O3:K6, revealed the need to include the organism in microbiological surveillance and to re-examine control programs for shellfish harvesting areas and ready-to-eat seafood.[20] *V. parahaemolyticus* infections were also documented around Europe such as Denmark, Finland, France, Italy, Norway, United Kingdom, and Sweden; of those, some infections were related to consumption of raw or lightly cooked shellfish.[12,21]

V. cholerae consists of about 200 serogroups, with only the serogroups O1, O139, O75, and O141 responsible for human illness. In particular, the serogroups O1 and O139 cause cholera, while the other serogroups cause diarrheal syndromes but not cholera. In the past, only the serogroup O1 has been historically implicated in cholera outbreaks, but the serogroup O139 (non-O1) was identified as the cause of one of the great cholera outbreaks that began in Madras (India, Asia) and spread throughout India, Thailand and Bangladesh in October 1992.[22] In the summer of 1994, *V. cholerae* O1 likely caused an outbreak of 12 cholera cases in Hong Kong, linked with seafood consumption, including shellfish, mantis shrimps and crabs.[23] Throughout the decade of the 1980s, *V. cholerae* O1 was isolated from patients who consumed crab meat in Maryland, Texas, and Louisiana in the United States.[24] In 2011 an outbreak associated with the consumption of undercooked steamed oysters harvested in Apalachicola Bay, FL, United States, contaminated with serogroup O75 was reported.[25] From 1984 to 2014, 52 vibriosis cases were recorded in the United States because of the consumption of particularly raw or undercooked oysters, clams, shrimp, and crabs contaminated with toxigenic *V. cholerae* serogroups O75 and O141.[26] Of those, the infections of serogroup O75 were linked with the consumption of raw oysters from Florida; those of serogroup O141 were linked with oysters from Florida and clams from New Jersey while some infections were linked with exposure of the patients to freshwater in Arizona, Michigan, Missouri, and Texas.[26] In Europe, raw and undercooked fish and shellfish, particularly mussels, have been implicated in the transmission of *V. cholerae* in Germany (due to fish from Nigeria), Italy, and Portugal.[27] To understand the sources of the illness, vibriosis, researchers placed much focus on studying pathogenic *Vibrio* spp in seafood (Table 32.1).

32.2.2 Salmonella

Salmonella causes foodborne illness. To date, over 2500 serotypes or serovars are known within two species; *Salmonella bongori* and *Salmonella enterica*. *S. enterica* serotype Enteritidis and *S. enterica* serotype Typhimurium have been recognized as the most important serotypes of *Salmonella* transmitted from animal to human.[71] *Salmonella* causes 1 million foodborne illnesses and approximately 30% of total foodborne deaths every year in the United States.[72,73] Salmonellosis has been linked with the consumption of, for example, cucumbers, chicken, eggs, raw tuna, pistachios, precut melon, and a variety of low-moisture foods. From 1998 to 2004, *Salmonella* was the most frequent cause of seafood-related outbreaks in the United States, mostly associated with the consumption of crustaceans including shrimp.[74] From 2007 to 2019, several outbreaks were documented in the United States due to fish consumption[75–78]:

1. an outbreak of *Salmonella* Sandiego linked to eating tuna salad at a restaurant in Washington State in 2007,
2. an outbreak of *Salmonella* Barranquilla linked to eating raw tuna or bass fish at a restaurant in Massachusetts in 2008,
3. an outbreak of *Salmonella* Paratyphi B linked to the consumption of raw ahi tuna imported from Asia in Hawaii in 2010,
4. a multi-state outbreak of *Salmonella* Bareilly and *Salmonella* Nchanga linked to consumption of frozen raw yellowfin tuna products in 2012,
5. an outbreak of *Salmonella* Paratyphi B variant L (+) tartrate (+) and *Salmonella* Weltevreden suspected of being linked to the consumption of frozen raw tuna in 2015,
6. a multistate outbreak of *Salmonella* Paratyphi linked to tuna loins in 2017,
7. an outbreak of *Salmonella* Paratyphi B infections linked to consumption of raw tuna in 2018–19 and
8. a multistate outbreak of *Salmonella* Newport infections linked to consumption of sushi made with frozen raw tuna in 2019.

In Japan, where most illnesses from seafood are caused by *V. parahaemolyticus*, *Salmonella* is another main source of illness. From 1987 to 1996, 69 *Salmonella* outbreaks and 3951 cases associated with fish and shellfish consumption were reported.[79] Seafood-borne illness outbreaks and cases related to *Salmonella* are limited in the EU and Canada.[80–82] In the EU, 1.4% (7 outbreaks) of total salmonellosis outbreaks are related to the consumption of fish and fish products, while only 1% (5 outbreaks) are linked to the consumption of crustaceans, shellfish, mollusks, and their products.[80] An outbreak of *Salmonella* Paratyphi B associated with a fish-and-chip shop[83] and an outbreak of *Salmonella* Enteritidis phage type 19 infection associated with cockles[84] occurred in the United Kingdom. In August 1991, an outbreak of *Salmonella* Paratyphi B and *Salmonella* Litchfield associated with the consumption of smoked halibut was recorded in five rural areas in Leipzig, Germany.[85] Moreover, outbreaks (60 cases, 3 deaths) of *Salmonella* Livingstone were linked to the consumption of

TABLE 32.1 The most important foodborne *Vibrio* spp and *Salmonella enterica* serovars detected in seafood worldwide.

Potential pathogen	Source	Origin	References
Vibrio parahaemolyticus	Oysters	China	28
		Korea	29
		Taiwan	30,31
		Long Island Sound, United States	32
		Chesapeake Bay, Maryland, United States	33
		Mexico's Gulf coast	34
		Sydney	35
		New Zealand	36
		Netherlands	37
	Clams	Malaysia	38
		Taiwan	31
		China	28
		North Carolina, United States	39
		Long Island Sound, United States	32
	Shrimp and fish	China	40
		China	41
		Singapore	42
	Shrimp	Malaysia	38
	Mediterranean mussels	Italy	43–45
	Blue mussels	German Wadden Sea, Germany	46
		Netherlands	37
	Greenshell mussels	New Zealand	36
	Mussels and clams	Italy	47
	Bivalves and fish fillet	Switzerland	48
	Blue crabs	Maryland, United States	49
Vibrio vulnificus	Oysters	Long Island Sound	32
		Louisiana, United States	50
	Blue crabs	Maryland, United States	49
	Clams, giant tiger prawn, mantis shrimp	China	51
	Mediterranean mussels	Italy	44,45
	Blue mussels	German Wadden Sea	46
Vibrio cholerae (containing virulence genes such as *toxR*, *rtxA*, *hlyA*, *opmU*, non-containing cholera toxin genes)	Oysters and fish	Apalachicola Bay, Florida, USA	52

(Continued)

TABLE 32.1 (Continued)

Potential pathogen	Source	Origin	References
Vibrio cholerae (noncholera virulence factors)	Fish fillets and squid	Switzerland	48
Salmonella Newport	Oysters	Thirty-six US bays of West, East and Gulf coasts	53
Salmonella Newport, Mbandaka, Braenderup, Cerro, Meunchen, I:4,12:i:2		Arizona, United States	54
Salmonella Infantis Typhimurium, Schwarzengrund, and Manhattan		Japan	55
Salmonella Paratyphi B, Seremban and Kentucky		Phang Nga Bay, Thailand	56
Salmonella Typhimurium, Enteritidis, Weltevreden and other serovars	Oysters, shrimp, freshwater fish, saltwater fish	China	57
Salmonella Weltevreden	Black tiger prawn (imported)	Japan	58
Salmonella Newport and Weltevreden	Harvested and farmed shrimp	North Western Province, Sri Lanka	59
Salmonella Potsdam, Bareilly, Braenderup, Hvittingfoss, Typhimurium, Wandsworth, Bovismorbificans, Derby, Give, Lexington, Newport, Rissen, Saintpaul, Stanley, Thompson, Aberdeen, Agona, Anatum, Havana, Heidelberg, Indiana, Javiana, Kiambu, Kottbus, Mbandaka, Urbana, Virchow, Weltevreden, 4: b:-, 3,10:r:-	Farmed freshwater fish	Vietnam	60
Salmonella Braenderup, Chester, Bareilly, Kentucky, Give, Virchow, Agona, Anatum, Corvallis, Enteritidis, Lexington, Newport, Saintpaul, Stanley, Tennessee, Thompson, Typhimurium, Urbana, Wandsworth, and Weltevreden	Shrimp	Vietnam	60
Salmonella Enteritidis (mostly PT4), Typhimurium, Bredeney, Virchow, and others for example, Stanley, Agona, Newport, San-diego, Wien, Ohio,	Bivalve molluscs such as cockles, mussels, scallops and oysters	United Kingdom	61
Salmonella Weltevreden, Anatum, Wandsworth, and Potsdam	brackishwater cultured tropical prawns	United Kingdom	62
Salmonella Blockley, and Kentucky	Mussels	Coast of Agadir, Morocco	63
Salmonella Waycross, and Salamae	Nile perch,	Lake Victoria, Tanzania	64
Salmonella Typhimurium	Sardines	Lake Victoria, Tanzania	65
Salmonella Senftenberg, Typhimurium, and Agona	Clams, cockles, mussels, oysters	Spain	66
Salmonella	Clams	Portugal	67
	Sea bass, shrimp, oysters, blood cockles	Thailand	68
	Shrimp	Thailand	69
	Shrimp (farmed) and clams	India	70

processed fish products in Norway and Sweden, and two separate outbreaks of *Salmonella* Enteritidis phage type 14b were linked to the consumption of frozen sesame prawn toast. These outbreaks occurred in Europe due to contaminated eggs used as an ingredient in the products. In Canada, an outbreak of *S.* Typhi infection (11 patients) was associated with the consumption of imported lappas (limpets, an aquatic snail[82]). *S. enterica* serotypes or serovars have been isolated mainly from fish and shellfish, including oysters, mussels, shrimp, prawns, sardines, and perch (Table 32.1).

32.2.3 Aeromonas

Aeromonas hydrophila, *Aeromonas caviae*, and *Aeromonas veronii* biovar sobria are the most important pathogens of the genus *Aeromonas*. These microorganisms can cause clinical infections for example, gastrointestinal tract diseases, infections of tissue, skin, respiratory tract, and urogenital tract, and septicemia, in humans. *Aeromonas*, especially *A. hydrophila*, have been isolated from food sources for example, raw red meat, seafood, poultry, dairy products, vegetables, and from asymptomatic and immunocompromised food-handlers.[85–87] Although it has a high incidence in fish such as whiting, trout, plaice, and salmon in European countries,[89] in grass carp in South China,[90] in fish and shrimps in Chennai, India,[91] in domestic processed catfish fillets in the United States,[92] pathogenic *A. hydrophila* does not always constitute a serious foodborne hazard.[93] In 1982, 472 cases of gastroenteritis were recorded in Louisiana due to the consumption of raw oysters harvested from the Sister Lake area in Terrebonne Parish and St. Mary's Point area in Jefferson Parish. One year later, seven more cases of gastroenteritis were reported in St. Petersburg Florida, in which oysters originated from the same area in Louisiana. Similar *A. hydrophila* bacteria were implicated in both outbreaks.[94] In Europe, outbreaks associated with *A. hydrophila* are due to the consumption of fish and meat products reported in Sweden,[95,] and raw fermented fish in Norway (Daskalov, 2006;[96]).

32.2.4 Listeria

The genus *Listeria* is composed of 8 subspecies: *L. monocytogenes, L. innocua, L. welshimeri, L. seeligeri, L. grayi, L. ivanovii, L. marthii, and L. rocourtiae.*[97] *L. monocytogenes* is the microorganism responsible for most (99%) listeriosis cases.[98] *L. monocytogenes* has been differentiated into 13 serovars with 95% of strains isolated from humans or foods being either 1/2a, 1/2b, and 4b.[99] Serovar 1/2 is most commonly associated with food.[100] Although rare, listeriosis is considered a significant public health concern because of its high mortality rate which ranges between 20%–40%.[99]

In the United States, Mead et al.[73] estimated 2518 cases of listeriosis occur annually. Symptoms of listeriosis can occur 3 days to 3 weeks after consumption. Highly susceptible individuals include the elderly, pregnant women, newborns, and the immunocompromised. According to the US National Outbreak Reporting System (NORS) there were 50 outbreaks between 2013–18, with 417 illnesses, 369 hospitalizations, and 64 deaths. The largest listeriosis outbreak, which occurred in South Africa in 2017–18, resulted in over 900 people falling ill and at least 180 deaths. The implicated product was an RTE processed meat product, called polony[101] and the identified strain was sequence type 6. Whilst none of these outbreaks occurred due to contaminated seafood consumption, both smoked fish and seafood have been named among the foods most frequently implicated elsewhere.[102,103]

In Europe, a multi-country outbreak of *L. monocytogenes* sequence type 8 linked to the consumption of salmon products, was identified through whole-genome sequencing (WGS) analysis.[104] Ready-to-eat salmon products, such as cold-smoked and marinated salmon, are the likely sources of listeriosis cases in Denmark, Germany, and France since 2015.[105] From 1995 to 2004, vacuum-packed, cold-smoked, or cold-salted fish products might be responsible for at least one-quarter of listeriosis cases (78/315) that were caused by a certain sero-genotype or closely related genotypes in Finland.[106] Vacuum-packed, cold-smoked rainbow trout was also associated with febrile gastroenteritis in Finland,[107] while another outbreak of listeriosis was linked to the consumption of rainbow trout in Sweden.[108]

The control of this pathogen is of particular concern for ready-to-eat seafood such as cooked and peeled shrimp, cold and hot smoked salmon, or seafood used for sashimi because of its ability to survive and grow at refrigeration temperatures (2°C–4°C), at high salinity (10%) levels, under both low and high pH levels (4.5–9) and osmotic pressures for example, stresses.[98,103,109,110] Contamination can occur through cross-contamination with raw materials, during processing or post-processing contamination of RTE foods. In addition, *L. monocytogenes* can create biofilms on food contact surfaces, equipment, floors, and drains. Its biofilming ability gives it a high tolerance to disinfectants and other stressors. Allen et al.[100] suggested that strains persistently established within the food processing environment, for example, niche and harborage sites, may create conditions favorable for the exchange of genetic material among different strains of *Listeria* or between *Listeria* spp. and other genera of bacteria. They also proposed that stresses persistent populations are exposed to may facilitate disinfectant tolerance and unrelated antimicrobial tolerance. Kovacevic et al.[99] reported that many strains (45%) recovered from RTE foods have a mutation that creates a premature stop codon in the *inlA* gene, which encodes a membrane-bound protein that facilitates invasion into nonprofessional phagocytes. As a result, the membrane-bound protein produced by these strains with a mutated *inlA* genotype is not fully formed and the strains, therefore as measured *in vitro*, exhibit an attenuated virulence. Kovacevic et al.[99] hypothesized that mutability of the 1/2a strains may give it a competitive advantage under stressor conditions created by food processing and may also be the reason it is recovered more frequently in food production environments than the 4b strains which are "overrepresented" in clinical cases of listeriosis. In their study, they surveyed the British Columbia food supply and found that 35% of the isolates ($n = 54$) collected contained the premature stop codon. Specifically, for fish processing facilities examined ($n = 5$), three of the facilities had isolates that did not have the premature stop codon. However, two facilities had the premature stop codon in all of their isolates. Authors also found a 3-codon deletion in 13 strains from fish processing facilities. They reported all but one (an exception was a 1/2a strain) was a 4b serotype strain and that although they had the 3-codon deletion, they did not have the premature stop codon. They further reported that in an analysis of invasiveness using Caco-2 cells, one of the 4b isolates and the 1/2a isolate with the 3-codon deletion were 4.7 and 7.1 times more invasive than a control clinical isolate. Finally, they observed that 4b strains were able to more quickly adapt to temperature shifts than 1/2a isolates. They suggest "this implies that 4b strains present in foods may quickly adapt to host temperature" and thereby be more likely to cause disease. The mutability of *L. monocytogenes* strains, such as 1/2a, makes it more resistant to stresses such as disinfectants. Although mutability is correlated with reduced virulence, it does not make it non-virulent. Since symptoms with the mutated strains of *L. monocytogenes* are arguably milder, it suggests that cases of *L. monocytogenes* outbreaks related to fish may be undercounted since they are less likely to make it to the clinical stage.

32.2.5 Clostridium

C. botulinum and *Clostridium perfringens* are spore-forming pathogenic bacteria that are significant pathogens of concern for seafood because their spores are found in the water or mud of aquatic environs. Bryan[111] also reported that small numbers of these organisms can be found in the intestines of fish and then spread to flesh during cleaning. *C. botulinum* is a gram-positive, anaerobic bacillus that forms spores. It produces a heat-labile neurotoxin under anaerobic and low acid conditions, called botulin. The consumption of foods contaminated with such toxins can cause a serious illness called botulism. The toxin attacks the body's nerves and causes paralysis of motor and autonomic nerves (usually beginning with cranial nerves), difficulty breathing, and in severe cases, death. Because of the extremely toxic nature of the toxin produced by *C. botulinum*, the potential hazard is significant in foods under anaerobic storage conditions or reduced oxygen packaging (e.g., vacuum or modified atmosphere packaging—MAP without or with low oxygen) and strategies for controlling pathogen growth shall be applied (FDA, 2020).

Seven different types of neurotoxin have been identified (A, B, C, D, E, F, and G); however, types A, B, and E cause the most human illnesses.[112] In the aquatic environment, *C. botulinum* type E is the most prevalent in fish, water, and sediments of temperate waters, while types C and D usually dominate in those of tropical waters.[113,114] Several botulism outbreaks have been linked with the consumption of raw, undercooked, smoked, stale, or fermented seafood. The FDA's Fish and Fishery Products Hazards and Control Guidance (FDA, 2020) suggests that about 10 outbreaks of foodborne botulism occur in the United States every year. In a recent review by Sheng and Wang,[115] they reported from data collected from the US NORS a total of 14 outbreaks of *C. botulinum* in a twenty-year span (1998–2018) associated with seafood. These outbreaks resulted in 38 illnesses and 23 hospitalizations. Although outbreaks and illnesses represented only 2% and 1%, respectively, of all fish-associated outbreaks in the United States in that time span, the hospitalizations from *C. botulinum* illnesses represented 7.4% of all hospitalizations. Mortality is high as a result of *C. botulinum* intoxication and death is likely if antitoxin and respiratory support are not provided (FDA, 2020). Unfortunately, in the United States, most botulism cases are associated with home-canned, fermented, or smoked foods; however, fermented and salted seafood is also amongst the foods commonly associated with outbreaks.[111,116,117] From 1971 to 1984, seafood for example, raw, parboiled, or fermented meats from marine mammals, and fermented salmon eggs or fish, were also related to 61 outbreaks of food-borne botulism in Canada (122 cases, 21 deaths). Of these, 58 outbreaks were associated with *C. botulinum*, with type E dominating (52 outbreaks) among them.[118] In Europe, five cases of botulinum neurotoxin type E associated with the consumption of dried salted fish were reported in Germany and Spain in November 2016.[119] In 1964 fermented trout was the source of 16 outbreaks in Norway. From 1951 to 1984, 80% of the outbreaks in Denmark were caused by type E, almost all associated with fish consumption. In Sweden, five incidents were linked with fish consumption since 1969.[120] In South Africa, for the first time in 2002 two children died from consuming commercially produced tinned fish in tomato sauce, contaminated with a type A botulinum toxin.[121] The canning process was followed correctly; however, the cans were discarded and therefore exposed to the elements, after which pinholes developed and the organism gained entrance, where it produced the toxin. In 1991 18 individuals also died due to the consumption of a fish product called *faseikh* (uneviscerated, salted mullet fish) contaminated with E botulinal toxin, in Egypt.[122] To prevent foodborne botulism, vegetative cells, which are responsible for toxin production, and spores, are inactivated during thermal processing of foods in hermetically sealed containers. Additionally, growth and toxin formation by *C. botulinum* types A, B, E, and F can be prevented by controlling the level of acidity (pH) in the finished product to 4.6 or below, water activity to 0.85 or below by drying, and the amount of salt in the product to 20% water phase salt or more (FDA, 2020).

C. perfringens is an anaerobic gram-positive spore-forming bacterium. It is found naturally in soil and the intestinal tract of humans and warm-blooded animals. In general, it is known that the isolates of this type of *Clostridium* are defined by the production of alpha and iota toxins, however, there is a lack of knowledge about the pathogenesis of *C. perfringens* type E infections in humans.[123] *C. perfringens* thrives in high protein foods because of a preference for amino acids.[124] Onset of intoxication occurs within 8–16 h because toxins are produced in the gastrointestinal tract.[125,126] Since the duration of symptoms for *C. perfringens* is short, usually less than 24 h, it often goes undiagnosed. There are few reports on the presence of *C. perfringens* in seafood.[111] Bryan[111] suggests that mishandling and mistreatment of seafood is a common reason for *C. perfringens* illnesses. He explains that the spores of *C. perfringens* can reach fish and shellfish in water habitats (near sewage outfalls especially) from surfaces of holds in vessels, and surfaces of equipment and utensils used for processing. Although *C. perfringens* spores are highly heat resistant, exposure to high temperatures for example, at 90°C–100°C for 10–30 min, can reduce the number of *C. perfringens* spores by more than 90%.[127] Vegetative cells from germinated spores can multiply in cooked products when temperatures fall below 50°C and growth is very rapid at 46°C. Illness occurs at 10^6 or higher CFU/g. As a result, *C. perfringens* illnesses usually occur because of inadequate processing or preparation conditions such as improper cooling (rapidly cool <4.4°C/40F) or hot-holding at the wrong temperatures.[111] Examples of correct hot holding temperatures are ≥57°C (135F) for a maximum of 8 h or 60°C (140F) indefinitely.[128,129]

32.2.6 Viruses

Viruses are small acellular structures consisting of RNA or DNA with a protein coat. Enteric viruses replicate in the intestinal tract and are excreted through feces.[130] According to Butt et al.,[117] about half of all seafood-related outbreaks with confirmed etiology are caused by viruses in the United States each year. Khora,[130] reported viral disease associated with seafood being ~5% for hepatitis A (HAV) and 12%–47% for norovirus (NoV). Viruses in seafood typically come from raw or undercooked seafood harvested from waters contaminated with human feces or contaminated during post-harvest handling as a result of person-to-person spread through the fecal-oral route. Filter-feeding shellfish can accumulate viruses at a higher level than their natural occurrence in seawater.[130] These include oysters, clams, crabs, and lobsters.[130] Viruses can be destroyed by cooking; their inactivation occurs faster at temperatures ≥50°C than at temperatures ≤50°C.

Noroviruses (originally referred to as Norwalk-like viruses) were discovered from an outbreak in Norwalk, Ohio (United States) and are a type of human calicivirus. Noroviruses are the most frequent cause of nonacute gastroenteritis in the United States.[117] The infectious dose has been estimated to be as low as 100 particles[117] and the incubation period is 18–48 h. Thermal inactivation to achieve a 5-log reduction of murine NoV (a typical surrogate for human NoV studies) in shellfish meat has been demonstrated at 72°C in 10 s.[131] Duration of illness typically lasts 24–48 h. Sources are typically raw shellfish that have been exposed to human waste in harvest areas. NoV infection occurs most frequently from the consumption of raw oysters, but also mussels, cockles, and clams.[117] Outbreaks are associated mostly with the elderly in institutional settings, restaurants, schools, and vacation settings.[117]

HAV outbreaks associated with the consumption of shellfish have been recorded since 1956. In particular, the first reported seafood-related outbreak worldwide, occurred in Sweden and was associated with oyster consumption.[117] In the United States, the first such outbreak was in 1961 also due to the consumption of raw oysters in Mississippi Alabama[132] and raw clams in New Jersey.[133] Other outbreaks were associated with the consumption of raw or undercooked oysters, clams, cockles, whelks, mussels, prawns, and scallops, around the globe, from 1956 to 2016.[134] Contamination typically occurs from the pollution of aquatic habitats but can also result from contamination from workers, equipment or the processing environment. HAV is more resistant to chlorination than many other enteric viruses.[117] Iwamato et al. (2010) also reported that HAV is relatively heat resistant and can withstand steaming (such as what is used for clams) for short periods. Studies have demonstrated that in a protein environment (shellfish meat) it can take more than 15 min to achieve a 5-log reduction at 80°C.[135] Shellfish concentrate the virus several-fold due to filtration activities. The infectious dose is estimated to be between 10 and 100 particles. Incubation is 3–6 weeks and is then followed by fatigue, nausea, and upper abdominal discomfort.[117] Aside from HAV and NoV, other reported viruses with documented associations to seafood include calciviruses (shellfish), astroviruses (mussels, oysters), enterically transmitted non-A non-B hepatitis (shellfish), aichivirus (oysters), coxsackieviruses (shellfish), hepatitis E (shrimp, salmon, cod, mussels, hake, and squid), parvovirus (source not reported), poliovirus (shellfish), rotavirus (sewage), sapovirus (oysters, cockles, and smooth clams).[130]

32.3 Algae

Seaweed or marine macro algae are different from plants because they lack specialized tissues such as a root system and vascular structures.[136] The past decade has seen an increase in the commercialization of macro algae for food, especially as they are viewed as ecologically friendly,[137] using relatively fewer resources for their production and adding oxygen to seawater. The top seven most cultivated seaweed taxa are used either to produce carrageenan (*Eucheuma* spp., *Kapphycus alvarezii*), agar (*Gracilaria* spp), or human food (*Saccharina joponic*, *Undaria pinnatifida*, *Pyropia* spp, and *Sargassum fusiforme*). The top producers of aquacultured macro algae are China and Indonesia and for wild harvested macro algae, Chile, China, and Norway lead the way with kelp being the species most often targeted.[138]

In the aquatic environment, it has been established that the macro algal surface hosts a diverse group of bacteria with densities of 10^2 to 10^7 cells/cm^2.[136] Community patterns have been established as more species are conspecific[139] and not as tightly tied to the geography of their growth. This means that algae of the same species in different growing waters still seem to have more in common with their bacterial communities than dissimilar macroalgae growing in the same waters.[139] There is also evidence that macroalgal-associated bacteria contribute to host defenses against unwanted biofilm fouling and provide antimicrobial activities.[136] There is limited information, however, concerning pathogens associated with seaweed cultivation. In a risk assessment of product-related undesirable compounds, Stévant et al. [140] indicated that seaweed may accumulate heavy metals (lead, mercury, cadmium, and arsenic) or toxic levels of certain minerals (iodine, manganese, and zinc). They do note that there are few studies linking consumption to negative consequences other than perhaps the effects of high iodine content in some brown algae. They also note that the government of Norway is working on establishing a regulatory framework for the consumption of seaweed as human or animal food. A risk assessment conducted on seaweed by the National Food Institute in Denmark was released on July 31, 2019. The conclusions they came to were that seaweed consumption by the general population would be of low health risk for mercury, cadmium, and lead.[141] A similar assessment for food safety, however, was even more recently published by Banach et al.[142] The authors reviewed the literature, interviewed food safety experts, and conducted a workshop to better identify key standards to ensure safe food and feed from seaweed. From this work, they identified knowledge gaps which included physical hazards (ropes, plastics), effects of processing on seaweed, contamination transfer rate to seaweed, and the effect of antifouling or protective coatings on structures near seaweed cultivation, as well as seaweed type, adaptation, and farming practices.

32.4 Source of fish microbial contamination

32.4.1 Preharvest (prefarm gate)

Fish can be contaminated from inland sources with a wide range of bacterial and viral pathogens since the aquatic environment is strongly linked to the land. Rapid urbanization and industrialization coupled with an increase in human population have caused the degradation of aquatic environments around the world. Human settlements, industries, and agriculture are the major causes of contamination of water, sediment, and seafood in the coastal areas, rivers, estuaries, and lakes. In high-income countries, agriculture is the most important source of contamination of rivers, streams, wetlands, lakes, and coastal waters as opposed to human settlements and industries.[143]

32.4.1.1 Cropping systems

Tile drains or artificial subsurface drainage are used to drain agricultural fields of crop production. In Iowa (United States), tile drainage takes place extensively in cropland where artificial drainage has been characterized as the major pathway for *Enterobacter* to contaminate surface waters.[144] In general, tile drainage can serve as a means of transporting enteric pathogens for example, *Salmonella*, *Enterococcus*, and *E. coli* O157:H7, from the field to the broader surface water and further in rivers, lakes, and seas. The presence of these bacteria in surface waters usually occurs after manure application in the field.[144,145] Surface runoffs from agricultural fields are also a potential source of pathogen contamination to surrounding watersheds, usually during rainstorms.[146] Agricultural runoff is a dynamic environmental polluter when agricultural fields have been fertilized with liquid manure which often includes foodborne pathogens such as Shiga toxin-producing *E. coli* (STEC), *Salmonella*, *Campylobacter*, *Enterococcus*, and *Listeria*.[147,148]

Moreover, it occurs when irrigation water contaminated with human sewage or minimally treated biosolids has been applied in the field.[146] *E. coli* O157:H7 has been found in plant tissue because of the application of contaminated manure or irrigation of the crop with contaminated water in the field.[149] Potential pathogens such as *Staphylococcus, Klebsiella, Listeria*, and *Salmonella* have also been found in polluted river water, for example, the Plankenburg and Eerste Rivers in the Western Cape, South Africa. Contamination was due to the presence of informal settlements in the vicinity.[150] In artificial experiments, *E. coli* O157, *L. monocytogenes*, *Campylobacter jejuni*, and *Salmonella* (Typhimurium and Enteritidis) have survived in stored slurry and dirty water for months. This makes the application of organic waste products a potential source of pathogens entering the food chain.[151]

32.4.1.2 Livestock systems

Livestock production has increased dramatically, particularly in the urban areas of developing countries. The increase in animal production together with the high animal densities in livestock systems has led to the concentration of high manure quantities on the land. It has been estimated that 1.1 billion tons of manure in the United States were produced from 2.2 billion heads of livestock and poultry in 2007.[152] About one-third of livestock waste (cattle, pigs, poultry, and sheep) includes at least one pathogen such as *Escherichia coli* O157:H7, *Listeria, Salmonella*, or *Campylobacter*.[153] The production of waste in livestock systems sometimes exceeds the buffering capacity of surrounding systems, thus polluting surface and ground water.[143] Therefore livestock waste carrying foodborne pathogens, including enteric bacteria and viruses, can enter the aquatic environment and contaminate fish. Such pathogens have been isolated mainly from bivalves such as oysters, mussels, and clams, but also crustaceans such as shrimp and crabs. Also, foodborne pathogens such as *Salmonella* and antibiotic-resistant bacteria, have been found in the water of various fishponds in China, where many of the ponds were contaminated with human- and pig-associated fecal bacteria.[154]

32.4.1.3 Human settlements

Pathogens can be transferred from human settlements into the aquatic environments via the fecal-oral route by sewage, overflow, discharge, and groundwater. Fifty percent of the human population lives in urban areas, which are mostly located close to the sea or rivers. In megacities where over 10 million people live, sewage is the main source of contamination of rivers and seas. Sewage effluent contains municipal waste, water, and waste from domestic toilets, food and feed waste, fecal matter from pets and urban wildlife for example, birds, bats, and mammals. The surface and groundwater are often contaminated with pathogenic bacteria such as *Salmonella* and *E. coli* O157:H7 and viruses from the digestive tracts of wild animals, including food animals such as poultry, pigs, cattle, sheep and deer, and domestic animals (cats, dogs, birds, and horses) in urban and rural areas.[155,156] Indeed, similarities in bacterial diversity between fecal samples (chicken, pig, and human) and water samples have indicated fecal contamination from animals and humans in several locations around the major inflow rivers (Tiaoxi River) of Taihu Lakes in China.[157]

In Africa, Lake Victoria which borders the three East African countries of Uganda, Tanzania, and Kenya, is heavily polluted with microbial pathogens, chemicals, and suspended solids, mainly due to direct activities on the lake, untreated raw sewage, industrial effluent, runoff and storm water inflow. Serious waterborne diseases such as cholera, typhoid, and dysentery, are the main health problems for people in the Lake Victoria region. These problems are usually associated with the exposure of people to the lake's water for example, for fishing, swimming, and washing (Karanja, 2006). Pathogens and potentially emerging pathogens such as *L. monocytogenes, V. parahaemolyticus, E. coli, Klebsiella pneumoniae, S. enterica, Yersinia enterocolitica, Serratia mercescens, Provindencia rettgeri, Enterobacter aerogenes, Enterobacter cloacae, Morganella morganii, Proteus vulgaris, Proteus mirabilis* have also been isolated from both the water and freshwater fish of the lake for example, Nile tilapia. Such pathogens are also present in fish worldwide but at lower frequencies and abundances.[158] Similarly, raw domestic and industrial effluents from surrounding urban areas are the main sources of water and fish contamination with *E. coli* O157:H7 in Lake Chivero in Zimbabwe.[159]

In freshwater fish farms, inflow water from rivers can be a major source of fish contamination with *Salmonella* and multidrug-resistant bacteria.[160] The wastewater treatment plants cannot always manage the large quantities of waste resulting from the discharge of non-treatment wastes into water bodies, thus transporting pathogens into the aquatic environments. Various opportunistic human pathogens such as *A. hydrophila*, and *V. cholerae* have been isolated from wild fish harvested from locations up to 12 km from the point of treated wastewater discharge.[161] Storm water runoff and sewer overflows/floods in urban areas are also leading causes of transporting pathogenic bacteria and viruses from soil and road surfaces to rivers and coastal waters.

32.4.1.4 Industries

Wastewater from slaughterhouses is also involved in environmental contamination with various enteric pathogenic bacteria and viruses. Pathogens such as *S. enterica, Y. enterocolitica,*

E. coli including STEC, hepatitis E virus, and bovine enterovirus from animal processing wastewaters (cattle and sheep)[162–164] can escape into the surrounding environment, enter the water bodies, end up in the aquatic environment and contaminate seafood.[163] Fish can be contaminated with such pathogens as well as multidrug-resistant bacteria, from inflow water during farming.[160] In their study, the above researchers detected such bacteria in the water, sediment, feed, and trout samples (including marketed trout).

32.4.2 Postharvest (postfarm gate)

In the processing of fish, contamination can occur from the environment for example, air, workers, unsanitary equipment and working surfaces, insects, birds, washing water, ice, boxes, and vehicles, due to inadequate hygiene practices. Enteric pathogens of human or animal origin for example, *E. coli*, *Salmonella*, *Enterococcus*, *Enterobacter*, *Klebsiella*, *Shigella* as well as viruses and bacteria associated with workers' nose, throat, and skin for example, *S. aureus*, bacteria associated with unsanitary equipment and working surfaces for example, *L. monocytogenes*, and bacteria associated with skin, gills and digestive tract of fish for example, *C. botulinum* can enter the post-harvest process and contaminate seafood. Bacteria such as *Acinetobacter, Bacillus, Brevundimonas, Comamonas, Escherichia, Enterococcus, Enterobacter, Klebsiella, Legionella, Listeria, Staphylococcus, Stenotrophomonas, Sphingomonas*, and *Shigella*, have been found in seafood such as gilt-head seabream,[165] blue crabs[166] and rose shrimp.[167] The above-mentioned researchers linked the presence of those taxa in fish with inadequate hygiene practices during fishing/harvesting, handling, and/or packaging in ice, on fishing boats. Such bacteria for example, *E. coli*, *Enterococcus*, and *S. aureus* can sometimes be present in ice used for fish preservation in marketplaces.[168] It is therefore important to make ice from acceptable drinking water.

32.5 Fish, antibiotic resistance, and other public health concerns

Antibiotic resistance is rising to dangerously high levels around the world.[169] The close contact of bacteria with the antibiotic-contaminated domestic, hospital, industrial, or agricultural wastes may apply selective pressure to those bacteria that live in the environment resulting in increased antibiotic resistance. Pathogenic bacteria carrying antimicrobial resistance genes (ARGs) are often released with wastewater discharges into aquatic environments[170] and contaminate seafood. The presence of antibiotic-resistant bacteria in foods threatens the efficacy of human drugs when they colonize humans.[171]

Over the past few decades, antibiotic resistance has increased globally in animal farms as a result of the use of antibiotics for animal health and productivity.[172,173] In cattle farming, various antibiotics for example, amoxicillin, ceftiofur, cephapirin, cloxacillin, hetacillin, penicillin, ampicillin, ceftiofur, and pirlimycin are used against streptococcal or staphylococcal mastitis. In poultry farming, tetracycline, tylosin, salinomycin, bacitracin, virginiamycin, and bambermycin are often used.[174] In addition, antibiotics are also used as antimicrobial growth promoters in some countries. These include tetracyclines, ionophores, and penicillins. Antibiotics and antibiotic-resistant bacteria can move from farms through the water to natural ecosystems, including the aquatic environment and fish-growing waters. Moreover, the vigorous growth of aquaculture activity all over the world to meet increasing food demand for global population growth has been accompanied by a rapid increase in the use of antimicrobials, including those commonly used in human therapy. Antibiotics for example, oxytetracycline, sulphadiazine, florfenicol, sulfadimethoxine, erythromycin, amoxicillin, and enrofloxacin are usually used in aquaculture in Vietnam, China, and Bangladesh being the greatest users.[175] In the United States, antibiotics (approximately 80%) are used for livestock growth or prophylactic purposes in agriculture and aquaculture, while other countries have banned antibiotic use for animal growth.[176,177] The excessive use of antibiotics in aquaculture has led to a plethora of concerns for agencies, authorities, and researchers in the fields of environment, food safety, and public health, globally.[169,178] The 80% of antimicrobials used in aquaculture enter the environment and permit the increase of antibiotic-resistant bacteria amongst the susceptible bacteria, thereby affecting biodiversity in aquatic environments and the fish and shellfish microbiomes.[170] *Vibrio*, *Salmonella*, *E. coli*, *Enterobacter*, *Aeromonas*, and *L. monocytogenes* isolated from aquaculture water, raw or processed wild or farmed fish, and fish processing plants, have been found to present antibiotic resistance to various antimicrobial agents.[179–181] For example, in oyster aquaculture sites in Korea, *V. parahaemolyticus* was found to present resistance to vancomycin, ampicillin, and streptomycin.[181] *V. parahaemolyticus* isolated from the water of bivalve mollusks harvesting areas (Subaé river, Brazil) and the tissues of bivalve mollusks were resistant to ampicillin, cephalothin, chloramphenicol, and imipenem.[182] Resistance to antibiotics such as streptomycin, ampicillin, and cephalothin[41] or ampicillin, gentamicin, ciprofloxacin, levofloxacin, chloramphenicol, and tetracycline[183] was also observed in *V. parahaemolyticus* isolates collected from fish and shrimp from retail markets in China. Moreover, the majority of *A. hydrophila* isolates obtained from retailed grass carp were found to present resistance to ampicillin, tetracycline, and streptomycin.[90] *Salmonella* isolates from frozen imported freshwater fish originating from Thailand, India, Bahrain, Myanmar, and, Vietnam, to Saudi Arabia (supermarkets and grocery stores), were also found to be resistant to tetracycline, ampicillin, and amoxicillin-clavulanic acid.[184] In retail fish markets of Kerala, India, *L. monocytogenes* isolates from various fish products, presented resistance to ampicillin, penicillin, erythromycin, tetracycline, and clindamycin.[97] *L. monocytogenes* isolated from fish processing plants in Poland, were also found to be resistant to erythromycin, trimethoprim/sulfamethoxazole, penicillin, ampicillin, meropenem.[185] Additionally, antibiotic-resistant bacteria found in aquatic environments might originate from hospitals. Nosocomial antibiotic-resistant pathogens such as vancomycin-resistant enterococci (VRE) are often found in hospital-wastewater treatment plants. The ability of VRE to present high resistance to antimicrobials used in human therapy makes the treatment uncertain for the patient. Such pathogens can sometimes survive after waste processing and escape into the natural environment.[186] VRE have been isolated from both nonhuman sources, such as animals, birds and environmental samples, and from farmers and nonhospitalized humans.[187]

The widespread presence of microplastics in aquatic environments is an increasing concern for the spread of antibiotic-resistant bacteria. Potential pathogens such as *Aeromonas salmonicida, E. coli, V. parahaemolyticus, V. cholerae*, and *V. vulnificus*, that may contain antibiotic resistance genes, have been found on microplastics.[188] It is estimated that 5 trillion microparticles are floating on the waters, globally.[189] Plastic products, plastic pellets, and expanded polystyrene particles usually come from domestic, industrial, and fishing activity.[190] In the terrestrial environment, plastics contaminated with antibiotics from industrial, hospital, or agricultural wastes may cause resistance to the bacteria that colonize plastics. In the open sea, plastic serves as a new ecological habitat that promotes microbial colonization from the surrounding water and biofilm formation.[191] Potential pathogenic vibrios have been found in microplastic-associated biofilms among other bacterial species.[192] Winds and currents can transfer and dispense the plastic-attached bacteria across the open sea,[193] thus allowing pathogens, including antibiotic-resistant bacteria, to be transmitted to fish and shellfish and threatening the public's health.

32.6 New trends in the detection of microbial hazards

32.6.1 Detection methods

PCR-based methods such as traditional PCR, Real-time PCR, Multiplex PCR, and high-resolution melting (HRM) have been used to detect pathogens, including antibiotic-resistant bacteria. In foods, pathogenic bacteria usually present in very low cell numbers (1−100 cells). In such cases, enrichment steps are essential for pathogen detection before molecular analysis. In particular, the food matrix for example, fish tissue, has to be homogenated with a pre-enrichment medium or further with other enrichment media that allow stressed or injured cells to recover and the number of cells to increase to detectable population levels. Afterward, plating onto selective agar media and confirmation of the isolates can be followed by PCR-based methods (culture-dependent analysis). Alternatively, the culture-dependent approach is avoided, and samples can be taken directly from an enrichment step to be used for the molecular analysis (culture-independent analysis). Currently, researchers are attempting to develop intelligent culture-independent approaches to detect pathogens in an extremely short time using PCR-based analysis avoiding the time-consuming enrichment steps (no data publicly available yet).

32.6.1.1 PCR based methods

PCR-based methods have been recognized as the most important and reliable methods for pathogen detection. In seafood microbiology, PCR-based methods have been used as research tools to explore seafood microbiota, for example, potential pathogens and spoilers or to detect toxigenic/virulence genes or ARGs.

32.6.1.2 Traditional PCR

Traditional PCR has been used to study the presence of potential pathogens such as *V. parahaemolyticus*, based on toxigenic/virulence genes (e.g., *toxR*, *tlh*, *tdh*, *trh*), in shellfish such as mussels.[194,195] Additionally, traditional PCR has been combined with ELISA into a single analytical technique (PCR-ELISA) for the detection of *V. parahaemolyticus* and *C. botulinum* in seafood.[196,197]

There are also studies on the development of rapid protocols for pathogen detection based on traditional PCR in which researchers attempted to reduce the duration of the enrichment steps. For example, Kumar et al.[198] developed a rapid and sensitive 8-h PCR assay (8-h enrichment) for the detection of *Salmonella* serovars such as *S.* Typhi, *S.* Typhimurium, *S.* Enteritidis, *S.* Mbandaka, *S.* Bareilly, and *S.* Weltevreden in seafood, using samples of fish, shrimps, mussels, crabs, oysters and clams from local fish markets in Cochin (India). According to the aforementioned researchers, this method can give reliable results within one working day.

32.6.1.3 Real-time PCR

Real-time PCR is a fast and reliable molecular method for the detection and quantification of pathogens in foods, including seafood, in which the amplification of a targeted DNA region is monitored in real-time. In international literature, there is a multitude of publications focused on the detection of pathogens in seafood. Since the contaminated seafood may lead to serious health problems for the consumer, there is a need to develop rapid and reliable Real-Time PCR-based protocols for pathogen detection. Several real-time PCR protocols have been developed for the detection of the most important foodborne pathogens in seafood such as *V. vulnificus* in oysters[199] and clams,[200] *V. parahaemolyticus* in oysters[201] and shrimp,[202] *V. parahaemolyticus*, *V. cholerae* and *V. vulnificus* in Alaska pollock, striped catfish and Black tiger prawn[203] and in other various fish species and clams.[204] Scientists are attempting to develop intelligent ways to detect pathogens by avoiding an enrichment step before Real-time PCR analysis, using alternative approaches for example, spiking assays.[205] In their study, Taminiau et al.[205] used pathogenic bacteria such as *C. jejuni*, *Campylobacter coli*, enterohemorrhagic *E. coli*, *Salmonella* spp., *V. parahaemolyticus*, and *V. vulnificus* as reference strains in various populations and artificially contaminated raw shrimp, cooked shrimp, and raw mussels.[205] The researchers concluded that their real-time PCR protocols may be suitable alternative methods compared to the classical ones to ensure the absence of foodborne pathogens.

32.6.1.4 High-resolution melting

HRM analysis is a simple, highly sensitive, specific, closed-tube, and low-cost approach,[206] which has been used (1) to evaluate genetic diversity and subtype at species/subspecies level; (2) to recognize phylogenetic groupings; (3) to identify antimicrobial resistance; (4) to detect and screen for mutations related to drug-resistance; (5) to discriminate gene isoforms, in real-time.[207] HRM analysis has been applied for the detection of foodborne pathogens such as *Salmonella* spp.,[208–210] *Listeria* spp,[211] *L. monocytogenes*,[209,210] *Shigella*, *Staphylococcus aureus*, *Vibrio parahaemolyticus*,[210] *E. coli* O157,[209,212] diarrheagenic *E. coli*,[210] and *Bacillus cereus*.[213] Additionally, HRM has recently been proposed as a tool for rapid differentiation and cost-effective identification of bacterial species isolated from seafood.[214,215]

32.6.1.5 Multiplex PCR

Multiplex PCR is another PCR-based method for pathogen detection that uses multiple primers in one PCR. This method has been used for the detection of, for example, *V. parahaemolyticus* in octopus, manta ray pangasius, and boiled frozen mussels,[216] *V. vulnificus* in oysters,[217] *E. coli*, *S.* Typhimurium, *V. vulnificus*, *V. cholerae* and *V. parahaemolyticus* in oysters,[218] *V. parahaemolyticus*, *V. cholerae*, *V. vulnificus* in raw and cooked seafood,[219] *Salmonella* spp. and *Shigella* spp. in mussels,[220] *Salmonella* spp. in seafood and seafood handling environments,[221] *Yersinia enterocolitica* in mussels, shrimp and cephalopods,[222] antibiotic-resistant *V. parahaemolyticus* and *V. vulnificus* in oysters[223] and antibiotic-resistant *L. monocytogenes* in seafood.[224] Multiplex PCR has also been used for the development of a method for the detection of *V. parahaemolyticus, Salmonella* spp., and *L. monocytogenes* in raw shrimp without a prior enrichment step.[225] Additionally, multiplex PCR protocols have been developed for simultaneous detection of pathogens such as *Salmonella* spp. and *L. monocytogenes* in fish, vegetables, bivalves, cephalopods, crustaceans, ready-to-eat foods, byproducts, and environmental samples.[226] Multiplex PCR has been suggested as a suitable approach for the simultaneous and reliable detection of foodborne pathogens in food and environmental samples.

32.6.1.6 Next-generation sequencing

Over the last decade, the development of high-throughput technologies such as next-generation sequencing (NGS) is providing us with new ways to analyze microbial and functional diversity directly from the samples.[227–229] These technologies have reduced significantly the time and cost required for the in-depth analysis of microbial communities.

16S rRNA amplicon sequencing (16S NGS) analysis has been used to explore the composition of bacterial communities in seafood for example, gilt-head seabream,[165] Atlantic salmon,[230] Atlantic cod,[231] thawed European plaice, and South African hake, and deep-water Cape,[232] thawed common cuttlefish,[165] blue crab[166] and deepwater rose shrimp.[214] These studies revealed various potential spoilers and potential pathogens in such aquatic products. Of the potential pathogens, some came from the water column of fish harvesting or growing areas as natural microbiota of the water or contaminants from inland, while others came from various sources of contamination. Such sources include harvesting, handling, primary processing in aquaculture or fisheries facilities, and distribution. However, 16 S rRNA amplicon sequencing is not appropriate for pathogen detection since it is based on the phylogenetic 16 S rRNA gene. Therefore the 16 S rRNA amplicon sequencing analysis can only be used for the assessment of the bacterial communities up to a genus level by estimating the relative abundances of the bacteria.

On the other hand, *Shotgun metagenomics* can identify bacteria, viruses, and fungi at a higher resolution identification level (species or strain level) than the 16S rRNA amplicon sequencing. In food microbiology, Shotgun metagenomics has been used for the detection of STEC in spiked spinach samples[233] and other pathogens in the beef production chain.[234] Apart from the identification of species or strain level, Shotgun metagenomics can be used for the estimation of metabolic pathways and antibiotic resistance genes in various samples for example, fish gut.[235] Shotgun metagenomics could be a promising research tool for the detection of foodborne pathogens in seafood and in identifying sources of microbial contamination from farm-to-fork.

WGS can determine the whole genome of an organism (the order of bases in the genome of an organism). In foods, including seafood, WGS has been used to characterize and subtype the most important foodborne pathogens such as *L. monocytogenes*,[236,237] *S. enterica*,[222] *E. coli*[238,] and *V. parahaemolyticus*.[10,239–241] Moreover, the European Food Safety Authority (EFSA)[242] has been reporting the possible use of molecular typing methods for example, WGS, to assess antimicrobial resistance of pathogens such as *Salmonella*, *C. coli*, *C. jejuni*, *E. coli*, *Enterococcus faecalis*, *Enterococcus faecium* and methicillin-resistant *Staphylococcus aureus*. The food industry has begun discussing with scientists the application of WGS for microbial source tracking (MST) and pathogen detection, including virulence and antibiotic resistance genes.[243] The extensive application of WGS by the food industry might lead us to differentiate the strains that persist in processing facilities from those that enter from an outside source.[243]

32.6.2 Monitoring of microbial safety

MST is an environmental monitoring approach to monitor the sources of microbial contamination. In aquaculture, MST has been used to predict the presence of fecal pollution and estimate the level of hygiene and sanitation in water used for extensive and semi-intensive fish culture.[244] Microbiological, genotypic, phenotypic, molecular, and analytical methods have been applied in MST to detect and identify the host or the environment from which the microorganisms originate.[245,246] However, these approaches are not simple to apply for routine analysis for scientists to solve stakeholder problems rapidly (e.g., aquaculture sector, fish processing industry, retailers, and inspection authorities) that are associated with microbial safety of seafood along the production chain, during handling, in the processing continuum, during transportation and placing on the market.

Currently, HRM has been proposed as a promising tool for detecting the source of microbial contamination along the seafood chain, based on similarities of the HRM curve profiles between fish samples and samples from the potential contamination sources.[158,214,215] Parlapani[158] suggested HRM as a tool to monitor hygiene indicators and pathogens, including antibiotic-resistant bacteria, from farm to fork, based on the presence or absence and similarity of HRM curves of specific genes for example, toxigenic or antimicrobial resistance of pathogens. The new HRM-based hazard monitoring concept by Parlapani[158] can help seafood microbiologists rapidly solve problems that stakeholders have related to microbial fish quality or safety in aquaculture, fish processing, distribution, and placing on the market. This will contribute to minimizing food and economic losses in aquaculture and the fish industry as well as prevent future illness cases and deaths from these toxigenic strains that might be present in seafood.

32.7 Speculation on future challenges

32.7.1 Climate change and pathogens

The abundance and occurrence of pathogens are expected to increase in the future as a result of climate change. NASA has already reported in 'Bacteria Thrive as Ocean Warms'[1] in 2018 that the increasing sea surface temperatures can cause a rise in the abundance of *Vibrio* spp. and so cause an increase of vibriosis cases due to seafood consumption, particularly shellfish. Such bacteria also contain populations that are usually susceptible to various antibiotics of veterinary and human significance, characterizing them as contaminants of emerging concern. To tackle new challenges, the detection and monitoring of such contaminants along the seafood production chain, using cutting edge technologies such as NGS (e.g., Shotgun metagenomics) and WGS and PCR-based methodologies such as Real-time PCR, Multiplex PCR, and HRM, have to be established. Additionally, scientists are attempting to develop digital approaches as next-generation solutions for pathogen monitoring from farm-to-fork. Such technologies, methodologies, and approaches will contribute to creating a healthy aquatic environment and protecting public health in the context of climate change and antimicrobial resistance, to address the "Sustainable Development Goals" and the "One Health" approach.

References

1. National Aeronautics and Space Administration (NASA). Bacteria Thrive as Ocean Warms. 2018. <https://earthobservatory.nasa.gov>.
2. Food and Agriculture Organization (FAO). FAO and the 17 Sustainable Development Goals. 2015. <https://sustainabledevelopment.un.org/content/documents/2205FAO%20and%20the%2017%20SDGs.pdf>.
3. World Health Organization (WHO). One Health. 2017 <https://www.who.int/westernpacific/news/q-a-detail/one-health>.
4. U.S. Food and Drug Administration. Guidance for the Industry: Fish and Fishery Products Hazards and Controls Guidance, Fourth Edition. 2021. <https://www.fda.gov/media/80637/download>.

5. Food and Agriculture Organization (FAO) and World Health Organization (WHO), Risk assessment of *Vibrio vulnificus* in raw oysters. Microbiological Risk Assessment Series, No. 8. 2005a. pp. 114.
6. Vugia DJ, Tabnak F, Newton AE, Hernandez M, Griffin PM. Impact of 2003 state regulation on raw oyster-associated *Vibrio vulnificus* illnesses and deaths, California, USA. *Emerg Infect Dis*. 2013;19(8):1276–1280.
7. Hlady WG, Klontz KC. The epidemiology of *Vibrio* infections in Florida, 1981–1993. *J Infect Dis*. 1996;173:1176–1183.
8. Lee SH, Chung BH, Lee WC. Retrospective analysis of epidemiological aspects of *Vibrio vulnificus* infections in Korea in 2001–2010. *Japanese J Infect Dis*. 2013;66(4):331–333.
9. Heng SP, Letchumanan V, Deng CY, et al. *Vibrio vulnificus*: an environmental and clinical burden. *Front Microbiol*. 2017;8:997.
10. Baker-Austin C, Oliver JD. *Vibrio vulnificus*: new insights into a deadly opportunistic pathogen. *Environ Microbiol*. 2018;20:423–430.
11. Fujino T, Okuno Y, Nakada D, et al. On the bacteriological examination of shirasu food poisoning. *Med J Osaka Univ*. 1953;4:299–304.
12. Food and Agriculture Organization (FAO) and World Health Organization (WHO), 2020. Risk assessment tools for *Vibrio parahaemolyticus* and *Vibrio vulnificus* associated with seafood. Microbiological Risk Assessment Series No. 20. Rome.
13. Nair GB, Ramamurthy T, Bhattacharya SK, Dutta B, Takeda Y, Sack DA. Global dissemination of *Vibrio parahaemolyticus* serotype O3:K6 and its serovariants. *Clin Microbiol Rev*. 2007;20(1):39–48.
14. Dadisman TA, Nelson R, Molenda JR, Garber HJ. *Vibrio parahaemolyticus* gastroenteritis in Maryland. I. Clinical and epidemiologic aspects. *Am J Epidemiol*. 1972;96:414–426.
15. Molenda JR, Johnson WG, Fishbein M, Wentz B, Mehlman IJ, Dadisman Jr. TA. *Vibrio parahaemolyticus* gastroenteritis in Maryland: laboratory aspects. *Appl Microbiol*. 1972;24(3):444–448.
16. Centers for Disease Control and Prevention (CDC). Outbreak of *Vibrio parahaemolyticus* infection associated with eating raw oysters and clams harvested from Long Island Sound–Connecticut, New Jersey, and New York, 1998. *MMWR Morb Mortal Wkly Rep*. 1999;48(3):48–51.
17. Daniels NA, Ray B, Easton A, et al. Emergence of a new *Vibrio parahaemolyticus* serotype in raw oysters: a prevention quandary. *JAMA*. 2000;284(12):1541–1545.
18. García K, Torres R, Uribe P, et al. Dynamics of clinical and environmental *Vibrio parahaemolyticus* strains during seafood-related summer diarrhea outbreaks in southern Chile. *Appl Environ Microbiol*. 2009;75(23):7482–7487.
19. Harth E, Matsuda L, Hernández C, et al. Epidemiology of *Vibrio parahaemolyticus* outbreaks, southern Chile. *Emerg Infect Dis*. 2009;15(2):163–168.
20. Martinez-Urtaza J, Simental L, Velasco D, et al. Pandemic *Vibrio parahaemolyticus* O3:K6, Europe. *Emerg Infect Dis*. 2005;11(8):1319–1320.
21. Ottaviani D, Leoni F, Rocchegiani E, et al. First clinical report of pandemic *Vibrio parahaemolyticus* O3:K6 infection in Italy. *J Clin Microbiol*. 2008;46(6):2144–2145.
22. Sinha S, Chakraborty R, De K, et al. Escalating association of *Vibrio cholerae* O139 with cholera outbreaks in India. *J Clin Microbiol*. 2002;40(7):2635–2637.
23. Kam KM, Leung TH, Ho YY, Ho NK, Saw TA. Outbreak of *Vibrio cholerae* 01 in Hong Kong related to contaminated fish tank water. *Public Health*. 1995;109(5):389–395.
24. Lin FYC, Morris JG, Kaper JB, et al. Persistence of cholera in the United States: isolation of *Vibrio cholerae* 01 from a patient with diarrhea in Maryland. *J Clin Microbiol*. 1986;23(3):624–626.
25. Onifade, T.J. M., Hutchinson, R., Van Zile, K., Bodager, D., Baker, R., Blackmore, C., 2011. Toxin producing *Vibrio cholerae* O75 outbreak, United States. Eurosurveillance 16(20), pii = 19870.
26. Crowe SJ, Newton AE, Gould LH, et al. Vibriosis, not cholera: toxigenic *Vibrio cholerae* non-O1, non-O139 infections in the United States, 1984-2014. *Epidemiol Infect*. 2016;144(15):3335–3341.
27. Food and Agriculture Organization (FAO) and World Health Organization (WHO), 2005b. Risk assessment of choleragenic *Vibrio cholerae* 01 and 0139 in warm-water shrimp in international trade. Microbiological Risk Assessment Series, No. 9.
28. Han H, Li F, Yan W, et al. Temporal and spatial variation in the abundance of total and pathogenic *Vibrio parahaemolyticus* in shellfish in China. *PLoS One*. 2015;10(6):e0130302.
29. Mok JS, Ryu A, Kwon JY, Kim B, Park K. Distribution of *Vibrio* species isolated from bivalves and bivalve culture environments along the Gyeongnam coast in Korea: virulence and antimicrobial resistance of *Vibrio parahaemolyticus* isolates. *Food Control*. 2019;106:106697.
30. Chang HC, Chen ML, Su YC, Pai JY, Chiu TH. Molecular characterizations of pathogenic *Vibrio parahaemolyticus* isolated from Southern Taiwan oyster–growing environment. *Food Control*. 2011;22:245–251.
31. Yu WT, Jong KJ, Lin YR, Tsai SE, Tey YH, Wong HC. Prevalence of *Vibrio parahaemolyticus* in oyster and clam culturing environments in Taiwan. *Int J Food Microbiol*. 2013;160(3):185–192.
32. Jones JL, Lüdeke CH, Bowers JC, DeRosia-Banick K, Carey DH, Hastback W. Abundance of *Vibrio cholerae*, *V. vulnificus*, and *V. parahaemolyticus* in oysters (*Crassostrea virginica*) and clams (*Mercenaria mercenaria*) from Long Island sound. *Appl Environ Microbiol*. 2014;80(24):7667–7672.
33. Parveen S, Hettiarachchi KA, Bowers JC, et al. Seasonal distribution of total and pathogenic *Vibrio parahaemolyticus* in Chesapeake Bay oysters and waters. *Int J Food Microbiol*. 2008;128(2):354–361.
34. López-Hernández KM, Pardío-Sedas VT, Lizárraga-Partida L, et al. Environmental parameters influence on the dynamics of total and pathogenic *Vibrio parahaemolyticus* densities in *Crassostrea virginica* harvested from Mexico's Gulf coast. *Mar Pollut Bull*. 2015;91(1):317–329.
35. Eyles MJ, Davey GR, Arnold G. Behavior and incidence of *Vibro parahaemolyticus* in Sydney rock oysters (*Crassostrea commercialis*). *Int J Food Microbiol*. 1985;1(6):327–334.
36. Cruz CD, Hedderley D, Fletcher GC. Long-term study of *Vibrio parahaemolyticus* prevalence and distribution in New Zealand shellfish. *Appl Environ Microbiol*. 2015;81(7):2320–2327.
37. Schets FM, van den Berg HH, Rutjes SA, de Roda Husman AM. Pathogenic *Vibrio* species in dutch shellfish destined for direct human consumption. *J Food Prot*. 2010;73(4):734–738.
38. Malcolm TTH, Cheah YK, Wan Mohamed Radzi CWJ, et al. Detection and quantification of pathogenic *Vibrio parahaemolyticus*

in shellfish by using multiplex PCR and loop-mediated isothermal amplification assay. *Food Control*. 2015;47:664–671.

39. Froelich BA, Phippen B, Fowler P, Noble RT, Oliver JD. Differences in abundances of total *Vibrio* spp., *V. vulnificus*, and *V. parahaemolyticus* in clams and oysters in North Carolina. *Appl Environ Microbiol*. 2017;83:e02265–16.
40. Lei T, Jiang F, He M, et al. Prevalence, virulence, antimicrobial resistance, and molecular characterization of fluoroquinolone resistance of *Vibrio parahaemolyticus* from different types of food samples in China. *Int J Food Microbiol*. 2020;317:108461.
41. Xie TF, Wu QP, Zhang JM, Xu XK, Cheng JH. Comparison of *Vibrio parahaemolyticus* isolates from aquatic products and clinical by antibiotic susceptibility, virulence, and molecular characterisation. *Food Control*. 2017;71:315–321.
42. Huang Y, Ghate V, Phua L, Yuk HG. Prevalence of *Salmonella* and *Vibrio* spp. in seafood products sold in Singapore. *J Food Prot*. 2012;75(7):1320–1323.
43. Lamon S, Consolati SG, Fois F, et al. Occurrence, seasonal distribution, and molecular characterization of *Vibrio vulnificus*, *Vibrio cholerae*, and *Vibrio parahaemolyticus* in shellfish (*Mytilus galloprovincialis* and *Ruditapes decussatus*) collected in Sardinia (Italy). *J Food Prot*. 2019;82(11):1851–1856.
44. Normanno G, Parisi A, Addante N, et al. *Vibrio parahaemolyticus*, *Vibrio vulnificus* and microorganisms of fecal origin in mussels (*Mytilus galloprovincialis*) sold in the Puglia region (Italy). *Int J Food Microbiol*. 2006;106(2):219–222.
45. Ripabelli G, Sammarco ML, Grasso GM, Fanelli I, Caprioli A, Luzzi I. Occurrence of *Vibrio* and other pathogenic bacteria in *Mytilus galloprovincialis* (mussels) harvested from Adriatic Sea, Italy. *Int J Food Microbiol*. 1999;49(1-2):43–48.
46. Lhafi SK, Kühne M. Occurrence of *Vibrio* spp. in blue mussels (*Mytilus edulis*) from the German Wadden Sea. *Int J Food Microbiol*. 2007;116(2):297–300.
47. Suffredini E, Mioni R, Mazzette R, et al. Detection and quantification of *Vibrio parahaemolyticus* in shellfish from Italian production areas. *Int J Food Microbiol*. 2014;184:14–20.
48. Schärer K, Savioz S, Cernela N, Saegesser G, Stephan R. Occurrence of *Vibrio* spp. in fish and shellfish collected from the Swiss market. *J Food Prot*. 2011;74(8):1345–1347.
49. Rodgers C, Parveen S, Chigbu P, Jacobs J, Rhodes M, Harter-Dennis J. Prevalence of *Vibrio parahaemolyticus*, and *Vibrio vulnificus* in blue crabs (*Callinectes sapidus*), seawater and sediments of the Maryland Coastal Bays. *J Appl Microbiol*. 2014;117(4):1198–1209.
50. Staley C, Jones MK, Wright AC, Harwood VJ. Genetic and quantitative assessment of *Vibrio vulnificus* populations in oyster (*Crassostrea virginica*) tissues. *Environ Microbiol Rep*. 2011;3(5):543–549.
51. Yano Y, Yokoyama M, Satomi M, Oikawa H, Chen SS. Occurrence of *Vibrio vulnificus* in fish and shellfish available from markets in China. *J Food Prot*. 2004;67(8):1617–1623.
52. Fang L, Ginn AM, Harper J, Kane AS, Wright AC. Survey and genetic characterization of *Vibrio cholerae* in Apalachicola Bay, Florida (2012-2014). *J Appl Microbiol*. 2019;126(4):1265–1277.
53. Brands DA, Inman AE, Gerba CP, et al. Prevalence of *Salmonella* spp. in oysters in the United States. *Appl Environ Microbiol*. 2005;71(2):893–897.
54. Brillhart CD, Joens LA. Prevalence and characterization of *Salmonella* serovars isolated from oysters served raw in restaurants. *J Food Prot*. 2011;74(6):1025–1029.
55. Hara-Kudo Y, Konuma H, Kamata Y, et al. Prevalence of the main food-borne pathogens in retail food under the national food surveillance system in Japan. *Food Addit Contam Part A, Chem Anal Control Expos Risk Assess*. 2013;30(8):1450–1458.
56. Jeamsripong S, Chuanchuen R, Atwill ER. Assessment of bacterial accumulation and environmental factors in *Sentinel oysters* and estuarine water quality from the Phang Nga Estuary Area in Thailand. *Int J Environ Res Public Health*. 2018;15(9):1970.
57. Yang X, Wu Q, Zhang J, et al. Prevalence, enumeration, and characterization of *Salmonella* isolated from aquatic food products from retail markets in China. *Food Control*. 2015;57:308–313.
58. Asai Y, Kaneko M, Ohtsuka K, et al. *Salmonella* prevalence in seafood imported into Japan. *J Food Prot*. 2008;71(7):1460–1464.
59. Kamalika J, Ubeyratne H, Kleer J, et al. Prevalence of *Salmonella* in marketed *Penaeus monodon* shrimps in North Western Province, Sri Lanka. *Berl und Münchener Tierärztliche Wochenschr*. 2008;121(11-12):418–421.
60. Nguyen DT, Kanki M, Nguyen PD, et al. Prevalence, antibiotic resistance, and extended-spectrum and AmpC β-lactamase productivity of *Salmonella* isolates from raw meat and seafood samples in Ho Chi Minh City, Vietnam. *Int J Food Microbiol*. 2016;236:115–122.
61. Wilson IG, Moore JE. Presence of *Salmonella* spp. and *Campylobacter* spp. in shellfish. *Epidemiol Infect*. 1996;116(2):147–153.
62. Reilly PJ, Twiddy DR. *Salmonella* and *Vibrio cholerae* in brackish-water cultured tropical prawns. *Int J Food Microbiol*. 1992;16(4):293–301.
63. Setti I, Rodriguez-Castro A, Pata MP, et al. Characteristics and dynamics of *Salmonella* contamination along the coast of Agadir, Morocco. *Appl Environ Microbiol*. 2009;75(24):7700–7709.
64. Baniga Z, Mdegela RH, Lisa B, Kusiluka LJM, Dalsgaard A. Prevalence and characterisation of *Salmonella* Waycross and *Salmonella enterica* subsp. salamae in Nile perch (*Lates niloticus*) of Lake Victoria, Tanzania. *Food Control*. 2019;100:28–34.
65. Baniga Z, Dalsgaard A, Mhongole OJ, Madsen H, Mdegela RH. Microbial quality and safety of fresh and dried *Rastrineobola argentea* from Lake Victoria, Tanzania. *Food Control*. 2017;81:16–22.
66. Martinez-Urtaza J, Saco M, de Novoa J, et al. Influence of environmental factors and human activity on the presence of *Salmonella* serovars in a marine environment. *Appl Environ Microbiol*. 2004;70(4):2089–2097.
67. Anacleto P, Pedro S, Nunes ML, Rosa R, Marques A. Microbiological composition of native and exotic clams from Tagus estuary: effect of season and environmental parameters. *Mar Pollut Bull*. 2013;74(1):116–124.
68. Woodring J, Srijan A, Puripunyakom P, Oransathid W, Wongstitwilairoong B, Mason C. Prevalence and antimicrobial susceptibilities of *Vibrio*, *salmonella*, and *Aeromonas* isolates from various uncooked seafoods in Thailand. *J Food Prot*. 2012;75(1):41–47.
69. Minami A, Chaicumpa W, Chongsa-Nguan M, et al. Prevalence of foodborne pathogens in open markets and supermarkets in Thailand. *Food Control*. 2010;21(3):221–226.
70. Bhaskar N, Setty TMR, Reddy GVS, et al. Incidence of *Salmonella* in cultured shrimp *Penaeus monodon*. *Aquaculture*. 1995;138(1–4):257–266.

71. World Health Organization (WHO), 2020. *Salmonella* (non-typhoidal). <https://www.who.int/news-room/fact-sheets/detail/salmonella-(non-typhoidal)>.
72. Centers for Disease Control and Prevention (CDC), 2018. <https// www.cdc.gov/foodborneburden/2011-foodborne-estimates.html>.
73. Mead PS, Slutsker L, Dietz V, et al. Food-related illness and death in the United States. *Emerg Infect Dis*. 1999;5(5):607–625.
74. National Advisory Committee on Microbiological Criteria For Foods (NACMCF). Response to the questions posed by the food and drug administration and the national marine fisheries service regarding determination of cooking parameters for safe seafood for consumers. *J Food Prot*. 2008;71(6):1287–1308.
75. Centers for Disease Control and Prevention (CDC), 2012. Multistate outbreak of *Salmonella* Bareilly and *Salmonella* Nchanga infections associated with a raw scraped ground tuna product (Final Update). <https://www.cdc.gov/salmonella/bareilly-04-12/index.html>.
76. Centers for Disease Control and Prevention (CDC), 2015. Multistate outbreak of *Salmonella* Paratyphi B variant L(+) tartrate(+) and *Salmonella* Weltevreden infections linked to frozen raw tuna (Final Update). <https://www.cdc.gov/salmonella/paratyphi-b-05-15/index.html>.
77. Centers for Disease Control and Prevention (CDC), 2019. Outbreak of *Salmonella* infections linked to frozen raw tuna. <https://www.cdc.gov/salmonella/newport-04-19/index.html>.
78. Foodborne Illness Outbreak Database (2020). <http://www.outbreakdatabase.com/details/2007-outbreak-of-salmonella-sandiego-linked-to-tuna-salad-washington/?>.
79. Japan Ministry of Health and Welfare, 1987-1996. Number of incidents, patients and deaths from food poisoning by pathogenic substance and causative food. Tokyo, Japan, Veterinary Sanitation Division, Environmental Health Bureau.
80. European Food Safety Authority. Annual Report. Parma, Italy: EFSA; 2010. <https://www.efsa.europa.eu/en/corporate/pub/ar10>.
81. Food and Agriculture Organization (FAO) and World Health Organization (WHO), 1995. Collaborating centre for research and training in food hygiene and zoonoses. WHO surveillance programme for control of food-borne infections and intoxication's in Europe. Sixth Report, 1990-1992. Berlin, Germany, Federal Institute for Health Protection of Consumers and Veterinary Medicine.
82. Todd EC. Seafood-associated diseases and control in Canada. *Rev Scientifique et Tech (Int Office Epizootics)*. 1997;16(2):661–672.
83. Francis S, Rowland J, Rattenbury K, et al. An outbreak of paratyphoid fever in the UK associated with a fish-and-chip shop. *Epidemiol Infect*. 1989;103(3):445–448.
84. Greenwood M, Winnard G, Bagot B. An outbreak of *Salmonella enteritidis* phage type 19 infection associated with cockles. *Commun Dis Public Health*. 1998;1(1):35–37.
85. Kühn H, Gericke B, Klepp M, Fellmann G, Rabsch W. Ausbruch von *Salmonella* paratyphi B-Infektionen im Zusammenhang mit dem Genuss von Räucherfisch [Outbreak of *Salmonella* paratyphi B infections in connection with consumption of smoked fish]. *Gesundheitswesen*. 1994;56(4):211–214.
86. Daskalov H. The importance of *Aeromonas hydrophila* in food safety. *Food Control*. 2006;17(6):474–483.
87. Abeyta Jr C, Wekell MM. Potential sources of *Aeromonas hydrophila*. *J Food Saf*. 1988;9:11–22.
88. Palumbo S. The *Aeromonas hydrophila* Group in Food. In: Austin B, Altwegg M, Gosling PJ, Joseph S, eds. *The Genus Aeromonas*. John Wiley & Sons, Ltd; 1996:287–310.
89. Davies AR, Capell C, Jehanno D, Nychas GJE, Kirby RM. The importance of *Aeromonas hydrophila* in food safety. *Food Control*. 2006;17:474–483.
90. Yang Y, Miao P, Li H, Tan S, Yu H, Yu H. Antibiotic susceptibility and molecular characterization of *Aeromonas hydrophila* from grass carp. *J Food Saf*. 2018;38:e12393.
91. Illanchezian S, Jayaraman S, Manoharan MS, Valsalam S. Virulence and cytotoxicity of seafood borne *Aeromonas hydrophila*. *Braz J Microbiol*. 2010;41(4):978–983.
92. Wang C, Silva JL. Prevalence and characteristics of *Aeromonas* species isolated from processed channel catfish. *J Food Prot*. 1999;62(1):30–34.
93. Mateos D, Anguita J, Naharro G, Paniagua C. Influence of growth temperature on the production of extracellular virulence factors and pathogenicity of environmental and human strains of *Aeromonas hydrophila*. *J Appl Bacteriol*. 1993;74(2):111–118.
94. Abeyta Jr C, Kaysner CA, Wekell MM, Sullivan JJ, Stelma GN. Recovery of *Aeromonas hydrophila* from oysters implicated in an outbreak of foodborne illness. *J Food Prot*. 1986;49(8):643–646.
95. Krovacek K, Dumontet S, Eriksson E, Baloda SB. Isolation, and virulence profiles, of *Aeromonas hydrophila* implicated in an outbreak of food poisoning in Sweden. *Microbiol Immunol*. 1995;39 (9):655–661.
96. Granum PE, O'Sullivan K, Tomás JM, Ormen O. Possible virulence factors of *Aeromonas* spp. from food and water. *FEMS Immunol Med Microbiol*. 1998;21(2):131–137.
97. Basha K, Kumar N, Das V, et al. Prevalence, molecular characterization, genetic heterogeneity and antimicrobial resistance of *Listeria monocytogenes* associated with fish and fishery environment in Kerala, India. *Lett Appl Microbiol*. 2019;69:286–293.
98. Lasagabaster A, Jiménez E, Lehnherr T, Miranda-Cadena K, Lehnherr H. Bacteriophage biocontrol to fight *Listeria* outbreaks in seafood. *Food Chem Toxicol*. 2020;145:111682.
99. Kovacevic J, Sagert J, Wozniak A, Gilmour MW, Allen KJ. Antimicrobial resistance and co-selection phenomenon in *Listeria* spp. recovered from food and food production environments. *Food Microbiol*. 2013;34(2):319–327.
100. Menudier A, Bosiraud C, Nicolas JA. Virulence of *Listeria monocytogenes* serovars and *Listeria* spp. in experimental infection of mice. *J Food Prot*. 1991;54(12):917–921.
101. Thomas J, Govender N, McCarthy KM, et al. Outbreak of listeriosis in South Africa associated with processed meat. *N Engl J Med*. 2020;382(7):632–643.
102. Allen KJ, Wałecka-Zacharska E, Chen JC, et al. *Listeria monocytogenes*—an examination of food chain factors potentially contributing to antimicrobial resistance. *Food Microbiol*. 2016;54:178–189.
103. Vázquez-Boland JA, Kuhn M, Berche P, et al. *Listeria* pathogenesis and molecular virulence determinants. *Clin Microbiol Rev*. 2001;14(3):584–640.
104. Rapid Alert System for Food and Feed (RASSF), 2018. Food and feed safety alerts. <https://ec.europa.eu/food/safety/rasff_en>.
105. European Centre for Disease Prevention and Control and European Food Safety Authority (ECDC), 2018. Multi-country outbreak of *Listeria monocytogenes* sequence type 8 infections linked to consumption of salmon products. Stockholm and Parma, ECDC/EFSA. <https://www.ecdc.europa.eu/en/publications-data/multi-country-outbreak-listeria-monocytogenes-sequence-type-8-infections-linked>.

106. Lyytikäinen O, Nakari UM, Lukinmaa S, Kela E, Nguyen Tran Minh N, Siitonen A. Surveillance of listeriosis in Finland during 1995–2004. *Eurosurveillance*. 2006;11(6):82–85.
107. Miettinen MK, Siitonen A, Heiskanen P, Haajanen H, Björkroth KJ, Korkeala HJ. Molecular epidemiology of an outbreak of febrile gastroenteritis caused by *Listeria monocytogenes* in cold-smoked rainbow trout. *J Clin Microbiol*. 1999;37(7):2358–2360.
108. Ericsson H, Eklöw A, Danielsson-Tham ML, et al. An outbreak of listeriosis suspected to have been caused by rainbow trout. *J Clin Microbiol*. 1997;35(11):2904–2907.
109. Ribeiro VB, Mujahid S, Orsi RH, et al. Contributions of σ(B) and PrfA to *Listeria monocytogenes* salt stress under food relevant conditions. *Int J Food Microbiol*. 2014;177:98–108.
110. Vermeulen A, Gysemans KP, Bernaerts K, et al. Influence of pH, water activity and acetic acid concentration on *Listeria monocytogenes* at 7 degrees C: data collection for the development of a growth/no growth model. *Int J Food Microbiol*. 2007;114(3):332–341.
111. Bryan FL. Epidemiology of foodborne diseases transmitted by fish, shellfish and marine crustaceans in the United States, 1970–1978. *J food Prot*. 1980;43(11):859–876.
112. World Health Organization (WHO), 1999. *Clostridium botulinum*. <https://www.who.int/csr/delibepidemics/clostridiumbotulism.pdf>.
113. Huss HH. Distribution of *Clostridium botulinum*. *Appl Environ Microbiol*. 1980;39(4):764–769.
114. Lalitha KV, Gopakumar K. Distribution and ecology of *Clostridium botulinum* in fish and aquatic environments of a tropical region. *Food Microbiol*. 2000;17(5):535–541.
115. Sheng L, Wang L. The microbial safety of fish and fish products: recent advances in understanding its significance, contamination sources, and control strategies. *Compr Rev Food Sci Food Saf*. 2021;20:738–786.
116. Astaraki N, Akhtar S. The study of microbial contamination in seafood and fish. *Medbiotech J*. 2020;04(03):102–108.
117. Butt AA, Aldridge KE, Sanders CV. Infections related to the ingestion of seafood Part I: viral and bacterial infections. *Lancet Infect Dis*. 2004;4(4):201–212.
118. Hauschild AHW, Gauvreau L. Food-borne botulism in Canada, 1971-84. *Can Med Assoc J*. 1985;133:1141–1146.
119. EFSA (European Food Safety Authority) and ECDC (European Centre for Disease Prevention and Control), 2016. Type E botulism associated with fish product consumption – Germany and Spain. EFSA supporting publication 2016, EN-1157. 7 pp. doi:10.2903/sp.efsa.2016.EN1157.
120. Gombas DE. *Clostridium botulinum* ecology and control in foodsIn: Hauschild AHW, Dodds KL, eds. 270 Madison Ave., New York: Marcel Dekker, Inc; 1993:238–239.
121. Frean J, Arntzen L, van den Heever J, Perovic O. Fatal type A botulism in South Africa, 2002. *Trans R Soc Tropical Med Hyg*. 2004;98(5):290–295.
122. Weber JT, Hibbs Jr RG, Darwish A, et al. A massive outbreak of type E botulism associated with traditional salted fish in Cairo. *J Infect Dis*. 1993;167(2):451–454.
123. Uzal FA, Freedman JC, Shrestha A, et al. Towards an understanding of the role of *Clostridium perfringens* toxins in human and animal disease. *Future Microbiol*. 2014;9(3):361–377.
124. Poluru A, Sahu R, Nelapati K. Detection and characterization of *Clostridium perfringens* in seafoods. *Int J Livest Res*. 2017; 7(7):177–183. Available from: https://doi.org/10.5455/ijlr.20170513100616.
125. Iwamoto M, Ayers T, Mahon BE, Swerdlow DL. Epidemiology of seafood-associated infections in the United States. *Clin Microbiol Rev*. 2010;23(2):399–411.
126. Murtaza M, Yoshida T, Waheed Z, et al. Seafood poisoning symptom, treatment and prevention. *Borneo J Mar Sci Aquaculture*. 2018;2:64–69.
127. Wang G, Paredes-Sabja D, Sarker MR, Green C, Setlow P, Li YQ. Effects of wet heat treatment on the germination of individual spores of *Clostridium perfringens*. *J Appl Microbiol*. 2012;113:824–836.
128. Florida Department of Agriculture and Consumer Services (FDACS), 2016. Cooking and Hot Holding Food, Florida Department of Agriculture and Consumer Services, Division of Food Safety. FDACS-)-02084 Rev 9/16. <https://www.fdacs.gov/content/download/67385/file/Cooking-and-Hot-Holding-Food.pdf>.
129. Food Safety and Inspection Service (FSIS), 2002. Hot Holding Temperature. National Advisory Committee on Microbiological Criteria for Foods. U.S. Department of Agriculture Food Safety Inspection Service. <https://www.fsis.usda.gov/wps/portal/fsis/topics/regulations/advisory-committees/nacmcf-reports/nacmcf-report-hot-holding-2002>.
130. Khora SS. Risk from viral pathogens in seafood. *Diet, Microbiome Health*. 2018;439–481.
131. Bozkurt H, Leiser S, Davidson PM, D'Souza DH. Thermal inactivation kinetic modeling of human norovirus surrogates in blue mussel (*Mytilus edulis*) homogenate. *Int J Food Microbiol*. 2014;172:130–136.
132. Mason JO, McLean WR. Infectious hepatitis traced to the consumption of raw oysters. *Am J Hyg*. 1962;75:90–111.
133. Dougherty WJ, Altman R. Viral hepatitis in New Jersey 1960–1961. *Am J Med*. 1962;32:704–716.
134. Marler B., 2016. Hepatitis A in Shellfish – A Bit(e) of History. <https://www.marlerblog.com/legal-cases/hepatitis-a-in-shellfish-a-bite-of-history/>.
135. Croci L, Ciccozzi M, De Medici D, et al. Inactivation of hepatitis A virus in heat-treated mussels. *J Appl Microbiol*. 1999;87(6):884–888.
136. Egan S, Harder T, Burke C, Steinberg P, Kjelleberg S, Thomas T. The seaweed holobiont: understanding seaweed–bacteria interactions. *FEMS Microbiol Rev*. 2013;37(3):462–476.
137. Neori A. Essential role of seaweed cultivation in integrated multi-trophic aquaculture farms for global expansion of mariculture: an analysis. *J Appl Phycol*. 2008;20(5):567–570.
138. Buschmann AH, Camus C, Infante J, et al. Seaweed production: overview of the global state of exploitation, farming and emerging research activity. *Eur J Phycol*. 2017;52(4):391–406.
139. Lachnit T, Blümel M, Imhoff JF, Wahl M. Specific epibacterial communities on macroalgae: phylogeny matters more than habitat. *Aquat Biol*. 2009;5(2):181–186.
140. Stévant P, Rebours C, Chapman A. Seaweed aquaculture in Norway: recent industrial developments and future perspectives. *Aquaculture Int*. 2017;25:1373–1390.
141. National Food Institute. Analysis and risk assessment of seaweed Technical University of Denmark, Denmark, Sá Monteiro, M., Sloth, J., Holdt, S., Hansen, M *EFSA J*. 2019;17:e170915.

142. Banach JL, Hoek-van den Hil EF, van der Fels-Klerx HJ. Food safety hazards in the European seaweed chain. *Compr Rev Food Sci Food Saf.* 2020;19(2):332–364.

143. International Water Management Institute (IWMI) and Food and Agricultural Organization of the United Nations (FAO). *Water pollution from agriculture, a global review*. Rome: FAO; 2017. Available from: http://www.fao.org/3/a-i7754e.pdf%20.

144. Rieke EL, Moorman TB, Soupir ML, Yang F, Howe A. Assessing pathogen presence in an intensively tile drained, agricultural watershed. *J Environ Qual.* 2018;47(5):1033–1042.

145. Givens CE, Kolpin DW, Borchardt MA, Duris JW, Moorman TB, Spencer SK. Detection of hepatitis E virus and other livestock-related pathogens in Iowa streams. *Sci Total Environ.* 2016;566-567:1042–1051.

146. U.S. Department of Agriculture (USDA), 2012. Introduction to waterborne pathogens in agricultural watersheds. Nutrient Management Technical Note No. 9. <https://directives.sc.egov.usda.gov/OpenNonWebContent.aspx?content = 32935.wba>.

147. Hutchison ML, Walters LD, Avery SM, Munro F, Moore A. Analyses of livestock production, waste storage, and pathogen levels and prevalences in farm manures. *Appl Environ Microbiol.* 2005;71(3):1231–1236.

148. Ziemer CJ, Bonner JM, Cole D, et al. Fate and transport of zoonotic, bacterial, viral, and parasitic pathogens during swine manure treatment, storage, and land application. *J Anim Sci.* 2010;88(13 Suppl):E84–E94.

149. Solomon EB, Yaron S, Matthews KR. Transmission of *Escherichia coli* O157:H7 from contaminated manure and irrigation water to lettuce plant tissue and its subsequent internalization. *Appl Environ Microbiol.* 2002;68(1):397–400.

150. Britz T, Sigge G, Huisamen N, et al. Fluctuations of indicator and index microbes as indication of pollution over three years in the Plankenburg and Eerste Rivers, Western Cape, South Africa. *Water South Afr.* 2013;39(4):457–466.

151. Nicholson FA, Groves SJ, Chambers BJ. Pathogen survival during livestock manure storage and following land application. *Bioresour Technol.* 2005;96(2):135–143.

152. U.S. Environmental Protection Agency. 2013. Literature review of contaminants in livestock and poultry manure and implications for water quality." <http://water.epa.gov/scitech/cec/upload/LiteratureReview-of-Contaminants-in-Livestock-and-Poultry-Manure-and-Implications-for-WaterQuality.pdf>.

153. Hutchison ML, Walters LD, Avery SM, Synge BA, Moore A. Levels of zoonotic agents in British livestock manures. *Lett Appl Microbiol.* 2004;39(2):207–214.

154. Klase G, Lee S, Liang S, Kim J, Zo YG, Lee J. The microbiome and antibiotic resistance in integrated fishfarm water: implications of environmental public health. *Sci Total Environ.* 2019;649:1491–1501.

155. Chique C, Hynds P, Burke LP, Morris D, Ryan MP, O'Dwyer J. Contamination of domestic groundwater systems by verotoxigenic *Escherichia coli* (VTEC), 2003–2019: a global scoping review. *Water Res.* 2020;188:116496.

156. Mulvihill PR, Ali SH. Disaster incubation, cumulative impacts and the urban/ex-urban/rural dynamic. *Environ Impact Assess Rev.* 2007;27(4):343–358.

157. Vadde KK, McCarthy AJ, Rong R, Sekar R. Quantification of microbial source tracking and pathogenic bacterial markers in water and sediments of Tiaoxi River (Taihu Watershed). *Front Microbiol.* 2019;10:699.

158. Parlapani FF. Microbial diversity of seafood. *Curr OpFood Sci.* 2021;37:45–51.

159. Manjengwa F, Nhiwatiwa T, Nyakudya E, Banda P. Fish from a polluted lake (Lake Chivero, Zimbabwe): a food safety issue of concern. *Food Qual Saf.* 2019;3:157–167.

160. Antunes P, Campos J, Mourão J, Pereira J, Novais C, Peixe L. Inflow water is a major source of trout farming contamination with *Salmonella* and multidrug resistant bacteria. *Sci Total Environ.* 2018;642:1163–1171.

161. Topić Popović N, Kepec S, Kazazić SP, et al. The impact of treated wastewaters on fish bacterial flora: a public health perspective. *Croatian J Fish.* 2019;77(3):133–136.

162. Ayaz ND, Gencay YE, Erol I. Prevalence and molecular characterization of sorbitol fermenting and non-fermenting *Escherichia coli* O157:H7(+)/H7(-) isolated from cattle at slaughterhouse and slaughterhouse wastewater. *Int J Food Microbiol.* 2014;174:31–38.

163. Donnison AM, Ross CM. Animal and human faecal pollution in New Zealand rivers. *N ZealJ Mar Freshw Res.* 1999;33:119–128.

164. Um MM, Barraud O, Kérourédan M, et al. Comparison of the incidence of pathogenic and antibiotic-resistant *Escherichia coli* strains in adult cattle and veal calf slaughterhouse effluents highlighted different risks for public health. *Water Res.* 2016;88:30–38.

165. Parlapani FF, Michailidou S, Pasentsis K, Argiriou A, Krey G, Boziaris IS. A meta-barcoding approach to assess and compare the storage temperature-dependent bacterial diversity of gilt-head sea bream (*Sparus aurata*) originating from fish farms from two geographically distinct areas of Greece. *Int J Food Microbiol.* 2018;278:36–43.

166. Parlapani FF, Anagnostopoulos DA, Koromilas S, et al. Bacterial communities and potential spoilage markers of whole blue crab (*Callinectes sapidus*) stored under commercial simulated conditions. *Food Microbiol.* 2019;82:325–333.

167. Parlapani FF, Ferrocino I, Michailidou S, et al. Microbiota and volatilome profile of fresh and chill-stored deepwater rose shrimp (*Parapenaeus longirostris*). *Food Res Int.* 2020;132:109057.

168. Teixeira P, Brandão J, Silva S, et al. Microbiological and chemical quality of ice used to preserve fish in Lisbon marketplaces. *J Food Saf.* 2019;39:e12641.

169. World Bank. *Pulling together to beat superbugs knowledge and implementation gaps in addressing antimicrobial resistance (English)*. HNP/Agriculture Global Antimicrobial Resistance Initiative Washington, D.C., World Bank Group; 2019.

170. Cabello F, Godfrey HP, Tomova A, et al. Antimicrobial use in aquaculture re-examined: its relevance to antimicrobial resistance and to animal and human health. *Environ Microbiol.* 2013;15:1917–1942.

171. Smith DL, Harris AD, Johnson JA, Silbergeld EK, Morris Jr. JG. Animal antibiotic use has an early but important impact on the emergence of antibiotic resistance in human commensal bacteria. *Proc Natl Acad Sci U S A.* 2002;99(9):6434–6439.

172. Cabello FC. Heavy use of prophylactic antibiotics in aquaculture: a growing problem for human and animal health and for the environment. *Environ Microbiol.* 2006;8:1137–1144.

173. Van Boeckel TP. Global trends in antimicrobial resistance in animals in low- and middle-income countries. *Science*. 2019;365. Available from: https://doi.org/10.1126/science.aaw1944.
174. Mehdi Y, Létourneau-Montminy MP, Gaucher ML, et al. Use of antibiotics in broiler production: global impacts and alternatives. *Anim Nutr*. 2018;4(2):170–178.
175. Lulijwa R, Rupia EJ, Alfaro AC. Antibiotic use in aquaculture, policies and regulation, health and environmental risks: a review of the top 15 major producers. *Rev Aquac*. 2020;12:640–663.
176. Manyi-Loh C, Mamphweli S, Meyer E, Okoh A. Antibiotic use in agriculture and its consequential resistance in environmental sources: potential public health implications. *Molecules*. 2018;23(4):795.
177. Vincent AT, Gauthier J, Derome N, Charette SJ. The rise and fall of antibiotics in aquaculture. In: Derome N, ed. *Microbial Communities in Aquaculture Ecosystems*. Cham: Springer; 2019.
178. Marshall BM, Levy SB. Food animals and antimicrobials: impacts on human health. *Clin Microbiol Rev*. 2011;24(4):718–733.
179. Elmahdi S, DaSilva LV, Parveen S. Antibiotic resistance of *Vibrio parahaemolyticus* and *Vibrio vulnificus* in various countries: a review. *Food Microbiol*. 2016;57:128e134.
180. He Y, Tang Y, Sun F, Chen L. Detection and characterization of integrative and conjugative elements (ICEs)-positive *Vibrio cholerae* isolates from aquacultured shrimp and the environment in Shanghai, China. *Mar Pollut Bull*. 2015;101:526–532.
181. Kang CH, Shin Y, Jang S, et al. Characterization of *Vibrio parahaemolyticus* isolated from oysters in Korea: resistance to various antibiotics and prevalence of virulence genes. *Mar Pollut Bull*. 2017;118:261–266.
182. Silva IP, de Sousa OV, Saraiva MAF, Evangelista-Barreto NS. *Vibrio cholerae* non-O1 in bivalve mollusks harvesting area in Bahia, Brazil. *Afr J Microbiol Res*. 2016;10(26):1005–1010.
183. Li Y, Xie T, Pang R, et al. Food-Borne *Vibrio parahaemolyticus* in China: prevalence, antibiotic susceptibility, and genetic characterization. *Front Microbiol*. 2020;11:1670.
184. Elhadi N. Prevalence and antimicrobial resistance of *Salmonella* spp. in raw retail frozen imported freshwater fish to eastern province of Saudi Arabia. *Asian Pac J Trop Biomed*. 2014;4(3):234–238.
185. Skowron K, Wiktorczyk N, Grudlewska K, et al. Phenotypic and genotypic evaluation of *Listeria monocytogenes* strains isolated from fish and fish processing plants. *Ann Microbiol*. 2019;69:469–482.
186. Keen PL, Patrick DM. Tracking change: a look at the ecological footprint of antibiotics and antimicrobial resistance. *Antibiotics*. 2013;2:191–205.
187. Hammerum AM. *Enterococci* of animal origin and their significance for public health. *Clin Microbiol Infect*. 2012;18:619–625.
188. Bowley J, Baker-Austin C, Porter A, Hartnell R, Lewis C. Oceanic hitchhikers – assessing pathogen risks from marine microplastic. *Trends Microbiol*. 2021;29(2):107–116.
189. Eriksen M, Lebreton LCM, Carson HS, et al. Plastic pollution in the World's oceans: more than 5 trillion plastic pieces weighing over 250,000 tons afloat at sea. *PLoS One*. 2014;9:e111913.
190. Tziourrou P, Megalovasilis P, Tsounia M, Karapanagioti HK. Characteristics of microplastics on two beaches affected by different land uses in Salamina Island in Saronikos Gulf, east Mediterranean. *Mar Pollut Bull*. 2019;149:110531.
191. Zettler ER, Mincer TJ, Amaral-Zettle LA. Life in the "Plastisphere": microbial communities on plastic marine debris. *Environ Sci Technol*. 2013;47:7137–7146.
192. Kesy K, Oberbeckmann S, Kreikemeyer B, Labrenz M. Spatial environmental heterogeneity determines young biofilm assemblages on microplastics in Baltic Sea mesocosms. *Front Microbiol*. 2019;10:1665.
193. Kiessling T, Gutow L, Thiel M. Marine litter as habitat and dispersal vector. In: Bergmann M, Gutow L, Klages M, eds. *Marine Anthropogenic Litter*. Cham: Springer; 2015.
194. Di Pinto A, Ciccarese G, De Corato R, Novello L, Terio V. Detection of pathogenic *Vibrio parahaemolyticus* in southern Italian shellfish. *Food Control*. 2008;19:1037–1041.
195. Ottaviani D, Santarelli S, Bacchiocchi S, Masini L, Ghittino C, Bacchiocchi I. Presence of pathogenic *Vibrio parahaemolyticus* strains in mussels from the Adriatic Sea, Italy. *Food Microbiol*. 2005;22:585–590.
196. Di Pinto A, Terio V, Di Pinto P, Colao V, Tantillo G. Detection of *Vibrio parahaemolyticus* in shellfish using polymerase chain reaction–enzyme-linked immunosorbent assay. *Lett Appl Microbiol*. 2012;54:494–498.
197. Fach P, Perelle S, Dilasser F, et al. Detection by PCR–enzyme-linked immunosorbent assay of *Clostridium botulinum* in fish and environmental samples from a coastal area in Northern France. *Appl Environ Microbiol*. 2002;68(12):5870–5876.
198. Kumar R, Surendran PK, Thampuran N. An eight-hour PCR-based technique for detection of *Salmonella* serovars in seafood. *World J Microbiol Biotechnol*. 2008;24:627–631.
199. Campbell MS, Wright AC. Real-time PCR analysis of *Vibrio vulnificus* from oysters. *Appl Environ Microbiol*. 2003;69(12):7137–7144.
200. D'Souza C, Prithvisagar KS, Deekshit VK, Karunasagar I, Karunasagar I, Kumar BK. Exploring the pathogenic potential of *Vibrio vulnificus* isolated from seafood harvested along the Mangaluru Coast, India. *Microorganisms*. 2020;8(7):999.
201. Blackstone GM, Nordstrom JL, Vickery MC, Bowen MD, Meyer RF, DePaola A. Detection of pathogenic *Vibrio parahaemolyticus* in oyster enrichments by real time PCR. *J Microbiol Methods*. 2003;53(2):149–155.
202. Cao X, Zhao L, Zhang J, et al. Detection of viable but nonculturable *Vibrio parahaemolyticus* in shrimp samples using improved real-time PCR and real-time LAMP methods. *Food Control*. 2019;103:145–152.
203. Eschbach E, Martin A, Huhn J, et al. Detection of enteropathogenic *Vibrio parahaemolyticus*, *Vibrio cholerae* and *Vibrio vulnificus*: performance of real-time PCR kits in an interlaboratory study. *Eur Food Res Technol*. 2017;243:1335–1342.
204. Gdoura M, Sellami H, Nasfi H, et al. Molecular detection of the three major pathogenic *Vibrio* species from seafood products and sediments in Tunisia using real-time PCR. *J Food Prot*. 2016;79(12):2086–2094.
205. Taminiau B, Korsak N, Lemaire C, Delcenserie V, Daube G. Validation of real-time PCR for detection of six major pathogens in seafood products. *Food Control*. 2014;44:130–137.
206. Vossen RH, Aten E, Roos A, den Dunnen JT. High-resolution melting analysis (HRMA): more than just sequence variant screening. *Hum Mutat*. 2009;30(6):860–866.
207. Tamburro M, Ripabelli G. High resolution melting as a rapid, reliable, accurate and cost-effective emerging tool for genotyping pathogenic bacteria and enhancing molecular epidemiological surveillance: a comprehensive review of the literature. *Annali di Igiene*. 2017;29(4):293–316.

208. Liu Y, Singh P, Mustapha A. Multiplex high resolution melt-curve real-time PCR assay for reliable detection of *Salmonella*. *Food Control*. 2018;91:225–230.
209. Omiccioli E, Amagliani G, Brandi G, Magnani M. A new platform for Real-Time PCR detection of *Salmonella* spp., *Listeria monocytogenes* and *Escherichia coli* O157 in milk. *Food Microbiol*. 2009;26(6):615–622.
210. Pei Hua N, Chen Z, Ji W, Wen Jie T, Xue Jun M. Detection and identification of six foodborne bacteria by two-tube multiplex real time PCR and melting curve analysis. *Biomed Environ Sci*. 2014;27(10):770–778.
211. Jin D, Luo Y, Zhang Z, et al. Rapid molecular identification of *Listeria* species by use of real-time PCR and high-resolution melting analysis. *FEMS Microbiol Lett*. 2012;330(1):72–80.
212. Liu Y, Singh P, Mustapha A. High-resolution melt curve PCR assay for specific detection of *E. coli* O157:H7 in beef. *Food Control*. 2018;86:275–282.
213. Forghani F, Singh P, Seo K-H, Oh D-H. A novel pentaplex real time (RT)- PCR high resolution melt curve assay for simultaneous detection of emetic and enterotoxin producing *Bacillus cereus* in food. *Food Control*. 2016;60:560–568.
214. Parlapani FF, Syropoulou F, Tsiartsafis A, et al. HRM analysis as a tool to facilitate identification of bacteria from mussels during storage at 4°C. *Food Microbiol*. 2020;85:103304.
215. Syropoulou F, Parlapani FF, Bosmali I, Madesis P, Boziaris IS. HRM and 16S rRNA gene sequencing reveal the cultivable microbiota of the European sea bass during ice storage. *Int J Food Microbiol*. 2020;327:108658.
216. Garrido A, Chapela M-J, Ferreira M, et al. Development of a multiplex real-time PCR method for pathogenic *Vibrio parahaemolyticus* detection (*tdh* and *trh*). *Food Control*. 2012;24:128–135.
217. Han F, Ge B. Multiplex PCR assays for simultaneous detection and characterization of *Vibrio vulnificus* strains. *Lett Appl Microbiol*. 2010;51:234–240.
218. Brasher CW, DePaola A, Jones DD, Bej AK. Detection of microbial pathogens in shellfish with multiplex PCR. *Curr Microbiol*. 1998;37(2):101–107.
219. Messelhäusser U, Colditz J, Thärigen D, Kleih W, Höller C, Busch U. Detection and differentiation of *Vibrio* spp. in seafood and fish samples with cultural and molecular methods. *Int J Food Microbiol*. 2010;142(3):360–364.
220. Vantarakis A, Komninou G, Venieri D, Papapetropoulou M. Development of a multiplex PCR detection of *Salmonella* spp. and *Shigella* spp. in mussels. *Lett Appl Microbiol*. 2000;31:105–109.
221. Sahu B, Singh SD, Behera BK, Panda SK, Das A, Parida PK. Rapid detection of *Salmonella* contamination in seafoods using multiplex PCR. *Braz J Microbiol*. 2019;50(3):807–816.
222. Li C, Gölz G, Alter T, Barac A, Hertwig S, Riedel C. Prevalence and antimicrobial resistance of *Yersinia enterocolitica* in retail seafood. *J Food Prot*. 2018;81(3):497–501.
223. Elmahdi S, Parveen S, Ossai S, et al. *Vibrio parahaemolyticus* and *Vibrio vulnificus* recovered from oysters during an oyster relay study. *Appl Environ Microbiol*. 2018;84(3):e01790–17.
224. Cetinkaya F, Elal Mus T, Yibar A, Guclu N, Tavsanli H, Cibik R. *L. monocytogenes* in raw and ready-to-eat foods. *J Food Saf*. 2014;34:42–49.
225. Zhang Z, Liu H, Lou Y, et al. Quantifying viable *Vibrio parahaemolyticus* and *Listeria monocytogenes* simultaneously in raw shrimp. *Appl Microbiol Biotechnol*. 2015;99(15):6451–6462.
226. Garrido A, Chapela M-J, Román B, et al. A new multiplex real-time PCR developed method for *Salmonella* spp. and *Listeria monocytogenes* detection in food and environmental samples. *Food Control*. 2013;30:76–85.
227. Edwards RA, Rodriguez-Brito B, Wegley L, et al. Using pyrosequencing to shed light on deep mine microbial ecology. *BMC Genomics*. 2006;7:57.
228. Novais RC, Thorstenson YR. The evolution of Pyrosequencing® for microbiology: from genes to genomes. *J Microbiol Methods*. 2011;86:1–7.
229. Quince C, Lanzen A, Curtis TP, et al. Accurate determination of microbial diversity from 454 pyrosequencing data. *Nat Methods*. 2009;6:639–641.
230. Jääskeläinen E, Jakobsen LMA, Hultman J, Eggers N, Bertram HC, Björkroth J. Metabolomics and bacterial diversity of packaged yellowfin tuna (*Thunnus albacares*) and salmon (*Salmo salar*) show fish species-specific spoilage development during chilled storage. *Int J Food Microbiol*. 2019;293:44–52.
231. Kuuliala L, Al Hage Y, Ioannidis A-G, et al. Microbiological, chemical and sensory spoilage analysis of raw Atlantic cod (*Gadus morhua*) stored under modified atmospheres. *Food Microbiol*. 2018;70:232–244.
232. Zotta T, Parente E, Ianniello RG, De Filippis F, Ricciardi A. Dynamics of bacterial communities and interaction networks in thawed fish fillets during chilled storage in air. *Int J Food Microbiol*. 2019;293:102–113.
233. Leonard SR, Mammel MK, Lacher DW, Elkins CA. Application of metagenomic sequencing to food safety, detection of Shiga toxin-producing *Escherichia coli* on fresh bagged spinach. *Appl Environ Microbiol*. 2015;81(23):8183–8191.
234. Yang X, Noyes NR, Doster E, et al. Use of metagenomic Shotgun sequencing technology to detect foodborne pathogens within the microbiome of the beef production chain. *Appl Environ Microbiol*. 2016;82(8):2433–2443.
235. Tyagi A, Singh B, Billekallu Thammegowda NK, Singh NK. Shotgun metagenomics offers novel insights into taxonomic compositions, metabolic pathways and antibiotic resistance genes in fish gut microbiome. *Arch Microbiol*. 2019;201(3):295–303.
236. Chen J-Q, Regan P, Laksanalamai P, Healey S, Hu Z. Prevalence and methodologies for detection, characterization and subtyping of *Listeria monocytogenes* and *L. ivanovii* in foods and environmental sources. *Food Sci Hum Wellness*. 2017;6(3):97–120.
237. Palma F, Brauge T, Radomski N, et al. Dynamics of mobile genetic elements of *Listeria monocytogenes* persisting in ready-to-eat seafood processing plants in France. *BMC Genomics*. 2020;21:130.
238. Martin CC, Svanevik CS, Lunestad BT, Sekse C, Johannessen GS. Isolation and characterisation of Shiga toxin-producing *Escherichia coli* from Norwegian bivalves. *Food Microbiol*. 2019;84:103268.
239. Chung HY, Lee B, Na EJ, et al. Potential survival and pathogenesis of a novel strain, *Vibrio parahaemolyticus* FORC_022, isolated from a soy sauce marinated crab by genome and transcriptome analyses. *Front Microbiol*. 2018;9:1504.
240. Trinh SA, Leyn SA, Rodionov ID, Godzik A, Satchell KJF. Draft genome sequences of two *Vibrio parahaemolyticus* strains associated with gastroenteritis after raw seafood ingestion in Colorado. *Genome Announc*. 2018;6(3):e01387–17.

241. Yang C, Zhang X, Fan H, et al. Genetic diversity, virulence factors and farm-to-table spread pattern of *Vibrio parahaemolyticus* food-associated isolates. *Food Microbiol.* 2019;84:103270.
242. European Food Safety Authority (EFSA). Whole genome sequencing and metagenomics for outbreak investigation, source attribution and risk assessment of food-borne microorganisms. *EFSA Journal.* 2019;17(12):5898. Available from: https://doi.org/10.2903/j.efsa.2019.5898.
243. Rantsiou K, Kathariou S, Winkler A, et al. Next generation microbiological risk assessment: opportunities of whole genome sequencing (WGS) for foodborne pathogen surveillance, source tracking and risk assessment. *Int J Food Microbiol.* 2018;287:3–9.
244. de Donno A, Montagna MT, de Rinaldis A, Zonno V, Gabutti G. Microbiological parameters in brackish water pond used for extensive and semi-intensive fish-culture: acquatina. *Water Air Soil Pollut.* 2002;134:205–214.
245. Parveen S, Hodge NC, Stall RE, Farrah SR, Tamplin ML. Phenotypic and genotypic characterization of human and non-human *Escherichia coli. Water Res.* 2001;35(2):379–386.
246. Scott TM, Rose JB, Jenkins TM, Farrah SR, Lukasik J. Microbial source tracking: current methodology and future directions. *Appl Environ Microbiol.* 2002;68(12):5796–5803.

Chapter 33

The evolution of molecular methods to study seafood-associated pathogens

Craig Baker-Austin[1] **and Jaime Martinez-Urtaza**[1,2]

[1]*Centre for Environment, Fisheries and Aquaculture (CEFAS), Weymouth, United Kingdom,* [2]*Department of Genetics and Microbiology, Faculty of Biosciences, Autonomous University of Barcelona, Barcelona, Spain*

Abstract

A variety of different pathogenic bacteria, viruses, and harmful algal biotoxin-producing organisms can accumulate in shellfish and other seafoods and cause a variety of human diseases. Worldwide, seafood is responsible for an important proportion of foodborne illnesses and associated outbreaks. The study of these pathogens has evolved markedly over the last two decades with the advent of molecular and genomic-based methods. Here we provide a brief overview of the most important human pathogens associated with seafood—focusing on bivalve shellfish while outlining how methods to study these pathogens have been applied and evolved in tandem with the revolution in genomic and molecular-based techniques. Certain methods, such as rapid identification methodologies including polymerase chain reaction (PCR), real-time PCR, and loop-mediated isothermal amplification, and whole-genome sequencing of pathogens of interest, have greatly altered our understanding of the pathogens responsible for seafood-associated illness. We present here some pertinent examples of how methods have evolved—particularly in the last decade—using shellfish-associated outbreak investigations that have utilized both traditional as well as "next generation" subtyping approaches. Finally, we outline novel approaches to study seafood-associated pathogens and discuss which of these techniques may be applied to study these organisms in the future.

Keywords: *Vibrio vulnificus*; *Vibrio parahaemolyticus*; oysters; norovirus; genome; MLST

33.1 Introduction

Seafood is part of a healthy diet, but seafood consumption is not risk-free.[1] For over 200 years, ingestion of seafood, and in particular shellfish, has been recognized as a cause of outbreaks of bacterial and viral infections.[2,3] Raw and partially cooked molluscan shellfish (clams, oysters, and mussels) have a long history as vectors of infectious agents and marine biotoxins.[4] Some seafood commodities are inherently more risky than others owing to many factors, including the nature of the environment from which they come, their mode of feeding, the season during which they are harvested, and how they are prepared and served.[1] Since shellfish can accumulate a range of human pathogens, in particular bacterial, viral, parasitic, and harmful biotoxin-producing organisms and their associated toxins, this food commodity is at particular risk. This diverse array of biological pathogens results in a wide variety of clinical syndromes, each with its own distinct epidemiology. Recently, the rapid growth of seafood production, such as bivalve shellfish, may greatly amplify human health risks. For instance, global aquaculture production more than tripled in live-weight volume from 34 million tons (Mt) in 1997 to 112 Mt in 2017.[5] Since the early 1970s the global consumption of shellfish has increased considerably—and with it, the reports of outbreaks of infections.[2] Changes in epidemiology will also amplify disease risk: an increasingly aging population, coupled to individuals with underlying risk conditions, can make certain pathogens more likely to result in hospitalization and death.[6] Illnesses are typically attributed to bacterial and viral agents that are associated either with human wastes (delivered to estuarine and marine environments in sewage effluents that have received variable levels of treatment) or to bacterial pathogens indigenous to coastal marine environments (e.g., *Vibrio* spp.).[4] As such, from a risk perspective, microbial risks associated with shellfish consumption can broadly be defined as naturally occurring and human-mediated. Of these, viral pathogens such as norovirus, hepatitis A, and the bacterial pathogen genera vibrios are globally the most important, and as such represent the main focus of this chapter. We briefly outline some of the major foodborne pathogens associated with seafood consumption globally and discuss recent epidemiological trends associated with these pathogen risks:

Present Knowledge in Food Safety. DOI: https://doi.org/10.1016/B978-0-12-819470-6.00004-4

33.2 Naturally occurring microbial risks

A wide variety of pathogenic bacteria, viruses, and harmful biotoxin-producing organisms are present naturally in marine waters. Because filter feeding shellfish are capable of filtering large volumes of water, they can accumulate these naturally occurring microbial constituents present in the water column. Various historical studies have shown that certain pathogens such as *Vibrio* densities in oysters can exceed 100 times that observed in the overlying water column.[7] We outline here the main naturally occurring seafood pathogens that are present in shellfish.

33.3 Pathogenic vibrios

Vibrio spp. are ubiquitous bacteria found in low salinity waters around the world.[8] Approximately a dozen *Vibrio* species are known to cause disease in humans,[9] and infection is usually initiated from exposure to seawater or consumption of raw or undercooked seafood.[10] Vibrios are responsible for a number of severe infections both in humans and animals.[11] Vibriosis is characterized by diarrhea, primary septicemia, wound infections, or other extra-intestinal infections. Select strains of *Vibrio cholerae*, *Vibrio parahaemolyticus*, *Vibrio vulnificus*, and *Vibrio alginolyticus* are perhaps considered the most serious human pathogens from this genus, yet two *Vibrio* species in particular, *V. vulnificus* and *V. parahaemolyticus* are significant foodborne human pathogens, and most frequently infections occur via the consumption of naturally contaminated shellfish produce. Typical clinical characteristics of *V. parahaemolyticus* infections include abdominal cramps, diarrhea, nausea, headaches, fever, and chills, but typically resolve in 2–3 days without medical intervention.[12] *V. vulnificus* infections are typically more severe, and alongside fever, chills, can lead to secondary lesions, sepsis, and death. This pathogen is responsible for over 95% of seafood-related deaths in the United States and carries the highest fatality rate of any foodborne pathogen.[6] The epidemiology associated with these two pathogens is also quite distinct: *V. parahaemolyticus* tends to cause outbreaks of seafood-associated gastroenteritis, while *V. vulnificus* sporadic infections.[8] It is worth noting that these pathogens represent a significant cause of morbidity and mortality. For example, an estimated 80,000 people contract *Vibrio* infections each year in the United States, with a sizeable fraction originating from foodborne sources such as consumption of raw or undercooked seafood produce. Epidemiological data from the Centers for Disease Control in the United States have indicated that there has been a significant increase in reported infections associated with vibrios, particularly in the last two decades. Annual incidence of reported vibriosis per 100,000 population has increased significantly in the United States from 1996 to 2010,[13] highlighting the importance of these pathogens from a clinical context. Unfortunately, a global burden on shellfish-associated vibriosis is unclear.[8] Calculations based upon probable incidence of vibriosis have estimated that *V. vulnificus* and *V. parahaemolyticus* are the first and third most costly marine-borne pathogens, costing $233 and $20 million, respectively.[14] Because the growth of pathogenic vibrios in the natural environment is largely dictated by ambient temperature, this group of pathogens represents an important and tangible barometer of climate change in marine systems.[15] Given warming of coastal regions, coupled to increasing consumption of seafood and at-risk groups for *Vibrio* infections (e.g., the elderly, individuals with conditions that make infections more likely to progress such as diabetes, liver, and immune disorders), it is likely that seafood-associated *Vibrio* infections may increase rapidly in the future.

The other main naturally occurring risk present in shellfish are marine biotoxins. Marine phytoplankton are single-celled algae that are autochthonous constituents of marine waters. A number of marine phytoplankton species can produce toxins that can accumulate in the flesh of shellfish and can pose a risk to human health if consumed. These harmful algal blooms are generally caused by the rapid growth of phytoplankton that may contain highly toxic chemicals, capable of causing illness and even death to both aquatic organisms and humans.[16] When environmental conditions are favorable, these toxin-producing phytoplankton can rapidly increase in abundance. The main harmful algal biotoxins (HAB) genera of concern for human health in Europe are the dinoflagellates *Alexandrium*, which are typically associated with the production of toxins responsible for paralytic shellfish poisoning, *Dinophysis* toxins associated with diarrhetic shellfish poisoning, and the diatom *Pseudo-nitzschia* toxins associated with amnesic shellfish poisoning (ASTs).[17] The dinoflagellates *Azadinium* (azaspiracid toxins, AZA), *Protoceratium reticulatum*, *Lingulodinium polyedra*, and *Gonyaulax spinifera* (yessotoxins, YTX) are less of an issue in the UK waters, although AZA has caused significant problems for the Irish shellfish industry.[18] There has been recent concern regarding the emergence of the potent neurotoxin tetrodotoxin in European shellfish produce;[19,20] however, the source of this toxin remains elusive. Although not the focus of this chapter, there have been several studies recently utilizing molecular methods to both detect and quantify HABs-producing organisms in environmental samples.[21–23]

33.4 Human-introduced pathogens

Fecal contamination of surface waters can originate from many sources including agricultural runoff, wild animals and birds, as well as human inputs from sewage. Because a variety of human pathogens, including bacteria (e.g., *Salmonella*, *V. cholerae*), viruses (e.g., norovirus, hepatitis

A, rotavirus, and astrovirus), and parasites, are present in fecal waste such as sewage, they represent an important and well-established route through which pathogens can be introduced into the environment and subsequently enter the food chain. In particular, the contamination of bivalve shellfish with norovirus from human and hepatitis A from fecal sources is recognized as a major human health risk.[24] Globally, epidemiological evidence gathered in recent years suggests that human enteric viruses are the most common pathogens transmitted by bivalve shellfish,[2,24] with norovirus (NoVs) the most commonly implicated infection. NoVs are the most common viral agents of acute gastroenteritis in humans, and high concentrations of NoVs are discharged into the environment.[25] The typical incubation period of norovirus infections is 24–48 h and symptoms include vomiting, diarrhea, abdominal pain, low-grade fever, headache, and myalgia.[26] Norovirus infections are typically self-limiting and resolve within a few days. Conversely, hepatitis A virus (HAV) are significantly more serious. HAV infection is considered the most serious viral infection linked to shellfish consumption, causing a debilitating disease and, occasionally, death.[2] Although infections associated with HAV are rare in the developed West (where HAV endemicity in the community is low), HAV has been implicated in large shellfish-associated outbreaks. An outbreak of HAV infection in Shanghai, China, in 1988, in which almost 300,000 cases was linked to the consumption of clams harvested from a sewage-polluted area, demonstrates that this pathogen can cause devastating human health impacts.[2,27] To date, this outbreak represents the largest virus-associated foodborne incident ever reported, highlighting its importance as a foodborne pathogen. Certain bacterial species such as *Campylobacter*, *Salmonella*, *Shigella* species, and *Escherichia coli*, which are commonly implicated in gastroenteritis, are only occasionally traced to seafood.[2] Historically, *Salmonella typhi* (the causative agent of typhoid fever) was once a significant cause of illness associated with seafood consumption. With improvements in sanitation over the past several decades, *Salmonella* serotype Typhi went from being the leading cause of *Salmonella* infection to becoming relatively uncommon.[1]

33.5 The evolution of methods—norovirus and hepatitis A virus

Over the last two decades, the tools used in the laboratory to study the above pathogen (e.g., viruses and bacterial pathogens) are almost unrecognizable to those initially utilized in the 1980s and early 1990s. Much of this progress has been facilitated by the advent of molecular microbiological approaches such as polymerase chain reaction (PCR) and more recently, real-time PCR (RT-PCR). Molecular methods employing PCR for the detection of viruses in shellfish have been published since the mid-1990s.[24,28] It is important to note that all published methods with demonstrable ability to detect viruses in bivalve shellfish or other foods have generally utilized PCR-based approaches. This is because methods based on other detection systems utilized for clinical diagnostic samples (e.g., current ELISA methods and scanning electron microscopy) have not been demonstrated to have adequate performance (sensitivity) for environmentally contaminated samples such as bivalve shellfish or other foods.[29] A significant limitation to study viral pathogens in shellfish has been the lack of successful cultivation-based techniques, although some methods have been proposed recently.[30] Coupled to this, PCR-based approaches target the genome of the pathogen in question, which may overestimate the risks posed. These limitations are important because they have direct impacts on the application of PCR-based methods to foodstuffs. To circumvent some of these issues, the utilization of bacteriophage cultivation alongside RT-PCR detection of NoV has been suggested as a potential approach. Lowther et al.[31] combined RT-PCR testing with a test for infectious F-RNA phage to better estimate health risks associated with NoV in oysters, and found this combination of approaches better predicted the presence of infectious NoV than RT-PCR testing alone.[31]

Over the last two decades significant progress has been made in the establishment of sensitive and robust molecular approaches to detect and quantify NoV in shellfish. A standard validated method for the detection of norovirus in molluscan shellfish was developed in the early 2010s, leading to the publication of a two-part technical specification for determination of HAC and NoV in food matrices (ISO/TS 15216:2013), which was published jointly by the European Committee for Standardisation and the International Organization for Standardization in 2013.[32] A full ISO standard method (ISO 15216–1:2017) including validation data was subsequently published for the quantification of levels of HAV and norovirus genogroup I (GI) and II (GII) RNA, from test samples of foodstuffs (soft fruit, leaf, stem and bulb vegetables, bottled water, Bilvalve molluscan shellfish (BMS)) or food surfaces. This testing methodology has been widely used internationally and was recently used as part of a European Food Safety Authority (EFSA)-led harmonized monitoring across Europe to establish data on the prevalence of NoV in European oysters.[33] It should be noted that the development of virological methods using PCR and applied to shellfish represent among the first standardized methods of their kind applied in food microbiology. More recently, a set of novel approaches have been applied to study NoV in shellfish. For example, applications such as digital PCR (dPCR) have been successfully applied to study the prevalence of NoV in oysters.[34] Because of the sensitivity of dPCR, the application of this methodology could be as an early warning system, which is useful for further risk analysis studies. A recent comparison of RT-PCR versus dPCR suggests that dPCR can be a suitable method for the precise quantification of NoV in oysters.[35] There is now increasing interest in using high-throughput sequencing approaches to understand NoV abundance and genetic diversity in environmental samples. A study analyzed NoV diversity and evaluated strain-dependent accumulation patterns in three oyster samples using a metagenomic methodology. The study allowed the sequencing of full NoV genomes from contaminated oyster samples, even at relatively low concentrations.[36]

33.6 Evolution of approaches—pathogenic vibrios

A variety of approaches have been developed for the isolation, detection, enumeration, and characterization of vibrios from environmental matrices and food samples.[37] As with the study of pathogenic viruses implicated in shellfish-associated outbreaks, the advent of molecular methods in the late 1980s onward heralded a clear step change in how laboratories studied these pathogenic bacteria. Laboratories carrying out downstream confirmatory testing of vibrios from shellfish samples typically use species-specific PCR methods. Currently, tests are available for all major *Vibrio* pathogens with associated conventional PCR[38,39] and RT-PCR assays[40–42] for species-level confirmation. PCR of the virulence genes for *Vibrio* pathogens, for example, *tdh/trh* analysis of *V. parahaemolyticus*,[41] as well as a variety of virulence-associated PCR tests for *V. vulnificus*[43,44] are frequently carried out during in-depth clinical investigations.[8] More recently, the use of loop-mediated amplification-based methods (loop-mediated isothermal amplification) have been successfully applied to detect *V. parahaemolyticus* and *V. vulnificus* from environmental, clinical, and food sources.[45,46] Perhaps, where the most rapid evolution of approaches has been observed have been in the more in-depth subtyping methodologies required during outbreak investigations. Until around a decade ago, methods such as multilocus sequence typing (MLST),[47] pulsed-field gel electrophoresis (PFGE),[48] and serotyping were the mainstay methodologies utilized in outbreak investigations. Despite the publication of the full genome sequences of the *Vibrio* species *V. parahaemolyticus* and *V. vulnificus* almost 20 years ago,[49,50] the routine use of Sanger method in the early 2000s was prohibitive for most microbiology laboratories. Sequencing based on this technology was expensive, cumbersome, and time-consuming, restricting the use of whole-genome sequencing (WGS). However, the availability of information about the sequence and organization of the totality of the genes in the genome sequences created a new framework for sequencing-based studies of bacterial populations based on the sequence of a limited number of genes. This approach—MLST—typically used sequences of seven housekeeping genes defined for each bacterial species and distributed along the chromosome, which were used to analyze bacteria at population level, defining the population structure and identifying the distinctive contribution mutation and recombination as driving forces of evolution. Contrary to other typing techniques used before, sequencing data could be easily shared about networks of collaborators and deposited in a single, centralized, and publicly accessible repository of data. Based on the publicity available data from the genomic sequencing, MLST schemes were developed for the three big pathogenic *Vibrio* (https://pubmlst.org/databases/),[47,51,52] and with the help of the first generation of bioinformatic tools, scientists were able for first time to compare isolates from different sources and regions, and contribute to obtain a global picture of *Vibrio* populations and their incredible diversity in environmental sources. Likewise, PFGE, which using restriction enzymes to digest and following polyacrylamide-gel electrophoresis produce a defined fingerprint of a microbial genome, was used extensively for outbreak investigations[48,53] (Fig. 33.1). Both methods were extremely useful in more fully understanding the evolution of epidemic clones within a regional or global context and being able to place.

33.7 Understanding past outbreaks

It has become evident with the advent of WGS that these older methodologies (e.g., PFGE, MLST, and serotyping) lacked granularity and resolution, particularly where closely related strains were implicated in outbreaks (Fig. 33.1). One of the most exciting developments in the study of vibrios has been in the ability to utilize WGS approaches to retrospectively study outbreaks. However, the ability to piece together the phylogenetic and evolutionary history of bacterial pathogens from outbreak situations using high-throughput sequencing is relatively new concept.[54,55] Recent studies using WGS have been invaluable in piecing together the elusive spread of these pathogenic foodborne bacteria, and these in general use the same concepts as MLST and PFGE but with larger, more robust, and finely scaled datasets (Fig. 33.2). In 2012 a large foodborne outbreak of *V. parahaemolyticus* was reported in northern Spain and the East coast of the United States, linked to seafood produce.[56] At the time, the outbreaks appeared to be driven by the same strain of *V. parahaemolyticus* (ST36), a highly pathogenic strain

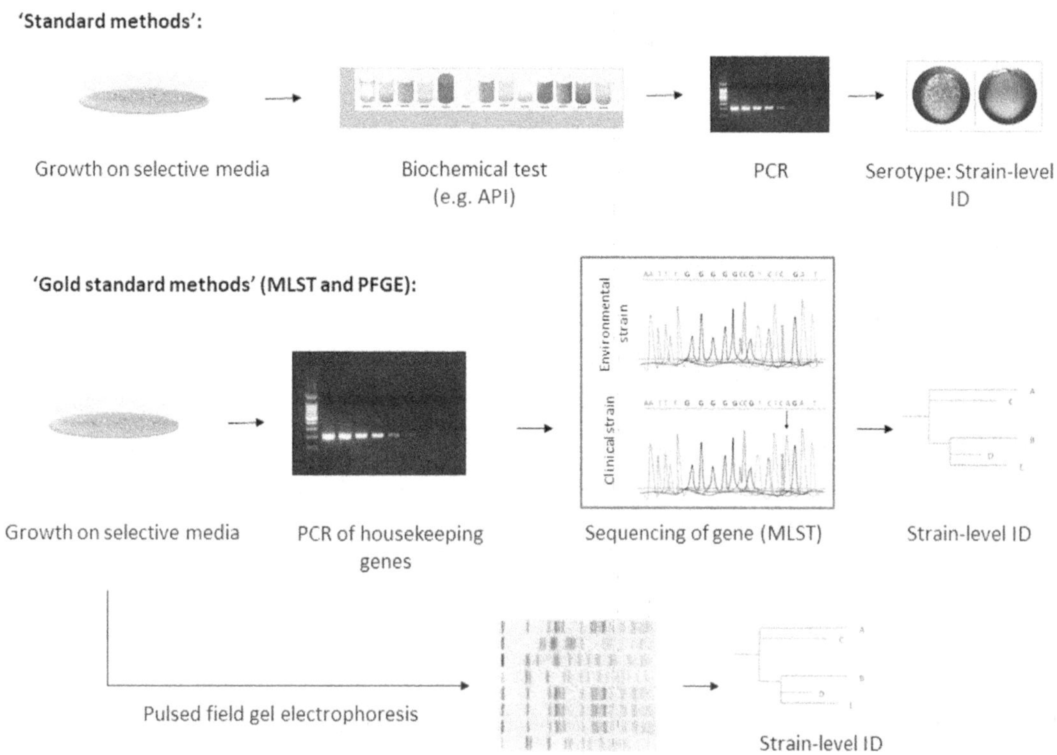

FIGURE 33.1 Methods such as PCR, biochemical testing, and serotyping are still used routinely and will probably remain important tools to identify strains involved in outbreaks. Subtyping methods such as PFGE and MLST represent the "gold standard" approaches for determining the sources of bacterial outbreaks associated with shellfish. The methods were gradually supplanted in the last decade by WGS-enabled methodologies. *MLST*, multi-locus sequence typing; *PCR*, polymerase chain reaction; *PFGE*, pulsed-field gel electrophoresis; *WGS*, whole-genome sequencing.

that now appeared to be circulating pandemically. Martinez-Urtaza et al. used genome-wide analyses of *V. parahaemolyticus* to reconstruct the evolutionary history of a highly pathogenic clone (ST36) over the course of its geographic expansion across the United States and into Europe.[57] Previous work using PFGE, MLST, and serotyping had indicated that the strains responsible for these outbreaks were indistinguishable. Utilizing WGS the origin of this lineage was estimated to be in ~1985. They noted that by 1995, a new variant emerged in the region and quickly replaced the old clone, which has not been detected since 2000.[57] The authors also suggested that after several introductions into the northeast coast of the United States, a new clone differentiated into a highly dynamic group that continues to cause illness on the northeast coast of the United States. Surprisingly, the strains detected in Europe in 2012[56] diverged from this ancestral group around 2000. More recently, an analysis of ST36 strains that have emerged in Peru[58] and have shown the potential timeframe and route of the transcontinental expansion of ST36 *V. parahaemolyticus* into South America. The identification of ST36 strains in both clinical and environmental sources is suggestive that these pathogens have now established themselves in Latin America, with potential for ongoing foodborne risk. In all of these studies, the unparalleled granularity afforded by WGS (compared to older subtyping methods) has allowed researchers to provide a more cohesive and integrated view of these pathogens in both time and space.

Virus testing of outbreak samples has greatly improved our understanding regarding the levels of virus likely to cause human infections; however, this understanding is still incomplete. Using collaboration with industry partners Lowther et al. used illness complaints by customers to determine illness reporting rates for batches of oysters provided by a single depuration center compared to shellfish not implicated in disease. These samples were compared with rates with NoV levels in batches as determined by RT-PCR. A statistically significant difference between NoV levels in the two sets of samples was observed. The geometric mean of the levels in outbreak samples (1048 copies per gram) was almost one order of magnitude higher than for positive nonoutbreak-related samples (121 copies per gram).[59]

33.8 Future directions

The rate of technological change with regards to studying shellfish pathogens—particularly in the last decade—has opened up new and exciting opportunities to study these

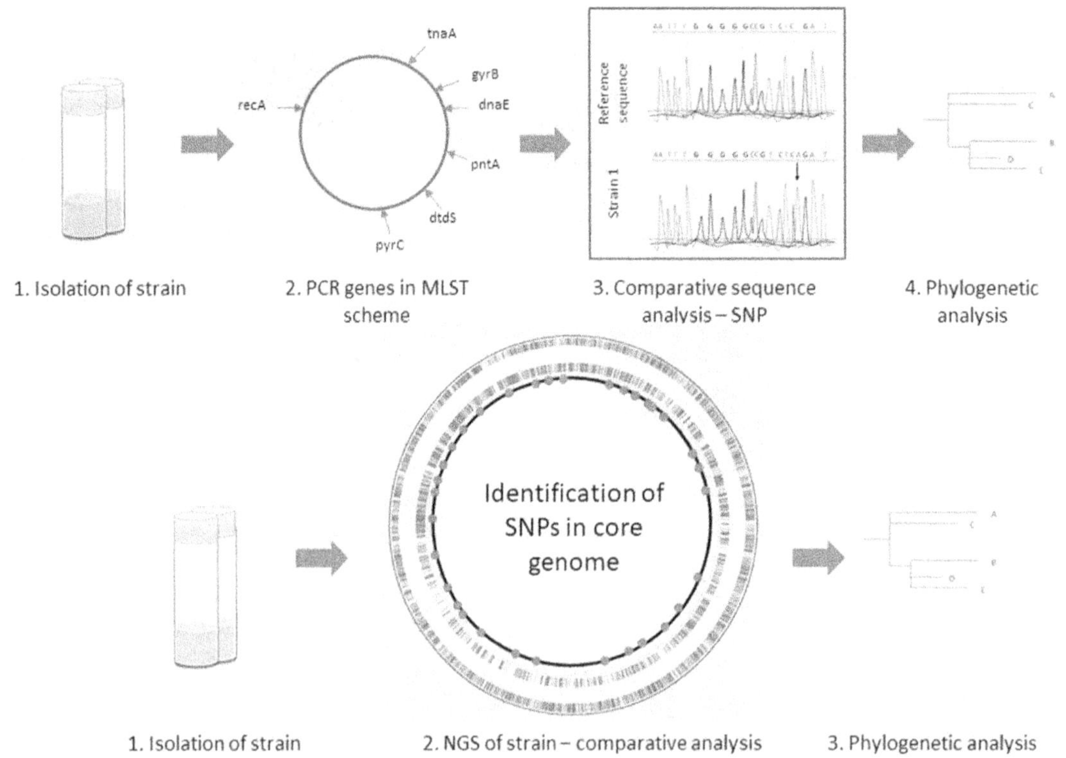

FIGURE 33.2 In the last decade (2012 onward) WGS-enabled methods have superseded many of the older bacteriological subtyping methods used to study shellfish-associated outbreaks caused by bacteria. The ability to identify small variations in the genomes of strains implicated in outbreaks (SNPs) allows closely related isolates to be distinguished. These methods are cheaper, faster, and provide greater resolution and granularity compared to subtyping approaches such as MLST and PFGE. *MLST*, multilocus sequence typing; *PFGE*, pulsed-field gel electrophoresis; *SNPs*, single nucleotide polymorphisms; *WGS*, whole-genome sequencing.

important human pathogens. In particular, numerous recent studies have shown that WGS can be used creatively for a variety of applications that are relevant in the field of epidemiology, clinical diagnosis and ecology, among others. For example, *Vibrio* infections such as *V. vulnificus* have a rapid onset of symptoms and can subsequently develop into necrotizing fasciitis and secondary septicemia in a matter of hours. Unfortunately, routine examinations may fail to identify a pathogen, which was the case in a study by Li et al., in 2019, where a suspected *Vibrio vulnificus* infection examined using routine wound and blood culture work did not lead to a correct clinical diagnosis. WGS was used for fast and accurate identification of *V. vulnificus*, with the use of PCR to confirm the subsequent results. This study demonstrates the effectiveness of WGS as a diagnostic method when routine examinations should fail.[60,61] A key limitation for the current testing methods used for viruses in shellfish is based around the lack of cultivation methods for viruses as well as the ability to discriminate between infectious and noninfectious viral particles (which cannot be differentiated by current PCR methods). The use of specific treatments to samples (e.g., which can intercalate with nucleic acids, such as via propidium monoazide) has been suggested as a potential approach to distinguish between infectious and noninfectious NoV by PCR.[62,63] The use of surrogates such as Porcine Gastric Mucin Binding Assay and bacteriophages to accurately reflect the presence of potentially infectious NoV in environmental and food samples is an area of ongoing research,[31,64] but is garnering important insights into this current limitation in virological research.

Advances in molecular methods, in particular sequencing technologies, are moving at breakneck speed, and so too are analysis tools to scrutinize these datasets. Many of these approaches can now be achieved in almost real time. One of the most exciting developments is nanopore sequencing technologies—which can produce long read length sequences quickly and cheaply. Because these instruments are also portable, there is now the potential to use these methods in field-based applications, such as during outbreak situations.[65] Data visualization approaches are also evolving quickly, to keep pace with the exponential increase in sequencing data and the inherent complexity therein. These approaches when applied to shellfish pathogens offer the potential to revolutionize the field of infectious diseases and microbiology by allowing us to unravel key aspects related to the evolution and spread of infections. Such approaches are incredibly exciting, and will open a variety of applications, bridging the gaps between genomics, environmental microbiology, clinical infectious diseases, and epidemiology.

References

1. Iwamoto M, Ayers T, Mahon BE, Swerdlow DL. Epidemiology of seafood-associated infections in the United States. *Clin Microbiol Rev*. 2010;23:399–411.
2. Potasman I, Paz A, Odeh M. Infectious outbreaks associated with bivalve shellfish consumption: a worldwide perspective. *Clin Infect Dis*. 2002;35:921–928.
3. Pasquier JPA. Essai medicale sur les huitre. *Paris Fac Med*. 1816.
4. Rippey. Infectious diseases associated with molluscan shellfish consumption. *Clin Microbiol Rev*. 1994;7:419–425.
5. Naylor RL, et al. A 20-year retrospective review of global aquaculture. *Nature*. 2021;591:551–563.
6. Baker-Austin C, Oliver JD. *Vibrio vulnificus*: new insights into a deadly opportunistic pathogen. *Environ Microbiol*. 2018. Available from: https://doi.org/10.1111/1462-2920.13955.
7. Depaola A, Hopkins LH, Peeler JT, Wentz B, McPhearson RM. Incidence of *Vibrio parahaemolyticus* in U.S. coastal waters and oysters from shellfish-growing areas. *Appl Environ Microbiol*. 1990;56:2299–2302.
8. Baker-Austin C, et al. *Vibrio* spp. infections. *Nat Rev Dis Prim*. 2018;4:1–20. Available from: https://doi.org/10.1038/s41572-018-0005-8.
9. Austin B. *Bacteria pathogens of marine fish. Ocean Health: Pathogens in Marine Environment*. 2005391–413.
10. Altekruse SF, et al. *Vibrio gastroenteritis* in the US Gulf of Mexico region: the role of raw oysters. *Epidemiol Infect*. 2000;124:489–495.
11. Vezzulli L, Colwell RR, Pruzzo C. Ocean warming and spread of pathogenic vibrios in the aquatic environment. *Microb Ecol*. 2013;65:817–825.
12. Baker-Austin C, Stockley L, Rangdale R, Martinez-Urtaza J. Environmental occurrence and clinical impact of *Vibrio vulnificus* and *Vibrio parahaemolyticus*: a European perspective. *Environ Microbiol Rep*. 2010;2:7–18.
13. Newton A, Kendall M, Vugia DJ, Henao OL, Mahon BE. Increasing rates of vibriosis in the United States, 1996–2010: review of surveillance data from 2 systems. *Clin Infect Dis*. 2012;54:391–395.
14. Ralston EP, Kite-Powell H, Beet A. An estimate of the cost of acute health effects from food- and water-borne marine pathogens and toxins in the USA. *J Water Health*. 2011;9:680–694.
15. Baker-Austin C, Trinanes J, Gonzalez-Escalona N, Martinez-Urtaza J. Non-Cholera vibrios: the microbial barometer of climate change. *Trends Microbiol*. 2017;25:76–84.
16. Visciano P, et al. Marine biotoxins: occurrence, toxicity, regulatory limits and reference methods. *Front Microbiol*. 2016;7:1–10.
17. Davidson K, Bresnan E. Shellfish toxicity in UK waters: a threat to human health? *Environ Health*. 2009;8:2–5.
18. Chevallier OP, et al. New insights into the causes of human illness due to consumption of azaspiracid contaminated shellfish. *Sci Rep*. 2015;5:1–8.
19. Turner AD, Powell A, Schofield A, Lees DN, Baker-Austin C. Detection of the pufferfish toxin tetrodotoxin in European bivalves, England, 2013 to 2014. *Euro Surveill*. 2015;21009.
20. Turner AD, et al. Detection of Tetrodotoxin Shellfish Poisoning (TSP) toxins and causative factors in bivalve molluscs from the UK. *Mar Drugs*. 2017;15.
21. Lee HG, et al. An advanced tool, droplet digital PCR (DdPCR), for absolute quantification of the red-tide dinoflagellate, *Cochlodinium polykrikoides* Margalef (Dinophyceae). *Algae*. 2017;32:189–197.
22. Hatfield RG, et al. Development of a TaqMan qPCR assay for detection of *Alexandrium* spp. and application to harmful algal bloom monitoring. *Toxicon X*. 2019;2.
23. Durán-Vinet B, et al. Potential applications of CRISPR/Cas for next-generation biomonitoring of harmful algae blooms: a review. *Harmful Algae*. 2021;103:102027.
24. Lees DN. Viruses and bivalve shellfish. *Int J Food Microbiol*. 2000;59:81–116.
25. Le Guyader FS, et al. Detection and quantification of noroviruses in shellfish. *Appl Environ Microbiol*. 2009;75:618–624.
26. Prato R, et al. Norovirus gastroenteritis general outbreak associated with raw shellfish consumption in South Italy. *BMC Infect Dis*. 2004;4:1–6.
27. Tang YW, et al. A serologically confirmed, case-control study, of a large outbreak of hepatitis A in China, associated with consumption of clams. *Epidemiol Infect*. 1991;107:651–657.
28. Lees DN, Henshilwood K, Green J, Gallimore CI, Brown DWG. Detection of small round structured viruses in shellfish by reverse transcription-PCR. *Appl Environ Microbiol*. 1995;61:4418–4424.
29. Lees D. International standardisation of a method for detection of human pathogenic viruses in molluscan shellfish. *Food Environ Virol*. 2010;2:146–155.
30. Estes MK, et al. Human norovirus cultivation in nontransformed stem cell-derived human intestinal enteroid cultures: success and challenges. *Viruses*. 2019;11:9–11.
31. Lowther JA, Cross L, Stapleton T, et al. Use of F-specific RNA bacteriophage to estimate infectious norovirus levels in oysters. *Food Environ Virol*. 2019;11:247–258.
32. Lowther JA, et al. Validation of EN ISO method 15216 – part 1 – quantification of hepatitis A virus and norovirus in food matrices. *Int J Food Microbiol*. 2019;288:82–90.
33. European Food Safety Authority. Technical specifications on the harmonised monitoring and reporting of antimicrobial resistance in *Salmonella*, *Campylobacter* and indicator *Escherichia coli* and *Enterococcus* spp. bacteria transmitted through food. *EFSA J*. 2012;10:1–64.
34. Polo D, et al. Digital PCR for quantifying norovirus in oysters implicated in outbreaks, France. *Emerg Infect Dis*. 2016;22: 2189–2191.
35. Persson S, Eriksson R, Lowther J, Ellström P, Simonsson M. Comparison between RT droplet digital PCR and RT real-time PCR for quantification of noroviruses in oysters. *Int J Food Microbiol*. 2018;2:73–83.
36. Strubbia S, Schaeffer J, Besnard A, et al. Metagenomic to evaluate norovirus genomic diversity in oysters: impact on hexamer selection and targeted capture-based enrichment. *Int J Food Microbiol*. 2020;323.
37. Hartnell RE, et al. A pan-European ring trial to validate an International Standard for detection of *Vibrio cholerae*, *Vibrio parahaemolyticus* and *Vibrio vulnificus* in seafoods. *Int J Food Microbiol*. 2018. Available from: https://doi.org/10.1016/j.ijfoodmicro.2018.02.008.

38. Panicker G, Call DR, Krug MJ, Bej AK. Detection of pathogenic *Vibrio* spp. in shellfish by using multiplex PCR and DNA microarrays. *Appl Environ Microbiol.* 2004;70:7436–7444.
39. Hill WE, et al. Polymerase chain reaction identification of *Vibrio vulnificus* in artificially contaminated oysters. *Appl Environ Microbiol.* 1991;57:707–711.
40. Campbell MS, Wright AC. Real-time PCR analysis of *Vibrio vulnificus* from oysters. *Appl Environ Microbiol.* 2003;69:7137–7144.
41. Nordstrom JL, Vickery MCL, Blackstone GM, Murray SL, DePaola A. Development of a multiplex real-time PCR assay with an internal amplification control for the detection of total and pathogenic *Vibrio parahaemolyticus* bacteria in oysters. *Appl Environ Microbiol.* 2007;73:5840–5847.
42. Taiwo M, et al. Comparison of toxR and tlh based PCR assays for *Vibrio parahaemolyticus. Food Control.* 2017;77:116–120.
43. Baker-Austin C, et al. PilF polymorphism-based real-time PCR to distinguish *Vibrio vulnificus* strains of human health relevance. *Food Microbiol.* 2012;30:17–23.
44. Baker-Austin C, et al. Rapid in situ detection of virulent *Vibrio vulnificus* strains in raw oyster matrices using real-time PCR. *Environ Microbiol Rep.* 2010;2:76–80.
45. Han F, Ge B. Evaluation of a loop-mediated isothermal amplification assay for detecting *Vibrio vulnificus* in raw oysters. *Foodborne Pathog Dis.* 2008;5:311–320.
46. Yamazaki W, Kumeda Y, Uemura R, Misawa N. Evaluation of a loop-mediated isothermal amplification assay for rapid and simple detection of *Vibrio parahaemolyticus* in naturally contaminated seafood samples. *Food Microbiol.* 2011;28:1238–1241.
47. Gonzalez-Escalona N, et al. Determination of molecular phylogenetics of *Vibrio parahaemolyticus* strains by multilocus sequence typing. *J Bacteriol.* 2008;190:2831–2840.
48. Kai MK, et al. Evaluation and validation of a PulseNet standardized pulsed-field gel electrophoresis protocol for subtyping *Vibrio parahaemolyticus*: an International Multicenter Collaborative study. *J Clin Microbiol.* 2008;46:2766–2773.
49. Chen CY, et al. Comparative genome analysis of *Vibrio vulnificus*, a marine pathogen. *Genome Res.* 2003;13:2577–2587.
50. Makino K, et al. Genome sequence of *Vibrio parahaemolyticus*: a pathogenic mechanism distinct from that of *V. cholerae. Lancet.* 2003;361:743–749.
51. Bisharat N, et al. Hybrid *Vibrio vulnificus. Emerg Infect Dis.* 2005;11:30–35.
52. Octavia S, et al. Population structure and evolution of non-O1/non-O139 *Vibrio cholerae* by multilocus sequence typing. *PLoS One.* 2013;8.
53. Martinez-Urtaza J, et al. Characterization of pathogenic *Vibrio parahaemolyticus* isolates from clinical sources in Spain and comparison with Asian and North American pandemic isolates. *J Clin Microbiol.* 2004;42:4672–4678.
54. Köser CU, et al. Routine use of microbial whole genome sequencing in diagnostic and public health microbiology. *PLoS Pathog.* 2012;8.
55. Harris SR, et al. Evolution of MRSA during hospital transmission and intercontinental spread. *Science.* 2010;327:469–474.
56. Martinez-Urtaza J, et al. Spread of Pacific Northwest *Vibrio parahaemolyticus* strain. *N Engl J Med.* 2013;369:1573–1574.
57. Martinez-Urtaza J, et al. Genomic variation and evolution of *Vibrio parahaemolyticus* ST36 over the course of a transcontinental epidemic expansion. *mBio.* 2017;8:1–17.
58. Abanto M, Gavilan RG, Baker-Austin C, Gonzalez-Escalona N, Martinez-Urtaza J. Global expansion of Pacific Northwest *Vibrio parahaemolyticus* sequence type 36. *Emerg Infect Dis.* 2020;26:323–326.
59. Lowther JA, Gustar NE, Hartnell RE, Lees DN. Comparison of norovirus RNA levels in outbreak-related oysters with background environmental levels. *J Food Prot.* 2012;75:389–393.
60. Li L, Wang L, Zhang C, Chen P, Luo X. A case of *Vibrio vulnificus* related wound infection diagnosed by next-generation sequencing. *IDCases.* 2019;15:e00497.
61. Alekseyev YO, et al. A next-generation sequencing primer—how does it work and what can it do? *Acad Pathol.* 2018;5. 2374289518766521.
62. Gensberger ET, et al. Evaluation of quantitative PCR combined with PMA treatment for molecular assessment of microbial water quality. *Water Res.* 2014;67:367–376.
63. Kim SY, Ko G. Using propidium monoazide to distinguish between viable and nonviable bacteria, MS2 and murine norovirus. *Lett Appl Microbiol.* 2012;55:182–188.
64. Li X, Chen H. Evaluation of the porcine gastric mucin binding assay for high-pressure-inactivation studies using murine norovirus and tulane virus. *Appl Environ Microbiol.* 2015;81: 515–521.
65. Quick J, et al. Real-time, portable genome sequencing for Ebola surveillance. *Nature.* 2016;530:228–232.

Section VII

Changes in pathogenic microbiological contamination of food throughout the various stages of the food chain post-processing

Chapter 34

Microbiological safety in food retail

Karen Job[1], Karin Carstensen[2] and Lucia E. Anelich[3]

[1]*The Food Brain Consultancy, Melbourne, VIC, Australia,* [2]*Woolworths South Africa (Pty) Ltd, Cape Town, Western Cape, South Africa,* [3]*Anelich Consulting, Pretoria, South Africa*

Abstract

The role and responsibilities of a food retailer in providing safe food for the consumer, are unique and complex. Retailers must cover the risks in the whole supply chain from "field to fork" or from the safety of raw materials to influencing consumer behavior, across a diverse range of product types and processes. Food retailers need to understand the nature of the products they sell, their selling operation procedures, and their customers, as well as the hazards that may affect their food. Several other aspects must be considered, including shelf-life, date marking, own brands versus branded goods, cooking/handling instructions on the packaging, ensuring that the chill (cold) chain is not compromised, managing food waste, participating in food recalls, conducting food safety audits on their suppliers and more.

In-store hospitality units such as cafes or restaurants, or unpackaged food such as loose produce, in-store bakeries, delicatessen counters, or rotisserie chickens in a retail environment can introduce diverse microbiological hazards that must be managed accordingly. Similarly, counters offering sliced cooked and cured meats, cheeses, and salads are a common feature of retail stores and bring with them special considerations on pathogen control.

The rapid growth of online and home deliveries in recent years has brought an additional set of challenges to retail risk management.

Keywords: Retailer; consumer; food safety; risk management; *Listeria monocytogenes*; *Campylobacter*; food waste; date marking or labeling

34.1 Introduction

A retail food store is defined as any establishment or section of an establishment where food and food products are offered to the consumer and intended for off-premises consumption.[1] A food retailer is essentially the point in the food chain between the end of food manufacturing and distribution and the consumer receiving that food. The consumer therefore expects and trusts that the food purchased is safe for human consumption if ready-to-eat (RTE). If the food requires further cooking before consumption, the expectation is that the food will be rendered safe to consume. Retailer accountability must, therefore, uniquely cover the risks in the whole supply chain from "field to fork" or from the safety of raw materials to influencing consumer behavior, across a diverse range of product types and processes but with the ultimate focus on protecting the consumer and also their brand.

This chapter explores the role and responsibilities of a food retailer in microbiological food safety risk management.

34.2 The importance of defining and agreeing on "What makes food safe" in the eyes of a retailer

Food safety at retail begins with good procurement practices and ends with good recall procedures, should a food safety matter arise.[2]

To ensure that the food and beverage on sale in a retailer is safe the collaboration of the retailer with its brand manufacturing partners and national brand producers is essential. In several countries, food-related legislation states that the brand owner is ultimately accountable for the sale of safe products, but the manufacturer who makes own-label products is responsible for a significant amount of product safety with their day-to-day operations.[3] Yet in some others, the retailer is responsible for both the sale of own-brand and national brand products.[4,5] The understanding and agreement of 'what makes a product safe?' must be discussed from the outset of any product development process and agreed upon in a commercial contract, such as a product specification.

Food retailers need to know and understand the nature of the products that they sell, their selling operation procedures and customers, and the hazards that may affect

Present Knowledge in Food Safety. DOI: https://doi.org/10.1016/B978-0-12-819470-6.00077-9

their food. For basic food retailers selling prepacked food, basic good housekeeping may be sufficient to address food safety.[6]

From a microbiological safety point of view, there are two things to consider. Is the hazard from the *growth* of an organism or the *survival* of an organism? In a HACCP-based food safety management system the identification of a microbiological hazard should not be a generic microbiological risk, instead, it must consider and state the specific pathogens, including viruses and parasites, of concern. Furthermore, a clear distinction should be made between what constitutes a true risk to human health, when an identified hazard is present.[7]

The reason for this is that the subsequent controls may be different; if for example, one is concerned about the survival of *Salmonella* spp. then a process such as heat, or pressure may be required to reduce the hazard to an acceptable level. Growth of *Salmonella* is less relevant in an RTE product as mere presence is enough to render the food unacceptable and potentially unsafe. Even a small quantity of *Salmonella*, less than 10 CFU/g, especially in low moisture foods, has been shown through epidemiological evidence to have caused illness.[8]

In contrast, there are some species of potentially pathogenic bacteria where one is concerned about their growth. If this is the case one's HACCP-based food safety management system must contain processes, or hurdles that prevent the multiplication and growth of the target pathogens. These could be intrinsic factors such as pH or water activity (a_w), or a packaging format that creates an aerobic or anaerobic environment, depending on the pathogens of concern. For example, in an RTE food such as a dip such as hummus, the growth of *Listeria monocytogenes* is prevented by lowering the pH to a level below which the organism cannot grow, that is <4.4 by the addition of acidic ingredients such as lemon juice, or additives such as citric acid.[9,10]

Whilst for bacteria such as *L. monocytogenes* the growth of the vegetative cells is a consideration, there are other foods for which preventing the growth of spore formers and toxin producers is critical for achieving food safety. Examples are *Bacillus cereus*; unless the heat process is sufficient to deliver commercial sterility by obtaining a minimum F_0 of 3, the destruction of bacterial spores is rarely achieved through pasteurization temperatures used in chilled food manufacture.[11] The germination and outgrowth of spores usually have a longer lag phase than the replication of vegetative cells. There is therefore a risk that *B. cereus* spores may be present in chilled foods if these foods have a long shelf life (over 20 days) and are stored in consumers' refrigerators (which are likely to be over the 3°C needed to prevent growth for some spore formers). For *B. cereus*, it can germinate and grow to levels sufficient for the production of potentially harmful toxins if the food does not have an intrinsic factor or an additive that would prevent such growth. As an example, a foodstuff such as filled pasta contains a risk from the germination, growth to high enough levels, and subsequent toxin production of *B. cereus*. The spores are potentially present in the wheat flour ingredient. When micromodeled using online tools such as CB Premium[12] then *B. cereus* could grow to levels greater than 10^5 CFU/g from a starting point of 10 cells in just 21 days. These products typically have shelf lives above 50 days. Therefore, to prevent this hazard from occurring at levels that can result in toxin production, products such as fresh-filled pasta should have an intrinsic factor such as a water activity of below 0.970 throughout the product to prevent the risk of toxin production occurring. Alternatively, the retailer could choose to shorten the shelf life of the product or reduce the a_W by adding salt, provided that the salt levels in the final product comply with relevant legislation. However, reducing the shelf life of such products is commercially undesirable and can even make the product commercially unfeasible as the quantity of food that cannot be sold, also known as "in-store waste levels", becomes too high; it is, therefore, important for a retail technologist to balance the commerciality of a product with its safety and regulatory compliance.

The length of shelf life based on a microbial hazard and its control is often overlooked from a HACCP-based food safety manufacturing plan as the determination of shelf-life occurs during the product development phase. Therefore, it is not something that is routinely measured or monitored by the manufacturer in the same way as temperature, time, pH, or a_W is monitored on each production run. However, it is the role of a retail food technologist to ensure that shelf-life is set at a safe number of days, considering all the potential microbiological hazards, to manage risk to consumer health by ensuring that an acceptable level of the particular hazard is not exceeded.

An important consideration for both the retailer and manufacturer in defining what makes food safe is the definition and understanding of the ultimate consumer. This is often referred to in HACCP-based food safety management systems as "intended use," where the use of the final product, as well as the target consumer/s, are considered. Such assessments must be based on validated shelf-life studies as well as provide proper storage and usage instructions. For many products, this will be a mainstream adult consumer, but if a product is marketed at a specific population group, for example, food for children, then the vulnerability of that group must be considered. Baby food is an obvious example of this and in most countries, additional regulations and controls exist for the production of safe food for babies. However, a retailer must still responsibly market a range of foods to children, or even potentially to an older demographic who over a certain age (older than 65), are defined as more vulnerable to foodborne illness. In this regard, retailers must consider their marketing information or message and method, product type, and safety standards. This is an area open to some interpretation and is difficult to regulate, but one for serious consideration when defining an acceptable level of risk in a modern HACCP-based food safety management system.

34.3 The role of HACCP-based food safety management systems and due diligence in retail

HACCP has come a long way since it was first conceived in the 1960s as part of Pillsbury designing and manufacturing the first foods for space flight, but its purpose remains unchanged. It is internationally recognized as a logical tool for identifying and defining significant hazards and their subsequent management.[6]

As retailers, reviewing the HACCP documentation with their manufacturing partners is an important part of developing new products and managing their ongoing safe production and sale. However, as innovation in food sold in retailers has accelerated over the past decade and products have become more complex, it has brought with it the need for a broader, more all-encompassing food safety management system.

Given that a retailer's role is to protect the safety of its consumers, a key part is a proactive rather than a reactive approach to food safety management. Whilst HACCP is intended to be a proactive food safety tool by predicting and preventing significant hazards and their risks, implementation has, in many instances, become reactive. An example of such reactive behavior is the heavy focus placed on microbiological testing of the end product for safety rather than using end-product microbiological testing as verification of the effectiveness of the HACCP plan.[6]

Fresh produce has historically and continues to be associated with many foodborne illness outbreaks. Recent examples are the Shiga-toxin *Escherichia coli* (STEC) infections in the United States in 2011 and again in 2018; the latter outbreak resulted in a 45%–60% drop in the price of romaine lettuce and hundreds of people sickened.[13] In products such as salads that are eaten raw, where there is no "kill step" such as cooking to destroy potential pathogens, they may be unsafe due to potential contamination by pathogens. Examples are STEC or *Salmonella*; therefore ensuring that such products are not contaminated during growing and harvesting is essential. Recognizing this fact drove many retailers in the 2000s, to either develop their own or through the formation of industry groups, create fresh produce growing standards. These new standards that demanded control of fundamental points such as irrigation water quality, restricting the use of untreated organic fertilizers, and managing the health and hygiene of field workers are now commonplace requirements to supply to large retailers. This proactive, preventative approach to what happens in the field, before the factory gate, means that control measures, such as decontamination by washing with biocides, have a much greater success rate of reducing the hazard to an acceptable level, which for fresh salad items to be eaten raw, must be an absence of STEC and *Salmonella*, and other soil-borne pathogens.

The evolution of HACCP into a food safety management system has progressed significantly related to the increasing complexity of food and product ranges, for example, minimally processed fresh produce and chilled prepared foods consisting of several ingredients. Furthermore, it has also progressed in areas where previously, rendering a food safe, relied on the consumer cooking the product before consumption. A retailer's aspirational goal for the microbiological safety of its products is to sell food with the highest level of safety based on the principle of continuous improvement. The example of using good agricultural practices in the primary sector of the supply chain to minimize the level of pathogens entering a fresh produce factory is not the only area that retailers have strived to improve upon.

Camplylobacter species are the main cause of foodborne human bacterial gastroenteritis in the developed world. In the United Kingdom it was thought to affect an estimated 280,000 people a year. Chicken is considered the most important vehicle for transmission of this organism and even though proper hygienic handling and thorough cooking will eliminate this hazard, the UK Food Standards Agency (FSA) joined forces with the food industry with the aim of reducing the prevalence in raw chicken over time in order to reduce the public health impact of *Campylobacter*. A study by the FSA in 2008 showed 27% of chicken samples were 'highly contaminated' (defined as greater than 1000 CFU/g of chicken skin) with *Campylobacter* spp. A joint FSA and industry target was set to reduce the prevalence of the most contaminated chickens to below 10% at the end of the slaughter process by the end of 2015. This target deadline was extended to 2016 after an FSA survey in 2014–15 found that *Campylobacter* spp. was found in 73.3% of fresh chickens at the retail level, of which 19.4% had >1000 CFU/g of chicken skin.[14] The target was eventually achieved, and in year four of the annual FSA sampling survey of fresh chickens at retail, the level of highly contaminated samples had reduced to under 7%.[15] Achieving this reduction in pathogen levels in United Kingdom chicken sold to consumers by retail required a collaborative and complete supply chain approach. Competitors both in processing and in retail came together to conduct trials and share data and research findings to achieve the jointly agreed targets. This style and scale of collaboration was unprecedented, and was not without its challenges as commercially competitive businesses came together to explore a wide variety of interventions ranging from biosecurity on farms to novel processing innovations in slaughterhouses and leak-proof finished products packaging as well as improved consumer handling messages. The determination and drive for the UK poultry industry and United Kingdom retailers to continue to reduce the prevalence of *Campylobacter* spp. in raw whole chickens continues today. This precompetitive, total supply chain and cross-industry approach to significantly reduce the hazard and subsequent risk to consumers from consuming chicken in the United Kingdom, remains an inspiring and world-leading approach that reiterates a retailer's aim to reduce the prevalence of the pathogen in consumers' kitchens. This underscores the importance of continuously seeking improvements even though cooking instructions are in place.

For a retailer selling safe food, an important concept within a HACCP-based food safety management system is one of due diligence. A fundamental part of proving due diligence is the concept of reducing the risk to, or maintaining it at an "acceptable level." This is in case of a legal challenge; however, due diligence can also be a useful way of balancing the level of controls and interventions needed to sell a safe, but also organoleptically desirable and commercially viable product.

The work on both the produce growing standards and the UK *Campylobacter* campaign demonstrate that setting an acceptable level can and should change with time. A culture of continuous improvement is a vital part of ensuring safe foods as new products and innovations are developed and launched.[16] The UK campaign on *Campylobacter* reduction in raw chicken demonstrates this approach and culture on a grand and extensive scale, but it can also be implemented at a much more local level within the individual retailers and their manufacturing partners.

It is vital to remember that in food production and retailing, microbiological risk can never be eliminated; that is the concept of "zero risk" in food safety does not exist.[17] Even in the well-established and understood process of canning that targets a minimum of a 12 log reduction in proteolytic *C. botulinum* spores, this only reduces the probability of the presence of a spore to 1 in a trillion cans. This level of risk of the presence of the hazard and potential toxin production is unimaginably small and is widely accepted by both industry and regulators to be low enough to be acceptable; however, it is important to note that it is still not total elimination. The definition and agreement of an acceptable level for less severe processing or less established processes, as opposed to canning, for example, depends on many factors; a key one being the harm that the food-borne illness could potentially cause. For *C. botulinum*, the mortality rate of botulism is high (20%–50%) with only a very small dose of the botulinum toxin. The production of the botulinum toxin is considered a much more severe hazard than toxins produced by *B. cereus* for example, which usually only cause self-limiting, short-lived gastrointestinal illness.[18]

The role of a retailer in deciding its level of acceptable risk will depend somewhat on the level of food safety that the retailer wishes to achieve and the country in which it operates. The local regulator will define this in law to some extent, but legislation often states that the food must not cause harm and must comply with specified microbial levels often stated as microbiological criteria with associated sampling plans.[19]

Another important factor in determining an acceptable level will be the number of potential consumers exposed to a particular hazard. Major nationwide retailers are the source of food for a much greater proportion of a country's population than small artisan producers selling at a farmer's market, for example. With that sizeable market share comes enormous responsibility. Such retailers must take more extensive precautions to sell food that carries a negligible risk of food-borne illness. This naturally translates into the resources in quality and food safety teams that exist in retailers to define and deliver safe food. In the UK, following the significant reduction in *Campylobacter* spp. incidence in chickens sold at large retailers, the expected positive public health impact did not directly translate into a proportional reduction in cases of food-borne illness. This demonstrates that improvements made, needed to be translated and communicated to the smaller retailers and butchers to have the desired public health benefits. It also highlights the behaviors and hygiene practices in the kitchen by consumers. Awareness of hazards associated with foods and the responsibility that consumers must take to protect themselves and minimize their own risk of suffering from food-borne illness still carries great significance. Even with a culture of continuous improvement and the aspiration of retailers to consistently sell safe food, one remains aware that even with an "absence" requirement, total pathogen elimination from food is not possible.

34.4 Manufacturing standards—driving food safety or confusion?

Whilst lack of knowledge of a hazard or lack of awareness of risk can sometimes be the root cause of mistakes in food manufacturing and retailing, more often the cause of events that lead to outbreaks or recalls are inexperience, complacency, and assumptions.

As referred to earlier in this chapter, the development of innovation in products and processes, particularly in chilled food, has been of great benefit to the consumer and to the growth of the food industry. With innovation, however, comes new and different ingredients, products, and processes which are accompanied by ever-increasing rules, regulations, and standards to comply with. To protect their consumers, retailers globally define their level of acceptable risk for their due diligence. In doing this, many will also define the standards with which manufacturers must comply, to produce their brand products, and/or they may insist on the use of independent globally-recognized standards, such as those bench-marked by the Global Food Safety Initiative (GFSI).[20] This is necessary as individual retail brands have a responsibility to define and manage their level of risk. However, with the advent of multiple standards that one manufacturing site must comply with, came the risk of overcomplicating the food safety management systems. This over-complication has resulted in a loss of sight of the importance of the fundamentals discussed in section one about 'what makes food safe'. In addition, these extremely prescriptive standards, whilst so often built on lessons learned from past mistakes, are not conducive to building a deep understanding and knowledge of food safety, driving improvements, innovation, and change.

The GFSI, which is part of the Consumer Goods Forum has attempted to address this by benchmarking food safety certification programs.[21] However retailers still want and need to produce their standards, particularly when own-brand products are involved, where reputation and a high level of trust by consumers, must be protected and maintained. The historical result of retailers' bespoke standards being in the format of an extensive list of highly prescriptive and specific requirements has resulted in a manufacturer resorting to a paper-based gap analysis against all the retailer standards. The danger comes from subsequently basing their factory systems and monitoring on this gap analysis, instead of observing, reviewing, and defining the actual specifics of their unique factory and processes. This is understandable given that the passing of a retailer specified audit is usually the commercial gateway to supply them. However, this can also mean that fundamental hazards associated with their unique process and environment have not been risk-assessed, which can lead to mistakes and, in the worst case, harm to the consumer. There is a solution to this issue and one that progressive and innovative retailers and large FMCG brands are beginning to explore and implement. It is a move from highly prescriptive manufacturing standards to outcome-driven standards. In this scenario, a manufacturer must be able to demonstrate that they are in control of a specific aspect of food safety, but crucially *how* they do this, is up to them. There will still be a place for some clear mandatory requirements which reflect the brand (e.g., a premium, a more trusted retailer might ask for additional controls to protect their more valuable brand reputation than a discounter whose customers have a greater tolerance for inconsistency related to the price they pay for the goods), but more broadly enables manufacturers to show how they meet those requirements through their systems, risk assessments, mitigations, and controls. What is also important is that the learnings from past issues and incidents which have made some of the existing standards so unwieldy are not lost. Guidance-style documents to ensure that these learnings are cascaded and shared are crucial. They not only communicate the benefits of lessons learned but also support the reality that not all manufacturers have the same size and capability of technical teams, and so some will need additional guidance on how they could achieve the control of the specified aspect of food safety. This system, therefore, allows for greater flexibility at the manufacturer level.

Another disadvantage of the common-place prescriptive standards is that they can be a barrier to process innovations. An example in the management of microbiological food safety could be the application of produce decontamination. The basic principles of washing salad products in water containing biocides such as chlorine have long been used to safely produce a ready-to-eat (RTE) finished product, such as a preprepared sandwich containing that fresh salad item. A lettuce leaf is almost always eaten raw, so using a more absolute reduction mechanism such as heat to reduce the presence of any soil-borne pathogens such as *Salmonella* or STEC that may inadvertently be in the leaves from field contamination, is not an option. The physicality of washing the leaves in the industrial washing equipment dislodges the bacteria from the leaf surface and the biocide in the wash water injures or kills the bacteria, both pathogenic and nonpathogenic, in the water so it cannot re-contaminate the leaf. A historical, prescriptive standard for producing decontamination may, for example, define the time, type, and level of biocide used. It does not consider the bacterial loading of the raw material which now, with much-improved field-based agricultural food safety standards, may be lower than when the manufacturing standard was originally developed. It also assumes biocide-containing water is the only mechanism by which salad produce could be made safe to consume without cooking. The advent of new technologies such as vertical farms using hydroponic technology rather than soil to grow the salad items means the need for water and biocides is much reduced and indeed if the vertical farm is designed so that the growing takes place in a high care standard environment, then there is likely no need to wash the produce. Current prescriptive standards would mean that a supplier would not pass the audit if they did not wash their produce in specified biocides at specific concentrations, even if the produce was grown in such a way that achieving the acceptable level of risk did not require this treatment.

Another, more specific example showing how a traditional prescriptive manufacturing standard caused an error that led to a potential food safety issue, is the industrial cooking of frozen prawns. The cooking time and temperature for the process were subject to extensive validation, where extra safety margins were added to ensure exposure of a minimum of 70°C for 2 min.[22] This was done to account for circumstances such as the potential overloading of the cooker or overlapping prawns. The cooling process postcook was also defined and validated. The validated process and its daily verification checks had worked well producing a safe, good quality product for many years. One day a retailer initiated a promotion with short notice and the orders doubled overnight. The operative in the factory took the frozen prawns from the freezer as done for every other production day but found that there was a lack of space to defrost them in the chiller, so six bags rather than four were placed in each container to defrost. The due diligence paperwork for the batches was completed accurately and in full. A Quality Assurance manager completed a routine taste panel before the product was shipped to the retailer's distribution center. The taste panel noticed a gray-blue color on some of the prawns, in one of the packs sampled. The entire day's production was put into quarantine so that it did not leave the factory. A full investigation followed. A retrospective review of the paperwork showed no issues, all cooking and cooling temperature checks were within specification, there were no engineering issues recorded, the operative running the line was experienced and well trained and they had worked on that line for years. Many more packs were sampled, and a small number of packs were found with visibly gray/blue prawns inside. The costly, but correct decision was taken to reject the entire day's production. The supplier complied with all the prescriptive manufacturing standards provided by their retail customers and had a very good track record of high audit scores. However, because the process had been designed based on cooking raw protein items, requirements from the retailers had focused on the cooking process and failsafe of the oven section as well as the cooling process to obtain chilled temperatures after cooking. They neglected to explore their defrosting process and the capacity of their facilities. This type of process step is very specific to the individual factory's layout and facilities; it is therefore highly unlikely to be documented in a retailer manufacturing standard or that of other food safety certification bodies. The only requirement was that defrosting should take place in a chilled environment. There was no continuous precook temperature recording activity. During the HACCP validation and associated data gathering, the company had recorded the ingoing temperature, but did not do so continuously; the prawns were simply defrosted and kept chilled below 5°C.

After interviewing the operative involved who gave a detailed account of what had been done that day, the managers finally realized what had happened; the overloaded containers of defrosting prawns in the chiller had meant that the in-going temperature of the prawns was more than likely sub-zero, rather than the 1°C–2°C that had been documented in the product's HACCP validation process. This coupled with the fact that the cooker was operating at maximum capacity throughout the production day, meant that a few of the prawns did not reach their minimum core cooking temperature and therefore the minimum time/temperature requirement of 70°C for 2 min was not achieved.

In this example, no consumers were harmed, but it was a costly mistake that could easily have been prevented if the process had been observed on the factory floor from start to end, as part of the determination of the HACCP plan and the bottleneck of the chiller and defrosting container capacity had been noted. The corrective action in this scenario was that a record would be kept of the temperature of the prawns going into the cooking process, to spot any minor deviation and trend toward a lower temperature than the requirement. Furthermore, a limit on the number of bags of prawns per container was determined as a control point for the factory operative to adhere to.

The reality is that retailers make commercial decisions that can dramatically increase or decrease order volumes, sometimes at very short notice. Normally, most manufacturers will do everything they can not to short supply a product, so incidents like the ones described here can happen. For this reason, the HACCP-based food safety manufacturing plans must not only be based on the retailer's documentation but should also take into account the very specific layout, capacities, and facilities of their production environment. A move from retailer prescriptive standards and that of other food safety certification bodies to adopt a more outcome-based structure and format of its manufacturing standards is a positive one.

Culturally within organizations, there will likely be initial resistance to moving to an outcome-based manufacturing standard. The latter is harder to audit and score as it requires the auditor and retailer to listen and understand the explanation of the manufacturer on why they consider their product safe, what their process is, and the method they have undertaken to ensure safety, rather than simply ticking a box on whether they comply with a specifically defined clause. Such an audit also requires a qualitative judgment to be made, which is more difficult than a quantitative judgment and therefore requires appropriately skilled and experienced food safety auditors in a particular sector.

Such an outcome-based approach can be a great complement to a company that is exploring defining and measuring its food safety culture. The positive benefits of enabling innovation, of upskilling a broader number of people to objectively and critically review their process and fundamentally watch and observe real factory practices should drive an attitude and culture of continuous improvement and ultimately result in safer, more cost-effective products.[23]

34.5 Testing doesn't make food safe

Testing has long been relied upon as a fundamental way of proving that a product is safe. A test certificate from an accredited laboratory showing the absence of a pathogen can provide false reassurance that all is well with the product and its process. However, such a result only indicates regulatory compliance. One must ask whether this sense of security is justified and whether the importance one gives to the result is proportionate to the rest of the HACCP-based food safety plan.

One cannot test safety into food. Furthermore, microbiological end-product testing can be a significant expense for a food business and it is therefore important that testing is done with a specific purpose in mind. If the purpose for conducting a particular test cannot be defined, then the analysis should probably not be done.[24]

There are several other issues related to sole reliance on end-product testing for pathogens that is the target pathogen is rarely distributed homogenously in the product, therefore there is a significant probability that a defective batch would be released into the market, regardless of whether the result complied with legislation.[25] This is also dependent on the microbiological criterion adopted. Testing within a HACCP-based food safety management system, where process controls are in place and implemented, together with several well-designed and defined microbiological criteria at important locations in the food chain, provides one with a greater level of reassurance that the risk-based approach taken, is effective.[24] This in turn suggests that the validated process to reduce the target organism to an acceptable level has functioned as intended. However, for presence/absence testing as opposed to enumeration, it is accepted that there is no guarantee that the pathogen is not present, because to be certain of complete absence, the entire batch would need to be tested, which is naturally impractical. Hence, the importance of selecting appropriate microbiological criteria.[25]

Selection of appropriate testing methods is key to providing the target microorganism with the best possible chance to grow, if present, particularly where sub-lethal injury to microbial cells is expected. If the method does not provide for resuscitation of sub-lethally injured cells, false-negative results may occur, which will increase the likelihood of releasing a contaminated batch into commerce.[25] There is also a growing hypothesis that some species of pathogens such as *Salmonella* or *Campylobacter* could become viable nonculturable (VNC) after exposure to biocides used to wash fresh produce.[26] This means that they are still present and potentially virulent, but are unable to grow on laboratory media. This reiterates the importance of integrating appropriate microbiological criteria into a well-designed HACCP-based food safety management system, to prevent, eliminate or reduce the target pathogen to acceptable levels in the food.

34.6 Managing food safety risks in a store environment and the impact that the growth of online and home delivery has on retail risk management

For food retailers selling only prepacked food, basic good housekeeping may be sufficient to address food safety.[6] However, in certain instances, additional control measures should be applied.

34.6.1 Temperature controls

Whilst all the factors of food safety risk must be considered for the retail environment when selling fully packaged food, the main concern from a microbiological food safety risk perspective, is often temperature control, which is predominantly associated with chilled and frozen food. The temperature must also be managed for ambient food products, but this is more related to maintaining quality parameters rather than food safety.

The cold chain, involving refrigerated storage depots and refrigerated distribution was first developed in the 1960s in the United Kingdom to bring fresh, chilled chicken to the consumer. It is now a well-understood concept and established across the world. It is not complex as a principle, but it is fundamental to ensuring the stated shelf lives of many products. A retailer would therefore always consider the risk of the cold chain being broken across the supply chain in their risk assessments. Temperature is monitored and recorded throughout the supply chain, from the distribution vehicles to storage depots and on arrival at the store. The distribution depots are chilled warehouses, so the risk to the product from a temperature management point of view when being allocated to stores and loaded on or off chilled trucks is low. It is the arrival at the store and transfer to chilled storage areas backstage, or straight onto the display in the chiller cabinets for the consumer where the break in the cold chain is first likely to occur. Rather than just checking the temperature of the delivery vehicle or display cabinets, the temperature of actual products should be probed and recorded. In addition, an early warning system that monitors air temperatures in display fridges could provide an additional warning system that loss of chilling is at risk. To avoid chill chain breakage, a backup power supply should be in place to prevent unnecessary food wastage. Where product checks identify a break in the cold chain, appropriate corrective actions must be implemented.

As with a manufacturing environment, HACCP-based food safety management plans are also developed for the retail environment.[6] Mirroring the principles of a HACCP plan for a factory, these plans mustn't be overcomplicated. Furthermore, when developing controls and mitigations, retailers should consider the reality of trading in a busy store environment with the impact of staff knowledge on food safety likely to be at a basic level.

Chilled food products will spend some time out of chilled storage when being taken to the retail shop floor to be put on display. The time estimate for this is usually in the region of 20–30 min. During this time the temperature that food will increase to, will likely not exceed 10°C, provided that the initial temperature of the food was below 5°C and then, this would likely be for only a few minutes. At these times and temperatures, there is little time for bacteria to multiply to levels that could cause harm. Whilst the replication time of the fastest-growing bacteria, such as *E. coli*, is often quoted as 20 min, this is at their optimal growth conditions.[27] The optimal growth temperature for most food-borne pathogens, is closer to 30°C–40°C. Therefore this short period of time outside of chilled storage, from a practical point of view, is deemed to be acceptable, even in the case of *L. monocytogenes* which is an acknowledged psychrotrophic pathogen. It is also relatively cool on a retail store refrigerated aisle due to the air conditioning and the refrigerator units in operation, which both add another level of confidence to the risk of potentially breaking the cold chain.

The second point at which the cold chain may break is with the consumer after they have removed the product from the refrigerator in the retail store, taken to the till point for purchase, and then taken home via a mode of transport whether that is walking, driving in a car or some form of public transport. This amount of time before the consumer then places the item in their domestic refrigerator can vary widely, but the often-used time from a risk assessment point of view is two hours. In temperate climates such as Europe, the temperature abuse level reached for this period of time is commonly 20°C–22°C, which is a comfortable room temperature.[28] In hotter climates this will likely be different as higher temperatures may be reached in a shorter period of time. In some countries, consumers will be aware of the fact they are transporting chilled food in hot climates and so would consciously aim to have their chilled products home and into their refrigerator in a shorter time period. However, in many other countries, this level of awareness does not exist and therefore, the product may be compromised. Retailers in the latter environments should take these differences into consideration, with a view to local conditions.

The final step where the cold chain alters is in a domestic refrigerator. There is still a surprising lack of robust and extensive data for the realistic consumer domestic refrigerator temperature. A large proportion of global consumers in developed countries would know if questioned that they are supposed to store chilled food below 5°C, but in reality, even with modern refrigerators, temperatures are closer to 8°C and in some cases, even higher. In studies conducted between 1991 and 2016, the mean, minimum and maximum temperatures of domestic refrigerators ranged from <5°C–8.1°C, −7.9°C to 3.8°C, and 11.4°C–20.7°C, respectively.[29] Additionally, in 2018 Campden BRI in the United Kingdom undertook a test of 35 fridges over 30 days, the results showed that 53% of them were above 5°C and a further 16% were above 8°C.[28] However, conducting shelf-life studies at too high a temperature, such as even 10°C, could dramatically and unnecessarily, reduce the organoleptic shelf life of products for the majority of consumers and thereby increase the amount of food waste. As mentioned elsewhere, this is not considered the correct action, therefore choosing a more realistic temperature of 8°C is often settled on for a risk-based shelf life validation study,[30] which aligns well with the mean maximum temperature cited by[29] as 8.1°C.

The exact protocol of temperatures and times when validating chilled products' shelf life will vary between retailers, and this should be the case as the retailers are all managing their brands and as referred to in the introduction, each brand will have an associated level of trust, value, and expectation attached to it.[28] A common protocol in a temperate climate, developed country with a geographical distribution that has less than one day's transportation time from the manufacturing site to the retail depot and another day to a retail store could be as shown in Fig. 34.1.

The impact of the 20–30 min out of the cold chain in a retail store is not typically included in the validation model for shelf-life as it would have such a low impact on any bacterial growth in the product as explained above. However, different climates and different efficiencies in the distribution chain may reflect a different scenario, which should be considered.

The shelf life validation study will consider the organoleptic properties of the product and would involve some

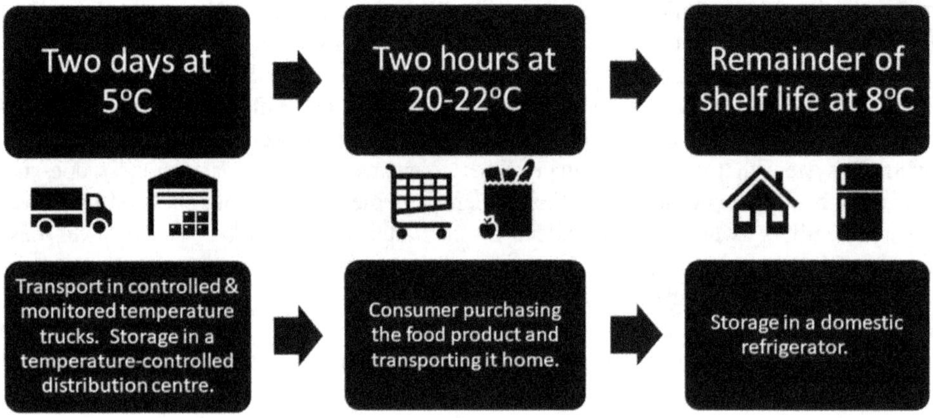

FIGURE 34.1 Protocol for transportation of chilled food products.

microbiological testing, both for the pathogens of concern identified in the manufacturer's HACCP plan and the most relevant process hygiene indicator organisms. In chilled foods that contain salads, or other uncooked produce, a process hygiene criterion would typically be *E. coli* and for food that is fully cooked, would likely include Enterobacteriaceae as a more useful indicator to test for.

Historically a retailer would also have considered including a total viable count (TVC) in a chilled product. The shelf life would end when the TVC and/or the Enterobacteriaceae or *E. coli* levels hit a certain predetermined threshold. Studies done by UK retailers in the mid-2000s changed this mindset and showed that food spoilage was very rarely linked to a specific count of these types of organisms. This was a positive step forward in shelf-life extension to aid both commercialities of products and the reduction of unnecessary food waste.

34.6.2 Date marking

The total shelf life of a product is established during the development phase, considering both food safety and eating quality.

Food products are either labeled with a Best Before or Use By date for consumers.[31]

> *"Best Before Date" or "Best Quality Before Date" means the date which signifies the end of the period, under any stated storage conditions, during which the unopened product will remain fully marketable and will retain any specific qualities for which implied or expressed claims have been made. However, beyond the date, the food may still be acceptable for consumption.*

> *"Use-by Date" or "Expiration Date" means the date which signifies the end of the period under any stated storage conditions, after which the product should not be sold or consumed due to safety and quality reasons.*

The European Food Safety Authority (EFSA) developed a science-based decision tree tool to assist food businesses to determine which date marking is appropriate (selecting Best Before or Use By) based on pathogen survival and/or potential growth.[32]

Stock rotation and the management of product date marking in retail stores is an important consumer protection step, as consumers trust the retailer to manage product date marking, and will seldom check date marking when buying food. As part of their food safety process, retailers need to have procedures to manage food shelf life. The retail store needs a process to remove products from shelves on Sell By date, or Best Before and Use By.[33]

To minimize food waste and ensure food security, retailers need to responsibly and safely handle food products removed from shelves at the end of their shelf life. Whilst products which have reached their Use By date must be destroyed, products that have reached their Best Before may go to 'salvage shops' or be donated to charities, such as food banks.[34,35]

34.6.3 Other considerations in a retail store environment

Having hospitality units such as cafes or restaurants, or unpackaged food such as loose produce displays, in-store bakeries, delicatessen counters, or rotisserie chickens in a retail environment can add great theater and freshness for consumers. However, all of these introduce more microbiological risks that must be considered as part of the store's HACCP-based food safety plans. The most crucial part of control for all of these offerings is the store retail employee's knowledge and understanding of food hygiene and food safety. Appropriate training and recognizing the complexity and accountability of the staff members responsible for handling raw poultry or slicing cooked meat in such kitchen environments is greater than the one who is working to replenish the shelves with prepackaged goods. The retailer can prevent potential process failure by staff by procuring equipment such as ovens for rotisserie chicken that can be loaded at low risk and unpacked on a high-risk consumer-facing counter.

Consumers may demand that they are served by staff wearing gloves. Consumers can be advised via in-store messages that the use of gloves gives a false sense of security, and explain that staff rather regularly wash their hands to ensure food safety.

Counters offering sliced cooked and cured meats, cheeses, and salads have become a common feature of large retail stores and bring with them special considerations on control of *L. monocytogenes* in particular. These counters do not only offer a theater and freshness cue to the consumer, but they also allow for consumers to purchase the exact quantities they need rather than larger prepacked items in these product groups, which can reduce unnecessary food waste in the home. Many retail stores now handle and carry out minor processing tasks such as slicing RTE products, cutting, and wrapping cheeses into portions, and mixing salads in a deli area of the store, usually open to the customer view. These product types can carry a risk of a low level of presence of *L. monocytogenes*, either from cross-contamination in the factory they were processed in or in the case of unpasteurized cheeses and salad ingredients as inherent low-level contamination from raw materials. For this reason, extra diligence related to handling procedures, cleaning and disinfection as well as staff training should be in place in these in-store environments. The principles of listeria controls from a manufacturing environment can be successfully translated to retail in-store environments.[36] These principles include:

1. sanitary design principles of equipment to prevent harborage of bacteria, such as listeria, and also enable ease of cleaning;
2. use of appropriate cleaning chemicals, detergents, and sanitizers suitable for breaking down biofilms and providing a lethality for listeria for all areas of the environment and equipment used for RTE foods; and
3. staff training on the risks of listeria contamination and the need to ensure that cross-contamination from raw to RTE products in the deli area is prevented.[36]

The recent backlash by consumers against single-use plastics and the subsequent move to more unpackaged food in the retail environment brings additional risks, which are easily managed with an in-store HACCP system that runs on the same principles as described in the Section 34.1. Managing and minimizing cross contamination from raw to RTE unpackaged foods is the most fundamental area of control. However, a full risk assessment of technologies such as misting fresh produce to keep it from drying out must be done, again avoiding assumptions and involving appropriately experienced and knowledgeable people in the risk assessment.

34.6.4 Online shopping and home delivery

The rise of online and home delivery in recent years has seen a marked increase that is set to continue. The SARS-CoV-2 pandemic, which began in 2020, accelerated this growth of home delivery and it is predicted to continue to be a significant proportion of how consumers shop for their food in the future.[37,38] This could carry with it less risk than the consumer shopping in the retail store, especially where the food and the chill chain are under the control of the retailer to the consumer's front door. This maintenance of the chill chain and lowering of risk increases further still if the allocation of products to fulfill the consumer's online order is done from a chilled depot rather than shopped by a retail employee in the store. The business model that determines this will be dependent on the retailer, but as online shopping and home delivery become an increasing volume of the retailers' business, it encourages the 'direct from depot' delivery model, which will have a positive impact on maintaining longest possible spoilage-free and safe shelf lives. As this transition to home delivery increases, the shelf life studies described earlier in this section become worst-case scenarios as temperature abuse at 20°C–22°C is highly unlikely to occur in the life of the product. Therefore, if the retailer fulfills only an online rather than a physical store model, which some globally do already, then this abuse stage of any own-brand products in the shelf life studies could potentially be removed. This, in turn, should lead to increased shelf life for the products which, as discussed previously, is always a priority for a retail technologist to deliver, that is the longest possible appropriate shelf life.

An additional risk of home delivery is the provision of products that are sold by weight such as fresh meat and fish or sliced cooked meats which in-store would be purchased by engaging with a retail employee across a clear and highly visible counter format. Where this operation is done in a distribution center, rather than in front of the customer audience in-store, it must be the focus of retailers to ensure that the same controls of temperature, personal hygiene, and cross-contamination risks are understood, the staff is adequately trained and correct measures adhered to.

34.7 Consumer-facing communication, from packaging to marketing, and its role in maintaining food safety, including product recalls

34.7.1 Consumer preparation instructions

There is another often forgotten area of potential risk when creating a manufacturing HACCP-based food safety management system. This is the role that the information on the packaging and the retailer team plays.

Regarding packaging, in the case of raw or partially heat-treated products such as crumbed chicken, a retailer will take steps as described in Section 34.2 to reduce the presence of pathogens, even on raw products to as low as possible. However, it is still the handling and cooking in the consumer's home that is the final hurdle in ensuring the product is safe to eat. How can one ensure that minimum cooking time and temperature combinations to ensure product safety, are reached in the consumer's kitchen?

In reality for raw products, despite the fact that the validation of cooking instructions is fundamental in delivering this hurdle to the overall safety controls for that product, it is rarely a feature in a manufacturer's HACCP plan. It should be treated in the same way as any other mitigation or control step for an identified hazard, and have a well-thought-through plan with failsafes and safety margins built-in. The risk of it not being carried out sufficiently can increase if the responsibility lies with the product development team instead of with the technical team. The perception may be created that the cooking instructions are part of how the customer experiences the quality of the food and not as an important safety control.

As with all areas of HACCP-based food safety management, assumptions must be identified and considered. A basic principle of a good customer/consumer cook validation is the use of a calibrated oven or at least the use of a calibrated temperature probe that continuously measures the actual oven temperature as opposed to just following the setting on the thermostat. Further consideration should be given to "worst case" products and other parameters such as the largest piece size in the pack (usually based on the raw material specification and verified by measuring weight and dimensions during factory trials), and the coldest possible product going into the oven. An example of the latter is a product being taken straight from a 5°C fridge and placed directly in the oven, unless the cooking instructions specifically instruct the customer to take another specific action, such as taking a joint of meat from the fridge 30 min before placing in the oven.

The size of the oven, different types of foods in it as well as the volume of foods in the oven are important factors too. Products that have a 'cook from frozen' instruction will decrease the temperature of a preheated oven, initially from its set point. The more frozen or chilled a food is, the lower the set temperature of the oven will fall. This is important when a pack contains multiple items that could either be cooked individually or the packet in its entirety. For example, if an individual portion from a pack of four frozen breaded fish portions, is cooked, then the oven temperature will fall far less and the portion will cook faster than if all four were placed in the oven at the same time. This follows the second law of thermodynamics.[39] The cooking validation trials must explore these aspects and determine if the length of time needed for one can be the same as all four, or whether there should be different cooking times given on a pack for one, two, three, or four portions. This mentality of oven loading affecting cook time would be commonplace in a factory-based cook validation but could be overlooked in the validation for customer cooking instructions.

Cooking instructions will only ever be a guide, as all ovens vary and one cannot guarantee that consumers will follow the instructions exactly as intended, especially around areas such as preheating an oven. However, this should not be regarded as an excuse to not have a fully considered instruction, as it could still form a part of a due diligence defense.

A close relationship between the marketing and technical teams at the retailer level can be particularly useful as the marketing and packaging design teams influence consumer behavior around food safety, even if not realized. A good example is not showing raw and cooked items nearby on the pack photography. Most importantly in terms of influencing consumer behavior, is when a retailer uses a chef or celebrity as part of its advertising campaigns. Here, retailers should always ensure that these persons implement good personal hygiene and cross-contamination practices at all times and in all media, whether it's a social media post or recipe or menu card in an in-store magazine. A responsible retailer must play its role in consumer education on good food safety practices such as keeping raw and cooked food separate and keeping hot food hot, and cold food cold.

34.7.2 Consumer storage instructions

When consumers open food product packaging (e.g., cans, MAP packed, UHT, etc.) or thaw frozen products, the nature of the product may change and it may be exposed to microbes. It is therefore important to provide consumers with science-based information on how to store products and guidance on how long the food will remain safe.[40]

34.7.3 Customer complaints

Another key consumer communication aspect is customer complaints and product returns. As the retailer is the consumer's point of contact with the food industry, consumers are a key feedback loop giving both the retailer and producer valuable information that systems and processes may be out of control.

34.7.4 Recalls

Retail's last and very key responsibility in food safety is a product recall. As the final link to the consumer, it is the retailer who will either initiate a recall or be the implementer of recalls initiated by the product's producers, when food products prove to be potentially unsafe. As such, retailers must have an effective, well-practiced recall procedure in place and this should constitute an important part of a HACCP-based food safety management system at the retailer level.

34.8 Conclusions

Retailers should ask two important questions. "Is the food safe?" "Can the manufacturer prove it?" Both have been explored in this chapter. Risk is rarely something one can eliminate in the food industry as zero risk does not exist. However, retailers must manage risk by reducing hazards to an acceptable level, all whilst balancing other social risks such as food insecurity, food waste, product quality, and commercial sustainability of a business.

Technological innovations such as new processes to reduce the microbiological load or improve efficiencies by reducing the energy needed for thermal or cooling processes will all play an increasing role in the challenges for a food technologist over the coming decade. A retailer's responsibility is to drive standards and behaviors that maximize these opportunities, and in doing so maintain and ultimately continue improving the safety of food for consumers.

References

1. Law Insider. Retail food store/grocery definition. <https://www.lawinsider.com/dictionary/retail-food-storegrocery>; 2021 Accessed 20.12.21.
2. Farber J, Crichton J, Snyder Jr. OP. Chapter 1: an introduction to retail food safety. In: Farber J, Crichton J, Snyder Jr OP, eds. *Retail Food Safety*. Springer; 2014:1–2.
3. EC. European Commission Regulation No 178/2002 laying down the general principles and requirements of food law, establishing the European Food Safety Authority and laying down procedures in matters of food safety. <https://eur-lex.europa.eu/legal-content/EN/ALL/?uri = celex%3A32002R0178>; 2002 Accessed 20.02.22.
4. SA Govt. South African Government. Foodstuffs, Cosmetics and Disinfectants Act 54 of 1972. <https://www.gov.za/documents/foodstuffs-cosmetics-and-disinfectants-act-2-jun-1972-000>; 1972 Accessed 20.12.21.
5. SA Govt. South African Government. Consumer Protection Act 68 of 2008. <https://www.gov.za/documents/consumer-protection-act>; 2008 Accessed 20.12.21.
6. CAC. Codex Alimentarius Commission. General principles of food hygiene CXC 1-1969.; 2020 Accessed 15.12.21.
7. Anelich. Microbiological hazards and risks in food safety. Food and Beverage Reporter, August 2021, pp. 18-19. <https://fbreporter.co.za/fbr-digital-edition-august-2021/>; 2021 Accessed 05.11.21.
8. Beuchat LR, Komitopoulou E, Beckers H, et al. Low-water activity foods: Increased concern as vehicles of foodborne pathogens. *J Food Prot*. 2013;76(1):150–172. Available from: https://doi.org/10.4315/0362-028X.JFP-12-211.
9. FZANZ. Compendium of Microbiological Criteria for Food. <https://www.foodstandards.gov.au/publications/pages/compendium-of-microbiological-criteria-for-food.aspx>; 2018 Accessed 12.11.21.
10. NZ Govt. New Zealand Government. Guidance for the control of *Listeria monocytogenes* in ready-to-eat foods part 1: listeria management and glossary. Ministry for Primary Industries. <https://www.mpi.govt.nz/dmsdocument/16300-guidance-for-the-control-of-listeria-monocytogenes-in-ready-to-eat-foods-part-1-listeria-management-and-glossary>; 2017 Accessed 22.12.21.
11. Campden BRI (2008) Guideline No. 56, Heat Processing of packaged foods: guidelines for establishing the thermal process <https://www.campdenbri.co.uk/publications/publication.php?publicationId = a603ddf2-bde6-e411-80db-0050569719df>; May 2008 Accessed 20.02.22.
12. CB Premium. Computational Biology Premium; Predictive food safety. <https://www.cbpremium.org/>; 2021 Accessed 20.12.21.
13. Gray. Financial impact of the Romaine Lettuce *E. coli* outbreak isn't over – fortune. <https://fortune.com/2018/05/30/romaine-lettuce-e-coli-outbreak-impacts/>; 2018 Accessed 20.02.22.
14. FSA. Food Standards Agency. A microbiological survey of Campylobacter contamination in fresh, whole UK-produced chilled chicken at retail sale. <https://www.food.gov.uk/research/eggs-and-poultry/a-microbiological-survey-of-campylobacter-contamination-in-fresh-whole-uk-produced-chilled-chicken-at-retail-sale>; 2015 Accessed 20.12.21.
15. FSA. Food Standards Agency. A microbiological survey of Campylobacter contamination in fresh, whole UK-produced chilled chicken at retail sale. FSA project FS 102121, Year 4 report. <https://webarchive.nationalarchives.gov.uk/ukgwa/20200803152234/https://www.food.gov.uk/sites/default/files/media/document/fs102121-year-4-campylobacter-report.pdf>; 2019 Accessed 20.12.21.
16. ISO. International Standards Organization, ISO 22000:2018. Food Safety Management Systems – Requirements for any organization in the food chain. <https://www.iso.org/iso-22000-food-safety-management.html>; 2018 Accessed 20.12.21.
17. Zwietering MH, Garre A, Wiedmann M, Buchanan RL. All food processes have a residual risk, some are small, some very small and some are extremely small: zero risk does not exist. *Curr OpFood Sci*. 2020;36:83–92.
18. ICMSF International Commission on Microbiological Specifications for Foods. Microorganisms in Foods 5: Characteristics of Microbial Pathogens. Blackie Academic & Professional, 1996.
19. EC. European Commission Regulation No 2073/2005 on microbiological criteria for foodstuffs. <https://eur-lex.europa.eu/legal-content/EN/ALL/?uri = CELEX%3A32005R2073>; 2005 Accessed 20.12.21.
20. Anelich, L.E, Swoffer, K.P. Chapter 4: The applications and uses of GFSI-benchmarked food safety schemes in relation to retail. In: Retail Food Safety; eds: J. Farber, J. Crichton, O.P. Snyder Jr. 37-41. Springer, 2014.
21. GFSI. Global Food Safety Initiative. <https://mygfsi.com/>; 2021 Accessed 20.12.21.
22. Gaze. Campden BRI: Guideline No. 51, Pasteurisation: A food industry practical guide, ed 2. <https://www.campdenbri.co.uk/publications/pdfs/g51.pdf> 2006.

23. GFSI A culture of food safety; a position paper from the global food safety initiative. V 1.0 4/11/18 GFSI-Food-Safety-Culture-Full.pdf (mygfsi.com), 2018 Accessed 20.02.22.
24. ICMSF International Commission on Microbiological Specifications for Foods. Microorganisms in Foods 8: Use of Data for Assessing Process Control and Product Acceptance. Springer, 2011.
25. ICMSF. *International commission on microbiological specifications for foods. Microorganisms in Foods 7: Microbiological Testing in Food Safety Management.* 2nd ed Springer; 2018.
26. Warner, J. Novel techniques for the in situ detection of bacteria on salad leaf surfaces. PhD thesis. School of Biological Sciences, Faculty of Medicine, Health and Life Sciences, University of Southampton. <https://www.semanticscholar.org/paper/Novel-techniques-for-the-in-situ-detection-of-on-Warner/4273562104de4b9f437a05bd3c061b06d29bbd22>; 2009 Accessed 20.12.21.
27. Fossum S, Crooke E, Skarstad K. Organization of sister origins and replisomes during multifork DNA replication in *Escherichia coli. Eur Mol Biol Organ.* 2007;26(21):4514–4522. Available from: https://doi.org/10.1038/sj.emboj.7601871.
28. Everis. Campden BRI Blog: Can we assume consumers' fridges are at a safe temperature? <https://www.campdenbri.co.uk/blogs/consumers-fridges-safe.php>; 2020 Accessed 20.02.22.
29. EFSA. European Food Safety Authority. *Listeria monocytogenes* contamination of ready-to-eat foods and the risk for human health in the EU. *EFSA J.* 2018;. Available from: https://doi.org/10.2903/j.efsa.2018.5134.
30. Everis. Campden BRI Guideline No. 46, Evaluation of microbiological shelf life of foods 2nd ed. <https://www.campdenbri.co.uk/publications/pdfs/g46_2.pdf>; 2019 Accessed 20.12.21.
31. CAC. Codex Alimentarius Commission. General standard for the labelling of prepackaged foods CXS 1-1985.; 2018 Accessed 15.12.21.
32. EFSA. European Food Safety Authority. 'Use by' or 'best before'? New tool to support food operators. <https://www.efsa.europa.eu/en/news/use-or-best-new-tool-support-food-operators>; 2020 Accessed 03.11.21.
33. EC. European Commission notice. EU guidelines on food donation. <https://eur-lex.europa.eu/legal-content/EN/TXT/?uri = CELEX:52017XC1025(01)>; 2017 Accessed 03.11.21.
34. WRAP. Food date labelling. <https://wrap.org.uk/taking-action/food-drink/actions/date-labelling>; 2019 Accessed 06.08.21.
35. FMI. Guidance for the control of *Listeria monocytogenes*, risks in retail stores. <https://www.fmi.org/forms/store/ProductFormPublic/guidance-for-the-control-of-listeria-monocytogenes-free-pdf-download>; 2008 Accessed 20.12.21.
36. Australian Bureau of statistics. Online sales, June 2021, – supplementary COVID-19 analysis. <https://www.abs.gov.au/articles/online-sales-june-2021-supplementary-covid-19-analysis>; 2021 Accessed 20.02.22.
37. Statista. Online grocery shopping in the United Kingdom (UK) – statistics and facts. <https://www.statista.com/topics/3144/online-grocery-shopping-in-the-united-kingdom/#dossierKeyfigures>; 2022 Accessed 20.02.22.
38. Encyclopaedia Britannica. The second law of thermodynamics. <https://www.britannica.com/science/thermodynamics/The-second-law-of-thermodynamics>; 2002 Accessed 20.02.22.
39. EFSA European Food Safety Authority. Guidance on date marking and related food information: part 2 (food information). <https://www.efsa.europa.eu/en/efsajournal/pub/6510> 2021. doi.org/10.2903/j.efsa.2021.6510.
40. EC. European Commission Notice providing guidance of food safety management systems for retail activities, including food donations. <https://eur-lex.europa.eu/legal-content/EN/TXT/?uri = OJ%3AJOC_2020_199_R_0001>; 2020 Accessed 12.12.21.

Chapter 35

Reduction of the microbial load of food by processing and modified atmosphere packaging

Elna M. Buys[1], B.C. Dlamini[2], James A. Elegbeleye[1] and N.N. Mehlomakulu[1]

[1]*Department of Consumer and Food Sciences, Faculty of Natural and Agricultural Sciences, University of Pretoria, Pretoria, South Africa,* [2]*Department of Biotechnology and Food Technology, Faculty of Science, University of Johannesburg, Johannesburg, South Africa*

Abstract

Microbial spoilage of food is a leading cause of food spoilage, which can lead to considerable losses besides the morbidity and/or mortality that accompany outbreaks associated with foodborne pathogens. This may impact the sustainable development goals negatively if not sufficiently tackled. Efforts are being made toward minimizing the disruptive effects of microbes in food and in the production of food, which is safe and nutritious with an extended shelf-life. Novel food processing technologies have been developed to address the challenge of microbial reduction in food and by extension, the production of safe foods. Examples of such nonthermal processing technologies are the application of modified atmosphere packaging (MAP), high-pressure processing, and cold plasma. This chapter explores the efficacy of several processing technologies, with a main focus on MAP, in reducing the microbial load in some foods as well as benefits and drawbacks on the food value chain.

Keywords: Microbial load; packaging; foodborne pathogens; processing

35.1 Introduction

Food processing, in its fundamental definition, is the conversion of raw materials into a finished product with optimal quality attributes, that is, microbiological, nutrition, and sensory, which render the product safe, nutritious, and acceptable for consumption.[1] To ensure optimum quality, food processing focuses on the whole food chain, from farm to fork. Failure to monitor activities before and during processing to achieve optimal quality or reduction in microbial load can lead to foodborne illnesses on consumption of that food.[2] Hence, food processing technologies are adopted under stringent conditions to reduce or eliminate foodborne hazards.

One of the major biological hazards in food processing is the presence and/or growth of pathogenic microorganisms during and after processing. Thus food processing is aimed at preserving the quality attributes of food by destroying pathogens and inhibit or control their proliferation. Indeed, currently applied food processing technologies can retain the sensory and nutritional quality of food as well as inhibit the growth of pathogenic microorganisms.[1] However, pathogenic microorganisms continue to be a cause for concern throughout the food chain due to their role in reported foodborne outbreaks.[3]

Pathogenic bacteria cause either food infections or intoxications due to the consumption of viable bacterial cells or secreted toxin, respectively.[4] Foodborne outbreaks result in the loss of lives, extended hospitalizations, lawsuits, and economic loss to the food industry. In the United States alone, the estimated economic cost for all foodborne illnesses is between \$60.9 and \$90.2 billion with an approximate 600 million cases globally and 420,000 deaths in 2010.[5,6] According to the Centers for Disease Control and Prevention, *Salmonella*, *Clostridium perfringens*, *Campylobacter*, and *Staphylococcus aureus* are the leading pathogens responsible for foodborne disease outbreaks.[7] On a global scale, these foodborne diseases are associated with a variety of food source exposure routes. The persistence of foodborne pathogens throughout the food chain is attributed to multiple factors at varying degrees of occurrence. Notably, improper handling and storage of raw material, inadequate processing of food, unhygienic food processing facilities, and poor application of Good Manufacturing Practices and Food Safety Standards are contributory factors.[8] The failure or nonadherence to either one or more of these factors presents

Present Knowledge in Food Safety. DOI: https://doi.org/10.1016/B978-0-12-819470-6.00064-0

a favorable environment for foodborne pathogens to proliferate. These pathogens establish their dominance by developing adaptation responses to the processing stresses through genetic and physiological adjustments, which render the bacteria resistant to food processing–related stresses.[9,10]

Microbial inactivation through thermal processing technologies such as pasteurization and sterilization are established based on two premises: (1) heat resistance of microorganisms for each specific product formulation and composition and (2) the heating rate of the specific product.[1,11] On the other hand, microbial inactivation by nonthermal processing technologies such as high-pressure processing (HPP), sonication, microwave, irradiation, ohmic heating, ozonation, pulsed electric fields (PEF), and cold plasma (CP) is chiefly based on the resistance of the microorganism to the processing hurdle or stress and processing conditions (Table 35.1). These factors, however, do not render the technologies insufficient as they meet the aim of commercial sterilization technologies used in food processing, at ambient or sublethal temperatures, thereby minimizing negative effects on nutritional and quality parameters of food.[12,13]

These technologies are either applied before packaging or postpackaging based on the nature of the technology or can be used in combination with other food processing or preservation technologies and methods.[2,14]

This chapter focuses on the use of nonthermal processing technologies and modified atmosphere packaging (MAP) in inactivating pathogenic microorganisms during processing. The concept of hurdle technology when using these processing technologies is discussed with the view of whether a reduction in the microbial population is achievable.

35.2 Microbial load reduction in food through hurdle technology

Unit operations applied in food processing exert hurdles that pathogenic microorganisms must overcome to survive in a food product. Hurdle technology is the use of a combination of different preservation factors or techniques as hurdles against the microorganism to achieve a multitarget, mild but reliable preservation effect on the food product.[15] These hurdles can act in unison or in a sequential manner, can be inclusive of intrinsic and extrinsic parameters, can be processed based or implicit to a food product (Table 35.1). As such, the hurdles can be either derived from microbial activity or be physical or physicochemical attributes (Table 35.2).

The synergistic effect of the hurdles on the microbial cells can target the cell wall, cell membrane, DNA, enzymes, and/or intracellular proteins, thus disturbing the internal pH, oxidation-reduction potential, and morphology of microorganisms.[12,17] However, it is the effect of the hurdle on the microorganism that determines the

TABLE 35.1 Factors to be considered for optimum microbial inactivation and food quality during food processing.

Treatment condition	Target microorganism characteristics	Food product characteristics	Effect on food product
Strength (dose) of treatment, type and procedure of treatment, treatment duration, temperature	Initial microbial load, resistance to treatment, interaction with other microorganisms, mechanism for treatment resistance	Solid or liquid state, viscosity, packaged or not, conductivity of product	Shelf life, quality, and organoleptic characteristics

Source: Adapted from Bahrami A, Moaddabdoost Baboli Z, Schimmel K, Jafari SM, Williams L. Efficiency of novel processing technologies for the control of Listeria monocytogenes in food products. Trends Food Sci Technol. 2020[12]; and Fellows PJ, Introduction. In: Food Processing Technology. Elsevier; 2017: xv–xxiii.[1]

TABLE 35.2 Food preservation hurdles.

Type of hurdle	Examples
Microbially derived	Antibiotics, bacteriocins, competitive flora, protective cultures
Physical	Packaging (aseptic, vacuum, modified atmosphere, active, films, and coatings), radiation (microwave, UV, and irradiation), temperature (high or low), photodynamic inactivation, high pressure, sonication, electric current
Physico-chemical	Carbon dioxide, ethanol, lactic acid, lactoperoxidase, low pH, low redox potential, low water activity, Maillard reaction products, organic acids, oxygen, ozone, phenols, phosphates, salt, smoking, sodium nitrite/nitrate, sodium or potassium sulfite, spices and herbs, surface treatment agents

Source: Ohlsson T, Bengtsson N. Minimal Processing Technologies in the Food Industries. Woodhead Publishing Limited; 2002.[16]

lethality and hurdle intensity.[11,13] These factors are, however, dependent on the selection of hurdles suitable for a specific food product, the target microorganism, and the mode of action of the hurdle as shown in Table 35.2. Even though nonthermal technologies are deemed to be mild product type-specific preservation technologies compared to thermal processing technologies, they can destroy viable pathogenic cells and bacterial spores.[1]

35.3 Homeostatic disturbance of pathogenic bacteria

The ability of microorganisms to maintain a uniform and stable internal status renders a homeostatic environment that is suitable for cell division and multiplication. However, disturbance of this status hinders cell multiplication. Microorganisms live within narrow internal pH limits; thus, changes in this intrinsic parameter result in the cells pumping electrons out of the intracellular environment to maintain this homeostatic balance. Another type of homeostatic balance is maintaining a positive pressure by retaining the osmolarity of the cytoplasm higher than that of the cell environment.[11,13] These changes are demanding on the cells since energy expenditure is directed toward repair mechanisms rather than replication mechanisms. Therefore the cells remain in the lag phase of growth and with prolonged exposure to a hurdle or a subsequent hurdle, the cell never fully recovers and eventually dies.[17]

35.4 Stress shock protein of pathogenic bacteria

When a microorganism is exposed to a stressful environment, for example, multiple hurdles, as a mode of survival mechanism, the genes coding for stress shock proteins are activated. Notably, the exposure does not generate a multistress response instead of a specific stress response. Thus a particular hurdle will evoke a known and identifiable stress response (Table 35.3). Reported

TABLE 35.3 Bacterial stress response to food processing hurdles.

Environmental condition	Stage in the food system	Bacterial stress response	Reference organisms
Low temperature	Freezing/refrigeration	Expression of cold shock domain proteins (e.g., CspA, CspB, and CspD)	*Listeria, Bacillus, Pseudomonas*
High temperature	Temperature abuse, food processing	Heat-shock proteins acting as molecular chaperones are induced that repairs damaged proteins, e.g., DnaK, GroEL, ClpAP	*Geobacillus, Bacillus subtilis*
Low pH	Fermentation (competitive flora), food acidification	Production of acid shock proteins (ASP), enzymes that raise the intracellular pH, efflux system that pumps protons	*Listeria, Clostridium*
Bile stress	Consumption	Transcriptional regulators, efflux pump, repair proteins for DNA and cell membrane	
Osmotic pressure (NaCl, glucose, etc.)	Food additives	Uptake systems for potassium, transport of solutes (e.g., betaine, proline, carnitine)	
Oxidative stress	Exposure to oxidative compounds or air during processing	Production of repair proteins such as superoxide dismutase and endonuclease IV	
High pressure	Food processing	Production of pressure-induced proteins (PIPs)	
Drying (freeze, vacuum and air)	Food processing		
Radiation (UV, gamma and X-rays)	Food processing	Production of photoreactivation enzymes (e.g., photolyase), alkyl group removal, base excision repair	*Escherichia coli*
Food preservatives (benzoic acid, sorbic acid, etc.)	Food processing	Induction of acid-tolerance response, production of degrading enzymes, for example, methyl para(4)-hydroxybenzoate in efflux system, etc.	*Pseudomonas, Listeria, Saccharomyces*
Sanitizers, for example, quaternary ammonium compounds (QACs), chlorine		Expression of genes against biocides such as QACs (e.g., *qacE, qacEΔ1, qacF, qacG, and qacH*)	*Pseudomonas, Aeromonas, Shewanella*, and *Listeria*

stress responses in food processing are induced by either heat, pH, water activity (a_w), ethanol, oxidative compounds, or starvation in addition to other hurdles.[9] These stress responses render the microorganisms resistant to the effect of the hurdle, compromising the quality of the food product. However, the application of multiple hurdles in the processing chain inhibits the growth and/or proliferation of the microorganism through metabolic exhaustion.[15]

In the case of *Listeria monocytogenes*, it is resistant to mild heat treatment and can adapt to environmental stresses such as decreasing a_w, increasing salt, decreasing fat and fiber content, and higher acidity. Heat tolerance of *L. monocytogenes* is attributed to the upregulation of *ClpE*, *ClpB* genes with *ClpL* as the predictor of this resistance.[12] Microorganisms can also exhibit "cross-tolerance" or tolerance for other stresses after exposure to a single stress. Cross-tolerance may likely occur when the stress is not applied simultaneously to cause metabolic exhaustion of the unwanted microorganisms.[17] *L. monocytogenes*, for instance, has been observed to have the same re-growth potential as normal cells after induced stress of acid (pH 4.2), osmotic pressure (10% NaCl), and heat (55°C for 30 min).[18] The same has been observed in other well-known pathogens associated with foodborne outbreaks such as *Salmonella* and *Escherichia coli* O157:H7.[10] This tolerance is because of stress adaptation and alteration in gene expression of the bacteria during food processing. Stress proteins are produced against stresses such as heat, oxidative stress, bile, low pH, and high salt concentration, which are the characteristic conventional hurdles used during food processing.[9] Table 35.3 shows the responses of bacteria to different stresses during food processing while Table 35.4 reveals the important spoilage and pathogenic microorganisms that must be controlled, whose presence in food can negatively affect the food or the health of consumers.

35.5 Metabolic exhaustion of pathogenic bacteria

Microbial cells exposed to a mild hurdle can be sublethally injured as observed in thermally treated bacterial cells.[11] This defeats the purpose of eliminating the microorganism to meet the 5-log reduction for most pathogenic bacteria as the bacteria will initiate recovery mechanisms.[2] However, sequential application of one or more hurdles allows attack of the already injured cells to prevent their growth.[13] Thus the synergistic effect of the hurdles ensuring energy consumption and expenditure by microorganisms does not follow the course of cell replication and maintenance of energy balance. The cells exhaust all energy toward repair mechanisms and eventually die.[21]

In the case of nonthermal technologies, the effect of the hurdle determines whether cells are sublethally injured or completely inactivated based on their growth phase, sensitivity to the processing technology hurdle and cell morphology. The effect of high-pressure sublethally injured cells is similar to that of thermally injured cells, albeit differing cell repair mechanisms.[11,14] After decompression in HPP, cells in the exponential phase cannot repair pressure-damaged membranes, while stationary phase cells can repair their membranes.[22] The application of other hurdles in a sequential manner post-HPP allows for a synergistic effect to destroy injured vegetative cells. However, the barosensitivity of the bacteria must be taken into consideration. Barosensitivity of bacteria follows the order (pressure resistance > pressure sensitivity): bacterial spores > Gram-positive bacteria > Gram-negative bacteria. However, to destroy bacterial spores, a synergistic effect of pressure (400–900 MPa) and heat (90°C–120°C) is required. The same synergistic effect is observed with irradiation followed by heat, with Gram-negative bacteria being more sensitive than Gram-positive bacteria, while irradiation with MAP requires a low radiation dose to achieve the same result.[1] Bacterial spores in food products are resistant to PEF with Gram-positive bacteria being less resistant than Gram-negative bacteria. PEF bacterial inactivation increases when a synergistic effect of either high temperature, low ionic strength, or low pH hurdle is applied.[23]

Thus even though some of the nonthermal technologies can alone destroy a bacterial pathogen, there must be a threshold to reach the desired food quality. Metabolic exhaustion through the application of sequential "mild" intensity hurdles, for example, oxidation-reduction potential, MAP, or reduced a_w, can achieve bactericidal effects without affecting product quality.

35.6 Reductions of microbial load by modified atmosphere packaging

For centuries, smoking has been used in the processing and preservation of perishable foods such as meat and fish, presumably shortly after the discovery of fire. Besides the heat applied during the smoking of food, the process itself is the closest to MAP because it involves the reduction of oxygen and microbes by the various compounds produced from the reaction.[24] It was not until the 1930s that the usefulness of changing or altering the atmosphere around stored fresh produce was linked with an extension of its shelf life. Its adoption has grown widely, especially in Europe, since it was first introduced to the United Kingdom in 1979 for extending the shelf-life of some processed meat.[25,26]

The purpose of food packaging is to provide improved quality of a product that is stable, fresh-like, and with an

TABLE 35.4 Important microorganisms that must be controlled during food processing.

Category	Major microorganisms	Food sources	Effects
Pathogen	*Bacillus cereus*	Meat, stews, gravies	Abdominal cramps, watery diarrhea, nausea
	Brucella spp.	Raw milk and soft cheeses from unpasteurized milk	Sweating, joint, and muscle pain
	Campylobacter jejuni	Contaminated water, raw or undercooked poultry, unpasteurized milk	Diarrhea, cramps, fever, and vomiting
	Clostridium botulinum	Hermetically sealed or canned foods such as fermented fish, baked potatoes, and meats	Diarrhea, nausea, vomiting blurred vision, difficulty swallowing, muscle weakness; can result in respiratory failure and death
	Clostridium perfringens	Meats, poultry, gravy, dried or precooked foods, time and/or temperature-abused foods	Severe abdominal cramps and watery diarrhea
	Diarrheagenic *Escherichia coli* (ETEC, EHEC, EPEC)	Contaminated foods such as meat, juice, vegetables, and water	Watery or bloody diarrhea, fever, abdominal cramps
	Hepatitis A	Sea-foods and contaminated foods	Jaundice, lethargy, loss of appetite, fever, nausea, vomiting
	Listeria monocytogenes	Raw milk, soft cheeses from unpasteurized milk, ready-to-eat foods especially from meat	Meningitis, bacteremia, fever, nausea, muscle aches, diarrhea, stillbirth, or premature delivery in pregnant women, death may occur in children and immunocompromised patients
	Mycobacterium bovis	Raw milk and soft cheeses from unpasteurized milk	Symptoms of tuberculosis
	Norovirus	Raw produce, contaminated foods, and water	Nausea, vomiting, abdominal cramping, diarrhea, fever, headache, vomiting
	Salmonella spp.	Eggs, poultry, meat, unpasteurized milk or juice, cheese, contaminated foods, fruits, and vegetables	Abdominal cramps, fever, and vomiting
	Shigella spp.	Raw foods, contaminated foods, and water	Abdominal cramps, fever and vomiting, diarrhea with feces containing blood and mucus
	Rotavirus	Raw foods, contaminated foods, and water	Diarrhea, vomiting, fever, belly pain, and dehydration in infants
	Toxoplasma gondii		Swollen lymph glands, muscle aches and pains, fever
Spoilage	LAB[a] (*Brochothrix thermosphacta, Enterococcus, Lactococcus, Lactobacillus, Leuconostoc, Weissella*)	Different types of food such as meat, vegetables, and beverages including low pH food	Greening of meat, gas formation in cheeses (blowing), pickles (bloater damage), and canned or packaged meat and vegetables. Off-flavors described as mousy, cheesy, malty, acidic, buttery, or liver-like may be detected in wine, meats, milk, or juices spoiled by these bacteria, production of exopolysaccharide causing slime formation in meats and ropiness in some beverages

(Continued)

TABLE 35.4 (Continued)

Category	Major microorganisms	Food sources	Effects
	Enterobacteriaceae (*Salmonella*, *Vibrio*, *Klebsiella*, *Proteus*, etc.)	Highly proteinaceous foods such as meat, milk, cheese, seafoods, cured meat, and beer	Production of enzymes that break down amino acids into volatile compounds like foul-smelling diamines and sulfur compounds
	Pseudomonas spp. (*P. fluorescens*, *P. putida*, *P. fragi*)	Spoilage of refrigerated food meat, seafood, poultry, milk, etc.	
	Aerobic spore-forming bacteria such as *Bacillus subtilis*, *Bacillus velezensis*, *B. cereus*, and *Geobacillus stearothermophilus*	Dairy products such as extended shelf life (ESL) and ultra-high temperature (UHT) milk, bakery products, and canned food	The psychrotrophs can spoil refrigerated dairy products; others such as *Bacillus subtilis* are mesophilic and can spoil bakery products, whereas others such as *G. stearothermophilus* are thermophilic and spoil foods that are canned or in hermetically sealed packages
	Clostridium spp. (*C. algidicarnis*, *C. sporogenes*, *C. estertheticum*, *C. perfringens*, *Clostridium butyricum*, *Clostridium gasigenes*)	Vacuum-packed chilled meat, semihard (Gouda) cheese, and other low pH hermetically sealed foods and canned bean-sprouts	Spoilage causing softening, dripping, and an offensive odor especially of meat. *C. gasigenes* and others produce gas causing a type of spoilage known as "blown or burst packs."
	Alicyclobacillus spp.	Low acid, pasteurized foods such as fruit juice, e.g., apple juice	Cloudiness and sediment, production of compounds such as guaiacol and by 2,6-dibromophenol and 2,6-dichlorophenol causing an antiseptic flavor
	Leuconostoc	Low pH fermented beverages	Oily consistency of foods makes it undesirable
	Zygosaccharomyces spp. (*Z. bailii*, *Z. bisporus*, *Z. rouxii*)	High sugar and salt food such as fruit juices, concentrates, sirups, honey, jams, confectionery, sauces, and alcoholic beverages	Fermentative spoilage, haziness, production of carbon dioxide, which may result in leakage or explosion of packed foods that can cause the container to leak or, in extreme cases, explode. Metabolite production such as acetic acid, esters, and alcohols can cause a change in flavor that is undesirable
	Saccharomyces spp.	Fermented foods and beverages	Production of metabolites that alters the flavor of foods such as ethanol, esters, ketones, aldehydes, alcohols, and sulfur compounds
	Candida spp.	Different types of foods	Enzymatic spoilage and production of metabolites
	Dekkera spp.	Wine	Enzymatic spoilage and production of metabolites such asphenolic causing a mousy flavor in the wine

[a]*Lactic acid bacteria.*
Source: Adley CC, Ryan MP. The nature and extent of foodborne disease. In: Antimicrobial Food Packaging. Elsevier; 2016:1–10[19]; Petruzzi L, Corbo MR, Sinigaglia M, Bevilacqua A. Microbial spoilage of foods. In: The Microbiological Quality of Food. Elsevier; 2017:1–21.[20]

increased shelf-life in such a way that the product is easily stored, transported, and delivered to consumers. The rising desire of consumers for a minimally processed, fresh-like product with a long shelf-life has created innovative packaging techniques such as MAP. Therefore MAP as well as packaging is generally tailored toward meeting these demands of consumers by protecting such products from mechanical impairment and deterring chemical and biochemical changes in the product as well as preventing microbial spoilage.[27] Besides these major roles of food packaging, it also serves as material on which information about composition, caloric value, shelf-life, and other relevant information on the food product is printed.[28]

MAP involves the alteration in the gaseous atmosphere around or enclosing food products with the sole purpose of preserving the integrity of the food and extending its shelf life. This modification is achieved by either removing the gaseous contents from the headspace of a food package or by the variation of the oxygen, nitrogen, and carbon dioxide gases in the headspace to inhibit the growth of spoilage and pathogenic microbes in the packed food. For fresh produce, MAP reduces the rate of tissue respiration and browning reaction thereby extending product shelf-life and esthetics in the case of freshly cut products.[26,29,30] MAP has found a wide application in different products such as meat, vegetables, fruits, and freshly cut products such as apples. This chapter highlights the fundamental principles of MAP, its efficacy, and uniqueness compared with other technologies. Furthermore, in the chapter, its limitations, recent trends, and potential future advancements in its application are explored.

35.7 Fundamental principles of modified atmosphere packaging

The earth's atmosphere consists of a different mixture of gases that sustains all living things, including microbial life, which is predominantly responsible for spoilage associated with food and foodborne diseases. Any alteration in the ratio of these gases either accelerate or decrease the rate of respiration in both the cells of the product as well as contaminating microbes. As an example, the respiration rate of both the tissues of fresh produce and microbial flora can be reduced by increasing the concentration of CO_2 and decreasing that of O_2. This, in turn, extends the shelf-life of the product, due to the CO_2 surrounding the tissues, which reduces some biochemical reactions involved in tissue respiration, ripening, and senescence.[31,32] Specific biochemical pathways that are inhibited by using high CO_2 and low O_2 include those involving the synthesis of ethylene as well as pigments (chlorophyll, carotenoids, anthocyanins, etc.), volatile compounds and aroma, components of the cell wall and organic acids (citric acid, carboxylic acid, etc.). These are processes that determine the sensory properties of fruit such as appearance, texture, taste, flavor, and aroma.[33]

In MAP, the process of gaseous modification is taken a notch higher by selecting a gas or combination of gases enclosed within a selective packaging material that is designed for such a purpose. The gases can also be inert gases that slow down the respiration rate of fresh produce to a large extent and consequently prevent the deterioration of the product as it pertains to the color, sensory, and nutritional properties. Nitrogen (N_2), oxygen (O_2), and carbon dioxide (CO_2) are the three gases frequently used in MAP. Other gases that are not so commonly used include inert gases such as argon (Ar) and helium (He), nitrous oxide or di-nitrogen monoxide (N_2O), and superatmospheric O_2. The goal of MAP is to replace entrapped gases (mostly atmospheric gases) within a packaged food product to produce an equilibrium of gases that either inhibit or slow down the growth of aerobic and anaerobic microorganisms without any adverse biochemical effect on the food. The ratio of the gases used is dependent on the type of packaged food to which the technique is applied. As an example, freshly cut apples turn brown in the presence of oxygen and the enzyme polyphenol oxidase, which makes it undesirable even without any spoilage. The same oxygen is desired for the characteristic bright pink color of fresh meat upon exposure to oxygen, which causes the myoglobin in the meat to be oxidized to oxymyoglobin. There is a difference that must be noted between MAP and controlled atmosphere (CA) as the two can easily be confused. CA is used in the bulk storage or transportation of fresh produce to slow down the ripening process specifically targeted at suppressing the production of ethylene gas, which speeds up the ripening process. Just as the name suggests, CA does not involve the packaging of the produce but attempts to control the atmospheric conditions at which the produce is stored or being transported.[34] Unlike in MAP, the concentrations of gases in the atmosphere in CA must be closely monitored and rectified accordingly. For these to be achieved, CA is fitted with an airtight storage environment, analyzers, removal, and injection mechanisms for the gases (O_2 and CO_2) to maintain the desired ambient condition.[35] This means that for CA the desired atmospheric condition can be achieved faster than for MAP. CA can be used in combination with low temperature or refrigeration to achieve the best result by slowing down the respiration rate of a fresh product further.[31]

35.8 Passive versus active modified atmosphere packaging

There are two general approaches used during MAP depending on the type of packaging material used whether high- or low-barrier material. These are known as passive and active MAP. While active MAP makes use of high-barrier materials that prevent an exchange of gases with the atmosphere, passive MAP makes use of low-barrier food packaging materials. This low-barrier food packaging material allows the exchange of gases until an equilibrium is reached between the respiration rate of the fresh produce and the permeability of the packaging material within the package, most especially during product storage.[36] These techniques are usually used in the preservation of ready-to-eat (RTE) foods, fresh produce, and horticultural goods under reduced temperature or in combination with other technologies such as ultrasound (US). Passive MAP is successfully applied to commodities such as lettuce, tomato, cabbage, and broccoli.[37–39]

In active packaging (AP), there is a deliberate inclusion of some active components either in the headspace or as part of the packaging material itself. These active compounds are usually targeted at scavenging gases such as O_2, CO_2, and ethylene gases. Recent developments in active MAP have seen the incorporation of antimicrobials and other compounds to inhibit the growth of microbes and for the regulated release of some flavor compounds as the case requires.[40,41]

35.9 The effect of gas mixtures on microorganisms/spores

Spoilage of food can be divided into microbial and non-microbial spoilage. Besides their ability to cause foodborne illnesses, microbes are the leading cause of food spoilage and reduction of shelf-life for most products. This is because of their ubiquity in nature and versatility concerning the environment that they can colonize and the production of degradative enzymes.[42,43] The main idea in MAP, as it relates to the control of microbes, is the removal or the substitution of gases generally required by microorganisms with another gas or mixture of gases. Largely, microorganisms that are associated with food can be classified into four groups based on their demand for O_2.[44] These categories are:

1. Obligate aerobes: These are microorganisms that require free O_2 for growth. During the metabolic process, O_2 is used as the terminal electron acceptor in the electron transport chain. Examples of obligate aerobes are *Pseudomonas* and *Bacillus* besides most yeasts and molds.
2. Obligate anaerobes: These groups of microbes are affected by the concentrations of O_2 present in the atmosphere or environment. The tolerance for O_2 differs between species and is in the range of 0.5%–8%. Examples of microbes in this group are *Clostridium*, *Actinomyces*, and *Bacteroides*.
3. Facultative anaerobes: Some good examples of this type of microbe are the well-known pathogens such as *Listeria*, *Salmonella*, *Staphylococcus*, and *E. coli* as well as fungi such as *Saccharomyces*. They can utilize O_2 when the gas is present. They easily resort to anaerobic respiration or fermentation in the absence of O_2 while using other terminal electron acceptors during the metabolism of organic substrates.

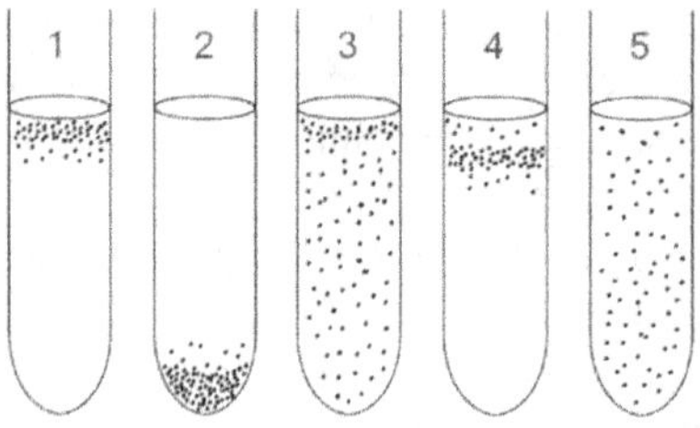

FIGURE 35.1 The response of microbes to O_2 when in thioglycolate broth: (1) Obligate aerobes grow at the air interface because they can grow without oxygen. (2) Obligate anaerobes can only survive without oxygen; hence they grow at the bottom of the tube that has the lowest oxygen penetration. (3) Facultative anaerobes both oxygen and anoxic conditions. (4) Microaerophiles require oxygen but at a lower concentration. (5) Aero-tolerant microbes neither require oxygen nor are they poisoned by it.

4. Microaerophiles: This group of microbes requires O_2 in the range of 5%–10% as well as CO_2 of between 8% and 10% for optimal growth. Examples of bacteria in this category include *Lactobacillus* and *Campylobacter*.
5. Aero-tolerant microbes: Aero-tolerant microbes, as the name suggests, do not need O_2 for their metabolism and they are neither affected after exposure to O_2. An example is *Streptococcus* spp.

Based on this demand for O_2, MAP can be designed to inhibit the growth of microorganisms commonly associated with a particular type of food that may cause either spoilage or foodborne illness when such contaminated food is consumed. The design of an effective MAP requires an understanding of several factors besides the nature of the associated microbial contaminants; these include gas permeability, characteristics, and atmospheric condition of the product, among others.[45] Such knowledge can inform the combination of gases that can be used during a MAP regime. Two types of gases are typically used in MAP; these are conventional versus nonconventional gases (Fig. 35.1).

35.10 Conventional and nonconventional gases used in modified atmosphere packaging

The gases used in MAP can be broadly classified into conventional and nonconventional gases. Examples of conventional gases are CO_2, N_2, and O_2 and nonconventional gases are Ar (Argon), nitrous oxide (NO_2), and ozone (O_3). These gases are used in different ratios depending on the types of food they are applied to. Conventional gases are commonly used with one or two gases used in a specific proportion depending on the type of food or product to be packed. To prevent the growth of spoilage microbes in nonrespiring packed food, a combination of CO_2, N_2, and O_2 is often used in such a way that CO_2 gas forms about a third or half of the gas combination. In general, during MAP, CO_2 is used for its bacteriostatic and fungistatic properties while O_2 is used to preserve the color, such as in the case of the bright-red coloration of oxymyoglobin in meat. N_2 is used as an inert filler to prevent the collapse of the pack and maintain the ratio of other gases in the combination.[46,47]

35.11 Functions of gases used in modified atmosphere packaging

35.11.1 Carbon dioxide

The application of CO_2 is more effective against aerobic microbes that usually cause the spoilage of food products; it thus extends the shelf-life of a product. Excluding the gas in vegetables and other plant-based products helps in slowing down the degradation of the pigment chlorophyll and thus preserves the sensory quality of the product. The gas also inhibits the production of ethylene in produce when used at optimum concentration, but its application must be consistent with the property of the specific food.[48] At a concentration above 20%, it slows down the growth of microbial contaminants, but at higher concentrations, it exhibits some bacteriostatic and fungistatic effects. The bacteriostatic effect is more obvious in Gram-negative bacteria such as *Pseudomonas*.[49] The disadvantage of using this gas at a higher concentration is that it may promote the growth of anaerobes such as *Clostridium*. The gas also exerts its influence by solubilizing in water and oil to produce an acid (H_2CO_3), which in turn lowers the pH and may affect the taste of the product, create a collapse of the packaging material, and result in drip loss. The gas is thus combined with a filler gas like N_2 to prevent this collapse. The low pH affects several metabolic pathways in the microbe causing a disturbance in its homeostasis and eventual death or increase in the lag phase depending on the concentration of the gas.[50] CO_2 exhibits some effect at 10% concentration, but the greatest effect is observed against most microbes between 20% and 50%, especially under chilled conditions.

35.11.2 Oxygen

Aerobic microbes as well as respiring plants (e.g., vegetables) or animals (e.g., shellfish) require O_2 for their activities. The gas also gives meat the characteristic freshness of the cherry-red oxymyoglobin. The disadvantage of the gas, when used at low concentration in MAP, is that it can promote the growth of some aerobic organisms resulting in an offensive aroma of spoilage and browning reaction in fresh-cut fruit. Notwithstanding, at a high concentration between 50% and 90% (super-atmospheric oxygen), both enzymatic browning and microbial growth are inhibited.[51] The presence of O_2 is toxic to obligate anaerobes such as *Clostridium botulinum*. The gas is used at either a low concentration (less than 10%) or a very high concentration (more than 50%). This is to prevent the growth of aerobes, which often occurs at more than 10% concentration. At less than 5% concentration, the growth of anaerobes is promoted and plant respiration is halted or slowed down, which is needed to maintain freshness and extend the shelf-life of vegetables. High Oxygen Atmospheres, which is a gas combination containing $>70\%$ O_2, was proven to be more effective than Equilibrium Modified Atmosphere packaging (EMAP). EMAP improves the preservation of fresh produce by using favorable levels of gases that remain constant for most of the packaging time and causes retardation of the lag phase in most spoilage and pathogenic organisms such as molds, yeasts, and *Listeria* in RTE food.[52]

35.11.3 Nitrogen

N_2 is applied in MAP as a filler gas to displace O_2 because of its inert nature and with no effect on the product. Since the gas is poorly absorbed by the food, it provides some mechanical protection to the food from abrasion and crushing. N_2 is cheap and commonly available; hence it is a cheaper alternative than the use of nonconventional gases such as helium (He) and argon (Ar). In general, N_2 is used to preserve the appearance of a product, whereas CO_2 is used for preservation of flavor.[53] Table 35.5 shows different types of foods and conventional gases required for MAP.

35.12 Nonconventional gases used in modified atmosphere packaging

Other gases that are used in MAP but not as commonly as the ones above are carbon monoxide (CO) and super-atmospheric O_2, argon (Ar), xenon (Xe), neon (Ne), sulfur dioxide (SO_2), helium (He), and nitrous oxide (N_2O). In the United States, CO is used with a low concentration of O_2 to give the cherry-red coloration in meat. The gas reacts with the oxymyoglobin of blood to give the deep red color. This color can be retained even if spoilage of the product occurs and thus might lead to poor judgment of the product, besides the fact that the gas is toxic. Hence, its use is not permitted in the European Union (EU). Nonconventional gases have been applied in combination with conventional gases, especially CO_2, in different packaged fresh-cut foods such as apples, potatoes, strawberries, cucumbers, and sardines.[54–58] By a mechanism yet to be understood, Ar as well as other nonconventional gases are able to preserve the antioxidant properties of some compounds such as beta-carotene and phenolics. They were observed to slow down the breakdown of

TABLE 35.5 Different food types and the conventional gases required for modified atmosphere packaging.

Food type	Gases (%)		
	Oxygen (O_2)	Carbon dioxide (CO_2)	Nitrogen (N_2)
Raw red meat	70–80	20–30	
Raw offal	80	20	
Raw poultry and game birds	0–20	30–40	60–70
Poultry, dark portion, and cuts	70–80	20–30	
Raw fish (low fat)	30	40	30
Raw fish (high fat)		40	60
Mollusks and crustaceans	30	40	30
Cooked and cured meats		30–40	60–70
Cooked and cured fish and seafood		30–40	60–70
Cooked and cured poultry and game		30–40	60–70
Ready meals		30	70
Combination products		30–40	60–70
Fresh pasta products		50	50
Bakery		30–70	0–70
Soft cheesesHard cheeseGrated hard cheeses		400–30	6010070–100
Dried food products			100
Cooked vegetables		30–40	60–70
Fresh fruit and vegetables	5	5	90
Liquid food and beverages			100
Carbonated soft drinks		100	

chlorophyll as well as promote tissue respiration in fresh-cut produce.[59] The use of noble gases (Ar, Ne, Xe, He) is gaining acceptance as N_2 replacements in minimally processed fruit and vegetables. This is because of their high solubility and diffusion, which makes them better at displacing O_2 and other dissolved gases, thus impacting negatively on microbial growth and inhibiting deleterious oxidative reaction.[60] A study by Wu et al.[61] observed that high-pressure argon (H-Ar) treatment of apples under chilled conditions for 2 weeks impeded browning reaction as well as the growth of mesophilic and psychrotrophic bacteria besides yeasts and molds. With a solubility twice that of N_2, H-Ar reacts with intracellular water to produce clathrate hydrates, which affects the reaction of enzymes (e.g., catalase and peroxidase) and a_w. Clathrate hydrates can also inactivate the spores of pathogenic *Bacillus cereus* under freezing conditions.[62] This treatment of H-Ar can keep fruit and vegetables for up to 2 weeks under refrigerated temperatures without losing much of the freshness.[63] Although Ar seems to be widely used among the nonconventional gases apart from super-atmospheric O_2, others such as He and N_2O have shown some potential application. N_2O can reduce the respiration and ripening of fruit by affecting the production of ethylene. He can be used to slow down the rate of fermentation of substrates by reducing the diffusion of O_2. Both He and N_2O increase the antioxidant content in fruits and vegetables and reduce the growth of microbes and senescence, thus extending product shelf-life.[64,65]

Ozone (O_3) is widely used in the preservation of fruits such as berries because of its strong oxidizing and antimicrobial properties. It can interfere and break down most cellular components such as enzymes, nucleic acids, proteins, peptide-glucan, and lipids and even the cell membrane of bacteria, spores, molds, and yeasts. Its application and exposure to microbes cause the leakage and lysis of cells and eventual cell death.[66] Pathogens such as *B. cereus, L. monocytogenes*, and *Salmonella enterica* are sensitive to the gas including spores of *B. cereus*. Most vegetative cells of pathogens are inactivated by 20 ppm of O_3 in water. Ozonation must be carried out daily unlike in other gases due to the highly unstable nature of the gas and its short half-life (20 min) in water.[67,68] Ozonation must be applied carefully and in moderation, because excessive application may promote the growth of aerobic microbes, as the gas readily breaks down into O_2 besides causing discoloration of the product. This is despite the fact that no observable damage has been noted on antioxidants in produce such as flavonoids and anthocyanins.[69] The use of O_3 is generally regarded as safe in the EU as well as by the FDA (United States) as a substitute for chlorine.

With the application of MAP in different products, shelf-life has been successfully extended between 50% and 500% while using little or no preservatives, as demanded by most consumers. MAP has also resulted in minimizing food waste as retailers can display products for longer periods of time on shelves with freshness still preserved. The advantage to the food industry is that the coverage for product distribution is expanded as MAP serves as an enabler for companies to reach wider markets beyond their geographical locations without compromising product quality and safety.

35.13 Limitations of modified atmosphere packaging

Concerns have been expressed about the effectiveness of MAP on both aerobic and anaerobic spore-formers such as *B. cereus* and *C. botulinum* in Refrigerated Processed Foods of Extended Durability (REPFEDs) especially when temperature is abused.[70–72] *C. botulinum* Group II is a major threat in chilled or refrigerated foods because of its ability to produce neurotoxin during storage under low O_2 MAP.[73] This is partly because of the failure of the redox potential created in food under low O_2 to inhibit the germination of spores and consequent secretion of botulinum neurotoxins under low O_2 MAP. Some of the nonproteolytic, psychrophilic strains of *C. botulinum* grow under conditions of about 10% O_2 to produce toxins, which are specifically debilitating when ingested with food.[74,75]

For *L. monocytogenes* in Queso Fresco (a type of cheese), Brown et al.[76] observed that MAP was effective with increasing % of CO_2 of gas combination when stored at 7°C for 35 days. The downside of this may be an increase in pH of the food due to the dissolution of the gas in aqueous content within the food matrix, which may prevent its adoption in foods with neutral or high pH. Depending on the combination of gases used, MAP can inhibit the germination and outgrowth of bacterial spores in products, especially when pretreated.[77] Psychrotrophic facultative anaerobes such as *L. monocytogenes* and *Yersinia enterocolitica* and some mesophiles such as strains of *Salmonella* as well as other spoilage microbes may grow when storage temperature is compromised or packaging material is tampered with; this could affect the safety and quality of such products.[78] This further reinforces the need for a strict temperature regime during storage of product and the pretreatment (hurdle) of product to reduce the initial microbial load before applying MAP.

In addition to the above limitation, MAP has been shown not to have a significant effect on enteric foodborne viruses such as hepatitis A virus (HAV) when present on the surface of produce using CO_2 and N_2, regardless of the proportion in which these gases are applied.[79] According to Hennechart-Collette et al.[80] HAV and norovirus are the leading causes of food-related outbreaks that result in nonbacterial gastroenteritis. These viruses maintain their activity to a considerable extent under freezing conditions, especially in RTE foods and have been the leading causes of foodborne illness in the EU in 2014 according to EFSA.[81]

The choice or type of packaging material plays a major role in the survival of microbes in all their different forms under MAP. MAP can also be combined with other processing technologies to ensure the safety of food and traceability after processing. Besides this, incorrect gas composition or leaks caused by defective temperature or pressure and contaminated equipment may compromise product safety; however, with improvement in MAP and other processing technologies, these risks can be minimized. Unlike the use of preservatives, in most cases, the gases are not absorbed by food and thus, do not change the nature or taste of the product. But there are exceptions to this rule. For example, a concentration of excessive CO_2 may be absorbed by the food, which makes it more acidic (sour). These effects can, however, be avoided with suitable gas mixtures. Furthermore, the high levels of oxygen in MAP can cause oxidative changes in meat, resulting in sensory deviations.

35.14 Nonthermal inactivation methods for reducing foodborne pathogens

Novel food processing technologies can be divided into thermal and nonthermal applications. Novel nonthermal food processing technologies are becoming more favored by the food industry. Their adoption is necessitated by the increased demand for safe and more nutritious food by consumers. Conventional thermal technology for food processing has improved over the years, particularly when combined with other hurdles.[82] However, there are still some limitations associated with the effect of heat on the organoleptic and nutritional quality of food.[83] As an alternative, novel food technologies provide minimal negative effects on the sensory and nutritional quality of food.

In this section, nonthermal technologies are discussed since they seem to have more future benefits than novel thermal technologies. An overview of the principles of these techniques is explained but importantly, the potential application of nonthermal technologies in combination with other techniques is explored. This is because when applied in synergy, nonthermal technologies may be used at low concentrations and thus potentially reduce application costs and the negative effects associated with some such technologies.

35.14.1 Ultrasound

US is a nonthermal treatment that uses longitudinal waves that are above 20 kHz. It is regarded as a "green technology" because of its eco-friendly and nontoxic nature.[84] The application of high-frequency US to food for long periods has been shown to achieve a sterilizing effect and ensures microbiological safety.[85] However, subjecting food to high intensity US for extended periods generates heat that can affect biological structures. Because of this, US is generally used with other techniques to ensure effective microbial inactivation with minimal loss in the nutritional and sensory properties of food.[86] US energy inactivates microorganisms through the formation and collapse of small air bubbles or cavities that produce high local pressures and temperatures that break down the cell walls of microorganisms. The extent of cell damage depends on the frequency of the US, duration of the process, microbial characteristics, and composition of the food.[87]

Successful application of US at low frequency, when combined with other treatments, has been reported in several studies. Shamila-Syuhada et al.[88] reported about 4 log CFU/mL reduction in various pathogens when US was used in combination with hydrogen peroxide (Table 35.6). These workers reported higher microbial inactivation and shorter treatment times at lower amplitude (62.5 μm) when compared with sonication alone. Elsewhere, up to 6.9 log CFU/mL reduction in *E. coli* O157:H7 was observed when US was combined with thyme essential oil nanoemulsions (TEON) for the treatment of cherry tomato surfaces, while US alone achieved 0.9 log CFU/g reduction. Low-frequency US achieved >5 log CFU/mL reduction of *Listeria innocua* (a surrogate for *Listeria monocyogenes*) when combined with zinc oxide (ZnO) while samples without ZnO showed <1 log CFU/mL reduction. Synergistic bactericidal efficacy of US when applied simultaneously with fumaric acid (FA) was also observed in apple juice.[89] These workers further reported that FA did not substantially reduce the pH of the juice to values outside those for fresh apple juice. They further associated the synergistic effect to damage of the cell membrane, which allowed FA to diffuse and subsequently reduce intracellular pH.

35.14.2 Pulsed electric fields

PEF is preferred in the food industry because of its minimal negative effects on the nutritional and sensory properties of food compared to conventional techniques.[106,107] The technology involves subjecting food to varying electric pulses (0.1–80 kV/cm) in a chamber. Inactivation of microorganisms occurs at high intensity (15–40 kV/cm) leading to the formation of pores (electroporation) in microbial cell membranes.[108] Consequently, leakage of intracellular material occurs and if the cell fails to repair itself, it loses viability.[109] Inactivation of foodborne pathogens such as *E. coli* and *Salmonella* Typhimurium and surrogate microorganisms such as *L. innocua* has been achieved with PEF. However, the lethal effect of PEF is dependent on the strength of the electric field, the type of pulse, the chamber used, apart from the food matrix and microbial characteristics.[110] The main disadvantage of PEF technology is that it is only suitable for the treatment of liquid and semisolid foods and not suitable for solid food products. In addition, it requires high costs for implementation, and this hinders its broad adoption by the food industry.[107,111,112] Also, PEF technology does not inactivate bacterial spores but can potentially reduce spores when combined with heat.[113]

Parallel treatment of whole fresh blueberries with PEF and peracetic acid caused up to 3.0 log CFU/g reduction in *L. innocua* and *E. coli* counts (Table 35.6).[114] Although the treatment did not negatively affect color and appearance, the blueberries were softer after treatment. Therefore more studies to minimize the effect on texture are needed for such treatments. Other workers have achieved 5 log CFU/mL reduction in *E. coli* O157:H7 when guava juice was treated with PEF and *Mentha piperita* L. (peppermint) nanoemulsions, while PEF alone resulted in only a 4.2 log CFU/mL inactivation.[99] Elsewhere, 1.5 log CFU/g reduction in *Campylobacter jejuni* was achieved when raw chicken was sequentially treated with PEF and oregano essential oil.[100] PEF has also been used in combination with mild heat (50°C) to achieve over 5 log CFU/mL reduction in *E. coli* and *Salmonella* Enteritidis in red apple juice.[115] The combined treatment did not significantly affect pH, titratable acidity, total soluble solids, and electrical conductivity of the juice compared to conventional thermal treatment.

35.14.3 High hydrostatic pressure

High hydrostatic pressure (HHP), also known as ultra-high pressure, is a relatively new food processing technology that is suitable for inactivating pathogens mainly in liquid food, but is also effective in some solid food. It involves treating food with high pressure (100–1000 MPa) for

TABLE 35.6 Novel technologies applied in the control of pathogens and the recommended treatment conditions.

Technology	Product	Target microorganisms	Treatment conditions	Log reduction	References
Ultrasound + H_2PO_2 (0.10%)	UHT milk-spiked	*Staphylococcus aureus*	62.5 μm amplitude, 10 min	3.9 log CFU/mL	88
		Listeria monocytogenes	62.5 μm amplitude, 10 min	4.2 log CFU/mL	88
		Salmonella Typhimurium	62.5 μm amplitude, 10 min	4.9 log CFU/mL	88
		Escherichia coli	62.5 μm amplitude, 10 min	4.9 log CFU/mL	88
Ultrasound + TEON (0.125 mg/L)	Cherry tomatoes	*E. coli* O157:H7	US (167 W/L) and TEON, 9 min	4.48–6.94 log CFU/sample	90
Ultrasound + ZnO (40 mM)	Deionized water	*Listeria innocua*	20 kHz, 43–45 W, 120 μm, 8 min, RT	>5 log CFU/mL	91
Ultrasound + mild heat	Chinese bayberry juice	*Bacillus subtilis*	200 W, 63°C, 14.18 min	5 log CFU/mL	92
			400 W, 63°C, 9.59 min	5 log CFU/mL	92
Ultrasound + lysozyme	Liquid whole egg	*Salmonella* Typhimurium	986 W/cm^2 at 35°C for 20 min	4.26 $\log_{10}$ cycles	93
Ultrasound + fumaric acid (0.15%)	Apple juice	*E. coli* O157:H7	40 kHz, 25 mm wavelength, 700 W, RT	5.67 log CFU/mL	89
		Salmonella Typhimurium	40 kHz, 25 mm wavelength, 700 W, RT	6.35 log CFU/mL	89
		L. monocytogenes	40 kHz, 25 mm wavelength, 700 W, RT	3.47 log CFU/mL	89
HPP + citral (1%)	Ground beef	*E. coli* O157:H7	380 MPa for 15 min, <40°C	>5.0 log CFU/g	94
		Uropathogenic *E. coli*	380 MPa for 15 min, <40°C	>5.0 log CFU/g	94
HPP + fermentation & drying	Fermented sausages	*E. coli* O157:H7	600 MPa for 3 min, ~14°C	4.8 log CFU/g	95
HPP + low pH	Açaí Juice	*L. monocytogenes*	400 MPa for 1 min, 5°C, pH 4.3 and 2.9°Brix	>6.0 log CFU/mL	96
		E. coli O157:H7	400 MPa for 1 min, 5°C, pH 4.3 and 2.9°Brix		
		Salmonella spp.	400 MPa for 1 min, 5°C, pH 4.3 and 2.9°Brix		
PEF + cauliflower & Mandarin by product infusion (10%)	Buffered peptone water	*Salmonella* Typhimurium	20 kV, −900 μs, 37°C	4.0 log cycles	97
PEF + peracetic acid (60 ppm)	Blueberries	*L. innocua*	2 kV/cm, 1 Ms pulse width, 100 pulses/s	Up to 3.0 log CFU/g	98
		E. coli K12	2 kV/cm, 1 Ms pulse width, 100 pulses/s	Up to 3.0 log CFU/g	98
PEF + *Mentha piperita* L. Nanoemulsion (0.31 μL/mL)	Guava Juice	*E. coli* O157:H7	30 kV/cm for 150 μs	5.0 log CFU/mL	99
PEF + *M. piperita* L. nanoemuslsion (0.16 μL/mL)	Mango juice	*E. coli* O157:H7	35 kV/cm for 150 μs	5.0 log CFU/mL	99
PEF + Oregano solution (15.625 ppm)	Raw chicken	*Campylobacter jejuni*	1 kV/cm, 20 μs pulse width, frequency of 1 Hz	1.5 $\log_{10}$ CFU/g	100

(Continued)

TABLE 35.6 (Continued)

Technology	Product	Target microorganisms	Treatment conditions	Log reduction	References
PEF + mild heat (50°C)	Red apple juice	*E. coli*	35 kV/cm for 258 μs	5.2 log CFU/mL	101
		Salmonella Enteritidis	35 kV/cm for 258 μs	6.0 log CFU/mL	101
CAP + nisin (35 IU/mL)	Food model system	*L. innocua*	He:O_2, 7 kV, ~7 W power at 15 kHz for 30 min	Approx. 2 log CFU	102
CAP + nisin-based sanitizer	Granny Smith apples	*L. monocytogenes*	Arc jet, 36 kV, 40 s followed by placement in antimicrobial solution for 3 min	3.4 log CFU/g	103
CP + aerosolized H_2O_2 (7.8%)	Romaine lettuce—upper leaf	*L. innocua*	17 kV, 7 psi, 30 s sprays, 30 min dwell time	5.2 log CFU/piece	104
	Cantaloupe rind	*L. innocua*	17 kV, 7 psi, 30 s sprays, 30 min dwell time	5. 1 log CFU/piece	104
	Tomato surface	*L. innocua*	17 kV, 7 psi, 8 sprays, 30 min dwell time	5. 2 log CFU/piece	104
CP + radio frequency (RF) thermal	Red pepper powder	*E. coli* O157:H7	FR—5 kW, 1500 W, 120 s	3.7 log CFU/g	105
			DBD—1000 W N_2:O_2 = 100:1, 4–10 kV, 20–60 kHz		
		Staphylococcus aureus	FR—5 kW, 1500 W, 120 s	3.2 log CFU/g	105
			DBD—1000 W N_2:O_2 = 100:1, 4–10 kV, 20–60 kHz		

varying times (min) and at room or mild-processing temperatures.[116,117] Water is usually used as a medium for transmitting pressure and the process is effective with or without packaging. However, the processing of packaged food with HPP is preferred because it limits postprocessing contamination. Microbial inactivation with HPP is attributed to several changes such as the unfolding of protein structure, cell membrane damage, changes in membrane fluidity, loss of intracellular pH, and subsequently cell death.[12] Dissociation of ribosomes in microbial cells can also be caused by pressure leading to a loss in viability.[118] Since HPP is applied at low temperatures, the technology does not cause significant changes in the nutritional and sensory properties of food.[116] However, several studies have indicated that HPP may not always cause cell death, which means sublethally injured cells may get repaired during storage when the pressure was not severe.[95,119,120] Because of this, the combination of HPP with other technologies has been investigated to ensure food safety.

Chien et al.[94] demonstrated that effective inactivation of *E. coli* (5 log CFU/g reduction, 15 min) in ground beef can be achieved at low pressure (380 MPa) when HPP treatment is combined with 1% citral. Without citral, the same log reduction was achieved at a higher pressure (500 MPa) after the same period of 15 min. HPP treatment of fermented sausages during drying has also been reported to enhance *E. coli* O157:H7 reduction by 4.8 log CFU/g compared to sausages without HPP treatment.[95] The use of low pressure can reduce food quality losses associated with treatments at high pressure. Gouvea et al.[96] reported that more than 6 log CFU/mL reduction in *L. monocytogenes*, *E. coli* O157:H7, and *Salmonella* spp. can be achieved at relatively low pressure (400 MPa, 1 min) when treating juice with a low pH (4.0) and low soluble solids (2.9°Brix). In general, 600 MPa for 3 min is recommended for the treatment of such products to ensure safety during storage.

35.14.4 Cold plasma

CP is a nonthermal technology that has gained the interest of food scientists because of its ability to rapidly inactivate microorganisms at atmospheric pressure. The technology generates "plasma," a quasi-neutral ionized gas that comprises reactive molecular species such as ions,

UV photons, electrons, atomic species, and charged particles.[121,122] Multiple antimicrobial mechanisms have been reported for CP treatment, but they all rely on one or more of the generated molecular species. Microorganisms can have a direct chemical interaction with the reactive species, while in some instances, generated UV causes damage to cellular components and membranes leading to DNA breakage and cell death.[87] The extent of microbial inactivation with CP is dependent on the composition of the feed gas, voltage, relative humidity, and duration of treatment. Importantly, CP treatment can be applied on packaged food products to prevent contamination after processing.[122–124]

Nisin has been shown to enhance (approximately 2 log CFU/mL reduction) antimicrobial activity of CAP against *L. innocua* in food model media compared to individual CP treatments[102] (Table 35.6). A higher inactivation of *L. monocytogenes* (3.4 log CFU/g reduction) was reported when CAP-treated apples were subjected to a nisin-based sanitizer.[103] These workers further suggested a major reduction with nisin-based antimicrobial treatment time (1 h to 3 min) with their method possibly due to the resultant high chemical susceptibility of the pathogen after CP treatment. More effective inactivation of *L. innocua* (5 log CFU/ piece) was reported when surfaces of fresh produce were treated with aerosolized H_2O_2 and CP.[104] Low *L. innocua* reductions (1.4–3.8 log CFU/piece) were obtained with H_2O_2 treatments alone. Other studies have investigated the combined effect of CP with thermal radiofrequency treatment for the inactivation of *E. coli* O157:H7 and *S. aureus* in red pepper powder.[105] The combined treatment achieved 3.2 and 3.7 log CFU/g reductions in *S. aureus* and *E. coli*, respectively, without significantly affecting the color or free radical scavenging activity of the powder.

35.15 Risk assessment, microbial modeling and bacterial community dynamic considerations in terms of modified atmosphere packaging

Risk-based food safety management and predictive microbiology evaluate the effect of processing, distribution, and storage operations on food safety in advance, contributing to safety assurance rather than food safety confirmation.[125] Risk-based food safety management is linked to identifying and controlling specified hazards rather than end-product controls to ensure the desired level of consumer protection. Translating risk-based food safety management concepts into practical settings are, however, complex.[126]

Only a limited number of risk assessments have been carried out related to pathogens associated with MAP food products. One such study evaluated the safety of vacuum packaging/MAP fresh red meat held at 3°C–8°C, concerning nonproteolytic *C. botulinum*. The exposure assessment and challenge test experiment both supported the safety of current industry practices as well as current shelf life. Important factors assuring the safety of these products were confirmed,[75] thus adding value to industry operating under the risk-based food safety management framework, rather than the end-product controls, which may have not been sufficient to protect the consumer.

Adaptation and evolution of microorganisms within a changing environment, such as MAP and other novel technologies, has the potential to affect the genotypes or lineages of pathogens. In their review, Metselaar et al.[127] found that genotype-specific risk assessment and cell-based modeling have the potential to reduce the uncertainty in risk characterizations.

Predictive microbiology uses mathematical models that correlate bacterial growth or death response to the environmental conditions in which food is found. Using this concept, we can evaluate the effect of processing, distribution, and storage operations on food safety in advance.[125] The industry can, therefore, determine the shelf life of a new product under modified environmental conditions, determine when the acceptable maximum level of bacteria will be reached in the product as well as the storage time it will take to reach that level.

Several research papers have focused on the development of models for MAP products[29,30] and provided an overview of MAP's factors that influence the quality of stored minimally processed fresh-cut fruit products. The focus was placed on apples and the development of mathematical models that can be useful for the prediction of their spoilage during storage and subsequently their shelf-life. Mathematical models used for MAP related to fruit usually target packaging, an extension of storage, control of microbiology, respiration physiology, postharvest conditions, and preservation of quality.[128] Recently, Hutchings et al.[129] proposed a model that determines the minimum permeability requirements to maintain the shelf-life of red meat in high oxygen MAP. The mathematical model was developed to predict the growth of *Pseudomonas* spp. and headspace gas dynamics, providing the basis for the development of a new packaging film. Instead of extensive experimentation to determine the exact permeability at which barrier properties exceed requirements, mathematical modeling, can offer a predictive tool and the capacity to adjust variables without experiments. Other food commodities for which predictive models have been proposed are MAP dandelion greens and MAP-gutted sea bass.[130,131]

Understanding spoilage associated with varying microbial metabolic pathways has been made possible with high-throughput DNA sequencing technology[132,133] combined the functional analysis of metagenomes with the physicochemical changes of MAP beef to understand the underlying mechanisms for meat microbiological deterioration. They are providing new insights into microbial succession and spoilage phenomena occurring in steaks under different MAP conditions, which will be beneficial for controlling the spoilage of MAP meat. This approach is novel and still needs to be validated.

35.16 Present technologies and future trends

MAP and other food processing technologies are not always used in isolation but in combination with other tools such as irradiation, ultraviolet radiation, ozone, essential oils, low temperature, intelligent packaging (IP), and AP.[134] MAP has been combined with irradiation, thermal treatment, and preservatives. Packaging plays an important role in the freshness, quality, integrity, and shelf-life of packaged food. Packaging serves as a barrier against contamination, mechanical damage, and spillage. It also serves as a medium of communication and identification, conveying information as well as nutritional information and product details to the consumer.[135,136]

AP involves the incorporation of active compounds to the packaging material, which confers on it other functions besides its original function as a mechanical barrier.[68] Some examples of AP scavengers are for ethylene, O_2, CO_2, and ethanol emitters. On the other hand, IP or smart packaging integrates innovative technologies that give real-time information of the packaged food that can facilitate an increase in shelf-life and quality, report on spoilage/freshness or breach of the packaging barriers, among others, along the distribution chain. Some of these monitoring devices can be integrated with smartphones as an application to monitor changes within a packaged food product including microbial contamination.[137] Nanotechnology has found important applications in the development of novel packaging materials that are biodegradable, sustainable with improved structure and functionality without placing a burden on the environment. There are nanobased thermoresponsive polymers as well those infused with added functionalities such as antimicrobial, improved barrier, and mechanical strength.[138] Besides its use as protective barrier, the use of food packaging as a communication system that integrates the ability to sense, identify, monitor, and track in real-time both external and internal changes that relate to product safety, is gaining traction. Innovations in sensors and biosensors have made possible the development of devices, sensing systems, and materials that enhance food safety and preserve the quality of MAP food.

IP can be categorized based on its intended use in the packaged food, that is, whether sensors, data carriers, or indicators (external or internal). Specific examples of these IP attributes are freshness indicators, ripeness indicators, leak indicators, pH indicators, and temperature indicators (critical temperature indicators, time-temperature indicators, and temperature-time integrators). For the traceability or the application of packaging material as a communication tool, intelligent barcodes and radio frequency identification tags have been used to store readable data containing the history of the food product, which enables both retailers and consumers to make choices during purchase by compiling the product history, which can be accessed by a scanner. They have been applied in dairy, bakery, and horticulture products.[139–141] Sensors are another form of IP and can be applied as chemical sensors, gas sensors, and biosensors with biological compounds as the analytes. Biosensors have been used to monitor spoilage of beef and chicken as well as to monitor residual pesticides in packaged foods.[142,143]

The operation of sensors is based on the detection and transformation of signals from one form to another using a transducer. They can either be conventional analytes that can detect changes in environmental signals such as pH, humidity, color, and innovative concepts such as edible sensors, which are aimed at nondestructive and visual detection of spoiled food. These detectors can be passive or active, with varied functions such as chemical and gas sensors and biosensors. Sensors and biosensors have been applied in detecting spoiled fish and as a freshness indicator in milk.[54,144] Sensors can either be an interaction between gaseous or chemical substrates with a specific analyte whereas biosensors make use of biological analytes. As an example, vinyl groups and tryptamine were incorporated into a nanofiber for the detection of biogenic amines in beer. The same principle is also used in the detection of volatiles such as amines in food as a freshness indicator especially in fish products.[145] The various sensors and nanosensors provide information on the food and the environment around it. This information can be communicated to consumers to aid in making a sound judgment on the food during purchase or before consumption. The application of intelligent systems represents a quantum leap in the improvement of traceability, authentication, chemical and pathogen contamination, spoilage, antitheft, and anticounterfeiting especially in the case of food fraud or when the integrity of the food has been compromised.[146]

A recent development in antimicrobial AP integrates the use of emitting sachets and absorbent pads as well as techniques to either elaborate their concentration or control it in hermetically packaged foods. Some antimicrobial compounds used in AP include ethanol, aldehydes, chlorine dioxide, allyl isothiocyanate (AITC), essential oils, or bioactive compounds, which are targeted at preventing the growth of pathogens and spoilage organisms.[147]

35.17 Conclusion

The future is bright for MAP as well as other processing technologies because innovative applications are constantly developed to solve the issue of food safety and safeguard the health of the consumers. It is recommended that these technologies could be applied in combination to enhance food safety. Therefore integrated advanced research in the field of thermal and nonthermal processing should be performed for the successful growth and wide adoption of these technologies.

References

1. Fellows PJ. *Introduction. Food Processing Technology*. Elsevier; 2017:xv–xxiii.
2. Barba FJ, Koubaa M, do Prado-Silva L, Orlien V, de Souza Sant'Ana A. Mild processing applied to the inactivation of the main foodborne bacterial pathogens: a review. *Trends Food Sci Technol*. 201766.
3. Tack DM, Marder EP, Griffin PM, et al. Preliminary incidence and trends of infections with pathogens transmitted commonly through food — Foodborne Diseases Active Surveillance Network, 10 U.S. sites, 2015–2018. *Am J Transpl*. 2019;19:1859–1863.
4. Bintsis T. Foodborne pathogens. *AIMS Microbiol*. 2017;3: 529–563.
5. Scharff RL. *The economic burden of foodborne illness in the United States. Food Safety Economics*. Springer International Publishing; 2018:123–142.
6. Devleesschauwer B, Haagsma JA, Mangen M-JJ, Lake RJ, Havelaar AH. *The global burden of foodborne disease. Food Safety Economics*. Springer International Publishing; 2018:107–122.
7. CDC. Foodborne germs and illnesses [WWW document]. http://www.cdc.gov/foodsafety. https://www.cdc.gov/foodsafety/foodborne-germs.html; 2016 Accessed 10.05.20.
8. Stein RA, Chirilă M. *Routes of transmission in the food chain. Foodborne Diseases*. Elsevier; 2017:65–103.
9. Begley M, Hill C. Stress adaptation in foodborne pathogens. *Annu Rev Food Sci Technol*. 2015.
10. Liao X, Ma Y, Daliri EB-M, et al. Interplay of antibiotic resistance and food-associated stress tolerance in foodborne pathogens. *Trends Food Sci Technol*. 2020;95:97–106.
11. Smelt JPPM, Brul S. Thermal inactivation of microorganisms. *Crit Rev Food Sci Nutr*. 2014.
12. Bahrami A, Moaddabdoost Baboli Z, Schimmel K, Jafari SM, Williams L. Efficiency of novel processing technologies for the control of *Listeria monocytogenes* in food products. *Trends Food Sci Technol*. 2020.
13. Khan I, Tango CN, Miskeen S, Lee BH, Oh DH. Hurdle technology: a novel approach for enhanced food quality and safety – a review. *Food Control*. 2017.
14. Zhang H, Tikekar RV, Ding Q, Gilbert AR, Wimsatt ST. Inactivation of foodborne pathogens by the synergistic combinations of food processing technologies and food-grade compounds. *Compr Rev Food Sci Food Saf*. 2020.
15. Leistner L. Basic aspects of food preservation by hurdle technology. *Int J Food Microbiol*. 2000;55:181–186.
16. Ohlsson T, Bengtsson N. *Minimal Processing Technologies in the Food Industries*. Woodhead Publishing Limited; 2002.
17. Tsironi T, Houhoula D, Taoukis P. Hurdle technology for fish preservation. *Aquac Fish*. 2020;5:65–71.
18. Sibanda T, Buys EM. Resuscitation and growth kinetics of sublethally injured *Listeria monocytogenes* strains following fluorescence activated cell sorting (FACS). *Food Res Int*. 2017;100: 150–158.
19. Adley CC, Ryan MP. *The nature and extent of foodborne disease. Antimicrobial Food Packaging*. Elsevier; 2016:1–10.
20. Petruzzi L, Corbo MR, Sinigaglia M, Bevilacqua A. *Microbial spoilage of foods. The Microbiological Quality of Food*. Elsevier; 2017:1–21.
21. Peleg M. The hurdle technology metaphor revisited. *Food Eng Rev*. 2020.
22. Alvarez-Ordóñez A, Broussolle V, Colin P, Nguyen-The C, Prieto M. The adaptive response of bacterial food-borne pathogens in the environment, host and food: implications for food safety. *Int J Food Microbiol*. 2015.
23. Timmermans RAH, Nierop Groot MN, Nederhoff AL, van Boekel MAJS, Matser AM, Mastwijk HC. Pulsed electric field processing of different fruit juices: impact of pH and temperature on inactivation of spoilage and pathogenic micro-organisms. *Int J Food Microbiol*. 2014.
24. Adeyeye SAO, Oyewole OB, Obadina OA, et al. Effect of smoking methods on quality and safety of traditional smoked fish from Lagos State, Nigeria. *J Culin Sci Technol*. 2017;15:17–35.
25. Aaron L. B. *A perspective on MAP products in North America and Western Europe. Principles of Modified-Atmosphere and Sous Vide Product Packaging*. Routledge; 2018:13–36.
26. Priyadarshi R, Deeba F, Sauraj, Negi YS. *Modified atmosphere packaging development. Processing and Development of Polysaccharide-Based Biopolymers for Packaging Applications*. Elsevier; 2020:261–280.
27. Galić K, Ščetar M, Kurek M. The benefits of processing and packaging. *Trends Food Sci Technol*. 2011;22:127–137.
28. Ghoshal G. *Recent trends in active, smart, and intelligent packaging for food products. Food Packaging and Preservation*. Elsevier; 2018:343–374.
29. Putnik P, Roohinejad S, Greiner R, Granato D, Bekhit AE-DA, Bursać Kovačević D. Prediction and modeling of microbial growth in minimally processed fresh-cut apples packaged in a modified atmosphere: a review. *Food Control*. 2017;80:411–419.
30. Putnik P, Bursać Kovačević D, Herceg K, et al. Modelling the shelf-life of minimally-processed fresh-cut apples packaged in a modified atmosphere using food quality parameters. *Food Control*. 2017;81:55–64.
31. Chien YW. Biochemical basis of the effects of modified and controlled atmospheres. *Stewart Postharvest Rev*. 2006;2:1–4.
32. Cukrov D, Brizzolara S, Tonutti P. *Physiological and biochemical effects of controlled and modified atmospheres. Postharvest Physiology and Biochemistry of Fruits and Vegetables*. Elsevier; 2019:425–441.
33. Plotto A, Bai J, Baldwin E. *Effect of CA/MA on sensory quality. Controlled and Modified Atmospheres for Fresh and Fresh-Cut Produce*. Elsevier; 2020:109–130.
34. Campbell A. *Modified atmosphere packaging (MAP) of foods and its combination with electron beam processing. Electron Beam*

Pasteurization and Complementary Food Processing Technologies. Elsevier; 2015:185–194.

35. Kirtil E, Oztop MH. *Controlled and modified atmosphere packaging. Reference Module in Food Science*. Elsevier; 2016.
36. Mangaraj S, Goswami TK, Mahajan PV. Applications of plastic films for modified atmosphere packaging of fruits and vegetables: a review. *Food Eng Rev*. 2009;1:133–158.
37. Sheikhi A, Mirdehghan SH, Ferguson L. Extending storage potential of de-hulled fresh pistachios in passive-modified atmosphere. *J Sci Food Agric*. 2019;99:3426–3433.
38. He Y, Huang H, Li L, et al. The effects of modified atmosphere packaging and enzyme inhibitors on protein oxidation of tilapia muscle during iced storage. *LWT - Food Sci Technol*. 2018;87:186–193.
39. Irazoqui M, Romero M, Paulsen E, et al. Effect of power ultrasound on quality of fresh-cut lettuce (cv. Vera) packaged in passive modified atmosphere. *Food Bioprod Process*. 2019.
40. Caleb OJ, Fawole OA, Mphahlele RR, Opara UL. Impact of preharvest and postharvest factors on changes in volatile compounds of pomegranate fruit and minimally processed arils - review. *Sci Hortic (Amst)*. 2015.
41. Janjarasskul T, Suppakul P. Active and intelligent packaging: the indication of quality and safety. *Crit Rev Food Sci Nutr*. 2018;58:808–831.
42. Azad ZRAA, Ahmad MF, Siddiqui WA. *Food spoilage and food contamination. Health and Safety Aspects of Food Processing Technologies*. Cham: Springer International Publishing; 2019:9–28.
43. Odeyemi OA, Alegbeleye OO, Strateva M, Stratev D. Understanding spoilage microbial community and spoilage mechanisms in foods of animal origin. *Compr Rev Food Sci Food Saf*. 2020;19:311–331.
44. Rolfe C, Daryaei H. *Intrinsic and extrinsic factors affecting microbial growth in food systems. Food Engineering Series*. Springer; 2020:3–24.
45. Reinas I, Oliveira J, Pereira J, Mahajan P, Poças F. A quantitative approach to assess the contribution of seals to the permeability of water vapour and oxygen in thermosealed packages. *Food Packag Shelf Life*. 2016;7:34–40.
46. Sivertsvik M, Jeksrud WK, Rosnes JT. A review of modified atmosphere packaging of fish and fishery products - significance of microbial growth, activities and safety. *Int J Food Sci Technol*. 2002;37:107–127.
47. Kerry JP, O'Grady MN, Hogan SA. Past, current and potential utilisation of active and intelligent packaging systems for meat and muscle-based products: a review. *Meat Sci*. 2006.
48. Lee DS. Carbon dioxide absorbers for food packaging applications. *Trends Food Sci Technol*. 2016;57:146–155.
49. Scifò GO, Randazzo CL, Restuccia C, Fava G, Caggia C. *Listeria innocua* growth in fresh cut mixed leafy salads packaged in modified atmosphere. *Food Control*. 2009;20:611–617.
50. Floros JD, Matsos KI. *Introduction to modified atmosphere packaging. Innovations in Food Packaging*. Elsevier; 2005:159–172.
51. López-Gálvez F, Ragaert P, Haque MA, Eriksson M, van Labeke MC, Devlieghere F. High oxygen atmospheres can induce russet spotting development in minimally processed iceberg lettuce. *Postharvest Biol Technol*. 2015.
52. Jacxsens L, Devlieghere F, Van der Steen C, Debevere J. Effect of high oxygen modified atmosphere packaging on microbial growth and sensorial qualities of fresh-cut produce. *Int J Food Microbiol*. 2001;71:197–210.
53. Bibi N, Khattak AB, Mehmood Z. Quality improvement and shelf life extension of persimmon fruit (*Diospyros kaki*). *J Food Eng*. 2007;79:1359–1363.
54. Shen X, Zhang M, Devahastin S, Guo Z. Effects of pressurized argon and nitrogen treatments in combination with modified atmosphere on quality characteristics of fresh-cut potatoes. *Postharvest Biol Technol*. 2019.
55. Van de Velde F, Méndez-Galarraga MP, Grace MH, Fenoglio C, Lila MA, Pirovani MÉ. Changes due to high oxygen and high carbon dioxide atmospheres on the general quality and the polyphenolic profile of strawberries. *Postharvest Biol Technol*. 2019.
56. Cortellino G, Gobbi S, Bianchi G, Rizzolo A. Modified atmosphere packaging for shelf life extension of fresh-cut apples. *Trends Food Sci Technol*. 2015;46:320–330.
57. De Aguiar Saldanha Pinheiro AC, Urbinati E, Tappi S, et al. The impact of gas mixtures of argon and nitrous oxide (N_2O) on quality parameters of sardine (*Sardina pilchardus*) fillets during refrigerated storage. *Food Res Int*. 2019;115:268–275.
58. Olawuyi IF, Park JJ, Lee JJ, Lee WY. Combined effect of chitosan coating and modified atmosphere packaging on fresh-cut cucumber. *Food Sci Nutr*. 2019;7:1043–1052.
59. de Siqueira Oliveira L, Eça KS, de Aquino AC, da Silva LMR. *Modified and controlled atmosphere packaging. Fresh-Cut Fruits and Vegetables*. Elsevier; 2020:151–164.
60. Ghidelli C, Pérez-Gago MB. Recent advances in modified atmosphere packaging and edible coatings to maintain quality of fresh-cut fruits and vegetables. *Crit Rev Food Sci Nutr*. 2018;58:662–679.
61. Wu ZS, Zhang M, Wang S. Effects of high pressure argon treatments on the quality of fresh-cut apples at cold storage. *Food Control*. 2012;23:120–127.
62. Fujii K, Ohtani A, Watanabe J, Ohgoshi H, Fujii T, Honma K. High-pressure inactivation of *Bacillus cereus* spores in the presence of argon. *Int. J. Food Microbiol*. 2002.
63. Meng X, Zhang M, Adhikari B. Extending shelf-life of fresh-cut green peppers using pressurized argon treatment. *Postharvest Biol Technol*. 2012;71:13–20.
64. Silveira AC, Araneda C, Hinojosa A, Escalona VH. Effect of non-conventional modified atmosphere packaging on fresh cut watercress (*Nasturtium officinale* R. Br.) quality. *Postharvest Biol Technol*. 2014;92:114–120.
65. Gouble B, Fath D, Soudain P. Nitrous oxide inhibition of ethylene production in ripening and senescing climacteric fruits. *Postharvest Biol Technol*. 1995;5:311–321.
66. Onopiuk A, Półtorak A, Moczkowska M, Szpicer A, Wierzbicka A. The impact of ozone on health-promoting, microbiological, and colour properties of *Rubus ideaus* raspberries. *CyTA - J Food*. 2017;15:563–573.
67. Rico D, Martín-Diana AB, Barat JM, Barry-Ryan C. Extending and measuring the quality of fresh-cut fruit and vegetables: a review. *Trends Food Sci Technol*. 2007;18:373–386.
68. De Corato U. Improving the shelf-life and quality of fresh and minimally-processed fruits and vegetables for a modern food industry: a comprehensive critical review from the traditional technologies into the most promising advancements. *Crit Rev Food Sci Nutr*. 2020;60:940–975.

69. Piechowiak T, Antos P, Józefczyk R, Kosowski P, Skrobacz K, Balawejder M. Impact of ozonation process on the microbiological contamination and antioxidant capacity of highbush blueberry (*Vaccinum corymbosum* L.) fruit during cold storage. *Ozone Sci Eng*. 2019;41:376–385.
70. Valero M, Leontidis S, Fernández PS, Martínez A, Salmerón MC. Growth of *Bacillus cereus* in natural and acidified carrot substrates over the temperature range 5–30°C. *Food Microbiol.* 2000.
71. Caleb OJ, Mahajan PV, Al-Said FAJ, Opara UL. Modified atmosphere packaging technology of fresh and fresh-cut produce and the microbial consequences—a review. *Food Bioprocess Technol.* 2013;6:303–329.
72. Lindström M, Kiviniemi K, Korkeala H. Hazard and control of group II (non-proteolytic) *Clostridium botulinum* in modern food processing. *Int J Food Microbiol.* 2006;108:92–104.
73. Del Torre M, Stecchini ML, Peck MW. Investigation of the ability of proteolytic *Clostridium botulinum* to multiply and produce toxin in fresh Italian pasta. *J Food Prot.* 1998;61:988–993.
74. Conner DE, Scott VN, Bernard DT, Kautter DA. Potential *Clostridium botulinum* hazards associated with extended shelf-life refrigerated foods: a review. *J Food Saf.* 1989;10:131–153.
75. Peck MW, Webb MD, Goodburn KE. Assessment of the risk of botulism from chilled, vacuum/modified atmosphere packed fresh beef, lamb and pork held at 3 °C–8 °C. *Food Microbiol.* 2020;91:103544.
76. Brown SRB, Forauer EC, D'Amico DJ. Effect of modified atmosphere packaging on the growth of spoilage microorganisms and *Listeria monocytogenes* on fresh cheese. *J Dairy Sci.* 2018;101:7768–7779.
77. Novak JS, Yuan JTC. The fate of *Clostridium perfringens* spores exposed to ozone and/or mild heat pretreatment on beef surfaces followed by modified atmosphere packaging. *Food Microbiol.* 2004;21:667–673.
78. Oliveira M, Usall J, Solsona C, Alegre I, Viñas I, Abadias M. Effects of packaging type and storage temperature on the growth of foodborne pathogens on shredded "Romaine" lettuce. *Food Microbiol.* 2010;27:375–380.
79. Bidawid S, Farber JM, Sattar SA. Survival of hepatitis a virus on modified atmosphere-packaged (MAP) lettuce. *Food Microbiol.* 2001;18:95–102.
80. Hennechart-Collette C, Martin-Latil S, Fraisse A, Niveau F, Perelle S. Virological analyses in collective catering outbreaks in France between 2012 and 2017. *Food Microbiol.* 2020;91:103546.
81. Sánchez G, Bosch A. *Survival of enteric viruses in the environment and food. Viruses in Foods.* Springer International Publishing; 2016:367–392.
82. Alexandre EMC, Pinto CA, Moreira SA, Pintado M, Saraiva JA. *Nonthermal food processing/preservation technologies. Saving Food.* Elsevier; 2019:141–169.
83. Tafti AG, Peighambardoust SH, Hesari J, Bahrami A, Bonab ES. Physico-chemical and functional properties of spray-dried sourdough in breadmaking. *Food Sci Technol Int.* 2013.
84. Majid I, Nayik GA, Nanda V. Ultrasonication and food technology: a review. *Cogent Food Agric.* 2015.
85. Sarkinas A, Sakalauskiene K, Raisutis R, et al. Inactivation of some pathogenic bacteria and phytoviruses by ultrasonic treatment. *Microb Pathog.* 2018;123:144–148.
86. Deng LZ, Mujumdar AS, Pan Z, et al. Emerging chemical and physical disinfection technologies of fruits and vegetables: a comprehensive review. *Crit Rev Food Sci Nutr.* 2020.
87. Hernández-Hernández HM, Moreno-Vilet L, Villanueva-Rodríguez SJ. Current status of emerging food processing technologies in Latin America: novel non-thermal processing. *Innov Food Sci Emerg Technol.* 2019;58:102233.
88. Shamila-Syuhada AK, Chuah L-O, Wan-Nadiah WA, et al. Inactivation of microbiota and selected spoilage and pathogenic bacteria in milk by combinations of ultrasound, hydrogen peroxide, and active lactoperoxidase system. *Int Dairy J.* 2016;61: 120–125.
89. Park J-S, Ha J-W. Ultrasound treatment combined with fumaric acid for inactivating food-borne pathogens in apple juice and its mechanisms. *Food Microbiol.* 2019;84:103277.
90. He Q, Guo M, Jin TZ, Arabi SA, Liu D. Ultrasound improves the decontamination effect of thyme essential oil nanoemulsions against *Escherichia coli* O157: H7 on cherry tomatoes. *Int J Food Microbiol.* 2021;337:108936.
91. Dolan HL, Bastarrachea LJ, Tikekar RV. Inactivation of *Listeria innocua* by a combined treatment of low-frequency ultrasound and zinc oxide. *LWT - Food Sci Technol.* 2018;88:146–151.
92. Li J, Cheng H, Liao X, et al. Inactivation of *Bacillus subtilis* and quality assurance in Chinese bayberry (Myrica rubra) juice with ultrasound and mild heat. *LWT - Food Sci Technol.* 2019;108:113–119.
93. Bi X, Wang X, Chen Y, Chen L, Xing Y, Che Z. Effects of combination treatments of lysozyme and high power ultrasound on the Salmonella typhimurium inactivation and quality of liquid whole egg. *Ultrason Sonochem.* 2020;60:104763.
94. Chien SY, Sheen S, Sommers C, Sheen LY. Modeling the inactivation of *Escherichia coli* O157:H7 and Uropathogenic *E. coli* in ground beef by high pressure processing and citral. *Food Control.* 2017.
95. Balamurugan S, Gemmell C, Lau ATY, et al. High pressure processing during drying of fermented sausages can enhance safety and reduce time required to produce a dry fermented product. *Food Control.* 2020;113:107224.
96. Gouvea FS, Padilla-Zakour OI, Worobo RW, Xavier BM, Walter EHM, Rosenthal A. Effect of high-pressure processing on bacterial inactivation in açaí juices with varying pH and soluble solids content. *Innov Food Sci Emerg Technol.* 2020.
97. Sanz-Puig M, Santos-Carvalho L, Cunha LM, Pina-Pérez MC, Martínez A, Rodrigo D. Effect of pulsed electric fields (PEF) combined with natural antimicrobial by-products against *S. Typhimurium. Innov Food Sci Emerg Technol.* 2016;37:322–328.
98. Jin TZ, Yu Y, Gurtler JB. Effects of pulsed electric field processing on microbial survival, quality change and nutritional characteristics of blueberries. *LWT - Food Sci Technol.* 2016;77: 517–524.
99. de Carvalho RJ, de Souza GT, Pagán E, García-Gonzalo D, Magnani M, Pagán R. Nanoemulsions of *Mentha piperita* L. essential oil in combination with mild heat, pulsed electric fields (PEF) and high hydrostatic pressure (HHP) as an alternative to inactivate *Escherichia coli* O157: H7 in fruit juices. *Innov Food Sci Emerg Technol.* 2018;48:219–227.
100. Clemente I, Condón-Abantoa S, Pedrós-Garrido S, Whyte P, Lyng JG. Efficacy of pulsed electric fields and antimicrobial

compounds used alone and in combination for the inactivation of *Campylobacter jejuni* in liquids and raw chicken. *Food Control.* 2020;107:106491.

101. Niu D, Zeng X, Ren E, et al. Review of the application of pulsed electric fields (PEF) technology for food processing in China. *Food Res Int.* 2020;137:109715.
102. Costello KM, Smet C, Gutierrez-Merino J, Bussemaker M, Van Impe JF, Velliou EG. The impact of food model system structure on the inactivation of *Listeria innocua* by cold atmospheric plasma and nisin combined treatments. *Int J Food Microbiol.* 2021.
103. Ukuku DO, Niemira BA, Ukanalis J. Nisin-based antimircobial combination with cold plasma treatment inactivate *Listeria monocytogenes* on Granny Smith apples. *LWT.* 2019.
104. Song Y, Fan X. Cold plasma enhances the efficacy of aerosolized hydrogen peroxide in reducing populations of Salmonella Typhimurium and *Listeria innocua* on grape tomatoes, apples, cantaloupe and romaine lettuce. *Food Microbiol.* 2020;87: 103391.
105. Choi EJ, Yang HS, Park HW, Chun HH. Inactivation of *Escherichia coli* O157:H7 and *Staphylococcus aureus* in red pepper powder using a combination of radio frequency thermal and indirect dielectric barrier discharge plasma non-thermal treatments. *LWT.* 2018;93:477–484.
106. Yang N, Huang K, Lyu C, Wang J. Pulsed electric field technology in the manufacturing processes of wine, beer, and rice wine: a review. *Food Control.* 2016;61:28–38.
107. Agcam E, Akyildiz A, Akdemir Evrendilek G. A comparative assessment of long-term storage stability and quality attributes of orange juice in response to pulsed electric fields and heat treatments. *Food Bioprod Process.* 2016.
108. Fernández A, Cebrián G, Álvarez-Ordóñez A, Prieto M, Bernardo A, López M. Influence of acid and low-temperature adaptation on pulsed electric fields resistance of *Enterococcus faecium* in media of different pH. *Innov Food Sci Emerg Technol.* 2018;45: 382–389.
109. Liu ZW, Zeng XA, Sun DW, Han Z, Aadil RM. Synergistic effect of thermal and pulsed electric field (PEF) treatment on the permeability of soya PC and DPPC vesicles. *J Food Eng.* 2015.
110. Knoerzer K, Buckow R, Trujillo FJ, Juliano P. Multiphysics simulation of innovative food processing technologies. *Food Eng Rev.* 2015;7:64–81.
111. Shahbaz HM, Kim JU, Kim SH, Park J. Advances in nonthermal processing technologies for enhanced microbiological safety and quality of fresh fruit and juice products. In: *Food Processing for Increased Quality and Consumption*; 2018.
112. Priyadarshini A, Rajauria G, O'Donnell CP, Tiwari BK. Emerging food processing technologies and factors impacting their industrial adoption. *Crit Rev Food Sci Nutr.* 2019.
113. Soni A, Oey I, Silcock P, Ross IK, Bremer PJ. Effect of pulsed electric field with moderate heat (80°C) on inactivation, thermal resistance and differential gene expression in *B. cereus* spores. *J Food Process Preserv.* 2020;44(e14503):1–12.
114. Jin TZ, Yu Y, Gurtler JB. Effects of pulsed electric field processing on microbial survival, quality change and nutritional characteristics of blueberries. *LWT.* 2017;77:517–524.
115. Katiyo W, Yang R, Zhao W. Effects of combined pulsed electric fields and mild temperature pasteurization on microbial inactivation and physicochemical properties of cloudy red apple juice (*Malus pumila* Niedzwetzkyana (Dieck). *J Food Saf.* 2017.
116. Zhao G, Zhang R, Zhang M. Effects of high hydrostatic pressure processing and subsequent storage on phenolic contents and antioxidant activity in fruit and vegetable products. *Int J Food Sci Technol.* 2017;52:3–12.
117. Kaur BP, Rao PS. Modeling the combined effect of pressure and mild heat on the inactivation kinetics of *Escherichia coli*, *Listeria innocua*, and *Staphylococcus aureus* in black tiger shrimp (Penaeus monodon). *Front Microbiol.* 2017.
118. Georget E, Sevenich R, Reineke K, et al. Inactivation of microorganisms by high isostatic pressure processing in complex matrices: a review. *Innov Food Sci Emerg Technol.* 2015;27:1–14.
119. Wang X, Uyttendaele M, Geeraerd A, Steen L, Fraeye I, Devlieghere F. Thermal inactivation kinetics of surface contaminating *Listeria monocytogenes* on vacuum-packaged agar surface and ready-to-eat sliced ham and sausage. *Food Res Int.* 2016.
120. Misiou O, van Nassau TJ, Lenz CA, Vogel RF. The preservation of *Listeria*-critical foods by a combination of endolysin and high hydrostatic pressure. *Int J Food Microbiol.* 2018.
121. Wan Z, Chen Y, Pankaj SK, Keener KM. High voltage atmospheric cold plasma treatment of refrigerated chicken eggs for control of *Salmonella* Enteritidis contamination on egg shell. *LWT - Food Sci Technol.* 2017;76:124–130.
122. Li X, Farid M. A review on recent development in non-conventional food sterilization technologies. *J Food Eng.* 2016; 182:33–45.
123. Ziuzina D, Patil S, Cullen PJ, Keener KM, Bourke P. Atmospheric cold plasma inactivation of *Escherichia coli*, *Salmonella enterica* serovar Typhimurium and *Listeria monocytogenes* inoculated on fresh produce. *Food Microbiol.* 2014; 42:109–116.
124. Misra NN, Yepez X, Xu L, Keener K. In-package cold plasma technologies. *J Food Eng.* 2019;244:21–31.
125. Isabelle L, André L. Quantitative prediction of microbial behaviour during food processing using an integrated modelling approach: a review. *Int J Refrig.* 2006;29:968–984.
126. Membré J-M, Boué G. Quantitative microbiological risk assessment in food industry: theory and practical application. *Food Res Int.* 2018;106:1132–1139.
127. Metselaar KI, Abee T, Zwietering MH, den Besten HMW. Modeling and validation of the ecological behavior of wild-type *Listeria monocytogenes* and stress-resistant variants. *Appl Env Microbiol.* 2016;82:5389–5401.
128. Belay ZA, Caleb OJ, Opara UL. Modelling approaches for designing and evaluating the performance of modified atmosphere packaging (MAP) systems for fresh produce: A review. *Food Packag Shelf Life.* 2016.
129. Hutchings N, Smyth B, Cunningham E, Mangwandi C. Development of a mathematical model to predict the growth of *Pseudomonas* spp. in, and film permeability requirements of, high oxygen modified atmosphere packaging for red meat. *J Food Eng.* 2021;289:110251.
130. Tsironi T, Ntzimani A, Gogou E, et al. Modeling the effect of active modified atmosphere packaging on the microbial stability and shelf life of gutted sea bass. *Appl Sci.* 2019.
131. Dermesonluoglu E, Fileri K, Orfanoudaki A, Tsevdou M, Tsironi T, Taoukis P. Modelling the microbial spoilage and quality decay

of pre-packed dandelion leaves as a function of temperature. *J Food Eng*. 2016;184:21–30.
132. Yang X, Zhu L, Zhang Y, Liang R, Luo X. Microbial community dynamics analysis by high-throughput sequencing in chilled beef longissimus steaks packaged under modified atmospheres. *Meat Sci*. 2018;141:94–102.
133. Zagorec M, Champomier-Vergès M-C. Lactobacillus sakei: a starter for sausage fermentation, a protective culture for meat products. *Microorganisms*. 2017.
134. Bodbodak S, Moshfeghifar M. *Advances in modified atmosphere packaging of fruits and vegetables. Eco-Friendly Technology for Postharvest Produce Quality*. Elsevier; 2016:127–183.
135. Sohail M, Sun D-W, Zhu Z. Recent developments in intelligent packaging for enhancing food quality and safety. *Crit Rev Food Sci Nutr*. 2018;58:2650–2662.
136. Biji KB, Ravishankar CN, Mohan CO, Srinivasa Gopal TK. Smart packaging systems for food applications: a review. *J Food Sci Technol*. 2015.
137. Coskun AF, Wong J, Khodadadi D, Nagi R, Tey A, Ozcan A. A personalized food allergen testing platform on a cellphone. *Lab Chip*. 2013;13:636–640.
138. Wilson MD, Stanley RA, Eyles A, Ross T. Innovative processes and technologies for modified atmosphere packaging of fresh and fresh-cut fruits and vegetables. *Crit Rev Food Sci Nutr*. 2019;59:411–422.
139. Costa C, Antonucci F, Pallottino F, Aguzzi J, Sarriá D, Menesatti P. A review on agri-food supply chain traceability by means of RFID technology. *Food Bioprocess Technol*. 2013.
140. Kalpana S, Priyadarshini SR, Maria Leena M, Moses JA, Anandharamakrishnan C. Intelligent packaging: trends and applications in food systems. *Trends Food Sci Technol*. 2019;93: 145–157.
141. Mahalik N, Kim K. The role of information technology developments in food supply chain integration and monitoring. In: *Innovation and Future Trends in Food Manufacturing and Supply Chain Technologies*, 2016.
142. Schumann B, Schmid M. Packaging concepts for fresh and processed meat – recent progresses. *Innov Food Sci Emerg Technol*. 2018;47:88–100.
143. Hsu C-P, Chen P-C, Wang Y-L. A novel and robust packaging technology for miniaturized FET-based biosensors with microfluidic channels. *ECS Trans*. 2016;72:33–35.
144. Kiryukhin MV, Lau HH, Goh SH, Teh C, Korzh V, Sadovoy A. A membrane film sensor with encapsulated fluorescent dyes towards express freshness monitoring of packaged food. *Talanta*. 2018.
145. Ramon-Marquez T, Medina-Castillo AL, Fernandez-Gutierrez A, Fernandez-Sanchez JF. Novel optical sensing film based on a functional nonwoven nanofibre mat for an easy, fast and highly selective and sensitive detection of tryptamine in beer. *Biosens Bioelectron*. 2016.
146. Dilmaçünal T. *Intelligent systems in the food packaging industry. Nanotechnology Applications in Food*. Elsevier; 2017: 287–306.
147. Lim LT. *Active and intelligent packaging materials. Comprehensive Biotechnology*. Elsevier; 2019:688–702.

Chapter 36

Food defense: types of threat, defense plans, and mitigation strategies

Louise Manning
Sustainable Agri-food Systems, Lincoln Institute for Agri-food Technology, University of Lincoln, United Kingdom

Abstract
Defending consumer, business, and national food supply from intentional malicious attack is an essential public health and business resilience strategy that must be appropriately developed, be agile enough to address all potential threats and be built on strong knowledge of the industry sector and the mitigation strategies available. This chapter considers the present knowledge on food defense strategies, how they are developed using a risk based approach and how they can be applied within the food chain. At international, national and business level, food defense plans need to be designed, implemented and verified to ensure that they remain current and effective. There is still a significant knowledge gap when organizations are seeking to implement food defense plans and a need for greater capacity building to ensure that risk managers understand the methodological approaches that are currently being used, their value but their particular limitations too.

Keywords: Food defense; threat; assessment; defense plan; mitigation strategy

36.1 Introduction

Food defense is widely discussed in the literature as concerning all forms of intentional malicious attack on a food batch, lot, or food supply chain.[1–6] This includes ideological attack[2]; or terrorism[4,6]; and where there is an intention by the perpetrators to cause wide scale public harm[7] or political harm to a given nation, or political party. As a result, a food defense attack can lead to compromised food materials and products, supply chain disruption,[8] and panic or fear.[9] Further, food defense can be described as an active process or strategy to protect food, organizations, and food supply chains.[2,10] Food defense is said to contribute to "the mitigation of potential risks in intentional contamination and food fraud, which can have a harmful effect on humans and public health, business, economy, etc." (p. 217).[11] Some sources state that food defense is distinct from food safety, food quality, and food fraud issues.[6] Others suggest that food defense includes all intentional acts of adulteration, including food fraud, tampering, food terrorism, cyber-attacks, and hacktivism too.[8,12] Indeed, it is important to articulate, and then differentiate, what the intentional versus unintentional element of adulteration means in practice.[4–6,13,14] This confused narrative means there is a lack of consistency in how adulteration is defined firstly in legislation between different countries, in academic literature, and also in supply chain standards (for a fuller explanation, see Ref.[14]). The United States Food and Drug Administration (FDA) makes a distinction between food safety and food defense:

> Food safety and food defence approaches consider contaminants differently. For food safety purposes, contaminants are often considered based on their historical association with a commodity and outbreaks of foodborne illness; whereas food defence considers intelligent adversaries who may attempt to contaminate food with a wide range of potential contaminants (p. 44).[7]

The European Union (EU) does not define food defense specifically, instead they differentiate in terms of intentional deliberate acts of adulteration and ideologically motivated intentional adulteration which they term "bioterrorism."[15] The potential for detection of the agent as well as the lethality of the agent material itself will be considered by the perpetrators when they determine the consequence of their actions, that is, perpetrators are "impact motivated."[4] This means when considering food defense issues, the agent (contaminant) and the profile of the perpetrator should be assessed together. Intentional ideologically motivated adulteration is "the deliberate contamination of food with a biological, chemical,

Present Knowledge in Food Safety. DOI: https://doi.org/10.1016/B978-0-12-819470-6.00001-9

radiological, or physical agent by an individual or group of individuals with the intent to cause wide scale public health harm" (p. 14).[7] In comparison, economically motivated adulteration (EMA) is associated with food fraud activities undertaken for economic or competitive gain rather than public health harm. However, the legal and moral line between competitively driven EMA, and the intentional sabotage of competitors' activities, for example, is quite nuanced.

This chapter will consider the different types of threat that can be considered as a food defense issue and the means for their mitigation. Case study examples will be used to illustrate the scope of food defense incidents and the challenges that occurred to identify appropriate defensive action once the incident was identified. The term "threat" is now considered more closely.

36.2 Food defense threat

36.2.1 Introduction

A threat is "something that can cause loss or harm which arises from the ill-intent of people" (p. 3).[8] Food defense threats involve a motivation to do harm to distinct, intended and targeted victim(s) with notions of personal benefit to the perpetrator in terms of underpinning an ideological statement, a means to gain objective impact, or more emotively drive outcomes such as notoriety, revenge, or restorative justice.[16–20] Spink et al.[9,21] pose that an offender can be characterized by either their profile (offender-based) or their activity (offense-based). Further, in a food defense incident the interaction between the perpetrator and the potential victim(s) is of particular interest. The influence of the relationship between the offender/perpetrator and the victim(s) is important because it can include elements of control and power and is affected by how the victim is perceived by the perpetrator as person, victim or object.[22,23] Studies have considered, for example, disgruntled employees[24]; employees more generally either within the business or working for suppliers or external contractors, or people with no connection to the business.[25] While offender profiling is not new, considering the profile of the perpetrator in order to develop appropriate and effective food defense mitigation strategies is still in its infancy. The food defense threat could be *personal* against a known group or individual, for example, religious group, and thus halal or kosher food may be a target, or the action may be driven because of an event that occurred in the perpetrator's own personal life, for example, a disgruntled employee who then commits an act against a particular business.[24]

Alternatively, the perpetrator may relate to the victims as a *vehicle* or target, for example, a crime directed at children through a targeted food (milk powder, baby food) means that the offender may see the target for the attack, not necessarily as the direct target, but instead the one most likely to deliver the best impact for their cause or intention. These activities can be influenced by affective or emotive drivers, for example, political or religious ideology, anger at society as a whole or simply a means to extort money from a food business. This type of crime can therefore have multiple victims and while the action is directed at a target individual or group, the overarching impact is intended to be on society at large. Finally, according to Canter,[22,23] if the victim is seen as an *object* by the perpetrator then there will be few emotional elements to the food crime. The perpetrator will as a result see the victim as having very little significance as a person in the process of delivering their overall objectives. At the wider criminal level, this is observable in crimes such as human trafficking.

36.2.2 The vocabulary associated with threat analysis and the development of mitigation strategies

PAS 96[8] differentiates between four types of threats in terms of the activity, that is, malicious contamination, extortion, espionage, and cyber-crime. FDA (2019) uses the terms credible threat, insider threat, and threat landscape. A *credible threat* is a threat that exists when a perpetrator has the ability, motivation, and opportunity to carry out that threat. A credible threat is thus a realistic concern for the target individual, business, supply chain or nation involved. *Insider threat* is determined to "be posed by an individual who exploits their position, credentials, or employment to achieve trusted access to the means, processes, equipment, material, location, facility, and/or target necessary to carry out [an ideologically motivated attack, intentional adulteration to cause harm or] a terrorist action" (p.38).[7] Here, as highlighted by Spink et al.,[9,21] the term threat is focused on the perpetrator. The *threat landscape* is the scope of food defense threats under consideration when developing a food defense plan. The threat landscape includes characterization of the threat agents, identifying the established threats themselves, and determining the potential for emerging threats.

The *agent material* is any chemical, biological, radiological, nuclear (CBRN) or physical material used in a food defense threat, that is, to maliciously and intentionally adulterate (contaminate) food where the action is then actively disclosed to organizations and the general public to derive personal, political or social impact.[7,26–30] Some examples of known agent materials are synthesized in Table 36.1. The *threat agent* is an individual or group that wishes to perpetrate the threat on the threat target.[31]

TABLE 36.1 Examples of agent materials used in intentional adulteration of supply chains 1950–2008.

Stage of supply chain	Agents materials used
Post harvest, and manufacturing	Glass, mercury, needles, rat poison
Preharvest	Cyanide, glyphosate, plant toxin, rodenticide
Retail and food service	Acetone, arsenic, atropine, cyanide, herbicide, insecticide, pesticide, physical contaminants incl. rodenticide, rohypnol, *Salmonella typhimurium*, thallium
Water supply	Cyanide, insecticide, pesticide, sarin, sheep dip, VX (a nerve agent)

Source: Adapted from Dalziel GR. Food defense incidents 1950–2008: a chronology and analysis of incidents involving the malicious contamination of the food supply chain. Report. Centre of Excellence for National Security (CENS). S Rajaratnam School of International Studies, Nanyang Technology University, Singapore; 2009.

TABLE 36.2 Examples of threat agents.

Internal organizational or supply chain threat agents	External threat agents	Internal and external threat agents
Contractors Customers Disgruntled employees Former employees Insider employees Suppliers Visitors	Activists Cults Cyber criminals Domestic terrorists Disgruntled competitor Extremists and Zealots Hacktivists International terrorists Racist groups Supremacist organizations	Extortionist Individuals seeking retribution or harboring a grudge Individuals with health issues–mental health, psychopaths, deranged individuals Saboteurs Spies

Source: Adapted from Manning L. Food defence: refining the taxonomy of food defence threats, Trends Food Sci Technol. 2019;85:107–115; Baybutt P. Assessing risks from threats to process plants: threat and vulnerability analysis. Process Saf Prog. 2002;21(4):269–275.

Examples of threat agents are evolving as more research is undertaken in this area (Table 36.2).[32] The *established threat can be described* as a combination of the known agent material and threat agent. These threats are known and have been identified in previous incidents. An *emergent threat* is a threat where there is a low level of understanding or evidence, but its significance and credibility is expected to increase. This threat is a combination of a potential agent material and the motivations of the threat agent(s).

The threat target can be identified either as a *direct threat target*, for example, a country, government, organization or individual that is the intended victim of the food defense threat or an *indirect threat* target. An indirect threat target is described here as a vehicle for the food defense threat (e.g., baby food) where the resultant threat impact is intended to be on the organization, nation or other direct threat target, but the indirect threat target, for example, baby food is chosen because it will create the greatest impact and concern. Indeed, Felson and Clarke,[33] in their routine activity approach, differentiate between the target (a person or an object) and the victim (a person) or in the context of food defense, the *threat victim* in the context of food defense would be an organization or nation state. When seeking to develop a new terminology the *threat attack* can be described as the intentional malicious attack itself on a given point, step or procedure. The attack can be a *single threat attack*, that is, a single instance and at a single point or can be a persistent attack where there are multiple instances and/or multiple points where the attack is perpetrated. This is explored further in the case studies.

Threat analysis describes how the risk manager(s) identify the threat agent and the agent material and then the likelihood of the threat being realized as well as the consequences should this threat occur.[32] Vulnerability is

TABLE 36.3 Motivations, goals, and threat targets for food defense threats.

Motivation	Goal	Threat target	
		Direct threat target	Indirect threat target
Economic failure	Deliver an economic impact on an organization, group or nation	Multiple	The specific organization, group or nation
Ideological	Deliver an impact according to an ideological motive	Multiple	Individuals or guardians that can drive an ideological change
Issue-orientated	Protect or end something the perpetrator believes is important	Multiple	Individuals connected to or guardians of the issue that can protect or make the change
Political	Change political beliefs or policies	Multiple	Governments
Religious	Deliver an impact according to a religion based motive	Multiple	Given religious group
Revenge and retribution	Seek to deliver justice as perceived by the perpetrator	Multiple	Individuals, groups or organizations specific to the issue
Social	Change a way of life	Multiple	Individuals, groups or organizations specific to the issue

Source: Adapted from Baybutt P. Assessing risks from threats to process plants: threat and vulnerability analysis. Process Saf Prog. 2002;21(4):269–275.

the susceptibility to intentional adulteration of a point, step, or procedure in a facility's food process (p. 11)[7] or in a wider supply chain. The potential for an intentional malicious attack on a food batch, lot, or food supply chain, where a vulnerability may be exploited *can be called the threat risk*. Threat risk is a calculation of the likelihood of the threat being realized and the severity of the impact of the threat, if it is realized. The *threat profile* is a summary of the qualitative estimate of the likelihood of credible threats being realized[32]; using existing information about known threats, and incidents.[34] Another term that is used is *threat intelligence*. Threat intelligence is the information that can be used to determine the credibility of a given agent material, threat agent or vulnerability. This includes information and knowledge about threat agents, their modus operandi, objectives, tactics, techniques, and procedures.[34] These terms, some of which are used widely in the literature and food supply chain standards and others relatively new sit within the vocabulary used when developing threat assessment, management, and threat mitigation strategies. *Threat mitigation strategies* are "those risk-based, reasonably appropriate measures that a person knowledgeable about food defense would employ to significantly minimize or prevent significant vulnerabilities identified at actionable process steps, and that are consistent with the current scientific understanding of food defense at the time of the analysis" (p. 11).[7] Key to determining appropriate mitigation strategies is to consider whether the threats are internal or external to the organization.

Internal threat agents include contractors, customers, disgruntled, former and insider employees, suppliers and visitors. Interpersonal stressors in the internal and contractual work environment can lead to alienation and attempts of sabotage, retaliatory action or efforts to obtain restorative justice[35]; or interactional justice where a lack of fairness or equity is perceived.[36] *External threat agents* represent a wide and diverse group (Table 36.2) and their perception as a credible threat will be situational to a given product, organization and national situation. It is important to not only identify the individual(s) of concern, but also their motivations, goals and threat targets (Table 36.3). There are multiple examples of threat agent, but five types of threat agents are considered in this chapter in more depth: industrial spies (espionage), and then extortionists, saboteurs, extremists, activists and cults, where although the mode of threat attack might be similar (tampering and sabotage of food products); the threat agent and their motives are different, and finally, the last type of threat agent is terrorists. However this review of threat agents does provide more generally a wider understanding of the range of threat agents outlined in Table 36.2 and their goals and motivations as described in Table 36.3.

36.2.3 Industrial spies (espionage)

Espionage, or industrial spying, involves the covert collection without the data owners' consent of personally held, rather than publically held, information or data.

This privately held data can include intellectual property such as copyrights, designs, blueprints or data that underpins brand value, patents, processing techniques, product formulations, recipes, software systems, trademarks, theories, for commercial advantage.[11,37–39] The characteristic activities of espionage include:

1. Breaking and entering into a competitor's premises to steal information or installing recording devices.
2. Contacting competitors using a fake identity, for example, pretending to be a potential customer or supplier.
3. Covert surveillance and recording through spy cameras and electronic eavesdropping.
4. Hiring private detectives to track competitor's staff.
5. Infiltrating competitor organizations with industrial spies and insider employees.
6. Infiltrating computerized and digital systems remotely.
7. Interviewing competitors' employees for a bogus job vacancy.
8. Pressuring the customers or suppliers of competitors to reveal sensitive information about their operations, and
9. Searching through a competitor's rubbish.[8,37,38]

Espionage is a key threat that needs to be considered within food defense mitigation strategies.

36.2.4 Extortionists

Extortion can be described as the actions undertaken to obtain something which the perpetrator values (e.g., money, assets, influence or impact) from a person or organization by force, intimidation, threat or illegal activity.[4] Examples of food related extortion incidents often involving a demand for money or a list of demands include:

1. The Heinz Baby Food incident in 1988 (see Fisher[40]).
2. The 2003 cyanide in sardines incident in South Africa.[41]
3. The 2014 Fonterra incident in New Zealand where anonymous threats targeted baby formula in order to threaten the dairy company and the wider dairy sector.[42–44]
4. The 2016 UK food cyanide extortion incident.[45]
5. The 2017 German extortion case with a demand for nearly £8.8 million.[46–48]
6. In December 2019, Heinz and Tesco voluntarily recalled all 7 + months "Heinz By Nature" baby food range after a single jar of baby food was identified as having been tampered with and two sharp metal fragments were found in the jar.[49]

36.2.5 Saboteurs

Sabotage is a wide term with regard to the activities and motivations it represents. Sabotage is the deliberate damage, disruptions or destruction of assets, infrastructure or intangible assets (brand); or a wish to subvert an organization's operations in order to weaken a competitor. Sabotage is also driven by a motive to draw personal attention through the act or make a protest or political point by creating unfavorable publicity, embarrassment, production delays or harming relationships, employees or customers.[50–53] Sabotage can be due to internal threat agents including employees often seeking to damage the organization itself.[54,55] There have been examples of food sabotage in food service as an active retribution for customer hostility or rudeness.[56,57]

Revenge or retribution can be a powerful motive for the initial threat attack. In 2018 in Australia, sewing needles were found by a consumer in strawberries in a pack purchased from a retail store. This incident is an example of alleged sabotage.[58] In the subsequent weeks from the original incident, there were 186 reports of sewing needles found in strawberries, some found to be hoaxes ($n = 15$), including multiple reports in Queensland ($n = 77$) with 68 strawberry brands affected.[59] A woman was seen putting a needle into a banana in what was believed to be a copycat act.[60] These copycat cases from other perpetrators influences the ability of investigators to identify the threat agent and the threat intelligence around the original alleged sabotage incident. Sewing needles have been used in a range of sabotage incidents often undertaken, or identified at the retail store (Table 36.4), some with associated extortion demands, others without any additional communication from the perpetrator. Food Standards Australia New Zealand in their subsequent report to government on the strawberry incident cited a need for further action to be able to give a coordinated response between regulators and industry in the event of a future suspected sabotage incident.[61] The series of recommendations is discussed later in this chapter in the wider context of food defense mitigation strategies.

36.2.6 Extremists, activists, and cults

Extremists have been linked to a number of food defense incidents (Table 36.5) including: anarchists, politically and ideologically motivated activists including hacktivists, extremists, and cults. Anarchists aim to bring about anarchy and a dismantling of existing political and social structures and hierarchies in favor of new structures and systems. In December 2016, Greek anarchists claimed on a website that they had contaminated several food and drink products linked with multinational companies such as Coca-Cola, Nestlé, Unilever and Delta Foods, and a Greek company and as a result products were withdrawn from shelves in supermarkets in Athens.[71,72] The claim that foods contaminated with chlorine and hydrochloric acid which were then put back on supermarket shelves

TABLE 36.4 Examples of suspected sabotage incidents involving the use of sewing needles and pins.

Year	Location	Description	Linked to published extortion attempt
2009	Canada	Seven deli products sold at a No Frills supermarket in Guelph, Ontario, were found to have sewing needles inside them.[62]	No
2010	Canada	Five incidents recorded in Toronto of needles being embedded in food products; two at a No Frills supermarket.[63]	No
2010	Japan	Employee at supermarket in Kitakyishu, Japan found three needles stuck to a plastic bag containing thinly sliced cabbage in April. A month before another supermarket in the same town discovered similar needles (three cases). Several products in another town were found with needles inserted into bread products. No link was identified at the time.[64]	No
2012	Canada	Needle found in Air Canada sandwich during a flight.[65]	No
2012	Europe	Needles used to tamper with yoghurt[66]	No
2015	Canada	Nails and needles found inserted into potatoes[67]	No
2016	Canada	Needle found inserted into children's candy[68]	No
2018	Canada	Sewing pins found in meat products (three separate incidents) purchased at grocery stores in Nanaimo, Vancouver[69]	No
2018	Australia	Strawberries and other fruits were found to contain sewing needles after an initial incident and then multiple copycat events[58]	No
2019	Australia	Needle in grapes purchased in Melbourne[70]	No

TABLE 36.5 Examples of suspected incidents involving activists, extremists, and cults.

Year	Country	Description
1952	Kenya	The Mau used African Bush Milk (a plant toxin) to poison cattle of the Kikuyu tribe.[29,73]
1978	Israel	In 1978, another Palestinian group, the "Arab Revolutionary Council," targeted Israeli citrus fruit, using liquid mercury as an agent material and in 1988, Israeli grapefruit exports were threatened with contamination.[74]
1981	United Kingdom	In 1981, an ecoactivist group, "Dark Harvest," threatened placing anthrax contaminated soil in places throughout the United Kingdom to highlight the ecological dangers of chemical and germ warfare.[75]
1984	United States	In September 1984, the Rajneeshee group (some described as a cult) intentionally contaminated salad bars in 10 restaurants in the town of The Dalles with *Salmonella*, in order to influence the voting in a local election. There were 751 cases of illness.[29,76]
1986	Sri Lanka	Tamil militants threatened to destroy the national economy either by using potassium cyanide or by bringing in nonindigenous diseases to devastate rubber and tea plantations.[29]
2014	United States	The hacktivist group Anonymous caused major disruption in hospital operations at Boston's Children's Hospital.[77]
2016	Italy	In June 2016, Italian anarchists threatened to contaminate foodstuff in supermarkets in Lombardy with herbicide.[71]
2016	Greece	In December 2016, Greek anarchists claimed they had contaminated several food and drink products of multinational companies.[71,72]

was seen as a "credible threat" by authorities. Delta Foods stated:

> This move affects a Greek company, which employs more than 1200 workers, has been working with 1400 Greek farmers for more than 60 years, and actively supports the Greek family, economy and region. Apart from the damage that it creates, it's directed against farmers and hundreds of affiliated stakeholders (distribution network, retail outlets, suppliers) and eventually it's turned directly against the Greek society itself.[72]

Activists are individuals or groups who organize with the aim of influencing public policy and/or an organization, social norms and values through a concerted action to achieve their specific goals, which may be political, economic, or social.[78,79] In order to achieve their goals they need to position themselves and legitimize their group and their ideas and build a membership base.[78] Hacktivism is the usually clandestine use of electronic hacking to help advance political or social causes.[80] Hacktivists are able to use strong and complex digital connections to target specific attacks on organizations, governments or individuals. Hacktivists undertake cyber-attacks against a target that are ideologically or politically motivated, for example, data exposure to highlight potential unethical practices by institutions or defacement of organizational websites.[81]

In creating a typology of food defense issues, it is difficult to distinguish between the forms of intentional contamination described here and incidents described as terrorism.

36.2.7 Terrorism

Terrorism at its simplest is the politically motivated violence or threat of such violence with the intention of causing fear.[82] In Title 22 Chapter 38 of US Code 2656f,[83] terrorism is defined as "premeditated, politically motivated violence perpetrated against noncombatant [civilian] targets by subnational groups or clandestine agents." Terrorist activities are enacted to attain a specific ideological or political goal,[84] engender fear, terror, panic and anxiety in the general population or a particular group and as a result reduce the level of confidence in the government, leading to uncertainty and political instability.[28,85] There are multiple definitions of food-related terrorism (Table 36.6). These focus on deliberate adulteration of food with an agent material to cause harm, injury or death.

Food terrorism can cause severe implications for the health of the population, weaken or destroy economic growth and cause significant trade disruption, and consequential loss to the local or national economy.[29] The resultant direct or indirect impact could lead to the culling of livestock, and the potential compensation paid to farmers and producers, collection and disposal of rejected food products and a loss of consumer and political confidence and the direct impact on public health services including hospitalization and illness related costs. Green et al.[91] argue that there is a typology of food terrorism starting with terrorism of which a subset is bioterrorism which may or may not be related to food; to food terrorism of which a subset is agroterrorism that relates specifically to primary production. Agroterrorism in itself could be driven by a range of threat agents and may prove an all-encompassing theme that includes: (1) militant activists and animal rights groups; (2) international terrorists; (3) domestic terrorists; (4) disgruntled insider employees or industry specialists; and (5) economic opportunists wishing to cause economic disruption and market volatility.[92] Agrodefense, the actions that can be taken to reduce the likelihood of an agroterrorism incident, specifically can be addressed by specific mitigation strategies and through the use of food testing methods, and farm security checks. However, convictions for planning of terrorism acts in the United Kingdom are often delivered through traditional policing/antiterrorism methods showing that routine

TABLE 36.6 Definitions of food related terrorism.

	Definition	Source
Agroterrorism	The deliberate introduction of a disease agent, either against livestock or into the food chain, for purposes of undermining stability and generating fear.	86
Agroterrorism	The deliberate use of biological or chemical means to depreciate, stunt, halt, or destroy an agricultural asset or set of assets.	87
Agroterorism	The deliberate introduction of an animal or plant disease with the goal of generating fear, causing economic losses, and/or undermining social stability.	88
Bioterrorism	The deliberate release of viruses, bacteria or other agents used to cause illness or death in people, but also in animals or plants.	89
Bioterrorism	The deliberate poisoning or contamination of the food supply to achieve some political goal.	84
Bioterrorism	The deliberate release of viruses, bacteria, or other germs (agents) used to cause illness or death in people, animals, or plants.	90
Food terrorism	An act or threat of deliberate contamination of food for the purpose of causing injury or death to civilian populations.	74
Food terrorism	The deliberate (or threat of) contamination of food with hazardous agents (biological, chemical, physical, or radionuclear) for the purpose of causing injury or death and/or disrupting social, economic, or political stability.	28

surveillance measures are as important as implementing prevention and mitigation strategies. The World Health Organization (WHO) in their 2002 Report *Terrorist threats to food: guidance for establishing and strengthening prevention and response systems* states that an essential means to preventing food terrorism is the development, validation, implementation, monitoring and effective verification of management programmes and their associated security measures. Further, the WHO report states that effective prevention requires food defense mitigation strategies that deliver a concerted defense approach between government and industry.

36.2.8 Food defense vulnerability and threat assessment

Food defense vulnerability assessment considers the potential public health impact of the agent material (a factor of severity and scale), and accessibility, that is, the potential for the threat agent to access and successfully adulterate the product if a contaminant were added.[7] Supply chain vulnerability has been suggested as being a combination of opportunity, the motivation of threat agents and what drives this motivation and the efficacy of control measures that have been adopted at all levels of the supply chain and national food supply (see van Ruth et al.[93]). The FDA suggests the use of Carver + SHOCK, an adapted military tool where Carver is an acronym for the six attributes used to evaluate the potential for an attack on a threat target: criticality, accessibility, recuperability, vulnerability, effect, and recognizability; SHOCK recognizes the combined economic, public health and psychological impacts of a given threat attack.[7] This approach can select given targets and risk rank them using a scoring system that helps to prioritize mitigation strategies.[25] The introduction in 2016 of the FDA Food Defense Plan Builder, supported creating standardization of the methodologies for US food operators and countries seeking to export into the United States.[4,24,25]

Horizon scanning is the thorough examination of potential threats and vulnerabilities in order to identify uncertainties or market forces that can influence food related crime, prioritize threats and the means for their effective mitigation and management, and provide early warning of particular established and emerging threats.[94–96] Therefore horizon scanning is a systematic approach to consider evidence of trends and scenarios in order to determine whether an organization is adequately prepared for established and emerging threats and if the organization has implemented, or can readily adopt adequate means for their elimination, mitigation or control.

The Global Food Safety Initiative[2] highlights food defense threat assessment tools such as threat analysis critical control point (TACCP). The application of TACCP in the PAS 96 process aims to identify the likelihood and consequences of a threat being realized. The scope of TACCP is wider in terms of the threats considered than simply food defense, as it also addresses food fraud, cyber-crime and so on (see PAS 96[8]). TACCP also considers the typology and impact of the perpetrators.[4] TACCP and Carver + SHOCK both have a risk based semi-quantitative element to prioritize threats[4] and then to inform food defense mitigation strategies. Vulnerability analysis critical control point (VACCP) focuses on vulnerability, exposure or susceptibility to an incident.[4,97]

36.3 Food defense mitigation strategies

In general, mitigation strategies are used in the food supply chain to manage risk. Mitigation strategies require the organization to take precautionary, and preventive actions to reduce risk and in doing so incur cost for a potential event that might never be realized.[98] For food defense attacks to be successful they rely on a lack of preparedness by the threat target or victim that then creates a vulnerability.[99,100] Increasingly, manufacturers, retailers and food service organizations are requiring formal food defense mitigation strategies as a prerequisite to supply.[99] These mitigation strategies include the active steps taken, the protection activities, process or procedures, often called security measures or countermeasures, that reduce the risk associated with food defense threats.[4,5,101]

Facility-wide security measures, may include the need to address a particular vulnerability at a given point but are usually: "general, nontargeted, protective measures that are implemented at the facility-wide level to protect personnel, property, or product" (FDA, 2019, p. 12). This means that security measures can be global in nature and may form part of general good manufacturing practice prerequisite programmes or can be specific and address a single vulnerability.[4] Mitigation strategies derived from a food defense vulnerability assessment form one element of a food defense plan along with validation, monitoring, corrective action, and verification procedures.[7] These terms among others are described in more detail in Table 36.7.

Guardians monitor and protect food, processes, organizations, supply chains and nations against food defense issues and the absence of effective guardians makes an attack more likely.[17] Guardians are visible individuals who have positions of authority in organizations combined with the relevant knowledge, skills and understanding and are able to implement, monitor and verify a food defense system.[103–105] *Hurdles* are the formal components in a food defense system that either reduce opportunity for intentional adulteration to occur by either

TABLE 36.7 Food defense plan definitions.

Term	Definition	Source
Food defense guardian	Guardians monitor and protect food, processes, organizations, supply chains and nations against food defense issues and the absence of effective guardians makes an attack more likely.	17
Food defense monitoring	Means to conduct a planned sequence of observations or measurements to assess whether mitigation strategies are operating as intended.	7
Food defense plan	A set of written documents that is based upon food defense principles and incorporates a vulnerability assessment, includes mitigation strategies, and delineates food defense monitoring, corrective action, and verification procedures to be followed.	7
Food defense system	The result of the implementation of the food defense plan.	7
Food defense validation	The activities undertaken to ensure that security measures (countermeasures) are functioning as intended, that is, within established predefined limits. Target levels and tolerances may be set to provide assurance that loss of security will be detected before vulnerability actually occurs.	102
Food defense verification	The application of methods, procedures, and other evaluations, in addition to food defense monitoring, to determine whether a mitigation strategy or combination of mitigation strategies is or has been operating as intended according to the food defense plan.	7
Hurdles	The formal components in a food defense system that reduce opportunity for intentional adulteration to occur by either assisting detection or by acting as a deterrent.	101
Hurdle gap	The vulnerability that occurs when a hurdle that is part of a mitigation strategy is either not in place or if it is in place is not effective.	101

Source: Adapted from FDA. *Mitigation Strategies to Protect Food Against Intentional Adulteration: Guidance for Industry*. US Department of Health and Human Services Food and Drug Administration Center for Food Safety and Applied Nutrition. Available at: <https://www.fda.gov/downloads/Food/GuidanceRegulation/GuidanceDocumentsRegulatoryInformation/UCM611043.pdf>; March 2019 Accessed 02.01.2020; Cohen L, Felson M. Social change and crime rate trends: a routine activity approach. *Am Sociol Rev*. 1979;44(4):588–608; Spink J, Moyer DC, Park H, et al. Introduction to Food Fraud including translation and interpretation to Russian, Korean and Chinese languages. *Food Chem*. 2015;189:102-107; and Manning L. Development of a food safety verification risk model. *Br Food J*. 2013;115(4):575–589.

assisting detection or act as a deterrent.[4,6,101,105,106] A *hurdle gap* is the vulnerability that can occur when a hurdle that is part of a mitigation strategy is either not in place, or if it is in place is not effective.[101]

The term hurdle or hurdle technology is not new in food science.[107] Hurdle technology is the combined methods, processes, security measures, techniques or barrier technologies to ensure safe food, thus the higher the hurdle the greater the effort needed to overcome it.[107] This approach considers the synergistic effect of combined hurdle strategies rather than individual discrete hurdles, and how this provides a higher level of security and confidence than an individual single security measure.[107,108] Hurdles can be described as either *physical hurdles or hard controls* in terms of active measures protecting structural assets (barriers, enclosed production systems, security systems), or *artefact-based hurdles or soft controls* such as passive measures including procedures, policies and protocols, for example, management practices, product recall and crisis management planning.[7,93,109] Indeed, van Ruth et al.[110] identify 21 control measures that address food fraud. These have been adapted at the facility level in the context of food defense (Table 36.8). In van Ruth et al.'s study of 42 businesses, 85% had a traceability system in place, 65% has whistle blowing measures but only half were undertaking employee integrity screening.

Bendovschi[111] determines three kinds of countermeasure: *preventive security controls* that aim to prevent the realization of a threat; *detective security controls* that assist in identifying a particular threat and *corrective security controls* that are implemented if nonconformity is identified. Other sources[93,101,110] and among others categorize countermeasures into four categories: two preventive (deterrence and prevention), another detective (detection), and the other corrective (disruption). Deterrence seeks to inhibit threat agent activity by limiting opportunity to act (prevention) and promoting the negative personal consequences of taking action, so detection activities can identify incidences of food defense activities and disrupt threat agent activities to minimize their impact.[105]

While preventive security measures at the facility and supply chain level have been considered in the literature (see Table 36.8), it is only after a food defense incident that the efficacy of detective security control and corrective security controls can be truly determined. However, de Abreu et al.[25] in their study in Brazil demonstrate the value of undertaking food defense related audits with an

TABLE 36.8 Examples of control measures in a food defense system.

		General measures	
		Hard	**Soft**
Preventive security measures	Design	Cyber-secure computer system and servers.	Information system (internal and external) Employee system access controls. Website controls
		Biometric or fingerprint checking equipment on entry to facility.	People integrity screening including criminal background and credit check tests. Designated colored clothing for specific areas. ID badges and visitor protocols Ethical code of conduct. Whistleblowing procedure. Insider attacker control procedure
		Physical material and product segregation in stores, production areas and on vehicles.	Tracking and tracing system (internal and external) inclusive of supplier. Risk assessment of all materials on site to determine potential internal agent materials
		Enclosed tanks and transfer systems to move materials and product to reduce the potential for an attacker to access the product. Locked access caps on all hoses and pipework especially external access points.	Tamper-evident seals protocols requiring resealing of ingredient storage containers when tamper-evident packaging has been opened and tamper evident sealing of all containers when not in use.
		Automated and enclosed equipment, such as automated computer-weighing, measuring, and addition equipment, to reduce human interaction with secondary ingredients or rework;	Weighing and handling procedures.
		Faculty design to minimize risk of attack (visibility and security). CCTV systems on the premises. Building design including adequate lighting and minimizing locations where individuals can access materials or product unseen. Restricted access and physical site zoning, locking doors and barriers. Enable vulnerable points with alarms and sirens if they are opened. Motion detection sensors in vulnerable areas.	Security controls. Site maps and access controls. Security personnel protocols with designated access to keys, swipe cards and access codes. Buddy system to prevent lone working. Increased supervision of highly vulnerable areas.
		Covered systems. Use of sight glasses. Use of cleaning in place systems to minimize the risk of intentional contamination during cleaning.	Protocols for staffing levels, lone worker protocols and worker procedures in sensitive areas Ensuring all protective clothing is without pockets so items cannot be concealed.
		Material segregation on arrival until goods inwards inspection.	Supplier approval protocols and contractual arrangements. Reference checks. Financial checks. Driver check-in and identification procedures. Drivers do not leave vehicles when on site.
		–	Product design procedures and identification of particular risk associated with ingredients, product identity or provenance
		–	Training protocols
	Validation	–	Validation protocol

(Continued)

TABLE 36.8 (Continued)

		General measures	
		Hard	**Soft**
Detective security measures	Monitoring system	Equipment and facilities Foreign body detection equipment, for example, metal and foreign body detection and x-ray.	Raw material protocol Finished product protocol Supplier protocol Stock inventories of harmful materials. Monitoring of hurdles and guardians
	Verification system	Equipment and facilities	Raw material protocol Finished product protocol Supplier protocol Verification of hurdles and guardians
Corrective security measures	Corrective action system	Quarantine facilities	Contingency plan Product recall plan Product disposal plan

Source: Adapted from FDA. *Mitigation strategies to protect food against intentional adulteration: guidance for industry*. US Department of Health and Human Services Food and Drug Administration Center for Food Safety and Applied Nutrition. Available at: <https://www.fda.gov/downloads/Food/GuidanceRegulation/GuidanceDocumentsRegulatoryInformation/UCM611043.pdf>; March 2019 Accessed 02.01.2020; Baybutt P. Assessing risks from threats to process plants: threat and vulnerability analysis. *Process Saf Prog*. 2002;21(4):269–275; Soon JM, Manning L, Smith R. Advancing understanding of pinchpoints and crime prevention in the food supply chain. *Crime Prev Community Saf*. 2019b;21(1):1–19; and Bendovschi A. Cyber-attacks—trends, patterns and security countermeasures. *Procedia Econ Financ*. 2015;28:24–31.

associated gap analysis. The gap analysis can then inform an action plan that individual businesses can develop and implement. A case study is now used in this chapter to consider the efficacy of food defense systems more specifically.

After the 2018 Australian strawberry incident, this report[61] highlighted a number of food defense vulnerabilities within the supply chain (preventive) and also the detective security control and corrective security controls (Table 36.9), and the lessons learned (Table 36.10). The major lessons learned from the incident were around clear and consistent messaging and an understanding of the positive and negative role of mainstream and social media in a food defense incident. Social media can play a role in accelerating copycat activities that mask the actual issue of concern. There also need to be better national coordination in the event of a food defense incident and relationships and networks need to be developed prior to crises.

The lack of registration of fruit businesses and the lack of discrete product lots and full traceability systems being in place hampered the response to the incident. There was also limited mapping ability for the supply chain, ineffective preparedness and a lack of resources to respond. Reflecting on this case study highlights that there need to be:

1. Clear and well communicated food defense incident response protocols and formal communication linkages between regulators, health departments, and police.
2. A central agency to ensure national coordination of messaging and information associated with a food defense incident and also better coordination of the terminology used so the messaging is constant. This is especially important where there are emotions such as fear or dread associated with the incident.
3. Police and enforcement bodies should play a headline role in national food incident debriefs with the media when intentional food tampering is believed to be involved.
4. Risk assessment that understands supply chain vulnerabilities and the approach should be co-created by government and industry and be broad, proportionate to the incident and scalable.
5. Notification and registration of food premises and horticultural production is essential so they can be identified and mapped during a food defense crisis.
6. Traceability (both tracking and tracing) and traceability protocols must be established that are universal and appropriate for a timely response in the event of a food defense incident.

This case study demonstrates the breadth of protocols, and response in the event of a food defense incident. A failure to address such an incident in a timely and proportionate manner could lead to public panic, total boycotting of certain foods with resultant economic loss and the realization of a food scare. In this context a food scare can be described as "the response to a food incident (real or perceived) that causes a sudden disruption to the food supply chain and to food consumption patterns"[112] (p. 133).

TABLE 36.9 Vulnerabilities identified in the 2018 Australian strawberry incident.

Factor	Vulnerabilities identified
Communication and coordination arrangements	Inconsistent public communication messages are damaging to the industry and to the investigations being undertaken by food regulators and police. The interface between multiple local regulators and national regulators can be weak if suitable protocols are not in place. The volume of communication during the crisis on multiple media channels was unexpected and difficult to manage for all actors. Communications on social media can play a role in instigating copycat incidents. There can be an impact on brands that are named in communications but are not part of the actual recall.
Crisis management	Assumption was made that industry had the capacity to respond in crises and this was not the case. Other horticultural organizations provided support and Queensland Strawberries employed a crisis communication expert.
Food safety culture	There was a suggestion of a lack of food safety culture at farm level.
Product recall process	There was some confusion about the terminology and wording used by all agencies during the incident relating to product recall, for example, product withdrawal from shelf, product recall from consumers, removed from sale. The mapping of the supply chain involved in the recall was problematic.
Supply chain vulnerability	Deliberate sabotage (tampering) can potentially occur at any stage in the supply chain and factors that increase this vulnerability are: too many opportunities for a potential attack; the seasonal nature of work and labor hiring practices creates challenges in ensuring people integrity; comingling of product from more than one farm (preventing traceability) and the packaging itself that may prevent tampering may reduce shelf-life. The use of metal detection too may mean the perpetrators could just change the agent material to plastic or other materials.
Traceability	Traceability to source was affected by a lack of regulatory requirements for business notification/registration. Locating farms and the nature of operations was an issue. Practices such as comingling of produce from more than one farm/supplier led to a loss of traceability and there was an inability to easily track and trace the product. The supply chain mapping to identify all actors and interactions was inadequate.

Source: Adapted from FSANZ (Food Standards Australia New Zealand). Strawberry tampering incident – report to government. Available at: <https://www.foodstandards.gov.au/publications/SiteAssets/Pages/Strawberry-tampering-incident/FSANZ%20Strawberry%20Report%20doc.pdf>; 2018 Accessed 02.01.2020.

TABLE 36.10 Lessons learned in the 2018 Australian strawberry incident.

Factor	Lessons learned
Communication and coordination arrangements	• Clear leadership structures and early and consistent messaging (by police and health agencies) is vital to successful public communication during a food defense incident. • When an incident becomes national, a single point of contact and a single website that provides real-time public information is required. • Communications on social media can play a role in instigating copycat incidents so during the corrective security phase communication protocols must include a social media strategy. However, social media can also have a positive impact in developing consumer support for the industry. • Clear communication is needed so that products that are not affected do not become part of the recall. • Communication activities need to ensure they do not interfere with criminal investigations and potential prosecutions. • There should be clear police/government/industry incident debrief protocols in place. • Communication protocols need to be in place to address the impact on export markets and trade.
Crisis management	• Industry bodies need to have access to crisis management resources and have a crisis management preparedness plan that can be used in the event of a food defense incident.
Product recall	• There is a need for better communication, collaboration and consistency in the terminology used during the product recall phase.
Regulatory control	• Regulatory and enforcement authorities require a strong contact list developed before a food defense crisis • There is a need for a formal reactive national coordination strategy in place with industry to address a crisis and the optimum methods of communication with mainstream media and social media.

(Continued)

TABLE 36.10 (Continued)

Factor	Lessons learned
Resilience	• Measures are needed to increase consumer confidence in the fresh produce sector. • Protocols need to be in place that allow for better crisis management preparedness measures and increase industry resilience during and after a crisis.
Risk assessment and mitigation	• Risk assessment is required that understands supply chain vulnerabilities. • This approach should be co-created by government and industry and be broad, scalable, proportionate and scalable.
Traceability	• Notification and registration of food premises and horticultural production is required. • Traceability along the supply chain needs to be better understood and measures identified and adopted to enhance supply chain integrity. The customary "one step forward, one step back" approach rather than field to fork full chain traceability may be inadequate. • Traceability protocols needs to be universal, address tracking and tracing and appropriate for a timely response and must encompass food defense issues.

Source: Adapted from FSANZ (Food Standards Australia New Zealand). Strawberry tampering incident – report to government. Available at: <https://www.foodstandards.gov.au/publications/SiteAssets/Pages/Strawberry-tampering-incident/FSANZ%20Strawberry%20Report%20doc.pdf>; 2018 Accessed 02.01.2020.

The motivation for such incidents is the scare, concern or fear factor and this is a challenge for all food regulators seeking to safeguard the food supply chain.

36.3.1 Research gaps and future direction

This chapter has considered food defense which is a contemporary topic in the food science and food supply chain literature. At international, national and business level, food defense mitigation strategies need to be designed, implemented and verified to ensure that they remain current and effective. There is still a significant knowledge gap when organizations are seeking to implement food defense plans and associated mitigation strategies and also to reduce vulnerability to such activities. There is also a need for greater capacity building to ensure that risk managers understand the methodological approaches that are currently being used, their value, but also their particular limitations too.

References

1. BRC (British Retail Consortium). *Global Standard Food Safety*; 2018. Issue 8 TSO Books ISBN 9781784903343.
2. GFSI (Global Food Safety Initiative). GFSI Benchmarking Requirements Version 7.2. Available at: <https://www.mygfsi.com/certification/benchmarking/gfsi-guidance-document.html>; 2017 Accessed 30.12.19.
3. GFSI (Global Food Safety Initiative). GFSI position on mitigating the public health risk of food fraud. July 2014. Available at: <http://www.mygfsi.com/news-resources/news/295-gfsi-position-paper-on-mitigating-the-public-health-risk-of-food-fraud.html>; 2014 Accessed 4.10.18.
4. Manning L. Food defence: refining the taxonomy of food defence threats. *Trends Food Sci Technol*. 2019;85:107–115.
5. Manning L, Soon JM. Food safety, food fraud and food defence: a fast evolving literature. *J Food Sci*. 2016;81(4):R823–R834.
6. Spink J, Moyer DC. Defining the public health threat of food fraud. *J Food Sci*. 2011;76(9):R157–R163.
7. FDA. Mitigation Strategies to Protect Food Against Intentional Adulteration: Guidance for Industry. US Department of Health and Human Services Food and Drug Administration Center for Food Safety and Applied Nutrition. Available at: <https://www.fda.gov/downloads/Food/GuidanceRegulation/GuidanceDocumentsRegulatoryInformation/UCM611043.pdf>; March 2019 Accessed 02.01.20.
8. PAS 96. *Guide Protecting Defending Food Drink Deliberate Attack*. London: BSI; 2017.
9. Spink J, Moyer DC, Park H, Heinonen JA. Defining the types of counterfeiters, counterfeiting and offender organizations. *Crime Sci*. 2013;2:8.
10. FDA. Food defense. Available at: <https://www.fda.gov/Food/FoodDefense/default.htm>; 2020a Accessed 02.01.20.
11. Bogadi NP, Banović M, Babić I. Food defence system in food industry: perspective of the EU countries. *J Verbraucherschutz Lebensmittelsicherheit*. 2016;11(3):217–226.
12. Davidson RK, Antunes W, Madslien EH, et al. From food defence to food supply chain integrity. *Br Food J*. 2017;119(1):52–66.
13. Bandal S, Singh A, Mangal M, Mangal AK, Kumar S. Food adulteration: sources, health risks, and detection methods. *Crit Rev Food Sci Nutr*. 2017;57(6):1174–1189. Available from: http://doi.org/10.1080/10408398.2014.967834.
14. Kowalska A, Soon JM, Manning L. A study on adulteration in cereals and bakery products from Poland including a review of definitions. *Food Control*. 2018;92:348–356.
15. European Commission. 2019 Annual report. The EU Food Fraud Network and the Administrative Assistance and Cooperation System. Available at: <https://ec.europa.eu/food/sites/food/files/safety/docs/ff_ffn_annual-report_2019.pdf>; 2019.

16. Walklate S. *Understanding Criminology*. Buckingham: Open University Press; 2007.
17. Cohen L, Felson M. Social change and crime rate trends: a routine activity approach. *Am Sociol Rev*. 1979;44(4):588–608.
18. Hirschauer N, Zwoll S. Understanding and managing behavioural risks: the case of malpractice in poultry production. *Eur J Law Econ*. 2008;26:27–60.
19. Hirschi T. *Causes of Delinquency*. Berkeley: University of California Press; 1969.
20. Pease, K. Rational choice theory. In, McLaughlin, E. and Muncie, J. (eds.). *The Sage Dictionary of Criminology*. London: Sage; 2006.
21. Spink J, Moyer DC, Park H, Heinonen JA. Development of a product-counterfeiting incident cluster tool. *Crime Sci*. 2014;3:3.
22. Canter DV. Offender profiling and criminal differentiation. *Leg Crim Psychol*. 2000;5(1):23–46.
23. Canter D. Offender profiles. *Psychologist*. 1989;2:12–16.
24. Lopes LO, Silva R, Guimarães JT, et al. Food defense: perceptions and attitudes of Brazilian dairy companies. *J Dairy Sci*. 2020;103(9):8675–8682.
25. de Abreu VLF, Silva R, Luchese R, Monteiro SS, Esmerino EA, Mathias SP. Impact assessment of the implementation of food defense plan in a Brazilian army military organization. *Food Control*. 2020;107288. Available from: https://doi.org/10.1016/j.foodcont.2020.107288.
26. Dalziel GR. Food defense incidents 1950–2008: a chronology and analysis of incidents involving the malicious contamination of the food supply chain. Report. Centre of Excellence for National Security (CENS). S Rajaratnam School of International Studies, Nanyang Technology University, Singapore; 2009.
27. Elad D. Risk assessment of malicious biocontamination of food. *J Food Prot*. 2005;68(6):1302–1305.
28. Fredrickson NR. Food security: food defense and biosecurity. *Encycl Agric Food Syst*. 2014;3:311–323.
29. Manning L, Baines RN, Chadd SA. Deliberate contamination of the food supply chain. *Br Food J*. 2005;107(4):225–245.
30. Meulenbelt S. Assessing chemical, biological, radiological and nuclear threats to the food supply chain. *Glob Security: Health Sci Policy*. 2018;3(1):14–27.
31. Banjari I. *Food and bioterrorism–the case of airline catering. Defence Against Bioterrorism*. Dordrecht: Springer; 2018:229–237.
32. Baybutt P. Assessing risks from threats to process plants: threat and vulnerability analysis. *Process Saf Prog*. 2002;21(4):269–275.
33. Felson. M & Clarke, RV. Opportunity makes the thief: practical theory for crime prevention police research series paper 98. London: Home Office. <https://pdfs.semanticscholar.org/09db/dbce90b22357d58671c41a50c8c2f5dc1cf0.pdf>; 1998.
34. Muckin M, Fitch SC. *A Threat-Driven Approach to Cyber Security*. Lockheed Martin Corporation. Available at: <https://pdfs.semanticscholar.org/dc7e/99de96c622dea52701a1a70172e532969b89.pdf>; 2019.
35. Ambrose ML, Seabright MA, Schminke M. Sabotage in the workplace: the role of organizational injustice. *Organ Behav Hum Decis Process*. 2002;89(1):947–965. Available from: https://doi.org/10.1016/S0749-5978(02)00037-7.
36. Moorman RH. Relationship between organizational justice and organizational citizenship behaviors: do fairness perceptions influence employee citizenship? *J Appl Psychol*. 1991;76(6):845. Available from: http://doi.org/10.1037/0021-9010.76.6.845.
37. Van Arnam RC. Business war: economic espionage in the United States and the European Union and the need for greater trade secret protection. *NCJ Int'l L & Com Reg*. 2001;27:95.
38. Crane A. In the company of spies: when competitive intelligence gathering becomes industrial espionage. *Bus Horiz*. 2005;48(3):233–240.
39. Budiono GL, Sawitri NN. Strategic business espionage: an ethics and business practices to gain opportunity or community problems. *Stud Bus Econ*. 2017;12(1):29–39.
40. Fisher D. New cases of tainted baby food plague Britons. Available at: <http://articles.latimes.com/1989-04-28/news/mn-1925_1_baby-food-new-cases-heinz-baby>; 1989 Accessed 01.01.20.
41. UPI. Woman eats poisoned fish in extortion plot. Available at: <https://www.upi.com/Top_News/2003/07/01/Woman-eats-poisoned-fish-in-extortion-plot/20021057097512/>; 2003 Accessed 01.10.20.
42. Manhire T. New Zealand prime minister says poison threat to milk powder 'ecoterrorism'. *The Guardian* 10th March 2015. Available at: <https://www.theguardian.com/world/2015/mar/10/new-zealand-prime-minister-poison-threat-milk-powder-ecoterrorism>; 2015 Accessed 01.01. 20.
43. BBC. New Zealand man jailed for milk formula 1080 threat. Available at: <https://www.bbc.co.uk/news/world-asia-35878645>; 2016 Accessed 01.01.20.
44. Cooney TP, Varelis P, Bendall JG. High-throughput quantification of monofluoroacetate (1080) in milk as a response to an extortion threat. *J Food Prot*. 2016;79(2):273–281.
45. Smith L. £2 million blackmail plotter claimed he had laced supermarket food with cyanide. Available at: <https://www.mirror.co.uk/news/trials/2million-blackmail-plotter-claimed-laced-8751269>; 2016 Accessed 01.01.20.
46. Licea M. Man charged with poisoning baby food in extortion plot. Available at: <https://nypost.com/2017/09/30/man-charged-with-poisoning-baby-food-in-extortion-plot/>; 2017 Accessed 01.01.20.
47. BBC. Poisoned baby food: German jailed for attempted murder. Available at: <https://www.bbc.co.uk/news/amp/world-europe-45951642>; 2018 Accessed 01.01.20.
48. Rojas N. Man puts lethal poison into baby food to blackmail supermarkets in €10 million extortion plot. Available at: <https://www.ibtimes.co.uk/man-puts-lethal-poison-into-baby-food-blackmail-supermarkets-10m-extortion-plot-1641233>; 2017 Accessed 01.01.20.
49. FSA (Food Standards Agency). Heinz and Tesco recall 7 + months Heinz By Nature baby food jars because a product purchased from Tesco has been tampered with.Available at: <https://www.food.gov.uk/news-alerts/alert/fsa-prin-52-2019>; 2019 Accessed 01.01.20.
50. Crino, MD. Employee sabotage: a random or preventable phenomenon? J Manag Issues, 311-330; 1994.
51. Fiorino M, Barone C, Barone M, Mason M, Bhagat A. *Chemical additives for foods. Impact of food-related quality system certifications on the management of working flows. Quality Systems in the Food Industry*. Cham: Springer; 2019:1–27.
52. Koc M, Jernigan C, Das R. Food security and food sovereignty in Iraq: the impact of war and sanctions on the civilian population. *Food Cult Soc*. 2007;10(2):317–348.
53. Robinson SL, Bennett RJ. A typology of deviant workplace behaviors: a multidimensional scaling study. *Acad Manag J*. 1995;38(2):555–572.

54. Krischer MM, Penney LM, Hunter EM. Can counterproductive work behaviors be productive? CWB as emotion-focused coping. *J Occup Health Psychol.* 2010;15(2):154.
55. Spector, PE & Fox, S. The stressor–emotion model of counterproductive work behaviour. In S. Fox & P. Spector (Eds.), Counterproductive Work Behavior: Investigations of Actors and Targets (pp. 151–174). Washington, DC: American Psychological Association; 2005.
56. Zhou X, Ma J, Dong X. Empowering supervision and service sabotage: a moderated mediation model based on conservation of resources theory. *Tour Manag.* 2018;64:170–187.
57. Huang YSS, Greenbaum RL, Bonner JM, Wang CS. Why sabotage customers who mistreat you? Activated hostility and subsequent devaluation of targets as a moral disengagement mechanism. *J Appl Psychol.* 2019;104(4):495.
58. Marsh J. Strawberry needle scare: woman allegedly spiked punnets for revenge. Available at: <https://edition.cnn.com/2018/11/12/australia/australia-strawberry-needle-intl/index.html>; 2018 Accessed 29.12.19.
59. Pearlman J. Australian woman accused of planting needles in strawberries 'motivated by spite'. Available at: <https://www.telegraph.co.uk/news/2018/11/12/australian-woman-accused-planting-needles-strawberries-motivated/>; 2018 Accessed 01.01.20.
60. Siddique H. Strawberry needle sabotage scare spreds to all six Australian states. Available at: <https://www.theguardian.com/australia-news/2018/sep/17/australian-police-say-needle-found-in-banana-as-strawberry-sabotage-spreads>; 2018 Accessed 02.01.20.
61. FSANZ (Food Standards Australia New Zealand). Strawberry tampering incident – report to government. Available at: <https://www.foodstandards.gov.au/publications/SiteAssets/Pages/Strawberry-tampering-incident/FSANZ%20Strawberry%20Report%20doc.pdf>; 2018 Accessed 02.01.20.
62. CTV News. CFIA adds three more products to needle list. Available at: <https://toronto.ctvnews.ca/cfia-adds-three-more-products-to-needle-list-1.381079>; 2009 Accessed 02.01.20.
63. Foodsafetyblog. Toronto Police Service issue public safety alert for food product tampering. Available at: <https://foodsafetychat.blogspot.com/2010/06/toronto-police-service-issue-public.html>; 2010 Accessed 02.01.20.
64. JapanTimes. Needles turning up in food items. Available at: <https://www.japantimes.co.jp/news/2010/04/02/national/needles-turning-up-in-food-items/#.Xg3QCkf7RRZ>; 2010 Accessed 02.01.20.
65. BBC. Needle found in Air Canada sandwich. Available at: <https://www.bbc.co.uk/news/world-us-canada-19081953>; 2012 Accessed 02.01.20.
66. RASFF (Risk Assessment for Food and Feed) Portal. Available at: <https://webgate.ec.europa.eu/rasff-window/portal/>; 2020 Accessed 02.01.20.
67. CFIA Canadian Food Inspection Agency. Food safety warning – suspected food tampering in potatoes. Available at: <https://www.inspection.gc.ca/food-recall-warnings-and-allergy-alerts/2015-05-21/eng/1432249577183/1432249579929>; 2015 Accessed 02.01.20.
68. Pace N. Police investigating two cases of food tampering in Halifax after thumbtack, needle found. Available at: <https://globalnews.ca/news/3120043/police-investigating-two-cases-of-food-tampering-in-halifax-after-thumbtack-needle-found/>; 2016 Accessed 02.01.20.
69. CBC News. Sewing pins found in meat products sold in Nanaimo grocery stores. Available at: <https://www.cbc.ca/news/canada/british-columbia/food-tampering-1.4642174>; 2018 Accessed 02.01.20.
70. Offer K. Woman claims to have found needle in grapes bought from Aldi supermarket in Melbourne's west. Available at: <https://www.news.com.au/lifestyle/food/food-warnings/woman-claims-to-have-found-needle-in-grapes-bought-from-aldi-supermarket-in-melbournes-west/news-story/7f34d9009161626ee6a945472d601dfd>; 2019 Accessed 02.01.20.
71. EUROPOL. European Union Terrorism Situation and Trend Report 2017. Available at: <https://www.europol.europa.eu/sites/default/files/documents/tesat2017_0.pdf>; 2017 Accessed 2.01.20.
72. Michalopoulos S. Food and drinks withdrawn from Greek supermarkets after poisoning threat. Available at: <https://www.euractiv.com/section/agriculture-food/news/food-and-drinks-withdrawn-from-greek-supermarkets-after-poisoning-threat/>; 2016 Accessed 02.01.20.
73. Wilson TM, Logan-Henfrey L, Weller R, Kellman B. Agroterrorism, biological crimes and biowarfare targeting animal agriculture. In: Brown C, Bolin C, eds. *Emerging Diseases of Animals.* Washington, DC: ASM Press; 2000:23–57.
74. World Health Organization. *Terrorist Threats to Food: Guidance for Establishing and Strengthening Prevention and Response Systems.* Food Safety Programme. World Health Organization; 2002. ISBN 9241545844.
75. Carus WS. *Bioterrorism and Biocrimes: The Illicit Use of Biological Agents in the 20th Century.* Washington, DC: Center for Counter-Proliferation Research, National Defense University; 1999.
76. Sobel J, Khan AS, Swerdlow DL. Threat of a biological terrorist attack on the US food supply: the CDC perspective. *Lancet.* 2002;359(9309):874–880.
77. Mohammed D. US healthcare industry: cybersecurity regulatory and compliance issues. *J Res Bus Econ Manag.* 2017;9(5):1771–1776.
78. Werder KP. Responding to activism: an experimental analysis of public relations strategy influence on attributes of publics. *J Public Relat Res.* 2006;18(4):335–356.
79. Grunig JE. *Excellence in Public Relations and Communication Management.* Hillsdale, NJ: Lawrence Erlbaum Associates, Inc; 1992.
80. Manion M, Goodrum A. Terrorism or civil disobedience: toward a hacktivist ethic. *ACM SIGCAS Comput Soc.* 2000;30(2):14–19.
81. Van Niekerk B. An analysis of cyber-incidents in South Africa. *Afr J Inf Commun (AJIC).* 2017;20:113–132.
82. Levy BS, Sidel VW. *Terrorism and Public Health: A Balanced Approach to Strengthening Systems & Protecting People.* 2nd ed. New York, NY: Oxford University Press Inc.; 2012.
83. US Code Title 22 Chapter 38 2656f – Annual country reports on terrorism. Available at: <https://www.law.cornell.edu/uscode/text/22/2656f>; Accessed 02.01.20.
84. Nestle M. *Safe Food: Bacteria, Biotechnology and Bioterrorism.* London: University of California Press Ltd; 2003.
85. Alvarez MJ, Alvarez A, De Maggio MC, Oses A, Trombetta M, Setola R. *Protecting the food supply chain from terrorist attack. International Conference on Critical Infrastructure Protection.* Berlin, Heidelberg: Springer; 2010, March:157–167.

86. Haleem A, Khan S, Khan MI. Traceability implementation in food supply chain: a grey-DEMATEL approach. *Inf Process Agric.* 2019;6:335–348.
87. Grieco, D.F. Closing the barn door: Interagency approaches to reduce agroterrorism threats. Interagency Journal. 2015;6(2), 10. Available at https://thesimonscenter.org/wp-content/uploads/2015/05/IAJ-6-2-Spring-2015-28-37.pdf
88. Monke J. *Agroterrorism: Threats and Preparedness.* Washington, DC: Library of Congress, Congressional Research Service; 2007.
89. Jansen HJ, Breeveld FJ, Stijnis C, Grobusch MP. Biological warfare, bioterrorism, and biocrime. *Clin Microbiol Infect.* 2014;20 (6):488–496. Available from: https://doi.org/10.1111/1469-0691.12699.
90. Public Health Emergency. Public Health and Emergency Support for a Nation prepared. Available at: <https://www.phe.gov/emergency/bioterrorism/Pages/default.aspx>; 2020 Accessed 01.01.20.
91. Green S, Ellis T, Jung J, Lee J. Vulnerability, risk and agroterrorism: an examination of international strategy and its relevance for the Republic of Korea. *Crime Prev Community Saf.* 2017;19(1): 31–45.
92. Thomas J. A quick glance at agroterrorism response. Available at: <https://papers.ssrn.com/sol3/papers.cfm?abstract_id = 3175579>; 2018 Accessed 02.01.20.
93. van Ruth SM, Huisman W, Luning PA. Food fraud vulnerability and its key factors. *Trends Food Sci Technol.* 2017;67:70–75.
94. Roy HE, Peyton J, Aldridge DC, et al. Horizon scanning for invasive alien species with the potential to threaten biodiversity in Great Britain. *Glob Change Biol.* 2014;20(12):3859–3871.
95. Smith K, Byrne R. Horizon scanning rural crime in England. *Crime Prev Community Saf.* 2019;1–15.
96. Stanley MC, Beggs JR, Bassett IE, et al. Emerging threats in urban ecosystems: a horizon scanning exercise. *Front Ecol Environ.* 2015;13(10):553–560.
97. Soon JM, Krzyzaniak SC, Shuttlewood Z, Smith M, Jack L. Food fraud vulnerability assessment tools used in food industry. *Food Control.* 2019;101:225–232.
98. Talluri S, Kull TJ, Yildiz H, Yoon J. Assessing the efficiency of risk mitigation strategies in supply chains. *J Bus Logist.* 2013; 34(4):253–269.
99. Wiśniewska MZ. HACCP-based food defense systems. *J Manag Financ.* 2015;13:106–119.
100. Olson D. Agroterrorism threats to America's economy and food supply. FBI Law Enforcement Bulletin; February 2012.
101. Spink J, Moyer DC, Park H, et al. Introduction to food fraud including translation and interpretation to Russian, Korean and Chinese languages. *Food Chem.* 2015;189:102–107.
102. Manning L. Development of a food safety verification risk model. *Br Food J.* 2013;115(4):575–589.
103. Hollis ME, Wilson JM. Who are the guardians in product counterfeiting? A theoretical application of routine activities theory. *Crime Prev Community Saf.* 2014;16(3):169–188.
104. Reynald DM. Guardianship in action: developing a new tool for measurement. *Crime Prev Community Saf.* 2009;1(1):1–20.
105. Soon JM, Manning L, Smith R. Advancing understanding of pinchpoints and crime prevention in the food supply chain. *Crime Prev Community Saf.* 2019;21(1):1–19.
106. Spink J, Chen W, Zhang G, Speier-Pero C. Introducing the Food Fraud Prevention Cycle (FFPC): a dynamic information management and strategic roadmap. *Food Control.* 2019;105: 233–241.
107. Leistner L, Gorris LG. Food preservation by hurdle technology. *Trends Food Sci Technol.* 1995;6(2):41–46.
108. Khan I, Tango CN, Miskeen S, Lee BH, Oh DH. Hurdle technology: a novel approach for enhanced food quality and safety–a review. *Food Control.* 2017;73:1426–1444.
109. Mitenius, N, Kennedy SP, Busta FF. *Food* Defense, Food Safety Management: A Practical Guide for the Food Industry. Motarjemi Y., & Lelieveld H., editors. 1st ed Academic Press, Elsevier, ISBN 9780123815040. p 937–958; 2014.
110. van Ruth SM, Luning PA, Silvis ICJ, Yang Y, Huisman W. Differences in fraud vulnerability in various food supply chains and their tiers. *Food Control.* 2018;84:375–381.
111. Bendovschi A. Cyber-attacks—trends, patterns and security countermeasures. *Procedia Econ Financ.* 2015;28:24–31.
112. Whitworth E, Druckman A, Woodward A. Food scares: a comprehensive categorisation. *British Food Journal.* 2017;119(1): 131–142. Available from: https://doi.org/10.1108/BFJ-06-2016-0263.

Chapter 37

Sampling, testing methodologies, and their implication in risk assessment, including interpretation of detection limits

Carolina Ripolles-Avila, Brayan R.H. Cervantes-Huamán and José Juan Rodríguez-Jerez

Area of Human Nutrition and Food Science, Departament de Ciència Animal i dels Aliments, Facultat de Veterinària, Universitat Autònoma de Barcelona, Barcelona, Spain

Abstract

One of the most important actions related to the prevention of foodborne diseases and implemented by all food industries with the aim of protecting the health of consumers is the continuous control of food pathogens and other microbial indicators in food products. Analytical determinations of the presence of pathogens in food serve to find a relationship between production systems and their level of food safety. This chapter focuses on addressing a problem often related to the design of food tests and the interpretation of results that aim to achieve an optimal assessment of the safety of commercially marketed foods. The intention is to show what food sampling consists of, to deepen on the existing analytical methodologies with an industrial perspective, and to present a simple statistical approach using examples which will help in the decision making of food companies concerned about the safety of the products they produce and wanting to perform well in their analytical costs.

Keywords: *Listeria monocytogenes*; sampling; analytical methods; pathogen control; results interpretation; descriptive statistics

37.1 Introduction

An important increase in food demand worldwide is expected by 2050 in the light of estimates that the world population will potentially reach around 9.8 billion.[1] A greater food production will likewise be expected and will absolutely be a key to satisfying this demand. This food should not only be nutritious, readily available, and simple to access, but it should also be innocuous for the consumer. In this regard, consumers' growing concern about food safety and quality, mainly due to scares like bovine spongiform encephalopathy, horse meat burgers instead of beef burgers, fipronil in eggs, the South African listeriosis outbreak have forced the public and private food sectors to develop higher standards in relation to food safety and quality.[2,3] Due to the pressure exerted by both consumers, who are increasingly concerned about health, and by the competent authorities responsible for ensuring that foodborne diseases do not occur, microbiological and chemical control from the production of food to its marketing will be essential. Notably, food products can easily become contaminated throughout the production chain via unsanitary surfaces, poor handling, and improper food processing.[4,5] If the food in question becomes contaminated, does not undergo exhaustive control by the food operator and ends up being marketed, outbreaks can occur followed by the associated public and economic burdens. To this effect, the control of pathogenic microorganisms and chemical hazards along the food chain would lead to significant reductions in the transmitted foodborne diseases resulting from the consumption of contaminated food.[6,7]

For microbial and chemical food control, both the sampling and the analytical techniques used become a key aspect for obtaining results and for the subsequent decision making process.[8] To this end, this chapter focuses on addressing a problem often related to the design of food analysis and the interpretation of results that aim to achieve an optimal assessment of the safety of the foods placed in the market. Sampling is considered as the mainstay of analysis and its interpretation as the basis of food safety, differentiating between quantitative and qualitative measures.[9] Sometimes when sampling, there are many errors that lead

Present Knowledge in Food Safety. DOI: https://doi.org/10.1016/B978-0-12-819470-6.00022-6

to poor management decisions. Among the most common are a smaller number of samples than are required, nonrepresentative samples (e.g., not random), badly labeled samples, improper storage, and storage not in accordance with the legislation, among others.[10] Each type of food is different and is not always homogeneous, and so the sampling plan must be adapted to the stated objectives. Firstly, regarding avoiding to commit these types of errors, and given that it must be guaranteed at all times, compliance with the legislation cannot be the sole objective. The main objective is to make a safe product and to do so, statistical resources that have not previously been considered and will be discussed further in the following sections must be used.

In parallel, it is also important to focus on the analytical methods for food control. To this end, conventional methods, rapid methods, and the perspective of the food industry when selecting one type or another will be discussed in this chapter. Research into detecting pathogenic microorganisms has led to countless articles and a significant investment by companies in the sector trying to introduce appropriate systems in the market.[8,11–13] To this effect, a week of laboratory work has traditionally been needed to achieve a good detection of pathogenic microorganisms through laboratory analysis. For years, research into new techniques has focused on reducing this time, obtaining at best a reduction of upto 24 h in obtaining analysis results, and always in specialized laboratories.[14] It is only recently that immune, genetic, electrical systems, and nanotechnology approaches, among others, have begun to combine for trying to give an earlier response.[8] Faced with the imminent need to obtain rapid results to be able to take decisions regarding releasing a lot or to apply more extensive cleaning and disinfection programs, the food industry must rely on rapid detection methodologies.[15] Food companies include this aspect as an important factor when choosing testing methodologies.

This chapter addresses the concepts of sampling, descriptive statistics, the conceptual difference between independent and repeated measures, the importance of the food safety objective (FSO), and interpretation of the frequency of presentation of a pathogen depending on the measure of the sample and the results history. Applicable testing methodologies are also discussed from a food industry perspective, and an example case is described to provide a practical view. It is hoped that this information will help the industry and facilitate decision making.

37.2 Importance of the hazard analysis and critical control points plan and legislation

In food safety, the implementation of the hazard analysis and critical control points (HACCP) plan guarantees the control of the processes, and the microbiological criteria allow their effectiveness to be validated.[16] In Europe, food regulations indicate that safety must be ensured through a preventive approach, with the implementation of prerequisites and the application of procedures based on the principles of HACCP as a crucial system.[17] Its implementation strengthens the positions of companies and improves their competitiveness. However, it is generally accepted that small and medium manufacturers find it difficult to implement food safety management systems.[18,19] Lack of knowledge and motivation, and confidence in food safety legislation together with scarce financial resources and human resource limitations are the main barriers to meeting the requirements demanded by official control.[20]

The importance of the HACCP plan is that it is a guarantee for food safety and is considered as the basis and the most effective tool for standardized schemes for food safety management[19] such as the International Standard ISO 22000, BRC, and IFS.[21,22] However, obstacles and barriers to its implementation and/or effective application have been identified and mainly include financial, technical, managerial, organizational, educational, and psychological limitations.[23] The bureaucratic aspects of HACCP, with its excessive and complicated documentation, has also been identified as one of the main barriers to its implementation.[21,23]

HACCP is a scientific and systematic program applied in the food sector to identify and control food hazards.[24] It covers two main components, hazard analysis and the critical limit control measures.[25] Hazard analysis is the process of identifying and evaluating potential food hazards that can negatively affect food safety, while control measures are designed to prevent and eliminate hazards or reduce them to an acceptable level.[26] The HACCP system has been widely implemented by developed countries due to its success in preventing food hazards. It is currently compulsory in many countries for food manufacturers to work in accordance with Codex HACCP principles,[27] hence there is a relevance of understanding the importance of sampling and its integration into the HACCP system. It is also important to know the analytical methods used to obtain results and how these are collected in historical laboratory analyses to create alerts that enable action to be taken when facing a critical performance and not unnecessarily. The generation of a historical record and other information to do with the performance of the applied processes, and the history of the product feeds the food safety management system and helps to keep food safety in finished products under control.[28] To this effect, those responsible for quality departments are required to be critical and take global perspectives.

37.3 Sampling program and plans

To determine food quality and safety, a sample must be taken and analyzed under the assumption that the results obtained from the sample will reflect the entire lot from which it was taken. The validity of this extrapolation will depend on the representativeness of the samples and the accuracy and precision of the analysis,[9] hence the importance of establishing an adequate sampling plan. A microbiological criterion is needed to determine if a food product is of good enough quality and is safe, and to follow up good manufacturing practices, shelf life, and the usefulness or suitability of a food or ingredient for a certain purpose.[29]

According to the International Commission for the Microbiological Specification of Foods,[30] the following five factors should be considered in the microbiological criterion: a description of the food to which the criterion applies since by differing in origin, composition, and processing, each foodstuff can have a different decomposition and safety problems; a description of the microorganisms or toxins capable of causing problems; details of analytical methods to detect or quantify microorganisms or toxins; the number and sample size that must be taken from a production lot; and the appropriate microbiological limits depending on the food and the microorganism to be evaluated.

It is recommended that food processing industries have a sampling program to verify the efficiency and effectiveness of their practices (i.e., GMP),[31,32] within which the sampling plan must be established, indicating the sample size and the evaluation criteria, which will depend on the aspect to be analyzed and the category of the quality characteristic to be observed or measured. Furthermore, an appropriate sampling plan must include a sampling procedure and decision criteria and be described by the following values: "*n*," which is the number of units to be analyzed, and "*c*," which is the maximum number of acceptable units between "*m*," which is the microbiological level that separates good quality from defective quality, and "*M*," which separates marginally acceptable from unacceptable quality. A sampling plan is stricter when higher the value of "*n*" and lower the value of "*c*."

37.3.1 Number and size of samples

There is no specific legislation establishing how many samples to take in accordance to statistical adequacy, or any rule that determines the exact number. However, there are working guides that can be of great help, including the "General guidelines on sampling CAC/GL 50–2004" of the *Codex Alimentarius*.

In food safety management, sampling plays an important role in verifying the microbial control. Valero et al.[33] concluded that the concentration of microorganisms in the sample affects the number of samples to be analyzed for some range of concentrations. Subtracting a large number of small units provides greater protection than subtracting the same total sample weight in fewer units. What is relevant is not the subtraction of a fraction of the lot, but the size of the sample taken at random and the acceptance and rejection criteria. Where there is increased risk, the number and size of the units should also be increased to minimize the probability of accepting a lot that should be rejected.[9] The lower the uniformity, the greater the number of samples that need to be subtracted. Sample size is critical in presence or absence analysis situations.

37.3.2 Selection based on attributes or variables: the decision making process

There are two different types of sampling plans, known as plans by attributes and plans by variables. In this regard, one-attribute, two-class, or three-class plans are used for microbiological examinations, while both attributes and variables are used for physical and chemical examinations.[10] These types of plans are defined according to FAO[34]:

- Attribute sampling plan: applied for qualitative determinations (i.e., absence or presence), the units are classified according to the quality characteristics of the product. In the case of microbiological controls, the quality characteristic would be "absence." An example of this is the case of *Salmonella* spp. in current legislation.
- Variable sampling plan: The concentrations of the parameters of interest, such as the specific level of a certain microorganism, are measured. By doing so, whether the microorganism is found within certain limits will be determined and the production batch under evaluation will be accepted or rejected. An example of this is the case of *Listeria monocytogenes* for ready-to-eat foods marketed during their shelf life.

The next question is whether to choose a plan by attributes or a plan by variables. At first glance, attribute plans are easier to implement since they are based on the presence or absence of a pathogen, whereby the lot is rejected if it is present and accepted if it is not detected. On the other hand, in the variables plan, small samples are needed and work is based on a mean and a standard deviation. Variable plans have been shown to be more effective with the same number of samples and the same acceptable quality level.[34]

Several factors must be considered when choosing a sampling plan: microbiological, epidemiological, and ecological factors, the probability of accepting or rejecting a lot, the limitations of the food industry (e.g., personnel and equipment, among others), and economic factors.[35] Since attribute plans are less efficient with a larger sample size required, they are more expensive.[10] When a parameter is not quantifiable an attribute plan is selected because, as mentioned above, it is a qualitative parameter. Likewise, when a parameter is quantifiable but there is doubt as to whether its distribution is within the normality, an attribute plan is chosen.[34] Contrarily, if we know that its distribution fits within the normality, the by variables sampling plan is selected. When the sample size is greater than 30 this can be ignored, but in many cases, companies do not want to analyze such a large number of samples because in practice this limits their decision making capacity.

37.3.3 Two-class sampling plans

In these plans, once the units have been analyzed, the sample is divided into two classes with the amount that divides acceptable from defective represented by "*m*." Units for which values between 0 and "*m*" are obtained are considered acceptable. Units for which values greater than "*m*" are obtained are considered defective.[36]

If a parameter poses a risk to the consumer, the sampling plan is much more rigorous. The treatment received by the product in the following phases must be considered since this may increase or decrease the risk.[10] In this case, there should be varying permissiveness since what is important is not the simple presence of a hazard, but the real risk to the health of potential consumers. For example, European legislation marks $n = 5$ for the general population, but when analyzing products aimed at a more sensitive population, such as babies or newborns, the n value rises to 10 or even 30. Similarly, if "*c*" decreases, the rigor of the plan increases (i.e., less permissive, less risk).[36]

37.3.4 Three-class sampling plans

These are plans in which the sample is divided into three classes after analysis of the units. The units for which values between 0 and *m* are obtained are considered acceptable. Units for which values between *m* and *M* are obtained are considered marginally acceptable. Units for which higher values of *M* are obtained are considered defective. There are various advantages of using the three-class plans. Firstly, based on practical experience, even observing GMP, some units can result in the marginally acceptable range without causing any problems, and can be accepted. Secondly, they are less affected by changes in the distribution of microorganisms within a flock due to unknown causes. And thirdly, they allow warning increases in risks if there is an increasing trend in the number of marginally acceptable units.

37.4 Testing methodologies: approaches to pathogen detection

The human cost of eating microbiologically unsafe food is the development of certain foodborne diseases which, in severe cases, can lead to death. Food products must therefore be controlled by the food industry and the competent authorities. One of the tools to do so is the microbiological analysis of food products, which is related to the application of methods for the detection, identification, and enumeration of microorganisms or chemical agents that may be present in food products.[8,35] Notably, failure to comply with the parameters set forth in Regulation 2073/2005 requires the immediate withdrawal of the product, including if it has already been distributed, and implies that microbiological analysis must be carried out prior to the release of any lot in the market.[36]

There are many methods to evaluate the microbiological content of food available to the food industry. They can be divided into conventional or traditional methods and rapid methods. Traditional or conventional methods for the microbiological analysis of food are those that have remained practically the same for many years, require the cultivation of the microorganism, and are normally included as ISO standards.[14] There are different strategies to achieve a reliable result more quickly, some of which are completely manual, which implies having sufficient human resources, while others allow a certain degree of automation, thereby increasing the laboratory's capacity to process a greater number of samples in less time. However, it also implies a significant economic investment to acquire the equipment.[37] Rapid methods for the microbiological examination of food can therefore be divided into two groups: (1) those that achieve a result more quickly than a traditional method; and (2) those that process more samples than a traditional technique in the same period.[38,39] Over the last two decades, these methods have been subject to constant advances, which have been accepted by the food industry and relied upon to make associated decisions regarding the release of a lot[8] or the appropriate measures to be taken, such as the cleaning and disinfection of industrial surfaces.[15]

All the stages in the food chain involved in any action related to food processing are responsible for the final safety and quality of the products, encompassing a "*from farm to fork*" perspective.[40] It is important to use reliable methods that involve as short an analysis time as possible to obtain rapid results, thus enabling decisions to be taken and public health problems prevented, in addition to accelerating the release of product batches in the market and consequently improving the product's availability and commercialization.

37.4.1 Conventional

Traditional microbial detection methods are still considered the "gold standard" by many food microbiology laboratories and regulatory agencies around the world.[14] These traditional methods are generally based on concepts and approaches developed in the early 20th century, and mostly examine the observable characteristics (i.e., phenotype) of microorganisms present in food. Nowadays, conventional methods appear to be unattractive methodologies, especially when compared with the novel technologies developed for the rapid detection of various pathogenic microorganisms in food products [41] or on industrial surfaces.[42] However, different food industries continue to rely on their use and on the official control of food made by the competent authorities, following the procedure indicated by the legislation (i.e., by the ISO reference). Food products can be released without risk and shelf life may be extended by some days if rapid results are obtained.[8] Furthermore, information on the efficient control of the process and how to avoid safety and quality issues can also be obtained if microbial detection is applied rapidly in the early stages of food processing.[43,44] Conventional methods would not fit with this objective.[8]

Traditional techniques for the microbiological analysis of food samples involve four different stages (Fig. 37.1). The first is the preenrichment stage, where enriched liquid media is generally fortified with determinate compounds useful to cultivate nutritionally demanding (stringent) microorganisms, such as meat extract. This stage allows the target microbes in a food sample to recover from the stress and/or damage that may have been caused by certain processing/conditions such as improper technology application and antimicrobial additives, among many others.[45] It also allows microorganisms to grow to detectable levels.[46] The second stage is considered as the selective enrichment phase, and the growth conditions applied are very restrictive so that only some microorganisms will be able to grow. This stage can be influenced by the presence of other microorganisms that can be resistant to the selective conditions of the media or limit the target pathogen so that it does not reach a minimum post-enrichment threshold level and goes undetected.[47] Hence, to diversify the change of a target microorganism to ensure its growth, different medias and cultivation conditions are sometimes created in parallel (e.g., the second step of the *Salmonella* spp. detection procedure, using conventional techniques). The third stage is the cultivation of the sample in a selective/differential medium. The inoculated medium is incubated under a defined set of conditions, including an appropriate temperature or gaseous environment, for a predetermined period, to allow distinctive colony formation by the target microbe. The final step of the detection procedure is the confirmatory testing, which requires the purification of the presumptive colony that needs to be tested for confirmation, making the procedure one day longer. In conventional methodologies, the confirmatory tests applied are those based on a biochemical perspective.[48]

As already pointed out, conventional methods have some limitations. In fact, the main limitations of these types of microbiological methods are that they are too slow, they are sometimes not totally reliable, they can fail to detect some microbes, they can be laborious, and they can also lack sensitivity and specificity.[8,14] These factors mean that traditional methods cannot deliver real time results and can therefore cause bottlenecks for the release of products from food companies. Hence, there is a need to develop more rapid but simpler, robust, and flexible methods for the detection and quantification of foodborne pathogens or indicator microorganisms (i.e., detection and quantification methodologies).

37.4.2 Rapid methods

There are several categories to classify commercially available rapid methods for the detection of foodborne pathogens, including but not limited to selective chromogenic media for the growth of the target pathogen, immunology-based assays, molecular assays, mass spectrometry (Fig. 37.2), and others that combine categories already mentioned with nanotechnology, sensors, etc. Research around the development of methods for rapid, accurate, and sensitive diagnosis to detect foodborne pathogens in food is ongoing because finding new

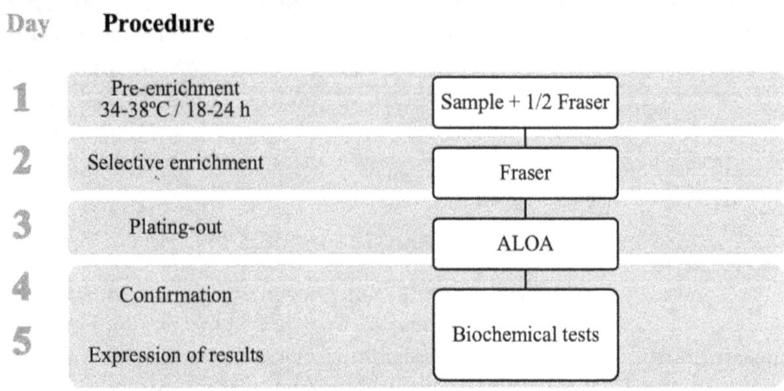

FIGURE 37.1 Diagram with the procedure steps for the detection of *Listeria* spp. and *Listeria monocytogenes* according to the EN ISO 11290–1:2017 standard.

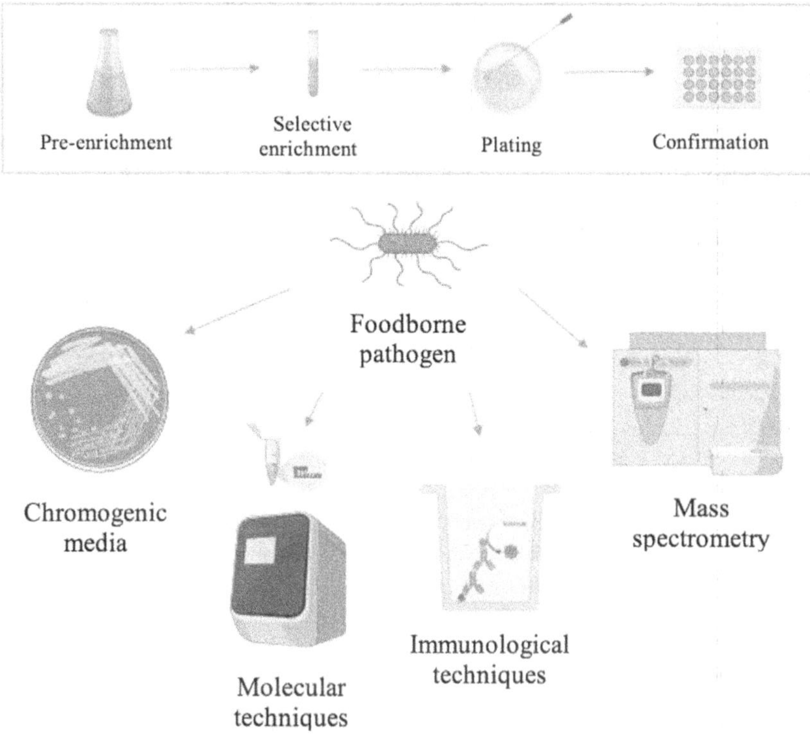

FIGURE 37.2 Overview of the conventional and alternative methods that can be employed for pathogen detection in food products.

methodologies would help the government to establish food safety policies or intervention strategies aimed at eliminating or mitigating the risk to the consumer, thus preventing outbreaks of foodborne illnesses.[8]

Starting with the first category, it is important to point out that culture media have evolved from basic to selective and differential, and include the use of chromogens for better selectivity and differentiation.[14] In their formulation, chromogenic media include chromogenic substrates that produce color when specific enzymatic activities for each microorganism are detected. Each color is characteristic of a specific microorganism, allowing for an easier and more precise differentiation than traditional culture media.[49] These culture media also enable the generalist and selective enrichment stages of the detection procedures to be merged in a single step, accelerating the time to obtain results. However, there are also disadvantages, the main one being that only species that are cultivable can be detected, meaning that it is not viable for the uncultivable ones, a microbial form with greater importance in recent times.[50] Immunoassays are based on specific mono or polyclonal antibodies used for the binding of somatic or flagellar antigens of the different foodborne pathogens. These assays have been widely used over time and are interesting as routine tests, partly due to their ability to detect pathogens in a viable but nonculturable state via a specific antigen-antibody interaction.[51] The problem is if these microbial species are not present at a sufficient level, making the previous enrichment stages still necessary since the detection limit of these methods is usually quite high, reaching upto 10^6-10^7 CFU/g.[8] Along this line of methodology, it is interesting to note that there has been intense research on the use of biotechnology to generate new forms of antibody preparation such as recombinant phage expression antibodies, and new recognition elements such as molecular imprinting polymers or aptamers.[52,53]

Rapid methods based on molecular detection using real-time PCR procedures allow the rapid and highly specific detection of most pathogens. Although the sensitivity of these techniques is usually greater than for the immunological ones, the interference of the matrix requires preenrichment procedures, although these are usually shorter than for procedures based on biochemical or immunological detection.[46,54] Following the discovery of PCR and fluorescence detection technology applications, the industry has opted for the constant development of new molecular tools that shorten detection time and are capable of providing a rapid response. In this context, it has opted for LAMP (*Loop-Mediated Isothermal Amplification*) technology, a system that relies on an isothermal nucleic acid amplification reaction directed at rRNA, using a specific endonuclease that works at medium temperature.[55] In the specific case of *L. monocytogenes*, rRNA is present in a much greater quantity in the cells of this pathogen than in conventional target DNA. This aspect implies that the enrichment stage can be greatly shortened. Detection occurs in real time, using a fluorescent molecular indicator.

Parallel to the detection of pathogens and as an integral part of the quality systems are the microbial quantification methods of certain indicator microorganisms. In this case, there are also fast and automated methodologies. One of the most used in the food industry is the Tempo system, based on estimation of the most probable count by number. The advantage it offers over a conventional plate count is the fact that the enumeration range is extended (for the plate count, the plates that obtain a count from 30 to 300 CFU/g, and for Tempo this limit is extended from 1 to 4900 CFU/g),[56] implying a reduction in the number of dilutions to obtain a count. At the same time, the quantification is carried out based on the fluorescence emitted after incubation since the reagents used are fluorogenic.[44] The results are automatically entered into a computer by means of a barcode reader, ensuring adaptation to the quality systems implemented in laboratories.

Lastly, it is important to highlight the fact that the use of a single analytical methodology for detection may not be enough for certain pathogens.[8] For example, in the case of the detection of *Campylobacter* spp., Hofreuter et al.[57] showed that this pathogen can vary from strain to strain, driven metabolically by the expression of virulence factors. This means that if the determination of these factors occurs at the molecular level, its detection will be problematic because it may not express such factors, despite molecular techniques being the most recommended for its evaluation. All this indicates that regardless of the very intense evolution of microbiological analysis methods in recent years, there is still a gap in terms of combining different methods with the aim of obtaining the most effective and efficient detection possible.

37.4.3 Industrial perspective

From the point of view of quality control, the microbiological contamination of food is one of the main concerns of most of the food industries in the world today.[42] It is therefore absolutely imperative to establish which microorganisms need to be detected or quantified, in which products, and with what reliability. To this effect, each region has a group of microorganisms that are of particular concern. Among them, at the EU level, is the control of *Salmonella* spp. and *L. monocytogenes*, in addition to *Campylobacter* spp. and *Escherichia coli*, and especially strains that fall within the enterotoxigenic group because these microorganisms have been described as the pathogens that cause the majority of foodborne diseases in the EU.[58] Campylobacteriosis and salmonellosis, in this order, correspond to the highest number of reported zoonoses, remaining stable since 2015. The third most frequent zoonosis is caused by Shiga toxin-producing *E. coli* (STEC), mainly associated with sources of beef and contaminated water. *Yersinia enterocolitica* infections, which may be associated with eating undercooked meat, are the fourth most frequently reported zoonosis in humans. Lastly, the number of confirmed cases of *L. monocytogenes* infections remained stable between 2015 and 2019, after a long period of increase, and continues to be the most serious zoonotic disease with the highest hospitalization (92%) and mortality rates (17.6%).[58] In other regions such as the United States, the pathogenic bacteria that cause most outbreaks are, in this order, *Salmonella* spp., followed by STEC, *Campylobacter* spp., and *Clostridium perfringens*.[59] Because of these differences, the food industry focuses on the analysis of one specific microbial target, which is why companies that develop analytical tests adapt to the needs of each region.

Regardless of the region, there is a common need among all types of food industries, namely the use of rapid methods to positively influence the speed of the associated decision making process.[8,12] To achieve fast and effective control, the techniques introduced in recent years have been the rapid methods. An important point from an industrial perspective when choosing a rapid method is to ensure that it has been subjected to comparative tests with the reference methods for their validation. On this regard, validation allows users of these procedures to be certain that the results will have the same validity as those obtained by the standard procedure.[12] Notably, however, the validation procedures are not universal for all food matrices, so there are alternative methods that can be validated to analyze specific matrices but not others.

Among the rapid techniques and from a food industry perspective, one that is extensively used is the immunological technique, together with molecular techniques. To this effect, molecular techniques require costly equipment and a properly equipped laboratory. Contrarily, immunological techniques can be applied in kit format in any situation and may not even require a specialized laboratory.[60,61] Techniques widely employed by immunological analysis protocols are the ELISA and the ELFA, which are not very effective in directly detecting pathogens in food. To achieve an optimal result, a preenrichment capable of increasing the number of viable microorganisms is essential to increase the signal and detect the presence of the pathogen.[8] In this case, a very relevant point for the food industry is the detection limits of the technique itself, which plays a fundamental role in the subsequent interpretation of results and the statistical study that must be carried out prior to making decisions related to the release of productive batches or other operations.

37.5 Risk assessment: the case of *Listeria monocytogenes* enumeration

37.5.1 Relevance of the pathogen and challenges for the food industry

L. monocytogenes is a Gram-positive bacterium that causes the disease known as listeriosis. Although its incidence is low,[58] it is seriously pathogenic, with the symptoms after infection ranging from febrile gastroenteritis in healthy individuals to serious infections such as septicemia, meningitis, encephalitis, or even death in groups considered at-risk.[62] In 98% of cases, the disease in humans is associated with strains of serotypes 1/2a, 1/2b, and 4b.[63] It should be noted that among the 13 serotypes identified so far, serotype 1/2a isolates are highly prevalent in food processing environments, while serotype 4b isolates have been shown to be more virulent.[64]

Regarding the infective dose, no clear relationship between dose and response has been able to be established, so its minimum infective dose has been fixed based on expert consultations, epidemiological data, and animal studies.[65] What has been demonstrated is that the minimum infective dose depends on individual factors such as age or the immune system, the most vulnerable population groups being the elderly, children, pregnant women, and immunosuppressed individuals.[66] Therefore the probability of a healthy person getting listeriosis depends on factors such as the vulnerability of the consumer, the virulence of the strain, the food matrix, and the concentration of the pathogen in it, establishing a direct relationship between the number of pathogenic cells and the probability of contracting the disease.[65] Once the bacteria has invaded the person, *L. monocytogenes* penetrates the intestine thus initiating an incubation period that can last between 1 and 90 days, complicating the identification of the origin of the infection.

The usual route of infection in humans is oral and the most common source is the ingestion of contaminated food. It should be noted that *L. monocytogenes* is capable of forming biofilms, which gives it resistance to adverse conditions and, consequently, makes it able to persist on food industry surfaces.[66,67] In fact, one of the main origins of its presence in food is cross-contamination from a contaminated food contact surface[42,68] (Fig. 37.3), making the implementation of integrated prevention systems combined with proper sanitation of food industries, especially surfaces and equipment, a requirement.[43]

Furthermore, it is essential to know what factors affect *L. monocytogenes* growth and survival to apply appropriate treatments to control the risk.[69] The factors capable of conditioning *L. monocytogenes* growth in food can be intrinsic or extrinsic. Its optimum growth temperature ranges between 30°C and 37°C, although it is also capable of growing at refrigeration temperatures of between 2°C and 4°C, and is able to reach high concentrations if the storage time is long.[70] In addition, it can survive at freezing temperatures of −18°C for several months, a factor that makes its control during storage periods essential. It has moderate heat resistance, making its elimination possible by applying a cooking process whereby a temperature of above 70°C is achieved in the center of the product for more than 2 min. The presence of the pathogen in products subjected to cooking processes is therefore usually due to recontamination after the cooking stage.[65] Furthermore, it has the ability to multiply within

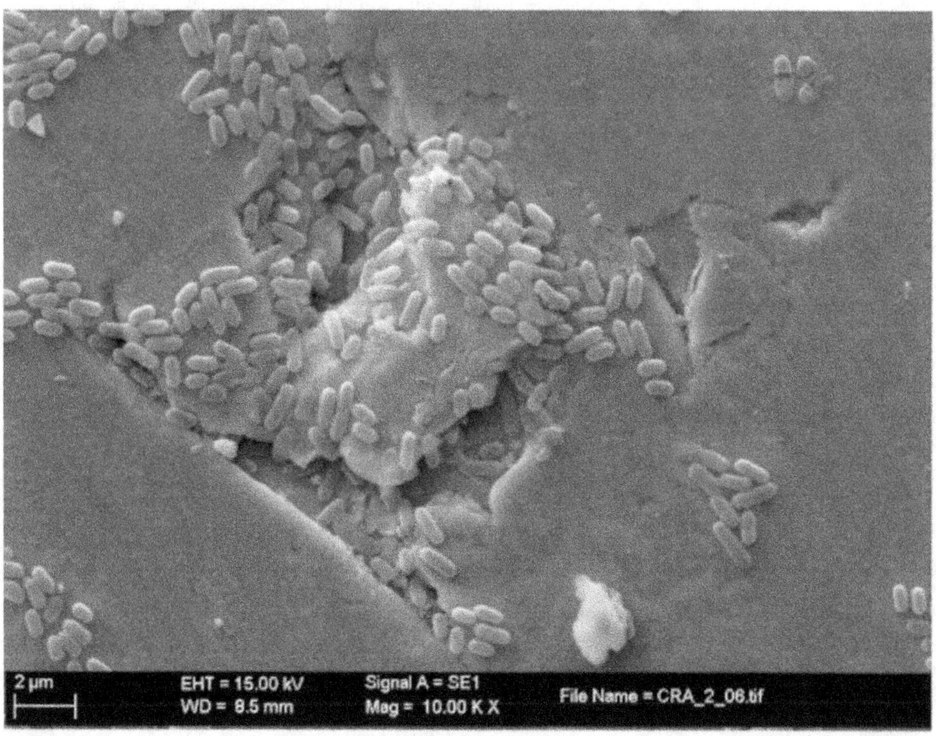

FIGURE 37.3 Scanning electron microscopy image of *Listeria monocytogenes* on a damaged stainless steel surface. Cells tend to enter the crack and thus protect themselves.

a wide pH range between 4.4 and 9.4, and to tolerate both low water activities of upto 0.92 and high osmotic pressures, reaching its maximum at 16%.[71]

37.5.2 Microbiological criteria in current legislation

Commission Regulation No. 2073/2005[36] regarding microbiological criteria applicable to food products establishes that food products that may favor *L. monocytogenes* growth must present absence of the target pathogen on 25 g of the food product, and that food products that do not favor *L. monocytogenes* growth can have a microbial count of the pathogen of upto a maximum of 100 CFU/g (Table 37.1). This figure is established because foods containing less than 100 colony forming units per gram (CFU/g) are considered to pose negligible risk for a healthy population.[72] Hence, the EU requires that foods that may pose a greater risk must demonstrate absence of the pathogen in 25 g when leaving the factory and have a maximum of 100 CFU/g during their shelf life. However, it is recommended that the at-risk population avoids the intake of the food products that most likely contain *L. monocytogenes* in high amounts.[73]

In this regard, the rigorousness of the sampling plans carried out depends on the susceptibility of the target population, establishing "zero tolerance" in the case of food products intended for infants or people with special medical uses. As can be observed in Table 37.1, the legislation discriminates by means of the number of samples to be analyzed from foods targeted at a population with special needs such as infants (i.e., for these products 10 samples are taken instead of 5, putting more pressure on the analyses and making to find a positive sample more probable). Ensuring compliance is the responsibility of the food industry that supplies the food to the food chain and therefore to the consumers.[36] Nonetheless, the analysis of the final product does not guarantee the food safety of the products, making it necessary to follow a preventive strategy based on good hygiene practices and the previously mentioned HACCP system.[74]

Regarding the products in which *L. monocytogenes* cannot grow, the legal limit is adjusted to 100 CFU/g in five samples from the beginning to the end of the commercial life. Consequently, the risk of the pathogen in food is not only linked to its presence, but also to a specific number of microorganisms. To address the matter of a food industry's decision to release a production lot in the market, and in the light of what has been discussed

TABLE 37.1 Microbiological criteria for *Listeria monocytogenes*.

Food product	Sampling plan		Limits		Reference analytical method	Phase where the criterion is applied
	n	*c*	*m*	*M*		
Ready-to-eat foods for infants and special medical uses	10	0	Absence in 25 g		EN/ISO 11290–1	Product marketed during its useful life
Ready-to-eat foods that may promote the development of *L. monocytogenes*, other than those intended for infants or for special medical uses	5	0	100 CFU/g		EN/ISO 11290–2	Product marketed during its useful life
	5	0	Absence in 25 g		EN/ISO 11290–1	Before the food is no longer under the control of the food company that produced it.
Ready-to-eat foods that cannot promote the development of *L. monocytogenes*, other than those intended for infants or for special medical purposes	5	0	100 CFU/g		EN/ISO 11290–2	Product marketed during its useful life

c, number of samples that give values between *m* and *M* (in this case *m* = *M*); *CFU*, colony forming units; *m*, limit value, satisfactory if all observed values are <*m*; *M*, maximum value, unsatisfactory if one or more observed values are >*M*; *n* = number of units that conform the sample.
Source: From EC. Regulation No 2073/2005. 2005.

above in terms of both sampling and analytical methods, the concept of statistics should be also retaken into consideration. In all cases, the problem revolves around the fact that we are observing a part of the population we are analyzing and we do not integrate the results of each sample over time. Not integrating our statistical knowledge and the associated decision making is a serious mistake.

37.5.3 Interpretation of the results of the sampling plan by variables with three classes for *L. monocytogenes*

Firstly, if the legal microbiological criteria of products in which *L. monocytogenes* cannot grow (i.e., 100 CFU/g) is converted into logarithms, the admissible quantity of these pathogen cells in the product is 2 log CFU/g ($n = 5$, $c = 0$, and $m = M = 100$ CFU/g). Therefore the sampling plan involves taking five random samples and analyzing them according to the UNE-EN ISO 11290–2 standard. However, neither the legislation nor the ISO standard establishes what statistical interpretation needs to be carried out, assuming that it must be known and so does not need to be defined. The problem is that even when it is known it is not usually applied and products that do not comply with the legislation might leave the food industry mistakenly believing that they do. For the statistical interpretation, it is important to take into consideration concepts such as normal population, mean calculation, standard deviation, and their corresponding interpretation.

Briefly, a normal distribution, as presented in Fig. 37.4, is one that homogeneously groups the analyzed population in specific percentages based on the mean, adding or subtracting the standard deviation several times. Therefore to establish if a sample that is representative of the population meets a microbiological criterion or not, the mean must be calculated and 1, 2 or 3 times the standard deviation added or subtracted. In the case of analyses performed on food samples, it is assumed that they always follow a normal distribution.

According to the previous figure, the value of the mean, adding and subtracting the standard deviation once, would encompass 62.2% of the population; adding and subtracting the standard deviation twice would encompass 95.4% of the population; and adding and subtracting the value three times would encompass 99.6% of the population. Therefore based on the estimate that involves analyzing five samples (i.e., sampling), the mean and the standard deviation obtained for the corresponding count needs to be calculated and a judgment based on a statistical assessment made to accept or reject a production batch (i.e., population).[29] Table 37.2 shows three different cases with series of three samples, each presenting different values and deviations, and showing that if a statistical assessment of the results is not adopted, then different outcomes can be considered and not the ones that will probably happen.

To understand the exemplification made in Table 37.2, the different samplings will now be discussed. Regarding sampling 1, the result of the mean would indicate that the lot is acceptable when really it is not. As previously mentioned, the maximum total population must be considered, so when three times the value of the standard deviation is added to the mean, it can be observed that the

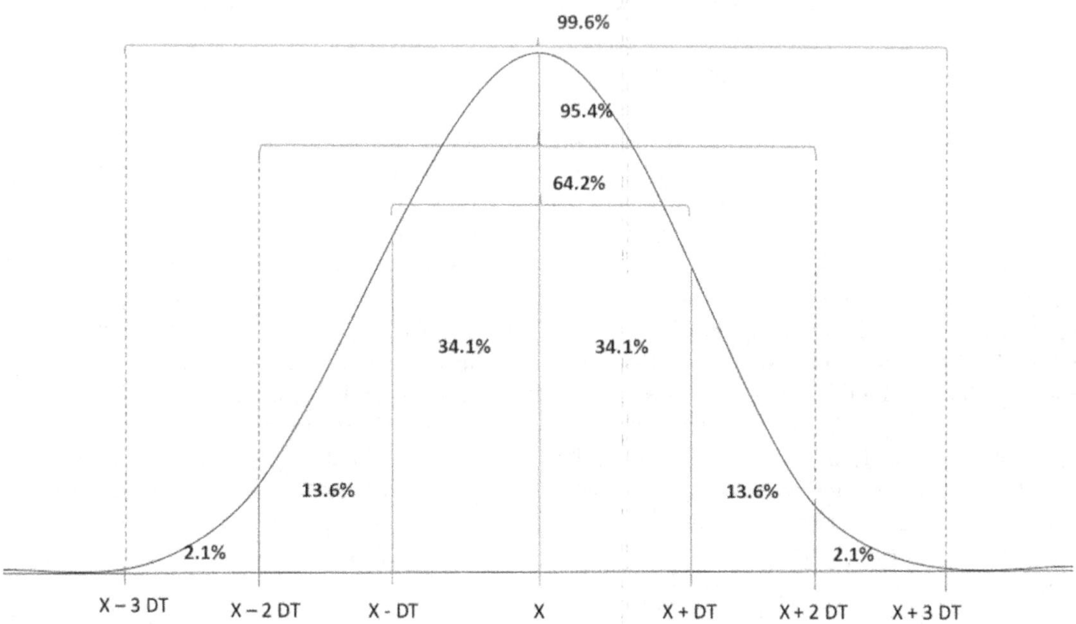

FIGURE 37.4 Scheme of a normal distribution necessary for the interpretation of results.

TABLE 37.2 Examples of results of microbiological analysis of food samples, for decision making process, regarding the acceptance or rejection of a food production batch.

Sample number	*Listeria monocytogenes* counts in CFU/g		
	Sampling 1	Sampling 2	Sampling 3
1	1	90	10
2	10	90	5
3	0	90	0
4	20	90	40
5	99	90	25
Mean	26	90	16
SD	41.6	0	16.4
X + 1SD	67.6	90	32.4
X + 2SD	109.2	90	48.7
X + 3SD	150.8	90	65.1

CFU, colony forming units; *SD*, standard deviation.

quantification of *L. monocytogenes* cells is 150.8 CFU/g, thus exceeding 100 CFU/g as the maximum acceptable level. Consequently, the hypothetical production lot must be rejected, despite of seeming that the lot can be released if observed independently.

On the other hand, if we take sampling 2, despite of the mean being higher than that of the first sampling, no variations among samples are obtained and, therefore, no standard deviation is obtained either. When considering the entire population, the result is 99 CFU/g, exceeding the maximum level allowed. Therefore the lot can be accepted despite of seeming that it is more contaminated than the previous one (i.e., sampling 1). Lastly, we look at sampling 3 which, like the previous one, is an acceptable lot. The standard deviation, in this case, is not as high as that of sampling 1 and is similar to the mean of the lot. When X + 3DT is calculated, the final level is less than 100 CFU/g and, therefore, acceptable.

Now let's consider the hypothetical case of a company with an internal control procedure that establishes a maximum limit of 80 CFU/g on the basis not to have any administrative problems with competent authorities and to not put the product at risk within the food company itself. Not only would the lot from the first sampling be rejected, but the second sampling would too. The important point here is what the food industry should do about this rejection. These values indicate that there is an error in the production and that those in charge of the food quality department must correct it. In the case of sampling 1, an evaluation of the entire installation starting with the prerequisites is needed because something is failing. As soon as the food industry detects the problem and rectifies the failing (e.g., cleaning and disinfection procedures, water control, pest control, or the food handlers, among others), the standard deviation will go down as the gap will be closed on the sample values, even though the mean remains the same. The decrease will be linked to the proper identification of the problem and the effectiveness of the measures taken. Following this example, in the case of sampling 2, the situation changes from having accepted the production lot to rejecting it. In this specific case, the fact that no standard deviation is observed indicates that the contamination comes from primary sources, because *L. monocytogenes* contamination is always the same. Therefore the prerequisite regarding the suppliers should be reviewed.

Likewise, it should be noted that if the number of samples (n) is increased, there is a higher probability that the standard deviation can be decreased, thereby achieving much more precise and representative values for the population. The legal limit of 100 CFU/g must always be respected with the inclusion of the corresponding statistical analysis. When calculating the mean and standard deviation of a production lot, first it should be verified that the mean does not exceed the FSO, which corresponds to the legal limit. If the mean is correct, the sum of the mean plus 3 times the standard deviation should be calculated which, if it does not exceed the FSO, indicates that the lot may be accepted. Thus, in food industries the limit must be less than 100 CFU/g for the mean plus three times the standard deviation, because the company limit must be less than the legal limit in case there is a failure in the production chain and conditions are no longer optimal. This can save the company from great financial losses caused by the loss of released food batches.

This interpretation of the results should not only serve to determine the safety of a production lot, but it should also allow the experts in food quality departments to consider where the problem in the production process is occurring to establish improvement measures. Firstly, the mean value of contamination by *L. monocytogenes* needs to be assessed. A high average value would indicate significant microbial contamination in the food industry. The degree to which this can be controlled throughout the production process will dictate how low the average will be. However, what the food industry really needs to be concerned about is the deviation on the results they obtain. A very narrow standard deviation usually indicates that the production process is very homogeneous since the contamination will come mainly from primary sources (i.e., from raw material suppliers or from the facility itself), usually making it easier to find the origin. Once controlled, the average contamination of the final product can normally be reduced.

37.5.4 Application in the food industry environment

Faced with this situation, it is important that food companies assimilate the discussed aspects at a management level to understand how they can affect the company in terms of competitiveness, responsibility, and risk. Firstly, a couple of basic statistical terms must be introduced since they are considered essential to understand the strategy described below. For that, it should be taken into consideration the analyses carried out in the companies, and if these analyses are being evaluated as independent measures or as repeated measures. According to the classical criterion, the analyses of food produced in the food industry are independent measures, clearly separating the batches from each other.[75] A production lot can be defined as a production unit that has been produced in a homogeneous way, so with the same raw materials, by the same personnel, and in the same plant, among other factors. The only stipulation is that there must be at least one daily batch. This leads the food industry to believe that production is carried out and, after cleaning and disinfecting, the production plant will be like it was on the first day in terms of hygiene. This is basically untrue. Every time a food industry is put into operation, there is a movement of microorganisms, which can find favorable conditions for their growth (i.e., water, nutrients, temperature, and time), taking a varying amount of time to grow. This leads to the fact that the longer the work shifts and the more moisture generated, the greater the microbiological risk.

When microorganisms grow in a plant, complex structures called biofilms, which allow their survival, are also frequently formed, resisting cleaning and disinfection tasks, thermal action, desiccation, and ultraviolet radiation.[42,76,77] A mature biofilm can contain more than 1 billion bacteria per square centimeter in a space smaller than the head of a pin. Consequently, their detection is almost impossible. If a unit of a few grams of product could carry just one tenth of a mature biofilm, there would be more than 100 million bacteria with the consequent risk that could pose in case a pathogen is present. Biofilms grow and expand throughout the food production plant,[69] and what at first affects only a few kilograms of product through a potential cross-contamination, can now affect tons of it. Therefore what happens on one day is not independent of what happens on another and therefore it cannot be considered that there is no connection. This leads to the consideration that the analysis of the samples should be thought of as repeated measures of the same reality.[9] Conceptually, the consequences of the interpretation of the analyses are very different, but a correct interpretation of the data can help to integrate the information obtained over time.

Moreover, with appropriate hygiene measures and the control and elimination of biofilms, it becomes clear how quickly and drastically the level of contamination is reduced. Therefore not only hygiene measures but also the frequency of sampling should be taken into account, together with their consideration as repeated measures. The problem with many food companies is that they do not carry out internal analyses and only official control analyses are being considered. This means that a company may only be analyzed once or twice a year. Therefore if a problem occurs in a target industry and the food company does not test their production batches often enough, the industry will not be able to know the real risk.

37.6 Research gaps and future directions

The microbiological analysis of food products must always be considered from a statistical perspective, and always bearing in mind that the result reflects a sampling on a population, which can be called a lot. If the sampling is done by variables, the result is numeric. In this case, the mean and standard deviation must be assessed, considering that the mean plus three times the standard deviation must be calculated to know if the entire lot is within the set limits. The sampling and subsequent analysis of the samples of a food plant should be understood as the result of the analysis of repeated measures. Historical monitoring of analytical results is essential to know the real presence of a pathogen in an industry and to determine the factors that affect it, such as seasonality, vacations, and periods of stoppage, among others. This is the basis for a good sampling by attributes, where the results obtained are qualitative. Once the risk level of a company is known, the FSO must be set as a way of limiting successive samplings, establishing the alert systems and implementing effective control and prevention measures. To this end, it is essential to have rapid analysis systems with as low detection limits as possible to be able to address decision making in relation to the release of production batches in the most efficient way possible.

References

1. United Nations. World population prospects. The 2017 revision; 2017.
2. Kotsanopoulos KV, Arvanitoyannis IS. The role of auditing, food safety, and food quality standards in the food industry: a review. *Compr Rev Food Sci Food Saf.* 2017;16(5):760–775. Available from: https://doi.org/10.1111/1541-4337.12293.
3. Trienekens J, Zuurbier P. Quality and safety standards in the food industry, developments and challenges. *Int J Prod Econ.* 2018; 113(1):107–122. Available from: https://doi.org/10.1016/j.ijpe.2007.02.050.

4. Barjaktarović-Labović S, Mugoša B, Andrejević V, et al. Food hygiene awareness and practices before and after intervention in food services in Montenegro. *Food Control*. 2018;85:466–471. Available from: https://doi.org/10.1016/j.foodcont.2017.10.032.
5. Ripolles-Avila C, Ríos-Castillo AG, Fontecha-Umaña F, Rodríguez-Jerez JJ. Removal of *Salmonella enterica* serovar Typhimurium and *Cronobacter sakazakii* biofilms from food contact surfaces through enzymatic catalysis. *J Food Saf*. 2019;1–10. Available from: https://doi.org/10.1111/jfs.12755. e12755.
6. Boelaert F, Amore G, Van der Stede Y, Hugas M. EU-wide monitoring of biological hazards along the food chain: achievements, challenges and EFSA vision for the future. *Curr Opin Food Sci*. 2016;12:52–62. Available from: https://doi.org/10.1016/j.cofs.2016.08.004.
7. Ramirez-Hernandez A, Galagarza OA, Álvarez Rodriguez MV, et al. Food safety in Peru: a review of fresh produce production and challenges in the public health system. *Compr Rev Food Sci Food Saf*. 2020;19(6):3323–3342. Available from: https://doi.org/10.1111/1541-4337.12647.
8. Ripolles-Avila C, Martínez-Garcia M, Capellas M, Yuste J, Fung D, Rodríguez-Jerez JJ. From hazard analysis to risk control using rapid methods in microbiology: a practical approach for the food industry. *Compr Rev Food Sci Food Saf*. 2020;19(4):1877–1907. Available from: https://doi.org/10.1111/1541-4337.12592.
9. Moreno-Torres Molina A, Ripolles-Avila C, Rodríguez-Jerez JJ. The importance of the analysis and interpretation of results in the control of pathogenic microorganisms in foods. The case of *Listeria monocytogenes. TECA Tecnol i Ciència dels Aliment*. 2020;19:10–19. Available from: https://doi.org/10.2436/20.2005.01.92.
10. NMKL. Guide on sampling for analysis of foods. Nordic Committee on Food Analysis no 12. <https://www.nmkl.org/index.php/en/publications/item/handbok-i-provetaking-av-naeringsmidlerhandbok-i-provetaking-av-naeringsmidler-nmkl-prosedyre-nr-12-2014>; 2014.
11. Valderrama WB, Dudley EG, Doores S, Cutter CN. Commercially available rapid methods for detection of selected foodborne pathogens. *Crit Rev Food Sci Nutr*. 2016;56(9):1519–1531. Available from: https://doi.org/10.1080/10408398.2013.775567.
12. Rohde A, Hammerl JA, Boone I, et al. Overview of validated alternative methods for the detection of foodborne bacterial pathogens. *Trends Food Sci Technol*. 2017;62:113–118. Available from: https://doi.org/10.1016/j.tifs.2017.02.006.
13. de Boer E, Beumer RR. Methodology for detection and typing of foodborne microorganisms. *Int J Food Microbiol*. 1999;50(1):119–130. Available from: https://doi.org/10.1016/S0168-1605(99)00081-1.
14. Fung D. Rapid methods and automation in microbiology. *Compr Rev Food Sci Food Saf*. 2002;1:3–22.
15. Ripolles-Avila C, Ríos-Castillo AG, Rodríguez-Jerez JJ. Development of a peroxide biodetector for a direct detection of biofilms produced by catalase-positive bacteria on food-contact surfaces. *CYTA - J Food*. 2018;16(1):506–515. Available from: https://doi.org/10.1080/19476337.2017.1418434.
16. Domenech E, Amorós JA, Escriche I. Effectiveness of prerequisites and the HACCP plan in the control of microbial contamination in ice cream and cheese companies. *Foodborne Pathog Dis*. 2013;10(3):222–228. Available from: https://doi.org/10.1089/fpd.2012.1305.
17. Amagliani G, Petruzzelli A, Omiccioli E, Tonucci F, Magnani M, Brandi G. Microbiological surveillance of a bovine raw milk farm through multiplex real-time PCR. *Foodborne Pathog Dis*. 2012;9(5):406–411. Available from: https://doi.org/10.1089/fpd.2011.1041.
18. Fielding L, Ellis L, Clayton D, Peters A. An evaluation of process specific information resources, aimed at hazard analysis, in small and medium enterprises in food manufacturing. *Food Control*. 2011;22(8):1171–1177. Available from: https://doi.org/10.1016/j.foodcont.2011.01.011.
19. Ricci A, Chemaly M, Davies R, et al. Hazard analysis approaches for certain small retail establishments in view of the application of their food safety management systems. *EFSA*. 2017;15. Available from: https://doi.org/10.2903/j.efsa.2017.4697.
20. Jianu C, Chiş C. Study on the hygiene knowledge of food handlers working in small and medium-sized companies in western Romania. *Food Control*. 2012;26(1):151–156. Available from: https://doi.org/10.1016/j.foodcont.2012.01.023.
21. Dzwolak W. Assessment of food allergen management in small food facilities. *Food Control*. 2017;73:323–331. Available from: https://doi.org/10.1016/j.foodcont.2016.08.019.
22. Soman R, Raman M. HACCP system - hazard analysis and assessment, based on ISO 22000:2005 methodology. *Food Control*. 2016;69:191–195. Available from: https://doi.org/10.1016/j.foodcont.2016.05.001.
23. Chen E, Flint S, Perry P, Perry M, Lau R. Implementation of nonregulatory food safety management schemes in New Zealand: a survey of the food and beverage industry. *Food Control*. 2015;47:569–576. Available from: https://doi.org/10.1016/j.foodcont.2014.08.009.
24. Meng L, Yang Q, Cheng J. Study on the application of HACCP system in ice-cream premix powder processing. *J Anhui Agric Sci*. 2011;39:6531–6533.
25. Nuchprayoon S, Sanprasert V, Kaewzaithim S, Saksirisampant W. Screening for intestinal parasitic infections among myanmar migrant workers in Thai food industry: a high-risk transmission. *J Immigr Minor Heal*. 2009;11(2):115–121. Available from: https://doi.org/10.1007/s10903-008-9169-8.
26. Hung YT, Liu CT, Peng IC, Hsu C, Yu RC, Cheng KC. The implementation of a hazard analysis and critical control point management system in a peanut butter ice cream plant. *J Food Drug Anal*. 2015;23(3):509–515. Available from: https://doi.org/10.1016/j.jfda.2015.02.005.
27. CAC. Code of hygienic practice for fresh fruits and vegetables. *WHO Guidelines Hand Hyg Health Care*. 2003;03(01):1–44.
28. Zwietering MH, Jacxsens L, Membré JM, Nauta M, Peterz M. Relevance of microbial finished product testing in food safety management. *Food Control*. 2016;60:31–43. Available from: https://doi.org/10.1016/j.foodcont.2015.07.002.
29. Whiting RC, Rainosek A, Buchanan RL, et al. Determining the microbiological criteria for lot rejection from the performance objective or food safety objective. *Int J Food Microbiol*. 2006;110(3):263–267. Available from: https://doi.org/10.1016/j.ijfoodmicro.2006.04.038.
30. ICMSF. Microorganisms in Foods 7. Microbiological testing in food safety. Kluwer Academic/Plenum Publishers. E.U.; 2002.
31. Amoa-Awua WK, Ngunjiri P, Anlobe J, et al. The effect of applying GMP and HACCP to traditional food processing at a semi-commercial

kenkey production plant in Ghana. *Food Control*. 2007;18(11): 1449–1457. Available from: https://doi.org/10.1016/j.foodcont.2006.10.009.
32. Spanu C, Jordan K. *Listeria monocytogenes* environmental sampling program in ready-to-eat processing facilities: a practical approach. *Compr Rev Food Sci Food Saf*. 2020;19(6):2843–2861. Available from: https://doi.org/10.1111/1541-4337.12619.
33. Valero A, Pasquali F, De Cesare A, Manfreda G. Model approach to estimate the probability of accepting a lot of heterogeneously contaminated powdered food using different sampling strategies. *Int J Food Microbiol*. 2014;184:35–38. Available from: https://doi.org/10.1016/j.ijfoodmicro.2013.12.032.
34. FAO. Directrices Generales Sobre El Muestreo (CAC/GL 50-2004).; 2004.
35. Zwietering MH, Ross T, Gorris LGM. *Food safety assurance systems: Microbiological testing, sampling plans, and microbiological criteria*. Vol 4. Elsevier Ltd; 2014. Available from: https://doi.org/10.1016/B978-0-12-378612-8.00363-2.
36. EC. Regulation No 2073/2005. 2005. Available from: https://doi.org/10.3969/j.issn.1673-8225.2009.50.026.
37. Croxatto A, Prod'hom G, Faverjon F, Rochais Y, Greub G. Laboratory automation in clinical bacteriology: what system to choose? *Clin Microbiol Infect*. 2016;22(3):217–235. Available from: https://doi.org/10.1016/j.cmi.2015.09.030.
38. Fung D. Rapid methods and automation in microbiology: a review. *Food Rev Int*. 1994;10:357–375. Available from: https://doi.org/10.1080/87559129409541006.
39. Nemati M, Hamidi A, Dizaj SM, Javaherzadeh V, Lotfipour F. An overview on novel microbial determination methods in pharmaceutical and food quality control. *Adv Pharm Bull*. 2016;6(3): 301–308. Available from: https://doi.org/10.15171/apb.2016.042.
40. EC. Regulation No 178/2002. 2002:1–24.
41. Hameed S, Xie L, Ying Y. Conventional and emerging detection techniques for pathogenic bacteria in food science: a review. *Trends Food Sci Technol*. 2018;81:61–73. Available from: https://doi.org/10.1016/j.tifs.2018.05.020.
42. González-Rivas F, Ripolles-Avila C, Fontecha-Umaña F, Ríos-Castillo AG, Rodríguez-Jerez JJ. Biofilms in the spotlight: detection, quantification, and removal methods. *Compr Rev Food Sci Food Saf*. 2018;17(5):1261–1276. Available from: https://doi.org/10.1111/1541-4337.12378.
43. Ripolles-Avila C, Ramos-Rubio M, Hascoët AS, Castillo M, Rodríguez-Jerez JJ. New approach for the removal of mature biofilms formed by wild strains of *Listeria monocytogenes* isolated from food contact surfaces in an Iberian pig processing plant. *Int J Food Microbiol*. 2020;323(March):108595. Available from: https://doi.org/10.1016/j.ijfoodmicro.2020.108595.
44. Ripolles-Avila C, Cervantes-Huaman BH, Hascoët A-S, Yuste J, Rodríguez-Jerez JJ. Quantification of mature *Listeria monocytogenes* biofilm cells formed by an *in vitro* model: a comparison of different methods. *Int J Food Microbiol*. 2019;289:209–214. Available from: https://doi.org/10.1016/j.ijfoodmicro.2018.10.020.
45. Ríos-Castillo AG, Ripolles-Avila C, Rodríguez-Jerez JJ. Detection of *Salmonella* Typhimurium and *Listeria monocytogenes* biofilm cells exposed to different drying and pre-enrichment times using conventional and rapid methods. *Int J Food Microbiol*. 2020;324 (January):108611. Available from: https://doi.org/10.1016/j.ijfoodmicro.2020.108611.
46. Law JWF, Mutalib NSA, Chan KG, Lee LH. Rapid methods for the detection of foodborne bacterial pathogens: principles, applications, advantages and limitations. *Front Microbiol*. 2015;5(Dec): 1–19. Available from: https://doi.org/10.3389/fmicb.2014.00770.
47. Dailey RC, Martin KG, Smiley RD. The effects of competition from non-pathogenic foodborne bacteria during the selective enrichment of *Listeria monocytogenes* using buffered *Listeria* enrichment broth. *Food Microbiol*. 2014;44:173–179. Available from: https://doi.org/10.1016/j.fm.2014.05.004.
48. Rajapaksha P, Elbourne A, Gangadoo S, Brown R, Cozzolino D, Chapman J. A review of methods for the detection of pathogenic microorganisms. *Analyst*. 2019;144(2):396–411. Available from: https://doi.org/10.1039/c8an01488d.
49. Manafi M. New developments in chromogenic and fluorogenic culture media. *Int J Food Microbiol*. 2000;60(2):205–218. Available from: https://doi.org/10.1016/S0168-1605(00)00312-3.
50. Castro AGSA Dorneles EMS, Santos ELS, et al. Viability of *Campylobacter* spp. in frozen and chilled broiler carcasses according to real-time PCR with propidium monoazide pretreatment. *Poult Sci*. 2018;97(5):1706–1711. Available from: https://doi.org/10.3382/ps/pey020.
51. Maciorowski KG, Herrera P, Jones FT, Pillai SD, Ricke SC. Cultural and immunological detection methods for *Salmonella* spp. in animal feeds—a review. *Vet Res Commun*. 2006;30(2): 127–137. Available from: https://doi.org/10.1007/s11259-006-3221-8.
52. Liu A, Shen L, Zeng Z, et al. A minireview of the methods for *Listeria monocytogenes* detection. *Food Anal Methods*. 2018;11 (1):215–223. Available from: https://doi.org/10.1007/s12161-017-0991-2.
53. Yang X, Zhou X, Zhu M, Xing D. Sensitive detection of *Listeria monocytogenes* based on highly efficient enrichment with vancomycin-conjugated brush-like magnetic nano-platforms. *Biosens Bioelectron*. 2017;91:238–245. Available from: https://doi.org/10.1016/j.bios.2016.11.044.
54. Váradi L, Luo JL, Hibbs DE, et al. Methods for the detection and identification of pathogenic bacteria: past, present, and future. *Chem Soc Rev*. 2017;46(16):4818–4832. Available from: https://doi.org/10.1039/c6cs00693k.
55. Hu L, Ma LM, Zheng S, et al. Development of a novel loop-mediated isothermal amplification (LAMP) assay for the detection of *Salmonella* ser. *Enteritidis* from egg products. *Food Control*. 2018;88:190–197. Available from: https://doi.org/10.1016/j.foodcont.2018.01.006.
56. Owen M, Willis C, Lamph D. Evaluation of the TEMPO® most probable number technique for the enumeration of Enterobacteriaceae in food and dairy products. *J Appl Microbiol*. 2010;109(5):1810–1816. Available from: https://doi.org/10.1111/j.1365-2672.2010.04810.x.
57. Hofreuter D, Novik V, Galán JE. Metabolic diversity in *Campylobacter jejuni* enhances specific tissue colonization. *Cell Host Microbe*. 2008;4(5):425–433. Available from: https://doi.org/10.1016/j.chom.2008.10.002.
58. EFSA-ECDC. The European Union one health 2019 zoonoses report. *EFSA J*. 2021;19(2):1–286. Available from: https://doi.org/10.2903/j.efsa.2021.6406.
59. Dewey-Mattia D, Manikonda K, Hall AJ, Wise ME, Crowe SJ. Surveillance for foodborne disease outbreaks—United States,

2009-2015. *Surveillance Summaries.* 2018;67:1–11. Available from: https://doi.org/10.15585/MMWR.SS6710A1.
60. Chen J, Park B. Label-free screening of foodborne *Salmonella* using surface plasmon resonance imaging. *Anal Bioanal Chem.* 2018;410(22):5455–5464. Available from: https://doi.org/10.1007/s00216-017-0810-z.
61. Lee KM, Runyon M, Herrman TJ, Phillips R, Hsieh J. Review of *Salmonella* detection and identification methods: aspects of rapid emergency response and food safety. *Food Control.* 2015; 47:264–276. Available from: https://doi.org/10.1016/j.foodcont.2014.07.011.
62. Ripolles-Avila C, Ríos-Castillo AG, Guerrero-Navarro AE, Rodríguez-Jerez JJ. Reinterpretation of a classic method for the quantification of cell density within biofilms of *Listeria monocytogenes*. *J Microbiol Exp.* 2018;6(2):70–75. Available from: https://doi.org/10.15406/jmen.2018.06.00190.
63. Ricci A, Allende A, Bolton D, et al. *Listeria monocytogenes* contamination of ready-to-eat foods and the risk for human health in the EU. *EFSA J.* 2018;16(1). Available from: https://doi.org/10.2903/j.efsa.2018.5134.
64. Ortiz S, López V, Villatoro D, López P, Dávila JC, Martínez-Suárez JV. A 3-Year surveillance of the genetic diversity and persistence of *Listeria monocytogenes* in an Iberian pig slaughterhouse and processing plant. *Foodborne Pathog Dis.* 2010;7(10): 1177–1184. Available from: https://doi.org/10.1089/fpd.2010.0535.
65. WHO-FAO. Risk assesment of *Listeria monocytogenes* in ready-to-eat foods. 2004;53.
66. Ripolles-Avila C, Hascoët A-S, Guerrero-Navarro AE, Rodríguez-Jerez JJ. Establishment of incubation conditions to optimize the *in vitro* formation of mature *Listeria monocytogenes* biofilms on food-contact surfaces. *Food Control.* 2018;92:240–248. Available from: https://doi.org/10.1016/j.foodcont.2018.04.054.
67. Mazaheri T, Ripolles-Avila C, Hascoët A-S, Rodríguez-Jerez JJ. Effect of an enzymatic treatment on the removal of mature *Listeria monocytogenes* biofilms: a quantitative and qualitative study. *Food Control.* 2020;114:107266. Available from: https://doi.org/10.1016/j.foodcont.2020.107266.
68. Mazaheri T, Cervantes-Huamán BRH, Bermúdez-Capdevila M, Ripolles-Avila C, Rodríguez-Jerez JJ. *Listeria monocytogenes* biofilms in the food industry: is the current hygiene program sufficient to combat the persistence of the pathogen? *Microorganisms.* 2021;9(1):1–19. Available from: https://doi.org/10.3390/microorganisms9010181.
69. Ripolles-Avila C, Hascoët A-S, Martínez-Suárez JV, Capita R, Rodríguez-Jerez JJ. Evaluation of the microbiological contamination of food processing environments through implementing surface sensors in an Iberian pork processing plant: an approach towards the control of *Listeria monocytogenes*. *Food Control.* 2019;(2018) 40–47. Available from: https://doi.org/10.1016/j.foodcont.2018.12.013.
70. AESAN. Informe del Comité Científico de la Agencia Española de Seguridad Alimentaria y Nutrición (AESAN) en relación a los estudios de vida útil para *Listeria monocytogenes* en determinados productos alimenticios. *Rev del Com Cientıfico la AESAN.* 2011;14:43–63. Available from: http://www.aecosan.msssi.gob.es/AECOSAN/docs/documentos/seguridad_alimentaria/evaluacion_riesgos/informes_comite/LISTERIA_M.VIDA_UTIL.pdf.
71. Rees CED, Doyle L, Taylor CM. *Listeria monocytogenes*. 3rd ed. Elsevier Inc; 2017. Available from: https://doi.org/10.1016/B978-0-12-385007-2.00012-7.
72. EFSA-ECDC. The European Union summary report on trends and sources of zoonoses, zoonotic agents and food-borne outbreaks in 2009. *EFSA J.* 2011;9(3):1–378. Available from: https://doi.org/10.2903/j.efsa.2011.2090.
73. AESAN. Informe del Comité Científico de la Agencia Española de Seguridad Alimentaria y Nutrición (AESAN) en relación a la evaluación del riesgo asociado a la presencia de *Listeria monocytogenes* en pescado fresco o congelado. *Rev del Com Cientıfico la AESAN.* 2009;10:27–40. Available from: http://www.aecosan.msssi.gob.es/AECOSAN/docs/documentos/seguridad_alimentaria/evaluacion_riesgos/informes_comite/LISTERIA_MONOCYTOGENES_PESCADO.pdf.
74. Das AK, Nanda PK, Das A, Biswas S. *Chapter 6. Hazards and safety issues of meat and meat products. Food Safety and Human Health.* Elsevier Inc; 2019:145–168. Available from: https://doi.org/10.1016/b978-0-12-816333-7.00006-0.
75. Røssvoll EH, Lavik R, Ueland Ø, Jacobsen E, Hagtvedt T, Langsrud S. Food safety practices among norwegian consumers. *J Food Prot.* 2013;76(11):1939–1947. Available from: https://doi.org/10.4315/0362-028X.JFP-12-269.
76. Hascoët AS, Ripolles-Avila C, Guerrero-Navarro AE, Rodríguez-Jerez JJ. Microbial ecology evaluation of an Iberian pig processing plant through implementing sch sensors and the influence of the resident microbiota on *Listeria monocytogenes*. *Appl Sci.* 2019;9(21):1–14. Available from: https://doi.org/10.3390/app9214611.
77. Fontecha-Umaña F, Ríos-Castillo AG, Ripolles-Avila C, Rodríguez-Jerez JJ. Antimicrobial activity and prevention of bacterial biofilm formation of silver and zinc oxide nanoparticle-containing polyester surfaces at various concentrations for use. *Foods.* 2020;9(442):1–15. Available from: https://doi.org/10.3390/foods9040442.

Section VIII

Current and emerging advances in food safety evaluation: chemicals

Chapter 38

The risk assessment paradigm for chemicals: a critical review of current and emerging approaches

John Doe
School of Pharmacy and Biomolecular Sciences, Liverpool John Moores University, Liverpool, United Kingdom

Abstract
The current paradigm for risk assessment developed in the 1970s–1980s. Critique of the system reveals that hazard identification and characterization uses many animals, takes a long time, costs much, and ties up much regulatory resource to assess each chemical. By focusing on endpoints, the system is always open to the criticism of missing something and will grow even larger as new concerns arise. Exposure assessment uses a tiered approach for assessing the use of a single chemical but has problems with concurrent exposures to more than one chemical. The automatic linking of classification to mandated risk management can cause problems. There is a great opportunity arising from: 50 years of study data, extensive in vitro data, and mathematics and computing power. Together they will allow a new structure for chemical safety decisions to be taken with confidence using less resource per assessment.

Keywords: Risk assessment; hazard identification and characterization; exposure assessment; hazard classification; adverse outcome pathway; tiered approach

38.1 Introduction

Chemicals have many uses which benefit society. A regulatory system has evolved over the last 50 years to meet the aim of allowing the use of chemicals to benefit society without causing harm to people. The system has evolved as knowledge of the potential adverse effects of chemicals has grown and it is now both *complex* (intrinsically, it has many parts which sometimes do not work seamlessly together) and *complicated* (extrinsically, it has external influences which act upon it to make it difficult to operate).

There has been huge investment by government, industry, and academia to develop new approach methodology. Technical progress has been made but fitting new technology into the existing system is proving to be difficult. There have been many programs heralding the need for reform fit for the 21st century (e.g., Tox21,[1] Risk21,[2] EU-ToxRisk[3]) but a fifth of the 21st century has now passed, and the old system is still in place.

There must be good reasons to make changes, which requires that the current system should be reviewed to determine its areas of weakness before new systems are developed.

38.1.1 Critique of the current system

There is only one way to use chemicals safely; exposure must not be higher than safe doses. In order to achieve this, potential adverse effects must be identified, the safe doses characterized, exposure must be assessed, and rules are required to decide whether a use is safe. We have a system which consists of three component subsystems:

- Hazard identification and characterization system
- Exposure assessment system
- Rules of use system

The current system can be analyzed against three factors:

- Does the system produce false negatives?—allowing potentially unsafe use
- Does the system produce false positives?—disallowing beneficial use
- Does the system require excess time and/or resources?—limiting the number of chemicals/uses which can be evaluated

38.1.2 Hazard identification and characterization

The current system uses a package of studies, mostly in laboratory animals, which is designed to detect a range of

Present Knowledge in Food Safety. DOI: https://doi.org/10.1016/B978-0-12-819470-6.00015-9

adverse effects or outcomes based on route of exposure, duration of exposure, or life stage being exposed—acute lethality, medium-term repeat dose toxicity, long-term toxicity, carcinogenicity, developmental toxicity, and reproductive toxicity. In addition, in vitro and in vivo studies assess genetic toxicity which is not an adverse outcome (AO) *per se* but may induce germ-line mutations, with the possibility of inherited disorders, and somatic mutations including those leading to cancer.

Each study maximizes the chances of detecting an adverse outcome by using high doses and testing to adverse effect or limit.

Apart from genetic toxicity studies, each study asks an open question: does this chemical cause an adverse effect in the situation in which it is tested, relying on the laboratory animal having the full range of biological processes which can be affected to produce an adverse outcome. The adverse outcomes are monitored by clinical observations of the animals, by clinical chemistry and hematology, by histopathology, and by direct observation of fetal and neonatal numbers and development.

Each of the studies uses a range of doses which are designed to explore the dose–response curve of any adverse outcome. Ideally, this should include the identification of a dose where no adverse outcome is observed (no adverse effect level, NOAEL). The way in which the hazard characterization is extrapolated to humans is part of the rules of use system.

38.1.3 Critique of hazard identification

38.1.3.1 False negatives

The system is designed to minimize false negatives. It uses a range of studies which mimic the range of human exposures in terms of duration and life stage. It uses a range of detection measures. It uses high doses. However, it is always open to the accusation that adverse effects could be missed by having a limited range of adverse outcomes being assessed. This has been the concern driving the inclusion of more endpoints and new study types. It is likely that left unchecked, the "full package" will continue to expand as new concerns emerge.

Following the dose response through the presence of adverse outcomes rather than assessing the underlying biological processes has the potential to be less precise in identifying chemicals which act on the same underlying mechanism, which would be required in concurrent exposure toxicity assessment.

38.1.3.2 False positives

As the system is designed to minimize false negatives it will be inherently susceptible to the presence of false positives. The study top doses are often many multiple orders of magnitude higher than those encountered by humans and it is doubtful if all the adverse outcomes detected at high doses would occur in practice. Some adverse effects have been shown to be rodent-specific and not relevant to humans, but the current system does not facilitate the elucidation of adverse outcome pathways (AOPs) to address human relevance and may require additional studies to investigate if adverse outcomes should be considered relevant.

38.1.3.3 Excess resources

For a full data package (agrochemicals,[4] biocides,[5] 1000 tons per annum chemicals[6]) the toxicity testing program takes a minimum of 4 years to complete, uses several thousand laboratory animals, and costs several million Euros. Elements of the full package are mandated under European regulation on registration evaluation, authorisation and restriction of chemicals (REACH)[6] with increasing requirements for higher annual tonnage production/use in Europe. Expense and time limit the number of chemicals which have been subjected to the full assessment. In addition, the number of animals and the laboratory resources which would be required to fully assess every chemical in use would be prohibitive. The full package demands the use of large amounts of expert resources by regulatory authorities because of the sheer volume of data which must be reviewed. Often additional studies are required to investigate the underlying mechanisms which result in the use of animals, take time to perform, are expensive, and use expert resource in regulatory authorities to review the data.

There is considerable redundancy in the process. Enough knowledge has been accumulated over 50 years to be able to often determine which adverse outcomes would result once a pathway has been identified. It is hardly ever necessary to do the full package of studies to identify the adverse outcomes which could result from different durations of exposure for repeat dose toxicity and for infertility. Adverse effects on fetal and neonatal development are not yet so readily predicted as, apart from endocrine-mediated effects, the underlying mechanisms are not well understood.

38.1.4 Exposure assessment

Exposure assessment is not as prescribed as hazard identification and characterization because of the wide range of potential situations in which people can be exposed to chemicals. A range of exposure models for each sector of use is available. In general a tiered strategy is used where the lowest tier (0) involves a semiquantitative assessment of all sources, pathways, and routes contributing to aggregate exposure to a substance, the next tier (1) tends to be a deterministic estimate with conservative assumptions, the penultimate tier (2) is a more realistic estimation of population exposure with increased use of measured data using probabilistic methods, and at the highest tier (3) exposure is modeled with a human-orientated approach using raw data sets.

38.1.5 Critique of exposure assessment

38.1.5.1 False negatives

The models used are primarily designed to assess exposure to a single chemical in a single use. There are challenges in assessing aggregate exposure—combined exposures to a single chemical across multiple uses, routes, and pathways, and concurrent exposure—exposure to multiple chemicals via multiple exposure pathways that affect a single biological target. These could lead to the underestimate of exposure and the probability of an adverse outcome. The current hazard identification and characterization process does not identify the underlying biological processes which makes it difficult to assess which chemicals should be included in concurrent risk assessment. In addition, on the exposure side, understanding of how to group chemicals based upon coexposure patterns is in its early stages.

38.1.5.2 False positives

Lower tier estimates of exposure are designed to be conservative, but unless higher tier estimates are available for the situation being considered, exposure can be overestimated. This overestimation would be compounded if conservative screening estimates are combined without additional refinement to generate aggregate or concurrent exposure predictions.

38.1.5.3 Excess resources

The need to move to higher tier studies can result in delay and considerable expenditure in performing specially designed studies.

38.1.6 Rules of use

The rules of use system encompass two approaches—classification and risk assessment. Both systems attempt to prevent situations occurring where exposure results in human doses which are above the safe level.

In classification,[7] chemicals are placed into different broad categories depending on the degree of hazard derived from the severity of effect and/or the dose level required to induce the effect. Currently chemicals are classified for acute lethality, dermal and eye irritation, dermal and respiratory sensitization, mutagenicity, single and repeat dose-specific organ toxicity, carcinogenicity, reproductive and developmental toxicity. Mutagenicity, carcinogenicity, and reproductive toxicity classifications are based only on hazard identification and not on hazard characterization. Each chemical within the category is deemed to have the same degree of hazard as all the others in that category. Classification can give guidance on whether all the substances in the category are suitable or unsuitable for certain uses.

In risk assessment, the degree of hazard is defined with more precision to a specific safe level based on the results of the safety studies. Risk assessment then goes on to compare the specific safe level for the substance with the specific exposures to make a safety decision. The results of the toxicology studies are used to derive safe doses (doses where effects would be very unlikely) for comparison with exposure levels for risk assessment. This is done by applying factors to the NOAEL which take into account conservatively assumed differences in susceptibility between laboratory animals and humans, and differences in susceptibility amongst the human population. Most commonly, a factor of 100 is used to divide the NOAEL to estimate a safe dose. A suite of safe doses for different durations of exposure ranging from single exposure to lifetime is developed. The appropriate safe dose is then compared with the estimated human exposure dose. This is an iterative process involving a tiered approach to exposure estimation until a decision can be made on whether the use is safe or not.

38.1.7 Critique of rules of use

38.1.7.1 False negatives

The major possibility of false negatives lies in the area of aggregate and concurrent assessment. The same chemical may be used in applications in different sectors or range of products and the potential for high aggregate exposure may not be explored. It is also a difficult judgment to know when a cumulative assessment is required based only on endpoint and this may be missed, especially when chemicals act on different parts of the same pathway.

38.1.7.2 False positives

It is not surprising that the rules of use for a safety system have several areas where false positives can occur. The major issue for this system is the use of conservative assumptions, which then cannot be removed when more information is available.

An extreme example is with plant protection products.[8] Registrants must provide an extensive dossier of studies on toxicity and extensive exposure data for each use of the substance. However, if the substance is classified as Category 1 for carcinogenicity or reproductive toxicity (based on hazard identification without consideration of the dose) all the required exposure data are ignored, and a blanket ban is imposed. This is based on an assumption that it is not possible to determine a safe dose for chemicals in Category 1 although for many chemicals when the underlying mechanism is known a safe dose can be determined. When this situation is compounded with the conservative nature of these tests, intentionally leading to a high false positive rate, the use of advantageous chemicals may be precluded.

The same concern is also seen with the use of Category 1 substances in mixtures, where complicated amendments to the guidelines for levels which can be included have been developed to take into account the lack of degree of dose consideration in the classification process for carcinogenicity and reproductive toxicity.

Other areas where false positives can occur include the use of overconservative factors in deriving safe doses and using overconservative estimates of exposure. It can prove difficult to get acceptance of refinement of the estimates for safe dose or exposure.

38.1.7.3 Excess resources

In general, the automatic linking of classification to automatic downstream risk management measures is a blunt instrument. Safe uses may not be permitted and if these have major commercial consequences the classification decisions will be challenged. This can result in registrants performing large numbers of studies using many animals and ties up large amounts of expert resource in regulatory authorities in reviewing data and submissions.

It would help if the guidelines for the required toxicity studies had a clear tiered approach similar to that which is required for exposure studies. For pesticides[4] and biocides,[5] the full package using 4000 animals must be done in the vast majority of cases. The guidelines for REACH[6] are based on tonnage rather than usage with a few exceptions. This means that a lot of animals may be used unnecessarily, and large amounts of redundant data must be reviewed by regulatory authorities.

The major points to emerge from the analysis of the current system were:

Hazard identification and characterization: The current system for hazard identification and characterization uses many animals, takes a long time to complete and review, costs much, and ties up a lot of regulatory resource for each chemical. By focusing on endpoints, it is always open to the criticism of missing something and will continue to grow as new concerns arise.

Exposure assessment: The current system for exposure assessment has a tiered approach for assessing the use of a single chemical in a particular use situation. Additional refinements in methods and data are needed to assess the risk of aggregate exposure to single chemicals and concurrent exposures to more than one chemical.

Rules of use system: The automatic linking of classification to downstream mandated risk management can cause situations which can increase the use of resources and can lead to the substitution of well-studied chemicals, for which safe use conditions can be determined, with untested chemicals. This problem arises from lack of hazard characterization in parts of the classification system and conflicts between the application of two systems at the same time: classification and risk assessment.

38.2 Ways forward

There are interlocking issues to be addressed in reaching the goal of the safe use of chemicals in the 21st century:

- By focusing on endpoints rather than underlying mechanisms, the current process is always open to the criticism of missing something and will continue to grow as new concerns arise.
- Extensive resources required to assess each chemical limit the number of assessments which can be made.
- Risks from aggregate and concurrent exposure remain challenging to assess.
- Conflict between classification and risk assessment.

Addressing these issues will require the overall framework to be revisited as well as attention being paid to the component parts. In order to do this, the best plan is to work backward from what is required to achieve chemical safety. Simply put, human exposure must not exceed safe dose levels. Exposure can become unsafe if safe dose levels are exceeded by one use of a chemical or from the use of the same chemical in different uses, or from high enough coexposure to chemicals which act on the same biological pathway.

Chemicals are rarely used only in one situation, so it is important to be able to assess safety in a range of uses and scenarios. This requires both hazard identification and characterization and exposure assessments which can be applied widely.

38.2.1 The way forward for hazard identification and characterization

The process of exposure assessment incorporates a tiered approach in which initial assessments contain conservative default values which are intended to overestimate exposure. If the expected human dose is below the safe dose, then the assessment concludes. However, if the safe dose is predicted to be exceeded, then the default values are replaced with usage and chemical specific values which reduce uncertainty until a safety conclusion can be drawn with confidence. This allows resources to be focused onto the situations of greatest concern.

In contrast, the hazard identification assessment process does not have an analogous tiered approach. There is a Tier 0 approach, the Threshold of Toxicological Concern (TTC),[9] which provides a default conservative estimate of safe dose based on the assumption that the chemical is as toxic as the most potent chemicals ever assessed. Once this safe dose is predicted to be exceeded, there is no recognized tiered approach in which resources can be focused where they are most needed.

The modern concept of the AOP[10] provides an opportunity for hazard identification and characterization to be done in a way which reduces uncertainty in a stepwise approach, which would result in fewer resources per chemical being required, and which would provide information on the biological pathway which is being perturbed.

We have now reached a stage where there is a great opportunity to develop a tiered approach which would provide increasing levels of certainty about adverse outcomes, safe doses, and the biological pathways involved. The opportunity arises from long-term investment in expertise by academia, industry, and government in three areas. We have over 50 years of study data on a large number of chemicals. These data are now available in databases with wide accessibility. We have a wide range of in vitro data on the effects of chemicals on key biological processes on many chemicals. We have mathematical and data handling capability, which allow the correlation of combinations of information sources to be made.

Most of the components required for this tiered approach are already in existence, but they need to be put into a framework. Inclusion in the framework should be based on performance criteria, not on mandated protocols, to allow for the framework to be developed as new methodology emerges. There will not be one for one replacement of existing studies, but data will be integrated from multiple sources to provide the required information to allow safety judgments to be made.

An outline for a tiered approach could be

Tier 0: TTC based on AO and chemistry

Does not identify AOP

Estimates safe dose with conservative default of up to seven orders of magnitude

Does not identify AO

Tier 1: In silico assessment based on structural alerts for key AOPs

Identifies some key AOPs

May provide an indication of safe dose

Identifies some key AOs

Tier 2: Range of in vitro assays designed to identify molecular initiating event (MIEs) and preliminary toxicokinetics

Identifies almost all key AOPs

Estimates of safe dose can be achieved by applying in vitro in vivo extrapolation with conservative defaults

Identifies key AOs

Tier 3: In vivo studies for repeat dose toxicity and developmental toxicity based on metabolomics/genomics

Identifies AOPs

Estimates safe dose with less conservative defaults

Identifies key AOs

The current suite of animal studies assessed in the same way

Identifies AOs

Estimates safe dose with less conservative defaults

Does not identify AOP

38.2.2 The way forward for exposure assessment

The current tiered approach for assessing single use of chemicals is working and will be refined as new technology becomes available. There is a need to develop more realistic models for higher tier assessments.

Another challenge is to know when aggregate risk assessment is necessary. Guidance is needed to indicate when higher tier aggregate assessments might be a priority. Considerations include relative contributions of different sources, level of conservatism in a screening single source assessment (e.g., a higher tier aggregate assessment may produce a lower exposure estimate than the maximum screening exposure predicted for a single use), and total exposure levels from representative biomonitoring studies.

Concurrent risk assessment also faces the same issues of lack of data when chemicals have been identified as acting on the same biological pathway and of the need for guidance on when cumulative risk assessment is a priority.

Databases are available which hold the required information, but they are not connected, they are of varied accessibility, and there are commercial sensitivity issues to be addressed.

38.2.3 The way forward for the rules of use

The major issue in the rules of use system is that there are two approaches at work at the same time within the system.

There are (1) risk-based approaches which follow the risk assessment process, and (2) hazard-based approaches which make conservative assumptions about hazard and exposure and lead directly to mandated risk management measures. There are problems when the two approaches are used in the same regulatory framework as the outcomes can contradict each other.

An issue with the risk assessment approach is that it is not possible at the moment to use a tiered approach for both hazard identification and characterization and exposure assessment. If the TTC is exceeded, a complete package of animal studies is required before exposure is assessed. Using a tiered approach for hazard identification and characterization would reduce the number of animals required, reduce the resources required to evaluate the data, and increase the number of chemicals and their uses which could be assessed.

A problem with the hazard-based approach (classification) is that it misses out stages in the process and thus is a blunt instrument. All chemicals in the hazard category are deemed to have the same degree of hazard. This could then be matched with use categories based on exposure, and this would avoid uses which would cause the safe dose to be exceeded. This can work if there are several categories for hazard and several categories for use. This is in effect a risk assessment with discrete variables (which can have only a limited number of values) for hazard and for exposure as opposed to traditional risk assessment which uses continuous variables. However, the fewer the categories the blunter the instrument. This means that it is difficult to discriminate between safe and unsafe uses which can lead to false positives and false negatives.

It is time that the categorization process for classification is reviewed to make the system more consistent and more applicable for use in making safety decisions. The system should be based on predicted human safe doses within each adverse outcome category.

There is no formal categorization scheme for chemical usage based on human exposure potential which could be matched up against a revised hazard categorization scheme. If one were developed, it would be simpler for downstream users to select the appropriate chemicals for their products and make it easier to communicate to users. It would also allow the tiered approach for hazard and exposure to be used if lower tier estimates of hazard and of exposure were low. If higher category uses were proposed, then higher tier assessments would be required.

38.3 Conclusions

The risk assessment paradigm for chemicals consists of three components: assessment of hazard (what can the chemical do and at what dose?), assessment of exposure (what is the dose?), and assessment of risk (is the dose enough to cause harm?).

The current paradigm for the assessment of hazard developed in the 1970s–1980s, and it is now due for a major overhaul. During the 1960s there was a growing realization that chemicals could cause adverse effects and that animal models could be used to detect and characterize these effects. Over time a series of studies was built up to cover a wide range of possible effects. For the most part, the studies took the form of trying to recreate in animals the situation of concern in humans.

The studies have been augmented as time has gone by as new concerns have arisen with additions to existing protocols, such as developmental landmarks in multigeneration studies to detect endocrine-mediated changes, and new studies such as developmental neurotoxicity which addressed concerns over the effects of chemicals on the developing neurological system. This has resulted in a process which requires large amounts of resources: time, animals, expenditure, and reviewing expertise. If the process remains focused on endpoints, it will continue to grow as new concerns arise.

Exposure assessment has developed a tiered approach which is focused on single chemicals. It needs to develop approaches for assessing the concurrent exposure to multiple chemicals.

Risk assessment suffers from an imbalance of having a tiered approach for exposure, but not for hazard which leads to inconsistency and concern over data gaps.

The rules by which the system operates suffer from complexities resulting from running two systems at once: risk assessment and hazard-based classification.

A tiered hazard assessment approach based on the AOP concept should be developed, which would be used alongside tiered exposure assessment to form an integrated risk assessment process which would reduce false positives and negatives and reduce the resources required for each assessment. This would allow more assessments to be made with the current level of resource expended by society on assessing the safety of chemicals.

We have now reached a stage where there is a great opportunity to develop a tiered approach which would provide increasing levels of certainty about adverse outcomes, safe doses, and the biological pathways involved. The opportunity arises from long-term investment in expertise by academia, industry, and government in three areas. We have over 50 years of study data on a large number of chemicals. These data are now available in databases with wide accessibility. We have a wide range of in vitro data on the effects of chemicals on key biological processes on many chemicals. We have mathematical and data handling capability, which allow the correlation of combinations of information sources to be made.

We have the opportunity to combine new approaches in hazard assessment and exposure assessment in a new structure to allow chemical safety decisions to be taken with confidence using less resource per assessment allowing more assessments to be made.

Acknowledgments

This chapter includes analysis carried out by the author as part of the initiation of ECETOC Transformational Programme 4: Development of an Integrated Approach for Chemicals Assessment (https://www.ecetoc.org/science-programme/transformational-programmes/). The views expressed are the author's and do not necessarily reflect ECETOC's position.

References

1. National Toxicology Program: Toxicology in the 21st Century. <https://ntp.niehs.nih.gov/whatwestudy/tox21/index.html>.
2. HESI Risk Assessment in the 21st Century (RISK21) Project. <https://risk21.org/about-risk21/>.
3. EU-ToxRisk – An Integrated European 'Flagship' Programme Driving Mechanism-based Toxicity Testing and Risk Assessment for the 21st Century. <https://www.eu-toxrisk.eu/>.
4. Commission Regulation (EU) No 283/2013 of 1 March 2013 Setting Out the Data Requirements for Active Substances, in Accordance with Regulation (EC) No 1107/2009 of the European Parliament and of the Council Concerning the Placing of Plant Protection Products on the Market Text with EEA Relevance.
5. European Chemical Agency (ECHA) Guidance on the Biocidal Products Regulation: Volume III: Human Health – Part A: Information Requirements Version 1.2. May 2018.
6. European Chemical Agency. <https://echa.europa.eu/regulations/reach/registration/information-requirements>.
7. European Chemical Agency Guidance on Labelling and Packaging in Accordance with Regulation (EC) No 1272/2008 Version 4.1. May 2020.
8. European Commission Scientific Advice Mechanism EU Authorisation Processes of Plant Protection Products Group of Chief Scientific Advisors Scientific Opinion 5/2018. <https://ec.europa.eu/research/sam/pdf/sam_ppp_report.pdf>.
9. European Food Standards Agency. Guidance on the use of the Threshold of Toxicological Concern approach in food safety assessment. *EFSA J.* 2019;17(6):5708.
10. OECD. *Users' Handbook Supplement to the Guidance Document for Developing and Assessing Adverse Outcome Pathways, OECD Series on Adverse Outcome Pathways (No. 1).* Paris: OECD Publishing; 2018. Available from: https://doi.org/10.1787/5jlv1m9d1g32-en.

Chapter 39

The use of artificial intelligence and big data for the safety evaluation of US food-relevant chemicals

Yuqi Fu[1], Thomas Luechtefeld[1,2], Agnes Karmaus[3] and Thomas Hartung[1,4]

[1]Center for Alternatives to Animal Testing (CAAT), Johns Hopkins Bloomberg School of Public Health, Baltimore, MD, United States, [2]ToxTrack Inc., Baltimore, MD, United States, [3]Integrated Laboratory Systems, LLC, Morrisville, NC, United States, [4]University of Konstanz, CAAT-Europe, Konstanz, Germany

Abstract

Environmental contaminants, naturally occurring toxicants, pesticide residues, and food additives are the four chemical-associated categories of six for food safety established by the Food and Drug Administration. The direct food additives, which are intentionally added to food, are the main focus of this case study, and the indirect food additives, such as pesticides, natural toxicants, and environmental residues will also be discussed. This study is attempting to investigate how artificial intelligence tools developed using big data could support the hazard evaluation of food additives.

Automated read-across technology, that is, the read-across-based structure activity relationships (RASAR) tool, was utilized to generate predictions, which were compared with traditional animal testing methods to assess utility for providing estimates of chemical toxicity for food-relevant substances. This was conducted using Underwriters Laboratories (UL) Cheminformatics Tool Kit followed by descriptive statistics and performance-based validation with datasets retrieved from sources such as the European Chemicals Agency, the US Environmental Protection Agency, the Occupational Safety and Health Administration, the European Food Safety Authority, and other literature.

In our analysis, the main findings indicate that more direct food additives than indirect food additives are in the training data and there were more non-toxicants than toxicants, which was expected for food-related substances. Most results were at "very strong" and "strong" reliability level. For 123 cases, where classifications could be retrieved from other sources for a preliminary validation, 83% of the RASAR results matched with the toxicological assessment results confirming that in silico tools can robustly generate predictions for informing on the potential of food-use chemical toxicity.

Keywords: Artificial intelligence; big data; food safety; additives

39.1 Introduction

39.1.1 Food safety and food additives

Food safety issues[1] concern how industrial and regulatory organizations manufacture, store, and deal food in order to prevent foodborne disease. In China, there is a proverb that says, "*illness finds its way in by the mouth*," which reflects the tight connection between food and human health and the importance of food safety in human life. In 1962 John F. Kennedy declared consumer safety as a fundamental right. Food safety has two fundamental aspects, that is, microbiological and chemical safety. More specifically, the Food and Drug Administration (FDA) established six categories of food safety hazards, which include microbial contamination, nutritional problems, environmental contaminants, naturally occurring toxicants, pesticides residues, and food additives. Food additives, and in part pesticide residues and other toxicants, are addressed in this research. Food safety regimens need to ensure every ingredient added to food is safe for human beings and therefore several organizations were established to test and evaluate the ingredients for possible toxicities including traditional animal testing and newly developed methods such as in silico testing.

During the process of manufacturing and storing food, the utilization of food additives is common for preservation, flavor, color, sugar substitutes, enzymes, acidulates, etc. FDA defines that food additives are not limited to things that are added to the food, which are named direct food additives, but also things that can contact and contaminate the food during the process of manufacturing and storing. Pesticides residues and packaging material

Present Knowledge in Food Safety. DOI: https://doi.org/10.1016/B978-0-12-819470-6.00061-5

are considered as indirect food additives.[2] Albeit some manufacturers have replaced food additives with natural ingredients, the trends of using food additive ingredients still increase globally, especially for artificial sweeteners.[3] According to a report, the year-on-year growth rate of seasoned and flavoring salt increased about 7% per year from 2016 to 2018 globally.[3] As the growing demands of food appearance, texture, flavor, and taste, the usage of different types of food additives continue to rise, it is important to come up with more effective methods to cope with those thousands of chemicals as food additives.[4]

39.1.2 Regulation of food additives

Regulations of food additives throughout the world have several similarities and dissimilarities. For example, the full extent of engineered nanomaterials that entered the United States is not known by FDA as most are considered as Generally Recognized as Safe (GRAS) substances, that is, considered safe by experts and exempted from the usual Federal Food, Drug, and Cosmetic Act (FFDCA). However, in Canada and the European Union (EU), any food containing engineered nanomaterials must be submitted to regulators before entering the market.[5] The global regulation of food additives is mainly led by a few safety assessment programs, which are the European Union Scientific Committee on Food, the European Food Safety Authority (EFSA), Food and Agriculture Organization (FAO) of the United Nations, and the US FDA.[6]

US food additive regulation for food additives or ingredients states that indirect food additives require review and yet exempt those generally recognized as safe by "qualified experts" as the substance had been sufficiently shown to be safe from premarket approval requirements[6]: The FDA needs to provide a regulation including any specifications and limitations to show the intended use of the additive is safe,[7] an estimation of dietary consumption, an assessment of likely toxicity and a risk management decision regarding safety. This process sometimes will also take nutritional habits and sensitive subpopulations into account. The FDA's assessment of new chemicals ought to be conducted based on sufficient available toxicological data and proper estimated dietary exposure. The process of addressing sufficient data will involve the consideration of testing according to the FDA Toxicological Principles for the Safety Assessment of Food Ingredients Redbook[8] conducted in compliance with good laboratory practice regulations.[7] The process of determining properly estimated dietary exposures is followed by the actual procedure of conducting the test and determining the point of departure, such as any adverse effects, no adverse effect levels, lowest effect levels, and other indications of toxicological concern.

Beginning in October 1999, FDA began to authorize food contact substances including indirect food additives through the food contact notification process. This notification process does not result in regulation. FDA does list information on "effective" (i.e., those that complete the authorization process) notifications for food contact substances on its internet site.[a] Additionally, FDA has operated an exemption process for listing indirect food additives in 21 CFR since 1995. See Code of Federal Regulations, Title 21, Section 170.39 (Threshold of regulation for substances used in food-contact articles) (2013).

Even though the FDA for GRAS states clearly that both food additives and GRAS ingredients require the same strength of evidence of safety, "currently, companies may determine substances are GRAS without FDA's approval or knowledge. However, a few substances previously considered GRAS have later been banned; and concerns have been raised about the safety of other GRAS substances, including those containing engineered nanomaterials, materials manufactured at a tiny scale to take advantage of novel properties..."[5]

The following approach has been proposed for GRAS evaluation[9]: (1) determining the GRAS eligibility of the substance; (2) collecting all available information on the substance separately for every information need; (3) considering a Threshold of Toxicological Concern approach;[10] (4) developing a test strategy; (5) carrying out the test strategy and the respective risk assessment; (6) considering mixture effects, sensitive subpopulation, and extreme use scenario; (7) evaluating metabolites, degradation products, and impurities; and (8) documenting the process and share the results with FDA, and the general public. As time goes by, an increasing number of new technologies will appear allowing to replace previous testing methods and to cope with chemicals, which could not be tested before.

In contrast to the US food additive regulation, the EU food additives regulation requires a mandatory premarket authorization rather than self-regulation by industry.[2] Also, cyclic reconsideration of the safety of additives is mandatory. The EU review for processing aids, i.e., the substances added for processing food and remaining in the finished product, does not legally require providing data to consumers as required for ingredients,[11] does not differ a lot from the regulation of GRAS except that it is more limited in scope. The Joint FAO/WHO Expert Committee on Food Additives (JECFA) for other countries also follows the same general approach for assessment.

39.1.3 Testing methods

The testing methods used for evaluating food additives include both traditional methods, such as animal testing, in vitro testing, and newly developed computational methods. In silico assessment is part of the new approach methods and is conducted through some computational programs and relies increasingly on big data, that is, large, diverse sets of information. Currently, alternatives to animal tests follow the philosophy known as the 3Rs—replacement, reduction, and refinement. This concept attempts to reduce or exclude animals from the tests, or alleviate the pain and distress posed on animals.[12]

Generally, animal testing is most common among the testing methods for food ingredients, though these tests can be costly, time-consuming, and results can sometimes be misleading. Due to the high demand for safety data prescribed in the FDA Redbook, there could be many animal tests conducted to test any specific chemical but typically a lot of testing is waived in the context of GRAS.[9] Individual tests can require large numbers of test animals. Easily, animal tests can amount to several million dollars for the full evaluation of a single substance. The process of food additives risk assessment attempts to determine a point of departure of adverse events such as the no-observed adverse effect level. Some animal tests can lead to ambiguous results, which requires follow-up testing that can significantly prolong the testing and registration process. Some tests take substantial time, for example, it can take easily five years to obtain the result of a cancer bioassay,[13] again slowing down the evaluation process, leading to the growing number of untested chemicals. Approximately 100 new petitions are submitted to the FDA annually for new food or color additives. GRAS determination, in contrast, requires only a (voluntary) notification. Neltner et al.[14] report that "Less than 38% of FDA-regulated additives have a published feeding study. For chemicals directly added to food, 21.6% have feeding studies necessary to estimate a safe level of exposure and 6.7% have reproductive or developmental toxicity data in FDA's database." The other important issue is that we need to extrapolate animal testing results to human beings. Due to ethical concerns, it is hard and often improper, to conduct human testing for food additives. Hence, experimental animals are used as surrogates for humans and extrapolation of the results by assessment or safety factors is required.

Earlier,[9] we discussed possible refinements of the animal studies due to scientific progress since the Redbook of 1983 (referring to the respective Organisation for Economic Co-operation and Development (OECD) test guidelines—TG):

1. Genotoxicity: Transgenic rodents TG488 with fewer false positives and possibly combined with repeated dose testing;
2. Short-term toxicity tests with rodents: Updated TG 407; combination with in vivo mutagenicity; combination with developmental toxicity screening assays (TG 422);
3. Subchronic toxicity studies with rodents: Updated TG 408;
4. Subchronic toxicity studies with nonrodents: Updated TG 409;
5. One-year toxicity studies with nonrodents (typically dogs): Possibly abandon based on pesticide experience;
6. Chronic toxicity or combined chronic toxicity/carcinogenicity studies with rodents: Updated TG 452, combined with carcinogenicity TG 453;
7. Carcinogenicity studies with rodents: Updated TG 451; TG 453 combined with chronic toxicity; consider abandoning completely based on poor performance; abandon mouse bioassay;
8. Reproduction studies: TG 443 (Extended One-Generation Reproductive Toxicity Study) instead of TG 416 (Two-Generation Reproduction Toxicity Study); consider abandoning completely based on poor performance;
9. Developmental toxicity studies: TG 421 or TG 422.

Alternatives to animal testing include in vitro data generation. We argued earlier[9] that a number of animal tests of FDA's Redbook could be changed due to technical progress to in vitro approaches:

1. Genotoxicity: Micronucleus test and Comet assay lacking. Reduction of false positives (maximum concentrations, p53 competent cells, etc.);
2. Carcinogenicity: Consider cell transformation assays (OECD guidance available) possibly with an Integrated Testing Strategy as currently being developed for pharmaceuticals.

Furthermore, a number of in vitro approaches are on the horizon for food safety testing use: This includes mutagenicity in skin models, microphysiological systems,[13] integrated testing strategies,[15] systems toxicology,[16,17] as well as for developmental and reproductive toxicity[18] zebrafish egg reproductive toxicity assays and in vitro embryotoxicity studies especially to replace second species. The ToxCast high-throughput screening (HTS) program,[b] is an open-access in vitro assay–based HTS program that provides a quick insight into the biochemical endpoints, cellular processes, and phenotypes for thousands of chemicals. A sizeable fraction of identified food-relevant chemicals are screened in this HTS program, namely 8659 food-relevant chemicals.[19] The ToxCast data have been used as the basis of some computational modeling projects to generate in silico predictive models, which can also be mined to predict chemical toxicity. The advantage of in silico models such as CERAPP[c] or COMPARA[d] is the ability to apply a model beyond the chemical inventory screened in the in vitro assays.

Another in silico alternative, read-across, is the most frequently used nonanimal alternative approach.[20,21]

Read-across predicts hazard from chemical analogs with known hazard data,[22] thus saving time and money especially when automated.[23,24] Another advantage of automated read-across is that it can be more accurate for predicting chemical-mediated toxicity, as shown by Luechtefeld et al.[25] For very large datasets, it is more convenient to input the data in a computational program to see the patterns, trends, and associations.

Read-across has been combined with machine learning approaches through quantitative structure–activity relationships resulting in the read-across-based structure activity relationships (RASAR) approach.[25] The model is used for predicting toxicological hazards such as skin sensitization, eye irritation, among others and is based on big data. As these are mainly industrial chemicals, a key question for our case study is how well they represent food-related chemicals. The database includes approximately 10 million chemicals and enables the identification of highly similar compounds. "This allows inference of respective properties in a process that is called read-across."[21] In conclusion, the cost- and time-effective nature of RASAR in addition to its accuracy means that this tool can be used to assess the toxicities and properties of chemicals based on structural similarity, determine the frequency of the hazards, evaluate the quality of previously conducted animal testing, and monitor the EU Registration, Evaluation, Authorisation and Restriction of Chemicals (REACH) registration.[22]

Food additive safety profiling utilizing artificial intelligence and big data could assist to cope with untested substances and impurities in food. Herein, the performance of RASAR is assessed for over a thousand food-relevant substances. This approach identified food-relevant substances that are noteworthy as potentially toxic or have discrepancies between actual and predicted properties. In the future, we would attempt an external validation by identifying chemicals with test results outside the read-across technology training set. With the expansion of the RASAR approach to more complex and systemic endpoints, this approach might help the development regulation of new and existing food additives.

39.2 Materials and methods

39.2.1 Datasets

The chemical list used for further statistical analysis was generated from the combination of three sources. Two were obtained from Karmaus et al.'s works published in 2016 and 2017 ("SuppFile2_SOMbins_SMILES" and "1,749 CPCat ToxCast details," respectively), and the last was ("Read-Across results") was generated by running the chemicals in "SuppFile2_SOMbins_SMILES" through the RASAR program (UL Cheminfomatics Toolkit 2.0, ULCT©). ULCT2.0.0 was the most recent version of the UL Cheminformatics Tool Kit at the time of this study. Relative to prior versions, it simplifies the modeling approach while increasing the amount of training data. The modeling approach is simplified by training a multitask single neural network on 40 separate UN Globally Harmonised System (GHS) hazard outputs rather than training a separate model for each endpoint. This approach also effectively increases the amount of training data for each endpoint through transfer learning. This rendition of the model represents a threefold increase in data (before curation there were 2,355,919 chemical-endpoint-value triplets in the source data) over the 2017 model.[25] The training set consists of 40 endpoints, 361,379 unique compounds, and 961,854 chemical-endpoint-value triplets. A simple shallow multitask neural network model architecture was used where the chemical input is passed through two large hidden layers and then a batch normalization layer before ending in 40 binary output layers representing each endpoint. This represents a hard parameter sharing multitask learning approach where every output directly shares the same input layers. A holdout validation set of 37,057 distinct compounds, 40 endpoints, and 63,839 chemical-endpoint-value triplets was used to evaluate model performance. On average, the nine predicted classifications were identified with 84% sensitivity and 73% specificity (79% balanced accuracy). For details, we have to refer to Underwriters Laboratories.

The compilation of a large inventory of food-use chemicals by Karmaus et al.[19] includes direct additives, indirect/food contact, and pesticide residue chemicals. Analyses in their work go on to limit the inventory to only those compounds that overlap with ToxCast. The subsequent Karmaus et al.'s[26] work then provided a comprehensive manual curation of the food-use chemicals in ToxCast, to refine the inventory to reflect food additives in current use in the United States specifically. This work excluded some chemicals that had originally been identified in the 2016 work as they had once been registered as food additives but in more recent years had been removed from use. In brief, the authors compiled 11,733 chemical entries from eight US food-relevant sources, which are six FDA inventories: Everything Added to Food in the United States (EAFUS), Generally Recognized as Safe (GRAS) Notice Inventory, Select Committee on GRAS Substance Database (SCOGS), List of Indirect Additives Used in Food Contact Substances, Inventory Effective Food Contact Substances, Threshold of Regulation (TOR) Exemptions, as well as the Flavor and Extract Manufacturers Association GRAS Inventory (FEMA) and the Aland Wood Pesticides database. After eliminating redundant and duplicate chemicals, 8965 distinct chemicals remained. Then, by distinguishing chemicals with discrete defined chemical structures, 8965 chemicals narrowed down to 4729 chemicals. These 4729 chemicals not only underwent further analysis to get the manual curation information, such as being direct food additives, indirect food additives, pesticides residues, and nonfood, but were also run in the present study through the RASAR technology (UL Cheminfomatics Toolkit 2.0, ULCT) to predict nine different health and environmental endpoints: acute toxicity, acute dermal irritation, acute dermal toxicity, acute aquatic toxicity, acute inhalation toxicity, chronic aquatic toxicity, eye irritation, mutagenicity, and skin sensitization. Finally, of the 4729 chemicals identified as food-relevant by Karmaus et al.,[19] a subset of 1530 were identified as being in the ToxCast HTS program inventory and thus had in vitro data available for analysis.

In Karmaus et al.[26] chemical use information was sought to build a larger inventory of potential food-use chemicals. To these means, 43,599 chemicals from CPCat (the EPA Chemical/Product Categories Database[27]) were originally sourced from 12 use-informative resource databases, which are: Aggregated Computational Toxicological Resources (ACToR) data sets and lists, ACToR UseBB, Design for the Environment (DfE), Dow Chemical Company (Dow), Drug Bank, US EPA 2006 Inventory Update Reporting (IUR) Modifications Rule and the 2012 Chemical Data Reporting (CDR) Rule, Swedish Chemicals Agency (Keml) National Industrial Chemicals Notification and Assessment Scheme (NICNAS), Retail Product Categories (RPC) database, Substances in Preparation in Nordic Countries (SPIN) database, and Human Toxome Project (HTP).[27] After isolating chemicals with the word "food" in use description fields, 43,599 chemicals narrowed down to 10,972 "food" chemicals. These 10,972 "food" chemicals then narrowed to 1749 "food" chemicals by requiring inclusion in the ToxCast HTS program as mining the in vitro HTS data was a focus of that study. Then, the list of 1530 food-relevant chemicals from the 2016 work was compared to these 1749 "food" chemicals identified from CPCat use annotations in the 2017 work identifying an overlap of 1276 food-use chemicals in ToxCast, which were subject to manual curation as part of the final 2017 analyses. This manual review provided the CASRNs (chemical abstract services (CAS) registration numbers, also referred to as CAS Number, is a unique numerical identifier assigned to every chemical substance described in the open scientific literature) and manual curation categorizations for corresponding chemicals. The study concluded that 65 of these chemicals were not currently food-use in the United States and thus the final inventory of food-use chemicals for analysis in ToxCast was 1211 chemicals for the Karmaus et al.'s[26] work.

The current RASAR analysis utilized the 4729 chemicals with chemical structure information from the Karmaus et al.'s[19] study. The chemical structures were defined by SMILES (simplified molecular input line entry system codes; SMILES are a line notation for describing the structure of chemical species using short ASCII strings), as SMILES are the required information to run a chemical analysis in the RASAR. Each of the 4729 chemicals was analyzed for nine different toxicological endpoints. The results provided 38,520 prediction results for 4729 chemicals. Prediction value of 0.5 was taken as the threshold for calling a chemical positive for a given hazard, that is, considered as toxic for the given hazard. Prediction values below 0.5 would be considered as negative, which means the tested chemical is predicted not to lead to the tested toxicity hazard. The reliability category, which is the confidence level of the prediction, for each prediction value was obtained as well. Reliability categories of "very strong" and "strong" reflect high confidence level of the prediction value. Reliability categories of "moderate" and "low" mean low confidence level of the prediction value. Reliability category "in training" means the chemical had data used for training the algorithm to build the prediction model. Reliability category "exclude" means the structure for the tested chemical does not fit the RASAR tool rules.

39.2.2 Statistics

In order to get the chemicals, which could be used for statistical analysis, the first step is assigning CASRNs identifiers for every chemical in the "Read-Across results" file generated by the RASAR tool. 38,520 results had been obtained for 4729 chemicals, to which first CASRN and then manual curation categorization[26] were mapped, not all of the inventory had manual curation use categories thus N/A was assigned to those chemicals. In total 1215 chemicals had SMILES identifiers, CASRNs, predictions of toxicity endpoints (i.e., acute aquatic toxicity and chronic aquatic toxicity), confidence levels of predictions, and manual curation categorizations (Fig. 39.1). Corresponding to this final inventory of 1215 chemicals suitable for statistical analyses were 10,935 RASAR prediction results.

These 1215 chemicals could be divided into eight manual curation categories, which were enumerated as follows: (1) direct food additive, (2) indirect food additive, (3) pesticide/residue, (4) nonfood, (5) chemicals which were not included in the manual curation, (6) chemicals mapped as both direct food additive + indirect food additive, (7) chemicals mapped as both direct food additive + pesticide/residue, and (8) chemicals mapped as both indirect food additive + pesticide/residue. The frequency of each new manual curation category in the 1215 chemicals list was calculated. To integrate the new manual curation categories, each manual curation category was further divided into subgroups based on the nine toxicity endpoints evaluated by RASAR. These subgroups could still be further divided into yet more subgroups based on the reliability levels.

39.2.3 Preliminary validation

The preliminary validation process compared a subset of the RASAR results with toxicological results from resources such as the European Chemicals Agency (ECHA),

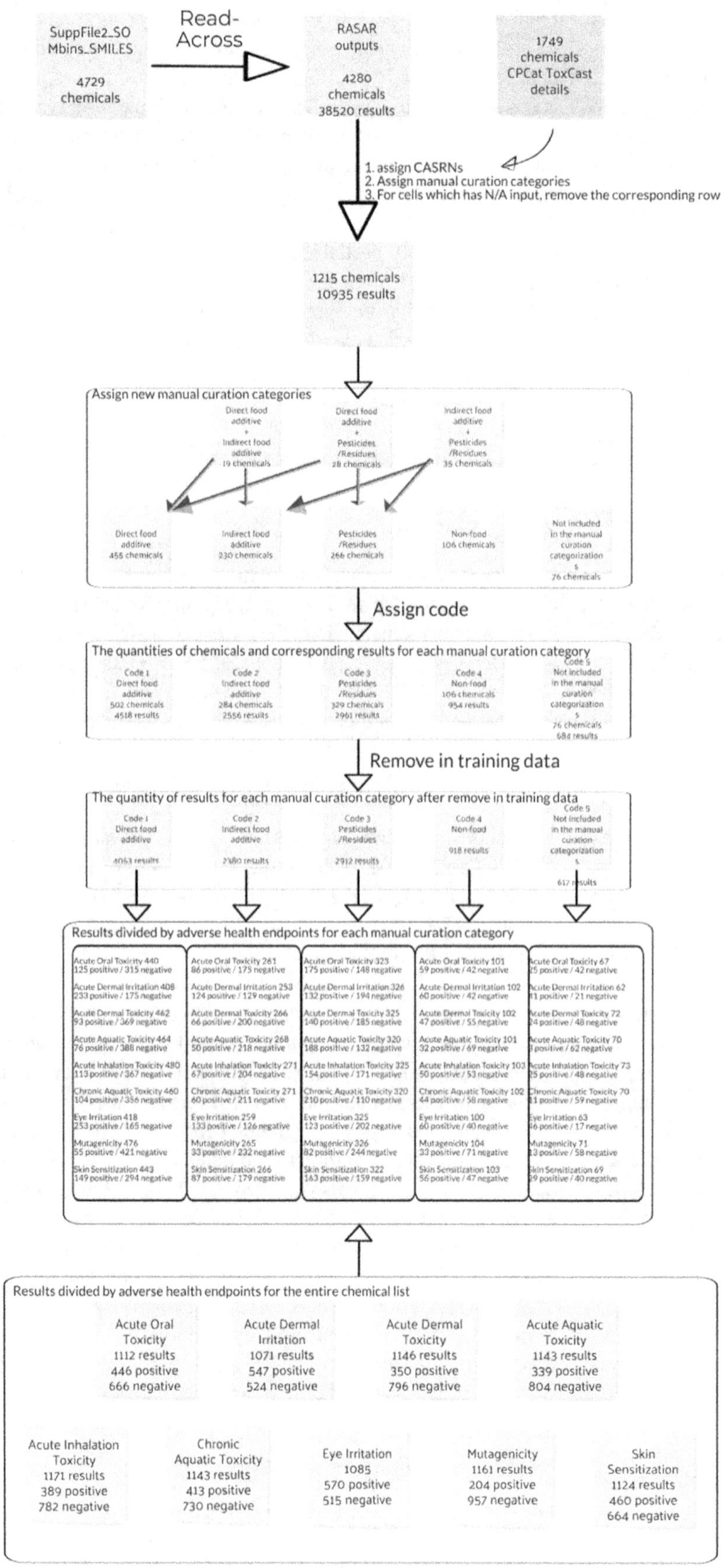

FIGURE 39.1 Workflow for the 1215 chemical list. A chemical list comprising 1215 chemicals and 10,935 RASAR results were divided into eight manual curation categories. The eight manual curation categories then condensed to five manual curation categories. After that, each category divided into nine subcategories based on toxicity hazards estimated by RASAR. In each subgroup, positive and negative results were counted, and the proportions are shown. *RASAR*, read-across-based structure activity relationships.

the Occupational Safety and Health Administration (OSHA), and other literature. It is important to know whether the RASAR results are accurate, so the toxicological information for selected 18 selected substances from other resources needs to be compared to show consistency. We choose high-confidence prediction as a best-case scenario, but it is noteworthy to state that the majority of predictions were of the "strong" and "very strong" reliability categories.

The selection of the 18 chemicals was based on the following steps: (1) chemicals were separated based on their manual curation categories; (2) chemicals were sorted to identify best prediction values. The highest five prediction values with "very strong" confidence levels were selected from each manual curation category. In total 25 results were picked. However, multiple results with different health endpoints could come from one chemical. For example, both eye irritation and acute dermal irritation for furfural are parts of the highest five prediction values in indirect food additive category. Hence, the 25 shortlisted results correspond to 18 unique selected chemicals. After deciding on the 18 chemicals, which would be used for validation purposes, all of their corresponding health endpoints, totally 162 results, were also retrieved to create a comprehensive comparison table facilitating review of the toxicity endpoint results from RASAR versus other sources (i.e., ECHA, US Environmental Protection Agency, OSHA, EFSA, and other literature).

39.3 Results

The purpose of the following comprehensive statistical analysis is testing the performance of RASAR when predicting whether the chemical is a toxicant, and identifying which manual curation subgroup has the highest positive rate for each toxicity endpoint; for each endpoint, the goal is testing the performance of RASAR when suggesting positive results (having a threshold equal to or above 0.5) and causing toxicity, or for negative results (having a threshold below 0.5) not causing toxicity. The aim is to show how accurate RASAR is in food additives evaluation to demonstrate the utility and robustness of the RASAR read-across platform in this chemical space.

39.3.1 Manual curation categorization

To determine the relative percentage of positive predictions within each manual curation category, 1215 chemicals were assigned a new manual curation. Since there are only few chemicals with two manual curations, the counting results of indirect food additive + pesticide/residue, direct food additive + pesticide/residue, direct food additive + indirect food additive were added to both applying categories direct food additive, indirect food additive, pesticide/residue, respectively, only slightly changing percentages but simplifying data evaluation (Table 39.1). For example,

TABLE 39.1 Five simplified manual curation categorization inventories for 1215 chemicals.

Manual curation categorization	Category number	Chemical count	Percentage
Direct food additive	1	502	39%
Pesticide/residue	3	329	25%
Indirect food additive	2	284	22%
Nonfood	4	106	8%
Not included in manual curation	5	76	6%
		1297[a]	100%

[a]*Note that simplification of including chemicals in both manual curation categories to which they were annotated results in some chemicals being included twice (in respective categories to which they were mapped; thus the total sum counts some chemicals twice.*

chemicals that are direct food additives but also indirect food additives represent only 2%. Therefore chemicals with two manual curation categories are not shown separately in the following tables (39.1-4) and graph (39.2) but were included in both categories they belong to.

39.3.2 In-training data

"In-training data" means these results were part of the training dataset to build the prediction model, or more specifically that these results are not predictions but originate from actual study data used to build the read-across program. Such data are also used for cross-validation as they have classifications based on animal studies. For example, 2-isobutyl-3-methoxypyrazine, $COC_1 = NC = CN = C_1CC(C)C$, labeled as "in-training" for eye irritation. This indicates that RASAR did not actually predict whether 2isobutyl-3-methoxypyrazine could trigger eye irritation, but rather knew since the data were provided and used to train the model. The actual classification has not yet been disclosed by UL as they are proprietary; their release for the purpose of validation is under negotiation. The sum of in-training data for each toxicity endpoint is summarized in Table 39.2. Ultimately, although RASAR provides predictions for the in-training data, these were excluded from further analysis (Table 39.3).

39.3.3 Health and environmental endpoints

The positive rate for each toxicity endpoint, per manual curation category, was evaluated to further characterize the performance of the RASAR technology (Table 39.4).

TABLE 39.2 Sum of in-training data for each toxicity endpoint by use category.

Positive + and negative in-training results for five manual curation divided by nine health endpoints

In-training data	Direct food additive	Indirect food additive	Nonfood	Pesticide/residue	Not included in manual curation	
Acute oral toxicity	62	23	5	6	9	105
Acute dermal irritation	94	31	4	3	14	146
Acute dermal toxicity	40	18	4	4	4	70
Acute aquatic toxicity	38	16	5	9	6	74
Acute inhalation toxicity	22	13	3	4	3	45
Chronic aquatic toxicity	42	13	4	9	6	74
Eye irritation	82	25	6	4	13	130
Mutagenicity	26	19	2	3	5	55
Skin sensitization	59	18	3	7	7	94
	465	176	36	49	67	

TABLE 39.3 Sum of results and in-training data per manual curation category.

Manual curation category	In-training results	Total results	Percentage of results in-training
Direct food additive	465	4518	10%
Indirect food additive	176	2556	7%
Nonfood	36	954	4%
Pesticide/residue	49	2961	2%
Not included	67	684	10%

The fractions of positive and negative results for each manual curation category per toxicity hazard are given. The total number for each toxicity endpoint has been used as the denominator when calculating the percentage.

A few trends become obvious: For example, when considering acute oral toxicity, in Table 39.3, the direct food additives, indirect food additives, and pesticides/residues have more results. Furthermore, negative results are more frequent than positive results for acute oral toxicity when considering direct food additives and indirect food additives (Table 39.4). Acute dermal toxicity, acute aquatic toxicity, acute inhalation toxicity, chronic aquatic toxicity, mutagenicity, and skin sensitization also have the similar distribution suggesting that negative results are more common across food-use chemicals in general than positive results. Table 39.4 shows that for acute oral toxicity, acute dermal toxicity, acute aquatic toxicity, acute inhalation toxicity, chronic aquatic toxicity, mutagenicity, and skin sensitization, pesticides/residues have more positive results. This is not altogether surprising as pesticide/residue chemicals are expected to be more bioactive than food ingredients. Interestingly, for acute dermal irritation and eye irritation, direct food additives have more positive results. For acute dermal irritation there were similar numbers of positive and negative results. However, for other health endpoints, negative rates are generally greater than positive rates, which should be expected for food-related substances.

39.3.4 Confidence level

Next, we analyzed how confident the program is when targeting different toxicity endpoints. There are three confidence levels, the first one is "very strong" and "strong," which means the program is confident about the prediction value. The second one is "moderate" and "weak," which means the program has low confidence about the prediction value. The last one is "exclude," which means the structure does not fit the RASAR rules, that is, outside of its applicability domain, and thus we cannot obtain the confidence level.

Fig. 39.2 provides the total positive and negative results at the different confidence levels for the specific toxicity endpoints.

High-confidence nontoxicant predictions are by far the highest percentage of the data. RASAR is also capable of

TABLE 39.4 Percentage of positive and negative results for each manual curation food-use category and toxicity endpoint.

Positivity rate and negativity rate										
	Direct food additive		Indirect food additive		Nonfood		Pesticide/residue		Not included in manual curation	
	Positive rate	Negative rate	Positive rate	Negative rate	Positive rate	Negative rate	Positive rate	Negative rate	Positive rate	Negative rate
Acute oral toxicity	28%	72%	33%	67%	58%	42%	54%	46%	37%	63%
Acute dermal irritation	57%	43%	49%	51%	59%	41%	40%	60%	66%	34%
Acute dermal toxicity	20%	80%	25%	75%	46%	54%	43%	57%	33%	67%
Acute aquatic toxicity	16%	84%	19%	81%	32%	68%	59%	41%	11%	89%
Acute inhalation toxicity	24%	76%	25%	75%	49%	51%	47%	53%	34%	66%
Chronic aquatic toxicity	23%	77%	22%	78%	43%	57%	66%	34%	16%	84%
Eye irritation	61%	39%	51%	49%	60%	40%	38%	62%	73%	27%
Mutagenicity	12%	88%	12%	88%	32%	68%	25%	75%	18%	82%
Skin sensitization	34%	66%	33%	67%	54%	46%	51%	49%	42%	58%

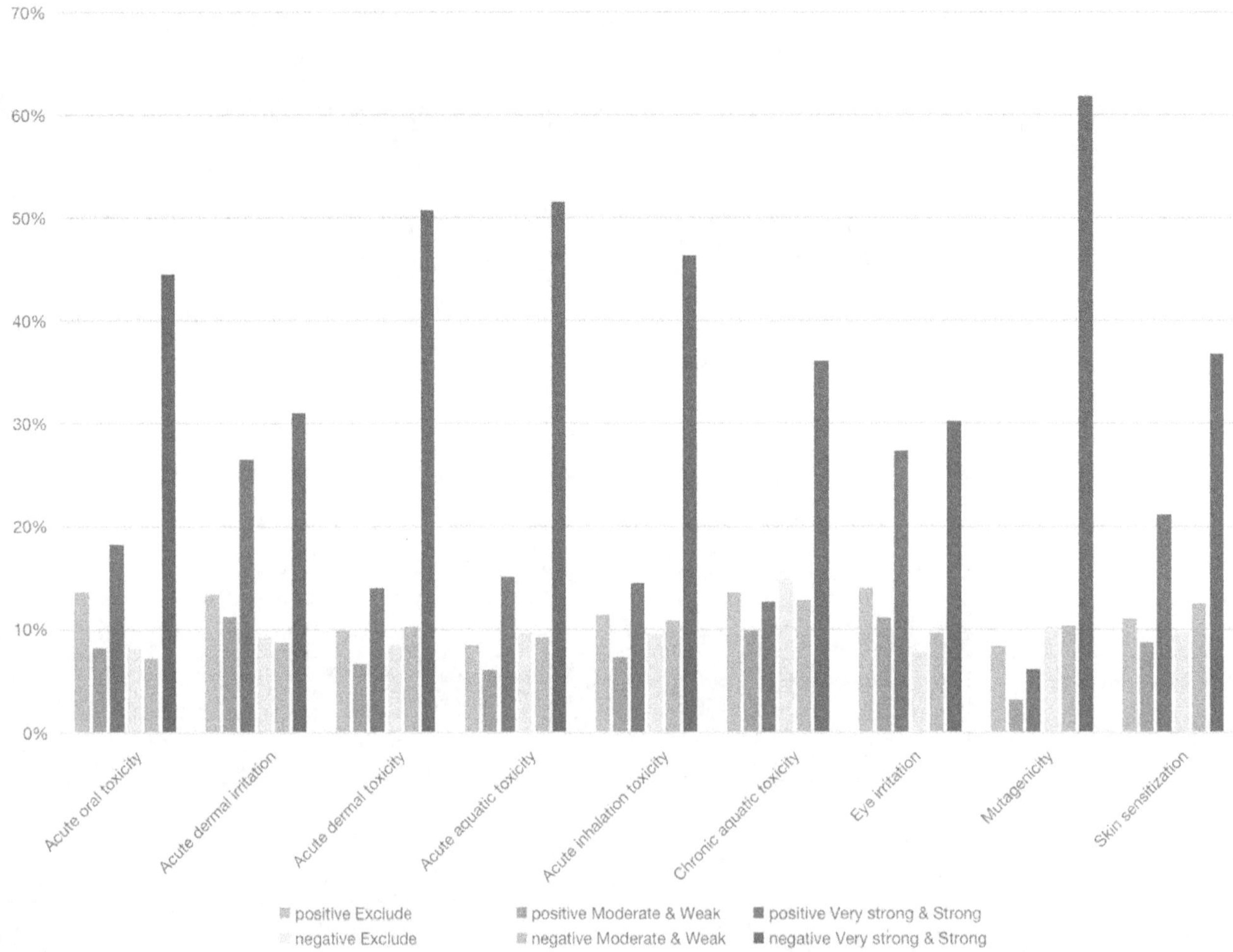

FIGURE 39.2 Confidence levels of positive and negative RASAR predictions for 1215 chemicals. For each toxicity endpoint, the first three (red) bars mean the results are positive (predicting a toxic effect), while the following three (blue) bars mean the results are negative (prediction indicates a nontoxicant). Darker color means the RASAR is more confident about the prediction results, while lighter color means RASAR prediction has lower confidence. *RASAR*, Read-across-based structure activity relationships.

identifying chemicals that could lead to toxicity endpoints with high confidence, but, in general, with better performance targeting nontoxicants than toxicants in this 1215 chemical inventory. Overall, there are much more results in "very strong" and "strong" positive and "very strong" and "strong" negative comparing to "moderate" and "weak" positive and "moderate" and "weak" negative, which suggests that RASAR could be a promising tool when predicting the toxicity endpoints for chemicals in this list (meaning for food-use chemistry in specific).

39.3.5 Performance assessment and preliminary validation

Preliminary validation was conducted by comparing the toxicological assessment results from RASAR and other sources. It is important to know whether the RASAR predictions were consistent with experimental results, so comparing the prediction results obtained from RASAR to toxicological assessment results from other sources, such as ECHA, OSHA, and other literature was conducted as a form of performance-based validation.

The five highest prediction values for RASAR outputs with "very strong" confidence level in each of the five manual curation categories (direct food additives, indirect food additives, pesticides/residues, nonfood, not included in manual curation categorization) were selected. There were 18 unique chemicals are corresponding to these 25 prediction values. Those 18 chemicals included allyl cyclohexanepropionate, α-phellandrene, methyl butyrate, 3-(methylthio)propyl isothiocyanate, pentachloropyridine, furfural, 2,4-diaminotoluene, dichlorobenzene, coumaphos, coumatetralyl, sulfotep, 2.4-D-1-butyl ester, terbufos, tefluthrin, deltamethrin, cypermethrin, fenvalerate, and 2,5-dimethulfuran. The final comprehensive listing, summarized in Table 39.4, includes all 18 chemicals with 162 toxicological assessment results whether the chemical is predicted to lead to the toxicity endpoints or not. For example, allyl cyclohexanepropionate has been identified as positive for acute aquatic toxicity in the RASAR, which means allyl cyclohexanepropionate is predicted to lead to acute aquatic toxicity based on RASAR results. In line, other sources also identify allyl cyclohexanepropionate as toxic to aquatic life and leading to acute hazard. Hence, both results match. Color codes for each result facilitate interpretation: green represents matching data (e.g., results from other sources are matching with the results from the RASAR), and red represents no-match (e.g., the results from other sources differ from the RASAR results). Colors also ranged from dark to light, reflecting the confidence level provided by RASAR.

Not all toxicity endpoints had complementary data found from other sources and literature. For example, α-phellandrene has a high confidence level RASAR prediction value for acute aquatic toxicity. However, in our search for other sources or literature, no data were available to confirm whether α-phellandrene would lead to acute aquatic toxicity to suggest its impact on aquatic life. This kind of results had been excluded from the preliminary validation process, and results marked as "exclude" in the RASAR were not used for this preliminary validation, either. Thus in total there were 123 results eligible for the preliminary validation evaluation (results summarized in Table 39.5). The percentage of data with match

TABLE 39.5 Comparison of RASAR predictions and complementary experimental data classification for high-confidence chemicals.

Chemical	CASRNs	Manual Curation Categorization	Acute Ora Toxicity	Acute Inhalatiion Toxicity	Acute Derma Toxicity	Acute Dermal Irritation	Eye Irritatioı	Skin Sensitizatioı	Acute Aquati Toxicity	Chronic Aquatic Toxicity	Mutagenicity
Allyl cyclohexanepropionate	2705-87-5	Direct food additive	(0.965) + √-√	(0.922) + √-√	(0.860) + √-√	(0.399) - /-√	(0.252) - x-/	(0.928) + √-√	(0.996) + √-√	(0.960) + √-√	(0.059) - x-x
α-phellandrene	99-83-2	Direct food additive	(0.025) - x-√	(0.093) - x-√	(0.039) - x-/	(0.127) - x-√	(0.048) - x-√	(0.905) + √-√	(0.994) + √-/	(0.829) + √-√	(0.060) - x-/
Methyl butyrate	623-42-7	Direct food additive	(0.034) - x-x	(0.185) - x-x	(0.140) - x-/	(0.991) + √-√	(0.993) + √-√	(0.132) - x-x	(0.076) - x-/	(0.130) - x-/	(0.161) - x-/
3-(Methylthio)propyl isothiocyanate	505-79-3	Direct food additive	(0.950) + √-√	(0.818) + √-√	(0.767) + √-√	(0.959) + √-√	(0.941) + √-√	(0.907) + √-/	(0.992) + √-√	(0.919) + √-√	(0.209) - x-/
Pentachloropyridine	2176-62-7	Indirect food additive	(0.822) + √-√	(0.980) + √-√	(0.969) + √-√	(0.969) + √-√	(0.945) + √-√	(0.924) + √-√	(0.991) + √-√	(0.902) + √-√	(0.174) - x-x
Furfural	98-01-1	Indirect food additive	(0.882) + √-√	(0.949) + √-√	(0.941) + √-√	(0.988) + √-√	(0.991) + √-√	(0.966) + √-√	(0.617) + /-√	(0.473) - /-√	(0.872) + √-√
2,4-Diaminotoluene	95-80-7	Indirect food additive	(0.934) + √-√	(0.937) + √-√	(0.990) + √-√	(0.901) + √-√	(0.822) + √-√	(0.983) + √-√	(0.824) + √-√	(0.810) + √-√	(0.987) + √-√
Dichlorobenzene	106-46-7	Indirect food additive Pesticides/residues	(0.758) + √-√	(0.796) + √-√	(0.925) + √-x	(0.989) + √-√	(0.974) + √-√	(0.713) + √-√	(0.539) + /-√	(0.290) - x-√	(0.903) + √-x
Coumaphos	56-72-4	Non-food	(0.827) + √-√	(0.937) + √-√	(0.892) + √-√	(0.354) - x-√	(0.278) - x-√	(0.811) + √-√	(0.996) + √-√	(0.857) + √-√	(0.515) + /-x
Coumatetralyl	5836-29-3	Non-food	(0.963) + √-√	(0.846) + √-√	(0.837) + √-√	(0.859) + √-√	(0.824) + √-√	(0.938) + √-x	(0.995) + √-√	(0.970) + √-√	(0.518) + /-√
sulfotep	3689-24-5	Non-food	(0.812) + √-√	(0.780) + √-√	(0.803) + √-√	(0.493) - /-√	(0.274) - x-√	(0.577) + /-√	(0.993) + √-√	(0.907) + √-√	(0.234) - x-x
2,4-D-1-butyl ester	94-80-4	Non-food	(0.973) + √-√	(0.984) + √-/	(0.971) + √-/	(0.703) + √-√	(0.590) + /-√	(0.976) + √-√	(0.984) + √-√	(0.902) + √-√	(0.245) - x-x
Terbufos	13071-79-9	Pesticides/residues	(0.648) + /-√	(0.626) + /-√	(0.557) + /-√	(0.490) - /-√	(0.225) - x-√	(0.617) + /-/	(0.998) + √-√	(0.922) + √-√	(0.299) - x-x
Tefluthrin	79538-32-2	Pesticides/residues	(0.644) + /-√	(0.822) + √-√	(0.691) + √-√	(0.031) - x-√	(0.015) - x-√	(0.065) - x-x	(0.997) + √-√	(0.971) + √-√	(0.063) - x-x
Deltamethrin	52918-63-5	Pesticides/residues	(0.831) + √-√	(0.715) + √-√	(0.658) + /-/	(0.763) + √-√	(0.587) + /-√	(0.940) + √-√	(0.997) + √-√	(0.907) + √-√	(0.346) - /-/
Cypermethrin	52315-97-8	Pesticides/residues	(0.556) + /-√	(0.454) - /-√	(0.284) - x-/	(0.059) - x-√	(0.039) - x-√	(0.310) - x-√	(0.996) + √-√	(0.939) + √-√	(0.043) - x-x
Fenvalerate	51630-58-1	Pesticides/residues	(0.466) - /-√	(0.039) - x-/	(0.020) - x-/	(0.022) - x-√	(0.016) - x-√	(0.157) - x-√	(0.994) + √-√	(0.948) + √-√	(0.021) - x-x
2,5-Dimethylfuran	625-86-5	Not included in manual curation	(0.933) + √-√	(0.979) + √-√	(0.975) + √-/	(0.996) + √-√	(0.996) + √-√	(0.975) + √-√	(0.595) + /-/	(0.514) + /-/	(0.821) + √-x

CASRNs, Chemical abstract services registration numbers; *RASAR*, read-across-based structure activity relationships.

versus not match between RASAR and other sources/literature are 83% and 17%, respectively.

For each chemical and given toxicity endpoint, prediction values are in brackets in the top line. The second line indicates RASAR prediction results with + for toxic (above the threshold 0.5) and − for nontoxic and slash (/) for "exclude" provided by RASAR for this toxicity endpoint. The third line represents the toxicological assessment results from other sources and literature: checkmark (√) represents other sources or literature do report this chemical will lead to this kind of toxicity hazard; cross (X) represents other sources or literature report this chemical is not leading to this kind of toxicity; slash (/) represents toxicological assessment results could not be found in other sources or literature. The color scheme for every pair of results: dark green represents the results from RASAR and other sources are consistent and that RASAR results had high confidence level for the prediction values; light green represents the results from RASAR and other sources match, but the RASAR shows low confidence level for the prediction; dark red represents the results do not match, but RASAR had high confidence for the prediction; light red represents the results do not match and the RASAR prediction had low confidence level; yellow represents the RASAR confidence level is marked as exclude; blue represents negative RASAR predictions for which toxicological assessment results cannot be found in other sources or literature; orange represents RASAR positive predictions for which toxicological assessment results cannot be found in other sources or literature. Numbers of results marked as yellow, blue, and orange, that is, not eligible for validation, are 23, 11, and 5, respectively.

39.4 Discussion

Artificial intelligence and big data are increasingly considered as an option for the safety evaluation of food additives. The increasing use of a variety of food additives mean more and more chemicals need to undergo safety assessment before adding to food and entering the market. Considering the materials, money, and time required for traditional animal testing, in silico alternatives such as RASAR become a promising method for safety evaluation given the time- and cost-effectiveness as well as accuracy. For this project, 38,250 predictions for 4729 food-relevant substances were made with an accuracy at the level of the reproducibility of the respective OECD guideline tests, which would amount to more than $200 million of testing costs and years of work.[2] The nine tests predicted cost more than $50,000 per chemical. This demonstrates the enormous potential of in silico tools to fill data-gaps, carry out plausibility checks or prioritize testing needs.

The current case study comprising 1215 food-use chemicals shows that descriptive statistical analysis supports the robust consistency of RASAR predictions compared to traditional toxicity testing data. Briefly, the 1215 chemicals are based on Karmaus et al.'s[19,26] works and RASAR results generated with the UL Cheminformatics Toolkit. Chemicals were analyzed in subgroups based on manual curation categories, toxicity endpoints, and confidence levels to comprehensively evaluate performance. Results showed that each chemical can be mapped to a manual curation category based on chemical use. The few chemicals with multiple manual curation categories typically have less in-training results, which could be explained as these chemicals are broadly used substances in a variety of fields with more available data. In-training chemicals predicted results, which are at the moment not accessible as proprietary, could be used for cross-validation once the data have been released. The majority of the 1215-chemical inventory was predicted to be nontoxicants as RASAR showed mostly negative predictions for toxicity endpoints. The analysis of confidence levels showed that RASAR has very high confidence levels for the nontoxicant predictions. In addition, the analysis of confidence level subgroups also provides high confidence level for toxicants, which shows the good performance of RASAR predictions compared to other sources and literature when considering toxicity safety evaluations.

During the preliminary validation process, a comparison table was made for 18 chemicals with 123 results eligible for our performance-based validation approach. Note that 23 results were labeled as "exclude" in RASAR and 16 results we could not find external data, so these 39 results were not included in the 123 results used for the preliminary validation process (Table 39.6).

In the 123 results which are eligible for validation, the evaluation from other sources for 102 results matched, while 21 results were no-match (83% and 17%, respectively). The results have also been separated by the 0.5 threshold (for predicted toxicant or nontoxicant, respectively) showing that more toxicants were predicted for our preliminary validation. Overall, good performance of RASAR was confirmed as the safety evaluation results from other sources and literature are highly matched with the generated predictions. It has to be noted though that substances were selected based on strong predicted effect and confidence for one endpoint, though we included all other eight toxicity endpoints of a given chemical as well for preliminary validation.

Notably, acute aquatic toxicity always had the highest prediction values for pesticide /residues. This is not unexpected as these chemicals are known to enter the environment and may contaminate the water system with toxic effects to aquatic life. Some chemicals categorized as direct food additive, indirect food additive, and nonfood

TABLE 39.6 Chemicals used for preliminary validation separated by color scheme.

Color	Color definition	Positive	Percentage	Negative	Percentage	Total	Percentage
Dark green	RASAR (high confidence predications) and other sources consistent	78	63%	8	7%	86	70%
Light green	RASAR (low confidence predications) and other sources consistent	12	10%	4	3%	16	13%
Dark red	RASAR (high confidence predications) and other sources inconsistent	3	2%	11	9%	14	11%
Light red	RASAR (low confidence predications) and other sources inconsistent	1	1%	6	5%	7	6%

The denominator used for calculating percentage is 123, which is the total of eligible endpoints for preliminary validation counts. *RASAR*, Read-across-based structure activity relationships.

also have highest prediction values for acute aquatic toxicity. Karmaus categorized chemicals which are not used in the United States anymore or foreign-use pesticides, drugs, components of cosmetics, and industrial chemicals as nonfood,[19] which means nonfood could contain pesticides too. It would be interesting to investigate the reason for the highest prediction values for the acute aquatic toxicity endpoint and further assess whether these chemicals should be prioritized for risk evaluation to aquatic species.

It is important to remember that chemicals mentioned in this research are mainly food-relevant chemicals currently used in the Unites States. Even though chemicals in nonfood manual curation category do include food-relevant chemicals used in foreign countries, there are likely far more food-relevant chemicals used worldwide. In addition, there are still data gaps. For RASAR, the detailed study information for in-training data, which could be used to conduct cross-validation, is not currently publicly available. Several chemicals also do not have too much information and available data outside the RASAR prediction, which prevented us from conducting preliminary validation on the prediction results for some toxicity endpoints. For example, 3-(methylthio)propyl isothiocyanate had about 0.9 prediction value in RASAR for skin sensitization. This high prediction value indicates 3-(methylthio)propyl isothiocyanate has a high likelihood for inducing skin sensitization as a direct food additive, in this case flavoring agent. However, during the process of searching information in other sources, there seems not too much research conducted on this chemical to allow evaluating its skin sensitization probability; while skin contact hazards are of lesser relevance in the context of food additives, they might still serve as proxy for food allergies and relevant for worker safety. Conflicting results also existed in data, which had high confidence level in the RASAR: α-Phellandrene was the only chemical that had more no-match results across toxicity endpoints than matched results: Five toxicity endpoints had prediction values less than 0.15, suggesting the chemical is a nontoxicant, but other sources suggested the chemical was fatal or harmful. Noteworthy, this screening level study is based on hazard identification and resulting risks cannot be estimated. Such in silico tools help narrow down possible health hazards, but ultimately it is important that exposure route and chemical amount be factored in to determine if there is truly any risk for adversity to arise from the food use, that is, is the amount in food, and the fact that we orally consume the chemical in that amount, posing a threat for these toxicities to be truly a risk?

39.5 Conclusions

This study demonstrates that RASAR could be a useful and trustworthy tool for food safety evaluation as more novel food additives are developed. It has to be noted, that the current implementation covers nine of the most frequently used toxicity endpoints; however, these are not necessarily endpoints suitable for comprehensive risk assessment. Ongoing work, in the context of the EU ONTOX project,[28] aims to integrate more endpoints relevant to risk assessment needs. Further parallel work aims for expansion to also assessing endocrine disruption. This is a significant step in benefitting public health from consuming ingredients which could have potential adverse health or environmental effects and achieve the goal of 3Rs (replacement, reduction, and refinement) of animal use in toxicological testing.

The toxicity endpoints evaluated herein have an enormous role in workplace safety and for transport regulations and are thus carried out for a large number of industrial chemicals including for food-related substances. Noteworthy, many of them also have nonfood applications and may be included in other formulations rendering them relevant for other industries to test. Future studies should focus on chemicals which have not been subjected to full in vivo toxicity testing for the nine toxicity endpoints included in our study (acute oral toxicity, acute dermal irritation, acute dermal toxicity, chronic aquatic toxicity, eye irritation, acute inhalation toxicity, acute aquatic toxicity, mutagenicity, skin sensitization) to gain more available data and broaden the chemical list eligible for performance-based validation. Cross-validation should also be done once the in-training data become available.

Taken together, this screening level case study supports the use of big-data/artificial intelligence (A.I.)-based methodologies to support the hazard assessment of food-relevant substances. Especially in the US system, where many substances lack publicly available data and the FDA has no premarketing authority, such screening tools could become extremely valuable. An independent performance evaluation of the tool is highly recommended but already now it may serve to help decisions on formulations and alternative chemistries in the sense of a Green Toxicology.[29,30] Especially, it appears to be suitable to identify testing needs for the large number of ill-characterized food-related chemicals on the US market.

Acknowledgment

ILS support for this work was funded with federal funds from the NIEHS, NIH under Contract No. HHSN273201500010C. Thomas Hartung is consultant for computational toxicology for UL and receives shares of their respective sales. Thomas Luechtefeld is founder and CEO of ToxTrack Inc., which implemented the RASAR approach for UL.

Endnotes

[a]https://www.fda.gov/food/food-ingredients-packaging.

[b]https://www.epa.gov/chemical-research/toxicity-forecasting.

[c]https://www.epa.gov/chemical-research/cerapp-collaborative-estrogen-receptor-activity-prediction-project-0.

[d]https://comptox.epa.gov/dashboard/chemical_lists/COMPARA/.

[e]https://ul-chemtoolkit.toxtrack.com.

References

1. Mitchell RE, Fraser AM, Bearon LB. Preventing food-borne illness in food service establishments: broadening the framework for intervention and research on safe food handling behaviors. *Int J Environ Health Res*. 2007;17(1):9–24. Available from: https://doi.org/10.1080/09603120601124371.
2. Meigs L, Smirnova L, Rovida C, Leist M, Hartung T. Animal testing and its alternatives – the most important omics is economics. *ALTEX*. 2018;35:275–305. Available from: https://doi.org/10.14573/altex.1807041.
3. Mordor Intelligence. Food Additives Market – growth, trends, and forecast (2020–2025). <https://www.mordorintelligence.com/industry-reports/global-food-additives-market-industry>; 2019.
4. Hartung T, Koeter H. Food for thought ... on alternative methods for food safety testing. *ALTEX*. 2008;25:259–264. Available from: https://doi.org/10.14573/altex.2008.4.259.
5. GAO. Food Safety: FDA should strengthen its oversight of food ingredients determined to be generally recognized as safe (GRAS). <http://www.gao.gov/products/GAO-10-246>; 2010.
6. Mitchell C. Global regulation of food additives. <https://pubs.acs.org/doi/pdf/10.1021/bk-2014-1162.ch001>; 2014.
7. Code of Federal Regulations, Title 21, Part 58: Good Laboratory Practice for Nonclinical Laboratory Studies; 2013.
8. FDA. *Toxicological Principles for the Safety Assessment of Food Ingredients Redbook 2000*; 2000.
9. Hartung T. Rebooting the generally recognized as safe (GRAS) approach for food additive safety in the US. *ALTEX*. 2018;3–25. Available from: https://doi.org/10.14573/altex.1712181.
10. Hartung T. Thresholds of toxicological concern – setting a threshold for testing below which there is little concern. *ALTEX*. 2017;331–351. Available from: https://doi.org/10.14573/altex.1707011.
11. Sakihara MC. Food ingredients with technological properties. *Eur Food Feed Law Rev*. 2018;13(5):392–402.
12. Macarthur Clark J. The 3Rs in research: a contemporary approach to replacement, reduction and refinement. *Br J Nutr*. 2017;120(s1):S1–S7. Available from: https://doi.org/10.1017/s0007114517002227.
13. Smirnova L, Kleinstreuer N, Corvi R, Levchenko A, Fitzpatrick SC, Hartung T. 3S – Systematic, systemic, and systems biology and toxicology. *ALTEX*. 2018;35:139–162. Available from: https://doi.org/10.14573/altex.1804051.
14. Neltner TG, Alger HM, Leonard JE, Maffini MV. Data gaps in toxicity testing of chemicals allowed in food in the United States. *Reprod Toxicol*. 2013;42:85–94. Available from: https://doi.org/10.1016/j.reprotox.2013.07.023.
15. Hartung T, Luechtefeld T, Maertens A, Kleensang A. Integrated testing strategies for safety assessments. *ALTEX*. 2013;30:3–18. Available from: https://doi.org/10.14573/altex.2013.1.003.
16. Hartung T, Van Vliet E, Jaworska J, Bonilla L, Skinner N, Thomas R. Systems toxicology. *ALTEX*. 2012;29:119–128. Available from: https://doi.org/10.14573/altex.2012.2.119.
17. Hartung T, Fitzgerald R, Jennings P, et al. Systems toxicology – real world applications and opportunities. *Chem Res Toxicol*. 2017;30:870–882. Available from: https://doi.org/10.1021/acs.chemrestox.7b00003.
18. Corvi R, Spielmann H, Hartung T. Alternative approaches for carcinogenicity and reproductive toxicity. In: The History of Alternative Test Methods in Toxicology, pp. 209–217. Academic Press, 2019. Available from: https://doi.org/10.1016/B978-0-12-813697-3.00024-X.
19. Karmaus AL, Filer DL, Martin MT, Houck KA. Evaluation of food-relevant chemicals in the ToxCast high-throughput screening program. *Food Chem Toxicol*. 2016;92:188–196. Available from: https://doi.org/10.1016/j.fct.2016.04.012.

20. Ball N, Cronin MTD, Shen J, et al. Toward Good Read-Across Practice (GRAP) guidance. *ALTEX*. 2016;33:149–166. Available from: https://doi.org/10.14573/altex.1601251.
21. Patlewicz G, Ball N, Becker RA, et al. Read-across approaches - misconceptions, promises and challenges ahead. *ALTEX*. 2014;31 (4):387–396. Available from: https://doi.org/10.14573/altex.1410071.
22. Hartung T. Making big sense from big data in toxicology by read-across. *ALTEX*. 2016;83–93. Available from: https://doi.org/10.14573/altex.1603091.
23. Luechtefeld T, Hartung T. Computational approaches to chemical hazard assessment. *ALTEX*. 2017;459–478. Available from: https://doi.org/10.14573/altex.1710141.
24. Luechtefeld T, Rowlands C, Hartung T. Big-data and machine learning to revamp computational toxicology and its use in risk assessment. *Toxicol Res*. 2018;7(5):732–744. Available from: https://doi.org/10.1039/c8tx00051d.
25. Luechtefeld T, Marsh D, Rowlands C, Hartung T. Machine learning of toxicological big data enables read-across structure activity relationships (RASAR) outperforming animal test reproducibility. *Toxicol Sci*. 2018;165(1):198–212. Available from: https://doi.org/10.1093/toxsci/kfy152.
26. Karmaus AL, Trautman TD, Krishan M, Filer DL, Fix LA. Curation of food-relevant chemicals in ToxCast. *Food Chem Toxicol*. 2017;103:174–182. Available from: https://doi.org/10.1016/j.fct.2017.03.006.
27. Dionisio KL, Frame AM, Goldsmith M-R, et al. Exploring consumer exposure pathways and patterns of use for chemicals in the environment. *Toxicol Rep*. 2015;2:228–237. Available from: https://doi.org/10.1016/j.toxrep.2014.12.009.
28. Vinken M, Benfenati E, Busquet F, et al. Safer chemicals using less animals: kick-off of the European ONTOX project. *Toxicology*. 2021;458:152846. Available from: https://doi.org/10.1016/j.tox.2021.152846.
29. Maertens A, Anastas N, Spencer PJ, Stephens M, Goldberg A, Hartung T. Green toxicology. *ALTEX*. 2014;31:243–249.
30. Maertens A, Hartung T. Green toxicology – know early about and avoid toxic product liabilities. *Toxicol Sci*. 2018;161:285–289. Available from: https://doi.org/10.1093/toxsci/kfx243.

Chapter 40

Potential human health effects following exposure to nano- and microplastics, lessons learned from nanomaterials

Hugo Brouwer, Femke L.N. Van Oijen and Hans Bouwmeester
Division of Toxicology, Wageningen University, Wageningen, The Netherlands

Abstract
A substantial part of the plastic produced worldwide ends up in the environment and degrades into nano- and microplastics. The particles are ubiquitously present in the air and enter the food production chain as contaminants. Ingestion of nano- and microplastics present in food and drinking water, or those present in swallowed lung mucus that contain trapped particles, represent the main route of human exposure. Yet much remains to be studied on the intestinal uptake by humans and the potential this exposure has to result in adverse health effects. Here we review the current knowledge and relate this to lessons learned from the field of nanotoxicology. We discuss how in vitro and in silico approaches can be used to support the risk assessment of nano- and microplastics.

Keywords: Nanoplastics; microplastics; toxicity; uptake; in vitro models; PBK models

40.1 Introduction

Worldwide the production and use of plastic is on the rise. The yearly production has now exceeded 360 million metric tons, of which around 40% is used for packaging.[1–3] A substantial part of the produced plastic ends up in the environment. The combined exposure to ultraviolet light and mechanical action in the environment causes the plastic material to become brittle and degrade into smaller-sized fragments.[4,5] Apart from these plastic fragments (often referred to as secondary particles), also primary nano- and microplastics can be found in the environment and human food products. Primary nano- and microplastics are intentionally manufactured for industrial purposes like pelleted precursors for plastic products, or have been used as abrasives in cleaning products.[4,6] Collectively these materials are called nano- and microplastics, where plastic fragments with a size range between 100 and 5 mm are commonly defined as microplastics, whereas particles with a size <100 nm are defined as nanoplastics.[7–9]

Micro and nanoplastics represent a highly diverse class of contaminants which can be found in a broad range of shapes and sizes.[7] Importantly the polymer composition of nano- and microplastics in environmental or food samples is very heterogenous with polyethylene (PE), polypropylene (PP), and polystyrene (PS) being the most abundant polymer types[10–12] though polyethylene terephtelate (PET) and poly-vinyl-chloride (PVC) are also frequently detected.[13–15] Additional complexity is introduced as micro and nanoplastics can contain a diversity of chemical mixtures comprised of compounds such as plasticizers, flame retardants, stabilizers, fillers and pigments to improve the functionality of the product.[16,17] Due to the relatively high surface area to volume ratio and hydrophobicity, micro and nanoplastics can adsorb chemicals from the environment. Well known examples of adsorbed chemicals are polychlorinated biphenyls, dioxins, polycyclic aromatic hydrocarbons, and polybrominated diphenyl ethers and pharmaceuticals.[18–27]

Humans can be exposed to micro and nanoplastics mainly via inhalatory or oral routes of exposure. Several studies have shown that micro and nanoplastics are present in the outdoor and indoor air.[28,29] From the inhalable (or respiratory) fraction of micro and nanoplastics at least a fraction will be trapped in the lung mucus and cleared via the mucociliary escalator. These trapped micro and nanoplastics are subsequently swallowed and enter the gastrointestinal tract. Direct ingestion of micro and nanoplastics, for instance via drinking water or consumed food also is an important source of human exposure.

Present Knowledge in Food Safety. DOI: https://doi.org/10.1016/B978-0-12-819470-6.00014-7

The presence of micro and nanoplastics in a great diversity of food items, ranging from bottled water, shell fish, honey and packaged food has been shown (and reviewed before[30,31]). Upon passage through the intestinal (or lung) epithelial barrier micro and nanoplastics may have the potential to cause adverse human health effects.[32] At this point parallels can be drawn with health effects observed after prolonged exposure to (ultra) fine dust that has been shown to trigger oxidative stress and inflammation ultimately resulting in cardiovascular and respiratory diseases.[33] In studying the hazards and risks of nano- and microplastics important lessons can also be learned from experiences with engineered nanomaterials.[34–36] The exposure to nanomaterials is similar to that of nano- and microplastics, since intestinal uptake represents an important potential route of entry of these materials.[37] Human exposure to nanomaterials can be both unintentional and intentional because of their deliberate addition to food, their widespread use in food packaging and other domestic products and the potential for their inadvertent ingestion from environmental contamination.[30] Engineered (nano)materials, including silicon dioxide (SiO_2), titanium dioxide (TiO_2) and silver (Ag) nanoparticles have been detected in food[38–41] which, together with nanomaterials present in products such as toothpaste, cosmetics and sun cream, have a clear potential for ingestion by humans.

Here we will review the potential mechanism by which nano- and microplastics can pass the intestinal epithelium, as well as available evidence for potential adverse health outcomes. The study of potential health effects of nano- and microplastics is in its infancy, although there is a surge in the number of recently published papers. We will discuss which parallels can be drawn between the studies of micro and nanoplastics and the development of the field of nanosafety.[34]

40.1.1 Effects of conditions in the gastrointestinal tract on nano- and microplastics

Nano- and microplastics that are swallowed are subjected to physical and biochemical conditions that are very different from those encountered via other exposure routes.[42] Upon entry into the stomach the materials encounter an environment that has an extremely low pH and a high ionic strength. Further pH changes in the small intestine, the presence of mucus and the resident microbiota in the GIT lumen add additional complexity to the physicochemical properties of the ingested nano- and microplastics[43,44] potentially resulting in differences in toxicokinetics and toxicodynamics of the micro and nanoplastics.

The dynamics in pH and ionic shifts that nano- and microplastics encounter during stomach and intestinal transit can affect the dispersity of the material, and could result in an agglomeration of the particles, as seen earlier for (silica) nanomaterials.[40] Particle agglomeration at high concentrations might result in a lower bioavailable concentration resulting in a nonlinear dose response curve (i.e., low effects at high nominal concentration administered orally), as observed following oral administration of silica nanomaterials.[45] Additionally the rich luminal environment results in coating of the nano- and microplastics with biomolecules,[43,44,46–49] that affect the uptake of micro and nanoplastics. Unlike metal(oxide) nanomaterials of which some dissolve under acidic conditions,[50] dissolution of micro and nanoplastics particles is unlikely to occur under physiological conditions.

A relatively unexplored area is the potential interaction of nano- and microplastics with the intestinal microbiome. The intestinal microbiome is known for its crucial role on human health in general[51] and its role in the metabolism of foodborne chemicals.[52,53] However the interactions between particles and the intestinal microbiome has to be better explored.[54] Only little can be learned from engineered nanomaterials[55] as, also there, the interactions with the intestinal microbiome have not been studied in detail (as recently reviewed[56]). Some evidence from rodents is appearing that high concentrations of intestinal nano- and microplastics can affect the diversity and composition of the gut microbiota,[57] however, the functional consequences need additional investigation. Many of the effects of metal nanomaterials on bacteria have been attributed to ions dissociated from nanomaterials,[56,58] thus it might be postulated that micro and nanoplastics have less effect on bacteria directly. However, micro and nanoplastics can contain cocktails of associated chemicals,[18–27] that potentially can affect the intestinal micro-organisms. Interestingly some studies have shown that nanomaterial exposure affects not only the composition of the microbial community (in the cecum), but also increased the production of the bacterial metabolite butyrate following a 21 day exposure of mice to chitosan particles loaded with copper sulfate,[59] while oral exposure of mice for 35 days to particulate matter (PM1) at 10 mg/g/day decreased intestinal butyrate concentrations.[60] Butyrate serves as a key energy source of intestinal cells[59] and as a critical mediator in other responses and might thus represent a vector of biological action following exposure to nanomaterials (and nanoplastics).[61,62] In vitro studies using human stools also confirmed that nanoparticles can affect intestinal metabolism. A 5-day incubation with CeO_2, TiO_2, ZnO nanomaterials in a model colon reactor resulted in a decreased butyrate production upon incubation with CeO_2 nanoparticles only.[63] No related studies on the interaction of nano- and microplastics have been identified so far.

In conclusion, the physicochemical properties of micro and nanoplastics like engineered nanomaterials can be affected by the biochemical conditions in the human gastrointestinal tract which in turn might affect the toxicokinetics and toxicodynamics of these materials. The effects micro and nanoplastics have on the intestinal microbiome and the microbial metabolism are yet largely unknown, but given the importance of the intestinal microbiome on human health this needs to be studied. It is important to note that there are differences between the human and rodent microbiome and that there are differences in microbiome diversity of communities collected from human stools and the communities in the intestine, complicating further studies. For instance, the microbial composition in the human small intestine was reported to be far less complex than that of the large intestine.[64] Thus a careful design of studies is needed.

40.1.2 Potential mechanisms of intestinal nano- and microplastics uptake

Mechanistic information on nanoparticle uptake processes across the intestinal epithelium has been almost exclusively derived from in vitro studies.[65,66] The used in vitro cell models attempt to emulate critical intestinal nano- and microplastics uptake functionality. The small intestine is mostly lined by enterocytes that bear a dense microvillus brush-border on the apical (lumen) side of the cells. The epithelium is sealed by tight junctions between the cells that prevent passage of most materials. Interspersed between enterocytes are goblet cells which secrete negatively charged mucus onto the gut epithelium. The mucus lining provides an additional barrier to the diffusion of particulates towards the epithelium, with smaller particles penetrating more easily through the mucus layer and positively charged particles getting trapped in the mucus.[67] The apical membrane of enterocytes is also covered with a complex glycocalyx which forms a size-selective barrier by the potential interaction of particulate material with surface molecules.[68,69] Lastly, so-called microfold cells (M-cells) can be found in specialized lymphoid-associated regions in the intestinal epithelium, the Peyer's patches and other gut-associated lymphoid tissues (GALT).[70] M-cells have a thinner apical glycocalyx and mucus layer and have the capacity to transport material, including inert particles, viruses and bacteria, and to deliver them to the underlying lymphoid cells.[71] Epithelial cells form a tight, dense monolayer and for that reason the paracellular route (i.e., between cells) of passage seems very unlikely for nano- and microplastics. Therefore it is often assumed that transcellular routes predominate, as also shown by in vitro experiments with epithelial cells.[72–78] It is likely that particles in the nano-size range are internalized through clathrin- and/or caveolin-dependent endocytosis, which operates in polarized epithelia,[79] while uptake of larger particles (>150 nm) occurs mainly by phagocytosis and micropinocytosis. The best characterized route for transcellular particle translocation is that through the aforementioned M-cells. However, transport through M-cells does not necessarily mean that the nanoplastics reach the bloodstream as M-cells are closely associated with immune cells. A study described that orally administered glucan and poly(lactic-*co*-glycolic acid) (PLGA) nanoparticles in mice were transported through M-cells and subsequently endocytosed by dendritic cells in the Peyer's patches and subsequently retained, thereby not reaching the bloodstream.[80] The close connection to the immune system also indicates that the intestinal immune homeostasis may be influenced by nanoplastics. This was also shown in a study in which it was observed that amorphous magnesium-substituted calcium phosphate nanoparticles enter the Peyer's patches via M-cells. These nanoparticles are spontaneously formed from calcium and phosphate ions that are naturally secreted into the lumen of the distal small intestine. These particles trap soluble macromolecules, such as bacterial peptidoglycan and orally fed protein antigens, which upon entering the Peyer's patches might result in interactions with the local immune system.[81] Despite their well-established transcystotic capacity, M-cells are scarce and other less efficient uptake routes via normal enterocytes may be quantitatively more important for nanoplastic uptake.[82] Indeed, significant uptake of particulate PLA-PEG nanomaterials (200 nm) has been reported in rat epithelial cells in vivo, with no preference for Peyer's patches compared to enterocytes in the villi.[67,83] To complicate this observation, in vitro results suggest different mechanism of uptake of these nanomaterials compared to 200 nm PS particles and 290 nm chitosan particles.[67,83] Earlier studies reported that while larger particles are preferentially taken up by rat Peyer's patches, uptake by enterocytes was significant and became more so as particle sizes of polymer nanoparticles decreased to 100 nm.[84–86] These data suggest that nano-sized particles may access additional uptake routes to those available for larger particles and support the concept that lower efficiency of nanoplastic uptake by enterocytes might be offset by its vastly larger presence in the intestinal epithelium compared with the specialized M-cells.

Paracellular transport is likely not a major route for nanoplastic passage through the healthy intestinal epithelium unless nanoplastics are small enough or have surface properties that increase tight junction permeability. However, there will not be such a strict limitation on paracellular transport in areas where the epithelium is damaged, during normal cell turnover at villus tips and in pathological states where intestinal epithelium translocation may be enhanced. For example, it is well known that bacterial translocation is enhanced by conditions such as trauma, inflammation, stroke, and chronic alcohol use.[87,88] This translocation is likely to be mirrored by increased uptake of particulate material. This concept is supported by in vitro studies demonstrating enhanced penetration of 2 μm PS particles across cultured CaCO-2 cells following alcohol treatment or irradiation, which enhance tight junction leakage.[89,90] Studies using in vitro models of the inflamed intestine have also reported increased cytotoxicity and inflammation after exposure to PE and PVC microplastics (but not following exposure to PS nanoplastics) compared to the healthy situation. Translocation could however not be measured since the size of the particles did not allow them to pass the transwell pores on which the intestinal cells were grown.[91,92] Nano- and microplastics come with a great diversity in size, shape, and polymer composition. How these variation contribute to different uptake profiles remains to be elucidated. Comparison of environmental plastic particles with engineered nanoplastics is challenging as differences in surface properties and shape might differentially govern uptake processes.

40.1.3 Nanomaterial uptake following ingestion by humans and rodents

Only very little human data is available on the potential systemic availability of nano- and microplastics. Recently a pilot study was published in which microplastic fragments were observed in the placentas from six patients with uneventful pregnancies.[93] Some of these fragments, with a size around 5 and 10 μm were observed on the fetal side of the placenta using Raman microspectroscopy.[93] Somewhat more information is available on particulate matter exposure in general. In a single dose study using human volunteers (n = 9) an oral exposure to 5 mg/kg body weight (315–620 mg person) of TiO_2 particles (10, 70, 1800 nm) did not result in a detectable concentration in urine 72 h postexposure. In addition, no values outside clinical ranges (whole blood erythrocytes) were observed.[94] However, in a comparable study where seven human volunteers ingested 100 mg food grade TiO_2 nanoparticles (mean size 260 nm), TiO_2 was observed in blood 2 h after administration, which peaked at 6 h following ingestion.[95] This study supported earlier findings where blood samples contained increased levels of TiO_2 after ingestion of 160 and 380 nm TiO_2 nanoparticles.[96] The presence of reflective particles in blood was interpreted as evidence of the presence of TiO_2 particles but this was not confirmed by direct analysis of particle composition (e.g., by single particle inductively coupled plasma mass spectrometry). Lastly, carbon black particles have been detected in human placentas in concentrations averaging (standard deviation between brackets) 0.95×10^4 (0.66×10^4) and 2.09×10^4 (0.9×10^4) particles/mm^3 placenta tissue for low and high exposed mothers, respectively. The authors showed that the placental carbon black load was positively associated with mothers' residential carbon black exposure during pregnancy (0.63–2.42 μg/m^3).[97]

Unfortunately, rodent studies do not provide much more data on the oral uptake of micro and nanoplastics. Earlier we estimated that only 0.2% of a single dose (administered via oral gavage) of 125 mg 50 nm PS particles was detected in the body after 6 h, which was increased to 1.7% for negatively charged PS particles of the same size.[98] Such low oral bioavailability of PS particles was recently confirmed in a study that used a single administration by gavage of desferrioxamine and radiolabeled plastic particles of various sizes (0.1 mg/animal of 20 nm, 220 nm, 1 μm, and 6 μm). For the smallest particles of 20 nm <0.001% was detected 48 h after administration.[98,99] We calculated[98] from earlier studies by Jani and colleagues (1990) that 6.6% of the administered 50 nm and 5.9% of 100 nm PS particles ended up in the body (1.25 mg/kg bw daily for 10 days).[85] Based on an extensive review of the literature the European Food Safety Authority[100] concluded that intestinal absorption of particles of 2–3 μm was not higher than 0.3%, based on rodent studies and ex vivo models using human tissues.[7] For 500 nm carboxylated particles administered by oral gavage for 5 days in a concentration of 12.5 mg/kg bw the total uptake was estimated to be 37.6%.[100] In another study rats were administered 20 nm rhodamine-labeled nanopolystyrene beads (2.64×10^{14} particles) via intratracheal instillation on gestational day (GD) 19. One day later, nanopolystyrene particles were detected in the maternal lung, heart, and spleen. PS nanoparticles were also observed in the placenta, fetal liver, lungs, heart, kidney, and brain suggesting maternal lung-to-fetal tissue nanoparticle translocation in late stage pregnancy.[101]

We conclude that there is a lack of data on uptake of micro and nanoplastics by humans, but based on the limited human data, systemic availability cannot be excluded. The limited amount of available data from animal studies is inconclusive as the reported uptake ranges from low (< 0001% for 20 nm particles) to high (37.6%) intestinal uptake depending on size and surface charge of the studied materials. Clearly more data is urgently needed on the uptake (rates) of micro and nanoplastics to which humans are exposed.

40.1.4 Effects of nano- and microplastics on gastrointestinal epithelium in vitro

The number of in vitro studies in which the potential effects of nano- and micro plastics are investigated is increasing rapidly. In Table 40.1, an overview of in vitro studies

TABLE 40.1 Results of in vitro studies using models for the human intestinal epithelium.

Material	Size	Concentration exposure duration	Significant effects in vitro	Assay	Cell model	References
Cytotoxicity						
PS	100 nm; 5 μm	0, 1, and 20 μg/mL for 96 h	100 nm 20 μg/mL increased LDH5 μm no effect	LDH	CaCO-2 cells (exposure with and without in vitro digestion)	104
PS	5 μm	0, 1 × 10^{-1}–10^{-8} mg/mL for 24 and 48 h	No effects	MTT	CaCO-2	105
PS	300 nm; 500 nm; 1 μm; 3 μm; 6 μm	0, 20, 50, 70, 90, and 120 μg/mL for 24 h	300 nm: all concentration 500 nm: 120 μg/mL 1 μm: 90 and 120 μg/mL 3 μm: 70, 90 and 120 μg/mL 6 μm: 50, 70, 90, and 120 μg/mL	MTT	CaCO-2	102
PS	50 nm;	0, 1, 5, 10, and 50 μg/cm² for 24 h	No effects	WST-1, LDH, number of nuclei	Normal mono and normal and inflamed cocultures CaCO-2/HT29-MTX-E12/THP-1	91
PS	50–100 nm	0, 25, 50, 100, 125, 150, 175, and 200 μg/mL for 24 and 48 h	175 and 200 μg/mL slight decrease in cell numbers after 48 h	Beckman counter method	CaCO-2 cells	106
PS	50–100 nm	0, 25, 50, 100, 125, 150, 175, and 200 μg/mL for 24 h	No effects	Beckman counter method	Coculture of CaCO-2/HT29 and a triple culture of CaCO-2/HT29 + Raji B	107
Carboxyl-modified PS	1, 4, and 10 μm	0, ~10^3, ~10^6, 10^7, ~10^8 particle/mL for 48 h	1 μm ~10^7 ~10^8 particle/mL 4 μm ~10^8 particle/mL	MTT	CaCO-2	108
Amine-modified PS	50 nm	0, 1, 5, 10, and 50 μg/cm² for 24 h	All concentration in CaCO-2, WST-1 (LDH in highest two concentrations) 10 and 50 μg/cm² in HT29MTX-E12: WST-1 and LDH 50 μg/cm² in triple cultures increased LDH	WST-1, LDH, number of nuclei	Normal and inflamed mono and cocultures CaCO-2/HT29-MTX-E12/THP-1	91
PET	<100 nm	0, 1, 5, 15, and 30 μg/mL for 24, 48, and 96 h	No effects	MTS and LDH	CaCO-2	109
PET	Polydisperse	0, 1, 5, 10, 25, 50, 75, and 100 mg/mL for 24 h	No effects	MTT	CaCO-2	110
PE	1–4 μm; 10–20 μm; polydisperse	1–4 μm: 0, 1, 5, 10, 25, and 50 mg/mL for 24 h10–20 μm; 0, 1, 5, 10, and 25 mg/mL for 24 h Polydisperse: 1, 5, 10, 25, 50, 75, and 100 mg/mL for 24 h	No effects	MTT	CaCO-2, reversed exposure	110

PA	<300 μm	0, 823.5–1380.0 μg/cm^2 for 6, 24, and 48 h	No effects	LDH	CaCO-2 + HT29-MTX + MDMs + MDDCs	111
PE	200–9900 nm	0, 10, and 50 μg/cm^2 for 24 h	50 μg/cm^2 in both stable and inflamed tricultures	LDH	Normal cocultures CaCO-2/HT29-MTX-E12/THP-1, normal exposure and reversed exposure. Inflamed cocultures Caco-2/HT29-MTX-E12/THP-1, reversed exposure	92
PP	Polydisperse	0, 1, 5, 10, 25, and 50 mg/mL for 24 h	Only significant effects the 10 mg/kg	MTT	CaCO-2, reversed exposure	110
PP	< 300 μm	0, 823.5–1380.0 μg/cm^2 for 6, 24, and 48 h	No effects	LDH	CaCO-2 + HT29-MTX + MDMs + MDDCs	111
PU (hard and ester)	<300 μm	0, 823.5–1380.0 μg/cm^2 for 6, 24, and 48 h	No effects	LDH	CaCO-2 + HT29-MTX + MDMs + MDDCs	111
PVC	<50 μm	0, 1, 5, 10, and 50 μg/cm^2 for 24 h	Only in inflamed triculture at 50 μg/cm^2 (reduced number of nuclei)	WST-1, LDH, number of nuclei	Normal and inflamed mono and cocultures CaCO-2/HT29-MTX-E12/THP-1	91
PVC	Polydisperse	0, 1, 5, 10, 25, 50, 75, and 100 mg/mL for 24 h	Cytotoxic at 75 and 100 mg/mL	MTT	CaCO-2	110
Barrier integrity						
PS	50 nm	0, 10, and 50 μg/cm^2 for 24 h	No effects	TEER	Normal and inflamed cocultures CaCO-2/HT29-MTX-E12/THP-1	91
PS	50–100 nm	0, 1, 25, 50, and 100 μg/mL for 24 h	No effects	TEER, LY transport	Coculture of CaCO-2/HT29 and a triple culture of CaCO-2/HT29 + Raji B	107
PS	100 nm; 5 μm	0, 1, and 20 μg/mL for 96 h	100 nm 20 μg/mL increased LY transport	LY transport	CaCO-2 cells (exposure with and without in vitro digestion)	104
			5 μm no effects			
Amine-modified PS	50 nm	0, 10, and 50 μg/cm^2 for 24 h	50 μg/cm^2 in healthy and inflamed triculture models	TEER	Normal and inflamed cocultures CaCO-2/HT29-MTX-E12/THP-1	91
PE	200–9900 nm	0, 10, and 50 μg/cm^2 for 24 h	No effects	TEER	Normal and inflamed cocultures CaCO-2/HT29-MTX-E12/THP-1, reversed exposure.	92
PVC	< 50 μm	0, 10, and 50 μg/cm^2 for 96 h	No effects	TEER	Normal and inflamed cocultures CaCO-2/HT29-MTX-E12/THP-1	91
ROS generation						
PS	300 nm; 500 nm; 1 μm; 3 μm; 6 μm	0 and 120 μg/mL for 24 h	300 nm 120 μg/mL	DCFH-DA	CaCO-2	102
			500 nm 120 μg/mL			
			1 μm 120 μg/mL			
			3 μm 120 μg/mL			
PS	50–100 nm	0, 1, 25, 50, and 100 μg/mL for 24 h	No effects	DCFH-DA	CaCO-2 cells	106
PS	50–100 nm		No effects			107

(*Continued*)

TABLE 40.1 (Continued)

Material	Size	Concentration exposure duration	Significant effects in vitro	Assay	Cell model	References
		0, 1, 25, 50, and 100 μg/mL for 24 h		DCFH-DA and DHE	Coculture of CaCO-2/HT29 and a triple culture of CaCO-2/HT29 + Raji B	
PET	<100 nm	0, 1, 5, 15, and 30 μg/mL for 24 h	No effects	DCFH-DA	CaCO-2	109
Inflammatory cytokine release						
PS	100 nm; 5 μm	0, 1, and 20 μg/mL for 96 h	Increased secretion of IL-8, MCP-1 of digested 100 nm 20 μg/mL 5 μm no effect	IL-8 and MCP-1	CaCO-2 cells (exposure with and without in vitro digestion)	104
PS	50 nm	0, 10, and 50 μg/cm^2 for 24 h	No effects	IL-1beta, IL-6, IL-8 and TNF-alpha release	Inflamed tricultures CaCO-2/HT29-MTX-E12/THP-1 and stable tricultures CaCO-2/HT29-MTX-E12/THP-1 (only IL-1beta and IL-8)	91
Amine-modified PS	50 nm	0, 10, and 50 μg/cm^2 for 24 h	No effects	IL-1beta, IL-6, IL-8 and TNF-alpha release	Inflamed tricultures CaCO-2/HT29-MTX-E12/THP-1 and stable tricultures Caco-2/HT29-MTX-E12/THP-1 (only IL-1beta and IL-8)	91
PVC	<50 μm	0, 10, and 50 μg/cm^2 for 24 h	50 μg/cm^2 Significant increased IL-1beta release, inflamed triculture, not significant for IL-6, IL-8 and TNF-alpha	IL-1beta, IL-6, IL-8 and TNF-alpha release	Inflamed tricultures CaCO-2/HT29-MTX-E12/THP-1 and stable tricultures CaCO-2/HT29-MTX-E12/THP-1 (only IL-1beta and IL-8)	91
PU (hard & ester)	<300 μm	0, 823.5–1380.0 μg/cm^2 for 6, 24, and 48 h	No effects	TNFα, IL-8, IL-1β	CaCO-2 + HT29-MTX + MDMs + MDDCs	111
PE	200–9900 nm	0, 10, and 50 μg/cm^2 for 24 h	50 μg/cm^2 significant increase IL-8 release stable triculture, not significant for IL-1beta, IL-6, and TNF-alpha	IL-1beta, IL-6, IL-8, TNF-alpha release	Normal and inflamed cocultures CaCO-2/HT29-MTX-E12/THP-1, reversed exposure	92
PP	<300 μm	0, 823.5–1380.0 μg/cm^2 for 6, 24, and 48 h	No effects	TNFα, IL-8, IL-1β	CaCO-2 + HT29-MTX + MDMs + MDDCs	111
PA	<300 μm	0, 823.5–1380.0 μg/cm^2 for 6, 24, and 48 h	No effects	TNFα, IL-8, IL-1β	CaCO-2 + HT29-MTX + MDMs + MDDCs	111
PET	<100 nm	0, 1, 5, 15, and 30 μg/mL for 24 h	No effects	IL-8 and MCP-1	CaCO-2	109
Altered gene expression						
PS	100 nm; 5 μm	0, 1, and 20 μg/mL for 96 h	Increased gene expression and secretion of IL-8, MCP-1 of digested 100 nm 20 μg/mL 5 μm no effect	Q-RT-PCR	CaCO-2 cells (exposure with and without in vitro digestion)	104

PS	5 μm	0, 12.5, and 50 mg/L for 24 h	NF-κB, MAPK signaling, cytokine-cytokine receptor interaction, and toll-like receptor were strongly influenced	RNA Seq	CaCO-2	105
PS	50–100 nm	0, 1, 25, 50, and 100 μg/mL for 24 h	No effects	RT PCR	Coculture of CaCO-2/HT29 and a triple culture of CaCO-2/HT29 + Raji B	107
PS	50–100 nm	0, 1, 25, 50, and 100 μg/mL for 24 and 48 h	No effects	RT-PCR	CaCO-2 cells	106
Mitochondrial membrane potential alterations						
PS	50–100 nm	0, 1, 25, 50, and 100 μg/mL for 24 h	Increased mitochondrial activity at concentrations ≥25 μg/mL	Mitoprobe TMRM assay	CaCO-2 cells	106
PS	300 nm; 500 nm; 1 μm; 3 μm; 6 μm	120 μg/mL for 24 h	500 nm 120 μg/mL 1 μm 120 μg/mL 3 μm 120 μg/mL 6 μm 120 μg/mL Reduced mitochondrial membrane potential	JC-1 assay kit	CaCO-2	102

PA, Polyamide; *PET*, polyethylene terephthalate; *PP*, polypropylene; *PS*, polystyrene; *PU*, polyurethane; *PVC*, polyvinyl chloride.

published in 2020 and the first half of 2021 that report the results of exposure studies using human intestinal epithelial cells is presented. Of the different polymer types studied, PS is the most frequently used. For the assessment of cytotoxicity different assays have been used, the MTT and WST-1 detect mitochondrial activity, while the LDH assay screens for membrane leakage. The MTT and WST-1 are more sensitive markers for cytotoxicity as can also be observed in Table 40.1 and larger sized particles are less cytotoxic than smaller ones[102] (Table 40.1). Interestingly also an effect on the mitochondrial membrane has been shown[102] (Table 40.1). Clearly, positively charged particles displayed increased cytotoxicity,[91] which has been observed previously.[103] For PET, PE, PA, and PP less data is available, but minimal cytotoxicity has been observed (Table 40.1). Cytotoxicity to the intestinal epithelial cells could result in a disrupted barrier function. Using TEER measurements this has not been shown, however using a longer exposure time in combination with a more sensitive approach in which the translocation of dextrans (Lucifer Yellow) was studied, increased translocation of Lucifer Yellow was observed following exposure to 100 nm PS particles.[104]

Increased production of reactive oxygen species (ROS) has been proposed as a common effect of both engineered nanomaterials and micro and nanoplastics.[112–114] Yet, from Table 40.1 the effects on ROS production following exposure of different sizes of PS to CaCO-2 cells are inconclusive. Immunotoxicity also is often mentioned as a potential adverse effect following exposure to micro and nanoplastics.[115] In some studies this was considered (Table 40.1), but in these studies only PS and PVC particles have been evaluated. A tendency that micro and nanoplastic exposure leads to increased cytokine excretion and gene expression has been noted in some studies, but not all (Table 40.1).

It is of interest to note that in vitro models of different complexity are being used, that is, monocultures of differentiated CaCO-2 cells, cocultures with mucus producing HT29-MTX cells and representative immune cells (i.e., Raij-B or THP-1 cells). From the noted effects (Table 40.1) it is difficult to recommend which cell model to use for which type of study. In previous work on silver nanoparticles we arrived at a similar conclusion.[116] As discussed above, pH dynamics, differences in ionic strengths and the dynamic biochemical conditions that nano- and micro particles encounter during gastrointestinal digestion could influence the uptake and local toxicity. Perhaps this is caused not so much by direct particle toxicity, but more dominantly as a consequence of the particle associated protein corona. This is exemplified by the increased secretion of IL-8 and MCP-1 of CaCO-2 cells exposed to 100 nm PS particles that have been incubated in different matrices.[104]

In most studies (Table 40.1) intestinal cells have only been exposed relatively short, while a realistic human exposure is chronic. It also appears that CaCO-2 cells are relatively unsensitive and have a poor endocytotic capacity compared to other cells, (i.e., THP-1 cells). In part this can be explained by the physiological role of these different cells, but also indicates the need to include cells that better emulate the human intestinal cell function. Potential models to consider in the future are human stem cell derived intestinal epithelial models.

40.1.5 Dosimetry in vitro and physiologically based kinetic models for nano- and microplastics

Extrapolation of results from in vitro studies using intestinal cells to the in vivo intestinal epithelium must be approached with caution. Apart from the caution in extrapolating the observations from cell-line-based models to the complex in vivo situation, concerns have also been raised about the concentration used in vitro and dosimetry of the nano- and microplastics (i.e., sedimentation of nano- and microplastics) in vitro. Meaningful interpretation and comparison of the results obtained using different in vitro experiments and extrapolation to in vivo data require reliable characterization of the nano- and microplastics and their agglomerates, as well as matrix-based influences on nano- and microplastics. For soluble chemicals it is reasonable to assume that the administered concentration (or nominal media concentration) is proportional to the cellular dose, and thus is a good measure of the concentration (or dose) at the target site.[117] However, micro and nanoparticles behave as colloid particles and the definition of a nano- and microplastics concentration in an in vitro system is far more complicated. From metal(oxide) nanomaterials we know that these materials can settle, diffuse, and agglomerate differentially which is determined by the properties of the nanomaterial itself (e.g., size, density, and surface chemistry) as well as by the solution matrix (e.g., viscosity, density, presence of proteins). Thus, nanoplastic dosimetry is affected not only by the concentration and used exposure time, but also by the nanoplastic characteristics and the environment.[117] Additionally in the case of nano- and microplastics and their aggregates, buoyancy of the materials needs to be considered. Buoyant nanoplastics rapidly move away from the cell surface in unagitated systems as is common in cell culture. As such the delivered dose of such particles will be exceedingly low, potentially underestimating true toxicity which has to be compensated by utilizing advanced in vitro models such as inverted cell culture,[92,118,119] semiwet culturing[111,120] or potentially the use of dynamically flowing systems such as cell-on-a-chip models.

To estimate the in vitro dosimetry computational dosimetry models such as the ISDD, ISD3 and DG models have been developed and refined.[121–124] These models apply to buoyant and nonbuoyant plastics (and nanomaterials) as in both cases only a fraction of the particles will reach the cell surface and robust methods for calculating the cellular dose are needed. Dosimetry models use a set of particle and matrix parameters to model particle sedimentation, aggregation, and also dissolution depending on the particles. Information which is commonly required includes information on the in vitro system, for example, the height of the liquid column, density and temperature of the medium as well as particle properties such as the average size, density and applied concentration. Information on particle aggregation can either be predicted in silico as is done in the ISDD algorithm[121] or determined experimentally by using dynamic light scattering measurements (DLS) to derive the hydrodynamic or aggregate sizes and volumetric centrifugal methods (to derive particle density) as is commonly done when working with the distorted grid and ISD3 algorithms.[123,124] The particle and aggregate properties are used to solve equations for the gravitational settling, drag force and Brownian diffusion which ultimately yields the time-dependent particle and aggregate concentrations at any given height in the liquid column.

Besides the quantitative description of the time-dependent nanoparticle concentration in vitro, efforts have also been made to predict in vivo nanomaterial concentrations based on results from in vitro studies using physiologically based kinetic (PBK) models. The generation of PBK models for nano- and microplastics is challenging due to the colloidal nature of nano- and microplastics and the lack of fundamental knowledge on nano- and microplastics ADME mechanisms (as discussed earlier in this chapter for intestinal uptake). Unlike small molecule compounds, nanoplastics are subjected to limited membrane permeability and PBK models assuming blood-flow limited transport yield less accurate nanoplastic concentrations.[125] The organ partitioning of nanoplastics is not dictated by the hydrophobicity of the compound and instead is largely governed by the phagocytotic capacity of organ-resident immune cells.[126,127] For this reason nanoparticle or micro and nanoplastic specific PBK-models commonly incorporate parameters that describe phagocytotic compartments that sequester nanoparticles within organs.[128] Despite the technical complexity, PBK models have been developed for quantum dots (20 nm),[129] metallic NPs such as silver (15–150 nm)[130] and titanium dioxide (15–150 nm),[131] nanocrystals and a handful of nanopolymers such as PLGA (50–135 nm).[132,133] While most PBK models only consider direct intravenous injection of nanoparticles, Bachler et. al. have included oral exposure of food-grade TiO_2 nanoparticles in their model to predict its ADME after oral ingestion.[131]

In conclusion, an estimation of dosimetry should be included in well-designed in vitro studies. Interesting developments are the use of semi–wet culturing protocols[111,120] or reversed exposure models aiming to increase the cellular contacts with the low density nano- and microplastics.[92,118,119] Reliable data on intestinal uptake are important to be able to predict in vivo uptake kinetics. Some studies have demonstrated the feasibility of nanoparticle (or plastic)-specific PBK models. Clearly, mechanistic knowledge on nanoplastic transport is very limited and current PBK models are still heavily depending on in vivo data for parameterization. The lack of in vitro parameterization of nanoplastic-PBK models hinders extrapolation to nanoplastic that lack in vivo organ concentrations and complicates extrapolation to humans where such data is exceedingly scarce. Nevertheless one promising study successfully showed interspecies extrapolation of a rodent and pig PBK models to the human situation.[134]

40.1.6 Effects of nano - and microplastics in vivo

The number of published oral exposure rodent in vivo studies increased rapidly in the past few years. Several studies focused on potential effects on the reproductive system of male[135–137] or female rodents,[138–140] potential cardiotoxicity,[141,142] and effects on the thyroid[140] and intestine.[142] Yet the results of these studies need to be interpreted with caution as mostly PS materials have been studied, and limited data on the characterization of the used microplastics is provided. Minimal characterization data needs from the field of engineered nanotoxicology[36] should be applied also in studying and reporting effects of nano- and microplastics. Most of these recent rodents studies have methodological issues in terms of the quality of the methods and approaches used in the histopathology, where essential controls are missing or blind scoring schemes appear not to be used by the authors. Yet data on increased cytokine production as observed in some of these studies might point toward adverse effects. Limited experimental data is available on the concentrations of the nano- and micro particles in tissues (as discussed above), which is needed to better relate the observed effects to the concentration of the microparticles in vivo.

Micro and nanoplastic toxicity studies thus far have used engineered nanospheres which have a monodisperse size, shape and single polymer composition. It is challenging to extrapolate these results to the real-life situation where humans are exposed to a highly heterogenous mixture of micro and nanoplastics' sizes, shapes, and composition. Interesting approaches have been proposed in which the reported environmental concentration of any given microplastic size range can be scaled to other size ranges by assuming that microplastic concentration follows a power-law function in relation to their size.[143] This method could be used to extrapolate microplastic concentrations used in toxicological studies to true environmental concentrations, that are more relevant for human exposure. Further research is needed to define methods to reliably relate single microplastic type toxicodynamic observations to the complex environmentally realistic exposure scenarios.

40.1.7 Conclusions and future outlook

Direct exposure to nano- and microplastics via ingestion (and indirectly via swallowed particles trapped in lung mucus) is an inevitable consequence of widespread occurrence of nano- and microplastics in the environment. However, the extent of ingestion and the potential risks this exposure affects humans remains poorly defined. The recently published rodent studies might be helpful to gain more insights into this, but studies of higher quality are needed. This mainly relates to an adequate characterization of the nano- and microplastics used, and the assessment of particle concentrations at the target organ.

To understand the mechanism of uptake of nano- and microplastics in vitro studies are useful. For this several in vitro models of the gastrointestinal epithelium have been developed, ranging from layers of a single cell type (often CaCO-2 cells) to more complex cocultures that for example incorporate M-cells and mucus secreting cells. While these models aim to reproduce the complex biology of the intestinal epithelium, the design and dosimetry of the nano- and microplastics exposure conditions needs careful attention.

We have observed interesting developments in novel designs of in vitro experiments, such as semiwet or reversed exposure study designs which can solve the issues related to limited nano- and microplastic cell contact due to low density and buoyancy of some nano- and microplastics. Recent innovations toward microfluidic experimental models might further improve the relevance of the exposure conditions. These experimental innovations need to be embedded in the design and data needs for particle kinetic and dynamic modeling of nano- and microplastics to extrapolate data from in vitro to in vivo.

Currently, reported in vivo rodent and human in vivo data suggests limited oral bioavailability of nano- and microplastics. However caution is needed here as only limited types of nano- and microplastics have been studied in vivo and reported intestinal uptake is highly variable. The limited human studies point towards the presence of nano- and microplastics in tissues, suggesting that uptake is possible. Also data humans exposed to (ultra) fine dust indicate that systemic uptake of particulate matter is possible especially following lifelong exposure.

The number of toxicological studies in which rodents have been exposed to nano- and microplastics is increasing rapidly. Potential effects on reproductive system, heart, thyroid and intestine have been reported. Most of these studies only used PS microplastics and often limited data on the characterization of the microplastics used is provided. Yet data on increased cytokine production as observed in some of the studies might point towards effects related to immunotoxicity. Clearly further toxicological studies are warranted and on a wider range of materials.

Lastly methodology needs to be developed in order to be able to extrapolate the observations from single nano- and microplastic types in vitro and in vivo studies to the complex environmental exposure conditions as seen in real life.

Acknowledgments

Funding for our research in this area has been provided by ZonMW (Project number: 458001001) and EU-H2020 Plasticheal (Grant agreement ID: 965196).

References

1. Geyer R, Jambeck JR, Law KL. Production, use, and fate of all plastics ever made. *Sci Adv*. 2017;3(7):e1700782. Available from: https://doi.org/10.1126/sciadv.1700782.
2. Rubio L, Marcos R, Hernandez A. Potential adverse health effects of ingested micro- and nanoplastics on humans. Lessons learned vivo vitro mammalian model. *J Toxicol Environ Health B Crit Rev*. 2020;23(2):51–68. Available from: https://doi.org/10.1080/10937404.2019.1700598.
3. PlasticsEurope. *Plastics—the Facts 2020*. Brussels: Association of Plastics Manufacturers; 2020.
4. Cole M, Lindeque P, Halsband C, Galloway TS. Microplastics as contaminants in the marine environment: a review. *Mar Pollut Bull*. 2011;62(12):2588–2597. Available from: https://doi.org/10.1016/j.marpolbul.2011.09.025.
5. Jambeck JR, Geyer R, Wilcox C, et al. Marine pollution. Plastic waste inputs from land into the ocean. *Science*. 2015;347 (6223):768–771. Available from: https://doi.org/10.1126/science.1260352.
6. Fendall LS, Sewell MA. Contributing to marine pollution by washing your face: microplastics in facial cleansers. *Mar Pollut Bull*. 2009;58(8):1225–1228. Available from: https://doi.org/10.1016/j.marpolbul.2009.04.025.
7. Alexander J, Barregard L, Bignami M, et al. Presence of microplastics and nanoplastics in food, with particular focus on seafood. *EFSA J*. 2016;14(6). Available from: https://doi.org/10.2903/j.efsa.2016.4501.
8. Bouwmeester H, Hollman PC, Peters RJ. Potential health impact of environmentally released micro- and nanoplastics in the human food production chain: experiences from nanotoxicology. *Environ Sci Technol*. 2015;49(15):8932–8947. Available from: https://doi.org/10.1021/acs.est.5b01090.

9. Cozar A, Echevarria F, Gonzalez-Gordillo JI, et al. Plastic debris in the open ocean. *Proc Natl Acad Sci U S A*. 2014;111(28):10239–10244. Available from: https://doi.org/10.1073/pnas.1314705111.
10. Kuhn S, van Oyen A, Bravo Rebolledo EL, Ask AV, van Franeker JA. Polymer types ingested by northern fulmars (*Fulmarus glacialis*) and southern hemisphere relatives. Article. *Environ Sci Pollut Res Int*. 2021;28(2):1643–1655. Available from: https://doi.org/10.1007/s11356-020-10540-6.
11. Kuhn S, van Oyen A, Booth AM, Meijboom A, van Franeker JA. Marine microplastic: preparation of relevant test materials for laboratory assessment of ecosystem impacts. *Artic Chemosphere*. 2018;213:103–113. Available from: https://doi.org/10.1016/j.chemosphere.2018.09.032.
12. Abidli S, Antunes JC, Ferreira JL, Lahbib Y, Sobral P, El Menif NT. Microplastics in sediments from the littoral zone of the north Tunisian coast (Mediterranean Sea). *Estuar Coast Shelf S*. 2018;205:1–9. Available from: https://doi.org/10.1016/j.ecss.2018.03.006.
13. Obbard RW, Sadri S, Wong YQ, Khitun AA, Baker I, Thompson RC. Global warming releases microplastic legacy frozen in Arctic Sea ice. *Earths Future*. 2014;2(6):315–320. Available from: https://doi.org/10.1002/2014ef000240.
14. Kanhai DK, Officer R, Lyashevska O, Thompson RC, O'Connor I. Microplastic abundance, distribution and composition along a latitudinal gradient in the Atlantic Ocean. *Mar Pollut Bull*. 2017;115(1–2):307–314. Available from: https://doi.org/10.1016/j.marpolbul.2016.12.025.
15. Horton AA, Svendsen C, Williams RJ, Spurgeon DJ, Lahive E. Large microplastic particles in sediments of tributaries of the River Thames, UK—abundance, sources and methods for effective quantification. *Mar Pollut Bull*. 2017;114(1):218–226. Available from: https://doi.org/10.1016/j.marpolbul.2016.09.004.
16. Zimmermann L, Dierkes G, Ternes TA, Volker C, Wagner M. Benchmarking the in vitro toxicity and chemical composition of plastic consumer products. *Environ Sci Technol*. 2019;53(19):11467–11477. Available from: https://doi.org/10.1021/acs.est.9b02293.
17. Hahladakis JN, Velis CA, Weber R, Iacovidou E, Purnell P. An overview of chemical additives present in plastics: migration, release, fate and environmental impact during their use, disposal and recycling. *J Hazard Mater*. 2018;344:179–199. Available from: https://doi.org/10.1016/j.jhazmat.2017.10.014.
18. Brennecke D, Duarte B, Paiva F, Cacador I, Canning-Clode J. Microplastics as vector for heavy metal contamination from the marine environment. *Estuar Coast Shelf Sci*. 2016;178:189–195. Available from: https://doi.org/10.1016/j.ecss.2015.12.003.
19. Koelmans AA, Bakir A, Burton GA, Janssen CR. Microplastic as a vector for chemicals in the aquatic environment: critical review and model-supported reinterpretation of empirical studies. *Environ Sci Technol*. 2016;50(7):3315–3326. Available from: https://doi.org/10.1021/acs.est.5b06069.
20. Li J, Zhang K, Zhang H. Adsorption of antibiotics on microplastics. *Environ Pollut*. 2018;237:460–467. Available from: https://doi.org/10.1016/j.envpol.2018.02.050.
21. Mato Y, Isobe T, Takada H, Kanehiro H, Ohtake C, Kaminuma T. Plastic resin pellets as a transport medium for toxic chemicals in the marine environment. *Environ Sci Technol*. 2001;35(2):318–324. Available from: https://doi.org/10.1021/es0010498.
22. Mendoza LMR, Jones PR. Characterisation of microplastics and toxic chemicals extracted from microplastic samples from the North Pacific Gyre. *Environ Chem*. 2015;12(5):611–617. Available from: https://doi.org/10.1071/En14236.
23. Rochman CM, Kurobe T, Flores I, Teh SJ. Early warning signs of endocrine disruption in adult fish from the ingestion of polyethylene with and without sorbed chemical pollutants from the marine environment. *Sci Total Environ*. 2014;493:656–661. Available from: https://doi.org/10.1016/j.scitotenv.2014.06.051.
24. Rodrigues JP, Duarte AC, Santos-Echeandia J, Rocha-Santos T. Significance of interactions between microplastics and POPs in the marine environment: a critical overview. *Trac-Trend Anal Chem*. 2019;111:252–260. Available from: https://doi.org/10.1016/j.trac.2018.11.038.
25. Wang W, Wang J. Different partition of polycyclic aromatic hydrocarbon on environmental particulates in freshwater: microplastics in comparison to natural sediment. *Ecotoxicol Environ Saf*. 2018;147:648–655. Available from: https://doi.org/10.1016/j.ecoenv.2017.09.029.
26. Wang Z, Chen M, Zhang L, et al. Sorption behaviors of phenanthrene on the microplastics identified in a mariculture farm in Xiangshan Bay, southeastern China. *Sci Total Environ*. 2018;628–629:1617–1626. Available from: https://doi.org/10.1016/j.scitotenv.2018.02.146.
27. Wu P, Huang J, Zheng Y, et al. Environmental occurrences, fate, and impacts of microplastics. *Ecotoxicol Environ Saf*. 2019;184:109612. Available from: https://doi.org/10.1016/j.ecoenv.2019.109612.
28. Wang Y, Huang J, Zhu F, Zhou S. Airborne microplastics: a review on the occurrence, migration and risks to humans. *Bull Environ Contam Toxicol*. 2021;. Available from: https://doi.org/10.1007/s00128-021-03180-0.
29. Rahman A, Sarkar A, Yadav OP, Achari G, Slobodnik J. Potential human health risks due to environmental exposure to nano- and microplastics and knowledge gaps: a scoping review. *Sci Total Environ*. 2021;757:143872. Available from: https://doi.org/10.1016/j.scitotenv.2020.143872.
30. Bouwmeester H, Brandhoff P, Marvin HJP, Weigel S, Peters RJB. State of the safety assessment and current use of nanomaterials in food and food production. *Trends Food Sci Tech*. 2014;40(2):200–210. Available from: https://doi.org/10.1016/j.tifs.2014.08.009.
31. Van Raamsdonk LWD, van der Zande M, Koelmans AA, et al. Current insights into monitoring, bioaccumulation, and potential health effects of microplastics present in the food chain. *Foods*. 2020;9(1):72. Available from: https://doi.org/10.3390/foods9010072.
32. Vethaak AD, Legler J. Microplastics and human health. *Science*. 2021;371(6530):672–674. Available from: https://doi.org/10.1126/science.abe5041.
33. Kelly FJ, Fussell JC. Toxicity of airborne particles-established evidence, knowledge gaps and emerging areas of importance. *Philos Trans A Math Phys Eng Sci*. 2020;378(2183):20190322. Available from: https://doi.org/10.1098/rsta.2019.0322.
34. Riediker M, Zink D, Kreyling W, et al. Particle toxicology and health—where are we? *Part Fibre Toxicol*. 2019;16(1):19. Available from: https://doi.org/10.1186/s12989-019-0302-8.
35. Bouwmeester H, Dekkers S, Noordam MY, et al. Review of health safety aspects of nanotechnologies in food production. *Regul*

Toxicol Pharmacol. 2009;53(1):52–62. Available from: https://doi.org/10.1016/j.yrtph.2008.10.008.

36. Bouwmeester H, Lynch I, Marvin HJ, et al. Minimal analytical characterization of engineered nanomaterials needed for hazard assessment in biological matrices. *Nanotoxicology.* 2011;5(1):1–11. Available from: https://doi.org/10.3109/17435391003775266.
37. Harisa GI, Badran MM, Alanazi FK, Attia SM. An overview of nanosomes delivery mechanisms: trafficking, orders, barriers and cellular effects. *Artif Cell Nanomed Biotechnol.* 2018;46(4):669–679. Available from: https://doi.org/10.1080/21691401.2017.1354301.
38. Weir A, Westerhoff P, Fabricius L, Hristovski K, Von Goetz N. Titanium dioxide nanoparticles in food and personal care products. *Environ Sci Technol.* 2012;46(4):2242–2250. Available from: https://doi.org/10.1021/es204168d.
39. Peters RJ, van Bemmel G, Herrera-Rivera Z, et al. Characterization of titanium dioxide nanoparticles in food products: analytical methods to define nanoparticles. *J Agric Food Chem.* 2014;62(27):6285–6293. Available from: https://doi.org/10.1021/jf5011885.
40. Peters R, Kramer E, Oomen AG, et al. Presence of nano-sized silica during in vitro digestion of foods containing silica as a food additive. *ACS Nano.* 2012;6(3):2441–2451. Available from: https://doi.org/10.1021/nn204728k.
41. Taboada-López MV, Alonso-Seijo N, Herbello-Hermelo P, Bermejo-Barrera P, Moreda-Piñeiro A. Determination and characterization of silver nanoparticles in bivalve molluscs by ultrasound assisted enzymatic hydrolysis and sp-ICP-MS. *Microchem J.* 2019;148:652–660. Available from: https://doi.org/10.1016/j.microc.2019.05.023.
42. Bellmann S, Carlander D, Fasano A, et al. Mammalian gastrointestinal tract parameters modulating the integrity, surface properties, and absorption of food-relevant nanomaterials. *Wiley Interdiscip Rev Nanomed Nanobiotechnol.* 2015;7(5):609–622. Available from: https://doi.org/10.1002/wnan.1333.
43. Walczak AP, Fokkink R, Peters R, et al. Behaviour of silver nanoparticles and silver ions in an in vitro human gastrointestinal digestion model. *Nanotoxicology.* 2013;7(7):1198–1210. Available from: https://doi.org/10.3109/17435390.2012.726382.
44. Abdelkhaliq A, van der Zande M, Punt A, et al. Impact of nanoparticle surface functionalization on the protein corona and cellular adhesion, uptake and transport. *J Nanobiotechnol.* 2018;16(1):70. Available from: https://doi.org/10.1186/s12951-018-0394-6.
45. Van Der Zande M, Vandebriel RJ, Groot MJ, et al. Sub-chronic toxicity study in rats orally exposed to nanostructured silica. *Part Fibre Toxicol.* 2014;11(1):8. Available from: https://doi.org/10.1186/1743-8977-11-8.
46. Lundqvist M, Stigler J, Elia G, Lynch I, Cedervall T, Dawson KA. Nanoparticle size and surface properties determine the protein corona with possible implications for biological impacts. *Proc Natl Acad Sci U S A.* 2008;105(38):14265–14270. Available from: https://doi.org/10.1073/pnas.0805135105.
47. Lesniak A, Fenaroli F, Monopoli MP, Aberg C, Dawson KA, Salvati A. Effects of the presence or absence of a protein corona on silica nanoparticle uptake and impact on cells. *ACS Nano.* 2012;6(7):5845–5857. Available from: https://doi.org/10.1021/nn300223w.
48. Docter D, Distler U, Storck W, et al. Quantitative profiling of the protein coronas that form around nanoparticles. *Nat Protoc.* 2014;9(9):2030–2044. Available from: https://doi.org/10.1038/nprot.2014.139.
49. Tenzer S, Docter D, Kuharev J, et al. Rapid formation of plasma protein corona critically affects nanoparticle pathophysiology. *Nat Nanotechnol.* 2013;8(10):772–781. Available from: https://doi.org/10.1038/nnano.2013.181.
50. Abdelkhaliq A, van der Zande M, Undas AK, Peters RJB, Bouwmeester H. Impact of in vitro digestion on gastrointestinal fate and uptake of silver nanoparticles with different surface modifications. *Nanotoxicology.* 2020;14(1):111–126. Available from: https://doi.org/10.1080/17435390.2019.1675794.
51. Fan Y, Pedersen O. Gut microbiota in human metabolic health and disease. *Nat Rev Microbiol.* 2021;19(1):55–71. Available from: https://doi.org/10.1038/s41579-020-0433-9.
52. van Dongen KCW, van der Zande M, Bruyneel B, et al. An in vitro model for microbial fructoselysine degradation shows substantial inter individual differences in metabolic capacities of human fecal slurries. *Toxicol In Vitro.* 2021;72:105078. Available from: https://doi.org/10.1016/j.tiv.2021.105078.
53. Jin J, Beekmann K, Ringo E, Rietjens IMCM, Xing FG. Interaction between food-borne mycotoxins and gut microbiota: a review. *Rev Food Control.* 2021;126107998. Available from: https://doi.org/10.1016/j.foodcont.2021.107998.
54. Bouwmeester H, Van Der Zande M, Jepson MA. Effects of food-borne nanomaterials on gastrointestinal tissues and microbiota. *Wiley Interdiscip Rev Nanomed Nanobiotechnol.* 2018;10(1):e1481. Available from: https://doi.org/10.1002/wnan.1481.
55. Pietroiusti A, Magrini A, Campagnolo L. New frontiers in nanotoxicology: gut microbiota/microbiome-mediated effects of engineered nanomaterials. *Toxicol Appl Pharmacol.* 2016;299:90–95. Available from: https://doi.org/10.1016/j.taap.2015.12.017.
56. Lamas B, Martins Breyner N, Houdeau E. Impacts of foodborne inorganic nanoparticles on the gut microbiota-immune axis: potential consequences for host health. *Part Fibre Toxicol.* 2020;17(1):19. Available from: https://doi.org/10.1186/s12989-020-00349-z.
57. Huang ZZ, Weng Y, Shen QC, Zhao Y, Jin YX. Microplastic: a potential threat to human and animal health by interfering with the intestinal barrier function and changing the intestinal microenvironment. *Sci Total Environ.* 2021;785. Available from: https://doi.org/10.1016/j.scitotenv.2021.147365.
58. Frohlich EE, Frohlich E. Cytotoxicity of nanoparticles contained in food on intestinal cells and the gut microbiota. *Int J Mol Sci.* 2016;17(4):509. Available from: https://doi.org/10.3390/ijms17040509.
59. Donohoe DR, Garge N, Zhang X, et al. The microbiome and butyrate regulate energy metabolism and autophagy in the mammalian colon. *Cell Metab.* 2011;13(5):517–526. Available from: https://doi.org/10.1016/j.cmet.2011.02.018.
60. Kish L, Hotte N, Kaplan GG, et al. Environmental particulate matter induces murine intestinal inflammatory responses and alters the gut microbiome. *PLoS One.* 2013;8(4):e62220. Available from: https://doi.org/10.1371/journal.pone.0062220.
61. Jin Y, Lu L, Tu W, Luo T, Fu Z. Impacts of polystyrene microplastic on the gut barrier, microbiota and metabolism of mice. *Sci Total Environ.* 2019;649:308–317. Available from: https://doi.org/10.1016/j.scitotenv.2018.08.353.
62. Lu L, Wan Z, Luo T, Fu Z, Jin Y. Polystyrene microplastics induce gut microbiota dysbiosis and hepatic lipid metabolism disorder in mice. *Sci Total Environ.* 2018;631–632:449–458. Available from: https://doi.org/10.1016/j.scitotenv.2018.03.051.

63. Taylor AA, Marcus IM, Guysi RL, Walker SL. Metal oxide nanoparticles induce minimal phenotypic changes in a model colon gut microbiota. *Environ Eng Sci.* 2015;32(7):602–612. Available from: https://doi.org/10.1089/ees.2014.0518.
64. Zoetendal EG, Raes J, Van Den Bogert B, et al. The human small intestinal microbiota is driven by rapid uptake and conversion of simple carbohydrates. *ISME J.* 2012;6(7):1415–1426. Available from: https://doi.org/10.1038/ismej.2011.212.
65. Braakhuis HM, Kloet SK, Kezic S, et al. Progress and future of in vitro models to study translocation of nanoparticles. *Arch Toxicol.* 2015;89(9):1469–1495. Available from: https://doi.org/10.1007/s00204-015-1518-5.
66. Lefebvre DE, Venema K, Gombau L, et al. Utility of models of the gastrointestinal tract for assessment of the digestion and absorption of engineered nanomaterials released from food matrices. *Nanotoxicology.* 2015;9(4):523–542. Available from: https://doi.org/10.3109/17435390.2014.948091.
67. Behrens I, Pena AI, Alonso MJ, Kissel T. Comparative uptake studies of bioadhesive and non-bioadhesive nanoparticles in human intestinal cell lines and rats: the effect of mucus on particle adsorption and transport. *Pharm Res.* 2002;19(8):1185–1193. Available from: https://doi.org/10.1023/a:1019854327540.
68. Szentkuti L, Lorenz K. The thickness of the mucus layer in different segments of the rat intestine. *Histochem J.* 1995;27(6):466–472.
69. Frey A, Giannasca KT, Weltzin R, et al. Role of the glycocalyx in regulating access of microparticles to apical plasma membranes of intestinal epithelial cells: implications for microbial attachment and oral vaccine targeting. *J Exp Med.* 1996;184(3):1045–1059. Available from: https://doi.org/10.1084/jem.184.3.1045.
70. Clark MA, Jepson MA, Hirst BH. Exploiting M cells for drug and vaccine delivery. *Adv Drug Deliv Rev.* 2001;50(1–2):81–106. Available from: https://doi.org/10.1016/s0169-409x(01)00149-1.
71. Neutra MR, Frey A, Kraehenbuhl JP. Epithelial M cells: gateways for mucosal infection and immunization. *Cell.* 1996;86(3):345–348. Available from: https://doi.org/10.1016/s0092-8674(00)80106-3.
72. Mahler GJ, Shuler ML, Glahn RP. Characterization of CaCO-2 and HT29-MTX cocultures in an in vitro digestion/cell culture model used to predict iron bioavailability. *J Nutritional Biochem.* 2009;20(7):494–502. Available from: https://doi.org/10.1016/j.jnutbio.2008.05.006.
73. Natoli M, Leoni BD, D'Agnano I, Zucco F, Felsani A. Good CaCO-2 cell culture practices. *Toxicol In Vitro.* 2012;26(8):1243–1246. Available from: https://doi.org/10.1016/j.tiv.2012.03.009.
74. Nkabinde LA, Shoba-Zikhali LN, Semete-Makokotlela B, et al. Permeation of PLGA nanoparticles across different in vitro models. *Curr Drug Delivery.* 2012;9(6):617–627. Available from: https://doi.org/10.2174/156720112803529819.
75. Koeneman BA, Zhang Y, Westerhoff P, Chen Y, Crittenden JC, Capco DG. Toxicity and cellular responses of intestinal cells exposed to titanium dioxide. *Cell Biol Toxicol.* 2010;26(3):225–238. Available from: https://doi.org/10.1007/s10565-009-9132-z.
76. Pereira DI, Bruggraber SF, Faria N, et al. Nanoparticulate iron(III) oxo-hydroxide delivers safe iron that is well absorbed and utilised in humans. *Nanomedicine..* 2014;10(8):1877–1886. Available from: https://doi.org/10.1016/j.nano.2014.06.012.
77. Song ZM, Chen N, Liu JH, et al. Biological effect of food additive titanium dioxide nanoparticles on intestine: an in vitro study. *J Appl Toxicol.* 2015;35(10):1169–1178. Available from: https://doi.org/10.1002/jat.3171.
78. Gaiser BK, Fernandes TF, Jepson M, Lead JR, Tyler CR, Stone V. Assessing exposure, uptake and toxicity of silver and cerium dioxide nanoparticles from contaminated environments. *Environ Health.* 2009;8(1):S2. Available from: https://doi.org/10.1186/1476-069X-8-S1-S2.
79. Howe SE, Lickteig DJ, Plunkett KN, Ryerse JS, Konjufca V. The uptake of soluble and particulate antigens by epithelial cells in the mouse small intestine. *PLoS One.* 2014;9(1):e86656. Available from: https://doi.org/10.1371/journal.pone.0086656.
80. De Jesus M, Ostroff GR, Levitz SM, Bartling TR, Mantis NJ. A population of Langerin-positive dendritic cells in murine Peyer's patches involved in sampling beta-glucan microparticles. *PLoS One.* 2014;9(3):e91002. Available from: https://doi.org/10.1371/journal.pone.0091002.
81. Powell JJ, Thomas-McKay E, Thoree V, et al. An endogenous nanomineral chaperones luminal antigen and peptidoglycan to intestinal immune cells. *Nat Nanotechnol.* 2015;10(4):361–369. Available from: https://doi.org/10.1038/nnano.2015.19.
82. Delon L, Gibson RJ, Prestidge CA, Thierry B. Mechanisms of uptake and transport of particulate formulations in the small intestine. *J Control Release.* 2022;343:584–599. Available from: https://doi.org/10.1016/j.jconrel.2022.02.006. 35149142.
83. McClean S, Prosser E, Meehan E, et al. Binding and uptake of biodegradable poly-DL-lactide micro- and nanoparticles in intestinal epithelia. *Eur J Pharm Sci.* 1998;6(2):153–163. Available from: https://doi.org/10.1016/s0928-0987(97)10007-0.
84. Hillery AM, Jani PU, Florence AT. Comparative, quantitative study of lymphoid and non-lymphoid uptake of 60 nm polystyrene particles. *J Drug Target.* 1994;2(2):151–156. Available from: https://doi.org/10.3109/10611869409015904.
85. Jani P, Halbert GW, Langridge J, Florence AT. Nanoparticle uptake by the rat gastrointestinal mucosa: quantitation and particle size dependency. *J Pharm Pharmacol.* 1990;42(12):821–826. Available from: https://doi.org/10.1111/j.2042-7158.1990.tb07033.x.
86. Jani PU, Mccarthy DE, Florence AT. Nanosphere and microsphere uptake via peyer patches - observation of the rate of uptake in the rat after a single oral dose. *Int J Pharm.* 1992;86(2–3):239–246. Available from: https://doi.org/10.1016/0378-5173(92)90202-D.
87. Berg RD. Bacterial translocation from the gastrointestinal tract. *J Med.* 1992;23(3–4):217–244.
88. Berg RD. Bacterial translocation from the gastrointestinal tract. *Adv Exp Med Biol.* 1999;473:11–30. Available from: https://doi.org/10.1007/978-1-4615-4143-1_2.
89. Moyes SM, Morris JF, Carr KE. Culture conditions and treatments affect CaCO-2 characteristics and particle uptake. *Int J Pharm.* 2010;387(1-2):7–18. Available from: https://doi.org/10.1016/j.ijpharm.2009.11.027.
90. Moyes SM, Killick EM, Morris JF, Kadhim MA, Hill MA, Carr KE. Changes produced by external radiation in parameters influencing intestinal permeability and microparticle uptake in vitro. *Int J Radiat Biol.* 2008;84(6):467–486. Available from: https://doi.org/10.1080/09553000802078388.
91. Busch M, Bredeck G, Kampfer AAM, Schins RPF. Investigations of acute effects of polystyrene and polyvinyl chloride micro- and

nanoplastics in an advanced in vitro triple culture model of the healthy and inflamed intestine. *Environ Res*. 2021;193:110536. Available from: https://doi.org/10.1016/j.envres.2020.110536.

92. Busch M, Kampfer AAM, Schins RPF. An inverted in vitro triple culture model of the healthy and inflamed intestine: adverse effects of polyethylene particles. *Chemosphere*. 2021;284:131345. Available from: https://doi.org/10.1016/j.chemosphere.2021.131345.
93. Ragusa A, Svelato A, Santacroce C, et al. Plasticenta: first evidence of microplastics in human placenta. *Environ Int*. 2021;146:106274. Available from: https://doi.org/10.1016/j.envint.2020.106274.
94. Jones K, Morton J, Smith I, Jurkschat K, Harding AH, Evans G. Human in vivo and in vitro studies on gastrointestinal absorption of titanium dioxide nanoparticles. *Toxicol Lett*. 2015;233(2):95–101. Available from: https://doi.org/10.1016/j.toxlet.2014.12.005.
95. Pele LC, Thoree V, Bruggraber SF, et al. Pharmaceutical/food grade titanium dioxide particles are absorbed into the bloodstream of human volunteers. *Part Fibre Toxicol*. 2015;12(1):26. Available from: https://doi.org/10.1186/s12989-015-0101-9.
96. Bockmann J, Lahl H, Eckhert T, Unterhalt B. Blood levels of titanium before and after oral administration of titanium dioxide. *Pharmazie*. 2000;55(2):140–143.
97. Bove H, Bongaerts E, Slenders E, et al. Ambient black carbon particles reach the fetal side of human placenta. *Nat Commun*. 2019;10(1):3866. Available from: https://doi.org/10.1038/s41467-019-11654-3.
98. Walczak AP, Hendriksen PJ, Woutersen RA, et al. Bioavailability and biodistribution of differently charged polystyrene nanoparticles upon oral exposure in rats. *J Nanopart Res*. 2015;17(5):231. Available from: https://doi.org/10.1007/s11051-015-3029-y.
99. Keinanen O, Dayts EJ, Rodriguez C, et al. Harnessing PET to track micro- and nanoplastics in vivo. *Sci Rep*. 2021;11(1):11463. Available from: https://doi.org/10.1038/s41598-021-90929-6.
100. Hussain N, Jani PU, Florence AT. Enhanced oral uptake of tomato lectin-conjugated nanoparticles in the rat. *Pharm Res*. 1997;14(5):613–618. Available from: https://doi.org/10.1023/a:1012153011884.
101. Fournier SB, D'Errico JN, Adler DS, et al. Nanopolystyrene translocation and fetal deposition after acute lung exposure during late-stage pregnancy. *Part Fibre Toxicol*. 2020;17(1):55. Available from: https://doi.org/10.1186/s12989-020-00385-9.
102. Wang Q, Bai J, Ning B, et al. Effects of bisphenol A and nanoscale and microscale polystyrene plastic exposure on particle uptake and toxicity in human CaCO-2 cells. *Chemosphere*. 2020;254:126788. Available from: https://doi.org/10.1016/j.chemosphere.2020.126788.
103. Walczak AP, Kramer E, Hendriksen PJ, et al. In vitro gastrointestinal digestion increases the translocation of polystyrene nanoparticles in an in vitro intestinal co-culture model. *Nanotoxicology*. 2015;9(7):886–894. Available from: https://doi.org/10.3109/17435390.2014.988664.
104. Liu S, Wu X, Gu W, Yu J, Wu B. Influence of the digestive process on intestinal toxicity of polystyrene microplastics as determined by in vitro CaCO-2 models. *Chemosphere*. 2020;256:127204. Available from: https://doi.org/10.1016/j.chemosphere.2020.127204.
105. Moyan H, Dušan P. Micro- and nano-plastics activation of oxidative and inflammatory adverse outcome pathways. *Redox Biol*. 2020;37:101620. Available from: https://doi.org/10.1016/j.redox.2020.101620.
106. Cortés C, Domenech J, Salazar M, Pastor S, Marcos R, Hernández A. Nanoplastics as a potential environmental health factor: effects of polystyrene nanoparticles on human intestinal epithelial CaCO-2 cells. *Environ Sci: Nano*. 2020;7(1):272–285. Available from: https://doi.org/10.1039/c9en00523d.
107. Domenech J, Hernandez A, Rubio L, Marcos R, Cortes C. Interactions of polystyrene nanoplastics with in vitro models of the human intestinal barrier. *Arch Toxicol*. 2020;94(9):2997–3012. Available from: https://doi.org/10.1007/s00204-020-02805-3.
108. Stock V, Bohmert L, Lisicki E, et al. Uptake and effects of orally ingested polystyrene microplastic particles in vitro and in vivo. *Arch Toxicol*. 2019;93(7):1817–1833. Available from: https://doi.org/10.1007/s00204-019-02478-7.
109. Magri D, Sanchez-Moreno P, Caputo G, et al. Laser ablation as a versatile tool to mimic polyethylene terephthalate nanoplastic pollutants: characterization and toxicology assessment. *ACS Nano*. 2018;12(8):7690–7700. Available from: https://doi.org/10.1021/acsnano.8b01331.
110. Stock V, Laurisch C, Franke J, et al. Uptake and cellular effects of PE, PP, PET and PVC microplastic particles. *Toxicol In Vitro*. 2021;70:105021. Available from: https://doi.org/10.1016/j.tiv.2020.105021.
111. Lehner R, Wohlleben W, Septiadi D, Landsiedel R, Petri-Fink A, Rothen-Rutishauser B. A novel 3D intestine barrier model to study the immune response upon exposure to microplastics. *Arch Toxicol*. 2020;94(7):2463–2479. Available from: https://doi.org/10.1007/s00204-020-02750-1.
112. Micro- and nano-plastics activation of oxidative and inflammatory adverse outcome pathways. 2020.
113. Brand W, Peters RJB, Braakhuis HM, Maslankiewicz L, Oomen AG. Possible effects of titanium dioxide particles on human liver, intestinal tissue, spleen and kidney after oral exposure. *Nanotoxicology*. 2020;14(7):985–1007. Available from: https://doi.org/10.1080/17435390.2020.1778809.
114. Boyes WK, Van Thriel C. Neurotoxicology of nanomaterials. *Chem Res Toxicol*. 2020;33(5):1121–1144. Available from: https://doi.org/10.1021/acs.chemrestox.0c00050.
115. Hirt N, Body-Malapel M. Immunotoxicity and intestinal effects of nano- and microplastics: a review of the literature. *Part Fibre Toxicol*. 2020;17(1):57. Available from: https://doi.org/10.1186/s12989-020-00387-7.
116. Walczak AP, Kramer E, Hendriksen PJ, et al. Translocation of differently sized and charged polystyrene nanoparticles in in vitro intestinal cell models of increasing complexity. *Nanotoxicology*. 2015;9(4):453–461. Available from: https://doi.org/10.3109/17435390.2014.944599.
117. Teeguarden JG, Hinderliter PM, Orr G, Thrall BD, Pounds JG. Particokinetics in vitro: dosimetry considerations for in vitro nanoparticle toxicity assessments. *Toxicol Sci*. 2007;95(2):300–312. Available from: https://doi.org/10.1093/toxsci/kfl165.
118. Stock V, Bohmert L, Donmez MH, Lampen A, Sieg H. An inverse cell culture model for floating plastic particles. *Anal Biochem*. 2020;591:113545. Available from: https://doi.org/10.1016/j.ab.2019.113545.
119. Watson CY, DeLoid GM, Pal A, Demokritou P. Buoyant nanoparticles: implications for nano-biointeractions in cellular studies. *Small*. 2016;12(23):3172–3180. Available from: https://doi.org/10.1002/smll.201600314.

120. Navabi N, McGuckin MA, Linden SK. Gastrointestinal cell lines form polarized epithelia with an adherent mucus layer when cultured in semi-wet interfaces with mechanical stimulation. *PLoS One*. 2013;8(7):e68761. Available from: https://doi.org/10.1371/journal.pone.0068761.
121. Hinderliter PM, Minard KR, Orr G, et al. ISDD: a computational model of particle sedimentation, diffusion and target cell dosimetry for in vitro toxicity studies. *Part Fibre Toxicol*. 2010;7(1):36. Available from: https://doi.org/10.1186/1743-8977-7-36.
122. DeLoid G, Cohen JM, Darrah T, et al. Estimating the effective density of engineered nanomaterials for in vitro dosimetry. *Nat Commun*. 2014;5:3514. Available from: https://doi.org/10.1038/ncomms4514.
123. DeLoid GM, Cohen JM, Pyrgiotakis G, et al. Advanced computational modeling for in vitro nanomaterial dosimetry. *Part Fibre Toxicol*. 2015;12:32. Available from: https://doi.org/10.1186/s12989-015-0109-1.
124. Thomas DG, Smith JN, Thrall BD, et al. ISD3: a particokinetic model for predicting the combined effects of particle sedimentation, diffusion and dissolution on cellular dosimetry for in vitro systems. *Part Fibre Toxicol*. 2018;15(1):6. Available from: https://doi.org/10.1186/s12989-018-0243-7.
125. Lee HA, Leavens TL, Mason SE, Monteiro-Riviere NA, Riviere JE. Comparison of quantum dot biodistribution with a blood-flow-limited physiologically based pharmacokinetic model. *Nano Lett*. 2009;9(2):794–799. Available from: https://doi.org/10.1021/nl803481q.
126. Deng L, Liu H, Ma Y, Miao Y, Fu X, Deng Q. Endocytosis mechanism in physiologically-based pharmacokinetic modeling of nanoparticles. *Toxicol Appl Pharmacol*. 2019;384:114765. Available from: https://doi.org/10.1016/j.taap.2019.114765.
127. Praetorius A, Tufenkji N, Goss KU, Scheringer M, Von Der Kammer F, Elimelech M. The road to nowhere: equilibrium partition coefficients for nanoparticles. *Environ Sci: Nano*. 2014;. Available from: https://doi.org/10.1039/c4en00043a.
128. Li M, Al-Jamal KT, Kostarelos K, Reineke J. Physiologically based pharmacokinetic modeling of nanoparticles. *ACS Nano*. 2010;. Available from: https://doi.org/10.1021/nn1018818.
129. Lin P, Chen JW, Chang LW, et al. Computational and ultrastructural toxicology of a nanoparticle, Quantum Dot 705, in mice. *Environ Sci Technol*. 2008;42(16):6264–6270. Available from: https://doi.org/10.1021/es800254a.
130. Bachler G, von Goetz N, Hungerbuhler K. A physiologically based pharmacokinetic model for ionic silver and silver nanoparticles. *Int J Nanomed*. 2013;8:3365–3382. Available from: https://doi.org/10.2147/IJN.S46624.
131. Bachler G, von Goetz N, Hungerbuhler K. Using physiologically based pharmacokinetic (PBPK) modeling for dietary risk assessment of titanium dioxide (TiO_2) nanoparticles. *Nanotoxicology*. 2015;9(3):373–380. Available from: https://doi.org/10.3109/17435390.2014.940404.
132. Carlander U, Li D, Jolliet O, Emond C, Johanson G. Toward a general physiologically-based pharmacokinetic model for intravenously injected nanoparticles. *Int J Nanomed*. 2016;11:625–640. Available from: https://doi.org/10.2147/IJN.S94370.
133. Li M, Panagi Z, Avgoustakis K, Reineke J. Physiologically based pharmacokinetic modeling of PLGA nanoparticles with varied mPEG content. *Int J Nanomed*. 2012;7:1345–1356. Available from: https://doi.org/10.2147/IJN.S23758.
134. Lin Z, Monteiro-Riviere NA, Kannan R, Riviere JE. A computational framework for interspecies pharmacokinetics, exposure and toxicity assessment of gold nanoparticles. *Nanomed (Lond)*. 2016;11(2):107–119. Available from: https://doi.org/10.2217/nnm.15.177.
135. Li S, Wang Q, Yu H, et al. Polystyrene microplastics induce blood-testis barrier disruption regulated by the MAPK-Nrf2 signaling pathway in rats. *Environ Sci Pollut Res Int*. 2021;324:75–85. Available from: https://doi.org/10.1007/s11356-021-13911-9.
136. Park EJ, Han JS, Park EJ, et al. Repeated-oral dose toxicity of polyethylene microplastics and the possible implications on reproduction and development of the next generation. *Toxicol Lett*. 2020;324:75–85. Available from: https://doi.org/10.1016/j.toxlet.2020.01.008.
137. Xie X, Deng T, Duan J, Xie J, Yuan J, Chen M. Exposure to polystyrene microplastics causes reproductive toxicity through oxidative stress and activation of the p38 MAPK signaling pathway. *Ecotoxicol Environ Saf*. 2020;190:110133. Available from: https://doi.org/10.1016/j.ecoenv.2019.110133.
138. Hou B, Wang F, Liu T, Wang Z. Reproductive toxicity of polystyrene microplastics: in vivo experimental study on testicular toxicity in mice. *J Hazard Mater*. 2021;405:124028. Available from: https://doi.org/10.1016/j.jhazmat.2020.124028.
139. An R, Wang X, Yang L, et al. Polystyrene microplastics cause granulosa cells apoptosis and fibrosis in ovary through oxidative stress in rats. *Toxicology*. 2021;449:152665. Available from: https://doi.org/10.1016/j.tox.2020.152665.
140. Amereh F, Eslami A, Fazelipour S, Rafiee M, Zibaii MI, Babaei M. Thyroid endocrine status and biochemical stress responses in adult male Wistar rats chronically exposed to pristine polystyrene nanoplastics. *Toxicol Res (Camb)*. 2019;8(6):953–963. Available from: https://doi.org/10.1039/c9tx00147f.
141. Wei J, Wang X, Liu Q, et al. The impact of polystyrene microplastics on cardiomyocytes pyroptosis through NLRP3/Caspase-1 signaling pathway and oxidative stress in Wistar rats. *Environ Toxicol*. 2021;36(5):935–944. Available from: https://doi.org/10.1002/tox.23095.
142. Li B, Ding Y, Cheng X, et al. Polyethylene microplastics affect the distribution of gut microbiota and inflammation development in mice. *Chemosphere*. 2020;244:125492. Available from: https://doi.org/10.1016/j.chemosphere.2019.125492.
143. Koelmans AA, Redondo-Hasselerharm PE, Mohamed Nor NH, Kooi M. Solving the nonalignment of methods and approaches used in microplastic research to consistently characterize risk. *Environ Sci Technol*. 2020;54(19):12307–12315. Available from: https://doi.org/10.1021/acs.est.0c02982.

Chapter 41

Exposure assessment: critical review of dietary exposure methodologies—from budget methods to stepped deterministic methods

Xiaoyu Bi
Exponent, Inc., Washington, DC, United States

Abstract
Dietary exposure assessments are a fundamental component in risk assessment. The process of quantifying dietary exposure in a population involves the use of models that vary in both complexity and detail. One group of models includes deterministic methods that are based on the of use a single value for the input parameters of food consumption and constituent concentration. Each method has advantages and limitations as well as varying degrees of resource expenditure. Therefore, when considering the most appropriate assessment method(s), it is critical to have a clear understanding of the purpose of the assessment and the available methods to which data can be obtained, applied, or further refined in a dietary exposure assessment.

Keywords: Dietary exposure; screening methods; model diets; deterministic methods

41.1 Introduction

Dietary exposure is an essential component for quantifying the potential risk associated with the consumption of dietary constituents and substances. It is calculated by combining estimates of food consumption and concentration of the dietary constituent or substance in the food under consideration by following the general equation:

$$\text{Dietary exposure} = \sum [\text{Food consumption} \times \text{Concentration}]$$

Numerous methodologies exist to evaluate dietary exposure and differ with respect to the underlying consumption and concentration data as well as the accompanying assumptions for the underlying data. Dietary exposure assessments range from the most conservative methods, often referred to as screening methods, to refined methods. The application of a given method largely depends on the dietary constituent or substance being evaluated, assessment purpose, and data availability. In general, the deterministic methods discussed in this chapter can be classified into three major groups: (1) screening methods, (2) model diets, and (3) refined methods. An overview for each method and advantages and limitations are provided herein. In addition, other refinement options as well as research gaps and future directions in dietary exposure are discussed. Probabilistic methods are discussed in detail in Chapter 48.

41.1.1 Screening methods

Screening methods offer a rapid and inexpensive approach to estimate exposure to a constituent or substance in the diet. These methods often utilize highly aggregated and conservative estimates for both consumption and concentration parameters to estimate exposure. Such data may include country-level production statistics as a proxy for consumption or the use of the maximum use rate of a given food additive in combination with other assumptions as described in more detail in the poundage and budget methods.

41.1.1.1 Poundage method

41.1.1.1.1 Method and application

The poundage method relies on national per capita production volume or sales data of foods or food constituents in a country over a specified period, usually on an annual

Present Knowledge in Food Safety. DOI: https://doi.org/10.1016/B978-0-12-819470-6.00070-6

basis. In the United States, the Economic Research Service (ERS) Food Availability (Per Capita) Data System (FADS) provides publicly available data on the annual food and nutrient availability for consumption. The FADS includes estimates for over 200 commodities including individual fruits, vegetables, grains, added sugars and sweeteners, dairy, and meats. These data serve as proxies for consumption estimates at the national level. The United Nations Food and Agriculture Organization's annual Food Balance Sheets are a standardized database compiled for over 150 countries and approximately 100 food commodity groups.[1]

In the poundage method, the mean per capita exposure estimate for a food additive is derived by dividing the total annual amount of the food additive available by the population size:

$$\text{Per capita mean dietary exposure to food additive} = \frac{\text{Annual volume of food additive}}{365 \text{ days} \times \text{population size}}$$

Standard body weight estimates are used to derive estimates a per kg body weight basis, if applicable. The method was applied, among others, by Kim et al.[2] to estimate the intake of 16 sweeteners for the Korean population. Assumptions are often used to refine the per capita estimates obtained from the poundage data. For instance, the Joint FAO/WHO Expert Committee on Food Additives (JECFA) used the poundage method to derive initial estimates of the intake of annatto for five countries, including Brazil and the United States,[3] and refined the estimated exposure estimate for Brazil by assuming that 28% of the population would consume annatto, and estimated the 90th percentile exposure for the US by multiplying the per capita mean by 2.

Food additive or other food constituent concentration can also be combined with poundage data to estimate exposure to the food constituent:

$$\text{Per capita mean dietary exposure} = \frac{\sum \text{Annual volume of food} \times \text{Concentration}}{365 \text{ days} \times \text{Population size}}$$

For example, Enig et al.[4] utilized the ERS production figures and disappearance data for fats and oils and published estimates of trans fatty acids concentrations in total fat to estimate trans fatty acid intakes. Food Balance Sheets have been utilized to estimate the global prevalence of inadequate zinc intake[5] and to characterize adherence to the Mediterranean diet of 41 countries over four decades.[6]

41.1.1.1.2 Advantages and limitations

The poundage method is rapid and inexpensive since it relies on available national statistics on food production rather than actual food consumption data. However, quality and accuracy of food production data can vary between commodities and countries. Since commodity data are for raw commodities and semiprocessed commodities, data that are often unaccounted for include food loss, food waste, processed foods, and noncommercial production. These limitations may lead to overestimation or underestimation of food availability, nutrient intake, and dietary exposure from the use of food supply data, especially for developing countries where data could be sparse.

While there are clear limitations to the underlying food production data that can be used in the poundage method, there are approaches to overcome the uncertainty in food production data. Such approaches include use of averaging of several years of data instead of relying on a single-year, comparing commodity data or country-specific data as percentage (of energy) or ratios (of total production), understanding the source of data in order to assess its quality (i.e., whether data are real or imputed), and application of relevant formulas and hypotheses to further refine the data.[7]

41.1.1.2 Budget method

41.1.1.2.1 The method and application

The budget method was developed in 1979 to derive screening estimates of the maximum food additive levels that can be used in a food and/or beverage supply without exceeding a food additive's acceptable daily intake (ADI).[8,9] This method has also been used to assess the theoretical maximum daily dietary exposure (TMDE) to food additives,[10] International Programme on Chemical Safety (IPCS), 2020 and is based on daily physiological limits of food and beverage consumption and default conservative assumptions. The estimation of the TMDE (mg/kg-bw/day) is as follows:

$$\begin{aligned}&\text{TMDE (mg/kg bw/day)}\\ &= \left[\begin{array}{l}\text{maximum level of additive in beverages (mg}/L) \times 0.1\ (L/\text{kg bw})\\ \times \text{ Percentage of beverages that many contain the additive}\end{array}\right]\\ &+ \left[\begin{array}{l}\text{maximum level of additive in solid foods (mg/kg)}\\ \qquad \times\ 0.05\ (\text{kg/kg bw})\\ \times \text{ Percentage of solid foods that many contain the additive}\end{array}\right]\end{aligned}$$

The default conservative assumptions include consumption estimates of solid foods of 0.05 kg food per kg body weight and nonmilk beverages of 0.1 L/kg body weight, the maximum concentration of the additive in foods and nonmilk beverages, and the proportion of solid foods and nonmilk beverages that may contain the additive. The consumption estimates of solid foods and nonmilk beverages assumed in the TMDE calculation are based on daily physiological limits.[8,11] The Joint FAO/WHO Expert Committee on Food Additives (JECFA)[9] and the European Commission[12] have applied the budget method as a screening method to assess food additives. Most recently, Barraj et al. (2021) utilized the budget method to estimate screening level intake estimates of low- and no-calorie sweeteners in Latin America.

The budget method can also be applied reversely and used to calculate the consumption amount of food that is necessary to reach the TMDE or the theoretical maximum allowable level of the chemical in foods or nonmilk beverages assuming all other components of the budget method calculation are known or assumed conservatively; this is referred to as the reverse budget method. The reverse budget method has been used to estimate the theoretical maximum concentration (TMC) of food colors[13] and low- and no-calorie sweeteners[14] in nonalcoholic beverages. In general, the TMC in solid foods or nonmilk beverages can be calculated using the following equation assuming all other components of the calculation, including the ADI-apportioned fraction for food or beverages, consumption rate for solid food or nonmilk beverage, and percentage of solid food or nonmilk beverages containing the food additive are known or assumed conservatively:

$$\begin{aligned}&\text{TMC}_{\text{Solid food or non-milk beverage}}\,(\text{mg/kg})\\&=\left[\text{ADI apportion}_{\text{Solid food or beverage}}\,(\text{mg/kg/day})\right]\\&\div\left[\begin{array}{l}\text{Consumption}_{\text{Solid food or non-milk beverage}}\,(L/\text{kg bw/day})\\\times\ (\text{Percent}_{\text{Solid food or non-milk beverage containing additive}})\end{array}\right]\end{aligned}$$

41.1.1.2.2 Advantages and limitations

Similar to the poundage method, the use of the budget method can also provide a rapid and inexpensive screening level estimate of the intake of a food additive or food constituent. Default consumption estimates as described above do not require actual food consumption data and are traditionally based on daily physiological limits of food and beverage consumption. The concentration of the additive in foods and nonmilk beverages is typically assumed to be the maximum reported use level of the additive, while the proportions of solid foods and nonmilk beverages that may contain the additive are set arbitrarily. All default assumptions to the budget method contribute to the conservativeness of the method. In more recent assessments, refinements to the default conservative assumptions in the budget method have been explored by using food consumption data from national surveys, sales data to approximate the fraction of the food supply that could contain the food additive, and/or concentration data obtained from product labels or food industry as performed by Barraj et al. (2021) and Tran et al.[13,14] These refinements reflect actual consumption and market data that would decrease the potential uncertainty in arbitrarily set default assumptions as well as the overall conservatism of the method.

41.1.2 Model diets

Estimates of exposure based on model diets rely on aggregated summary statistics for the consumption and/or concentration parameters. Model diets represent the consumption of or the concentration within a given food category or food commodity for a given population. Aggregated consumption summaries used in model diets can vary from the use of country-specific to clustered global food consumption data. Specifically described are the consumption data in the Global Environment Monitoring System/Food Contamination Monitoring and Assessment Program (GEMS/Food), Consumption Cluster Diets and nutrient and contaminant data collected from a total diet study (TDS).

41.1.2.1 Global Environment Monitoring System/Food Consumption Cluster Diets

41.1.2.1.1 Method and application

Initially developed in 1997 by the World Health Organization (WHO) GEMS/Food, the GEMS/Food Consumption Cluster Diets provide a summary of the global food consumption for 17 groups or clusters of countries. The 17 cluster diets were developed based on modeling of food supply data for raw and semiprocessed commodities from 2002 to 2007 in 179 countries.[15] For each cluster diet, the average per capita food consumption estimates are summarized for 18 broad categories and a total of 62 further refined food categories for the general population.

Cluster diets have been used to estimate dietary exposure to contaminants by applying concentration data for the chemical or compound of concern to the consumption estimates in the cluster diets.

41.1.2.1.2 Advantages and limitations

Cluster diets are most appropriate for an assessment at the regional or international level when national consumption data are not available. Cluster diets can allow developing countries to better implement regional food safety measures and basic dietary exposure assessments for various food hazards.[15] However, it should be noted that consumption patterns of clusters with larger populations may be more reflective of the consumption patterns within those countries due to the weighting method applied in the development of the cluster diets (Heraud et al., 2013). Therefore exposure assessments utilizing cluster diets may result in an overestimation particularly for countries with a smaller population than compared to other countries in the same cluster. An overestimation of consumption may also result since the underlying food supply data do not account for waste. Other limitations are that cluster diet estimates correspond only to raw and semiprocessed commodities and that intake variability among households and individuals or home production habits are not accounted for (Heraud et al., 2013).

41.1.2.2 Compiled summary consumption data

41.1.2.2.1 Method and application

Summary food consumption data obtained through the compilation and harmonization of existing individual food consumption surveys data collected by individual countries can also be used to estimate dietary exposure to food constituents. Examples of these databases include the European Food Safety Authority (EFSA) Comprehensive Food Consumption Database and the WHO Chronic individual food consumption database—summary statistics (CIFOCOss). The consumption data in both databases are standardized using the FoodEx2 classification scheme that aggregates individual food items into food groups and broader food categories in a hierarchical parent–child relationship. Data on per capita as well as per user basis, expressed on g/day or g/kg body weight/day for the total population as well as for select age and sex subpopulations are available from both databases. Summary statistics available include population size, number of consumers, means, and select percentiles. The EFSA database includes detailed data for a number of European Union (EU) countries. Data on chronic and acute food consumption are available at different refinement levels, ranging from Level 1 (least refined, e.g., Grains and grain-based products) to Level 7 (most refined, e.g., Cheese cream sponge cake). The WHO CIFOCOss database was created in 2012 and is periodically updated with data from member states. It currently includes data from 65 surveys conducted in 37 countries. Data in the CIFOCOss database are available at the FoodEx2 Level 4.

Estimated exposures are derived by combining the summary consumption estimates with assumed concentrations of the food constituent. Since only summary consumption data are available, assumptions are typically applied when estimating intake of food constituents that could be available in multiple food categories.

41.1.2.2.2 Advantages and limitations

The EFSA Comprehensive Food Consumption Database and the WHO CIFOCOss allow for estimating exposure estimates at the country level using consumption data that have been standardized using the same food classification scheme. Since the data are obtained from individual food consumption surveys conducted in the various countries, they are representative of actual food consumption. However, as mentioned above, since the data are only available in summary form, assumptions need to be made when the food constituent is available in multiple categories.

41.1.2.3 The total diet study or market basket method

41.1.2.3.1 Method and application

The TDS method combines the average concentration of nutrients or contaminants of interest from analytical testing of foods representative of the overall diet of a population with consumption estimates typically obtained from food consumption surveys. Foods undergoing analytical testing are collected from predefined areas according to the sampling plan, prepared in table-ready form (i.e., after they have been prepared for normal consumption and include only the edible portions of the food as consumed), and analyzed for the nutrient(s) or contaminant(s) of interest. Compositing of samples may be done either on an individual food basis or with more aggregated food categories. TDSs can be used as a screening tool for chemicals to identify foods or food groups and chemicals that may need detailed monitoring and can provide information on the concentration trend of a nutrient/contaminant and the dietary intake of the nutrient/contaminant over time.

The TDS approach has been used by the US Food and Drug Administration since 1961 and gained recognition in 1967 by the Joint Food and Agricultural Organization (FAO)/WHO.[16,17] The US TDS collects samples of approximately 280 foods in four regional market baskets per year and analyzes these foods for pesticides, industrial chemicals, radionuclides, toxic elements, and nutrient elements. The US TDS has been used to evaluate trends of sodium and lead[18] (Briguglio et al., 2015) as well as dietary exposures to lead and cadmium in conjunction with the food survey portion of the NHANES.[18–20] Ongoing TDSs are also conducted in other countries including the United Kingdom, Australia, France, Canada, Korea, Japan, and China.

41.1.2.3.2 Advantages and limitations

The TDS method can provide the most accurate measure of the average concentrations of nutrients and contaminants in foods because analytical testing is performed on the edible portion of the food sample and on the table-ready form or as consumed. Furthermore, the analysis of the sample takes into account any losses during food processing, preparation (e.g., washing, peeling, cooking), or storage (including migration from packaging, if any) and testing typically uses sensitive analytical methods. Foods collected and sampled are representative of the typical or usual diet of the population, and therefore, dietary exposure of nutrients or contaminants using the analytical results should not be calculated for specific individuals or groups with atypical food patterns. Estimates of dietary exposure from the TDS method are also not suitable on an acute basis or when contamination occurs. Moreover, since results of the analytical data provide the concentration at the mean only, the exposure distribution cannot be ascertained.

41.1.3 Refined methods

Refinements to the consumption and/or concentration estimates may often need to be considered to address uncertainty when these data are too conservative or nonrepresentative of the consumption amounts or concentration data. As a result of these possible issues, the resulting exposure estimate will be overly conservative and nonrepresentative. Moreover, due to the highly aggregated consumption and/or concentration data applied in both screening and model diet methods, estimates may often exceed the safety limits of the dietary constituent or substance. In such cases, refinement of the consumption data often involves utilizing data from reported consumption amounts of food and beverages by individuals collected in small population studies (e.g., the duplicate method) or large-scale national food consumption surveys.

41.1.3.1 The duplicate method

41.1.3.1.1 Method and application

The duplicate method (or duplicate portion method) involves the collection of duplicate amounts or portions for every food and beverage consumed for each participant over the duration of the study. Exposure estimates of the substance of concern are derived by multiplying the *actual* total daily amount of the food or beverage consumed with the concentration of the substance detected from analytical testing of the duplicate portion. This method is often used in epidemiological studies that estimate the intake of nutrients not available in food and nutrient composition databases or environmental contaminants and its correlation with a specific health effect or biomarker. For example, Julin et al.[21] studied the relationship between dietary cadmium assessed by the duplicate method and cadmium concentrations in urine and blood among 57 Swedish premenopausal women. It is suitable in developing countries, especially among population groups where the majority of meals are prepared at home as participants are tasked to make duplicate portions of their food. This method provides a direct exposure estimation whereas estimates from all other exposure methods are considered indirect.

41.1.3.1.2 Advantages and limitations

The strength of the duplicate method is undoubtably the ability to perform direct analysis of nutrients or environmental contaminants, where there is little to no food composition data from the actual duplicate food or beverage. However, this method is costly with respect to the preparation of duplicate portions and analytical testing of foods, demanding for participants due to a considerable amount of involvement to provide duplicate portions, and requires a significant amount of commitment from participants to complete the study. Due to these limitations, it is impractical to implement the duplicate method in a large-scale study population or to assess long-term intake.

41.1.3.2 Empirical distribution estimate using food consumption surveys

41.1.3.2.1 The methods

Consumption of foods, beverages, and dietary supplements can be estimated through data collected at an individual or household level from food consumption surveys. Data collected in food consumption surveys can be prospective (e.g., food diaries, duplicate portions) or retrospective (e.g., 24-h recall, food frequency) and the quality of data from such surveys highly depends on the survey design, methods, motivation, cooperation, and memory of survey participants. To estimate exposure to a food additive or food constituent, consumption data from these surveys are combined with concentration data. Survey methods including the 24-h recall and food frequency are discussed below.

41.1.3.2.2 24-h recall

Dietary recalls allow for the collection and estimation of absolute food and nutrient intake amounts. Subjects participating in a 24-h dietary recall are asked to recall detailed information on all foods and beverages (and dietary supplements) consumed in the past 24 h. Specifically, respondents are solicited by a trained interviewer to describe the food or beverage in detail including the type and amount of food and preparation method as well as time of day the food or beverage was consumed and source of food (e.g., grocery store, restaurant). In the United States, the National Health and Nutrition Examination Survey (NHANES) is a continuous survey that uses a complex multistage probability sample design and collects information about the health and diet of the civilian population. Within the program of studies in NHANES, the dietary component of the survey collects detailed information on all foods and beverages consumed by individual survey participants in the previous 24-h time period for up to two nonconsecutive days. The dietary component of the survey is conducted as a partnership between the US Department of Agriculture (USDA) and the US Department of Health and Human Services (DHHS). Well-known limitations to 24-h recall recalls are associated costs and administration time as well as misreporting that is influenced by participant eating habits (i.e., under reporting occurring among those with higher intake amounts), memory lapses (i.e., failure to recall foods consumed and the report of foods that were in fact not consumed for the recall day), and misrepresentation of portion sizes.[22]

41.1.3.2.3 Food frequency questionnaire

A food frequency questionnaire (FFQ) allows for the estimation of intake over a longer time frame and is commonly used in epidemiological studies to examine possible associations between long-term exposures and health outcomes. FFQs consist of a listing of individual foods and/or food groups for which survey respondents are asked to estimate the number of times, the food is consumed on a daily, weekly, monthly, or annual basis. FFQs are typically either completely qualitative and only ask about the frequency of consumption for the food items or semiquantitative collecting information on portion size. As part the dietary component of NHANES, information on the frequency of fish and shellfish consumption during the past 30 days were collected for every survey cycle. During NHANES 2003–2004 and 2005–2006 cycles, a FFQ containing 151 questions was used to collect information on the frequency of consumption of specific food and beverage categories based on participant consumption patterns over the past 12 months. Furthermore, frequency of consumption in the past 30 days was also collected for a small number of foods including milk, ready-to-eat foods, and frozen meals/pizza within the diet behavior and nutrition questionnaire. Advantages to FFQs include lower associated costs and administration time with a major limitations including participation burden and decreased accuracy associated with length of questionnaire and loss of detail on specific foods.

41.1.3.3 Deterministic estimates

41.1.3.3.1 Single-point estimates

In a dietary exposure assessment that utilizes single-point estimates, both the food consumption data and concentration data use point estimates as input parameters. Point estimates may correspond to the mean, median, or a high percentile from observed values. For concentration data, the maximum allowable concentration or the maximum observed concentration may also be considered for the single-point estimate used in the exposure calculation. Point estimates are often high-end values corresponding to conservative assumptions, which can result in a worst-case exposure estimate that may be most appropriate for a screening level assessment. However, the level of conservatism ultimately depends on the available information of the consumption and concentration data. Therefore it is important to understand and document assumptions and whether the point estimates identified for use in the assessment are representative of the underlying data and based on robust data. It is possible to refine deterministic estimates by using a distribution of values, if available, rather than point estimates for the input parameters.

41.1.3.3.2 Distribution estimates

Distribution estimates rely on empirical food consumption and/or concentration data. Most often, an empirical distribution for consumption and a concentration point estimate is used to calculate exposure. Since consumption amounts and food choices often differ on a day-to-day basis within and between individuals (i.e., intra- and interindividual variability), the distribution of consumption allows for this variability in consumption amounts. The distribution of consumption data may be obtained from individual dietary records from nationally representative food consumption surveys. Each value in the consumption distribution can be multiplied by the concentration point estimate to obtain a distribution of the total individual dietary exposure from which population summary statistics can be derived. If individual dietary records are unavailable, representative summary statistics on the consumption distribution can be multiplied by the concentration point estimate.

41.1.3.3.3 Other refinement options

For the consumption data used in the determination of exposure, other refinement options or adjustments to this input parameter may include obtaining data specific to sensitive subpopulations or subpopulations whose intake may be expected to be the highest or obtaining detailed data as to the specific foods or food groups expected to contain the food additive or food constituent of interest. If consumption data cannot be further refined and reflects a broad category of which only a subset of foods is anticipated to contain the food additive, it could be assumed that a fraction of foods contain the food additive. The fraction assumed could be an arbitrary yet conservative value or could be potentially obtained from market share data, product label data, or reported market trends in literature. For example, market-share adjustments have used to place weighting to beverage types uses of low- and no-calorie sweeteners[14] (Barraj et al., 2021) and food colors.[13]

With regard to the concentration of a food additive or food constituent, refinement options or adjustments may include use of maximum allowable concentration in foods which would result in highest exposures or the use of the maximum use level found in foods. The use of the maximum use level found in foods can also be assumed and is often referred to as exposures resulting from brand loyal consumers, where consumers are loyal to a brand that may always contain a high level of a food additive. Alternatively, the use of average or typical concentration values may correspond to the levels that consumers could or are actually exposed to. Other adjustments may include processing factors or portion of food that is actually consumed if data do not account for food loss due to spoilage or inedible components. When resources are available, surveys and analytical testing have been conducted to collect concentration data. For example, use level data on food colors has been collected from industry[23,24] and from analytical testing.[25] When individual analytical results are available, the treatment of nondetects should be considered since handling of nondetects could have an impact on exposure estimates. A summary of refinement options are presented in Table 41.1.

Refined assessments can also utilize more specific input data and sophisticated models that are able to provide more realistic exposure estimates. An example is the use of probabilistic modeling that combines the distribution of concentration for a food additive or food constituent and food consumption amounts to estimate exposure. The key difference is the use of distributions of consumption and concentration data instead of a single point value for each. A probabilistic model samples from each input distribution to produce an exposure distribution. More on probabilistic dietary exposure assessment is discussed in the next chapter.

41.2 Research gaps and future directions

As described earlier, there are many approaches to consider when conducting a dietary exposure assessment. Screening methods are simple and inexpensive in regard to resources needed and amount of time to conduct the assessment. However, similar to model diets, the data used in screening methods to calculate the consumption estimates are not reflective of actual consumption amounts and are often too conservative. In comparison, refined methods relying on dietary records are costly and complex, and require a significant amount of commitment from participants and administrators. Data collected from dietary records inherently have associated errors including reporting and measurement error. Given the various strengths and limitations that come with each dietary exposure method, method selection will need to be made in context of the purpose of the assessment. In general, when a dietary exposure assessment is being carried out for the purpose of assessing safety, it may be most efficient to start with simple screening methods and only move on to more refined and resource intensive approaches as necessary. That is, if a safety conclusion can be made based on conservative overestimate of exposure using screening model, then it is not necessary to carry out refined assessment. However, if safety cannot be determined based on screening model estimates, then more realistic exposure estimates based on refined methods would be warranted. On the other hand, when nutrient adequacy is the purpose of the dietary assessment, realistic dietary exposure based on refined methods would be needed. Therefore, when identifying the most appropriate

TABLE 41.1 Summary of refinement or adjustment options to the consumption and concentration parameters in the determination of exposure.

Refinement approaches	

Consumption data	• Obtain data specific to sensitive subpopulation or populations whose intake may be expected to be highest
	• Obtain data specific to foods or food groups expected contain the food additive or food constituent of interest
	• Adjust for fraction of total foods, specific foods, or food groups anticipated to contain the food additive or food constituent using
	  ◦ market share data
	  ◦ actual use by product label use
	• Use of mean, median, or high-end intakes among consumers

Concentration or use level data	• Highest brand-loyal exposure: use of maximum allowable or reported concentration in foods • Average or typical exposure: use of average or typical concentrations in foods • Apply adjustment factors to reflect processing of foods or the portion of food that is actually consumed • Obtain concentration data through a survey or sampling, if resources are available • Consider treatment of nondetects; assumption of nondetect = 0, nondetect = limit of detection, or other assumption

assessment method(s), it is critical to have a clear understanding of the purpose of the assessment, the available consumption and concentration data, areas of possible refinement or adjustment, and data limitations and uncertainties.

References

1. Food and Agriculture Organization of the United Nations (FAO). FAOSTAT: Food Balances. Available from: https://www.fao.org/faostat/en/#data/FBS; 2022.
2. Kim M, Lee G, Lim HS, et al. Safety assessment of 16 sweeteners for the Korean population using dietary intake monitoring and poundage method. *Food Addit Contam A Chem Anal Control Expo Risk Assess*. 2017;34(9):1500–1509.
3. Joint FAO/WHO Expert Committee on Food Additives (JECFA). Evaluation of national assessments of intake of annatto extracts (bixin). Available from: https://inchem.org/documents/jecfa/jecmono/v44jec15.htm; 2000.
4. Enig MG, Atal S, Keeney M, Sampugna J. Isomeric trans fatty acids in the U.S. diet. *J Am Coll Nutr*. 1990;9(5):471–486. Erratum in: *J Am Coll Nutr*. 1991;10(5):514. PMID: 2258534.
5. Wessells KR, Brown KH. Estimating the global prevalence of zinc deficiency: results based on zinc availability in national food supplies and the prevalence of stunting. *PLoS One*. 2012;7(11): e50568. Available from: https://www.ncbi.nlm.nih.gov/pmc/articles/PMC3510072/.
6. da Silva R, Bach-Faig A, Raidó Quintana B, Buckland G, Vaz de Almeida MD, Serra-Majem L. Worldwide variation of adherence to the Mediterranean diet, in 1961–1965 and 2000–2003. *Public Health Nutr*. 2009;12(9A):1676–1684. Available from: https://doi.org/10.1017/S1368980009990541.
7. Thar C, Jackson R, Swinburn B, Mhurchu CN. A review of the uses and reliability of food balance sheets in health research. *Nutr Rev*. 2020;78(12):989–1000. Available from: https://doi.org/10.1093/nutrit/nuaa023.
8. Hansen SC. Conditions for use of food additives based on a budget for an acceptable daily intake. *J Food Prot*. 1979;42(5):429–434.
9. Joint FAO/WHO Expert Committee on Food Additives (JECFA). Guidelines for the preparation of working papers on intake of food additives for the joint FAO/WHO expert committee on food additives. Available from: http://www.who.int/foodsafety/chem/jecfa/en/intake_guidelines.pdf; 2001.
10. Douglass JS, Barraj LM, Tennant DR, Long WR, Chaisson CF. Evaluation of the budget method for screening food additive intakes. *Food Addit Contam*. 1997;14(8):791–802.
11. Hansen SC. Acceptable daily intake of food additives and ceiling on levels of use. *Food Cosmet Toxicol*. 1966;4:427–432.
12. European Commission. Report on methodologies for the monitoring of food additive intake across the European union. Report of a working group on scientific cooperation on questions relating to food. In: *Task*. 4. Luxembourg (Germany): Office of Publications of the European Communities. SCOOP/INT/REPORT/; 2;1998.
13. Tran NL, Barraj LM, Hearty AP, Jack MM. Tiered intake assessment for food colours. *Food Addit Contam A Chem Anal Control Expo Risk Assess*. 2020;37(7):1118–1134. Available from: https://doi.org/10.1080/19440049.2020.1736341.
14. Tran NL, Barraj LM, Hearty AP, Jack MM. Tiered intake assessment for low- and no-calorie sweeteners in beverages. *Food Addit Contam A Chem Anal Control Expo Risk Assess*. 2021;38(2):208–222. Available from: https://doi.org/10.1080/19440049.2020.1843717.
15. Sy MM, Feinberg M, Verger P, Barré T, Clémençon S, Crépet A. New approach for the assessment of cluster diets. *Food Chem Toxicol*. 2013;52:180–187. Available from: https://doi.org/10.1016/j.fct.2012.11.005.
16. Pennington JA, Gunderson EL. History of the Food and Drug Administration's total diet study–1961 to 1987. *J Assoc Off Anal Chem*. 1987;70(5):772–782.
17. World Health Organization. Pesticide residues: report of the 1967 joint meeting of the FAO working party and the WHO expert committee. Geneva: FAO and WHO. Available from: http://apps.who.int/iris/bitstream/10665/40693; 1968.
18. Bolger PM, Carrington CD, Capar SG, Adams MA. Reductions of dietary lead exposure in the United States. *Chem Speciat Bioavailab*. 1991;3:31–35.
19. Gavelek A, Spungen J, Hoffman-Pennesi D, et al. Lead exposures in older children (males and females 7–17 years), women of childbearing age (females 16–49 years) and adults (males and females 18 + years): FDA total diet study 2014-16. *Food Addit Contam A Chem Anal Control Expo Risk Assess*. 2020;37(1):104–109.
20. Spungen JH. Children's exposures to lead and cadmium: FDA total diet study 2014–16. *Food Addit Contam A Chem Anal Control Expo Risk Assess*. 2019;36(6):893–903.
21. Julin B, Vahter M, Amzal B, Wolk A, Berglund M, Åkesson A. Relation between dietary cadmium intake and biomarkers of cadmium exposure in premenopausal women accounting for body iron stores. *Environ Health*. 2011;10:105.
22. Poslusna K, Ruprich J, de Vries JH, Jakubikova M, van't Veer P. Misreporting of energy and micronutrient intake estimated by food records and 24 hour recalls, control and adjustment methods in practice. *Br J Nutr*. 2009;101(Suppl 2):S73–S85. Available from: https://doi.org/10.1017/S0007114509990602.
23. Bastaki M, Farrell T, Bhusari S, Bi X, Scrafford C. Estimated daily intake and safety of FD&C food-colour additives in the US population. *Food Addit Contam A Chem Anal Control Expo Risk Assess*. 2017;34(6):891–904. Available from: https://doi.org/10.1080/19440049.2017.1308018. Erratum in: Food Addit Contam Part A Chem Anal Control Expo Risk Assess. 2017;34(6). PMID: 28332449.
24. Tennant DR. Screening potential intakes of colour additives used in non-alcoholic beverages. *Food Chem Toxicol*. 2008;46(6):1985–1993. Available from: https://doi.org/10.1016/j.fct.2008.01.051. 2008.
25. Doell DL, Folmer DE, Lee HS, Butts KM, Carberry SE. Exposure estimate for FD&C colour additives for the US population. *Food Addit Contam A Chem Anal Control Expo Risk Assess*. 2016;33(5):782–797. Available from: https://doi.org/10.1080/19440049.2016.1179536.

Chapter 42

Exposure assessment: modeling approaches including probabilistic methods, uncertainty analysis, and aggregate exposure from multiple sources

Marc C. Kennedy
Fera Science Ltd, York Biotech Campus, York, United Kingdom

Abstract

As part of a tiered risk assessment, it may be necessary to perform higher tier exposure modeling. Here, the more conservative assumptions of low tier models are progressively replaced with more sophisticated models and/or more detailed data in order to better approximate the true distribution of exposures within a population. To quantify variability in dietary exposure, consumption databases are typically combined with monitoring data for concentrations. This linking is done using random simulation. Uncertainty is interpreted differently, as it represents the limitation in knowledge. Probabilistic models are also well suited to quantifying the levels of exposure from nondietary sources. This chapter describes the methods available to perform probabilistic exposure modeling that quantify variability and uncertainty. It also highlights some recent international projects to harmonize the methods, software, and databases required to perform such assessments.

Keywords: Uncertainty; variability; Monte Carlo; chemical mixtures

Chapter points

- Methods for exposure modeling can vary in complexity depending on the assessment tier and the availability of data.
- Uncertainty is always present due to limitations in knowledge and data, but should be treated separately from variability where possible, and quantified as far as possible.
- Exposure to mixtures of chemicals from multiple sources requires careful treatment with more detailed data and specialist software.
- Recommended approaches have been specified in international guidance and implemented in standard software tools.
- Practical solutions that quantify uncertainty and variability might be provided through standard algorithms and software tools, but to assess the true level of conservatism requires careful analysis and judgment.

42.1 Introduction

Exposure assessment aims to characterize the levels of chemical exposure within a population of interest and is a key component of risk assessment. Risk is defined in terms of the likelihood of a hazardous exposure level, which requires an assessment of the variability of exposures and the uncertainty associated with that assessment. International guidelines[1] state that the variation in the populations should be considered and that uncertainty should be accounted for as far as possible. Within a population, variability arises from natural heterogeneity of individuals, their dietary choices, and random processes in food production. For some chemical classes, individuals may be exposed from both dietary and nondietary sources. Incorporating exposure sources beyond the diet introduces many more possible variations. Modeling the exposures arising from the combination of these factors is extremely challenging. Uncertainty arises from imperfect information about the true levels of exposure from multiple sources, including limited understanding of the true process (how well does the proposed model represent the real distribution of exposures in the population?) and limited datasets used to estimate model parameters. In low tier, or screening, assessments, variability and uncertainty

Present Knowledge in Food Safety. DOI: https://doi.org/10.1016/B978-0-12-819470-6.00032-9

are often accounted for jointly using a combination of conservative default values and safety factors. In most cases, these are *deterministic models* and will always produce identical results if evaluated repeatedly with the same inputs. Probabilistic models, on the other hand, use simulation to generate exposures randomly according to some measure of probability. Probabilistic approaches combine measured or simulated dietary records with measured or simulated chemical occurrence values randomly. By repeating the process, a simulated population of exposure values is generated, and these are then used to represent the distribution of exposures amongst individuals within the population. Deterministic models are simpler and more transparent. The impact of each parameter can be understood, and input values can be modified to investigate their impact on the exposure estimates. However, probabilistic models provide information about the proportion of individuals exceeding a given level of exposure. If the probabilistic model also includes an uncertainty quantification, then it gives information about how sure we are about the accuracy of the estimated proportion or about individual exposures. Furthermore, by combining multivariate data sources and submodels probabilistic models can capture realistic correlations between different components of population exposure that deterministic models cannot.

Whether it is deterministic or probabilistic, the model result should account for the variation of consumed items and variation of concentration levels within those items. In practice, a combination of deterministic and probabilistic methods is applied as part of an efficient strategy, in which initial simple model tiers are replaced by more complex tiers if necessary.

Probabilistic models are most commonly considered as part of higher tier assessments because in general they produce more realistic estimates but require more detailed inputs. Ultimately, a risk manager should be provided with information on the variation of exposures within the population, together with a separate assessment of uncertainty. Uncertainty is something that can in principle be reduced by obtaining additional information. Variability cannot be reduced with more information, although the true variability might be more accurately quantified. It is therefore important to calculate and present separately any uncertainty about those features of risk that are relevant in decision-making. The decision may be to collect more information, especially when uncertainty is large. In this chapter, we consider probabilistic models. Although more complex than deterministic models in general, practical solutions have been developed, which deal with individual model components separately (e.g., consumption, concentrations) and link them together using simulation. Probabilistic models provide convenient and flexible options and can be linked together mathematically to generate estimates of the overall risk that: (1) are more realistic than deterministic models; (2) identify the proportion of individuals exceeding a particular threshold; (3) include a measure of uncertainty in the risk quantity of interest.

Before probabilistic exposure assessment can be performed, the risk scenario should be carefully defined along with a clear understanding of the purpose of the risk assessment. The following questions should be addressed before selecting appropriate risk assessment models:

- What is the health effect of interest?
- Which population is to be considered in the risk assessment?
- What chemicals lead to the health effect?
- For which activities and exposure sources do these chemicals lead to exposure in the population of interest?
- What information is available for the selected combination of population, activities, and chemicals?
- What level of conservatism is appropriate, for decision-making? This should consider the protection goal of the risk assessment.

Answering the first 4 questions determines the risk scenario, whereas questions 5 and 6 help in selecting suitable modeling approaches. Methods of varying complexity and data requirements have been developed and will be described below. The final choice of method is often constrained due to a lack of good data or other information. In this case considering the impact of uncertainty is especially important.

The population and the unit of exposure are defined as part of the risk scenario. For example, populations of interest may be high-risk subgroups such as children, pregnant women, those with a restricted diet, or a wider population. Occupation-specific populations such as chemical spray operators could also be considered, depending on the purpose of the assessment. The unit of exposure could be expressed as an external or internal exposure, and the timescale must be comparable to the toxicological reference value associated with the health endpoint such as a chronic or acute threshold level. The unit is typically bodyweight scaled and expressed in terms of mg/kg-bw/day or μg/kg-bw/day, for example.

For a specific chemical or group of chemicals, the exposure level of any individual depends on the range of that individual's activities bringing them into contact with the chemical(s) and the pattern of occurrence of the chemical(s) in the contacted material. In dietary exposure, this corresponds to the combination of food and drink items consumed and the chemical concentrations in those individual items. Surveys and monitoring data provide information about selected food items, individuals, and daily consumptions, that can be combined to calculate exposure values (see chapter 41). In probabilistic modeling, the primary goal is to quantify the variability in each component as realistically as possible.

Aggregate exposure refers to the total exposure, per individual, from multiple sources. Examples that have been studied include exposures from crop spraying activities and in the diet, exposures from cosmetics, food packaging, children's toys, and environmental sources. The complexity increases when modeling exposure to more than one source of exposure. Firstly, this is due to the diversity of potential combinations of activities involved within the population. Often there is simply not enough information—whether models or measured data—on the combinations of activities or other parameters required to model the full distribution of aggregate exposures in detail. Another difficulty arises because different pathways of exposure such as dermal, oral (nondietary ingestion), or inhalation, involve different physiological processes and there is no simple method for accurately modeling the complex pathways .

In the remainder of this chapter various concepts and practical considerations associated with probabilistic exposure modeling are presented, starting with its use within the general tiered strategy for risk assessment, then introducing general algorithms to quantify variability or a combination of variability and uncertainty. Specific probabilistic models for the main aspects of dietary exposure will then be described, followed by aggregate exposure modeling from multiple sources. Practical challenges and ongoing work will then be highlighted, including international harmonization, available datasets and software to implement probabilistic methods. Finally, we point out some key research gaps and future directions.

42.2 Dietary exposure modeling of individuals

Probabilistic modeling allows for the quantification of the exposure distribution within a population of individuals or individual days. In this section, exposures of single individuals are first considered, expressed as functions of the primary person-specific factors (food intakes, concentrations, and bodyweight). The timescale of exposure is an important aspect of the risk scenario that depends on the chosen health effect. In the case of acute health effects, exposures of an individual on different days are important. For chronic health effects, a time-averaged exposure, or usual intake, is calculated.

Dietary exposure is estimated by combining individual consumption amounts with concentration amounts, for each item consumed, then aggregating to the level of an individual-day or an individual averaged over time. Mainly, this has been performed for single compounds assessed one at a time, but increasingly there is a move toward assessing mixture of multiple chemicals. We consider each case below.

42.2.1 Single compounds

For the acute case we are typically interested in the distribution, within the population, of total daily exposures per individual. For a hypothetical set of individuals $i = 1, 2, \ldots, I$, on days $j = 1, 2, \ldots, J$, realizations from this distribution are simulated using the following equation:

$$y_{ij} = \left(\sum_{k=1}^{p_{ij}} x_{ijk} c_{ijk}\right) / b_i \qquad (42.1)$$

where p_{ij} is the number of items consumed by individual i on day j, x_{ijk} is the amount (kg) of food item k consumed by individual i on day j, c_{ijk} is the concentration (mg/kg) in item k consumed by individual i on day j, and b_i is the bodyweight of individual i in kg. It is important to note that x_{ijk} represents an amount of a raw ingredient, as measured in c_{ijk}. Any preprocessing to account for recipes or processing effects must be performed first if necessary, so that x_{ijk} and c_{ijk} are compatible.

In the chronic case we assume here that the average *daily* intake is the appropriate measure, taking an average over a lifetime. Depending on the hazard assessment, measures averaged over other timescales could instead be used. The exposure realization corresponding to the ith individual is simulated as

$$y_i = \sum_{k=1}^{p_i} E(x_{ik}) E(c_{ik}) / b_i \qquad (42.2)$$

where $E(\cdot)$ denotes expectation over the required timescale. In this case various methods have been suggested to approximate the expected intake $E(x_{ik})$, which is also referred to as usual intake.[2] More on this will be discussed later in this chapter.

42.2.2 Multiple compounds

Chapter 49 deals with risk assessment of chemical mixtures. Probabilistic models can be extended when information about the intake of multiple chemicals per individual is available, using multivariate modeling. National monitoring data provide information about chemical concentrations in food. By sampling full records directly from the monitoring survey, for each item, the multivariate pattern of cooccurrence of chemicals is preserved in the same way that sampling dietary records keeps together realistic combinations of consumed items. In the acute case, the realizations become vectors $\boldsymbol{y}_{ij}$ with a component for each compound and Eq. (42.1) is replaced by

$$\boldsymbol{y}_{ij} = \left(\sum\nolimits_{k=1}^{p_{ij}} x_{ijk}\boldsymbol{c}_{ijk}\right)/b_i \tag{42.3}$$

where $\boldsymbol{c}_{ijk}$ is a vector of compound-specific concentrations in item k consumed by person i on day j. Similarly, the chronic case can be modified from Eq. (42.2) to give

$$\boldsymbol{y}_i = \left(\sum\nolimits_{k=1}^{p_i} E(x_{ik})E(\boldsymbol{c}_{ik})\right)/b_i \tag{42.4}$$

The collection of exposures $(\boldsymbol{y}_1, \ldots, \boldsymbol{y}_I)$, once generated, can be analyzed to identify important substance mixtures present in the diets of the population, taking account of the complex multivariate patterns of dietary consumption and residue concentrations occurring in the surveys. Taking the matrix of values formed from all individuals (in rows) and all substances (in columns), mathematical models are applied to identify distinct clusters[3] or to approximate the matrix using a low-dimensional projection.[4] Such an analysis can help to prioritize mixture testing on the most likely real exposure combinations as part of an efficient strategy. Each cluster would correspond to a distinct dietary grouping and the low-dimensional approximation filters out those substances and mixtures with low incidence. In the case of multiple compounds, the relative potencies of each compound may also be factored into the assessment. For example, a relative potency factor (RPF) of a compound can be multiplied by the corresponding component of the exposure.

42.2.3 Multiple food items per individual

As already mentioned, it is important to capture the multivariate structure of chemicals within food types, and the same applies for groups of food types per individual. For a single individual or individual person-day, it is convenient to denote the vector of consumptions (multiple foods) as $\boldsymbol{x}_{ij} = (x_{ij1}, \ldots, x_{ijp_i})$ for daily consumptions or $\boldsymbol{x}_i = (x_{i1}, \ldots, x_{ip_i})$ for time-averaged consumptions. The components of these vectors are the same elements used in Eqs. (42.1)–(42.4). This vector notation will be used later in the chapter when describing models for simulating variability and uncertainty in consumption amounts in a way that accounts for the multivariate structure.

42.3 Tiered approaches in exposure assessment

A tiered approach is recommended for risk assessments, as the most efficient and practical way of achieving the required balance of conservatism and realism when there is a limited budget.[5,6] The idea is to start with a simple estimate of exposure and hazard in the initial tier. Uncertainty and variability at this stage are generally accounted for by making multiple conservative assumptions. For example, in dietary exposure assessment the international estimate of short-term intake (IESTI) is used to calculate an acute exposure of a high-level consumer of a commodity to compare against an acute reference dose. Different versions of the IESTI are used for different types of commodity, but each uses a maximum field trial residue value and adjusts for unit-to-unit variability by multiplying a default variability factor. For simple initial cases this may also be referred to as the screening tier. It is designed to be highly precautionary but requires minimal data input and can quickly identify cases in which further assessment is unnecessary. If the initial tier leads to an exposure level exceeding the hazard reference value, then more refined tiers are used to achieve a more realistic estimate of exposure. Refinements can include the collection and inclusion of more relevant data, more refined or context-specific deterministic parameters, or by incorporating uncertainty and variability into the assessment using probabilistic modeling. Instead of estimating a single high-level exposure, probabilistic models provide a measure of the full range of exposures and their relative likelihood.

Deterministic models are simple to apply but have potential limitations. It is difficult to assess how conservative the results are. Probabilistic models have the potential to capture the real variability, as far as possible, and to quantify remaining uncertainty about the true distribution of exposures. They can also be used in one-off exercises to assess the actual conservatism of the default deterministic models.[7,8] In the European Food Safety Authority (EFSA) Opinion[8] (Section 3.1.1), assessments are included to measure the conservatism of the deterministic IESTI equation, relative to the "true" reference distribution defined by a probabilistic model. More detailed use of probabilistic models is also possible to investigate the impact of regulatory changes or public health advice. Examples include recommendations to consume a certain amount of oily fish[9] that uses probability to account for variability in existing consumption levels and possible health outcomes across all individuals. The indirect impact of a deterministic model from its effect on regulatory limits can also be studied. For example, the EFSA Opinion[8] used probabilistic modeling to assess the level of protection, defined as the proportion of individuals at or below the acute reference dose, under various scenarios. A series of probabilistic assessments were carried out in which the IESTI equation was used to determine maximum residue levels (MRLs). By testing different parameter values in the IESTI equation, the impact on the level of protection could be assessed after commodities above the hypothetical MRL were removed.

In the same way that probabilistic models can be considered a higher tier assessment than deterministic models, there are different levels of sophistication available when using probabilistic models. Empirical or parametric distributions can be used for individual parameters or submodels. An *empirical distribution* is the distribution of values in a data sample (Fig. 42.1). If these data were obtained by randomly sampling measured values directly from the true population of interest, the empirical distribution can be used as an approximation of this population. For probabilistic exposure modeling, random sampling from the empirical sample is carried out to approximate sampling from the true distribution. If the sample size is N, each point is assigned equal probability $1/N$ of selection, and the selection process is repeated to obtain as many simulations as required. The larger the sample size N used, the more accurately it represents the true population. Fig. 42.1 illustrates this with empirical distributions for $N=5$ and $N=100$ generated from the same theoretical distribution. The multivariate structure within individual sampling units (corresponding to real correlations) is automatically included when sampling full records per individual, which makes it a practical solution to capture complex multivariate structure. In dietary exposure this is particularly important to represent realistic consumption amounts of different consumed items or combinations of compounds occurring in purchased items, as explained earlier.

Parametric distributions are families of theoretical distributions such as normal or lognormal distributions that can be simulated from in the absence of measurement data of the appropriate quality. A typical example where this is required is when a small sample is measured but there is a need to estimate larger samples including extrapolation into the tails of the distribution. The location and shape of these distributions are defined by estimating their parameters. These may be fitted based on estimated summaries to match a real population. Where no data are available, expert opinions may be used to set suitable parameters.

Another possibility is to develop a probabilistic model but then use only a summary statistic within the final risk assessment. This option has the advantage that it can take account of uncertainty and/or variability using all available information, yet retain only the most important parameters in the final equation, and therefore produces a model that is simple to implement using spreadsheets or other standard software, and is quick to run.

These concepts will be developed further below to describe increasingly detailed possibilities for using empirical or parametric distributions for the separate components in Eqs. (42.1)–(42.4). The decision as to which of these are implemented depends on the level of information available and the selected model tier.

42.4 Quantifying variability

Random simulations from the true distribution of exposures can be generated by calculating. Eq. (42.1) repeatedly with different values of the component parameters x_{ijk}, $\boldsymbol{c}_{ijk}$, and b_i. These parameters are generated from the joint probability distribution $p(\boldsymbol{x}_{ij}, \boldsymbol{c}_{ijk}, b_i)$ that quantifies the true variation of these parameters. This approach, of approximating a sample from the distribution of a function by calculating its value repeatedly with simulated inputs, is known as Monte Carlo Sampling. The resulting values $(y_{11}, \ldots, y_{1J}, \ldots, y_{I1}, \ldots, y_{IJ})$ are realizations from a simulated population of person day exposures for IJ person days (Fig. 42.2). The same process can be generalized easily to include any extra parameters, such as processing factors and variability factors (introduced below) so the simulation model itself can be as complex as required.

It can generally be assumed that consumption amounts and concentrations (per kilogram consumed) are independent for a given food item. Therefore these can be

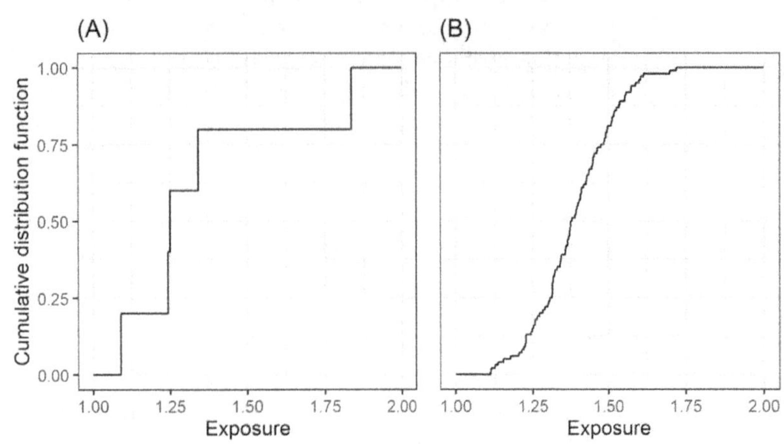

FIGURE 42.1 Empirical distributions with (A) $N=5$ points and (B) $N=100$ data points, simulated from the same underlying parametric distribution.

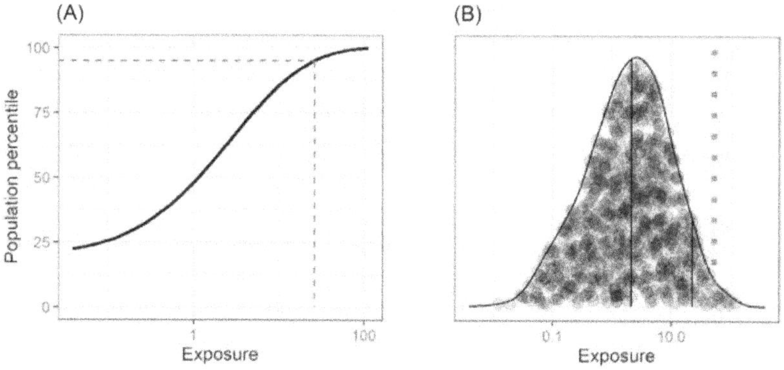

FIGURE 42.2 Example representations of probability distributions of exposure: (A) Estimate of the cumulative distribution function for population exposures. The vertical dashed red line represents a 95th percentile exposure within the population (26.1) obtained by reading off the simulated point at the 95th percentile; (B) probability density function with simulated points plotted under the curve. Black vertical lines are shown for the median and 95th percentile consumer. Red dotted line at exposure = 50 is a hypothetical hazard-based threshold dose.

modeled separately. It is often also assumed, for convenience, that consumption amount and bodyweight are independent.[a] With these assumptions the probability distribution $p(\boldsymbol{x}_{ij}, \boldsymbol{c}_{ijk}, b_i)$ can be expressed as the product $p(\boldsymbol{x}_{ij})p(\boldsymbol{c}_{ijk})p(b_i)$ and each component can be randomly generated from its own distribution. Examples of these and other types of probabilistic modeling are presented later.

The values $\boldsymbol{x}_{ij}$ and $\boldsymbol{c}_{ijk}$ can be generated from a parametric distribution or selected at random from a survey, that is, an empirical distribution. The consumption of different food items cannot be assumed to be independent. Personal dietary preferences and energy intake constraints mean that food items should be considered jointly. For example, some might prefer fruit and vegetables in preference to meat. Others may consume a large portion of fish or meat on a given day and be less likely to consume large amounts of both types together. For individual i on day j, the amounts consumed $\boldsymbol{x}_{ij} = (x_{ij1}, \ldots, x_{ijp_i})$ are therefore correlated. Dietary records contain realistic combinations of food at the individual level, so using these data is recommended to derive a realistic total exposure without requiring a more complex multivariate model of multiple foods. To estimate chronic intakes, the time-averaged mean consumption $E(x_{ik})$ must be estimated. The simplest solution is to use the averaged intake per person directly from the survey data, known as the observed individual mean (OIM) model. The OIM model tends to overestimate the high percentile average consumptions and underestimate the true proportion of consumers. This is because the highest observed consumptions in the short-term survey are unlikely to be representative of the longer-term average for the corresponding individual. Likewise, a zero consumption in the short survey does not necessarily mean the individual will never consume the item. Use of the short-term survey results alone can lead to biased estimates, but there are methods available, outlined below, to overcome this.

When designing a probabilistic model, care must be taken to identify and include substantial variations within the population of interest, and to question whether important subgroups have important differences in consumption patterns or characteristics. If using a parametric model, this means including parameters that correspond to the varying feature. Extensions to the basic models Eqs. (42.1)–(42.4) include the use of processing factors, day of the week effects, portion sizes and proportion of crop treated. If sampling from surveys is used, this also requires that enough individuals be represented in the data and that the sampling plan produces a balanced representative sample. It was mentioned in the previous section that some sampling plans are targeted or constrained in some other way. In these cases, sampling weights may be attached to each individual. The estimation should be adjusted to include these weights in the calculations Eqs. (42.1)–(42.4).

In this section uncertainty is not considered. The empirical or parametric distributions $p(\cdot)$ used to represent variation are assumed to be an adequate representation of the true distributions for the purpose of the risk assessment. When fitting a probabilistic model to represent variability, it is important to check the adequacy of the model fit against a range of plausible alternatives. Simple exploratory plots can be useful for confirming the fit of a distribution. Quantile–Quantile plots can be generated to compare the empirical data versus the equivalent ordered quantiles from a candidate theoretical distribution. Formal goodness-of-fit tests are also available in statistical software. For example, the Akaike Information Criterion (AIC) or Bayesian Information Criterion (BIC) can be calculated for each fitted model and compared when deciding amongst alternative models. The AIC and BIC penalize complex models, so help to avoid overfitting.

[a]When empirical consumption data are used correlation with an individual's bodyweight is automatically accounted for by keeping all consumed items together with that same individual. Then $p(\boldsymbol{x}_{ij}, \boldsymbol{c}_{ijk}, b_i) = p(\boldsymbol{x}_{ij}, b_i)p(\boldsymbol{c}_{ijk})$.

42.5 Quantifying variability and uncertainty

Even if it can be assumed that the model form is correct, it is unrealistic to presume that the parameters are estimated perfectly and the assumptions about the probability distributions $p(\cdot)$ are valid. For transparency it is important to quantify this uncertainty where possible, and to present it separately as explained in the introduction. Variability is due to real random variations in physical processes and individual behavior, whereas uncertainty is due to a lack of knowledge about a quantity. Uncertainty depends on the amount of relevant information available to a risk assessor at a given time, so it can vary between assessors and may be reduced by collecting more information. Information may come from a combination of sources including measurements, expert knowledge, or model results.

Variability and uncertainty can both be represented using probability distributions. For a variability distribution, the probability represents the relative frequencies of individual exposures within the population exceeding a given level or, equivalently, the probability that a random individual within the population exceeds that level. An uncertainty distribution instead represents strength of beliefs about a true but unobserved value.

At a fixed point in time within a given population and for a perfectly defined measure of exposure the true distribution of exposures has a fixed form. Uncertainty about this true distribution can be represented using a secondary probability distribution. In practice, the probability distribution for uncertainty is not expressed in mathematical form (parametric distribution) but is quantified implicitly by repeatedly simulating the collection of uncertain quantities and calculating an implied realization of the exposure (variability) distribution. This is the basis of a general purpose algorithm outlined below.

42.5.1 Simulating variability and uncertainty: two-dimensional Monte Carlo

The simulation algorithm generally implemented in probabilistic risk assessments to quantify variability and uncertainty separately is known as two-dimensional Monte Carlo (2DMC).[10,11] At the first level it involves generating multiple variability simulations, or variability loops, each of which represents an estimate of an individual exposure [e.g., as expressed in Eq. (42.1)]. The variability loops may also be referred to as inner loops and the uncertainty loops as outer loops to make clear the nested structure.

One uncertainty loop generates a full set of variability loops corresponding to a plausible distribution of individual exposures or individual-day exposures, for a given set of fixed uncertain parameters.

Repeating this for multiple uncertainty loops, each with a different set of parameters generated from the joint uncertainty distribution, generates multiple realizations of the exposure sets. The four steps are listed as follows.

- *Uncertainty loop*: Generate values for all uncertain parameters of the exposure model. Any parameters that are dependent must be generated jointly, either using a multivariate probability distribution or by first generating the independent variables then calculating the dependent variables, for example, with an equation, conditional on the independent variables.
- *Variability loop*: Generate an exposure value for a single individual-day (i,j) in Eq. (42.1) for acute exposure or individual (i) in Eq. (42.2) for chronic exposure, using fixed parameter values generated in Step 1 and any features of the corresponding individual in the simulated population.
- Repeat Step 2 for every individual in the simulated population.
- Repeat Step 1 for a large number of uncertainty realizations.

A selection of example outputs is demonstrated in Fig. 42.3. In panel (A) the full set of simulated points are shown from five uncertainty loops. From each uncertainty loop output, single summaries of the exposure distribution can be estimated directly from the corresponding points, and here we show five realizations of the unknown true p95 exposure. From 200 such realizations the uncertainty distribution of the p95 exposure can be characterized, as seen in Fig. 42.3D. Other distribution summaries could also be generated, and this flexibility along with the simplicity are the main advantages of the simulation approach. Reading off the 95% percentile in Fig. 42.3C, the median of the 95th percentile individual exposure is 26.1 (as also corresponding to the results shown in Fig. 42.2) and the p5, p95 uncertainty bounds are (17.65, 35). The percentage of simulated zeros is clear from the minimum y-axis values in Fig. 42.3B and C.

42.6 Probabilistic models for variability and uncertainty in dietary exposure

Within the general implementation framework of 2DMC, the identified variabilities and uncertainties should be simulated using appropriate distributions. Below we describe specific models that are currently used for the most important aspects.

42.6.1 Concentrations

Probabilistic dietary exposure models typically use empirical distributions of concentrations by sampling from data collected in national monitoring programs. The monitoring is

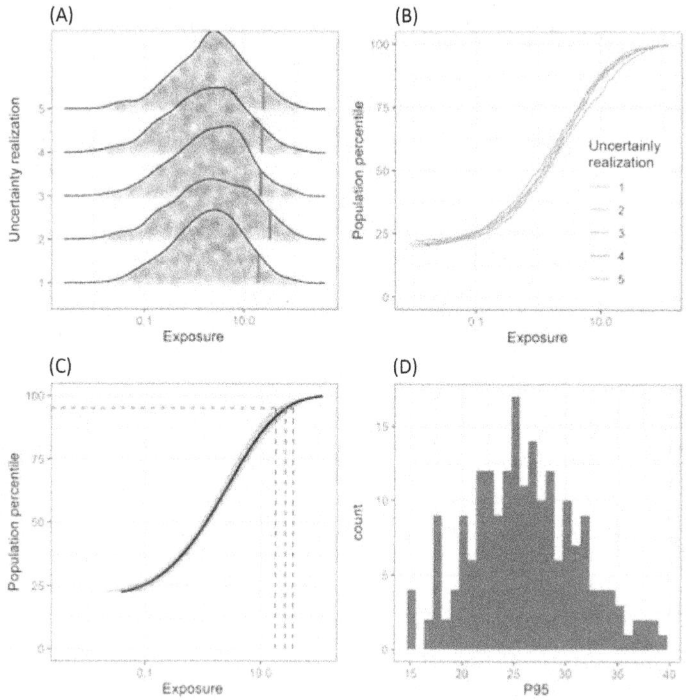

FIGURE 42.3 Example representation of the outputs from a two-dimensional Monte Carlo algorithm. (A) Density functions and simulated points from the first five uncertainty realizations (nonzero simulated exposures only). Red lines show the corresponding simulated 95th percentiles. (B) Cumulative distribution functions from the first five uncertainty realizations. (C) Summaries from all 200 uncertainty realizations. The gray band represent pointwise uncertainty intervals from 1000 uncertainty realizations, and the red dashed lines show how the median and (p5, p95) uncertainty intervals can be read off for a specific population percentile, here the 95th percentile exposure. (D) Histogram of 200 simulated p95 values, one from each uncertainty realization.

designed to cover important food types either because they are most commonly consumed or are believed to contain compounds of interest. In practice there is a limit to what can be measured, so some uncertainty derives from matching up the food as measured with food as consumed, in the intermediate step before computing exposure estimates such as Eqs. (42.1)–(42.4).

Each monitoring data point may correspond to a single consumable unit but more commonly represents a concentration in a composite sample that is formed from multiple units. For example, a batch of apples may yield a single composite measurement of concentration after combining several apples from a lot or batch. The distribution of composite values between multiple batches has less variation than the distribution of individual consumed units, so within a probabilistic exposure assessment it is necessary to consider the impact of the missing variation. Methods have been developed to adjust for this unit-to-unit variation within probabilistic modeling. In an EFSA Opinion on probabilistic modeling,[12] alternative approaches are described, referred to as lot-based and sample-based:

- Lot-based model: considering the distribution of lots, with the samples providing information about the unobserved mean and variance between lots and using further probabilistic modeling to simulate from the distribution of units within a lot.
- Sample-based model: considering the empirical distribution of samples and using additional simulation to recreate the units that made up each composite sample. This approach aims to recreate the data points that were sampled, in keeping with an empirical approach, rather than extrapolate to the full theoretical distribution.

One sample-based approach is to simulate unit values from a beta distribution $Beta(a, b)$ to represent the individual collected units. The rationale is that for a composite sample with known number of units n_u and mean concentration m, each individual unit within that composite has a minimum of 0 and maximum of $n_u m$. The parameters a and b are estimated from a coefficient of variation or a variability factor along with the mean value m.

A variability factor is defined as the ratio 97.5th percentile/mean for the distribution of units and is also used as a factor in the IESTI equation to extrapolate from a mean concentration to a default high level (97.5th percentile) concentration. Default variability factors have been established based on statistical analyses of single units.[13] These are crop-specific, depending on the size of the units. The fixed default variability factors can be used to estimate parameters to fit a unit concentration distribution of the required type (e.g., lognormal or beta). For example, assuming a lognormal distribution and variability factor v, the log-concentration is simulated from $N(\mu, \sigma)$ where $\mu = \ln(m) - \sigma^2/2$ and $\sigma = 1.96 - \sqrt{(1.96^2 - 2\log(v))}$. Whereas in the IESTI equation the variability factor is used to derive a point estimate of the 97.5th percentile, the fitted *distributions* are used for probabilistic simulation of unit concentrations. Details on fitted parameters for the beta distribution are given in documentation for the Monte Carlo Risk Assessment (MCRA) software.[14]

In chemical analysis of samples, there is always a limit to the level at which the measurement can be reliably reported. Values below the limit of detection or limit of reporting (LOR) lead to uncertainties about the censored values themselves and from subsequent modeling processes. For example, a common approach is the *substitution method*, which replaces the values with either 0, LOR, or LOR/2. Using the resulting imputed data to calculate risk empirically or parametrically by fitting a distribution has implications for the accuracy of the assessment overall. The substitution method overestimates the mean and underestimates the variability of the true distribution of concentrations. Often a more realistic approach is to assume a mixture distribution that assumes a proportion of censored values are true zeros. Values below the LOR are assigned a value of 0 with probability p_0 or a value between 0 and LOR with probability $1 - p_0$. The proportion of true zeros p_0 can be estimated from secondary data sources, such as proportions treated, or can be treated as an unknown parameter and estimated from the data. This will be referred to as the spiked-lognormal model, in which the spike is the probability of a true 0. Examples based on pesticide residues have also used agricultural usage statistics to estimate p_0 and these were found to improve the model fit, particularly in cases with large numbers of nondetects.[15]

For the nonzero concentrations, parametric methods can be applied with fixed families of distributions for positive random variables (e.g., lognormal, Weibull, or gamma distribution) and with parameters estimated by maximum likelihood estimation or Bayesian methods. The spiked lognormal is another example. Information from the values above the LOR can be used to estimate a parametric distribution and by extrapolation to predict the true values of the missing data. Nonparametric methods may also be used. These do not rely on parametric model forms, but instead use more robust statistical measures such as the median or order statistics. By not relying on a particular distribution shape, these methods are not affected by data outliers or incorrectly specified distributions. The trade-off is that they are less powerful in cases where the true distribution does follow the standard forms and they do not allow for probabilistic simulation that extrapolates beyond the available data. For nondetects, a suitable nonparametric method is the Kaplan–Meier (KM) method that uses the empirical cumulative distribution function. Estimated quantiles of the positive concentrations are not affected by the number of nondetects, provided that the quantiles of interest are greater than the proportion of nondetects. KM has been found to perform well for estimating the mean and high quantiles, provided the percentage of nondetects is not too high (<50%). Even with a high percentage of nondetects, it may perform better than parametric methods if the true distribution deviates from the assumed form. Four different methods have been tested with simulated data, assessing robustness under different amounts of censored data, sample size, and deviations from the assumed probability distributions.[16] In these simulation studies, the Weibull and Gamma distributions were found to be flexible enough to estimate the tested distributions well. The degree of censoring was found to have a large impact on the model bias.

42.6.2 Consumptions

Under the OIM model for average (usual) intake, the expected consumption amount of food item k for individual i is estimated as $E(x_{ik}) = \left(\sum_{j=1}^{J_i} x_{ijk}\right)/J_i$ where J_i is the number of survey days recorded for individual i. The OIM model has known biases as mentioned earlier. Over the very short period of a dietary survey many individuals have zero consumptions of a given item, even though their long-term average $E(x_{ik})$ is positive. Parametric methods can overcome these problems, by fitting the observed samples to a theoretical distribution, then simulating from the distribution instead of using the empirical estimates directly. Supplementary information can also be included, such as responses from food frequency questionnaires (FFQ), although these may also be subject to biases due to difficulty in recalling consumption events. For each food category, treating the frequency and amounts of consumption separately is recommended for those foods that are not eaten on a daily basis.[17,18] One implementation of this approach is the Beta-Binomial-Normal model.[19] The unknown frequency is assumed to follow a beta distribution, the number of positive consumption events is then generated from a binomial distribution, and finally each consumption amount is simulated from a fitted normal distribution. In general, the frequency and amount are positively correlated, and modeling these has been found to improve the estimation in the model developed by the National Cancer Institute.[20] Covariates such as age, sex, race, or FFQ information may be included in the model to account for variations between subgroups.

The bias affecting the usual intake estimation is not a problem for acute exposure, as there are enough individual days to capture the overall variation in daily exposure. For acute exposure the direct empirical simulation method is therefore generally applied. This method retains the information about real combinations of food consumed per individual, which is important in the acute exposure assessment but is not required in the chronic case Eqn. (42.2) or Eqn. (42.4).

42.6.3 Nondietary exposures

Variability and uncertainty distribution are dependent on the particular population of interest and the patterns of activities leading to exposure. When broadening the assessment to nondietary sources, many more variables need to be considered. The variability may be much higher than in the dietary case.

In any specific model, parameters to be factored in may include the proportion of items containing a chemical, frequency and duration of use, protective measures, breathing rates, and many others. One recent example used probabilistic simulations to estimate exposure to bisphenols from contact with thermal paper, various personal care products and dust.[21] Parameters included the frequency of handling thermal paper, skin area in contact, skin type, dust ingestion rates, and bisphenol occurrence rates. Probability distributions for these parameters can be obtained in broadly similar way as in the standard dietary exposure modeling case (through surveys, expert opinion, etc.). However, due to limited information the uncertainties involved will often be much higher for nondietary scenarios.

42.7 Quantifying uncertainty: alternative models

The previous section on quantifying variability and uncertainty was concerned with propagating uncertainty about input parameters and representing the implied impact in the risk assessment results, on the assumption that the uncertainty can be generated from a suitable distribution. Here we consider methods that can be used to quantify the uncertainty associated with the input parameters or data to provide the probability distributions for this purpose.

Uncertainties can be classified according to their source or type, and have been grouped into scenario, model and parameter uncertainties [as defined in guidance by the World Health Organization International Programme on Chemical Safety (WHO/IPCS)[22]] or similar groupings. Classifying sources of uncertainty in this way can be helpful when identifying and communicating the most relevant uncertainties in a given analysis. In general terms, scenario uncertainties arise from simplified assumptions made about the true risk scenario. Model uncertainties refer to the difference between reality and the model selected to approximate reality. Parameter uncertainties are associated with inaccuracies in the values used as model parameters or data values. Examples include measurement uncertainty, where the parameter or data value is inaccurately measured, censored data where the value is only known to be above/below a specific threshold and sampling uncertainty, which refers to uncertainty due to estimates being generated from a limited sample of data points relative to the population[b] size.

Bootstrapping is a method that can be applied to quantify sampling uncertainty.[23] If the sample size is n, bootstrapping works by repeatedly resampling (with replacement) n points from this sample. Repeating this B times generates B *bootstrap samples*. Sampling with replacement means that each point in a bootstrap sample is selected from the original sample, independently of the other points already sampled. A consequence is that some values of the original sample may be missing from a bootstrap sample and other values may be duplicated. Each bootstrap sample is then used to generate a new result. The collection of B results is an approximate sample from the sampling distribution of the calculated quantity, that can be used to quantify uncertainty. For example, a 95% confidence interval might be calculated directly from this sample. If the original sample is considered as an approximation to the true population, then each bootstrap-derived result is a realization from all the possible results that would be obtained using a sample of size n. As n increases, and if the sampling is random, the original sample approaches the underlying population, the B results all tend toward the true underlying quantity being estimated so the uncertainty interval shrinks. Bootstrapping is conceptually simple and can be applied in either the empirical or parametric case. For a parametric bootstrap, each bootstrap sample is used to generate a different parametric result in the same way that a single sample would be used. However, if the original sample is very small, it is not a realistic representation of the population. For very small sample size n, uncertainty can appear small because the same values are used repeatedly in each bootstrap, so this becomes an unreliable measure of uncertainty. For small samples, a Bayesian uncertainty calculation is more appropriate, as the uncertainty increases in a more realistic way for smaller samples. The Bayesian method requires a parametric likelihood function for the data, so requires additional information/assumptions about the data distribution. It also requires a specification of a prior distribution for unknown quantities.

Uncertainties can be quantitative or qualitative. Quantitative uncertainties are those that can be formulated in terms of uncertain numerical values. These can be handled using mathematical models of probability and statistics. Subjective expert opinion can also be elicited on the uncertain values. In many cases expert elicitation is the only available option, because measurements/models are not available or because the quantity being assessed is not measurable (e.g., some hypothetical future state). Structured elicitation methods have been developed that

[b]The population here refers to the total collection of entities for which the sample is representative. It may be a selected human population or a population of food items, for example.

aim to minimize the effect of known psychological biases when individuals try to express their beliefs about unknown quantities.[24] Qualitative uncertainties, such as those associated with the scenario or model choice, can be assessed by running alternative analyses and comparing the results. Each alternative analysis may include quantitative uncertainty modeling. This is the approach suggested in the EFSA Guidance[12] in which basic probabilistic models are defined for an optimistic and pessimistic scenario. The approach has been illustrated using alternative sets of input files and uncertainty model settings for the optimistic and pessimistic model scenarios, when calculating exposures to a group of pesticides.[25]

Bayesian models are suited to quantify the uncertainty in more complex distributions such as the spiked lognormal, because they allow for separate prior information about the proportion of true zeros to be accounted for and can be applied with the more complex two-part model.[26,27]

42.8 Aggregate exposure

Aggregate exposure is the result of combined exposure from multiple sources. In many countries and uses, there is a requirement that the combined effect should be assessed.[28,29] In probabilistic modeling, where the population distribution is assessed, the aggregation is considered for each individual in the population. The general Eqs. (42.3) and (42.4) can be extended to include the additional nondietary exposures. If we suppose, for example, that the nondietary exposures are comparable to the dietary exposures (compatible units and not scaled by bodyweight) then aggregate exposure can be expressed as

$$\mathbf{y}_{ij} = \left(\mathbf{z}_{ij}^{D} + \mathbf{z}_{ij}^{O} + \mathbf{z}_{ij}^{I} + \sum_{k=1}^{p_{ij}} x_{ijk}\mathbf{c}_{ijk}\right)/b_i \qquad (42.5)$$

for acute exposures and

$$\mathbf{y}_{i} = \left(\mathbf{z}_{i}^{D} + \mathbf{z}_{i}^{O} + \mathbf{z}_{i}^{I} + \sum_{k=1}^{p_{i}} E(x_{ik})E(\mathbf{c}_{ik})\right)/b_i \qquad (42.6)$$

for chronic exposures. The vector components $(\mathbf{z}_{ij}^{D}, \mathbf{z}_{ij}^{O}, \mathbf{z}_{ij}^{I})$ correspond to the dermal, oral, and inhalation exposures for individual i on day j and $(\mathbf{z}_{i}^{D}, \mathbf{z}_{i}^{O}, \mathbf{z}_{i}^{I})$ are time-averaged exposures for individual i. These three vectors are generally correlated, because for a given individual-day or individual the exposure sources and scenario are the same for all routes. Therefore the three routes should be calculated together within the nondietary model. As with the dietary source, exposures from multiple substances are included (hence the vectorized form). It is usual to include the effect of any absorption factors within the components of $(\mathbf{z}_{ij}^{D}, \mathbf{z}_{ij}^{O}, \mathbf{z}_{ij}^{I})$ or $(\mathbf{z}_{i}^{D}, \mathbf{z}_{i}^{O}, \mathbf{z}_{i}^{I})$. More generally, the components could also be generated as outputs from more complex toxicokinetic modeling, but it is important to ensure they are compatible with the dietary exposure components before using Eqs. (42.5) and (42.6) so that the summations are meaningful. The multisubstance exposures $\mathbf{y}_{ij}$ or $\mathbf{y}_i$ may be converted to a cumulative exposure after the sums Eqs. (42.5) or (42.6) are computed, for example using the RPFs.

Typical examples are the combination of dietary and residential or occupational exposures,[30] but other possible sources include consumer products, cosmetics and environmental exposures,[21] direct and indirect food additives.[31] Because regulation is usually restricted to individual areas (regulatory silos) exposure is generally considered separately for different sources. A more realistic assessment requires models that can combine exposures from all sources and there is an increasing interest to consider potential effects from mixtures even though the guidance and detailed methodology is not yet sufficiently developed for high tier assessments.[29,32] If an exposure model is intended to be compared with biomonitoring data, then aggregate exposures should be considered, as the recorded measurements will include multiple routes of exposure.[33]

The modeling methods used in dietary exposure assessment are also relevant for aggregated modeling, but the complexity is increased in many ways:

- The number of potential combinations of sources is large, and individuals within a population are subject to a different mix according to their circumstances and activity patterns.
- Individual sources of exposure are estimated using different methods and software. This is due to the diversity of exposure research and the varying availability of data covering different scenarios. It can lead to inconsistencies between the exposure sources and therefore bias in the aggregated assessment. This is discussed in the US Environmental Protection Agency (US EPA) general framework for aggregate exposures in screening assessments[34] in the context of aggregations of dietary, water, and residential exposures. The method outlined recognizes the potential for different levels of conservatism in each source, but this is considered suitable for a screening level assessment.
- Even if the chemicals in different sources have similar properties, the routes of exposure are often different. External to internal exposure modeling is required for each source to generate a single aggregate measure that can be assessed for hazard. For example, the timing of exposures and the process through time linking the original exposure to the target dose should be modeled. Simple standard solutions often used are to make simplified or conservative assumptions based on fixed absorption factors.

These complications require more careful modeling and quantification of the extra uncertainties and the combination of exposure routes.[35] Data can be extremely sparse for nondietary exposure sources, which means that uncertainty can be large but also difficult to quantify.

If data exist from a survey of relevant individuals, then randomly sampling those individuals is a good starting point for simulating exposure in a hypothetical population. This is typically most applicable for dietary exposure, because dietary intakes apply to all individuals, and populations are well represented in national surveys. The next stage is then to link those individuals with other exposure sources, resulting in an aggregate exposure per individual. Each individual may be exposed to multiple chemicals from each source, and exposure for dermal, oral, and inhalation should be computed.

For a realistic assessment, detailed information is required on the different combinations of activities that might lead to exposure or coexposure, for individuals within the population of interest. Ideally, this will include enough information to characterize the magnitude, frequency, and duration of exposure. For example, individuals use different cosmetic products during a day and the frequencies of use vary between individuals. The duration of exposure can depend on the length of an activity such as working with pesticides, but also the chemical properties and the nature of the product and its use (e.g., sprayed particles). When information is not available for each individual and their activities, a simpler approach is to model the relationship between general population characteristics and their activities. For example, within the MCRA software,[36] there is an option to assign different nondietary exposures to subpopulations stratified by sex or age range. In this case a different nondietary dataset is required for each distinct subgroup option.

- Uncertainty in the nondietary exposure sources may be computed using a bootstrap approach, as described above for the dietary case, or a more sophisticated approach that could include a statistical model or a purpose-built stochastic simulation model. To combine the uncertainty in nondietary exposure and uncertainty in dietary exposure the practical solution is to combine a single dietary realization with a single nondietary exposure realization within the variability loop. This is repeated for all surveyed individuals, within the variability loop, then the whole process is repeated for additional uncertainty realizations. Three broad strategies are available to link the dietary and nondietary individuals:

Option 1: Random Matching. Nondietary exposure selected purely at random.

Option 2: Random Matching Based on Identified Subgroups. Data are available from different subgroups, for example, categorized by age, sex, occupation, dietary preferences, or other grouping that might differentiate nondietary exposure. For example, residents (and their nondietary exposure distributions) could be grouped according to the type of sprayed fields they live adjacent to.[30] A nondietary exposure will be selected at random from the matching subgroup for each individual. Optionally, a proportion of individuals could also be assigned a zero nondietary exposure, which is appropriate if the nondietary exposure is known to affect only a subset of the population.

Option 3: Explicit Matching. Direct measurements are available from multiple exposure sources per individual, usually generated within a detailed study.

The matching algorithms are illustrated in Fig. 42.4. Given the simulated results, where each simulated record has an individual, chemical, and exposure source associated with it, relative contributions can be presented. Their uncertainties can also be shown if those have been simulated. The example shown in Fig. 42.5 includes dietary exposures of UK adult consumers and nondietary exposures resulting from crop spraying.[30]

42.9 Practical challenges

Probabilistic methods are more computationally demanding than deterministic methods and require additional data. Scaling up these methods to realistic numbers of chemicals is a computational challenge. Efforts are ongoing to increase the efficiency (see later section on future directions).

Insufficient data leads to large uncertainties, which may or may not be quantifiable, and can result in variability distributions required for probabilistic modeling that are not fully representative. This is particularly true when exposure potentially involves many exposure sources and mixtures of large groups of chemicals.

The concentrations or occurrence values c_{ijk} in Eqs. (42.1) or (42.3) may be estimated based on very few measurements, particularly for rarely consumed items or for chemicals that are not routinely monitored. This can lead to high uncertainty in the tails of the population exposure distribution. The average concentration $E(c_{ijk})$ used in a chronic assessment is less affected by this, as the impact of uncertainty is lower than for individual consumptions.

Some types of data are freely available, but others have restricted access.

Not all uncertainties can be calculated using statistical models, even when they are identified as being important. Sometimes data are not available, or the nature of the uncertainty means that data cannot be collected. Expert elicitation is an option when a parameter is well defined, important, and for which suitable experts can provide

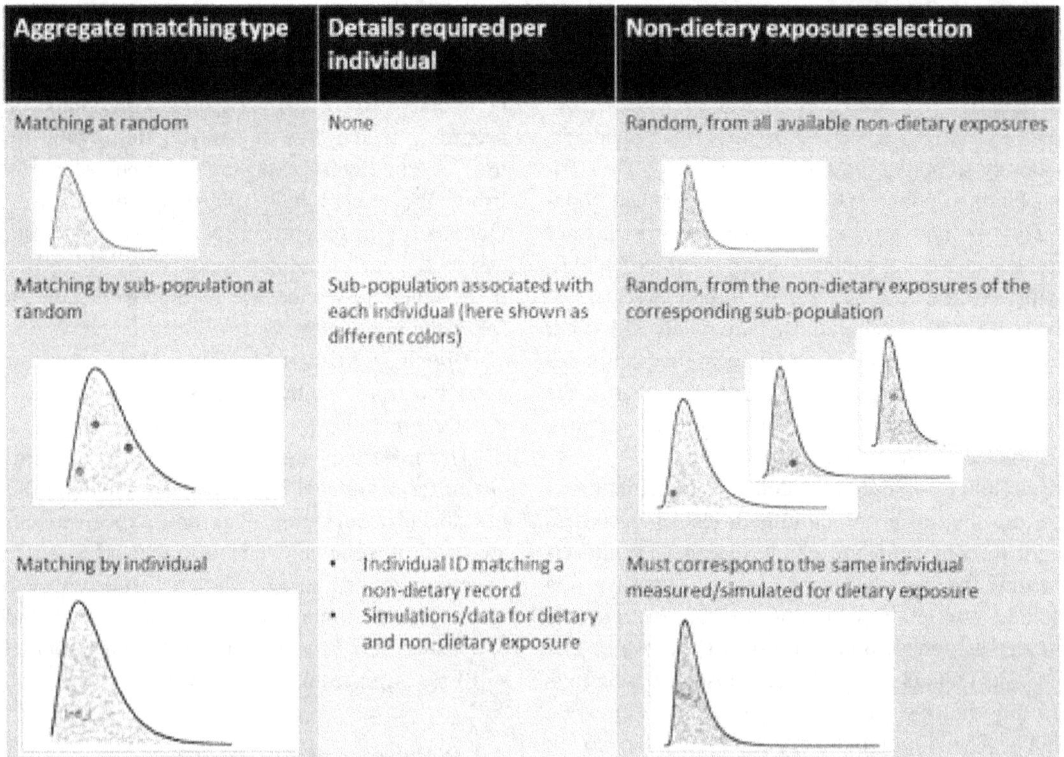

FIGURE 42.4 Three strategies for linking probabilistic dietary exposures (distributions in left panel) with probabilistic nondietary exposures (distributions in right panel) within an aggregate exposure simulation. Dietary and nondietary exposures must both be converted to the target dose before combining them. This may involve absorption factors for dermal, oral, and inhalation components, or more complex physiologically based pharmacokinetic (PBPK) modeling.

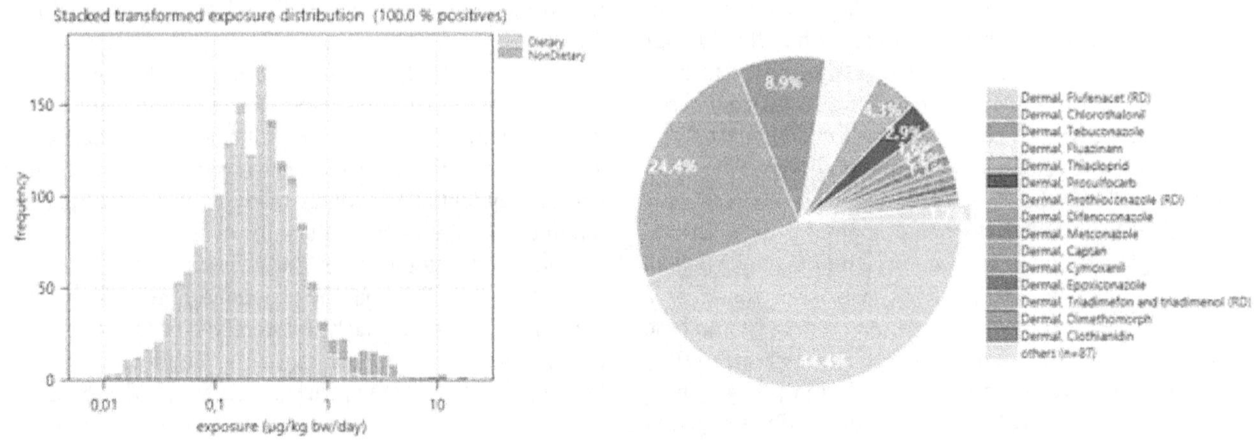

FIGURE 42.5 Summaries of aggregate exposure assessment based on the aggregate exposure analyses carried out in Kennedy et al.[30] The overall distribution of dietary and nondietary exposures (left panel) shows how most of the simulated population receive low levels from the diet, whereas a smaller proportion are simulated with higher exposures. The route of nondietary exposure and the relative contribution by pesticide and route can be generated using the simulated points (right panel).

opinions. Experts require training and facilitated workshops in order to elicit probabilities in a way that minimizes the effect of known psychological biases. Different experts have different knowledge and opinions. Ideally a group of experts will contribute to produce useful consensus distributions. There will also be cases where uncertainty cannot be quantified. Rather than ignoring the uncertainty in these cases it is important for transparency to document it clearly. Each unquantified source of uncertainty in theory has a different effect on the validity of the result. Furthermore, the different elements of the exposure assessment interact in complex ways and therefore the combined effect cannot be obtained simply by adding the individual effects. Guidance on best practice for communicating uncertainty associated with exposure assessments has been produced by EFSA[37] and European Chemicals Agency (ECHA).[38] These both emphasize the importance of documenting any assumptions, simplifications, or data quality issues that may lead to uncertainty in the results. The impacts of these uncertainties should also be quantified as far as possible, with the level of detail being appropriate to the context and proportionate to the possible consequences of the decision. Individual sources of uncertainty as well as combined uncertainty should be presented, so that if necessary further information could be gathered to reduce the most important sources. This process has been applied in the context of dietary exposure to pesticides.[25] Uncertainty quantification is an important tool within the tiered approach to risk assessment. At low tiers, uncertainty can be represented by conservative worst-case assumptions or safety factors. At more refined tiers, the uncertainties that are most critical can be iteratively updated using expert knowledge or statistical analysis of data if available. Proposals have been developed for dealing with these issues, with the different categories of uncertainty listed, as a way of ensuring that all aspects are considered in a systematic way.[39] Sensitivity analysis should be performed to understand model weaknesses and to identify critical parameters to refine. For example, extreme uncertainties arising from the pessimistic basic assessment might be iteratively replaced by more refined components or parameter values identified within a sensitivity analysis.

When linking dietary and nondietary exposure models within a probabilistic simulation, there is often a discrepancy in the quality of data, model, or level of conservatism associated with the different sources. This may lead to results being weighted unequally between the sources.

Probabilistic dietary and aggregate models are difficult to validate. Real measurements of aggregate exposures that correspond to the model scenario must be designed to avoid contamination from other sources. External exposures are more practical to obtain (e.g., measurements can be taken from outer or internal layers of clothing), but internal target doses are much more problematic. Human biomonitoring can include blood and urine. Small controlled studies might allow for direct linking of modeled and observed scenarios,[21] but the small sample sizes typically only allow for a crude assessment of the model accuracy. Larger biomonitoring studies have the problem that each individual may have multiple, and unknown, external exposure sources, making direct comparisons very difficult.[21,33]

42.10 International harmonization of methods and data

Several international organizations have been working toward harmonized approaches in relation to probabilistic methods for exposure assessment. The aim is to enable a more consistent approach to performing and interpreting assessments and more efficient use of resources. A clear and consistent approach is necessary for individual countries to meet their requirements for risk assessment under international trade agreements. While standardized deterministic methods have been applied for many years, additional work is required in relation to probabilistic methods as more varied and complex models are proposed.

The WHO/IPCS published a series of guidance documents as part of its harmonization project including 2 that relate to exposure modeling and associated uncertainty quantification.[22,40]

EFSA have also produced several guidance documents on probabilistic modeling and uncertainty analysis in exposure and risk assessment. This includes the guidance specifically related to probabilistic dietary exposure to pesticides.[12] For some of the main sources of variability and uncertainty, probabilistic models are described, including some of those outlined above. The areas covered by statistical methods included variations between lots/composite samples, additional unit-to-unit variability, sampling uncertainty due to limited sample sizes, residue values below the LOR, and parametric modeling of long-term consumption. For other sources of uncertainty, it is suggested that probabilistic modeling should be carried out only as part of a more refined assessment with specialist expertise. Instead, basic assessments are proposed to capture these uncertainties by conducting alternative model runs with optimistic and pessimistic assumptions.

In the United States, probabilistic models have been used in risk assessments conducted by the EPA since the release of policy and guidance information in 1997.[41,42] A wide range of tools and data including food and other routes of exposure are covered in the EPA expobox (http://www.epa.gov/expobox).

The Organisation for Economic Co-operation and Development (OECD) produced an overview of the methods available to assess risks from combined exposures to multiple chemicals and experience gained in the regulatory context.[43] Methodologies specific to aggregating exposure of individual chemicals are not included.

A recent guidance document from EFSA provides a more generalized overview, bringing together methods applied to human, animal, and ecological exposure assessment to multiple chemicals, and includes recommendations for uncertainty analysis.[44] These initiatives all share similar goals and generally arrive at similar conclusions in relation to probabilistic exposure modeling and uncertainty analysis. For example, they generally recommend a tiered approach similar to the WHO/IPCS Framework on Combined Exposures[5] with Tier 3 using probabilistic modeling.

European Union (EU)-funded projects have been conducted to collect data, and to improve and implement the latest models for probabilistic cumulative and aggregate exposure and risk assessment. Recent examples include the Acropolis project[45] and the more recent follow-up Horizon 2020 EuroMix project (euromixproject.eu), that used EU databases to develop probabilistic models for aggregate and cumulative (multicompound) exposure and risk assessment and applied these methods to cases studies.

Deterministic methods are currently used in the EU for pesticide risk assessment. EFSA guidance[12] recommends the use of probabilistic methods for higher tier assessments in cases where the deterministic approaches are not sufficient to reach a risk management decision. This recognizes that probabilistic methods require specialist treatment and additional resources that will not always be available. The EFSA guidance[12] provides suggested formats for outputs from probabilistic models, including a tabular format to document any unquantified uncertainties and their combined impact on the assessment. Alternative basic models are defined assuming an optimistic or pessimistic scenario. The idea is to provide practical model runs that would generate an interval of exposures containing the true levels. Options for refined assessments were also presented but should be carried out with professional statistical support.

Many of the methods outlined above sample records directly from consumption and concentration databases. Therefore much of the effort to harmonize approaches has been focused on standardized data formats with examples presented in the next section.

42.11 Available databases

The probabilistic modeling approaches described above will only provide a realistic representation of the true exposure if used with good quality data. For example, Monte Carlo approaches that randomly draw from consumption or concentration databases generally assume that the databases are representative of the population and risk scenario of interest. Even the most sophisticated models will lead to biased results when using inappropriate data, unless the bias is understood and is explicitly captured in the model.

In the United States, the Consolidated Human Activity Database (CHAD)[46] provides information from 23 human exposure studies and more than 54,000 individual days of human activity that can be freely downloaded. For each individual surveyed, demographic data and records from detailed hourly activity diaries are included. These provide essential data for cumulative and aggregate exposure models for population subgroups of interest. The updated version of CHAD is available online from US EPA[47] . Further relevant data sources are collected in the US EPA expobox.[48]

EFSA collects data from EU Member States on dietary consumption and contaminants required for harmonized risk assessments and to monitor the effectiveness of food safety programs. To aid Member States in providing data and to allow harmonized assessments, EFSA have developed FOODEX2, a standardized classification and description system to allow individual food items to be consistently recorded.[49] Summary statistics are made available as part of the EFSA Data Warehouse (https://www.efsa.europa.eu/en/science/data), which aims to improve public access to data. Also, raw data are made available in cases where these have already been published. The EFSA Comprehensive Database provides summary statistics of the dietary consumptions of individual countries, although these are not suitable for probabilistic modeling.

The European Centre for Ecotoxicology and Toxicology Of Chemicals (ECETOC) have developed the Human Exposure Assessment Tools Database (HEATDB; http://www.ecetoc.org/tools/ecetoc-heat-db/) that provides a directory of publicly available data and tools to carry out exposure assessments.[50] In addition to the main concentration and consumption data, other model parameters rely on good quality data sources. An example is the processing factors, applied to individual foods to account for processes such as cooking or peeling.[51]

42.12 Software

Development of methodology has been accompanied by software development to carry out standard probabilistic assessments at a national level. The US EPA has a long history of developing probabilistic exposure modeling software. These include the Stochastic Human Exposure and Dose Simulation (SHEDS) series of models, that implement a wide range of cumulative dietary and aggregate assessments from various sources and by different routes (inhalation, ingestion, dermal). The SHEDS-mutimedia software[52] includes the module SHEDS-dietary[53] for cumulative dietary exposure and SHEDS-residential[54] for aggregate residential exposure. Information on exposure factors and chemical concentrations are based on EPA field studies and literature. Bootstrapping is used to quantify sampling uncertainty associated with the data samples, and other types of uncertainties about model parameters can be quantified by selecting from a range of probability distributions. For variability, Monte Carlo simulations are performed in a 2DMC algorithm as described above. SHEDS-High throughput[55] is the latest edition in the series. It can handle many chemicals much more efficiently than SHEDS-Multimedia and may be used to prioritize research on the most relevant chemicals for toxicity testing and more refined exposure assessments.

As larger projects were conducted to harmonize approaches, web-based systems have been developed that aim to utilize standard file formats and are flexible enough to deal with many different types of exposure and risk problem. The MCRA software is a web-based system originally created as part of the EU MONTE CARLO project.[56] MCRA has been updated over several EU-funded and other projects. Recent extensions have been added in the EU FP7 project Acropolis to include cumulative and aggregate exposure sources, and in the H2020 project EuroMix to efficiently model larger groups of compounds and quantify uncertainty about their cumulative assessment group membership. The MCRA implementation is closely aligned with the latest relevant OECD and EFSA guidance documents.[43,44] The probabilistic models described earlier for consumption and concentrations are included as options and bootstrapping can be used along with these methods for uncertainty quantification.

A range of proprietary software tools has also been developed by Crème Global for aggregate and cumulative exposure modeling (http://www.cremeglobal.com, CARES-NG, http://caresng.org). This too allows for uncertainty quantification by the bootstrap method and includes options for combining nondietary sources. Flavorings, Additives, and food Contact materials Exposure Tool (FACET) is a software tool to model combined exposures to chemicals that migrate from food contact materials or are directly added to foods.[31] Associated data are available in the ExpoFacts Database.[57]

To generate nondietary exposures, software from many different fields has been developed, and here we mention a couple of examples that provide probabilistic outputs. ConsExpo is a program for exposure assessment developed by the Dutch National Institute for Public Health and the Environment (RIVM).[58] A recent update is the web-based ConsExpo Web (https://www.consexpo-web.nl/). Details of these tools and the default parameter values from safety factsheets are available at http://consexpo.nl/, including the factsheets that provide input parameter values and distributions to use for different situations. Probabilistic Aggregate Consumer Exposure Model (PACEM) provides higher tier probabilistic exposure assessments for chemicals in consumer products.[59] In a case study, PACEM outputs have been linked with dietary exposure results in MCRA.[21] This example relates to exposure to bisphenol chemicals in personal care products, thermal paper, and dust. Some models for other household and consumer products are mentioned in the guidance document of ECETOC.[50] Due to the broad range of different consumer products and scenarios that must be considered, lack of specific data and the need for conservative estimates, probabilistic models are rarely available. When they are used in aggregate assessments the model parameters tend to be conservative.

Although the probabilistic models used in aggregate and cumulative exposure software use broadly similar Monte Carlo approaches, there can be some differences due to model assumptions and parameter settings. This is exemplified by a study in which CARES, Calendex, ConsExpo, and SHEDS were compared using some standardized residential scenarios for aggregate exposure.[60]

To develop additional nondietary or dietary exposures outside of these existing systems, the mc2d R package[61] provides tools for generating and studying 2DMC results. More flexibility for research purposes is available within the R language itself.[62]

42.13 Research gaps and future directions

The models, databases, and software described above have been produced and applied in response to regulation in particular areas. To improve the realism of the assessment it will be important to consider combined exposure rather than in these regulatory silos. Multivariate modeling of different chemical *types* represents a further level of complexity, that has similarities to the modeling of multiple exposure sources in the aggregate case. Each type of chemical might require its own model, parameters, and data sources. These models/data/parameters will typically vary in the level of detail available. Cumulation of effects can be done separately as a final step, but different chemical types interact differently within the body (see also chapter 40).

Aggregating multiple exposure pathways should include consideration of the toxicodynamics, (how much of the substance reaches the target organ) and toxicokinetics (how long does the substance remain in the body) in a more realistic way. External doses must be converted to target doses and the dynamic time-course of the exposure must also be considered and compared to the critical exposure level (e.g., average or peak levels). The adverse outcome pathway approach provides a framework that could be analyzed using probabilistic models. Individual nodes and pathways are subject to different levels of uncertainty, but stochastic simulation provides a natural mechanism to propagate the uncertainty of exposure levels through the network.

As larger groups of chemicals and their mixtures are considered, new models and strategies are required to make the computations more efficient. One strategy is to preselect a small group of chemicals that will be included in the analysis and leave others out. EFSA have been developing cumulative assessment groups based on expert toxicological knowledge and studies. However, in the interests of transparency and the precautionary principle, reasons to exclude compounds that may contribute to the cumulative exposure need to be made explicit. Probabilistic modeling and uncertainty analysis offer possibilities to improve the process of cumulative exposure (and risk) assessment with large groups. The retain and refine method[63] developed in the EuroMix project is an iterative process that starts by including all possible chemicals in the analysis but quantifies uncertainty about any unknown parameters (including hazard). Default distributions are proposed to impute any missing information. The exposure and risk assessments quantify the uncertainties associated with the exposure and risk of individual chemicals relative to the overall cumulative effect, without excluding chemicals. Subsequent steps allow for iterative prioritization of smaller subsets, and uncertainty reduction, focused on the largest uncertainties. Further improvements and testing of this approach are required with larger groups of chemicals and uncertainty assessments for more sources of uncertainty.

Within a tiered approach, the level of conservatism is extremely difficult to assess when replacing the conservative assumptions with more realistic measurements or model components. Experience in Boon et al.'s[25] study shows that the pessimistic scenario can lead to extremely conservative exposure estimates and is not necessarily as straightforward to implement as originally envisioned. Therefore work is needed to define more realistic worst-case estimates that are practically useful.

Compared to the many sources of variation within the populations of interest, relatively few measurements can be obtained in practice due to limited resources. This inevitably leads to measurements that represent a few typical levels (or even a single level) rather than the full distribution. Total diet study (TDS) is a good example, where cooking practices and ranges of food types are combined within a single measured concentration level. Efforts have been made to combined these with supplementary data to learn about the true variation within consumed items.[64] An example is the use of composite samples of multiple items to measure concentrations. Use of composite samples captures the average concentration and is less costly than analyzing multiple foods of the same type, but information about the variation between single consumed units is lost. The modeling of unit-to-unit variation described earlier corrects for this but is based on general datasets of single units and is specific to pesticide residues in the sampled crops. The same principle could be applied in nonpesticide scenarios.

References

1. FAO and WHO. Working principles for risk analysis for application in the framework of the Codex Alimentarius. In: *Codex Alimentarius Commission – Procedural Manual*, 27 ed. Rome; 2019:254 pp.
2. Van Klaveren JD, Goedhart PW, Wapperom D, Van Der Voet H. A European tool for usual intake distribution estimation in relation to data collection by EFSA. <http://www.efsa.europa.eu/en/supporting/doc/300e.pdf>; 2012 Accessed 07.06.19.
3. Crépet A, Tressou J. Bayesian nonparametric model for clustering individual co-exposure to pesticides found in the French diet. *Bayesian Anal.* 2011;6:127–144.
4. Crépet A, Vanacker M, Sprong C, et al. Selecting mixtures on the basis of dietary exposure and hazard data: application to pesticide exposure in the European population in relation to steatosis. *Int J Hyg Environ Health.* 2019;222:291–306. Available from: https://doi.org/10.1016/j.ijheh.2018.12.002.
5. Meek ME(Bette), Boobis AR, Crofton KM, Heinemeyer G, Van Raaij M, Vickers C. Risk assessment of combined exposure to multiple chemicals: a WHO/IPCS framework. *Regul Toxicol Pharmacol.* 2011;60:S1–S14.
6. Kettler S, Kennedy M, McNamara C, et al. Assessing and reporting uncertainties in dietary exposure analysis – mapping of uncertainties in a tiered approach. *Food Chem Toxicol.* 2015;82:79–95.
7. Crépet A, Luong TM, Baines J, et al. An international probabilistic risk assessment of acute dietary exposure to pesticide residues in relation to codex maximum residue limits for pesticides in food. *Food Control.* 2021;121:107563. Available from: https://doi.org/10.1016/j.foodcont.2020.107563.
8. EFSA (European Food Safety Authority). Opinion of the Scientific Panel on Plant protection products and their Residues on acute dietary intake assessment of pesticide residues in fruit and vegetables. *EFSA J.* 2007;538:1–88. Available from: https://www.efsa.europa.eu/en/efsajournal/pub/538.
9. Hart A, Hoekstra J, Owen HL, et al. Qalibra: a general model for food risk-benefit assessment that quantifies variability and uncertainty. *Food Chem Toxicol.* 2013;54:4–17.
10. Hattis D, Burmaster DE. Assessment of variability and uncertainty distributions for practical risk analyses. *Risk Anal.* 1994;14:713–730.
11. Cullen A, Frey H. *Probabilistic Techniques in Exposure Assessment: A Handbook for Dealing with Variability and Uncertainty in Models and Inputs.* Springer; 1999.
12. EFSA (European Food Safety Authority) Panel on Plant Protection Products and their Residues (PPR). Guidance on the use of probabilistic methodology for modelling dietary exposure to pesticide residues. *EFSA J.* 2012;10(10):2839. Available from: https://doi.org/10.2903/j.efsa.2012.2839 (95 pp.).
13. EFSA (European Food Safety Authority). Opinion of the Scientific Panel on plant health, plant protection products and their residues on a request from Commission related to the appropriate variability factor(s) to be used for acute dietary exposure assessment of pesticides in fruit and vegetables. *EFSA J.* 2005;177:1–61.
14. MCRA. Monte Carlo Risk Assessment (MCRA) version 9.0. <https://mcra.rivm.nl>; 2019 Accessed 30.06.21.
15. Kennedy MC, Van Der Voet H, Roelofs VJ, et al. New approaches to uncertainty analysis for use in aggregate and cumulative risk assessment of pesticides. *Food Chem Toxicol.* 2015;79:54–64.
16. EFSA (European Food Safety Authority). Management of left-censored data in dietary exposure assessment of chemical

substances. *EFSA J.* 2010;8(3):96. Available from: https://doi.org/10.2903/j.efsa.2010.1557.

17. Slob W. Probabilistic dietary exposure assessment taking into account variability in both amount and frequency of consumption. *Food Chem Toxicol.* 2006;44:933–951.
18. Nusser SM, Carriquiry AL, Dodd KW, Fuller WA. A semiparametric transformation approach to estimating usual daily intake distributions. *J Am Stat Assoc.* 1996;91(436):1440–1449.
19. De Boer WJ, Van Der Voet H, Bokkers BGH, Bakker MI, Boon PE. A comparison of two models for estimating usual intake addressing zero consumptions and non-normality. *Food Addit Contam Part A.* 2009;26(11):1433–1449.
20. Tooze JA, Midthune D, Dodd KW, et al. A new method for estimating the usual intake of episodically consumed foods with application to their distribution. *J Am Diet Assoc.* 2006;106 (10):1575–1587.
21. Karrer C, De Boer W, Delmaar C, et al. Linking probabilistic exposure and pharmacokinetic modeling to assess the cumulative risk from the bisphenols BPA, BPS, BPF, and BPAF for Europeans. *Environ Sci Technol.* 2019;53(15):9181–9191. Available from: https://doi.org/10.1021/acs.est.9b01749.
22. WHO/IPCS. Uncertainty and data quality in exposure assessment. Part 1: Guidance Document on Characterizing and Communicating Uncertainty in Exposure Assessment (Harmonization Project Document No. 6). <https://www.who.int/ipcs/methods/harmonization/areas/exposure/en/>; 2008 Accessed 10.06.19.
23. Efron B, Tibshirani RJ. *An Introduction to the Bootstrap.* London: CRC Press; 1994.
24. EFSA (European Food Safety Authority). Guidance on expert knowledge elicitation in food and feed safety risk assessment. *EFSA J.* 2014;12(6):3734 (278 pp.). Available from: https://www.efsa.europa.eu/en/efsajournal/pub/3734.
25. Boon PE, Van Donkersgoed G, Christodoulou D, et al. Cumulative dietary exposure to a selected group of pesticides of the triazole group in different European countries according to the EFSA guidance on probabilistic modelling. *Food Chem Toxicol.* 2015;79:13–31. Available from: https://doi.org/10.1016/j.fct.2014.08.004.
26. Paulo MJ, Van Der Voet H, Jansen MJW, Ter Braak CJF, Van Klaveren JD. Risk assessment of dietary exposure to pesticides using a Bayesian method. *Pest Manag Sci.* 2005;61:759–766.
27. Kennedy M, Hart A. Bayesian modeling of measurement errors and pesticide concentration in dietary risk assessments. *Risk Anal.* 2009;2009(29):1427–1442.
28. FQPA (Food Quality Protection Act). Food Quality Protection Act. Public Law 104-170.<https://www.epa.gov/laws-regulations/summary-food-quality-protection-act>; 1996 Accessed 20.12.19.
29. Rotter S, Beronius A, Boobis AR, et al. Overview on legislation and scientific approaches for risk assessment of combined exposure to multiple chemicals: the potential EuroMix contribution. *Crit Rev Toxicol.* 2018;48(9):796–814.
30. Kennedy MC, Garthwaite DG, De Boer WJ, Kruisselbrink JW. Modelling aggregate exposure to pesticides from dietary and crop spray sources in UK residents. *Environ Sci Pollut Res.* 2019;26:9892–9907. Available from: https://doi.org/10.1007/s11356-019-04440-7.
31. Oldring PKT, O'Mahony C, Dixon J, et al. Development of a new modelling tool (FACET) to assess exposure to chemical migrants from food packaging. *Food Addit Contam Part A.* 2014;31 (3):444–465. Available from: https://doi.org/10.1080/19440049.2013.862348.
32. Kienzler A, Bopp S, Van Der Linden S, Berggren E, Worth A. Regulatory assessment of chemical mixtures: requirements, current approaches and future perspectives. *Regul Toxicol Pharmacol.* 2016;80:321–334.
33. Karrer C, Andreassen M, Von Goetz N, et al. The EuroMix human biomonitoring study: source-to-dose modeling of cumulative and aggregate exposure for the bisphenols BPA, BPS, and BPF and comparison with measured urinary levels. *Environ Int.* 2020;136:105397. Available from: https://doi.org/10.1016/j.envint.2019.105397.
34. US EPA (United States Environmental Protection Agency). Pesticide cumulative risk assessment: framework for screening analysis purpose. <https://www.regulations.gov/document?D = EPA-HQ-OPP-2015-0422-0019>; Published May 4, 2016. Accessed 30.06.21.
35. Karrer C, Roiss T, Von Goetz N, Skledar DG, Mašic LP, Hungerbühler K. Physiologically based pharmacokinetic (PBPK) modeling of the bisphenols BPA, BPS, BPF, and BPAF with new experimental metabolic parameters: comparing the pharmacokinetic behavior of BPA with its substitutes. *Environ Health Perspect.* 2018;126(7). Available from: https://doi.org/10.1289/EHP2739.
36. Van Der Voet H, De Boer WJ, Kruisselbrink JW, et al. The MCRA model for probabilistic single-compound and cumulative risk assessment of pesticides. *Food Chem Toxicol.* 2015;79:5–12. Available from: https://doi.org/10.1016/j.fct.2014.10.014.
37. EFSA (European Food Safety Authority). Guidance on uncertainty analysis in scientific assessments. *EFSA J.* 2018;16(1):5123. <https://www.efsa.europa.eu/en/efsajournal/pub/5123>.
38. ECHA (European Chemicals Agency). Guidance on information requirements and chemical safety assessment. Chapter 19 – uncertainty analysis. <https://echa.europa.eu/guidance-documents/guidance-on-information-requirements-and-chemical-safety-assessment>; 2012 Accessed 03.09.19.
39. Tennant D, Bánáti D, Kennedy MC, König J, O'Mahony C, Kettler S. Assessing and reporting uncertainties in dietary exposure analysis – part II: application of the uncertainty template to a practical example of exposure assessment. *Food Chem Toxicol.* 2017;109:68–80.
40. WHO/IPCS. Principles of characterizing and applying human exposure models (Harmonization Project Document No. 3). <https://www.who.int/ipcs/methods/harmonization/areas/exposure/en/>; 2005 Accessed 10.06.19.
41. US EPA (United States Environmental Protection Agency). Policy for use of probabilistic analysis in risk assessment at the U.S. Environmental Protection Agency. Washington, D.C. <https://www.epa.gov/risk/policy-use-probabilistic-analysis-risk-assessment-epa>; 1997 Accessed 30.06.21.
42. US EPA (United States Environmental Protection Agency). Guiding principles for Monte Carlo analysis. EPA/630/R-97/001. Washington, D.C. <https://www.epa.gov/risk/guiding-principles-monte-carlo-analysis>; 1997 Accessed 30.06.21.
43. OECD. Considerations for assessing the risks of combined exposure to multiple chemicals, Series on testing and assessment No. 296. Environment, Health and Safety Division, Environment Directorate. <http://www.oecd.org/chemicalsafety/risk-assessment/

considerations-for-assessing-the-risks-of-combined-exposure-to-multiple-chemicals.pdf>; 2018 Accessed 30.06.21.

44. EFSA Scientific Committee, More SJ, Bampidis V, Benford D, et al. Guidance on harmonised methodologies for human health, animal health and ecological risk assessment of combined exposure to multiple chemicals. *EFSA J.* 2019;17(3):5634 (77pp). <https://doi.org/10.2903/j.efsa.2019.5634>.
45. Van Klaveren JD, Kennedy MC, Moretto A, Verbeke W, Van Der Voet H, Boon PE. The ACROPOLIS project: its aims, achievements and way forward. *Food Chem Toxicol.* 2015;7:1–4. Available from: https://doi.org/10.1016/j.fct.2015.03.006.
46. McCurdy T, Glen G, Smith L, Lakkadi Y. The National Exposure Research Laboratory's consolidated human activity database. *J Expo Anal Environ Epidemiol.* 2000;10:566–578.
47. US EPA (United States Environmental Protection Agency). Consolidated Human Activity Database (CHAD) for use in human exposure and health studies and predictive models. <https://www.epa.gov/healthresearch/consolidated-human-activity-database-chad-use-human-exposure-and-health-studies-and>; Accessed 06.08.19.
48. US EPA (United States Environmental Protection Agency). EPA ExpoBox (A toolbox for exposure assessors). <https://www.epa.gov/expobox>; Accessed 30.06.21.
49. EFSA (European Food Safety Authority). The food classification and description system FoodEx2 (revision 2). EFSA Supporting Publication 2015:EN-804 (90 pp). <https://www.efsa.europa.eu/en/supporting/pub/804e>.
50. ECETOC. Guidance for effective use of human exposure data in risk assessment of chemicals. ECETOC Technical Report No. 126. <http://bit.ly/ecetoc-tr126>; 2016 Accessed 30.06.21.
51. Scholz R, Van Donkersgoed G, Herrmann M, et al. Database of processing techniques and processing factors compatible with the EFSA food classification and description system FoodEx 2. Objective 3: European database of processing factors for pesticides in food. EFSA Supporting Publication 2018:EN-1510. <https://doi.org/10.2903/sp.efsa.2018.EN-1508>.
52. Zartarian VG, Glen G, Smith I, Xue J. *SHEDS-Multimedia Model Version 3 (a) Technical Manual; (b) User Guide; and (c) Executable File to Launch SAS Program and Install Model.* EPA/600/R-08/118. Washington, DC: U.S. Environmental Protection Agency; 2008. <https://www.epa.gov/chemical-research/stochastic-human-exposure-and-dose-simulation-model-multimedia-multipathway-4> Accessed 07.08.19.
53. Xue J, Zartarian V, Nako S. *SHEDS-Dietary version 1. Technical Manual.* US EPA; 2012. <https://www.epa.gov/chemical-research/stochastic-human-exposure-and-dose-simulation-model-multimedia-multipathway-1>; Accessed 07.08.19.
54. Glen G, Zartarian V, Smith L, Xue J. *The Stochastic Human Exposure and Dose Simulation Model for Multimedia, Multipathway, Chemicals (SHEDS-Multimedia): Residential Module. SHEDS-Residential Version 4. Technical Manual.* US EPA Office of Research and Development; 2012. <https://www.epa.gov/chemical-research/stochastic-human-exposure-and-dose-simulation-model-multimedia-multipathway-4>; Accessed 07.08.19.
55. Isaacs KK, Glen WG, Egeghy P, et al. SHEDS-HT: an integrated probabilistic exposure model for prioritizing exposures to chemicals with near-field and dietary sources. *Environ Sci Technol.* 2014;48(21):12750–12759. Available from: https://doi.org/10.1021/es502513w.
56. Gibney MJ, Van Der Voet H. Introduction to the Monte Carlo project and the approach to the validation of probabilistic models of dietary exposure to selected food chemicals. *Food Addit Contam.* 2003;20(1):S1–S7.
57. Zenié A, Reina V. ExpoFacts Database. European Commission, Joint Research Centre (JRC). <http://data.europa.eu/89h/jrc-10114-10001>; 2007 Accessed 30.06.21.
58. Delmaar JE, Park MVDZ, Van Engelen JGM. ConsExpo 4.0, Consumer Exposure and Uptake Models. Program Manual. RIVM Report 320104004/2005. 2005.
59. Dudzina T, Delmaar CJE, Biesterbos JWH, et al. The probabilistic aggregate consumer exposure model (PACEM): validation and comparison to a lower-tier assessment for the cyclic siloxane D5. *Environ Int.* 2015;79:8–16.
60. Young BM, Tulve NS, Egeghy PP, et al. Comparison of four probabilistic models (CARES, Calendex, ConsExpo, and SHEDS) to estimate aggregate residential exposures to pesticides. *J Expo Sci Environ Epidemiol.* 2012;22:522–532.
61. Pouillot R, Delignette-Muller M-L. Evaluating variability and uncertainty in microbial quantitative risk assessment using two R packages. *Int J Food Microbiol.* 2010;142(3):330–340.
62. R. Core Team. *R: A Language and Environment for Statistical Computing.* Vienna: R Foundation for Statistical Computing; 2018. <https://www.R-project.org/>.
63. Kennedy MC, Hart ADM, Kruisselbrink JW, et al. A retain and refine approach to cumulative risk assessment. *Food Chem Toxicol.* 2020;138:111223. Available from: https://doi.org/10.1016/j.fct.2020.111223.
64. TDS-Exposure (Total Diet Study Exposure). Final Report Summary – Task 7.2. <https://cordis.europa.eu/project/id/289108/reporting>; Accessed 20.12.19.

Chapter 43

Exposure assessment: real-world examples of exposure models in action from simple deterministic to probabilistic aggregate and cumulative models

Cronan McNamara and Sandrine Pigat
Creme Global Ltd., Dublin, Ireland

Abstract

This chapter outlines probabilistic methods for assessing population dietary exposure. It discusses and makes recommendations on how to move from deterministic screening type calculations to higher tier, more refined calculations using probabilistic methods. The question of how to deal with variability and uncertainty in the exposure scenario input variables is covered. Probabilistic methods are more technically demanding but can overcome some of the challenges of aggregate and cumulative exposure assessment, whilst dealing effectively with variability and uncertainty. This results in a more refined and scientific approach to exposure. This chapter explains why it is important to document all model assumptions and qualitatively describe the potential effect of uncertainties. The evaluation of high-end exposures against toxicological endpoints is also briefly discussed. The type of data required for setting up the assessment and how to deal with data gaps are outlined and real-life case studies are included illustrating recommended approaches.

Keywords: Probabilistic modeling; probabilistic methods; uncertainty; variability; dietary exposure assessment; pesticide residues; optimistic; pessimistic assumptions; toxicological endpoints

Chapter points

- How calculating the level of exposure can be used to determine the possible health impact caused by the existence of chemical hazards in food.
- How the probabilistic Monte Carlo technique is used to evaluate exposure in a more refined and accurate way, using a probabilistic method and models.
- How probabilistic methods are frequently used in higher-tier evaluations as they give more realistic estimates.
- How a deterministic approach is typically used to initiate initial exposure assessments, including screening-level assessments.
- How before performing a probabilistic exposure assessment, the risk scenario and goal must be established.
- Why probabilistic approaches are more technically demanding than deterministic methods.
- How the exposure distribution among a population of individuals on specific days can be quantified, with confidence intervals, using probabilistic modeling.
- How exposure assessment can assist in determining the type, nature, incidence, and level of contact between the population and the pollutant under consideration.

43.1 Introduction

Chemical food safety requires the determination of the presence and levels of chemicals in food. These chemicals of interest include flavorings, additives, non-intentionally added substances (NIAS) from food processing, pesticides, contaminants, and so forth. The exposure evaluations, which take into consideration population consumption and presence and concentrations in foods consumed, estimate the distribution of exposure across the population and the percentage of the population that may be exposed to unsafe levels. Calculating the chance of a consumer being exposed to a substance and quantifying the extent of such exposure in comparison to health-based threshold values (or 'endpoints') is used to determine the safety of food and in particular chemical hazards in food.

Present Knowledge in Food Safety. DOI: https://doi.org/10.1016/B978-0-12-819470-6.00055-X

Exposure assessment is a major component of risk assessment, its goal is to characterize the levels of exposure to a substance within a population of interest. Risk can be loosely defined as Hazard times Exposure. A hazard is described as the inherent property of an agent having the potential to cause adverse effects in an organism exposed to the agent, whereas a risk is the probability of an adverse effect in an organism caused under specified circumstances by exposure to an agent. Overall risk assessment can be summarized in the below steps:

- Hazard Identification: adverse consequences of a substance
- Hazard Characterization: safe level of substance
- Exposure Assessment: how much gets into the body
- Risk Characterization: comparison of exposure level to hazard.

When looking at consumer safety, individual heterogeneity, dietary choices, and random processes in food production all contribute to the complexity of calculating exposure. Furthermore, individuals may be exposed to chemicals from both dietary and non-dietary sources and these 'aggregate exposures' must be evaluated to understand the full risk profile.

43.2 Probabilistic exposure modeling

To assess the population's exposure to a food contaminant or chemical, an initial approach is to use a screening method or a deterministic method. In certain cases, where the risk is low or the margin of exposure is high, it is sufficient to stop there. However when exposure results are nearing or exceeding a health-based guidance value, such as an Acceptable Daily Intake (ADI) or Tolerable Daily Intake (TDI) with this method, a more refined and less conservative approach is needed.

For the next stage in refined exposure models, a deterministic model can be used where food consumption surveys are used to provide detailed food intake data, and point value concentrations are set for the contaminant or chemical of interest in the foods. These concentrations are defined and matched carefully to the food codes in the consumption data. The point value could be the maximum concentration allowed in that food code, or set of food codes, for example. This method does produce a distribution of exposure (across the population) and therefore the results need to be expressed as statistics on that distribution (such as mean, median, or 95th percentile exposure).

The benefit of this method is that the distributional data can be analyzed to understand correlations and drivers of exposure, these could be variables such as age, sex, and food intake habits. The limitation of this approach, however, is that it assumes that all foods of a certain type contain the contaminant or chemical of interest and it is always at the highest level.

For the most refined results, probabilistic exposure assessment methods are used. These begin with the same underlying food consumption survey data, to represent the food intake habits of the population of interest but all other inputs can be probabilistic.

A tiered strategy is recommended to assess exposure. Tier 1-level analysis determines essential parameters for the exposure assessment; quantitative methodologies are used, beginning with a deterministic method (Tier 2) and progressing to a probabilistic approach (Tier 3), if necessary. Tier 2 is a deterministic technique that uses a collection of point values and correction factors to address the uncertainty in the particular sample, whereas Tier 3 is a probabilistic approach that uses a probability distribution function to characterize the uncertainty.[1,2]

A deterministic technique is typically used for initial exposure assessments, including screening-level assessments. This method generates a point estimate of exposure using point values and simple models (either high-end or typical exposure).[3] Deterministic assessments are simple, frequently use publicly available data, and produce easy-to-understand outcomes.

Probabilistic—higher tier—methods are used when more refined exposure results are required or when a more sophisticated understanding of the exposure scenarios is needed.

Probabilistic exposure modeling uses complex data or distributions as inputs instead of point values for important parameters. As a result, these models produce a more refined estimate of exposure and can assess the variability and uncertainty in the scenario.

A thorough study of probable sources and types of uncertainties in the model inputs (i.e., food consumption, chemical or contaminant presence, and concentrations) is carried out to ensure that those relevant uncertainties are captured and represented by the model.

Modeling guidelines distinguish between 'sources' of uncertainty, such as input data or exposure scenarios, and 'types' of uncertainty, such as measurement and sampling problems, as well as uncertainties related to default parameters, model structures, and associations.

43.2.1 Available outputs

Single values, or point estimates, are used as inputs to the exposure equation in a deterministic assessment. As a result, a deterministic assessment produces a point value for exposure as its output. Deterministic approaches can be employed for both screening-level, higher-tier assessments, and in components of multi-stressor and multi-pathway assessments.

The probabilistic evaluation uses data distributions from which several points or a valid range of values are identified as inputs to the exposure equation for numerous simulations. Therefore, the results of the probabilistic assessment can be expressed as statistics, expressed with confidence intervals, on those statistics. This is a key benefit of probabilistic modeling, the fact that all exposure statistics can be provided with confidence intervals that are based on the variability and uncertainties in the model scenario.

This is why probabilistic techniques are often intended for higher-level evaluations where a more scientific analysis of the situation is required.

In contrast, when employing deterministic methodologies, characterizing uncertainty and variability is challenging or limited. It can be very roughly approximated by assessing various deterministic scenarios, for example, a worst case, best case, and expected case model, but this is a very crude approach that gives the assessor very limited information on the relative likelihood of each scenario.

It is important to realize that with deterministic screening methods, there is a very large uncertainty around your understanding of the actual exposure. This uncertainty can often be assumed to be conservative (i.e., overestimating the exposure), but this is not always guaranteed to be the case, so a careful evaluation of uncertainties is important to carry out in each case.

43.2.2 Exposure methods and time frames of exposure

As discussed above, in order to get a more detailed understanding of exposure and its inherent uncertainty and/or variability, a probabilistic model is used that estimates exposure by addressing, at the very least, the variation in exposure owing to individual differences in consumption patterns.

Furthermore, the assessor may wish to analyze factors of exposure such as acute (or short-term) exposure, (typically 24 h, assessed against acute toxicity endpoints) and chronic (or long-term) exposure (related to chronic toxicity endpoints) which can be expressed as daily average intakes, based on the average intake across the number of food intake days in the survey for each consumer or extrapolated to longer-term intakes using methods such as the CARES NG n-day model[4] based on an extrapolated 365-day diary or the Iowa State University Method (ISUF)[5] or National Cancer Institute Method (NCI)[6] Long Term intake method.

These are the two main time frames of exposure models that can be identified based on the toxicity profile of the chemical of interest. Probabilistic models, such as Creme Food Safety[7,8] or CARES NG generally present options to the assessors to compute exposure to these types of time frames when running the model.

43.2.3 Assessing uncertainty

All uncertainties in the model should be assessed qualitatively, that is, the analyst should consider carefully whether a model assumption or a parameter's uncertainty is likely to lead to over-or underestimating of exposure, and to what degree. An understanding of the basics of the exposure model is key to determining this.

The probabilistic Monte Carlo technique is then used to evaluate exposure using a method that allows inputs to be expressed as distributions (which can be raw data, empirical distributions, or probabilistic expressions). In this technique, any input variable can be represented either as a number (point value) or as a complex mathematical or probabilistic expression (e.g., Uniform (10,20)), an empirical distribution (e.g., Histogram (0.2,21,0,4,12,0,6,17)) or a raw data set to be sampled from (e.g., Data (12,12,14,21,21,33,22)). Any of the above distribution types can be used to represent the uncertainty and/or variability in an input parameter.

Therefore Monte Carlo exposure systems support very significant complexity in the data sets that can be used as the model inputs, however, they also provide a simple, linear calculation for exposure evaluation, which is essentially adding up all of the exposures from each eating event for each subject in the population, working out the acute and/or chronic exposures for each person and then representing that as a distribution across the population which is then characterized by statistics such as mean and 95th percentile, for example.

The power of probabilistic models is that the uncertainties and variabilities expressed in the inputs are propagated through the model as the model samples these inputs multiple times and then repeats (iterates) through the model calculation multiple times in order to assess the entire exposure space. This results in a confidence range in the results of each statistic of interest.

Statistical methods such as bootstrapping on subjects and subject food intake diaries and custom methods to apply brand information such as market share and loyalty to the calculation of food and chemical intake can be included in these systems.

43.2.4 Cost-effectiveness

Although Monte Carlo simulations can be reasonably straightforward to set up if the software is well designed and organized, they are more time-consuming from a computational point of view, hence assessors may decide that using these more powerful methods is not essential in all circumstances. Typically, the most potentially harmful stressors, exposure pathways, and receptors are chosen for a probabilistic approach.[9]

The model output, whether deterministic or probabilistic, must account for variance in consumed items as well as variation in concentration levels within those items. In practice, a combination of deterministic and probabilistic approaches is used as part of a cost-effective strategy.[9]

Probabilistic models are frequently used in higher-tier evaluations as they give more realistic estimates but require more thought and care on the nature of the inputs.

It is a common myth to assume that probabilistic modeling requires the assessor to have lots of data for each input of interest. This is not the case. For example, expert opinion can be elicited to express an input as a plausible range. Often expressed as an "expected range" (characterized by, say, a Triangular (a,b,c) distribution) and an "extreme range" for an input variable. These can be quickly articulated and justified in order to run preliminary probabilistic models which will then assess the impact of those inputs. If they turn out to be very important - in that the key output statistics are sensitive to those inputs - it may well be worth refining those estimates by gathering more data for them, but if it turns out that the outputs are not sensitive to those inputs, then preliminary estimates (that you can justify) may well be sufficient.

Ultimately, information on the variation of exposures throughout the population should be presented to a risk manager, along with a separate assessment of uncertainty. Uncertainty can be reduced by acquiring more data, whereas variability may not be reduced by gathering more data, but could be quantified more precisely.

As a result, it's critical to assess and communicate any uncertainty about the risk characteristics that are relevant to making a decision individually. In case of high uncertainty, it may be best to acquire more data. Although more difficult than deterministic models in general, viable solutions have been created that deal with different model components (e.g., consumption, concentrations) independently and then link them together via simulation. Probabilistic models are easy and adaptable, and they can be logically connected to provide overall risk estimations as they have a higher level of realism than deterministic models; determine the percentage of people who exceed a certain criterion; and in the risk management, including a measure of uncertainty.[10]

43.3 Advantages of probabilistic exposure modeling

Exposure assessment can assist in determining the type, nature, incidence, and level of contact between the population and the pollutant under consideration. Traditional screening risk assessments (also known as the deterministic estimate or point estimate, or colloquially known as 'back of the envelope calculations) of hazardous compounds calculate a number that is assumed will safeguard the majority of the population.

Deviations from true values are accepted to assure consumer protection utilizing simple approaches by, in some situations, significantly overestimating actual exposure. Limit values are typically used in toxicology to describe risks. There should be no risk below a certain limit value; nevertheless, health impacts from cumulative chemical exposures or interactions cannot be ruled out above that number. This method is often debated. The question has been raised as to whether this method adequately accounts for transparent and accurate risk assessment. Probabilistic approaches could be used to emphasize this perceived lack of clarity, as well as to characterize and account for uncertainty in risk assessments.

- Probabilistic approaches provide for more accurate risk assessments, facilitating more effective risk management and leading to clearer risk communication.
- Separating variability from uncertainty provides more information.
- When simulating the overall production chain according to the "farm-to-fork" paradigm, the ability to estimate the success of intervention methods significantly improved.
- Probabilistic approaches reflect the complete picture of risk in the population, rather than just exceptional situations.
- When statistical approaches are used instead of subjective judgment, the estimates become more transparent and reliable.
- Aggregate and cumulative exposures can be computed and the risks associated with each evaluated in more detail.

Probabilistic risk modeling permits a wide variety of evidence-based decision-making, allowing the decision-maker to assess risks in both the short and long term, considering uncertainty.

43.4 Challenges of probabilistic exposure modeling

Probabilistic approaches require the right tools and are more scientifically and technically demanding than deterministic methods. It is something of a myth to say that probabilistic methods require more data, as there are alternative methods of characterizing uncertainties and variabilities in inputs that cover missing data that can be reliably used or scenario analysis can be used to explore the space of missing data.

It can be a computational problem to scale these algorithms up to realistic numbers of chemicals, but with the advent of cloud computing, these challenges can be overcome with the right expertise.

Inadequate data leads to huge uncertainties, which may or may not be quantified, and can result in variability distributions that are not entirely representative of probabilistic modeling. But it must be understood that these uncertainties are even more prevalent in the deterministic screening method calculations.

The complexity can increase when several exposure sources and mixtures of large groups of chemicals are involved in an exposure assessment.

Sometimes sparse data leads to concentration occurrence values being calculated on a very small number of measurements, especially for compounds that aren't consistently monitored.

This can result in the tails of the demographic exposure distribution being uncertain. It is always a challenge to estimate the tails of distribution as large numbers of iterations are needed in the computation. It requires an experienced statistician to understand the nuances of how to deal with this.

Because the influence of uncertainty is lower than for individual consumption levels, the average concentration employed in a chronic assessment is less affected by this. Even when they are determined as significant, not all uncertainties can be estimated using statistical models. Data is sometimes unavailable, or the nature of the uncertainty prevents data collection. When a parameter is well defined, significant, and suitable specialists can give opinions, expert interpretation is a possible solution.

To elicit probabilities in a way that reduces the effect of common psychological biases, experts require education and supervised workshops. Experts differ in their knowledge and viewpoints. There will be times when uncertainty is impossible to quantify. Rather than dismissing the uncertainty in these circumstances, it is critical to document it properly for transparency. In theory, each unsubstantiated source of uncertainty has a different impact on the result's validity. Furthermore, because the many components of the exposure assessment interact in sophisticated ways, the overall effect cannot be achieved by simply adding separate effects.

The repercussions of these uncertainties should also be quantified to the greatest extent possible, with a level of detail suitable to the context and proportionate to the decision's likely repercussions. Individual uncertainties, as well as aggregated sources of uncertainty, should be disclosed so that further information can be acquired if necessary, to reduce the most significant sources of uncertainty.

Within the tiered approach to risk assessment, an uncertainty quantification is an essential tool. Uncertainty can be expressed at the lowest tiers by conservative worst-case assumptions or safety levels. Expert knowledge or statistical analysis of data, if available, can be used to periodically update the most critical uncertainty at higher tiers. To comprehend model flaws and identify crucial parameters to improve, a sensitivity analysis should be carried out. Extreme uncertainties resulting from a pessimistic fundamental assessment, for example, could be iteratively substituted by more refined components or parameter values determined by a sensitivity study.

43.5 Data inputs

The exposure distribution among a population of individuals on specific days can be quantified using probabilistic modeling. Individual exposures are initially evaluated in this section, expressed as specific characteristics (food intakes, concentrations, and bodyweight). The duration of exposure is a crucial factor in the risk scenario, and it is determined by the desired health outcome. Individual exposures on different days are significant in the case of acute health impacts. A time-averaged exposure, or usual consumption, is calculated for chronic health impacts.

Individual consumption amounts are combined with concentration quantities for each item consumed to estimate dietary exposure.

In order to carry out a probabilistic exposure assessment, various data are needed. Commonly, besides in-depth expertise, data availability or accessibility are often the main determining factor when setting up such an assessment. Exposure can be calculated as follows:

$\sum$ = Amount of food consumed × frequency × concentration of containment × presence probability/ bodyweight (kg)

Some of the required input data are discussed below.

43.5.1 Data on individual consumption

Usually, national food consumption surveys are used for carrying out the assessment (see Chapter 37) These data can vary considerably by methodology applied, recency of the data, structure, level of detail (e.g., food descriptions, which could be multiple foods of the similar type represented by one generic food or foods recorded at a very granular level) as well as the completeness of the data. Examples of methodologies used to capture consumption data are 24-hour recall surveys or surveys based on food diaries. Consumption data is representative of a given population's diet. The databases usually comprise information on a couple of thousand participants representative of specific age groups and sociodemographics. The foods consumed within those surveys vary but usually span to a couple of thousand foods grouped into survey-specific food groups. For a given dietary exposure assessment, all foods containing the contaminant or chemical of interest have to be identified and are usually regrouped into a specific food category. This usually requires expert review and going through each food code one by one. For food additives and other regulated food ingredients, foods are usually categorized into defined food categories defining the recommended use levels, such as the Codex General Standard for Food Additives

(GSFA)[11] or the European Commission's food additive database.[12] These categories usually represent foods as consumed and can be more easily regrouped. For contaminants or chemicals measured in foods as an ingredient or Raw Agricultural Commodities (RAC) or Raw Primary Commodities (RPC), this can become more complex.

43.5.2 Recipe data or data on raw commodities

Oftentimes contaminant concentration levels are taken from sample data carried out on specific foods or ingredients. When trying to translate that into the food consumption data it can get very complex very quickly. For example, if a contaminant, like dioxins, is detected in pork meat, one has to account for all food sources consumed that contain pork meat. To account for pork as an ingredient, additional databases such as recipe databases or databases on raw commodities, including the What We Eat in America Food Commodity Intake Database (WWEIA FCID)[13] or EFSA's Raw primary Commodity Model[14] may be used. A recipe database is a food database that breaks each composite dish into its raw commodities and their ingredient fractions relative to that dish, for example, Food Standards Agency Standard Recipes Database.[15] Ideally those databases are already linked to the consumption surveys used, but in reality, this often isn't the case. Matching foods from those ingredient databases to the foods consumed in the survey can be done using expert judgment and in parallel to that, potentially a couple of automated techniques, such as flood mapping by key food descriptions and/or ontologies.

43.5.3 Data on chemical concentrations in food: point values, sample data, ranges/summary data

Chemical concentration data can come in different forms and at different levels of detail. Raw sample data may be retrieved from local, national, or international monitoring data or industry-specific monitoring data. Data from scientific reports or food safety authorities are another source of contaminant concentration data. These may already be summarized (across various products within a given food category), may be given as averages, minimum, maximum, and/or high percentile values, and usually, also show the number of samples taken including non-detects and positive samples. Maximum permitted levels (MPLs), as set by food authorities, may be used if no other data is available. Product-specific concentrations, that is, from a food safety incident from a food ingredient manufacturer may also be used when looking at more targeted exposure assessments.

To estimate exposure, depending on availability and complexity required for the assessment, concentrations may be averaged, the maximum may be used, and individual measurements may be used probabilistically at equal likelihood or weighted. Uncertainties of a given exposure assessment need to be addressed.

43.5.4 Data to define the presence of chemicals/additives

Once the contaminant data to be used in the exposure assessment has been identified, a possible and desired refinement is to look at the occurrence or presence probability of a given contaminant. If we assume that the contaminant is always present at a given concentration, it will result in an overestimate of exposure. In reality, a contaminant may not always be present, but due to the data available, it proves to be quite challenging to account for this refinement. In the case of sample data, zero concentrations may be recorded or the limit of quantification (LOQ) or limit of detection (LOD). This can be used to account for the percentage of the contaminant present in a given food or food product by (1) using a conservative approach using the LOD/LOQ if the concentration is below the LOD/LOQ, (2) using zero, or a defined fraction of the LOD/LOQ, (3) or even using a random value between zero and the LOD/LOQ.

Other possible sources of data to account for occurrence are market data like Mintel GNDP[16] or open food facts[17] or product-specific sales data or studies looking at products, for example containing a given chemical or not, and then deriving the occurrence based on this data. Some online databases such as Mintel GNPD list label information of nutrients and ingredients (however not contaminants) such as additives. This can be greatly helpful to derive a probability of the presence of a given ingredient per food category of a representative market.

43.6 Real-world examples of exposure models in action

The use of data science within food safety, including dietary exposure assessment, has become more prevalent and has been steadily complementing more traditional approaches. Probabilistic modeling for making informed decisions in product safety and consumer safety, business strategy has now demonstrated its value to stakeholders from industry, governments, and research organizations on many occasions, some of which are described below.

An exposure study on Acrylonitrile Butadiene Styrene (ABS),[18] an opaque polymer used in a variety of applications, including kitchen utensils, was carried out using a probabilistic approach and a multitude of data sources. During use chemicals, such as residual monomers like styrene, can migrate from ABS. Data on food consumption from the French national food consumption survey (INCA3)[19] was used and foods deemed to be prepared at home and coming into contact with kitchen utensils were identified. This experiment employed 17 regularly used kitchen utensils to estimate the population's exposure to styrene via repeated usage, building on pilot research that assessed styrene exposure from a mixing bowl. It was acknowledged that each homemade food in the French survey would only come into contact with a few ABS kitchen items throughout its preparation, rather than all 17 of them. As a result, the next stage was to pair each cooked meal and beverage with the ABS kitchen item(s) it would most likely come into contact with during its preparation. This was accomplished by going over the items recorded in the research and picking foods that required the use of a specific article. Some culinary items are only acceptable for use with specific ingredients, such as a vegetable peeler, which is only suitable for use with vegetables and fruits. In the INCA3 survey, several composite dishes (dishes made up of multiple different commodity ingredients) were matched to kitchen items that might be needed in their preparation. Where an article would not come into contact with all of the elements in the composite dish, a proportionality factor was assigned to each food-article coupling, i.e., a proportion of the dish that would come in contact with that particular article. To assign a "proportionality factor" representing the proportion of an ingredient found in the composite dish, recipe data from the UK[15] was used as a proxy due to no data being available for France. Another data source used was from a Euromonitor survey[20] on the kitchenware market and the availability of ABS kitchenware and was used as a guideline of the articles on the market as well as a data source for the market share (based on availability) of each article-type. These percentages were used in weighted distributions created to represent the probability of the article that the food was in contact with being made of ABS. Another set of input data consisted of styrene migration levels into various food kinds as a result of ABS food contact, according to a Fraunhofer IVV study. In comparison to a worst-case scenario exposure assessment, where individuals' body weights and food and beverage consumption are standardized, including real dietary data in an exposure assessment is a significant enhancement. In reality, a population is made up of people with a wide range of body weights and eating habits, therefore using survey data rather than making broad assumptions in an exposure assessment will bring the conclusions closer to reality.

Another case study using various data sources and coming up with a probabilistic exposure assessment is a study looking at children with phenylketonuria (PKU) and severe cow's milk protein allergy (CMPA), who eat a combination of prescribed, specially prepared foods for special medical purposes (FSMPs) and limited portions of regular meals. Artificial sweeteners are consumed by these individuals through a combination of free and prescribed diets. Young patients with PKU and CMPA are more likely than age-matched healthy children to exceed ADIs for additives. One of the challenges was the lack of data on consumption representing this cohort of patients. A high-tier exposure assessment of young children with PKU and CMPA to artificial sweeteners has been successfully assessed using a predictive modeling technique. The goal of this study was to anticipate possible steviol glycoside exposure in young children with PKU and CMPA, taking into account the possibility of future steviol glycoside supplies. Food consumption data were derived from the National Preschool and Nutrition Survey's food consumption survey data of healthy young children in Ireland. Specially developed amino acid-based FSMPs were utilized in the exposure model to substitute whole or milk protein diets and were included to replace limited foods. The FSMP consumption was calculated using the recommendations for ensuring adequate protein intake in these patients. According to the results of the exposure assessment, the maximum allowed level (MPL) for FSMPs should be carefully considered to avoid exposure to the ADI. These findings can be utilized to help the medical nutrition business make better decisions.[21]

The next example discusses an aggregate exposure assessment to Vitamin A via various routes, including cosmetic products such as body lotion, hand and face cream, rinse-off products, dietary supplements, food, and beverages.[22] The study aimed to estimate exposure distributions to vitamin A, in the form of retinol equivalents (REs), in pre-/post-menopausal and menopausal women in European and US populations compared to the EU Tolerable Upper Intake Limit. Due to a lack of data or know-how of possible methodologies, aggregate exposure assessments are not typically performed except for deterministic additive worst-case calculations. For setting up this aggregate exposure assessment some of the data components were:

- Data on cosmetic product use: A derivative in consumer products was investigated using the Mintel Global New Products Database (GNPD). Mintel GNPD (http://portal.mintel.com/) is an online database that tracks consumer product launches across the globe.
- Frequency of application and cosmetic product consumption. Frequency of application data was used as available from Kantar Worldpanel (http://www.kantarworldpanel.com)
- Amount per product use. Data in Creme Care and Cosmetics on the amount (mg)
- Retention factors for each product
- Distributions of RE concentrations for each product
- Different scenarios for cosmetic product use
- Dietary consumption data from the US and Europe and their food composition data
- The dermal and oral bioavailability of vitamin A
- Dermal penetration data
- Oral bioavailability.

The addition of habits and practice data and probabilistic modeling approaches to the exposure assessment for Vitamin A, described in this study as retinol and retinyl esters, retinyl acetate, and retinyl palmitate, resulted in a significant drop in exposure estimates. In 2016, the Scientific Committee on Consumer Safety (SCCS) issued an opinion on Vitamin A as retinol and retinyl esters, R acetate, and R palmitate, declaring the materials safe when used at their maximum concentrations in individual cosmetic products. The SCCS used a deterministic approach to calculate aggregated exposure to cosmetic items. This deterministic exposure evaluation assumes that all cosmetic products are applied at the highest possible frequency and quantity. Furthermore, it was considered that all products had the maximum amount of Vitamin A. (in RE equivalents). According to the SCCS, the exposure estimates were predicated on the worst-case scenario, resulting in an overestimation of vitamin A intake through cosmetic use. To offer a realistic estimate of aggregate exposure to individuals across a community, this study used the Creme Care and Cosmetics Exposure model,[23] a probabilistic (Monte Carlo) model, which calculates exposure from cosmetics and beauty products on a systematic, topical, oral, and inhalation level. In order to calculate aggregate exposure, the model and data were combined with the Creme Food Model.[7,8]

43.7 Practical considerations for exposure assessments

Before performing a probabilistic exposure assessment, the risk scenario and goal must be established. Risk assessment models shall be chosen after considering the following questions:

1. What is the impact of interest on one's health?
2. In the risk assessment, which population should be focused on?
3. What chemicals are responsible for the negative health effects?
4. To what activities and exposure sources do these substances cause exposure in the target population?
5. What information is available for the population, activities, and chemicals that have been chosen?
6. In terms of decision-making, what level of conservatism is acceptable? This must take into account the risk assessment's safety goal.

The risk scenario is determined by answering questions 1–4, while questions 5 and 6 aid in the selection of appropriate modeling methodologies. Methods with varying levels of complexity and data needs have been developed and will be described in the following sections. Due to a lack of credible data or other information, the ultimate method choice is frequently limited. In this scenario, it's extremely important to study the influence of uncertainty.

As part of the risk scenario, the population, and unit of exposure are determined. Populations of interest could include high-risk sub-groups including adolescents, pregnant women, people on a restricted diet, or the public at large.

Depending on the objective of the assessment, occupation-specific populations like chemical spray operators could also be addressed. The timeline must be comparable to the toxicological reference value associated with the health endpoint, such as a chronic or acute threshold level, and the unit of exposure could be external or internal.

Bodyweight scaled units, such as mg/kg-bw/day or μg/kg-bw/day, are commonly used. The exposure level of any individual to a specific chemical or set of chemicals is determined by the set of scenarios that bring them into contact with the chemical(s) and the pattern of occurrence of the chemical(s) in the related material. This is the mix of food and drinks taken and the chemical concentrations in those specific items in dietary exposure. As previously discussed, surveys and monitoring data provide information on specific foods, individuals, and daily consumption levels, which can be combined to generate exposure estimates. The basic purpose of probabilistic modeling is to measure the variability in each element as precisely as possible.

Aggregate exposure refers to a person's total exposure from several sources. Exposures through crop spraying activities and in the diet, as well as exposures from cosmetics, food packaging, children's toys, and environmental sources, can be included in an aggregate exposure assessment. When modeling exposure to several sources, the complexity grows.

This is attributable to the wide range of possible activity patterns among the population. There is frequently insufficient data—whether in the form of models or a complete set of measurable data—on the combinations of activities or other characteristics required to model the full range of aggregate exposures in detail. Combining data sources using probabilistic methods can overcome this lack of a comprehensive data set.

Another challenge derives from the fact that multiple exposure pathways, such as topical, oral (non-dietary intake), and inhalation, entail various physiological processes, and there is no simple mechanism for adequately modeling the diverse pathways.

43.8 General conceptual approach in probabilistic risk analysis (PRA)

PRA consists of several major steps that follow the standard method for assessing environmental health risks. These include (1) determining the problem and/or decision criteria; (2) gathering information; (3) interpreting the information; (4) identifying and implementing models and methods for evaluating variability and/or uncertainty; (5) quantifying interindividual or population uncertainty and risk in indicators relevant to decision-making; and (6) sensitivity data to assess key sources of variability.

Identifying the assessment endpoints or concerns that are pertinent to the decision-making process and stakeholders, and that can be treated in a scientific assessment process, is what problem formulation includes. Following problem formulation, information is required from stakeholders and professionals regarding the scenarios to quantify. The analysts select or develop models based on the scenarios and assessment endpoints, which involves the identification of model input data requirements and the collection of data or other information (e.g., expert judgment encoded as a result of a formal analysis stage) which can be used to quantify model inputs. In the process of creating probability distributions to represent variability, uncertainty, or both for a specific input, the data or other information for model inputs is analyzed.

The model output is estimated when a scenario, model, and inputs have been specified. Using Monte Carlo Analysis (MCA) or other probabilistic methodologies, generate samples from the probability distributions of each model input, run the model with one random value from each probabilistic input, and produce one matching estimate of the model outputs. To construct a synthetic statistical sample of model outputs, this technique is often performed hundreds or thousands of times. The probability distribution of the output of interest is interpreted from these output data.

43.9 Comparing exposure results to toxicological endpoints

The margin of exposure (MOE) is defined as the ratio between a defined end-point (e.g., NOAEL or BMDL) on the (animal) dose-response curve for the critical effect and an exposure estimate (which can be from a point estimate or probabilistic model) in a risk assessment. The MOE was recently proposed for genotoxic and carcinogenic chemical risk assessment. In contrast to the original MOE, we now define the individual margin of exposure (IMoE) as an image where both the denominator and the numerator pertain to human individuals. The integrated PRA's goal will be to examine the IMoE's distribution.

The following steps are included in the suggested probabilistic risk assessment:

1. Calculate the individual exposure (IEXP), individual critical effect dose (ICED), and then the individual margin of exposure (IMoE) distributions.
2. Derive population characteristics of interest from the latter distribution, such as the probability of critical exposure (PoCE) or a specific percentile of the IMoE distribution;
3. Quantify model input uncertainties and assess the associated uncertainty in the projected PoCE (or other characteristics).

The goal of presenting the results should be to highlight what the existing data and modeling can imply about the incidence of various levels of dietary exposure compared to the relevant toxic reference values, as well as a clear and fair statement of the results' limitations and uncertainties.

43.10 Research gaps and future directions

This chapter outlined how probabilistic methods are important for assessing dietary exposure and provides a roadmap on how to carry out these evaluations. Probabilistic exposure assessments are especially important when the exposure needs to be understood at a refined level and/or when aggregate or cumulative exposure estimates are required. These methods may be more technically challenging but can overcome the lack of refinement or confidence available from deterministic methods. Probabilistic methods deal more effectively with variability and uncertainty, especially when aggregate and cumulative exposure scenarios are required and result in a more refined and scientifically robust understanding of exposure.

Some gaps in being able to carry out an exposure assessment are data availability as well as having the right expertise to carry them out successfully. Data is normally taken from national food consumption surveys and lab data on chemicals or data derived from literature. However, some EU member states as well as other countries either don't have data available or are not willing to share their data in the required format (as opposed to summarized population statistics). Similarly, data on concentration levels and occurrence can be hard to source. In order to be able to carry out exposure assessment, knowledge of the data used, that is, the methodologies applied to obtain the input data on consumption and concentration levels are of importance. Similarly, understanding how to use and interpret the statistical outcomes of the exposure model requires in-depth expertise.

Future, and even present, opportunities, more and more consider the area of total aggregate exposure. Instead of looking at chemical exposure from a food intake perspective only, a more holistic approach can be taken. Industry associations are more and more exploring exposure from multiple routes, such as ingestion (food and other means), inhalation, dermal absorption, or occupational exposure some noteworthy examples are CARES NG or the Vitamin A exposure study[21] but also new ingredients of concern such as Cannabidiols (CBDs) will be more meaningful when looking at aggregate exposures. Although it may still be a challenge to navigate from a regulatory perspective, exposures to substances shouldn't be looked at in isolation anymore in order to assess consumer safety. When going beyond the science of assessment, some challenges facing the food industry right now are so complex that they cannot be solved by humans alone. Determining correlations between multiple interrelated parameters and how they influence each other and the outcome can be challenging, and this, unfortunately, is how most things occur in the real world. Trying to model and solve these scenarios with basic calculations and expert intuition can only get you so far. This is where the strength of machine learning and artificial intelligence (AI) comes to the fore. By building models and using AI, we can get closer to modeling the real world. The food industry is going through a revolution. From software models which aim to prevent contamination outbreaks that lead to product recalls and sometimes cost lives, to faster new product development to meet the ever-changing needs of consumers, to retailers using data for demand forecasting and customer engagement – AI and big data are essential tools for staying competitive in the food industry.

References

1. Kettler S, Kennedy M, McNamara C, et al. Assessing and reporting uncertainties in dietary exposure analysis: mapping of uncertainties in a tiered approach. *Food Chem Toxicol*. 2015;82:79–95. Available from: https://doi.org/10.1016/j.fct.2015.04.007.
2. EFSA Scientific Committee, Benford D, Halldorsson T, et al. The principles and methods behind EFSA's guidance on uncertainty analysis in scientific assessment. *EFSA J*. 2018;16(1):e05122. Available from: https://doi.org/10.2903/j.efsa.2018.5122.
3. Kennedy MC, Hart ADM, Kruisselbrink JW, et al. A retain and refine approach to cumulative risk assessment. *Food Chem Toxicol*. 2020;138:111223. Available from: https://doi.org/10.1016/j.fct.2020.111223.
4. The CARES NG development org: <https://caresng.org/>; Accessed July 2021.
5. Nusser SM, Carriquiry AL, Dodd KW, Fuller WA. A semiparametric transformation approach to estimating usual daily intake distributions. *J Am Stat Assoc*. 1996;91(436):1440–1449. Available from: https://doi.org/10.1080/01621459.1996.10476712.
6. Tooze JA, Midthune D, Dodd KW, et al. A new statistical method for estimating the usual intake of episodically consumed foods with application to their distribution. *J Am Diet Assoc*. 2006;106(10):1575–1587. Available from: https://doi.org/10.1016/j.jada.2006.07.003.
7. McNamara C, Naddy B, Rohan D, Sexton J. Design, development and validation of software for modelling dietary exposure to food chemicals and nutrients. *Food Addit Contam*. 2003;20(sup001):S8–S26. Available from: https://doi.org/10.1080/0265203031000152460.
8. The Creme Food Safety Model. <https://www.cremeglobal.com/creme-food-safety/>; Accessed July 2021.
9. EFSA Scientific Committee, Hardy A, Benford D, et al. Update: guidance on the use of the benchmark dose approach in risk assessment. *EFSA J*. 2017;15(1):e04658. Available from: https://doi.org/10.2903/j.efsa.2017.4658.
10. EFSA Panel on Additives and Products or Substances used in Animal Feed (FEEDAP), Rychen G, Aquilina G, et al. Guidance on the assessment of the safety of feed additives for the consumer. *EFSA J*. 2017;15(10):e05022. Available from: https://doi.org/10.2903/j.efsa.2017.5022.
11. Codex Alimentarius International Food Standards. Codex general standard for food additives (GSFA). General standard for food additives codex stan 192-1995. <http://www.fao.org/fao-who-codexalimentarius/codex-texts/dbs/gsfa/en/>; Accessed July 2021 European Commission. Food Additives Database. 2017 <https://webgate.ec.europa.eu/foods_system/main/?event = categories.search>; Accessed July 2021.
12. U.S. EPA. What we eat in America – food commodity intake database 2005–10. <https://fcid.foodrisk.org/>; Accessed July 2021.
13. EFSA (European Food Safety Authority), Dujardin B, Kirwan L. Technical report on the raw primary commodity (RPC) model: strengthening EFSA's capacity to assess dietary exposure at different levels of the food chain, from raw primary commodities to foods as consumed. *EFSA Support Public*. 2019;16(1). Available from: https://doi.org/10.2903/sp.efsa.2019.EN-1532. EN-1532. 30 pp.
14. MRC Human Nutrition Research. Food Standards Agency Standard Recipes Database, 1992–2012. UK Data Service. 2017; SN: 8159, <https://doi.org/10.5255/UKDA-SN-8159-1>.
15. Mintel Global New Products Database (GNPD). <http://portal.mintel.com/> Accessed July 2021.
16. Open Food Facts <https://world.openfoodfacts.org/> Accessed July 2021.
17. Flynn B, Pemberton M, Doyle J, McNamara C, Pigat S. Refined exposure assessment of migrated styrene from repeat-use ABS kitchen articles. 2021; Manuscript submitted for publication.
18. French Agency on Food, E. and O. H. and S. (ANSES), Dubuisson C, Carrillo S, et al. The French dietary survey on the general population (INCA3). *EFSA Support Publ*. 2017;14(12):1351E. Available from: https://doi.org/10.2903/sp.efsa.2017.EN-1351.
19. Euromonitor International. ABS/SAN in Kitchenware Equipment. Custom Methodology. 2016 (Unpublished report).
20. O'Sullivan AJ, Pigat S, O'Mahony C, Gibney MJ, McKevitt AI. Predictive modelling of the exposure to steviol glycosides in Irish patients aged 1-3 years with phenylketonuria and cow's milk protein allergy. *Food Addit Contam Part A Chem Anal Control Expo Risk Assess*. 2018;35(1):40–48. Available from: https://doi.org/10.1080/19440049.2017.1401737.
21. Tozer S, O'Mahony C, Hannah J, et al. Aggregate exposure modelling of vitamin A from cosmetic products, diet and food supplements. *Food Chem Toxicol*. 2019;131:110549. Available from: https://doi.org/10.1016/j.fct.2019.05.057.
22. Creme Care & Cosmetics: Aggregate Exposure from Real Consumer Data. <http://www.cremeglobal.com/products/cosmetics/>; Accessed July 2021.
23. Silva AV, Ringblom J, Lindh C, Scott K, Jakobsson K, Öberg M. A probabilistic approach to evaluate the risk of decreased total triiodothyronine hormone levels following chronic exposure to PFOS and PFHxS via contaminated drinking water. *Environ health Perspect*. 2020;128(7):076001.

Chapter 44

The role of computational toxicology in the risk assessment of food products

Timothy E.H. Allen[1], Steve Gutsell[2] and Ans Punt[3]

[1]*MRC Toxicology Unit, University of Cambridge, Cambridge, United Kingdom,* [2]*Unilever Safety and Environmental Assurance Centre, Colworth Science Park, Sharnbrook, United Kingdom,* [3]*Wageningen Food Safety Research, Wageningen, The Netherlands*

Abstract

Computational toxicology is a growing field with the aim of answering a diverse set of toxicological questions using computational algorithms. This includes questions such as: Can we predict the toxicity of a new chemical based on existing data points? How can we interpret large amounts of biological data? How does a chemical distribute itself inside the body? In this chapter, we aim to introduce general ideas around modeling techniques and couple this to cutting-edge research examples. We discuss the strengths of in silico toxicology and why they are coming to the forefront amongst new approach methodologies. Finally, we consider what the future holds, the importance of high-quality data, and the hurdles that must be overcome to see further regulatory acceptance of in silico models.

Keywords: Computational toxicology; in silico modeling; QSAR; PBK; machine learning; AOP; big data

Chapter Points

1. Computational toxicology is the use of computational and mathematical methods to aid understanding in the field of toxicology.
2. Computational toxicology, along with in vitro toxicology, is gaining additional attention as the field of toxicology looks to move away from in vivo methods.
3. Computational toxicology often involves the constructions of models from existing data,and can include data gathering, model training, and methodology validation.
4. These models can be used both to gain understanding of underlying toxicological mechanisms and as rapid tools to assist with decision-making or prioritization.

44.1 What is computational toxicology?

Computational toxicology involves the use of computer algorithms and mathematical relationships to better understand and predict adverse events in human health and the environment based on the use of existing data.[1] The field integrates understanding from medicine, biology, biochemistry, chemistry, mathematics, statistics, and computer science, making it a multidisciplinary area in which to work and study. This involves not only the development of new algorithms, but also the generation of best modeling practice, the deployment of models in safety evaluation and risk assessment, the integration and management of data, and the regulatory acceptance of computational methods.

Computational toxicology is a field gaining increasing importance across the safety evaluations of new food ingredients, chemical products, agrochemicals, and pharmaceuticals. This is at least partly due to the drive away from animal experiments in safety science,[2] but also because of the advantages computational methods afford. Computational power has increased dramatically over recent years and continues to do so. We now can generate, store, and model experimental data on a scale historically unheard of. These factors have combined with new computational methodologies and algorithms to create an explosion in the research into and deployment of computational toxicology methods.

This chapter involves a discussion on computational algorithms in toxicological food safety evaluations, including examples from other domains like high production volume chemicals, pharmaceuticals, and consumer products that are relevant to food safety. Computational toxicology is a wide field, encompassing a large amount of work involving the use of computers to help solve problems in toxicology. In this chapter, we focus on predictive models and the understanding of biological pathways, as these are areas we have the most experience in. As such, this chapter should not be considered all-encompassing, and areas we will not discuss in detail, such as experimental data interpretation, dose–response modeling, or high-throughput robotic assays, can also be considered computational toxicology.

Present Knowledge in Food Safety. DOI: https://doi.org/10.1016/B978-0-12-819470-6.00007-X

44.2 The role of computers in safety science

Toxicological risk assessment has been undergoing a paradigm shift, moving away from in vivo data generated using animal experiments and toward procedures and frameworks that incorporate nonanimal new approach methodologies (NAMs). Traditional in vivo toxicity studies still form the basis of the majority of global regulations relating to assuring human and environmental safety, but in recent times there have been shifts in societal, scientific, and regulatory mindsets toward the development of new ways to assure safety. New mechanistic toxicology frameworks rely on an understanding of how toxicity is caused by a chemical, which is thought to provide a more scientifically sound methodology on which to base safety decisions when compared to animal experiments.

The National Research Council (NRC) of the United States opened the field for discussion in 2007, in an attempt to make toxicity testing quicker, less expensive, and more relevant to human exposures.[2] This report pointed to several advances in the fields of biology and biotechnology that make it possible to feed data into new risk assessment approaches. This included an increased understanding of the underlying biological processes involved in toxicology and the holistic nature of biology, through mechanistic toxicity studies, -omics technologies, and systems biology.[3–5]

In silico methods also have their part to play in this paradigm shift. As we have seen, computational models can help make sense of large volumes of data, provide predictions to target necessary in vitro experiments more rapidly and effectively calculate the exposure or dose an individual is exposed to. These combined changes aim to move toxicology away from a science based on observation to one based on understanding,[6] while also reducing the community's reliance on in vivo experiments which some people consider to be unethical. The coordination of the international scientific community, including collaborations between industrial, academic, and regulatory groups, is of great importance for the advancement of toxicity testing, and the accomplishment of these goals.[7]

An increase in throughput due to NAMs, and particularly computational toxicology methods, is especially attractive in the food sector. Food toxicology studies are designed to establish how much of a chemical or food additive is safe to eat given current information, but that information is often lacking.[8] As of a 2013 study by Neltner et al. fewer than 38% of Food and Drug Administration (FDA)-regulated additives in the United States have a published feeding study, with even fewer meeting the level required to estimate a safe level of exposure or fully understand their reproductive or developmental toxicity potential. Additional data and understanding are required to help overcome this shortfall, and the prioritization of in vitro and in silico methods to complement existing data can help ensure the protection of consumers going forward. This is acknowledged for a variety of computational methods that will be outlined in this chapter, including physiologically-based kinetic (PBK), and quantitative structure−activity relationship (QSAR) models, with supporting case studies to make use of NAMs.[9]

A number of key regulatory and legislative changes have assisted in the NAMs paradigm shift already. The use of animal experiments in the risk assessments of cosmetic products has been illegal in the European Union (EU) since 2013 following the cosmetics directive.[10] This ban includes the testing of finished cosmetic products and cosmetic ingredients on animals and a ban on the sale of products (developed after 2004) and ingredients (since 2009) in the EU which were tested on animals. A further European guideline, ICH M7,[11] allows for the use of computational methodologies in the assessment of the mutagenicity of pharmaceutical impurities, given that two complementary methods are used to provide a good weight of evidence. Another EU Directive, 2010/63/EU,[12] aims to further the protection of animals used for scientific purposes, introducing new regulations and requirements to carry out such tests. The advancement of these regulations shows a desire for new methods which do not rely on animals, including information that can be provided by computational methods.

This has been followed up more recently by the commitment of the US Environmental Protection Agency (EPA) to phase out all animal tests on mammals by 2035.[13] The announcement included significant research funding for US universities to further develop nonanimal alternatives to current tests. Many welcome the ambitious program, but others suggest alternative methods are not well enough developed to replace animal experiments. While some of these concerns are valid and the EPA must be careful moving forward to ensure enough rigorous coverage is met by new approaches, legislative lead has proved itself important in previous examples, such as in the EU. This drive from the top can continue pushing toxicology toward the goals set by the NRC in 2007.

The strength of NAMs and changes to regulatory attitudes toward in vitro and in silico toxicology have led to several industry-led initiatives to improve the safety evaluation/risk assessment procedure. One significant contribution was the work of Baltazar et al. in 2020.[14] This study involved the consideration of two hypothetical consumer products containing the chemical compound coumarin. Coumarin is a well-studied chemical with a good understanding of its toxicological effects, but for the purpose of these case studies, this information was ignored. Instead, internal concentrations of coumarin were calculated using a PBK model considering the route of dermal exposure suitable for the products in question, a skin cream and a body lotion.[15] A collection of in vitro screens measuring bioactivity were combined with structural alert-based computational tools to generate a point of departure (POD) value, which could then be compared to the exposure previously calculated. Margins of safety were calculated and found to be greater than 100, which combined with the in silico and in vitro data showing coumarin to be neither genotoxic, an immunomodulator nor systemically toxic through the 44 biological targets considered demonstrates a significant weight of evidence for these products being safe. Case studies such as these are vital in supporting both in silico and in vitro methods and proving their value to the toxicology community as a genuine alternative to more traditional animal experiments.

44.3 Constructing a model

The vast majority of the computational models outlined in the later sections of this chapter are constructed with a basic framework in mind. To introduce readers to these models without an understanding of the modeling process is a disservice to the reader, as a basic understanding of this procedure will allow you to better understand why specific choices are made or how the models are evaluated. This section provides an overview of how the modeling procedure can be approached, but ultimately these are guidelines for good modeling practice and are not always followed verbatim, or in this order.

Model construction begins with the identification of the questions the algorithm should help to answer. The choice of question is very important and will undoubtedly be influenced by factors discussed below, including the kinds of modeling approaches the modeler wants to apply, the data they have available, and the interest of the individual/research team. Data for the task will then be obtained relevant to the question identified, and it must be suitable for the task at hand. For example, data such as a collection of animal LD50 values for pharmaceutical chemicals are likely to be unsuitable to build a model for exploring the mechanistic effects of food ingredients on humans. Generally, modelers want to collect as much data as possible that cover a wide area of chemical space, incorporating different molecular structural features, descriptors, and functionalities, and is reported in a way that makes it reliable, although this is often practically impossible. For this reason, the curation of data is often performed to ensure it is of suitable modeling quality.

Models can then be constructed, and for this purpose the gathered data are often split into a training set, for model construction, and a test set, for model evaluation. Sometimes a third set, often called a validation set, is used to select model parameters to ensure they are not biased toward the test set used in evaluation. Generally, several modeling procedures should be applied, or at least several differently tuned versions of the same approach to ensure the procedure is producing an optimal algorithm for making predictions (Fig. 44.1). The best produced algorithm can then be further evaluated by comparing it to other computational procedures, preferably those trying to make predictions using a similar dataset, in a procedure known as benchmarking. Ultimately it is good for modelers to also produce evaluations on truly external data for evaluation—that is, data produced from a different source to the training, validation, and test sets. This provides more information on how the algorithm will perform in real life, as even the use of the test set can be overoptimistic of model performance.

Final considerations of models are important in their deployment. For example, in which cases are the predictions of this algorithm valid? How can the model be obtained and used by toxicologists? How easy is it to use and understand? The first of these questions is often best answered using an applicability domain, a procedure for identifying how close the input chemical is to the chemicals in the training set. If the input chemical is similar to those in the training set, then the model prediction is far more likely to be accurate and useful than if it is different. That said, defining "similar" is often a challenge in itself, and can mean having similar chemical groups, physicochemical descriptors, or biological profiles. Releasing the model into the public domain helps answer the second query, although long-term maintenance of any released

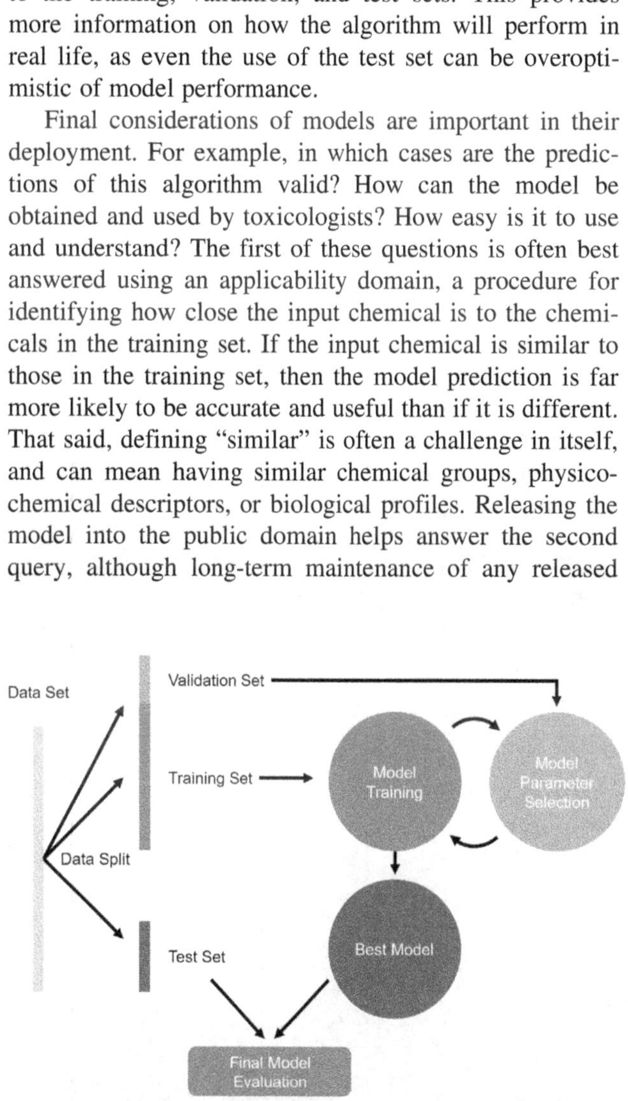

FIGURE 44.1 A general procedure for model construction. Collected data are split, sometimes into two parts, and sometimes three. Crucially, some data should always be kept away from the model training and parameter selection process for final evaluation and statistical performance reporting. *Adapted with permission from Wedlake AJ, Allen TEH, Goodman JM, et al. Confidence in inactive and active predictions from structural alerts.* Chem Res Toxicol. *2020;33(12):3010–3022. https://doi.org/10.1021/acs.chemrestox.0c00332. Copyright 2020 American Chemical Society.*

code is required to ensure it continues to work once development is finished. Finally, high-quality documentation is required to help with the third issue, including a thorough explanation of the modeling procedure, sharing of the training data, understanding of uncertainty and robustly calculated model performance statistics, and mechanistic understanding of the predictions, if appropriate.[16]

44.4 Computational techniques

QSARs are among the best known and well-established methods for linking chemical structure to activity in the chemical and biological sciences.[17] The "activity" that is referred to here can mean a variety of different things, from predicting biological activity which may be useful in assessing the toxic effects of chemicals to chemical properties which can be useful in determining exposures (these are sometimes referred to as quantitative structure−property relationships or QSPRs). At the heart of these relationships is a mathematical link between the representation of the chemical structure and the activity that needs to be predicted (Fig. 44.2A). Chemical structure itself is often represented mathematically through chemical descriptors or fingerprints, adding an additional level of complexity. QSARs have been used in both regression tasks (where the prediction required is a numerical value such as pKa or protein binding affinity) and classification tasks (where the prediction involves classifying the input molecule as active or inactive). One of the simplest and earliest examples of QSAR comes from the field of environmental toxicology, where acute fish toxicity was found to be well predicted by a linear relationship to the octanol−water partition coefficient, logP.[18]

Expert systems are another class of computational algorithms considered to have a high level of interpretability and reliability. Lhasa's Derek Nexus is a collection of such algorithms.[19] The SARs within Derek are coded by expert chemists based on their understanding of the biological interactions those types of molecules can make. These SARs often consist of structural alerts, features of a chemical considered to be important to its toxicological effects (Fig. 44.2B). This makes the model development phase very complex, involving a large amount of manual effort, but has the advantage of being able to provide additional information on why a certain prediction was made. Lhasa's expert chemists have put significant effort into explaining the justification for each structural alert that is linked to a toxicological outcome. By doing this when a prediction is used in safety evaluation the user has confidence in the algorithm and can understand why a prediction was made.

Machine learning algorithms have gained a lot of attention in several fields, including toxicology.[20−23] They encompass a wide variety of different techniques for allowing machines to learn from existing data without input from a human programmer. This can be considered the complete opposite from an expert system, where a human expert entirely codes the reasoning, with the machine just being pointed at large amounts of data and allowed to learn. As a result, machine learning algorithms are sometimes seen as analogous, or even directly related,

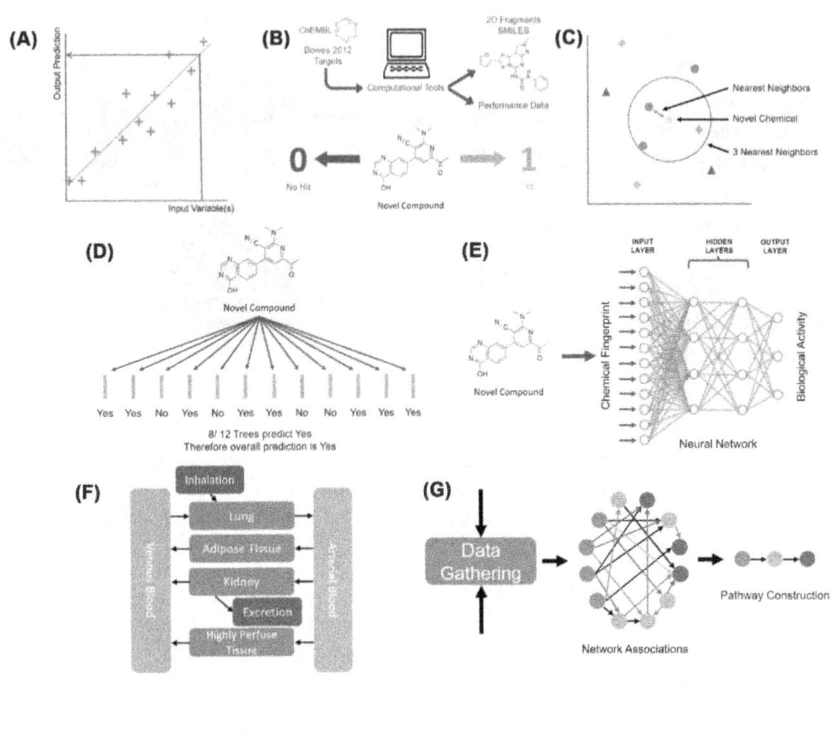

FIGURE 44.2 Graphical representations of some of the techniques outlined above, including (A) linear regression, (B) structural alert, (C) nearest neighbor, (D) random forest, (E) neural network, (F) physiologically based kinetic modeling, and (G) biological pathway construction.

to QSARs. Machine learning algorithms often involve a large number of input variables that allow the machines to learn by themselves and may be used in QSAR development. However, some QSARs are built using specific inputs chosen as important and related to the predicted output by the human model-building expert, which is not machine learning. The ability of these algorithms to learn from data and make use of high numbers of variables makes them extremely powerful predictors across a wide variety of tasks, including speech recognition and image classification. The weaknesses of these methods are that they generally require a large amount of input data, and are challenging to interpret.[17] A significant amount of work is ongoing to try to better understand the predictions of these powerful machines.[24–26]

Some examples of machine learning tools include nearest neighbor algorithms, random forests, and neural networks. Nearest neighbor algorithms use input variables to place existing data points on a surface or multitude of surfaces for comparison to new examples to identify which cases are closest (Fig. 44.2C). During training, principle component analysis is often used to identify suitable surfaces to differentiate training set examples, for example into different classes useful in the prediction process. The closest example or examples are then used to judge the new case against and make an evaluation. Random forests make use of an ensemble of different mathematical relationships, or trees, where the model input is varied at random between each one during the training procedure (Fig. 44.2D). This allows for the calculation of a large number of models which can then be combined into the final model decision. In a classification decision, each tree would vote on which class a novel input belonged in and a consensus used to provide an output for the overall model. Neural networks are computational networks based on the working of the human brain (Fig. 44.2E). Input features are linked to predicted outputs using a network of mathematical relationships which are adjusted during training to ensure the best fit during model training. Neural networks with multiple internal hidden layers are known as deep neural networks or deep learning. By using many layers of mathematical relationships and activation functions these models can learn nonlinearity in data and break down complex tasks. This allows them to be among the most powerful algorithms in use today.

Mechanistic models describe the stepwise behavior and effects of chemicals in a body as they would occur. The most well-known type of mechanistic models that are used within the field of toxicology are PBK models that simulate the absorption, distribution, metabolism, and elimination (ADME) of a chemical in a body and mimic each of these processes with differential equations (Fig. 44.2F). Likewise, toxicological pathways and biological response mechanisms can be obtained using computational tools such as data mining and statistical association (Fig. 44.2G). Extracting and organizing the enormity of scientific data contained within the public knowledge is a task computers are well suited to. Computationally produced networks of biological pathways can then be used as a starting point for human experts to accelerate our understanding of toxicological mechanisms.

44.5 Qualitative and quantitative modeling

"The dose makes the poison," or so the old adage says. This phrase is attributed to Paracelsus who is considered the father of the field of toxicology. The principle refers to the idea that all things—even essentials for life such as water or oxygen—can be toxic if exposure to them is too high. It is, therefore, crucial to also understand the dose levels at which these hazards are induced and to obtain concentration or dose–response curves to set a POD for risk assessment (Fig. 44.3). Classically the dose that does not lead to an observable effect in animal studies no observed adverse effect level (NOAEL) is used as a POD for setting a health-based guidance value like an acceptable daily intake or tolerable daily intake. Alternatively, a benchmark dose (BMD) causing 10% effect in animals or the lower confidence of this BMD (BMDL) as a POD by fitting the dose–response curves can be used. In vitro potencies of chemicals are generally expressed as the 50% active or effective concentration (AC50 or EC50), 10% or 50% benchmark concentrations (BMC10 or BMC50), or in case of an inhibitory effect the inhibitory constant (Ki). There are increasing efforts to develop quantitative computational models to make such potency predictions based on the molecular structure and/or physicochemical properties. Some of these numerical values lend themselves well to quantitative modeling, such as AC50, Ki, or BMD—while NOAELs are perhaps less useful as depending on the experiment you might be just under the adverse effect level, or quite far removed from it. Quantitative models in the field of kinetics like PBK modeling aim at predicting internal plasma and/or tissue concentrations that are related to the effective concentrations of a chemical. Such predictions are, for example, relevant to extrapolate in vitro effect concentrations to equivalent oral doses in humans or to provide better means to extrapolate high-dose animal experimental results to low-dose (individual) human exposure scenarios.

While quantitative modeling might be considered the ultimate objective for computational model use in a safety decision-making process, a wide variety of computational algorithms have been developed to classify

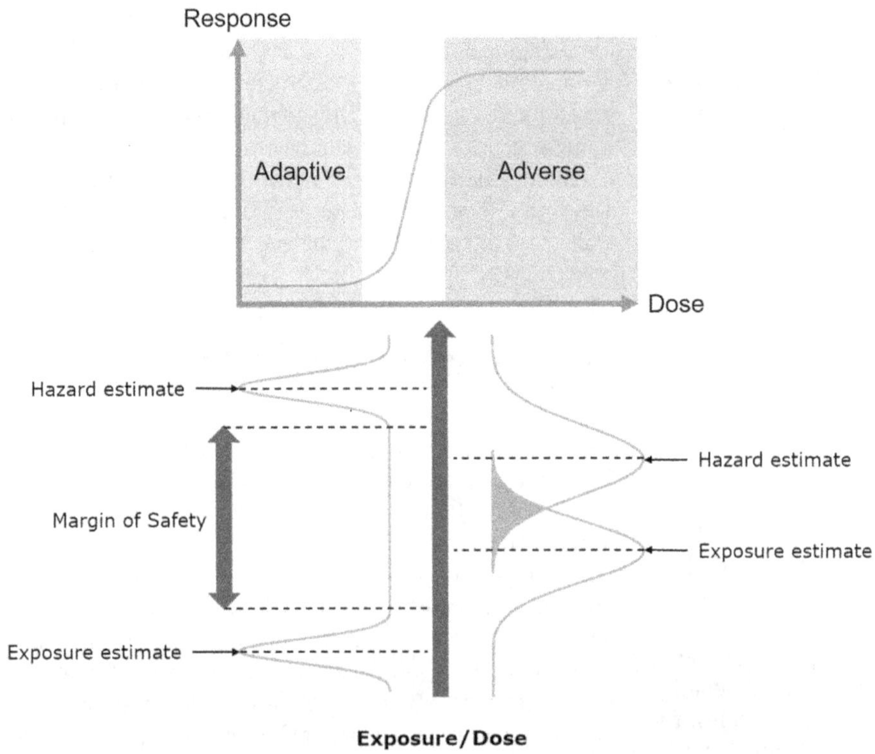

FIGURE 44.3 A cartoon of a dose–response curve showing how the biological response moves from adaptive at low exposure to adverse at high exposure and two examples of risk assessment scenarios. On the left, a large margin of safety is established between two distinct distributions, one for the exposure and one for the hazard. On the right overlap between such distributions suggests a potential for an adverse outcome.

chemicals depending on their predicted chemical activity. This qualitative or classification task is often less computationally complex and more approachable for the datasets available when compared to quantitative modeling. These algorithms often classify molecules as "active" or "inactive" but can also classify as "high activity," "moderate activity," or "low activity," based on a threshold corresponding to how active a molecule is. These algorithms see use in safety science during screening, when a large number of potential chemicals need to be narrowed down for further investigation, or risk prioritization, to identify the most likely hazard for additional testing, as the speed and high throughput of such algorithms are particularly important in these scenarios.

44.6 Exposure modeling

When making a safety decision a key consideration is how much of a chemical an individual, organ or cell is exposed to. A quantitative modeling computational tool that has gained much attention over the last decade to assist in answering this question is PBK modeling (Fig. 44.4).[27,28] In a PBK model the body is represented as a connected collection of compartments linked by blood flow. The models use differential mathematical relationships to describe the ADME processes that transport the chemical between the compartments. PBK models contribute to better extrapolations of animal experimental study results to humans. Traditionally such extrapolations rely upon default extrapolation factors (e.g., a multiplication factor of 10 for extrapolation between an animal and a human) to derive numerical values for health evaluation in humans from animals. PBK methods provide a more scientific approach to this. By simulating the plasma concentration of a chemical of interest in both the animal species of interest and humans, a so-called human equivalent dose can be obtained that can be used as a replacement of the default uncertainty factor for interspecies differences in kinetics. This approach has for example been applied in recent risk evaluations of bisphenol A, dioxins, and Perfluoroalkyl and Polyfluoroalkyl Substances (PFAS) by European Food Safety Authority (EFSA).[29–31] PBK modeling also has a key role to play in the replacement of animal experiments as it allows you to convert in vitro data into human dose–response or potency information. Louisse et al. showed with a range of examples that combining in vitro toxicity data with PBK modeling can lead to relevant predictions of potencies of chemicals in vivo that can be used as an alternative to animal testing.[28]

A selection of examples of such quantitative in vitro in vivo extrapolations (QIVIVE) in the field of food toxicology includes (1) the predictions of human-relevant estrogenic potencies of bisphenol A and different bisphenol A replacers,[32] (2) the prediction of liver toxicity by pyrrolizidine alkaloids,[33] and (3) predictions of DNA adduct formation by the plant toxin aristolochic acid[34]

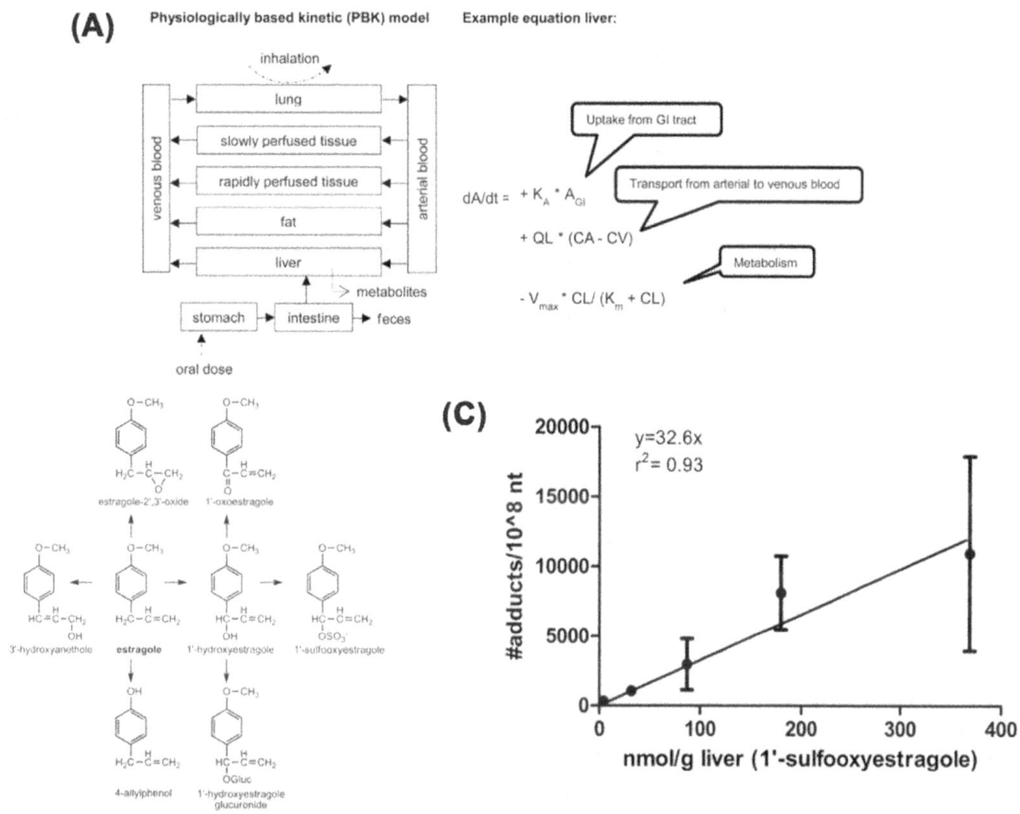

FIGURE 44.4 Graphics representing some key ideas outlined in this section. (A) PBK models are constructed by combining mathematical relationships. Metabolites must be considered when building such models (B), which can then be compared to (C) experimental results. *(A) Reprinted with permission from Louisse J, Beekmann K, Rietjens IMCM. Use of physiologically based kinetic modeling-based reverse dosimetry to predict in vivo toxicity from in vitro data.* Chem Res Toxicol. *2017;30:114–125. https://doi.org/10.1021/acs.chemrestox.6b00302. Copyright 2017 American Chemical Society. (B and C) Reprinted with permission from Punt A, Paini A, Spenkelink A, et al. Evaluation of interindividual human variation in bioactivation and DNA adduct formation of estragole in liver predicted by physiologically based kinetic/dynamic and Monte Carlo modeling.* Chem Res Toxicol. *2016;29:659–668. https://doi.org/10.1021/acs.chemrestox.5b00493. Copyright 2016 American Chemical Society.*

and natural flavorings like estragole[35] and α,β-unsaturated aldehydes.[36] PBK-based QIVIVE can also be used to predict human-relevant potencies for beneficial health effects. PBK-based QIVIVE has for example been applied to predict the potential of the flavonoid hesperidin[37] to affect protein kinase activity, endothelial cell migration, and pro-inflammatory molecules at relevant dietary intake levels.

As with all modeling procedures the effectiveness of a PBK model is heavily dependent on the quality of input data used to derive its internal parameters.[38,39] Whereas PBK models were originally developed by fitting input parameters to in vivo kinetic data, these input data are increasingly derived from in vitro experiments or with in silico tools. Metabolic clearance can for example be effectively measured by measuring the in vitro conversion by primary liver hepatocytes, S9 or microsomes (the latter by addition of relevant co-factors). Caco-2 permeability measurements can be used to estimate the uptake rate of a chemical. Distribution parameters, including the fraction unbound in plasma, plasma:tissue partition coefficients, and the blood:plasma ratio, can either be measured in vitro or calculated in silico. Excretion of a compound by the kidneys is generally simulated to depend on the glomerular filtration rate and fraction unbound in plasma. Transporter-dependent processes can also be included in a PBK model, though these are usually included in a later stage when initial model estimates based on the above parameters do not lead to satisfactory results when compared to in vivo findings.[40,41] Many modeling platforms are available to assist in the construction of PBK models, including the open-source High-Throughput Toxicokinetics (httk)-r package[42,43] IndusChemFate, a package developed by Cefic LRI,[44] QIVIVEtools a webtool developed by Wageningen Food Safety Research,[45] and PK-SIM.[46] Commercial software that are available include Certara's Simcyp PBPK Simulator and Gastroplus.

Another consideration regarding exposure relates to the potential biotransformations of chemicals in organisms. One problem in this area is the prediction of metabolites of a parent chemical; the parent chemical may not cause any adverse effects but can be metabolized into one that can. Example tools for this include FAME 3[47,48] and SMARTCyp[49] which provide predictions of the sites of metabolism and type of metabolites that are formed based on nearest neighbor algorithms. Lhasa's Meteor[50,51] produces metabolism predictions using a rule-based expert system programmed by expert scientists with knowledge of such transformations. Other examples of qualitative prediction models for kinetics are models that predict if a chemical is likely to be a substrate to a specific transporter or P450 enzyme. Examples of publicly available tools are ADMETlab,[52,53] SwissADME,[54,55] and Vienna LiverTox Workspace.[56] These tools were developed by model training against large datasets using machine learning techniques like random forests and support vector machines.

44.7 Predicting apical traditional toxicity endpoints

Many predictive toxicology algorithms are developed with the aim of predicting a specific toxicological effect that has historically been used in safety assessment. These traditional toxicity endpoints are mostly measured in vivo, and some in vitro. Some examples include modeling the in vitro Ames assay, which itself models mutagenicity, or modeling based on in vivo data corresponding to carcinogenicity, reproductive toxicity, or acute oral toxicity.

One of the most significant efforts in the deployment of computational toxicology is Lhasa's Derek Nexus.[19] Derek is an expert system coded by human experts to make toxicity predictions based on mechanistic and experimental knowledge (Fig. 44.5A). Lhasa makes use of partnerships with a number of sponsor companies to gather a large dataset of chemicals. Using this data, structural alerts and rules are coded for several toxicity endpoints in Derek, including carcinogenicity, mutagenicity, genotoxicity, skin and respiratory sensitization, teratogenicity, irritation, and reproductive toxicity. By containing rules devised and curated by expert scientists Derek can provide additional information when a prediction is made on the anticipated mechanism of toxicity and background information on why specific rules have been written. While this procedure is time-consuming it does make these predictions very useful in a safety evaluation. Recent work at Lhasa has led to the development of negative confidence intervals when predictions of inactivity are made. These predictions can be some of the most challenging to use when an algorithm is constructed around active structural alerts, as the absence of these features is often not enough to classify a molecule as inactive. In the realms of bacterial mutagenicity and skin sensitization, Derek is now able to give confidence in these decisions by considering how similar chemicals that are predicted negative are to training set negatives.[57]

Derek, along with several other methodologies, has been evaluated for their capacity to predict the bacterial mutagenicity of food contact ingredients.[58] Toxtree[59] contains structural alerts for the prediction of the in vitro Ames test and is therefore a good comparison for Derek. VEGA Consensus[60] is a weighted QSAR combining the predictions of three individual mathematical models for the prediction of the Ames test and is compared to another Lhasa tool, Sarah Nexus.[61] Sarah is a statistical-based QSAR, and together these tools allow for the comparison of structural alert decision trees (Derek and Toxtree) to statistical mathematical models (VEGA and Sarah). In this study, the statistical models were found to

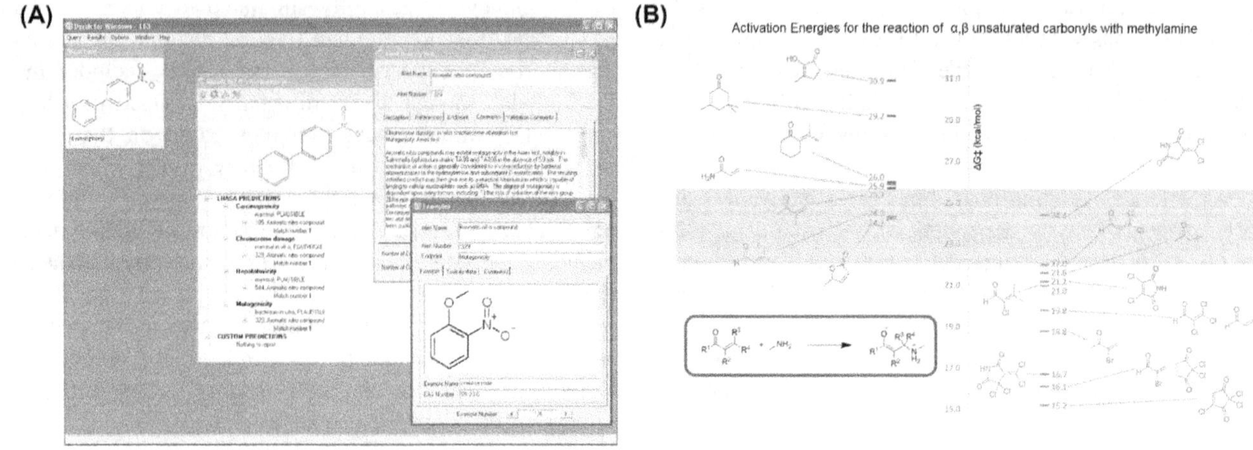

FIGURE 44.5 Graphics representing some key ideas outlined in this section. Lhasa's Derek provides expert comments to back up its toxicity predictions (A). (B) Chemical reaction mechanisms and activation energies can be linked to some toxicities such as mutagenicity. *(A) Reprinted with permission from Marchant CA, Briggs KA, Long A. In silico tools for sharing data and knowledge on toxicity and metabolism: Derek for Windows, Meteor, and Vitic.* Toxicol Mech Methods. *2008;18(2–3):177–187. (B) Reprinted from Allen TEH, Grayson MN, Goodman JM, Gutsell S, Russell PJ. Using transition state modeling to predict mutagenicity for Michael acceptors.* J Chem Inf Model. *2018;58:1266–1271. https://doi.org/10.1021/acs.jcim.8b00130.*

perform best, with Sarah having the highest accuracy of 96%. This is a very high level of performance, and it partially explained due to the fact that some compounds in the evaluation dataset are also present in the training data. When considering only the new compounds this figure drops to 87%, and the models particularly struggle to predict new experimental positives. The authors combine the Sarah and VEGA Consensus predictions, identifying a positive prediction by either model as an active prediction, which results in increased statistical performance. They also note that the use of applicability domains in Sarah and VEGA is important in raising the performance of these models, as well as understanding where their predictions are appropriate, and where they are not.

Other methodologies have also been applied to make qualitative predictions of bacterial mutagenicity. As mutagenicity can be caused by direct molecular DNA modification, computational modeling of these reactions can be considered a sensible strategy. Density functional theory quantum chemistry calculations provide insight into these reactions, as illustrated by Allen et al. in 2018[62] and Townsend et al. in 2019.[63] These works use the hypothesis that unreactive chemicals with high activation energy barriers cannot modify DNA and hence will not be found to be mutagenic in the Ames mutagenicity assay (Fig. 44.5B). Across these two studies, this association is confirmed and energy barriers that prevent direct DNA modification are established. This mechanistic understanding that can be gained through the in vitro Ames assay and computational models of it allows these models to fit between the traditional in vivo toxicity tests covered in this section and the mechanistic models in the next section.

Another popular QSAR endpoint, rat carcinogenicity, was evaluated by Valerio Jr. et al. considering chemicals found in the human diet in 2007.[64] The MDL QSAR modeling software[65] was used for model construction and a custom QSAR was trained on a total of 1201 chemicals spanning pharmaceuticals, industrial chemicals, and some dietary chemicals. Calculated chemical descriptors were used as an input to classify the chemicals as either high or low risk, based on experimental evidence. One hundred and one external dietary chemicals were then used to evaluate the model, showing 80% accuracy. This can be considered good performance, as the training data contained far more pharmaceutical and industrial chemicals than food chemicals and shows that even QSARs trained on those kinds of data points can be useful in food safety evaluation.

The collaborative acute toxicity modeling suite (CATMoS) tool is a free online resource for screening organic chemicals for acute oral toxicity.[66] The models provide both qualitative and quantitative predictions using a consensus QSAR approach modeling a combined publicly available database.[67] The predicted endpoints include LD50 values, which are less useful from a mechanistic perspective but sometimes required for regulatory purposes. The Interagency Coordinating Committee for the Validation of Alternative Methods organized the global effort to develop these predictive tools and continues to push for regulatory acceptance of these models as a replacement for animal experiments.[68] Further model evaluation is ongoing, aiming to establish the applicability domain of such tools, along with outreach and training programs to champion the use of computational methods.

The OECD QSAR Toolbox[69] is an open-source toxicological database and model repository, containing a selection of QSARs for the prediction of physicochemical properties, environmental exposure, and human and environmental hazards. The Toolbox also includes the capacity for making metabolic and mechanistic predictions. The Toolbox is designed to provide transparent and comprehensible toxicity predictions, and provide information on structural analogs for read-across, the practice of using existing data to fill gaps on a new similar chemical.[70] This data gap filling potential is of use across toxicology, by governments, the chemical industry and stakeholders, and by encouraging the use of QSARs and other computational procedures the Toolbox aims to promote the regulatory acceptance of such tools.[71]

Additional recent work into the computational prediction of specific responses includes modeling mitochondrial toxicity,[72,73] repeat dose toxicity,[74–76] and liver toxicity[77–79] using a variety of in silico techniques.

44.8 Mechanistic toxicity modeling

As toxicology has moved away from observation-based in vivo experiments and toward mechanistic understanding, computational methods have also made this shift. In vitro assays, omics technologies and mechanistic understanding, through modeling and data interpretation, mean computational toxicology has shifted to be inextricably linked with other areas of toxicology. A result of this is the development of models using data measuring the specific binding of a chemical with a biological target such as an enzyme or receptor. These models closely link the chemistry of a molecule to its interaction, relying on the hypothesis that binders at a specific target have some kind of common chemical features that a model can extract. Structural alerts have been used to try and identify these features and machine learning algorithms can pick out these features from large datasets.

Combining several computational approaches can often provide additional model performance and insight into a chemical's toxicity. Wedlake et al. presented such an approach combining a Bayesian structural alert model with a machine learning random forest model to increase confidence in predictions.[80] This methodology relies on the idea that structural alerts are easier to interpret and make predictions based on chemical structure (Fig. 44.6A) while being well coupled to random forest models, which are more complex and in this case were constructed using physicochemical properties. A total of 90 biological targets were assessed using this methodology and statistical performance was found to increase when a consensus was reached compared to using either model individually. These predictions can also be supported by an understanding of chemical structure from the structural alert and which physicochemical properties are important from the random forest.

Structural alerts are primarily considered as a methodology for qualitative prediction tasks or classification, as the presence of a molecular substructure indicates activity while the absence indicates inactivity. Allen et al. were able to link structural alerts to quantitative predictions for molecules fitting into categories defined by structural alerts.[81] By considering the mean and range of the inhibitory constant (Ki) of the training set chemicals containing a particular structural alert a quantitative range of the Ki could be obtained. This has been done across a variety of biological targets, including G-protein coupled receptors, nuclear receptor, enzymes, ion channels, and transporters. Where these categories contain chemicals with similar activity levels this may be able to guide an activity estimate, while more spread values may require further follow-up calculations or experiments. By making use of the highly predictive structural alert procedure this method allows for rapid chemical assessment and activity estimation based on a robust and transparent algorithm.

This chemical categorization can be followed up by more detailed calculations to give finer estimates of molecular activity.[82] Allen et al. used comparative molecular field analysis, a 3D QSAR methodology

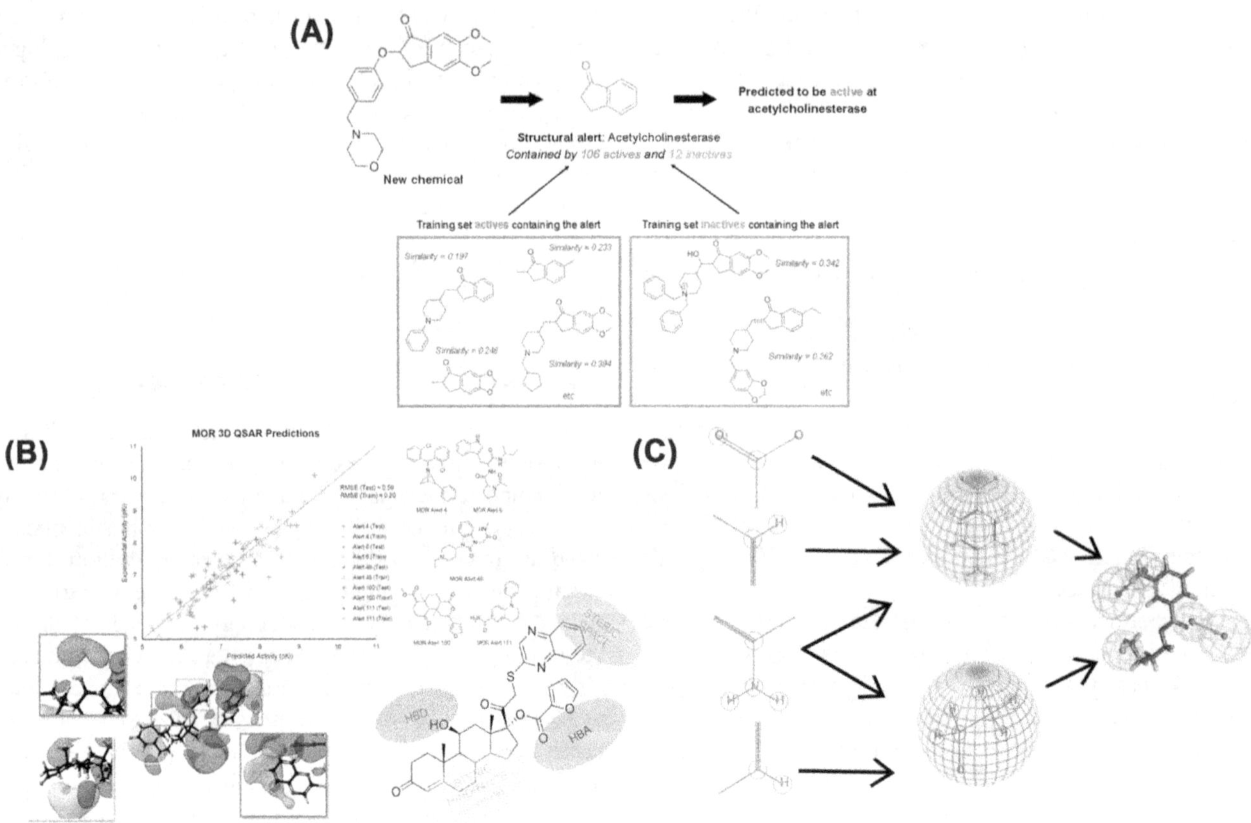

FIGURE 44.6 Graphics representing some key ideas outlined in Section 44.8. (A) Structural alerts are considered interpretable as their chemistries can be linked to existing molecules in the training data easily. (B) Using structural alerts for molecular categorization can be followed by more complex 3D QSAR calculations. (C) Deep learning breaks down chemical fingerprints to make predictions, which can be recombined to learn about the molecular features responsible. *(A) Reprinted with permission from Wedlake AJ, Folia M, Piechota S, et al. Structural alerts and Random forest models in a consensus approach for receptor binding molecular initiating events.* Chem Res Toxicol. *2020. https://doi.org/10.1021/acs.chemrestox.9b00325. Copyright 2019 American Chemical Society. (B) Adapted with permission from Allen TEH, Goodman JM, Gutsell S, Russell PJ. Quantitative predictions for molecular initiating events using three-dimensional quantitative structure-activity relationships.* Chem Res Toxicol. *2019;33(2):324–332. https://doi.org/10.1021/acs.chemrestox.9b00136. Copyright 2019 American Chemical Society. (C) Reprinted with permission from Unterthiner T, Mayr A, Klambauer G, Hochreiter S. Toxicity prediction using deep learning. 2015. http://arxiv.org/abs/1503.01445.*

(Fig. 44.6B), to overlap the steric and electronic fields generated from molecular structures to calculate biological activity across a variety of human biological targets (i.e., glucocorticoid receptor, mu opioid receptor, cyclooxygenase-2 enzyme, human ether-à-go-go related gene channel, and dopamine transporter). This methodology is considerably more complex than using 2D structural alerts but allows the model to gain a greater understanding of the 3D shape of molecules and provides insights into which parts of the chemical structure are involved in interactions with the biological target and why. A small-scale study was conducted and concluded that using the 2D alerts to group molecules for the 3D QSAR increased efficiency and provided molecular activity estimates within one log unit.

Deep neural networks or deep learning are a sophisticated class of machine learning algorithm which have recently been used effectively in computational toxicology classification tasks. The Tox21 Data Challenge was won by DeepTox, a deep neural network approach (Fig. 44.6C).[23] The challenge presented training data for 12 toxic effects, including nuclear receptor and stress response pathways, and evaluated models based on hidden test data. DeepTox scored the highest performance overall and in six of the individual tasks, outperforming more traditional computational approaches and other machine learning algorithms including naive Bayes, support vector machines, and random forests. Following this success, deep learning has been applied to other classification tasks, including the prediction of specific toxicity responses including drug-induced liver injury,[83] drug-target prediction,[84] and cardiotoxicity.[85]

Deep learning algorithms have been shown to perform excellently in prediction tasks but their inner workings and decision-making are extremely challenging, if not impossible, to interpret, a key requirement when it comes to toxicological decision-making.[17] More transparent algorithms such as structural alerts, particularly when coupled with expert knowledge provided by expert systems like Derek, hold a significant advantage here. Computational toxicologists must try to ensure other scientists and industry regulators can interpret the evidence used for a safety decision. To assist in this some groups have been investigating methods for interpreting neural networks, including the neural network activation similarity measure,[25] a measure for identifying similar chemicals through a trained neural network. This methodology relies on the idea that the neural network, a computational brain, "thinks" about similar molecules in similar ways, resulting in its decision-making pathways being activated in a similar way. Methodologies such as this can be used to identify candidates for read-across, allowing the algorithm to support its prediction hypothesis with evidence from existing data in an interpretable manner.

Additional recent work into the prediction of molecular interactions is performed using a variety of computational methods, including chemical structure,[86,87] molecular modeling,[88–90] and machine learning.[91,92]

44.9 Toxicity pathway construction

We have seen that computational models can provide information on how a food ingredient chemical can interact with molecular biological targets. To provide greater mechanistic understanding, we need to define the pathways that can lead to toxic effects. Adverse outcome pathways (AOPs) are of particular interest in this area.[93] AOPs are conceptual constructs linking a molecular initiating event, the chemical interaction which starts the pathway, to high-level adverse outcomes at an organ or organism level. Since their initial description in 2010 AOPs have been well adopted by the toxicology community, and the AOP Wiki,[94] an open-source platform for AOP development and dissemination contains a wide variety of developed pathways. AOPs require significant effort to develop but provide mechanistic understanding of how adverse effects occur, giving them and the in silico methodologies that feed into them an advantage when being implemented. The large level of effort required has often left gaps in AOP knowledge, particularly in areas such as food additives,[95] but the potential advantage of moving toward AOP-based toxicology evaluation cannot be understated.[96] Luckily, computational and data science approaches can provide help in this area.

AOP construction requires significant effort, gathering and curating data, analyzing effects, and linking pieces of information. Within the public domain, a large amount of knowledge remains undiscovered because of how labor and time-intensive this process is. Computational algorithms can help sift through this information, helping to set up computationally predicted AOPs to be evaluated and built upon by expert scientists (Fig. 44.7).[97,98] To investigate this, frequent itemset mining, a rule-based machine learning procedure for discovering links between databases, was used to find associations between ToxCast assay target genes and disease data from the comparative toxicogenomics database by identifying chemicals common to both datasets. This procedure provided a large network for investigation, which was conducted with two specific case studies in mind—considering fatty liver disease and the aryl hydrocarbon receptor. An interesting subnetwork link was established between the aryl hydrocarbon receptor and glaucoma, and while literature evidence exists linking these the link had not been captured in either database alone. Additional groups have built upon this framework, using data mining and mutual information statistics to link adverse outcomes reported in the FDA Adverse Event Reporting System to assay outcomes in ToxCast, with the aim of furthering understanding of cardiotoxicity.[99] The availability of data limited the

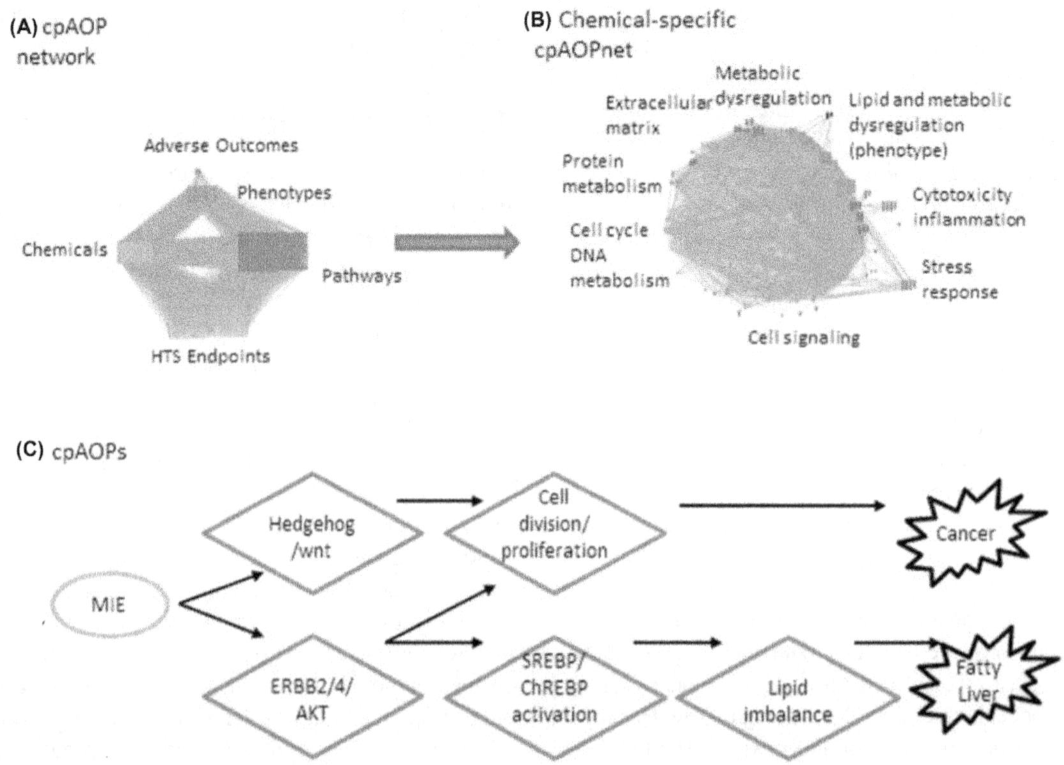

FIGURE 44.7 A computationally produced adverse outcome pathway (AOP) network (A) from which an AOP network was extracted for the chemical carbon tetrachloride (B). (C) Information in this network was then used to manually construct AOPs leading to cancer and fatty liver. *Reproduced from Bell SM, Angrish MM, Wood CE, Edwards SW. Integrating publicly available data to generate computationally predicted adverse outcome pathways for fatty liver.* Toxicol Sci. *2016;150(2):510–520. https://doi.org/10.1093/toxsci/kfw017.*

number of associations that could be found but a number were identified that echoed previous findings in the literature. These works provide a good basis for the continuation of computational AOP development alongside those efforts directed by expert scientists, to speed up the procedure and identify new informative links.

As has been mentioned already, an important requirement in risk assessment is a quantitative understanding of molecular activity, hazard, and exposure. As a result of this qualitative AOPs have only so much use. Quantitative AOPs (qAOPs) are required to provide this understanding and are starting to see development. These are particularly important for computational models as they allow predictions of molecular activity at a molecular or cellular level to be extrapolated to an organ or individual level more appropriate for the calculation of a POD. Linking quantitative in silico predictions to qAOPs combines the advantage of additional mechanistic understanding and quantitative adverse outcome predictions. Unlike directly modeling data which provide information on organ effects or survivability (e.g., predictions of lethal dose 50 values) mechanistic models linked to qAOPs do not skip over areas of important biological complexity. qAOPs are discussed in more detail in a 2020 review by Spinu et al.[100]

44.10 Integration of data and data sources

Many of the approaches we have outlined in this chapter require significant investment in data collection, either from existing sources in public databases or industry collections or through large-scale data collection. Computational approaches of almost any kind require training and validation data, and the quality of this data can have a significant effect on the models and algorithms generated. A common phrase in computational modeling encapsulates this idea perfectly—"garbage in, garbage out"—the idea that no modeling procedure can overcome the issues caused by bad data, no matter how sophisticated.

Bad data can come in a variety of flavors. Sometimes datasets are too small, meaning algorithms and models cannot fit to their trends properly. Sometimes they do not properly represent the breadth of chemical space, causing the generated models to be unsuitable for their desired use. Algorithms in food safety often come across these particular problems, as the number of tested food ingredient chemicals can be relatively low and (for obvious reasons) lack the bioactivity required to make predictive models.[95] Supplementing the existing data points with additional data points, from pharmaceutical studies, for example, can cause the second issue—making the models less relevant for food ingredients. Other problems in datasets come from quality assurance and data standardization, a procedure which often can be time-consuming, if not impossible, to overcome after an experiment has been completed. Can we ensure that every data point in a database has been conducted with exactly the same high level of good laboratory practice? No, but perhaps this expectation is unrealistic. Lowering the uncertainty in our data and hence our methods should be the end goal of computational toxicology, and for the data this can be achieved by collecting a large number of reliable examples covering a wide area of chemical space and checking the data quality.

To aid in this endeavor, individuals and industrial companies must make significant efforts to use best laboratory practice during data collection and to report all data points they can, including those that do not provide the expected or desired output. This issue has been encountered before when using public databases, where large numbers of biologically active chemicals are reported in the literature but the majority of the negative or inactive molecules are not reported.[101] Also, variation between laboratories as a result of generally small differences in protocols can have a large impact on the obtained data quality.[28] This makes computational modeling extremely challenging, as validating against experimental negatives or variable and uncertain data becomes very challenging. This problem can be overcome by examining chemical space on a larger scale to identify models which overpredict or by combining data from several sources, including those with more negatives.[25,80] While these solutions can provide datasets that can be modeled, the generation and release of additional high-quality data are always desirable to computational toxicologists.

One notable effort in the collection and distribution of a wide variety of toxicological data points in the US EPA's ToxCast program,[102] which uses rapid high throughput screening technology to efficiently collect data on thousands of chemicals of interest to the EPA. This dataset is considered useful due to the standardized nature of its collection and the wide variety of tested chemicals. As chemicals are chosen because they are of interest to the EPA the dataset is not biased toward a large number of active chemicals. The data are widely used both inside and outside the Agency, who make the data publicly available for other modelers to use, to both support safety decisions through techniques such as read-across and construct computational models for human and environmental toxicity prediction.[76,103] Moving forward the EPA is incorporating new technologies in high throughput screening into their work, including transcriptomics, metabolomics, and proteomics, which offer potential new sources of information on how cells respond to chemical insults.[104] Linking these responses to adverse outcomes using computational methods such as machine learning is certainly a potential opportunity here in the future. However, challenges still lie in standardized high-quality data collection, and the ability of computational algorithms to differentiate between the signal, the true response due to a toxicological insult, and the noise, the natural variation in such large datasets. While the ToxCast database is not focused on food-relevant chemicals, it does provide data and mechanistic information that can be of use in procedures such as read-across and data gap filling at this time.[105]

44.11 The future of computational toxicology

Computational modeling clearly has a larger role to play in the safety evaluation of new food ingredients moving forward (Fig. 44.8). The decreased time and monetary cost when compared to experimental approaches and increased pressure regarding the ethical and scientific shortcomings of in vivo animal methods present an opportunity for those wishing to develop and deploy more computational tools. Furthermore, an increase in computational power will speed up calculations and increased data sharing will enable greater model performance, particularly in the areas of machine learning and artificial intelligence. More experimental data will inevitably become available over time but the progression of projects to provide large batteries of consistently collected high throughput screening data, such as the aforementioned ToxCast database[102] help especially in providing data most suitable for computational modeling. While it will undoubtedly be some time before a true general intelligence from a computer becomes a reality, the models that can be generated using current classifiers and regressors are undeniably useful in safety decision-making.

These strengths do not mean the adoption of in silico toxicology will be an easy process. Computational toxicology models have existed for a considerable amount of time, and yet do not hold the same standing among regulators and decision-makers as in vitro or in vivo experiments. Many industries and regulators want further adoption of in silico models but rigorous evidence is required to ensure protection standards do not drop, and this will take time. As such, simply developing models and evaluating them in isolation will not help to overcome this issue. Academic, industrial, government, and regulatory scientists will need to work together, to establish what needs to be shown and how it can be for these methods to be more widely accepted. Developed models need to provide relevant

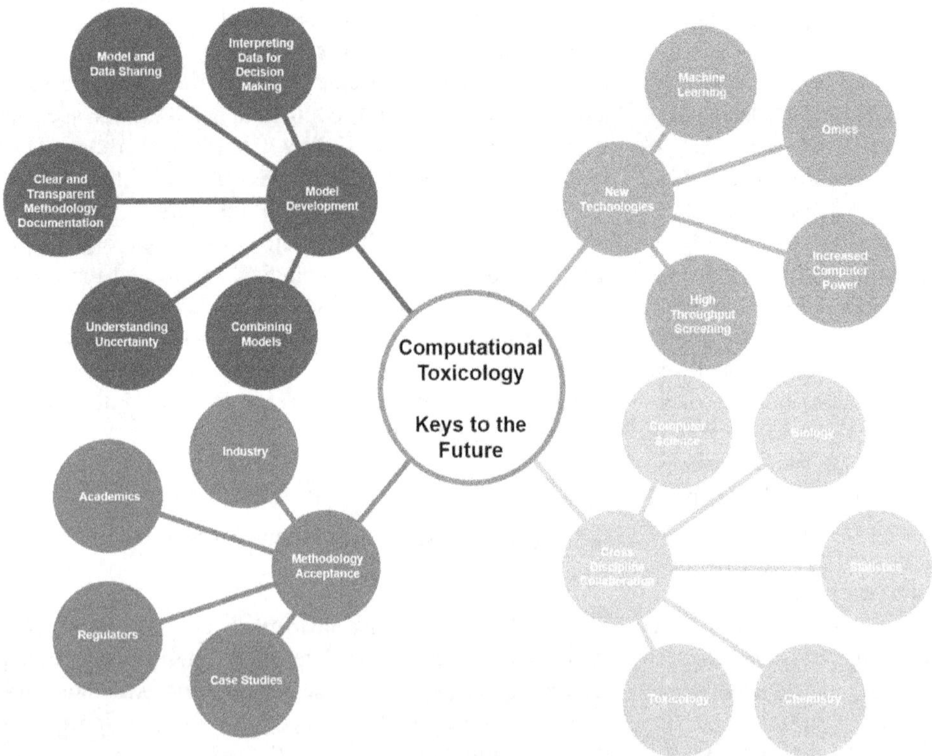

FIGURE 44.8 Some grouped ideas regarding the future of computational toxicology.

toxicological information for the best decisions to be made. Case studies will be a key step forward, as where industry can establish their chemicals meet safety standards with in silico calculations alongside the more regulatorily accepted experimental methods, the regulators will be able to see how and where these methods work. In the case of food ingredients, further integration of computational approaches into the safety assessment procedure,[9] including those presented here on the subjects of biotransformation, mechanistic toxicity prediction, and AOP construction, could prove extremely helpful.

To further drive computational toxicology in the future there are clear steps that can be taken whenever new models are developed. The sharing of methodology and data through online repositories must be at the forefront. Modelers should also endeavor to make their methodology as clear and transparent as possible, through documentation as well as choice of method, to convince others of its value. Finally, collaboration and combination of approaches across disciplines and scientific areas will be key to making an algorithmic procedure that can replace the need for animal testing while ensuring the protection of human health. Whose model performs the best is often not the most important question, as combining the results of several models almost always increases their performance, impact, and ability to convince decision-makers that they are right. Ultimately, a continued effort from cross-discipline expert scientists from across sectors will continue to push computational toxicology forward, and the use of these tools and models will see more acceptance in 21st century toxicology.

References

1. Raies AB, Bajic VB. In silico toxicology: computational methods for the prediction of chemical toxicity. *Wiley Interdiscip Rev Comput Mol Sci*. 2016;6(2):147–172. Available from: https://doi.org/10.1002/wcms.1240.
2. Committee on Toxicity Testing and Assessment of Environmental Agents and National Research Council. *Toxicology Testing in the 21st Century: A Vision and a Strategy*. Washington, DC: The National Academies Press; 2007.
3. Aardema MJ, MacGregor JT. Toxicology and genetic toxicology in the new era of "toxicogenomics": impact of "-omics" technologies. *Mutat Res*. 2002;499(1):13–25. Available from: http://www.ncbi.nlm.nih.gov/pubmed/11804602.
4. Kitano H. Systems biology: a brief overview. *Science*. 2002;295 (5560):1662–1664. Available from: https://doi.org/10.1126/science.1069492.
5. Henry CJ. Evolution of toxicology for risk assessment. *Int J Toxicol*. 2003;22(1):3–7. Available from: https://doi.org/10.1080/10915810305078.
6. Leist M, Hartung T, Nicotera P. The dawning of a new age of toxicology. *ALTEX*. 2008;25(2):103–114.
7. Hartung T. A toxicology for the 21st century—mapping the road ahead. *Toxicol Sci*. 2009;109(1):18–23. Available from: https://doi.org/10.1093/toxsci/kfp059.

8. Neltner TG, Alger HM, Leonard JE, Maffini MV. Data gaps in toxicity testing of chemicals allowed in food in the United States. *Reprod Toxicol*. 2013;42:85–94. Available from: https://doi.org/10.1016/j.reprotox.2013.07.023.
9. Blaauboer BJ, Boobis AR, Bradford B, et al. Considering new methodologies in strategies for safety assessment of foods and food ingredients margin of exposure. *Food Chem Toxicol*. 2016;91:19–35. Available from: https://doi.org/10.1016/j.fct.2016.02.019.
10. The 7th Amendment to the Cosmetics Directive. <http://ec.europa.eu/consumers/sectors/cosmetics/files/doc/antest/(2)_executive_summary_en.pdf>; Published 2003.
11. Amberg A, Beilke L, Bercu J, et al. Principles and procedures for implementation of ICH M7 recommended (Q)SAR analyses. *Regul Toxicol Pharmacol*. 2016;77:13–24. Available from: https://doi.org/10.1016/j.yrtph.2016.02.004.
12. European Union Directive 2010/63/EU. <https://ec.europa.eu/environment/chemicals/lab_animals/pdf/guidance/inspections/en.pdf>.
13. Grimm D. U.S. EPA to eliminate all mammal testing by 2035. *Science*. 2019. Available from: https://doi.org/10.1126/science.aaz4593.
14. Baltazar MT, Cable S, Carmichael PL, et al. A next-generation risk assessment case study for coumarin in cosmetic products. *Toxicol Sci*. 2020;176(1):236–252. Available from: https://doi.org/10.1093/toxsci/kfaa048.
15. Moxon TE, Li H, Lee M, et al. Application of physiologically based kinetic (PBK) modelling in the next generation risk assessment of dermally applied consumer products. *Toxicol In Vitro*. 2020;63:104746. Available from: https://doi.org/10.1016/j.tiv.2019.104746.
16. Cronin MTD, Richarz AN, Schultz TW. Identification and description of the uncertainty, variability, bias and influence in quantitative structure-activity relationships (QSARs) for toxicity prediction. *Regul Toxicol Pharmacol*. 2019;106:90–104. Available from: https://doi.org/10.1016/j.yrtph.2019.04.007.
17. Cherkasov A, Muratov EN, Fourches D, et al. QSAR modeling: where have you been? Where are you going to? *J Med Chem*. 2014;57(12):4977–5010. Available from: https://doi.org/10.1021/jm4004285.
18. Könemann H. Quantitative structure-activity relationships in fish toxicity studies. Part 1: Relationship for 50 industrial pollutants. *Toxicology*. 1981;19(3):209–221. Available from: https://doi.org/10.1016/0300-483X(81)90130-X.
19. Marchant CA, Briggs KA, Long A. In silico tools for sharing data and knowledge on toxicity and metabolism: Derek for Windows, Meteor, and Vitic. *Toxicol Mech Methods*. 2008;18(2–3):177–187.
20. Dahl GE, Jaitly N, Salakhutdinov R. Multi-task neural networks for QSAR predictions. 2014:1–21. <http://arxiv.org/abs/1406.1231>.
21. Wu Y, Wang G. Machine learning based toxicity prediction: from chemical structural description to transcriptome analysis. *Int J Mol Sci*. 2018;19(8). Available from: https://doi.org/10.3390/ijms19082358.
22. Unterthiner T, Mayr A, Klambauer G, Hochreiter S. Toxicity prediction using deep learning, 2015. http://arxiv.org/abs/1503.01445.
23. Mayr A, Klambauer G, Unterthiner T, Hochreiter S. DeepTox: toxicity prediction using deep learning. *Front Environ Sci*. 2016;3(80):1–15. Available from: https://doi.org/10.3389/fenvs.2015.00080.
24. Preuer K, Klambauer G, Rippmann F, Hochreiter S, Unterthiner T. Interpretable deep learning in drug discovery. In: Samek W, Montavon G, Vedaldi A, Hansen LK, Müller K-R, eds. *Explainable AI: Interpreting, Explaining and Visualizing Deep Learning*. Cham: Springer International Publishing; 2019:331–345. Available from: http://doi.org/10.1007/978-3-030-28954-6_18.
25. Allen TEH, Wedlake AJ, Goodman JM, et al. Neural network activation similarity: a new measure to assist decision making in chemical toxicology. *Chem Sci*. 2020;11:7335–7348. Available from: https://doi.org/10.1039/d0sc01637c.
26. Luechtefeld T, Marsh D, Rowlands C, Hartung T. Machine learning of toxicological big data enables read-across structure activity relationships (RASAR) outperforming animal test reproducibility. *Toxicol Sci*. 2018;165(1):198–212. Available from: https://doi.org/10.1093/toxsci/kfy152.
27. Paini A, Leonard JA, Joossens E, et al. Next generation physiologically based kinetic (NG-PBK) models in support of regulatory decision making. *Comput Toxicol*. 2019;9:61–72. Available from: https://doi.org/10.1016/j.comtox.2018.11.002.
28. Louisse J, Beekmann K, Rietjens IMCM. Use of physiologically based kinetic modeling-based reverse dosimetry to predict in vivo toxicity from in vitro data. *Chem Res Toxicol*. 2017;30:114–125. Available from: https://doi.org/10.1021/acs.chemrestox.6b00302.
29. EFSA. Scientific Opinion on the risks to public health related to the presence of bisphenol A (BPA) in foodstuffs. *EFSA J*. 2015;13(1):3978. Available from: https://doi.org/10.2903/j.efsa.2015.3978.
30. Knutsen HK, Alexander J, Barregård L, et al. Risk for animal and human health related to the presence of dioxins and dioxin-like PCBs in feed and food. *EFSA J*. 2018;16(11). Available from: https://doi.org/10.2903/j.efsa.2018.5333.
31. Schrenk D, Bignami M, Bodin L, et al. Risk to human health related to the presence of perfluoroalkyl substances in food. *EFSA J*. 2020;18(9). Available from: https://doi.org/10.2903/j.efsa.2020.6223.
32. Punt A, Aartse A, Bovee TFH, Gerssen A, Van Leeuwen SPJ. Quantitative in vitro-to- in vivo extrapolation (QIVIVE) of estrogenic and anti-androgenic potencies of BPA and BADGE analogues. *Arch Toxicol*. 2019;93(7):1941–1953. Available from: https://doi.org/10.1007/s00204-019-02479-6.
33. Ning J, Chen L, Strikwold M, Louisse J, Wesseling S, Rietjens IMCM. Use of an in vitro-in silico testing strategy to predict inter-species and inter-ethnic human differences in liver toxicity of the pyrrolizidine alkaloids lasiocarpine and riddelliine. *Arch Toxicol*. 2019;93(3):801–818. Available from: https://doi.org/10.1007/s00204-019-02397-7.
34. Abdullah R, Wesseling S, Spenkelink B, Louisse J, Punt A, Rietjens IMCM. Defining in vivo dose-response curves for kidney DNA adduct formation of aristolochic acid I in rat, mouse and human by an in vitro and physiologically based kinetic modeling approach. *J Appl Toxicol*. 2020;1–14. Available from: https://doi.org/10.1002/jat.4024.
35. Punt A, Paini A, Spenkelink A, et al. Evaluation of interindividual human variation in bioactivation and DNA adduct formation of estragole in liver predicted by physiologically based kinetic/dynamic and Monte Carlo modeling. *Chem Res Toxicol*. 2016;29:659–668. Available from: https://doi.org/10.1021/acs.chemrestox.5b00493.
36. Kiwamoto R, Spenkelink A, Rietjens IMCM, Punt A. An integrated QSAR-PBK/D modelling approach for predicting detoxi fi cation and DNA adduct formation of 18 acyclic food-borne α, β-unsaturated aldehydes. *Toxicol Appl Pharmacol*. 2015;282(1):108–117. Available from: https://doi.org/10.1016/j.taap.2014.10.014.
37. Boonpawa R, Spenkelink A, Punt A, Rietjens IMCM. Physiologically based kinetic modeling of hesperidin metabolism and its use to predict in vivo effective doses in humans. *Mol Nutr Food Res*. 2017;61:1–14. Available from: https://doi.org/10.1002/mnfr.201600894.

38. Louisse J, Alewijn M, Peijnenburg AACM, et al. Towards harmonization of test methods for in vitro hepatic clearance studies. *Toxicol In Vitro*. 2020;63:104722. Available from: https://doi.org/10.1016/j.tiv.2019.104722.
39. Punt A, Bouwmeester H, Blaauboer BJ, et al. New approach methodologies (NAMs) for human-relevant biokinetics predictions: meeting the paradigm shift in toxicology towards an animal-free chemical risk assessment. *ALTEX*. 2020;37(4):607–622. Available from: https://doi.org/10.14573/altex.2003242.
40. Jones HM, Rowland-Yeo K. Basic concepts in physiologically based pharmacokinetic modeling in drug discovery and development. *CPT Pharmacometrics Syst Pharmacol*. 2013;2(8):1–12. Available from: https://doi.org/10.1038/psp.2013.41.
41. Jorga K, Chavanne C, Frey N, et al. Bottom-up meets top-down: complementary physiologically based pharmacokinetic and population pharmacokinetic modeling for regulatory approval of a dosing algorithm of valganciclovir in very young children. *Clin Pharmacol Ther*. 2016;6(12):761–769. Available from: https://doi.org/10.1002/cpt.449.
42. Pearce RG, Setzer RW, Strope CL, Sipes NS, Wambaugh JF. httk: R package for high-throughput toxicokinetics. *J Stat Softw*. 2017;79(4). Available from: https://doi.org/10.18637/jss.v079.i04.
43. Wambaugh JF, Pearce RG, Ring C, et al. httk: high-throughput toxicokinetics. <https://cran.r-project.org/web/packages/httk/index.html>.
44. Cefic-LRI. IndusChemFate. <http://cefic-lri.org/toolbox/induschemfate/>.
45. Punt A, Pinckaers N, Nicole Peijnenburg A, Louisse J. Development of a web-based toolbox to support quantitative in vitro-to-in vivo extrapolations (QIVIVE) within non-animal testing strategies. *Chem Res Toxicol*. 2021;34:460–472.
46. PK-SIM. <http://www.open-systems-pharmacology.org/>.
47. FAME 3. <https://nerdd.zbh.uni-hamburg.de/fame3/>.
48. Šícho M, Stork C, Mazzolari A, et al. FAME 3: predicting the sites of metabolism in synthetic compounds and natural products for Phase 1 and Phase 2 metabolic enzymes. *J Chem Inf Model*. 2019;59(8):3400–3412. Available from: https://doi.org/10.1021/acs.jcim.9b00376.
49. SMARTCyp. <https://smartcyp.sund.ku.dk/mol_to_som>.
50. Meteor Nexus. <https://www.lhasalimited.org/products/meteor-nexus.htm>.
51. Nagaraju R, Prathusha AP, Kaza R, Bharathi K, Valerio LG, Long A. The in silico prediction of human-specific metabolites from hepatotoxic drugs. *Curr Drug Discov Technol*. 2010;7(3):170–187.
52. ADMETlab. <http://admet.scbdd.com/>.
53. Dong J, Wang NN, Yao ZJ, et al. AdMETlab: a platform for systematic ADMET evaluation based on a comprehensively collected ADMET database. *J Cheminform*. 2018;10(1):1–11. Available from: https://doi.org/10.1186/s13321-018-0283-x.
54. SwissADME. <http://www.swissadme.ch/>.
55. Daina A, Michielin O, Zoete V. SwissADME: a free web tool to evaluate pharmacokinetics, drug-likeness and medicinal chemistry friendliness of small molecules. *Sci Rep*. 2017;7:1–13. Available from: https://doi.org/10.1038/srep42717.
56. Vienna LiverTox Workspace. <https://livertox.univie.ac.at/>.
57. Williams RV, Amberg A, Brigo A, et al. It's difficult, but important, to make negative predictions. *Regul Toxicol Pharmacol*. 2016;76:79–86. Available from: https://doi.org/10.1016/j.yrtph.2016.01.008.
58. Bossuyt MVan, Hoeck EVan, Raitano G, Benfenati E, Mertens B, Rogiers V. Performance of in silico models for mutagenicity prediction of food contact materials. *Toxicol Sci*. 2018;163(2):632–638. Available from: https://doi.org/10.1093/toxsci/kfy057.
59. Toxtree. <http://www.toxtree.sourceforge.net>.
60. VEGA HUB. <http://www.vegahub.eu>.
61. Sarah Nexus. <https://www.lhasalimited.org/products/sarah-nexus.htm>.
62. Allen TEH, Grayson MN, Goodman JM, Gutsell S, Russell PJ. Using transition state modeling to predict mutagenicity for michael acceptors. *J Chem Inf Model*. 2018;58:1266–1271. Available from: https://doi.org/10.1021/acs.jcim.8b00130.
63. Townsend PA, Grayson MN. Density functional theory transition-state modeling for the prediction of Ames mutagenicity in 1,4 Michael acceptors. *J Chem Inf Model*. 2019;59(12):5099–5103. Available from: https://doi.org/10.1021/acs.jcim.9b00966.
64. Valerio LG, Arvidson KB, Chanderbhan RF, Contrera JF. Prediction of rodent carcinogenic potential of naturally occurring chemicals in the human diet using high-throughput QSAR predictive modeling. *Toxicol Appl Pharmacol*. 2007;222(1):1–16. Available from: https://doi.org/10.1016/j.taap.2007.03.012.
65. MDL QSAR. <http://www.mdli.com>.
66. CATMoS tool for predicting acute oral toxicity. <https://ntp.niehs.nih.gov/iccvamreport/2019/technology/comp-tools-dev/catmos/index.html#:~:text = CATMoS%20is%20a%20free%20online,%3C50%20mg%2Fkg%20vs>.
67. Mansouri K, Grulke CM, Judson RS, Williams AJ. OPERA models for predicting physicochemical properties and environmental fate endpoints. *J Cheminformatics*. 2018;10(1):1–19. Available from: https://doi.org/10.1186/s13321-018-0263-1.
68. Kleinstreuer NC, Karmaus AL, Mansouri K, Allen DG, Fitzpatrick JM, Patlewicz G. Predictive models for acute oral systemic toxicity: a workshop to bridge the gap from research to regulation. *Comput Toxicol*. 2018;8:21–24. Available from: https://doi.org/10.1016/j.comtox.2018.08.002.
69. The OECD QSAR Toolbox. <http://www.oecd.org/chemicalsafety/risk-assessment/theoecdqsartoolbox.htm>.
70. Schultz TW, Diderich R, Kuseva CD, Mekenyan OG. *The OECD QSAR Toolbox starts its second decade*. In: *Computational Toxicology*; 2018:55–77.
71. Dimitrov SD, Diderich R, Sobanski T, et al. QSAR toolbox – workflow and major functionalities. *SAR QSAR Environ Res*. 2016;27(3):203–219. Available from: https://doi.org/10.1080/1062936X.2015.1136680.
72. Nelms MD, Mellor CL, Cronin MTD, Madden JC, Enoch SJ. Development of an in silico profiler for mitochondrial toxicity. *Chem Res Toxicol*. 2015;28(10):1891–1902. Available from: https://doi.org/10.1021/acs.chemrestox.5b00275.
73. Zhang H, Yu P, Ren JX, et al. Development of novel prediction model for drug-induced mitochondrial toxicity by using naïve Bayes classifier method. *Food Chem Toxicol*. 2017;110:122–129. Available from: https://doi.org/10.1016/j.fct.2017.10.021.
74. Nelms MD, Ates G, Madden JC, et al. Proposal of an in silico profiler for categorisation of repeat dose toxicity data of hair dyes. *Arch Toxicol*. 2015;89:733–741. Available from: https://doi.org/10.1007/s00204-014-1277-8.
75. Liu J, Patlewicz G, Williams AJ, Thomas RS, Shah I. Predicting organ toxicity using in vitro bioactivity data and chemical structure. *Chem Res Toxicol*. 2017;30(11):2046–2059. Available from: https://doi.org/10.1021/acs.chemrestox.7b00084.

76. Pradeep P, Paul Friedman K, Judson R. Structure-based QSAR models to predict repeat dose toxicity points of departure. *Comput Toxicol*. 2020;16:100139. Available from: https://doi.org/10.1016/j.comtox.2020.100139.
77. Zhang C, Cheng F, Li W, Liu G, Lee PW, Tang Y. *In silico* prediction of drug induced liver toxicity using substructure pattern recognition method. *Mol Inform*. 2016;35(3–4):136–144. Available from: https://doi.org/10.1002/minf.201500055.
78. Zhang H, Ding L, Zou Y, et al. Predicting drug-induced liver injury in human with Naïve Bayes classifier approach. *J Comput Aided Mol Des*. 2016;30(10):889–898. Available from: https://doi.org/10.1007/s10822-016-9972-6.
79. He S, Ye T, Wang R, et al. An in silico model for predicting drug-induced hepatotoxicity. *Int J Mol Sci*. 2019;20(8):1–17. Available from: https://doi.org/10.3390/ijms20081897.
80. Wedlake AJ, Folia M, Piechota S, et al. Structural alerts and random forest models in a consensus approach for receptor binding molecular initiating events. *Chem Res Toxicol*. 2020. Available from: https://doi.org/10.1021/acs.chemrestox. 9b00325.
81. Allen TEH, Goodman JM, Gutsell S, Russell PJ. Using 2D structural alerts to define chemical categories for molecular initiating events. *Toxicol Sci*. 2018;165(1):213–223.
82. Allen TEH, Goodman JM, Gutsell S, Russell PJ. Quantitative predictions for molecular initiating events using three- dimensional quantitative structure – activity relationships. *Chem Res Toxicol*. 2020;33(2):324–332. Available from: https://doi.org/10.1021/acs.chemrestox.9b00136.
83. Xu Y, Dai Z, Chen F, Gao S, Pei J, Lai L. Deep learning for drug-induced liver injury. *J Chem Inf Model*. 2015;55(10):2085–2093. Available from: https://doi.org/10.1021/acs.jcim.5b00238.
84. Mayr A, Klambauer G, Unterthiner T, et al. Large-scale comparison of machine learning methods for drug target prediction on ChEMBL. *Chem Sci*. 2018;9(24):5441–5451. Available from: https://doi.org/10.1039/c8sc00148k.
85. Cai C, Guo P, Zhou Y, et al. Deep learning-based prediction of drug-induced cardiotoxicity. *J Chem Inf Model*. 2019;59(3):1073–1084. Available from: https://doi.org/10.1021/acs.jcim.8b00769.
86. Mellor CL, Steinmetz FP, Cronin MTD. Using molecular initiating events to develop a structural alert based screening workflow for nuclear receptor ligands associated with hepatic steatosis. *Chem Res Toxicol*. 2016;29(2):203–212. Available from: https://doi.org/10.1021/acs.chemrestox.5b00480.
87. Allen TEH, Nelms MD, Edwards SW, et al. In silico guidance for in vitro androgen and glucocorticoid receptor ToxCast assays. *Environ Sci Technol*. 2020;54(12):7461–7470. Available from: https://doi.org/10.1021/acs.est.0c01105.
88. Ebbrell DJ, Madden JC, Cronin MTD, Schultz TW, Enoch SJ. Development of a fragment-based in silico profiler for Michael addition thiol reactivity. *Chem Res Toxicol*. 2016;29(6):1073–1081. Available from: https://doi.org/10.1021/acs.chemrestox.6b00099.
89. Ebbrell DJ, Madden JC, Cronin MTD, Schultz TW, Enoch SJ. Validation of a fragment-based profiler for thiol reactivity for the prediction of toxicity: skin sensitization and *Tetrahymena pyriformis*. *Chem Res Toxicol*. 2017;30(2):604–613. Available from: https://doi.org/10.1021/acs.chemrestox.6b00361.
90. Tsakovska I, Al Sharif M, Alov P, et al. Molecular modelling study of the PPARγ receptor in relation to the mode of action/adverse outcome pathway framework for liver steatosis. *Int J Mol Sci*. 2014;15(5):7651–7666. Available from: https://doi.org/10.3390/ijms15057651.
91. Zhang C, Zhou Y, Gu S, et al. In silico prediction of hERG potassium channel blockage by chemical category approaches. *Toxicol Res (Camb)*. 2016;5(2):570–582. Available from: https://doi.org/10.1039/c5tx00294j.
92. Gadaleta D, Manganelli S, Roncaglioni A, Toma C, Benfenati E, Mombelli E. QSAR modeling of ToxCast assays relevant to the molecular initiating events of AOPs leading to hepatic steatosis. *J Chem Inf Model*. 2018;58(8):1501–1517. Available from: https://doi.org/10.1021/acs.jcim.8b00297.
93. Ankley GT, Bennett RS, Erickson RJ, et al. Adverse outcome pathways: a conceptual framework to support ecotoxicology research and risk assessment. *Environ Toxicol Chem*. 2010;29(3):730–741. Available from: https://doi.org/10.1002/etc.34.
94. European Commission Institute for Health and Consumer Protection. AOP Wiki. <http://ihcp.jrc.ec.europa.eu/our_activities/alt-animal-testing-safety-assessment-chemicals/improved_safety_assessment_ chemicals/adverse-outcome-pathways-aop>.
95. Kramer NI, Hoffmans Y, Wu S, et al. Characterizing the coverage of critical effects relevant in the safety evaluation of food additives by AOPs. *Arch Toxicol*. 2019;93(8):2115–2125. Available from: https://doi.org/10.1007/s00204-019-02501-x.
96. Vinken M, Kramer N, Allen TEH, et al. The use of adverse outcome pathways in the safety evaluation of food additives. *Arch Toxicol*. 2020;94(3):959–966. Available from: https://doi.org/10.1007/s00204-020-02670-0.
97. Oki O, Edwards SW. An integrative data mining approach to identifying adverse outcome pathway signatures. *Toxicology*. 2016;352:49–61. Available from: https://doi.org/10.1016/j.tox.2016.04.004.
98. Bell SM, Angrish MM, Wood CE, Edwards SW. Integrating publicly available data to generate computationally predicted adverse outcome pathways for fatty liver. *Toxicol Sci*. 2016;150(2):510–520. Available from: https://doi.org/10.1093/toxsci/kfw017.
99. Svensson F, Zou A, Mahmoud S, et al. Information-derived mechanistic hypotheses for structural cardiotoxicity. *Chem Res Toxicol*. 2018;31:1119–1127. Available from: https://doi.org/10.1021/acs.chemrestox.8b00159.
100. Spinu N, Cronin MTD, Enoch SJ, Madden JC, Worth AP. Quantitative adverse outcome pathway (qAOP) models for toxicity prediction. *Arch Toxicol*. 2020;94(5):1497–1510. Available from: https://doi.org/10.1007/s00204-020-02774-7.
101. Cheng T, Hao M, Takeda T, Bryant SH, Wang Y. Large-scale prediction of drug-target interaction: a data-centric review. *AAPS J*. 2017;19(5):1264–1275. Available from: https://doi.org/10.1208/s12248-017-0092-6.
102. ToxCast Database. <https://www.epa.gov/chemical-research/toxicity-forecasting>.
103. Richard AM, Judson RS, Houck KA, et al. ToxCast chemical landscape: paving the road to 21st century toxicology. *Chem Res Toxicol*. 2016;29(8):1225–1251. Available from: https://doi.org/10.1021/acs.chemrestox.6b00135.
104. Thomas RS, Bahadori T, Buckley TJ, et al. The next generation blueprint of computational toxicology at the U.S. Environmental Protection Agency. *Toxicol Sci*. 2019;169(2):317–332. Available from: https://doi.org/10.1093/toxsci/kfz058.
105. Punt A, Firman J, Boobis A, et al. Potential of ToxCast data in the safety assessment of food chemicals. *Toxicol Sci*. 2020;174(2):326–340. Available from: https://doi.org/10.1093/toxsci/kfaa008.

Chapter 45

Risk-benefit assessment

Jeljer Hoekstra[1], Maarten Nauta[2,3] and Morten Poulsen[2]

[1]RIVM, The National Institute for Public Health and the Environment, Bilthoven, The Netherlands, [2]National Food Institute, Technical University of Denmark (DTU), Kgs. Lyngby, Denmark, [3]Statens Serum Institut, Copenhagen S, Denmark

Abstract

Risk-benefit assessment assesses and compares risks and benefits in a food or substance to facilitate informed decision-making regarding food and public health policies. In the assessment, exposure scenarios are compared on risks and benefits. In some cases, advice on favorable exposure scenarios can be given by assessing risks and benefits separately but sometimes there is a need for a quantitative assessment expressing risks and benefits in a common health metric.

This chapter describes a methodology to perform a risk-benefit assessment and highlights the most important issues an assessor runs into.

Keywords: Risks; benefits; food policy; health metrics

Chapter Points

Most important for risk-benefit assessment is the problem definition in terms of exposure scenarios for the food(s) or substance(s) in question and the population of interest. A tiered approach allows for some of the questions to be answered semi-quantitatively, others need a full quantitative approach in which health metrics are calculated. Then dose-response functions have to be found either from human or animal data. Communication of the results is essential because the final policy decision may not depend only on maximization of health.

45.1 Introduction

45.1.1 History (background)

For a long-time risk assessment and benefit assessment of foods have been separate processes. However, these different assessments may give conflicting messages on the health effects of foods, which made food safety decision-makers increasingly aware of the need for an integrated approach. Therefore the European Food Safety Authority (EFSA) organized a scientific colloquium on risk-benefit analysis of foods in July 2006 to have an open scientific debate on the methods and approaches for risk-benefit analysis of foods. As a result several projects within the European framework such as BRAFO,[1,2] QALIBRA,[3] BENERIS,[4] and BEPRAIREBEAN[5,6] were started to integrate risk and benefits. Those projects produced, among others, guidance and methodologies for performing risk-benefit assessment. The following years showed an ever growing literature on case studies and refinements of methods. Good reviews can be found in Boué et al.,[7] Tijhuis et al.,[5] Nauta et al.,[8] Pires et al.,[9] and Assunção et al.,[10] Membre et al.,[11] and Verhagen et al.[12]

45.1.2 Structure and terminology

The EFSA Scientific Colloquium 2006 concluded that a risk-benefit analysis should mirror the approach agreed upon for risk analysis.[13] This implies that risk-benefit analysis includes a risk-benefit assessment, risk-benefit management, and risk-benefit communication. Here, the risk-benefit assessment is the scientific process where the potential adverse health effects are weighed against the potential beneficial health effects. The purpose of risk-benefit assessment is to offer scientific decision support to the risk-benefit manager. Initially, it was proposed to apply the steps in risk assessment (i.e., hazard identification, hazard characterization, exposure assessment, and risk characterization) in the benefit assessment as well, and in a last step combine them in a risk-benefit characterization, where the risks and benefits are integrated into a final estimate of the overall health impact. This provided a strong basis for the development of the methodology,[5] but later the proposed approach to risk benefit was specified in more detail to allow a better integration of demands of the different underlying disciplines: nutrition, toxicology, and microbiology.[8,14,15] For example, the proposal to define "benefit" as the counterpart of both "hazard" and "risk"[13] was confusing when terminology is

Present Knowledge in Food Safety. DOI: https://doi.org/10.1016/B978-0-12-819470-6.00039-1

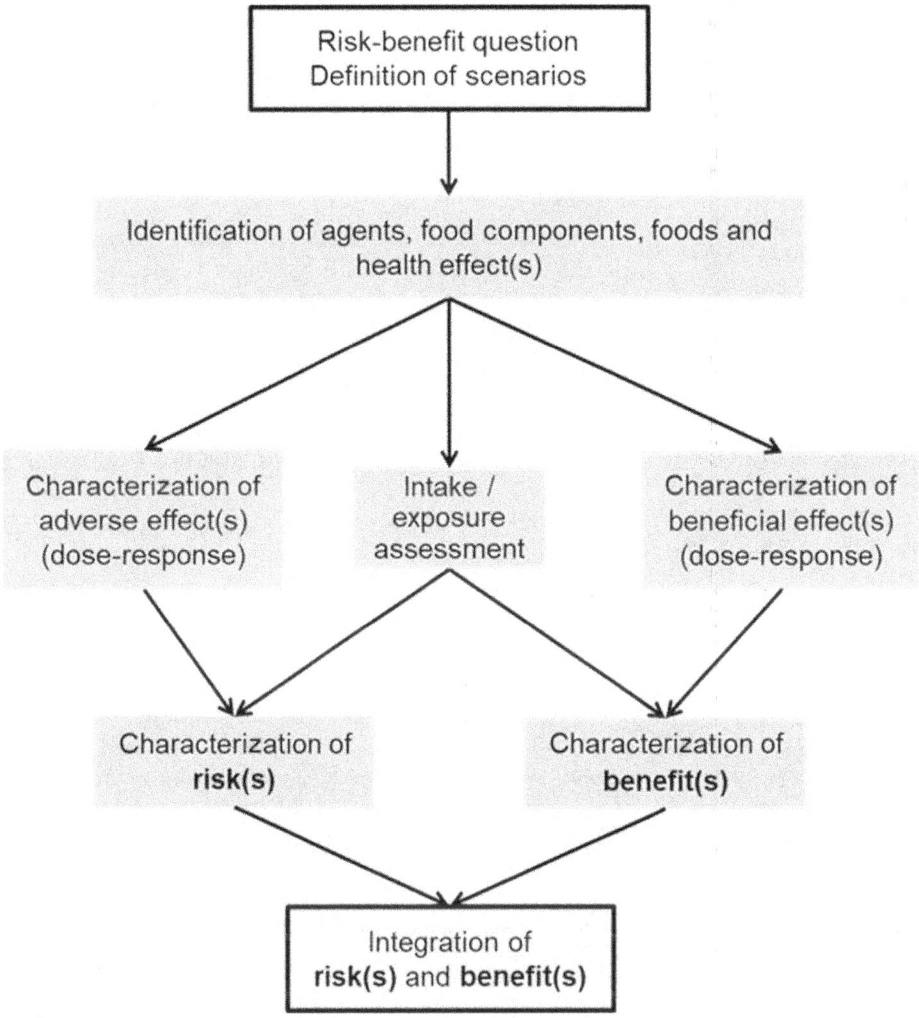

FIGURE 45.1 Steps in risk-benefit assessment.

worked out in more detail. Also with "hazard" being defined as either the "agent" with the potential to cause an adverse health effect[16] or the "inherent property of an agent" to cause adverse effects,[17] the meaning of "hazard identification" became unclear as well. Therefore we propose to define the steps in risk-benefit assessment as shown in Fig. 45.1, and to use the terminology presented in Box 47.1.

45.2 Problem definition

45.2.1 Risk-benefit questions

The initial phase of the risk-benefit assessment is of crucial importance to define the question and the approach taken, and to agree on them with the risk-benefit manager. The question should clarify the objective, scope, and limitations of the risk-benefit assessment in terms of what is (not) included in the assessment. On a high aggregate level a risk-benefit question is whether a potential policy measure, resulting in a changed exposure, is better, in terms of health, than some reference, usually the status-quo or zero. This means that in the end the risk-benefit question is about comparing different intake scenarios. An important element of the risk-benefit question is to clarify whether the answer should indicate the risk-benefit balance per se (i.e., whether the overall risk is larger than the benefit or vice versa) or should characterize the risk-benefit balance by stating how much larger the risk is than the benefit or vice versa. In general, the first question would be easier to answer, as a quantitative assessment may not be needed (see 45.3.1.2). However, the quantitative information may have added value that is of relevance for the risk manager, if other arguments than health impact (such as economical impact or sustainability) are part of the decision-making process (see 45.3.1.3).

45.2.2 Scenarios

The intake scenarios that are to be compared in the risk-benefit assessment should be explicitly stated. Often, the

BOX 45.1 Terminology for risk-benefit assessment as applied in this chapter.

Adverse health effect: A change in the morphology, physiology, growth, development, reproduction, or life span of a human or (sub)population, that results in an impairment of functional capacity, an impairment of the capacity to compensate for additional stress, or an increase in susceptibility to other influences.[18] An adverse health effect may be a disease or another health outcome that reduces quality of life or causes loss of life.

Beneficial health effect: A health effect with the opposite health impact of an adverse health effect. It increases quality of life, lowers a reduction in quality of life, or reduces the probability of loss of life.

Hazard: A biological, chemical, or physical agent in, or condition of, food with the potential to cause an adverse health effect.

Beneficial component: A biological, chemical or physical agent in, or condition of, food with the potential to cause a beneficial health effect.

Risk: A function of the probability of an adverse health effect and the severity of that effect, consequential to a hazard(s) in food, or the food product itself.

Benefit: A function of the probability of a beneficial health effect and the consequences of that effect, due to a beneficial component(s) in food, or the food product itself.

Health impact: The combined health consequences of the risks and benefits studied in one or more intake scenarios, expressed either qualitatively or quantitatively, by one common health metric or a combination of metrics.

reference scenario reflects the current intake of the food product(s) considered in the risk-benefit assessment, for which a change is expected or proposed. This change is defined in one or more alternative intake scenarios. The risk-benefit assessment studies whether there is an overall risk or benefit of following the alternative scenario as compared to the reference and/or what the health impact of the change in scenario is.

45.2.3 Choice of health effects, food components, and foods

A crucial step in the risk-benefit assessment is the decision on the included food components (i.e., chemicals, (micro-)nutrients, microorganisms, or other constituents present in food[14]) and foods, and to choose the relevant health effects associated with these food components and foods. Relevant health effects are usually selected on the basis of the strength of evidence (see 45.2.5). It is however difficult, as methods differ between research disciplines involved in risk-benefit assessment and between the types of health effects studied.

Also, the specific risk-benefit question, and the interest of the risk-benefit manager, may demand the inclusion of specific health effects, even though the evidence may be poor. This may happen when uncertainty of an effect is large but the potential health impact is also large. In such cases, transparent characterization of the uncertainty is crucial.

One should be aware that the level of scientific evidence needed for identifying negative and/or positive health effects is not consistent,[2] because the presence of benefits and the absence of risks need to be guaranteed.[5,19] As a consequence, risk may be more easily included in the risk-benefit assessment than benefits, which may result in a biased result.[8] For the selection of health effects to be included in the risk-benefit assessment, this implies that it is important to be consistent within the risk-benefit assessment, and be transparent of the selection in the communication of the results.

What to include is a challenging step, as the health impact of changes in intake often does not only depend on the intake of foods and/or food components referred to in the risk-benefit question, but also on the rest of the diet. Still, a selection is necessary to keep the assessment feasible.

A diagram as shown in Fig. 45.2 can be used to get an overview of the choices made. This lists the food, food components, and the health effects included in the risk-benefit assessment, and the relation between them.

45.2.4 Population of interest

Health effects and/or data related to health effects may be population-specific, for example if they are (predominantly) known to occur in women or men, elderly, or young children. The populations of interest associated with the different health effects considered in the risk-benefit assessment should therefore be indicated. If this population of interest is the same for all health effects, the risks and benefits apply to this specific population and the risk-benefit assessment can support decision-making for this population. If the populations are different, the risk-benefit manager may have the additional challenge of weighing the interest of different population groups, for example if the risk dominates in one population and the benefit dominates in another.[20]

45.2.5 Strength of the evidence

The selection of health effects associated with the intake of foods or food components should be a careful process, preferably based on a through literature review. Often, a large set of health effects can be considered, with varying degrees of evidence. In principle, only health effects for which convincing evidence is found should be included in the risk-benefit assessment. A generic classification of

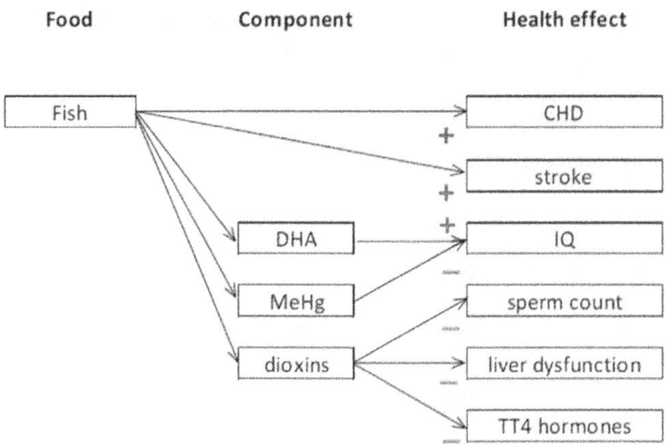

FIGURE 45.2 Overview of the food, food components, and health effects chosen to be included in the risk-benefit assessment performed by Hoekstra et al.[19] The arrows link the health effects to the different food(s) and food component(s) and whether they are considered to have a positive (+) or negative (−) health impact. *This figure is reproduced from Nauta et al.*[8]

evidence is used in risk-benefit assessment, as for example as applied for carcinogens.[21,22]

45.2.6 Biomarkers, intermediate health effects

Ideally, the health effects identified in the risk-benefit assessment are expressed as a specific disease or another well-described health outcome for which it has been described how it reduces or increases the quality of life. These health effects allow the characterization of the health impact, which is essential to compare risks and benefits in a risk-benefit assessment. However, health effects of foods and food components may also be characterized at an intermediate level, such as a change in the level of a biomarker. For example, a dose−response relation is available for vitamin D intake and the 25(OH) D serum level, but not for vitamin D and the incidence of hip fracture.[23] This is challenging because, for risk-benefit assessment, the health impact should be expressed for hip fractures. In general, biomarkers and intermediate health effects can only be applied if their relation with the health endpoint is described, or if an incomplete, descriptive risk-benefit assessment is performed.

45.3 Approaches for risk-benefit assessment

45.3.1 Tiered approach

Tiered approaches have been suggested for doing risk-benefit assessments (e.g., EFSA,[24] EFSA Scientific Colloquium 6 Summary Report) because a comprehensive quantitative risk-benefit is costly in terms of expertise and data. In many cases, a simple (qualitative) assessment may be sufficient for the risk manager to make a decision. The tiered approach developed in the European Union-project BRAFO is the most elaborate to date.[1,2]

This tiered approach assesses the benefits and risks when changing from a reference scenario to an alternative scenario. It results in a statement about the differences between the scenarios in terms of health benefits and risks for specific (sub)populations and whether there is a net health benefit of one scenario over the other. The tiered approach is illustrated by the flowchart shown in Fig. 45.3. The assessment starts with problem formulation, (see Section 45.2) and is ultimately expressed in exposure distributions for at least two scenarios, reference and alternative. Then, a sequence of four tiers allows progressively refined comparisons of benefits and risks, with their integration in the higher tiers. At any time in the process, the formulation of the risk-benefit question can be readdressed in consultation with the risk manager. This is indicated by the dashed arrows at the left side of the figure.

45.3.1.1 Separate risk and benefit assessment

Tier 1 is a separate risk assessment and benefits assessment with the objective of analyzing whether only benefits, only risks, both, or neither will occur. It is sufficient to consider only the relative effects, that is whether a beneficial or adverse change in effect between the reference and alternative scenarios is expected. For many effects, only brief consideration will be needed. If there is clear evidence on whether beneficial or adverse changes can be expected between the two scenarios, such evidence may take various forms, for example, comparing worst-case exposure with tolerable daily intake (TDI) shows no appreciable risk when judged against established criteria. If both risks and benefits occur the assessment progresses to the second tier, otherwise the assessment stops. However, there are generally both benefits and risks, generating the need for further assessment.

45.3.1.2 Qualitative integration of risk and benefit

In Tier 2, benefits and risks are compared with each other and integrated qualitatively. Health effects are evaluated based on incidence (number of people affected), severity of the health effects, duration of the disease, and additional mortality resulting from the effect. If either risks or benefits clearly dominate, then the appropriate scenario can be advised; else the assessment progresses to Tier 3. Tier 2 is often the decisive step in the assessment.

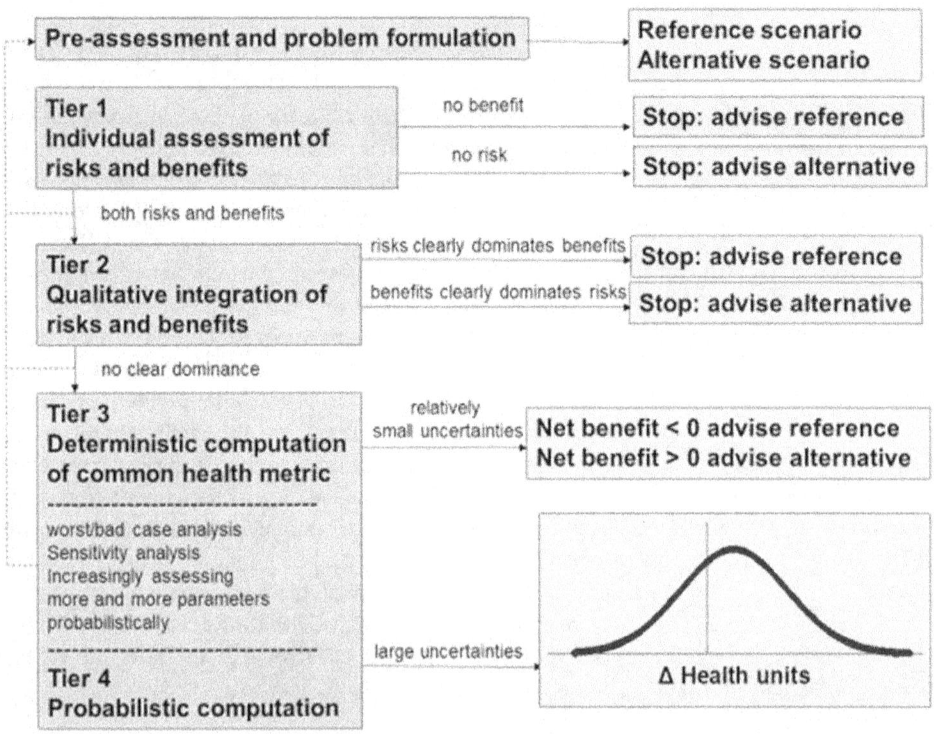

FIGURE 45.3 A flowchart of the BRAFO tiered approach.[1]

45.3.1.3 Quantitative integration of risk and benefit

In Tier 3, benefits and risks are calculated quantitatively in a deterministic way. Common metrics such as quality-adjusted life years (QALYs)/disability-adjusted life years (DALYs) (see Section 45.7.2) have been developed and are available for the process of integration. Finally, if necessary in Tier 4, uncertainty is addressed. This can be done in increasingly more sophisticated ways where finally a probabilistic approach is applied, using the same common metrics as in Tier 3.

45.3.2 Quantitative risk-benefit assessment

Quantitative risk-benefit assessment need not only be performed if Tier 3 of the tiered approach is reached, that is if there is no clear dominance of the risk over the benefit or vice versa. It can also be decided to do a quantitative risk-benefit assessment from the start, if the risk-benefit manager wants a quantitative estimate of the overall health impact. The advantage of such an estimate is that the magnitude of the overall health risk or benefit is known, and can be weighed against, for example, the associated costs, environmental impact, food quality or taste.

A quantitative risk-benefit assessment requires that the health impact of change from reference to alternative scenario, for each individual health effect, is quantified on a common scale of measurement. Such a common scale can be disease incidence or mortality, but it can also be an integrated composite health metric like the DALY. The choice for DALY is often made in risk-benefit assessments as it allows inclusion of incidence and duration of disease, severity of disease, and mortality, for all health endpoints considered.

When doing a quantitative risk-benefit assessment, a probabilistic approach including the variability is preferred, especially when the dose–response relation used is nonlinear. In that case the low and/or high doses associated with the largest risks and benefits may drive the final health impact estimate, and the use of point estimates may lead to misleading results. Uncertainty can be included by a probabilistic approach as well, as explained in Section 45.9.

45.4 Risks and benefits

Risks and benefits both deal with health effects as the result of intake of a substance, nutrient, or food item. Risks are usually associated with exposure to a substance that is not needed and where higher intakes/exposure are associated with a higher probability of adverse health effect. Usually there is an exposure level below which adverse health effects are considered negligible. The dose–response between exposure and probability of adverse health effect is an increasing function.

Benefits are often associated with intakes of food, substances that people cannot do without. There usually is a minimum intake at which no adverse health effects are expected and very often there is also an upper level above which adverse health effects are considered to occur. Exposure to substances or foods where a higher intake results in better health, generally a lower probability of adverse effects, are called benefits. However, everything is toxic when the dose is high enough. And then reduction of risk of substances that are realistically unavoidable or part of a normal diet are very often also called benefits. Reduction of transfat intake would be an example.

45.4.1 Chemicals

Food-associated chemicals include both man-made and those originating from nature. It is a very large and diverse group and the health effects of food-associated chemicals can range from completely harmless to highly toxic. In general, chemicals included in risk-benefit assessment are associated with risks. In risk-benefit assessment of foods like fish, nuts and seeds, chemicals that represent the risk part in the risk-benefit equation are often contaminants. In other cases, the adverse effects following food intake are due to chemicals like natural inherent toxins in the food, for example glycoalkaloids in potatoes and cyanogenic glycosides in linseeds.

45.4.2 Nutrients

Nutrients are substances that an individual needs to survive. As such they are associated with benefits. A too low intake should be avoided.

Micronutrients such as vitamins and minerals have minimum intake levels to avoid deficiencies but many also have upper levels at which negative health effects occur. Therefore, in a risk-benefit assessment people at the low intake extremes as well as those with high intake need to be taken into account.

Macronutrients such as fat and carbohydrates provide energy. In the context of risk-benefit assessment, usually a too low caloric intake is not relevant. Macronutrients are not associated with deficiencies but with the occurrence of disease, for example, heart disease or cancer. Here less is better as it results in a lower probability of developing the disease, as with toxicological risks but here the safest level is not zero.

Intake level of nutrients is often directly linked to a disease and therefore can be relatively easy expressed in a health metric such a as the DALY.

45.4.3 Microorganisms

Microorganisms (e.g. bacteria, viruses, and parasites) can be present in food and may be included in risk-benefit assessment as they can be associated with both adverse and beneficial health effects. Adverse health effects can come from foodborne pathogens such as *Salmonella* spp. and *Listeria monocytogenes*. For these, microbiological risk assessment methods have been incorporated in risk-benefit assessment. However, the beneficial effects of, for example, fermented foods and probiotics have to our knowledge not been included in published risk-benefit assessments.

Microorganisms are different from chemicals and nutrients in many respects that are relevant for risk-benefit assessment. The most frequently occurring health effects of microorganisms are related to gastrointestinal complaints which implies they are usually acute (i.e., they occur directly after intake) and short-term. However, serious sequelae, resulting in chronic illness or even death may occur as well. Also, exposure to foodborne pathogens may be prevented by good food hygiene and proper storage and thorough heating of the food.

Incorporation of microorganisms in risk-benefit assessment requires specific expertise and may fall outside the scope of the risk-benefit managers' request. Therefore they are not frequently incorporated in risk-benefit assessments so far. Examples where they have been included are a risk-benefit assessment on drinking water disinfection,[25] cold smoked salmon,[26] and infant formula.[27] However, inclusion of microorganisms in risk-benefit assessment is still considered as one of the challenges in risk-benefit assessment.[8]

45.4.4 Guidance values

Guidance values give quantitative information to the regulatory system that enables it to protect human health.[28] To establish health-based guidance values (HBGVs) such as acceptable daily intakes and TDI or tolerable weekly intake information about the no-observed adverse effect level (NOAEL) obtained from animal studies is often used as the point of reference.[29] Information on HBGVs can be of value when assessing risk and benefit of a given food, but should not be used in an integrated quantitative risk-benefit assessment where the real risks should be compared with the real benefits.

Within nutrition, some essential nutrients have a dual risk relationship with risks occurring at both the upper end ("excess") and lower end ("deficiency") of the intake range. The tolerable upper intake level is the maximum level of chronic daily nutrient intake from all sources judged to be unlikely to pose a risk of adverse health effects to humans.[30]

45.5 Intake and exposure assessment

Risk, benefits, and subsequent health effects depend on the level of exposure. Exposure can be calculated from intake data collected with, for example, food frequency questionnaires or total diet studies combined with concentration data from, for example, food composition tables and contamination databases, just as it is done for standard risk or benefit assessment.

Exposure assessment is needed for each food component or food item that is associated with a health effect that is considered relevant, and for every scenario. For chronic effects habitual long-term intake is needed, for acute effects maximum intake. Both depend on the variation in exposure per serving.

For risk-benefit assessments, especially a quantitative one (Tier 3), a few aspects need special attention, such as exposure assessment for food and food components, substitution, and background exposure.

45.5.1 Food versus food component

The method applied for exposure assessment will depend on whether a health effect incorporated in the risk-benefit assessment is linked to a food or to a food component. If the effect is directly linked to a food (such as coronary heart disease (CHD) or stroke to fish; Fig. 45.2), risk-benefit assessment requires an intake assessment of fish, based on representative intake data. If the effect is linked to a food component (such as docosahexaenoic acid (DHA) or methylmercury (MeHg) linked to the IQ of a newborn child), an exposure assessment is needed, which not only requires an intake assessment of the food, but also data on the concentrations of the food component in the food. Hence, an exposure assessment for substances, nutrients, and microorganisms requires more data.

45.5.2 Substitution

Foods are part of a diet. When one food is eaten more (e.g., fish) another one (e.g., meat) is eaten less or not at all. The mostly unspecified other food is often also associated with risks and benefits. Therefore the assessment has to be clear whether substitution of one food for another is considered to be part of the assessment or not. This aspect is often ignored and sometimes mentioned in the discussion as a caveat. Even if a food is not substituted then the extra calories result in health effects. Obviously, the assessment is more realistic when substitution is taken into account. However, that is not straightforward. It is very often not known which foods to choose as substitution, so several scenarios are investigated. Furthermore, with every substitute food an extra risk-benefit assessment is added which comes with a cost in extra effort and data, and introduces extra uncertainty.

Recently, Thomsen et al.[14,31] discussed substitution in great detail.

45.5.3 Background exposure

Exposure is not only the result of the intake of the food of interest but may come from various other sources, such as other foods and the environment. For a risk-benefit assessment, such background exposure from sources not considered in the risk-benefit assessment may be important as critical exposure levels for specific substances may be more easily reached.

Furthermore, some substances accumulate in the body which means that internal exposure is the effect of historic food intake.

45.6 Dose–response

Dose–response functions describe the relationship between a specific internal or external exposure or intake (dose) with a positive or negative health effect (response) and are necessary for a health impact calculation which often forms an important part of a risk-benefit assessment.

45.6.1 Human data

Beneficial effects in risk-benefit assessments are often derived from human epidemiological studies. Benefits are usually the decreased risk of developing a chronic disease when intake of a food or nutrient increases, such as the reduced risk in cardiovascular disease (CVD) due to fish (oil) intake. But also risk is sometimes based on human data, for example, MeHg intake of pregnant women which lowers IQ of their babies. Often this data comes from observational studies which has the advantage that it is relevant because it pertains to humans but has the disadvantage that the experimental setting is not controlled.

For instance, intakes may not be properly distributed and may be measured with substantial errors. Furthermore, there are covariables for which statistical adjustments have to be made. For quantitative risk-benefit assessments, dose–response relations are necessary. Unfortunately, from the perspective of a risk-benefit assessment, epidemiological studies are not primarily set up to establish dose–response functions and these are not always derived. Although a more extensive reporting would make it possible, risk-benefit assessors have to make do with what is available. Metaanalysis can be helpful. But the assessor must often deal with studies with different study designs, covariables that are only sometimes adjusted for. Data to extract a dose–response are not always reported and it can be difficult to combine results from different studies in one dose–response.

45.6.2 Animal data

Whereas information on beneficial effects in the risk-benefit assessment often is based on human data, information on adverse health effects is usually based on data from animal studies. However, such animal data will need an animal to human extrapolation before they can be used in a risk-benefit assessment.[2] The data obtained from the animal studies and used in the risk-benefit assessment are on dose–response relationships and reflect the quantitative estimate of the magnitude or incidence of effect caused by a given exposure level. To extrapolate from experimental animals to humans, detailed toxicokinetic and toxicodynamic information on the compound would be needed.

45.7 Risk-benefit characterization

45.7.1 Comparing risks and benefits

In a risk-benefit assessment generally different health states or disease associated with the risks and benefits, respectively, must be compared with each other. Risks and benefits can be integrated if they are expressed in a common unit. Each health effect (beneficial as well as adverse) is expressed in the same common metric so that different effects can be balanced on the same scale. The choice of metric depends on the complexity of the assessment. In a situation where different components affect the same health effect in an individual both positively and negatively, a net effect for the health outcome can be calculated, and integrated measures might not be needed (e.g., Fransen et al.[32] and Zeilmaker et al.[33]). However, usually the challenge is how to add up different kinds of health effects. How to compare, for example, one incidence of liver cancer with hundreds of cases of gastrointestinal infection? Or, how to compare death with a decline in cognitive functioning? The clue is to weigh or value these different health effects using a valuation function that rates all health effects on the same scale. Ideally, this measure of health includes all relevant aspects of health, such as mortality, morbidity, and quality of life.

45.7.2 Metrics

Various metrics have been suggested for quantitative integration of adverse and beneficial health effects.[34] Examples include disease incidence, life expectancy, willingness to pay (WTP) to avoid an adverse health outcome and DALYs or QALYs.

Implicitly when we use a metric like this, we assume that health maximization (in terms of the metric) is our goal. Ethical and equity issues do play a role in policy decisions, but are not accounted for in a health metric.[35,36] An example would be food fortification with folic acid[20] where the health benefits of the policy end up in one population group whereas the health risks end up in another.

45.7.2.1 Disability-adjusted life year and quality-adjusted life year

DALYs[37] and quality-adjusted life years (QALYs) are heath metrics that measure health in years corrected for health. Both metrics combine elements that characterize the magnitude of the health impact: number of people affected, severity, duration, and mortality. QALY and DALY are conceptually similar metrics.[34,38] One DALY represents the loss of one year of equivalent full health. Thus a DALY can be seen as the inverse of a QALY. QALYs measure the health gained compared to not living at all, when someone lives, with or without disease. DALYs measure the health loss compared to some ideal life expressed in years lost because of premature death and health loss because someone lives with a disease. In the terminology of Gold et al.,[34] both measures are health-adjusted life years. Traditionally, QALYs have been used to compare public health treatment options at a micro-scale, whilst DALYs have been more frequently used to estimate aggregate burdens of disease across national and regional populations. In risk-benefit assessments, DALYs are the most commonly used health metric.[7]

Fig. 45.4 shows graphically how in a risk-benefit assessment the health impact can be calculated. The graph shows the health of a person in the two scenarios, a reference and an alternative. In the reference scenario, the person develops a disease and then dies. In the alternative, he/she develops other diseases later in life and then dies at an older age. The yellow area is a measure of the difference in health between the scenarios, which happens to be the absolute difference in QALYs or DALYs (depending on whether one uses QALY or DALY weights).

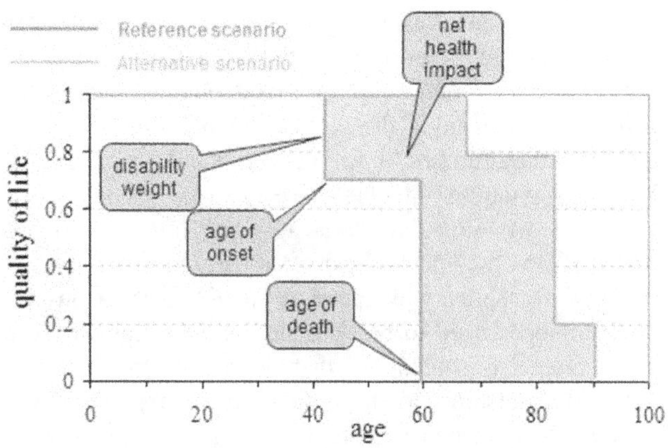

FIGURE 45.4 Representation of the health impact when a person changes his/her exposure from the reference to the alternative.

Alternatively, one can calculate the yellow area using the age of onset of the diseases, age of death, and disease weights in both scenarios. For a population, the individual health impact of every person is summed.

Quantifying beneficial health effects in terms of QALYs mean that we need to find or estimate the necessary variables. The disease weights may be found directly in the scientific literature or at websites from, for example, the WHO and the Institute for Health Metrics and Evaluation. However, in some cases—and this is particularly relevant to a context such as food-related health conditions—the precise nature of the impacts is not sufficiently defined so as to be able to define weights. For example, when animal experiments are performed with toxic substances, endpoints are measured that have no direct clinical counterpart. Sometimes this is also true for human epidemiological studies. Examples are epididymal sperm counts in rats that are exposed to dioxins or IQ tests for children whose mothers have been exposed to methylmercury via fish consumption. In order to compare these effects with other (beneficial) health effects they need to be converted in a common health measure. Obviously, this cannot be done without crude assumptions and the introduction of large and possibly unquantified uncertainties. As a result, the conversion to a clinical endpoint for which disease weights exist is not straightforward and the conversion needs to be explained.

Duration and mortality due to the disease are also demanding in their estimation and can become problematic if they depend on intake. Adverse health effects due to toxic substances are usually established through animal experiments. The first problem that needs to be solved is how the measured pathological effect in a laboratory animal can be converted to a human health effect, a health state for which we can find a quality of life weight. An ever bigger problem is that in animal experiments, age of onset and age at death are seldom measured. If it is measured we must decide how these variables can be converted to humans. Generally, it is not measured and this is a real problem. Presumably, in some cases, one can assume that the duration of a disease depends solely on the disease itself and not on, for example, the dose of the substance that causes the disease. In that case, one can estimate the duration from disease statistics from the human population. In other cases, it may be a chronic effect on offspring that starts at birth. Solutions to this problem are case-specific and often there may be no other option than using a wide range of possible ages of onset.

Incidences need to be estimated and for this we need dose–response functions that describe the relation between exposure and the probability of experiencing a health effect. In general, this is not trivial. From several epidemiological studies through a metaanalysis sometimes an association between intake and hazard ratios can be estimated, which must be converted to absolute probabilities of developing a disease. For toxicological studies with animals, usually dose–response data are available but there we have the problem that the measured endpoint must be converted to a human health effect for which we need to find a disability weight.

The assumptions have to be made clear and motivated. It is advised to perform sensitivity tests to investigate the influence of the assumptions on the final results.

45.7.2.2 Willingness to pay and willingness to accept

The WTP approach has its basis in the premise that changes in individuals' economic welfare can be valued according to what they are willing (and able) to pay to achieve that change. An alternative value measure based on the assumption of substitutability in preferences is the willingness to accept (WTA), which can be defined as the minimum amount of money the individual would require to voluntarily forgo an improvement that otherwise would be experienced.[39] In the context of risk-benefit this would be the amount of money someone would like to pay to avoid a negative health outcome. In the case of cost-benefit analysis health state is often expressed in a monetary value such as WTP or WTA. Ponce et al.[40] and Wong et al.[41] provide a general review of such metrics.

According to this assumption, individuals treat health like a special consumption good (commodity) and reveal their preferences through the choices that involve changes in the risk of health outcomes and the consumption of other economic goods whose values can be measured in monetary terms. That is, in many situations individuals act as if their preference functions include health risks as arguments, and make a variety of choices that involve trading off changes in their risk for other economic goods. When what is being changed can be measured in monetary terms, the individual WTP is revealed by these choices, which are the basis of the economic value of reductions in the risk of adverse health outcomes.

In the health economics literature, some methods for empirical estimation of WTP measures have been utilized, each providing a means to derive measures for individuals making trade-offs between risks to life and health and other consumption goods and services. The methods developed fall into two categories. The first involves inferring values for public goods through related markets, and thus relying on revealed preferences. Examples of this approach in environmental economics include travel cost models[42] and hedonic pricing.[43] The second category relies instead on constructed or hypothetical markets. These approaches are often termed, stated preference methods, with the contingent valuation method and choice experiments being currently the most popular in applied work. Environmental economists have made increasing use of stated preference methods in recent years, particularly in the fields of cost-benefit analysis, policy appraisal, and natural resource damage assessment. These methods have gained increased acceptance amongst both academic economists and policy-makers. The metric is sensitive to income and wealth. In risk-benefit assessments these metrics have hardly if at all been used.

45.7.2.3 Multicriteria analysis

There are well-established techniques to do multicriteria analysis, for example, the analytic hierarchy process methodology.[44] Typically, multicriteria methods are not used nor needed in risk-benefit assessment when the assessment is limited by heath issues only. However, when other effects are also important that are not easily incorporated in a health or monetary value, such as sustainability, then rudimentary forms of multicriteria decision analysis (MCDA) have been used, for example, Seves et al.[45] and Hollander et al.[46] Ruzante et al.[47] have proposed a framework to apply more systematically MCDA to risk-benefit assessments in foods.

45.8 Case studies

45.8.1 Fish

Fish contain various contaminants such as MeHg and dioxins, potentially causing adverse effects to human health but they also contain beneficial unsaturated fatty acids that can lower the risk of CVDs. Addressing the overall health impact of fish consumption in a risk-benefit assessment is therefore pertinent, and many publications have already addressed this dual role on human health.[14,19,26,31,33,48–52] In most of the risk-benefit publications on fish intake the same endpoints within toxicology and nutrition have been used. Some publications have also included microbiological endpoints. Increased consumption of fish is expected to lead to a decrease in the consumption of other foods, and the issue of substitution has been addressed in a few of these publications.[14,31,53] In the publications, the current consumption of fish and red and processed meat was compared with alternative scenarios in which red and processed meat were substituted with different fish species and the health impact quantified using DALYs as a common health metric. The overall findings from the mentioned publications showed an overall beneficial effect on human health from consumption of fish but also that if the intake of large predatory fish, containing high concentrations of contaminants, is proportionately high, an overall health loss can be expected. Emerging new risks in fish, such as perfluoroalkylated compounds, can also influence the risk-benefit balance.

45.8.2 Nuts

Risk-benefit assessments for an increased consumption of nuts have been performed in Denmark[54] and Sweden.[55] Nuts are often considered as a healthy and sustainable protein source.[56] The beneficial health effect is primarily found in a reduced risk of CVDs, such as coronary heart disease and strokes, but also as reduced risk for all-cause mortality and some types of cancer.[57] On the other hand, nuts may be contaminated with aflatoxin, where increased nut intake may imply exposure to unacceptable levels of this mycotoxin that increase the risk of liver cancer. Although they used somewhat different methods, both studies (Mejborn et al.[54] and Eneroth et al.[55]) assessed the health impact of increased nut consumption in terms of DALYs and found that the estimated benefits would be larger than the risks. The predicted number of cases of liver cancer is much lower than the number of CVD cases saved. As liver cancer is a serious (often fatal) disease, it is stressed that, despite the overall benefit of nut consumption, aflatoxin should be taken seriously and control measures against it remain important. As larger amounts of aflatoxin are found in some types of nuts, such as pistachios and brazil nuts, it might, for example, be recommended to limit the intake of these.

45.9 Uncertainty

In risk-benefit assessment, the available evidence is analyzed and health risks and benefit are compared, often on a common quantitative scale. Given the complexity of the underlying question and the lack of knowledge that we have in many parts of the assessment, it is inevitable that there is uncertainty associated with the conclusions of a risk-benefit assessment. In general, there are uncertainties related to the data and uncertainties related to the assessment methodologies. A major source of uncertainty lies, for example, in the dose–response relation, which, in the case of adverse health effects, can rarely be derived from experimental human data and where variation between human responses complicates the analysis of available data. In risk assessment, worst-case scenarios can be assumed, but in risk-benefit assessment the choice for such scenarios complicates a fair weighing of risks and benefits.

Consideration of uncertainty is important in risk-benefit assessment as it is in food safety risk assessment in general; the scientific assessment of the assessor should be transparent and clear to the manager, so (s)he can make a well informed decision. This has for example been recognized by EFSA, who published several documents to guide uncertainty analysis of their assessments.[58] In the tiered approach that is frequently used in risk-benefit assessment (Section 45.3.1), uncertainty is an important element in Tier 4, when the likelihood that the overall risk is larger than the benefit or vice versa has to be assessed. The QALIBRA tool has been developed as an aid to analyze the uncertainty in risk-benefit assessment.[3]

45.10 Ethics

Implicitly when we use a health metric, we assume that health maximization (in terms of the metric) is our goal. Ethical and equity issues do play a role in policy decisions, but are not accounted for in a health metric.[35,36] For example, when calculating QALYs or DALYs, the elderly are at a disadvantage, because by definition they have less life years left and thus have less opportunity to increase (health adjusted) life years. When using WTP, it may favor the rich because WTP reflects income distribution. Also, benefits and risks incorporated in one integrated measure may occur in different populations. Folic acid is a very good example[20] where the health benefits of the fortification policy end up in one population group whereas the health risks end up in another.

These are artifacts of the chosen metric and decision-makers need to be made aware of this. Thus it is important to be clear about the implicit choices that are made and always accompany the health metric with the distribution of separate adverse and beneficial health effects in subgroups expressed as incidence, mortality, and so on, and not only the overall value in some predefined metric.

45.11 Communication

Communicating the rationale behind performing a risk-benefit assessment is straightforward as it is intuitively perceived as the right thing to do. Including and combining both beneficial and adverse health effects when determining the overall health effect of a nutrient, food or diet just make very good sense.

Even though the idea of doing a risk-benefit assessment is easy to communicate, the outcome can be more difficult to disseminate to the public.[59] This is mainly due to the use of metrics, like DALY, QALY, and WTP in the risk-benefit assessment but also the uncertainty associated with the assessment. A metric like DALY is often applied for populations and it can be difficult to explain how DALY has been calculated and what it means to the individual person.[8] Furthermore, DALY is a comparative metric and to communicate a specific number of DALYs lost due to a defined intervention does not per se indicate whether this is a significant effect or not.

The uncertainty associated with the risk-benefit assessment should be identified, quantified, and communicated together with information regarding the limitations in available data and the assumptions made.[9] Nevertheless, when the outcome of the risk-benefit assessment is reported in popular media, information about uncertainty, limitations, and assumptions is often not reported. Despite issues with metrics and uncertainty, outcome based on a risk-benefit health assessment is straightforward to communicate as the assessment is only focusing on health. Expanding the risk-benefit assessment to include endpoints within economy and sustainability will certainly make the communication more challenging.

45.12 Future directions: sustainability, economy, and consumer perception

Risk-benefit assessments are often performed to answer a political or food managerial question. However, in policymaking other factors than health, like economy and sustainability are usually also taken into account. The decision whether to include, for example, economy and sustainability should be taken together with food managers and included in the risk-benefit question. Sustainability can be measured by different indicators such as CO_2 emission, land use, biodiversity, and so on, and the choice of indicator should be clearly communicated in the risk-benefit question. Similarly, economy and consumer perception can be measured in many different ways. Incorporation of data from new disciplines in the risk-benefit assessment is challenging as it makes the assessment more complex and less transparent.[9] Such incorporation is difficult using the present methodology in health-based risk-benefit assessment as more than one metric is involved. A way to overcome this is to use MCDA, where effects from different disciplines can be compared in a transparent way. An MCDA will be able to cover health, sustainability, economy, and consumer perception. However, increasing the number of disciplines and effect endpoints will inevitably lead to increased uncertainty.

References

1. Hoekstra J, Hart A, Boobis A, et al. BRAFO tiered approach for benefit-risk assessment of foods. *Food Chem Toxicol*. 2012;50(suppl 4):S684–698.
2. Boobis A, Chiodini A, Hoekstra J, et al. Critical appraisal of the assessment of benefits and risks for foods. BRAFO Consensus Working Group. *Food Chem Toxicol*. 2013;55:659–675. Available from: http://doi.org/10.1016/j.fct.2012.10.028.
3. Hart A, Hoekstra J, Owen H, et al. Qalibra: a general model for food risk–benefit assessment that quantifies variability and uncertainty. *Food Chem Toxicol*. 2013;54:4–17. Available from: http://doi.org/10.1016/j.fct.2012.11.056.
4. Tuomisto JT. Integrated benefit and risk analysis for assessing food safety and health benefit; results from QALIBRA and BENERIS. Foreword. *Food Chem Toxicol*. 2013;54:1–2.

5. Tijhuis MJ, de Jong N, Pohjola MV, et al. State of the art in benefit-risk analysis: food and nutrition. *Food Chem Toxicol.* 2012;50:5–25. Available from: http://doi.org/10.1016/j.fct.2011.06.010.
6. Verhagen H, Tijhuis MJ, Gunnlaugsdóttir H, et al. State of the art in benefit-risk analysis: introduction. *Food Chem Toxicol.* 2012;50:2–4.
7. Boué G, Guillou S, Antignac J-P, Bizec B, Membré J-M. Public health risk-benefit assessment associated with food consumption – a review. *Eur J Nutr Food Saf.* 2014;5(1):32–58. Available from: https://doi.org/10.9734/EJNFS/2015/12285.
8. Nauta MJ, Andersen R, Pilegaard K, et al. Meeting the challenges in the development of risk-benefit assessment of foods. *Trends Food Sci Technol.* 2018;76:90–100.
9. Pires SM, Boué G, Boobis A, et al. Risk benefit assessment of foods: key findings from an international workshop. *Food Res Int.* 2019;116:859–869.
10. Assunção R, Alvito P, Brazão R, et al. Building capacity in risk-benefit assessment of foods: lessons learned from the RB4EU project. *Trends Food Sci Technol.* 2019;91:541–548. Available from: https://doi.org/10.1016/j.tifs.2019.07.028.
11. Membre JM, Farakos SS, Nauta M. Risk-benefit analysis in food safety and nutrition. *Curr Opin Food Sci.* 2021;39:76–82. Available from: https://doi.org/10.1016/j.cofs.2020.12.009.
12. Verhagen H, Alonso-Andicoberry C, Assunção R, et al. Risk-benefit in food safety and nutrition–outcome of the 2019 Parma Summer School. *Int Food Res J.* 2021;141. Available from: https://doi.org/10.1016/j.foodres.2020.110073.
13. EFSA. EFSA Scientific Committee. Guidance on human health risk-benefit assessment of foods. *EFSA J.* 2010;8:1673. Available from: https://doi.org/10.2093/j.efsa.2010.1673.
14. Thomsen ST, de Boer W, Pires SM, et al. A probabilistic approach for risk-benefit assessment of food substitutions: a case study on substituting meat by fish. *Food Chem Toxicol.* 2019;126:79–96. Available from: https://doi.org/10.1016/j.fct.2019.02.018.
15. Boue G, Cummins E, Guillou S, Antignac J-P, Le Bizec B, Membré J-M. Development and application of a probabilistic risk-benefit assessment model for infant feeding integrating microbiological, nutritional, and chemical components. *Risk Anal.* 2017;37:2360–2388.
16. Codex Alimentarius Commission (CAC). *Procedural Manual.* 26th ed. Rome: FAO; 2018, Joint FAO/WHO Food Standards Programme. Available from: http://www.fao.org/3/i8608en/I8608EN.pdf.
17. IPCS. *Harmonization Project Document No. 1: IPCS Risk Assessment Terminology.* Geneva: WHO; 2004. http://www.inchem.org/documents/harmproj/harmproj/harmproj1.pdf.
18. FAO/WHO. *Food Safety Risk Analysis: A Guide for National Authorities. FAO Food and Nutrition Paper 87.* Rome: FAO; 2006. ISBN 978-92-5-105604-2.
19. Hoekstra J, Hart A, Owen H, et al. Fish, contaminants and human health: quantifying and weighing benefits and risks. *Food Chem Toxicol.* 2013;54:18–29. Available from: http://doi.org/10.1016/j.fct.2012.01.013.
20. Hoekstra J, Verkaik-Kloosterman J, Rompelberg C, et al. Integrated risk–benefit analyses: method development with folic acid as example. *Food Chem Toxicol.* 2008;46(3):893–909. Available from: http://doi.org/10.1016/j.fct.2007.10.015.
21. IARC. *IARC Monographs on the Identification of Carcinogenic Hazards to Humans (Preamble).* Lyon: IARC; 2019. Available from: https://monographs.iarc.who.int/wp-content/uploads/2019/01/Preamble-2019.pdf.
22. WHO/FAO. *Diet, Nutrition and the Prevention of Chronic Diseases. Report of the WHO/FAO Expert Consultation. WHO Technical Report Series, No. 916.* Geneva: WHO; 2003, ISBN 92 4 120916 X. Available from: https://apps.who.int/iris/bitstream/handle/10665/42665/WHO_TRS_916.pdf;jsessionid = 27ABC034CDBC5312B09F42B2932DEB74?sequence = 1.
23. Berjia FL, Hoekstra J, Verhagen H, Poulsen M, Andersen R, Nauta M. Finding the optimum scenario in risk-benefit assessment: an example on vitamin D. *Eur J Nutr Food Saf.* 2014;4(4):558–576.
24. EFSA. *EFSA Scientific Colloquium Summary Report: Risk-Benefit Analysis of Foods: Methods and Approaches.* Parma: EFSA; 2007.
25. Havelaar AH, De Hollander AEM, Teunis PFM, et al. Balancing the risks and benefits of drinking water disinfection, disability adjusted life-years on the scale. *Environ Health Perspect.* 2000;108(4):315–321.
26. Berjia FL, Andersen R, Hoekstra J, Poulsen M, Nauta M. Risk-benefit assessment of cold-smoked salmon: microbial risk vs nutritional benefit. *Eur J Food Res Rev.* 2012;2(2):49–68.
27. Boue G, Cummins E, Guillou S, Antignac J-P, Le Bizec B, Membré J-M. Public health risks and benefits associated with breast milk and infant formula consumption. *Crit Rev Food Sci Nutr.* 2018;58:1–20.
28. IPCS. *Chapter 5: Dose-response assessment and derivation of health-based guidance values. Environmental Health Criteria 240: Principles and Methods for the Risk Assessment of Chemicals in Food.* Geneva: WHO; 2009. ISBN 978 92 4 157240 8.
29. EFSA. EFSA Scientific Committee. Update: guidance on the use of the benchmark dose approach in risk assessment. *EFSA J.* 2017;15(1):4658. Available from: https://doi.org/10.2903/j.efsa.2017.4658.
30. EFSA Scientific Committee on Food and Scientific Panel on Dietetic Products, Nutrition and Allergies. *Tolerable Upper Intake Levels for Vitamins and Minerals.* EFSA; 2006. ISBN 92-9199-014-0. <https://www.efsa.europa.eu/sites/default/files/efsa_rep/blobserver_assets/ndatolerableuil.pdf>.
31. Thomsen ST, Pires SM, Devleesschauwer B, et al. Investigating the risk-benefit balance of substituting red and processed meat with fish in a Danish diet. *Food Chem Toxicol.* 2018;120:50–63. Available from: https://doi.org/10.1016/j.fct.2018.06.063.
32. Fransen H, de Jong N, Hendriksen M, et al. A tiered approach for risk-benefit assessment of foods. *Risk Anal.* 2010;30:808–816.
33. Zeilmaker MJ, Hoekstra J, van Eijkeren JCH, et al. Fish consumption during child bearing age: a quantitative risk-benefit analysis on neurodevelopment. *Food Chem Toxicol.* 2013;54:30–34. Available from: https://doi.org/10.1016/j.fct.2011.10.068.
34. Gold M, Stevenson D, Fryback DG. HALYs and QALYs and DALYs, Oh My: similarities and differences in summary measures of population health. *Annu Rev Public Health.* 2002;23:115–134.
35. Anand S, Hanson K. DALYs: efficiency vs equity. *World Dev.* 1998;26:307–310. Available from: https://doi.org/10.1016/S0305-750X(97)10019-5.
36. Brouwer W, van Exel J, Baker R, Donaldson C. The new myth: the social value of the QALY. *Pharmacoeconomics.* 2008;26:1–4. Available from: https://doi.org/10.2165/00019053-200826010-00001.
37. Murray CJ. Quantifying the burden of disease: the technical basis for disability-adjusted life years. *Bull World Health Organ.* 1994;72:429–445.

38. Sassi F. Calculating QALYs, comparing QALY and DALY calculations. *Health Policy Plan.* 2006;21:402–408.
39. Freeman AM. Economic valuation: what and why. In: Champ PA, Boyle KJ, Brown TC, eds. *A Primer on Nonmarket Valuation. The Economics of Non-Market Goods and Resources, Series 3.* Dordrecht: Springer; 2003. Available from: https://doi.org/10.1007/978-94-007-0826-6_1.
40. Ponce RA, Wong EY, Faustman EM. Quality adjusted life years (QALYs) and dose-response models in environmental health policy analysis – methodological considerations. *Sci Total Environ.* 2001;274:79–91. Available from: https://doi.org/10.1016/s0048-9697(01)00731-8.
41. Wong EY, Ponce RA, Farrow S, Bartell SM, Lee RC, Faustman EM. Comparative risk and policy analysis in environmental health. *Risk Anal.* 2003;23:1337–1349. Available from: https://doi.org/10.1111/j.0272-4332.2003.00405.x.
42. Ward FA, Beal D. *Valuing Nature with Travel Cost Models. New Horizons in Environmental Economics Series.* Cheltenham: Edward Elgar Publishing Ltd; 2000. ISBN 978 1 84064 078 6.
43. Palmquist RB, Israngkura A. Valuing air quality with hedonic and discrete choice models. *Am J Agric Econ.* 1999;81:1128–1133. Available from: https://doi.org/10.2307/1244096.
44. Saaty TL. Relative measurement and its generalization in decision making: why pairwise comparisons are central in mathematics for the measurement of intangible factors, the analytic hierarchy/network process. *Rev R Acad Cien Ser A Mat.* 2008;102:251–318. Available from: https://doi.org/10.1007/BF03191825.
45. Seves SM, Temme EHM, Brosens MCC, Zijp MC, Hoekstra J, Hollander A. Sustainability aspects and nutritional composition of fish: evaluation of wild and cultivated fish species consumed in the Netherlands. *Clim Change.* 2016;135:597–610. Available from: https://doi.org/10.1007/s10584-015-1581-1.
46. Hollander A, De Jonge R, Biesbroek S, Hoekstra J, Zijp MC. Exploring solutions for healthy, safe, and sustainable fatty acids (EPA and DHA) consumption in The Netherlands. *Sustain Sci.* 2019;14:303–313. Available from: https://doi.org/10.1007/s11625-018-0607-9.
47. Ruzante JM, Grieger KD, Woodward W, Lambertini E, Kowalcyk B. The use of multi-criteria decision analysis in food safety risk-benefit assessment. *Food Prot Trends.* 2017;37:132–139.
48. Domingo JL. Nutrients and chemical pollutants in fish and shellfish. Balancing health benefits and risks of regular fish consumption. *Crit Rev Food Sci Nutr.* 2016;56:979–988. Available from: https://doi.org/10.1080/10408398.2012.742985.
49. EFSA. EFSA Scientific Committee. Statement on the benefits of fish/seafood consumption compared to the risks of methylmercury in fish/seafood. *EFSA J.* 2015;13(1):3982. Available from: https://doi.org/10.2903/j.efsa.2015.3982 (36 pp).
50. Gao YX, Zhang HX, Li JG, et al. The benefit risk assessment of consumption of marine species based on Benefit-Risk Analysis for Foods (BRAFO)-tiered approach. *Biomed Environ Sci.* 2015;28:243–252. Available from: https://doi.org/10.3967/bes2015.035.
51. Hellberg RS, Dewitt CAM, Morrissey MT. Risk-benefit analysis of seafood consumption: a review. *Compr Rev Food Sci Food Saf.* 2012;11:490–517. Available from: https://doi.org/10.1111/j.1541-4337.2012.00200.x.
52. Sirot V, Leblanc J-C, Margaritis I. A risk-benefit analysis approach to seafood intake to determine optimal consumption. *Br J Nutr.* 2012;107:1812–1822. Available from: https://doi.org/10.1017/S0007114511005010.
53. Thomsen ST. *Risk-Benefit Assessment of Food Substitutions.* PhD Thesis. National food Institute, Technical University of Denmark; 2019. <https://orbit.dtu.dk/en/publications/risk-bene%EF%AC%81t-assessment-of-food-substitutions>.
54. Mejborn H, Jakobsen LS, Olesen PT, et al. *Helhedssyn på nødder – en risk-benefit vurdering* (in Danish). Søborg: DTU Food Institute; 2015. <http://www.food.dtu.dk//media/Institutter/Foedevareinstituttet/Publikationer/Pub-2015/Rapport_Helhedssyn-paa-noedder.ashx?la = da>.
55. Eneroth H, Wallin S, Leander K, Nilsson Sommar J, Åkesson A. Risks and benefits of increased nut consumption: cardiovascular health benefits outweigh the burden of carcinogenic effects attributed to aflatoxin B1 exposure. *Nutrients.* 2017;9(12):1355. Available from: https://doi.org/10.3390/nu9121355.
56. Willett W, Rockström J, Loken B, et al. Food in the Anthropocene: the EAT-Lancet Commission on healthy diets from sustainable food systems. *Lancet.* 2019;393(10170):447–492. Available from: https://doi.org/10.1016/S0140-6736(18)31788-4.
57. Aune D, Keum N, Giovannucci E, et al. Nut consumption and risk of cardiovascular disease, total cancer, all-cause and cause-specific mortality: a systematic review and dose-response meta-analysis of prospective studies. *BMC Med.* 2016;14(1):207. Available from: https://doi.org/10.1186/s12916-016-0730-3.
58. EFSA. EFSA Scientific Committee. Guidance on uncertainty analysis in scientific assessments. *EFSA J.* 2018;16(1):5123 (39 pp). Available from: https://doi.org/10.2903/j.efsa.2018.5123.
59. Frewer LJ, Fischer ARH, Brennan M, et al. Risk/benefit communication about food – a systematic review of the literature. *Crit Rev Food Sci Nutr.* 2016;56(10):1728–1745. Available from: https://doi.org/10.1080/10408398.2013.801337.

Chapter 46

Exposure-driven risk management strategies for chemicals in food

Samuel Benrejeb Godefroy[1,2]

[1]*Food Risk Analysis and Regulatory Excellence Platform (PARERA), Institute of Nutrition and Functional Foods (INAF), Québec, QC, Canada,*
[2]*Department of Food Sciences, Faculty of Agriculture and Food Sciences, Laval University, Quebec City, QC, Canada*

Abstract

The attribution of food-related diseases to a given chemical contaminant is difficult to establish given the lack of strong evidence documenting the negative impacts chemical substances—when present at levels of concern in food—may have on human health. This chapter reviews risk management strategies for foodborne contaminants, building on guidance developed and adopted by the Codex Alimentarius Commission (Codex), the international food standard setting body. These strategies include preventive measures and position the reliance on maximum levels (MLs), as part of a broader approach focused on contributing to reduce the exposure to target chemical contaminants. This chapter also examines guidance issued by Codex for food chemical management and attempts to discuss the introduction of performance indicators in order to assess the effectiveness of the applied management measures, including their ability to produce the sought-after outcomes. These indicators are components of a proposed logic model and are showcased with examples of interventions with the intention to reduce exposure to food chemical contaminants of environmental origin, of natural sources, and induced by food processing. Management approaches amounting to chasing low levels of contamination—which may in fact have little to no human health significance—or to focusing on enforcement of MLs in final products are not only disruptive to the food production system but yield limited impacts. Mechanisms aimed to identify and remove points of introduction or to reduce the level of contamination through targeted processing are preventive, more effective, and should be preferred.

Keywords: Chemicals in food; food chemical contamination; maximum level; performance indicators; risk management decision trees; risk ranking

46.1 Food chemical safety as an important determinant of health

Food impacts the daily life of all individuals. Issues surrounding food and health have continuously been the focus of increased public attention and public policy circles, nationally and internationally. Considerable research has been devoted to establishing the relationship between the incidence of chemicals, pathogens and nutrients in food and disease.

In the general context, where health care costs are rising rapidly in many developed economies, and where the growth of health expenditures is often higher than the growth of the gross domestic product, it is important to attempt and reduce or eliminate the costs associated with preventable diseases. Food and diet-related disease fall into this category and have been reported to constitute a considerable financial burden for all Organisation for Economic Co-operation and Development (OECD) countries.

Some examples of prominent foodborne disease are

- *Campylobacte*r, *Salmonella*, *Escherichia coli* O157 intoxications;
- variant Creutzfeldt–Jakob disease;
- chronic diseases: obesity, diabetes, cancer, heart diseases;
- immune suppression;
- allergies;
- anaphylaxis;
- neurological/developmental disorders.

The World Health Organization (WHO) has attempted to estimate the burden of disease related to food and foodborne hazards.[1] Thirty-one foodborne hazards, causing 32 distinct ailments, were included in the WHO's global estimates, that is, 11 diarrheal disease agents (1 virus, 7 bacteria, 3 protozoa), 7 invasive infectious disease agents (1 virus, 5 bacteria, 1 protozoon), 10 helminths, and 3 chemicals. Together, these 31 hazards were estimated to cause 600 million foodborne illnesses and 420,000 deaths in 2010. Among chemical hazards, aflatoxins were listed as one of the major sources of foodborne death; and, a high-burden

Present Knowledge in Food Safety. DOI: https://doi.org/10.1016/B978-0-12-819470-6.00043-3

hazard in Africa, Western Pacific, and South-East Asia. The WHO[1] estimates are regarded as conservative, due to underreporting, but also by reason of the fact that certain chronic diseases—for example, cancer, kidney failure, liver failure—resulting from contaminated food, only appear long after food ingestion; thus the causal link is rarely established. It appears, from this evaluation, that contribution of chemicals to this burden of disease is incomplete or limited on account of methodological challenges in estimating the contribution of disease and health conditions that may be negatively influenced by several possible chemical hazards.

Food has in fact been identified as a major vehicle of exposure, and in multiple instances, as the primary route of exposure to various chemical contaminants present in the environment.

Foodborne contaminants of chemical origin have been linked to health impacts, potentially affecting:

- neurological development,[2–4]
- classroom behavior,[5]
- IQ,[6–8]
- birth defects,[9]
- dementia in old age,[10]
- sexual and reproductive development,[11,12]
- kidney and liver function,[13]
- thyroid,[14,15]
- hormone balance,[16,17]
- hypertension,[18] and
- the immune system.[19]

These contaminants have also been, directly and indirectly, linked to cancer, osteoporosis, Parkinson's disease, and arthritis.

The magnitude foodborne chemical effects on morbidity and mortality in Canada, for example, has been the subject of various studies.[20,21] For instance, exposure to a single foodborne chemical such as methylmercury has been estimated to cost Canadians roughly 0.8 billion dollars annually.[22] It is also estimated that one in two Canadians will get cancer during their lifetime.[23] For both men and women, lung cancer remains the leading cause of cancer death; colorectal cancer is second, with documented foodborne chemical links in a significant number of cases.

Chronic diseases such as obesity, as well diabetes, can be influenced by chemicals like phthalates (entering in the composition of some plasticizers used in food containers), which interfere with endocrine function or homeostatic mechanisms. Hypothyroidism can be influenced by perchlorate, polychlorinated biphenyls (PCBs), and other chemicals. Unlike foodborne microbial agents, leading to acute effects, most health impacts related to chemicals in food are chronic in nature and often appear years after exposure (short and long term) to the chemical of interest. Statistics to corroborate foodborne illnesses linked to chemical contaminants are therefore much more difficult to establish given that it is difficult to single out one chemical for attribution as the unique cause of the adverse health effect. The diversity of endpoints for chemical contaminants and the cumulative/synergetic nature of potential health impacts, renders it difficult to establish the causality and therefore to develop intervention strategies with measurable outcomes on public health.

For the purposes of this chapter, *a chemical contaminant* is defined in a manner that paraphrases the definition used by the Codex Alimentarius Commission: "any chemical substance that may be present in food or feed that has **not** been added intentionally as part of any step of food production, and that could impact the overall safety or quality of the product."

46.2 Risk management measures: reduction of human exposure to target foodborne chemicals

A strategy aimed at improving health and enhancing protection through safer foods must target exposure reduction to a wide variety of chemicals entering the food supply from environmental sources or human activity.

As previously discussed, reducing exposure to foodborne chemicals will likely result in reducing the effects of four major health impacts: possible impairment of neurological development, hormonal disruption, cancer, and immune modulation. These health outcomes are in fact linked to each other. The endocrine system regulates all body functions and associations have been reported between hormones and the incidence of some types of cancer, such as breast cancer. Endocrine system imbalances affect the body's ability to defend itself against disease and are linked to disruption of the immune system. The endocrine system also impacts the development of the fetus; direct evidence has linked thyroid disorders during pregnancy with premature birth. Some chemicals such as lead, mercury, and PCBs directly impact neurological development.

Reduction of chemicals in food such as foodborne environmental contaminants, natural toxicants, and chemicals induced through food processing has become a priority for several food regulators around the world, as part of their contribution to the public health outcomes related to consumer protection and the reduction of the foodborne disease burden.

Risk management strategies were also designed to account for food production and trade considerations, ensuring that they are achievable, implementable by food business operators (FBOs), would not lead to undue food loss, and would not pose impediments to trade, internationally.

Risk management measures are generally driven by the guidance of Codex as expressed in the *General*

Standard for Contaminants and Toxins in Food and Feed, CXS 193-1995[24] which is regularly updated under the leadership of the Codex Committee on Contaminants in Food. This standard recommends to ensure that contaminant levels in food and feed be kept As low as reasonably achievable (ALARA), "through best practice such as Good Agricultural Practice (GAP) and Good Manufacturing Practice (GMP), following appropriate risk assessment." Following certain specific interventions is advocated as part of efforts to reduce contaminants in food and feed such as:

- prevention of food and feed contamination at the source, for example, by reducing environmental pollution;
- application of control measures, including technologies used in food and feed production at the various stages of the food/feed value chain; and
- application of measures to decontaminate food and feed and prevent the introduction of contaminated food and feed products to consumption.

Emphasis is made on preventive interventions, in contrast to chasing contamination in end-products. In this regard, early identification of possible points of introduction for contamination of food and feed is a key measure food producers, at every level of the production system, must apply.

Codex developed further guidance in the form of a *Code of Practice Concerning Source Directed Measures to Reduce Contamination of Food with Chemicals* (CAC/RCP 49-2001). The code raises awareness of possible sources of contamination of food and feed and of source-directed measures to prevent such contamination. These interventions are meant to drive reduction of exposure to chemicals in food and should result in a reduced reliance on the development and maintenance of MLs for contaminants in food, a subject that will be further discussed later in this chapter.

The Code of Practice offers examples to achieve ALARA, with the adoption of measures to eliminate or control the source of contamination, processing measures to reduce contaminant levels, and the identification and separation of contaminated supply from food fit for human consumption. Contaminated food is meant to be rejected for food use unless it can be reconditioned and made fit for human consumption, through acceptable processing practices. In doing so, mixing contaminated products with others that are considered acceptable is prohibited, as it would constitute a deliberate addition of a point of introduction for such chemical contamination.

As stipulated by the Code of Practice, applying preventive controls, the analysis of production and processing operations for the purposes of identifying hazards and assessing risks, is strongly encouraged. "This should lead to a determination of critical control points and the establishment of a system to monitor production at these points" as per the Hazard Analysis and Critical Control Point (HACCP) approach. Every effort should be made to not rely solely on measures of control at the end of the chain, that is, at the level of the end-product.

In some instances, and where the food supply's source of contamination appears to be unavoidable, such as sources resulting from heavy environmental contamination, leading to unacceptable level of chemical contaminants of environmental origin, it may be indispensable to take drastic measures such as "blacklisting" or banning areas of production, due to the accumulation of substances through environmental pollution that would not be possible to remove or to control with reasonable measures. "Prohibiting the production and/or sale of foods derived from such polluted areas and advising against the consumption of such foods," may be the most effective risk management approach (CAC/RCP 49-2001).

Risk management measures may need to be taken very much upstream in the food production system (CAC/RCP 49-2001) if they are to have an impact on the chemical safety of food, such as:

- control of pollutants' emissions from industry such as the chemical, mining, paper, and metal production industries;
- control of emission from sources of energy generation and use, such as power plant production, including nuclear plants and various means of transportation with high emission and particle production level; and
- control of the production, sale, use, and disposal of certain toxic, environmentally persistent substances—for example, organohalogen compounds (PCBs, brominated flame retardants) and heavy metals (lead, mercury, and cadmium).

These measures may be the only effective approach for such contaminants with an environmental source, yet, for which food is major source of exposure.

For other chemicals, such as acrylamide, which results directly from food processing conditions, the control is very much exercised during the food production stage, through the identification of the condition of formation of such chemicals—for example, ingredients that may react: asparagine and starch for acrylamide—and conditions that may favor such reactions—for example, temperature or pH. Controlling measures of production has resulted in significant reduction of process-induced chemicals, such as acrylamide.[25,26]

46.3 Managing chemicals in food beyond setting maximum levels

Effects of chemicals on human health are very much dependent on the level of exposure to these chemicals and the exposure period (chronic or acute). The level of the chemicals occurring in food and the amount and frequency of food consumed are the factors that drive exposure levels. Managing the risk of chemicals in food should therefore not be dictated by the presence of the hazard, but rather by the estimation of the possible health risks resulting from exposure. With today's analytical methods, it is possible to detect the lowest levels of chemicals, even in complex matrices such as food. Acting on the basis of such detection without understanding the source of the chemical, but more importantly their likely health impact, results in resource-intensive yet ineffective measures. When there are indications of the possible introduction of a chemical hazard into the food production system, a risk assessment is necessary to characterize the possible risks that humans consuming such food may be encountering. A thorough evaluation of management options follows and should account for their effectiveness in reducing exposure, their achievability, their cost implications, and the conditions for their sustainable application—for example, the ability of the industry to reliably comply with the measures of exposure reduction imposed.

It may be necessary to establish levels that serve as sentinels for reaching and maintaining the required threshold of exposure reduction. These levels may be used as guidance levels by industry or be set as regulatory limits or maximum levels (MLs).

Codex has developed principles that must be applied for establishing such MLs in food and feed (CXS 193-1995). These principles encompass following the Policy of the Committee on Contaminants in Food for Exposure Assessment of Contaminants and Toxins in Food and Food Groups (Section IV of the Codex Procedural Manual).[27]

MLs are to be established *only* for food in which the contaminant may be found in an amount that is significant for the total exposure of the consumer. These MLs are set in such a way that consumers are adequately protected, that is, resulting from the outputs of a health risk assessment, where health-based guidance values (HBGVs) such as tolerable daily intakes can be established for threshold chemicals.

The application of the MLs is meant to drive down exposure to the targeted chemical(s), through intervention measures identified as part of food production practices. Reduction of exposure would result in enhancing the protection of consumers and increasing the margin of exposure estimated as: Tolerable intake divided by the probable intake for a given period of time (day, week, month). The higher this level, the higher the margin of safety for consumers.

For nonthreshold chemicals, such as lead or genotoxic carcinogens, the same objective of exposure reduction is pursued. The margin of exposure can be estimated by relying on a benchmark dose identified for the chemical contaminant as part of its hazard characterization. The margin of exposure will be used to prioritize risk management activities for this chemical in food.

As described in CXS 193-1995, several considerations are made to derive MLs for chemicals in food. These include the following risk assessment outputs:

- Toxicological information: effects on human health, toxicokinetics, toxicodynamics; possible carryover of the toxic substance from feed to food;
- Analytical data: including validated qualitative and quantitative data and sampling protocols to be followed;
- Intake data: identification of food representing the major source of exposure, results of occurrence in various monitoring programs such as the total diet study (TDS) and other sources;
- Technological information: processes that support management, reduction of points of introduction or decontamination of the food, and feed supply;
- Achievability: such as costs of application and accessibility of control measures to the majority of FBOs.

It is important that reduction measures set to help achieve the MLs are available for application by FBOs, prior to imposing MLs, particularly if they are set using the regulatory instrument.

It is for this reason that Codex generally proceeds with the development of a Code of Practice, to support the reduction of exposure to a given contaminant in a food source, prior to imposing an ML.

The misunderstanding that the absence of a ML is equivalent to the absence of management requirements for a given chemical contaminant in a food continues.

Most recent food safety legislation and regulations put the onus on identifying food hazards and taking the appropriate action to mitigate risk on FBOs.[28,29]

Added guidance may be needed to help prioritize such interventions, particularly for emerging chemicals such as process-induced chemicals. Fig. 46.1 outlines a proposed risk-based approach, guiding decision-making in the management of these possible contaminants in food developed by Hanlon et al.[30] The approach calls for the development of criteria of risk ranking, availability of occurrence data, and toxicological information to support informed decisions and following a systematic decision tree to consider actions that may be required for risk mitigation.

The proposed approach calls for a holistic consideration of risk reduction, driven by the hazard characterization information used to prioritize the chemical, including by exposure levels, as well as exposure reduction that may be achievable. Although developed for process-induced chemicals, this approach has the potential to be further applied to other substances such as mycotoxins or other emerging chemicals of environmental origin.

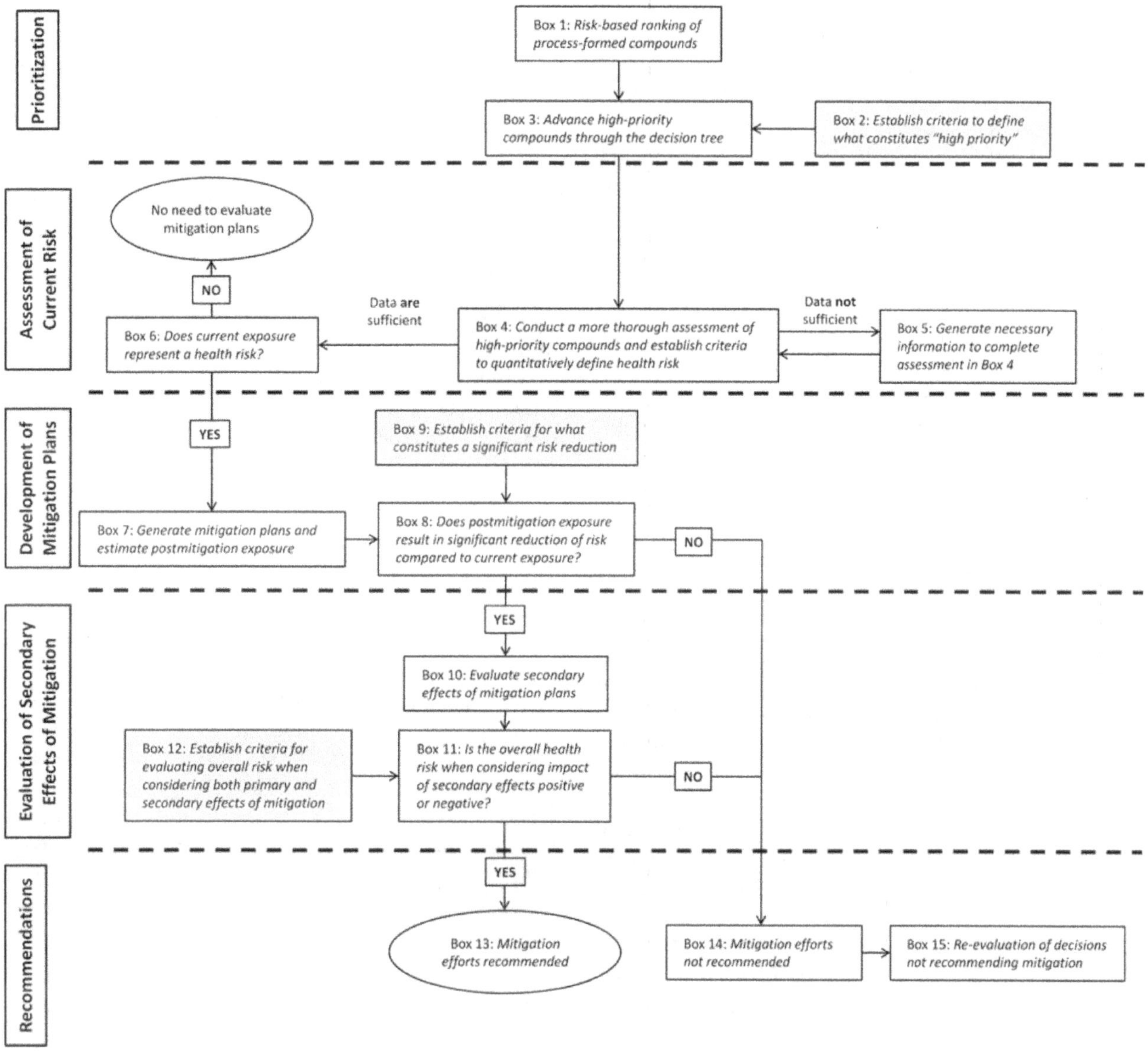

FIGURE 46.1 Final decision tree for a risk-based process for mitigation of process-formed compounds in food.[30]

Similarly, regulatory interventions should not be limited to establishing and enforcing MLs for chemicals in food. Rather, the development and implementation of food monitoring programs tracking contaminants in food, domestically produced and imported, is an important instrument of management that food regulators use for chemicals in food.

Planning and implementing Total Diet Studies (TDS) and other targeted food monitoring initiatives result in an indispensable source of data documenting the occurrence of chemicals in the food supply. The identification of unusual spikes in contaminant occurrence creates a signal for investigation and intervention by regulators. Such interventions do not necessitate the establishment of a ML but rely on risk assessments characterizing the potential health impact for a given food safety investigation involving contaminants in food.

Action can be taken in accordance with the "Guidelines for Rapid Risk Analysis Following Instances of Detection of Contaminants in Food, Where There is No Regulatory Level" or CXG 92-2019.[31]

These guidelines were established mainly for the purposes of supporting actions in the context of food import/export control and incorporate a rapid risk analysis approach using a cutoff value of 1 part per billion (ppb) or 1 μg/kg and the threshold of toxicological concern (TTC) to assess low levels of chemical exposures, and to identify if further data are required to assess human health risk. The scope of application excludes certain contaminant categories that were found unsuitable for rapid risk assessment given their chemical or toxicological properties, and in accordance with the TTC approach. Excluded chemicals encompass categories such as high potency carcinogens (i.e., aflatoxin-like, azoxy- or *N*-nitroso-compounds, benzidines), chemicals of unknown or unique structure, inorganic chemicals, metals and organometallics, proteins, steroids, nanomaterials, radioactive substances, organo-silicon compounds, and chemicals that are known or predicted to be persistent and bioaccumulate (CXG 92-2019).

Conversely, substances that would be subjected to this guideline include "contaminants that may occur in materials used or created during processing of food and that may be inadvertently present in the food (e.g., printing inks, oils/lubricants/resins used as manufacturing maintenance compounds, cleaning compounds, traces of chemicals used in the manufacturing facility); or chemicals used to mitigate specific environmental, sustainability and climate change issues, (e.g., nitrification and urease inhibitors), which have not been anticipated to be present in food" (CXG 92-2019).

The proposed approach aims primarily to develop a substantiated decision for a food consignment where a chemical is detected and where a regulatory decision is required. As such, the cutoff of 1 ppb was identified, as a trigger for action, based on the fact that a given consignment, "within a population, would only form a tenth of the standard adult daily diet, based on access to a varied diet that may contain the same food from other sources and a range of other food groups" (CXG92-2019). This cutoff value would not be suitable and would need to be further considered, for products constituting a major source of nutrition or a sole source food (e.g., infant formula).

A rapid risk assessment approach follows next, using the information available and with the required approximation needed, such as using structural properties of the chemical to predict possible HBGVs used as an appropriate threshold of no concern or reference value against which exposure levels would be compared.

A decision tree annexed to CXG 92-2019, and represented in Fig. 46.2, offers guidance for interventions by risk assessors and risk managers. Throughout the implementation of this process, it is indispensable to maintain communication between stakeholders, in particular the FBO(s) and food competent authorities that may be involved in the management of the food contaminant occurrence incident, including their risk assessment and risk management teams.

Risk assessment approaches and various levers of decision-making—for example, hypotheses, approximations—should be fully documented and made available if requested by stakeholders.

Although quite useful, it is not sure to what extent this approach is being applied in developing countries. Capacities and experience in conducting rapid chemical risk assessments need to be available and operational to carry out such functions. For this purpose, capacity building in chemical risk assessment must be developed and propagated internationally.

46.4 Performance indicators associated with reduction of exposure to chemicals in food

The simultaneous prevalence in the diet for the majority of these chemicals signals the difficulty to link the impact of an individual chemical or class of chemicals to a specific health outcome. Hence, reduction of exposure to chemicals in food cannot be easily linked to a positive impact on the ultimate public health outcomes previously described—for example, reduction of chronic diseases, IQ, incidence of cancers.

In developing a food safety strategy with the intent of reducing exposure to chemicals in food, performance indicators must be identified to better track outputs and short-/medium-term outcomes associated with interventions applied by various actors.

Fig. 46.3 presents a logic model that can be used to outline interventions, outputs, immediate-term and medium-term outcomes, as well as performance indicators used to track progress of stakeholders in their efforts to reduce exposure to target chemicals in food. This section will attempt to present some examples of performance indicators that may be considered with respect to the development of exposure and risk reduction strategies for chemical contaminants in food.

46.5 Foodborne environmental contaminants

Environmental contaminants are chemicals that accidentally or deliberately enter the environment, often, but not always, as a result of human activities. Some of these contaminants may have been manufactured for industrial use and because they are very stable they do not break down easily. If released into the environment, these contaminants may enter the food chain. Other environmental contaminants are naturally occurring chemicals, but industrial activity may increase their mobility or increase the amount available to circulate in the environment, allowing them to enter the food chain at higher levels than would otherwise occur.

A wide variety of environmental contaminants have been detected in food. These range from metals and "ionic" species like perchlorate to organic (carbon-based) substances, including the so-called "persistent organic pollutants" or POPs (named for their ability to exist in the

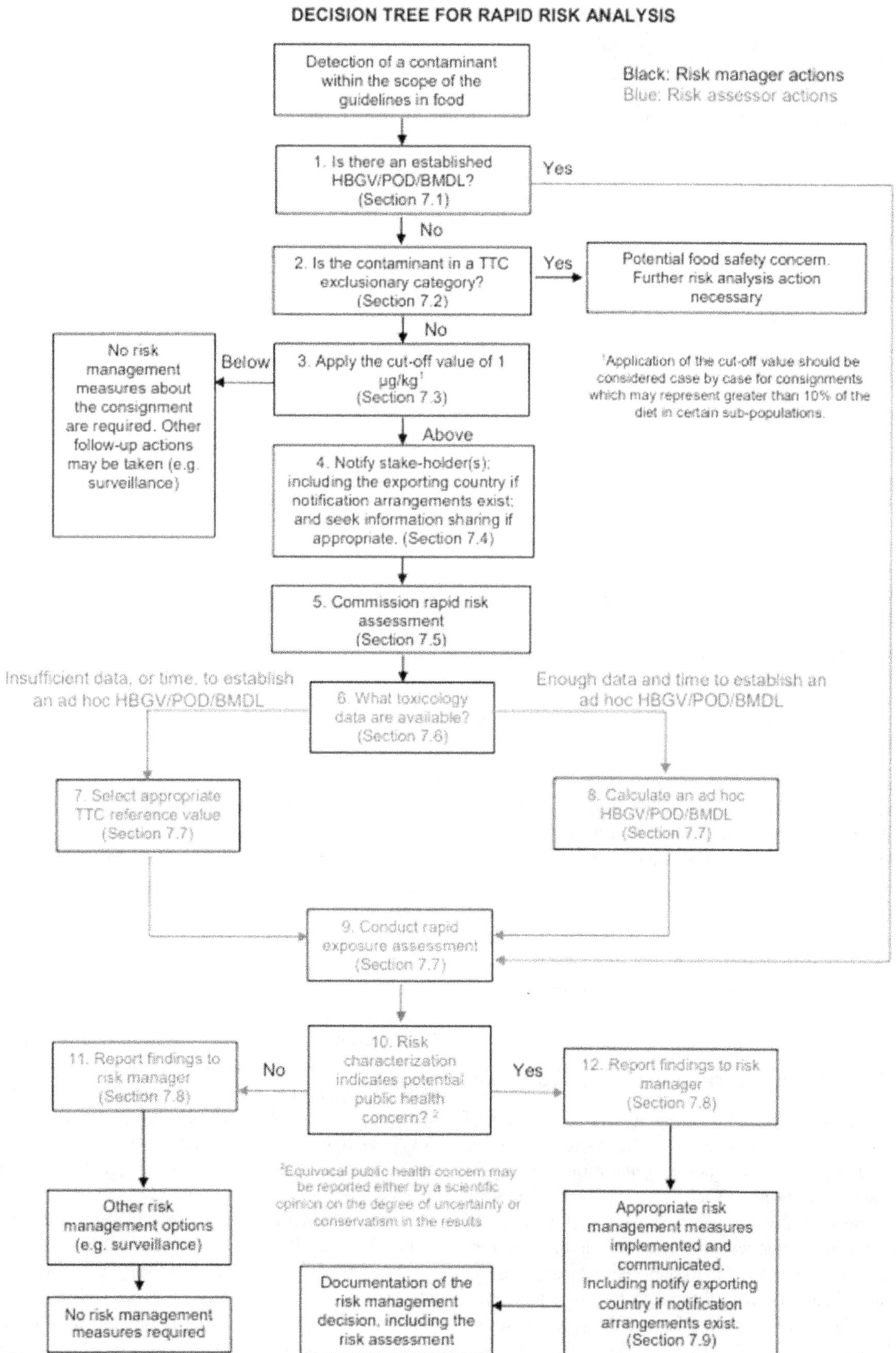

FIGURE 46.2 Decision tree for rapid risk analysis.[31]

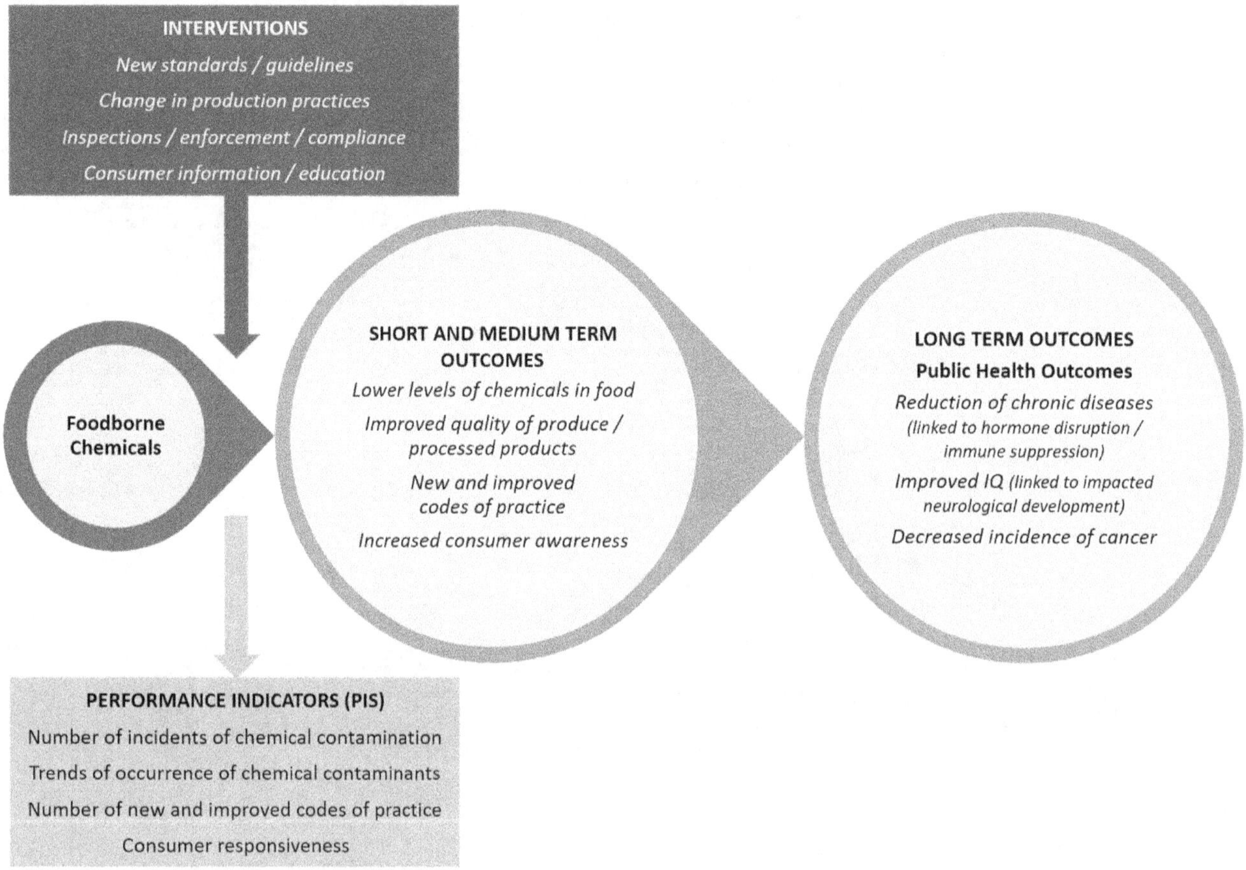

FIGURE 46.3 Logic model to support the reduction of exposure to chemicals in food.

environment for prolonged periods without breaking down). Legacy POPs such as PCBs have been banned from industrial or agricultural use in several countries, for many years, but remain in the food chain. Other POPs have been more recently identified, having been found in the environment and subsequently throughout the food chain—for example, brominated flame retardants, such as polybrominated diphenyl ethers or PBDEs.

Several chemicals constitute this category of foodborne contaminants:

46.5.1 Traditional persistent organic pollutants

Dioxins and furans are the common names for a group of chemicals that are formed during combustion processes such as waste incineration, power generation, metal production, and fuel burning. These compounds are found in small amounts in the air, water, and soil. As a result of their chemical persistence and presence in the environment, they also enter the food chain. Human exposure to dioxins and furans is mainly through the diet. PCBs are man-made chemicals that were banned from manufacture in North America in 1977. They are very persistent and can be transported over long distances. As a result, they are found throughout the environment. Humans are still exposed to small amounts of PCBs, primarily through some of the foods that we eat. Food surveillance and monitoring efforts have enabled to determine human exposure levels to these chemicals through food sources. Various risk management efforts have been underway to ensure that humans' exposure to these chemicals is continuously minimized. Specifically, the use of these substances has been banned for over 20 years in North America and other parts of the world.

Additional control measures have also been specifically designed for food sources, namely MLs, have been adopted by various food regulatory agencies to ensure that levels of PCBs and dioxins in food do not reach levels of health concern. These MLs seem to have minimum effectiveness when the intervention measures to reduce foodborne exposure are predominantly upstream in the food production system and therefore not under the control of the FBO.

Food surveillance and monitoring activities, aiming to measure and follow levels of these substances in food, tend to be far more effective to support the identification of higher areas of contamination and take measures to exclude certain sources of ingredients or food from the production cycle (reduction through identification of points of introduction and exclusion where possible). The TDS, a comprehensive food surveillance activity conducted in various countries, generally includes dioxins, furans, and PCBs as part of the targeted chemicals regularly measured in food making up the diets being surveyed. Data stemming from TDS conducted in Canada over the last 10 years have demonstrated a steady decrease in intake of legacy POPs, showing the effectiveness of risk mitigation strategies at the point of introduction (i.e., bans and limiting use of these chemicals).[32]

Given that these chemicals tend to accumulate in the fatty portions of animal-derived foods, additional measures are also taken in the form of targeted advice to consumers where needed. For example, food preparation instructions may be developed for meat and fish in ways that minimize exposure to fat. Additional consumption advice may also be issued for sport fish, where there is a presumption of accumulation of these chemicals in fish tissue in lakes and rivers. However, and in general, following a balanced diet with consumption of a variety of foods from each food group constitutes the best risk mitigation strategy to minimize human exposure to these chemicals from food sources, for the general population.

46.5.2 Emerging persistent organic pollutants—examples of polybrominated diphenyl ethers and perfluorinated chemicals

PBDEs are commercially produced substances that are used as flame retardants in a wide variety of consumer products. These compounds are very persistent in the environment. Available information indicates that the primary sources of human exposure to PBDEs are indoor air, indoor dust, and food, including human milk. Evaluation of the risks associated with the levels of PBDEs in foods consumed by populations—for example, in Canada,[33] China,[34] Nigeria,[35] and Europe[36]—concluded that these levels are not considered to pose a risk to human health. Nevertheless, continued surveillance and monitoring activities have been maintained to measure this class of chemicals in the environment and food and to support the development of additional measures, if required, to further minimize human exposure to this class of chemicals through food sources.

Perfluorinated chemicals (PFCs) are also man-made chemicals, used in commercial and consumer products and various industrial applications. Perfluorooctane sulfonate (PFOS) is perhaps the most well-known PFC and has been used, among other things, as a water, stain, and oil repellent for textiles, carpet, and food packaging, a surfactant in the electroplating industry, and an additive in fire-fighting foams. Due to their persistence and widespread use, PFCs have also been detected at low concentrations in the environment, food, and in human blood in different countries.

Interventions to reduce exposure to these classes of environmental contaminants will likely continue to be mostly related to terminating industrial production of certain flame retardants such as PBDEs or water repellents such as PFOS, as well as the safe disposal of current identified reservoirs. They may also encompass further recommendations or actions related to food production practices such as improved control of these contaminants in feed and by consequence in animal-derived foods.

Performance indicators must be developed to measure the impacts of such interventions. It is expected that tracking the reduction of occurrence for major representatives of flame retardants such as PBDEs will be easier than dioxins and furans since they have shorter half-lives. Food monitoring and surveillance activities need to be developed and maintained for food and feed sources where these chemicals have been mostly reported (i.e., animal-derived food). These monitoring activities may be extended to reach the earliest stages of food production, that is, animal feed. Biomonitoring activities such as measuring these chemicals in samples of blood serum or human milk will also be useful to measure the extent of overall exposure to these classes of chemicals from all sources. It would also enable, where possible, to attribute effects of reduction of exposure through food sources. Some of the monitoring parameters will therefore be:

- trends of reduction of levels of PBDEs in feed/food of animal origin over time;
- trends of reduction of PBDEs and PFCs in human milk and blood, over time.

46.5.3 Heavy metals such as mercury (and methylmercury)

Mercury is a naturally occurring metal in soil, rocks, and water bodies. It can also be released into the environment as a result of human activities involving combustion processes such as coal-fired power generation, metal mining, and waste incineration. The most common source of human exposure to mercury is the consumption of certain types of fish.

Mercury exists in different chemical forms. Metallic mercury or elemental mercury is the silvery, shiny liquid that was once commonly used in, for example, thermometers. Other forms of mercury can be classified as either "inorganic" or "organic." Inorganic mercury includes inorganic mercury salts such as mercuric chloride (chemical symbol: $HgCl_2$). Mercury is classified as organic when it is bound to a chemical species that is largely comprised of carbon. For example, ethylmercury (chemical symbol: $CH_3CH_2Hg^+$) is the active ingredient in a preservative used in vaccines. Methylmercury (chemical symbol: CH_3Hg^+) is another organic form of mercury that can be found in the aquatic environment, although normally at much lower levels than inorganic mercury.

Mercury is not locked permanently in each of its different forms. Rather, various processes result in environmental cycling of mercury among its different chemical forms. For example, microbial activity is one process that can transform inorganic mercury to methylmercury.

With respect to the types of mercury found in fish, both inorganic and organic mercury may be present. However, methylmercury is the predominant form of mercury in fish. Its chemical properties allow it to rapidly diffuse and tightly bind to proteins in aquatic biota, including the proteins in the muscle tissue of fish. This leads to bioaccumulation in the fish, with the mercury level increasing with age of the fish. In turn, biomagnification along the food chain leads to higher mercury levels in piscivorous fish that are higher in the food chain than in fish and other organisms that are low in the food chain. Inorganic mercury can also bioaccumulate but to a far lesser extent than methylmercury.

When ingested, organic mercury such as methylmercury, unlike elemental or inorganic forms, is almost completely absorbed from the gastrointestinal tract and distributed to all tissues. Methylmercury also readily crosses both the blood–brain barrier and the placenta. Some of the distributed methylmercury can be converted to inorganic mercury, mainly by microflora in the intestines.[37] A wide range of adverse health effects has been observed in humans following methylmercury exposure. The severity of these effects is largely dependent upon the magnitude of the dose and the duration of exposure. The central and peripheral nervous systems are generally considered to be the target organs of organic mercury-induced toxicity in humans.

Risk assessments related to the health effects of foodborne mercury [38–41] concluded that the major source of exposure to foodborne mercury is fish. Regular consumption by women of child-bearing age, of certain fish species such as predatory species, for example, barracuda, escolar, marlin, sea bass, shark, swordfish, bigeye tuna, and "fresh" tuna would lead to the provisional tolerable daily intake established for methylmercury to be exceeded by this subset of the population.

It was also found that it is possible to maintain an acceptable level of exposure to mercury by excluding certain fish, that may be highly contaminated from the regular consumption of the general population. Adopting a ML for mercury in fish was deemed to be a feasible and effective approach of risk management.[38] Not only does it drive exposure down, but it is also achievable, as most fish available in international markets were shown to achieve the set MLs by Codex.

Continued scrutiny of the level of mercury in fish through monitoring programs is needed to ensure that human exposure to this contaminant through food sources is maintained at low levels and to ensure the continued effectiveness of the imposed MLs amongst other risk management measures.

In establishing performance indicators for such efforts of reduction of food chemical exposure, examples of measures include:

- number and scope of compliance programs;
- percentage of compliance of food products (particularly fish and seafood) with standards/guidelines;
- measure of awareness of the food industry of the MLs allowed throughout the production chain;
- measure of consumer awareness of the advice offered;
- trends of reduction of levels of mercury in food (fish and seafood commodities in particular).

46.6 Natural toxicants

These chemicals are also broad and varied in nature—for example, mycotoxins, seafood toxins, phytotoxins. For some of these toxins, the main concern is related to adverse effects associated with acute exposure but, in most cases, the main focus of concern is related to potential disease outcomes resulting from long-term or chronic exposure to specific natural toxins.

Mycotoxins are toxic secondary metabolites that are naturally produced by certain types of fungi and that are associated with health disorders in animal and human beings. Most mycotoxins are chemically stable and survive food processing. Several hundred different mycotoxins have been identified, but the most commonly observed mycotoxins in food and feed, which present a concern for human health and livestock, include: aflatoxins, ochratoxin A, patulin, fumonisins, zearalenone, and nivalenol/deoxynivalenol.

Mycotoxins appear in the food chain as a result of molds infection of crops both before and after harvest. Consequently, mycotoxins can be found on numerous foodstuffs such as cereals, dried fruits, nuts, and spices.

Phycotoxins are complex chemicals produced by eukaryotic and prokaryotic algal organisms. Like mycotoxins, phycotoxins are secondary metabolites. These metabolites may be toxic to other living organisms, including humans. They will bioaccumulate in tissues when ingested by higher trophic animals all along the food chain. Besides, these compounds can undergo modifications all along the food chain which complicates their identification/quantification. Major phycotoxins include:

- domoic acid that causes amnesic shellfish poisoning;
- saxitoxins, causing paralytic shellfish poisoning;

- okadaic acid, one of the primary causes of diarrhetic shellfish poisoning;
- ciguatoxins, causing ciguatera, is present in tropical waters;
- brevitoxins, maitotoxins, and so on.

As is the case for most chemicals described above, it is difficult to accurately quantify the specific effects of intervention strategies on decreased morbidity and mortality due to numerous other confounding factors.

Depending on the nature of the toxin of interest and the food commodities of focus, intervention strategies will target:

- the introduction and application of codes of practice to reduce/eliminate conditions of toxin formation and persistence at the producer level (on-farm HACCP-like programs),
- the development of standards and guidelines or tolerances both at the point of production and the point of food sale;
- advice to consumers on food storage and handling.

Example of such interventions were applied to manage patulin in apples (and derived products: juices, etc.), ochratoxins in cereals, fumonisins in cereals and animal-derived foods, and biotoxins in seafood.

Performance indicators applied to reduction of exposure to selected natural toxicants could therefore focus on

- reduction of incidents of acute exposure to natural toxins, including seafood toxins;
- rate of compliance with any newly developed standard and guideline;
- number of codes of practice developed and applied (e.g., patulin in apples, ochratoxins in cereal);
- trend of reduction of levels of selected natural toxins in food commodities;
- industry awareness of codes of practice and their application at the various stages of the food continuum; and
- consumer awareness and uptake of advice developed.

46.7 Chemicals induced by food processing

In recent years, increasing concerns have been raised regarding the potential formation of certain chemicals as a result of normal cooking, heating, fermentation, or other food processing operations. Examples of such chemicals include acrylamide, furan, and chloropropanols.

For some of these substances, risk mitigation strategies have been developed and are being implemented at the national and international level (chloropropanols). For some others, significant gaps remain to better characterize hazards and risks. A proactive approach is therefore favored to mitigate potential risks (e.g., risks associated with acrylamide, a suspected genotoxic carcinogen) involving all stakeholders and consumers.

Interventions generally focus on the identification of the conditions of formation of these process-induced chemicals in food. Measures are then developed to better control production conditions to reduce such occurrence. These measures vary from considering better selection of sourced ingredients (e.g., specific species of potatoes destined to produce industrially made French fries or potato chips), or the introduction of new additives such as asparaginase, which is an enzyme that "quenches" the Maillard reaction, responsible for the production of acrylamide at high temperatures in corn-based chips—for example, updated cooking temperatures, or pH conditions—have also been identified as potential intervention measures to reduce acrylamide in food, including in home preparation settings.

As a result, performance indicators of exposure reduction may be considered as follows:

- trend of reduction in the level of acrylamide found in foods, considered to be the major contributors to exposure;
- trends of awareness by targeted food industry (manufacturers of commodities considered to be the largest contributors to exposure);
- industry workplans to reduce acrylamide in foods;
- change of consumer behavior as a result of increased awareness of risks associated to acrylamide in foods and suggested mitigation options.

46.8 Conclusion

Managing the risks associated with the occurrence of chemicals in food continues to be a public health priority. Risk management measures generally follow the guidance issued by Codex with the intent to drive to contaminants level in food ALARA. Preventive measures need to be applied through best practice propagated by GAP and GMP at all stages of food production. Preventing points of introduction of chemicals in food should remain a focus in conjunction with some interventions required significantly upstream in the food production system due to the nonfood production–related nature of the occurrence of such contaminants. As such, food production systems must adapt to such possible occurrences with appropriate preventive measures.

Because of the ubiquitous nature of chemical contamination in food, it is imperative that risk management strategies are not driven by the mere presence of the hazard through detection using increasingly sophisticated analytical technologies. When there is the indication of the possible introduction of a chemical hazard into the food production system, a risk assessment is necessary to characterize the possible risks posed to humans consuming such food. A thorough evaluation of management options should follow in consideration of their achievability, cost implication, and sustainability of application (i.e., the ability of FBOs to reliably comply with the measures of exposure reduction imposed).

Imposing MLs for contaminants in food, when certain conditions are fulfilled, may be an effective measure to drive exposure to chemical contaminants down. But the absence of a ML should not be perceived as equivalent to the absence of risk management requirements for a given chemical contaminant in a food. Preventive controls imposed by most recent food legislation such as the United States Food Safety Modernization Act (FSMA) or the Safe Food for Canadians Act (SFCA) puts the onus on the FBOs to identify and manage hazards that are likely to be introduced into food, including all potential chemical contaminants.

Guidance continues to be developed to adopt risk-based approaches in ranking chemical hazards and developing associated mitigation strategies by FBOs. Performance indicators need to accompany such measures to support the review of their effectiveness and the enhancement of their performance. Investing in capacity building programs is also a must, to further support food regulators in adopting Codex-aligned strategies for risk management of chemicals in food. More specifically, investments are needed in building competencies capable to apply the guidance on rapid risk analysis as part of incident management strategies related to the occurrence of chemicals in food.

References

1. WHO. WHO estimates of the global burden of foodborne diseases: foodborne disease burden epidemiology reference group 2007–2015. Available at <https://apps.who.int/iris/bitstream/handle/10665/199350/9789241565165_eng.pdf?sequence = 1>; 2015.
2. Grandjean D, Landrigan PJ. Developmental neurotoxicity of industrial chemicals. *Lancet*. 2006;368:2167–2178. Available at <https://www.sciencedirect.com/science/article/abs/pii/S0140673606696657>.
3. MacLusky NJ, Hajszan T, Leranth C. The environmental estrogen Bisphenol A inhibits estradiol-induced hippocampal synaptogenesis. *Environ Health Perspect*. 2005;113:675–679.
4. Schantz SL, Gardiner JC, Gasior DM, et al. Much ado about something: the weight of evidence for PCB effects on neuropsychological function. *Psychol Schs*. 2004;41:669–679. Available at <https://onlinelibrary.wiley.com/doi/abs/10.1002/pits.20008>.
5. Khan K, Factor-Litvak P, Wasserman GA, et al. Manganese exposure from drinking water and children's classroom behavior in Bangladesh. *Environ Health Perspect*. 2011;119(10):1501–1506. Available at <https://ehp.niehs.nih.gov/doi/full/10.1289/ehp.1003397>.
6. Sharma DC. Manganese in drinking water. Higher doses may hamper intellectual function. *Environ Health Perspect*. 2006;114:A50.
7. Stewart PW, Lonky E, Reihman J, et al. The relationship between prenatal PCB exposure and intelligence (IQ) in 9-year-old children. Environ. Health Perspect. 2008;113:1416–1422. Available at <https://ehp.niehs.nih.gov/doi/full/10.1289/ehp.11058>.
8. Carrington C, Devleesschauwer B, Gibb HJ, et al. Global burden of intellectual disability resulting from dietary exposure to lead, 2015. 2019. Available at <https://www.sciencedirect.com/science/article/abs/pii/S0013935119300957>.
9. Brender JD, Weyer PJ. Agricultural compounds in water and birth defects. *Water Health*. 2016;3:144–152. Available at <https://link.springer.com/article/10.1007/s40572-016-0085-0>.
10. Lee DH, Porta M, Lind L, et al. Neurotoxic chemicals in adipose tissue: a role in puzzling findings on obesity and dementia. *Neurology*. 2018;90:176–182. Available at <https://n.neurology.org/content/90/4/176.abstract>.
11. Main KM, Mortensen GK, Kaleva MM, et al. Human breast milk contamination with phthalates and alterations of endogenous reproductive hormones in infants three months of age. *Environ Health Perspect*. 2006;114(2):270–276. Available at <https://ehp.niehs.nih.gov/doi/full/10.1289/ehp.8075>.
12. Swan SH, Main KM, Liu F, et al. Decrease in anogenital distance among male infants with prenatal phthalate exposure. *Environ Health Perspect*. 2005;113:1056–1061.
13. Selmanoglu G, Karacaoglu E, Kilic A, et al. Toxicity of food contaminant furan on liver and kidney of growing male rats. *Environ Toxicol*. 2011;27(10):613–622. Available at <https://onlinelibrary.wiley.com/doi/abs/10.1002/tox.20673>.
14. Dahl R. NAS reports of perchlorate safety. *Environ Health Perspect*. 2005;113:A449.
15. Duntas LH, Chemical contamination and the thyroid. Endocrine. 2015;48:53–64. Available at <https://link.springer.com/article/10.1007/s12020-014-0442-4>.
16. Barrett JR. Pancreatic effects of EDCs. Low doses can impair glucagon secretion. *Environ Health Perspect*. 2005;113:A544.
17. Casals-Casas C, Desvergne B. Endocrine disruptors: from endocrine to metabolic disruption. *Annu Rev Physiol*. 2011;73:135–162. Available at <https://www.annualreviews.org/doi/abs/10.1146/annurev-physiol-012110-142200>.
18. Cheng Y, Schwartz J, Sparrow D, et al. Bone lead and blood lead levels in relation to baseline blood pressure and the prospective development of hypertension: the Normative Aging Study. *Am J Epidemiol*. 2001;153(2):164–171.
19. Quinete N, Hauser-Davies RA. Drinking water pollutants may affect the immune system: concerns regarding COVID-19 health effects. *Environ Sci Pollut Res*. 2021;28:1235–1246. <https://link.springer.com/article/10.1007/s11356-020-11487-4>.
20. Donaldson SG, Van Oostdam J, Tikhonov C, et al. Environmental contaminants and human health in the Canadian Arctic. *Sci Total Environ*. 2010;408:5165–5234. Available at <https://www.sciencedirect.com/science/article/abs/pii/S0048969710004559>.
21. Muir T, Zegarac M. Societal costs of exposure to toxic substances: economic and health costs of four case studies that are candidates for environmental causation. *Environ Health Perspect*. 2001;109:885–903.
22. Trasande L, Landrigan PJ, Schechter C. Public health and economic consequences of environmental methyl mercury toxicity to the developing brain. *Environ Health Perspect*. 2005;113:590–596.

23. Canadian Cancer Society/National Cancer Institute of Canada. Canadian Cancer Statistics 2019. ISSN 0835-2976. Available at: https://cdn.cancer.ca/-/media/files/research/cancer-statistics/2019-statistics/canadian-cancer-statistics-2019-en.pdf.
24. Codex Alimentarius. General standard for contaminants and toxins in food and feed, CXS 193-1995. Available at <http://www.fao.org/fao-who-codexalimentarius/sh-proxy/en/?lnk = 1&url = https%253A%252F%252Fworkspace.fao.org%252Fsites%252Fcodex%252FStandards%252FCXS%2B193-1995%252FCXS_193e.pdf>; 2019.
25. FAO/WHO. Joint FAO/WHO Expert Committee on food additives. Available at <http://www.fao.org/3/at877e/at877e.pdf>; 2005.
26. Taeymans D, Wood J, Ashby P, et al. A review of acrylamide: an industry perspective on research, analysis, formation, and control. *Crit Rev Food Sci Nutr.* 2010;44(5):323–347. Available at <https://www.tandfonline.com/doi/abs/10.1080/10408690490478082>.
27. Codex Alimentarius. Procedural manual. Available at <http://www.fao.org/3/i5079e/i5079e.pdf>; 2015.
28. SFCR. Safe food for Canadians regulations. Available at <https://laws-lois.justice.gc.ca/eng/regulations/SOR-2018-108/index.html>; 2019.
29. US FSMA. Food Safety Modernization Act. Available at <https://www.fda.gov/food/food-safety-modernization-act-fsma/full-text-food-safety-modernization-act-fsma>; 2011.
30. Hanlon P, Brorby GP, Krishan M. A risk-based strategy for evaluating mitigation options for process-formed compounds in food: workshop proceedings. *Int J Toxicol.* 2016;35:358–370. <https://journals.sagepub.com/doi/10.1177/1091581816640262>.
31. Codex Alimentarius. Guidelines for rapid risk analysis following instances of detection of contaminants in food where there is no regulatory level, CXG 92-2019. Available at <http://www.fao.org/fao-who-codexalimentarius/sh-proxy/en/?lnk = 1&url = https%253A%252F%252Fworkspace.fao.org%252Fsites%252Fcodex%252FStandards%252FCXG%2B92-2019%252FCXG_092e.pdf>; 2019.
32. Health Canada. Total diet study concentrations. Available at <http://www.hc-sc.gc.ca/fn-an/surveill/total-diet/concentration/index-eng.php>; 2009.
33. Gill U, Chu I, Ryan JJ, Feeley M. Polybrominated diphenyl ethers: human tissue levels and toxicology. *Rev Environ Contam Toxicol.* 2004;183:55–97.
34. Zhang L, Li J, Zhao Y, et al. Polybrominated diphenyl ethers (PBDEs) and indicator polychlorinated biphenyls (PCBs) in foods from China: levels, dietary intake, and risk assessment. *J Agric Food Chem, 2013.* 2013;61:6544–6551. Available at <https://pubs.acs.org/doi/abs/10.1021/jf4006565>.
35. Babalola BA, Adeyi AA. Levels, dietary intake and risk of polybrominated diphenyl ethers (PBDEs) in foods commonly consumed in Nigeria. *Food Chem.* 2018;265:78–84. Available at <https://www.sciencedirect.com/science/article/abs/pii/S0308814618308823>.
36. EFSA. Scientific Opinion on polybrominated diphenyl ethers (PBDEs) in food. *EFSA J.* 2011;9:2156–2430. Available at <https://efsa.onlinelibrary.wiley.com/doi/abs/10.2903/j.efsa.2011.2156>.
37. Clarkson TW, Magos L, Myers GJ. The toxicology of mercury—current exposures and clinical manifestations. *N Engl J Med.* 2003;349(18):1731–1737.
38. Health Canada. Human health risk assessment of mercury in fish and health benefits of fish consumption. Available at <https://www.canada.ca/content/dam/hc-sc/migration/hc-sc/fn-an/alt_formats/hpfb-dgpsa/pdf/nutrition/merc_fish_poisson-eng.pdf>; 2007.
39. Juric AK, Batal M, David W, et al. A total diet study and probabilistic assessment risk assessment of dietary mercury exposure among First Nations living on-reserve in Ontario, Canada. *Environ Res.* 2017;158:409–420. Available at <https://www.sciencedirect.com/science/article/abs/pii/S0013935117307545>.
40. Kwon YM, Lee HS, Yoo DC, et al. Dietary exposure and risk assessment of mercury from the Korean Total Diet Study. *J Toxicol Environ Health, Part A Curr.* 2009;72:1484–1492. Available at <https://www.tandfonline.com/doi/abs/10.1080/15287390903213061>.
41. Cheng Z, Wang HS, Du J, et al. Dietary exposure and risk assessment of mercury via total diet study in Cambodia. *Chemosphere.* 2013;92:143–149. Available at <https://www.sciencedirect.com/science/article/abs/pii/S0045653513003159>.

Chapter 47

Role of human epidemiology in risk assessment and management

Alfons Ramel
Faculty of Food Science and Nutrition, University of Iceland, Reykjavik, Iceland

Abstract
Conventions for assessing human health risks for contaminants, food additives, and other regulated products have largely centered around using animal experiments. Under this framework, epidemiological studies in humans, particularly observational studies, are often considered a secondary source of evidence. In this chapter, it is argued that the major strength of both observational and experimental studies in humans lies in their high external validity. That is if properly used and integrated with other lines of evidence the uncertainty of the animal to human extrapolation can be reduced or even eliminated. The limitations of assessing evidence by study design are explained with different examples. Areas of uncertainty associated with characterizing risk based on a few selected studies, judged to be of high quality, are also discussed. It is concluded that to allow for better integration of human epidemiology in risk assessment further development of evidence-based medicine should provide more room for expert judgment and mechanistic understanding.

Keywords: Epidemiology; toxicology; nutrition; evidence-based medicine; risk assessment

Chapter points

- The methodological principles and approaches for conducting epidemiological studies in humans and studies in animals are in general more comparable than different. The main difference relates to less controlled settings when studying free-living humans.
- The use of human studies greatly reduces or eliminates the need of animal to human extrapolation. This advantage comes at the expense of a higher risk of bias in both human observational and experimental studies.
- Adopting methodology from evidence-based medicine, such as ranking studies by design and appraising studies in terms of risk of bias, is both systematic and transparent. This methodology does, however, have its limitations and it should not replace expert judgment.
- All studies, both experimental and observational, suffer from different sources of bias. Emphasis should be placed on extracting relevant information from different studies, taking advantage of their designs, and weighing the evidence appropriately. The *Method of Triangulation* is one good example of such an approach.
- Developing more flexible frameworks for evidence synthesis using the benefits of evidence-based medicine while taking advantage of methods where expert judgment and biology play the main role is needed. This would lead to a more robust use of epidemiology in food safety assessment.

47.1 Introduction

Epidemiology is "*the study of the distribution and determinants of health states or events in specified populations and the application of this study to control of health problems*".[1] This definition covers both experimental and observational studies and the word "population" can equally refer to other species than humans. However, different terminology used by those working with animals and humans makes the methodological differences across the two disciplines often seem greater than it is. Failure to understand these differences may hamper evidence integration in food safety assessments.[2]

In food safety, observational studies are often used when assessing biological hazards,[3] deriving tolerable upper intake levels for nutrients[4] and for assessing the safety of chemicals in veterinary medicine in target species.[5] However, for assessing the risk of regulated products and contaminants, the methodological approach used has largely centered around controlled animal

Present Knowledge in Food Safety. DOI: https://doi.org/10.1016/B978-0-12-819470-6.00062-7

experiments. For assessing new substances this framework is logical as human experiments cannot be performed and observational studies can only be conducted post-authorization. Once human observational studies become available they are, however, often considered a secondary source of evidence.

Although studies in experimental animals are strong on causality, the interspecies extrapolation is subject to considerable uncertainty[6] and it is in this context that human epidemiology plays a major role. Epidemiological studies in humans are, however, prone to certain types of biases[a] and they are characterized by large between-subject variability.[b] It can be argued that these methodological complexities reflect the cost of observing or experimenting on free-living humans. Using conventions developed for toxicological studies may therefore not be the most optimal way to assess and interpret those studies. Still, previous work focusing on the integration of epidemiological studies in food safety is often centered on how "*tailoring epidemiologic studies to the risk assessment procedures*" can be achieved[7]; or highlighting their numerous limitations seen from the perspective of regulatory toxicology.[8,9] Although such work provides useful insight, many of the solutions proposed in such papers are impossible to implement in praxis.

Instead of focusing on how to fit epidemiological studies into the existing risk assessment paradigm, recent developments include an emphasis on evidence-based medicine[10] and a weight of evidence approach.[11] Both approaches require a transdisciplinary approach for assessing risk and, if used for guidance instead of replacing expert judgment, these methodologies may offer some way forward. This chapter aims to reflect on why human epidemiological studies are important to consider in any food safety assessment and how they could be more effectively integrated.

47.2 External validity – nice to have or needed?

The main strength of using evidence from experimental and observational studies in humans is that any effect or association observed, respectively, is observed in the target species. Although observational studies are prone to confounding, to a varying degree, proper evaluation of such studies may still reduce uncertainty and in some cases eliminate the need for an animal to human extrapolation. This strength is often overlooked by risk assessors, that are more concerned with certainty on causality and having unbiased effect estimates, to derive a health-based guidance value. The resulting accuracy[c] of the animal to human extrapolation is on the other hand often given less weight. That is, external validity touches on two key issues that any risk assessment has to address, namely establishing (1) if the agent being assessed is causally related to adverse health outcomes in humans; and (2) deriving as accurate a threshold of exposure as possible where no meaningful risk to health will occur.

In terms of establishing causality, human studies generally perform worse than animal studies, as there are far more limitations on what type of experimental conditions can be used, i.e., duration of the study, ensuring compliance, and performing examinations such as histopathology or measuring organ weights. On the other hand, a causal effect in a certain animal species may not necessarily be reproducible or relevant for humans. Although a thorough understanding of the mode of action and biological differences between the two species may reduce that uncertainty, it can never be fully eliminated. On this front, results from the pharmaceutical industry provide some insight into this dilemma. This can be achieved by comparing results from preclinical studies in animals, assessing the safety of potential candidate drugs, with results from randomized controlled trials (RCTs) in humans for the same drugs that have passed the preclinical stage. One such comparison of preclinical and clinical studies[6] estimated that around half of the candidate drugs that passed preclinical trials, failed to proceed after human clinical trials due to unanticipated human toxicity (see Fig. 47.1). For this particular comparison, the use of the term "human toxicity" may not necessarily reflect the complete failure of the preclinical testing to detect toxicity as other factors may influence the decision on which candidate drugs are taken further. Still, a similar picture also emerges when looking at adverse events of pharmaceuticals post-marketing. In a review of 93 serious adverse reactions post-marketing, related to 43 small molecule drugs, only 19% of these events were initially identified in animal studies during the preclinical stage.[12] Although more optimistic[13] and pessimistic[14] conclusions have been drawn, existing evidence indicates that the external validity of animal models is far from perfect.

To be fair the above examples may not accurately reflect the ability of toxicological studies within food safety to filter out or establish safe levels for new substances, as in those cases signs of adversity are often examined in several studies over large dose ranges combined with the use of uncertainty factors. While this approach may be robust in terms of safety in most cases, the resulting limitations are that many chemicals that are perfectly safe for humans at the intended use levels, maybe unnecessarily filtered out; or that the derived safe exposure levels are far more restrictive than needed, which is not necessarily beneficial for society or consumers.

To demonstrate how overly protective values might be derived when relying only on animal experiments, the

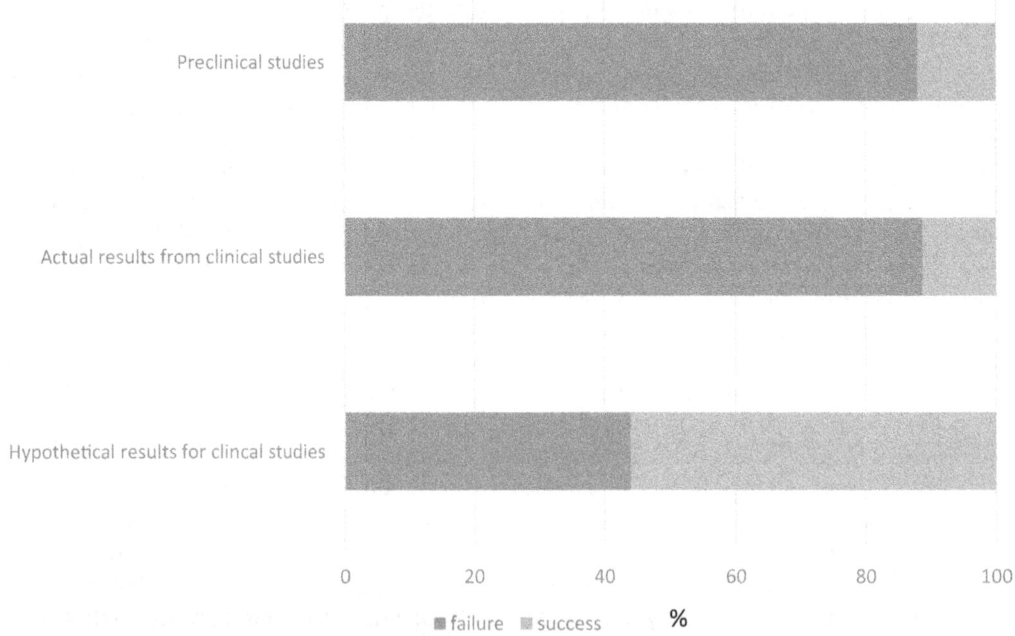

FIGURE 47.1 The column at the top shows the percentage of drugs that succeeded or failed during preclinical testing (this includes failure to identify benefits or indications of toxicity in animals). The middle column shows the percentage of drugs that failed during clinical testing in humans either due to toxicity or lack of efficacy. The lowest column shows what the expected failure rate for human clinical trials would be if animal testing would accurately predict human toxicity (the failure rate would be reduced by half (44% vs 88%)). *Adapted from Van Norman GA. Limitations of animal studies for predicting toxicity in clinical trials: is it time to rethink our current approach? JACC Basic Transl Sci. 2019;4(7):845.*

data-rich case of caffeine is just one example. For caffeine, the no observed adverse effect level (NOAEL) for reprotoxic effects in parental rats and mice in the presence of general toxicity, has been observed at around 22 mg/kg bw. Fetotoxicity has been observed at around half that level.[15] Assuming that no human studies were available, and these NOAELs would be used as reference points, using a standard uncertainty factor of 100, the resulting health-based guidance values would be around 7–14 mg/day for a 70 kg adult (~1/10th of a cup of coffee). This is at least ~15 and up to ~60 times below the level of no safety concern of 200 mg/day for pregnant women and 400 mg/day for adults set by EFSA, respectively.[16] Although the EFSA level of no safety concern is derived based on human interventions, a review of existing observational studies in humans would still provide compelling evidence that no adversity can be expected from a few mg of caffeine being consumed daily.

In summary, high external validity is one of the main strengths of human epidemiology. Despite the higher risk of bias and lack of controlled settings compared to animal experiments, the use of evidence from human studies may greatly reduce uncertainties in hazard identification and result in more accurate estimates being derived in risk characterization.

47.3 Hazard identification – rules for evidence grading versus expert judgment

In the previous section, it was argued that the use of human epidemiology may substantially reduce uncertainty in hazard identification due to high external validity. The limitation on the other hand is that the evidence from epidemiological studies that risk assessors are often confronted with, can be diverse, complex, and far from perfect when compared with experimental studies conducted under ideal conditions. One approach to confronting such a complex evidence base has been to rank (or grade) the evidence in terms of pre-defined rules. This includes ranking studies based on their design and evaluating individual attributes of study conduct for risk of bias. In one publication from the early 1990s, when this methodology was gaining momentum, the justification for this approach was formulated as follows:

"Evidence-based medicine de-emphasizes intuition, unsystematic clinical experience, and ***pathophysiologic rationale*** *as sufficient grounds for clinical decision making and stresses the examination of evidence from clinical research. Evidence-based medicine requires new skills of the physician, including efficient literature searching and the application of formal rules of evidence evaluating the clinical literature.".*[17]

TABLE 47.1 Grades of evidence for the purported quality of study design as formulated by the US Preventive Services Task Force.[18]

I	Evidence obtained from at least one properly *randomized, controlled trial.*
II-1	Evidence obtained from *well-designed controlled trials without randomization*
II-2	Evidence obtained from *well-designed cohort or case-control analytic studies*, preferably from more than one center or research group.
II-3	Evidence was obtained from multiple time series with or without the intervention. Dramatic results in uncontrolled experiments (such as the results of the introduction of penicillin treatment in the 1940s) could also be regarded as this type of evidence.
III	Opinions of respected authorities, based on clinical experience; *descriptive studies* and *case reports*; or reports of expert committees.

One example of such "formal rules" for grading evidence by design is given in Table 47.1. This example is based on the proposed evidence grading by the US Preventive Services Task Force.[18] Here the highest grade of evidence is assigned when there exists at least one properly conducted RCT. The next grade below refers to evidence from well-conducted non-randomized interventions; followed by evidence from well-conducted prospective cohort studies or case-control studies. Descriptive studies, which include cross-sectional studies, ecological studies, and case reports, are assigned the lowest ranking. A similar ranking has also been proposed in other versions of such an evidence pyramid[19] where evidence from meta-analyses and systematic reviews rank above RCTs and case-control studies sometimes rank below cohort studies. A similar hierarchy of experimental and observational studies has also been proposed in animal epidemiology.[20]

Although pre-defined rules on how to rank evidence have some advantages, including greater transparency in decision making and a systematic approach, this methodology has its limitations, particularly if applied too generally. The main criticism of evidence-based medicine is that it places too much emphasis on rules at the expense of understanding mechanisms and clinical experience; and that it is too restrictive in terms of evidence inclusion.[21] Regardless of how rules for evidence synthesis are laid out, there are always exceptions and in such cases, deviations from any pre-defined rule based on expert judgment are crucial to avoid spurious conclusions.

Another point to consider is that evidence-based medicine and conventions for grading studies have been developed for a clinical setting where the primary aim is to improve people's health through medical intervention. This is not the aim of most studies conducted within the remit of food safety and public health research.[d] The proposed ranking of study designs, and other rules developed for a clinical setting, may not always be equally relevant or applicable.

In summary, in this section, it has been argued that strict rules for evidence grading may not be directly applicable for studies conducted within the remit of food safety and other areas of public health. Overconfidence in formal rules for evidence assessment has its limitations as all studies suffer from different types of biases so that such rules often cannot be universally applied to assess study quality. By being aware of the strengths and weaknesses of different designs and by identifying exceptions, more robust conclusions can be drawn. The discussion and examples provided in the next two sections try to shed some light on this issue for experimental and observational studies, respectively.

47.4 Strengths and limitations of human interventions

Rules for grading studies by design were initially developed for ranking evidence related to clinical care and patient treatment. In those settings, experimental studies can be performed to test the efficacy of treatments in subjects that have an underlying disease or health condition that can be improved. By design, net benefit rather than net harm is the expected outcome, although there might be a trade-off between benefit and risk in some circumstances. In such cases performing experiments under controlled conditions (RCTs or other non-randomized interventions) is ethically justifiable and participants are often highly motivated, which usually translates into a high rate of compliance due to expected benefits. In food safety and other areas of public health, all interventions that do not have the potential of being directly beneficial are simply ruled out. Most chemicals used in food are intended to have an indirect benefit, hence their proposed use. For example, a preservative reduces bacterial spoilage. Therefore the only human experimental studies providing information relevant for risk assessors are

1. studies that were initially designed for other purposes but can be used to rule out harm at certain exposure levels or exposure contrast.

2. studies that were designed to improve health but unexpectedly resulted in an adverse event.

Both are further explained through the examples below.

As an example, the International Agency for Research on Cancer (IARC) concluded in 2015 that red meat is "probably carcinogenic to humans" and processed meat is "carcinogenic to humans".[22] This conclusion was based on reviewing more than 800 observational studies. One counterargument to the IARCs conclusion has been to use evidence from RCTs where participants have been assigned diets that consist of lower vs. higher (controls) meat consumption. A review of such studies has not found any indications for effects on cancer or mortality, leading one study to the confident conclusion that evidence from RCTs highlights *"the uncertainty regarding causal relationships between red meat consumption and major cardiometabolic and cancer outcomes"*.[23] There is no denying that uncertainty exists, but the problem with such interpretation of these RCTs is that none of them was designed to examine health benefits of low meat consumption. Instead, they involved multiple lifestyle components including changes in several dietary factors in the treatment arm. The exposure contrast observed in these studies was generally modest and the duration was often, perhaps, too short for making any meaningful conclusion on factors affecting cancer risk and mortality. Although varying opinions exists, another equally valid conclusion is that the only inference on causality these RCTs can with certainty make is: *that there is limited evidence for a causal effect on cancer and longevity when middle-aged study participants are asked to change their dietary and lifestyle habits*. That is, despite the potentially lower risk of bias from RCTs, it is important to carefully consider what a given study was designed for and to evaluate if sufficient exposure contrast and compliance were achieved, before drawing strong conclusions.

Compared to lifestyle interventions, supplement trials are generally more specific, which reduces the risk of bias in terms of poor compliance. One reason is that it is easier for participants to take supplements in the form of pills or capsules, compared to making major dietary or other lifestyle changes. It is also easier in such studies to achieve a greater exposure contrast. Supplement trials for individual nutrients often provide important information for setting tolerable upper limits. As an example, for vitamin D,[e] an RCT giving six 2-monthly oral doses of 3 mg of vitamin D to middle-aged adults, provides some evidence of the safety of such occasional bolus doses.[24] On the other hand, another RCT aimed at assessing the efficacy of vitamin D supplementation on the risk of falls and fractures in older men, giving a single bolus dose of 12.5 mg of vitamin D per year (over 3–5 years), observed higher propensity for falls as a result of treatment.[25] Evidence from these two studies suggests that the use of bolus doses, in general, may not be without risk. Based on evidence from human interventions conducted for different purposes, a tolerable upper limit for vitamin D of 100 μg/day, based on NOAEL of 250 μg/day for hypercalcemia, has been set with some precision.[26] Such data-rich cases are however, scarce.

As an example of (b), some supplement trials have shown unexpected results, that provided information on the safety of supplements, such as a slightly higher cancer and mortality risk among male smokers randomized to beta carotene[27] or higher prostate cancer risk in participants randomized to vitamin E supplementation (borderline significant, 28). The results from these trials do however, hold limited information on cancer risk when consuming antioxidant-rich foods, such as fruits and vegetables, where observational evidence consistently shows lower cancer rates with higher consumption.[f,28] One reasonable conclusion, a controversial Nobel laurate made in his review on antioxidants and cancer, was that *"Blueberries best be eaten because they taste good, not because their consumption will lead to less cancer."*[29] The antioxidant story is by no means the only example of trials generating unexpected results that contradict observational evidence. In the late 1970s a high protein supplementation (40 g of casein in liquid form) aimed at improving fetal growth and birth outcomes among poor African American Women in New York, resulted in an excess of very early premature births and associated neonatal deaths.[30] The total amount of protein from the diet and the supplement was no greater than what can be achieved through diet alone, where no indication of adversity has later been observed in large prospective cohorts.[31] This particular study has had much influence emphasizing the need for being cautious when doing experiments on vulnerable populations. One conclusion that can be drawn from these two examples is that the effects of supplements taken in isolation may be very different from those expected when the same nutrients are consumed through a balanced diet.

Finally, although RCTs are well suited to provide evidence on a causal link between nutrient supplementation and health, the limitation of many such studies is that they often recruit relatively healthy subjects, sometimes due to ethical reasons. Many such trials have been conducted to test the efficacy of supplementation with different nutrients for lowering the risk of depression,[32] cancer,[33] and pregnancy complications,[34] usually resulting in limited or no benefits. One reason for such NULL findings, apart from the lack of causality, is that contrary to the researcher's belief, there are in most cases no benefits to be expected from nutrient supplementation among relatively well-nourished and healthy study participants. That is, the choice of how the experiment is designed in terms of who is recruited is much more important than just making "blind" conclusions on causality based on study design alone.

47.5 Strengths and limitations of observational studies

Observational studies generally recruit subjects from the target population that one wishes to study. As such, they often have higher external validity compared to intervention studies, and the exposure is assessed under real-life conditions. The limitation of these studies is that they are prone to confounding and other biases to various degrees meaning drawing strong conclusions on causality from a single study, in the absence of other evidence, is subject to uncertainty. It is not the aim of this section to explain possible biases or confounding in detail and the reader is referred to other reading material for further explanation.[1,2] Instead, this section reflects on the limitations of assessing observational studies judged to be most reliable. Considerable attention is also given to the quality of exposure assessment, which apart from the lack of a controlled setting, distinguishes observational studies from experimental studies.

47.5.1 Is it sufficient to rely on "gold standard" methods in evidence assessment?

In observational studies, exposure is assessed but not administered (i.e., no dosing). Therefore the accuracy and reliability of the method used is a key issue to look for when assessing study quality and interpreting its results. Exposure can be assessed using objective or subjective measures and although the former is often considered more precise and reliable, excluding evidence based on subjective or less precise measures may lead to less robust conclusions.

As an example, several studies have examined the associations between serum perfluoroalkyl acids (PFAS) and birth weight. For assessing exposure to long-chain PFAS ($\geq$ 6 carbons), blood concentrations are generally considered "gold standard" as PFAS have a long-elimination half-life and are stable in blood.[35] However, during pregnancy, concentrations are less stable due to physiological changes that occur to support fetal growth, including blood volume expansion and increased glomerular filtration rate.[g,36] These changes may confound the relationship between PFAS and birth weight. For example, when the first relatively large (n$\sim$400 to 1400) studies in 2007 suggested an inverse association between perfluorooctanoic acid (PFOA) concentrations in blood and birth weight,[h,37,38] this mechanism for confounding had been postulated.[39] A later study from the large C8-cohort, provided some evidence to address the plausibility of such confounding.[40] That study recruited subjects who had been exposed to PFOA through contaminated drinking water around *DuPont* facilities in Little Hocking, Ohio. The study retrospectively extracted information on $\sim$4500 previous births occurring before the contamination became known. The study estimated past pregnancy exposure to PFOA using pharmacokinetic modeling linked to self-reported residential history and estimates of past drinking water concentrations.[41] The predictions from this modeling showed a high correlation between modeled and measured serum samples drawn from participants at recruitment (r$\sim$0.67). Based on this modeled exposure, which is invariant to physiological changes, no association with birth weight was observed. The modeled exposure contrast for PFOA in the C8 cohort was much larger (range: $\sim$1 to 700 ng/mL) compared to the measured concentrations in the other two studies (range: $\sim$0 to 50 ng/mL). One would therefore also expect to see something in the direction of an inverse association with birth weight in the C8 cohort if a causal relationship existed. Still, this study does not on its own prove that a causal association does not exist (no single study is perfect and in the C8 study, the retrospective exposure assessment rests on several assumptions). The study does, however, provide a reasonable argument against causality that needs reflection in any weighing of the evidence. However, one study appraising available evidence using the Navigation Guide systematic review methodology excluded the C8 cohort from its quantitative synthesis citing a high risk of bias for the exposure. That review concluded, based on meta-analyses of nine studies measuring exposure in maternal serum, that PFOA is adversely associated with birth weight.[42] On the other hand, another review considering the C8 study, reached a different conclusion.[43] For this particular sample the jury may still be out.

47.5.2 Restricting the evidence to "low risk of bias" studies can create bias

In their 2019 opinion on a dietary reference value for sodium, EFSA evaluated observational and intervention studies examining the link between sodium intake and cardiovascular disease outcomes.[44] Using a systematic review approach, the evidence was assessed using the OHAT-NTP critical appraisal tool,[i] categorizing each study in terms of risk of bias as either "*low*", "*moderate*", or "*high*". Studies judged to be at low risk of bias received more weight when weighing the overall evidence. Only RCTs and prospective cohort studies were included. For the cohort studies, only those assessing exposure using at least one 24-hour urinary collection were evaluated "*to minimize the risk of bias*". All other observational studies were excluded. As expected, the opinion concluded, based on evidence from RCTs, that sodium reduction significantly reduces blood pressure, which is a strong risk factor for stroke.[45] With no RCTs available,[j] the relationship with stroke was evaluated based on three prospective cohort studies that met the exposure-inclusion criteria. All other observational evidence was excluded. Two studies[46,47] were judged to be of '*moderate*' risk of bias and found no association with stroke. One study, judged to be of '*low*' risk of bias, found a lower incidence of stroke among those with high 24-h urinary sodium excretion.[48] The overall conclusion weighing these three studies was that "*There is some evidence for an inverse association between sodium urinary excretion and risk of stroke*".[k]

The low risk of bias study[48] responsible for this confident conclusion, whose findings have limited support by biology, requires some discussion. In this well-conducted study, two 24-urine samples were collected at baseline (1997–1999) and two more samples were collected at later follow-up (2001–2003). The study included 7330 individuals who were followed up over a median of 12.5 years, during which 183 stroke cases occurred. Although managing to collect 4 × 24-urine samples in over 7000 participants is impressive, each measurement only reflects sodium intake during the previous day. Between days sodium can vary greatly.[49] With more than 12 years of follow-up in subjects of whom many would be experiencing age-related weight and health changes, one can expect some changes in diet and lifestyle over the follow-up period. A key question to answer is, if an accurate assessment of sodium excretion for the previous day on 4 occasions, years before an event is likely to have contributed to the risk of stroke? Furthermore, it is highly plausible that the burden of collecting 24-hour urine, ideally collecting every drop into one storage tank over 24 h, may have led to biased exposure assessment. That is, the burden of collection may have resulted in participants being more prone to collect urine in the privacy of their homes instead of going about their daily life as normal. This may have affected their normal dietary habits and physical routine (leading to measures not representative of their normal dietary habits). Even in patients that should, for medical reasons, be more motivated to collect 24-hour urine, the limitations of this method are well known.[50] That is, even though each 24-hour urinary collection quantifies total sodium intake during the previous day, there are less accurate (in terms of absolute quantification) dietary assessment methods that may better reflect long-term habitual intake, which would have been justifiable to include in the assessment. Such studies have suggested a positive association between sodium and stroke,[51] which is consistent with biology and other lines of evidence.[45]

Before excluding evidence in this particular example, it would have been reasonable to answer the question of how other imprecise measures of sodium intake may lead to a biased association with stroke, and in which direction? The take-home message is that it does not increase confidence in any conclusion to pick the most accurate exposure or best studies for evidence assessment (and feel confident of the outcome simply because some methodological approach was followed by the book). A low risk of bias does not exclude bias and vice versa. The duration of exposure covered by the method relative to the disease progression cannot be ignored, and even studies judged to be a '*low*' risk of bias may not necessarily live up to their labeling. The '*high*' risk alternative may occasionally represent reality better.

47.5.3 Looking beyond the risk of bias

The two examples above highlighted some of the potential pitfalls of failing to acknowledge the limitations of "gold standard" methods, relying on too strict inclusion/exclusion criteria, and disproportional weighing of evidence using "high quality" studies. The question is then, what other alternatives exist.

One proposed solution has been to take advantage of different methods in terms of the risk of bias. As in the two examples above, measured concentrations of PFOA during pregnancy are to some extent affected by the state of pregnancy, which external exposure estimates may bypass. Similarly, 24-hour urine collection only reflects exposure during the previous day and the burden of collecting 24-hour urine may lead to departures from the normal behavior that one aims to measure. The use of repeated spot urine samples or dietary assessment methods provides a less robust assessment of absolute intake, but may still be sufficient to rank subjects according to long-term intake. These different approaches often do not share the same source of potential biases. This way of integrating results from different approaches, where each approach has different sources of potential bias that are unrelated to each other, is called the *Method of Triangulation*.[52,53] This method of assessing evidence has been proposed as an alternative to the more dogmatic approach used in evidence-based medicine and has the potential to bypass some of its flaws. To be fair, the *Method of Triangulation* may not have as clear a structure for decision making, as each study has to be evaluated, using expert judgment, relative to other studies that differ in terms of potential biases. A reasonable way forward, taking advantage of both approaches would be some sort of integration of the two methodologies. Given the fact that many within evidence-based medicine are aware of its potential limitations, and many improvements have been made over the years, further improvements may be expected.[54]

47.5.4 Use and integration of different study designs

Making use of all available evidence appropriately is one hallmark of a thorough risk assessment. Such use is perhaps more likely to occur in data-poor assessments, where any information provides some value, as opposed to data-rich assessments, where reducing the burden of assessing volumes of studies often tilts risk assessors towards focusing only on "the more reliable studies". The case of sodium mentioned above is one such example. In the case of nutrients, there are also good examples of the appropriate use of existing evidence which are not overly focused on the study design hierarchy. This is the case in many previous assessments for establishing tolerable upper intake levels for vitamins and minerals, which follow the same principles as for any other chemical risk assessment.[55] The important difference for nutrients, however, is that there is a dual risk, associated with both inadequate and high intake. The margin between the two extremes is often so small that the uncertainty associated with the animal-to-human extrapolation limits the use of animal experiments.

One example of making appropriate use of a study considered to be of inferior design, are recommendations provided by the Committee on Toxicity in the UK in 1997 for vitamin B6,[56] and later establishment of a tolerable upper intake level by EFSA in 2006.[4] For vitamin B6 the current recommended intake[l] is 1.6 mg/day, with the 95th percentile for dietary intake generally being below 5 mg/day.[4] However, supplement use or high intakes of foods fortified with vitamin B6 (i.e., certain soft drinks) may greatly increase the risk of exceeding the upper limit.[57,58] At such intakes, possible adverse effects on the central nervous system may occur, whose severity depends on both dose and duration of exposure. In rats, neuron damage has been observed at doses as low as 600 mg/kg bw/day after ~1 week of treatment and more subtle neurological effects have been detected at lower, but highly varying doses (0.3–84 mg/kg bw/day), after several weeks of treatment.[4] In humans several case reports of neuropathy have been documented relating to long-term use of vitamin B6 supplements, but establishing a threshold is difficult due to large heterogeneity in reported dose and duration.[4] More information could be extracted from an essentially cross-sectional study of 172 women who attended a private practice, specializing in premenstrual syndrome.[59] The women were asked if they were taking vitamin B6 supplements[m] and if so, their serum B6 levels were measured. Of these 172 women, 103 reported neurological symptoms. The women reporting neurological symptoms reported daily supplement use ranging from less than 50 mg up to ~500 mg/day (median of ~100 mg) with duration ranging between 1 to 5 years. Those without symptoms generally had a shorter duration of use and took more modest doses. After discontinuing use, most women with symptoms reported full recovery a few months later. On the basis of this study, EFSA established a tolerable upper intake limit of 25 mg/day by applying an uncertainty factor of 4 to the median intake of 100 mg from that study[4]; and the Committee of Toxicity recommended that the maximum daily supplement use should not exceed 10 mg.[56]

The interesting aspect of this risk characterization is that despite the existence of controlled animal experiments and a few intervention studies, the cross-sectional study conducted in self-referred patients using subjective measures of exposure and outcome provided the most relevant information. Not surprisingly the use of this study and the resulting recommendation was questioned as being based on the "slimmest of evidence".[60] No attempt was however, made to explain what biases might have occurred and how they could plausibly explain the result of the study as coincidental. One argument in defense of this study would simply be that there is no reason why supplement users would not be able to give an accurate description of the amount and duration of their past use and report their neurological symptoms with relatively high precision without any meaningful bias to occur. As in this example, once some certainty on causality has been established, for example with support from animal data and case reports, cross-sectional studies or other study designs can provide valuable input in terms of characterizing risk.

More generally, cross-sectional studies can provide more robust information on possible effect size compared to RCTs, as they are generally conducted in more representative populations and they may also be available for sensitive subpopulations, including children, the elderly, and pregnant women, that are important to consider for characterizing risk. To illustrate this, the relationship between sodium intake and blood pressure can again be taken as an example. In this data-rich case, one meta-analysis showed near-identical effect estimates for the decrease in blood pressure as a result of a reduction in sodium intake, when comparing results from RCTs on the one hand, and results from mostly cross-sectional observational studies on the other.[61] Similar observations between effect sizes, reported in RCTs and observational studies, have been reported for other outcomes in the medical literature.[62] For many risk assessments, RCTs may not be available and in such cases, there is no reason why cross-sectional studies should not be used for hazard identification[63] and risk characterization. This should of course be done on a case-by-case basis, carefully assessing limitations and possible risk of biases that may occur in parallel.

The above examples, mostly focusing on cross-sectional versus RCT designs, are by no means exceptional. There are good examples, such as for the case of

PFAS in the C8 cohort mentioned above, of how ecological design can be used to rule out bias that may occur from associations established using biomarker analyses.[64] To give another example, retrospective case-control studies, which may suffer from recall bias but have the advantages of recruiting a high number of cases as well as being easier to conduct often provide added support to findings from prospective cohort studies, that are more difficult to conduct and may suffer from potential biases associated with loss to follow-up. One such example is the consistent findings of retrospective case-control and prospective cohort studies for the association between trans-fatty acids and cardiovascular disease.[65] The evidence from these studies and others contributed to the discontinuation of the use of these fatty acids in food and legal restrictions being set on their use in Europe.

In summary, if interpreted based on their limitations and strengths, observational evidence from various study designs often provides a much stronger basis for hazard identification and risk characterization than just focusing on selected study designs presumed to be "low risk of bias". The examples above highlighting these limitations have by no means focused on rare exceptions. Similarly, there are also many circumstances, not addressed in this chapter, where the exclusion of studies can be fully justified. All such decisions have to be taken on a case-by-case basis. The challenge when excluding evidence *a priori* is to justify such decisions clearly with well-formulated reasoning. Such reasoning often requires that the evidence that one considered too uncertain and justifiable to exclude must be evaluated to some degree. If this is not done properly, the users of that assessment (i.e., risk managers, scientists, or the interested public) are less likely to accept its conclusions.

47.6 Research gaps and future direction

In this chapter, the role of human epidemiology in risk assessment has been argued for by highlighting its high external validity, which may reduce the uncertainty associated with the animal to human extrapolation. Although the discussion on the use of evidence-based medicine to assess evidence in risk assessment has been partly critical and directed towards pointing out its limitations, it is by no means the suggestion that the use of this methodology should be reduced or abolished. The existence of evidence-based medicine was in part driven by a lack of transparency and consistency in how evidence was previously assessed and as such the methodology has led to many positive improvements. This has, however, not been without flaws. One is that rules can often be used as an excuse for not relying on expert judgment or they can lead to ignoring important evidence when it does not fit into a certain box.

The purpose of this chapter has also been to give some directions on how human epidemiology can be used for chemical risk assessment and highlight areas where work is needed to adapt the evidence-based methodology to the risk assessments paradigm (for which the original methodology was not designed). The method of triangulation or other more expert-knowledge-guided approaches combined with a clear, transparent structure of reporting, which is the hallmark of evidence-based medicine, offers some way forward. Another aspect that has been highlighted in this chapter is that different study designs and methods used for exposure assessment all have their place, to some degree, in any risk assessment. The nature of studying free-living humans is such that one cannot just rely on one best method for exposure assessment or something that one considers the most reliable study. Therefore simply calling for better studies,[8,9] which is often voiced among risk assessors, is perhaps not always the right way forward. The biomedical literature, not just human epidemiology, is saturated with studies of modest to poor quality along with the occasional well-conducted studies. Studies whose findings are likely to be coincidental[n] are usually easy to identify by expert judgment. What future work needs to focus on, instead of only wishing for better studies, is how results from several lines of evidence can be used to identify and characterize risk taking the strengths and limitations of these different sources of evidence into consideration.

The use of epidemiological studies for characterizing risk has in the past often been done in the same way as for toxicological studies, using the presumed "single best study" to establish health-based guidance values.[66,67] Such an approach may not be the most appropriate for the same reason that no single study is perfect, and information provided by several studies generally reduces uncertainty. That is, due to the large between human variability and the fact that all studies suffer from methodological limitations, more sophisticated or flexible approaches for characterizing risk are needed. For this purpose, future work would need to address the adaptation of the benchmark dose methodology so it can be appropriately used for human epidemiological studies and more specific, (less generic) guidance to be developed for the weight of evidence approach for integrating human studies with other lines of evidence. How this can be achieved in praxis is beyond the scope of this chapter.

Endnotes

[a]i.e., confounding in observational studies and departures from intended treatment in human interventions.

[b]at least compared to studies in inbred experimental animals.

[c]Accuracy here may both refer to health-based guidance values that are not protective enough or overly protective. Although use of default uncertainty factors may more often result in values that are overly protective the resulting accuracy is still poor and not optimal.

[d]For example in public health research, interventions are often conducted with the aim of preventing adverse health outcomes, but not improving underlying disease condition. The former is often more complex and difficult to achieve and may require a different experimental setup.

[e]another example of a) above.

[f]Which is not the same as saying that the antioxidant is the causal link, if one assumes that these observational studies are unbiased and high consumption of fruit and vegetables at the expense of other foods may reduce the risk of developing cancer.

[g]Particularly for the carboxylic acids (including PFOA) higher glomerular filtration rate will result in higher excretion rate, thereby lowering concentrations as pregnancy progresses.

[h]If confounding by physiological change does occur, one would expect greater influence in late pregnancy where these changes have peaked. In the two cited studies, stronger association was observed in the lone study relying on cord blood[37] compared with the other studies where maternal serum was drawn early in pregnancy.[38]

[i]https://ntp.niehs.nih.gov/ntp/ohat/pubs/riskofbiastool_508.pdf.

[j]In contrast to RCTs on blood pressure, such studies would require interventions stretching over many month and optimally several years.

[k]High 24-hour sodium urinary excretion reflects high sodium intake during the previous 24 hours.

[l]Or population reference index.

[m]Vitamin B6 supplements have sometimes been recommended for relieving premenstrual symptoms, including anxiety and depression.

[n]Such findings are not only confined to "poor" or "high risk of bias" studies.

References

1. Porta MS. 5th ed. *International Epidemiological Association. A Dictionary of Epidemiology*. 289. Oxford; New York: Oxford University Press; 2008. xxiv.
2. Committee ES, More S, Bambidis V, et al. Draft for internal testing scientific committee guidance on appraising and integrating evidence from epidemiological studies for use in EFSA's scientific assessments. *EFSA J*. 2020;18(8):e06221.
3. Hazards EPoB. Role played by the environment in the emergence and spread of antimicrobial resistance (AMR) through the food chain. *EFSA J*. 2021;19(6):176.
4. Authority EFS. Tolerable upper intake levels for vitamins and minerals 2006.
5. Welfare EPoAHa. Statement on the use of animal-based measures to assess the welfare of animals. *EFSA J*. 2012;10(6):29.
6. Van Norman GA. Limitations of animal studies for predicting toxicity in clinical trials: is it time to rethink our current approach? *JACC Basic Transl Sci*. 2019;4(7):845–854.
7. van den Brandt P, Voorrips L, Hertz-Picciotto I, et al. The contribution of epidemiology. *Food Chem Toxicol*. 2002;40(2-3):387–424.
8. Products EPoPP, Their R, Ockleford C, et al. Scientific opinion of the PPR panel on the follow-up of the findings of the external scientific report 'literature review of epidemiological studies linking exposure to pesticides and health effects'. *EFSA J*. 2017;15(10): e05007.
9. Hernandez AF, Tsatsakis AM. Human exposure to chemical mixtures: challenges for the integration of toxicology with epidemiology data in risk assessment. *Food Chem Toxicol*. 2017;103:188–193.
10. Whaley P, Halsall C, Agerstrand M, et al. Implementing systematic review techniques in chemical risk assessment: challenges, opportunities and recommendations. *Environ Int*. 2016;92-93:556–564.
11. Committee ES, Hardy A, Benford D, et al. Guidance on the use of the weight of evidence approach in scientific assessments. *EFSA J*. 2017;15(8):e04971.
12. van Meer PJ, Kooijman M, Gispen-de Wied CC, Moors EH, Schellekens H. The ability of animal studies to detect serious post marketing adverse events is limited. *Regul Toxicol Pharmacol*. 2012;64(3):345–349.
13. Olson H, Betton G, Robinson D, et al. Concordance of the toxicity of pharmaceuticals in humans and in animals. *Regul Toxicol Pharmacol*. 2000;32(1):56–67.
14. Bailey J, Thew M, Balls M. An analysis of the use of animal models in predicting human toxicology and drug safety. *Altern Lab Anim*. 2014;42(3):181–199.
15. OECD-SIDS. Initial Assessment Report for SIAM 14: Caffeine. Report. Paris, France: OECD; 2002 March.
16. EFSA Panel on Dietetic Products NaAN. Scientific opinion on the safety of caffeine. *EFSA J*. 2015;13(5).
17. Evidence-Based Medicine Working G.. Evidence-based medicine. A new approach to teaching the practice of medicine. *JAMA*.. 1992;268(17):2420–2425.
18. Force PST. *Guide to Clinical Preventive Services: Report of the US Preventive Services Task Force*. 2nd ed. Baltimore, MD: Williams & Wilkins; 1996.
19. Murad MH, Asi N, Alsawas M, Alahdab F. New evidence pyramid. *Evid Based Med*. 2016;21(4):125–127.
20. Sargeant JM, Kelton DF, O'Connor AM. Study designs and systematic reviews of interventions: building evidence across study designs. *Zoonoses Public Health*. 2014;61(Suppl 1):10–17.
21. Cohen AM, Stavri PZ, Hersh WR. A categorization and analysis of the criticisms of evidence-based medicine. *Int J Med Inf*. 2004;73 (1):35–43.
22. Bouvard V, Loomis D, Guyton KZ, et al. Carcinogenicity of consumption of red and processed meat. *Lancet Oncol*. 2015;16 (16):1599–1600.
23. Zeraatkar D, Johnston BC, Bartoszko J, et al. Effect of lower versus higher red meat intake on cardiometabolic and cancer outcomes: a systematic review of randomized trials. *Ann Intern Med*. 2019;171(10):721–731.
24. Martineau AR, MacLaughlin BD, Hooper RL, et al. Double-blind randomised placebo-controlled trial of bolus-dose vitamin D3 supplementation in adults with asthma (ViDiAs). *Thorax*. 2015;70(5):451–457.
25. Sanders KM, Stuart AL, Williamson EJ, et al. Annual high-dose oral vitamin D and falls and fractures in older women: a randomized controlled trial. *JAMA*.. 2010;303(18):1815–1822.
26. EFSA Panel on Dietetic Products NaAN. Scientific opinion on the tolerable upper intake level of vitamin D. *EFSA J*. 2012;10(7).
27. Alpha-Tocopherol BCCPSG. The effect of vitamin E and beta carotene on the incidence of lung cancer and other cancers in male smokers. *N Engl J Med*. 1994;330(15):1029–1035.
28. Aune D, Giovannucci E, Boffetta P, et al. Fruit and vegetable intake and the risk of cardiovascular disease, total cancer and all-cause mortality-a systematic review and dose-response meta-analysis of prospective studies. *Int J Epidemiol*. 2017;46(3):1029–1056.
29. Watson J. Oxidants, antioxidants and the current incurability of metastatic cancers. *Open Biol*. 2013;3(1):120144.

30. Rush D, Stein Z, Susser M. A randomized controlled trial of prenatal nutritional supplementation in New York City. *Pediatrics*. 1980;65(4):683–697.
31. Halldorsson TI, Birgisdottir BE, Brantsaeter AL, et al. Old question revisited: are high-protein diets safe in pregnancy? *Nutrients*.. 2021;13(2).
32. Makrides M, Gibson RA, McPhee AJ, et al. Effect of DHA supplementation during pregnancy on maternal depression and neurodevelopment of young children: a randomized controlled trial. *JAMA*.. 2010;304(15):1675–1683.
33. Lippman SM, Klein EA, Goodman PJ, et al. Effect of selenium and vitamin E on risk of prostate cancer and other cancers: the selenium and vitamin e cancer prevention trial (SELECT). *JAMA*.. 2009;301(1):39–51.
34. Olsen SF, Halldorsson TI, Li M, et al. Examining the effect of fish oil supplementation in chinese pregnant women on gestation duration and risk of preterm delivery. *J Nutr*. 2019;149(11):1942–1951.
35. Wu XM, Bennett DH, Calafat AM, et al. Serum concentrations of perfluorinated compounds (PFC) among selected populations of children and adults in California. *Environ Res*. 2015;136:264–273.
36. Sanghavi M, Rutherford JD. Cardiovascular physiology of pregnancy. *Circulation*. 2014;130(12):1003–1008.
37. Fei C, McLaughlin JK, Tarone RE, Olsen J. Perfluorinated chemicals and fetal growth: a study within the danish national birth cohort. *Environ Health Perspect*. 2007;115(11):1677–1682.
38. Apelberg BJ, Goldman LR, Calafat AM, et al. Determinants of fetal exposure to polyfluoroalkyl compounds in Baltimore, Maryland. *Environ Sci Technol*. 2007;41(11):3891–3897.
39. Savitz DA. Guest editorial: biomarkers of perfluorinated chemicals and birth weight. *Environ Health Perspect*. 2007;115(11):A528–A529.
40. Savitz DA, Stein CR, Elston B, et al. Relationship of perfluorooctanoic acid exposure to pregnancy outcome based on birth records in the mid-Ohio Valley. *Environ Health Perspect*. 2012;120(8):1201–1207.
41. Shin HM, Vieira VM, Ryan PB, Steenland K, Bartell SM. Retrospective exposure estimation and predicted versus observed serum perfluorooctanoic acid concentrations for participants in the C8 health project. *Environ Health Perspect*. 2011;119(12):1760–1765.
42. Johnson PI, Sutton P, Atchley DS, et al. The navigation guide – evidence-based medicine meets environmental health: systematic review of human evidence for PFOA effects on fetal growth. *Environ Health Perspect*. 2014;122(10):1028–1039.
43. Steenland K, Barry V, Savitz D. Serum perfluorooctanoic acid and birthweight: an updated meta-analysis with bias analysis. *Epidemiology*. 2018;29(6):765–776.
44. Efsa Panel on Nutrition NF, Food A, Turck D, et al. Dietary reference values for sodium. *EFSA J*. 2019;17(9):e05778.
45. Appel LJ, Frohlich ED, Hall JE, et al. The importance of population-wide sodium reduction as a means to prevent cardiovascular disease and stroke: a call to action from the american heart association. *Circulation*.. 2011;123(10):1138–1143.
46. Stolarz-Skrzypek K, Kuznetsova T, Thijs L, et al. Fatal and nonfatal outcomes, incidence of hypertension, and blood pressure changes in relation to urinary sodium excretion. *JAMA*.. 2011;305(17):1777–1785.
47. Tuomilehto J, Jousilahti P, Rastenyte D, et al. Urinary sodium excretion and cardiovascular mortality in Finland: a prospective study. *Lancet*.. 2001;357(9259):848–851.
48. Kieneker LM, Eisenga MF, Gansevoort RT, et al. Association of low urinary sodium excretion with increased risk of stroke. *Mayo Clin Proc*. 2018;93(12):1803–1809.
49. Liu K, Stamler J. Assessment of sodium intake in epidemiological studies on blood pressure. *Ann Clin Res*. 1984;16(Suppl 43):49–54.
50. Xiang A, Nourian A, Ghiraldi E, Friedlander JI. Improving compliance with 24-H urine collections: understanding inadequacies in the collection process and risk factors for poor compliance. *Curr Urol Rep*. 2021;22(8):38.
51. Strazzullo P, D'Elia L, Kandala NB, Cappuccio FP. Salt intake, stroke, and cardiovascular disease: meta-analysis of prospective studies. *BMJ*.. 2009;339:b4567.
52. Pearce N, Vandenbroucke JP, Lawlor DA. Causal inference in environmental epidemiology: old and new approaches. *Epidemiology*. 2019;30(3):311–316.
53. Lawlor DA, Tilling K, Davey Smith G. Triangulation in aetiological epidemiology. *Int J Epidemiol*. 2016;45(6):1866–1886.
54. Djulbegovic B, Guyatt GH. Progress in evidence-based medicine: a quarter century on. *Lancet*.. 2017;390(10092):415–423.
55. Committee ES, More S, Bampidis V, et al. Statement on the derivation of health-based guidance values (HBGVs) for regulated products that are also nutrients. *EFSA J*. 2021;19(3):e06479.
56. Committee on Toxicity of Chemicals in Food Cpate. Statement on vitamin B6 (pyridoxine) toxicity. 1997 June.
57. Pieszko C, Baranowska I, Flores A. Determination of energizers in energy drinks. *J Anal Chem*. 2010;65:7.
58. Sista SRS, Lozowska D, Katzin LW, Vu TH. Multivitamin supplements and energy drinks in pyridoxine megavitaminosis. *Neurol Clin Pract*. 2015;5(6):509–511.
59. Dalton K, Dalton MJ. Characteristics of pyridoxine overdose neuropathy syndrome. *Acta Neurol Scand*. 1987;76(1):8–11.
60. Still time for rational debate about vitamin B6. *Lancet*. 1998;351 (9115):1523.
61. Leyvraz M, Chatelan A, da Costa BR, et al. Sodium intake and blood pressure in children and adolescents: a systematic review and meta-analysis of experimental and observational studies. *Int J Epidemiol*. 2018;47(6):1796–1810.
62. Golder S, Loke YK, Bland M. Meta-analyses of adverse effects data derived from randomised controlled trials as compared to observational studies: methodological overview. *PLoS Med*. 2011;8(5):e1001026.
63. Spector PE. Do not cross me: optimizing the use of cross-sectional designs. *J Bus Psychol*. 2019;34:12.
64. Gallo V, Leonardi G, Genser B, et al. Serum perfluorooctanoate (PFOA) and perfluorooctane sulfonate (PFOS) concentrations and liver function biomarkers in a population with elevated PFOA exposure. *Environ Health Perspect*. 2012;120(5):655–660.
65. Mozaffarian D, Katan MB, Ascherio A, Stampfer MJ, Willett WC. Trans fatty acids and cardiovascular disease. *N Engl J Med*. 2006;354(15):1601–1613.
66. Chain EPoCitF, Knutsen HK, Alexander J, et al. Risk for animal and human health related to the presence of dioxins and dioxin-like PCBs in feed and food. *EFSA J*. 2018;16(11):e05333.
67. Chain EPoCitF, Schrenk D, Bignami M, et al. Risk to human health related to the presence of perfluoroalkyl substances in food. *EFSA J*. 2020;18(9):e06223.

Chapter 48

Risk-based approaches in food allergy

Geert Houben[1,2], W. Marty Blom[1,2] and Marjolein Meijerink[1]

[1]Netherlands Organisation for Applied Scientific Research TNO, Utrecht, The Netherlands, [2]University Medical Center Utrecht, Utrecht, The Netherlands

Abstract

Food allergy has been recognized already in early history as a condition triggered in some individuals upon consumptions of specific foods. However, its recognition as an essential element to be addressed in food safety management is of much more recent date. As a consequence, risk assessment and risk management practices for food allergy are less well established and harmonized and significantly lag behind those for chemical and microbiological hazards. Nevertheless, in most regions of the world, assessment and management of risks of allergens in food are nowadays regulatory required, while the science underlying the assessment of allergenic hazards and risks has developed well during last decades. In this chapter, a brief history, state-of-the-art, and possible future improvements of the allergenicity risk analysis are described, with a focus on ingredients and residues from allergenic foods intentionally or unintentionally present in food, and allergenicity of proteins in novel food supply.

Keywords: Food allergy; risk assessment; risk management; ingredients; residues; thresholds; reference doses; novel food; sustainable food; allergenicity scaling

48.1 Introduction

Undesired reactions to extrinsic substances can develop through various mechanisms (Fig. 48.1). While in principle, all individuals are susceptible to toxic substances, hypersensitivity affects only a proportion of the population. In case the immune system does not play an initiating role in hypersensitivity reactions, we speak of intolerance, while in case of allergy, the primary mechanism is immune mediated.[1] There are four main types of allergic reactions.[1] The Type 1 allergic reactions are the most important type in food allergy.[2] Type 1 food allergies are Immunoglobulin E (IgE) mediated and only occur in people who have become sensitized and have developed IgE antibodies against specific proteins (allergens) in food. Upon renewed ingestion of these proteins, cell-bound IgE antibodies in our blood and tissues may bind to the allergenic proteins or fragments of these, which activates these cells and triggers cascades of inflammatory processes. This leads to a broad range of allergic symptoms, ranging from mild local symptoms to severe systemic multiorgan effects that may be life threatening and sometimes fatal.[3]

One of the earliest descriptions of what likely was food allergy can be found in the works of Hippocrates. He described for cheese that "there are some who can take it to satiety without being hurt by it in the least, but, on the contrary, it is wonderful what strength it imparts to those it agrees with; but there are some who do not bear it well, their constitutions are different, and they differ in this respect, that what in their body is incompatible with cheese, is roused and put in commotion by such a thing; and those in whose bodies such a humor happens to prevail in greater quantity and intensity, are likely to suffer the more from it. But if the thing had been pernicious to of man, it would have hurt all. Whoever knows these things will not suffer from it" (from: On Ancient Medicine, By Hippocrates, Written 400 BCE, Translated by Francis Adams, Part 20, in The Genuine Works of Hippocrates, Baltimore, Williams, 1939).[4] But despite the

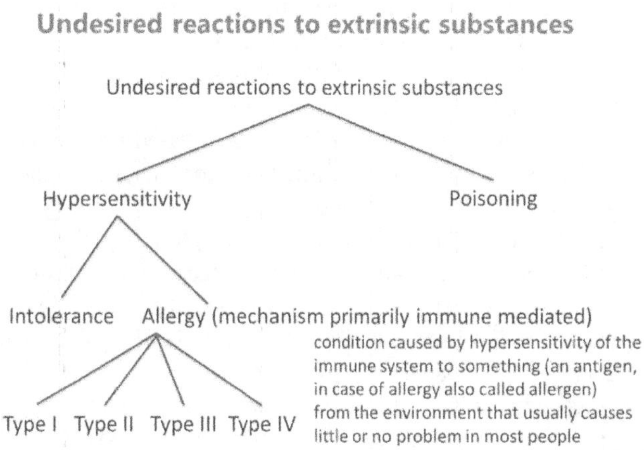

FIGURE 48.1 Distinct types of undesired reactions to extrinsic substances.

Present Knowledge in Food Safety. DOI: https://doi.org/10.1016/B978-0-12-819470-6.00010-X

early description of food allergy, its recognition as an essential element also to be addressed in food safety management is of much more recent date. As a consequence, hazard and risk assessment and risk management practices for food allergy are less well established and harmonized and actually significantly lag behind those for chemical and microbiological hazards.

It should be realized that proteins are an essential nutritional element of our diet and that almost all foods contain proteins. Furthermore, most, if not all proteins in our diet have some allergenic potency. As a consequence, almost all foods will in principle be allergenic. Nevertheless, the majority of food allergies are caused by a relatively small group of foods: milk, egg, peanut, tree nuts, fish, crustacean shellfish, wheat, and soy (US Food and Drug Administration (FDA). Food Allergies: What you need to know. https://www.fda.gov/Food/IngredientsPackagingLabeling/FoodAllergens/ucm079311.htm).

Food allergic consumers need to avoid or strongly restrict ingestion of the foods they are allergic to, which may be not too difficult in case of for instance a glass of milk or a bowl of peanuts. However, the presence of allergenic foods, or protein-containing ingredients derived from these, in other, processed foods is not always easy to note. Legislations have therefore developed in most regions of the world that prescribe the declaration of major allergenic foods and ingredients if added to food. However, the allergenic foods to which these regulations apply differ between the various jurisdictions[5] and the basis for the selections is not always clear. Allergenic proteins may also unintentionally end up in food products, for instance due to agricultural comingling, contamination during storage or transport at any stage of the production chain, or cross-contact at the production site. During the last decades, food suppliers increasingly apply precautionary allergen labeling (PAL) to warn consumers for the potential risks of unintended allergen presence (UAP). However, harmonized regulatory guidance for the use of PAL is lacking.[5] The science underlying the assessment of allergenic hazards and risks has developed well during last decades and allows further development, improvement, and harmonization of risk-based management of allergenic protein exposure of consumers.

Our current, generally mainly animal-based protein supply has an enormous environmental impact and increasing the sustainability of our food protein supply is urgently needed. But, as most if not all proteins are allergenic, new food protein sources will pose new allergenic risks, and premarket assessment and approval of these are important to prevent unnecessary increase of the burden of food allergy.[6,7] Approaches for the premarket assessment of allergenicity of new food proteins initially mainly started to come to development for the assessment of foods derived from genetically modified organisms (GMOs), but have also slowly come to development for proteins in novel food supply the last decade. However, the tools for the premarket assessment of allergenicity of new food proteins are still poor in methods with proven high predictive value.[8]

In this chapter, some history, state-of-the-art, and possible future improvements of the allergenicity risk analysis are described, with a focus on ingredients and residues from allergenic foods intentionally or unintentionally present in food, and allergenicity of proteins in novel food supply.

48.2 Risk analysis of ingredients and residues from allergenic foods

Ingredients and residues from allergenic foods can intentionally or unintentionally be present in food. Risk management efforts in all cases are mainly focused on avoiding or reducing unnecessary allergen presence in food products and on properly informing the consumer on the presence of allergenic foods or ingredients, or on potential UAP. The risk analysis situations for the intentional and the unintentional presence of allergens, however, differ considerably, as do the challenges and needs for improving the situations. Major current issues are the selection of allergenic foods, and ingredients derived from these, that should be regulated, and the criteria for applying, as well as for not applying PAL.

48.2.1 Intentional use of allergenic ingredients

Several major allergenic foods and ingredients derived from these are important elements of our food supply and are also present as added ingredients in numerous processed foods. Food allergic consumers need to avoid or strongly restrict ingestion of the proteins they are allergic to, and this is only possible if they are well informed about the presence of allergenic substances in food. Legislation that prescribes the declaration of major allergenic foods and ingredients if added to food is the most important instrument that enables consumers to avoid food that contains these allergenic foods and ingredients. Such legislation is in force in most regions of the world and generally is hazard-based, that is, simply the addition of specified allergenic foods or ingredients derived from these to food products obliges to label the presence of these, irrespective of the risk these pose. Examples of such regulations are the European Union (EU) Directives 2003/89/EC and 2007/86/EC[9,10] and the US Food Allergen Labeling and Consumer Protection Act.[11] These regulations also provide in the possibility to apply for an exemption from labeling requirement. In the EU, the European Food Safety Authority (EFSA), and in the United States, the FDA, are the Competent Authorities to review such application and if sufficiently substantiated that certain ingredients or substances derived from regulated allergenic foods are not likely to cause adverse reactions in susceptible individuals, an exemption may be granted. It is to be noted that, while the labeling requirement regulations are hazard-based, these exemption regulations in principle are risk-based: based on the substantiation that adverse reactions are not likely, that is, the risk is negligible. Yet the substantiation of a negligible risk currently often relies on proof of absence of the hazard, making the application of the criterion in practice still hazard-based. Nevertheless, a quantitative risk assessment (QRA)-based approach may be applied as specified for instance by FDA's Food Allergen Labeling Exemption Petitions and Notifications Guidance for Industry.[12] QRA methods in food allergy and databases containing the data needed for such risk assessment have been developed during the past one-and-half decade and may increasingly be applied in future in the evaluation of labeling exemption applications. QRA methods for food allergens were mainly developed because of the need to assess and manage the risks of UAP and will be addressed in more detail in Section 48.2.2.1 of this chapter.

48.2.1.1 Risk-based criteria for the selection of allergenic foods for regulation

In all regions of the world, allergen labeling legislation, if applied, only prescribes such labeling for specified selected allergenic foods and ingredients, while the allergenic foods to which these regulations apply differ between the various jurisdictions.[5] The basis for the selections is not always clear. A decision to include or to not include a specific allergenic food in such regulation has an enormous impact, not only for the ones it primarily personally affects—the allergic individuals—but also for food business operators, healthcare workers, authorities, and many others. Therefore, Expert Groups of the Food Allergy Taskforce of the International Life Sciences Institute (ISLI) Europe investigated and proposed an improved science-based selection of allergenic foods for labeling regulation based on public health importance.

Björkstén et al.[13] proposed that the identification of allergenic foods of public health importance should be based on the establishment of involvement of an IgE-mediated mechanism in adverse effect induction, but also on a proof of actual occurrence of adverse effects caused by an IgE-mediated mechanism. Furthermore, they considered the prevalence of allergy to the foods, the potency of the foods for triggering allergic symptoms, and the severity of such symptoms important criteria. Their publication also addresses quality of evidence aspects for these criteria: what type of data give what level of evidence on each of the criteria? Van Bilsen et al.[14] performed an evaluation of the criteria proposed by Björkstén et al. and proposed several modifications for assessing the quality of evidence. Chung et al.[15] subsequently reported on an international workshop held in 2010 in which external stakeholders and experts evaluated the quality of evidence criteria published by van Bilsen et al., by applying these in several case studies to existing study results on several allergenic foods. Chung et al. also discussed how to combine quality of evidence information from study data and public health importance information about allergenic foods based on the data itself. Yet, one key challenge remained: how to judge, express, and compare public health importance of allergenic foods? The latter was addressed by Houben et al.,[16] who proposed to establish or rank allergenic foods according to their public health relevance, based on the prevalence of allergy to the foods and the potency of these foods to trigger allergic symptoms. They also presented a proof of concept illustration for prioritizing allergenic foods for regulation based on these parameters. The data selected for the proof of principle illustration in the publication by Houben et al. were intentionally biased to illustrate how to deal with variability in prevalence, potency as well as quality of evidence of data.[16] In 2020 Remington et al.[17] and Houben et al.[18] published results of analyses from the world's largest threshold database giving detailed insight into the potency of 14 major allergenic foods to trigger allergic symptoms. They published eliciting dose (ED) values for objective symptom elicitation by these foods derived via state-of-the-art evaluation and statistical modeling of results from low-dose oral challenges of allergic individuals using discrete as well as cumulative dose datasets. These data can be used to design a proof of principle for the prioritization as done in Houben et al.,[16] but this time using real potency and prevalence figures for allergenic foods. Therefore the ED50 values for milk, soy, egg, peanut, wheat, fish, and shrimp from the discrete dose datasets in Houben et al.[18] were combined with estimated overall point prevalence values based on positive food challenges or convincing history of allergy for these allergenic foods as published by Nwaru et al.,[19] to illustrate the ranking and comparison of allergenic foods according to these parameters based on actual highest quality data (Fig. 48.2). For shrimp, the estimated overall point prevalence for shellfish allergy from Nwaru et al. was used. Ranking according to ED50 values from the cumulative dose datasets from Houben et al.[18] would give in the same order of ranking of these foods as for the discrete dose dataset ED50 values.

The availability of reliable ED50 values for seven other allergenic foods (cashew, celery, hazelnut, lupin, mustard, sesame, walnut; Houben et al.[18]) and extensive data from literature searches and reviews on the prevalence of allergy to various foods allows development of a benchmark of such scaling of allergenic foods according to their public health importance as input for application of risk-based prioritization of allergenic foods for labeling legislation, as proposed by Houben et al.[16]

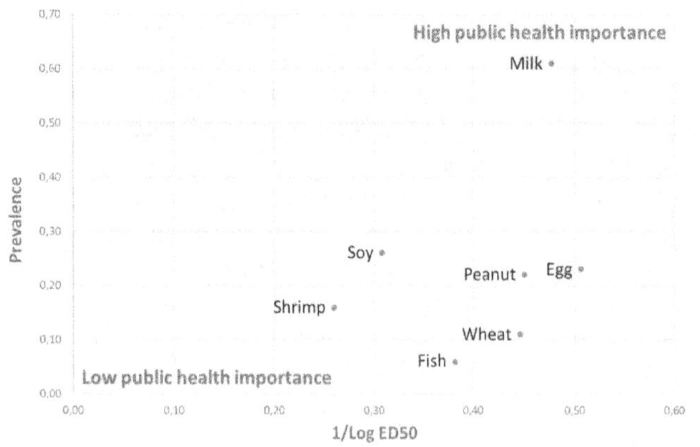

FIGURE 48.2 Illustration of public health importance ranking of allergenic foods according to the prevalence of allergy to the foods and ED50 values of these foods triggering objective allergic symptoms in 50% of the allergic individuals (based on ED50 values of discrete dose datasets from Houben et al.[18] and estimated overall point prevalence values based on positive food challenges or convincing history of allergy from Nwaru et al.[19]; for shrimp, the estimated overall point prevalence for shellfish allergy from Nwaru et al. was used).

48.2.2 Unintended allergen presence

The broad use of major allergenic foods and ingredients derived from these in our food supply and their presence all over in food production chains and facilities inevitably poses the risk of UAP. When the ingredient labeling legislation in Europe came to development in the second half of the nineties of last century, it was realized that such legislation someday would also trigger a need for information about the risks of UAP. As it was also clear that complete absence of any UAP seldom or never can be guaranteed, a hazard-based approach was unlikely to provide a solution for managing UAP. In those days, risk assessment approaches for food allergens, however, were not yet well explored. Dr. Geert F. Houben from the Netherlands Organisation for Applied Scientific Research (TNO) was the first to start exploring a QRA modeling approach for allergens based on probabilistic techniques in the late nineties, and first presented the concept at the First International Food Allergy Forum, held on April 15 and 16, 2002, in The Netherlands.[20] Probabilistic QRA (PQRA) is nowadays considered the most appropriate method of allergen risk assessment for population risk management purposes.[21] However, as also acknowledged by Houben back in 2002, data needed for applying this approach were lacking at the beginning of this century and had to be generated.

Risk assessment is based on a comparison of the exposure to a hazard and the potency of that hazard to cause harm. In most cases, a deterministic approach is used, in which a single value of the expected or measured exposure, often the P90, P95, or maximum exposure of the population, is compared to a single value of the potency to cause harm in the population, often a no-observed-adverse-effect-level or a lowest observed adverse effect level in the sensitive population, divided by a safety factor. If the value for the exposure exceeds that for the potency, a risk is assumed. The outcome thus is a binary one: a risk is assumed or not. In contrast, in a probabilistic risk assessment, not only single values from the exposure and potency data are used, but all information from the full range of datapoints and distributions of the population's exposure to a hazard and the potency of the hazard to cause harm in the population can be used and compared. This gives insight into the chance on an adverse reaction as well as in the variability and uncertainty in the estimates.[20] Simply worded and visualized, with food allergen PQRA, the proportion of eating occasions at which individuals' allergen intakes exceed the individuals' thresholds can be calculated (Fig. 48.3).

The allergen intake is determined by the level of the allergen in a food product and the amount of that food product consumed. For assessing the risk of certain levels of allergens in food products, the most important datasets thus required are the amounts of food products consumed by allergic individuals and the distribution of thresholds for effect elicitation in allergic individuals by the various allergenic foods. Since 2002, TNO in collaboration with many partners continued to develop the food allergen PQRA approach as well as the datasets required for such risk assessment. Now, by the year 2021, the food allergen PQRA methodology as well as our understanding of and datasets on thresholds for effect elicitation for various allergenic foods and on food intake by allergic individuals have reached a mature state and allow broad and reliable application for quantifying risks of (unintended) allergen presence in food. In Section 48.2.2.1, food allergen PQRA will be addressed in more detail.

PQRA of food allergens requires advanced expert knowledge, experience with probabilistic modeling, and access to suitable tools and datasets. Although it is considered the most appropriate method of risk assessment for population risk management purposes, performing a PQRA is not feasible for everyone, but also not always the only approach for getting relevant information. There may be circumstances in which a deterministic risk assessment (DRA) may be useful. As indicated above, complete absence of any UAP can never or seldom be guaranteed. This has motivated food business operators to apply PAL, to warn food allergic consumers or those buying or preparing food for food allergic individuals for the possible risk of allergen presence. However, there is no harmonized guidance or practice for when and when not to warn for the possible presence of allergens, and various studies have shown that there is little or no correlation between the presence and absence of a precautionary statement and the actual risk of allergen presence.[22–24]

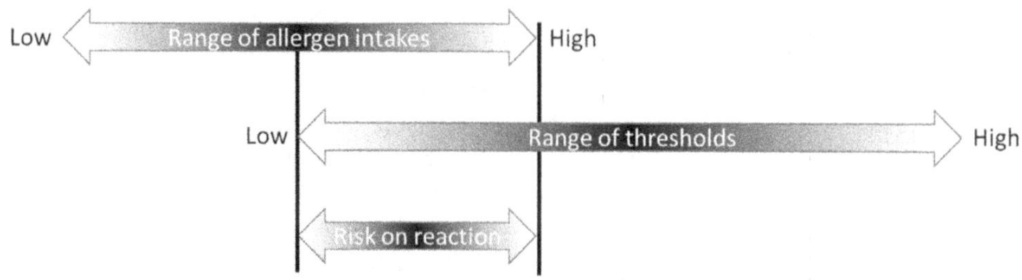

FIGURE 48.3 Food allergen probabilistic quantitative risk assessment is based on a comparison of the range of allergen intakes per eating occasion by allergic individuals and the range of thresholds for effect elicitation in the allergic population, which gives quantitative information on the chance on an allergic reaction, that is the proportion of eating occasions at which the individuals' allergen intakes exceeds the individuals' thresholds for that allergen. The shading intensity represents the distribution in the population: the darker the shade, the larger the proportion of the occasions in that range. *Based on Spanjersberg MQI, Kruizinga AG, Rennen MAJ, Houben GF Risk assessment and food allergy: the probabilistic model applied to allergens. Food Chem Toxicol. 2007;45(1):49. https://doi.org/10.1016/j.fct.2006.07.018.*

The same data and methodological principles as developed for food allergen PQRA can also be used for a DRA and to provide quantitative guidance for PAL. These aspects are further addressed in Sections 48.2.2.2 and 48.2.2.3, respectively.

48.2.2.1 Probabilistic quantitative risk assessment of food allergens

48.2.2.1.1 The history of probabilistic quantitative risk assessment of food allergens

The first publication by TNO on the application of PQRA modeling to food allergens[20] was a proof of principle, as reliable datasets for broad application were still lacking. But the authors sketched various potential applications that could take away important hurdles for the application of risk-based food safety management to allergens. In a follow-up paper in 2008, Kruizinga et al.[25] reported on sensitivity analyses performed to identify which parts of the PQRA model most influence the output, to get insight into the reliability of PQRA and guide future data gathering for improving the application opportunities of PQRA of allergens in food. The sensitivity analyses demonstrated that a shift in the distribution of the EDs reflecting a more potent allergen, and an increase in the proportion of the population consuming a food, increased the number of estimated allergic reactions considerably. In contrast, the number of estimated allergic reactions hardly changed when the EDs were based on a more severe response, or when the amount of food consumed was increased.[25] In 2009, Spanjersberg et al.[26] elaborated on the principles and various potential applications of probabilistic approaches in food allergen risk analyses. In the same year, Madsen et al.[21] reported on a workshop organized by the EU project EuroPrevall in which various approaches for food allergen risk assessment were assessed. Probabilistic modeling was considered to be the most promising approach for use in population risk assessment, among others because it does not rely on low-dose extrapolations with its inherent issues. Meanwhile, generation and collection of datasets considered most important to be enriched for the further development and application of food allergen PQRA came to development.

48.2.2.1.2 Development and validation of eliciting dose-distribution datasets

In 2010, Blom et al.[27] presented for the first time on a threshold database build by TNO. This was done at the symposium Frontiers in Food Allergen Risk Assessment, held in Nice, France, jointly organized by ILSI Europe, the EU project EuroPrevall, ILSI Health and Environmental Sciences Institute, the UK Food Standards Agency, and the Food Allergy Research and Resources Program (FARRP) of the University of Nebraska, United States (https://hesiglobal.org/wp-content/uploads/sites/11/2016/06/ILSI_Eur_Symposium102210.pdf). The TNO database contained results from low-dose challenges of allergic individuals with allergenic substances. At the symposium, Dr. Geert F. Houben from TNO and Dr. Steve Taylor from FARRP met and recognized the opportunities of joining forces and data and entered into a partnership. This led to what is still the world's largest threshold database, in 2020 containing low-dose challenge data from almost 3500 allergic individuals.[17,18]

In 2014, in the framework of elaborating reference doses (RDs) for PAL (see also Section 48.2.2.3), TNO and FARRP together with others first published results from statistical analyses from their joint threshold database. Doses predicted to elicit mild objective allergic symptoms in 1% or 5% of the allergic individuals were published for 10 allergenic foods.[28,29] Although the database contains results from low-dose challenges with various allergenic foods from many patients, many clinics, multiple regions of the world, and various processed forms of challenge materials, and so on, and is likely to capture much of the sources of inter- and intraindividual variability that may influence EDs, the question arose how well the ED-distributions account for variability in

EDs in daily life. Therefore several studies were conducted to validate predicted ED values and to investigate the influence of sources of variability and uncertainty. Zurzolo et al.[30] and Hourihane et al.[31] conducted and published perhaps the most important validation study. In a multicenter study involving three geographically diverse regions in Cork, Boston, and Melbourne, 378 children aged 1–18 years were dosed with peanut protein at the dose predicted to elicit mild objective symptoms in 5% of the allergic population (ED05) according to Taylor et al.[28] Only eight subjects (2.1% instead of predicted 5%) met the prefixed criteria for mild objective symptoms. All reactions were mild; only four patients received any medications (antihistamines), while none needed adrenaline/epinephrine.[31] This result indicates that the dataset and modeling approach used by Taylor et al.[28] resulted in a somewhat conservative estimate, slightly overestimating the risk, and confirms the safety of the ED05 estimate. In the framework of the EU project Integrated Approaches to Food Allergen and Allergy Risk Management (iFAAM: https://cordis.europa.eu/project/id/312147), similar single-dose studies were started on milk, egg and hazelnut in four different clinical centers. Although none of these iFAAM studies reached the statistical power needed for formally validating the respective ED05 values, the results obtained did at least not falsify the safety of the ED05 values for these allergenic foods, while confirming the safety of the hazelnut ED05 with reasonable statistical certainty. The single dose challenges undertaken for hazelnut and milk have provided important pilot data and indicate that further validation using additional subjects will enable the ED05 values to be fully validated. However, none of the 75 children recruited into the study reacted to the ED05 for egg. This could be interpreted to suggest the estimated and tested ED05 is lower than the actual ED05.[32] Dua et al.[33] investigated the possible influence of cofactors on EDs, by studying the effect of sleep deprivation and exercise on reaction thresholds in peanut allergic individuals. They found that these cofactors might influence reaction thresholds, but the group ED01 value under the stressed conditions was still above the ED01 value for peanut obtained from the most recent analyses of the TNO-FARRP threshold database.[17,18] These cofactors thus might influence thresholds, but apparently not beyond the variability already captured in the database from which ED-values can be calculated, containing data from multiple patients, clinics, regions of the world, and processed forms of challenge materials, and likely also covering differences in health status (such as underlying infections, hormonal variations), seasonal influences, lack of sleep due to anxiousness because of the scheduled challenge test, and so on. Furthermore, cofactors do not play a role for every patient and will not be present during all unintended allergen exposure occasions,[34] and their possible influence on population ED-distributions in normal life will therefore be small. Versluis et al.[35] also found no evidence for an association between potential cofactors examined and reaction severity. In various multistakeholder conferences, it was considered appropriate to account for a potential role of cofactors in individual patient allergy management and not in allergen management programs.[36,37] As analyses of EDs derived from studies in different age groups, different geographic locations or with differently processed challenge materials found no difference in ED-distributions attributable to these variables,[17,18,29,38] the available ED datasets allow broad, worldwide application in risk assessment.

With all the achievements described above, considerable insight has been gained into the variability in potencies of allergenic foods, the distribution of the EDs for effect elicitation for the major allergenic foods, and the reliability of such ED-distribution as one of the important inputs for food allergen PQRA according to sensitivity analyses of Kruizinga et al.[25] Although the sensitivity analyses showed that the number of estimated allergic reactions by PQRA hardly changed when the EDs were based on a more severe response, for harmonization purposes, it is of major importance to carefully consider how to use results from low-dose challenges and on what symptoms to base ED-distributions. Westerhout et al.[39] therefore developed and published guidance for this based on consensus among a broad range of international experts, thereby further contributing to an optimal harmonization of input parameters for PQRA of food allergens.

Data used so far for ED-distribution modeling are mainly derived from double-blind placebo-controlled food challenges (DBPCFCs),[17,18,28,40–42] but recent analyses indicate that data from open challenges are comparably reliable for population threshold distribution modeling.[43] While collecting data from DBPCFCs, TNO and FARRP therefore also started capturing data on open challenges and addition of these data to the TNO-FARRP threshold database will likely increase the number of datapoints from low-dose challenges of allergic individuals with various allergenic foods with approximately another thousand. This may particularly be of importance for allergenic foods for which relatively few or no datapoints from DBPCFCs are available. For several allergenic foods, (far) over 100 datapoints are available, but for some, only a limited or no dataset is available. For assessing the reliability of limited datapoints and guiding prioritization for the generation or collection of additional data from low-dose challenges, Klein Entink et al.[44] performed an evaluation of the influence of the number of oral food challenge datapoints on the accuracy of threshold dose distribution modeling and concluded that the largest relative gains in accuracy are obtained when sample sizes increase up to 60. This indicates that challenge data from

60 patients or more may result in acceptably reliable ED-distributions, closely matching those of larger datasets. Nevertheless, if risk management decisions are needed, decisions may be made on sample sizes with less than 60 individuals and sometimes even less than 30 individuals, depending on the distribution of datapoints along the ED-distribution curve.[44] With the addition and use of data from open challenges, acceptably rich datasets and elaboration of ED-distributions may become feasible for more major allergenic foods the coming years.

A source of variability of PQRA-outcomes not yet mentioned, is the choice of statistical models. For instance, ED-distributions for many years were modeled using various statistical models, mostly based on Loglogistic, Lognormal, and Weibull distributions.[45] This, however, results in different predictions of risks or ED-values for single datasets, which may give rise to distinct interpretations and decisions. Taylor et al.[28] applied expert judgment based on the fit of the predicted ED-distribution with the original datapoints from the low-dose challenges and discarded models that showed a poor fit. Statistical model averaging would be a more transparent way to achieve unambiguousness of modeling results,[46] but a model averaging method was not available for the type of data available for food allergen ED-distribution modeling.[17,18,47] TNO and FARRP in collaboration with external experts therefore developed a model averaging method suitable for this goal.[47] This method was used to analyze the data contained in the 2020 version of the TNO-FARRP threshold database, using the international consensus guidance for the evaluation and use of results from low-dose challenges as published by Westerhout et al.[39] Results of these analyses were published by Remington et al.[17] and Houben et al.[18]

48.2.2.1.3 Development and validation of food intake-distribution datasets

As explained before, for assessing the risk of certain levels of allergens in food products, besides ED-distribution data from the various allergenic foods, data on the amounts of food products consumed by allergic individuals are essential. Food intake data are available from food consumption surveys from many countries.[48] However, most of these surveys have been conducted for nutritional or toxicological assessment purposes. For these purposes, generally long-term average intake amounts are the most important measure of food intake and most published information from these surveys are on this measure. In contrast, because IgE-mediated food allergic reactions generally develop within minutes to half an hour after intake of the allergenic protein, intake amounts at single eating occasions is the relevant measure of food intake for food allergy risk assessment and risk management. Data from food consumption surveys do contain information on this latter, acute food intake amounts, but this information usually is not published or even not assessed. For use in food allergen risk assessment, this information therefore usually has to be extracted from the original survey data records and needs to be processed specifically for the purpose of food allergen risk analysis. In parallel with the development of ED-distribution datasets, food intake datasets specifically attuned to the requirements of food allergen risk analyses have been developed.[20,23] However, these datasets are all based on surveys among the general population or specific age groups of the general population, and not specifically among food allergic individuals. In parallel with the development of food intake datasets for food allergen risk analyses, studies were conducted to investigate the suitability of datasets from the general population for use in allergen risk analysis for the food allergic population.[49]

The sensitivity analyses by Kruizinga et al. showed that an increase in the proportion of the population consuming a food increased the number of estimated allergic reactions considerably.[25] It is likely that food allergic individuals avoid specific foods and thus may have a tendency of more often choosing other, alternative food products. For some food products, the proportion of the population eating these thus will likely differ between the general and the allergic population. As this proportion significantly influences the number of estimated allergic reactions, it is recommended to avoid using the proportion of users in the risk assessment and to express risk assessment outcomes for instance as the chance on allergic symptoms in case an allergic individual eats a food product containing a certain level of allergenic protein. This way, the proportion of the population using the product, a figure that may not be available specifically for the allergic subpopulation, is not needed.

If the proportion of the population using the product is left out of the risk assessment equation, only the amounts consumed of a product by the allergic user population at single eating occasions is needed. The sensitivity analyses of Kruizinga et al. showed that the number of estimated allergic reactions hardly changed when the amount of food consumed was changed.[25] This indicates that the amount consumed of a product is a less critical factor. Furthermore, in case allergic individuals decide to eat a specific food product, it may be assumed that there are not really reasons why, on a group level, the amounts consumed would differ from nonallergic users. This, however, is an assumption that preferably should be verified, to support the suitability of general population food intake data for food allergen risk assessment. Blom et al.[49] therefore conducted food intake surveys in two cohorts of food allergic individuals and compared the food intake with that by matched samples from the Dutch National Food Consumption Survey and found no statistically significant differences between either of the two allergic populations and the general population. Consequently, only small variations in estimated risks of allergen levels in food products were found, that would not result in different risk management decisions. They concluded that food intake data from the general population can be used for food allergen risk assessment and will not lead to a relevant under- or overestimation of the risk for the food allergic population.[49] As food intake data from the general population have been surveyed in many countries, food intake data suitable for food allergen risk assessment therefore are available from surveys in many countries. But, as indicated before, this needs to concern acute food intake information, which generally has to be extracted from the original survey data records and needs to be processed specifically for the purpose of food allergen risk analysis.

48.2.2.1.4 Application of probabilistic quantitative risk assessment of food allergens

In 2010, the first two studies of actual application of PQRA of food allergens appeared. Spanjersberg et al. published on a study triggered by a case of a cow's milk protein allergic patient that experienced a severe allergic reaction to a dark chocolate product containing undeclared milk proteins and showed that milk protein concentrations in unlabeled products can reach levels that may elicit allergic reactions in up to 68% of the adult allergic consumers.[23] In the same year, Rimbaud et al.[50] published a probabilistic model applied to peanut in chocolate, which was later broadened to various food products.[51] With the further development of datasets on ED-distributions for various allergenic foods and food intake datasets suitable for food allergen risk assessment, broad application became feasible and Remington et al.[22] and Blom et al.[24] published results of risk analysis studies on proteins from a range of allergenic foods in multiple food products on the market in the United Kingdom and the Netherlands, respectively.

A complex aspect inherent to the methodological principles of the PQRA models used is that any level of an allergen in a food product, even the lowest level, will be predicted to pose a (tiny) risk. This is due to the statistical distributions of the datasets used. The probabilistic model selects samples from the ED and the food intake distributions, which sometimes coincidentally may combine a value at the high end tail of the food intake distribution and the low-end tail of the ED-distribution, which even may be values beyond the rage actually occurring in practice. This was nicely illustrated by Blom et al.,[52] who assessed risks from residual peanut protein present in highly refined vegetable oils due to cross-contact with refined peanut oil, and showed that the low incidence of predicted allergic reactions concerned reactions predicted to occur for doses of peanut protein which were at least a factor of 10 below the lowest individual clinical threshold dose in the large threshold dataset for peanut. They also presented a way of analyzing this, allowing the conclusion that the health risk from cross-contact between vegetable oils and refined peanut oil is negligible, despite a small risk mathematically predicted by PQRA. A similar analysis was previously applied by Remington et al.[53]

48.2.2.2 Deterministic risk assessment of food allergens

Although PQRA is considered the most appropriate method of risk assessment for population risk management purposes, there may be circumstances in which a DRA may be useful.[18] Within the framework of the EU project iFAAM (https://cordis.europa.eu/project/id/312147), in which TNO led the food allergen risk assessment and risk management work packages, DRA was incorporated in a tiered risk analysis approach to perform a first quick check on possible risks. In case the DRA indicates a possible risk, risk mitigation measures or a more refined risk assessment, and if needed a PQRA with expert support, should be considered.[37]

Although the amount consumed of a food product appeared a less critical factor in PQRA of food allergens,[25] use of appropriate food intake values nevertheless is important, particularly in case of a DRA, in which not the whole distribution of food intake amounts in the population, but only one single value of food intake is used. Under- or overestimation of the intake of food products may result in inaccurate judgments and can result in riskfull situations or in unnecessary measures and recall and destruction of batches of food products assumed unsafe. Selection of appropriate single intake values of food intake appears difficult for many, as found out at several workshops (co)organized by TNO. Groups of risk assessors and quality managers from food companies were presented with several case descriptions together with various options for selecting food intake values for risk assessment. Prior to the exercises, each group was quite convinced to know which type of data was appropriate. Yet, considerable differences occurred between the various groups in the selection of food intake values considered appropriate (Fig. 48.4). If these different choices would be used for exposure assessment in DRA or for assessing the need for PAL, with for instance a difference of a factor of 8 for crisps between group 1 and 6, these would result in considerable differences in assessed risks or in decisions regarding the need for PAL for one and the same food product.

Further guidance for the selection of appropriate food intake data thus is important for assuring correct DRA of food allergens and harmonization of PAL practices.

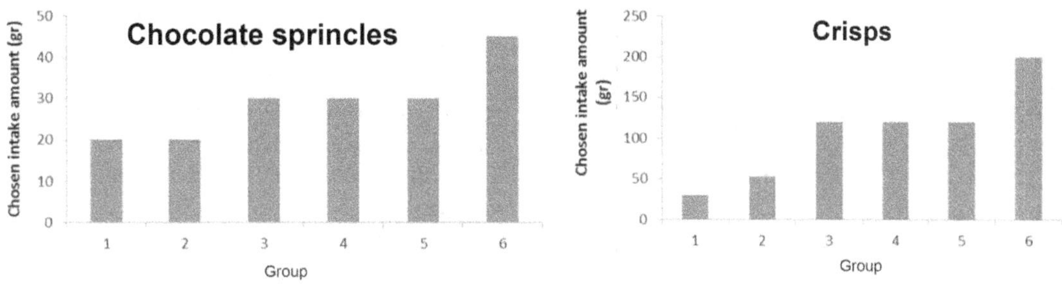

FIGURE 48.4 Examples illustrating the difficulty of selecting appropriate food intake values for use in food allergen risk assessment. In workshops with groups of risk assessors and quality managers from food companies, several case descriptions were given together with various options for selecting food intake values for use in risk assessment. Considerable differences occurred in the selection of food intake values considered appropriate between the groups.

Therefore, in the framework of the iFAAM project, Blom et al.[54] conducted sensitivity analysis to derive a food consumption point estimate for DRA of food allergens. They simulated scenarios of presence of protein from 10 different allergenic foods in food products of 48 food groups, at eight different concentrations, ranging from 1 to 1000 mg protein from the allergenic food/kg food product. For each scenario, they calculated the intake of protein from the allergenic food using 13 different measures for the food product intake amount on a single eating occasion, ranging from the P50 up to the P100 (max) from the population intake distribution. Each of these intakes of protein from the allergenic food was used to perform a DRA, which was compared with a PQRA for the same scenario. For 99% of the food groups, the P50 consumption resulted in a safe DRA, while the P75 did so for 100% of the food groups. The authors concluded that the P75 of the general population food intake at single eating occasions is optimal for use in DRA of food allergens and is adequately conservative for DRA of food allergens in a public health context to comply with an ED01 safety objective. More recently, Blom et al. (in preparation) updated these analyses and showed that intake values based on the P50 to P65 of the general population distribution of the single eating occasion intake of foods result in compliance with a broad range of safety objectives (including the ED01 and ED05) without being overconservative. Based on these results, they recommend to use this P50 as food intake value for DRA. If the P50 is not available, the mean would be a good alternative, as analyses of the intake data showed that the mean generally is between p50 and p65.

To be able to conduct a DRA, besides appropriate food intake values, insight into the risk posed by various doses of allergenic protein from allergenic foods is need. To support risk assessors, to assure the use of the best available up-to-date data, and to stimulate harmonization of food allergen risk assessment and risk management and PAL practices, Houben et al.[18] in 2020 published full population ED-distribution information for 14 priority allergenic foods. Additionally, they gave several recommendations for the use of the published ED information as well as regarding the selection of appropriate food intake data and the conduct of food allergen DRA in general.

48.2.2.3 Quantitative guidance for precautionary allergen labeling

The importance and broad use of several major allergenic foods and ingredients derived from these in our current food supply, pose the risk of UAP in food products. All companies in the food chain, from breeding and harvest, through transport and processing, to end product and retail companies, have a role in mitigating the risk of UAP. However, for certain chains and products, the risk of UAP cannot be reduced to a zero or negligible risk. To warn allergic consumers or those buying or preparing food for allergic consumers for the possible risks of UAP, food business operators have introduced the use of PAL. However, many incidents and studies have shown that the use and absence of PAL show little or no correlation with the actual risks of UAP.[23,24,55–60] These studies have shown that, depending on the study and the product categories and allergens investigated, products with PAL appeared to actually contain the allergen warned for in 7%–93% of the products. This implies that also 7%–93% did not contain the allergen warned for. Products without a warning appeared to contain major allergens not warned for in 11%–53% of the cases. To investigate to what extent labeling issues play a role in the occurrence of unexpected allergic reactions, Blom et al.[24] and Michelsen-Huisman et al.[61] conducted a prospective study in which 157 food allergic individuals were followed during one year and were requested to report every case of unexpected allergic reaction and to collect the culprit food products. Half of the subjects had 1 or more, on average 2, unexpected allergic reaction during the one-year follow-up. These reactions generally were mild to severe and 4% of the subjects ended up in a hospital

Emergency Room. In the majority of the cases, a prepacked food product was the culprit food. Samples of all food products collected were analyzed for the presence of the allergens the respective allergic patient was allergic to, but only for allergens not declared to be an ingredient of the food product. In 38% of the products, 1–4 culprit noningredient allergens were present. PAL info and allergen presences were in agreement in 57% of the products, and thus not in agreement in 43% of the products, while sometimes there was a PAL for other allergens than those found at analysis. Levels of noningredient allergens were comparable for products with or without PAL.[24] The results of this prospective study clearly illustrate that food allergic consumers cannot rely on the presence or absence of PAL and that the current situation daily puts millions of food allergic consumers at risk. There thus is an urgent need to improve allergen information on food. Several aspects need to be addressed to achieve this, but most important and the first is the implementation and harmonization of quantitative guidance for when and when not to apply PAL.

There are two countries that already in the early years of this century decided to prescribe a quantitative criterion for obligatory labeling of UAP. In Japan, for all allergens present at levels above 10 mg/kg food product, mandatory disclosure applies, while in Switzerland, levels above 1000 mg/kg require disclosure.[5] However, these quantitative criteria do not take into consideration differences in amounts consumed of the various foods and the fact that allergenic foods vary considerably in their potency to induce allergic symptoms. For instance, the proteins from mustard are a factor of 460 to 640 more potent in triggering allergic symptoms than those from shrimp, based on a comparison of ED50 values as published by Houben et al.[18] ED50 values are considered an appropriate value for comparing potencies of allergenic foods.[16] The cutoff chosen by Switzerland is so high that proteins from most major allergenic foods may be present in many foods (depending on the amounts consumed of the food) at levels that may trigger allergic symptoms in up to 50% of the allergic consumers without requirement to be labeled, while for several allergenic foods, the Japanese cutoff may be very conservative and perhaps overprotective, as nicely illustrated in Madsen et al.[62]

The Allergen Bureau of Australia and New Zealand developed a quantitative guidance accounting for the differences in potency of the various allergen foods to induce allergic symptoms and for differences in food intake. In their Voluntary Incidental Trace Allergen Labeling (VITAL) program,[63] different action levels (ALs) are recommended for proteins from the various major allergenic foods, depending on the intake of the food containing residues of an allergenic food and the allergenic food's potency to induce allergic symptoms. This potency is reflected in RDs, which were elaborated by TNO and FARRP though statistical analysis of data from the TNO-FARRP threshold database and recommended by the VITAL Scientific Expert Panel (VSEP). The RDs are used to calculate the ALs for PAL accounting for the intake of the food containing residues of the allergenic food (VITAL ® Voluntary Incidental Trace Allergen Labellingl Allergen Bureau). The first version of these RDs was implemented in the VITAL program in 2012.[28,29] Since then, many conferences, expert groups, and projects worldwide discussed and evaluated these RDs for suitability to guide PAL decisions.

Between 2010 and 2013, an Expert Group of the Food Allergy Task Force of ILSI Europe evaluated the reliability and suitability of the data underlying the RDs as well as the RDs derived by Taylor et al.[28] for food allergen risk assessment and risk management. The RDs as well as the data underlying these were considered appropriate for these goals. One particular aspect was specifically investigated. That was the question whether ALs based on the RDs would also be sufficiently protective for scenario's in which two different food items, eaten by an allergic consumer during one meal, would both have a risk of incidental unintended presence of the same allergenic protein. In Crevel et al.,[64] these analyses are described and the authors conclude that the ALs and RDs are also sufficiently protective in such scenarios. The results of the work of the Expert Group were presented and discussed at an international workshop in Reading, United Kingdom, 2012, organized by ILSI Europe in collaboration with FARRP, Health Canada, ILSI Japan, ILSI North America, and the University of Nebraska. The participating representatives from patient organizations, industry, government, clinicians, dieticians, and science, from all continents of the world, agreed that a consistent, transparent set of RDs, as a basis for ALs, would be a desirable outcome, and that data from food challenge studies, as used for the RDs proposed by Taylor et al.,[28] are the appropriate foundation from which RDs and ALs can be derived. They also agreed that sufficient data exist to move forward and that the proposed RDs constitute a reasonable first pass to minimize risks to the allergic consumer while maintaining food choices. Finally, they emphasized that introduction of RDs should be accompanied by appropriate training, education, and communication (Advances in the Risk Management of Unintended Presence of Allergenic Foods in Manufactured Food Products—An Overview. https://ilsi.eu/webinar-on-allergen-risk-assessment/).

During the last decade, many food companies have started to use the RDs proposed by Taylor et al.[28] as a benchmark for managing UAP and deciding on PAL. Also several authorities, particularly those in northwestern Europe, accepted the concept of using RDs and moved away from a zero-risk approach for the management of UAP.[62] They also accepted the type of data and the modeling approaches to derive RDs and made use of the TNO-FARRP data and analyses published in Taylor et al.[28] However, they make different choices regarding the level of conservatism.[62] Further effort to promote consensus and harmonization apparently is needed. The efforts conducted and the results obtained were already summarized in Section 48.2.2.1 of this book chapter and mainly consisted of the further development and validation of population ED-distribution datasets. All these results were used to derive updated ED01 and ED05 values for 14 different major allergenic foods, based on over 3400 individual patient threshold datapoints.[17] These ED-values were used by the VSEP to recommend updated RDs, based on the ED01 values, for the VITAL program of the Allergen Bureau of Australia and New Zealand, which were adopted in a 2019 update of the VITAL program as VITAL version 3.0 RDs.[65] These updated RDs, combined with the results of Blom et al.[54] and Blom et al (in preparation) on the most appropriate food intake value to use as a point estimate for food allergen risk assessment, that is, the P50 or mean of the general population food intake at single eating occasions, provide unambiguous guidance for establishing ALs for PAL and hopefully contribute to further consensus and harmonization of food allergen risk assessment and risk management practices.

ALs calculated using RDs based on for instance the ED01 and the P75 of the general population food intake at single eating occasions can be used to further illustrate the difference between using one single regulatory limit as done by Switzerland and Japan and an approach accounting for the differences in potency in symptom elicitation of various allergenic foods and differences in food intake. Fig. 48.5 shows the AL for all combinations of iFAAM food groups (food groups ordered according to increasing P75 value from top to bottom; iFAAM food group P75 values from Birot et al.[66]) and protein from allergenic foods potentially unintendedly present in food products in these food groups (allergenic foods ordered according to increasing potency, that is, decreasing RD, from left to right; RDs from VITAL 3.0).[65] In color, it is indicated how the single Japanese or Swiss regulatory thresholds compare with the food group and allergenic food-specific VITAL ALs. As can be seen, the Swiss regulatory threshold results in a higher risk (>>1%) for almost all combinations of food groups and allergenic foods. This is also the case for the Japanese threshold in about half of the combinations of food groups and allergenic foods, but in a considerable number of combinations of food groups and allergenic foods, the Japanese threshold is more protective (over-protective) compared to the VITAL AL.

Another comparison often considered is that of the ALs resulting from the application of RDs and sensitivities of analytical methods. Many are concerned that ALs derived from the RDs are too low to allow verification of compliance by analytical monitoring, particularly for food products of which high quantities are consumed at a single meal, for which relatively low concentrations of allergenic protein may already result in high allergen intakes. However, case studies have shown that analytical sensitivities are sufficient to analyze at an appropriate level for most food product–allergen combinations, if analyses are conducted targeted. In Fig. 48.6, this approach is illustrated using similar tables as for the comparison of VITAL ALs with the Japanese and Swiss regulatory thresholds. The left table in Fig. 48.6 shows the same

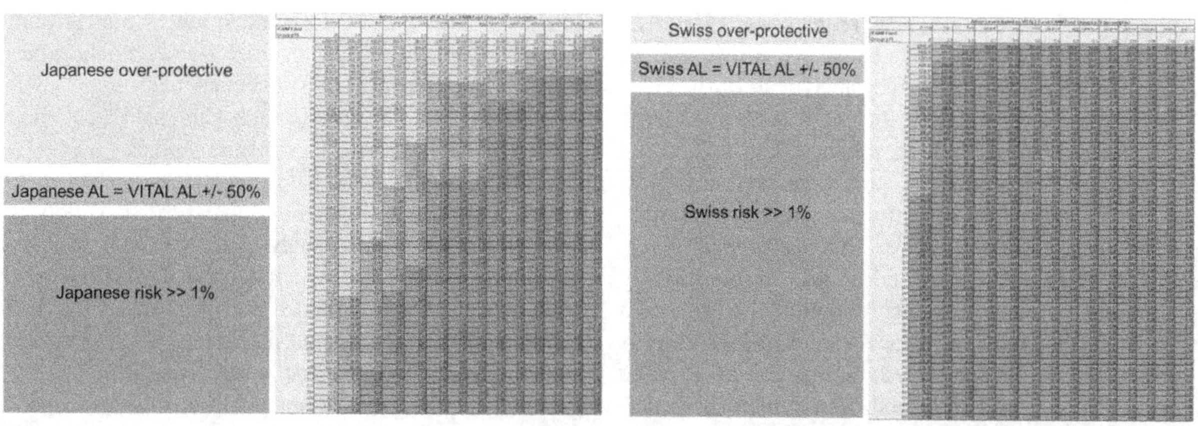

FIGURE 48.5 Illustration of the difference between using one single regulatory threshold as done by Switzerland and Japan and an approach accounting for the differences in food intake and in potency in symptom elicitation of various allergenic foods. Tables show action levels (ALs) for precautionary allergen labeling for all combinations of population P75 intakes of iFAAM food groups[66] and Voluntary Incidental Trace Allergen Labeling (VITAL) version 3.0 reference doses for allergenic foods.[65] The single Japanese or Swiss regulatory threshold is comparable with VITAL AL (within VITAL AL ± 50%) for part of the food products-allergen combinations; The Japanese or Swiss regulatory threshold is over-protective in comparison with VITAL AL in part of the combinations; The Japanese or Swiss regulatory threshold results in a risk higher (>>1%) than that with VITAL AL in the majority of combinations.

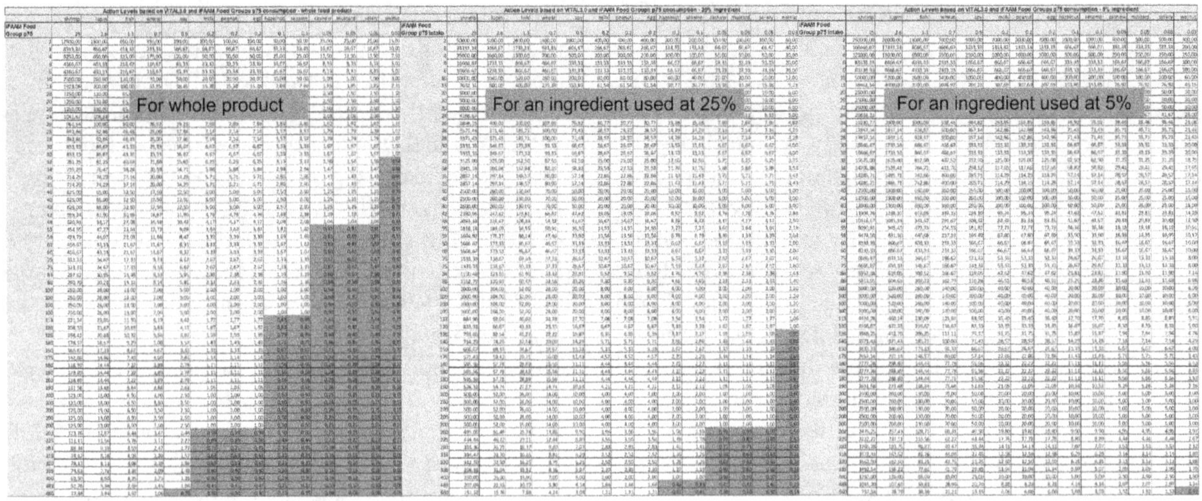

FIGURE 48.6 Illustration of the adequacy of sensitivity of analytical methods for verification of compliance of food products with reference doses (RDs). Tables show action levels for precautionary allergen labeling for all combinations of population P75 intakes of iFAAM food groups[66] and Voluntary Incidental Trace Allergen Labeling (VITAL) version 3.0 RDs for allergenic foods[65] (left table) and corresponding levels for ingredients used at a level of 25% (middle table) and 5% (right table) in a food product. An analytical limit of determination of 1 mg/kg food is assumed. Uncolored cells: analytical sensitivity adequate; colored cells: analytical sensitivity of 1 mg/kg food insufficient.

ALS for all combinations of population P75 intakes of iFAAM food groups and VITAL version 3.0 RDs for allergenic foods as in Fig. 48.5. Most analytical methods can reliably quantify proteins from allergenic foods at levels down to below 1 mg/kg food product. If conservatively, a Limit of Determination of 1 mg/kg food is assumed, analytical sensitivities are sufficient for most food group-allergenic food combinations (uncolored combinations in left table of Fig. 48.6). However, for some food groups, ALs for protein from several allergenic foods are too low to verify (red-colored combinations). Yet, in most cases, such food products are composed of several ingredients, which provide the opportunity to analyze the ingredients prior to use or purchase. The ALs that apply for the end product as consumed can be used to calculate corresponding required analytical sensitivities for ingredients. For instance, for ingredients used at a level of 25% or 5% in a food product, 4 and 20 times higher limits in the ingredients apply, respectively. This results in an enormous reduction in the food product-allergenic food combinations for which analytical sensitivity may be insufficient (middle and right table in Fig. 48.6). This illustrates that analysis of ingredients often is a feasible solution in case analytical sensitivity is insufficient for an end product. It further has to be noted that sensitivities of analytical methods for allergens generally allow analyses at levels below 1 mg/kg food, implying that the number of combinations for which the analytical sensitivity is too low is actually lower that assumed in Fig. 48.6.

It should be realized that in case of incidental presence of allergens, monitoring and control through sampling and analysis generally are extremely inefficient and insufficient for protecting the allergic consumer. A careful risk analysis to identify potential allergenic hazards and their entry points and validation and verification of appropriate control of these, by the food business operator but also by authorities, is a much better guarantee of optimal protection of the allergic consumer. If identified that an ingredient or a raw material is an unavoidable potential incidental source of an allergen, then income specifications for such ingredient or raw material are needed (i.e., the provider of the ingredient or a raw material needs to assess and declare the maximum level of UAP), to assure that the maximal incidental UAP will not lead to a level in excess of the AL for that allergen in the end product. It then is much more efficient to monitor the ingredient or raw material for compliance, particularly if this poses less analytical challenges.

Overall, the above illustrates that analytical methods often may be adequate to verify compliance of food products with ALs for PAL based on RDs derived from ED01 values. For cases in which the analytical sensitivity is not sufficient or borderline, analyses as presented in Fig. 48.6 can guide for required specifications for improvement of analytical methods. It finally has to be noted that in food safety standard setting, establishment of a health-based standard usually is done first, on the basis of which the targets and requirements of analytical methods are specified, and in case additional methods or improvement of methods is needed, time to achieve these improvements may be allowed prior to coming into effect and enforcement of the standard. It should preferably not work the other way around, that analytical methods are thought to be needed prior to establishing a safety standard.

As will be obvious from the above, reliable methodologies and datasets have become available during the last decade that would enable establishment of internationally harmonized RDs for PAL. However, absence of agreement on what risk is tolerable has made it difficult to set such quantitative limits to manage food allergen risks and effectively protect allergic consumers. An Expert Group of ILSI Europe proposed a framework built around the criteria suggested by Murphy and Gardoni[67] for approaches to defining tolerable risks.[62] Applying these criteria to food allergy, the Expert Group concluded that sufficient knowledge exists to implement the framework, including sufficient expertise across the whole range of stakeholders to allow opinions to be heard and respected, and a consensus to be achieved.[62]

48.2.3 The way forward

In the previous sections of this chapter, the history, advancements, and state-of-the-art regarding the risk analysis of ingredients and residues from current, existing allergenic foods have been described. During the second decade of this century, methodologies and datasets have grown to maturity and with the publication of the full range of population ED values for 14 priority allergenic foods by Houben et al.[18] in 2020, final pieces of crucial detailed input data for the risk analysis of these priority allergenic foods have become available and accessible for all. Also, in many stakeholder meetings, consensus was found that it is time to move forward with implementing a risk-based approach to allergen management. All pieces seemed to come together with a perfect timing to optimally inform an ad hoc Joint FAO/WHO Expert Consultation on Risk Assessment of Food Allergens, to address the various aspects of risk analysis of food allergens in 2020 and 2021.[68] Hopefully, somewhen in the first half of the current twenties, we will have version 2.0 of risk analysis of ingredients and residues of allergenic foods: a real risk-based management of food allergens.

48.3 Allergenicity of proteins in novel food supply

Our current nutritional protein supply heavily relies on animal-based proteins. Animal-based food protein production, however, has an enormous environmental impact and increasing the sustainability of our food protein supply is urgently needed. New protein sources and yield, processing and application of protein-rich fractions from existing sources that currently are not used may provide an important contribution to the required innovations. However, as most, if not all proteins are allergenic, new protein products will pose new allergenic risks, and premarket assessment and approval of these is important to not unacceptably increase the burden of food allergy. Approaches for the assessment of allergenicity of new food protein products initially mainly came to development for the assessment of foods derived from GMOs, but have also slowly come to development for proteins in novel food supply the last decade.[69] Allergenic risks of new food proteins may result from potential cross-reactivity in individuals allergic to related proteins or from development of new allergies due to de novo allergenicity. There may be practical issues that hamper the assessment of risks due to cross-reactivity that need to be addressed on a case by case basis, but in general, the approaches for assessing cross-reactivity seem to perform well and are well applicable.[7] However, particularly the tools for the premarket assessment of de novo allergenicity of new food proteins are still poor in methods with proven high predictive value.[7,8]

48.3.1 History and current approaches for assessing allergenicity of new food protein products

Over the last decades, several approaches and recommendations for evaluating the potential allergenicity of new food protein products were published, which were mainly focused on the assessment of transgenic proteins in genetically modified (GM) crops.[70] The first systematic approach was published by the International Food Biotechnology Council (IFBC), in collaboration with the Allergy and Immunology Institute (AII) of the ILSI in 1996.[71] This approach addressed the potential allergenic concerns of GM crops and suggested the use of a decision tree and introduced the use of bioinformatics and pepsin resistance for the assessment.[72] An important starting point for the assessment was the consideration of the source of the transgene, that is, whether this concerns an allergenic or a nonallergenic source. In case of an allergenic source, an IgE-binding study using sera from well-characterized patients allergic to the source was suggested, followed, if necessary, by additional clinical studies such as skin-prick testing or food challenge studies. In case of a nonallergenic source, a homology search for eight or more contiguous identical amino acids and a pepsin resistance study were suggested. If a significant bioinformatics match occurred, an IgE-binding study and additional clinical studies were recommended by the IFBC/ILSI.[70]

Approximate five years later, the Joint Food and Agriculture Organization/World Health Organization of the United Nations (FAO/WHO) Consultation on Foods Derived from Biotechnology developed a new approach including additional recommendations.[73] Like IFBC/ILSI, FAO/WHO recommended to consider the source of the transgene (allergenic or nonallergenic) and subsequent bioinformatics and pepsin resistance analysis. Also, specific IgE-binding studies using sera from well-characterized individuals allergic to an identified allergenic source were recommended. However, the FAO/WHO eliminated human testing and modified the bioinformatics parameters, that is, they decreased the threshold from eight or more to six or more contiguous identical amino acids and introduced a new parameter of >35% amino acid identity over an 80 amino acid window to identify potential cross-reactive allergenic proteins.[70] Later studies have indicated that the decreased threshold (six or more contiguous identical amino acids) occurs too commonly across proteins, which resulted in a high number of false-positive findings and should therefore not be utilized.[74–77] In 2007 Ladics et al. reported that a conventional analysis (overall sequence alignments) produced fewer false-positive findings (i.e., fewer nonallergenic proteins identified as allergens) and equivalent false-negative rates (i.e., allergenic proteins identified as nonallergens) compared to the 80 amino acid window search suggested by FAO/WHO.[70,78]

The FAO/WHO also included a few new recommendations in addition to the sliding-window parameter, including (1) targeted serum screening (assessment of IgE binding in sera from subjects with allergic responses to broadly related categories of foods) of proteins from nonallergenic sources; (2) targeted serum screening of proteins with no amino acid sequence homology to known allergens; and (3) use of animal models.[70] The FAO/WHO recommendation was adopted by Codex Alimentarius.[79] Later, further guidance was published by the EFSA's GMO Panel[80] and an update in 2011.[81] Herein, a weight-of-evidence approach was proposed, which involved an integrated case-by-case approach to be used in the allergenicity risk assessment of newly expressed proteins in GM feed and foods.

In comparison to the assessment of foods derived from GM species, the allergenicity assessment of new food protein sources usually poses several additional challenges. In the latter case, high, nutritionally relevant levels of proteins will be present and the products generally will contain a complex mixture of many different proteins. Therefore, TNO in collaboration with the UMC Utrecht developed a more broadly (not only for GM products) applicable approach for the allergenicity assessment of new food proteins and protein sources.[69] This approach was applied in an extensive study on the allergenicity of insect proteins as potential new protein source for human consumption.[82]

In the following paragraphs, the main aspects and methods for the allergenicity assessment of new food proteins and protein sources are discussed.

48.3.1.1 History of use of the new protein(s) and/or source

An evaluation of the history of use—or more broadly put, the history of exposure—is aimed at establishing a possible allergenic potential based on historical human exposure to a protein or its source. An early example of the relevance of this evaluation is the establishment of allergenicity in Brazil nut allergic individuals of a GM soybean that contained a gene from Brazil nut. This gene appeared to code for an allergenic protein in Brazil nut.[83] The evaluation of a possible allergenic potential based on historical human exposure can be extended to an evaluation of possible allergenicity of taxonomically related species. This way, insect proteins were identified as being allergenic to individuals with shrimp allergy.[84,85] History of exposure can also provide direct evidence for a de novo sensitizing potency or even de novo allergenicity, as also was demonstrated for insect proteins.[86] The results of the evaluation of possible allergenicity apparent from a history of use or exposure can give direction for the selection of sera for targeted testing of possible binding of new protein(s) to IgE from allergic individuals and thus potential (cross-reactive) allergenicity for such individuals. Further direction for the selection of sera for targeted testing of IgE binding can be obtained from evaluating amino acid sequence homology with known allergens. If no potential risk groups are identified based on historical human exposure or amino acid sequence homology screening, nontargeted IgE-binding tests can be performed using a broad panel of sera from individuals with different spectra of allergies. The combination of the evaluation of these three aspects (history of exposure, amino acid sequence homology, and IgE binding) is mainly meant to give insight into potential allergenic risks for existing allergic individuals due to cross-reactivity. In the following paragraphs, the methods and approaches for evaluating amino acid sequence homology with known allergens and IgE binding are addressed in more detail.

48.3.1.2 Amino acid sequence homology with known allergens

It is well known that only a minority of all proteins identified so far display relevant allergenic activity and these can be assigned to approximately 2% of all known protein families.[87] A full and detailed in silico search for allergen IgE cross-reactivity based on amino acid sequence homology requires a comprehensive, well-curated allergen database. During the last decade, efforts have been undertaken to set up a number of allergen databases collecting and curating the existing data of allergen sequences such as the International Union of Immunological Societies (IUIS) allergen database (http://www.allergen.org), AllergenOnline (http://www.allergenonline.org), Allergome (http://www.allergome.org/), ALLFam (http://www.meduniwien.ac.at/allfam/), and the COMPARE database (http://comparedatabase.org/).[88] The IUIS database provides the systematic nomenclature for allergens and is supervised and updated by a specific committee.[89] AllergenOnline provides access to a peer-reviewed allergen list and sequence searchable database intended for the identification of proteins that may present a potential risk of allergenic cross-reactivity. The Allergome database provides a comprehensive, nonpeer-reviewed collection of information on allergenic proteins, while in the ALLFam database allergens are grouped according to their protein family characteristics. The COMPARE database built by the Health and Environment Science Institute (HESI) is available since February 2017 and has been updated annually since then, which is a new transparent resource for the identification of protein sequences including known and putative allergens.[88] Allergenic risk assessment using these databases requires the analysis of the primary sequence from the target protein(s) and the assessment of potential sequence similarity to known allergens.[80]

The existing bioinformatics approaches can aid to identify potential cross-reactivity of a protein new to the diet with known allergens. When a significant primary sequence alignment is obtained in silico, it is interpreted as a possibility that the new protein could be recognized by IgE in consumers with the corresponding, cross-reactive allergy. In this case, a next step in the allergenicity assessment can be in vitro testing of the new protein with patient serum for verification of the cross-reactivity. In practice, it is most likely that the protein will not be used in a commercialized product.[8]

However, several studies have shown that the official bioinformatic criteria (>35% identity over an 80 amino acid sliding-window and an eight or more exact-match) set by regulatory agencies[73] for comparing the amino acid sequence of a new protein with that of known allergens falsely predict many nonallergenic proteins as posing an allergenic risk.[90–94] These studies also showed the potential of alternative bioinformatic algorithms. For instance, the 1:1 FASTA approach, developed and published by Song et al.,[92] was found to be equally sensitive to the sliding-window search for detecting true allergens, but showed much better selectivity (i.e., lower frequency of prediction of low-risk protein sequences as being allergenic).[90–92] Furthermore, a study by Mirsky et al. in 2013 showed that multifactor bioinformatic criteria result in improved selectivity for detecting known allergens and represent an additional avenue for evaluating the allergenic risk of new food proteins.[95] They determined the sensitivities and specificities resulting from the use of two established methods and hundreds of possible methods (in 17 categories) to assess 27,243 Viridiplantae transgenic proteins, in silico, for their potential allergenicity. The authors showed that they were able to lower the current percentage of false positives without raising the current percentage of false negatives—at best, a reduction in the percentage of false positives from ~10% to ~6% was achieved without any increase in the percentage of false negatives and with only minor changes to the existing criteria.

New bioinformatics approaches, such as potentially the 1:1 FASTA approach, can be used to supplement the amino-acid sequence identity and >35% identity over 80 amino acids criteria and can serve as a second tier to detect potential biologically irrelevant homology hits generated by the FAO/WHO/CODEX criterion.[91]

48.3.1.3 Binding of the new protein(s) to IgE from allergic individuals

When there is a high degree of sequence homology of a new protein with a known allergen or when the source of the gene/protein or taxonomically related species commonly causes allergies, specific serum screening is recommended by Codex/EFSA.[96–98] Sera from patients with a clinical food allergy to the related allergen/food are tested to determine whether the new protein(s) may be cross-reactive with a known allergen. There are different types of IgE-binding studies such as targeted or broad IgE-binding screens, functional IgE-binding testing, and identification of IgE-binding proteins.[69]

Targeted IgE-binding screens are used to identify putative allergen(s) using sera from clinically proven allergic patient.[69] The bioinformatics data as well as observations from the history of exposure can be used for a smart selection of allergic patients that might be at risk. For instance, sera from individuals previously sensitized against phylogenetically related foods, (e.g., serum from shrimp allergic patients, when testing for allergenicity of insect proteins) can be used. Also, negative controls, preferably sera from individuals with nonphylogenetically related allergies should be used (e.g., peanut, when testing insect proteins) to exclude nonspecific IgE binding. A panel of sera obtained from patients with different allergy profiles [such as allergies to pollen (birch/grass, mite), plant (e.g., peanut, soy, tree nuts, wheat), and animal (egg, milk, fish, crustaceans)] can be used for broad screening to identify possible cross-reactive activity that is not suspected based on the evaluation of a history of exposure or amino acid sequence assessments. It is preferred to use individual sera from patients with a well-documented allergy rather than pooled sera to optimize the sensitivity of the test. As patient selection can have a big impact on the outcome of the test, it is important to consider the amount of patient sera to be used and the selection of sera should be critically evaluated.[69]

There are multiple techniques that can be used for testing IgE binding, such as enzyme-linked immuno sorbent assay (ELISA), Radioallergosorbent-test (RAST), and immunoblot.[99] The immunoblot has some advantages over the other techniques, as multiple proteins can be visualized simultaneously and it gives more information on the presence of different allergenic proteins and differences between patients.[100] However, a drawback is that proteins will lose their natural structure (denaturing buffers) and thus false-negative results can be obtained.[100] Therefore ELISA or RAST, in combination with the immunoblot, is preferred.

It is necessary to test the clinical relevance of possibly detected in vitro IgE binding with functional IgE-testing strategies, as IgE binding as such does not automatically indicate that a clinically relevant reaction will take place.[69] A DBPCFC is generally regarded as the "gold standard" in food allergy diagnosis, and would be preferred for confirming relevant IgE binding.[99] However, the DBPCFC is quite impactful for the patient, an approval of a medical ethical committee is needed, and the test has to be performed in a specialized clinical and safe setting. Alternatively to the DBPCFC or as a prescreening, a basophil activation test (BAT) and skin prick tests (SPT) can be used.[99,101] The SPT is often used and widely accepted in clinical diagnosis of food allergy. The BAT is not used in routine diagnostics and the predictive value is not proven yet; however, the advantage over the SPT is that different protein extracts, including stringent buffers such as urea can be used. An alternative for the BAT with human cells is the rat basophilic leukemia cells assay, which uses cells transfected with the Fcε receptor type I which is primed with human IgE.[69,102]

48.3.1.4 Resistance to digestive breakdown

Resistance to pepsin digestion is proposed as a key part of the current allergenicity assessment of (transgenic) proteins.[81,96,103] This is based on the postulate and preliminary observations that resistance to gastric digestion differed between two sets of proteins derived from foods: commonly allergenic and rarely allergenic.[104] Thus such resistance might be an intrinsic feature of allergens and therefore a new protein that is resistant to gastric digestion, or is partially degraded into stable fragments of sufficient size, is assumed to have the potential to interact with the immune system, whereas a protein that is rapidly and completely degraded is assumed to unlikely interact and evoke an immune response.[104]

Degradation of a protein will likely influence the effective dose and severity of reaction in the elicitation phases. However, it has been established that no absolute correlation exists between pepsin resistance and allergenicity.[105–108] Currently, stability in a pepsin resistance test is one of the main pillars for assessing the allergenic potential of new proteins, though its predictive value remains unknown. In 2017, COST Actions ImpARAS and INFOGEST jointly organized a workshop addressing the relevance and applicability of the pepsin resistance test in allergenicity assessment of proteins and how to improve the test. The main conclusions of this workshop were published by Verhoeckx et al. in 2019, and they concluded that protein digestion is relevant for allergenicity of some proteins, but not for all.[109] According to the authors, many other factors in addition to digestion in the stomach might play more pivotal roles and some of these factors may have a great impact on digestion and should be included in the digestion assay strategy.[109] However, these factors were indicated to complicate the design and implementation of a simple, suitable, and predictive digestion assay/strategy enormously, especially because it is not clear yet how these factors exactly influence digestion as well as allergenicity, and how these factors could be included. Moreover, as the authors state, there is no rationale on which to base a clear readout that is predictive for allergenicity exclusively and the exact route of exposure and mechanisms behind food sensitization and food allergy are not fully understood yet. Therefore they suggest to omit the digestion test from the allergenicity assessment strategy for now and put an effort into filling the knowledge gaps.[109]

48.3.1.5 Assessment of de novo sensitizing and allergenic potency

There are no broadly accepted predictive and validated methods available to accurately predict the de novo allergenicity of new food proteins. Most assays focus on cross-reactivity and fail to identify or exclude de novo allergenic activity. For example, the traditional bioinformatics approach identified 4 out of 208 known mealworm proteins as allergenic (cross-reactivity to mites), but failed to identify proteins that were responsible for de novo sensitization to mealworm which led to clinically relevant food allergic responses.[84,86]

Several studies have been described on physicochemical and biochemical property-based predictive approaches for allergenicity,[110] for instance AllerTop,[111,112] proAP/PREAL,[113,114] and another machine learning technique described by Mohabatkar et al.[115] The AllerTop model is including multiple machine learning techniques for predicting the allergenicity of food, inhalant, and toxin allergens based on 29 principal physicochemical properties of amino acids combined into three descriptors (hydrophobicity, molecular size, and polarity). The model performance measures with AllerTop were good (≥90%), but were based on a relatively small dataset containing 684 allergenic food proteins and 684 nonallergenic proteins. The nonallergenic proteins were selected based on having no homology with known allergens, introducing a potential bias in the negative control dataset. Other nonallergenic proteins might have been unnecessarily excluded due to these criteria. Moreover, inherent to the selection criterion for nonallergenic proteins (having no homology with known allergens), the method possibly only well detects cross-reactive proteins.[110]

Wang and colleagues have developed two web tools, proAP and PREAL, where proAP predicts protein allergenicity based on predicted secondary structure and PREAL predicts protein allergenicity based on 25 protein features (e.g., subcellular location and amino acid composition).[113,114] Both these models are also machine learning technique-based and showed good model performances with values of ≥ 89% for datasets of 989 allergenic proteins and 989 nonallergenic proteins for proAP and 1176 allergenic proteins and 1176 nonallergenic proteins for PREAL. However, proteins with >30% homology with known allergens were excluded from the nonallergen dataset, potentially providing the same drawbacks as the AllerTop model.[110] Mohabatkar and colleagues applied a machine learning technique for predicting the allergenicity of proteins based on only six properties [hydrophobicity, hydrophilicity, side chain mass, acid dissociation constant (pka) of the α-COOH group, pka of the α-NH3 + group and inhibitory concentration (pI)] and by using a pseudo amino acid composition. The pseudo amino acid composition included information on the amino acid composition and sequence order correlation. The model performance measures were good (≥89%) but were also based on a relatively small dataset including 460 allergenic proteins and 560 nonallergenic proteins. The nonallergenic proteins with textual information indicating potential allergenicity were excluded, indicating that their negative control dataset was somewhat biased.[110]

Westerhout et al. in 2019 published a random forest model developed using another selection criterion for allergenic and nonallergenic proteins, that is, being or being not included in the COMprehensive Protein Allergen Resource (COMPARE) database (http://www.comparedatabase.org).[110] For this study, they used a dataset of 525,745 unique proteins, of which 1673 were considered allergenic. From these, 27,005 nonallergenic proteins and 824 allergenic proteins were used for training the model, and 49,535 other nonallergenic proteins and 849 other allergenic proteins were used for validation and testing. Bias checks indicated that the skewed proportion of allergenic/nonallergenic proteins did not influence the performance measures. The random forest model was trained, validated, and tested on distinguishing allergenic from nonallergenic proteins based on calculated physicochemical and biochemical properties of the proteins. The final prediction model described by the authors was based on 29 calculated variables (not the same as the 29 as used by the AllerTop model) and predicted the allergenicity of a random protein from the animal, fungi, or plant kingdom with a sensitivity, specificity, and overall accuracy of each between 85% and 91%. A model as described by Westerhout et al. may complement the weight-of-evidence approach as suggested by Codex/EFSA to further improve the assessment of the allergenic potential of new proteins and to predict the de novo allergenicity of new food proteins.[110]

48.3.1.6 Animal models

Many attempts have been conducted to develop suitable animal models to evaluate the potential sensitizing capacity of novels foods.[6,116] However, none have been validated or widely accepted. The performance of animal models is highly dependent on the choice of animals, as well as the experimental design including the selection of appropriate endpoint parameters, which is often leading to contradictory results. Børgh et al. suggested that a good model should asses multiple doses of the protein and the proteins should be tested preferably in a relevant food matrix and not as an isolated protein to control for matrix effects.[116] To accurately determine allergenicity, additional endpoint parameters should be measured in addition to IgE induction, such as mucosal responses (e.g., cell infiltration) or serum inflammatory mediators (e.g., mast cell products) and assessment of in vivo responses to protein challenge (such as change in temperature or ear swelling).[6] As indicated before also for the optimization of the bioinformatic approaches, it is important to include a large set of appropriate positive and negative reference proteins, when developing, optimizing, and validating an in vivo model. Furthermore, Verhoeckx et al. suggested to perform a ring trial across multiple laboratories, to identify factors that might impact the stability and transferability of the animal model.[6] Recently, Castan et al. published a review regarding the identification of the optimal ex vivo and in vivo disease endpoint parameters and their relevance when assessing potential allergenicity of novel foods in experimental animal models,[117] including the use of temperature, level of immunoglobulins, phenotyping of cell infiltrate, and cytokine production, and stated that these endpoints provide information about the allergic reaction and the degree of sensitizing capacity of the allergen.[6] However, the clinical parameters of food allergic reactions that are described for the available mouse food allergy models reviewed by Schülke et al. in 2019,[118] showed that the models are still incomplete. While anaphylactic reactions (which, in the mouse, are often additionally mediated via IgG1 antibodies), local inflammation in the area of the mouth, throat, and face, as well as diarrhea can be relatively consistently induced in different mouse models, skin reactions (resulting in itching and ruffed fur) which are commonly associated with food allergic reactions, as well as other local symptoms of the gastrointestinal inflammation [nausea, abdominal pain, and vomiting (anatomically not possible in mice)], can so far not be reproduced or monitored in objective and quantitative ways by the available models.[118] Furthermore, it is important to known that the frequency of allergen-specific antibodies upon usage of adjuvants in mouse models is often significantly higher than the frequencies usually observed in allergic patients as shown by Kanagaratham et al. The authors reported frequencies of allergen-specific IgE antibodies of up to 80% in the mouse when using alum as an adjuvant, while allergen-specific IgE frequencies in allergic patients to a single food allergen were reported to be only approximately 0.1%–15%.[119] Overall, it must be concluded that, despite many efforts over the previous two to three decades, no animal models have been presented that reliably can assess the allergenic potency of new food proteins. Although the developed and possible improved future models may be of value for studying specific aspects of the Adverse Outcome Pathways in food allergy, it remains questionable whether animal models may be a feasible way to improve allergenicity assessment approaches for new food proteins, while posing significant ethical constraints.

48.3.2 The future of allergenicity assessment of new food protein products

Allergenicity assessment is one of the most challenging aspects in the safety assessment of new protein-containing foods, as there is no single regulatory accepted predictive and validated method to assess the allergenicity of new proteins, new sources, or new protein-containing products. Therefore a weight-of-evidence approach as currently recommended by for instance EFSA for the assessment of allergenicity of GM products is applied, but inherently to such approach, this does not give clear black-white outcomes. Information from the history of exposure to the proteins, their sources or taxonomically related sources, sequence homology testing, and targeted and broad IgE-binding screening and, if indicated, testing for biologically relevance of detected IgE-binding have been proven successful in predicting potential cross-reactivity in existing allergy sufferers. Inclusion of a method such as the 1:1 FASTA approach may enrich the methodological repertoire for assessing cross-reactivity risks. However, broadly accepted predictive and validated methods to assess the de novo sensitizing and allergenic potency of new food proteins at premarked stages are lacking. Animal models and digestion susceptibility testing have been shown to be of limited predictive value. In silico methods such as the random forest model developed by Westerhout et al. are promising but may need further case studies and substantiation to become broadly accepted.[110] There thus is a need for improvement of the methodological repertoire, particularly for assessing the potential de novo allergenic potential of new food proteins.

In 2019, Houben et al. published a discussion paper arguing that new method development should be guided by the information requested by risk managers for their risk management decision-making.[7] Without such guidance, any investment in method development potentially is a waste of time and resources, and perhaps even an unethical use of animal experimentation, as it may not adequately target the relevant parameters and criteria ultimately requested by risk managers. To trigger a process toward formulation of a clear risk management request, the authors made an inventory of possible parameters and criteria that theoretically could be used for accepting or not accepting a new food protein product in view of allergenic risks. Additionally, they made an inventory of the consequences of each possible parameter and criterion in terms of what these would mean for society and what method development would be required. Improvements in methodological repertoire will only be achieved and implemented if accepted by stakeholders and scientifically and technologically feasible within acceptablem timeframe and investments. The inventory of the consequences of the theoretically possible parameters and criteria as listed by Houben et al. indicates that most options will be difficult to accept by stakeholders, will jeopardize food innovations, or would not be scientifically or technologically feasible within acceptable timeframe and investments. Nevertheless, some (combinations) of parameters, criteria, and methods may be acceptable as well as feasible and may provide a way forward. For example, Houben et al. suggested to investigate the possibility of developing a threshold of allergenic concern (TAC) concept,[7] comparable to the threshold of toxicological concern concept in toxicology. Such approach, if working, could help to make a selection of proteins present at potentially relevant levels and could exempt many proteins present in new protein sources from further assessment because of an expected exposure below the TAC. This would increase the applicability of an approach such as the Random Forest model developed by Westerhout et al.,[110] that is able to distinguish allergenic from nonallergenic proteins. This latter model requires amino acid sequence information from the proteins to be assessed. Full characterization of the amino acid sequences of all proteins may be difficult to achieve in case of intended new nutritional protein sources, because these may contain many different unknown or unidentified proteins at the same time. However, many of these unknown or unidentified proteins may be present at low levels and exempting these from further assessment based on a TAC concept would limit the effort needed for applying the Random Forest model developed by Westerhout et al. This latter model was shown to be able to identify previously unidentified allergens in insects that were demonstrated to have sensitized humans.[110] This model therefore can be an important future addition to the weight-of-evidence approaches such as that proposed by EFSA or the more broadly applicable allergenicity assessment approach for new food proteins as proposed by Verhoeckx et al.,[69] particularly in cases where there is no information from relevant historical exposure. Combination of these approaches with the application of the concept of TAC, if substantiated, may be a feasible way forward. Yet, as indicated before, the way forward should preferably be guided by risk managers through a specification of the information requested for their risk management decision-making.

References

1. Abbas AK, Lichtman AH, Pillai S, Baker DL, Baker A. Cellular and Molecular Immunology: Antigen Presentation to T Lymphocytes and the Functions of Major Histocompatibility Complex Molecules. 2018.
2. Van Bilsen JHM, Szłapka ES, Ojalvo DL, et al. Application of the adverse outcome pathway (AOP) concept to structure the available in vivo and in vitro mechanistic data for allergic sensitization to food proteins. *Clin Transl Allergy*. 2017;1–18. Available from: https://doi.org/10.1186/s13601-017-0152-0.
3. Skypala IJ. Food-induced anaphylaxis: role of hidden allergens and cofactors. *Front Immunol*. 2019;. Available from: https://doi.org/10.3389/fimmu.2019.00673.
4. Book Review: The Genuine Works of Hippocrates. Translated from the Greek by Francis Adams. 384 pp. Baltimore: Williams & Wilkins Co., 1939. $3.00. *N Engl J Med*. 1939. doi:10.1056/nejm193908242210821.
5. Allen KJ, Turner PJ, Pawankar R, et al. Precautionary labelling of foods for allergen content: are we ready for a global framework? *World Allergy Organ J*. 2014;7(1):10. Available from: https://doi.org/10.1186/1939-4551-7-10.
6. Verhoeckx K, Lindholm Bøgh K, Constable A, et al. COST action "ImpARAS": what have we learnt to improve food allergy risk assessment. A summary of a 4 year networking consortium. *Clin Transl Allergy*. 2020;10(1):1–12. Available from: https://doi.org/10.1186/s13601-020-00318-x.
7. Houben G, Blom M, Alvito P, et al. Defining the targets for the assessment of IgE-mediated allergenicity of new or modified food proteins. *Food Chem Toxicol*. 2019;127:61–69. Available from: https://doi.org/10.1016/j.fct.2019.02.036.
8. Remington BC, Broekman HCH, Blom WM, et al. Approaches to assess IgE mediated allergy risks (sensitization and cross-reactivity) from new or modified dietary proteins. *Food Chem Toxicol*. 2018;112:97–107. Available from: https://doi.org/10.1016/j.fct.2017.12.025.
9. The European Parliament and the Council. Directive 2003/89/EC of the European Parliament and of the Council of 10 November 2003 amending Directive 2000/13/EC as regards indication of the ingredients present in foodstuffs. *Off J Eur Union*. 2003;(12):2003–2006.
10. Council Regulation (EC). Commission Directive 2007/68/EC. *Off J Eur Union*. 2007;OJ 310(10):1–4.
11. FALCPA. Food Allergen Labeling and Consumer Protection Act. Public Law 108-282. 905–911. <https://www.fda.gov/food/food-allergensgluten-free-guidance-documents-regulatory-information/food-allergen-labeling-and-consumer-protection-act-2004-falcpa>; 2004.
12. FDA. Guidance for industry: Food allergen labeling exemption petitions and notifications. <https://www.fda.gov/regulatory-information/search-fda-guidance-documents/guidance-industry-food-allergen-labeling-exemption-petitions-and-notifications>; 2015.
13. Björkstén B, Crevel R, Hischenhuber C, et al. Criteria for identifying allergenic foods of public health importance. *Regul Toxicol Pharmacol*. 2008;51(1):42–52. Available from: https://doi.org/10.1016/j.yrtph.2008.01.002.
14. van Bilsen JHM, Ronsmans S, Crevel RWR, et al. Evaluation of scientific criteria for identifying allergenic foods of public health importance. *Regul Toxicol Pharmacol*. 2011;60(3):281–289. Available from: https://doi.org/10.1016/j.yrtph.2010.08.024.
15. Chung YJ, Ronsmans S, Crevel RWR, et al. Application of scientific criteria to food allergens of public health importance. *Regul Toxicol Pharmacol*. 2012;64(2):315–323. Available from: https://doi.org/10.1016/j.yrtph.2012.07.009.
16. Houben G, Burney P, Chan CH, et al. Prioritisation of allergenic foods with respect to public health relevance. Report from an ILSI Europe Food Allergy Task Force Expert Group. *Food Chem Toxicol*. 2016;89:8–18. Available from: https://doi.org/10.1016/j.fct.2015.12.028.
17. Remington BC, Westerhout J, Meima MY, et al. Updated population minimal eliciting dose distributions for use in risk assessment of 14 priority food allergens. *Food Chem Toxicol*. 2020;139:111259. Available from: https://doi.org/10.1016/j.fct.2020.111259.
18. Houben GF, Baumert JL, Blom WM, et al. Full range of population Eliciting Dose values for 14 priority allergenic foods and recommendations for use in risk characterization. *Food Chem Toxicol*. 2020;146:111831. Available from: https://doi.org/10.1016/j.fct.2020.111831.
19. Nwaru BI, Hickstein L, Panesar SS, et al. Prevalence of common food allergies in Europe: a systematic review and meta-analysis. *Allergy*. 2014;69(8):992–1007. Available from: https://doi.org/10.1111/all.12423.
20. Spanjersberg MQI, Kruizinga AG, Rennen MAJ, Houben GF. Risk assessment and food allergy: the probabilistic model applied to allergens. *Food Chem Toxicol*. 2007;45(1):49. Available from: https://doi.org/10.1016/j.fct.2006.07.018.
21. Madsen CB, Hattersley S, Buck J, et al. Approaches to risk assessment in food allergy: report from a workshop "developing a framework for assessing the risk from allergenic foods". *Food Chem Toxicol*. 2009;47(2):480–489. Available from: https://doi.org/10.1016/j.fct.2008.12.001.
22. Remington BC, Baumert JL, Blom WM, et al. Unintended allergens in precautionary labelled and unlabelled products pose significant risks to UK allergic consumers. *Allergy Eur J Allergy Clin Immunol*. 2015;70(7):813–819. Available from: https://doi.org/10.1111/all.12625.
23. Spanjersberg MQI, Knulst AC, Kruizinga AG, et al. Concentrations of undeclared allergens in food products can reach levels that are relevant for public health. *Food Addit Contam Part A Chem Anal Control Expo Risk Assess*. 2010;27(2):169–174. Available from: https://doi.org/10.1080/19440040903317513.
24. Blom WM, Michelsen-Huisman AD, van Os-Medendorp H, et al. Accidental food allergy reactions: products and undeclared ingredients. *J Allergy Clin Immunol*. 2018;142(3):865–875. Available from: https://doi.org/10.1016/j.jaci.2018.04.041.
25. Kruizinga AG, Briggs D, Crevel RWR, et al. Probabilistic risk assessment model for allergens in food: sensitivity analysis of the minimum eliciting dose and food consumption. *Food Chem Toxicol*. 2008;46(5):1437–1443. Available from: https://doi.org/10.1016/j.fct.2007.09.109.

26. Spanjersberg MQ, Luijckx NBL, Houben GF Risk analysis of food allergens. In: Jedrychowski L., Wichers H.J., (eds.) *Chemical and Biological Properties of Food Allergens*. CRC Press, Boca Raton, FL; 2009:387-397.
27. Blom WM, Dubois AEJ, Kruizinga AG, et al. Food allergy: threshold distribution curves for major food allergens. In: Proceedings of the Symposium on "Frontiers in Food Allergen Risk Assessment," 20–22th October, 2010. Nice, France; 2010. Available from: https://doi.org/10.1016/j.jaci.2012.10.034.
28. Taylor SL, Baumert JL, Kruizinga AG, et al. Establishment of reference doses for residues of allergenic foods: report of the VITAL Expert Panel. *Food Chem Toxicol*. 2014;63:9–17. Available from: https://doi.org/10.1016/j.fct.2013.10.032.
29. Allen KJ, Remington BC, Baumert JL, et al. Allergen reference doses for precautionary labeling (VITAL 2.0): clinical implications. *J Allergy Clin Immunol*. 2014;133(1):156–164. Available from: https://doi.org/10.1016/j.jaci.2013.06.042.
30. Zurzolo GA, Allen KJ, Taylor SL, et al. Peanut Allergen Threshold Study (PATS): validation of eliciting doses using a novel single-dose challenge protocol. *Allergy Asthma Clin Immunol*. 2013;9 (1):35. Available from: https://doi.org/10.1186/1710-1492-9-35.
31. Hourihane JO, Allen KJ, Shreffler WG, et al. Peanut Allergen Threshold Study (PATS): novel single-dose oral food challenge study to validate eliciting doses in children with peanut allergy. *J Allergy Clin Immunol*. 2017;139(5):1583–1590. Available from: https://doi.org/10.1016/j.jaci.2017.01.030.
32. IFAAM. Project coordinator C. Mills. Project Final Report IFAAM GA 312147. Manchester. <https://cordis.europa.eu/result/rcn/208641_en.html>; 2018.
33. Dua S, Garcia MR, Bond S, et al. Reaction thresholds in in peanut-allergic adults and the influence of exercise and sleep deprivation: a randomised controlled trial. *J Allergy Clin Immunol*. 2019;143(2): AB202. Available from: https://doi.org/10.1016/j.jaci.2018.12.617.
34. Versluis A, van Os-Medendorp H, Kruizinga AG, Blom WM, Houben GF, Knulst AC. Cofactors in allergic reactions to food: physical exercise and alcohol are the most important. *Immunity Inflamm Dis*. 2016;4 (4):392–400. Available from: https://doi.org/10.1002/iid3.120.
35. Versluis A, van Os-Medendorp H, Blom WM, et al. Potential cofactors in accidental food allergic reactions are frequently present but may not influence severity and occurrence. *Clin Exp Allergy*. 2018;49 (2):207–215. Available from: https://doi.org/10.1111/cea.13282.
36. Roberts G, Allen K, Ballmer-Weber B, et al. Identifying and managing patients at risk of severe allergic reactions to food: report from two iFAAM workshops. *Clin Exp Allergy*. 2019;. Available from: https://doi.org/10.1111/cea.13516.
37. DunnGalvin A, Roberts G, Schnadt S, et al. Evidence based approaches to the application of Precautionary Allergen Labelling: report from two iFAAM workshops. *Clin Exp Allergy*. 2019;. Available from: https://doi.org/10.1111/cea.13464.
38. Remington BC, Westerhout J, Campbell DE, Turner PJ. Minimal impact of extensive heating of hen's egg and cow's milk in a food matrix on threshold dose-distribution curves. *Allergy*. 2017;72:1816–1819.
39. Westerhout J, Baumert JL, Blom WM, et al. Deriving individual threshold doses from clinical food challenge data for population risk assessment of food allergens. *J Allergy Clin Immunol*. 2019;. Available from: https://doi.org/10.1016/j.jaci.2019.07.046.
40. Ballmer-Weber BK, Fernandez-Rivas M, Beyer K, et al. How much is too much? Threshold dose distributions for 5 food allergens. *J Allergy Clin Immunol*. 2015;135(4):964–971. Available from: https://doi.org/10.1016/j.jaci.2014.10.047.
41. Blom WM, Vlieg-Boerstra BJ, Kruizinga AG, Van Der Heide S, Houben GF, Dubois AEJ. Threshold dose distributions for 5 major allergenic foods in children. *J Allergy Clin Immunol*. 2013;131 (1):172–179. Available from: http://doi.org/10.1016/j.jaci.2012.10.034.
42. Taylor SL, Crevel RWR, Sheffield D, Kabourek J, Baumert J. Threshold dose for peanut: risk characterization based upon published results from challenges of peanut-allergic individuals. *Food Chem Toxicol*. 2009;47(6):1198–1204. Available from: https://doi.org/10.1016/j.fct.2009.02.011.
43. Remington BC, Westerhout J, Dubois AEJ, et al. Suitability of low-dose, open food challenge data to supplement double-blind, placebo-controlled data in generation of food allergen threshold dose distributions. *Clin Exp Allergy*. 2020;1–4. Available from: https://doi.org/10.1111/cea.13753.
44. Entink RHK, Remington BC, Blom WM, et al. Food allergy population thresholds: an evaluation of the number of oral food challenges and dosing schemes on the accuracy of threshold dose distribution modeling. *Food Chem Toxicol*. 2014;70:134–143. Available from: https://doi.org/10.1016/j.fct.2014.05.001.
45. Crevel RWR, Briggs D, Hefle SL, Knulst AC, Taylor SL. Hazard characterisation in food allergen risk assessment: the application of statistical approaches and the use of clinical data. *Food Chem Toxicol*. 2007;45(5):691–701. Available from: https://doi.org/10.1016/j.fct.2006.09.005.
46. EFSA Scientific Committee. Update: use of the benchmark dose approach in risk assessment. *EFSA J*. 2017;15(1):1–41. Available from: https://doi.org/10.2903/j.efsa.2017.4658.
47. Wheeler MW, Westerhout J, Baumert JL, Remington BC. Bayesian stacked parametric survival with frailty components and interval censored failure times. *Risk Anal*. 2021;41:56–66. Available from: http://arxiv.org/abs/1908.11334.
48. de Keyzer W, Bracke T, McNaughton SA, et al. Cross-continental comparison of national food consumption survey methods—a narrative review. *Nutrients*. 2015;7(5):3587–3620. Available from: https://doi.org/10.3390/nu7053587.
49. Blom WM, van Os-Medendorp H, Bijlsma S, et al. Allergen risk assessment: food intake levels of the general population represent those of food allergic patients. *Food Chem Toxicol*. 2020;146. Available from: https://doi.org/10.1016/j.fct.2020.111781.
50. Rimbaud L, Heraud F, La Vieille S, et al. Quantitative risk assessment relating to adventitious presence of allergens in food: a probabilistic model applied to peanut in chocolate. *Risk Anal*. 2010;30(1):7–19. Available from: https://doi.org/10.1111/j.1539-6924.2009.01322.x.
51. Rimbaud L, Heraud F, La S, Leblanc J-C, Crepet A. Quantitative risk assessment relating to the inadvertent presence of peanut allergens in various food products. *Int Food Risk Anal J*. 2013;3(4):1. Available from: https://doi.org/10.5772/56646.
52. Blom WM, Kruizinga AG, Rubingh CM, Remington BC, Crevel RWR, Houben GF. Assessing food allergy risks from residual peanut protein in highly refined vegetable oil. *Food Chem Toxicol*. 2017;106:306–313. Available from: https://doi.org/10.1016/j.fct.2017.05.072.
53. Remington BC, Taylor SL, Marx DB, Petersen BJ, Baumert JL. Soy in wheat – contamination levels and food allergy risk assessment. *Food Chem Toxicol*. 2013;62:485–491. Available from: https://doi.org/10.1016/j.fct.2013.09.013.

54. Blom WM, Remington BC, Baumert JL, et al. Sensitivity analysis to derive a food consumption point estimate for deterministic food allergy risk assessment. *Food Chem Toxicol.* 2019;125:413–421. Available from: https://doi.org/10.1016/j.fct.2019.01.025.
55. Allen KJ, Taylor SL. The consequences of precautionary allergen labeling: safe haven or unjustifiable burden? *J Allergy Clin Immunol Pract.* 2018;6(2):400–407. Available from: https://doi.org/10.1016/j.jaip.2017.12.025.
56. VWA. Onderzoek naar de declaratie van allergenen op levensmiddelen – Fact sheet. 2007.
57. Pele M, Brohee M, Anklam E, et al. Peanut and hazelnut traces in cookies and chocolates: relationship between analytical results and declaration of food allergens on product labels. *Food Addit Contam.* 2007;24(12):1334–1344. Available from: https://doi.org/10.1080/02652030701458113.
58. Food Safety Authority of Ireland. Food allergens and labelling survey. <http://www.fsai.ie/resources_publications/allergen_labelling_2011.html.html>; June 2011 Accessed 09.04.13.
59. Remington BC. Risk Assessment of Trace and Undeclared Allergens in Processed Foods. Dissertations, Theses, & Student Research in Food Science and Technology. <http://digitalcommons.unl.edu/foodscidiss/32>; 2013.
60. Waiblinger H-U, Schulze G. Action levels for food allergens: an approach for official food control in Germany. *J AOAC Int.* 2018;101(1):17–22. Available from: https://doi.org/10.5740/jaoacint.17-0383.
61. Michelsen-Huisman AD, van Os-Medendorp H, Blom WM, et al. Accidental allergic reactions in food allergy: causes related to products and patient's management. *Allergy.* 2018;1–5. Available from: https://doi.org/10.1111/all.13560.
62. Madsen CB, van den Dungen MW, Cochrane S, et al. Can we define a level of protection for allergic consumers that everyone can accept? *Regul Toxicol Pharmacol.* 2020;117. Available from: https://doi.org/10.1016/j.yrtph.2020.104751.
63. Brooke-Taylor S, Christensen G, Grinter K, Sherlock R, Warren L. The Allergen Bureau VITAL Program. *J AOAC Int.* 2018;101(1):1–6. Available from: https://doi.org/10.5740/jaoacint.17-0392.
64. Crevel RWR, Baumert JL, Baka A, et al. Development and evolution of risk assessment for food allergens. *Food Chem Toxicol.* 2014;67:262–276. Available from: https://doi.org/10.1016/j.fct.2014.01.032.
65. Allergen Bureau. Summary of the VITAL Scientific Expert Panel recommendations (9 pp.). <http://www.allergenbureau.net/downloads/vital/VSEP-Summary-Report-Oct-2011.pdf>; 2019.
66. Birot S, Madsen CB, Kruizinga AG, Crépet A, Christensen T, Brockhoff PB. Food groups for allergen risk assessment: combining food consumption data from different countries in Europe. *Food Chem Toxicol.* 2018;118:371–381. Available from: https://doi.org/10.1016/j.fct.2018.05.042.
67. Murphy C, Gardoni P. The acceptability and the tolerability of societal risks: a capabilities-based approach. *Sci Eng Ethics.* 2008;. Available from: https://doi.org/10.1007/s11948-007-9031-8.
68. FAO/WHO. Ad hoc Joint FAO/WHO Expert Consultation on risk assessment of food allergens (7 pp.).<http://www.fao.org/3/ca7121en/ca7121en.pdf>; 2020.
69. Verhoeckx K, Broekman H, Knulst A, Houben G. Allergenicity assessment strategy for novel food proteins and protein sources. *Regul Toxicol Pharmacol.* 2016;79:118–124. Available from: https://doi.org/10.1016/j.yrtph.2016.03.016.
70. Ladics GS, Selgrade MJK. Identifying food proteins with allergenic potential: evolution of approaches to safety assessment and research to provide additional tools. *Regul Toxicol Pharmacol.* 2009;. Available from: https://doi.org/10.1016/j.yrtph.2008.10.010.
71. Metcalfe DD, Astwood JD, Townsend R, Sampson HA, Taylor SL, Fuchs RL. Assessment of the allergenic potential of foods derived from genetically engineered crop plants. *Crit Rev Food Sci Nutr.* 1996;36(suppl):S165–S186.
72. Herman RA, Storer NP, Gao Y. Digestion assays in allergenicity assessment of transgenic proteins. *Environ Health Perspect.* 2006;. Available from: https://doi.org/10.1289/ehp.8803.
73. FAO/WHO. Evaluation of allergenicity of genetically modified foods. Report of a Joint FAO/WHO Expert Consultation on Allergenicity of Foods Derived from Biotechnology. January 22–25, 2011.
74. Hileman RE, Silvanovich A, Goodman RE, et al. Bioinformatic methods for allergenicity assessment using a comprehensive allergen database. *Int Arch Allergy Immunol.* 2002;. Available from: https://doi.org/10.1159/000063861.
75. Michael S. Allergenicity prediction by protein sequence. *FASEB J.* 2003;17:1141–1143.
76. Ladics GS, Bardina L, Cressman RF, Mattsson JL, Sampson HA. Lack of cross-reactivity between the *Bacillus thuringiensis* derived protein Cry1F in maize grain and dust mite Der p7 protein with human sera positive for Der p7-IgE. *Regul Toxicol Pharmacol.* 2006;. Available from: https://doi.org/10.1016/j.yrtph.2005.11.005.
77. Silvanovich A, Nemeth MA, Song P, Herman R, Tagliani L, Bannon GA. The value of short amino acid sequence matches for prediction of protein allergenicity. *Toxicol Sci.* 2006;. Available from: https://doi.org/10.1093/toxsci/kfj068.
78. Ladics GS, Bannon GA, Silvanovich A, Cressman RF. Comparison of conventional FASTA identity searches with the 80 amino acid sliding window FASTA search for the elucidation of potential identities to known allergens. *Mol Nutr Food Res.* 2007;. Available from: https://doi.org/10.1002/mnfr.200600231.
79. Codex Alimentarius Commission. Alinorm 03/34: Joint FAO/WHO Food Standard Programme, Codex Alimentarius Commission, Twenty-Fifth Session, Rome, Italy, 30 June–5 July, 2003. Appendix III: Guideline for the conduct of food safety assessment of foods derived from recombinant-DNA plants. 2003.
80. European Food Safety Authority. Scientific opinion on the assessment of allergenicity of GM plants and microorganisms and derived food and feed. *EFSA J.* 2010;8(7):1700. Available from: https://doi.org/10.2903/j.efsa.2010.1700.
81. EFSA Panel on Genetically Modified Organisms. Guidance for risk assessment of food and feed from genetically modified plants. *EFSA J.* 2011;9(5):2150. Available from: https://doi.org/10.2903/j.efsa.2011.2150.
82. Hustinx-Broekman HCHP. Allergenic Risks of Mealworm and Other Insects: An Approach to Assess the Risks of New Food Proteins in Allergic Patients. (Ph.D. dissertation). Utrecht University; 2017.
83. Hefle SL, Nordlee JA, Taylor SL. Allergenic foods. *Crit Rev Food Sci Nutr.* 1996;. Available from: https://doi.org/10.1080/10408399609527760.
84. Verhoeckx KCM, Van Broekhoven S, Den Hartog-jager CF, et al. House dust mite (Der p 10) and crustacean allergic patients may react to food containing Yellow mealworm proteins. *Food Chem Toxicol.* 2014;65:364–373. Available from: https://doi.org/10.1016/j.fct.2013.12.049.

85. Broekman H, Verhoeckx KC, Den Hartog Jager CF, et al. Majority of shrimp-allergic patients are allergic to mealworm. *J Allergy Clin Immunol.* 2016;137(4):1261–1263. Available from: https://doi.org/10.1016/j.jaci.2016.01.005.
86. Broekman HCHP, Knulst AC, den Hartog Jager CF, et al. Primary respiratory and food allergy to mealworm. *J Allergy Clin Immunol.* 2017;5(2):600–603.e7. Available from: https://doi.org/10.1016/j.jaci.2017.01.035.
87. Radauer C, Bublin M, Wagner S, Mari A, Breiteneder H. Allergens are distributed into few protein families and possess a restricted number of biochemical functions. *J Allergy Clin Immunol.* 2008;. Available from: https://doi.org/10.1016/j.jaci.2008.01.025.
88. Mazzucchelli G, Holzhauser T, Cirkovic Velickovic T, et al. Current (food) allergenic risk assessment: is it fit for novel foods? Status quo and identification of gaps. *Mol Nutr Food Res.* 2018;. Available from: https://doi.org/10.1002/mnfr.201700278.
89. Pomés A, Davies JM, Gadermaier G, et al. WHO/IUIS Allergen Nomenclature: providing a common language. *Mol Immunol.* 2018;. Available from: https://doi.org/10.1016/j.molimm.2018.03.003.
90. Cressman RF, Ladics G. Further evaluation of the utility of "sliding window" FASTA in predicting cross-reactivity with allergenic proteins. *Regul Toxicol Pharmacol.* 2009;54(3):S20–S25.
91. Song P, Herman R, Kumpatla S. 1:1 FASTA update: using the power of E-values in FASTA to detect potential allergen cross-reactivity. *Toxicol Rep.* 2015;. Available from: https://doi.org/10.1016/j.toxrep.2015.08.005.
92. Song P, Herman RA, Kumpatla S. Evaluation of global sequence comparison and one-to-one FASTA local alignment in regulatory allergenicity assessment of transgenic proteins in food crops. *Food Chem Toxicol.* 2014;. Available from: https://doi.org/10.1016/j.fct.2014.06.008.
93. Herman RA, Song P. Allergen false-detection using official bioinformatic algorithms. *GM Crop Food.* 2020;. Available from: https://doi.org/10.1080/21645698.2019.1709021.
94. Herman RA, Song P. Validation of bioinformatic approaches for predicting allergen cross reactivity. *Food Chem Toxicol.* 2019;. Available from: https://doi.org/10.1016/j.fct.2019.110656.
95. Mirsky HP, Cressman RF, Ladics GS. Comparative assessment of multiple criteria for the in silico prediction of cross-reactivity of proteins to known allergens. *Regul Toxicol Pharmacol.* 2013;. Available from: https://doi.org/10.1016/j.yrtph.2013.08.001.
96. Codex. *Foods Derived from Modern Biotechnology.* 2nd ed Rome: Food and Agriculture Organization of the United Nations, Codex Alimentarius Commission; 2009. 2nd ed.
97. EFSA Panel on Genetically Modified Organisms (GMO). Guidance for risk assessment of food and feed from genetically modified plants. *EFSA J.* <https://doi.org/10.2903/j.efsa.2011.2150>; 2011.
98. EFSA Panel on Genetically Modified Organisms (GMO Panel). Scientific Opinion on the assessment of allergenicity of GM plants and microorganisms and derived food and feed. EFSA J. 2010. <https://doi.org/10.2903/j.efsa.2010.1700>.
99. Ansotegui IJ, Melioli G, Canonica GW, et al. IgE allergy diagnostics and other relevant tests in allergy, a World Allergy Organization position paper. *World Allergy Organ J.* 2020;. Available from: https://doi.org/10.1016/j.waojou.2019.100080.
100. Ghosh R, Gilda JE, Gomes AV. The necessity of and strategies for improving confidence in the accuracy of western blots. *Expert Rev Proteomics.* 2014;. Available from: https://doi.org/10.1586/14789450.2014.939635.
101. Hoffmann HJ, Santos AF, Mayorga C, et al. The clinical utility of basophil activation testing in diagnosis and monitoring of allergic disease. *Allergy Eur J Allergy Clin Immunol.* 2015;. Available from: https://doi.org/10.1111/all.12698.
102. Rashid A, Sadroddiny E, Ye HT, et al. Review: diagnostic and therapeutic applications of rat basophilic leukemia cells. *Mol Immunol.* 2012;. Available from: https://doi.org/10.1016/j.molimm.2012.05.019.
103. Goodman RE, Vieths S, Sampson HA, et al. Allergenicity assessment of genetically modified crops – what makes sense? *Nat Biotechnol.* 2008;. Available from: https://doi.org/10.1038/nbt1343.
104. Astwood JD, Leach JN, Fuchs RL. Stability of food allergens to digestion in vitro. *Nat Biotechnol.* 1996;. Available from: https://doi.org/10.1038/nbt1096-1269.
105. Parenti MD, Santoro A, Del Rio A, Franceschi C. Literature review in support of adjuvanticity/immunogenicity assessment of proteins. *EFSA Support Publ.* 2019;. Available from: https://doi.org/10.2903/sp.efsa.2019.en-1551.
106. Bannon GA, Goodman RE, Leach JN, Rice E, Fuchs RL, Astwood JD. Digestive stability in the context of assessing the potential allergenicity of food proteins. *Comments Toxicol.* 2002;. Available from: https://doi.org/10.1080/08865140214384.
107. Clare Mills EN, Marsh JT, Johnson PE, et al. Literature review: 'in vitro digestibility tests for allergenicity assessment.'. *EFSA Support Publ.* 2017. Available from: https://doi.org/10.2903/sp.efsa.2013.en-529.
108. Moreno FJ. Gastrointestinal digestion of food allergens: effect on their allergenicity. *Biomed Pharmacother.* 2007;. Available from: https://doi.org/10.1016/j.biopha.2006.10.005.
109. Verhoeckx K, Bøgh KL, Dupont D, et al. The relevance of a digestibility evaluation in the allergenicity risk assessment of novel proteins. Opinion of a joint initiative of COST action ImpARAS and COST action INFOGEST. *Food Chem Toxicol.* 2019;. Available from: https://doi.org/10.1016/j.fct.2019.04.052.
110. Westerhout J, Krone T, Snippe A, et al. Allergenicity prediction of novel and modified proteins: not a mission impossible! Development of a Random Forest allergenicity prediction model. *Regul Toxicol Pharmacol.* 2019;. Available from: https://doi.org/10.1016/j.yrtph.2019.104422.
111. Dimitrov I, Bangov I, Flower DR, Doytchinova I. AllerTOP v.2 – a server for in silico prediction of allergens. *J Mol Model.* 2014;20(6):2278. Available from: https://doi.org/10.1007/s00894-014-2278-5.
112. Dimitrov I, Flower DR, Doytchinova I. AllerTOP – a server for in silico prediction of allergens. *BMC Bioinform.* 2013;14(suppl 6):S4 (Epub Apr 17, 2013).
113. Wang J, Zhang D, Li J. PREAL: prediction of allergenic protein by maximum Relevance Minimum Redundancy (mRMR) feature selection. *BMC Syst Biol.* 2013;. Available from: https://doi.org/10.1186/1752-0509-7-S5-S9.
114. Wang J, Yu Y, Zhao Y, Zhang D, Li J. Evaluation and integration of existing methods for computational prediction of allergens. *BMC Bioinform.* 2013;. Available from: https://doi.org/10.1186/1471-2105-14-S4-S1.
115. Mohabatkar H, Mohammad Beigi M, Abdolahi K, Mohsenzadeh S. Prediction of allergenic proteins by means of the concept of

Chou's pseudo amino acid composition and a machine learning approach. *Med Chem.* 2012;. Available from: https://doi.org/10.2174/157340613804488341.

116. Bøgh KLK, Van Bilsen J, Głogowski R, et al. Current challenges facing the assessment of the allergenic capacity of food allergens in animal models. *Clin Transl Allergy.* 2016;6(1):21. Available from: https://doi.org/10.1186/s13601-016-0110-2.

117. Castan L, Bøgh KL, Maryniak NZ, et al. Overview of in vivo and ex vivo endpoints in murine food allergy models: suitable for evaluation of the sensitizing capacity of novel proteins? *Allergy Eur J Allergy Clin Immunol.* 2020;. Available from: https://doi.org/10.1111/all.13943.

118. Schülke S, Albrecht M. Mouse models for food allergies: where do we stand? *Cells.* 2019;. Available from: https://doi.org/10.3390/cells8060546.

119. Kanagaratham C, Sallis BF, Fiebiger E. Experimental models for studying food allergy. *Cell Mol Gastroenterol Hepatol.* 2018;. Available from: https://doi.org/10.1016/j.jcmgh.2018.05.010.

Chapter 49

Risk assessment of mixtures in the food chain

Angelo Moretto
Department of Cardio-Thoraco-Vascular and Public Health Sciences, University Hospital, Padua, Italy

Abstract
Many chemicals are present in food as a result of involuntary contamination or resulting from voluntary addition, for example, pesticide or veterinary drug residues, or additives. Assessment of the health risk associated with combined exposure to multiple chemicals from food presents many issues. From the toxicological side, the main question is the identification of the compounds to include in a group for which to assess combined risk. Different criteria have been developed that resulted in groups of compounds of different sizes. Intake can be assessed with increasing levels of refinement, which require increasing levels of resources, in order to identify the occurrence of combined exposures. Assessments have been carried out so far for a number of groups of pesticide residues which resulted in estimated intakes that did not raise concern. However, there is a need for international harmonization of methodologies, especially in those fields where international food trade is involved.

Keywords: Cumulative; index compound; hazard quotient; hazard index; margin of exposure; probabilistic; harmonization

49.1 Introduction

Humans are continuously exposed, via different routes, to chemicals of both natural origin or derived from human activities. With respect to food, chemicals may be naturally present in the crop and their concentration may change during processing to obtain the food we eat. Concentrations may increase or decrease, or new substances may develop during processing, but these are generally considered safe based on evidence of lack of adverse effects after normal use. There are exceptions to this, but they are not considered in this chapter. This chapter will focus on the risk assessment of chemicals that do not "naturally" belong to a crop or a food item but appear as a consequence of voluntary addition, as in the case of pesticides, additives, veterinary drugs, or food contact materials, or as contaminants accidentally or unavoidably present in the crop or in a food item. The latter include for example, dioxins deposited in fields where animals graze, polycyclic aromatic hydrocarbons (PAH) deriving from cooking, metals present in the ground where plants grow, and mycotoxins deriving from fungal infection of certain cereals.

Moreover, certain chemicals are present not only in food but also in other environmental compartments and, hence, human exposure can occur via a number of other pathways (e.g., residential, occupational) and routes (inhalation, dermal deposition). Generally, different exposure pathways are evaluated and are under the responsibility of different national or international/sovranational regulatory bodies or different departments within the same body, that act under specific and, at times, not consistent or complimentary regulation; this is particularly true in the case of combined exposure to chemicals.[1]

In any case, it is the totality of exposure, via all pathways and routes, that is, aggregate exposure, that matters in the determination of the risk. This has already been recognized in 1996 by the United States with the Food Quality Protection Act (FQPA),[2] and later by WHO[3] and the European Union,[4] among others. However, this issue has not been yet fully addressed in existing regulations, except in certain instances including pesticides by the Environmental Protection Agency (EPA),[5] but efforts are underway.

The risk assessment of contaminants in food has been traditionally addressed on a compound-by-compound basis, except for some exceptions for groups of compounds that generally occur or are formed together: this is the case of the dioxins (polychlorinated dibenzo-para-dioxins, PCDD)/furans [polychlorinated dibenzo-para-furans (PCDF)]/dioxin-like PCBs (polychlorobiphenyls), of the PAHs, of the aflatoxins. In other situations, more

Present Knowledge in Food Safety. DOI: https://doi.org/10.1016/B978-0-12-819470-6.00054-8

compounds are present in the same medium (e.g., food or specific crops) and the mixture might be poorly defined. In this case, the "whole mixture approach" can be applied; especially, but not only, when the mixture is poorly defined the mixture is assessed as if it were a single chemical. This holistic approach has the advantage of taking into account the overall toxicological activity of the mixture, including interactions.[6–8]

49.2 Types of combined actions

The toxicological effects of combined exposures to more than one compound can be classified into three types which are variously named[9,10]:

1. Independent, response addition, simple dissimilar action, independent joint action, simple independent action: the toxicological effects of each individual compound are the consequence of different, separate mechanisms or modes of action; as such the type of effect and the target organ/system may differ between compounds. In essence, the effects seen can each be reproduced by the exposure to each individual compound alone, because they do not influence each other's biological/toxicological activity. Hence, there is a response or effect addition.
2. Additive, dose-addition, simple similar action, relative dose-addition, similar joint action: this occurs when the compounds share the same mechanism or mode of action (MoA). In this case, the only notable difference will be in the potency: that is, different doses will be required to obtain the same effect. To simplify, this effect is based on the theory that compounds bind to a receptor that triggers a cascade of events leading to the final adverse phenotypic outcome. The relative affinity determines the extent of occupancy of the receptor at any given concentration; the higher the affinity the lower the concentration required to trigger/modulate the effect. Hence, the relative potency among different compounds or, better, their potency-normalized concentration will predict the fraction of the biological response attributable to each compound. These are the compounds for which an assessment of the combined exposure is deemed relevant. More details will be provided below when discussing the criteria for grouping compounds.
3. Interactive: this includes a form of effect that deviates from either response- or dose-addition. This refers to the instances when the combined effect of more than one chemical is either lower (antagonistic, inhibitory, and infra-or sub-additive) or higher (synergistic, potentiating, and supra-additive) than that expected on the basis of response-addition (1) or dose addition (2).

49.3 When to assess the risk of combined exposures from chemicals in food

While it is conceivable that combined exposures to chemicals present in food may result in any of the types of combined effects described above, quantitative exposure considerations need to be introduced before embarking on complex and resource-intensive experiments, calculations and considerations. In fact, certain classes of chemicals, such as pesticides, food additives, veterinary drugs, and food contact materials, are strictly regulated and require authorization prior to use. Such authorization depends, among others, on the assessment of the risk for the consumer and the consequent identification of appropriate management measures to ensure that the intake for humans is below the established safe exposure limits. These limits are such that the maximum allowed exposure is lower than the human equivalent no-observable-adverse-effect-level (NOAEL) for the critical toxicological effect. The margin of exposure (MoE) from the NOAEL or the safety/uncertainty factor (UF) to be applied in setting the reference values (RVs) (e.g., the Acceptable Daily Intake, ADI, the Acute Reference Dose (ARfD), the Tolerable Daily Intake, TDI) can vary between about 10 to over 1000-fold, depending on various considerations, including data availability, data quality, the severity of the effect. For these groups of compounds, which are regulated and monitored to ensure that exposure is within the limits and hence no toxic effect is expected, combined effects deriving from independent action [described in (1) above] are not generally expected.

Among the different types of interaction [described in (3) above], those relevant for risk assessment are those that result in a higher-than-expected effect based on either response- or dose addition. In any case, it should be borne in mind that exposure via food is generally low and there is pragmatic information that this kind of interaction is unlikely to occur at these low exposure levels, or, at least, the deviation for the expected effect is of minor size. Available studies with quantitative estimates of interaction at low doses (i.e., doses between the NOAEL and the LOAEL) with a determination of the dose-response curve are not many. In particular, in the evaluation of the six studies that provided useful quantitative estimates of synergy, the magnitude of synergy at low doses did not exceed the levels predicted by additive models by more than a factor of four.[6] A more recent review of the experimental studies with mixtures[11] did not find additional in vivo studies in mammals but reviewed also a number of studies in vitro or in vivo in lower species. The conclusion was that there is support for the default assumption that dose-additivity is appropriate for addressing the risk assessment of combined exposures, with the awareness that there might be specific cases where this does not correctly apply. In fact, any deviation from dose-additivity was small (up to fourfold as described by ref.[6]) so it might also be within the experimental variability. It is also to be noted that in a number of the cases the deviation from additivity was observed only at the higher doses used in the study. Martin et al.[11] also noted that a large proportion of studies that claimed synergistic effects were discounted as not different from dose-additivity, upon proper reappraisal of the data. Therefore for exposures deriving from chemicals present in food, the approach is to address interaction on a case-by-case basis. For instance, the European Chemicals Agency (EChA) proposed that only a deviation between dose addition predictions and measured combined toxicities by a factor of five or more needs to be regarded as synergistic/antagonistic and should be explicitly addressed in the assessment of combined exposure risks.[12]

On the contrary, those interactions resulting in lower-than-expected effects will be of low or no concern and need to be addressed only in very specific situations where such a "beneficial" combined effect will result in protection of public health not otherwise obtainable.

In summary, the approach for risk assessment of mixture exposure from chemicals in food is to combine those chemicals for which dose additivity is expected.

49.4 Which substances should be evaluated in a cumulative risk assessment? Common mechanism groups and cumulative assessment groups

The approach to group substances (present in food) for which to carry out a cumulative risk assessment (CRA) differs between the United States (EPA) and EU European Food Safety Authority (EFSA). The activity has been mainly carried out on pesticide residues, but it is now being applied to other classes of chemicals that can be found in food.

EPA issued a "Guidance For Identifying Pesticide Chemicals and Other Substances that have a Common Mechanism of Toxicity[13] and a "Guidance on Cumulative Risk Assessment of Pesticide Chemicals That Have a Common Mechanism of Toxicity" in 2002[5] with an updated framework in 2016.[15] EPA concluded that CRA should be carried out for those compounds for which a common mode/mechanism of action, leading to a common toxic effect, has been established and proposed criteria to identify the compounds that should belong to a cumulative assessment group (CAG). These criteria include:

1. chemical structural similarity: this is considered a starting point since in many cases a shared chemical structure may translate to a shared toxicophore (i.e., a chemical group that is associated with the toxic effect). The chemical structure needs to be looked at in combination with other considerations since it is not sufficient to support by itself the inclusion in a Common mechanism group (CMG);
2. hazard profile: target organ(s), adverse effects/apical outcomes, and pharmacokinetics properties are evaluated and compared among compounds in order to assess commonalities. In particular, effects at lower doses, driving the definition of the point of departure (PoD) (NOAEL or BMD(L)) are considered more relevant. Effects should be related to specific targets (e.g., an enzymatic activity, hormonal level) rather than being non-specific (e.g., changes in body weight or food consumption). In most cases, a common apical outcome will not be used as the sole factor in determining a candidate's CMG for screening purposes. For instance, it is considered inappropriate to include all neurotoxic pesticides in a single candidate group, or those causing liver or kidney toxicity since these generally derive from repeated high doses and multiple pathways. So the latter need to be evaluated in the context of knowledge of mammalian MoA/ Adverse Outcome Pathway (AOP) and chemical structure.
3. MoA/AOP/Common Mechanism of Toxicity: this knowledge is considered the strongest information and is the foundation for establishing the CMG. EPA indicates the criteria to organize, evaluate and assess the data in order to reach the conclusion, which includes the identification of the key events within an MoA or AOP, considering strength, consistency, dose-response, temporal concordance, and biological plausibility in a weight of evidence (WoE) analysis. In this context, pesticidal MoA may provide useful starting information, when data on mammals are missing or scanty.

On this basis, EPA indicates the following final options:

1. Conclusion of No Common Mechanism, no further CRA work is necessary. This includes two possibilities: either some groups of pesticides do not share a similar toxicological profile or the toxicological database does not support a testable hypothesis for a common MoA.
2. Candidate CMG can be formed and screening-level exposure analysis is conducted: these candidate CMGs have shared characteristics that suggest a common pathway or support a testable hypothesis for a common MoA. In this case a screening-level, highly conservative, exposure analysis is conducted with tiers of increased refinement. This analysis includes an evaluation of toxicological and exposure data based on

available information with a minimal resource approach; if in this way the screening risk does not exceed the level of concern, no further detailed elaborations are required. If the level of concern is exceeded, additional data to better describe the MoA/AOP may be needed to confirm the compounds belonging to the CMG, or more detailed exposure refinements might be carried out, resulting in a formal and full CRA of what will be called a CAG.

3. CMG can be established: available mechanistic data support the definition of an MoA/AOP. Then a formal and full CRA will be carried out.

In this respect, EPA indicates that the best use can be made of data on mammalian MoA/AOP for the group and pharmacokinetics data for individual members of the prospective group, which will provide the strongest foundation for establishing a CMG. This will be based on the framework proposed by a WHO working group and others where criteria are presented to organize the data and describe the key events, and their dose-response and temporal concordance, which lead to the adverse health outcome.[16–20] EPA clearly states that "non-specific toxic effects, unless tied to an MoA/AOP or testable hypothesis related to a potential MoA/AOP, would not support a candidate CMG."[15] Non-specific effects, such as body weight changes or food consumption alterations, are those that are not related to specific target sites (e.g., an enzyme or hormone) or target tissue (e.g., thyroid or blood), and, therefore are unlikely to derive from a common toxic pathway. EPA underlines that a common apical (phenomenological) adverse outcome will not be generally used by itself to identify a CMG, even for screening purposes because this needs to be evaluated in the context of the information on MoA/AOP.

EPA has, so far, established five CMGs, namely: organophosphorus esters (OPs), N-methyl carbamates (NMCs), chloracetanilides, triazines, and naturally occurring pyrethrins and synthetic pyrethroids, for which a CRA has been carried out (see below). In addition, EPA considered thiocarbamates and dithiocarbamates but concluded that these pesticides did not share a common mechanism (see: http://epa.gov/pesticides/cumulative/thiocarb.pdf; http://epa.gov/oppsrrd1/cumulative/dithiocarb.pdf).

For EPA, a further step is needed in order to select which chemicals from a specific CMG should be assessed. As a consequence, a subset of the CMG denominated CAG is set up by excluding those compounds that provide minimal contribution either because of low toxic potency or because of limited use (i.e., low exposure) or both.

The 2002 CRA guidance from ref.[5] notes that not all cumulative assessments need to be of the same depth and scope and that it is important to determine the need for a comprehensive risk assessment by considering the exposure profile. For instance, only those pesticides whose uses, routes, and pathways of exposure will present sufficient exposure and hazard potential will be included in the CAG for the quantitative estimates of risk. In fact, based on exposure data the evaluation of the CMG triazines (atrazine, simazine, and propazine) in 2006 resulted in an actual CAG including only atrazine and simazine because exposures to propazine are not anticipated via any of the relevant exposure pathways.[14,21]

EFSA is actively working on CRA, initially for pesticide residues[22] and lately also for other chemicals in food and the environment.[23] The approach taken by EFSA provides for the identification of toxicological target organs and organ systems as a first grouping criterion (CAG level 1, CAG-1). This is then refined by identifying a specific phenomenological effect on the target organ/system (CAG level 2, CAG-2). If data allow, the grouping can be further refined by identifying a common mode or mechanism of action (CAG level 3 and 4, CAG-3, CAG-4).

The initial screening of toxic effect(s) on target organ/organ systems (CAG-1) done by EFSA resulted in many of the substances being included in more than one CAG-1 because they showed effects on several organ/organ systems.[24,25]

Upon further refinement, CAG-2 was proposed to include compounds causing a specific phenomenological effect on the target organ/organ system in question without considering the MoA. A number of compounds were found to cause several specific phenomenological effects in a given target organ/organ system. The reason for this is that the proposed different specific effects could be considered as representing a continuum of pathological findings for a given target organ/organ system. EFSA took the position that some effects, which would be considered in single substance assessment as being non-adverse (e.g., if seen below a certain limit of magnitude) should be considered as being potentially adverse (i.e., relevant) within the context of CRA. Similarly, effects that are transient (i.e., observed after a short period of exposure, only, but not later) might be considered adaptive for single substance assessment, but EFSA could not exclude that the capacity for adaptation of an organism will be exhausted if there is exposure to several substances simultaneously, hence becoming relevant for CRA.

CAG-3 was proposed when information or a hypothesis was available on a common MoA behind a specific effect. This could be applied to only a limited number of compounds acting for example, on certain parts of the endocrine system and the nervous system.

CAG-4 was proposed for some of the active substances for which data, also from the open literature, could support the identification of a specific mechanism of action: for example, acetylcholinesterase inhibitors (and thus modulate the cholinergic system; CAG-3) or antagonists to the androgen receptor (and thus affecting, for example, the male reproductive organs via an anti-androgenic MoA; CAG-3).

While the approach taken in the USA can be viewed as based on inclusion criteria, that is, relatively stringent toxicological information on MoA/AOP is required for defining a CMG and including compounds into it, the approach in the European Union starts with very broad CAGs essentially based on organs as targets of (any) toxicity; CAGs are then refined to the extent possible with identification of increasingly detailed information to exclude compounds from a CAG or to form more specific CAGs out of a broader CAG. In the latter approach, lower weight is given to the MoA, and emphasis is on the commonality of the apical outcome or some late key events within different, apparently or putatively, converging AOPs. This EFSA approach follows the EU Commission recommendations that, in the absence of information, a precautionary approach should be followed that is, an "exclusion approach," so, with the lack of relevant data about modes of action and pathways leading to common adverse effects, common target organs can be used as a proxy. So substances may be included in a CAG, although they might exert their effects through MoAs that are not relevant for that CAG, resulting in an overestimation of the risk.

In addition, contrary to the EPA approach, EFSA considered that a compound should be included in a CAG regardless of whether the common toxic effect represented the critical effect (i.e., the effect that drives its risk assessment from which health-based guidance values such as ADI or ARfD are derived), or that the effect occurs only at higher doses. This is because EFSA believed that pesticides with common toxicity pathways will elicit relevant common toxic effects in an additive fashion, regardless of the occurrence of other effects at lower doses.

49.5 Methods for cumulative risk assessment

49.5.1 Component-based approach

A number of methods can be used for CRA that need to be carried out keeping in mind that compounds in the same CAG cause the same effects but have different potencies in causing such an effect. Therefore to estimate the combined risk, either the different potencies need to be normalized or the exposure needs to be normalized to the potency in order to have a common scale to compare. Some methods deal with toxicity and exposure separately, while others elaborate the information at the same time. The Hazard Index (HI), the Cumulative Risk Index (CRI), the Reference point index (RfPI), and the Combined margin of exposure or Margin of Exposure Total (MOET) belong to the latter category, while the relative potency factor (RPF) and toxic equivalency factor (TEF) methods, which involve essentially the same approach, deal with toxicity separately from exposure.

49.5.1.1 Relative potency factor/toxic equivalency factor

With this method, the potency of each compound is normalized to the potency of a so-called "index compound" (IC): this method was initially developed for dioxins and called TEF[26] and was proposed by US EPA for the CRA of pesticides. This method is also known as potency equivalency factor (PEF) or relative potency factor (RPF) method.[5] The following steps are applied in this method: (1) determine the toxic potency of each compound, (2) select a compound as reference for all other compounds, the "index compound", (3) calculate the potency of each compound in the CAG relative to the IC, (4) determine the point of departure or RV for the IC.

The 2002 EPA CRA guidance,[5] recommends that the IC should: (1) have high-quality dose-response data; (2) have a toxicological/biological profile for the common toxicity that is representative of the common toxic effect (s); and (3) be well-characterized for the common mechanism of toxicity. This means that the IC does not necessarily need to be the most potent, but it is important that it has the most robust toxicological database for the common toxic effect via the routes of interest so that the identified NOAEL is the least uncertain or, better, the benchmark dose (BMD) has the narrowest confidence interval.

EPA later indicated that RPFs and PoDs/RfPs can be derived at the screening level using NOAELs when criteria are less stringent and leave room for refinements in cases where the screening level assessment indicates some level of concern.[27]

In principle, the potencies should be derived from a consistent and uniform dataset. However, this is not always possible, especially for chemicals that are not pesticides. In fact, for pesticide approval, an extensive number of studies are submitted to regulatory bodies, but this is not the case for other chemicals that can be found in food. Once the relevant studies have been identified, more accurate potencies can be derived from dose-response modeling. This is a rather resource-intensive exercise since it requires modeling of the available data that are usually reported with NOAELs and LOAELs, and not modeled. Using the BMD is the approach taken by EPA for CRA of pesticide residues in food[13] while EFSA essentially used the NOAELs although the use of BMDs or a combination of NOAELs and BMDs is foreseen.[23] Different UFs can be applied to the individual RfP

(BMD or NOAEL/LOAEL) before calculating the RPF either because additional UFs are required or some UFs need not be applied to some compounds (e.g., when human data are available).

When calculating the RPF one assumption is that compounds have parallel dose-response curves, which is not necessarily true, and hence this is a source of uncertainty. This might somehow be ascertained by comparing the slopes of the dose-response curves when BMDs are used.[29] When using NOAELs, we should also be aware that NOAELs/LOAELs may be distributed at varying levels along the dose-response relationship curve and, in particular, at various distances from the "true" NAEL (no adverse effect level), depending for example, on dose-spacing and the sensitivity of the end-point used.

In the end, the toxicity of the mixture is calculated by adding the potency-normalized doses and expressed as IC equivalents. This IC-equivalent dose is then compared to the RV or the RfP (or PoD) of the IC, and the same risk consideration is applied as if it were as a single compound; that is, if using the RfP the MoE is calculated (see below) and if using the RV the hazard quotient (HQ) is used.

49.5.1.2 Hazard index

The HI is the sum of the HQs for each component. The HQ is the ratio between exposure and the RV (e.g., ADI, ARfD, and TDI). An HQ of less than 1 means that the estimated/measured exposure is lower than the RV and hence acceptable, also an HI lower than 1 means that the combined risk is considered acceptable.

$$\mathrm{HI} = \frac{\mathrm{Exp1}}{\mathrm{RV1}} + \frac{\mathrm{Exp2}}{\mathrm{RV2}} + \ldots \frac{\mathrm{Exp}n}{\mathrm{RV}n}$$

That is

$$\mathrm{HI} = \mathrm{HQ1} + \mathrm{HQ2} + \ldots \mathrm{HQ}n$$

The HI relates directly to the RV, which is a common, readily available, and well-understood parameter of acceptable risk. Consequently, besides being transparent and understandable, HI methodology is (relatively) rapid and simple since RVs are readily available and it can serve as a useful screening method. In particular, the HI can be refined, if needed, when the RV of one or more compounds within the CAG is based on an effect that is not the common toxic effect or the assessment factor applied to establish the RV from the RfP or PoD includes additional adjustments not related to the endpoint of concern. In this case, an adjusted HI (aHI) will be obtained.

49.5.1.3 Reference point index

The RfPI is the sum of the exposures to each compound expressed as a fraction of their respective RfPs (PoDs) for the relevant common effect. To take into account the safety/assessment/ UFs, the RfPI should be multiplied by the chosen factor and when the result is lower than 1, the combined risk is considered acceptable.

$$\mathrm{RfPI} = \frac{\mathrm{Exp1}}{\mathrm{RfP1}} + \frac{\mathrm{Exp2}}{\mathrm{RfP2}} + \ldots \frac{\mathrm{Exp}n}{\mathrm{RfP}n} \times \mathrm{UF}$$

As for the HI, the RfPI is mathematically rather simple and transparent, however, there is a difference to the HI in that a common UF is applied to the RfPI and the possible need for different UFs is not taken into account. However, if needed, accommodation for chemical-specific UFs can be made earlier in the calculation but this can result in a less readily transparent process.

49.5.1.4 The combined margin of exposure

For an individual compound, the MoE is the ratio of the RfP or PoD to the measured or estimated exposure in humans: in fact, it is the inverse calculation made for the RfPI, before the application of the UF. The MOE is then compared to the chosen UF, and if the MOE is higher than the UF then exposure is considered acceptable. The combined MOE is called the MOET, and is calculated as the reciprocal of the sum of the reciprocals of the individual MOEs (see equation below).

$$\mathrm{MOE} = \frac{\mathrm{BMD10(or\ NOAEL)}}{\mathrm{Exposure}}$$

$$\mathrm{MOET} = \frac{1}{(1/\mathrm{MOE1}) + (1/\mathrm{MOE2}) + \ldots (1/\mathrm{MOE}n)}$$

Similar to the MOE, when the MOET is greater than the chosen UF (usually 100, but an alternative value can be specified by the risk manager) the combined risk is considered acceptable. As for the RfPI, adjustments of individual UFs, if needed, should be done early in the process. Since the MOE is in widespread use, expressing the results of the assessment as MOET can facilitate communication with the public.

This approach is taken by the EPA which considers aggregate (food, drinking water, and residential exposure) in its CRA. In doing so, each pathway of exposure has its own MOE that is then combined in the MOET.[5]

49.5.1.5 Cumulative risk index

The reciprocal of the HQ (i.e., the ratio between the RV and the exposure) is called the risk index (RI). A ratio higher than 1 means that the estimated/measured exposure is lower than the RV. The CRI is the reciprocal of the sum of the HQs. As such, when the CRI is greater than 1, the combined risk is considered acceptable. While the CRI is simply a different way of expressing the HI, it is not as transparent or understandable as the HI and involves a more complex calculation.

$$RI = \frac{RfP}{Exposure \times UF} = \frac{RV}{Exposure} = \frac{1}{HQ}$$

49.5.2 Whole mixture approach

The whole mixture approach may be appropriate for certain contaminants (e.g., mineral oil mixtures) or food and feed additives that are added as whole mixtures (e.g., essential oils from botanical extracts). The different whole mixtures might be characterized with different precision and completeness of the toxicological data. If the whole mixture is poorly characterized, use of in silico and read-across is extremely limited since information on the chemical structures of components is required to apply these methods. In cases when availabile information on the source of the mixture provides an indication that certain types of chemicals (e.g., carcinogens) are not present, then it might be possible to apply tools such as the threshold of toxicological concern (TTC) to the mixture, which will be then considered as a single compound.[30–32] If more data are available, either for the whole mixture of concern or for similar whole mixture(s), the RfP/PoD (e.g., the BMDL, the NOAEL) might be identified from which to derive the RV by applying an UF, considered appropriate by expert judgment.

49.6 Assessment of exposure

Assessment of exposure via food can be performed via different methods and data[33] which can provide different levels of accuracy and provide different levels of conservativism. In the case of combined exposures, the situation is even more complex and possibly resource intensive. Both EPA and EFSA have developed methods to address CRA. While EFSA has so far limited the assessment to dietary intake, EPA has developed methods for aggregate cumulative exposure (i.e., dietary, residential, and via drinking water).

Both methodologies include tiered approaches depending on the level of refinement required for the assessment.

EPA exposure evaluation starts with the identification of the use patterns of the chemicals within a candidate CMG, which include registered crops and residential use (if any). Different levels of refinement can be reached for every single pesticide depending on the type of data used to define the food residues (i.e., tolerance levels, field trial or Pesticide Data Program (PDP) data), and other considerations such as percent crop treated, processing data. EPA distinguishes between screening level and complete CRA, the latter being performed if the outcome of the screening level CRA is not reassuring. Different tiers are proposed for screening levels that range from assuming complete co-occurrence in both food and drinking water (Tier 1) to consideration of the probability of high-end residue values in drinking water (Tier 2) and consideration of the probability of co-occurrence of food residues, taking into account only the compound that yields the highest exposure (corrected by the RPF) (Tier 3). Tier 3 still does not include monitoring data for foods and hence is an overestimation of the exposure. These tiers represent the screening steps and the assessment may stop at any of these tiers if the outcome is reassuring.

In the more refined approach of EPA duration, frequency, and seasonality of exposure are included. Moreover, overlapping exposure scenarios and co-occurrence, and populations of concern are identified. Refined exposure estimates for food are based on residue monitoring data from the USDA's PDP supplemented with information from the Food and Drug Administration's (FDA) Pesticide Residue Monitoring Program and Total Diet Study. The PDP provides also an indication of the co-occurrence of residues in the same food. In addition, EPA treats samples with non-detectable residues as "zero" values. This approach was taken because it was found that it does not significantly under-estimate exposures, in particular at the upper percentiles of exposure, which are those more relevant for regulation.

In general, EPA addresses food consumption of different age groups that may include, not necessarily in all CRA: Infants less than 1-year-old, Children 1–2 years old, Children 3–5 years old, Children 6–12 years old, Youths 13–19 years old, Adults 20–49 years old, Adults 50 + years old, Females 13–49 years old.

Although deterministic models are routinely adopted for conducting dietary exposure assessments for the regulatory approval of pesticides, EFSA used probabilistic models for conducting CRA.[34,35]

Presently EFSA uses monitoring data collected by the Member States under their official monitoring programs in selected years and individual food consumption data from 10 populations of consumers from different countries and different age groups. Foods selected included 30 raw, widely consumed in Europe, primary commodities of plant origin, water, and foods for infants and young children. The approach was based on tiers of different refinement levels. Tier I applies very conservative assumptions that allow efficient screening of exposure with a likely significant overestimation. For instance, measurements below the LOQ are imputed as 1/2 LOQ if the residue was found at measurable levels in at least one substance-commodity combination, otherwise, they were treated as "zero."

Tier II includes assumptions that are more refined but still intended to be conservative. For instance, an estimation of use frequencies is made according to the agricultural use patterns, which allowed the estimation of true "zeros." This is still an overestimate but more refined that the one described in Tier I.

EFSA observed that randomly assigning active substances to unspecific measurements (i.e., a measurement that may comprise multiple active substances) and imputing left-censored data (i.e., measurements below the limit of quantification) had a significant impact on the calculations. In addition, EFSA cannot yet further refine the assessment, as EPA did, based on the use frequency of pesticides because this information is not available in the EU. Also, the limitation of data on the effect of processing prevents another possible refinement. However, the absence of such information leads to an important overestimation of the exposure.

49.7 Cumulative risk assessment conducted so far in United States and EU

Due to the different approaches to the definition of CAGs, except, to some extent, for inhibitors of AChE, the pesticide groups evaluated by EPA and EFSA differ. In fact, EPA CAGs are, initially, based on the chemical structure while EFSA CAGs are based on the final apical adverse effect with different levels of refinement. Both EPA and EFSA performed a probabilistic assessment indicating the percentiles of the (sub)population associated with a specific MOE.

49.7.1 Inhibitors of acetylcholinesterase (European Food Safety Authority and Environmental Protection Agency)

EPA and EFSA took different approaches because, based on toxicodynamic (TD) considerations, EPA established a CAG with organophosphorus esters (OPs),[36] that are irreversible AChE inhibitors, and a different CAG with carbamates,[37] that are rapidly (hours) reversible inhibitors, while EFSA considered that even for chronic exposure both OPs and carbamates should be assessed together.[39]

For OPs, EPA[36] selected methamidophos as the IC since it had high-quality dose-response data for all routes of exposure. EPA used brain cholinesterase inhibition in female rats measured at 21 days of exposure or longer. This is because a steady-state AChE inhibition is reached after 3–4 weeks of exposure to any OP. The relative potencies were estimated from the BMD_{10} (the dose causing a 10% effect) for brain AChE inhibition derived from the application of an exponential dose-response model. The BMD_{10} was also used to define the PoD for methamidophos. Moreover, the additional UF for children required by the FQPA was either waived or reduced for the 13 OPs that had relevant studies. For all other OPs, an FQPA factor of 10X was retained. The compound-specific FQPA safety factor was directly applied to the RPF for each OP. In this way, the target MOET of 100 could be applied for OP CRA.

The cumulative dietary intake of OPs was based on a refined estimation of the distribution of exposures across the United States because they are based on residue monitoring data from the USDA's PDP with the integration of information derived from the FDA Surveillance Monitoring Programs and Total Diet Study. The PDP data includes data on the major children's foods and provide surrogate information for crops not included in the survey. The PDP also indicates the co-occurrence of OP pesticides in the same sample.

EPA concluded that the CRA for food was driven by a few uses of OP pesticides on food crops, namely methamidophos/acephate on beans, watermelon, and tomato; and phorate on potatoes. In any case, the cumulative MOEs from exposure to OPs for the highest percentile (99.9th) of the population do not raise concern since they ranged from 99 for the most exposed subgroup (children 3–5) to 300 for youths 13–19.

For carbamates, EPA[37] used the BMD_{10} (i.e., the dose causing 10% AChE inhibition) to estimate the potency and the relative potency. In particular, for those compounds for which there were no studies in juvenile animals an additional 10 × UF was added as required by the United States FQPA,[2] and for those compounds for which there were acceptable studies in humans, the 10 × UF for an animal to human extrapolation was not applied. Oxamyl was chosen as the IC and for it, the $BMDL_{10}$ (the lower 95% confidence limit of the BMD_{10}) was used as PoD for each route of exposure (oral, dermal, inhalation).

EPA evaluation also considered aggregate exposure to OPs or carbamates, which included not only food but also drinking water and residential exposure.[36,37]

EFSA conducted the CRA for acute and chronic AChE inhibition from pesticide residues in food for 10 European populations of consumers, from different countries and age groups. The CAG included 47 compounds, 36 OPs, and 11 carbamates.[38,39]

To derive potencies, EFSA used the NOAEL for a statistically significant 20% reduction of AChE activity compared to controls.[40] In addition, cases where the NOAEL for AChE inhibition was higher than the critical NOAEL (i.e., the NOAEL from which the ADI or the ARfD were derived) were flagged.

The IC chosen for acute effects was oxamyl because of the robustness of the database while for the chronic effects omethoate was selected mainly because of the consistency of findings across species, including mouse, rat, rabbit, and dog.

EFSA noted that AChE inhibition by individual compounds has, generally, a NOAEL that is, sometimes significantly, lower than that for clinical effects on the motor, sensory and autonomic divisions of the nervous system, or on neuropathological effects that form the basis for other CAGs on which OPs and carbamates are also included (see below point 49.7.6).

EFSA applied probabilistic modeling using monitoring data obtained by the Members States in 2016–18. EFSA concluded, that based on uncertainty analysis (35 sources of uncertainty have been identified and analyzed) and other methodological considerations, cumulative exposure to acetylcholinesterase inhibitors does not exceed the threshold for regulatory consideration for any of the population groups considered with a certainty ranging from 50- > 90% in the different populations considered, for both acute and chronic exposure. The acute exposure was driven by exposure to chlorpyrifos, triazophos, and omethoate, and to a minor extent dichlorvos, formetanate, and carbofuran. The chronic exposure, at the high end, was driven by a few combinations of substance-commodity (i.e., omethoate and dimethoate in olives for oil production, pirimiphos-methyl in wheat, chlorpyrifos in oranges, and, to a lesser extent, monocrotophos and dichlorvos in drinking water).

49.7.2 Triazines (Environmental Protection Agency)

EPA identified a common mechanism of toxicity for the chlorotriazine herbicides, atrazine, propazine, and simazine.[14] The identified mechanism relates to a neuroendocrine activity that results in both reproductive and developmental effects. Three major chlorinated metabolites, desethyl-s-atrazine (DEA), desisopropyl-s-atrazine (DIA), and diaminochlorotriazine (DACT) have also been found to share the same effects. Hence, the CMG includes the three pesticides and their three chlorinated metabolites. Based on the lack of these effects following treatment with other triazines, such as ametryn, prometryn, prometon, metsulfuron methyl, trisulfuron, chlorsulfuron, and DPX-M631, these herbicides were not included in the CMG and no CRA was conducted on them. No common acute effects have been identified for triazine herbicides.[41] Therefore only chronic exposure was evaluated for CRA. Based on toxicological considerations, EPA utilized 4-day dietary exposure data since the PoDs do not differ between 4-day and chronic exposure studies, and because 4-day exposure scenarios are expected to be higher than the chronic ones, hence resulting in a more conservative assessment. In addition, EPA conducted a screening level aggregate CRA, for nonfood exposures which resulted in a conservative assessment. For the derivation of the PoDs, EPA applied PBPK (physiologically based pharmacokinetic) models that provided the most conservative value. In addition, based on the PBPK modeling, the UF for interspecies toxicokinetic (TK) extrapolation was waived resulting in a final UF of 30, instead of the standard 100.

The conclusion was that there were no risks of concern for the 4-day cumulative dietary (food only) or cumulative dietary aggregate (food + drinking water) scenarios for the chlorotriazines. EPA found that residential exposure was quantitatively more relevant than dietary or drinking water exposure.

49.7.3 Pyrethrins and synthetic pyrethroids (Environmental Protection Agency)

EPA[42] conducted a screening level CRA for pyrethrins and synthetic pyrethroids that resulted in no concerns for cumulative aggregate (dietary, drinking water, and residential) exposure to these compounds.

The naturally occurring pyrethrins and synthetic pyrethroids form a CMG based on "(1) shared structural characteristics; and (2) shared ability to interact with voltage-gated sodium channels (VGSC), resulting in disruption of membrane excitability in the nervous system, ultimately leading to neurotoxicity characterized by two different toxicity syndromes."[42] Disruption of the activity of the VGSC leads to an alteration of action potentials, that represent the basis for the clinical neurotoxicity present in pyrethroid poisoning.[43,44] The common structural characteristics are represented by the acid and alcohol moieties joined by an ether linkage. The interaction with VGSC has been demonstrated in vitro, with alterations in membrane excitability and firing potential, the compounds differing in their potency, and some dynamic properties. These data support the link between modification of the VGSC and the clinical signs.[43]

Pyrethroids may cause two different syndromes, that are named after the predominant signs and defined as Type I and Type II, in rodents. These Types may be related to the different effects on the VGSC.[43] Type I pyrethroids cause progressive fine whole-body tremor, exaggerated startle response, uncoordinated twitching of the dorsal muscles, and hyperexcitability. This is associated in vitro with a modest increase in the activation (channel opening) of VGSC followed by a decay described by a single exponential. Type II pyrethroids cause repetitive chewing, nosing, and washing, excessive salivation, coarse whole-body tremor, increased extensor tone in the hind limbs, choreiform movements of the limbs and tail, and convulsions. Because of the predominant choreiform movements and salivation, this syndrome is called CS syndrome. These compounds in vitro cause a large increase of the activation of VGSC followed by a decay described by a fast and a slow exponential component.[45] The presence of the alpha-3-cyano-3-phenoxybenzyl group in the molecule is predictive of Type II (CS) syndrome. However, some compounds do not fit the definition of either type since they show mixed, intermediate symptomatology.[44,46] In addition, in humans, these two syndromes cannot be easily identified, possibly because most of the human poisonings reported in the literature occurred after ingestion or high exposure to Type II pyrethroids, which are the more potent.[47–49]

On this basis, EPA[50] concluded that should refinements of the CRA be needed, pyrethrins and pyrethroids might be divided into two sub-groups in relation to the presence or lack thereof of the alpha-cyano group.

In the 2011 CRA, EPA excluded from the CAG compounds with very low toxicity (i.e., no neurotoxicity at 5000 mg/kg in rats) (tetramethrin and sumithrin), compounds that did not show residues in crops in the USA PDP, compounds that were used in residential settings. which do not have the potential for significant exposure or insignificant amount of use. This resulted in 15 compounds remaining in the CAG. EPA considered that measures of behavior in animals were appropriate for extrapolating risk to humans and an adequate proxy for VGSC interaction given the lack of an in vivo biomarker for such an effect.

EPA noted that studies submitted for pesticide registration were not adequate for establishing the RPFs. In fact, because of the short temporal nature of pyrethroid effects that have a short half-life and rapid reversibility, potencies should be determined by measuring the effects at or near the peak concentration. Only some published studies provided this information, which also included gavage administration and comparable vehicle and volume of administration, and were used to define the RPFs.[46,51,52]

The IC chosen was deltamethrin because it had the most robust database and lower variability around the BMD central estimate: these characteristics minimize the error or uncertainty in the CRA estimates. The RPFs were all derived from a complex evaluation of the data leading to the definition of BMD_{20} for the behavioral observations made in the animal studies. The PoD for deltamethrin was the 95% lower confidence interval for the BMD_{20}. In establishing the RV, EPA applied an additional UF of 3 for TK for children less than 6 years of age to those compounds that did not have specific studies in juvenile animals. EPA decided to incorporate the additional UF into the target MOE and not as a chemical-specific adjusted RPF.

Dietary consumption data used for the CRA included the USDA's Continuing Survey of Food Intakes by Individuals and the pesticide residue monitoring data collected by the USDA PDP. With regard to dietary assessment, for pyrethroids some conservative assumptions (e.g., processing factors were not applied) were made with respect to the full methodology, in view of the screening level of the CRA. Nevertheless, no dietary risk of concern was identified for pyrethroids. In fact, the MOET was well above 1000 for all age groups at the 99.9th percentile.

49.7.4 Chloroacetanilide pesticides (Environmental Protection Agency)

EPA[53] included in the CAG chloroacetanilide pesticides that have a common MoA for the production of tumors of the nasal olfactory epithelium in rats. This mechanism entails the generation of a common tissue reactive metabolite that causes cytotoxicity and subsequent regenerative proliferation in the nasal epithelium. Following sustained cytotoxicity and proliferation neoplasia may develop. Alachlor, acetochlor, and butachlor share this mechanism and have been included in the CMG, but based on exposure considerations, since butachlor is not registered in the United States, the actual CAG only includes acetochlor and alachlor. Since the tumors of the nasal olfactory epithelium arise through a non-mutagenic, non-linear, MoA, the use of the MoE approach was considered appropriate. Alachlor was chosen as IC with acetochlor having an RPF of 0.05. For both compounds, NOAELs and not BMDs have been used to define the RPF and the RV.

Since there is no residential use for these compounds, EPA decided to evaluate dietary exposure with a limited degree of refinement. In fact, values in food were not derived from residue monitoring data but rather the anticipated residues available from the registration dossier of alachlor and the tolerance value (corrected for processing factors) of acetochlor were used instead. All estimates were adjusted for the values of percent crop treated that were available to EPA. In this way, exposure is certainly overestimated.

Even using this high-end deterministic exposure estimate and the NOAELs instead of the BMDs, the MOET was in excess of 13,000.

49.7.5 Compounds affecting the thyroid

The EFSA[28,35,54] CRA for effects on thyroid started from a database that included information on all pesticides that caused effects possibly related to thyroid toxicity. After analysis of this database, two effects were found to meet the criteria established for consideration in CRA.[30,55] These two specific effects were hypothyroidism, and parafollicular cell (C-cell) hypertrophy/hyperplasia/neoplasia. For other effects, such as thyroid-mediated impaired neurodevelopment, there was insufficient information to address the combined effects of pesticides. The compounds included in the two CAGs were 128 for hypothyroidism and 17 for C-cell hypertrophy, hyperplasia, and neoplasia. For the former CAG, EFSA assessed the uncertainty related to its composition by expert knowledge elicitation (EKE)[56] which resulted in a median estimate of 71 (as opposed to 128) for the number of substances to be included in this CAG. The same exercise was not conducted for the other CAG because the CRA was estimated to be smaller than that for the CAG for hypothyroidism.

Other identified sources of uncertainty were related to the toxicological characterization of the compounds, the characteristics of the dose−response relationship, the contribution of metabolites and degradation products, the adequacy of the dose-addition model, and the inter- and intra-species differences in toxicological sensitivity.

Although it was recommended[23] to characterize the potency of the compounds included in the CAGs using, as reference points, the BMDL, the potencies, and related RPFs have been estimated using the NOAELs for the most sensitive indicator of effect in the relevant study.

The dietary intake assessment was independently performed for ten population groups, including adults, children (3−9 years), and toddlers (1−3 years) in the web-based probabilistic Monte Carlo Risk Assessment (MCRA) (more details can be found in Ref.[57]) or the EFSA SAS software.[35] Using SAS software, Tier I (occurrence based on authorized uses) and Tier II (occurrence based on monitoring data) modeling approaches have been used, both conservative with Tier II being more refined. The cumulative exposure was expressed as the total margin of exposure (MOET) at the 50th to 99.9th percentile of the exposure distribution, the latter being the percentile of the exposure distribution considered relevant for regulatory actions. At Tier II, for the CAG thyroid parafollicular cells, the MOET at the 99.9th percentile of exposure in the ten population groups was between 1468 and 3978; for the CAG hypothyroidism, it was between 100 and 199 for toddlers and children, and between 267 and 314 for adults. Very minor differences were observed using MCRA.

The main drivers for exposure to CAG hypothyroidism were bromide ion, followed by propineb, thiabendazole, ziram, mancozeb, pyrimethanil, chlorpropham, and cyprodinil, while thiram and ziram drove the exposure to CAG parafollicular cells

Sensitivity analyses on the 31 identified possible sources of uncertainty showed that the MOET in tier II may be two-to-four times higher than that calculated.

49.7.6 Other effects on the nervous system (European Food Safety Authority)

In addition, to brain and/or erythrocyte acetylcholinesterase (AChE) inhibition, EFSA identified another four specific nervous system effects that could lead to the establishment of CAGs.[40] These effects were functional alterations of three divisions of the nervous system ((1) motor, (2) sensory, and (3) autonomic functions, respectively), and (4) histological neuropathological changes in neural tissues. EFSA did not address other effects such as cognitive alteration and developmental neurotoxicity because the available information was not deemed sufficient. Compounds were included in a CAG based on either the chemical structure that could be associated with a MoA linked to the effect or on toxicological endpoints related to the specific effect.

These CAGs were based on

1. evidence of a functional alteration of the motor division of the nervous system because of reduced motor activity, increased motor activity, alteration of muscle strength or coordination;
2. evidence of a functional alteration of the sensory division of the nervous system because of decreased reactivity, increased reactivity, or proprioception and sensory deficits;
3. evidence of a functional alteration of the autonomic division of the nervous system because of miosis, mydriasis, increased salivation, lacrimation, piloerection, urination;
4. evidence of histologic neuropathological effects such as axonal degeneration, myelin degeneration, or neuronal degeneration/necrosis.

On this basis, a compound could be included in more than one CAG. Besides the 47 compounds included in CAG brain/blood AChE inhibition, 119 compounds were included in CAG (1), 101 in each of CAG (2) and CAG (3), and 19 in CAG (4). Potencies were defined on the basis of the NOAELs for the most sensitive indicator of effect from short- or long-term studies. ICs were chosen to derive the RPFs. EFSA recognized that the effects that describe different CAGs may involve targets and MoA that are common to different CAGs. Therefore for example, compounds targeting gamma-aminobutyric acid (GABA) receptors can induce motor and sensory signs of toxicity because of the physiological role of these GABA-ergic neurons. As a consequence many compounds affect all 3 functional divisions of the nervous system and, hence, can be included in CAG (1), (2), and (3). EFSA concluded that considering both the composition of the CAGs and the relative NOAELs, the CRA of each CAG would be covered by performing CRAs with the CAGs for brain and/or erythrocyte AChE inhibition and functional alterations of the motor division.

The uncertainty in the composition of the CAG for functional alterations of the motor division (1) was addressed using the WoE and EKE techniques.[56]

EFSA chose as IC oxamyl based on the robustness of data and the number of endpoints affected in the acute neurotoxicity study.

The acute CRA for this CAG applying the same criteria and methodology used for acute AChE inhibition (see above) resulted in similar conclusions, that there is no exceedance of the threshold for regulatory concern. Triazophos and deltamethrin were the main drivers of the exposure, followed by beta-cypermethrin, omethoate, thiram, chlormequat, and acrinathrin.

The chronic CRA has not yet been performed, but EFSA already indicated emamectin benzoate as IC because the data were robust and the effects were consistently seen across studies and animal species (rat, dog, and mouse).

49.8 Future directions

CRA requires multidisciplinary expertise that needs to integrate and develop new methods and approaches. Sources of information and data on hazard, exposure, and risk to multiple compounds are available in different places, use different metrics and models, and even definitions may be different.[1,32,33,58,59] This situation poses challenges at national and international levels. Research projects and other activities have been and are being conducted to identify data gaps and provide recommendations to further development of CRA, in general, and from exposures deriving from food in particular.[60–62]

49.8.1 Methodological improvements

The possibility of occurrence of synergy and potentiation is considered low based on a few studies that identified modest, if any, evidence for an approximately <fourfold increase in toxicity in studies with mixtures ranging from 2 to 18 chemicals.[6,63] It should be noted that in the studies that suggested some synergy, the doses of the individual components exceeded their respective PoDs or RfPs. Therefore the conclusion on possible synergy at lower (at or below the PoD/RfP) doses was extrapolated but not measured. Hence the conclusion is not firm.[32] In addition, in mixture studies the application of statistical and other mathematical methods is not simple because the dose-response curves of the individual compounds may not be parallel which complicates the mathematical elaboration and increases the uncertainty of the conclusions.[29]

Another issue to consider relates to the assessment of data-poor compounds. For instance, at the screening level, the TTC approach is being explored in conjunction with the default assumption of dose additivity, as a means to prioritize or even conclude the assessment of compounds or mixtures.[6,31,64]

Other non-animal methods may also help in defining CAGs. For instance, structural similarity between two or more chemical substances may indicate the inclusion in a CAG by using expert judgment, read-across, and/or the help of in silico approaches and software, in particular when there are data-rich members of a CAG ([23,65]; EChA at https://echa.europa.eu/support/registration/how-to-avoid-unnecessary-testing-on-animals/grouping-of-substances-and-read-across[66];)

More consistent integration of TK data with TD data should be developed to better identify compounds to be grouped or to be included in existing CAGs.[23,67,68] In addition, information on TK could also improve the CRA by refining potency estimation and RPFs.[69,70] To this end, not only in vitro/in vivo data can be used, but software has been and is being, developed to predict the likelihood that a particular reaction takes place for a specific chemical.[69,71] These are more advanced in the pharmaceutical industry but for the chemical space relevant to food and feed safety, such as biocides, pesticides, additives, and contaminants, more work needs to be done.

Linked to TK information are the biomonitoring data that might help in identifying the likelihood and extent of co-exposures if appropriately linked to monitoring data in a given population (see below).

Progress in mechanistic understanding of toxicological effects will allow more informed decisions in grouping substances for CRA. Especially, the development of more quantitative AOPs[72–74] will resolve some or most of the uncertainties related to groupings and, possibly, reconcile the two contrasting approaches taken by EPA and EFSA.

Probabilistic exposure assessment methodologies and guidance for aggregate exposure assessment methodologies for single and multiple chemicals need to be developed and implemented. This is in conjunction with the development and accessibility of databases for exposure assessment that would include production, use, and occurrence in different media. In addition, data should be structured in harmonized templates so that international cooperation will be facilitated (see below).

Given the fact that there can likely be a high number of chemicals, sources, and routes of exposure to be considered, prioritization methods need to be further developed to be applied to make the best use of resources. Criteria for prioritization can be exposure-driven or risk-based. Exposure-driven approaches allow for assessment of co-exposure even in the absence of toxicological information and, based on the probability or extent of exposure, the need for CRA can be prioritized or even discounted. Risk-based criteria make use of both hazard information and exposure estimation to identify the most relevant co-exposures for a given population.[75] A methodology based on sparse non-negative matrix underapproximation has been proposed by Crepet et al.[76] and applied to different populations.[76–79] This methodology is based on the identification of a CAG at any level of refinement followed by the calculation of the exposure for each pesticide belonging to the selected CAG. Each substance concentration will be normalized using the respective RPF. Then the statistical method is applied to determine the components of the main mixtures to which the studied population is exposed. This may reduce the number of compounds for which to conduct the CRA and eventually refine the assessment which is always a resource-consuming exercise. Other approaches have also been used.[75]

In addition, further work is needed to take into account the fact that the real exposure of humans to various chemical substances occurs via different routes, simultaneously or in sequence, and from different sources. EPA is already assessing aggregate exposure to pesticides, and thoughts should be given to how to consistently apply this approach to other chemical classes and in other parts of the world.

49.8.2 International harmonization

There are substantial differences in both the legal requirements for CRA, in food and in general, and the methodologies for carrying it out between countries and even across regulatory sectors in the same country.[1] Effort needs to be consistently put towards harmonization of the CRA which has been identified as a priority since as a result of these differences there might be different levels of standard settings which in turn could affect international trade. In this respect, a recent Expert consultation convened by WHO under the auspices of the Horizon 2020 project Euromix indicated in the area of food a relevant role in international harmonization can be played by the FAO/WHO Joint Meeting on Pesticide Residue (JMPR) and Joint Expert Committee on Food Additives (JECFA), which deals with food additives, contaminants, and residues of veterinary drugs, ([3] available at https://www.who.int/foodsafety/areas_work/chemical-risks/Euromix_Report.pdf). The report provided a set of recommendations with actions to take to identify needs and means to develop an approach that can be adopted by JECFA and JMPR. In fact, since WHO with FAO and through the Codex Alimentarius, is responsible for setting international norms and standards that regulate the international trade of food, an internationally harmonized approach would be essential. It has been recommended that suitable tools and any associated computational facilities for probabilistic modeling of combined exposures to multiple chemicals should be made available to JECFA/JMPR experts.

The report of the WHO Expert consultation indicates a pragmatic approach to focusing on relevant compounds and exposures. The proposal is based on the assessment of the estimated dietary exposure for a single compound: the compounds will be considered for CRA if the estimated exposure is higher than 10 percent of the relevant health-based guidance value (such as ADI and ARfD) or, if not available, the calculated MoE is less than 10 fold of the MoE considered adequate for that a compound. These values should be reviewed following a foreseen pilot test by JECFA and JMPR. A similar approach is used by EPA although precise values are not given. Also in this case international harmonization should be pursued.

References

1. Rotter S, Beronius A, Boobis AR, et al. Overview on legislation and scientific approaches for risk assessment of combined exposure to multiple chemicals: the potential EuroMix contribution. *Crit Rev Toxicol.* 2018;48(9):796–814. Available from: https://doi.org/10.1080/10408444.2018.1541964.
2. FQPA (Food Quality Protection Act). *US Public Law 104–170, Aug. 3, 110 STAT.* 1996. *1489–1538.* <https://www.epa.gov/laws-regulations/summary-food-quality-protection-act> Accessed 17.08.21.
3. WHO (World Health Organization). *Exposure Assessment for Chemicals in Food, Report of the FAO/WHO Workshop, Annapolis, Maryland, USA, 2–6 May 2005.* <https://apps.who.int/iris/handle/10665/44027>. 2008. Accessed 17.08.21.
4. European Union. *Regulation (EC) No. 396/2005 of the European Parliament and of the Council of 23 February 2005 on maximum residue levels of pesticides in or on food and feed of plant and animal origin and amending Council Directive 91/414/EEC (OJ L 70, 16.3.2005, p. 1).* <https://eur-lex.europa.eu/legal-content/EN/ALL/?uri = celex%3A32005R0396>. 2005. Accessed 17.08.21.
5. EPA (Environmental Protection Agency). *Guidance on Cumulative Risk Assessment of Pesticide Chemicals that have a Common Mechanism of Toxicity.* <https://www.epa.gov/pesticide-science-and-assessing-pesticide-risks/guidance-cumulative-risk-assessment-pesticide>. 2002. Accessed 02.10.21.
6. Boobis A, Budinsky R, Collie S, et al. Critical analysis of literature on low-dose synergy for use in screening chemical mixtures for risk assessment. *Crit Rev Toxicol.* 2011;41(5):369–383. Available from: https://doi.org/10.3109/10408444.2010.543655.
7. Kortenkamp A, Backhaus T, Faust M. *State of the Art Report on Mixture Toxicity.* Report 391. <http://ec.europa.eu/environment/chemicals/effects/pdf/report_mixture_toxicity.pdf>. 2009. Accessed 02.10.21.
8. OECD (Organisation for Economic Co-operation and Development). *Guidance on Grouping of Chemicals, Second Edition*, Paris, OECD Publishing; 2017. OECD Series on Testing and Assessment, No. 194. <https://www.oecd.org/publications/guidance-on-grouping-of-chemicals-second-edition-9789264274679-en.htm>. 2017. Accessed 02.10.21.
9. Feron VJ, Groten JP. Toxicological evaluation of chemical mixtures. *Food Chem Toxicol.* 2002;40:825–839.
10. Wilkinson CF, Christoph GR, Julien E, et al. Assessing the risk of exposures to multiple chemicals with a common mechanism of toxicity: how to cumulate? *Regul Toxicol Pharmacol.* 2000;31:31–43.
11. Martin O, Scholze M, Ermler S, et al. Ten years of research on synergisms and antagonisms in chemical mixtures: A systematic

review and quantitative reappraisal of mixture studies. *Environ Int.* 2021;146:106206. Available from: https://doi.org/10.1016/j.envint.2020.106206.

12. ECHA (European Chemicals Agency). Guidance on the Biocidal Products Regulation. Volume IV Environment – Assessment and Evaluation (Parts B + C) Version 2.0 October 2017. <https://echa.europa.eu/documents/10162/23036412/bpr_guidance_ra_vol_iv_-part_bc_en.pdf/e2622aea-0b93-493f-85a3-f9cb42be16ae>. 2017. Accessed 19.08.21.
13. EPA (Environmental Protection Agency). *Guidance For Identifying Pesticide Chemicals and Other Substances that have a Common Mechanism of Toxicity.* <https://www.epa.gov/pesticide-science-and-assessing-pesticide-risks/guidance-identifying-pesticide-chemicals-and-other>. 1999. Accessed 25.07.21.
14. EPA (Environmental Protection Agency). *The Grouping of a Series of Triazine Pesticides Based on a Common Mechanism of Toxicity.* <https://www.regulations.gov/document/EPA-HQ-OPP-2005-0481-0011>. 2002. Accessed 07.08.21.
15. EPA (Environmental Protection Agency). *Pesticide Cumulative Risk Assessment Framework Final.* <https://www.regulations.gov/document/EPA-HQ-OPP-2015-0422-0019>. 2016. Accessed 17.09.21.
16. Boobis AR, Doe JE, Heinrich-Hirsch B, et al. IPCS framework for analyzing the relevance of a noncancer mode of action for humans. *Crit Rev Toxicol.* 2008;38:87–96.
17. EPA (Environmental Protection Agency). *Guidelines for carcinogen risk assessment.* Risk Assessment Forum, Washington, DC; <https://www.epa.gov/risk/guidelines-carcinogen-risk-assessment> 2005. Accessed 05.10.21.
18. Meek ME, Boobis A, Cote I, et al. New developments in the evolution and application of the WHO/IPCS framework on mode of action/species concordance analysis. *J Appl Toxicol.* 2014;34:1–18.
19. Seed J, Carney EW, Corley RA, et al. Overview: using mode of action and life stage information to evaluate the human relevance of animal toxicity data. *Crit Rev Toxicol.* 2005;35(8 – 9): 664–672.
20. Sonich-Mullin C, Fielder R, Wiltse J, et al. IPCS conceptual framework for evaluating a mode of action for chemical carcinogenesis. *Regul Toxicol Pharmacol.* 2001;34:146–152.
21. EPA (Environmental Protection Agency). *Triazine Cumulative Risk Assessment.* <https://www.regulations.gov/document/EPA-HQ-OPP-2005-0481-0003>. 2006. Accessed 1709.21.
22. EFSA (European Food Safety Authority). Opinion of the Scientific Panel on Plant Protection products and their Residues to evaluate the suitability of existing methodologies and, if appropriate, the identification of new approaches to assess cumulative and synergistic risks from pesticides to human health with a view to set MRLs for those pesticides in the frame of Regulation (EC) 396/2005. *EFSA J.* 2008;704:1–84. Available from: http://www.efsa.europa.eu/en/efsajournal/pub/705.htm.
23. EFSA Scientific Committee, More SJ, Bampidis V, et al. Guidance on harmonised methodologies for human health, animal health and ecological risk assessment of combined exposure to multiple chemicals. *EFSA J.* 2019;17(3):5634. Available from: https://doi.org/10.2903/j.efsa.2019.5634. 77 pp.
24. RIVM, ICPS, ANSES. Toxicological data analysis to support grouping of pesticide active substances for cumulative risk assessment of effects on liver, on the nervous system and on reproduction and development. *EFSA Suppor Public.* 2013;10(1):EN-392. Available from: https://doi.org/10.2903/sp.efsa.2013.en-392. Published 2013. Accessed August 17, 2021.
25. RIVM, ICPS, ANSES. Toxicological data collection and analysis to support grouping of pesticide active substances for cumulative risk assessment of effects on the nervous system, liver, adrenal, eye, reproduction and development and thyroid system. EFSA Suppor Public;13(2):EN-999, 184 pp. https://doi.org/10.2903/sp.efsa.2016.EN-999. 2016. Accessed 17.08.21.
26. Van den Berg M, Birnbaum LS, Denison M, et al. The 2005 World Health Organization reevaluation of human and mammalian toxic equivalency factors for dioxins and dioxin-like compounds. *Toxicol Sci.* 2006;93:223–241.
27. EPA (Environmental Protection Agency). *Framework for Cumulative Risk Assessment.* <https://www.epa.gov/sites/default/files/2014-11/documents/frmwrk_cum_risk_assmnt.pdf>. 2003. Accessed 04.10.21.
28. EFSA (European Food Safety Authority), Crivellente F, Hart A, et al. Scientific report on the establishment of cumulative assessment groups of pesticides for their effects on the thyroid. *EFSA J.* 2019;17(9):5801. Available from: https://doi.org/10.2903/j.efsa.2019.5801. 50 pp.
29. Slob W, Setzer RW. *Shape and steepness of toxicological dose–response relationships of continuous endpoints. Crit Rev Toxicol.* 44. 2014270–297.
30. EFSA. International framework dealing with human risk assessment of combined exposure to multiple chemicals (European Food Safety Authority)*EFSA J.* 2013;11(7):3313. Available from: https://doi.org/10.2903/j.efsa.2013.3313.
31. EFSA (European Food Safety Authority). EFSA scientific colloquium 24 –'omics in risk assessment: state of the art and next. *EFSA Support Public.* 2018;EN-1512. Available from: https://doi.org/10.2903/sp.efsa.2018.EN-1512.
32. Tralau T, Oelgeschläger M, Kugler J, et al. A prospective whole-mixture approach to assess risk of the food and chemical exposome. *Nat Food.* 2021;2:463–468. Available from: https://doi.org/10.1038/s43016-021-00316-7.
33. Bopp SK, Kienzler A, Richarz AN, et al. Regulatory assessment and risk management of chemical mixtures: challenges and ways forward. *Crit Rev Toxicol.* 2019;49(2):174–189. Available from: https://doi.org/10.1080/10408444.2019.1579169.
34. EFSA Panel on Plant Protection Products and their Residues (PPR). Guidance on the use of probabilistic methodology for modelling dietary exposure to pesticide residues. *EFSA J.* 2012;10(10):2839. Available from: https://doi.org/10.2903/j.efsa.2012.2839 [95 pp.].
35. EFSA (European Food Safety Authority), Dujardin B, Bocca V. Scientific report on the cumulative dietary exposure assessment of pesticides that have chronic effects on the thyroid using SAS® software. *EFSA J.* 2019;17(9):5763. Available from: https://doi.org/10.2903/j.efsa.2019.5763. 49 pp.
36. EPA (Environmental Protection Agency). *Organophosphorus Cumulative Risk Assessment.* <https://www.regulations.gov/document/EPA-HQ-OPP-2006-0618-0002>. 2006 (update). Accessed 16.09.21.
37. EPA (Environmental Protection Agency). *Revised N-methyl Carbamate Cumulative Risk.* <https://www.regulations.gov/document/EPA-HQ-OPP-2008-0347-0029>. 2007. Accessed 17.09.21.
38. EFSA (European Food Safety Authority), Craig PS, Dujardin B, et al. Scientific report on cumulative dietary risk characterisation

of pesticides that have acute effects on the nervous system. *EFSA J.* 2020;18(4):6087. Available from: https://doi.org/10.2903/j.efsa.2020.6087. 79 pp.
39. EFSA (European Food Safety Authority), Anastassiadou M, Choi J, et al. Scientific report on the cumulative dietary risk assessment of chronic acetylcholinesterase inhibition by residues of pesticides. *EFSA J.* 2021;19(2):6392. Available from: https://doi.org/10.2903/j.efsa.2021.6392. 151 pp.
40. EFSA (European Food Safety Authority), Crivellente F, Hart A, et al. Scientific report on the establishment of cumulative assessment groups of pesticides for their effects on the nervous system. *EFSA J.* 2019;17(9):5800. Available from: https://doi.org/10.2903/j.efsa.2019.5800. 115 pp.
41. EPA. *Chlorotriazines: Cumulative Risk Assessment - Atrazine, Propazine, and Simazine.* <https://downloads.regulations.gov/EPA-HQ-OPP-2013-0266-1160/content.pdf>. 2018. Accessed 02.10.21.
42. EPA (Environmental Protection Agency). *Pyrethrins/Pyrethroid Cumulative Risk Assessment.* <https://www.regulations.gov/docket/EPA-HQ-OPP-2011-0746/document>. 2011. Accessed 17.10.21.
43. Ray DE, Moretto A. Organochlorine and pyrethroid insecticides. In: McQueen C, ed. *Comprehensive Toxicology.* vol. 6–15. Elsevier; 2018:242–258.
44. Wolansky MJ, Harrill JA. Neurobehavioral toxicology of pyrethroid insecticides in adult animals: a critical review. *Neurotoxicol Teratol.* 2008;30:55–78.
45. Choi JS, Soderlund DM. Structure-activity relationships for the action of 11 pyrethroid insecticides on rat Na v 1.8 sodium channels expressed in Xenopus oocytes. *Toxicol Appl Pharmacol.* 2006;211(3):233–244. Available from: https://doi.org/10.1016/j.taap.2005.06.022. 15.
46. Weiner ML, Nemec M, Sheets L, et al. Comparative functional observational battery study of twelve commercial pyrethroid insecticides in male rats following acute oral exposure. *Neurotoxicology.* 2009;30(SUPPL):S1–S16.
47. He F, Wang S, Liu L, et al. Clinical manifestations and diagnosis of acute pyrethroid poisoning. *Arch Toxicol.* 1989;63:54–58.
48. Joy RM, Albertson TE, Ray DE. Type I and type II pyrethroids increase inhibition in the hippocampal dentate gyrus of the rat. *Toxicol Appl Pharmacol.* 1989;98:398–412.
49. Ray DE, Fry JR. A reassessment of the neurotoxicity of pyrethroid insecticides. *Pharmacol Ther.* 2006;111:174–193.
50. EPA (Environmental Protection Agency). *Common Mechanism Grouping for the Pyrethrins and Synthetic Pyrethroids.* <https://www.regulations.gov/document/EPA-HQ-OPP-2011-0746-0045>. 2013. Accessed 05.10.21.
51. Herberth MF. An oral (gavage) acute neurotoxicity comparison study in rats. WIL Research Laboratories, LLC. Laboratory report WIL-118041, December 20, 2010. MRID 48333801 (unpublished, as quoted by EPA, 2011).
52. Wolansky M, Gennings C, Crofton K. Relative potencies for acute effects of pyrethroids on motor function in rats. *Toxicol Sci.* 2006;89(1):271–277.
53. EPA (Environmental Protection Agency). *Cumulative risk from chloroacetanilide pesticides.* <https://www.regulations.gov/document/EPA-HQ-OPP-2006-0202-0002>. 2006. Accessed 17.09.21.
54. EFSA (European Food Safety Authority), Craig PS, Dujardin B, et al. Scientific report on the cumulative dietary risk characterisation of pesticides that have chronic effects on the thyroid. *EFSA J.* 2020;18(4):6088. Available from: https://doi.org/10.2903/j.efsa.2020.6088. 71 pp.
55. EFSA Panel on Plant Protection Products and their Residues (PPR). Scientific opinion on the identification of pesticides to be included in cumulative assessment groups on the basis of their toxicological profile. *EFSA J.* 2013;11(7):3293. Available from: https://doi.org/10.2903/j.efsa.2013.3293 (updated 2014).
56. EFSA. Guidance on expert knowledge elicitation in food and feed safety risk assessment (European Food Safety Authority)*EFSA J.* 2014;12(6):3734. Available from: https://doi.org/10.2903/j.efsa.2014.3734.
57. Van Klaveren JD, Kruisselbrink, de Boer WJ, et al. Cumulative dietary exposure assessment of pesticides that have chronic effects on the thyroid using MCRA software. *EFSA Suppor Public.* 2019; EN-1707. Available from: https://doi.org/10.2903/sp.efsa.2019.en-1707. Published 2019. Accessed August 17, 2021.
58. Evans RM, Martin OV, Faust M, et al. Should the scope of human mixture risk assessment span legislative/regulatory silos for chemicals? *Sci Total Environ.* 2016;543(Part A):757–764. Available from: https://doi.org/10.1016/j.scitotenv.2015.10.162.
59. Fischer BC, Rotter S, Schubert J, et al. Recommendations for international harmonisation, implementation and further development of suitable scientific approaches regarding the assessment of mixture effects. *Food Chem Toxicol.* 2020;141:111388. Available from: https://doi.org/10.1016/j.fct.2020.111388.
60. Bopp SK, Barouki R, Brack W, et al. Current EU research activities on combined exposure to multiple chemicals. *Environ Int.* 2018;120:544–562. Available from: https://doi.org/10.1016/j.envint.2018.07.037.
61. Kienzler A, Bopp SK, van der Linden S, et al. Regulatory assessment of chemical mixtures: requirements, current approaches and future perspectives. *Regul Toxicol Pharmacol.* 2016;80:321–334.
62. Price PS, Jarabek AM, Burgoon LD. Organizing mechanism-related information on chemical interactions using a framework based on the aggregate exposure and adverse outcome pathways. *Environ Int.* 2020;138:105673. Available from: https://doi.org/10.1016/j.envint.2020.105673.
63. Zoupa M, Zwart EP, Gremmer ER, et al. Dose addition in chemical mixtures inducing craniofacial malformations in zebrafish (Danio rerio) embryos. *Food Chem Toxicol.* 2020;137:111117. Available from: https://doi.org/10.1016/j.fct.2020.111117.
64. Price PS, Hollnagel HM, Zabik JM. Characterizing the noncancer toxicity of mixtures using concepts from the TTC and quantitative models of uncertainty in mixture toxicity. *Risk Anal.* 2009;29:1534–1548.
65. Helman G, Shah I, Williams AJ, et al. Generalized read-across (GenRA): a workflow implemented into the EPA CompTox chemicals dashboard. *ALTEX.* 2019;36(3):462–465. Available from: https://doi.org/10.14573/altex.1811292.
66. Williams AJ, Lambert JC, Thayer K, et al. Sourcing data on chemical properties and hazard data from the US-EPA CompTox chemicals dashboard: a practical guide for human risk assessment. *Environ Int.* 2021;154:106566. Available from: https://doi.org/10.1016/j.envint.2021.106566.
67. Beronius A, Zilliacus J, Hanberg A, et al. Methodology for health risk assessment of combined exposures to multiple chemicals. *Food Chem Toxicol.* 2020;143:111520. Available from: https://doi.org/10.1016/j.fct.2020.111520.
68. Braeuning A, Marx-Stoelting P. Mixture prioritization and testing: the importance of toxicokinetics. *Arch Toxicol.* 2021;95

(5):1863–1864. Available from: https://doi.org/10.1007/s00204-021-03026-y.

69. van der Voet H, Kruisselbrink JW, de Boer WJ, et al. The MCRA toolbox of models and data to support chemical mixture risk assessment. *Food Chem Toxicol.* 2020;138:111–185. Available from: https://doi.org/10.1016/j.fct.2020.111185.
70. Yang C, Cronin MTD, Arvidson KB, et al. COSMOS next generation – a public knowledge base leveraging chemical and biological data to support the regulatory assessment of chemicals. *Comput Toxicol.* 2021;19:100175. Available from: https://doi.org/10.1016/j.comtox.2021.100175.
71. Cheng S, Bois FY. A mechanistic modeling framework for predicting metabolic interactions in complex mixtures. *Environ Health Perspect.* 2011;119:1712–1718.
72. Perkins EJ, Ashauer R, Burgoon L, et al. Building and applying quantitative adverse outcome pathway models for chemical hazard and risk assessment. *Environ Toxicol Chem.* 2019;38(9):1850–1865. Available from: https://doi.org/10.1002/etc.4505.
73. Spinu N, Cronin MTD, Enoch SJ, et al. Quantitative adverse outcome pathway (qAOP) models for toxicity prediction. *Arch Toxicol.* 2020;94(5):1497–1510. Available from: https://doi.org/10.1007/s00204-020-02774-7.
74. Vinken M, Benfenati E, Busquet F, et al. Safer chemicals using less animals: kick-off of the European ONTOX project. *Toxicology.* 2021;30:458. Available from: https://doi.org/10.1016/j.tox.2021.152846. 152846.
75. Lee WC, Fisher M, Davis K, et al. Identification of chemical mixtures to which Canadian pregnant women are exposed: the MIREC study. *Environ Int.* 2017;99:321–330. Available from: https://doi.org/10.1016/j.envint.2016.12.015.
76. Crepet A, Tressou J, Graillot V, et al. Identification of the main pesticide residue mixtures to which the French population is exposed. *Environ Res.* 2013;126:125–133.
77. Mancini FR, Frenoy P, Fiolet T, et al. Identification of chemical mixtures to which women are exposed through the diet: results from the French E3N cohort. *Environ Int.* 2021;152:106467. Available from: https://doi.org/10.1016/j.envint.2021.106467.
78. Traoré T, Béchaux C, Sirot V, et al. To which chemical mixtures is the French population exposed? Mixture identification from the second French total diet study. *Food Chem Toxicol.* 2016;98(Pt B):179–188. Available from: https://doi.org/10.1016/j.fct.2016.10.028.
79. Traoré T, Forhan A, Sirot V, et al. To which mixtures are French pregnant women mainly exposed? A combination of the second French total diet study with the EDEN and ELFE cohort studies. *Food Chem Toxicol.* 2018;111:310–328. Available from: https://doi.org/10.1016/j.fct.2017.11.016.

Section IX

Current and emerging advances in food safety evaluation: pathogenic microorganisms including prions

Chapter 50

Prions: detection of bovine spongiform encephalopathy and links to variant Creutzfeldt–Jakob disease

Timm Konold[1], **Mark Arnold**[2] **and Amie Adkin**[3]

[1]*Department of Pathology and Animal Sciences, APHA Weybridge, Addlestone, United Kingdom,* [2]*Department of Epidemiological Sciences, APHA Weybridge, Addlestone, United Kingdom,* [3]*Risk Assessment Unit, Food Standards Agency, London, United Kingdom*

Abstract

Bovine spongiform encephalopathy (BSE) is a naturally occurring prion disease that was first discovered in Great Britain and has since been detected in many other countries. Epidemiological studies soon established that it was a foodborne disease caused by feeding of contaminated meat and bone meal, although the source of the agent remains unresolved to this day. The BSE agent is transmissible to various other species and is the cause of variant Creutzfeldt–Jakob disease (vCJD) in humans. Risk assessments were imperative to control the epidemic, and legislative measures were introduced to protect animal and human health. The decline of the number of BSE and vCJD cases has led to calls to review and relax some of these measures. New challenges are the more recent discoveries of novel or existing prion diseases with different phenotypes. Research into the origin of BSE, tissue distribution, and persistence in the environment should continue.

Keywords: Bovine spongiform encephalopathy; variant Creutzfeldt–Jakob disease; prion; transmission studies; risk assessment; disease prevention

50.1 Discovery of bovine spongiform encephalopathy in cattle

When in 1987 an article appeared in the British journal *The Veterinary Record* to describe a novel progressive spongiform encephalopathy in 10 cattle[1] nobody could have foreseen the consequences it would have worldwide in subsequent years, with more than 180,000 cattle affected in the United Kingdom alone and more than 5000 cattle in other countries.[2] The disease reported by British veterinarians from the then Central Veterinary Laboratory and the Ministry of Agriculture, Fisheries and Food was characterized by bilateral symmetrical vacuolation of neuropil and neurones in the gray matter of the brainstem and presence of fibrils visualized by electron microscopy. This bovine spongiform encephalopathy (BSE) resembled a disease in sheep and goats that was known in the country for centuries: scrapie, a transmissible spongiform encephalopathy (TSE) with similar vacuolar changes and scrapie-associated fibrils in the brain. Other known naturally occurring diseases were chronic wasting disease (CWD) in captive mule deer and rocky mountain elk, transmissible mink encephalopathy, and human encephalopathies, such as Kuru and Creutzfeldt–Jakob disease (CJD). The disease produced neurological signs in adult cattle and first signs associated with this disease were observed in a cow in April 1985. Affected cattle would become apprehensive and fearful, hyperesthetic to external stimuli, and developed incoordination, which eventually resulted in recumbency (Fig. 50.1).

The disease reached epidemic proportions in Great Britain: by 1990 the disease had already affected more than 17,000 cattle and the most frequent clinical signs were apprehension, hyperesthesia, and ataxia, with at least one of these signs present in 97% of cases.[3] It was suggested that a combination of these signs and loss of body weight or condition should trigger suspicion of BSE. The rapid increase in cases since its first report in 1987 led to an epidemiological investigation of its cause, which was not associated with the use of veterinary pharmaceuticals or agricultural chemicals, such as herbicides or pesticides, but the distribution of cases, onset of disease, and greater incidence in dairy cattle suggested a foodborne origin instead. The risk of exposure was 30 times more likely in calves compared to adults, exposure commenced in the winter 1981/82 and incubation periods ranged from 2.5 to

Present Knowledge in Food Safety. DOI: https://doi.org/10.1016/B978-0-12-819470-6.00042-1

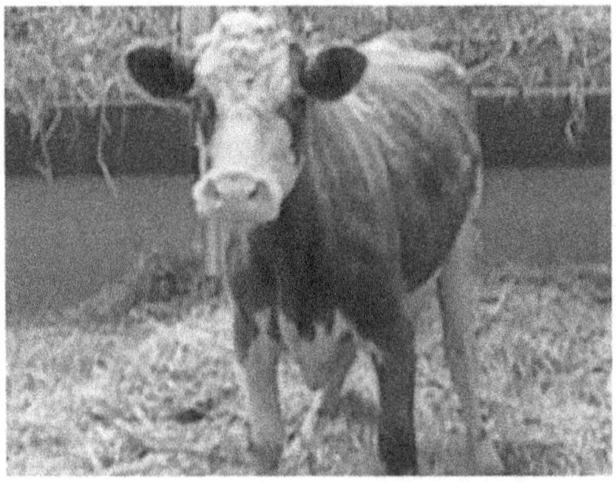

FIGURE 50.1 Natural case of BSE with rigid, wide-based stance and high head carriage suggestive of increased alertness. The visible rib cage is also evidence of a poorer body condition.

at least eight years. The occurrence of cases was linked to the consumption of concentrate rations containing meat and bone meal (MBM) and changes in the production of MBM during the 1970s and 1980s. A dramatic increase in the sheep population, increased inclusion of material from casualty and condemned sheep to produce MBM, lower rendering temperatures, and the discontinued practice of fat extraction in the rendering process were all considered factors to expose cattle to a TSE agent pathogenic for cattle via cattle feedstuffs.[4] It remains unknown to this day which agent was responsible for the epidemic. It is now commonly accepted that TSEs are caused by misfolding of a naturally occurring protein in mammals, the cellular prion protein PrP^C, which by misfolding changes its conformation from an α-helix to a β-sheet and thereby becomes resistant to proteolytic digestion,[5] increasingly accumulates in the brain (PrP^d or PrP^{Sc}) and is associated with disease. Different protein conformations may explain the strain phenomenon but the origin of the BSE strain remains unresolved. It may be a selection of a scrapie strain or strains that either remained unchanged or changed during recycling in cattle to become pathogenic for cattle, a spontaneous genetic mutation within the prion protein gene in cattle and subsequent recycling in cattle, or a TSE agent originating from another, possibly exotic species that was incorporated in MBM.[6] Although it has been shown that classical scrapie is transmissible to cattle by the intracerebral route, the disease does not resemble BSE,[7–11] and it did not appear to be transmissible by the oral route.[12,13]

Whilst BSE was initially considered a British problem, it was soon discovered in other countries, such as Northern Ireland[14] and Switzerland,[15] with single cases in other countries linked to the import of cattle from Great Britain[16–18] or feedstuffs from the United Kingdom. In 2001 the European Union (EU) introduced active monitoring for BSE in adult healthy slaughter cattle and fallen stock, which detected indigenous BSE cases in countries, where BSE had previously only been found in imported cattle, for example Italy[19] or Germany.[20] It turned out that reliance on reporting of clinical suspects alone, which formed the basis of BSE surveillance in most countries at the time, was too unreliable to estimate BSE prevalence in a country.[21]

50.2 Discovery of variant Creutzfeldt–Jakob disease and link to BSE

When BSE was first discovered and compared with scrapie in sheep, it was not expected that the disease in cattle was transmissible to humans because scrapie in sheep and goats or any animal TSE known at the time had never been associated with human cases of TSEs. The most common human TSE, CJD, was first described in the 1920s and exists as familial (genetic), iatrogenic, and sporadic CJD. Sporadic CJD is found worldwide and usually affects 1 per million people, with 80% between 50 and 70 years of age.[22] It occurs even in Australia, which is considered free from the endemic form of scrapie. Indeed, a working party to examine and advise on the implications of BSE in relation to both animal health and any possible human health risks led by Sir Richard Southwood concluded in February 1989 that "the risk of transmission of BSE to humans appears remote and it is therefore most unlikely that BSE will have any implications for human health. It points out that the related disease scrapie in sheep has been present in the UK for over 200 years and there has been no evidence of transmission to man." However, it was acknowledged that "if their assessment proves incorrect the implications would be serious." [23] A case-control study of risk factors of CJD in Europe published later in 1998 found little evidence for an association between the risk of CJD and either animal exposure or consumption of processed bovine meat or milk products for the period 1993–95.[24] In May 1990 John Gummer, the British Minister of Agriculture, Fisheries and Food, was shown on television eating a hamburger to assure the public that British beef was safe to eat. At around the same time, surveillance for CJD in the United Kingdom was reinstituted to identify patterns in CJD that may be linked to BSE. In 1996, 10 cases of CJD with a clinical onset between 1994 and 1995 were reported, which were considered unusual in terms of neuropathology and the relative young age of onset (under 45 years of age) compared to sporadic CJD. The disease was termed variant CJD (vCJD) and although the authors suggested that exposure to BSE was the most likely explanation for this new disease, it needed to be proven by animal transmission studies and continued epidemiological vigilance.[25] Cases of vCJD were also reported in continental Europe.[26] Evidence that supported the hypothesis that BSE was the origin of vCJD soon started to arrive: prion glycoform profiles obtained by Western blots of proteinase K-treated brain homogenates were similar in wild-type mice, cats, and macaques infected with the BSE agent and vCJD patients and distinct from sporadic CJD.[27] Transmission of BSE in cattle to wild-type mice showed the same disease phenotype as vCJD, which was distinct from scrapie in sheep and sporadic CJD.[28] In transgenic mice expressing only human prion protein, BSE and vCJD showed similarities with regards to incubation period, clinical signs, and brain pathology, which were different to other human TSEs transmitted to these mice.[29] BSE transmission to macaques resulted in disease with clinical, molecular, and neuropathological features that were similar to vCJD.[30] BSE is now widely regarded as an animal prion disease that is zoonotic, and the most likely route of infection is dietary exposure although iatrogenic infection may account for some of the cases such as blood transfusion.[31] Whilst the first predictions of a vCJD epidemic fortunately proved to be untrue they have nevertheless been 178 cases of vCJD in the United Kingdom up to May 2, 2022.[32] The possible presence of subclinical carriers is, however, a problem and one of the reasons why continued human surveillance is still important.[33]

50.3 Studies to determine infectivity in bovine tissues from BSE-affected cattle

After the discovery of BSE in Great Britain studies about the pathogenesis were soon commissioned where cattle were orally inoculated with a brainstem pool from naturally infected cattle and tissues harvested throughout the incubation period. Tissues were then inoculated into wild-type mice to determine which transmitted the BSE agent. After the link between BSE and vCJD had been demonstrated it became even more important to establish which tissues harbor infectivity to safeguard public health by removing and disposing of this specified risk material (SRM). These studies established that the BSE prion was mainly confined to the central nervous system: prions and infectivity were present in brain, spinal cord, dorsal root ganglia, trigeminal ganglia but also in distal ileum, presumably the entry point of prions before migrating to the central nervous system.[34,35] Infectivity was, however, also detected in 6 of 16 mice inoculated with bone marrow from cattle culled 38 months post inoculation (mpi) although not from cattle culled 40 mpi.[36] It soon became evident that wild-type mice were not as susceptible to BSE as cattle and consequently groups of five cattle were inoculated by the intracerebral route with a range of tissues harvested from the same oral pathogenesis study mentioned above or confirmed BSE field cases. Animals were monitored clinically until the development of clinical signs or study end-point at 7 years post inoculation and examined by postmortem TSE tests. These studies established, in addition to the mouse studies, infectivity in the palatine tonsil taken from orally inoculated cattle at 10 mpi but also pooled nictitating membrane taken from confirmed field cases (one of five cattle succumbed in each group).[37,38] There was no evidence of infectivity in bone marrow collected from cattle at 22, 26, 32, or 36 mpi.[39] A summary of the cattle bioassay study results is given in Table 50.1.

Several pathogenesis studies were carried out subsequently, making use of the development of more sensitive prion detection methods in tissue, such as immunohistochemistry and Western immunoblot to detect disease-associated prion protein, and better mouse models, such as bovine transgenic mice, which carried the bovine prion protein gene and were more sensitive than wild-type mice to test for tissue infectivity. These all came to the same conclusion: the BSE agent enters the body via the small intestine, predominantly the ileum, and then follows the splanchnic (sympathetic) route via the spinal cord and vagal (parasympathetic) route to the brainstem.[40–44] There is no evidence of neuroinvasion via the circumventricular organ, which lacks a blood–brain barrier.[45] Detection of prions by immunohistochemistry in sensory ganglia after detection in brainstem and spinal cord suggests a retrograde transport of the BSE agent that occurs fairly late in the disease stage and is the rationale for the age-dependent removal and disposal of spinal cord at slaughter.[40] Peripheral nervous tissue that had not been previously investigated such as facial, vagal, phrenic, and sciatic nerve was also found to be infectious.[46,47] Low-level infectivity was also reported for semitendinosus muscle from a terminal naturally infected cow with BSE and adrenal gland from orally inoculated, clinically affected cattle, which may be attributable to the innervation of these tissues. By comparing number and PrP immunolabeling in lymphoid follicles between distal ileum (SRM) and jejunum/ duodenum (not SRM) of cattle orally inoculated with BSE brain, it was concluded that infectivity was considerably less in jejunum and duodenum, particularly at low dose exposure, which mimics natural exposure.[48]

Most importantly, there is currently no evidence for infectivity or presence of prions in milk or blood from BSE-affected cattle.[49–52] In one study, addition of labeled PrP^{Sc} aggregates to serum from six BSE cattle at clinical end-stage resulted in fibril formation detectable by flow cytometry, which was not detected in four controls[53] and suggested that PrP in the serum from the BSE cattle acted as seed for fibril formation but it has not been established whether the aggregates were infectious.

TABLE 50.1 Cattle bioassay of tissue or fluid from experimentally challenged and naturally infected cattle.

	Time of death of orally challenged cattle (months post challenge)							Natural infection
Tissue	6 (*N* = 3)	10 (*N* = 3)	18 (*N* = 3)	22 (*N* = 3)	26 (*N* = 1)	32 (*N* = 2)	36 (*N* = 3)	*N* = 10
Caudal medulla/spinal cord pool (C2–3, T10–11, L3–4)	86			86	85	**23 (22–24)**		
Caudal medulla	86	84	88 (87–88)		90 (84–90)			
Spinal cord pool (C2–3, T10–11, L3–4)	86	84 (63–84)	88 (36–88)		90 (83–90)			
Skeletal muscle pool (masseter, semitendinosus, longissimus dorsi)	84		95 (26–98)		88 (80–88)	99		
Sciatic/radial nerves	84 (64–84)		86		89	96 (70–96)		
Parotid/submandibular salivary gland			87		89 (54–89)			
Distal ileum	**27 (25–30)**	**22 (22–23)**	**24 (24–25)**		89 (88–89)	86		
Liver	84		98 (80–98)		89	98		
Spleen	85	84	87		89 (69–89)			
Thymus	86 (67–84)	84						
Tonsil	85 (85–86)	84, **45**[a]	88 (56–88)		90 (86–90)			
Mesenteric lymph node	85 (81–85)		87		89			
Superficial cervical/ popliteal lymph node	84		87		88 (50–88)			
Buffy coat	85		87		89 (77–89)	98 (74–98)		
Bone marrow				91	91 (70–91)	88 (80–91)	90	
Skin			87 (76–87)		89 (81–89)	84		
Kidney	84		98 (93–98)		89 (86–89)	97		
Urine			87 (78–87)					
Nictitating membrane								84 (53–84), **33**[a]

Groups of five were inoculated intracerebrally with material from orally challenged cattle (*N*, number of cattle indicated in the top row) that were culled at predetermined time points or from naturally infected cattle (one group only). Cattle were culled upon display of neurological signs consistent with bovine spongiform encephalopathy (BSE) or due to intercurrent diseases. Times are given as median survival times in months and range in parentheses (if applicable). BSE diagnosis was based on histopathology, immunohistochemistry, Western immunoblot, and rapid test ELISA. Positive results are displayed in bold. Two groups of saline solution-inoculated cattle served as controls with a median survival time of 85 (31–85) and 99 (97–99) months, respectively. For more details on methods refer to previous publications.[37,38]

[a]*Denotes one animal only.*

A list of distribution of prions or infectivity in tissues from BSE-affected cattle was published by the World Health Organization,[54] which separated high infectivity tissues (brain, spinal cord, retina, optic nerve, ganglia) from lower infectivity tissues (some lymphoid tissue and alimentary tract tissue and other tissue shown to produce some infectivity in cattle or moue bioassays) and tissues with no detected infectivity or prions. This list needs to be updated regularly as more sensitive prion detection methods are developed and new research findings published. For example, protein misfolding cyclic amplification (PMCA) mimics in vitro the conversion process from PrP^C to PrP^{Sc} that takes place in vivo by adding substrate containing PrP^C to the test sample and running alternate cycles of incubation and sonication, which will amplify PrP^{Sc} if present in the test sample and make it detectable by TSE post-mortem tests.[55] Whilst the presence of PrP^{Sc} is not necessarily equivalent to infectivity, which is detectable by bioassay, PMCA had a comparable sensitivity to the bioassay in bovine transgenic mice when diluted BSE brain samples were tested. However, it was unable to detect PrP^{Sc} in nasal mucosa and tongue tissue from two clinically affected BSE field cases whereas infectivity was detected by transgenic mouse bioassay.[56] Japanese researchers reported detection of PrP^{Sc} by PMCA in submandibular and parotid glands of orally infected cattle.[49] It is probable that the range of tissues or fluids with detectable prions or infectivity may increase as new research findings are published, even though there is considerable variation in the results in tissues with low level of infectivity and the route of inoculation and dose may also affect the outcome and may represent a worst-case scenario.

50.4 Transmission studies in other species to assess susceptibility and likelihood of occurrence in other species

As epidemiological studies demonstrated that BSE in cattle was a foodborne disease through feeding of contaminated MBM, it was obvious that the risk of disease in other species could not be ignored and transmission studies were soon initiated (summarized in 2008[57]). Indeed, one of the hypotheses of the origin of BSE was that it represented a TSE strain in sheep. In addition, many farm animal species, including fish, were fed MBM prior to the BSE outbreak, which may have also ingested contaminated MBM.[58] TSEs started to occur naturally in other ruminant species kept in zoos, such as nyala (*Tragelaphus angasi*), gemsbok (*Oryx gazelle*), Arabian and Scimitar-horned oryx (*Oryx leucoryx*, *Oryx dammah*), eland (*Taurotragus oryx*), greater kudu (*Tragelaphus strepsiceros*), and American bison (*Bison bison*), which was attributed mainly to the feeding of contaminated MBM but may have been subsequently transmitted vertically or horizontally, which may explain the relatively higher number of affected cases in the greater kudu where infectivity could also be demonstrated in peripheral tissues.[59] Similarly, a TSE was diagnosed in exotic cats held in zoos, such as cheetah (*Acinonyx jubatus*), puma (*Felis concolor*), tiger (*Panthera tigris*), lion (*Panthera leo*), ocelot (*Felis pardalis*), and Asian golden cat (*Catopuma temminckii*),[60] which was most likely introduced by feeding meat from slaughtered cattle with BSE. Domestic cats were first found to be affected by this feline spongiform encephalopathy in 1990[61] and the agent had the same "signature" as the BSE strain in wild-type mice.[62] Cases that occurred outside Great Britain often originated from England but indigenous cases have also been described in countries that had cases of BSE like Switzerland[63] and France.[64]

The successful experimental transmission to sheep and goats was first reported in 1993, and both intracerebral and oral inoculation with BSE brain homogenate from cattle resulted in infection.[65] Multiple studies were carried out subsequently, using either cattle-derived or goat- or sheep-passaged BSE brain homogenate, to investigate the influence of dose, route, breed, and prion protein genotype on susceptibility, incubation period, pathogenesis, PrP^{Sc} tissue distribution, and infectivity.[66–72] The peripheral distribution of PrP^{Sc} in BSE-infected sheep and goats, and particular presence of infectivity in blood,[73] even in subclinical animals, was concerning in terms of food safety if BSE was to be found in the small ruminant population. In addition, studies in human transgenic mice, which are used to mimic susceptibility of humans to TSEs, showed that sheep- and goat-passaged BSE had higher transmission efficiency than cattle-derived BSE and produced the same vCJD phenotype.[74] EU-wide scrapie surveillance of fallen stock and healthy slaughter animals that was introduced to detect BSE in small ruminants has not found evidence for the disease present in sheep,[75] whereas BSE has been found retrospectively in a slaughtered goat in France,[76] and a clinically affected goat in Scotland,[77] which confirmed that the threat of crossing species was real.

Red deer (*Cervus elaphus*), which are the most commonly farmed cervid species in the United Kingdom and were likely to have been exposed to contaminated MBM in proprietary feeds, were susceptible to infection with the BSE agent by the intracerebral[78] and oral route.[79] Incubation period and attack rate were significantly different in parenteral (6/6, 794–1260 days) versus oral infection (1/6, 1740 days). Compared to experimental oral infection of red deer with the CWD agent from elk, PrP^{Sc} was not detected in lymphoid tissue and may suggest a low risk of environmental contamination as seen with BSE in cattle.[79] It is unknown whether lack of peripheral distribution is a consistent finding in BSE-infected red deer because this is also not consistent in natural CWD infection discovered subsequently: PrP^{Sc} may[80] or may not[81] be detectable in lymphoid tissue.

Transmission studies in pigs demonstrated that the BSE agent produced clinical disease if inoculated parenterally, and infectivity was not only found in brain but also in some alimentary tissues.[82] Similar findings were reported for pigs inoculated intracerebrally with sheep-adapted BSE where infectivity was found in a range of lymphoid tissue, nerves, and muscle.[83] By contrast, feeding three doses of BSE-infected brain in amounts equivalent to the maximum daily intake of MBM used in commercial pig rations at that time did not produce evidence of infection,[82] which indicated a considerable species barrier. Pathological examinations of pig brains taken during the BSE epidemic revealed the presence of vacuolar changes predominantly in the rostral colliculus, which were strikingly similar to the neuropil vacuolation seen in TSEs. The presence of a TSE, however, could not be substantiated when pigs were inoculated parenterally with these brains and monitored for disease.[84]

Intracerebral and oral inoculation of chickens with BSE brainstem homogenate failed to produce a TSE: no PrP^{Sc} was detected by immunohistochemistry, and infectivity studies in mice and subsequent passage in further chickens gave negative results.[85]

In the only study so far documented in fish, gilthead sea breams were orally challenged with BSE brain homogenates, and whilst they did not show clinical disease there were signs of neurodegeneration and plaque-like protein aggregates in the brain, particularly in the cerebellum, with a pattern similarly seen in mammalian TSEs although no vacuolation was observed.[86] It remained unclear whether this novel fish amyloidosis was a prion disease and no further results from transmission studies in bovine transgenic mice have been reported. In 2013 the EU relaxed the feeding ban on processed animal protein (PAP) to farmed animals, which had been in place since 2001, and allowed the inclusion of PAP from nonruminants in aquatic feed, provided that it is derived entirely from Category 3 material (i.e., material approved for human consumption at the point of slaughter) that has been specially treated to render it suitable for direct use as feed material or for any other use in feedstuffs. In August 2021, the European Union re-authorized the use of PAP from nonruminants in pig and poultry feed whilst retaining the segregation by species, that is, permitting pig PAP to poultry and poultry PAP to pigs.

50.5 Risk assessments and controls

50.5.1 Controlling the disease in cattle (1988–2001)

There have been a number of measures aimed at controlling BSE, some aimed at eliminating transmission in cattle and others aimed at preventing transmission to humans. In terms of those aimed at eliminating transmission in cattle, the first control measure for BSE was introduced in the United Kingdom in June 1988. This prohibited the inclusion of MBM in ruminant feed, following the discovery that the key route of transmission was the inclusion of contaminated MBM in cattle rations.[4] While this ruminant feed ban produced a marked reduction in cattle cases in the United Kingdom, it was insufficient on its own to eliminate cases, and so was supplemented in September 1990 with the specified bovine offal (SBO) ban, which removed those tissues from inclusion in the feed chain which were thought most likely to contain infectivity. Subsequent epidemiological analyses both in United Kingdom[87] and elsewhere, including Northern Ireland, France, Switzerland, and Spain,[88–91] showed a correlation between the risk of BSE cases and the presence of pigs and poultry from the same area. Thus it was concluded that there was cross-contamination between feed produced for pigs and poultry, where MBM was permissible, and feed for ruminants. This led to a reinforced feed ban in the United Kingdom in April 1996, which prohibited the use of mammalian MBM for any farmed animal, a measure subsequently introduced across the EU from January 2001. In terms of measures aimed primarily at reducing human exposure to BSE, there were two key controls. Firstly, the SBO ban (November 1989 in the United Kingdom), which prohibited the use of cattle tissues suspected of being potentially infectious from inclusion in the food chain. Secondly, following the detection of the link between vCJD and cattle, cattle over the age of 30 months were excluded from the food chain in the United Kingdom.

As the outbreak spread to Europe, controls were gradually introduced in EU member states. In terms of measures aimed specifically at reducing human exposure, there were two key controls. The timing of control measures and thus the year of the peak of the epidemic differed between those European countries with significant numbers of cases. It peaked earliest, in the 1988 birth cohort in the United Kingdom where control measures were implemented earliest. Other EU countries also introduced ruminant feed bans in the late 1980s (e.g., The Netherlands, 1989) or early 1990s (e.g., France and Ireland, 1990) and it was banned across the EU in July 1994. EU-wide controls were introduced on minimum temperature and humidity requirements for MBM production in April 1997 and the removal of bovine tissues considered to be infectious (SRM ban) in October 2000, although some EU member states had already introduced equivalent legislation (e.g., France in 1994, and The Netherlands and Ireland in 1995). Other EU countries had their peak birth cohort risk estimated to be at its highest in 1995 (France), 1996 (Ireland), 1997 (Italy and Germany), and 1998 (The Netherlands).[92]

In the face of growing concerns for the international spread of the disease and to facilitate trade, efforts to categorize the risk status of trading countries were initiated in 1995 with the adoption of the World Organisation for Animal Health (WOAH) International Animal Health Code chapter on BSE. Some monitoring was required, and a risk status was associated with a countries level of incidence or the absence of clinical disease. By May 1998 a revised BSE chapter was agreed where the country status was based on the combined results of a risk assessment (release, exposure, and consequence assessment, culminating in a risk estimate) and the results of prescribed active surveillance, designed to achieve a certain confidence in freedom from disease. At the European level, in 1998 the Scientific Steering Committee of the EU Commission began to develop the basis of a geographical BSE risk (GBR) assessment.[93] The assessment provided a framework to estimate a qualitative indicator of the likelihood of the presence of one or more cattle being infected with BSE, at a given point in time, in a country or region. It was noted that the GBR had no direct bearing on likely vCJD numbers linked to BSE exposure. By 2000 23 GBR assessments were finalized grading 23 countries from I (unlikely) to IV (confirmed) at a higher level.[93] These assessments were revised as further surveillance and scientific knowledge was accumulated.

50.5.2 Monitoring the epidemic and deregulation in the face of decline (2001 to present)

Following the implementation of the control measures and the beginning of the decline of BSE cases, there was a greater focus on active surveillance to monitor the decline of the outbreak (and potentially detect any re-emergence) and on modeling studies/risk assessments to inform policy makers as to the effectiveness of existing controls, whether additional controls are needed or whether controls can be lifted.

In terms of surveillance, during the early years of BSE when the cases were rising, detection relied upon clinical suspects being notified to the veterinary authorities by farmers and veterinarians, that is, passive surveillance. Passive surveillance has been found to be an ineffective measure for detection of BSE cases.[21] Therefore for monitoring of the outbreak, active surveillance was introduced across the EU in July 2001.[94] In addition to passive surveillance, this consisted of the testing of risk animals (emergency slaughter and animals that die on farm) over 24 months of age and healthy slaughtered animals over 30 months of age. This would provide a considerable data source with which to inform subsequent risk and modeling studies.

The world trade guidelines from WOAH on active surveillance stipulated an approach which assigned points to each sample taken based on the likelihood of detecting infected cattle in that subpopulation. The total points accumulated can then periodically be compared to the target points for that country.[95] A country must reach its points target and adhere to either Type A or B surveillance. Type A surveillance consists of testing to reach a threshold of at least 1 case per 100,000 in the adult population to a level of confidence of 95%. Type B surveillance is testing to reach threshold of at least 1 case per 50,000, and may be carried out by countries of negligible risk status or those of controlled risk following achievement of the relevant points target using Type A surveillance. Various cohort-based models were designed to estimate the power of different surveillance systems including BSurvE,[96,97] which was based on a point system. The point values consist of the ratio of the exit probability of an infected and detected animal, to the exit probability of an uninfected animal into the different exit streams.

Shortly after the discovery of the link between BSE in cattle and vCJD in humans, mathematical models were developed to estimate the size of the outbreak of vCJD. These models were based on comparisons of the BSE and vCJD outbreaks, inferring the amount of infectivity entering the food chain, and projecting forward from the limited vCJD case numbers based on the observed BSE outbreak. There were a large number of uncertain parameters in these models including the human incubation period of vCJD, the impact of the SBO bans on infectivity in the food chain, with ranges of human cases varying from 100,000 in 20-years' time[98] to up to 1,000,000 by 2080. Subsequent modeling studies benefitted from more vCJD case data, owing to the results of testing approximately 8000 appendix tissues.[99] The later studies showed a much narrower range of further vCJD deaths up to the end of 2080 (10–2600), and a subsequent study showed an even narrower range, up to 263 by end of 2080.[100]

While these statistical modeling approaches to predict vCJD outbreak size could make attempts at predicting the number of human cases from the size of the BSE outbreak and the number of human cases early in the vCJD outbreak, they could not effectively quantify the impact of control measures to limit human exposure. This was able to be done through the use of quantitative risk assessments (QRAs), which combined estimates of the number of infected BSE animals entering the food chain from statistical models,[101,102] the infectivity of cattle tissues, and estimates of the impact of certain control measures on the amount of infectivity getting through, to produce estimates of human exposure to BSE infectivity through food.

The first BSE control to be reviewed was the Over Thirty Month (OTM) rule in cattle in 2003, by which time the number of cases in the United Kingdom had decreased substantially from its peak. This rule prevented beef from cattle aged over 30 months entering the food chain and was a substitute for a cohort cull. A combination of statistical modeling (to estimate the number of infected cattle entering the food chain) and QRA (to estimate the infectivity per cattle carcass) was used to review the impact of a number of potential changes to the OTM rule on human exposure to contaminated food. The risk assessment showed that the SBO ban of November 1989 would have reduced the infectivity from a bovine carcass entering the food chain by approximately 90%.[103] It also showed that the main contributors to human exposure up to 2001 were mechanically recovered meat, head meat, and dorsal root ganglia in meat. Combining estimates of infectivity per animal with a modeling study to estimate the number of infected animals entering the food chain[101] enabled the human exposure at the time of the review of the OTM Scheme in 2003 to be estimated at 1/10,000 that of the peak of the epidemic, and allowed an informed decision to be made to relax the OTM rule to allow animals of all ages born after July 1, 1996 (the timing of the reinforced feed ban) into the food chain, given the low estimates of human exposure from relaxing it.

The future approach for reducing multiple controls across Europe was proposed in 2005 in the first TSE Roadmap.[104] This report presented the possible options between 2005 and 2014 in a stepwise approach the EU was planning to take, supported by scientific evidence, and mapping out measures holistically ensuring that a change in one control was not considered independently of others. A second TSE Roadmap was issued in 2010 to outline future possible amendments from 2010 to 2015 whilst ensuring deregulation was accompanied by a review of current measures and taking into account technical issues and enforcement.[105] During the epidemic, European countries put in place more stringent SRM bans, and therefore as part of the amendments, a number of tissues have been delisted to further align the EU SRM list with the world WOAH SRM list. In many instances, QRAs were commissioned or undertaken by the European Food Safety Authority (EFSA) and individual countries to provide risk estimates prior to relaxation of controls. For example, the EFSA's continuing use of the QRA of the BSE risk posed by PAP[106,107]; the development of the TSE infectivity model—TSEi[108,109] to accompany the EU's re-introduction of bovine intestines and mesenteries into the food chain followed and the United Kingdom's use of the BSE control model[110] and scrapie control model.[111]

One of the challenges in the use of QRAs to measure difference in human exposure to changing controls is to translate estimates of infectivity entering the food chain into estimates of human cases. In the modeling study of the review of the OTM rule[101] an assumption was made that there would be 5000 total deaths from vCJD arising from exposure up to 2003, and an estimate of bovine oral ID50s per human death was estimated. This estimate was then used to predict the future number of vCJD deaths arising from changes to the OTM rule review. This showed less than 1 vCJD case arising from changes to the OTM rule, but was based on assumptions on the number of vCJD deaths, which was very uncertain. There have been attempts made to estimate the cattle–human species barrier elsewhere[112] based on estimates of the total number of cattle ID50s entering the food chain and the exposure per person, resulting in a species barrier estimate of 100–4000. However, this is also highly uncertain and subsequent risk assessments of cattle infectivity entering the food chain have tended to provide estimates in terms of bovine oral ID50s (Adkin et al.[110] and other EFSA QRAs) rather than estimates of human cases.

In addition to the review of BSE control measures across the EU, there have been a number of assessments of surveillance as the epidemic has declined. A review in 2008[113] showed that less than one case would be missed across the EU in each of the healthy slaughter and fallen stock streams if the age of sampling was increased to 48 months, and from January 2009, the member states from the EU-15, which could show a declining or low prevalence of BSE and had implemented the EU surveillance for at least six years, could apply for the increased age of testing. The most recent review of surveillance in the EU involved the assessment of the number of healthy slaughter animals to be tested in order to detect a prevalence of 1 in 100,000 in the standing population, aiming to align EU surveillance with WOAH recommendations for BSE surveillance. For this work, a model was developed specifically to estimate the power of surveillance in the EU (C-TSEMM), both at member state and EU level[114] and to estimate how long it would take to detect re-emergence of BSE should it occur.[115]

50.6 Future predictions

The measures to eradicate BSE or minimize risk of exposure to humans, such as investigation, slaughter, and compensation in case of disease detection, disposal of carcasses, active surveillance, disposal of cattle over 30 months in the United Kingdom between 1996 and 2005 and collection and disposal of SRM from abattoirs,[116] are expensive, and legislative changes have already been introduced to reduce costs. With the decline of BSE cases it is likely that active surveillance will be reduced further. A study using data from the United Kingdom indicated that increasing the age at which fallen stock cattle are tested was less cost-effective than reducing the proportion of fallen stock.[117] As most of the EU member states are recognized as having a negligible BSE risk (currently Greece with a controlled BSE risk as of June 2022) in accordance with Chapter 11.4. of the Terrestrial Code,[95] the EU has also removed the prohibition on the import and export of PAP derived from ruminants, although certain conditions apply to ensure that the exported products do not contain higher BSE risk like MBM. The requirement for strict controls and reliable tests to detect infringements are important aspects to consider if the MBM ban is to be reviewed in future.

It is difficult to predict when no further classical BSE cases will be detected. The effectiveness and speed of control measures introduced varied between European countries and consequently the shape of the decline in risk between cohorts differed between countries.[92] A modeling study predicted a 0.02% probability of having a BSE case confirmed in the United Kingdom as late as 2026, which is later than in EU countries because of the initial higher BSE prevalence and the relatively large cattle population compared to EU member states.[118] Indeed, a classical BSE case was confirmed in England in September 2021. The decline in cases will certainly affect future surveillance activities, although for the recently diagnosed individual cases in France, Ireland, or Scotland more than 10 years after the ruminant feed ban it is often impossible to find a definite source of infection.[119,120] Residual contaminated food from a feed silo used since the 1980s was believed to be the most likely source of the infection in the most recent case in the UK.[121] Researchers in Japan predicted an end to their BSE epidemic by 2012[122] and the last case in Japan was reported in 2009. Proposals have been made in 2019 to revise the WOAH BSE standards for risk assessment and mandated surveillance. The proposals potentially place more focus on evidence of measures taken to prevent BSE agents being recycled in the cattle population, rather than adherence to surveillance thresholds. However, no changes have yet been agreed.

Whilst BSE and scrapie have declined over time, naturally occurring prion diseases have been detected in other species (prion disease in camelids in North Africa in 2018[123]) or in countries not previously known to harbor the disease (CWD in Scandinavia since 2016[81,124,125]). Prion diseases in cervids were previously only known to occur in North America and South Korea from imported cases. Movement of animals and trade of cervid products with other countries increase the risk of spread to other countries. Whilst there is currently no indication that prion diseases in cervids are zoonotic,[126,127] some of the cases in Norway differ from the North American cases in their phenotype,[128] and whilst transmission studies of the cases in Norway and Finland to transgenic mice and bank voles are ongoing to characterize the disease,[125] first results confirm that the isolates are different from North America and also different dependent on species, reindeer, or moose.[129] Camelid prion disease was first discovered in slaughtered dromedary camels in Algeria and may be more common than expected based on the number of camels presented with neurological signs at slaughter.[123] It is not yet known whether this disease poses a threat to humans.

There is a continuous need for CJD surveillance in humans to confirm gradual decline of the number of vCJD cases and to assess efficacy of control measures. Different surveillance streams have been suggested, such as surveillance of children with progressive intellectual and neurological deterioration[130] or screening of donated banked brain tissue.[131] Cases of vCJD were most frequent in the United Kingdom, with more than 170 cases diagnosed.[132] The detection of cases caused by blood transfusion, including an asymptomatic 129 MV heterozygous patient whereas all clinical cases have been in 129 MM homozygous patients, raised concerns about a second epidemic wave, and it was estimated that cases are likely to continue in the United Kingdom with a low-level annual incidence of around 11 cases for a lengthy period of years to decades.[133]

50.7 Research gaps

Although millions have been spent on research into TSEs worldwide to address important questions on epidemiology, pathology, and pathogenesis of naturally occurring TSEs, the reduction in cases has subsequently led to a reduction in funding, even though some questions have remained unresolved and new TSEs have emerged.

In 2004 researchers reported two new BSE types,[134,135] which was novel because there was no previous evidence for diversity of BSE isolates based on mouse studies.[136] The pathological changes seen in the cases in Italy led to the name of bovine amyloidotic spongiform encephalopathy (BASE). Proteinase-treated brain samples from these new cases differed in their migration pattern in a Western blot, with the lowest unglycosylated protein band being either lower (L-type, as seen in BASE) or higher (H-type) than conventional BSE, which was subsequently termed classical or C-type BSE. These cases occurred in cattle aged 8 years or older at a frequency of 1–2 per million tested, which was comparable to sporadic CJD in humans, and also in countries with low risk of foodborne BSE.[137,138] This suggested that H- and L-type BSE may be sporadic diseases in older cattle. Transmission studies in cattle using the intracerebral route demonstrated that the molecular profile is maintained,[139–142] even after second passage.[143,144] This is different to serial transmission studies in mice, which demonstrated that an atypical BSE agent may develop characteristics indistinguishable from classical BSE.[145–147] This led to the hypothesis that atypical BSE may have been the agent responsible for the BSE epidemic if it was transmitted to a nonbovine host and subsequently recycled in MBM. Possible intermediate hosts are sheep or goats but transmission of L-type BSE to these species did not result in a phenotype change resembling classical BSE.[148,149] If atypical BSE represents a sporadic disease originating from the brain, experimental models using the intracerebral route should be appropriate to study pathogenesis and tissue distribution of prions, which is relevant to food safety. There is some evidence that the PrP^{Sc} distribution in peripheral tissues seems to follow the same pattern as for classical BSE,[41] which implies that the current controls to protect the consumer from classical BSE are also adequate for atypical BSE but more studies on the tissue distribution of atypical BSE prions and their infectious titer are needed, which has also been highlighted by the EFSA.[150] This is particularly important since transmission of L-type BSE to transgenic mice expressing the human prion protein gene produced disease,[151,152] which suggested that humans are susceptible. Indeed, transmission of L-type BSE was also successful by the intracerebral and oral route in nonhuman primates.[153] These transmission studies even implied that atypical BSE may be more pathogenic to humans than classical BSE. The phenotype of BASE in cattle had some similarities to the MV2 subtype of sporadic CJD[135] and—when transmitted to macaques—some similarities to the MM2 cortical subtype of sporadic CJD.[154] However, when transmitted to mice there was no evidence that this form of BSE was responsible for the known forms of sporadic CJD.[155]

A more recent study demonstrated that isolates of atypical scrapie, a supposedly sporadic TSE in sheep, can display properties indistinguishable from classical BSE when transmitted to transgenic mice expressing the bovine prion protein gene, and low levels of classical BSE prions were also detectable in ovine atypical scrapie isolates subjected to PMCA.[156] More recently, minipigs intracerebrally inoculated with atypical scrapie brain homogenate were shown to harbor classical BSE prions by PMCA, even though they were asymptomatic and negative for TSEs by other tests and mouse bioassay.[157] Whilst it has previously been reported that atypical scrapie can switch properties within sheep,[158] it was unexpected to find a classical BSE phenotype in bovine transgenic mice or asymptomatic minipigs. This supported the hypothesis that TSE isolates consist of several PrP^{Sc} conformers, of which one stable strain is selected upon cross-species transmission ("cloud model"[159]). Whether an atypical scrapie isolate could have been the agent recycled in MBM and the ultimate cause of the classical BSE epidemic is still not known. Transmission studies in cattle would be required to determine whether cattle are susceptible to atypical scrapie by the parenteral and, in particular, oral route and whether the resulting disease resembles classical BSE. Given that multiple classical scrapie strains exist,[160,161] it is equally possible that a scrapie strain not yet transmitted or characterized in cattle or bovine transgenic mice could be propagated as BSE strain in cattle. The important aspect of all these studies is the ability of strains to change properties when transmitted to the same species with different genetic makeup (e.g., prion protein genotype) or different species. Relaxation of TSE control measures, such as the reintroduction of feeding of PAP to nonruminant species, reduced monitoring for TSEs, and exclusion of scrapie from the list of notifiable diseases, has been implemented or is under consideration and may increase the risk of exposure to potentially zoonotic strains. Thus it is important to understand how prion strains can diverge if transmitted to other species.

Despite many studies to determine the pathogenesis of BSE in cattle, which were imperative to inform on tissue infectivity distribution in BSE, compared to scrapie in sheep and CWD in deer surprisingly little has been done with regards to infectivity or prion detection in body secretions or excretions (saliva, feces, urine), which may contribute to disease transmission or environmental contamination. With the development of ultrasensitive tests that make use of the ability of disease-associated prion protein to convert normal prion protein in a test tube, such as PMCA and Real-Time Quaking-induced Conversion,[162] it is possible to screen more samples collected from naturally or experimentally infected cattle and also samples where microbiological contamination is prohibitive for animal bioassays. The vast majority of existing studies utilized single time-point samples, which is appropriate if prion shedding is indeed continuous but may not be the case as shown for saliva and urine from deer experimentally infected with the CWD agent.[163] In this species, PrPSc tissue distribution is considerably greater compared to BSE in cattle, so prion shedding in cattle may even be more infrequent if it occurs at all. Whilst there is no epidemiological evidence that transmission of BSE between cattle is a major contributor to infection, maternal transmission particularly in the clinical phase is likely,[164] and more studies are needed to rule out milk as a source of infection as there has been no evidence for infectivity in embryos or semen.[165] Similarly, the detection of prion seeding activity by PMCA in salivary glands and saliva[49] requires further attention. The study of possible excretion of BSE prions via feces in cattle has also been neglected despite PrPSc and infectivity being detected in cattle in the gut-associated lymphoid tissue of the small intestine. It is noteworthy that the detection of PrPSc by PMCA in feces from scrapie-affected sheep was attributed mainly to shedding via the gut-associated lymphoid tissue.[166] Shedding of prions may not only result in immediate transmission to other cattle in the vicinity but, equally important, may lead to environmental contamination, which is a concern because of the considerable resistance of prions to inactivation by heat or other inactivation procedures normally fully effective for other pathogens. It has been shown that BSE infectivity persisted in sewage[167] for at least 8 months and in buried bovine heads spiked with BSE brain for at least five years, which may also spread to watercourses via rain water drainage.[168] The binding of prions to soil (reviewed by Smith et al.[169]) and wheat grass roots and leaves[170] has also been demonstrated. Further research in measuring environmental contamination in a farm setting is desirable. This may become more important in future years if classical BSE continues to be diagnosed in cattle born after the MBM feeding ban. In an opinion on the occurrence of these cases after the ban, the EFSA summarized that the most likely origin was a common source, consistent with a feed source, with other causes possibly maternal transmission or environmental contamination. However, considerable uncertainty remained about the origin of disease in individual animals.[120] The fact that an oral dose of 1 mg of BSE brainstem homogenate was still able to produce BSE in cattle[171,172] highlights the risk of infection through contamination of feedstuffs with prions.

Acknowledgments

We thank the APHA lead scientist for critical reading of this chapter. Writing this chapter was partly funded by the UK Department for Food, Environment and Rural Affairs (SE1961). The animal study described in Table 1 was funded by Defra (SE1824-25) and the FSA (M03006-7) and managed by Mr. Stephen Hawkins.

References

1. Wells GA, Scott AC, Johnson CT, et al. A novel progressive spongiform encephalopathy in cattle. *Vet Rec*. 1987;121:419–420.
2. Worldmapper. BSE cases 1987–2016. https://worldmapper.org/maps/bse-cases-1987-2016/; 2022 Accessed 24.05.22.
3. Wilesmith JW, Hoinville LJ, Ryan JB, et al. Bovine spongiform encephalopathy: aspects of the clinical picture and analyses of possible changes 1986–1990. *Vet Rec*. 1992;130:197–201.
4. Wilesmith JW, Wells GA, Cranwell MP, et al. Bovine spongiform encephalopathy: epidemiological studies. *Vet Rec*. 1988;123:638–644.
5. Prusiner SB. The prion diseases. *Sci Am*. 1995;272:48–57.
6. Prince MJ, Bailey JA, Barrowman PR, et al. Bovine spongiform encephalopathy. *Rev Sci Tech*. 2003;22:37–60.
7. Bolea R, Hedman C, López-Pérez Ó, et al. Experimental transmission to a calf of an isolate of Spanish classical scrapie. *J Gen Virol*. 2017;98:2628–2634.
8. Clark WW, Hourrigan JL, Hadlow WJ. Encephalopathy in cattle experimentally infected with the scrapie agent. *Am J Vet Res*. 1995;56:606–612.
9. Cutlip RC, Miller JM, Lehmkuhl HD. Second passage of a US scrapie agent in cattle. *J Comp Pathol*. 1997;117:271–275.
10. Konold T, Lee YH, Stack MJ, et al. Different prion disease phenotypes result from inoculation of cattle with two temporally separated sources of sheep scrapie from Great Britain. *BMC Vet Res*. 2006;2:31.
11. Konold T, Nonno R, Spiropoulos J, et al. Further characterisation of transmissible spongiform encephalopathy phenotypes after inoculation of cattle with two temporally separated sources of sheep scrapie from Great Britain. *BMC Res Notes*. 2015;8:312.
12. Cutlip RC, Miller JM, Hamir AN, et al. Resistance of cattle to scrapie by the oral route. *Can J Vet Res*. 2001;65:131–132.
13. Konold T, Spiropoulos J, Chaplin MJ, et al. Unsuccessful oral transmission of scrapie from British sheep to cattle. *Vet Rec*. 2013;173:118.
14. Denny GO, Hueston WD. Epidemiology of bovine spongiform encephalopathy in Northern Ireland 1988 to 1995. *Vet Rec*. 1997;140:302–306.
15. Cachin M, Vandevelde M, Zurbriggen A. Ein Fall von spongiformer Enzephalopathie ("Rinderwahnsinn") bei einer Kuh in der Schweiz [A case of spongiform encephalopathy ("cattle madness") in a cow in Switzerland]. *Schweiz Arch Tierheilkd*. 1991;133:53–57.
16. Carolan DJP, Wells GAH, Wilesmith JW. BSE in Oman. *Vet Rec*. 1990;126:92.
17. Chen SS, Charlton KM, Balachandran AV, et al. Bovine spongiform encephalopathy identified in a cow imported to Canada from the United Kingdom – a case report. *Can Vet J*. 1996;37:38–40.
18. Agerholm JS, Krogh HV, Nielsen TK, et al. A case of bovine spongiform encephalopathy in Denmark. *Acta Vet Scand*. 1993;34:99–100.
19. Caramelli M, Acutis P, Bozetta E, et al. Bovine spongiform encephalopathy in Italian herds. *Vet Rec*. 2003;153:711–712.
20. Buschmann A, Conraths FJ, Selhorst T, et al. Imported and indigenous BSE cases in Germany. *Vet Microbiol*. 2007;123:287–293.
21. Ducrot C, Arnold M, de Koeijer A, et al. Review on the epidemiology and dynamics of BSE epidemics. *Vet Res*. 2008;39:15.
22. Weihl CC, Roos RP. Creutzfeldt-Jakob disease, new variant Creutzfeldt-Jakob disease, and bovine spongiform encephalopathy. *Neurol Clin*. 1999;17:835–859.
23. UK Parliament. BSE: Southwood report. https://api.parliament.uk/historic-hansard/written-answers/1989/feb/28/bse-southwood-report; 1989 Accessed 24.05.22.
24. van Duijn CM, Delasnerie-Laupretre N, Masullo C, et al. Case-control study of risk factors of Creutzfeldt-Jakob disease in Europe during 1993–95. European Union (EU) Collaborative Study Group of Creutzfeldt-Jakob disease (CJD). *Lancet*. 1998;351:1081–1085.
25. Will RG, Ironside JW, Zeidler M, et al. A new variant of Creutzfeldt-Jakob disease in the UK. *Lancet*. 1996;347:921–925.
26. Streichenberger N, Jordan D, Verejan I, et al. The first case of new variant Creutzfeldt-Jakob disease in France: clinical data and neuropathological findings. *Acta Neuropathol*. 2000;99:704–708.
27. Collinge J, Sidle KCL, Meads J, et al. Molecular analysis of prion strain variation and the aetiology of 'new variant' CJD. *Nature*. 1996;383:685–690.
28. Bruce ME, Will RG, Ironside JW, et al. Transmissions to mice indicate that 'new variant' CJD is caused by the BSE agent. *Nature*. 1997;389:498–501.
29. Hill AF, Desbruslais M, Joiner S, et al. The same prion strain causes vCJD and BSE. *Nature*. 1997;389:448–450.

30. Lasmézas CI, Deslys JP, Demaimay R, et al. BSE transmission to macaques. *Nature*. 1996;381:743–744.
31. Hewitt PE, Llewelyn CA, MacKenzie J, et al. Three reported cases of variant Creutzfeldt-Jakob disease transmission following transfusion of labile blood components. *Vox Sang*. 2006;91:348.
32. National CJD Research & Surveillance Unit. Creutzfeldt-Jakob disease in the UK (By calendar year). <https://www.cjd.ed.ac.uk/sites/default/files/figs.pdf>; 2022 Accessed 24.05.22.
33. Watson N, Brandel J-P, Green A, et al. The importance of ongoing international surveillance for Creutzfeldt–Jakob disease. *Nat Rev Neurol*. 2021;17:362–379.
34. Wells GAH, Dawson M, Hawkins SAC, et al. Preliminary observations on the pathogenesis of experimental bovine spongiform encephalopathy. In: Gibbs CJJ, ed. *Bovine Spongiform Encephalopathy – The BSE Dilemma*. New York: Springer Verlag; 1996:28–44.
35. Wells GAH, Hawkins SAC, Green RB, et al. Preliminary observations on the pathogenesis of experimental bovine spongiform encephalopathy (BSE): an update. *Vet Rec*. 1998;142:103–106.
36. Wells GAH, Hawkins SAC, Green RB, et al. Limited detection of sternal bone marrow infectivity in the clinical phase of experimental bovine spongiform encephalopathy (BSE). *Vet Rec*. 1999;144:292–294.
37. Wells GAH, Spiropoulos J, Hawkins SAC, et al. Pathogenesis of experimental bovine spongiform encephalopathy: preclinical infectivity in tonsil and observations on the distribution of lingual tonsil in slaughtered cattle. *Vet Rec*. 2005;156:401–407.
38. Konold T, Sayers AR, Sach A, et al. Relationship between clinical signs and postmortem test status in cattle experimentally infected with the bovine spongiform encephalopathy agent. *BMC Vet Res*. 2010;6:53.
39. Sohn HJ, Lee YH, Green RB, et al. Bone marrow infectivity in cattle exposed to the bovine spongiform encephalopathy agent. *Vet Rec*. 2009;164:272–273.
40. Simmons MM, Spiropoulos J, Webb PR, et al. Experimental classical bovine spongiform encephalopathy: definition and progression of neural PrP immunolabeling in relation to diagnosis and disease controls. *Vet Pathol*. 2011;48:948–963.
41. Balkema-Buschmann A, Fast C, Kaatz M, et al. Pathogenesis of classical and atypical BSE in cattle. *Prev Vet Med*. 2011;102:112–117.
42. Terry LA, Marsh S, Ryder SJ, et al. Detection of disease-specific PrP in the distal ileum of cattle exposed orally to the agent of bovine spongiform encephalopathy. *Vet Rec*. 2003;152:387–392.
43. Hoffmann C, Ziegler U, Buschmann A, et al. Prions spread via the autonomic nervous system from the gut to the central nervous system in cattle incubating bovine spongiform encephalopathy. *J Gen Virol*. 2007;88:1048–1055.
44. Kaatz M, Fast C, Ziegler U, et al. Spread of classic BSE prions from the gut via the peripheral nervous system to the brain. *Am J Pathol*. 2012;181:515–524.
45. Sisó S, Martin S, Konold T, et al. Minimal involvement of the circumventricular organs in the pathogenesis of spontaneously arising and experimentally induced classical bovine spongiform encephalopathy. *J Comp Pathol*. 2012;147:305–315.
46. Masujin K, Matthews D, Wells GAH, et al. Prions in the peripheral nerves of bovine spongiform encephalopathy-affected cattle. *J Gen Virol*. 2007;88:1850–1858.
47. Buschmann A, Groschup MH. Highly bovine spongiform encephalopathy-sensitive transgenic mice confirm the essential restriction of infectivity to the nervous system in clinically diseased cattle. *J Infect Dis*. 2005;192:934–942.
48. Stack MJ, Moore SJ, Vidal-Diez A, et al. Experimental bovine spongiform encephalopathy: detection of PrP(Sc) in the small intestine relative to exposure dose and age. *J Comp Pathol*. 2011;145:289–301.
49. Murayama Y, Yoshioka M, Masujin K, et al. Sulfated dextrans enhance in vitro amplification of bovine spongiform encephalopathy PrP^{Sc} and enable ultrasensitive detection of bovine PrP^{Sc}. *PLoS One*. 2010;5:e13152.
50. Bannach O, Reinartz E, Henke F, et al. Analysis of prion protein aggregates in blood and brain from pre-clinical and clinical BSE cases. *Vet Microbiol*. 2013;166:102–108.
51. Everest SJ, Thorne LT, Hawthorn JA, et al. No abnormal prion protein detected in the milk of cattle infected with the bovine spongiform encephalopathy agent. *J Gen Virol*. 2006;87:2433–2441.
52. Fast C, Keller M, Kaatz M, et al. Low levels of classical BSE infectivity in rendered fat tissue. *Vet Res*. 2018;49:122.
53. Trieschmann L, Navarrete Santos A, Kaschig K, et al. Ultrasensitive detection of prion protein fibrils by flow cytometry in blood from cattle affected with bovine spongiform encephalopathy. *BMC Biotechnol*. 2005;5:26.
54. World Health Organization. WHO tables on tissue infectivity distribution in transmissible spongiform encephalopathies. <https://www.who.int/publications/m/item/WHO-EMP-QSM-2010.1>; Published 2010 Accessed 24.05.22.
55. Barria MA, Gonzalez-Romero D, Soto C. Cyclic amplification of prion protein misfolding. *Methods Mol Biol*. 2012;849:199–212.
56. Balkema-Buschmann A, Eiden M, Hoffmann C, et al. BSE infectivity in the absence of detectable PrP^{Sc} accumulation in the tongue and nasal mucosa of terminally diseased cattle. *J Gen Virol*. 2011;92:467–476.
57. Simmons MM, Spiropoulos J, Hawkins SA, et al. Approaches to investigating transmission of spongiform encephalopathies in domestic animals using BSE as an example. *Vet Res*. 2008;39:34.
58. Matthews D, Cooke BC. The potential for transmissible spongiform encephalopathies in non-ruminant livestock and fish. *Rev Sci Tech*. 2003;22:283–296.
59. Cunningham AA, Kirkwood JK, Dawson M, et al. Distribution of bovine spongiform encephalopathy in greater kudu (*Tragelaphus strepsiceros*). *Emerg Infect Dis*. 2004;10:1044–1049.
60. Kirkwood JK, Cunningham AA. Epidemiological observations on spongiform encephalopathies in captive wild animals in the British Isles. *Vet Rec*. 1994;135:296–303.
61. Wyatt JM, Pearson GR, Smerdon T, et al. Spongiform encephalopathy in a cat. *Vet Rec*. 1990;126:513.
62. Bruce ME. TSE strain variation. *Br Med Bull*. 2003;66:99–108.
63. Demierre S, Botteron C, Cizinauskas S, et al. Feline Spongiforme Enzephalopathie: Erster klinischer Fall in der Schweiz. [Feline spongiform encephalopathy: first clinical case in Switzerland]. *Schweiz Arch Tierheilkd*. 2002;144:550–557.
64. Bencsik A, Debeer S, Petit T, et al. Possible case of maternal transmission of feline spongiform encephalopathy in a captive cheetah. *PLoS One*. 2009;4:e6929.
65. Foster JD, Hope J, Fraser H. Transmission of bovine spongiform encephalopathy to sheep and goats. *Vet Rec*. 1993;133:339–341.
66. McGovern G, Martin S, Jeffrey M, et al. Influence of breed and genotype on the onset and distribution of infectivity and disease-associated

prion protein in sheep following oral infection with the bovine spongiform encephalopathy agent. *J Comp Pathol*. 2015;152:28–40.

67. McGovern G, Martin S, Jeffrey M, et al. Minimum effective dose of cattle and sheep BSE for oral sheep infection. *PLoS One*. 2016;11:e0151440.
68. Fast C, Goldmann W, Berthon P, et al. Protecting effect of PrP codons M142 and K222 in goats orally challenged with bovine spongiform encephalopathy prions. *Vet Res*. 2017;48:52.
69. Foster JD, Parnham D, Chong A, et al. Clinical signs, histopathology and genetics of experimental transmission of BSE and natural scrapie to sheep and goats. *Vet Rec*. 2001;148:165–171.
70. Aguilar-Calvo P, Fast C, Tauscher K, et al. Effect of Q211 and K222 PRNP polymorphic variants in the susceptibility of goats to oral infection with goat bovine spongiform encephalopathy. *J Infect Dis*. 2015;212:664–672.
71. Houston F, Goldmann W, Foster J, et al. Comparative susceptibility of sheep of different origins, breeds and PRNP genotypes to challenge with bovine spongiform encephalopathy and scrapie. *PLoS One*. 2015;10:e0143251.
72. Jeffrey M, Witz JP, Martin S, et al. Dynamics of the natural transmission of bovine spongiform encephalopathy within an intensively managed sheep flock. *Vet Res*. 2015;46:126.
73. Houston F, Foster JD, Chong A, et al. Transmission of BSE by blood transfusion in sheep. *Lancet*. 2000;356:999–1000.
74. Padilla D, Béringue V, Espinosa JC, et al. Sheep and goat BSE propagate more efficiently than cattle BSE in human PrP transgenic mice. *PLoS Pathog*. 2011;7:e1001319.
75. Stack M, Jeffrey M, Gubbins S, et al. Monitoring for bovine spongiform encephalopathy in sheep in Great Britain, 1998–2004. *J Gen Virol*. 2006;87:2099–2107.
76. Eloit M, Adjou K, Coulpier M, et al. BSE agent signatures in a goat. *Vet Rec*. 2005;156:523–524.
77. Spiropoulos J, Lockey R, Sallis RE, et al. Isolation of prion with BSE properties from farmed goat. *Emerg Infect Dis*. 2011;17:2253–2261.
78. Dagleish MP, Martin S, Steele P, et al. Experimental transmission of bovine spongiform encephalopathy to European red deer (*Cervus elaphus elaphus*). *BMC Vet Res*. 2008;4:17.
79. Martin S, Jeffrey M, Gonzalez L, et al. Immunohistochemical and biochemical characteristics of BSE and CWD in experimentally infected European red deer (*Cervus elaphus elaphus*). *BMC Vet Res*. 2009;5:26.
80. Schwabenlander MD, Culhane MR, Hall SM, et al. A case of chronic wasting disease in a captive red deer (*Cervus elaphus*). *J Vet Diagn Invest*. 2013;25:573–576.
81. Vikøren T, Våge J, Madslien KI, et al. First detection of chronic wasting disease in a wild red deer (*Cervus elaphus*) in Europe. *J Wildl Dis*. 2019;55:970–972.
82. Wells GAH, Hawkins SAC, Austin AR, et al. Studies of the transmissibility of the agent of bovine spongiform encephalopathy to pigs. *J Gen Virol*. 2003;84:1021–1031.
83. Hedman C, Otero A, Douet J-Y, et al. Detection of PrP^{res} in peripheral tissue in pigs with clinical disease induced by intracerebral challenge with sheep-passaged bovine spongiform encephalopathy agent. *PLOS One*. 2018;13:e0199914.
84. Konold T, Spiropoulos J, Chaplin MJ, et al. Transmissibility studies of vacuolar changes in the rostral colliculus of pigs. *BMC Vet Res*. 2009;5:35.
85. Moore J, Hawkins SA, Austin AR, et al. Studies of the transmissibility of the agent of bovine spongiform encephalopathy to the domestic chicken. *BMC Res Notes*. 2011;4:501.
86. Salta E, Panagiotidis C, Teliousis K, et al. Evaluation of the possible transmission of BSE and scrapie to gilthead sea bream (*Sparus aurata*). *PLoS One*. 2009;4:e6175.
87. Stevenson MA, Morris RS, Lawson AB, et al. Area-level risks for BSE in British cattle before and after the July 1988 meat and bone meal feed ban. *Prev Vet Med*. 2005;69:129–144.
88. Abrial D, Calavas D, Jarrige N, et al. Poultry, pig and the risk of BSE following the feed ban in France – a spatial analysis. *Vet Res*. 2005;36:615–628.
89. Schwermer H, Heim D. Cases of bovine spongiform encephalopathy born in Switzerland before and after the ban on the use of bovine specified risk material in feed. *Vet Rec*. 2007;160:73–77.
90. Sheridan HA, McGrath G, White P, et al. A temporal-spatial analysis of bovine spongiform encephalopathy in Irish cattle herds, from 1996 to 2000. *Can J Vet Res*. 2005;69:19.
91. Allepuz A, López-Quílez A, Forte A, et al. Spatial analysis of bovine spongiform encephalopathy in Galicia, Spain (2000–2005). *Prev Vet Med*. 2007;79:174–185.
92. Ducrot C, Sala C, Ru G, et al. Modelling BSE trend over time in Europe, a risk assessment perspective. *Eur J Epidemiol*. 2010;25: 411–419.
93. Scientific Steering Committee. Final opinion of the Scientific Steering Committee on the geographical risk of bovine spongiform encephalopathy (GBR). <https://ec.europa.eu/food/system/files/2020-12/sci-com_ssc_out113_en.pdf>; 2000 Accessed 24.05.22.
94. European Council. Council Decision of 4 December 2000 concerning certain protection measures with regard to transmissible spongiform encephalopathies and the feeding of animal protein (2000/766/EC). <https://eur-lex.europa.eu/LexUriServ/LexUriServ.do?uri = OJ:L:2000:306:0032:0033:EN:PDF>; Published 2000 Accessed 24.05.22.
95. WOAH. Chapter 11.4: Bovine spongiform encephalopathy. In: *Terrestrial Animal Health Code*. Paris: World Organisation for Animal Health; 2021: 1–16.
96. Prattley DJ, Cannon RM, Wilesmith JW, et al. A model (BSurvE) for estimating the prevalence of bovine spongiform encephalopathy in a national herd. *Prev Vet Med*. 2007;80:330–343.
97. Prattley DJ, Morris RS, Cannon RM, et al. A model (BSurvE) for evaluating national surveillance programs for bovine spongiform encephalopathy. *Prev Vet Med*. 2007;81:225–235.
98. Cousens SN, Vynnycky E, Zeidler M, et al. Predicting the CJD epidemic in humans. *Nature*. 1997;385:197–198.
99. Ghani AC, Donnelly CA, Ferguson NM, et al. Updated projections of future vCJD deaths in the UK. *BMC Infect Dis*. 2003;3:4.
100. Clarke P, Ghani AC. Projections of the future course of the primary vCJD epidemic in the UK: inclusion of subclinical infection and the possibility of wider genetic susceptibility. *J R Soc Interface*. 2005;2:19–31.
101. Ferguson NM, Donnelly CA. Assessment of the risk posed by bovine spongiform encephalopathy in cattle in Great Britain and the impact of potential changes to current control measures. *Proc R Soc Lond Ser B Biol Sci*. 2003;270:1579–1584.
102. Arnold M, Wilesmith J. Modelling studies on bovine spongiform encephalopathy occurrence to assist in the review of the over 30 months rule in Great Britain. *Proc R Soc Lond B*. 2003;270:2141–2145.

103. Comer PJ, Huntly PJ. TSE risk assessments: a decision support tool. *Stat Methods Med Res*. 2003;12:279–291.
104. European Commission. The TSE roadmap. <https://ec.europa.eu/food/system/files/2016-10/biosafety_food-borne-disease_tse_road-map1.pdf>; 2005 Accessed 24.05.22.
105. European Commission. The TSE roadmap 2. <https://ec.europa.eu/food/system/files/2016-10/biosafety_food-borne-disease_tse_road-map2.pdf>; 2010 Accessed 24.05.22.
106. EFSA Panel on Biological Hazards. Scientific opinion on the revision of the quantitative risk assessment (QRA) of the BSE risk posed by processed animal proteins (PAPs). *EFSA J*. 2011;9:1947.
107. EFSA Panel on Biological HazardsRicci A, Allende A, et al. Updated quantitative risk assessment (QRA) of the BSE risk posed by processed animal protein (PAP). *EFSA J*. 2018;16:5314.
108. Adkin A, Simons R, Arnold M. TSE infectivity model (TSEi) in animal tissues: bovine intestines and mesenteries. <https://www.efsa.europa.eu/en/supporting/pub/en-559>; 2014 Accessed 24.05.22.
109. EFSA BIOHAZ Panel. Scientific Opinion on BSE risk in bovine intestines and mesentery. *EFSA J*. 2014;12:3554.
110. Adkin A, Webster V, Arnold ME, et al. Estimating the impact on the food chain of changing bovine spongiform encephalopathy (BSE) control measures: the BSE control model. *Prev Vet Med*. 2010;93:170–182.
111. Adkin A, Horigan V, Rajanayagam B, et al. Estimating the impact on food and edible materials of changing scrapie control measures: the scrapie control model. *Prev Vet Med*. 2018;158:51–64.
112. EFSA. Opinion of the Scientific Panel on Biological Hazards of the European Food Safety Authority on the "Quantitative assessment of the human BSE risk posed by gelatine with respect to residual BSE risk.". *EFSA J*. 2006;312:1–29.
113. EFSA BioHAZ Panel. Scientific opinion of the panel on biological hazards on a request from the European Commission on the risk for human and animal health related to the revision of the BSE monitoring regime in some member states. *EFSA J*. 2008;762:1–47.
114. Adkin A, Simons R, Arnold M. Assessing the sensitivity of European surveillance for detecting BSE in cattle according to international standards. *Prev Vet Med*. 2016;135:113–122.
115. Simons RRL, Arnold ME, Adkin A. Assessing the time taken for a surveillance system to detect a re-emergence of bovine spongiform encephalopathy in cattle. *Prev Vet Med*. 2017;138:48–54.
116. Simmons M, Ru G, Casalone C, et al. DISCONTOOLS: identifying gaps in controlling bovine spongiform encephalopathy. *Transbound Emerg Dis*. 2018;65:9–21.
117. Wall BA, Arnold ME, Radia D, et al. Evidence for more cost-effective surveillance options for bovine spongiform encephalopathy (BSE) and scrapie in Great Britain. *Eurosurveillance*. 2017;22:22–30.
118. Arnold ME, Simons RRL, Hope J, et al. Is there a decline in bovine spongiform encephalopathy cases born after reinforced feed bans? A modelling study in EU member states. *Epidemiol Infect*. 2017;145:2280–2286.
119. O'Connor JT, Byrne JP, More SJ, et al. Using an epidemiological framework and bovine spongiform encephalopathy investigation questionnaire to investigate suspect bovine spongiform encephalopathy cases: an example from a bovine spongiform encephalopathy case in Ireland in 2015. *Vet Rec*. 2018;182:168.
120. EFSA BIOHAZ PanelRicci A, Allende A, et al. Bovine spongiform encephalopathy (BSE) cases born after the total feed ban. *EFSA J*. 2017;15:4885.
121. APHA. Report on the epidemiological investigation of a single BSE case in Somerset, England (RBSE 2021:00002). <https://assets.publishing.service.gov.uk/government/uploads/system/uploads/attachment_data/file/1041282/Report_on_the_epidemiological_investigation_of_a_single_BSE_case_in_Somerset.pdf> 2021 Accessed 24.05.22.
122. Sugiura K, Kikuchi E, Onodera T. Updated prediction for the BSE epidemic in dairy cattle in Japan. *Prev Vet Med*. 2009;89:272–276.
123. Babelhadj B, Di Bari MA, Pirisinu L, et al. Prion disease in dromedary camels, Algeria. *Emerg Infect Dis*. 2018;24:1029–1036.
124. Benestad SL, Mitchell G, Simmons M, et al. First case of chronic wasting disease in Europe in a Norwegian free-ranging reindeer. *Vet Res*. 2016;47:88.
125. EFSA BIOHAZ Panel (EFSA Panel on Biological Hazards) Koutsoumanis K, Allende A, et al. Scientific opinion on the update on chronic wasting disease (CWD) III. *EFSA J*. 2019;17:5863.
126. Race B, Williams K, Chesebro B. Transmission studies of chronic wasting disease to transgenic mice overexpressing human prion protein using the RT-QuIC assay. *Vet Res*. 2019;50:6.
127. Race B, Williams K, Orrú CD, et al. Lack of transmission of chronic wasting disease to cynomolgus macaques. *J Virol*. 2018;92. e00550-18.
128. Pirisinu L, Tran L, Chiappini B, et al. Novel type of chronic wasting disease detected in moose (*Alces alces*), Norway. *Emerg Infect Dis*. 2018;24:2210–2218.
129. Nonno R, Di Bari MA, Pirisinu L, et al. Studies in bank voles reveal strain differences between chronic wasting disease prions from Norway and North America. *Proc Natl Acad Sci USA*. 2020;117:31417–31426.
130. Verity C, Winstone AM, Will R, et al. Surveillance for variant CJD: should more children with neurodegenerative diseases have autopsies? *Arch Dis Child*. 2019;104:360–365.
131. Peden AH, Kanguru L, Ritchie DL, et al. Study protocol for enhanced CJD surveillance in the 65 + years population group in Scotland: an observational neuropathological screening study of banked brain tissue donations for evidence of prion disease. *BMJ Open*. 2019;9:e033744.
132. Seed CR, Hewitt PE, Dodd RY, et al. Creutzfeldt-Jakob disease and blood transfusion safety. *Vox Sang*. 2018;113:220–231.
133. Garske T, Ghani AC. Uncertainty in the tail of the variant Creutzfeldt-Jakob disease epidemic in the UK. *PLoS One*. 2010;5:e15626.
134. Biacabe AG, Laplanche JL, Ryder S, et al. Distinct molecular phenotypes in bovine prion diseases. *EMBO Rep*. 2004;5:110–114.
135. Casalone C, Zanusso G, Acutis P, et al. Identification of a second bovine amyloidotic spongiform encephalopathy: molecular similarities with sporadic Creutzfeldt-Jakob disease. *Proc Natl Acad Sci U S A*. 2004;101:3065–3070.
136. Green R, Horrocks C, Wilkinson A, et al. Primary isolation of the bovine spongiform encephalopathy agent in mice: agent definition based on a review of 150 transmissions. *J Comp Pathol*. 2005;132:117–131.
137. Tranulis MA, Benestad SL, Baron T, et al. Atypical prion diseases in humans and animals. *Top Curr Chem*. 2011;305:23–50.
138. Iulini B, Costassa EV, Corona C, et al. Classical and atypical bovine spongiform encephalopathy: epidemiology, pathogenesis and diagnosis. In: Tutar Y, ed. *Prion*. London: IntechOpen; 2017:3–25.

139. Balkema-Buschmann A, Ziegler U, McIntyre L, et al. Experimental challenge of cattle with German atypical bovine spongiform encephalopathy (BSE) isolates. *J Toxicol Environ Health A*. 2011;74:103–109.
140. Fukuda S, Iwamaru Y, Imamura M, et al. Intraspecies transmission of L-type-like bovine spongiform encephalopathy detected in Japan. *Microbiol Immunol*. 2009;53:704–707.
141. Konold T, Bone GE, Clifford D, et al. Experimental H-type and L-type bovine spongiform encephalopathy in cattle: observation of two clinical syndromes and diagnostic challenges. *BMC Vet Res*. 2012;8:22.
142. Lombardi G, Casalone C, D'Angelo A, et al. Intraspecies transmission of BASE induces clinical dullness and amyotrophic changes. *PLoS Pathog*. 2008;4:e1000075.
143. Okada H, Iwamaru Y, Kakizaki M, et al. Properties of L-type bovine spongiform encephalopathy in intraspecies passages. *Vet Pathol*. 2012;49:819–823.
144. Konold T, Phelan LJ, Clifford D, et al. The pathological and molecular but not clinical phenotypes are maintained after second passage of experimental atypical bovine spongiform encephalopathy in cattle. *BMC Vet Res*. 2014;10:243.
145. Torres JM, Andréoletti O, Lacroux C, et al. Classical bovine spongiform encephalopathy by transmission of H-type prion in homologous prion protein context. *Emerg Infect Dis*. 2011;17:1636–1644.
146. Bencsik A, Leboidre M, Debeer S, et al. Unique properties of the classical bovine spongiform encephalopathy strain and its emergence from H-type bovine spongiform encephalopathy substantiated by VM transmission studies. *J Neuropathol Exp Neurol*. 2013;72:211–218.
147. Capobianco R, Casalone C, Suardi S, et al. Conversion of the BASE prion strain into the BSE strain: the origin of BSE? *PLoS Pathog*. 2007;3:e31.
148. Simmons MM, Chaplin MJ, Konold T, et al. L-BSE experimentally transmitted to sheep presents as a unique disease phenotype. *Vet Res*. 2016;47:112.
149. Vallino Costassa E, D'Angelo A, Mazza M, et al. Clinical, pathological, and molecular features of classical and L-type atypical-BSE in goats. *PLoS One*. 2018;13:e0198037.
150. European Food Safety Authority. Protocol for further laboratory investigations into the distribution of infectivity of atypical BSE. *EFSA J*. 2014;12:3798.
151. Béringue V, Herzog L, Reine F, et al. Transmission of atypical bovine prions to mice transgenic for human prion protein. *Emerg Infect Dis*. 2008;14:1898–1901.
152. Kong Q, Zheng M, Casalone C, et al. Evaluation of the human transmission risk of an atypical bovine spongiform encephalopathy prion strain. *J Virol*. 2008;82:3697–3701.
153. Mestre-Francés N, Nicot S, Rouland S, et al. Oral transmission of L-type bovine spongiform encephalopathy in primate model. *Emerg Infect Dis*. 2012;18:142–145.
154. Comoy EE, Casalone C, Lescoutra-Etchegaray N, et al. Atypical BSE (BASE) transmitted from asymptomatic aging cattle to a primate. *PLoS One*. 2008;3:e3017.
155. Jaumain E, Quadrio I, Herzog L, et al. Absence of evidence for a causal link between bovine spongiform encephalopathy strain variant L-BSE and known forms of sporadic Creutzfeldt-Jakob disease in human PrP transgenic mice. *J Virol*. 2016;90:10867–10874.
156. Huor A, Espinosa JC, Vidal E, et al. The emergence of classical BSE from atypical/Nor98 scrapie. *Proc Natl Acad Sci U S A*. 2019;116:26853–26862.
157. Marín B, Otero A, Lugan S, et al. Classical BSE prions emerge from asymptomatic pigs challenged with atypical/Nor98 scrapie. *Sci Rep*. 2021;11:17428.
158. Simmons MM, Moore SJ, Lockey R, et al. Phenotype shift from atypical scrapie to CH1641 following experimental transmission in sheep. *PLoS One*. 2015;10:e0117063.
159. Makarava N, Baskakov IV. The evolution of transmissible prions: the role of deformed templating. *PLoS Pathog*. 2013;9:e1003759.
160. Thackray AM, Hopkins L, Lockey R, et al. Propagation of ovine prions from "poor" transmitter scrapie isolates in ovine PrP transgenic mice. *Exp Mol Pathol*. 2012;92:167–174.
161. Bruce ME, Boyle A, Cousens S, et al. Strain characterization of natural sheep scrapie and comparison with BSE. *J Gen Virol*. 2002;83:695–704.
162. Atarashi R, Sano K, Satoh K, et al. Real-time quaking-induced conversion: a highly sensitive assay for prion detection. *Prion*. 2011;5:150–153.
163. Henderson DM, Denkers ND, Hoover CE, et al. Longitudinal detection of prion shedding in saliva and urine by chronic wasting disease-infected deer by real-time quaking-induced conversion. *J Virol*. 2015;89:9338–9347.
164. Donnelly CA, Ferguson NM, Ghani AC, et al. Analysis of dam-calf pairs of BSE cases: confirmation of a maternal risk enhancement. *Proc R Soc Lond B*. 1997;264:1647–1656.
165. Wrathall AE, Brown KFD, Sayers AR, et al. Studies of embryo transfer from cattle clinically affected by bovine spongiform encephalopathy (BSE). *Vet Rec*. 2002;150:365–378.
166. Terry LA, Howells L, Bishop K, et al. Detection of prions in the faeces of sheep naturally infected with classical scrapie. *Vet Res*. 2011;42:65.
167. Maluquer de Motes C, Espinosa JC, Esteban A, et al. Persistence of the bovine spongiform encephalopathy infectious agent in sewage. *Environ Res*. 2012;117:1–7.
168. Somerville RA, Fernie K, Smith A, et al. BSE infectivity survives burial for five years with only limited spread. *Arch Virol*. 2019;164:1135–1145.
169. Smith CB, Booth CJ, Pedersen JA. Fate of prions in soil: a review. *J Environ Qual*. 2011;40:449–461.
170. Pritzkow S, Morales R, Moda F, et al. Grass plants bind, retain, uptake, and transport infectious prions. *Cell Rep*. 2015;11:1168–1175.
171. Wells GAH, Konold T, Arnold ME, et al. Bovine spongiform encephalopathy: the effect of oral exposure dose on attack rate and incubation period in cattle. *J Gen Virol*. 2007;88:1363–1373.
172. Konold T, Arnold ME, Austin AR, et al. Bovine spongiform encephalopathy: the effect of oral exposure dose on attack rate and incubation period in cattle – an update. *BMC Res Notes*. 2012;5:674.

Chapter 51

Role of real-time DNA analyses, biomarkers, resistance measurement, and ecosystem management in *Campylobacter* risk analysis

Jasmina Vidic[1], Sandrine Auger[1], Marco Marin[1], Francesco Rizzotto[1], Nabila Haddad[2], Sandrine Guillou[2], Muriel Guyard-Nicodème[3], Priya Vizzini[4], Alessia Cossettini[4], Marisa Manzano[4], Zoi Kotsiri[5], Efstratia Panteleli[5] and Apostolos Vantarakis[5]

[1]*MICALIS Institut, Univerisité Paris-Saclay, INRAE, AgroParisTech, Jouy en Josas, France,* [2]*SECALIM, INRAE, Oniris, Nantes, France,* [3]*ANSES – Ploufragan-Plouzané-Niort Laboratory, Ploufragan, France,* [4]*Dipartimento di Scienze AgroAlimentari, Ambientali e Animali, Università di Udine, Udine, Italy,* [5]*Environmental and Microbiology Unit, Department of Public Health, Medical School, University of Patras, Patras, Greece*

Abstract

Campylobacter is one of the four most important pathogens that cause foodborne disease in humans, with symptoms as fever, diarrhea, abdominal cramps, and vomiting. In some cases, the illness can evolve toward more severe pathologies or leads to patient death. The main source of transmission is generally believed to be via contaminated undercooked meat, meat products, and raw milk. Food safety is fundamental to assure consumers safety. A risk control could be achieved using analysis methods that can reduce the time required for results still maintaining specificity and sensitivity. Here we describe advanced methods for *Campylobacter* detection that reduce the time needed for a response which may reduce risks of foodborne outbreaks.

Keywords: Foodborne pathogen; food analysis and screening; biosensor; molecular methods; lipooligosaccharide; LAMP; NGS; RT-PCR; ddPCR

51.1 Introduction

Listeria, *Salmonella*, *Campylobacter*, *Escherichia coli*, and *Bacillus cereus* are among the most important pathogens that cause foodborne disease in humans, with symptoms as fever, diarrhea, abdominal cramps, and vomiting. In some cases, the illness can evolve toward more severe pathologies or lead to patient death. Food safety is fundamental to assure consumers health. Even though microbiological analysis is performed on food from production to market, there are still cases of foodborne outbreaks.

The world population is increasing over the years and is expected to be 8.5 billion in 2030.[1] According to the data reported by the World Health Organization (WHO), 600 million persons fall ill (about 1 out of 10 people in the world) every year, due to the ingestion of contaminated foods or water, containing bacteria, viruses, parasites, chemical substances, or toxins. This implies 420,000 deaths, of which 230,000 are related to diarrheal agents, the most frequent causes of foodborne illness.[2] Moreover, various cases of zoonoses are related to low-income countries.

Susceptibility to foodborne diseases is higher in specific population categories: children, elderly, pregnant women, and immunosuppressed.[3] In an observational study conducted in New Zealand, 74,454 notifications and 3192 hospitalizations were due to nonviral gastroenteritis in children, of which almost half are credited to be caused by *Campylobacter*.[4] However, during the 19 years of this study, results demonstrated a decline in the number of notifications for the majority of foodborne diseases, which could be related to upgraded food safety practices.

People over 65 years are also highly vulnerable to foodborne diseases. Different factors can influence the situation: immune system (characterized by a general decline in cell function), medical status (related to the

Present Knowledge in Food Safety. DOI: https://doi.org/10.1016/B978-0-12-819470-6.00026-3

presence of other pathologies or conditions as diabetes), and use of antibiotics, nutrient deficiency, chronic illness, lifestyle (including dietary habits), hospitalizations, and living in long-term facilities.[5] A study performed on the Dutch population estimated that the percentage of people over 65 years will increase from 16% in 2011 to 25% in 2060, with a peak of 26% in 2040. This increase of the elderly group in the population directly entailed an amplification of the proportion of foodborne diseases.[6] In 2040 the proportion of illness caused by *Campylobacter* and *Salmonella* is expected to increase by around 10%.

The WHO led a recent research to show regional differences in the burden of foodborne diseases. The highest burden per population was observed in Africa with 91 million cases and 137,000 deaths, followed by the South-East Asia. In a study carried out in Eastern Cape, South Africa, the highest prevalence of foodborne diseases was determined in rural provinces, surrounded by many low-income and semirural villages.[7] In a total of 399 people almost one-third fell ill because of foodborne disease during the period 2012–14. In the same period, only four cases were reported in clinic registers, despite 19 participants have benefited from treatment in primary healthcare clinics. This demonstrated the lack in the health surveillance system. Furthermore, the same study stated that there was a significant correlation between education levels (no education levels, tertiary education levels, or higher education levels) and food safety concern levels: people with any form of education were more aware of the food safety risks, whereas 52.9% of the participants were not concerned about the safety of the food prepared away from home or sold by traders or supermarkets. Despite these achievements, almost 60% of the participants thought that a good solution to decrease foodborne disease could be to increase the number of inspections in food outlets. These results show the need to improve monitoring systems in the preparation of food and to increase the health education and food safety awareness. From the data collected by WHO, from January to September 2020 there were 104 food safety incidents, of whom 56 were biological hazard incidents, involving countries from Europe, Americas, Africa, Western Pacific, Eastern Mediterranean and South-East Asia.

As a result of numerous foodborne disease outbreaks and food scandals, the consumer concerns and interest in food safety increased. In 2016 through an online survey conducted in Australia,[8] 489 participants indicated their agreement with different statements linked to the importance of modalities of food production, transport, and storage, to the knowledge and confidence on the traceability system. The Australian consumers required information on food production along the supply chain, but not all the distributers thought that traceability was a good way to express this information. In particular, there was a strong resistance toward the traceability system from the older or from consumers with a low level of education, due to their lower knowledge of what traceability means and includes. On the contrary, younger participants, with a better understanding of the system, were associated with a higher level of willingness to accept to pay more. Hence, to be able to use traceability as an instrument for food safety to increase the consumer confidence, it is necessary to educate buyers and elaborate adequate communication systems.

Another study[9] aimed to investigate the most important food values for consumers, in relation to imported fruit and vegetables in Japan, Taiwan, and Indonesia. The feedback of 1350 participants were collected: >50% were highly educated (university level) and the average age of the participants from all three countries was below 50 years. Seven different food values associated to the imported fruit and vegetables were presented to participants, including labeling product origin, food safety certification, high-quality appearance, domestic rarity, plantation methods and freshness, and the importance of all of these was assessed in relation to another fundamental food value, the price. Based on the probability class share for each country three major types of consumer group were obtained including consumers with similar preferences toward food values in each group. The results indicated that the Majority Group, the biggest group including consumers from all the three countries, selected "food safety certified" as the most important characteristic in the selection of imported fruit and vegetables.

Several studies performed on consumers' choices showed that consumers were willing to pay a premium for *Campylobacter*-free chicken.[10,11]

51.2 *Campylobacter* spp.

Campylobacter is an important foodborne pathogen. According to the data collected by the European Food Safety Authority (EFSA), since 2005 campylobacteriosis is the most frequently reported foodborne disease, with more than 246,000 cases in Europe in 2018.[12] The majority of infections are sporadic, that is, not associated with outbreaks.

The genus *Campylobacter* belongs to the bacterial family Campylobacteriaceae; within this family, 32 species and 12 subspecies are currently recognized. The four species of *Campylobacter* most commonly associated with human infections are *Campylobacter jejuni* and *Campylobacter coli*, which cause about 90% of human campylobacteriosis, *Campylobacter lari* and *Campylobacter upsaliensis*.[13] They show a characteristic corkscrew-like motility due to the presence of a single or polar flagellum to one or both end of cell (Fig. 51.1). This pathogen is a thin spirally curved (0.2–0.8 μm × 0.5–5 μm) Gram-negative bacteria and

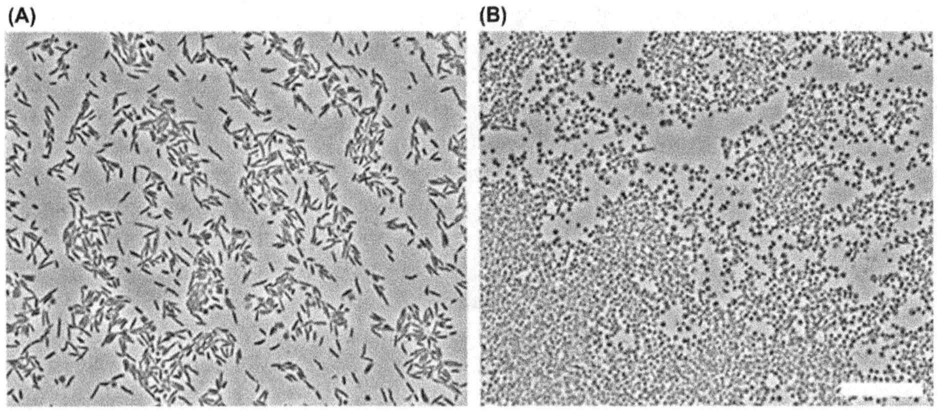

FIGURE 51.1 Optical microscopy visualization of *Campylobacter jejuni* Bf strain changing their cell shape from a typically spiral (A) to a coccoid in the presence of oxygen (B). Bar, 5 μm.

oxidase-positive, characterized by its capability to grow under microaerophilic conditions (10% CO_2 and 5% O_2). Due to their ability to grow between 37°C and 42°C (optimum at 41.5°C), but inability to grow below 30°C, these pathogens are described as thermotolerant species. Other environmental conditions that not allow their growth are water activity (W_A) below 0.987, NaCl concentration above 2% w/v, and pH < 4.9 or >9.0.[14]

Campylobacter can be got by the ingestion of several contaminated foods. A minor source is unpasteurized milk and its products including cheese, unwashed fruits, and vegetables contaminated through contact with soil or water (lakes and streams) containing feces from infected cows, birds, or other animals. Studies have shown that the main source is undercooked poultry meat such as broiler and turkey.[15] Indeed, each step of meat production from primary production, transport, slaughter, and meat processing to product and consumption have an important role in the transmission of *Campylobacter* spp. At the level of primary production, the risk factors are related to the season, age of poultry, use of extended breeding, nondrinking water supply, and use of antimicrobials, while the subsequent steps are related to possible cross-contamination episodes.[15]

The campylobacteriosis may be categorized as a traveler disease. Mughini-Gras et al. investigated the characteristics of campylobacteriosis as a traveler disease in the Dutch population.[16] On the basis on an earlier case-control study, the participants were divided into two main groups (cases and controls), and they were asked to fill out a questionnaire regarding traveling abroad and food habits. From the outcomes, the destination was known for 325 diseased travelers and 238 healthy travelers that were all included in the examination, limiting the cases on probable exotic origin. The regions associated with a high risk for campylobacteriosis were Southern Europe, Asia, Africa, South America, and the Caribbean. The factors positively linked to this travel campylobacteriosis were different, including healthy factors (use of antacids, chronic enteropathies), food habits (consume of salad outside Europe, handle/eat raw or undercooked pork or chicken, drink bottled water), and seasonality (most riskily periods are those related to popular holidays in the Netherlands). It was also estimated that over 3% of domestic cases were linked to *Campylobacter*'s introduced strains from exotic destinations, probably spread through person-to-person transmission.

Recently, Schmutz et al. estimated the annual Swiss healthcare cost of 2012 associated with acute gastroenteritis, including campylobacteriosis.[17] Patients were included into four groups: patients consulting a physician without stool testing (A), patients consulting a physician with negative *Campylobacter* stool test result (B), patients with a positive *Campylobacter* stool test result (C), and patients hospitalized due to campylobacteriosis (D). The range of costs, encompassing groups A, B, C, and D, went from €30 to €4828, and the estimated average healthcare cost for every patient with confirmed campylobacteriosis, comprehending also the required hospitalization, is €975. The estimated total cost needed for treating the conditions of the four groups of patients was €29−€45 million, among which €8.3 million/year were required to heal campylobacteriosis, and this high amount is attributable to the hospital stay, that could vary from 2 to 11 nights. A decrease of the numbers could be achieved using analysis methods that can reduce the time required for results still maintaining specificity and sensitivity.

Campylobacteriosis mainly occurs in the small intestine of humans due to flagella-mediated motility, bacterial adherence to the intestinal mucosa, invasive ability, and toxins production. Tribble et al. showed that the minimum infection dose is 100 cells with an incubation time from 2 to 5 days.[18] As reported in Hansson et al.'s study the major symptoms caused by campylobacteriosis are self-limiting gastroenteritis and acute diarrhea, fever, abdominal cramps, and vomiting that can last from 2 to 10 days.[13] The infection may evolve in several complications such as acute colitis, acute appendicitis, colorectal cancer, and Barrett's esophagus. *Campylobacter* are also implicated in various human systemic infections including endocarditis, neonatal sepsis, pneumonia, and bloodstream infections. Other major postinfections added to campylobacteriosis disease include severe neuropathy, Guillain–Barré syndrome (GBS), and Miller–Fisher syndrome. In small group of patients, *Campylobacter* spp. have also been reported to be associated with extragastrointestinal infections such as brain abscesses, meningitis, lung infections, bacteremia, and arthritis.

The European Commission Regulation No. 2073/2005 which establishes microbiological criteria for specific food categories was amended with the commission regulation (European Union, EU) 2017/1495 introducing a hygiene criterion process for *Campylobacter*. This modification was based on the scientific opinion published on EFSA 2010, 2011, and 2012 on a public health hazard and risk from the consumption of broiler meat which identifies *Campylobacter* as of high public health relevance. Starting from 2018, the criteria for *Campylobacter* spp. are set as ≤ 1000 colony forming units (CFU)/g in the carcass of broiler after chilling (EU 2017/1495). The pressure on slaughterhouses to deliver chicken carcasses with low *Campylobacter* contamination to the EU market will increase in future. Currently the slaughterhouse has to collect five neck skin samples every week after cooling of the carcasses. If during a period of 10 weeks, 20 neck skin samples out of 50 are tested positive for *Campylobacter* numbers higher than 1000 CFU/g, the slaughterhouse must take actions to improve the slaughter hygiene. Since last year, this process hygiene criterion has become modified, with a limit of 15 neck skin samples out of 50, while starting from 2025, the number allowed will decrease further, to only 10 positive neck skin samples per 50.

51.3 Methods for *Campylobacter* detection

51.3.1 Official methods for *Campylobacter* detection

The current gold standard method used for the detection and enumeration of *Campylobacter* spp. is the ISO 10272:2017 (Fig. 51.2). It is applied on products for the human consumption and animal feeding, on environmental samples from production and transport area, and on samples from the primary production stage such as animal feces, swabs, and dust. The ISO 10272:1-2017 establishes three detection procedures for several food matrices depending on the estimated level of *Campylobacter* spp. and background microflora (Fig. 51.2A). Therefore the protocols include a selective enrichment step in Bolton broth or in Preston broth or a direct plating on modified charcoal cefoperazone (mCCDA) agar plates for samples with low number of *Campylobacter* and microflora; for samples with low number of *Campylobacter* and high microflora; and for samples with high number of *Campylobacter*, respectively. Instead, the ISO 10272:2-2017 establishes the enumeration method for the number

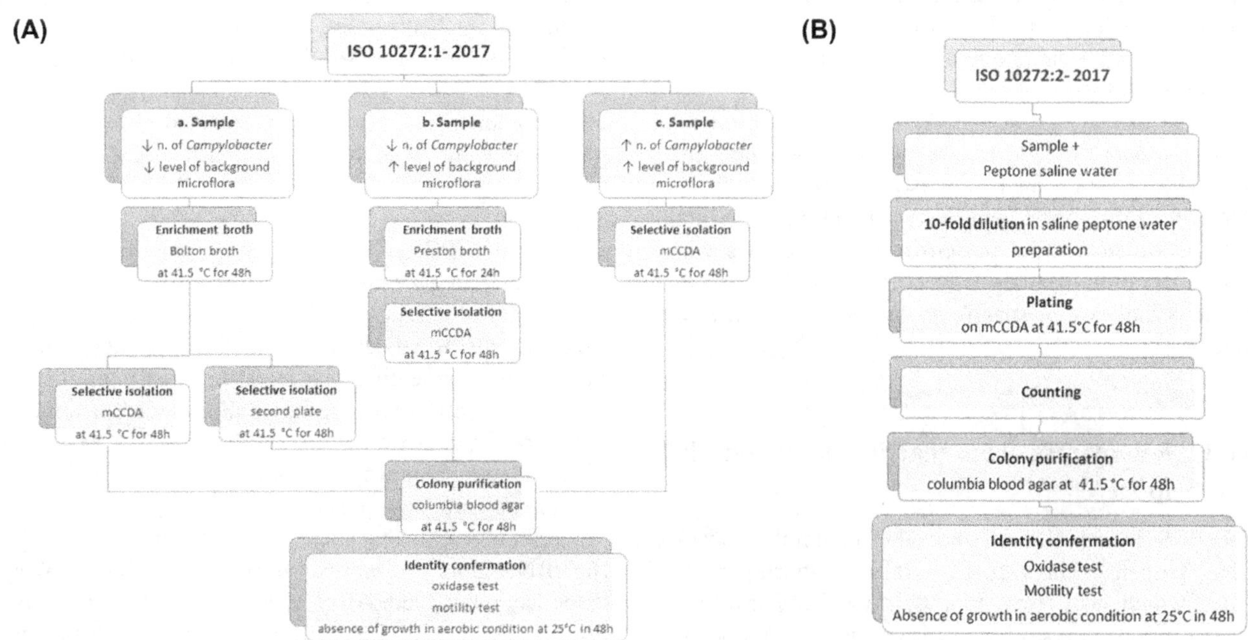

FIGURE 51.2 Schematic presentation of (A) the ISO 10272:1-2017 and (B) the ISO 10272:2-2017 methods for *Campylobacter* cells identification and quantification in food samples. Arrows indicate low or high level of *Campylobacter* and background microflora in the sample.

of *Campylobacter* CFU by plating in single the serial dilution of samples homogenized in peptone-salt solution. Fig. 51.2B illustrates the standard ISO 10272:2-2017 protocol for *Campylobacter* detection in poultry meat.

The official identification and quantification of *Campylobacter* spp. rely thus on culture-based methods, and bacterial biochemical/phenotypical characterization.[19] Taking into account the very low infective doses of *Campylobacter* (100 cells), an enrichment step in Preston or Bolton broth for 24–48 h before the isolation of the suspected colonies by culturing onto selective agar plates incubated in chambers for microaerophilic conditions, requiring additional 48–72 h, is needed. *Campylobacter* is usually present in low numbers in chicken meat and skin when compared to coliforms and Enterobacteriaceae making its isolation on common agar media difficult. The official method is, thus, time-consuming and expensive and does not meet the need of the food industry. Moreover, the complex official method for *Campylobacter* detection may provide false negative results as a consequence of its capability to enter in a viable but not culturable (VBNC) state in food matrices, making difficult its detection by culture-based methods.[19,20]

Classical microbiological methods for identification of *Campylobacter* by the optical microscope are not simple. As illustrated in Fig. 51.1, the bacterium can change its spiral distinctive shape into spherical or coccoid. Such morphological modifications are typical for *Campylobacter* cells under thermal or oxygen stress, condition of refrigerated chicken carcasses. Finally, the current problem of official methods is the lack of a high selective medium, and the emergence of bacterial resistance against the antibiotic added to make selective the enrichment broths.

Therefore we describe here rapid methods for *Campylobacter* detection like polymerase chain reaction (PCR), loop-mediated isothermal amplification (LAMP), biosensors, and next-generation sequencing (NGS). Molecular and biosensor-based methods which reduce the time of analysis in comparison to traditional methods and ensure specificity are needed by the food industry.

51.3.2 Polymerase chain reaction detection of *Campylobacter*

The PCR is a molecular tool able to amplify specific DNA sequences in vitro in a relative short period of time, which was first proposed by Kary Mullis in 1985.[21] Food analyses with PCR consist of (1) food sampling, (2) DNA extraction, (3) PCR amplification, and (4) result visualization. The amplification of the initial target DNA occurs through multiple cycles; each PCR cycle leads to a logarithmic base 2 increase of the number of the initial number of DNA molecules (2^n with n cycles). Three main steps are needed: denaturation of double-stranded DNA, annealing of primers to a single-stranded DNA, and extension of the new sequence due to the action of the DNA polymerase. Each PCR cycle composed of these three steps is repeated for 30–40 times.

A mixture composed of the following reagents: buffer solution, DNA polymerase, deoxyribonucleotide triphosphates (dNTPs), a couple of primers (forward and reverse), $MgCl_2$, and the DNA target to be amplified. Fig. 51.3A shows the PCR steps that lead to the production of millions of copies of the template.[22] To evaluate the success or failure of the PCR assay, the PCR product (amplicon) is run in an agarose gel. The length of the amplicons (bp number) is determined, to verify the correct amplification.

Mateo et al.[23] applied a PCR-based method for the detection of *Campylobacter* in poultry samples and compared the results with those obtained from the cultural method. Seventy-three samples (68 raw and 5 cooked chicken products) were purchased from supermarkets in Spain.[23] The detection of *Campylobacter* in the naturally contaminated samples, was based on the amplification of the 16S rRNA gene, with the production of an expected amplicon of 857 bp for its amplification. The limit of detection (LoD) of 5 and 40 CFU/mL was achieved with the plate count method and PCR, respectively. Furthermore, the time required to perform the PCR test even adding 24 h of enrichment, was of two days while the cultural method needed five days. Fontanot et al. used a pair of sensitive and specific primers for the detection of *C. jejuni* and *C. coli* in poultry meat samples.[24] The 24 h enrichment in Preston broth enabled to successfully apply the PCR protocol and to reach a LoD of 5and 1.5×10^2 cells/g of chicken meat for *C. jejuni* and *C. coli*, respectively.

Multiplex PCR allows the detection of more than one target sequence in only one reaction, thanks to the use of multiple sets of primers per reaction. To optimize the performance of this method, primers should have close annealing temperatures and amplicons should be of different lengths to allow their differentiation after the agarose gel electrophoresis.[25] A multiplex PCR was developed by Alves et al.[26] for detection of *Salmonella* spp. and *Campylobacter* spp. in naturally contaminated chicken meat samples. Primers for the 16S rRNA gene in *Campylobacter*, amplifying a 287 bp sequence, were used. After 24 h enrichment, it was possible to detect 10^2 CFU/mL of *C. jejuni*; while after 48 h of selective enrichment the LoD of 1 CFU/mL was achieved.

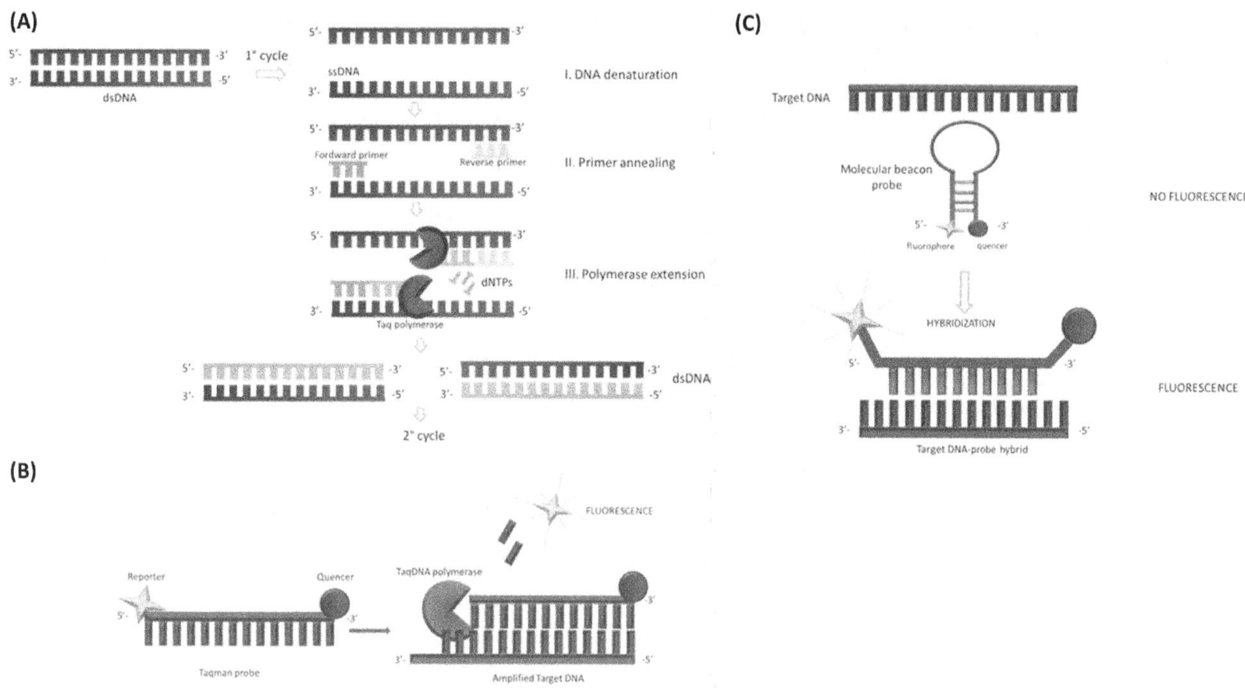

FIGURE 51.3 (A) Representation of the cyclic process of the polymerase chain reaction. (B) Structure and mechanism of action of TaqMan probe. (C) Schematic presentation of DNA detection using molecular beacon probe.

51.3.3 Real-time polymerase chain reaction detection of *Campylobacter*

Real-time PCR (RT-PCR), also called quantitative PCR (qPCR), differs from the classical PCR because it enables a quantitative analysis of specific DNA targets. The principle of qPCR is the quantification of the amount of the target DNA through the emission of fluorescence produced during the amplification cycles. The quantification is obtained by creating a calibration curve for testing serial decimal dilutions of the target analyte DNA by plotting fluorescence values versus number of cycles.[27,28] This method allows high sensitivity and low response time, but requires specialized personnel to be performed.[28] In addition, the method cannot distinguish between live and dead cells. To overcome the problem of detecting dead cells, a dye propidium-monoazide (PMA) can be used. PMA selectively penetrates the membrane of dead cells (compromised cells), and covalently binds the DNA, preventing the PMA-bound DNA to be amplified. The addition of PMA must be performed before the extraction of the DNA used as template.[29]

In RT-PCR, the fluorescence emission which allows a direct quantification of the target, can be obtained by using a DNA intercalator, such as SyBrGreen, or specific DNA labeled probes. The molecules of intercalating dyes (IDs) are able to bind reversibly to single- or double-stranded DNA producing signal proportional to the increase of intercalated IDs in the amplicons.[27] The main issue when intercalant molecules are used in RT-PCR is that they can intercalate any double-stranded DNA present in the reaction with no specificity. To eliminate such nonspecific signals, which would require a high-resolution melting analysis to verify result, specific labeled DNA probes were introduced in RT-PCR, in order to increase the specificity of the results.[30]

Specific probes (single-stranded oligonucleotide sequences) designed to be only complementary to the target DNA, contain two fluorescent molecules (fluorophores), a quencher at 5′ end of the sequence and a reporter at 3′ end. The energy emitted from the reporter after excitation by a laser is absorbed by the quencher. Once the reporter and the quencher are distanced the fluorescence emitted from the reporter is detected by the detection system present in the device. Hydrolysis and hybridization probes are used in RT-PCR. The hydrolysis probes (like TaqMan probes) enable a mechanism based on the $5' \rightarrow 3'$ exonuclease activity (Fig. 51.3B). These probes are designed to have the two fluorophores at a defined distance, which allows the absorption of reporter emitted light from quencher. During amplification, the TaqMan probe binds the target sequence, and during extension step, the DNA polymerase displaces the reporter bound at the first nucleotide of the probe through its $5' \rightarrow 3'$ exonuclease activity. Once the reporter is far from the quencher its fluorescence can be detected. The utilization of a specific probe avoids the use of the high melting curve analysis.[31]

Also, RT-PCR uses mRNA as template in place of DNA, to avoid the possible amplification of DNA from dead cells. Lv et al. integrated PMA with qPCR targeting the *rpoB* gene to detect and quantify *C. jejuni* in the VBNC state, obtained by an exogenously applied osmotic stress (i.e., 7% NaCl).[32] The PMA-qPCR test was highly specific for *C. jejuni* with a LoD of 2.43 log CFU/mL in pure bacterial culture, and 3.12 log CFU/g for VBNC *C. jejuni* from chicken breasts. Hybridization probes such as beacon probes[31] emit a fluorescent signal during annealing and extension phase (Fig. 51.3C) following the same principle of TaqMan. A nucleic acid sequence–based amplification assay based on molecular beacons was used for real-time detection of *C. jejuni* and *C. coli* in samples of chicken meat.[33] Molecular beacons were utilized also in a multiplex RT-PCR for simultaneous detection of eight foodborne pathogens in a single reaction in clinical samples.[34] This assay took advantage of modified molecular beacons and the multicolor combinational probe coding strategy to discriminate *C. jejuni* from other pathogens with the detection limits of about 5×10^3 CFU/g stool.

Although, RT-PCR is fast, sensitive, specific, and quantitative, it relies on enzymes which can be inhibited by contaminants present in food or enrichment broth providing false-negative results. To avoid inhibition of the test, and the detection of dead cells, Wolffs et al. applied RT-PCR in combination with a discontinuous buoyant density gradient method, called flotation.[35] Studying the buoyant densities of different *Campylobacter* spp., authors observed that densities changed during growth but all varied among ranges from 1.065 to 1.109 g/mL. These data enabled development of a flotation assay to distinguish viable and VBNC cells from dead cells. RT-PCR applied after the flotation enabled *Campylobacter* detection with the LoD as low as 8.6×10^2 CFU/mL without culture enrichment. The quantification was possible with the LoD of 2.6×10^3 CFU/mL. Furthermore, the flotation method was validated using samples containing VBNC and dead cells after their storage at 4°C or 20°C for 21 days. A similar amount of the VBNC cells was detected using RT-PCR and 5-cyano-2,3-ditolyl tetrazolium chloride-4′,6′-diamidino-2-phenylindole staining.

51.3.4 Droplet digital polymerase chain reaction detection of *Campylobacter*

The digital PCR (dPCR) technology has emerged as a powerful tool for precise quantification of nucleic acids with higher sensitivity and reproducibility compared to qPCR. One of major advantages of dPCR is the absolute quantification with no calibration curve required. It is based on dividing the studied sample into a large number of partitions in order to perform a multitude of PCR reactions simultaneously. The sample is serially diluted to achieve a limiting dilution, where each partition contains, at most, one target DNA molecule. Recently, droplet digital PCR (ddPCR) has been introduced in food microbiology analysis.[36] ddPCR includes the use of aqueous droplets (containing the target DNA and the reaction mixture required for PCR) dispersed in oil to compartmentalize PCR reactions. After encapsulation of the DNA molecules in microdroplets (10,000–20,000), the latter are injected into a thermal cycler in order to carry out the PCR reaction. The droplets are then reinjected into a reader which measures the fluorescence (fluorescent probes or molecules intercalating in DNA) of each of the droplets at the end point of the PCR reaction. Counting the number of positive droplets in relation to their total number makes it possible to directly calculate a number of target DNA copies/μL, after readjustment according to Poisson statistics. Compared to qPCR, dPCR is less sensitive to the presence of inhibitors, possibly through the effect of dilution and compartmentalization. Recently, Peruzy et al. evaluated the presence of *Campylobacter* spp. in different food samples by RT-PCR and ddPCR.[37] In this work, ddPCR allowed the quantification of low numbers of target molecules (10 CFU/mL). The authors proposed a novel analytic approach based on an initial screening of the samples with RT-PCR and then on rapid and precise quantification of *Campylobacter* spp. with a ddPCR on those samples resulted positive.

51.3.5 Loop-mediated isothermal amplification detection of *Campylobacter*

The development and advent of PCR in the early 1980s, found widespread application in all areas of life science and transformed molecular biology. PCR became the most powerful tool in molecular diagnostics due to the ability of the technique to amplify a target nucleic acid sequence in large numbers. However, PCR-based methods require highly skilled personnel, expensive equipment and facilities, in order to test at any given location. To overcome these limitations, several different nucleic acid amplification methods have been developed over that last 30 years. The one method that attracted the most scientific interest is LAMP method. The simplicity, robustness, and low cost of the method are what have attracted the most attention.[38] LAMP exhibits excellent specificity because of the use of 4–6 specific primers that bind to 6 (or 8) different regions of the target sequence. The use of three primer sets, namely, an inner primer set (FIP and BIP), an outer primer set (F3 and B3), and a loop primer set (LF and LB), results in highly specific, sensitive, and rapid reactions,[39] as illustrated in Fig. 51.4. The

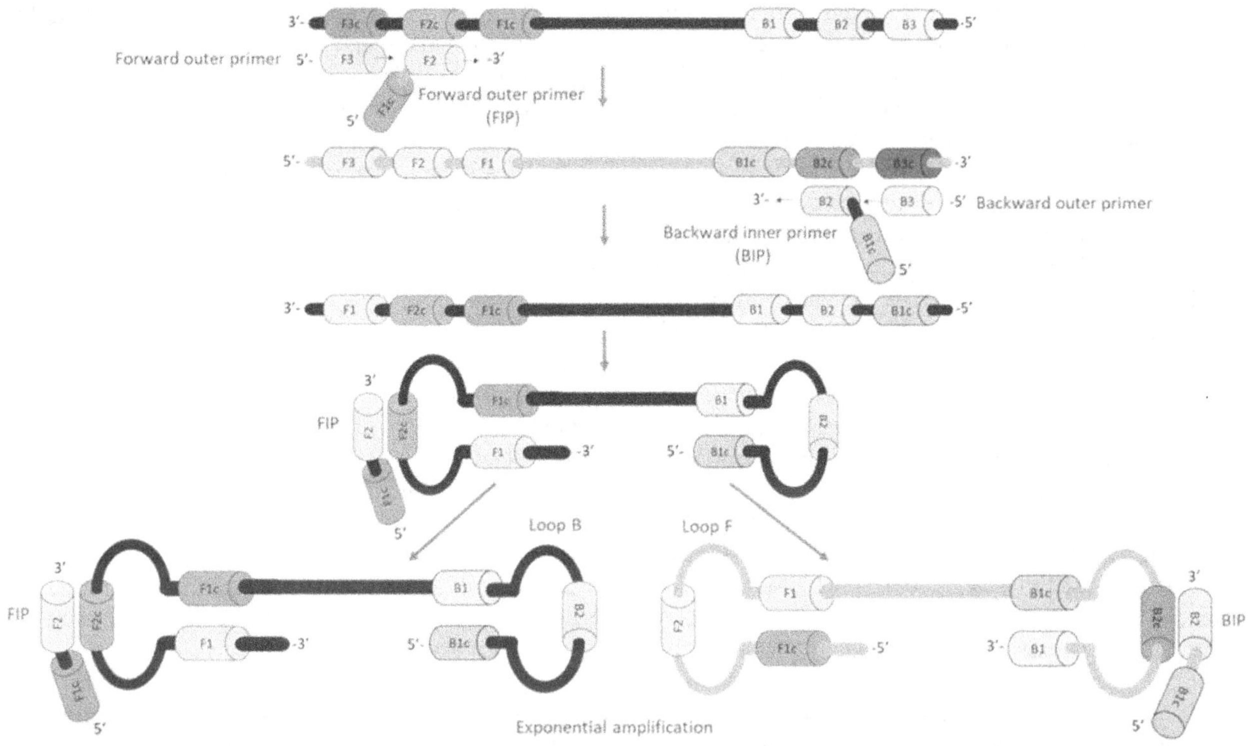

FIGURE 51.4 Illustration of loop-mediated isothermal amplification principle.

amplification of nucleic acid can be simply achieved under isothermal conditions ranging from 60°C to 65°C by using Bst DNA polymerase, an enzyme that demonstrates highly displacement activity. In addition, the Bst DNA polymerase provides superior tolerance to inhibitory substances that could typically hinder a PCR-based method.[40]

During the first stage of LAMP reaction the two sets of primers, the inner primer set and the outer primer set, hybridizing to their target sequences and strand-displacing Bst DNA polymerase initiate complementary strand synthesis resulting in the formation of a stem-loop structure. At the second stage of LAMP the third primer set, the loop primer set, can be added and elongation reactions are consecutively repeated by using the stem-loop regions as a stage. The addition of loop primers results in exponential amplification of LAMP amplicons in a short period of time. The end product of LAMP repeats of a short target sequence linked together with the loop structure resulting in large cauliflower-like structures. This method is based on the principle of the high production of a large quantity of DNA amplification products.

Many advancements and variations of the LAMP have occurred since its initial description in 2000.[39] In 2002 Nagamine et al. presented the third set of LAMP primers, the loop primers, which accelerated the LAMP reaction and allowed production of very large amounts of DNA in a short period of time.[41] Subsequently, the conventional LAMP was combined with other methods and different forms of LAMP were developed, including RT-LAMP, multiplex LAMP, real-time LAMP, and others.

DNA resulting from LAMP method is not suitable for downstream applications. The amount of DNA produced by this method, however, is so large that allows visualization of the end product in numerous modes which makes this DNA amplification method so appealing. The naked eye detection of LAMP amplicons or under ultraviolet (UV) light eliminates the need for expensive apparatuses, as well as, providing an excellent point of test method.[42] Simple end-point detection methods of the LAMP amplicons include observing changes in the turbidity, colorimetric detection visible by the naked eye, or detection under UV light. During LAMP reactions apart from large amount of DNA produced also large amounts of byproducts are released, which can be used for detecting positive results in the reaction tube. For example, pyrophosphate ions released as dNTPs are integrated into the DNA strands and produce a white precipitate when it binds to magnesium present in the reaction mixture. This precipitate is produced in large amounts and its presence is proportional to the amount of DNA produced during the reaction. The white precipitate can be easily visualized by observing changes in the turbidity of the reaction tube or by the formation of a white pellet after centrifuging the tube. Alternative, the precipitate formation can be measured in real time by measuring the turbidity in the reaction tube at certain time intervals. Similarly, the hydroxynaphthol blue dye can be used, which changes color from violet to blue when depletion of magnesium ions occurs in the reaction mixture. Thus instead of observing a change in turbidity a very obvious color change will appear when DNA amplification will occur in the reaction tube. Calcein dye also produces a distinct color change, from orange to yellow-green, when the manganese ion from the dye forms a complex with pyrophosphate produced during DNA polymerization. The color change is visible by naked eye as well as bright fluorescence under UV light. Fluorescent DNA stains, such as SYBR green and EvaGreen, have also been used for LAMP detection that directly identifies double-stranded DNA formation in the reaction tube. Fluorescent dyes can be added at the beginning or at the end of the reaction depending on the dye chosen, since some DNA dyes seem to inhibit DNA formation. Fluorescent dyes have also been used to develop real-time LAMP assays.

Lateral flow assay is about special technique because of the low cost, user-friendly, simplicity, rapidity, and portability. The sample is applied at one end of the strip (sample pad), which has been combined with LAMP buffer mix because of plenty of advantages that these two techniques combine. A suitable background for interaction with the detection system that gave the opportunity for a development of a mobile biosensor with LAMP technology application. The progress of sensors leads to the detection of pathogens directly from an environmental sample which brings vast benefits, especially in foodborne diseases.[42]

During the LAMP reaction, high amounts of white magnesium pyrophosphate precipitate and DNA amplicon about 400 ng/μL in 0.2 mL PCR reaction vials permitted a simpler and inexpensive means for detection.[43] It can therefore be detected even by naked eyes when using appropriate DNA staining techniques[44] or fluorescence,[45] either in end point or real-time formats by using water bath or commercial RT-PCR instrument.[43] Amplification times of typically vary between 30 and 90 min, depending on the starting DNA template.[46]

The resulting LAMP amplicons can be visualized by the naked eye, or using colorimetric and lateral flow biosensors, obviating the need for expensive apparatuses. However, there is a susceptibility to obtain false positives due to cross-contamination, nonspecific amplification, or primer dimerization.[42] The use of various compounds such as dimethyl sulfoxide (DMSO),[47] pullulan,[48] betaine,[39] increased LAMP sensitivity and specificity. With these advantages, LAMP has currently emerged as a promising candidate for reliable identification of *Campylobacter* spp.[49]

A portable device was proposed in the detection of *C. jejuni* and *C. coli* in poultry products. LAMP products were detected using a small, low-cost portable commercial blue LED trans-illuminator and a direct visual detection strategy was demonstrated. The analytical sensitivity of 50 CFU/mL was achieved for testing of *C. jejuni* and *C. coli* in spiked chicken feces without enrichment. The whole procedure needed 60–70 min including the time for amplification to the final results. The results showed that the method is specific, sensitive, and is suitable to develop for rapid detection of *Campylobacter* spp. at poultry production.[50]

A very interesting approach was proposed by Thongphueak et al. in 2019. The detection of *Campylobacter* spp. in meat samples which was developed by using LAMP combined with DNA-based bioassay methods, including a lateral flow dipstick (LFD) and gold nanoparticles (AgNPs)-DNA probe assay.[51] The primers were designed from the conserved nucleotide regions of *Campylobacter* spp. The LoD of the LAMP-LFD and LAMP-AuNPs analysis was 360 fg/μL.

The LAMP amplification was applied in bovine specimens spiked with *Campylobacter fetus*. The simple and rapid LAMP assay proposed the surveillance of *C. fetus* in screening of bovine liver and vaginal mucus specimens. The investigations are focusing on the determination of causative agents of food poisoning.[52]

The rapidness of this method enables the identification of *Campylobacter* in two different conditions: flocks in slaughter before and after a freezing/heating treatment, in order to check for the effective slaughterhouses control strategy for preventing campylobacteriosis. A LAMP assay for the direct screening of naturally contaminated chicken cloacal swabs for *C. jejuni*/*C. coli* was conducted to compare the result with conventional quantitative culture methods. The results showed that high sensitivity, specificity, positive predictive value, and negative predictive value. In this study, the LAMP assay lasted less than 90 min from the arrival of the fecal samples in the laboratory until final results. This work showed that LAMP is an accurate, rapid, and easy-to-perform tool to prevent the spread of *Campylobacter* contamination between broiler flocks at the farm level or in slaughterhouses before slaughtering.[53]

The need to prevent and secure the poultry products in a short time leads to today's fast-paced food supply chain. The comparative advantage of this research is that it does not require bacterial culture or DNA purification and the results obtained in just an hour. The detection of *Campylobacter* with LAMP in slaughterhouses, showed 100% positive results of swabs with an enumeration result of 800 CFU/swab, and 98.6% (69 out of 70) of samples reported as negative by enumeration (10 CFU/swab) compared with conventional culture-based enumeration methods. This test could also be used in boot swabs from poultry houses, and in that way it represents a convenient screening tool that can be implemented on farm and at slaughterhouses in order to reinforce the control of *Campylobacter* contamination throughout the food supply chain.[54]

The challenges in diagnosing infectious disease permit the advent of portable, easy-to-use diagnostic tools capable of detecting a wide range of microbes. A microfluidic platform that combined ultrasensitive immunoassay and LAMP method was proposed. A disposable disk with automatic sampling inlets is paired with a noncontact heating system and precise rotary control system to yield an easy-to-use platform. The detection of pathogens showed an analytical sensitivity of about 1−30 cells in stool matrix in an hour. The specific advantage of radiative heating is the ability to introduce optical elements to control temperature by modulating incident radiation with an opaque barrier or neutral density filters for intermediate temperature states. In addition, changing the rotational speed of the disc during heating in order to manipulate convective cooling can also help modulate temperature. This heating system, when combined with a precision rotary control system and a high-sensitivity optical detection system, yields a versatile, portable technology capable of providing accurate diagnostic data for myriad purposes, such as guiding the treatment of individual patients, helping combat the increasing levels of antimicrobial resistance, aiding in outbreak tracking and routine public health surveillance, and driving targeted vaccination programs.[55]

A detailed work reported 10 *Campylobacter* strains and 13 non-*Campylobacter* bacterial species based on immunomagnetic separation and LAMP. Swab samples were analyzed by using LAMP method in 90 min duration without enrichment or DNA purification. It had 74% probability of detecting 10^4 CFU/mL of a boot swab suspension. The analysis in poultry farms showed 100% correlation with parallel results obtained by standard microbiological methods.[54]

An intersecting approach was developed by Alamer et al.[56] They developed a cotton swab detection system that involves all the steps into an integrated bacterial collection, preconcentration, and detection on Q-tips.[56] The platform was based on a sandwich assay that detects different pathogens visually by color changes. To concentrate and collect pathogens, lactoferrin was immobilized on cotton and used as capturing tool from surfaces. The procedure follows by the immersion of the cotton conjugated with antibodies to different colored nanobeads. The target cell captured between the lactoferrin and the specific antibody-conjugated beads resulted in a change of color due to the beads aggregation. The results indicated that the developed method can be applied not only for qualitative determination, but also for semiquantitative detection because of the difference in color intensity with increasing the concentration of the pathogenic bacteria. The analytical limitation was 10 CFU/mL on chicken meat surfaces.[56]

51.3.6 DNA dot blot detection of *Campylobacter*

The DNA dot blot test is a simple technique that enables to detect unfractionated genomic DNA after its immobilization on a nitrocellulose or nylon membrane. Hybridization with a specific labeled DNA probe is carried out on the paper to analyze the presence and relative abundance of target sequences in the blotted DNA sample. DNA dot blot sensors are usually associated with a PCR step, including LAMP, to allow for detection of pathogens in low titers in food samples. In contrast to PCR-based methods, dot blot tests are not sensitive to inhibitor molecules from food matrices as they are based on hybridization.

Fontanot et al. applied the dot blot method to detect *C. jejuni* and *C. coli in* poultry meat samples.[24] The target DNA were extracted from the Preston enrichment broth at 24 h, immobilized on nylon membrane, and hybridized with specific digoxigenin-labeled ssDNA probe. Upon subsequent addition of the phosphatase-conjugated antidigoxigenin antibody a colorimetric read-out provided the bacterial quantification. The LoD of 25 ng/μL was obtained from the analyzed contaminated samples.

Recently, the proof-of-concept of the highly sensitivity, cost-effective, specific, and easy-to-perform dot blot assay for *Campylobacter* spp. detection was demonstrated.[57] The sensitivity was improved by newly designed highly specific DNA probe that recognizes several points in the 16S rRNA gene of the most prevalent *Campylobacter* spp. causing infections *C. jejuni*, *C. coli*, *C. lari*, and *C. upsaliensis*. After hybridization with the biotin-labeled probe, silica nanoparticles (Si-NPs) carrying multiple biotin tags were attached to the detection probe via streptavidin molecules. In the next step, the Si-NPs enabled to attach multiple streptavidin−horseradish peroxidase molecules. Utilization of biotin-Si-NPs boosted the strepatavidin−horseradish chemiluminescent signal read-out over 30 times compared to a single streptavidin molecule and enabled direct bacterial detection in naturally contaminated chicken meat samples without any preamplification step. A LoD of 3 pg/μL of DNA, similar to those obtained by RT-PCR, was achieved (Fig. 51.5A). Compared to RT-PCR this enhanced dot blot sensor is cheaper, easier, and insensitive to inhibition of DNA polymerase by molecules from the food matrices.

51.3.7 Immunochromatographic assay for *Campylobacter*

Lateral flow assay, also known as lateral flow immunochromatographic assay, is a paper-based method, which allows an easy, rapid, and cost-less bacterial biomarker detection. He et al. developed a rapid and specific paper-based immunochromatographic assay for *Campylobacter*

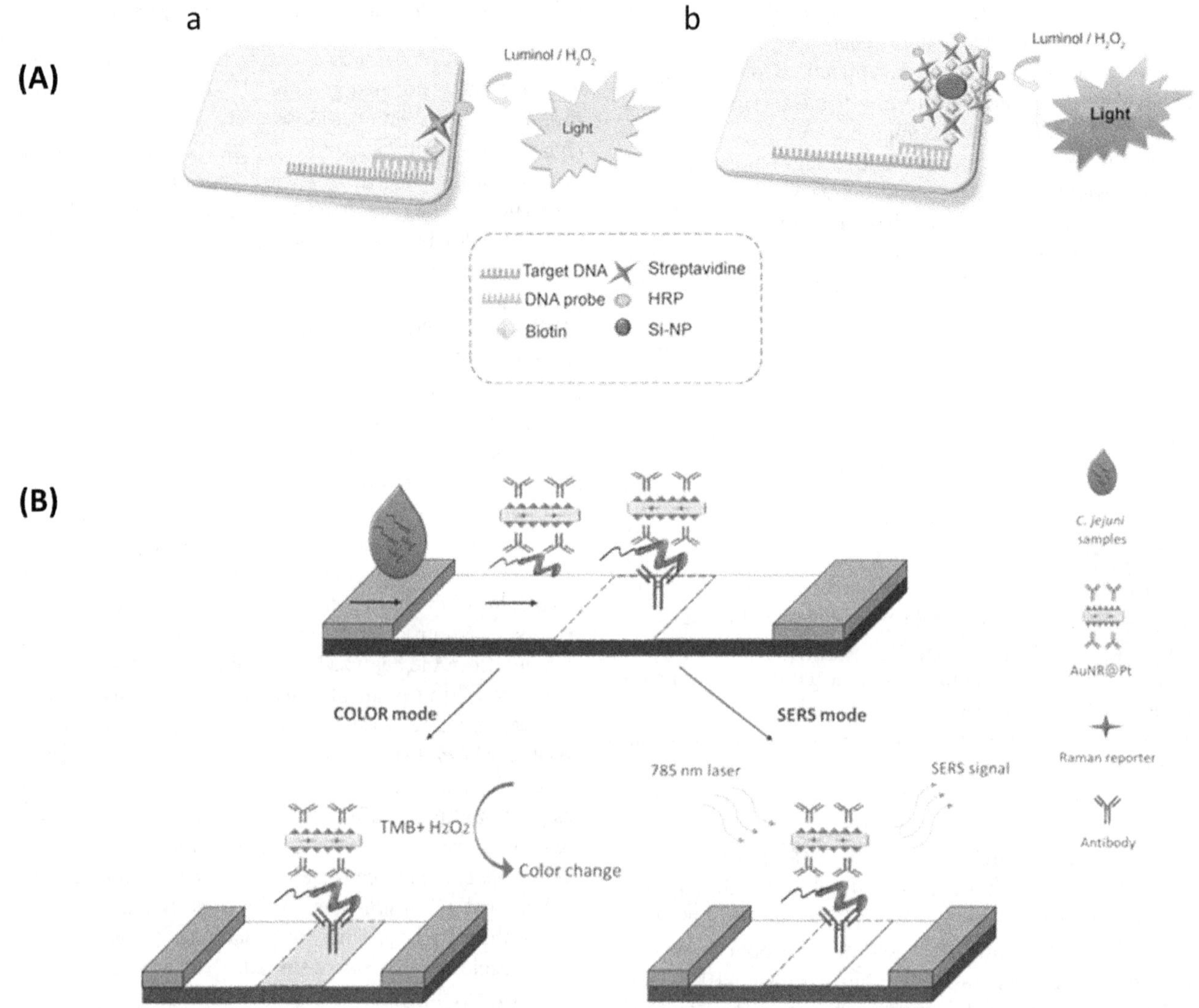

FIGURE 51.5 (A) Schematic representation of *Campylobacter* detection on paper-based DNA hybridization with a complementary biotinylated DNA probe, and a streptavidin-HRP read-out through dot blot (a). The signal was amplified using highly functionalized biotin-Si-NPs instead of a single biotin (b). (B) Lateral flow assay for detection of *C. jejuni* by colorimetric and surface-enhanced Raman scattering mode using AuNR@Pt. *HRP*, The enzyme horseradish peroxidase. *(A) With permission from Vizzini P, Manzano M, Farre C, et al. Highly sensitive detection of* Campylobacter *spp. in chicken meat using a silica nanoparticle enhanced dot blot DNA biosensor.* Biosens Bioelectron. *2021;171: 112689. (B) Adapted from He D, Wu Z, Cui B, Xu E, Jin Z. Establishment of a dual mode immunochromatographic assay for* Campylobacter jejuni *detection.* Food Chem. *2019;289:708–713.*

detection with a wide detection range, low detection limit, high specificity and sensitivity.[58] The assay was implemented with nanoenzyme technology and the bacterium was detected using simultaneously the color signal and surface-enhanced Raman scattering (SERS) signal, in order to increase the assay sensitivity. Platinum-coated gold nanorods (AuNR@Pt), used as signal amplifier, were synthesized and conjugated with Raman reporter and anti-*Campylobacter* specific antibodies. After the addition of the sample, it flowed longitudinally by capillarity (Fig. 51.5B). Upon *C. jejuni* cells binding to the antibodies attached to the AuNR@Pt NPs, the formed complex continued to flow until conjugate with the capture antibodies immobilized at the test line. When 3′,3′,5,5′-tetramethylbenzidine (TMB) substrate and H_2O_2 are added, AuNR@Pt generated a strong emission of blue color. The product obtained due to the rapid catalytic oxidation, provided SERS spectra under laser excitations at 785 nm. Both color and SERS signal intensity were proportional to *C. jejuni* concentration in the range of 10^2–10^6 and 10^2–5×10^6 CFU/mL with LoD of 75 and 50 CFU/mL, respectively.[58]

51.3.8 Electrochemical biosensors for *Campylobacter* detection

Electrochemical biosensors are frequently chosen for bacterial detection because of their advantages: low cost, sensitive, and easy to miniaturize.[19,59,60] They also offer a rapid analysis and they can be used with turbid samples.[61] One of the principal reasons that make these sensors widely used is the easy implementation with antibody-based techniques, DNA probes and aptamers, and solutions that can reduce low selectivity problems.[20,59] The main electrochemical biosensor techniques are the amperometric/voltammetric, impedimetric, and conductimetric.[62]

Amperometric biosensors are usually based on a three-electrode system (working electrode, reference electrode, and counter electrode) and the most widely used mode with it are the cyclic voltammetry, linear sweep voltammetry, and amperometry.[63] Amperometric biosensors exploit the proportional relation between the concentration of the analyte and its reduction/oxidation current peak at a specific potential.[64] These sensors are typically implemented with DNA base pairing, antibody–antigen or enzyme–reagent interactions.[61] Ivintski et al. developed a technique based on the electron transfer through a bilayer lipid membrane using antibodies specific for *Campylobacter* spp.[65] Another example is the antibody-bacteria-antibody strategy used by Viswanathan et al.: antibodies specific for *Campylobacter* spp. were immobilized on a screen-printed electrode.[66] After exposure to bovine milk spiked with *Campylobacter*, the electrode was immersed in a solution containing antibody-conjugated Pbs nanocrystals. The signal obtained by the square-wave anodic stripping voltammetry and correlated to the number of cells, had a LoD of 4×10^2 CFU/mL.

Unlike amperometric biosensors, impedimetric biosensor always functions close to the equilibrium state. This enables to obtain highly stable responses that can be averaged over a long-time range to yield a precise measurement. The current–voltage relation can be used around the equilibrium potential indicated by the current-over potential equation and can be carried out over a wide frequency range, such as 10^6-10^{-4} Hz.[63] Huang et al. studied an impedimetric biosensor based on a glassy carbon electrode with modified Fe_3O_4 NPs for the detection of *C. jejuni*.[67] The detection was performed by measuring relative impedance change before and after *C. jejuni* addition to the electrode carrying a specific anti-*Campylobacter* antibody. Under the optimized conditions, the relative change in impedance was proportional to the logarithmic value of *C. jejuni* concentrations ranging from 1.0×10^3 to 1.0×10^7 CFU/mL in diarrhea patients' stool samples without an enrichment step.

Another promising approach was based on the measurement of the change in conductance carried by microorganism' metabolites between a pair of electrodes. The main advantage of this technique is that no labeling is needed. However, the method suffers from a high variability, as observed for *C. jejuni* detection.[68] To detect *C. jejuni*, the conductimetric analysis was performed on numerous basal medium components to develop a growth-enhancing broth medium for detection of freeze-injured bacterial cells. Using stressed *Campylobacter* cultures, a direct linear relationship was observed between detection times and the initial inoculum level with the LoD of 10, 100, 1000, and 10,000 CFU/mL after 28.6, 24.9, 21.4, and 17.0 h of inoculation, respectively.

51.3.9 Optical biosensors for *Campylobacter* detection

Optical biosensors exploit the interaction between a light and a biorecognition element, giving a signal proportional to the concentration of the analyte. They are the most common type of biosensor. They offer multiple advantages, such as high specificity and sensitivity, a real-time and nondestructive detection, and cost-effectiveness. In the last decades, an intense development has been made thanks to this technology in the approach to different disciplines including microelectronics, micro/nanotechnologies, chemistry, molecular biology, and biotechnology.[69] Several optical sensors have been reported for *Campylobacter* detection. A surface plasmon resonance (SPR) biosensor was firstly developed by Sista et al. for real-time detection of *Campylobacter* spp. with a detection range from 10^2 to 10^9 CFU/mL.[70] The SPR sensing strategy is based on the reflected light intensity or the resonance angle shifts evaluation occurred when a light source is reflected after passing through a prism covered by a thin metal layer. More in depth, at the « resonance angle » level, once the light pass by the glass prism and arrives at the metal surface, light is absorbed by the electrons on the metal field causing their resonation. This phenomenon (SPR) causes a decrease in the intensity of the reflected light, resulting in shifts in the reflectivity curves. The curve shift depends on the bound or unbound status of the immobilized molecule onto the metal surface with the target analyte.

The specificity of detection can be obtained by immobilization of the specific anti-*Campylobacter* antibody[71] or the receptor-binding protein of *Campylobacter* bacteriophage NCTC 12673[72] on the gold surface of the sensor chip. Although SPR biosensors are widely used due to their rapidity and sensitivity, total internal reflection can occur, given the restricted degree of penetration of the evanescent film. To solve this problem Masdor et al. have developed a subtractive inhibition assay-SPR (SIA-SPR) for the detection of *C. jejuni*.[73] This method is based on two antibody binding reactions. For this, a primary antibody (a rabbit polyclonal antibody specific for *C. jejuni*) was added to the chicken sample matrix and mixed with an increasing concentration of *C. jejuni*, going from 1×10^1 to 1×10^7 CFU/mL. After 1 h, unbound molecules of antibody were separated from the cell-bound antibodies through a sequential centrifugation step. The authors performed also tried a filtration step, but they highlighted a limitation of this technique that the filter entrapped the antibody, and therefore its final concentration was not correct. Meanwhile, the secondary antibody, a goat F(ab) antirabbit IgG, was immobilized on the golden biosensor surface. By now, the supernatant obtained from the centrifugation (containing the free unbounded antibodies) was injected on the immobilized antibody on the SPR sensor surface to quantify the concentration of *C. jejuni* detected. The SPR signal was maximum in the absence of the target and decreased for contaminated samples. The LoD resulting from the use of this SIA-SPR was 131 ± 4 CFU/mL.

Shams et al. studied a ssDNA-GNRs (gold nanorods) nanobiosensor for the specific detection of *C. jejuni* and *C. coli*. GNRs were prepared and characterized by using UV-vis spectrophotometer (400–900 nm) to obtain the SPR characteristics.[74] The biorecognition element used was a ssDNA probe specific to the *cadF* gene of *Campylobacter*. The probe was synthesized with a thiol group (–SH) at its 5′ to allow surface functionalization due to the covalent binding of the ssDNA with the gold surface. After the formation of the complex ssDNA-GNRs (with different concentrations of the probe) UV-vis spectroscopy was used for its monitoring. First, the biosensor properties were evaluated using recombinant plasmid (pTG19-T/cadF), used as positive control, and a synthetic single-stranded probe (95 bp). Second, the samples used for a direct evaluation were collected directly from 283 stool samples of children with suspected campylobacteriosis. An immediate change in SPR absorbance was recorded by UV-vis spectrophotometry in presence of the target gene. The specificity of the test was 100%, the sensitivity 88% and the LoD was 10^2 copy number/L of stool. Wei et al. developed a SPR biosensor based on polyclonal antibodies that detected *C. jejuni* with a LoD of 10^3 CFU/mL in a pure culture and rinse water of spiked broiler meat within 30–45 min.[75] However authors pointed out that further improvements of the sensor are needed because of the significant interfering of meat proteins and lipids to the signal. Optical SPR sensors may have a multiplex format to enable simultaneously real-time detection of different bacteria. Taylor et al. detected *E. coli* O157:H7, *Salmonella* typhimurium, *Listeria monocytogenes*, and *C. jejuni*, in both phosphate buffered saline (PBS) and spiked apple juice using a multichannel SPR.[71] Results showed a LoD of 1.1×10^5 CFU/mL for *Campylobacter*. Substituting antibodies by the receptor-binding protein of *Campylobacter* bacteriophage NCTC 12673 resulted in a selective and sensitive detection of *C. jejuni* with a LoD of 10^2 CFU/mL.[72] The protein was immobilized on the gold surface of the sensor chip by the oriented immobilization of glutathione S-transferase-Gp48 protein using glutathione self-assembled monolayers. Furthermore, it was shown the feasibility of phage receptor-binding proteins to be immobilized onto magnetic beads for bacteria preconcentration purposes, allowing a faster performance of the sensor even with a large sample volume compared to whole phages.

Another example of optical sensor is the total internal reflection fluorescence array biosensor, a technique that allows detection through the excitement of a fluorophore conjugated to bio-probes specific for the analyte, such as antibodies. Sapsford et al. developed an array biosensor implemented with a sandwich immunoassay complex for the detection of *C. jejuni* and other pathogens in a complex food matrix.[76]

Fluorescence resonance energy transfer (FRET) is another common optical technique, based on the energy transfer that occurs between a photo-excited donor chromophore and an acceptor fluorescent molecule which is located at a distance of less than 10 nm. An example is the miniaturized AgNPs-based FRET probe developed by Darbha et al. for the detection of *Campylobacter* DNA.[77]

Organic light-emitting diode/device (OLED) is a technology that uses a fluorescence excitation source in different optical detection techniques. It can be implemented in a protein-microarray. OLED scans the microarray surface and the fluorescence signal is then detected by a charcoal cefoperazone deoxycholate (CCD) camera and processed.[78] Manzano et al. developed a biochip for *Campylobacter* spp. detection based on OLED which allowed to reveal the presence of a hybrid generated by annealing between a DNA probe labeled with a fluorophore and the DNA target.[79] This led to a short time and highly sensitive detection (0.37 ng/μL of genomic DNA).

51.3.10 Colorimetric assays for *Campylobacter* detection

Amid the biosensors for *Campylobacter* detection, colorimetric sensors based on AuNPs are particularly interesting because they enable real-time and *in situ* detection without any instrumentation. AuNPs colorimetric assay owns a peculiar physical phenomenon called localized SPR (LSPR). The optical phenomenon occurs due to the particles' small sizes (2–100 nm). Different color shades can be obtained depending on the particles size, shape, and distance. The AuNPs detection strategy is commonly based on a color change due to the aggregation of the NPs in the presence of the target once salt is added as a breaking agent of the attractive and repulsive forces involved. The importance of this type of assay arose due to AuNPs simple surface functionalization with different recognition elements (such as proteins, ssDNA, antibodies, aptamers), high specificity and sensitivity. Depending on the recognition element with, it is possible to detect biomarker molecules, DNA sequence, or even whole bacteria cells. For instance, aptamers are frequently used instead of antibodies with the aim to detect the entire bacterial cell due to their specificity, lower cost, and easier production. Furthermore, these types of sensors require small amount of reagents or samples and do not need specific high skilled personnel or sophisticated instrumentations, which allow them to be a cost-effective biosensor.[80] These advantages, together with the naked eye visualization, enhanced the AuNPs colorimetric sensor to be a really competitive technology in comparison with the commonly used ones.

Kim et al. developed a two-stage label-free assay for *Campylobacter* detection in chicken carcasses using AuNPs and specific aptamers that recognized the whole bacterial cells (Fig. 51.6A).[81] Red solution of stabilized AuNPs changed the color to purple in the presence of the bacterial cells. The LoD as low as 7.2×10^5 and 5.6×10^5 CFU/mL was obtained for *C. jejuni* and *C. coli*, respectively, in chicken carcass rinse within 30 min. The assay was optimized by adding adenine base to the aptamer sequence in order to improve its adsorption to the gold surface. Other factors, such as the AuNPs/aptamer ration, pH of the solution, and type and concentration of salt, were explored and optimized to enhance the sensor efficiency. The authors pointed out different outcomes depending on the pathogens growth phase. The main limitation of the assay came from its inefficacy to detect stressed *Campylobacter* cells. The aptamer used as a recognition element was selected to bind spiral *Campylobacter* cells but not those of spherical or coccoid morphology.

Other strategies using enzyme or enzyme-like activity exploited by the NPs, were elaborated in order to provoke a visible color change in the presence of the target pathogen. Dehghani et al. took advantage of the peculiar peroxidase-like activity of palladium (Pd) to develop a gold-coated NP (Au@Pd) colorimetric aptasensor for *C. jejuni* detection in milk (Fig. 51.6B).[82] The visible color change was dependent on the amount of aptamers adsorbed onto the metal surface; the more the aptamers were, the more peroxidase-like activity was inhibited and more substrate (TMB) oxidation decreased. As depicted in Fig. 51.5, the color change was dependent on the TMB oxidation which desorb from Au@Pd surface in the presence of bacterial cells. The LoD of only 100 CFU/mL was detected in spiked milk. This technology allowed to identify the whole *C. jejuni* cells in less than 2 h.

With a different approach, McVey et al. used the RNase H enzymatic activity to detect *C. jejuni* DNA extracted from contaminated chicken meat.[83] AuNPs were functionalized with RNA that specifically hybridized with the selected *C. jejuni* DNA fragment. Once the complex RNA-DNA formed, the RNA was enzymatically cleaved to allow the DNA to hybridize with another RNA strand. Once all RNA fragments onto the AuNPs surface were cleaved, the addition of the NaCl enabled the color change by the NPs aggregation. In the absence of the target DNA, no cleavage occurred due to the absence of RNA-DNA structure and the RNA on the AuNPs surface acted as a steric hindrance for AuNPs aggregation, so no color change was observed after NaCl addition. This assay allowed to detect 1.2 pM and 18.0 fM of the target DNA by means of UV-Vis spectroscopy and dynamic light scattering, respectively, in food matrix in less than 3 h.

Gold nanorods were used to detect genomic DNA of *C. jejuni* and *C. coli*.[74] A specific ssDNA probe of *cadF* gene was immobilized by adsorption to Au nanorods. The color change occurred upon hybridization of the *cadF* gene with the immobilized probe on the gold surface. The nanobiosensor outcomes were compared with PCR and RT-PCR results in order to evaluate the assay efficiency. Despite some false-negative results, the detection limit of biosensor was 10^2 copy number/mL which was similar to the one obtained with the RT-PCR and lower compared to the PCR one.

51.3.11 Piezoelectric biosensors for *Campylobacter* detection

Piezoelectric biosensors are characterized by a piezoelectric crystal which vibrates at a certain frequency when induced by an electrical signal. The recognition elements are immobilized on the crystal and once the target binds to them, the event causes a measurable oscillation in the vibrational frequency of the crystal, directly correlated with the added mass on the crystal surface.[84] Quartz-Crystal Microbalance (QCM) is the major type of piezoelectric biosensors used for pathogen detection, in light of their advantages, such as real-time monitoring and ease of use. A QCM-immunosensor was developed by Masdor et al. for *C. jejuni* detection.[85] The sensor performances were evaluated for a direct, sandwich, and gold-NPs amplified setup using a fully automated QCM. This device allowed the measurement of oscillation in the vibrational frequency at the active and control surfaces, presented as two spots on the prism. In the direct assay, different concentrations of *C. jejuni* were injected on either the surface immobilized rabbit polyclonal antibodies or mouse monoclonal antibodies, resulting in a LoD of 2.0×10^5 and 2.0×10^6 CFU/mL, respectively. In the sandwich assay, the capture antibody used was the rabbit polyclonal antibody, whereas the detection antibodies

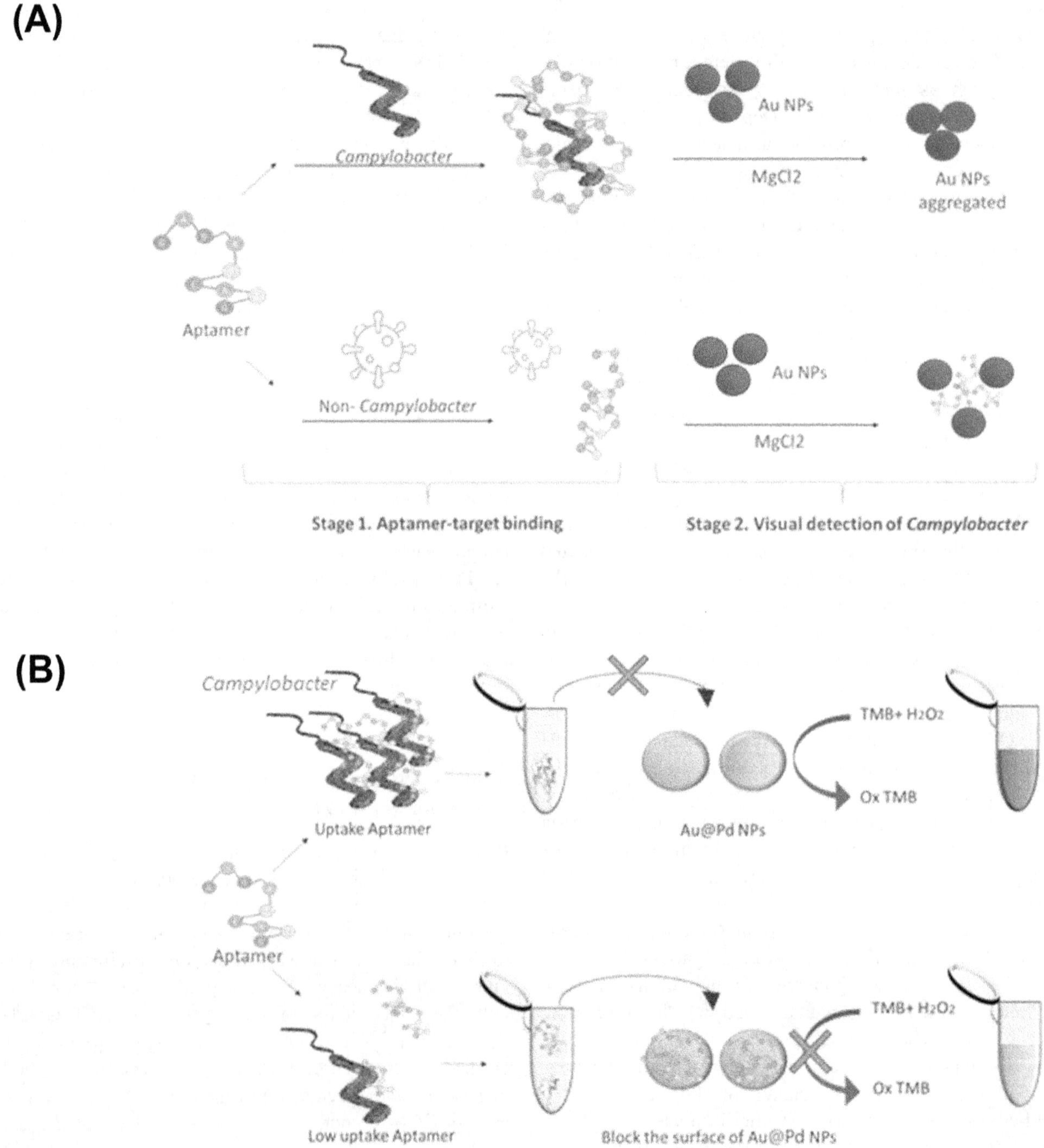

FIGURE 51.6 (A) Schematic illustration showing the detection principle of the colorimetric platform for *Campylobacter* detection, and (B) schematic illustration of colorimetric aptasensor for *Campylobacter* cells detection using Au@Pd nanoparticles. *(A) Adapted from Kim Y-J, Kim H-S, Chon J-W, Kim D-H, Hyeon J-Y, Seo K-H. New colorimetric aptasensor for rapid on-site detection of* Campylobacter jejuni *and* Campylobacter coli *in chicken carcass samples.* Anal Chim Acta. *2018;1029:78–85. (B) Adapted from Dehghani Z, Hosseini M, Mohammadnejad J, Bakhshi B, Rezayan AH. Colorimetric aptasensor for* Campylobacter jejuni *cells by exploiting the peroxidase like activity of Au@ Pd nanoparticles.* Microchim Acta. *2018;185(10):448.*

were *C. jejuni* monoclonal or polyclonal antibodies. The LoD of this method was 2.4×10^4 CFU/mL. In the AuNPs-based assay, the capture element was a polyclonal antibody against *C. jejuni*, while the detection element was composed of an antibody conjugated to AuNPs to increase the mass. The LoD was 1.5×10^2 CFU/mL.

51.3.12 *Campylobacter* detection by next-generation sequencing

High-throughput sequencing, also known as NGS, has allowed a significant advance in the genetic study of *Campylobacter*. It allows the parallel sequencing of billions of nucleotides per experiment (or "run") in one short and relatively inexpensive step. The development of new sequencing technologies now makes the genomic study accessible to many laboratories, leading to extensive studies for epidemiology characterizations including surveillance and outbreak detection, as well as phylogenetic antimicrobial resistance analyses. The use of whole genome sequencing (WGS) has become the preferred diagnostic and surveillance approach for global food safety regulatory agencies.[86] For example, in combination with epidemiological methods, WGS is used to identify both sources and transmission pathways during diseases outbreak investigations leading to improve detection and management of *C. jejuni* infections.[87] By focusing on allelic variation and differentiation between isolates, scientists can trace outbreaks with significant discriminatory power. Data from WGS have been used to identify biomarkers to develop diagnostic assays. Furthermore, 165 sequenced genomes of *C. jejuni* were used to identify biomarkers specifically associated to clinical strains.[88] A diagnostic tool for *C. jejuni* isolates that encode cstII or cstIII-sialyltransferase was developed by combining WGS and mutiplex qPCR.[89]

Moreover, the applications of NGS have increased the understanding of the evolutionary and epidemiological dynamics of *Campylobacter*. WGS is particularly interesting for the comparative study of bacterial whole genomes and the identification of virulence factors and antibiotic resistance markers within the genus *Campylobacter*. For example, the identification of islands of pathogenicity in *C. fetus*, a species responsible for sepsis in human pathology, allows the study of the associated virulence factors and their roles in adaptation to host, horizontal gene transfer, or cell protection.[90] WGS analysis for resistance genes is also used to predict the antibiotic resistance phenotype. The four priority antimicrobial drug resistance of *C. jejuni* and *C. coli* are ciprofloxacin, erythromycin, tetracycline and, since June 2016, gentamicin.[12] New resistance genes are regularly described and high correlations between genotype and antibiotic resistance are observed.[91–94]

Nevertheless, there are still some limitations to the genotypic prediction of antibiotic resistance. This is based on in-depth knowledge of the various mechanisms of resistance to concerned antibiotics and required available databases of known resistance genes. WGS does not allow the formal identification of resistance mechanisms that have not yet been elucidated. In addition, NGS technology allows to obtain a fragmented genome, which is then assembled in contigs which can make difficult to determine the chromosomal or plasmid location of the resistance genes. Finally, the level of gene expression as well as the synergistic effects of various resistance mechanisms cannot be evaluated by WGS, although they can have a great influence on the levels of antibiotics' minimum inhibitory concentration.

51.4 Toward biomarkers identification to predict *Campylobacter* behavior

According to the US National Institute of Health, a biomarker is "a biological entity assessed as an indicator relating to normal biological processes, pathogenic processes, or pharmacological responses to a therapeutic intervention, which can be objectively measured."[95] Proteins, genes, metabolites, or minerals are all cellular constituents that can be considered as biomarkers. Therefore advances in omics technologies such as genomics, transcriptomics, proteomics, and metabolomics contribute to biomarker identification.

Biomarkers are widely used in the medical field and in particular biomarkers associated with cancer. Cancer is an abnormal, uncontrolled proliferation of cells in the body, due to mutation occurring on genes that control cell division or tumor repressor genes involved in particular in the reduction of the cell division rate, DNA repair, or in the cell death process (apoptosis). Genetic alterations of cancer cells, as point mutation, gene rearrangement or amplifications, and subsequent disturbances of cell division and proliferation will be manifested by release of biomarkers of such changes in majority of patients with a specific type of cancer. Therefore they can be used as biomarkers for the cancer detection, but also to measure the risk of cancer development or progression in a specific tissue or to predict responses to various treatments. The recent revolution in molecular biology, with the rise of high-throughput sequencing and increased molecular characterization of tumor tissue, has led to an exponential increase in attempts to measure and target aberrant pathways at the molecular level, improving cancer biomarker development.

Phenotypic diversity of foodborne pathogens resides in many features: (1) their adequation with specific hosts, habitats, or environments; (2) their ability to grow or survive to food processing steps; and (3) their virulence capability, that is, their probability to induce a disease into the host. The discovery of biomarkers enabling to predict one or several of these features would improve the identification of strains at high risk potential and potentially associated with specific human populations, strains persistent through time and space, and conditions favorable to the establishment of pathogens in specific environments or food facilities. The prediction of phenotypic behavior using cellular indicators is a key area of research in the field of foodborne pathogens, spoilage organisms, and organisms used in functional food applications.[96–98] These cellular indicators also called biomarkers of adaptive stress response would enable to predict the impact of stress conditions on subsequent bacterial robustness, and could be exploited to adapt processing conditions to control microbial hazards. Focusing on food safety application, it could then be possible to transpose biomarker concept to the food sector in order to improve the detection of foodborne pathogens in food or food environment but also to predict the impact of stress on the pathogen behavior (survival, inactivation, virulence) (Fig. 51.7).

One of the challenges for the use of biomarkers in food safety resides in the integration of omics data into quantitative microbial risk assessment (QMRA) models in order to better control hazards in food.[99–102] Biomarker development is relevant in the different components of QMRA, that is, hazard identification, exposure assessment, and hazard characterization. Discovering biomarkers enabling the prediction of bacterial behavior would be useful to refine current microbial exposure assessment. Indeed, there is important behavior variability among strains and even among individual cells. This variability may result in differences regarding resistance and adaptation to food processes, growth–no growth boundaries, growth rate and duration of the lag phase, ability to enter into the VBNC state and then to regrow under more favorable conditions.[103] This variability affects the level of contamination of the foodborne pathogen at each step of the food process, and ultimately at the time of consumption. Currently, QMRA is based upon mean behaviors of pathogens regarding for instance thermal inactivation, resistance to physicochemical conditions (salt, aw, additives, etc.), growth characteristics, and so on. It is expected that in some situations, the level of bacterial contamination might be over- or underestimated.[104] Technological developments in omics methods through the application WGS have considerably improved detection of pathogens in food. Our understanding of the behavior of microorganisms in response to diverse environmental conditions has progressed and revealed general and specific stress response features that could lead to identification of cellular indicators for stress adaptive behavior.[101,105,106] Most of the omics studies performed so far have not been designed for food safety risk assessment.[107,108] However, several studies have sought to integrate omics data to predict or better characterize the behavior of bacteria in the context of food safety by the identification of potential cellular markers involved in bacterial survival, virulence, or resistance to stress.[99,101,109–111]

One of the main challenges to biomarker development will be to quantitatively correlate the microbial responses at the molecular level (and the massive amount of data generated by omics technologies) to the phenotypic analysis to identify robust indicators.[99,112] In addition, biomarker concept will gain in emphasis if it can be used as

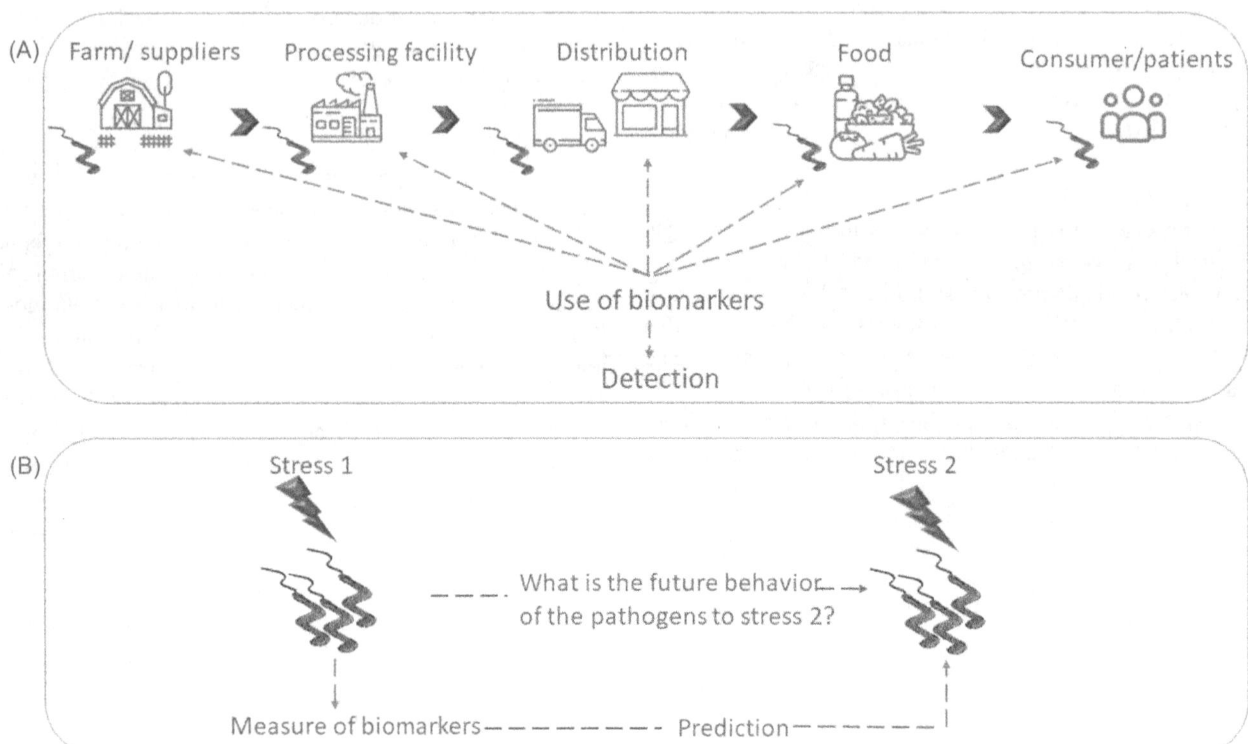

FIGURE 51.7 Schematic representation of biomarkers relevance in (A) detection and (B) prediction of foodborne pathogens behavior such as growth, inactivation, or virulence features.

decision-making tools to improve food safety and quality issues.

Increasingly affordable due to recent advances in NGS, functional genomics represent great promises for the discovery of molecular-based biomarkers of phenotypes like adaptation to host and environment, behavior (growth, lag phase duration, stress resistance, and persistence) or virulence.[113] WGS analysis is currently used in several countries in real-time surveillance of foodborne pathogens, including *Campylobacter* spp.[114] In addition, most national public health reference laboratories in the EU have now access to WGS-based typing of microbial pathogens for surveillance of infectious diseases and drug resistance transmission.[115] Surveillance of *Campylobacter* has been investigated by EFSA in Italy for the development of risk assessment tools based on molecular typing and WGS (EFSA).[116] Tracking the sources of microbial contamination (source attribution) and thus understanding the pathogen association with reservoirs or habitats, delineating transmission routes, and predicting functional properties of isolates such as antibiotic resistance, through the integration of WGS data, are some objectives pursued by these strategies. Some WGS studies on *C. jejuni* and *C. coli* have for example shown potential insights on *Campylobacter* antimicrobial resistance and host adaptations.[93,117–119]

There are very few studies aiming at identifying biomarkers of bacterial behavior. For example, candidate biomarkers of a genetic, enzymatic, or protein nature have been selected for *B. cereus* on the basis of its adaptive behavior and its robustness following exposure to four mild stress conditions (mild heat, acid, salt, and oxidative stress) by comparing genome-wide transcriptome profiles.[101] Regarding *C. jejuni*, although it cannot grow given its stringent growth requirements (microaerophilic conditions and narrow temperature range: 30°C–42°C), it can survive to slaughterhouse environments but must deal with stressful conditions encountered during poultry processing and storage. Duqué et al. showed that the inactivation of *C. jejuni* during storage was strain-dependent but also depended on the steps previously undergone by the bacteria, that is on its cell history.[120] Gene expression biomarkers were therefore sought within selected core genes of *C. jejuni* commonly associated with stress, in order to possibly predict the future behavior of *C. jejuni* following application of stress conditions.[121,122] Correlation analysis between the expression of candidate gene biomarkers and survival rates of *C. jejuni* following storage enabled to identify 10 potential gene biomarkers, including genes encoding regulators and chaperone proteins.[121] *C. jejuni* is also known to enter into the VNBC state, a stress-induced phenotype, and more quickly in biofilms.[123] Cells in the VNBC state have been shown to resuscitate, recovering their virulence potential and infectivity, in various conditions.[124–126] Bacteria in the VBNC state cannot be detected by conventional cultural methods, while they can still represent a risk after resuscitation, predicting the conditions triggering the reversal of this dormant state would be therefore very useful for decision makers.

Another challenge that identifying biomarkers could address is predicting disease severity and host adaptation to improve hazard characterization. It could help in building mechanistic dose–response models.[102] Current dose–response models of *C. jejuni*[127,128] should be extended to include strain variability and host immunity factors.[129] The identification of biomarkers associated with virulence of *C. jejuni* or susceptibility of some populations could help to predict high risk exposure situations.

51.5 Lipooligosaccharide of *Campylobacter* strains as a biomarker of its pathogenicity

In addition to be responsible for the major cause of bacterial gastroenteritis in developed countries, *Campylobacter* can also be responsible for the development of postinfection diseases. GBS is the leading cause of acute flaccid paralysis in the world. GBS is an autoimmune disorder of the peripheral nervous system characterized by limb weakness and areflexia. Various antecedent infections can trigger GBS, for example cytomegalovirus, Epstein–Barr virus, Haemophilus influenzae, Hepatite E virus, ZIKA virus, or *Mycoplasma pneumoniae*, but *C. jejuni* is generally recognized as the most common antecedent agent.[130,131] Indeed, epidemiological association between *C. jejuni* infection and GBS is established and case-control studies report that *C. jejuni* infection precede GBS in 22%–66% of the patients.[132–135] Moreover, it is estimated that approximately 1 in 1000 patients with *C. jejuni* infection develops GBS.[136] In those cases with a preceding *C. jejuni* infection, molecular mimicry between lipooligosaccharides (LOS) present in the *C. jejuni* outer cell membrane and gangliosides present in peripheral nerves plays a crucial role in the pathogenesis of GBS.[137] Due to these epitopes on *C. jejuni* cell surfaces, antibodies produced against the LOS during the bacterial infection not only recognized LOS structures, but also human neuronal gangliosides. In susceptible host, this autoimmune reactivity can trigger the GBS or its variant the Miller–Fisher Syndrome (MFS) that is characterized by ophthalmoplegia, ataxia, and areflexia.[137–139] Only certain *C. jejuni* LOS has structural similarities to the human gangliosides GM1, GD1a, and GQ1b present in peripheral nerve axons.[131]

The LOS presents in the outer membrane of *C. jejuni* lacks the O-antigen that contains the repeating oligosaccharide polymer of the outer core of LPS of many bacteria. *C. jejuni* LOS is constituted with a lipid A backbone, an inner core composed by two heptose and two glucose units, and an LOS outer core composed of a short oligosaccharide. The LOS outer core structure is highly diverse among the strains and this diversity reflects the LOS biosynthesis locus complexity. Twenty-three distinct classes of LOS biosynthesis loci are described so far, based on major genetic differences, gene content, and organization. Hameed et al.[140] recently proposed to simplify the classification grouping them in the four different groups as initially described by Karlyshev et al.[141] based on sharing similar gene contents. Only certain LOS classes are considered as important risk factors in development of postinfectious neurological complications, and sialylation of the LOS core has been associated with ganglioside mimicry in GBS or its variant MFS related to *Campylobacter* strains.[131,142] So far, five LOS classes, A, B, C, M, R, and V belonging to the group 1, harbor sialyltransferase genes (*cstII or cstIII*) and *N*-acetylneuraminate biosynthesis genes (*neuABC*) involved in incorporating sialic acids into the LOS.[140,143–145] It was shown that 96% of GBS-associated strains had LOS locus classes A, B, or C, compared to 70% of enteritis-associated strains.[131] However, the LOS class A is more frequently associated with the GBS-associated strains.[131,142] Godschalk et al.[142] reported that MFS was associated with LOS class B strains, but it was later demonstrated that it was in fact the *cstII* gene polymorphism that directs the clinical features.[131] Indeed, two different alleles of this gene lead to a different produced enzyme with a threonine (Thr) or an asparagine (Asp) at the position 51 resulting in variability in the LOS.[145] Koga et al. demonstrated that the MFS was mainly associated to the presence of strains with *cstII* (Asn51) genotype and most of the LOS class B strains had this genotype.[131]

Determination of the LOS class to characterize *C. jejuni* strains circulating in patients or in the food chain, was generally performed by PCR-based screening of LOS gene contents in numerous studies.[146–149] Due to the complexity of the gene content of the different LOS locus classes, a single PCR was not sufficient to determine the LOS class but needed the targeting of several specific genes. For example, LOS class A isolates can be distinguished from class B isolates because amplification will be obtained by PCR primers targeting genes common to class A and B (*cstII*) but not after successive screening by a class B-specific primer (*cgtA-IIb*).[146–149] In 2018 Neal-McKinney et al. developed a multiplex PCR (qPCR) method using primers and fluorescent probes to detect in a single step, the two sialyltransferase genes (*cstII* or *cstIII*) from a collection of *C. jejuni* strains from food and environmental samples. This method is faster than the previous ones but it would not permit the precise determination of the LOS class.[89] WGS data can also be used to study the potential for LOS sialylation of *C. jeuni* isolates. Genome sequencing data from public databases were screened to detect the *Campylobacter* sialyltransferase genes[89] and recently,[150] analyzed WGS data to determine the LOS class of *C. jejuni* strains isolated from patients with diarrhea.[150]

Hameed et al. compared the distribution of LOS locus classes in all *C. jejuni* populations (clinical, enteritis, and poultry) from previous studies and concluded that approximately 50%–75% of the strains belong to class A, B or C.[140] Poultry implication is generally recognized in human campylobacteriosis and several studies compared LOS classes from *C. jejuni* strains isolated from poultry and from humans. These studies reported similar distributions of the sialylated LOS locus classes among the human and chicken isolates[149,151–153]; however, Thépault et al. in 2017 found significantly more isolates harboring LOS class A, B, or C in human isolates compared to the poultry isolates.[154] In poultry, the LOS locus class A is generally underrepresented compared to LOS class B or C and can vary from 1.4% to 13.2% depending on the studies. LOS class B and C isolates represent together, almost 50% of the total number of the isolates.[149,151–154]

The vast majority of *Campylobacter*-related GBS cases is attributed to *C. jejuni* but several studies reported that other thermophilic *Campylobacter* species have been associated with GBS, in particular *C. coli* and *C. upsaliensis*.[133,155–158] However, their role in promoting the disease remain unclear. Funakoshi et al.[156] and van Belkum et al.[155] could not demonstrate the ganglioside mimicry in the LOS of *C. coli* strains isolated from GBS patients. Genomic comparative analysis of the LOS and capsular polysaccharide (CPS) gene clusters revealed that certain strains of *C. coli* and *C. upsaliensis* possess genes homologous to the sialic acid but they were found external of the LOS.[159] In *C. coli*, those genes were found in the CPS indicating that the CPS might also be involved in ganglioside mimicry.[158,159] More recently, a comprehensive investigation about the presence, frequency, and distribution of the molecular machinery for the biosynthesis of sialylated LOS structures in *C. coli* population was performed using the whole genome sequences deposited in a public database.[160] This work revealed considerable evidence supporting the expression of ganglioside-like LOS in *C. coli*, as 16 (over 27). LOS locus classes were shown to contain the essential molecular machinery to potentially express sialylated LOS (i.e., a *cst* homolog and *neuABC*). However, those strains carrying *C. jejuni*-like LOS locus represent approximately 1% of sequenced strains, which might explain the low incidence of *C. coli*-related GBS.[160]

LOS sialylation and molecular mimicry with ganglioside are not the only factors to cause postinfectious neurological complications, other host and/or bacterial factors are required. However, LOS sialylation could be used as a biomarker to characterize strains circulating along the food chain and could permit to better assess the risk for the consumer. It could also be required to develop specific control measures to limit the exposure of the consumer to these potentially neuropathic strains.

51.6 Risk analysis and detection methods

Besides having a health aspect, food poisoning affects the economy due to the costs of hospitalization, work absence, financial losses associated with consumers' concerns of food quality, and the cost of legal proceedings. Schmutz et al. estimated the annual Swiss healthcare cost of 2012 associated with acute gastroenteritis, including campylobacteriosis.[17] The US Department of Agriculture estimated that the country spends in specific for campylobacteriosis \$1,928,787,166 a year. The campylobacteriosis cases and a large proportion of these costs could be avoided by adopting analysis methods that can reduce the time required for results maintaining specificity and sensibility, improving how food is handled from farm to fork. The risk management and prevention of campylobacteriosis urgently need a fast, cheap, and highly accurate detection method for timely removing and effective tracing of contaminated foods.

Until now, methods used for food analysis still rely on the traditional cultural growth. The conventional methods are considered as a golden standard and most ISO methods are based on them. However, their main disadvantage is the time required to obtain results. For this reason in the last 30 years the many efforts have been devoted to develop and optimize rapid alternative methods. However, the LoD of alternative methods rarely exceed 10^2-10^3 CFU/mL in a direct detection (in almost all the examples reported the analysis were performed on 25 g of food matrix artificially contaminated with the pathogen of interest) remaining above the values critical for human health for some bacterial pathogens. To increase the sensitivity a preenrichment step has to be performed. Even with this additional step, the pathogen detection with rapid methods is achieved in shorter time compared to traditional. Another peculiar feature of these methods is the possibility to detect more pathogens simultaneously while maintaining high levels of specificity.

The PCR is a method allowing amplification in vitro of DNA in low concentrations, making it suitable for the detection of any microorganism. In addition, some PCR methods provide a quantitative response. Despite their rapidity, specificity, and selectivity, PCR methods still exhibit some drawbacks. A direct PCR method cannot distinguish dead and viable cells (except from RT-PCR) resulting in an incorrect detection. Moreover, PCR requires some preparation steps prior to amplification. In addition the PCR performance can be affected by components of food. For instance, fat and proteins from food sample may make difficult DNA extraction or inhibit DNA polymerase.

Biosensors are easy-to-use devices that do not need a specific training to be applied. In some cases, they do not require preparation steps and can be directly applied for on-site detection. However, as *Campylobacter* can be present in a very low amount, in most cases an enrichment step is necessary. Due to the complexity and inhomogeneity of a food matrix, the result may be not accurate. Furthermore, the binding affinity between the target and recognition element may change in the time which highlights the biosensor instability.[84]

One of the tasks of the food technologist is to ensure the production of safe food safeguarding of consumers health. Traditional cultural methods are techniques used for the pathogen detection that assure a high sensitivity and efficiency, but they are time-consuming and this is the biggest limitation in testing foods. In fact, it may happen that an unsafe food product is commercialized and consumed by the consumers, leading to a foodborne illness before having obtained the results of the analyses.

It is also possible that the results of the exceeding of a microbiological limit in a food product are obtained when the products are on the market, asking for a withdrawal or recall of the products, a very expensive procedure. Consequently, the application of rapid methods can certainly reduce the times of analysis and therefore solve all the correlated problems, particularly related to food with a short shelf-life (of about 30–45 days), as ready-to-eat products, fresh vegetable and fruit, fresh meat and fish. However, it should be taken into account the complexity of a food matrix and its high heterogeneity, which require of pretreatments to make the product compatible with the analytical methods; these extra procedures can increase the time of analysis. In addition, another feature of the food matrix is the target bacteria not uniformly distributed and its presence in low concentrations. Hence, these rapid methods are efficient tools toward pathogen detection but they have to be also suitable for the food matrix to which they are applied.

This review reports and compares the features of rapid methods, PCR, NGS, and biosensors, highlighting important features such as high specificity and sensitivity, and low time to provide the results of analysis. The numerous examples reported demonstrate the rapid development of these techniques, given the necessity to solve the problem of the time-requiring cultural approach. Although rapid detection methods are under expansion worldwide, they are slowly adopted by the food industry and regulatory policies. The challenges that are yet to be solved include adaptation of protocols and detection performance in specific food systems. To be used outside research laboratories, a rapid method usually needs optimization for implementation in field conditions in order to reduce the risk of obtaining false-positive or negative results. Furthermore, development of reference materials, harmonization of sampling methods, mobile analysis, and data networking significantly support developing highly sensitive and selective biosensors for real-time in situ monitoring. Finally, to reach food industry rapid methods should be robust compared to traditional technologies, and professional control analysis should be encouraged to replace the traditional methods with the novel ones that offer significant benefits.

The development of rapid methods for pathogen detection is necessary regarding the needs of the food industry. Methods presented in this review, PCR, NGS, and biosensors, may match the features of cultural methods, but by improving them, the application of these techniques could not only reduce the risk of foodborne outbreaks and consumers health problems, but also lead to a decrease of direct and indirect healthcare costs. Comparing advantages and disadvantages of these two methods, biosensors seem to be the better candidate to replace cultural methods. Even though both techniques provide results in reduced times, only biosensors provide all: the detection of pathogens in foods in a couple of hours, possibility for on situ monitoring, and a low LoD without preenrichment steps. In order to achieve full integration of biosensors in food safety control a standardization of these devices is necessary taking into account the complexity of food matrix, before they will be fully adapted by the foodborne outbreaks.

References

1. UN. *Population 2030: Demographic Challenges and Opportunities for Sustainable Development Planning*. New York: UN Department of Economic and Social Affairs; 2015.
2. WHO. *WHO Estimates of the Global Burden of Foodborne Diseases: Foodborne Disease Burden Epidemiology Reference Group 2007–2015*. World Health Organization; 2015.
3. Franz CM, den Besten HM, Boehnlein C, Gareis M, Zwietering MH, Fusco V. Reprint of: microbial food safety in the 21st century: emerging challenges and foodborne pathogenic bacteria. *Trends Food Sci Technol*. 2019;84:34–37.
4. Jeffs E, Williman J, Brunton C, Gullam J, Walls T. The epidemiology of listeriosis in pregnant women and children in New Zealand from 1997 to 2016: an observational study. *BMC Public Health*. 2020;20(1):1–8.
5. IUFoST. Foodborne disease and vulnerable groups. *Sci Inf Bull (SIB)*. 2015;1–12.
6. Bouwknegt M, Van Pelt W, Havelaar AH. Scoping the impact of changes in population age-structure on the future burden of foodborne disease in the Netherlands, 2020–2060. *Int J Environ Res Public Health*. 2013;10(7):2888–2896.
7. Bisholo KZ, Ghuman S, Haffejee F. Food-borne disease prevalence in rural villages in the Eastern Cape, South Africa. *Afr J Prim Health Care Family Med*. 2018;10(1):1–5.
8. Zhang A, Jakku E. Australian consumers' preferences for food attributes: a latent profile analysis. *Foods*. 2021;10(1):56.
9. Yang T, Dharmasena S. Consumers preferences on nutritional attributes of dairy-alternative beverages: hedonic pricing models. *Food Sci Nutr*. 2020;8(10):5362–5378.
10. Yeung RM, Morris J. Food safety risk: consumer perception and purchase behaviour. *Br Food J*. 2001;103:170–187.
11. Christensen T, Morkbak M, Hasler B, Lundhede T, Porsbo L, Christoffersen L. Information, risk perception and consumer behaviour: a choice experiment on food safety and animal welfare. Rapport/Fodevareokonomisk Institut, No. 180; 2006.
12. EFSA. The European Union summary report on trends and sources of zoonoses, zoonotic agents and food-borne outbreaks in 2017. *EFSA J*. 2018;16(12):e05500.
13. Hansson I, Sandberg M, Habib I, Lowman R, Engvall EO. Knowledge gaps in control of *Campylobacter* for prevention of campylobacteriosis. *Transbound Emerg Dis*. 2018;65:30–48.
14. Silva J, Leite D, Fernandes M, Mena C, Gibbs PA, Teixeira P. *Campylobacter* spp. as a foodborne pathogen: a review. *Front Microbiol*. 2011;2:200.
15. FAO. Food safety risk profile for *Campylobacter* species in broiler (young) chickens. <http://www.fao.org/tempref/codex/Meetings/CCFH/CCFH40/fh40rpcb.pdf>; 2007.
16. Mughini-Gras L, Smid J, Wagenaar J, et al. Campylobacteriosis in returning travellers and potential secondary transmission of exotic strains. *Epidemiol Infect*. 2014;142(6):1277–1288.
17. Schmutz C, Mäusezahl D, Bless P, Hatz C, Schwenkglenks M, Urbinello D. Estimating healthcare costs of acute gastroenteritis and human campylobacteriosis in Switzerland. *Epidemiol Infect*. 2017;145(4):627–641.
18. Tribble DR, Baqar S, Scott DA, et al. Assessment of the duration of protection in *Campylobacter jejuni* experimental infection in humans. *Infect Immun*. 2010;78(4):1750–1759.
19. Vizzini P, Braidot M, Vidic J, Manzano M. Electrochemical and optical biosensors for the detection of *Campylobacter* and *Listeria*: an update look. *Micromachines*. 2019;10(8):500.
20. Vidic J, Manzano M, Chang C-M, Jaffrezic-Renault N. Advanced biosensors for detection of pathogens related to livestock and poultry. *Vet Res*. 2017;48(1):11.
21. Mullis K, Faloona F, Scharf S, Saiki R, Horn G, Erlich H. *Specific enzymatic amplification of DNA in vitro: the polymerase chain reaction. Cold Spring Harbor Symp Quant Biol*. 51. Cold Spring Harbor Laboratory Press; 1986:263–273.
22. Chuang L-Y, Cheng Y-H, Yang C-H. Specific primer design for the polymerase chain reaction. *Biotechnol Lett*. 2013;35(10):1541–1549.
23. Mateo E, Cárcamo J, Urquijo M, Perales I, Fernández-Astorga A. Evaluation of a PCR assay for the detection and identification of *Campylobacter jejuni* and *Campylobacter coli* in retail poultry products. *Res Microbiol*. 2005;156(4):568–574.
24. Fontanot M, Iacumin L, Cecchini F, Comi G, Manzano M. Rapid detection and differentiation of important *Campylobacter* spp. in poultry samples by dot blot and PCR. *Food Microbiol*. 2014;43:28–34.
25. Shi X-M, Long F, Suo B. Molecular methods for the detection and characterization of foodborne pathogens. *Pure Appl Chem*. 2010;82(1):69–79.
26. Alves J, Marques VV, Pereira LFPH, Yoko E, de Oliveira TCRM. Multiplex PCR for the detection of *Campylobacter* spp. and *Salmonella* spp. in chicken meat. *J Food Saf*. 2012;32(3):345–350.
27. Fedorov A, Sochivko D, Varlamov D. Model of fluorescent signal generation from an intercalating dye in the course of a polymerase chain reaction. *Tech Phys*. 2020;65(9):1516–1520.
28. Fraga D, Meulia T, Fenster S. Real-time PCR. *Curr Protoc Essent Lab Tech*. 2014;8(1). 10.13.11-10.13.40.
29. Wang B-B, Wang Q, Jin Y-G, Ma M-H, Cai Z-X. Two-color quantum dots-based fluorescence resonance energy transfer for rapid and sensitive detection of Salmonella on eggshells. *J Photochem Photobiol A Chem*. 2015;299:131–137.

30. Fedorov A, Sochivko D, Varlamov D, Kurochkin V. Simulation of kinetic curves of polymerase chain reaction obtained using fluorescent oligonucleotide probes. *Tech Phys*. 2018;63(10):1430–1434.
31. Navarro E, Serrano-Heras G, Castaño M, Solera J. Real-time PCR detection chemistry. *Clin Chim Acta*. 2015;439:231–250.
32. Lv R, Wang K, Feng J, Heeney DD, Liu D, Lu X. Detection and quantification of viable but non-culturable *Campylobacter jejuni*. *Front Microbiol*. 2020;10:2920.
33. Churruca E, Girbau C, Martinez I, Mateo E, Alonso R, Fernandez-Astorga A. Detection of *Campylobacter jejuni* and *Campylobacter coli* in chicken meat samples by real-time nucleic acid sequence-based amplification with molecular beacons. *Int J Food Microbiol*. 2007;117(1):85–90.
34. Hu Q, Lyu D, Shi X, et al. A modified molecular beacons–based multiplex real-time PCR assay for simultaneous detection of eight foodborne pathogens in a single reaction and its application. *Foodborne Pathog Dis*. 2014;11(3):207–214.
35. Wolffs P, Norling B, Hoorfar J, Griffiths M, Rådström P. Quantification of *Campylobacter* spp. in chicken rinse samples by using flotation prior to real-time PCR. *Appl Environ Microbiol*. 2005;71(10):5759–5764.
36. Gobert G, Cotillard A, Fourmestraux C, Pruvost L, Miguet J, Boyer M. Droplet digital PCR improves absolute quantification of viable lactic acid bacteria in faecal samples. *J Microbiol Methods*. 2018;148:64–73.
37. Peruzy MF, Proroga YTR, Capuano F, et al. Detection and quantification of *Campylobacter* in foods: new analytic approaches to detect and quantify *Campylobacter* spp. in food samples. *Ital J Food Saf*. 2020;9(2):8591.
38. Poon LL, Wong BW, Ma EH, et al. Sensitive and inexpensive molecular test for falciparum malaria: detecting *Plasmodium falciparum* DNA directly from heat-treated blood by loop-mediated isothermal amplification. *Clin Chem*. 2006;52(2):303–306.
39. Notomi T, Okayama H, Masubuchi H, et al. Loop-mediated isothermal amplification of DNA. *Nucleic Acids Res*. 2000;28(12):e63.
40. Kaneko H, Kawana T, Fukushima E, Suzutani T. Tolerance of loop-mediated isothermal amplification to a culture medium and biological substances. *J Biochem Biophys Methods*. 2007;70(3):499–501.
41. Nagamine K, Hase T, Notomi T. Accelerated reaction by loop-mediated isothermal amplification using loop primers. *Mol Cell Probes*. 2002;16(3):223–229.
42. Mukama O, Wu J, Li Z, et al. An ultrasensitive and specific point-of-care CRISPR/Cas12 based lateral flow biosensor for the rapid detection of nucleic acids. *Biosens Bioelectron*. 2020;112143.
43. Mori Y, Notomi T. Loop-mediated isothermal amplification (LAMP): a rapid, accurate, and cost-effective diagnostic method for infectious diseases. *J Infect Chemother*. 2009;15(2):62–69.
44. Xie L, Wang T, Huang T, Hou W, Huang G, Du Y. Dew inspired breathing-based detection of genetic point mutation visualized by naked eye. *Sci Rep*. 2014;4:6300.
45. Chen S, Ge B. Development of a toxR-based loop-mediated isothermal amplification assay for detecting *Vibrio parahaemolyticus*. *BMC Microbiol*. 2010;10(1):41.
46. Seyrig G, Ahmad F, Stedtfeld RD, Tourlousse DM, Hashsham SA. *Simple, powerful, and smart: using LAMP for low-cost screening of multiple waterborne pathogens. Environmental Microbiology: Current Technology and Water Applications*. Caister Academic; 2011:103–125.
47. Watts MR, James G, Sultana Y, et al. A loop-mediated isothermal amplification (LAMP) assay for *Strongyloides stercoralis* in stool that uses a visual detection method with SYTO-82 fluorescent dye. *Am J Trop Med Hyg*. 2014;90(2):306–311.
48. Gao X, Sun B, Guan Y. Pullulan reduces the non-specific amplification of loop-mediated isothermal amplification (LAMP). *Anal Bioanal Chem*. 2019;411(6):1211–1218.
49. Niessen L, Luo J, Denschlag C, Vogel RF. The application of loop-mediated isothermal amplification (LAMP) in food testing for bacterial pathogens and fungal contaminants. *Food Microbiol*. 2013;36(2):191–206.
50. Linh Quyen T, Nordentoft S, Chidambara Vinayaka A, et al. A sensitive, specific and simple loop mediated isothermal amplification method for rapid detection of *Campylobacter* spp. in broiler production. *Front Microbiol*. 2019;10:2443.
51. Thongphueak D, Chansiri K, Sriyapai T, Areekit S, Santiwatanakul S, Wangroongsarb P. Development of the rapid test kit for the identification of *Campylobacter* spp. based on loop-mediated isothermal amplification (LAMP) in combination with a lateral flow dipstick (LFD) and gold nano-DNA probe (AuNPs). *Sci Technol Asia*. 2019;24:63–71.
52. Yamazaki W, Taguchi M, Ishibashi M, Nukina M, Misawa N, Inoue K. Development of a loop-mediated isothermal amplification assay for sensitive and rapid detection of *Campylobacter fetus*. *Vet Microbiol*. 2009;136(3–4):393–396.
53. Sabike II, Uemura R, Kirino Y, et al. Use of direct LAMP screening of broiler fecal samples for *Campylobacter jejuni* and *Campylobacter coli* in the positive flock identification strategy. *Front Microbiol*. 2016;7:1582.
54. Romero MR, Cook N. A rapid LAMP-based method for screening poultry samples for *Campylobacter* without enrichment. *Front Microbiol*. 2018;9:2401.
55. Phaneuf CR, Mangadu B, Tran HM, et al. Integrated LAMP and immunoassay platform for diarrheal disease detection. *Biosens Bioelectron*. 2018;120:93–101.
56. Alamer S, Eissa S, Chinnappan R, Herron P, Zourob M. Rapid colorimetric lactoferrin-based sandwich immunoassay on cotton swabs for the detection of foodborne pathogenic bacteria. *Talanta*. 2018;185:275–280.
57. Vizzini P, Manzano M, Farre C, et al. Highly sensitive detection of *Campylobacter* spp. in chicken meat using a silica nanoparticle enhanced dot blot DNA biosensor. *Biosens Bioelectron*. 2021;171:112689.
58. He D, Wu Z, Cui B, Xu E, Jin Z. Establishment of a dual mode immunochromatographic assay for *Campylobacter jejuni* detection. *Food Chem*. 2019;289:708–713.
59. Vidic J, Vizzini P, Manzano M, et al. Point-of-need DNA testing for detection of foodborne pathogenic bacteria. *Sensors*. 2019;19(5):1100.
60. Manzano M, Viezzi S, Mazerat S, Marks RS, Vidic J. Rapid and label-free electrochemical DNA biosensor for detecting hepatitis A virus. *Biosens Bioelectron*. 2018;100:89–95.
61. Shah J, Wilkins E. Electrochemical biosensors for detection of biological warfare agents. *Electroanalysis*. 2003;15(3):157–167.
62. Allen JB, Larry RF. *Electrochemical Methods: Fundamentals and Applications*. John Wiley & Sons; 2001.
63. Bard AJ, Faulkner LR. Fundamentals and applications. *Electrochem Methods*. 2001;2(482):580–632.

64. Yang X, Kirsch J, Simonian A. *Campylobacter* spp. detection in the 21st century: a review of the recent achievements in biosensor development. *J Microbiol Methods*. 2013;95(1):48–56.
65. Ivnitski D, Wilkins E, Tien H, Ottova A. Electrochemical biosensor based on supported planar lipid bilayers for fast detection of pathogenic bacteria. *Electrochem Commun*. 2000;2(7):457–460.
66. Viswanathan S, Rani C, Ho J-aA. Electrochemical immunosensor for multiplexed detection of food-borne pathogens using nanocrystal bioconjugates and MWCNT screen-printed electrode. *Talanta*. 2012;94:315–319.
67. Huang J, Yang G, Meng W, Wu L, Zhu A. An electrochemical impedimetric immunosensor for label-free detection of *Campylobacter jejuni* in diarrhea patients' stool based on O-carboxymethylchitosan surface modified Fe_3O_4 nanoparticles. *Biosens Bioelectron*. 2010;25(5):1204–1211.
68. Line JE, Pearson KG. Development of a selective broth medium for the detection of injured *Campylobacter jejuni* by capacitance monitoring. *J Food Prot*. 2003;66(10):1752–1755.
69. Damborský P, Švitel J, Katrlík J. Optical biosensors. *Essays Biochem*. 2016;60(1):91–100.
70. Sista S, Wei D, Oyarzabal O, Simonian A. Sensitive surface plasmon resonance biosensor for the near-real time detection of *Campylobacter jejuni*. *ECS. ECS Meeting Abstracts*. 2006;1468:39.
71. Taylor AD, Ladd J, Yu Q, Chen S, Homola J, Jiang S. Quantitative and simultaneous detection of four foodborne bacterial pathogens with a multi-channel SPR sensor. *Biosens Bioelectron*. 2006;22(5):752–758.
72. Singh A, Arutyunov D, McDermott MT, Szymanski CM, Evoy S. Specific detection of *Campylobacter jejuni* using the bacteriophage NCTC 12673 receptor binding protein as a probe. *Analyst*. 2011;136(22):4780–4786.
73. Masdor NA, Altintas Z, Shukor MY, Tothill IE. Subtractive inhibition assay for the detection of *Campylobacter jejuni* in chicken samples using surface plasmon resonance. *Sci Rep*. 2019;9(1):1–10.
74. Shams S, Bakhshi B, Moghadam TT, Behmanesh M. A sensitive gold-nanorods-based nanobiosensor for specific detection of *Campylobacter jejuni* and *Campylobacter coli*. *J Nanobiotechnol*. 2019;17(1):1–13.
75. Wei D, Oyarzabal OA, Huang T-S, Balasubramanian S, Sista S, Simonian AL. Development of a surface plasmon resonance biosensor for the identification of *Campylobacter jejuni*. *J Microbiol Methods*. 2007;69(1):78–85.
76. Sapsford KE, Rasooly A, Taitt CR, Ligler FS. Detection of *Campylobacter* and *Shigella* species in food samples using an array biosensor. *Anal Chem*. 2004;76(2):433–440.
77. Darbha GK, Lee E, Anderson YR, Fowler P, Mitchell K, Ray PC. Miniaturized sensor for microbial pathogens DNA and chemical toxins. *IEEE Sens J*. 2008;8(6):693–700.
78. Marcello A, Sblattero D, Cioarec C, Maiuri P, Melpignano P. A deep-blue OLED-based biochip for protein microarray fluorescence detection. *Biosens Bioelectron*. 2013;46:44–47.
79. Manzano M, Cecchini F, Fontanot M, Iacumin L, Comi G, Melpignano P. OLED-based DNA biochip for *Campylobacter* spp. detection in poultry meat samples. *Biosens Bioelectron*. 2015;66:271–276.
80. Yadav N, Chhillar AK, Rana JS. Detection of pathogenic bacteria with special emphasis to biosensors integrated with gold nanoparticles. *Sens Int*. 2020;1:100028.
81. Kim Y-J, Kim H-S, Chon J-W, Kim D-H, Hyeon J-Y, Seo K-H. New colorimetric aptasensor for rapid on-site detection of *Campylobacter jejuni* and *Campylobacter coli* in chicken carcass samples. *Anal Chim Acta*. 2018;1029:78–85.
82. Dehghani Z, Hosseini M, Mohammadnejad J, Bakhshi B, Rezayan AH. Colorimetric aptasensor for *Campylobacter jejuni* cells by exploiting the peroxidase like activity of Au@ Pd nanoparticles. *Microchim Acta*. 2018;185(10):448.
83. McVey C, Huang F, Elliott C, Cao C. Endonuclease controlled aggregation of gold nanoparticles for the ultrasensitive detection of pathogenic bacterial DNA. *Biosens Bioelectron*. 2017;92:502–508.
84. Sharma H, Mutharasan R. Review of biosensors for foodborne pathogens and toxins. *Sens Actuators B Chem*. 2013;183:535–549.
85. Masdor NA, Altintas Z, Tothill IE. Sensitive detection of *Campylobacter jejuni* using nanoparticles enhanced QCM sensor. *Biosens Bioelectron*. 2016;78:328–336.
86. Taboada EN, Graham MR, Carriço JA, Van Domselaar G. Food safety in the age of next generation sequencing, bioinformatics, and open data access. *Front Microbiol*. 2017;8:909.
87. Llarena A-K, Taboada E, Rossi M. Whole-genome sequencing in epidemiology of *Campylobacter jejuni* infections. *J Clin Microbiol*. 2017;55(5):1269–1275.
88. Brzozowska N, Gourlay J, O'Sullivan A, et al., 2018. Characterizing genetic circuit components in *E. coli* towards a *Campylobacter jejuni* biosensor. BioRxiv, 290155.
89. Neal-McKinney JM, Liu KC, Jinneman KC, Wu W-H, Rice DH. Whole genome sequencing and multiplex qPCR methods to identify *Campylobacter jejuni* encoding cst-II or cst-III sialyltransferase. *Front Microbiol*. 2018;9:408.
90. Ali A, Soares SC, Santos AR, et al. *Campylobacter fetus* subspecies: comparative genomics and prediction of potential virulence targets. *Gene*. 2012;508(2):145–156.
91. Redondo N, Carroll A, McNamara E. Molecular characterization of *Campylobacter* causing human clinical infection using whole-genome sequencing: virulence, antimicrobial resistance and phylogeny in Ireland. *PLoS One*. 2019;14(7):e0219088.
92. Zhao S, Mukherjee S, Chen Y, et al. Novel gentamicin resistance genes in Campylobacter isolated from humans and retail meats in the USA. *J Antimicrob Chemother*. 2015;70(5):1314–1321.
93. Zhao S, Tyson GH, Chen Y, et al. Whole-genome sequencing analysis accurately predicts antimicrobial resistance phenotypes in *Campylobacter* spp. *Appl Environ Microbiol*. 2016;82(2):459–466.
94. Chen Y, Mukherjee S, Hoffmann M, et al. Whole-genome sequencing of gentamicin-resistant *Campylobacter coli* isolated from US retail meats reveals novel plasmid-mediated aminoglycoside resistance genes. *Antimicrob Agents Chemother*. 2013;57 (11):5398–5405.
95. Biomarkers Definitions Working GroupAtkinson Jr AJ, Colburn WA, et al. Biomarkers and surrogate endpoints: preferred definitions and conceptual framework. *Clin Pharmacol Ther*. 2001;69 (3):89–95.
96. Van De Guchte M, Serror P, Chervaux C, Smokvina T, Ehrlich SD, Maguin E. Stress responses in lactic acid bacteria. *Antonie Van Leeuwenhoek*. 2002;82(1–4):187–216.
97. Brul S, Schuren F, Montijn R, Keijser B, Van der Spek H, Oomes S. The impact of functional genomics on microbiological food quality and safety. *Int J Food Microbiol*. 2006;112(3):195–199.

98. Zomer A, van Sinderen D. Intertwinement of stress response regulons in Bifidobacterium breve UCC2003. *Gut Microbes*. 2010;1(2):100–102.
99. Pielaat A, Boer MP, Wijnands LM, et al. First step in using molecular data for microbial food safety risk assessment; hazard identification of *Escherichia coli* O157: H7 by coupling genomic data with in vitro adherence to human epithelial cells. *Int J Food Microbiol*. 2015;213:130–138.
100. Cocolin L, Mataragas M, Bourdichon F, et al. Next generation microbiological risk assessment meta-omics: the next need for integration. *Int J Food Microbiol*. 2018;287:10–17.
101. Den Besten HM, Arvind A, Gaballo HM, Moezelaar R, Zwietering MH, Abee T. Short-and long-term biomarkers for bacterial robustness: a framework for quantifying correlations between cellular indicators and adaptive behavior. *PLoS One*. 2010;5(10):e13746.
102. Haddad N, Johnson N, Kathariou S, et al. Next generation microbiological risk assessment—potential of omics data for hazard characterisation. *Int J Food Microbiol*. 2018;287:28–39.
103. Membre J-M, Guillou S. Latest developments in foodborne pathogen risk assessment. *Curr Opin Food Sci*. 2016;8:120–126.
104. den Besten HM, Amézquita A, Bover-Cid S, et al. Next generation of microbiological risk assessment: potential of omics data for exposure assessment. *Int J Food Microbiol*. 2018;287:18–27.
105. Desriac N, Coroller L, Sohier D, Postollec F. An integrative approach to identify *Bacillus weihenstephanensis* resistance biomarkers using gene expression quantification throughout acid inactivation. *Food Microbiol*. 2012;32(1):172–178.
106. Desriac N, Postollec F, Coroller L, Sohier D, Abee T, Den Besten H. Prediction of *Bacillus weihenstephanensis* acid resistance: the use of gene expression patterns to select potential biomarkers. *Int J Food Microbiol*. 2013;167(1):80–86.
107. Pielaat A, Barker G, Hendriksen P, Hollman P, Peijnenburg A, Ter Kuile B. A foresight study on emerging technologies: state of the art of omics technologies and potential applications in food and feed safety. *EFSA Support Publ*. 2013;10(10):495E.
108. Brul S, Bassett J, Cook P, et al. 'Omics' technologies in quantitative microbial risk assessment. *Trends Food Sci Technol*. 2012;27(1):12–24.
109. Desriac N, Broussolle V, Postollec F, et al. *Bacillus cereus* cell response upon exposure to acid environment: toward the identification of potential biomarkers. *Front Microbiol*. 2013;4:284.
110. Fritsch L, Guillier L, Augustin J-C. Next generation quantitative microbiological risk assessment: refinement of the cold smoked salmon-related listeriosis risk model by integrating genomic data. *Microb Risk Anal*. 2018;10:20–27.
111. Lindsey RL, Pouseele H, Chen JC, Strockbine NA, Carleton HA. Implementation of whole genome sequencing (WGS) for identification and characterization of Shiga toxin-producing *Escherichia coli* (STEC) in the United States. *Front Microbiol*. 2016;7:766.
112. Franz E, Gras LM, Dallman T. Significance of whole genome sequencing for surveillance, source attribution and microbial risk assessment of foodborne pathogens. *Curr Opin Food Sci*. 2016;8:74–79.
113. Rantsiou K, Kathariou S, Winkler A, et al. Next generation microbiological risk assessment: opportunities of whole genome sequencing (WGS) for foodborne pathogen surveillance, source tracking and risk assessment. *Int J Food Microbiol*. 2018;287:3–9.
114. FDA. Whole genome sequencing (WGS) program. <https://www.fda.gov/food/science-research-food/whole-genome-sequencing-wgs-program>; 2020.
115. European Centre for Disease Prevention and Control. In: *Monitoring the use of whole-genome sequencing in infectious disease surveillance in Europe*. Stockholm: ECDC; 2018.
116. Istituto Zooprofilattico Sperimentale dell'Abruzzo e del Molise "G. Caporale", T., ItalyArdelean A, Calistri P, et al. Development of food safety risk assessment tools based on molecular typing and WGS of *Campylobacter jejuni* genome. *EFSA J*. 2019;17:e170903.
117. Painset A, Day M, Doumith M, et al. Comparison of phenotypic and WGS-derived antimicrobial resistance profiles of *Campylobacter jejuni* and *Campylobacter coli* isolated from cases of diarrhoeal disease in England and Wales, 2015–16. *J Antimicrob Chemother*. 2020;75(4):883–889.
118. Rokney A, Valinsky L, Vranckx K, et al. WGS-based prediction and analysis of antimicrobial resistance in *Campylobacter jejuni* isolates from Israel. *Front Cell Infect Microbiol*. 2020;10:365.
119. Dutta V, Altermann E, Olson J, Wray GA, Siletzky RM, Kathariou S. Whole-genome sequences of agricultural, host-associated *Campylobacter coli* and *Campylobacter jejuni* strains. *Genome Announc*. 2016;4(4). e00833-16.
120. Duqué B, Haddad N, Rossero A, Membré J-M, Guillou S. Influence of cell history on the subsequent inactivation of *Campylobacter jejuni* during cold storage under modified atmosphere. *Food Microbiol*. 2019;84:103263.
121. Duqué B. *Innovative Methodology Combining Transcriptomics, Statistics, and Modelling to Evaluate the Capacity of Campylobacter jejuni to Survive Stress* [Ph.D. thesis]. Oniris; 2020.
122. Duqué B, Rezé S, Rossero A, Membré J-M, Guillou S, Haddad N. Quantification of *Campylobacter jejuni* gene expression after successive stresses mimicking poultry slaughtering steps. *Food Microbiol*. 2021;98:103795.
123. Magajna BA, Schraft H. *Campylobacter jejuni* biofilm cells become viable but non-culturable (VBNC) in low nutrient conditions at 4 C more quickly than their planktonic counterparts. *Food Control*. 2015;50:45–50.
124. Bovill R, Mackey dB. Resuscitation of 'non-culturable'cells from aged cultures of *Campylobacter jejuni*. *Microbiology*. 1997;143(5):1575–1581.
125. Cappelier J, Minet J, Magras C, Colwell R, Federighi M. Recovery in embryonated eggs of viable but nonculturable *Campylobacter jejuni* cells and maintenance of ability to adhere to HeLa cells after resuscitation. *Appl Environ Microbiol*. 1999;65(11):5154–5157.
126. Baffone W, Casaroli A, Citterio B, et al. *Campylobacter jejuni* loss of culturability in aqueous microcosms and ability to resuscitate in a mouse model. *Int J Food Microbiol*. 2006;107(1):83–91.
127. Teunis P, Havelaar A. The beta Poisson dose-response model is not a single-hit model. *Risk Anal*. 2000;20(4):513–520.
128. Teunis P, Van den Brandhof W, Nauta M, Wagenaar J, Van den Kerkhof H, Van Pelt W. A reconsideration of the *Campylobacter* dose–response relation. *Epidemiol Infect*. 2005;133(4):583–592.

129. Teunis PF, Marinović AB, Tribble DR, Porter CK, Swart A. Acute illness from *Campylobacter jejuni* may require high doses while infection occurs at low doses. *Epidemics*. 2018;24:1–20.
130. Wachira VK, Peixoto HM, de Oliveira MRF. Systematic review of factors associated with the development of Guillain–Barré syndrome 2007–2017: what has changed? *Trop Med Int Health*. 2019;24(2):132–142.
131. Koga M, Gilbert M, Takahashi M, et al. Comprehensive analysis of bacterial risk factors for the development of Guillain-Barré syndrome after *Campylobacter jejuni enteritis*. *J Infect Dis*. 2006;193(4):547–555.
132. Rees JH, Soudain SE, Gregson NA, Hughes RA. *Campylobacter jejuni* infection and Guillain–Barré syndrome. *N Engl J Med*. 1995;333(21):1374–1379.
133. Ho T, Mishu B, Li C, et al. Guillain-Barre syndrome in northern China. Relationship to *Campylobacter jejuni* infection and anti-glycolipid antibodies. *Brain*. 1995;118(3):597–605.
134. Islam Z, Jacobs B, van Belkum A, et al. Axonal variant of Guillain-Barre syndrome associated with Campylobacter infection in Bangladesh. *Neurology*. 2010;74(7):581–587.
135. Jacobs BC, van Doorn PA, Tio-Gillen AP, et al. *Campylobacter jejuni* infections and anti-GM1 antibodies in Guillain-Barré syndrome. *Ann Neurol*. 1996;40(2):181–187.
136. Allos BM. Association between *Campylobacter* infection and Guillain-Barré syndrome. *J Infect Dis*. 1997;176(suppl 2): S125–S128.
137. Ang CW, Jacobs BC, Laman JD. The Guillain–Barré syndrome: a true case of molecular mimicry. *Trends Immunol*. 2004;25 (2):61–66.
138. Yuki N, Susuki K, Koga M, et al. Carbohydrate mimicry between human ganglioside GM1 and *Campylobacter jejuni* lipooligosaccharide causes Guillain–Barré syndrome. *Proc Natl Acad Sci U S A*. 2004;101(31):11404–11409.
139. Nachamkin I, Allos BM, Ho T. *Campylobacter* species and Guillain-Barre syndrome. *Clin Microbiol Rev*. 1998;11(3):555–567.
140. Hameed A, Woodacre A, Machado LR, Marsden GL. An updated classification system and review of the lipooligosaccharide biosynthesis gene locus in *Campylobacter jejuni*. *Front Microbiol*. 2020;11:677.
141. Karlyshev AV, Ketley JM, Wren BW. The *Campylobacter jejuni* glycome. *FEMS Microbiol Rev*. 2005;29(2):377–390.
142. Godschalk PC, Heikema AP, Gilbert M, et al. The crucial role of *Campylobacter jejuni* genes in anti-ganglioside antibody induction in Guillain-Barre syndrome. *J Clin Investig*. 2004;114(11):1659–1665.
143. Parker CT, Gilbert M, Yuki N, Endtz HP, Mandrell RE. Characterization of lipooligosaccharide-biosynthetic loci of *Campylobacter jejuni* reveals new lipooligosaccharide classes: evidence of mosaic organizations. *J Bacteriol*. 2008;190(16):5681–5689.
144. Parker CT, Horn ST, Gilbert M, Miller WG, Woodward DL, Mandrell RE. Comparison of *Campylobacter jejuni* lipooligosaccharide biosynthesis loci from a variety of sources. *J Clin Microbiol*. 2005;43(6):2771–2781.
145. Gilbert M, Karwaski M-F, Bernatchez S, et al. The genetic bases for the variation in the lipo-oligosaccharide of the mucosal pathogen, *Campylobacter jejuni* biosynthesis of sialylated ganglioside mimics in the core oligosaccharide. *J Biol Chem*. 2002;277(1):327–337.
146. Revez J, Hänninen M-L. Lipooligosaccharide locus classes are associated with certain *Campylobacter jejuni* multilocus sequence types. *Eur J Clin Microbiol Infect Dis*. 2012;31 (9):2203–2209.
147. Serichantalergs O, Wassanarungroj P, Khemnu N, et al. Distribution of genes related to Type 6 secretion system and lipooligosaccharide that induced ganglioside mimicry among *Campylobacter jejuni* isolated from human diarrhea in Thailand. *Gut Pathog*. 2020;12:1–10.
148. Guyard-Nicodème M, Rivoal K, Houard E, et al. Prevalence and characterization of *Campylobacter jejuni* from chicken meat sold in French retail outlets. *Int J Food Microbiol*. 2015;203:8–14.
149. Habib I, Louwen R, Uyttendaele M, et al. Correlation between genotypic diversity, lipooligosaccharide gene locus class variation, and caco-2 cell invasion potential of *Campylobacter jejuni* isolates from chicken meat and humans: contribution to virulotyping. *Appl Environ Microbiol*. 2009;75(13):4277–4288.
150. Fiedoruk K, Daniluk T, Rozkiewicz D, Oldak E, Prasad S, Swiecicka I. Whole-genome comparative analysis of *Campylobacter jejuni* strains isolated from patients with diarrhea in northeastern Poland. *Gut Pathog*. 2019;11(1):1–10.
151. Elhadidy M, Arguello H, Álvarez-Ordóñez A, et al. Orthogonal typing methods identify genetic diversity among Belgian *Campylobacter jejuni* strains isolated over a decade from poultry and cases of sporadic human illness. *Int J Food Microbiol*. 2018;275:66–75.
152. Ellström P, Hansson I, Nilsson A, Rautelin H, Engvall EO. Lipooligosaccharide locus classes and putative virulence genes among chicken and human *Campylobacter jejuni* isolates. *BMC Microbiol*. 2016;16(1):116.
153. Hardy CG, Lackey LG, Cannon J, Price LB, Silbergeld EK. Prevalence of potentially neuropathic *Campylobacter jejuni* strains on commercial broiler chicken products. *Int J Food Microbiol*. 2011;145(2–3):395–399.
154. Thépault A, Méric G, Rivoal K, et al. Genome-wide identification of host-segregating epidemiological markers for source attribution in *Campylobacter jejuni*. *Appl Environ Microbiol*. 2017;83(7).
155. van Belkum A, Jacobs B, van Beek E, et al. Can *Campylobacter coli* induce Guillain-Barré syndrome? *Eur J Clin Microbiol Infect Dis*. 2009;28(5):557–560.
156. Funakoshi K, Koga M, Takahashi M, Hirata K, Yuki N. *Campylobacter coli* enteritis and Guillain–Barré syndrome: no evidence of molecular mimicry and serological relationship. *J Neurol Sci*. 2006;246(1–2):163–168.
157. Goddard E, Lastovica A, Argent A. Campylobacter 0: 41 isolation in Guillain-Barre syndrome. *Arch Dis Child*. 1997;76(6):526–528.
158. Bersudsky M, Rosenberg P, Rudensky B, Wirguin I. Lipopolysaccharides of a *Campylobacter coli* isolate from a patient with Guillain-Barré syndrome display ganglioside mimicry. *J Peripher Nerv Syst*. 2000;5(4):240.
159. Richards VP, Lefébure T, Bitar PDP, Stanhope MJ. Comparative characterization of the virulence gene clusters (lipooligosaccharide [LOS] and capsular polysaccharide [CPS]) for *Campylobacter coli*, *Campylobacter jejuni* subsp. *jejuni* and related *Campylobacter* species. *Infect Genet Evol*. 2013;14:200–213.
160. Culebro A, Machado MP, Carriço JA, Rossi M. Origin, evolution, and distribution of the molecular machinery for biosynthesis of sialylated lipooligosaccharide structures in *Campylobacter coli*. *Sci Rep*. 2018;8(1):1–9.

Chapter 52

Identification and assessment of exposure to emerging foodborne pathogens using foodborne human viruses as an example

Robert L. Buchanan

Center for Food Safety and Security Systems, Department of Nutrition and Food Science, University of Maryland, College Park, MD, United States

Abstract

The past 80 years has seen the emergence of a variety of foodborne diseases caused by contamination of foods with emerging bacterial, viral, fungal, algal, protozoan, and parasitic disease agents, including potential metabolites. Control of these emerging pathogens requires the rapid acquisition of knowledge related to the microorganism's characteristics, ecology, etiology, and survival within food matrices. This, in turn, depends on our ability to rapidly mobilize public health, research, and industry resources. Such capability is key to getting a rapid response to a new threat. The emergence of human viruses provides an excellent example of emerging foodborne threats. Current knowledge indicates fecal/oral transmission favors nonenveloped foodborne viruses, and their control is likely to provide even greater control of enveloped viruses, since the latter are more susceptible to tools used to eliminate the former.

Keywords: Norovirus; hepatitis A virus; preventive controls; risk mitigation

52.1 Introduction to emerging foodborne diseases

Prior to World War II, there were relatively few pathogenic microorganisms where foods were considered a major vehicle for transmission. This included a relatively small number of bacteria (e.g., *Salmonella* spp.),[1] *Clostridium botulinum*,[2] *Staphylococcus aureus*,[3] *Shigella dysenteriae*,[4] *Vibrio cholerae*,[5] protozoa (*Entamoeba histolytica*)[6], parasites such as *Taenia solium*[7] and *Trichinella spiralis*,[8] and likely human viruses [e.g., hepatitis A virus (HAV)[9]]. In part due to the conditions associated with World War II, there was a significant expansion of knowledge of infectious diseases and their epidemiology, including those transmitted by food and water that would have previously been considered "exotic" diseases.

After the war, there was a large investment in microbiological research and public health epidemiology that led to the identification of new microbiological threats that had not been widely recognized as major contributors to foodborne microbiological disease. For example, in the mid-1940s, *Clostridium perfringens* (previously *Clostridium welchii*) began to be implicated in outbreaks of diarrheal disease associated with contaminated foods[10,59]. This appeared to be limited to *C. perfringens* Type A strains, but this was initially controversial since the disease could not be reproduced consistently. Ultimately it was determined that certain strains produced endospores, with substantially greater thermal resistant endospores, that produced an enterotoxin during sporulation.[11] A similar situation occurred with *Bacillus cereus* which began to be implicated with foodborne disease outbreaks in the 1950s, which ultimately led to identification of both diarrheal and emetic strains that are now internationally recognized as important foodborne pathogenic bacteria (Hobbs, 1974). This was the same era that saw the status of *Escherichia coli* as a nonpathogenic bacterium weaken as outbreaks of infantile diarrhea and travelers' diarrhea were linked to enteropathogenic *E. coli* and enterotoxigenic *E. coli.*[12] The initial outbreaks of *Vibrio parahaemolyticus* associated with seafood were observed in the 1950s[5] and *Aeromonas hydrophila* in the early 1960s.[13] The emergence of new food safety concerns was not limited to bacteria. For example, an outbreak of "Turkey X" disease in 1960 led to the identification of aflatoxins, and the role of mycotoxins as food safety concerns.

Present Knowledge in Food Safety. DOI: https://doi.org/10.1016/B978-0-12-819470-6.00057-3

Since the emergence of new foodborne hazards described above, there has been almost a continual series of emerging foodborne threats to public health. This includes emergence of *Vibrio vulnificus* in 1976,[5] *Listeria monocytogenes* in 1981,[14] enterohemorrhagic *E. coli* in 1982,[15] *Cronobacter sakazakii* in 1990[60]. This is not limited to bacterial hazards. The emergence of norovirus (NoV) in 1969 has since led to it being considered one of the most frequent causes of foodborne outbreaks.[16] The protozoan species *Cyclospora cayetanensis* began to be recognized in international foodborne outbreaks in 1993.[17] Human cases of prion-associated Bovine Spongiform Encephalopathy were added to the list of foodborne hazards in 2004.[18] In addition to initial emergence, we saw the re-emergence of previously recognized pathogens such as the establishment of *C. botulinum* as the causes of infantile botulism.[19,20] The apparent increase and emergence of new microbiological threats to food safety appear to reflect several factors such as improvements in our understanding of disease mechanisms, the globalization of the food supply, international sharing of outbreak reporting, and ongoing consumer apprehensions related to the safety of food supply.

The history of emerging diseases has demonstrated that in stable environments and communities, the rate of new diseases occurs at a slow rate, and its spread limited to specific regions. Often when an emergence occurs, it can be traced to a significant change in climate, diet, movement of animal or human populations, or changes in technology. A pertinent historical example of a food associated emergence is the outbreaks of ergotism in Europe beginning in CE 857. The condition was originally referred to as Saint Anthony's Fire and caused outbreaks in Europe during the Middle Ages. Centuries later, the cause of ergotism was determined to be a group of mycotoxins produced by the fungus *Claviceps purpurea*. The emergence of this mycotoxicosis was coincident with the introduction of rye into European diets. *C. purpurea* is a field fungus disease associated with this cereal grain. On an even larger scale, our history is replete with the emergence of devastating outbreaks associated with increased rate of European exploration of the world to establish new trading opportunities. This was accompanied by disastrous dissemination of diseases such as smallpox, tuberculosis, and leprosy, particularly to North America, South America, and the Polynesian islands.

The overall goal of this chapter is to describe the general process of dealing with emerging foodborne pathogens and the process by which their risks to the consuming population are established and ultimately controlled. This will be followed in a more detailed examination using foodborne human viruses as examples.

52.2 Knowledge needed to control an emerging foodborne concern

The identification of a new foodborne microbiological hazard starts a process focused on acquiring key information needed to assess the risk to public health and develop control strategies for mitigating those risks. The effectiveness of the process is highly dependent on mobilizing multiple public health, scientific, engineering, and industry resources. Key to developing effective control strategies is acquiring and understanding areas such as the:

- Identity of the microbiological agent
- Methods for the detection, differentiation, and enumeration of the hazard
- Epidemiology of the hazard and its array of adverse effects
- Mechanism of pathogenicity
- Potential for immune-based protection
- Identification of human subpopulations at increased risk
- Modes and vehicles of transmission
- Normal habitat and reservoirs of the agent
- Identification of potential prevention strategies
- Identification of potential intervention strategies
- Survival characteristics of the agent
- Potential for growth or amplification of the hazard in foods
- Survival potential of the hazard in foods

This often requires bringing together expertise from around the world. In foodborne disease this is a role that is often played by two United Nations' agencies, World Health Organization (WHO) and Food and Agriculture Organization (FAO), working in cooperation with national government agencies. The WHO and FAO are also the lead agencies for the international food standards-setting body, Codex Alimentarius. This organization has played an important role in trying to harmonize standard setting for foods globally, in part, as a means of ensuring that such standards are based on scientific evidence and consider alternative methods and technologies for achieving those standards.

As indicated above, gaining control of an emerging foodborne microbiological threat as rapidly as possible is dependent on being able to gather key data and conduct targeted research. This often requires that teams of experts must be rapidly mobilized and coordinated to ensure a timely response. However, this is a challenge because this also means that researchers will have to halt their current activities to focus on the emerging pathogen. Traditionally, this has proven difficult because of our inability to predict what the next emerging pathogen will be and the cost of maintaining expertise and facilities needed to address each of the numerous potential threats.

Traditionally, this has fallen to national government agencies to maintain expertise and facilities that can be rapidly mobilized. For example, in response to concerns about potential food defense threats, the US Food and Drug Administration (FDA), Center for Disease Control and Prevention, US Department of Agriculture/Food Safety and Inspection Service, and State agencies initiated the Food Emergency Response Network (FERN) that has subsequently expanded to include a range of food safety and food defense concerns.[21] However, often such cooperative programs continue to deal with the last threat. This can lead to a loss of focus on being prepared to deal with the next threat.

In most countries, the greatest food safety research resources are associated with academia. These resources play an important role in the middle phase of addressing and emerging foodborne disease threat. This largely reflects the availability of funds to support new research. This typically reflects the process of acquiring funding from government agencies at both the national and state levels, from philanthropic foundations, and industrial/trade organizations. This typically involves "calls for proposals," submission and review of submitted proposals, and administrative finalization of proposals, and initiation of active research. In most cases this process would take approximately 2–3 years to scale up a new research effort. There are exceptions that historically reduce this time frame. The most common is the establishment of formal cooperative research agreements between government or industry entities and academic institutions. This has proven to be an effective way of accelerating acquisition of needed scientific information related to the emerging food safety threat. There are examples of several public/private partnerships in the area of food safety that have made contributions over several decades, often focusing on a specific aspect of food safety. Similar to the government consortia above, the limiting factor for public/private programs is again the continuity of such efforts. In particular, efforts focused on future needs in relation to emerging foodborne threats that focus on prevention programs often have limited life spans once a threat is controlled. The typical justification is "Why should we continue to fund this project, when there is no current threat and many other research areas are more deserving of funding?" This will be discussed later in the chapter.

52.2.1 Role of risk assessment

The underlying purpose of rapid data and research undertaken when a new microbiological threat emerges (or when a known microbiological threat re-emerges in a new form) is to acquire the knowledge needed to assess the risk posed to the consuming population and evaluate the potential effectiveness of prevention/intervention approaches for mitigating those risks. Prior to the 1990s, this was largely done by bringing together scientists, regulators, industry representatives, and public health officials. Now the process is likely to be augmented using new microbial risk assessment techniques developed in the past 20 years, which were, in turn, realized as a result of the prior 10-year international investment in predictive food microbiology modeling during the 1990s. Beginning in the 1970s, the evaluation of the microbiological safety of food manufacturing facilities has been conducted through hazard analysis as an initial step in developing Hazard Analysis Critical Control Point programs.[22] A critical step during a traditional hazard analysis is after listing all of the potential hazards, the "significant hazards" are identified and become the focus of the critical control point phase of ongoing HACCP programs. The process of determining the significant hazards is in effect the conduct of a risk assessment. The purpose is to determine (1) the probability that a hazard will reach a level where it will lead to adverse effects in the consuming population, (2) the magnitude and likely consequences when such adverse events occur, and (3) the ability of a food safety plan to prevent or mitigate such events.[22–25]

The term microbiological risk assessment covers a broad array of types, techniques, and purposes. Such risk assessments range from relatively simple qualitative risk assessments, through semiquantitative risk assessments, to complex quantitative risk assessments. The quantitative risk assessments are further divided into simpler deterministic assessments to substantially more complex stochastic assessments. The increasing use of the more complex stochastic quantitative microbial risk assessments has been fostered by the availability of various software applications that allow researchers to run sophisticated modeling programs from their personal computers. This includes the ability to run "what-if" scenarios to assess the impact of potential mitigation strategies.[26] Microbiological risk assessment can have several different formats depending on the risk managers' needs. The three most common are (1) risk ranking risk assessments where the relative risks among food classes, pathogens, geographical locations, technologies, etc. need to be compared; (2) product/pathogen pathway risk assessments where the risk factors contributing to the production, distribution, marketing, and preparation are used to assess mitigation alternatives; and (3) attribution assessments when dealing with a pathogen that has multiple pathways for infecting a population. Much of the early work developing microbiological risk assessments and risk assessment techniques were performed by government agencies[23,27–29] and intergovernmental organizations such as the FAO/WHO Joint Expert Meeting on Microbiological Risk Assessment (JEMRA) (https://www.who.int/foodsafety/micro/jemra/en/). Since then, microbiological risk assessments, including sophisticated stochastic modeling, are routinely done by academicians, consulting services, larger corporations, and many governments around the world.

While different formats for conducting a microbiological risk assessment have been proposed, the one most widely used for foods, after being adopted by a number of national governments and Codex Alimentarius, consists of four phases: Hazard Identification (HI), Exposure Assessment (EA), Hazard Characterization (HC), and Risk Characterization (RC).[24]

The HI provides a summary of the current state of knowledge regarding the biological agent, the adverse effects associated with the biological agent, the foods currently implicated, how these foods are produced, processed, and consumed, and other potential sources of the hazard. In the latter case, it is not unusual for foodborne pathogens to include agents that are also disseminated by water and person-to-person transmission. The HI section is also where the scope of the risk assessment is established, including the specific "risk management questions" that the risk assessment has been asked to address.

The EA establishes exposure of the public to the biological agent and/or its toxic metabolites. This phase evaluates the probability that the hazard is present in the food, both in terms of levels and frequency of occurrence. This can be difficult since the analyses of foods for a pathogen are typically done earlier in the food chain, whereas the measurement of risk is dependent on estimating the level of the agent actually being consumed. This can be quite complex, particularly for bacteria and fungi that can multiply in a food, and for almost all biological agents that can be inactivated by cooking or other food processing steps. This is the primary reason why quantitative microbiological risk assessment was hampered until the development of predictive microbiology modeling techniques. This is further complicated by the limited sensitivity of most microbiological testing of foods and the need to be able to extrapolate to low levels of contamination. Finally, there is limited knowledge concerning what consumers eat, how often they eat it, how they prepare the food, and the amount they actually consume. Most of this type of information is derived from nutritional status studies performed by a limited number of national governments and/or estimates of food sales by food manufacturers.

The HC is the phase that establishes the dose–response relationships associated with the elicitation of an adverse effect caused by the hazard. As with the EA, this can be a complex process since there is typically a great degree of diversity that has to be considered in selecting the adverse effect caused by the hazard and relative susceptibility of the consuming population. It is well established that infectious microorganisms can vary substantially in terms of their relative virulence. Likewise, it is well known that certain subpopulations are likely to be more susceptible to a pathogen or more likely to have life threatening sequelae. In general, the very young, the elderly and individuals with underlying conditions such as diabetes, cancer, or immunosuppressive therapies and pregnant women are more susceptible. On the other hand, for a number of infectious diseases (e.g., HAV) prior exposure can provide lifetime immunity unless the immune system is severely suppressed. This type of diversity leads to dose–response relationships that have huge variances. Risk assessments have gotten around this difficulty by using multiple dose–response relationships. For example, the FDA/FSIS risk assessment for *L. monocytogenes* developed dose–response models for three groups, healthy individuals, the elderly, and neonatal infants[30] and the subsequent FAO/WHO *L. monocytogenes* developed relative risk dose–response models for 13 subpopulations at increased risk.[31]

The RC involves the combination of the HC and the EA to determine the risk associated with the ingestion of the biological agent in the food(s) being considered in the risk assessment. Depending on the specific design of the risk assessment, the RC addresses the risk management questions posed by the requestor. Typically the results of an RC will provide two types of risk metrics, the risk per serving of the contaminated food and the annual risk to the country. The first provides the risk to individual consumers each time they partake of a serving of the food, while the latter estimates the overall public health burden to the country. A quantitative RC model also allows the consideration of "What-If" scenarios to provide estimates of how medical advances (e.g., development of a vaccine) or changes in the supply chain, food processing, food distribution, and home preparation are likely to mitigate the risks. The opportunities to perform sensitivity analyses that examine the relative importance of risk factors, and perform uncertainty analyses to separate uncertainty from inherent variability are among the features that can be realized by performing stochastic quantitative microbial risk assessments.

52.3 Emergence of foodborne viruses

With the 2019-novel Corona Virus (nCOVID-19) pandemic affecting public health globally, there has been renewed interest in foodborne viruses as potential hazards in foods and food ingredients. However, viral diseases were recognized long before there were methods for their detection and characterization. The earliest evidence of primate-associated virus infections is Herpes viruses found in the fossil records 80,000,000 years ago. Since the beginning of record keeping by ancient civilizations through the Middle Ages, outbreaks and even pandemics were associated with smallpox, influenza, rabies, polio, and measles viruses. However, physical proof that these agents existed was not confirmed until the early application of electron microscopy in 1939[61], and quantitation of viral load by the use of plaque assays in 1952.[32,33]

Viruses can be divided into two broad categories, enveloped and nonenveloped. The former has an outer "envelope" consisting in large part of the previous host cell's plasma membrane as the new virus particle buds off from the host cell. The viral envelope appears to help facilitate the dissemination of the virus from one host cell to another, and allows it to avoid the host's immune response. The nonenveloped viruses lack this structure, likely due to their life cycle involving the production of an enzyme that mediates lysis of the host cell. Thus a nonenveloped virus consists of an outer protein capsid which protects the viral genetic material (DNA or RNA). In general, foodborne human viruses are nonenveloped; a characteristic that is associated with the viral particle being more resistant to adverse conditions such as heating or desiccation.[16] Foodborne viruses are typically those that are transmitted by an oral/fecal route, where ingestion of intact virions is the predominant route of transmission.[16,34] However, it is important to note that foods are not their only route of transmission. Their transfer via fecal material can include foods, water, and person-to-person[34] (see Table 52.1). The two most important of the foodborne viruses are HAV and NoV. NoV is considered one of the major foodborne pathogens in terms of number of cases and number of hospitalizations per year, but is generally nonfatal. Hepatitis A infections are primarily a childhood disease in developing countries related to water consumption, while it is a more serious pathogen in developed countries where it can be a cause of serious infections in immunologically naïve adults and have a higher incidence of being transmitted via foods. However, in developed countries, the number of hepatitis A infections has been declining substantially with the introduction of highly effective vaccines. Similarly, prior to the 1950s polio virus was a concern from food, water, and person-to-person dissemination, but thanks to a global vaccination effort, is almost totally eradicated as a human disease.

Foodborne outbreaks with HAV and NoV are typically associated with foods prepared by infected food workers, consumption of ready-to-eat foods that receive no or minimal cooking, and food harvested or prepared with contaminated water. Examples includes foods such as shellfish harvested from feces-contaminated growing waters,[35,36] frozen berries (e.g., raspberries, blackberries, and strawberries),[37] and possible asymptomatic food workers.[38] Several risk assessments have been conducted on various factors associated with both NoV[39–43] and HAV.[36,44] Most of the other foodborne viruses have not had formal risk assessments performed with the exception of Hepatitis E which has been linked to hepatitis cases transmitted from pigs.[45,46]

52.3.1 Estimating exposure to foodborne viruses

As discussed above, making informed decisions about the level of control needed to safeguard foods from a microbiological threat is ideally based on scientific understanding of the disease and the factors related to the occurrence of the biological agent in foods and how different foods affect the frequency and the levels in a food. Several factors have to be considered when trying to conduct a reasonably accurate exposure assessment that could be used in conjunction with a dose–response curve (HA) to develop the RC.

TABLE 52.1 Characteristics of foodborne viral infections.

Frequency of transmission	Virus name	Virus family	Genome	Routes of transmission		
				Oral/ fecal–food	Person - to-person	Water/ environment
High	Hepatitis A	*Picornaviridae*	ssRNA	X	X	X
	Norovirus	*Caliciviridae*	ssRNA	X	X	X
Low/unknown	Hepatitis E	*Hepeviridae*	ssRNA	X		X
Rare	Aichi	*Picornaviridae*	ssRNA	X		X
	Astro	*Astroviridae*	ssRNA	X	X	X
	Rota	*Reoviridae*	dsRNA	X	X	
	Sapo	*Caliciviridae*	ssRNA	X	X	
Historic	Polio	*Picornaviridae*	ssRNA	X	X	X

Source: Adapted from Miranda RC, Schaffner DW. Virus risk in the food supply chain. Curr. Opin. Food Sci. 2019;30:43–48, and graciously provided with their permission.

52.3.1.1 Quantifying virus levels in foods

Traditional methods for quantifying the levels of a virus in a food have been done using plaque assays where the food is diluted and the dilutions are used to inoculate an appropriate confluent monolayer of cells, and estimate the original level of virions by the number of plaques observed. While there are issues such as viral clumping that can underestimate the viral load, this has long been a standard method for determining viral counts.[47] However, the approach becomes more challenging when assessing viral loads in foods. The assays must suppress the growth of bacteria and fungi in the foods that would contaminate the cell culture plates. This typically would require the maceration of the food, followed by centrifugation or ultrafiltration to remove bacteria and food debris or alternatively providing antimicrobials that suppress bacterial growth without interfering with the target virus. A limiting factor is the duration of the incubation times needed, which can range up to 8 days. Another limiting factor is that it is limited to lytic viruses. This is not a problem with most known foodborne viruses which are lytic, nonenveloped viruses.

The traditional plaque assays cannot be routinely used for the two most important foodborne viruses, NoV and HAV. An effective cell line has not been identified for NoV.[48] While a limited number of specialized cell culture techniques have been developed for the cultivation of HAV, such as fetal rhesus monkey kidney cell line (Frhk-4),[49] they are not routinely used in the detection of HAV in foods. Instead, HAV and HAE detection has increasingly relied on antibody-based or genomic-based detection systems,[50–53] Reliance on immunologic and genomic methods is also true for NoV.[54–56]

Another important attribute associated with quantifying viruses is determining how many of the virions are actually capable of entering a host cell and initiate reproduction of new viruses. Early in virus research it was noted that when viral particles in an inoculum were counted by electron microscopy or flow cytometer the number observed was generally substantially higher than the number of plaques noted with plaque assay or a similar method based on virus replication. Originally in phage and then human virus research these observations were referred to a host's "multiplicity of infection." The metric used to describe this phenomenon was initially interpreted as the number of times a single host cell could be infected.[57,58] However, this interpretation of the phenomenon has been challenged. The metric currently used for measuring this effect is the P/IU ratio where P is the number of viral particles and IU is the infectious units as determined by a plaque assay or similar measure of infectivity. Klasse[57] cited a number of examples of P/IU values such as polio virus (30–1000), herpes simplex virus (50–200), dengue virus (3000–70,000), and papilloma virus (10,000). These values are interpreted as having a substantial portion of the viruses released not being capable of causing an infection or the loss of infectivity as the viruses are stored. The variability within a virus is interpreted as "strain" differences.[57] The actual entry into a host cell in culture has been found to be complex, involving the likelihood of the viral particle coming in contact with the host cell, the mechanism of absorption, the number of receptor sites per cell, the fidelity of the reverse transcriptase activity in the host cell, and the number of capsids formed without their nucleic acid.[57] These factors could interfere with methods to quantify the levels and frequency of virus in foods and development of dose–response relationships. For example, if a detection method was antibody-based, if there was a large number of capsid without a nucleic acid, this would lead to an overestimation of virus levels. Similar concerns would be occurring if a portion of the nucleic acid molecules contains replication errors.

52.3.1.2 Estimating the levels of infectious viruses ingested by consumers

The determination of consumers' exposures to a foodborne pathogen is dependent on knowing the dose that the individual actually ingests during eating occasions. However, this value is almost impossible to determine directly since pathogen levels in foods are determined at some point prior to consumption. Changes can take place between initial measurements and consumption in a relatively short time span, increasing by orders of magnitude if the pathogen can grow in the food (not applicable to viruses) or decreasing rapidly if the food is subjected to an intervention technology such as cooking. As mentioned earlier, the technological advances that allowed barriers to be overcome was the investment in predictive microbiology modeling of the events that take place during the cultivation, processing, distribution, marketing, and preparation of foods. This allows the risk assessment to estimate the levels of pathogens or their toxic metabolites being ingested.

The estimation of the levels actually ingested for foodborne viruses is somewhat simplified by the fact that human viruses do not grow in foods. Thus the predictive microbiology modeling needed is limited to survival models, inactivation models, and risk ranking models. However, generating the data to develop such models is generally considered more complicated due to the increased complexity of working with viruses in foods. The development of inactivation models is relatively straightforward for treatments such as thermal processing, but can be more complex for alternative technologies. The development of survival models is more complex due to the ability of the viruses to withstand adverse environments and the complexities of assessing the percentage of infectious units over time and environmental conditions. However, with a concerted effort EA and HC phases of a microbial risk assessment can be accomplished.

The completion of a quantitative microbial risk assessment allows the selection of risk management strategies to be evaluated, with long-term focus being highly dependent on the availability of medical advances. The most effective control of foodborne pathogens has been viruses that are amendable to vaccines that provide long-term immunity, as is the case with polio virus and HAV. Alternatively, when the virus does not lend itself to the development of a vaccine, as is the case with NoV to date, then the strategy for control will involve the development of a series of preventive and intervention controls that are put into place to mitigate the risks.

52.4 Concluding remarks

The periodic emergence of new foodborne pathogenic microorganisms is a threat that has been faced by mankind over the entire course of its history. Earlier in our history the combination of geographic distancing and slow rate of interactions among human populations, such emergences tended to be limited to specific regions. As discussed earlier, a classic example is the explosion of smallpox among the indigenous populations in North and South America. Since the industrial revolution, the speed at which both food and people move around the world has steadily increased such that the COVID-19 pandemic spread around the world in months instead of decades.

The lament too often heard is "how can you know what is the next emerging pathogen going to be." While one cannot predict with certainty what the next emerging foodborne disease will be, public health and food safety experts have long preached that it is not a matter of if, but a matter of when. While we may not know the identity of a new emerging foodborne biological threat, we have substantial experience in knowing the types of information that would be needed to identify the threat, characterize its epidemiology and etiology, the potential types of processes and practices that would be needed to control the pathogen, and the communication systems needed to get this information out to the farmers, food manufacturers, distributors, retail companies, and consumers need to protect themselves and their businesses. The focus needs to be how to acquire this knowledge as quickly and efficiently as possible. An example that I like to cite when it comes to emerging diseases is the formation of the US Public Health Service in the early days of the United States to respond to the emergence of a yellow fever outbreak in Philadelphia, which at the time was the nation's capital. I consider this a good model for maintaining a cadre of highly trained scientists and physicians that can respond to a national need within 24 h. Such capability is key to getting a rapid response to a new threat. However, that is not sufficient by itself and typically requires the effort to take advantage of the expertise that is available in our universities, medical schools, and the food industry. In such a scenario, past experience has indicated that ongoing public/private partnerships are an effective way of being able to rapidly focus on a new public health concern. Such partnerships may also be a means of coordinating the work that needs to be accomplished. Too often in an emerging emergency, there is a great deal of redundancy in the research that is being done. While some redundancy is at the heart of the scientific method, it should be planned for if at all possible. Finally, sustained efforts of this nature too often face an inability to attract long-term support while waiting for the next emerging pathogen. Thus emergency planning requires the organizations supporting such an effort have meaningful research to return to while continuing to expand our ability to control current and future microbial threats to our food supply.

References

1. Li H, Wang H, D'Aoust J-Y, Maurer J. *Salmonella* species. In: Doyle MP, Buchanan RL, eds. *Food Microbiology: Fundamentals and Frontiers.* 4th ed. Washington, DC: ASM Press; 2013:225–261.
2. Johnson EA. Clostridium botulinum. In: Doyle MP, Buchanan RL, eds. *Food Microbiology: Fundamentals and Frontiers.* 4th ed. Washington, DC: ASM Press; 2013:441–463.
3. Seo KS, Bohach GA. Staphylococcus aureus. In: Doyle MP, Buchanan RL, eds. *Food Microbiology: Fundamentals and Frontiers.* 4th ed. Washington, DC: ASM Press; 2013:547–573.
4. Binet R, Lampel KA. *Shigella* species. In: Doyle MP, Buchanan RL, eds. *Food Microbiology: Fundamentals and Frontiers.* 4th ed. Washington, DC: ASM Press; 2013:377–399.
5. Oliver JD, Pruzzo C, Vezzulli L, Kaper JB. *Vibrio* species. In: Doyle MP, Buchanan RL, eds. *Food Microbiology: Fundamentals and Frontiers.* 4th ed. Washington, DC: ASM Press; 2013:401–439.
6. Schaudinn F. Untersuchungen über die Fontpflauzung einigen Rhizopoden (Vorlaufige Mittheilung). *Arb K Gsudhtsamte.* 1903;19:547–576.
7. Del Bruttoa OH, García HH. *Taenia solium* cysticercosis—the lessons of history. *J Neurol Sci.* 2015;359:392–395.
8. Campbell WC. History of trichinosis: Paget, Owen and the discovery of *Trichinella spiralis. Bull Hist Med.* 1979;53(4):520–552.
9. Cuthbert JA. Hepatitis A: old and new. *Clin Microbiol Rev.* 2001;14(1):38–58.
10. Hobbs BC, Smith ME, Oakley CL, Warrack GH, Cruickshank JC. *Clostridium welchii* food poisoning. *J Hyg.* 1953;51:75–101.
11. McClane BA, Robertson SL, Li J. Clostridium perfringens. In: Doyle MP, Buchanan RL, eds. *Food Microbiology: Fundamentals and Frontiers.* 4th ed. Washington, DC: ASM Press; 2013:465–489.

12. Clarke SC, Haigh RD, Freestone PPE, Williams PH. Enteropathogenic *Escherichia coli* infection: history and clinical aspects. *Br J Biomed Sci.* 2002;59(2):123–127.
13. Galindo CL, Chopra AK. *Aeromonas* and *Plesiomonas.* In: Doyle MP, Beuchat LR, eds. *Food Microbiology: Fundamentals and Frontiers.* 3rd ed. Washington, DC: ASM Press; 2007.
14. Ryser ET, Buchanan RL. Listeria monocytogenes. In: Doyle MP, Buchanan RL, eds. Food Microbiology: Fundamentals and Frontiers. 4th ed. Washington, DC: ASM Press; 2013:503–545.
15. Meng J, LeJeune JT, Zhao T, Doyle MP. Enterohemorrhagic *Escherichia coli.* In: Doyle MP, Buchanan RL, eds. *Food Microbiology: Fundamentals and Frontiers.* 4th ed. Washington, DC: ASM Press; 2013:287–309.
16. Jaykus L-A, D'Souza DH, Moe CL. Foodborne viral pathogens. In: Doyle MP, Buchanan RL, eds. *Food Microbiology: Fundamentals and Frontiers.* 4th ed. Washington, DC: ASM Press; 2013:619–649.
17. Ortega YR. Protozoan parasites. In: Doyle MP, Buchanan RL, eds. *Food Microbiology: Fundamentals and Frontiers.* 4th ed. Washington, DC: ASM Press; 2013:713–733.
18. Brown PW, Detwiler LA. Bovine spongiform encephalopathy. In: Doyle MP, Buchanan RL, eds. *Food Microbiology: Fundamentals and Frontiers.* 4th ed. Washington, DC: ASM Press; 2013:651–671.
19. Buchanan RL. Preparing for emerging and unknown threats: public health. NABC Report 23: Food Security: The Intersection of Sustainability, Safety and Defense. Ithaca, NY: National Agricultural Biotechnology Council; 2011.
20. Shapiro RL, Hatheway C, Swerdlow DL. Botulism in the United States: a clinical and epidemiologic review. *Ann. Intern. Med.* 1998;128 (3):221–228.
21. FDA. Food safety and the coronavirus disease 2019 (COVID-19). <https://www.fda.gov/food/food-safety-during-emergencies/food-safety-and-coronavirus-disease-2019-covid-19>; 2020 Accessed 09.10.20.
22. Buchanan RL, Williams EN. Hazard analysis and critical control point system: use in managing microbiological food safety risks. In: Doyle MP, Buchanan RL, eds. *Food Microbiology: Fundamentals and Frontiers.* 4th ed. Washington, DC: ASM Press; 2013:1039–1057.
23. ICMSF (International Commission on Microbiological Specifications for Foods). Potential application of risk assessment techniques to microbiological issues related to international trade in food and food products. *J Food Prot.* 1998;61:1075–1086.
24. Ruzante JM, Whiting RC, Dennis SB, Buchanan RL. Microbial risk assessment. In: Doyle MP, Buchanan RL, eds. *Food Microbiology: Fundamentals and Frontiers.* 4th ed. Washington, DC: ASM Press; 2013:1023–1037.
25. Whiting RC, Buchanan RL. Predictive microbiology, HACCP, and risk assessment. In: *Proceedings of the 1997/2 Conference on Predictive Microbiology Applied to Chilled Food Preservation.* International Institute of Refrigeration; 1999:105–112.
26. Carrington CD, Dennis SB, Whiting RC, Buchanan RL. Putting a risk assessment model to work: *Listeria monocytogenes* 'what-if' scenarios. *J Assoc Food Drug Off.* 2004;68:5–19.
27. NACMCF (National Advisory Committee on Microbiological Criteria for Foods). Principles of risk assessment for illness caused by foodborne biological agents. *J Food Prot.* 1998;61:1071–1074.
28. Buchanan RL, Dennis SB. Microbial risk assessment: a tool for regulatory decision making. *J Assoc Food Drug Off.* 2001;65 (3):36–46.
29. Whiting RC, Buchanan RL. Development of a quantitative risk assessment mode for *Salmonella enteritidis* in pasteurized liquid eggs. *Int J Food Microbiol.* 1997;36:111–125.
30. FDA/FSIS. *Quantitative Risk Assessment on the Public Health Impact from Foodborne Listeria monocytogenes among Selected Categories of Ready-to-Eat Foods.* Washington, DC: U.S. Food and Drug Administration; 2003. Available from: https://www.fda.gov/food/cfsan-risk-safety-assessments/quantitative-assessment-relative-risk-public-health-foodborne-listeria-monocytogenes-among-selected. Accessed 04.10.20.
31. FAO/WHO. *Risk Assessment of Listeria monocytogenes in Ready-to-Eat Foods.* Microbiological Risk Assessment Series No. 6. Rome, Italy: Food and Agricultural Organization; 2004.
32. Cooper PD. The plaque assay of animal viruses. *Adv Virus Res.* 1961;8:319–378.
33. Dulbecco R, Vogt M. Some problems of animal virology as studied by the plaque technique. *Cold Spring Harb Symp Quant Biol.* 1953;18:273–279.
34. Miranda RC, Schaffner DW. Virus risk in the food supply chain. *Curr Opin Food Sci.* 2019;30:43–48.
35. Baker K, Morris J, McCarthy N, et al. An outbreak of norovirus infection linked to oyster consumption at a UK restaurant, February 2010. *J Public Health (Bangkok).* 2011;33: 205–211.
36. Pinto RM, Costafreda MI, Bosch A. Risk assessment in shellfish-borne outbreaks of hepatitis A. *Appl Environ Microbiol.* 2009;75:7350–7355.
37. Nasheri N, Vester A, Petronella N. Foodborne viral outbreaks associated with frozen produce. *Epidemiol Infect.* 2019;147:e291.
38. Newman KL, Moe CL, Kirby AE, et al. Norovirus in symptomatic and asymptomatic individuals: cytokines and viral shedding. *Clin Exp Immunol.* 2016;184(3):347–357.
39. Duret S, Pouillot R, Fanaselle W, et al. Quantitative risk assessment of norovirus transmission in food establishments: Evaluating the impact of intervention strategies and food employee behavior on the risk associated with norovirus in foods. *Risk Anal.* 2017;. Available from: https://doi.org/10.1111/risa.12758.
40. Masago Y, Katayama H, Watanabe T, et al. Quantitative risk assessment of noroviruses in drinking water based on qualitative data in Japan. *Environ Sci Technol.* 2006;40(23):7428–7433.
41. Mok H-F, Barker SF, Hamilton AJ. A probabilistic quantitative microbial risk assessment model of norovirus disease burden from wastewater irrigation of vegetables in Shepparton, Australia. *Water Res.* 2014;54:347–362.
42. Van Abel N, Schoen ME, Kissel JC, Meschke JS. Comparison of risk predicted by multiple norovirus dose–response models and implications for quantitative microbial risk assessment. *Risk Anal.* 2016;. Available from: https://doi.org/10.1111/risa.12616.
43. Vergara GGRV, Rose JB, Gin KYH. Risk assessment of noroviruses and human adenoviruses in recreational surface waters. *Water Res.* 2016;103:276–282.
44. FDA. Risk profile: hepatitis A virus infection associated with consumption of fresh and fresh-cut produce. <https://www.fda.gov/science-research/peer-review-scientific-information-and-assessments/peer-review-report>; 2018 Accessed 06.10.20.

45. Crotta M, Lavazza A, Mateusa A, Guitiana J. Quantitative risk assessment of hepatitis E virus: modelling the occurrence of viraemic pigs and the presence of the virus in organs of food safety interest. *Microb Risk Anal*. 2018;9:64–71.
46. Ogawa H, Hirayama H, Tanaka S, et al. Risk assessment for hepatitis E virus infection from domestic pigs introduced into an experimental animal facility in a medical school. *J Vet Med Sci*. 2019;81:1191–1196.
47. Baer A, Kehn-Hall K. Viral concentration determination through plaque assays: using traditional and novel overlay systems. *J Vis Exp*. 2014;93:52065.
48. Duizer E, Schwab KJ, Neill FH, Atmar RL, Koopmans MPG, Estes MK. Laboratory efforts to cultivate noroviruses. *J Gen Virol*. 2004;85:79–87.
49. Flehmig B. Hepatitis A-virus in cell culture: I. Propagation of different hepatitis A virus isolates in a fetal rhesus monkey kidney cell line (Frhk-4). *Med Microbiol Immunol*. 1980;168:239–248.
50. Jean J, Blais B, André Darveau A, Fliss I. Detection of hepatitis A virus by the nucleic acid sequence-based amplification technique and comparison with reverse transcription-PCR. *Appl Environ Microbiol*. 2001;67:5593–5600.
51. Shan XC, Wolffs P, Griffiths MW. Rapid and quantitative detection of hepatitis A virus from green onion and strawberry rinses by use of real-time reverse transcription-PCR. *Appl Environ Microbiol*. 2005;71:5624–5626.
52. Williams-Woods J, Hartman G, Burkhardt III W. Chapter 26B: Detection of hepatitis A virus in foods. In: *FDA Bacteriological Analytical Manual*. <https://www.fda.gov/food/laboratory-methods-food/bam-chapter-26b-detection-hepatitis-virus-foods>; 2014 Accessed 08.10.20.
53. Zhang J, Ge SX, Huang GY, et al. Evaluation of antibody-based and nucleic acid-based assays for diagnosis of hepatitis E virus infection in a Rhesus monkey model. *J Med Virol*. 2003;71:518–526.
54. Park YB, You-Hee Cho Y-H, Jee YM, Ko GP. Immunomagnetic separation combined with real-time reverse transcriptase PCR assays for detection of norovirus in contaminated food. *Appl Environ Microbiol*. 2008;74:4226–4230.
55. Tian P, Mandrell R. Detection of norovirus capsid proteins in faecal and food samples by a real time immuno-PCR method. *J Appl Microbiol*. 2005;100:564–574.
56. Vinje J. Advances in laboratory methods for detection and typing of norovirus. *J Clin Microbiol*. 2015;53:373–381.
57. Klasse PJ. Molecular determinants of the ratio of inert to infectious virus particles. *Prog Mol Biol Transl Sci*. 2015;129:285–326.
58. Shabram P, Aguilar-Cordova E. Multiplicity of infection/multiplicity of confusion. *Mol Ther*. 2000;2(5):420–421.
59. Hobbs BC. *Clostridium welchii and Bacillus cereus. Postgraduate Medical Journal*. 1974;50:597–602.
60. Pagotto FJ, Abdesselem K. Cronobacter Species. in M.P. Doyle and R.L. Buchanan Food Microbiology: Fundamentals and Frontiers, 4th ed. ASM Press, Washington D.C. Book Chapter. 2013;311–337.
61. Goldsmith CS, Miller SE. Modern uses of electron microscopy for detection of viruseS. *Clinical Microbiology Reviews*. 2009;22:552–563.

Chapter 53

Transfer of viruses implicated in human disease through food

Kiran N. Bhilegaonkar[1] and Rahul P. Kolhe[2]

[1]*ICAR—Indian Veterinary Research Institute, Regional Centre, Pune, Maharashtra, India,* [2]*KNP College of Veterinary Science, MAFSU, Shirwal, Maharashtra, India*

Abstract

Viruses involved in human foodborne illness due to the consumption of contaminated foods and water are typically referred to as foodborne viruses. Foodborne viruses such as hepatitis A and norovirus are highly contagious, prevalent globally, and responsible for community outbreaks. Some other foodborne viruses include rotavirus, hepatitis E, adenovirus, tick-borne encephalitis, avian influenza, sapovirus, Aichivirus, and nipah viruses. Some foodborne viruses are zoonotic and harbored by animals and birds. Foodborne viruses have typical fecal-oral transmission cycles but other routes of transmission such as direct person-to-person contact, indirect contact with fomites, and airborne through droplets/aerosols have also been reported. The fecal-oral route of transmission is typical and consumption of contaminated foods and water or use of contaminated water in food preparation is responsible for foodborne viral outbreaks. The epidemiology of foodborne viruses is complex and a comprehensive strategy such as the "One Health" approach is important for managing the risk of foodborne viruses.

Keywords: Viruses; hepatitis A; norovirus; zoonotic

53.1 Introduction

Viruses have been recognized as important causes of foodborne diseases. In many developed countries, viruses are now recognized to be common causes of foodborne illness, however, in developing countries, they are rarely diagnosed, as the diagnostic facilities for detection of foodborne viruses are not widely available. Viruses are very small microorganisms (0.02−0.4 uM) with diverse structural and biological properties and require a host cell for replication. The genomic composition varies among different viruses; it can be either DNA or RNA, single-stranded or double-stranded and some viruses have a segmented genome. The structure of some viruses is relatively simple with a single protein coat that is, capsid, whereas others may have complex protein coats with an enveloped membrane surrounding the capsid.[1] The stability and environmental resistance of the viral particle depends on the viral structure; viruses with simple structures are more stable and resistant to environmental conditions in comparison to complex structured viruses.[2] Most foodborne viruses have a simple structure without an envelope and are thus quite stable outside of their host.[3] They demonstrate resistance extremes of pH (acid and alkaline), drying, and radiation.[3,4] These viruses are also able to resist mild food production processes routinely used to inactivate or control bacterial pathogens in contaminated foods.[5]

Viruses can be transmitted in different ways for example, respiratory route (droplets/aerosols), fecal-oral route, direct contact (contact with infected selcretions/excretions/blood, sexual intercourse, contact with infected animals in case of zoonotic viruses), via vectors (mosquitoes or ticks), indirect (vehicles/fomites – cloths/other inanimate objects contaminated with a virus). Viruses involved in human foodborne illness due to consumption of contaminated foods and water are typically referred to as foodborne viruses. Foodborne viruses like Hepatitis A (HAV) and Noroviruses (NoV) are highly contagious, prevalent globally, and responsible for community outbreaks. Fecal-oral route of transmission is typical for foodborne viruses; they are excreted in feces and sometimes in the vomitus. Poor hygiene and sanitation are predisposing factors responsible for the contamination of food with viruses. Consumption of contaminated foods and water or use of contaminated water in food preparation is responsible for foodborne viral outbreaks.[6] Viruses most frequently involved in foodborne infections are NoV and HAV, but other viruses such as Human Rotavirus (HRV), Hepatitis E virus (HEV), Astrovirus, Aichivirus,

Present Knowledge in Food Safety. DOI: https://doi.org/10.1016/B978-0-12-819470-6.00060-3

Sapovirus, Enterovirus, Parvovirus, and Adenovirus can also be transmitted by food. In addition, some other viruses may occasionally be transmitted to humans via food, although their typical mode of transmission is different and they may not cause actual foodborne illnesses for example, Nipah, tick-borne encephalitis, Coronaviruses (SARS/MERS CoV), and Avian Influenza[7,8] (Fig. 53.1). Clinical manifestations recorded in humans due to foodborne viruses may vary and depend on the group of viruses infecting the human host system. Typically, NoV, HRVs, Astroviruses, Aichivirus, Sapo, and Adenoviruses cause gastroenteritis. Viruses like HAV and HEV cause hepatitis and therefore, infect the liver. Enteroviruses, though fecally transmitted, exhibit different pathogenesis and they affect the central nervous system.

In 2008 the Food and Agriculture Organization (FAO) and the World Health Organization (WHO) published a Microbiological Risk Assessment (MRA) report called: "Viruses in Food: Scientific Advice to Support Risk Management Activities".[5] This report can be considered as a tool to be used in the management of risks posed by foodborne viruses, including the elaboration of standards for food in international trade. Important characteristics of foodborne viruses and associated illnesses as per the MRA report are, (1) a living host cell is essential for virus replication and viruses don't replicate on/in food and neither do they deteriorate or spoil food; compositional and organoleptic attributes of foods remain unchanged, even if the food is contaminated with virus particles; (2) few virus particles, as low as one particle, can cause human illness; (3) fecal shedding of foodborne viruses occurs and infected individuals may excrete large amounts of virus particles in stool (10^7-10^{11} per gram); (4) foodborne viruses are generally resistant to environmental conditions and are persistent in the environment, and they can tolerate extreme pH, radiation and drying; (5) the role of animals in the zoonotic transmission of foodborne viruses is significantly lower except for a few like HEV; (6) NoV and HAV are priority foodborne viruses, highly contagious and are spread from person-to-person; secondary transmission via food contaminated by food handlers is commonly associated with foodborne outbreaks of NoV and HAV; (7) characteristics of foodborne viruses present new challenges for food safety risk managers and thus, new guidelines and different approaches need to be implemented when dealing with foodborne viruses.

Foodborne viruses have a typical fecal-oral transmission cycle, and foodborne outbreaks are mostly associated with the consumption of contaminated shellfish, water, vegetables, and fruits.[9,10] It is desirable to have food safety guidelines validated for foodborne viruses. Our understanding of the current control measures for foodborne viruses is limited and there are no indicator organisms for viruses in foods, which can be monitored as is the case for indicator bacteria. Therefore, preventive approaches to avoid contamination at primary and secondary levels of food production and processing are warranted and these need to be integrated with sound HACCP-based food safety management systems. Virus numbers remain static in food as they cannot replicate on/in food; however, certain processes like heating and High-Pressure Processing (HPP) can reduce their numbers. The risk of contamination at primary production is more related to NoV and HAV, especially from infected food handlers, who work with raw products. Rarely does indirect food contamination occur from aerosols or respiratory droplets where viruses like Nipah, SARS, avian influenza, and SARS-CoV-2 are concerned.

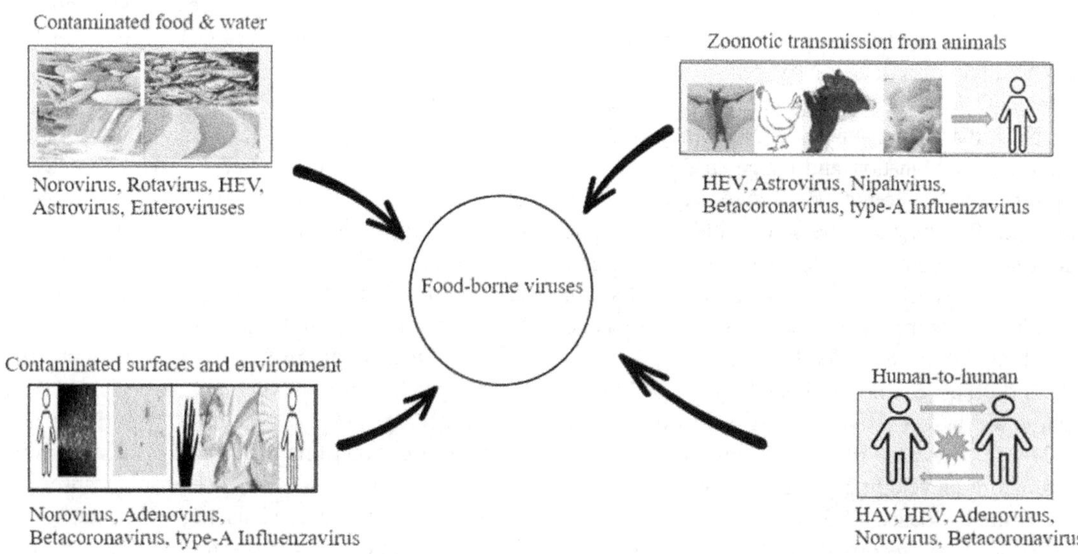

FIGURE 53.1 Transmission of foodborne viruses.

53.2 Foodborne viruses

The list of viruses infecting humans is extensive and they can be grouped into 24 families. Of all known viruses, nearly 10 viral agents are known to be transmitted through foods. Some of the foodborne viruses are zoonotic in nature and can be transmitted through animals and birds.[9] Poor hygiene and sanitation are predisposing factors responsible for viral food contamination. Important foodborne viruses and their public health significance are described in Tables 53.1 and 53.2.

53.3 Norovirus

NoV are one of the predominant enteric viruses causing acute gastroenteritis globally. These viruses belong to the genus Norovirus of the family *Caliciviridae*. These are small, non-enveloped, single-stranded positive-sense RNA viruses measuring approximately 27 nm. The RNA genome size of norovirus is ~ 7.6 kb and it comprises three open reading frames (ORFs) which encode eight viral proteins. There are six non-structural proteins encoded by ORF1, whereas ORF2 and ORF3 are translated to produce structural proteins VP1 and VP2, respectively.[31] Based on amino acid diversity in the VP1 and ORF1 proteins, NoV are classified into different genogroups and genotypes.[12,32] In 2019, Norovirus classification was updated and they now comprise ten genogroups (GI–GX) and 48 genotypes. Similarly, new nomenclature typing has also been proposed for NoV in which after reporting of genotype, P-type is mentioned in brackets [e.g., GI.1 (P1)]. This is known as dual typing nomenclature.[33] Most human illnesses are associated with genogroups I, II, and IV. According to the Centers for Disease Control and Prevention (CDC), Norovirus genotype GII.4 is a predominant circulating strain causing NoV gastroenteritis worldwide.[34] In addition, genotypes I and IV are also associated with human illness. NoV genotype III is present in bovines and genotype IV may infect pigs.[35] Genetic diversity of NoV exists in nature and NoV may undergo point mutations. Recombination and antigenic drift in NoV can give birth to new NoV genotypes of an emerging nature. The human population may then be susceptible to emerging NoV due to a lack of immunity. The presence of the GII.4-like NoV strain in livestock and GII.4-like noroviral RNA in meat samples highlights the significance of indirect zoonotic transmission of NoV through the food chain.[36,37]

NoV is ubiquitous and approximately 18% of human diarrheal cases are associated with NoV infection. Every year over 213 000 deaths, mostly in children under 5 years of age from developing countries, are associated with NoV.[38] The incidence of NoV infection and diarrheal disease has been recorded in diverse populations namely, children, the immunocompromised, restaurant patrons, military persons, travelers, cruise ship passengers, health care facilities, nursing homes, and schools. This virus is also referred to as the cruise ship virus and recurrent outbreaks in cruise ship passengers are often recorded.[39] The global burden of NoV diarrheal disease is believed to be much higher than the current estimates, particularly in poorly resourced countries. NoV differential diagnosis and detection are challenging as reinfection does occur and it is difficult to differentiate between clinical and asymptomatic cases. Similarly, NoV is excreted in the stool of infected persons for several weeks.[40] Thus personal hygiene and sanitation are essential for the prevention of NoV infection.

Transmission and spread of NoV are possible by various routes, especially through direct contact with fecal matter and vomitus of infected persons. Persons with clinical illness and even asymptomatic carriers may shed billions of norovirus particles in their feces. As for other foodborne pathogens, NoV has a typical fecal-oral mode of transmission. Contaminated water and food as well as contaminated hands can spread the virus rapidly.[41,42] It has been shown that even after recovery from an infection, a person can still shed NoV for up to two weeks.[40,43] The infectious dose of NoV is low and less than 100 virus particles can produce illness in humans, whilst very high levels are excreted by individuals per gram of feces.[44] Similarly, prolonged shedding of NoV by infected persons coupled with their environmental resistance increases the risk of norovirus infection several times. Person-to-person transmission through airborne fomites has also been recorded. The risk of norovirus infection is higher in closed dwellings, daycare centers, nursery schools, and refugee camps where sanitary conditions are poorly maintained. Foodborne outbreaks of NoV infection have most often been associated with seafood, especially oysters eaten raw. Foodborne genotypes of NoV are diverse and mostly belong to genotypes GII.4, GI.4, GI.1, and GI.2. Food handlers working in kitchens, restaurants, and food processing facilities may contaminate foods directly or indirectly. Ready-to-eat (RTE) salads, vegetables, and seafood like clams, mussels, oysters, shellfish, mashed potato, chicken, and beef have been associated with NoV outbreaks through the involvement of food handlers.[45]

The incubation period for NoV infection is very short and it may vary from 1.1 to 2.2 days (~24 to 48 h). Symptoms may include diarrhea, vomiting, and abdominal pain in general. However, some patients may experience headaches, fever, chills, and photophobia. Immunocompromised persons may have prolonged and more severe infections than those of healthy individuals.[12] For laboratory diagnosis, Reverse Transcription PCR (RT-PCR) is recognized as the gold standard technique for the detection of NoV. Stool and vomit samples collected within 48–72 h post-infection are preferred clinical

TABLE 53.1 Characteristics of viruses transmitted through food and water, causing foodborne illness.

Sr. no.	Name of the virus	Transmission	Infectious dose or $TCID_{50}$	Incubation period	Clinical symptoms	Major foods involved in outbreaks	Availability of vaccine	References
1	Norovirus	Fecal-oral, direct contact	~18–2800 virus particles	12–48 h	Vomiting, diarrhea, nausea, abdominal pain	Shellfish, bakery products, salad, sandwich, etc.	Under phase II clinical trial	11–13
2	Hepatitis A	Fecal-oral, direct contact, blood transfusion	~10–100 virus particles	2–6 weeks	Jaundice, fulminant hepatitis	Water, seafood, salads, meat, juice	Available	14
3	Hepatitis E	Fecal-oral, direct contact, zoonotic from pigs	Unknown	2–8 weeks	Hepatitis, abortion, meningitis, pancreatitis	Pig liver sausage, water, oyster, vegetables grown on pig slurry	Only for use in China	15–17
4	Rotavirus	Fecal-oral, zoonotic from animals	~100–1000 virus particles	Less than 48 h	Watery diarrhea, fever, vomiting	Water, shellfish, vegetables, ice cream	Available	18–20
5	Human Adenovirus (HAdVs)	Fecal-oral, direct contact	~150 PFU	10–24 days	Respiratory illness	Water, shellfish, fruits and vegetables	Only available for US military	13,21
6	Astrovirus	Fecal-oral, direct contact	Unknown	3–4 days	Gastroenteritis	Shellfish, fruits and vegetable, water	Not available	13,22
7	Enterovirus/ Poliovirus	Fecal-oral, and respiratory	~2–20 Plaque forming particles	Variable (3–35 days)	Poliomyelitis	Water	Available	13,23
8	Sapovirus	Fecal-oral, direct contact	~1000–2800 virus particles	1–4 days	Nausea, chills, headache, myalgia	Shellfish, oysters, lunch boxes contaminated by food handlers, water	Not available	24
9	Aichivirus	Fecal-oral, direct contact	Unknown	1–2 days	Mild to asymptomatic	Water and shellfish	Not available	25,26

TABLE 53.2 Characteristics of viruses potentially transmitted through food, but not necessarily causing illness via this route.

Sr. no.	Name of the virus	Transmission	Infectious dose or $TCID_{50}$	Incubation period	Clinical symptoms	Major foods involved in outbreaks	Availability of vaccine	Reference
1	Nipah virus	Contact with bats saliva, urine, feces, airborne, occupational exposure	$\sim 10^3$ to 10^6 PFU in experimental animals	4–14 days	Fever, headache, sore throat, encephalitis	Fruits, date palm sap	Under clinical trial	27
2	Coronaviruses SARS, MERS and SARS CoV-2	Aerosols and respiratory droplets, personal contact and contact with contaminated inanimate surfaces	Unknown	2–14 days	Fever, sore throat, cough, pneumonia	Not regarded as a foodborne virus	Only intended for respiratory-acquired COVID-19	28
3	Influenza type A /H5N1	Direct contact, occupational exposure from infected poultry	$1-8 \times 10^4$ $TCID_{50}$	2–5 days	Fever, cough, acute respiratory distress syndrome (ARDS)	Duck blood and duck meat, not a typical food-borne virus	Only intended for outbreaks of H5N1 in humans	29
4	TBEV	Tick bite, unpasteurized milk and milk products	Unknown	7–14 days	Fever, malaise, nausea, headache, muscle pain, meningitis, encephalitis	Raw goat milk and cheese	Available in some endemic countries	30

samples for diagnosis. Similarly, enzyme immunoassays (EIAs) are commercially available for the detection of NoV antigens in stool samples. Lateral flow immunochromatographic assays are also commercially available for rapid detection of NoV. In many settings, laboratory diagnosis is not possible due to the lack of access to specialized laboratories. Thus, Kaplan's criteria for clinical diagnosis are used,[46] which include four major observations for the epidemiological investigation of NoV as mentioned below:

1. Vomiting in more than half of symptomatic cases
2. Mean (or median) incubation period of 24–48 h
3. Mean (or median) duration of illness of 12–60 h
4. No bacterial pathogen isolated in stool culture.

For detection of NoV from foods, PCR-based methods that is ISO15216-1 and ISO 15216-2,[47,48] are standardized qualitative and quantitative methods which are extensively used for NoV detection and quantification in food matrices including bivalve mollusks, berries, leafy greens, vegetables, bottled water, and food surfaces.

Prevention and control of NoV infection can be achieved through personal and environmental hygiene and the adoption of food safety measures in the food chain. Washing of hands with soap after using the toilet and after changing diapers as well as proper washing of fruits and vegetables with clean potable water is essential. As NoV is relatively resistant to temperature, thorough cooking of food is also essential. NoV can remain stable in the environment for lengthy periods and can survive on food surfaces stored at 4°C without a reduction in titer. Survival studies of NoV on artificially inoculated foods revealed that NoV can survive at refrigeration temperature in lettuce (7°C/10 days), minced meat (6°C/2 days), marinated mussels (4°C/28 days), strawberries (4°C/7 days), raspberries (4°C/7 days) and turkey for 10 days at 7°C.[49–52] It can also remain viable in water, food, and on solid surfaces like ceramic, steel, glass, and carpets for lengthy periods of time, for example, it may persist in water for up to 728 days.[53] For fruit and vegetables, less than 1 log reduction was found after two weeks. For its inactivation, available disinfectants for food or food contact surfaces are hypochlorite, chlorine with a pH above 8, UV radiation, HPP, and high-temperature processing. Temperatures above 140°F (60°C) are sufficient to inactivate NoV in foods. There are several EPA registered antimicrobial chemical agents commercially available that are effective against NoV. Household chlorine bleach at 1000–5000 ppm per gallon of water can be used effectively for surface disinfection against NoV. Currently, a vaccine is not available for the prevention of NoV infection. Certain challenges limiting norovirus vaccine development include mutation and genetic diversity of circulating strains, poor knowledge of natural immunity, and lack of immune correlation and protection. Several attempts have been made to develop a candidate NoV vaccine, and currently, 3 types of vaccines are under various stages of development. These include vaccines prepared from non-replicating virus-like particles, protruding (P) particles, and recombinant adenovirus.[54] NoV vaccines need to be broad-spectrum multivalent, which could give protection against currently circulating genotypes.

53.4 Hepatitis A virus

Hepatitis A viruses (HAVs) are non-enveloped, icosahedral, single-stranded positive-sense RNA viruses (27–32 nm) belonging to the genus *Hepatovirus* of the family Picornaviridae. The genome size is ~7.5 kb, and out of six genotypes (I–VI), three genotypes (I–III) infect humans, and the other three infect simians (IV–VI).[55] The most prevalent genotypes in humans are I and III, and there are subgenotypes such as IA and IB prevalent in the USA, Europe, China, and Japan.[56] This virus is a predominant cause of viral hepatitis in humans and it was identified in 1973 by Feinstone and colleagues[57] through immune electron microscopy in fecal samples. A single serotype of HAV exists and lifelong immunity is developed after infection. According to the WHO, an estimated 1.4 million human cases and seven thousand deaths are recorded per year due to HAV.[58] An increase in cases of HAV has been recorded in the USA from 2013 to 2018. Out of the 10 most important foodborne pathogens, HAV is in the sixth position and it is a reportable pathogen in the USA and Canada.[59,60]

Transmission and spread of HAV occur through consumption of contaminated food, water, close contact with an infected person, and blood transfusions. Food- and water-borne HAV outbreaks are recorded across the world and contaminated water, juice, milk, salads, meat, and seafood are important vehicles of HAV transmission.[59,61] HAV can survive for months in experimentally contaminated fresh water, seawater, marine sediments, wastewater, soils, and oysters.[62] Cross-contamination of food in the kitchen is also possible if food is handled by infected food handlers. HAV is more heat resistant than NoV and the temperature required for adequate heating of food to inactivate it is more than 85°C.[63] Lower temperatures will require longer heating times, for example, Bidawid et al.[64] found that 0.68 min were required at 80°C to achieve a 5-log reduction in HAV titer in skimmed and homogenized milk, as opposed to <0.5 min at 85°C to achieve a similar log reduction. After a person is infected with HAV, the virus is excreted in feces two weeks before the development of symptoms, and virus shedding continues for several weeks after exhibiting symptoms.[55] Usually, the incubation period for HAV infection is 28 days, however, it may range from 15 to 50 days. The exact dose of HAV is not known; however, it is presumed that very low numbers of virus particles (10–100 particles) can cause infection.[65] Compared to adults, children and infants shed HAV for longer periods.[66]

The pathogenesis of HAV includes the migration of the virus to the liver from the gastrointestinal tract (GIT) within a few hours of ingestion and its replication in hepatocytes. After the liver is affected, HAV is transported back to the GIT through bile. HAV is often detected at very high levels in stool samples, up to 10^9 particles/gram. Viral load is higher in infected persons with jaundice during the early stages of viremia and HAV can then be detected in blood samples. HAV infection may induce jaundice or it may be asymptomatic without showing symptoms of jaundice. In adults, anicteric or icteric hepatitis is commonly observed whereas, in children, infection is mostly subclinical. Relapsing of infection is possible and fulminant hepatitis with death is recorded occasionally in patients above 50 years of age.[67]

A large outbreak of HAV infection associated with the consumption of undercooked food prepared by infected food handlers was recorded by the Kentucky health department, in the USA in 1994. Suspected foods responsible for the outbreak were pineapple, vegetable dip, and cheese.[68] The hygienic production and handling of food are essential to prevent the presence of HAV in food processing establishments. Foodborne transmission is very common in the epidemiology of HAV and it has been detected in a variety of foods like shellfish, oysters, vegetables, dairy products, juices, ice cream, fruits, and bakery products. Fecally contaminated water, soil, sewage, food processing equipment, and hands are the main sources of food contamination.[63,69] Proper cooking of food before consumption and avoiding eating undercooked or partially cooked foods are recommended to prevent foodborne outbreaks of HAV. Heating is the most effective measure for HAV inactivation. Heat inactivation can be efficiently achieved above 85°C–90°C within 1.5 min.[70,71] Similarly, gamma irradiation is also effective for the inactivation of HAV on fruit and vegetables.[72]

HAV can survive in bottled water for up to one year[73] and is also able to remain infective in dried fecal matter for several days. In a study, it was observed that HAV remained viable for 30 days dried feces stored under 42% relative humidity and 25°C temperature, and experimental inoculation of treated fecal matter in the marmosets could establish seroconversion to HAV antibodies after 28–35 days with HAV detection in the fecal matter of experimentally inoculated marmosets.[74] This virus can survive for four hours on contaminated human hands as compared to other enteric pathogens.[75] HAV is resistant to several environmental conditions and remains viable for months on surfaces.[76] HAV can survive at low pH (1) and low relative humidity (25%), but can be inactivated by chlorine (10–15 ppm residual chlorine concentration) after 30 min or free residual chlorine of 2.0 mg/L for 15 min.[77] Generally, HAV is not inactivated by alcohol-based hand sanitizers.

Diagnosis of HAV infection can be done effectively by using serological assays. IgM and IgG antibodies are detected in the serum, urine, stool, and saliva of infected persons. The level of IgM antibody declines after 3–6 months, however, IgG is detectable for years and provides lifelong immunity.[78] Saliva screening is considered an alternative to serum antibody testing. Several commercial kits are available for the serological diagnosis of HAV. Molecular techniques are highly sensitive and specific for the detection of HAV nucleic acids in clinical, food, and environmental samples. These include RT-PCR, RFLP, sequencing, and Southern blotting.[66]

As for NoV, PCR-based methods are primarily used for the detection of HAV from foods. ISO 15216-1[47] and ISO 15216-2[48] are the standardized qualitative and quantitative methods used for the detection and quantification of HAV in different food matrices.

Prevention and control of HAV are possible through the adoption of general principles of hygiene and sanitation. Food hygiene is critical in this context, followed by vaccination of food handlers. Effective vaccines are available against HAV and in countries where HAV vaccination is introduced in the national immunization program, cases of HAV infection have reduced dramatically. The HAV vaccine can be administered in two doses to any person above the age of 12 months. Currently available HAV vaccines are formalin-inactivated vaccines derived from HM 175/GBM strains and live attenuated vaccines derived from the H2 strain.[79]

53.5 Hepatitis E virus

Globally, the HEV is considered a leading cause of acute viral hepatitis infecting the liver. This virus belongs to the genus *Hepevirus* and the *Hepeviridae* family. It is a single-stranded positive-sense RNA virus, non-enveloped with icosahedral symmetry and a virion size of roughly 27–32 nm diameter. The genome size of HEV is approximately 7.2 kb and this virus was first visualized under the electron microscope by Russian investigators in 1983.[80] The RNA genome of HEV is composed of partially overlapping discontinuous three ORF1, ORF2, ORF3, and ORF4 has recently been discovered in HEV genotype 1. ORFs encode for different proteins, for example, ORF1 encodes for non-structural proteins, ORF2 encodes for capsid proteins and ORF3 is responsible for releasing virions.[81] There are eight known genotypes of HEV, but only four genotypes are of human health significance. Some of the genotypes are zoonotic in nature and can be transmitted by domestic and wild animals, especially wild boar and deer. HEV genotypes 1 and 2 are non-zoonotic and are primarily transmitted through water, whereas genotypes 3 and 4 have diverse host ranges and are present in humans, pigs, cattle, goats, deer, camels, and yak. Meatborne transmission of HEV genotypes 3 and 4 is also recognized.[82,83] In wild boars, HEV genotypes 5 and 6 have been detected, but these genotypes are not pathogenic to humans. Similarly, HEV genotypes 7 and 8 were identified in camels, and HEV genotype 7 was detected in a clinical case where it was associated with the consumption of camel meat and milk.[84,85]

The global burden of disease for HEV is not exactly known but the disease is more endemic in the Eastern and Southern regions of the world. Approximately 20 million infections, 3.3 million symptomatic cases, and 70,000 deaths per year are attributed to HEV infection.[86] Recent meta-analysis of the global burden of HEV revealed a very high incidence of HEV and ~939 million people are thought to have experienced this infection, and 15–110 million have ongoing HEV infections.[87] The global pattern of distribution of HEV genotypes and the endemic nature of infection may vary. There are four distinct zones of disease prevalence or occurrence namely, hyper-endemic, endemic, distinctive pattern, and sporadic zones. Countries of South and East Asia, and East and West Africa are under the hyper-endemic zone. Middle Eastern and South American countries are in endemic zones. Egypt falls under the distinctive pattern and European countries are under the sporadic zone. In hyper-endemic and endemic regions, most of the cases are due to genotypes 1 and 2, and in the sporadic zone, genotype 3 is more prevalent.[88] Socio-economic conditions, access to quality drinking water, hygiene and sanitation, and zoonotic prevalence are some of the important factors determining the geographical pattern of HEV.

Transmission of HEV occurs mostly through contaminated water and food; however, direct person-to-person contact, blood transfusions, solid organ transplants, and indirect infections from pets like cats, dogs, and rabbits are also possible. Fecal contamination of drinking water is the predominant risk factor in HEV outbreaks compared to other enteric pathogens. The risk of contracting an infection is more likely in military camps, refugee camps, war zones, and disasters where basic hygiene and sanitation are challenged. Genotype 3 is usually transmitted through the ingestion of undercooked meat or meat products derived from infected animals like pork and liver.[89,90] Zoonotic transmission of HEV is possible through consumption of contaminated foods of animal origin, contact with animals, and feces/manure mixed with water and agricultural runoff.[91] HEV has been detected in raw liver, sausages, vegetables, strawberries, and raspberries cultivated using pig slurry.[88] In China, milking cows were found to excrete HEV genotype 4 RNA in milk samples with a very high titer.[92] Even though foodborne transmission of HEV through pork liver has been documented, it is not as common as for HAV. In France, pig liver sausage was reported as a source of HEV transmission to humans.[93] HEV genotype 3 was also confirmed in pork and in infected persons who ate the pork in Barcelona, Spain.[94] Seafood is also at risk of contamination by HEV if water is contaminated by sewage or fecal matter and it has been detected in shellfish, mussels, and oysters.[95,96] In Colombia HEV was detected in environmental samples collected from drinking water treatment plants and in sewage.[97] HEV genotypes 3 and 4 are zoonotic and they are widely distributed in the pig population, globally. Zoonotic HEV viruses can also be transmitted through water contaminated with animal fecal matter.[98]

The incubation period of HEV is in the range of 2–10 weeks with an average of 5–6 weeks, and fecal shedding of the virus starts a few days before symptoms appear and continues 4 weeks post-infection.[89] Adult persons in the age group of 15–40 years are susceptible and are mostly symptomatic. During the initial stages of infection, typical symptoms are anorexia, nausea, vomiting, skin rash, and abdominal pain. Later, jaundice develops and the liver becomes enlarged. Acute liver failure is a risk and death may occur in fulminant hepatitis cases. If HEV infection is contracted in advanced pregnancy, there is a higher risk of acute liver failure, abortion, and death. In chronic immune-deficient patients, infection with genotype 4 has been recorded.[58] Occasionally, HEV infection may be associated with extra-hepatic involvements, and certain disorders like Guillain-Barre syndrome, pancreatitis, meningitis, and myocarditis are possible.[84]

Diagnosis of HEV infection is largely dependent on the serological detection of anti HEV antibodies in the blood serum and viral RNA by RT-PCR. IgM antibodies may be detected up to four months after exposure and RNA can be detected after three weeks of exposure in blood samples. Titers of IgG antibodies will also decrease over time and infection doesn't provide lifelong immunity. Fecal shedding of HEV by infected persons may continue for up to six weeks. In chronic cases of HEV infection, serology has several limitations and false-negative results may be encountered; therefore, along with serology, the use of RT-PCR for the detection of viral RNA in stool and blood samples is more reliable. For detection of HEV in meat and meat products, RT-PCR and RT-qPCR methods are useful.[99–101]

Prevention and control of HEV infection are possible through combinations of efforts towards improvement of hygiene, sanitation, access to potable drinking water, inactivation of viruses in food by proper cooking of particularly meat, control of environmental sources, vaccination (where available), and surveillance for the pathogen.

Food and water must be boiled to over 90°C for HEV inactivation. Similarly, washing fruits and vegetables with a chlorine concentration of 200 ppm may inactivate the virus. Only one vaccine is currently commercially available for use in China named Hecolin and three intramuscular doses are recommended for use in people above 16 years of age. However, the vaccine is not yet available elsewhere (https://www.who.int/news-room/fact-sheets/detail/hepatitis-e). In 2016 the WHO in its World Health Assembly adopted the decision to reduce the global burden of new viral hepatitis infections and deaths by 90% and 65%, respectively, by 2030.[102]

53.6 Rotaviruses

One of the important causes of diarrheal illness in children less than 5 years of age is infection with rotaviruses. The structure of the virus resembles that of a wheel with inner spokes and an outer smooth rim, therefore the name "rotavirus". The genus Rotavirus belongs to the family Reoviridae. These are segmented double-stranded RNA viruses with 11 segments, non-enveloped, about 70 nm in diameter with icosahedral symmetry. Each segment represents one gene, and these genes encode six structural viral proteins (VP1–VP4, VP5, VP7) and six non-structural (NSP1–NSP6) proteins. Segment 11 of the rotavirus encodes for two proteins namely NSP5 and NSP6. These viruses are further divided into various groups (A–J). Human and animal rotaviruses comprise groups A, B, C, and H, whereas groups D, E, F, and G are present only in animals. Similarly, group E is only present in swine.[103,104] Birds associated with rotaviruses are from groups D, F and G.[105] Group A rotaviruses are important in the epidemiology of human infection. However, groups B and C may infect humans to a lesser extent. Two structural proteins namely, VP4 (P protein) and VP7 (G protein) are very important in the nomenclature and vaccine development for rotaviruses. Based on variations in the glycoprotein (G) and protease-cleaved protein (P), about 36G and 51P genotypes are identified in animals and humans. Group A rotavirus genotypes predominantly circulating globally include six G and three P genotypes viz, G1, G2, G3, G4, G9, G12, and P4, P6, and P8, respectively. All six G types in combination with P6 and P8 are the more specific genotypes currently circulating globally. Among all the known DNA viruses, the rate of the point mutation in rotaviruses is much higher, which is approximately 5×10^{-5} per nucleotide.[106] In nature, several G and P genotype combinations may occur due to genetic re-assortment; however, all the possible genotypes cannot equally infect and cause illness in humans and animals. In humans, predominant genotypes responsible for more than 90% of rotavirus diarrhea cases are combinations of P (8) and G1, G2, G3, and G4. More diverse rotavirus genotypes and serotypes are present in animals and birds and their zoonotic potential cannot be ruled out. Interspecies transmission of rotaviruses from animals to humans could be responsible for the emergence of new strains. Some of the strains of animal origin are found infecting humans in certain regions of the world like G6 (P9), G6 (P13), and G5, G8, and G10 strains.[107] Similarly, G3 and G9 strains from animals have also been detected in humans.

The global burden of rotavirus-associated infection and diarrhea is higher in developing countries such as Asia and Sub-Saharan Africa. It is mostly associated with malnutrition, poor immunity, and lack of personal hygiene. According to the WHO, rotaviruses are the predominant agents responsible for deaths in children globally.[102] Approximately 215,000 deaths in children below 5 years of age are attributed to rotavirus infections globally and in India alone, contributes to about 26% of such global deaths.[108] The transmission cycle of rotavirus is fecal-oral in nature and infected persons can excrete large numbers of virus particles in their feces, approximately 10^{10} per gram, whereas less than 10 rotavirus particles are needed to induce illness.[109] Prolonged shedding of rotaviruses through stool may occur for over 50 days. In close settings and compromised hygiene and sanitary conditions, chances of infection are higher. Rotavirus can be transmitted from human to human through direct contact such as contaminated hands, mechanically through physical objects, or fecally-contaminated food and water.

A study from Pakistan revealed the prevalence of rotavirus with free-living amoebae in drinking water supplies.[110] Rotaviruses were detected in oysters and vegetables studied in Mexico and the G2 [P4] genotype was the predominant type of rotavirus in kitchens due to poor hygiene and cross-contamination during food preparation as a result of infected food handlers.[111] Poor kitchen hygiene may contaminate prepared foods and such food handlers could be the predominant source of household transmission of infection to children.[112] Foods associated with rotavirus outbreaks have been described globally and served foods like salads, lettuce, ice, water, shellfish, and strawberries were found to be contaminated with rotaviruses.[113–115]

The incubation period of rotavirus is relatively short (less than 48 h) in humans and it infects enterocytes of the small intestine. After virus entry into the host cells, new virions are produced within 10–12 h. Rotavirus cases may be symptomatic or asymptomatic, and the severity of infection depends on re-infection or whether an infection was acquired for the first time. Typical gastrointestinal symptoms comprise watery diarrhea, vomiting, and fever. Severe diarrhea may cause dehydration, electrolyte imbalance, shock, and death in infants. Other than gastroenteritis, occasionally rotaviruses can cause extra-intestinal infections like meningitis, biliary atresia, and antigenaemia.[116]

Diagnosis of rotavirus can be done by serological, virus culture, and molecular techniques. The presence of rotavirus-specific IgA antibodies in the serum of infected people and even in vaccinated children is used as a marker for assessing rotavirus protection. In clinical patients, differential diagnosis is needed for adenovirus, norovirus, *Salmonella*, and *Escherichia coli* associated gastroenteritis. Seasonal outbreaks of diarrhea, particularly in winter, can often be correlated with rotavirus infection. Laboratory confirmation is possible through the detection of rotavirus antigen in stool samples by ELISA and immunochromatography. RT-PCR and real-time RT-PCR assays are highly sensitive in confirmatory diagnosis and genotyping of rotaviruses. Polyacrylamide Gel Electrophoresis of Rotavirus RNA (RNA-PAGE) is the gold standard routinely used for the detection of rotaviruses based on the electrophoretic pattern of their RNA. Since rotaviruses have a segmented RNA genome, their RNA can be easily visualized with silver staining of SDS-polyacrylamide gels. Rotaviruses of mammalian and non-mammalian origin may exhibit different migration patterns on RNA-PAGE. For the cultivation and propagation of human and animal rotaviruses in the laboratory, primary and continuous cell lines prepared from rhesus monkey kidneys like MA104 are used. Adaption of HRVs to cell culture is generally lower than for animal rotaviruses. For handling and culturing of rotaviruses, Biosafety Level 2 (BSL-2) facilities are required.[117]

Prevention and control of rotavirus infection in humans needs an integrated approach comprising personal and environmental hygiene, sanitation, hand washing, education, and vaccination. Rotaviruses are stable in different environmental conditions such as low temperature and wide pH (3–10) range but are sensitive to chemical disinfectants such as ethanol, phenolic compounds, sodium hypochlorite, and formaldehyde.[118,119] In daycare centers, a report showed that rotavirus could be isolated from several environmental samples.[120] Vaccination is by far the most effective preventive strategy against rotavirus infection. WHO emphasizes the inclusion of rotavirus vaccination for children in endemic countries as a part of the national immunization program.[102,108] It is encouraging to note that about 90 countries have included rotavirus vaccination in their national immunization programs. India became the first Asian country to include the rotavirus vaccine in its universal immunization program in 2016. Available rotavirus vaccines are safe and effective and according to the WHO, the first dose should be given along with the DTP vaccine after 6 weeks of age in children. Broadly used rotavirus vaccines globally are the RV5 vaccine, RotaTeq manufactured by Merck, USA, and the RV1 vaccine, Rotarix manufactured by GlaxoSmithKline, Belgium.[108]

53.7 Adenoviruses

These are non-enveloped viruses with double-stranded linear DNA and icosahedral symmetry. Virion size is roughly 80–110 nm, and Human Adenoviruses (HAdVs) are large in size, about 150 MDa. They belong to the family *Adenoviridae*, which is a broad family of adenoviruses comprising five genera namely, *Mastedenovirus*, *Aviadenovirus*, *Atadenovirus*, *Ichtadenovirus*, and *Siadenovirus*. Adenoviruses infecting humans and other mammals like bovines, equines, bats, primates, canines, pigs, dolphins, shrews, and squirrels are from the genus *Mastedenovirus*, whereas, other genera comprise adenoviruses that infect birds, cattle, sheep, ducks, fish, and reptiles.[18,121] The adenovirus was first detected in human adenoid tissue in 1953 by Wallace Rowe and colleagues and currently, 67 HAdVs serotypes and over 70 genotypes have been identified.[18] These are further classified into seven species, namely HAdVs A, B, C, D, E, F, and G. Adenoviruses currently infecting humans and circulating globally are A, B, C, D, E, and F species. Most common infections are recorded in children.[122,123] The potential for inter-species transmission of adenoviruses of animals and birds to humans has been explained and thus adenoviruses are significant in the context of zoonosis and the One Health concept.[18]

Adenoviruses are a diverse group of viruses transmitted through various routes like airborne droplets, the fecal-oral route, food handlers, organ transplants, and fomites. Furthermore, adenoviruses may be transmitted indirectly through sharing of goggles and towels at the swimming pool. Contaminated food and water are also possible vehicles of transmission. Children and immunocompromised persons are at a greater risk of acquiring symptomatic infection. In other cases, mild or asymptomatic infection is often seen. To date, 103 HAdVs genotypes are documented and some of the genotypes namely, HAdV-3, 4, 5, 7, 11, 14, 21 cause respiratory infection in healthy adults.[124] Adenoviruses are excreted in feces in large numbers, usually 10^{11} particles/gram and they can survive well in the environment, and due to fecal contamination, HAdV-F 40 and 41 are transmitted via the fecal-oral route, which causes gastroenteritis in humans.[125] A study revealed the emergence of HAdV-B76, which is identical to simian adenoviruses, thus zoonotic emergence of adenoviruses cannot be neglected.[126] Adenoviruses have been detected in food, water, and environmental samples, however, foodborne outbreaks are not documented. Due to the frequent occurrence of adenoviruses in the aquatic environment, they are part of a candidate contaminant list of the United States Environmental Protection Agency (USEPA) since 1998. As compared to other enteric RNA viruses, adenoviruses are highly resistant (60 times) to UV radiation.[125] A study from Michigan revealed a very high prevalence of adenoviruses in wastewater, surface water, and combined sewer overflow (CSO) samples by real-time PCR. All the CSO samples were positive for adenoviruses and the DNA concentration found was 1.15×10^6 viruses/liter and in sewage, 5.35×10^5 viruses/liter. Some of the river samples showed adenovirus DNA concentrations above the detection limit of real-time PCR. Adenovirus Serotype 41 was found to be predominant in primary effluent and raw sewage.[127] A study in Spain also revealed the potential occurrence of porcine adenoviruses, bovine adenoviruses, and bovine polyomaviruses in rivers, slaughterhouses, and sewage samples.[128] Adenovirus has been detected in ground water and vegetable samples from South Korea.[129]

The global prevalence of adenoviruses associated with childhood gastroenteritis is very high and it is considered a priority agent after rotaviruses. Infected persons can excrete adenoviruses in feces and urine for lengthy periods of time. They cause diverse symptoms like gastroenteritis, respiratory illness, kerato-conjunctivitis, and meningoencephalitis. HAdVs 40 and 41 are major causes of gastroenteritis whilst HAdV 4 is associated with respiratory diseases.[130,131] Adenovirus may persist on fresh fruit and vegetables for several days at refrigeration temperatures. Survival of Ad2 on lettuce, strawberries, and raspberries was studied for 10 days at 4°C, and a decrease in the recovered Ad2 levels by 1.97 $\log_{10}$, 2.38 $\log_{10}$, and 1.14 $\log_{10}$, respectively, were recorded after 10 days.[132]

Even though adenoviruses that infect humans are prevalent globally, the exact burden of the disease is unknown. About 2%–5% of all respiratory infections could be due to HAdVs. Infection may occur throughout the year, however, the incidence is higher in winter and the early summer months.[133] In most cases, the severity of infection is low, and mild self-limiting clinical symptoms may develop, however, in immunocompromised persons, clinical illness may progress to severe respiratory complications. In healthy individuals, infection is milder and self-limiting and the prevalence of respiratory illness due to adenoviruses is higher in crowded clusters like military camps, schools, day care centers, and hospitals. The incubation period of infection is generally up to 10 days and may extend to 24 days. The infective dose of adenovirus is less than 150 plaque-forming units (PFU). Enteric adenoviruses can survive in water for long periods. Rigotto et al.[134] studied the survival of Ad2 and Ad41 in surface and ground waters incubated at 10°C and 19°C for up to 301 days. Concentrations of Ad2 and Ad41 were relatively stable in all waters at 10°C for at least 160 days and in some instances up to 301 days. Therefore, sewage-contaminated water should be considered an important source of infection in endemic regions. Adenovirus pharyngoconjunctival fever associated with swimming pools has been documented in several countries.[102]

Laboratory diagnosis of adenoviruses is done by employing numerous techniques. It can be detected in a variety of samples like nasal and throat swabs, conjunctival swabs, stool, blood, cerebrospinal fluid, and biopsy tissue. For isolation of adenoviruses, various cell lines are used that is, A549, HeLa, HEp-2, KB, MRC-5, and Graham-293 Ad5-transformed secondary HEK.[135] Electron microscopy is used for observing the viruses. Adenovirus antigen detection, directly in specimens, can be achieved by ELISA, latex agglutination test, and immunohistochemistry. Hemagglutination inhibition and complement fixation tests are also used in the serodiagnosis of adenoviruses. Molecular diagnosis is done by detection of viral DNA by multiplex PCR, real-time PCR, and sequencing. For typing of adenoviruses, the serum neutralization test is the gold standard method. Molecular techniques are also used for typing of adenoviruses targeting hexon or fiber genes. With the advent of sequencing technology, next-generation sequencing (NGS) is being used for a better understanding of the genomic structure of adenoviruses.[135]

Management of adenovirus infection is critical in infants and children. A basic infection control protocol includes frequent hand washing with soap, especially after contact with an infected person and contaminated material, avoidance of close contact with symptomatic persons, adequate chlorination of swimming pool water, and access to potable drinking water. Inactivation of adenoviruses can be achieved by the use of heat, sodium hypochlorite, chlorine, and formaldehyde.[136,137] Currently, the HAdVs type 4 and 7 vaccines are approved by the US Food and Drug Administration (FDA); however, it is only available for the US military and not for the general public.[21]

53.8 Astroviruses

These are small non-enveloped, single-stranded positive-sense RNA viruses from the *Astroviridae* family with icosahedral symmetry and virion size of roughly 28–30 nm diameter. The RNA genome of astroviruses is in the range of 6–8 kb. The RNA genome has three ORFs viz. ORF1a and ORF1b encode non-structural proteins and ORF2 encodes for structural proteins. These viruses were separated from *Picornaviridae* and *Caliciviridae* by the International Committee on Taxonomy of Viruses (ICTV) in 1995 and were classified under the genus *Astrovirus* of the family *Astroviridae*.[138] Further research revealed the classification of astroviruses into two separate genera that is, *Mamastrovirus* (astroviruses of mammals) and *Avastrovirus* (astroviruses of avian species) by ICTV in 2005.[139] Astroviruses were first recognized in 1975 in human stool samples using electron microscopy by Appleton and Higgins.[140] The name astrovirus was given by Madeley and Cosgrove due to its star-like appearance as in Greek, astron means star.[141] Standard abbreviations were given by ICTV for referring to astrovirus species, for example, human astrovirus is abbreviated as HAstV and avian astroviruses AAstV. Mammalian astroviruses are found in the feces of a wide number of species namely, cattle, cats, dogs, wild canids and felids, sheep, pigs, rabbits, and sea lions; avian astroviruses are present in chickens, turkeys, pigeons, guinea fowl and several aquatic species of birds.[139] There are eight known human serotypes of astroviruses (HAstV-1 to HAstV-8) and they cause diarrheal illness in humans. However, two novel human astroviruses have recently been described and named HAstV-MBL1 (Melbourne) and HAstV-VA (Virginia). These novel astroviruses are further divided into several genotypes.[142]

The global burden of disease due to human astroviruses is unknown but community-acquired astroviruses are found in 3%–6% of children with infectious gastroenteritis.[141] Infection is not limited to children and may be seen in all age groups. The risk of infection is higher in cases of close dwellings and under poor hygiene and sanitary conditions. Astrovirus gastroenteritis is prevalent throughout the year; however, its incidence is higher in autumn and winter. Although all eight genotypes of HAstV are globally prevalent, HAstV-1 is predominantly associated with human infection.[143]

Transmission and spread of astroviruses occur mainly through contaminated water and food; it has a typical fecal-oral transmission cycle. Person-to-person transmission by direct contact is another route of transmission. Cross-species transmission of mammalian astroviruses is possible in nature, however, zoonotic transmission to humans is rare. Astroviruses have been detected in more than 80 mammalian and avian hosts and their intra-species and cross-species transmission has been recently reviewed.[22] Astroviruses found in pigs and bats are more diverse and simultaneous co-infection of several mammalian astroviruses in a single host may give emergence to new strains. Astroviruses undergo recombination which has been previously detected in humans, cattle, swine, and non-human primates. Genetic diversity, multiple hosts, and the potential for cross-species transmission make astroviruses a possible candidate for emerging zoonoses.[144,145] Sero-positivity to turkey Astrovirus TAstV-2 was detected in about 26% of workers having exposure to turkeys at a farm or an abattoir, highlighting the possibility of cross-species transmission of these viruses.[146] Interestingly, astrovirus infection in humans is found mostly in combination with other enteric viruses like rotaviruses and NoV.

Water is an important vehicle in the epidemiology of human astrovirus infection. Infected persons can excrete astroviruses in huge numbers ($\sim 10^{13}$ per gram of feces), therefore, untreated and fecally-polluted water is a risk factor for humans. A large foodborne outbreak of astrovirus infection in more than 4700 people was recorded in Osaka, Japan in 1991. All the affected people were exposed to contaminated food supplied by a common vendor.[147] Astroviruses are highly stable in unchlorinated water and residual infectivity was detected in the presence of free chlorine for a few hours.[148] Persistence of human astrovirus has also been studied in fresh and marine water.[149] Human astrovirus RNA was detected in oysters collected from Chiba bay, in Japan.[150] Epidemiological investigation of large gastroenteritis outbreaks in France associated with shellfish consumption revealed detection of astrovirus in shellfish and fecal samples.[151] Shellfish contamination by astrovirus and other enteric viruses was also reported in China.[114] Shellfish cultivated in contaminated water and fruits and vegetables grown using sewage-contaminated water for irrigation provide a high risk for HAstV infection. In Ghana, the HAstV genome was detected in tap water used for drinking purposes.[152]

Variation in the pathogenesis and development of symptoms in infected individuals may exist with human astroviruses. The incubation period may vary between 3–4 days and an infected person can shed $10^{10}-10^{11}$ particles/g of feces. Typically, symptoms include watery diarrhea, abdominal pain, fever, vomiting, and anorexia. However, most of the time, astrovirus infection is asymptomatic and its epidemiology is not clear. Extra-intestinal association of HAstV, such as meningitis, was also recorded in immunocompromised patients.[153]

Diagnosis of astrovirus infection is done by detecting virus RNA in fecal, food, and water samples. Cell culture is used for propagation, using host-specific cell lines, but some of the viruses are poorly adapted to cell lines and also lose their infectivity over subsequent passages. Human embryonated kidney cells and human intestinal cells Caco-2 are used for its propagation. EIAs are commercially available for the detection of HAstV in stool samples. RT-PCR and quantitative real-time RT-PCR are the most reliable and sensitive techniques.

Prevention of astrovirus infection is possible through the implementation of measures directed toward the prevention of water pollution, drinking water chlorination, heat inactivation, sanitation, and food hygiene. The role of the food handler in restaurants, food establishments, and catering services is critical to avoiding cross-contamination. Food contact surfaces must be cleaned routinely to avoid the risk of astrovirus spread via fomites and inanimate objects like knives, kitchen utensils, choppers, and similar.[139] Astroviruses are highly resistant to environmental conditions, and their stability and release into the environment is a matter of concern. They are resistant to alcohols, bleach, detergents, UV light (up to 100 mJ/cm^2), and heating at 50°C for an hour or 60°C for 5 min.[141] They remain stable at a pH of 3 and freezing temperatures; heat inactivation can be achieved above 60°C. The use of 90% alcohol is effective against HAstV and water disinfection using chlorine concentrations above 1 mg/mL of free chlorine is possible. At present, a vaccine is not commercially available for its prevention.

53.9 Sapovirus

Sapovirus belongs to the genus *Sapovirus* of the *Caliciviridae* family. This virus was detected in human fecal samples in 1976 in the United Kingdom as a new pathogen. In 1982 a prototype strain of sapovirus was detected in Japan and it was referred to as "Sapporo-like viruses." However, in 2002, ICTV classified them in the genus *Sapovirus* and the family *Caliciviridae*.[154] These are small non-enveloped, single-stranded positive-sense RNA viruses, roughly 30–38 nm in diameter with icosahedral symmetry and a genome size of ~7 to 7.77 kb. There are three ORFs viz ORF1, ORF 2, and ORF3 in human sapoviruses. ORF1 encodes for six non-structural proteins (NS1, NS2, NS3, NS4, NS5, NS6-7) and VP1 capsid protein, whilst ORF2 is thought to encode for minor structural proteins, and the function of ORF3 is unknown.[24] Sapoviruses are classified into five genogroups, of which GI, GII, GIV, and GV affect humans and GIII infects porcine species. Similarly, human sapoviruses are further sub-grouped into 17 genotypes. The prevalence of sapovirus genogroups GI and GII is higher in low to middle-income countries.[155]

It is regarded as a global viral agent causing episodes of gastroenteritis in association with other enteric viruses like rotavirus, norovirus, and adenovirus in children under 5 years of age. However, infection is not limited to children and it may cause gastroenteritis in adults and immunocompromised persons as well. Transmission of sapovirus occurs through the fecal-oral route and contaminated water, food, and food handlers as well as direct person-to-person contact.[156] Sapoviruses may contaminate water reservoirs like rivers, ponds, and lakes, therefore, access to clean potable water is essential. Asymptomatic people can shed sapoviruses in their feces, thus food handlers should always adopt the highest standards of food hygiene.

The incubation period of infection is 1–4 days and typical symptoms may include gastroenteritis, nausea, vomiting, abdominal cramps, and myalgia. The risk of spread is higher in close settings like child care centers, schools, and wedding ceremonies. Most of the time symptoms will subside within a week and mortality is rare. Sapovirus excretion in feces continues even after recovery and it may be excreted for up to 1–4 weeks. Both symptomatic and asymptomatic persons can shed virus particles in large numbers, usually 10^5–10^{11} particles/g of fecal matter.[24]

The largest outbreak of sapovirus gastroenteritis was in 2010 and was associated with lunch boxes supplied by the catering company from Aichi, Gifu, and Mie Prefectures of Japan. Molecular studies revealed the confirmation of Sapovirus GI.2 and the strains detected in ill persons after consumption of the contaminated food and in food handlers were identical.[157] An outbreak of sapovirus strain GI.3 was recorded in school students from Gyeonggi-do, Korea in 2018. Sapovirus was detected in stool samples but it could not be detected in environmental samples.[158] Another investigation from Japan linked a human outbreak of sapovirus and norovirus with the consumption of shellfish.[159] A sapovirus outbreak of the genogroup IV was detected in people who had attended a wedding and had a common food exposure.[160] Human enteric viruses including sapovirus were detected during the surveillance of oyster-associated gastroenteritis outbreaks in Osaka city, Japan.[161]

Diagnosis of sapovirus principally depends upon the use of molecular techniques like RT-PCR and quantitative real-time RT-PCR. Recently, *in vitro* replication and propagation of human sapovirus were successfully demonstrated using human cell lines prepared from the testicle and duodenal cells. Sapoviruses could be replicated more efficiently (~6 log increase) in the duodenal cell line.[162] Wang et al.[163] studied the stability of porcine sapovirus (SaV) as a surrogate for human norovirus (HuNoV). Similar resistance to heat (56°C) and chlorine was observed in SaV and HuNoV, but SaV showed more resistance to ethanol than HuNoVs. SaV remained stable at pH 3.0–8.0. Preventive approaches for sapovirus infection should be directed towards basic hygiene, sanitation, cleaning, and disinfection. Drinking water purification, chlorination, hand hygiene, thorough cooking of food, and heat inactivation are recommended practices. Currently, there is no vaccine and no antiviral drug available for sapovirus prevention.

53.10 Aichivirus

Aichivirus is a new enteric virus isolated from a person with non- bacterial gastroenteritis due to the consumption of oysters from Aichi, Japan in 1989. Aichiviruses are small (~30 nm), non- enveloped, single-stranded positive-sense RNA (8280 nucleotides and poly (A) tail) viruses from the genus *Kobuvirus* of the *Picornaviridae* family. The genus *Kobuvirus* consists of six species of human and animal Aichiviruses (Aichivirus A, B, C, D, E, F). Aichivirus A is further divided into six subspecies including human Aichivirus genotypes A, B, and C.[164,165] The virus genome consists of a single ORF (7.3 kb) which encodes for structural proteins (VP0, VP3, VP1) and non-structural proteins (2A, 2B, 2C, 3A, 3B, 3C, 3D), which play an important role in virus replication.[166] The

Aichivirus is also an enteric pathogen and spreads through contaminated food and water. Typically, the Aichivirus follows a fecal-oral route of transmission and its prevalence is very high compared to other enteric viruses. This virus is routinely detected in combination with other enteric viruses in water, sewage, and other foods like shellfish.[165] Due to its great abundance in the environment, Aichivirus may be referred to as an indicator of environmental enteric viral contamination.[25] Fecally-contaminated water is one of the risk factors for Aichivirus infection. Consequently, contaminated water used for drinking, shellfish cultivation, recreational activities, and irrigation is important in its epidemiology.

Aichivirus is prevalent in Asia and it may be the predominant cause of gastroenteritis in infants and children, as it was detected in fecal samples of infants and children with diarrhea in Japan, Bangladesh, Thailand, and Vietnam. All the fecal specimens were negative for other enteric viruses namely, rotavirus, norovirus, adenovirus, astrovirus, and sapovirus.[167] Aichivirus infection is mostly mild and symptoms will generally last for 2–4 days. The virus replicates in intestinal enterocytes and symptomatic patients experience abdominal pain, diarrhea, nausea, and vomiting.

Even though the Aichivirus is important as a public health pathogen, its epidemiology is not well studied. Other than Japan, the Aichivirus was detected in Germany and Brazil, and several other countries in stool samples, sewage, water, and various foods.[168–170] A molecular study in the Netherlands showed a very high prevalence in surface water and sewage samples examined during 1987–2012. The dominance of genotype B was recorded, although Aichivirus A was also prevalent.[171] Extensive molecular characterization of Aichivirus in effluent and river water samples studied in Japan revealed a greater prevalence of Aichivirus A in the aquatic environment.[26]

Achiviruses are stable under environmental conditions and can survive varying pH values of 2–10, high hydrostatic pressure (600 Mpa), and refrigerated storage and they exhibit resistance to 90% isopropanol and ethanol for 5 min.[171–173] Over 4 $\log_{10}$ reduction of Aichivirus was achieved after heat treatment at 56°C for 20 min.[172] Application of UV light (240 mWs/cm^2) to Aichivirus achieved reductions of 4.5–4.6 log $TCID_{50}/mL$, 2.5–5.6 log $TCID_{50}/mL$, and 1.9–2.6 log $TCID_{50}/mL$ in contaminated lettuce, green onions, and strawberries, respectively.[174] Infectivity of AiV was observed after 21 days in cranberry juice kept at refrigerated storage conditions and cranberry cocktail at a pH of 3.0.[175] Diagnosis of Aichivirus infection is done by electron microscopy, detection of virus RNA particles by RT-PCR and real-time PCR, serology, and detection of antigen in stool by ELISA. Virus-specific IgG, IgM, and IgA antibodies can be detected by ELISA and virus neutralization tests in the patients' paired sera.[176] Virus isolation can be attempted using cell lines like BSC-1 and Vero cells with cytopathic effects. Modern molecular tools like LAMP, digital RT-PCR, and pyrosequencing are highly sensitive. Personal hygiene, hand washing, food safety, chlorination of water, and decontamination of inanimate surfaces help prevent Aichivirus infection.

53.11 Other viruses that may infect food

Most foodborne viruses display a fecal-oral transmission pattern where they are excreted in large numbers in animal/human feces and they then contaminate food, water, and environmental reservoirs, thereby increasing the risk of human infection. Some viruses are not typically enteric or foodborne in nature, however, their spread through food packaging material and inanimate objects coming into contact with food may occur. Some respiratory viruses like Influenza type A viruses (Highly Pathogenic Avian Influenza-HPAI, e.g., H5N1), severe acute respiratory syndrome causing coronaviruses such as SARS-CoV, MERS CoV, SARS-CoV-2 and neurotropic viruses like nipah virus, poliovirus, and tick-borne encephalitis (TBE) virus may accidentally get introduced into the food chain.[177]

The poliovirus belongs to the genus Enterovirus of Picornaviridae family. It causes poliomyelitis and is transmitted through the fecal-oral route. Environmental monitoring of poliovirus is essential for wild type and vaccine-derived polioviruses, as wild polioviruses are endemic in Afghanistan, Pakistan, and Nigeria and the risk of poliovirus importation from endemic countries to other polio-free countries cannot be ruled out.[178] Experimental inoculation of poliovirus on fresh produce (lettuce, onion, cabbage, raspberry, and strawberry) stored at household refrigeration temperatures revealed virus persistence in fresh vegetables and fruits for several days (8.4–14.2 days) highlighting the potential food safety risk of poliovirus.[179] The earliest report on the survival of poliovirus 1 in soil flooded with sewage and effluent containing the virus revealed its detection in soil and on vegetables such as lettuce and radishes; in the winter season, the virus was detected for up to 96 days.[180]

The nipah virus is an emerging zoonotic virus prevalent in most Asian countries. It belongs to the genus *Henipavirus* of the *Paramyxoviridae* family and was first detected in the Nipah village of Malaysia in 1998.[181] It is transmitted by fruit bats to intermediate animals like pigs and humans. Human to human transmission is commonly reported for nipah virus. Foodborne transmission of nipah virus may be possible if fruits and vegetables are contaminated with the saliva, urine, and feces of bats carrying the virus.[128] Although there are no human outbreaks or confirmed cases reported due to consumption of infected fruit, this route is considered a potential source of nipah virus infection. In the first reported outbreak of nipah virus disease in 1998 in Malaysia, human infection was associated with close contact with infected pigs, which were exposed to partially eaten fruits dropped by bats in the pig sty.[182,183] In other outbreaks in Bangladesh in 2001 and 2005, consumption of raw date palm sap contaminated with bat saliva and excreta of bats was implicated as the source of infection, and symptoms of fever, seizures, and altered mental status were recorded in 124 cases.[184] In 2018 a nipah virus outbreak was reported in the Kerala state of India and over 91% mortality was recorded in this outbreak.[185] An occupational risk of infection to humans is also associated with abattoir work during the slaughtering and dressing of infected animals.[27]

Coronaviruses are respiratory pathogens and some of them are zoonotic in nature like SARS-CoV and MERS-CoV. The current pandemic of SARS-CoV-2 (COVID-19) is highly devastating and this viral infection is principally transmitted through person-to-person contact and via aerosols and respiratory droplets. Transmission via contaminated surfaces, although possible, is not regarded as a primary route of transmission. Since SARS-CoV-2 remains stable in air and on inanimate surfaces like stainless steel, cardboard, copper, and plastic for several hours,[186–189] its possible mechanical transmission by food packaging material cannot be ruled out.[190] Concerns over the risk of SARS-CoV-2 to food safety have been raised, however foodborne outbreaks of SARS-CoV-2 have not been reported and it is unlikely that the virus is foodborne.[28,191,192] High-touch surfaces should be cleaned and sanitized regularly, to prevent an occupational health hazard from arising.[191] If contamination by SARS-CoV-2 occurs, it is important to note that it cannot multiply in food (as for other viruses) and the viral load will likely decrease during storage. For decontamination from surfaces, the use of 0.1% sodium hypochlorite, 0.5% H_2O_2, and 70% ethanol is effective. For air disinfection of the food processing environment, air filters and UV light are effective.[28]

Tick-borne encephalitis virus (TBEV) is another foodborne virus of minor significance from the genus *Flavivirus* and the *Flaviviridae* family. It is transmitted mainly by tick bite, however, foodborne transmission through consumption of unpasteurized milk and milk products prepared from goat's milk has been documented.[182,193]

53.12 Management of foodborne virus infections

Risk analysis is integral to food safety management systems and the ultimate goal of risk analysis is the protection of human health through the production of safe and wholesome food. Microbial Risk Assessment (MRA), risk management, and risk communication are fundamental interacting components of food safety risk analysis.[194] Risk assessment is the first step of risk analysis and it is solely a scientific process responsible for generating technical information used by risk managers in food establishments. Scientific information in terms of exposure assessment of the likelihood of occurrence, estimates of populations exposed to hazards, infectious dose, survival, multiplication, and numbers of organism/cells consumed through contaminated food is key for the management of risk. Based upon the scientific findings of risk assessment, further policy and regulatory decisions are taken to manage identified risks, that is, risk management. The last step in the process of risk analysis is risk communication, which is interactive. The information gathered through risk assessment and risk management must be shared among various stakeholders involved in the food chain.[195,196]

Risk assessment of viruses present in foods is highly challenging due to the poor understanding of food virology. Some of the known difficulties are quantification of virus particles in food, their identification, isolation, assessment of the level of contamination, and possibilities of heterogeneous distribution of viruses on food matrices. Most foodborne viruses are detected in food by targeting viral nucleic acids, however, this technique doesn't provide reliable information on viral infectivity. Similarly, for viruses in food or water, reliable indicator organisms are not specified and thus the presence of viruses in food and water is difficult to forecast. Survival of enteric foodborne viruses on different surfaces and their environmental stability are further challenges in conducting an effective risk assessment.

Although risk assessment of viruses in food and water is challenging, prevention of contamination of water bodies with human stool, sewage, and animal feces must be given priority. Most enteric viruses are acquired through the consumption of shellfish harvested from contaminated water, vegetables grown using sewage or fecally-contaminated irrigation water, and fruits and other food items exposed to contaminated water used during washing and other processing operations. Enteric viruses may persist in sewage, manure, and other biomaterials for several days. Therefore the use of contaminated water for agricultural irrigation is not advocated. Secondary transmission of foodborne viruses is possible through infected or asymptomatic human carriers while handling foods, therefore, cross-contamination is likely to happen if personal hygiene is compromised, as infected persons can shed millions of virus particles in the stool.

Globally, most studies have focused on the MRA of viruses in irrigation water, drinking water, and foods like raspberries, berries, lettuce, pork liver, chicken, eggs, oysters, and other seafood. Comprehensive overviews of risk assessments of foodborne viruses have been published,[4,197,198] which provide greater insight into the MRA of viruses in food. As per the joint FAO and WHO meeting report,[5] food and water-borne viruses of public health concern that should receive priority are HAV, HEV, NoV, HRVs, and other emerging viruses like HAPI-H5N1, SARS-CoV, and Nipah virus. Based on available scientific information and risk assessment studies, some food commodities as described below should be given priority in terms of food commodities and the associated risk of viruses.[5]

1. Bivalve molluscan shellfish including oysters, clams, cockles, and mussels for HAV and NoV.
2. Fresh produce (leafy vegetables and fruits) for HAV and NoV.
3. Prepared foods for HAV and NoV.
4. Water for food preparation for HRVs and
5. Emerging viruses; poultry for HPAI, porcine origin products for HEV, and fruits for Nipah virus.

Food products that have limited shelf life and foods which are being consumed raw/partially cooked like salads and molluscan shellfish demand more stringent preharvest risk management options for foodborne pathogens, as post-harvest management has limitations for such commodities. For highly prevalent enteric viruses like NoV, HAV, and HRV, their inactivation in sewage and prevention of water bodies engaged in shellfish farming from becoming contaminated is essential, through collaborative efforts and integration of several departments/agencies like agriculture, animal husbandry, fisheries, pollution control, and health. Post-harvest techniques are largely dependent on the processing, decontamination, and preservation of foods. To avoid cross-contamination through food handlers and contaminated surfaces, quality control systems must be integrated with Good Hygiene Practices (GHP), Good Manufacturing Practices (GMP), Hazard Analysis and Critical Control Point (HACCP) approach, and Total Quality Management (TQM). Several gaps exist in terms of available technological solutions and their utility for the prevention and control of foodborne viruses. Therefore, consideration must be given to the challenges faced by the food industry while validating and implementing strategies directed toward the control of viruses in foods.[4] Table 53.3 outlines the perseverance of foodborne viruses in the environment as well as their prevention and inactivation. Generally, strategies directed towards bacterial control in terms of change in pH, moisture, and low temperature are inadequate to arrest the risk of viruses in foods. Moreover, viruses are more stable at low chilling and freezing temperatures. Thermal inactivation is the most effective method of control of foodborne viruses and several time-temperature combinations have been studied for the inactivation of viruses in different types of foods like shellfish, lettuce, spinach, freeze-dried berries, and strawberries. Almost all the major enteric viruses like NoV, HAV, and HEV are inactivated completely at temperatures above $\geq 90°C$ for >90 s including shellfish matrix.[194] For example, NoV, HAV, and enteroviruses in boiling water can be reduced by 4 $\log_{10}$. In other food matrices like milk, cream, spinach, raspberry puree, onion, basil, and pet foods, a $\log_{10}$ reduction in the range of $\geq 3-4.4$ has been reported at a temperature range of 71°C–80°C.[64,113,199] Steam blanching of vegetables above 95°C for 2.5 min will inactivate HAV and heating of pork to an internal temperature above 71°C for 20 min will take care of HEV.

HPP also inactivates NoV and HAV in shellfish at 600 MPa pressure at 6°C for 5 min.[211] In another study, a 4.3 $\log_{10}$ reduction of HAV was recorded in strawberry puree and onion slices subjected to 375 MPa for 5 min at 22°C.[212] Irradiation of food is another promising technology for food preservation and control of foodborne pathogens, however, viruses are more resistant than bacteria and parasites to the process of gamma irradiation due to their smaller genome size. In the food processing industry, the use of sanitizing agents and disinfectants for surface cleaning is practiced. Similarly, chlorine-based compounds like sodium hypochlorite, calcium hypochlorite, and hypochlorous acid may reduce foodborne virus load on surfaces.

53.13 Conclusions

Foodborne enteric viruses constitute a global challenge to food safety and their surveillance needs to be strengthened in developing countries. The exact burden of human illness associated with viruses in foods remains unclear at the global level and their role in extra-intestinal infections other than gastroenteritis needs to be explored. Enteric viruses can survive for a very long time (even years) at temperatures below 5°C and especially in the absence of UV light. There is good evidence that the inactivation of viruses in the environment is less effective if they are absorbed onto or embedded within suspended solid matter that is not dried out. Viruses like HAV, NoV, and HEV can resist complete inactivation in the environment for a very long time.[213] GHP, improvement in sanitation, sewage treatment, and implementation of the highest standards of food hygiene should minimize the incidence of food-related virus outbreaks. Studies on the environmental stability of food viruses in different agro-ecological climates, on foods, soil, and food contact surfaces will help in developing effective control measures. The

TABLE 53.3 Stability of foodborne viruses.

Sr. no	Virus, structure, size, and disease	Zoonotic risk	Environmental stability	Inactivation	Chemical inactivation	Prevention	References
1	*Hepatitis A virus*, non–enveloped, ssRNA, + ve sense, 27–32 nm, causes hepatitis	No. Other than the fecal-oral route, HAV is spread through blood transfusions	Resistant to free chlorine, and if organic matter is high, it persists in dried feces; food contact surfaces; environment, and mussels for up to one month at room temperature; in frozen raspberries can survive up to 90 days;	Heating above 85°C for one minute, UV, HPP	Formalin, ozone, concentrated chlorine	Good Hygiene Practices (GHP), personal hygiene, HPP, irradiation, washing of fruits and vegetables; washing with potable water can achieve 1–2 log reduction	177,200
2	*Hepatitis E virus*, non-enveloped, ssRNA, + ve sense, 27–34 nm, causes hepatitis	Yes, can be transmitted from wild and domestic animals especially pigs, food and water	Highly stable at acidic and alkaline pH; survives up to 10 years in frozen conditions; highly infective	Heat inactivation > 65°C for 5 min and > 80°C for 1 min for genotypes 3 and 4. Complete inactivation in food at an internal temperature of 71°C for 20 min	Chlorine	Water quality standards, proper disposal of human and animal feces, thorough cooking of foods, GHP	201,202
3	*Human Adenovirus*, non–enveloped, dsDNA, 70–90 nm, causes respiratory illness, pneumonia, croup, bronchitis, gastroenteritis, and meningitis, respiratory infections	No	Survive on a plastic surface in an environment with low relative humidity for up to 35 days; Thermally stable at 10°C–85°C and pH 4–8; resistant to chemicals like peracetic acid, provodine iodine and formaldehyde	Gamma irradiation of water; HPP	Chlorine, chlorine dioxide, ozone	GHP, cooking, use of chlorine, chlorine dioxide and ozone for disinfection of food contact surfaces and surface disinfection of fruits	203
4	*Rotaviruses*, non–enveloped, dsRNA, 70 nm, cause diarrheal illness	Yes	Survive for many weeks in the environment; survive on fruits and vegetables stored at refrigerated temperatures for 2–3 weeks; Highly stable in feces, survive in the air for up to 9 days at 20°C	UV, HPP	8% formaldehyde for 5 min; 70% ethanol for 30 min; 2% Lysol and phenol for 1 h	GHP, cooking, use of chlorine, chlorine dioxide and ozone for disinfection of food contact surfaces and surface disinfection of fruits	118,204,205
5	*Norovirus*, non–enveloped, ssRNA, + ve sense, 27–40 nm, causes gastroenteritis	Genogroup I	Survive on foods and food contact surfaces for several days	UV, HPP, > 60°C, pH 2.7 > 10^4 loss 1 min in boiling water	Chlorine	GHP, cooking, use of chlorine, chlorine dioxide and ozone for disinfection of food contact surfaces and surface disinfection of fruits	53,177,206

6	*Astroviruses*, non–enveloped, ssRNA, + ve sense, 28–30 nm, causes gastroenteritis	Not clearly recognized	Stable at pH 3; thermally stable 5 min at 60°C; Classic HAstV survive for long periods in water (up to 90 days); genogroup B is more resistant to chlorine disinfection than genogroup A	Disinfection treatments of 2 h with 1 mg/mL of free chlorine are effective;	Astrovirus survival and inactivation in food matrices have not been extensively studied; disinfection of contaminated fomites with 90% alcohol has proven useful	Chlorination, boiling, GHP	139
8	*Sapovirus*, non-enveloped, ssRNA, + ve sense, 30–38 nm, causes gastroenteritis	No	Porcine sapovirus is stable at pH 3.0 to 8.0 at room temperature for 1 h;	UV	Sensitive to 60%–70% ethanol at room temperature for 30 s; 200 mg/L sodium hypochlorite at room temperature for 30 min; heating at 56°C for 2 h	GHP food and environmental hygiene	24,207
9	*Aichiviruses*, non–enveloped, ssRNA, + ve sense, 30 nm, cause gastroenteritis	Interspecies transmission of non-human Kobuviruses in animals is possible	AiV-1 is stable at a wide range of pH (2–10) and resistant (<0.5 log_{10} inactivation) to 90% isopropanol or ethanol for up to 5 min; AiV-1 on stainless steel disks seems to be insensitive to chlorine treatment (1.3 log_{10} inactivation by 1000 ppm for 5 min)	HPP; heat treatment at 56°C for 20 min inactivate AiV-1 (>4 log_{10} inactivation)	Inactivated within a day by dairy manure-based composting	GHP, food hygiene, water disinfection, sewage treatment and disposal	25,165
10	*Poliovirus*, non–enveloped, ssRNA, + ve sense, 40–50 nm, causes poliomyelitis	No	Survives 1 h at 50°C; resistant to chlorine; incomplete inactivation by formaldehyde	Heat, UV	Chlorine dioxide	GHP, vaccination, hygiene and sanitation	208
11	*Nipah virus*, enveloped, ssRNA,—ve sense, 150–500 nm, causes fever, headache, respiratory infection, encephalitis	Yes	> 10 h on surfaces; RNA found on hospital surfaces; heat-sensitive; can survive in urine and contaminated fruit juice for days; survival characteristics in an environment not well known;	Moderately stable in an environment (tolerates heat up to 60°C, pH 4.0–10.0)	Susceptible to most soaps and disinfectants; sodium hypochlorite, ether and alcohol	Avoid consumption of raw date palm sap; prevent contact with bats; use of PPE, GHP, protection during slaughtering operations of pigs; NiV testing of exposed people; strict biosecurity at swine farms	209,210

development of more effective food-grade disinfectants for foodborne viruses is another area for focused research and development. Most viruses recognized in the recent past are emerging zoonotic viruses and their epidemiology is very complex. Thus, more emphasis on the zoonotic nature of viruses is warranted in the context of One Health. The role of the aquatic environment, particularly shellfish cultivated and harvested from polluted water is critical in the epidemiology of foodborne enteric viruses. Application of novel methods like HPP and cold plasma technologies before food packaging and preservation will be beneficial in terms of virus inactivation without affecting the nutritional and compositional quality of food.

References

1. Lodish H, Berk A, Zipursky SL, et al. *Molecular Cell Biology*. 4th ed New York: W. H. Freeman; 2000, Section 6.3, Viruses: Structure, Function, and Uses. Available from: https://www.ncbi.nlm.nih.gov/books/NBK21523/.
2. Seymour IJ, Appleton H. A review, foodborne viruses and fresh produce. *J Appl Microbiol*. 2001;91:759–773.
3. Koopmans M, Duizer E. Foodborne viruses: an emerging problem. *Int J Food Microbiol*. 2004;90(1):23–41. Available from: https://doi.org/10.1016/s0168-1605(03)00169-7.
4. Bosch A, Gkogka E, Le Guyader FS, et al. Foodborne viruses: detection, risk assessment, and control options in food processing. *Int J Food Microbiol*. 2018;285:110–118. Available from: https://doi.org/10.1016/j.ijfoodmicro.2018.06.001.
5. FAO/WHO (Food and Agriculture Organization of the United Nations/World Health Organization). Microbiological hazards in fresh leafy vegetables and herbs: Meeting Report. Microbiological Risk Assessment Series No. 14. Rome. 2008, 151 p.
6. Shukla S, Cho H, Kwon OJ, Chung SH, Kim M. Prevalence and evaluation strategies for viral contamination in food products: risk to human health-a review. *Crit Rev Food Sci Nutr*. 2016;1–15. Available from: https://doi.org/10.1080/10408398.2016.1182891.
7. EFSA. Panel on Biological Hazards (BIOHAZ) Scientific opinion on an update on the present knowledge on the occurrence and control of food-borne viruses. *EFSA J*. 2011;9(7):2190. Available from: https://doi.org/10.2903/j.efsa.2011.2190, www.efsa.europa.eu/efsajournal. 96. Available at. (accessed December 2011).
8. Greening GE. Human and animal viruses in food (including taxonomy of enteric viruses). In: Sagar G, ed. *Viruses in Foods*. vol. XVIII. New York: Springer; 2006:5–42. (In: Food MicroBiology and Food Safety).
9. Koopmans M. *Food-borne viruses from a global perspective. Institute of Medicine (US). Improving Food Safety Through a One Health Approach: Workshop Summary*. Washington (DC): National Academies Press (US); 2012:A9. https://www.ncbi.nlm.nih.gov/books/NBK114484/.
10. Scallan E, Hoekstra RM, Angulo FJ, et al. Foodborne illness acquired in the United States—major pathogens. *Emerg Infect Dis*. 2011;17(1):7–15.
11. Mattison CP, Cardemil CV, Hall AJ. Progress on norovirus vaccine research: public health considerations and future directions. *Expert Rev Vaccines*. 2018;17(9):773–784. Available from: https://doi.org/10.1080/14760584.2018.1510327.
12. Robilotti E, Deresinski S, Pinsky BA. Norovirus. *Clin Microbiol Rev*. 2015;28(1):134–164. Available from: https://doi.org/10.1128/CMR.00075-14.
13. Yezli S, Otter JA. Minimum infective dose of the major human respiratory and enteric viruses transmitted through food and the environment. *Food Environ Virol*. 2011;3(1):1–30. Available from: https://doi.org/10.1007/s12560-011-9056-7.
14. Franco E, Meleleo C, Serino L, Sorbara D, Zaratti L. Hepatitis A: epidemiology and prevention in developing countries. *World J Hepatol*. 2012;4(3):68–73. Available from: https://doi.org/10.4254/wjh.v4.i3.68.
15. Pavio N, Merbah T, Thébault A. Frequent hepatitis E virus contamination in food containing raw pork liver, France. *Emerg Infect Dis*. 2014;20(11):1925–1927. Available from: https://doi.org/10.3201/eid2011.140891.
16. Webb GW, Dalton HR. Hepatitis E: an underestimated emerging threat. *Therap Adv Infect Dis*. 2019;6. Available from: https://doi.org/10.1177/2049936119837162.
17. Wu X, Chen P, Lin H, Hao X, Liang Z. Hepatitis E virus: current epidemiology and vaccine. *Hum Vaccin Immunother*. 2016;12(10):2603–2610. Available from: https://doi.org/10.1080/21645515.2016.1184806.
18. Borkenhagen LK, Fieldhouse JK, Seto D, Gray GC. Are adenoviruses zoonotic? A systematic review of the evidence. *Emerg Microbes Infect*. 2019;8(1):1679–1687. Available from: https://doi.org/10.1080/22221751.2019.1690953.
19. Hart CA, Cunliffe NA, Nakagomi O. Diarrhoea caused by viruses. *Manson's Trop Dis*. 2009;815–824. Available from: https://doi.org/10.1016/B978-1-4160-4470-3.50049-5.
20. Ward RL, Bernstein DI, Young EC, Sherwood JR, Knowlton DR, Schiff GM. Human rotavirus studies in volunteers: determination of infectious dose and serological response to infection. *J Infect Dis*. 1986;154(5):871–880. Available from: https://doi.org/10.1093/infdis/154.5.871.
21. Radin JM, Hawksworth AW, Blair PJ, et al. Dramatic decline of respiratory illness among US military recruits after the renewed use of adenovirus vaccines. *Clin Infect Dis*. 2014;59(7):962–968. Available from: https://doi.org/10.1093/cid/ciu507.
22. Roach SN, Langlois RA. Intra-and cross-species transmission of astroviruses. *Viruses*. 2021;13:1127. Available from: https://doi.org/10.3390/v13061127.
23. Patel M, Cochi S. Addressing the challenges and opportunities of the polio endgame: lessons for the future. *J Infect Dis*. 2017;216(suppl_1):S1–S8. Available from: https://doi.org/10.1093/infdis/jix117.
24. Oka T, Wang Q, Katayama K, Saif LJ. Comprehensive review of human sapoviruses. *Clin Microbiol Rev*. 2015;28(1):32–53. Available from: https://doi.org/10.1128/CMR.00011-14.
25. Kitajima M, Gerba CP. Aichivirus 1: environmental occurrence and behavior. *Pathog (Basel, Switz)*. 2015;4(2):256–268. Available from: https://doi.org/10.3390/pathogens4020256.
26. Kitajima M, Haramoto E, Phanuwan C, Katayama H. Prevalence and genetic diversity of Aichiviruses in wastewater and river water in Japan. *Appl Environ Microbiol*. 2011;77(6):2184–2187. Available from: https://doi.org/10.1128/AEM.02328-10.

27. Singh RK, Dhama K, Chakraborty S, et al. Nipah virus: epidemiology, pathology, immunobiology and advances in diagnosis, vaccine designing and control strategies-a comprehensive review. *Vet Q.* 2019;39(1):26–55. Available from: https://doi.org/10.1080/01652176.2019.1580827.
28. Anelich L, Lues R, Farber JM, Parreira VR. SARS-CoV-2 and risk to food safety. *Front Nutr.* 2020;7:580551. Available from: https://doi.org/10.3389/fnut.2020.580551.
29. Zou S, Guo J, Gao R, et al. Inactivation of the novel avian influenza A (H7N9) virus under physical conditions or chemical agents treatment. *Virol J.* 2013;10:289. Available from: https://doi.org/10.1186/1743-422X-10-289.
30. Offerdahl DK, Clancy NG, Bloom ME. Stability of a tick-borne flavivirus in milk. *Front Bioeng Biotechnol.* 2016;4:40. Available from: https://doi.org/10.3389/fbioe.2016.00040.
31. Green KY. Caliciviridae: the noroviruses. In: Knipe DM, Howley PM, eds. *Fields Virology*. Philadelphia, PA: Lippincott, Williams & Wilkins; 2013.
32. Jiang X, Wang M, Wang K, Estes MK. Sequence and genomic organization of norwalk virus. *Virology.* 1993;195:51–61. Available from: https://doi.org/10.1006/viro.1993.1345.
33. Chhabra P, de Graaf M, Parra GI, et al. Updated classification of norovirus genogroups and genotypes. *J Gen Virol.* 2019;100(10):1393–1406. Available from: https://doi.org/10.1099/jgv.0.001318. Erratum in: J Gen Virol. 2020 Aug;101(8):893.
34. CDC [Centres for Disease Control and Prevention]. Norovirus: virus classification. <https://www.cdc.gov/norovirus/lab/virus-classification.html>; 2021 Accessed 01.11.21.
35. Parra GI. Emergence of norovirus strains: a tale of two genes. *Virus Evol.* 2019;5(2):vez048. Available from: https://doi.org/10.1093/ve/vez048.
36. Mattison K, Shukla A, Cook A, et al. Human noroviruses in swine and cattle. *Emerg Infect Dis.* 2007;13(8):1184–1188. Available from: https://doi.org/10.3201/eid1308.070005.
37. Villabruna N, Koopmans M, de Graaf M. Animals as Reservoir for Human Norovirus. *Viruses.* 2019;11(5):478. Available from: https://doi.org/10.3390/v11050478.
38. Pires SM, Fischer-Walker CL, Lanata CF, et al. Aetiology-specific estimates of the global and regional incidence and mortality of diarrhoeal diseases commonly transmitted through food. *PLoS One.* 2015;10(12):e0142927. pmid:26632843; PubMed Central PMCID: PMCPMC4668836.
39. Isakbaeva ET, Widdowson MA, Beard RS, et al. Norovirus transmission on cruise ship. *Emerg Infect Dis.* 2005;11(1):154–158. Available from: https://doi.org/10.3201/eid1101.040434.
40. Atmar RL, Opekun AR, Gilger MA, et al. Norwalk virus shedding after experimental human infection. *Emerg Infect Dis.* 2008;14(10):1553–1557. Available from: https://doi.org/10.3201/eid1410.080117.
41. Lopman B, Gastanaduy P, Park GW, Hall AJ, Parashar UD, Vinje J. Environmental transmission of norovirus gastroenteritis. *Curr Opin Virol.* 2012;2:96–102.
42. Teunis PF, Moe CL, Liu P, et al. Norwalk virus: how infectious is it? *J Med Virol.* 2008;80:1468–1476.
43. Shah MP, Hall AJ. Norovirus illnesses in children and adolescents. *Infect Dis Clin North Am.* 2018;32(1):103–118. Available from: https://doi.org/10.1016/j.idc.2017.11.004.
44. CDC [Centres for Disease Control and Prevention]. Norovisus illness: hey facts. <https://www.cdc.gov/norovirus/downloads/key-facts.pdf>; 2021, Accessed 01.11.21.
45. Hardstaff JL, Clough HE, Lutje V, McIntyre KM, Harris JP, Garner P, O'Brien SJ. Foodborne and Food-Handler Norovirus Outbreaks: A Systematic Review. *Foodborne Pathogens and Disease.* 2018;15(10):589–597. Available from: https://doi.org/10.1089/fpd.2018.2452.
46. Kaplan JE, Gary GW, Baron RC, et al. Epidemiology of norwalk gastroenteritis and the role of norwalk virus in outbreaks of acute nonbacterial gastroenteritis. *Ann Intern Med.* 1982;96(6 Pt 1):756–761. Available from: https://doi.org/10.7326/0003-4819-96-6-756.
47. ISO 15216-1:2017 Microbiology of the food chain — Horizontal method for determination of hepatitis A virus and norovirus using real-time RT-PCR — Part 1: Method for quantification, 2017.
48. ISO 15216-2:2019 Microbiology of the food chain — Horizontal method for determination of hepatitis A virus and norovirus using real-time RT-PCR — Part 2: Method for detection, 2019.
49. Hewitt J, Greening GE. Survival and persistence of norovirus, hepatitis A virus, and feline calicivirus in marinated mussels. *J Food Prot.* 2004;67(8):1743–1750.
50. Lamhoujeb S, Fliss I, Ngazoa SE, Jean J. Evaluation of the persistence of infectious human noroviruses on food surfaces by using realtime nucleic acid sequence-based amplification. *Appl Environ Microbiol.* 2008;74:3349–3355.
51. Mormann S, Dabisch M, Becker B. Effects of technological processes on the tenacity and inactivation of norovirus genogroup II in experimentally contaminated foods. *Appl Environ Microbiol.* 2010;76:536–545.
52. Verhaelen K, Bouwknegt M, Carratalà A, et al. Virus transfer proportions between gloved fingertips, soft berries, and lettuce, and associated health risks. *Int J Food Microbiol.* 2013;166(3):419–425. Available from: https://doi.org/10.1016/j.ijfoodmicro.2013.07.025.
53. Cook N, Knight A, Richards GP. Persistence and elimination of human norovirus in food and on food contact surfaces: a critical review. *J Food Prot.* 2016;79(7):1273–1294. Available from: https://doi.org/10.4315/0362-028X.JFP-15-570.
54. Esposito S, Principi N. Norovirus vaccine: priorities for future research and development. *Front Immunol.* 2020;11:1383.
55. Lemon SM, Ott JJ, Van Damme P, Shouval D. Type A viral hepatitis: a summary and update on the molecular virology, epidemiology, pathogenesis and prevention. *J Hepatol.* 2018;68:167–184.
56. Robertson BH, Jansen RW, Khanna B, et al. Genetic relatedness of hepatitis A virus strains recovered from different geographical regions. *J Gen Virol.* 1992;73(Pt 6):1365–1377.
57. Feinstone SM. History of the discovery of hepatitis A virus. *Cold Spring Harb Perspect Med.* 2019;9(5):a031740. Available from: https://doi.org/10.1101/cshperspect.a031740.
58. WHO (2020), Hepatitis E. WHO News Room/Fact sheet updated on 27 July 2020. <https://www.who.int/news-room/fact-sheets/detail/hepatitis-e>.
59. Foster MA, Hofmeister MG, Kupronis BA, et al. Increase in hepatitis A virus infections-United States, 2013–2018. *MMWR Morbidity Mortal Wkly Rep.* 2019;68(18):413–415. Available from: https://doi.org/10.15585/mmwr.mm6818a2.

60. Wu J, Zou S, Giulivi A. Current hepatitis A status in Canada. *Can J Infect Dis = J Canadien des Maladies Infectieuses.* 2001;12 (6):341–344. Available from: https://doi.org/10.1155/2001/834670.
61. Frank C, Walter J, Muehlen M, et al. Major outbreak of hepatitis A associated with orange juice among tourists, Egypt, 2004. *Emerg Infect Dis.* 2007;13(1):156–158. Available from: https://doi.org/10.3201/eid1301.060487.
62. Venter JM, van HJ, Vivier JC, Grabow WO, Taylor MB. Hepatitis A virus in surface water in South Africa: what are the risks? *J Water Health.* 2007;5:229–240.
63. Sattar SA, Jason T, Bidawid S, Farber J. Foodborne spread of hepatitis A: recent studies on virus survival, transfer and inactivation. *Can J Infect Dis.* 2000;11(3):159–163. Available from: https://doi.org/10.1155/2000/805156.
64. Bidawid S, Farber JM, Sattar SA, Hayward S. Heat inactivation of hepatitis A virus in dairy foods. *J Food Prot.* 2000;63:522–528.
65. FDA [U.S. Food and Drug Administration]. *Hepatitis A Virus. In: Bad Bug Book, Foodborne. Pathogenic Microorganisms and Natural Toxins.* 2nd ed 2012:173–177.
66. Nainan OV, Xia G, Vaughan G, Margolis HS. Diagnosis of hepatitis a virus infection: a molecular approach. *Clin Microbiol Rev.* 2006;19(1):63–79. Available from: https://doi.org/10.1128/CMR.19.1.63-79.2006.
67. Phan C, Hollinger FB. Hepatitis A: natural history, immunopathogenesis, and outcome. *Clin Liver Dis.* 2013;2(6):231–234. Available from: https://doi.org/10.1002/cld.253.
68. Massoudi MS, Bell BP, Paredes V, Insko J, Evans K, Shapiro CN. An outbreak of hepatitis A associated with an infected foodhandler. *Public Health Rep (Washington, DC: 1974).* 1999;114 (2):157–164. Available from: https://doi.org/10.1093/phr/114.2.157.
69. Cliver DO. Virus transmission via food. *World Health Stat Q.* 1997;50:90–101.
70. Bozkurt H, D'Souza DH, Davidson PM. Determination of thermal inactivation kinetics of hepatitis A virus in blue mussel (Mytilusedulis) homogenate. *Appl Environ Microbiol.* 2014;80 (10):3191–3197. Available from: https://doi.org/10.1128/AEM.00428-14.
71. Deboosere N, Pinon A, Delobel A, et al. A predictive microbiology approach for thermal inactivation of hepatitis A virus in acidified berries. *Food Microbiol.* 2010;27:962–967. Available from: https://doi.org/10.1016/j.fm.2010.05.018.
72. Bidawid S, Farber JM, Sattar SA. Inactivation of hepatitis A virus in fruits and vegetables by gamma irradiation. *Int J Food Microbiol.* 2000;57:91–97.
73. Biziagos E, Passagot J, Crance JM, Deloince R. Long-term survival of hepatitis A virus and poliovirus type 1 in mineral water. *Applied and Environmental Microbiology.* 1988;54(11):2705–2710. Available from: https://doi.org/10.1128/aem.54.11.2705-2710.1988.
74. McCaustland KA, Bond WW, Bradley DW, Ebert JW, Maynard JE. Survival of hepatitis A virus in feces after drying and storage for 1 month. *J Clin Microbiol.* 1982;16(5):957–958. Available from: https://doi.org/10.1128/jcm.16.5.957-958.1982.
75. Mbithi JN, Springthorpe VS, Boulet JR, Sattar SA. Survival of hepatitis A virus on human hands and its transfer on contact with animate and inanimate surfaces. *J Clin Microbiol.* 1992;30 (4):757–763. Available from: https://doi.org/10.1128/jcm.30.4.757-763.1992.
76. Mbithi JN, Springthorpe VS, Sattar SA. Effect of relative humidity and air temperature on survival of hepatitis A virus on environmental surfaces. *Appl Environ Microbiol.* 1991;1991 (57):1394–1399.
77. van der Poel, W., Rzezutka, A. Hepatitis A. In: J.B. Rose and B. Jiménez-Cisneros, (eds) Water and Sanitation for the 21st Century: Health and Microbiological Aspects of Excreta and Wastewater Management (Global Water Pathogen Project). (J.S Meschke, and R. Girones (eds), Part 3: Specific Excreted Pathogens: Environmental and Epidemiology Aspects – Section 1: Viruses), Michigan State University, E. Lansing, MI, UNESCO. 2017. <https://doi.org/10.14321/waterpathogens.12>.
78. Foster MA, Penina H, Nelson NP. Hepatits A. Pink Book on Epidemiology and Prevention of Vaccine-Preventable Diseases. Centres for Disease Control and Prevention. 2021. <https://www.cdc.gov/vaccines/pubs/pinkbook/downloads/hepa.pdf>.
79. Verma R, Khanna P. Hepatitis A vaccine should receive priority in national immunization schedule in India. *Hum Vaccin Immunother.* 2012;8(8):1132–1134. Available from: https://doi.org/10.4161/hv.20475.
80. Balayan MS, Andjaparidze AG, Savinskaya SS, et al. Evidence for a virus in non-A, non-B hepatitis transmitted via the fecal-oral route. *Intervirology.* 1983;20:23–31.
81. Mirazo S, Ramos N, Mainardi V, Gerona S, Arbiza J. Transmission, diagnosis, and management of hepatitis E: an update. *Hepatic Med Evid Res.* 2014;6:45–59. Available from: https://doi.org/10.2147/HMER.S63417.
82. Purdy MA, Harrison TJ, Jameel S, et al. ICTV virus taxonomy profile: hepeviridae. *J Gen Virol.* 2017;98(11):2645–2646.
83. Zhou J-H, Li X-R, Lan XI, et al. The genetic divergences of codon usage shed new lights on transmission of hepatitis E virus from swine to human. *Infect Genet Evol.* 2019;68:23–29.
84. Aslan AT, Balaban HY. Hepatitis E virus: epidemiology, diagnosis, clinical manifestations, and treatment. *World J Gastroenterol.* 2020;26(37):5543–5560. Available from: https://doi.org/10.3748/wjg.v26.i37.5543.
85. Lee GH, Tan BH, Teo EC, et al. Chronic infection withcamelid hepatitis E virus in a liver transplant recipient who regularly consumes camel meat and milk. *Gastroenterology.* 2016;150:355–357.e3.
86. Rein DB, Stevens GA, Theaker J, Wittenborn JS, Wiersma ST. The global burden of hepatitis E virus genotypes 1 and 2 in 2005. *Hepatology.* 2012;55(4):988–997. Available from: https://doi.org/10.1002/hep.25505.
87. Li P, Liu J, Li Y, et al. The global epidemiology of hepatitis E virus infection: A systematic review and meta-analysis. *Liver Int Off J Int Assoc Study Liver.* 2020;40(7):1516–1528. Available from: https://doi.org/10.1111/liv.14468.
88. Khuroo MS, Khuroo MS, Khuroo NS. Hepatitis E: Discovery, global impact, control and cure. *World J Gastroenterol.* 2016;22 (31):7030–7045. Available from: https://doi.org/10.3748/wjg.v22.i31.7030.
89. Kamar N, Dalton HR, Abravanel F, Izopet J. Hepatitis E virus infection. *Clin Microbiol Rev.* 2014;27(1):116–138. Available from: https://doi.org/10.1128/CMR.00057-13.
90. Song YJ, Park WJ, Park BJ, et al. Hepatitis E virus infections in humans and animals. *Clin Exp Vaccine Res.* 2014;3(1):29–36. Available from: https://doi.org/10.7774/cevr.2014.3.1.29.

91. Doceul V, Bagdassarian E, Demange A, Pavio N. Zoonotic hepatitis E virus: classification, animal reservoirs and transmission routes. *Viruses*. 2016;8:270. Available from: https://doi.org/10.3390/v8100270.
92. Huang F, Li Y, Yu W, et al. Excretion of infectious hepatitis E virus into milk in cows imposes high risks of zoonosis. *Hepatology*. 2016;64:350–359. Available from: https://doi.org/10.1002/hep.28668.
93. Colson P, Borentain P, Queyriaux B, et al. Pig liver sausage as a source of hepatitis E virus transmission to humans. *J Infect Dis*. 2010;202(6):825–834. Available from: https://doi.org/10.1086/655898.
94. Riveiro-Barciela M, Mínguez B, Gironés R, Rodriguez-Frías F, Quer J, Buti M. Phylogenetic demonstration of hepatitis E infection transmitted by pork meat ingestion. *J Clin Gastroenterol*. 2015;49(2):165–168. Available from: https://doi.org/10.1097/MCG.0000000000000113.
95. Grodzki M, Schaeffer J, Piquet JC, et al. Bioaccumulation efficiency, tissue distribution, and environmental occurrence of hepatitis E virus in bivalve shellfish from France. *Appl Environ Microbiol*. 2014;80(14):4269–4276. Available from: https://doi.org/10.1128/AEM.00978-14. Epub 2014 May 2. PMID: 24795382; PMCID: PMC4068666.
96. O'Hara Z, Crossan C, Craft J, Scobie L. First report of the presence of hepatitis E virus in Scottish-harvested shellfish purchased at retail level. *Food Environ Virol*. 2018;10:217–221.
97. Baez PA, Lopez MC, Duque-Jaramillo A, Pelaez D, Molina F, Navas MC. First evidence of the hepatitis E virus in environmental waters in Colombia. *PLoS One*. 2017;12(5):e0177525. Available from: https://doi.org/10.1371/journal.pone.0177525.
98. Fenaux H, Chassaing M, Berger S, Gantzer C, Bertrand I, Schvoerer E. Transmission of hepatitis E virus by water: an issue still pending in industrialized countries. *Water Res*. 2019;151:144–157. Available from: https://doi.org/10.1016/j.watres.2018.12.014. Epub 2018 Dec 18. PMID: 30594083.
99. Harrison L, Ramos TD, Wu X, DiCaprio E. Presence of hepatitis E virus in commercially available pork products. *Int J Food Microbiol*. 2021;339:109033. Available from: https://doi.org/10.1016/j.ijfoodmicro.2020.109033.
100. Martin-Latil S, Hennechart-Collette C, Delannoy S, Guillier L, Fach P, Perelle S. Quantification of hepatitis E virus in naturally-contaminated pig liver products. *Front Microbiol*. 2016;7:1183. Available from: https://doi.org/10.3389/fmicb.2016.01183.
101. Moor D, Liniger M, Baumgartner A, Felleisen R. Screening of ready-to-eat meat products for hepatitis E virus in Switzerland. *Food Environ Virol*. 2018;10(3):263–271.
102. WHO, UNICEF, World Bank. *State of the World's Vaccines and Immunization*. 3rd ed. Geneva: World Health Organization; 2009.
103. Crawford SE, Ramani S, Tate JE, et al. Rotavirus infection. *Nat Rev Dis Primers*. 2017;3:17083. Available from: https://doi.org/10.1038/nrdp.2017.83.
104. Santos N, Hoshino Y. Global distribution of rotavirus serotypes/genotypes and its implication for the development and implementation of an effective rotavirus vaccine. *Rev Med Virol*. 2005;15:29–56.
105. Deol P, Kattoor JJ, Sircar S, et al. Avian group D rotaviruses: structure, epidemiology, diagnosis, and perspectives on future research challenges. *Pathogens (Basel, Switz)*. 2017;6(4):53. Available from: https://doi.org/10.3390/pathogens6040053.
106. Rahman M, Sultana R, Podder G, et al. Typing of human rotaviruses: nucleotide mismatches between the VP7 gene and primer are associated with genotyping failure. *Virol J*. 2005;2:24. Available from: https://doi.org/10.1186/1743-422X-2-24.
107. Mukherjee A, Chawla-Sarkar M. Rotavirus infection: a perspective on epidemiology, genomic diversity and vaccine strategies. *Indian J Virol Organ Indian Virol Soc*. 2011;22(1):11–23. Available from: https://doi.org/10.1007/s13337-011-0039-y.
108. MoHFW. Ministry of Health & Family Welfare Government of India, operational guidelines introduction of rotavirus vaccine in the universal immunization programme. *Immun Div*. 2019;1–88.
109. Graham DY, Dufour GR, Estes MK. Minimal infective dose of rotavirus. *Arch Virol*. 1987;92:261–271.
110. Yousuf FA, Siddiqui R, Khan NA. Presence of rotavirus and free-living amoebae in the water supplies of Karachi, Pakistan. *Rev do Inst de Medicina Tropical de Sao Paulo*. 2017;59:e32. Available from: https://doi.org/10.1590/S1678-9946201759032.
111. Quiroz-Santiago C, Zquez-Salinas Cv́, Natividad-Bonifacio I, N-Romero BLB́, Ones-RamiŕRez EIQ. Rotavirus G2P[4] detection in fresh vegetables and oysters in Mexico City. *J Food Prot*. 2014;77(11):1953–1959. Available from: https://doi.org/10.4315/0362-028X.JFP-13-426.
112. de Wit MA, Koopmans MP, van Duynhoven YT. Risk factors for norovirus, Sapporo-like virus, and group A rotavirus gastroenteritis. *Emerging Infectious Diseases*. 2003;9(12):1563–1570. Available from: https://doi.org/10.3201/eid0912.020076.
113. CDC CDC fact sheet for healthy drinking water: drinking water treatment methods for backcountry and travel use [WWW Document] 2009. <https://www.cdc.gov/healthywater/pdf/drinking/Backcountry_Water_Treatment.pdf>.
114. Ming HX, Fan JF, Wu LJ, Liang YB. Prevalence of human enteric viruses and a potential indicator of contamination in shellfish in China. *J Food Saf*. 2013;33:209–214. Available from: https://doi.org/10.1111/jfs.12041.
115. Sattar SA, Tetro JA. Other foodborne viruses. In foodborne disease handbook. In: 2nd edn, Hui YH, Sattar SA, Murrell KD, Nip WK, Stanfield PS, eds. *Viruses, Parasites, Pathogens and HACCP*. Vol. 2. New York: Marcel Dekker; 2001:127–136.
116. Blutt SE, Matson DO, Crawford SE, et al. Rotavirus antigenemia in children is associated with viremia. *PLoS Med*. 2007;4(4):e121. Available from: https://doi.org/10.1371/journal.pmed.0040121.
117. Arnold M, Patton JT, McDonald SM. Culturing, storage, and quantification of rotaviruses. *Curr Protoc Microbiol*. 2009. Available from: https://doi.org/10.1002/9780471729259.mc15c03s15. *Chapter 15*, Unit–15C.3.
118. Meng ZD, Birch C, Heath R, Gust I. Physicochemical stability and inactivation of human and simian rotaviruses. *Appl Environ Microbiol*. 1987;53(4):727–730. Available from: https://doi.org/10.1128/aem.53.4.727-730.1987.
119. Sattar SA, Jacobsen H, Rahman H, Cusack TM, Rubino JR. Interruption of rotavirus spread through chemical disinfection. *Infect Control Hosp Epidemiol*. 1994;15(12):751–756. Available from: https://doi.org/10.1086/646852.
120. Keswick BH, Pickering LK, DuPont HL, Woodward WE. Survival and detection of rotaviruses on environmental surfaces in day care centers. *Appl Environ Microbiol*. 1983;46(4):813–816. Available from: https://doi.org/10.1128/AEM.46.4.813-816.1983.

121. Greening GE, Cannon JL. Human and animal viruses in food (including taxonomy of enteric viruses). *Viruses Foods*. 2016;5–57. Available from: https://doi.org/10.1007/978-3-319-30723-7_2.
122. Crenshaw BJ, Jones LB, Bell CR, Kumar S, Matthews QL. Perspective on adenoviruses: epidemiology, pathogenicity, and gene therapy. *Biomedicines*. 2019;7(3):61. Available from: https://doi.org/10.3390/biomedicines7030061.
123. Lynch 3rd JP, Kajon AE. Adenovirus: epidemiology, global spread of novel serotypes, and advances in treatment and prevention. *Semin Respir Crit Care Med*. 2016;37(4):586–602. Available from: https://doi.org/10.1055/s-0036-1584923.
124. Cai R, Mao N, Dai J, et al. Genetic variability of human adenovirus type 7 circulating in mainland China. *PLoS One*. 2020;15(4): e0232092. Available from: https://doi.org/10.1371/journal.pone.0232092.
125. Fong TT, Lipp EK. Enteric viruses of humans and animals in aquatic environments: health risks, detection, and potential water quality assessment tools. *Microbiol Mol Biol Rev MMBR*. 2005;69 (2):357–371. Available from: https://doi.org/10.1128/MMBR.69.2.357-371.2005.
126. Dehghan S, Seto J, Liu EB, et al. A zoonotic adenoviral human pathogen emerged through genomic recombination among human and nonhuman simian hosts. *J Virol*. 2019;93(18):e00564-19. Available from: https://doi.org/10.1128/JVI.00564-19.
127. Fong TT, Phanikumar MS, Xagoraraki I, Rose JB. Quantitative detection of human adenoviruses in wastewater and combined sewer overflows influencing a Michigan river. *Appl Environ Microbiol*. 2010;76(3):715–723. Available from: https://doi.org/10.1128/AEM.01316-09.
128. Epstein JH, Field HE, Luby S, Pulliam JR, Daszak P. Nipah virus: impact, origins, and causes of emergence. *Curr Infect Dis Rep*. 2006;8(1):59–65.
129. Cheong S, Lee C, Song SW, Choi WC, Lee CH, Kim SJ. Enteric viruses in raw vegetables and groundwater used for irrigation in South Korea. *Appl Environ Microbiol*. 2009;75(24):7745–7751. Available from: https://doi.org/10.1128/AEM.01629-09.
130. Crabtree KD, Gerba CP, Rose JB, Haas. CN. Waterborne adenovirus: a risk assessment. *Water Sci Technol*. 1997;35:1–6.
131. Cruz JR, Cáceres P, Cano F, Flores J, Bartlett A, Torún B. Adenovirus types 40 and 41 and rotaviruses associated with diarrhea in children from Guatemala. *J Clin Microbiol*. 1990;28:1780–1784.
132. Yépiz-Gómez MS, Gerba CP, Bright KR. Survival of respiratory viruses on fresh produce. *Food Environ Virol*. 2013;5 (3):150–156. Available from: https://doi.org/10.1007/s12560-013-9114-4. Advance online publication.
133. Hon KL, Leung AK. Severe childhood respiratory viral infections. *Adv Pediatr*. 2009;56(1):47–73. Available from: https://doi.org/10.1016/j.yapd.2009.08.019.
134. Rigotto C, Hanley K, Rochelle PA, De Leon R, Barardi CR, Yates MV. Survival of adenovirus types 2 and 41 in surface and ground waters measured by a plaque assay. *Environ Sci Technol*. 2011;45(9):4145–4150. Available from: https://doi.org/10.1021/es103922r.
135. Gray GC, Erdman DD. Adenovirus vaccines. *Plotkin's Vaccin*. 2018;121–133. Available from: https://doi.org/10.1016/B978-0-323-35761-6.00010-9. e8.
136. Lin Q, Lim J, Xue K, et al. Sanitizing agents for virus inactivation and disinfection. *View*. 2020;e16. Available from: https://doi.org/10.1002/viw2.16.
137. Thurston-Enriquez JA, Haas CN, Jacangelo J, Gerba CP. Chlorine inactivation of adenovirus type 40 and feline calicivirus. *Appl Environ Microbiol*. 2003;69(7):3979–3985. Available from: https://doi.org/10.1128/AEM.69.7.3979-3985.2003.
138. Monroe SS, Carter MJ, Herrmann JE, Kurtz JB, Matsui SM. Astroviridae. In: Murphy FA, Bishop DHL, Ghabrail SA, Jarvis AW, Martielli GP, Mayo MA, Summers MD, eds. *Virus Taxonomy: Classification and Nomenclature of Viruses. Sixth Report of the International Committee on Taxonomy of Viruses*. Vienna, Austria: Springer-Verlag; 1995:364–384.
139. Bosch A, Pintó RM, Guix S. Human astroviruses. *Clin Microbiol Rev*. 2014;27(4):1048–1074. Available from: https://doi.org/10.1128/CMR.00013-14.
140. Appleton H, Higgins PG. Viruses and gastroenteritis in infants. *Lancet*. 1975;1297.
141. Moser L, Schultz-Cherry S. Astroviruses. *Encycl Virol*. 2008;204–210. Available from: https://doi.org/10.1016/B978-012374410-4.00348-4.
142. Wohlgemuth N, Honce R, Schultz-Cherry S. Astrovirus evolution and emergence. *Infect Genet Evol J Mol Epidemiol Evolut Genet Infect Dis*. 2019;69:30–37. Available from: https://doi.org/10.1016/j.meegid.2019.01.009.
143. Schultz-Cherry S. Astroviruses. *Ref Module Biomed Sci*. 2014. Available from: https://doi.org/10.1016/B978-0-12-801238-3.02539-3.
144. Fischer K, Pinho Dos Reis V, Balkema-Buschmann A. Bat astroviruses: towards understanding the transmission dynamics of a neglected virus family. *Viruses*. 2017;9(2):34. Available from: https://doi.org/10.3390/v9020034.
145. Vu DL, Bosch A, Pintó RM, Guix S. Epidemiology of classic and novel human astrovirus: gastroenteritis and beyond. *Viruses*. 2017;9(2):33. Available from: https://doi.org/10.3390/v9020033.
146. Meliopoulos VA, Kayali G, Burnham A, et al. Detection of antibodies against turkey astrovirus in humans. *PLoS One*. 2014;9. Available from: https://doi.org/10.1371/journal.pone.0096934.
147. Oishi I, Yamazaki K, Kimoto T, et al. A large outbreak of acute gastroenteritis associated with astrovirus among students and teachers in Osaka, Japan. *J Infect Dis*. 1994;170(2):439–443. Available from: https://doi.org/10.1093/infdis/170.2.439.
148. Abad FX, Pintó RM, Villena C, Gajardo R, Bosch A. Astrovirus survival in drinking water. *Appl Environ Microbiol*. 1997;63 (8):3119–3122. Available from: https://doi.org/10.1128/AEM.63.8.3119-3122.1997.
149. Bosch A, Pinto RM, Villena C, Abad FX. Persistence of human astrovirus in fresh and marine water. *Water Sci Technol*. 1997;35:243–247. Available from: https://doi.org/10.1016/S0273-1223(97)00266-7.
150. Kitahashi T, Tanaka T, Utagawa E. [Detection of HAV, SRSV and astrovirus genomes from native oysters in Chiba City, Japan]. *KansenshogakuZasshi*. 1999;73(6):559–564. Available from: https://doi.org/10.11150/kansenshogakuzasshi1970.73.559. Japanese.
151. Le Guyader FS, Le Saux JC, Ambert-Balay K, et al. Aichivirus, norovirus, astrovirus, enterovirus, and rotavirus involved in clinical cases from a French oyster-related gastroenteritis outbreak. *J Clin Microbiol*. 2008;46(12):4011–4017. Available from: https://doi.org/10.1128/JCM.01044-08.

152. Dongdem JT, Damanka S, Asmah R. Molecular isolation of human norovirus and astrovirus in tap water by RT-PCR. *Int Res J Biochem Bioinformat*. 2011;1:131–138.
153. Johnson C, Hargest V, Cortez V, Meliopoulos VA, Schultz-Cherry S. Astrovirus pathogenesis. *Viruses*. 2017;9(1):22. Available from: https://doi.org/10.3390/v9010022.
154. Mayo MA. A summary of taxonomic changes recently approved by ICTV. *Arch Virol*. 2002;147(8):1655–1663. Available from: https://doi.org/10.1007/s007050200039.
155. Magwalivha M, Kabue JP, Traore AN, Potgieter N. Prevalence of human sapovirus in low and middle income countries. *Adv Virol*. 2018;2018:5986549. Available from: https://doi.org/10.1155/2018/5986549.
156. Hergens MP, NederbyÖhd J, Alm E, et al. Investigation of a food-borne outbreak of gastroenteritis in a school canteen revealed a variant of sapovirus genogroup V not detected by standard PCR, Sollentuna, Sweden, 2016. *Euro Surveill*. 2017;22(22):30543. Available from: https://doi.org/10.2807/1560-7917.ES.2017.22.22.30543.
157. Kobayashi S, Fujiwara N, Yasui Y, Yamashita T, Hiramatsu R, Minagawa H. A foodborne outbreak of sapovirus linked to catered box lunches in Japan. *Arch Virol*. 2012;157(10):1995–1997. Available from: https://doi.org/10.1007/s00705-012-1394-8. Epub 2012 Jun 30. PMID: 22752792.
158. Cho SR, Yun SJ, Chae SJ, et al. An outbreak associated with sapovirus GI.3 in an elementary school in Gyeonggi-do, Korea. *J Korean Med Sci*. 2020;35(34):e281. Available from: https://doi.org/10.3346/jkms.2020.35.e281.
159. Iizuka S, Oka T, Tabara K, et al. Detection of sapoviruses and noroviruses in an outbreak of gastroenteritis linked genetically to shellfish. *J Med Virol*. 2010;82(7):1247–1254. Available from: https://doi.org/10.1002/jmv.21791.
160. Yamashita Y, Ootsuka Y, Kondo R, et al. Molecular characterization of Sapovirus detected in a gastroenteritis outbreak at a wedding hall. *J Med Virol*. 2010;82(4):720–726. Available from: https://doi.org/10.1002/jmv.21646. Erratum in: J Med Virol. 2010 May;82(5):909. PMID: 20166168.
161. Iritani N, Kaida A, Abe N, et al. Detection and genetic characterization of human enteric viruses in oyster-associated gastroenteritis outbreaks between 2001 and 2012 in Osaka City, Japan. *J Med Virol*. 2014;86(12):2019–2025. Available from: https://doi.org/10.1002/jmv.23883. Epub 2014 Jan 10. PMID: 24415518.
162. Takagi H, Oka T, Shimoike T, et al. Human sapovirus propagation in human cell lines supplemented with bile acids. *Proc Natl Acad Sci U S A*. 2020;117(50):32078–32085. Available from: https://doi.org/10.1073/pnas.2007310117. Epub 2020 Nov 30. PMID: 33257564; PMCID: PMC7749338.
163. Wang Q, Zhang Z, Saif LJ. Stability of and attachment to lettuce by a culturable porcine sapovirus surrogate for human caliciviruses. *Appl Environ Microbiol*. 2012;78:3932–3940. Available from: https://doi.org/10.1128/AEM.06600-11.
164. Ambert-Balay K, Lorrot M, Bon F, et al. Prevalence and genetic diversity of Aichivirus strains in stool samples from community and hospitalized patients. *J Clin Microbiol*. 2008;46(4):1252–1258. Available from: https://doi.org/10.1128/JCM.02140-07.
165. Rivadulla E, Romalde JL. A comprehensive review on human Aichivirus. *Virol Sin*. 2020;35(5):501–516. Available from: https://doi.org/10.1007/s12250-020-00222-5.
166. Zhu L, Wang X, Ren J, et al. Structure of human Aichivirus and implications for receptor binding. *Nat Microbiol*. 2016;1:16150. Available from: https://doi.org/10.1038/nmicrobiol.2016.150.
167. Pham NT, Khamrin P, Nguyen TA, et al. Isolation and molecular characterization of Aichiviruses from fecal specimens collected in Japan, Bangladesh, Thailand, and Vietnam. *J Clin Microbiol*. 2007;45(7):2287–2288. Available from: https://doi.org/10.1128/JCM.00525-07.
168. Alcalá A, Vizzi E, Rodriguez-Diaz J, Zambrano JL, Betancourt W, Liprandi F. Molecular detection and characterization of Aichiviruses in sewage-polluted waters of Venezuela. *Appl Environ Microbiol*. 2010;76:4113–4115. Available from: https://doi.org/10.1128/AEM.00501-10.
169. Oh DY, Silva PA, Hauroeder B, Diedrich S, Cardoso DD, Schreier E. Molecular characterization of the first Aichiviruses isolated in Europe and in South America. *Arch Virol*. 2006;151(6):1199–1206.
170. Sdiri-Loulizi K, Hassine M, Aouni Z, et al. First molecular detection of Aichivirus in sewage and shellfish samples in the Monastir region of Tunisia. *Arch Virol*. 2010;155:1509–1513. Available from: https://doi.org/10.1007/s00705-010-0744-7.
171. Lodder WJ, Rutjes SA, Takumi K, de RodaHusman AM. Aichivirus in sewage and surface water, the Netherlands. *Emerg Infect Dis*. 2013;19(8):1222–1230. Available from: https://doi.org/10.3201/eid1908.130312.
172. Cromeans T, Park GW, Costantini V, et al. Comprehensive comparison of cultivable norovirus surrogates in response to different inactivation and disinfection treatments. *Appl Environ Microbiol*. 2014;80:5743–5751. Available from: https://doi.org/10.1128/AEM.01532-14.
173. Yamashita T, Sakae K, Tsuzuki H, et al. Complete nucleotide sequence and genetic organization of Aichivirus, a distinct member of the Picornaviridae associated with acute gastroenteritis in humans. *J Virol*. 1998;72:8408–8412. Available from: https://doi.org/10.1128/JVI.72.10.8408-8412.1998.
174. Fino VR, Kniel KE. UV light inactivation of hepatitis A virus, Aichivirus, and feline calicivirus on strawberries, green onions, and lettuce. *J Food Prot*. 2008;71(5):908–913. Available from: https://doi.org/10.4315/0362-028x-71.5.908.
175. Sewlikar S, D'Souza DH. Survival of hepatitis A virus and Aichi virus in cranberry-based juices at refrigeration (4°C). *Food Microbiology*. 2017;62:251–255. Available from: https://doi.org/10.1016/j.fm.2016.10.003.
176. Yamashita T, Ito M, Tsuzuki H, Sakae K. Identification of Aichivirus infection by measurement of immunoglobulin responses in an enzyme-linked immunosorbent assay. *J Clin Microbiol*. 2001;39(11):4178–4180. Available from: https://doi.org/10.1128/JCM.39.11.4178-4180.2001.
177. Roos YH. Water and pathogenic viruses inactivation—food engineering perspectives. *Food Eng Rev*. 2020;1–17. Available from: https://doi.org/10.1007/s12393-020-09234-z. Advance online publication.
178. de Oliveira Pereira JS, da Silva LR, de MeirelesNunes A, de Souza Oliveira S, da Costa EV, da Silva EE. Environmental surveillance of polioviruses in Rio de Janeiro, Brazil, in support to the activities of global polio eradication initiative. *Food Environ Virol*. 2016;8(1):27–33. Available from: https://doi.org/10.1007/s12560-015-9221-5.

179. Kurdziel AS, Wilkinson N, Langton S, Cook N. Survival of poliovirus on soft fruit and salad vegetables. *J Food Prot.* 2001;64 (5):706–709. Available from: https://doi.org/10.4315/0362-028x-64.5.706.
180. Tierney JT, Sullivan R, Larkin EP. Persistence of poliovirus 1 in soil and on vegetables grown in soil previously flooded with inoculated sewage sludge or effluent. *Appl Environ Microbiol.* 1977;33(1):109–113. Available from: https://doi.org/10.1128/AEM.33.1.109-113.1977.
181. Chua KB, Bellini WJ, Rota PA, et al. Nipah virus: a recently emergent deadly paramyxovirus. *Science.* 2000;288 (5470):1432–1435. Available from: https://doi.org/10.1126/science.288.5470.1432.
182. Chua KB. Nipah virus outbreak in Malaysia. *J Clin Virol.* 2003;26:265–275. Available from: https://doi.org/10.1016/S1386-6532(02)00268-8.
183. Pillai VS, Krishna G, ValiyaVeettil M. Nipah virus: past outbreaks and future containment. *Viruses.* 2020;12(4):465. Available from: https://doi.org/10.3390/v12040465.
184. Luby SP, Rahman M, Hossain MJ, et al. Foodborne transmission of nipah virus, Bangladesh. *Emerg Infect Dis* 2006;12(12):1888–1894. Available from: https://doi.org/10.3201/eid1212.060732.
185. Arunkumar G, Chandni R, Mourya DT, et al. Outbreak investigation of nipah virus disease in Kerala, India, Nipah Investigators People and Health Study Group. *J Infect Dis.* 2018;219 (12):1867–1878. Available from: https://doi.org/10.1093/infdis/jiy612.
186. Chin A, Chu J, Perera M, et al. Stability of SARS-CoV-2 in different environmental conditions. *Lancet Microbe.* 2020;1:e10.
187. Kratzel A, Steiner S, Todt D, et al. Temperature-dependent surface stability of SARS-CoV-2. *J Infect.* 2020;81:452–482.
188. Liu Y, Li T, Deng Y, Liu S, et al. Stability of SARS-CoV-2 on environmental surfaces and in human excreta. *J Hosp Infect.* 2021;107:105–107.
189. Riddell S, Goldie S, Hill A, et al. The effect of temperature on persistence of SARS-CoV-2 on common surfaces. *Virol J.* 2020;17:1–7.
190. FSA [Food Standards Agency UK]. Qualitative risk assessment on the risk of food or food contact materials as a transmission route for SARS-CoV-2. <https://www.food.gov.uk/research/research-projects/qualitative-risk-assessment-on-the-risk-of-food-or-food-contact-materials-as-a-transmission-route-for-sars-cov-2>; 2020. Accessed 22.11.21.
191. ICMSF. ICMSF Opinion on SARS-CoV-2 and its relationship to food safety. International Commission on Microbiological Specifications for Foods. 2020 pp. 1–8.
192. Yekta R, Vahid-Dastjerdi L, Norouzbeigi S, Mortazavian AM. Food products as potential carriers of SARS-CoV-2. *Food Control.* 2021;123:107754. Available from: https://doi.org/10.1016/j.foodcont.2020.107754.
193. Holzmann H, Aberle SW, Stiasny K, et al. Tick-borne encephalitis from eating goat cheese in a mountain region of Austria. *Emerg Infect Dis.* 2009;15(10):1671–1673. Available from: https://doi.org/10.3201/eid1510.090743.
194. CAC *Principles and Guidelines for the Conduct of Microbiological Risk Assessment* (2012 revised edition). CAC/GL-30 – 1999, Codex Alimentarius Commission, 1999.
195. FAO/WHO. *Food Safety Risk Analysis: A Guide for National Food Safety Authorities.* Geneva, Switzerland: World Health Organization, Food and Agricultural Association of the United Nations; 2006 [PubMed].
196. Jaykus L, Dennis S, Bernard D, et al. *Issue Paper: Using Risk Analysis to Inform Microbial Food Safety Decisions.* Ames, Iowa: Council for Agricultural Science and Technology (CAST); 2006. Issue Paper 31.
197. Bradshaw E, Jaykus LA. Risk assessment for foodborne viruses. *Viruses Foods.* 2016;471–503. Available from: https://doi.org/10.1007/978-3-319-30723-7_17.
198. De RodaHusman AM, Bouwknegt M. Quantitative risk assessment for food-and waterborne viruses. *Viruses Food Water.* 2013;159–175. Available from: https://doi.org/10.1533/9780857098870.2.159.
199. Baert L, Uyttendaele M, Vermeersch M, Van Coillie E, Debevere J. Survival and transfer of murine norovirus 1, a surrogate for human noroviruses, during the production process of deep-frozen onions and spinach. *J Food Prot.* 2008;71:1590–1597.
200. Govaris A, Pexara A. Inactivation of foodborne viruses by high-pressure processing (HPP). *Foods (Basel, Switz).* 2021;10(2):215. Available from: https://doi.org/10.3390/foods10020215.
201. Barnaud E, Rogée S, Garry P, Rose N, Pavio N. Thermal inactivation of infectious hepatitis E virus in experimentally contaminated food. *Appl Environ Microbiol.* 2012;78(15):5153–5159. Available from: https://doi.org/10.1128/AEM.00436-12.
202. Imagawa T, Sugiyama R, Shiota T, et al. Evaluation of heating conditions for inactivation of hepatitis E virus genotypes 3 and 4. *J Food Prot.* 2018;81(6):947–952. Available from: https://doi.org/10.4315/0362-028X.JFP-17-290.
203. Nauheim RC, Romanowski EG, Araullo-Cruz T, et al. Prolonged recoverability of desiccated adenovirus type 19 from various surfaces. *Ophthalmology.* 1990;97:1450–1453. Available from: https://doi.org/10.1016/sO161-6420(90)32389-8.
204. Moe K, Shirley JA. The effects of relative humidity and temperature on the survival of human rotavirus in faeces. *Arch Virol.* 1982;72:179–186.
205. Sattar SA, Ijaz MK, Johnson-Lussenburg CM, Springthorpe VS. Effect of relative humidity on the airborne survival of rotavirus SA11. *Applied and Environmental Microbiology.* 1984;47 (4):879–881. Available from: https://doi.org/10.1128/aem.47.4.879-881.1984.
206. Takahashi H, Ohuchi A, Miya S, Izawa Y, Kimura B. Effect of food residues on norovirus survival on stainless steel surfaces. *PLoS One.* 2011;6(8):e21951. Available from: https://doi.org/10.1371/journal.pone.0021951.
207. Becker-Dreps S, González F, Bucardo F. Sapovirus: an emerging cause of childhood diarrhea. *Curr OpInfect Dis.* 2020;33 (5):388–397. Available from: https://doi.org/10.1097/QCO.0000000000000671.
208. Shaffer PT, Metcalf TG, Sproul OJ. Chlorine resistance of poliovirus isolants recovered from drinking water. *Appl Environ Microbiol.* 1980;40(6):1115–1121. Available from: https://doi.org/10.1128/aem.40.6.1115-1121.1980.
209. Fogarty R, Halpin K, Hyatt AD, Daszak P, Mungall BA. Henipavirus susceptibility to environmental variables. *Virus Res.* 2008;132(1-2):140–144. Available from: https://doi.org/10.1016/j.virusres.2007.11.010.
210. Hassan MZ, Sazzad H, Luby SP, et al. Nipah virus contamination of hospital surfaces during outbreaks, Bangladesh, 2013–2014.

Emerg Infect Dis. 2018;24(1):15–21. Available from: https://doi.org/10.3201/eid2401.161758.

211. Leon JS, Kingsley DH, Montes JS, et al. Randomized, double-blinded clinical trial for human norovirus inactivation in oysters by high hydrostatic pressure processing. *Appl Environ Microbiol*. 2011;77:5476–5482.

212. Kingsley DH, Guan D, Hoover DG. Pressure inactivation of hepatitis A virus in strawberry puree and sliced green onions. *J Food Prot*. 2005;68:1748–1751.

213. Pesaro F, Sorg I, Metzler A. In situ inactivation of animal viruses and a coliphage in nonaerated liquid and semiliquid animal wastes. *Appl Environ Microbiol*. 1995;62:92–97.

Further reading

Bendinelli M, Pistello M, Maggi F, Fornai C, Freer G, Vatteroni ML. Molecular properties, biology, and clinical implications of TT virus, a recently identified widespread infectious agent of humans. *Clin Microbiol Rev*. 2001;14(1):98–113. Available from: https://doi.org/10.1128/CMR.14.1.98-113.2001.

Chitambar SD, Joshi MS, Sreenivasan MA, Arankalle VA. Fecal shedding of hepatitis A virus in Indian patients with hepatitis A and in experimentally infected Rhesus monkey. *Hepatol Res*. 2001;19(3):237–246. Available from: https://doi.org/10.1016/s1386-6346(00)00104-2.

Codex Alimentarius. Codex Committee on Food Hygiene; Rome: 2012. CAC/GL 79-2012 Guidelines on the Application of General Principles of Food Hygiene to the Control of Viruses in Food. (p. 13).

Fisher D, Reilly A, Kang EngZheng A, Cook AR, Anderson DE. Seeding of outbreaks of COVID-19 by contaminated fresh and frozen food. *BioRxiv [Prepr]*. 2020. Available from: https://doi.org/10.1101/2020.08.17.255166.

Greenberg HB, Estes MK. Rotaviruses: from pathogenesis to vaccination. *Gastroenterology*. 2009;136(6):1939–1951. Available from: https://doi.org/10.1053/j.gastro.2009.02.076.

Gutiérrez-Aguirre I, Steyer A, Boben J, Gruden K, Poljsak-Prijatelj M, Ravnikar M. Sensitive detection of multiple rotavirus genotypes with a single reverse transcription-real-time quantitative PCR assay. *J Clin Microbiol*. 2008;46(8):2547–2554. Available from: https://doi.org/10.1128/JCM.02428-07.

Liu X, Bates D, Grove SF, Lee A. *International Association for Food Protection Annual Meeting*. 2009. Effect of antimicrobial sanitizers and high power ultrasound on murine norovirus on romaine lettuce. T8-01.

Martin A, Lemon SM. Hepatitis A virus: from discovery to vaccines. *Hepatology*. 2006;43(2):S164–S172. Suppl. 1.

Maunula L, Rönnqvist M, Åberg R, Lunden J, Nevas M. The presence of norovirus and adenovirus on environmental surfaces in relation to the hygienic level in food service operations associated with a suspected gastroenteritis outbreak. *Food Environ Virol*. 2017;9(3):334–341. Available from: https://doi.org/10.1007/s12560-017-9291-7.

Mullis L, Saif LJ, Zhang Y, Zhang X, Azevedo MSP. Stability of bovine coronavirus on lettuce surfaces under household refrigeration conditions. *Food Microbiol*. 2012;30:180–186. Available from: https://doi.org/10.1016/j.fm.2011.12.009.

Newell DG, Koopmans M, Verhoef L, et al. Food-borne diseases—the challenges of 20 years ago still persist while new ones continue to emerge. *Int J Food Microbiol*. 2010;139:S3–S15.

Sharapov UM, Kentenyants K, Groeger J, Roberts H, Holmberg SD, Collier MG. Hepatitis A infections among food handlers in the United States, 1993-2011. *Public Health Rep (Washington, DC: 1974)*. 2016;131(1):26–29. Available from: https://doi.org/10.1177/003335491613100107.

Süss J. Epidemiology and ecology of TBE relevant to the production of effective vaccines. *Vaccine*. 2003;21(Suppl 1):S19–S35. Available from: https://doi.org/10.1016/S0264-410X(02)00812-5.

Tan M, Jiang X. Norovirus P particle: a subviral nanoparticle for vaccine development against norovirus, rotavirus and influenza virus. *Nanomedicine (London, Engl)*. 2012;7(6):889–897. Available from: https://doi.org/10.2217/nnm.12.62.

World Health Organization (WHO. *Water Recreation and Disease. Plausibility of Associated Infections: Acute Effects, Sequelae and Mortality by Kathy Pond*. London, UK: Published by IWA Publishing; 2005:191–231. ISBN: 1843390663.

World Health Organization Hepatitis A fact sheet. 2020. <https://www.who.int/news-room/fact-sheets/detail/hepatitis-a>.

World Health Organization. Global Health Sector Strategy on Viral Hepatitis 2016–2021. <https://www.who.int/hepatitis/strategy2016-2021/ghss-hep/en/>; 2016.

Chapter 54

Role of gut microbiota in food safety

Sik Yu So[1,2], Qinglong Wu[1,2] and Tor Savidge[1,2]

[1]*Department of Pathology and Immunology, Baylor College of Medicine, Houston, TX, United States,* [2]*Department of Pathology, Texas Children's Microbiome Center, Texas Children's Hospital, Houston, TX, United States*

Abstract

The human gastrointestinal tract is colonized by a complex microbial community known as the gut microbiota which has coevolved with humans over millennia. Emerging evidence connects gut microbiota to food safety as they play an important detoxification role, yet enhance retention and toxicity of certain food components in the host. Food components previously recognized as inert may impact host health through interactions with gut microbiota. At the same time, defined microbial consortia incorporated into food production processes may improve food safety. Here we review what is currently known about the relationship between gut microbiota and food safety, as well as address existing limitations and challenges.

Keywords: Probiotics; gut microbiota; foodborne pathogens; microbial community; microbes

Chapter points

- Gut microbiota may enhance retention and toxicity of food compounds through activation or reactivation of toxins, and/or modulation of hepatic metabolism.
- Gut microbiota protect against foodborne pathogens and toxins by detoxification and/or enhancing colonization resistance.
- Dietary components including food additives and toxins modulate gut microbiota composition, which may lead to undesirable health outcomes.
- Defined microbial consortium can be applied to improve food safety through replacement of antibiotics in agriculture, bio-preservation of food products and detoxification of food.
- Advancement in experimental setup and analytic tools facilitate evaluation of the role of microbiota in food safety, but is still constrained by a number of limitations.

54.1 Introduction

The human gastrointestinal (GI) tract is colonized by a complex microbial community known as the gut microbiota which has coevolved with humans over millenia. Bacteria represent the best studied microbes in the human GI tract, and while the major phyla are usually *Bacteroidetes*, *Firmicutes*, *Actinobacteria*, and *Proteobacteria*, the gut microbiota varies among individuals and is shaped during host development and environmental factors, including diet.

Over the past decades, it has been recognized that gut microbiota play several fundamental roles in maintaining human health. The commensal bacterial community is adapted to reside in the intestines, and is capable of protecting against colonization by pathogens. The gut microbiome also significantly impacts host physiology, for example, xenobiotic metabolism and toxicity, nutrient bioavailability, immune responses, etc. Dysbiosis, the imbalance of gut microbial community, can enhance our susceptibility to food poisoning. Although poorly defined and understood, dysbiosis is also implicated in the development of various human diseases, including metabolic syndrome, inflammatory bowel disease and cancer. Several large consortia projects such as the Human Microbiome Project (HMP) and Human Intestinal Tract (MetaHIT) have explored the composition of the human gut microbiome and provide insight into their significance in human health. Additionally, microbial metabolites such as short chain fatty acids (SCFAs) and bile acids are associated with the host health status.

After food consumption, dietary components interact and influence with the gut microbiota in the GI. As a result, food safety hazards in diet including food additives, foodborne pathogens, and toxins from pathogens or chemical reactions pose threat not only to the host but also to the gut microbial community. Considering the close association between the gut microbiota, diet and health, characterizing the role of gut bacteria in the food safety field is a priority need. To achieve this, there are

Present Knowledge in Food Safety. DOI: https://doi.org/10.1016/B978-0-12-819470-6.00012-3

several questions that need to be addressed: (1) How do gut microbiota influence the health impact of specific food components and pathogens which often constitute a natural pathobiont component of the GI ecosystem? (2) How do food components influence gut microbiota composition and function? (3) How can gut microbiota-related knowledge be applied to food safety practices? (4) How do we best study gut microbiota in food safety evaluation? This chapter will explore these topics and summarizes current knowledge on the role of the gut microbiota in food safety.

54.2 Role of gut microbiome in mediating effect of food components on host health

54.2.1 Metabolism of dietary components into toxic substances

Gut microbiota metabolize xenobiotics and influence host metabolism thus modulating the toxicity of ingested compounds. Gut microbiota adversely influence xenobiotic metabolism via multiple mechanisms. Firstly, gut microbiota may directly metabolize and bioactivate xenobiotics, resulting in activation of toxic compounds and production of toxic metabolites. Several types of enzymes have been identified for microbial biotransformation of xenobiotics, including azoreductases, nitroreductases, β-glucuronidases, sulfatases and β-lyases.[1] Melamine which causes renal failure was illegally added to infant formula to boost protein content. *Klebsiella* converts melamine into cyanuric acid, a key component of melamine-induced kidney stones. Rats given antibiotics were resistant to melamine, while rats colonized with *Klebsiella terrigena* showed exacerbated melamine-induced nephrotoxicity.[2] Polycyclic aromatic hydrocarbons (PAHs) are found in grilled meat and are known for their carcinogenic and estrogenic properties. Parent PAH compounds are not estrogenic, but biotransformation by the intestinal microbiota produces estrogenic hydroxy-PAH metabolites.[3] Other examples of microbial bioactivation of toxic compounds include reduction of Sudan dyes into potentially carcinogenic substances,[4,5] conversion of the sweetener cyclamate into toxic cyclohexylamine[6] and elevation of genotoxicity of 2-amino-3-methylimidazo[4,5-*f*]quinolone (IQ).[7,8]

Secondly, the gut microbiota may reactivate host-detoxified chemicals through deconjugation. In liver, phase II metabolism detoxifies xenobiotics through conjugation with glucuronic acid, sulfate or glutathione, the modified compounds are then released into the intestine where they interact with the gut microbiota. Gut bacteria are capable of deconjugation, resulting in regeneration of the original compounds or formation of new toxic metabolites. The resulting compounds are also nonpolar and with lower molecular weight thus are readily absorbed and returned to liver.[1] This results in enterohepatic cycling and delays elimination of toxic xenobiotics. For example, propachlor, a herbicide, is conjugated with glutathione by the liver for detoxification, yet subsequent deconjugation by gut microbiota enhances its toxicity in body.[9]

Thirdly, the gut microbiota may interfere with xenobiotic detoxification, by influencing host expression of metabolizing enzymes or producing metabolites that compete for metabolizing enzymes. The liver plays a major role in xenobiotic metabolism. At the same time, the gut-liver axis connects the intestine and gut microbiota to the liver. Germ-free and conventional mice have distinct expression of target genes related to xenobiotic metabolism by the liver.[10–12] Gut bacteria influence the expression of nuclear receptors such as constitutive androstane receptor and Pregnane X receptor which regulate expression of multiple metabolic enzymes and transporters. Enzymes involved in Phase I and Phase II metabolism such as Cytochromes P450 enzymes (CYPs) and sulfotransferases are also largely regulated by the gut microbiota. Furthermore, microbial metabolites may compete for enzymes involved in detoxification. For example, the microbial metabolite *p*-cresol sulfate competes for sulfotransferase SULT1A1 with acetaminophen, disrupting the detoxification process of the latter drug.[13] Although evidence shows that the gut microbiota influences host metabolism, few studies have evaluated the impact of such alteration on detoxification metabolism of specific dietary components. Further studies would be required to confirm the mechanism of action in relation to food toxicity (Fig. 54.1).

54.2.2 Healthy gut microbiome as a host defense mechanism against food toxins and foodborne illnesses

Although gut microbiota may enhance toxicity of certain compounds, they also play an important role in protecting the host from foodborne pathogens and toxins through several different mechanisms.

54.2.2.1 Detoxification of toxic compounds

As mentioned in the previous section, the gut microbiota metabolize dietary compounds in the intestine. Although some compounds will gain toxicity through the process, some will be converted into nontoxic or protective compounds. Gut microbiota may also directly bind with dietary toxins and reduce their bioavailability. One example is heterocyclic amines (HCAs) which are formed during the Maillard reaction. 2-Amino-1-methyl-6-phenylimidazo(4,5-*b*)pyridine (PhIP), one of the HCAs commonly

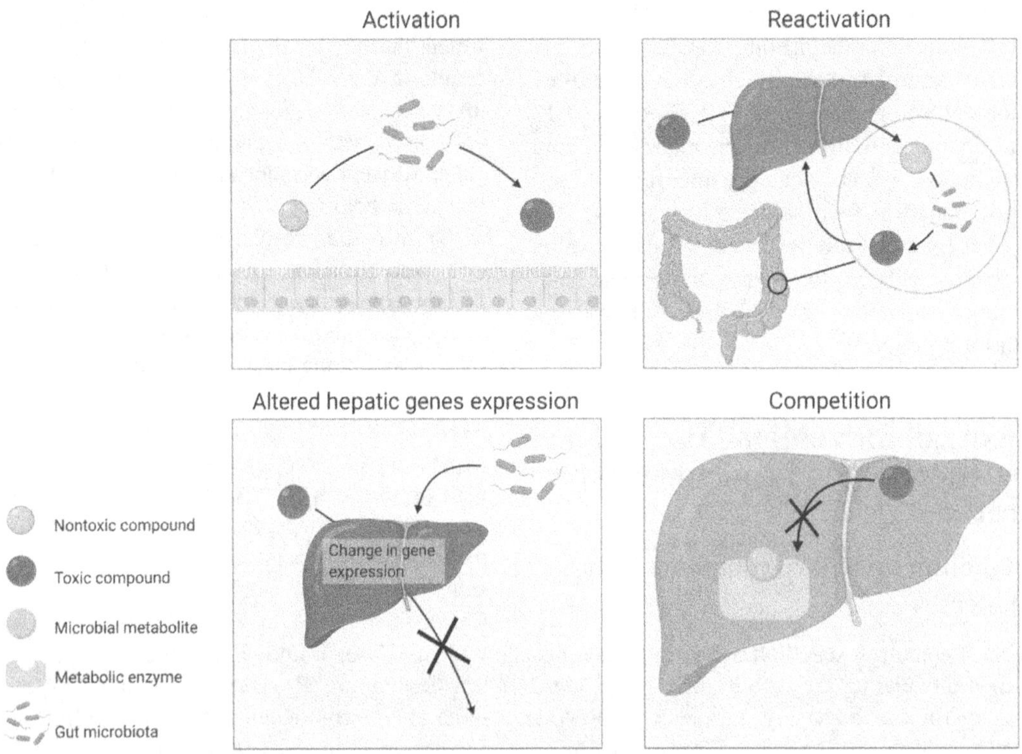

FIGURE 54.1 Mechanisms of gut microbiota adversely influences xenobiotic metabolism.

found in cooked red meat, is activated by CYP450 enzymes in the liver to form unstable metabolites that bind with DNA. Gut microbiota mediate the conversion of the harmful metabolites into less mutagenic PhIP-M1 via beta-glucuronidase (GUS) and glycerol/diol dehydratase (GDH) activity.[14] In vitro studies also found that gut microbiota, particularly lactic acid bacteria, bind with PhIP and other HCAs to reduce their mutagenicity.[15,16] Gut microbiota also protect against heavy metal toxicity as outlined above. Gut microbiota bind and sequester metals and enhance metal excretion. Alteration in gut microbiome function causes an inability to excrete mercury (Hg), Cd, and Pb.[17] Additionally, Hg toxicity is reduced by gut microbiota through demethylation of methylmercury (MeHg) and reduction of inorganic mercury to its least toxic elemental form.[1,18]

54.2.2.2 Direct mechanisms of colonization resistance against foodborne pathogens

Intestinal microbiota also restrict exogenous microbial colonization and expansion of pathogens. This ability is known as colonization resistance and is achieved directly through secretion of inhibitory or bactericidal molecules.[19] For example, Thuricin CD, a bacteriocin produced by *Bacillus thuringiensis*, specifically kills *Clostridiodes difficile* without influencing other commensals.[20] *Clostridium scindens* also protects against *C. difficile* infection through synthesizing secondary bile acids, although recent work has put into question the protective role of secondary bile acids in *C. difficile* infection.[21] Propionate produced by *Bacteroides* inhibits growth of *Salmonella*, by disrupting intracellular pH homeostasis.[22] Fengycins, a class of *Bacillus* lipopeptides, interferes quorum sensing signaling system of *Staphylococcus aureus* and abolish their colonization.[23]

Another direct mechanism for colonization resistance is competition for nutrients or niche. One example is carbon source limitation. Commensal bacteria are usually capable of catabolizing complex carbohydrates that are nondigestible by the host or other bacteria. Conversely, pathogens generally are restricted to utilize nutritious sources offered by commensal species such as monosaccharides, and those that cannot utilize the sources are eliminated.[24] In diets rich in simple sugars, commensal *Bacteroides thetaiotaomicron* is forced to metabolize monosaccharides and inhibits the growth of the pathogen *C. rodentium* by competing for available monosaccharides.[25] Furthermore, commensals are capable of outcompeting pathogens with similar metabolic niche. Commensal *Escherichia coli* have similar restrictions in carbohydrate utilization and metabolic niche as the closely related pathogen enterohaemorrhagic *E. coli* (EHEC). A combination of two commensal *E. coli* strains that utilize all types of sugars that are metabolizable by EHEC, completely occupy the metabolic niche and prevent colonization of EHEC by outcompeting this pathogen.[26] In addition to carbohydrates, commensals also compete with pathogens for other macro- and micronutrients including amino acids and iron.[27,28]

54.2.2.3 Indirect mechanisms of colonization resistance

Gut microbiota also mediate colonization resistance indirectly through enhancing intestinal barrier function and innate immune responses. There are several mechanisms of action where the microbiome influences and shapes the intestinal immune system. The physical intestinal barrier consists of the unstirred mucus layer, intestinal epithelial barrier and gut vascular barrier (GVB). The colonic mucus layer is formed by an outer layer which allows microbes to reside, and an inner layer that is often impenetrable to separate the epithelial layer from bacteria. The mucus layer selectively enhances the growth of microbes which can bind or digest mucin glycans. A thinner mucus layer is often associated with increased susceptibility to pathogen colonization. Commensal gut microbiota have profound effects on the thickness and integrity of the mucus layer. This is demonstrated by the reduced mucus layer thickness and increased penetrability in germ-free mice, as well as the restoration by supplementation of commensals or microbial products.[29,30] Under the mucus layer lies the epithelium, where epithelial cells are bound tightly by tight junctions, adherens junctions, desmosomes and gap junctions. Gut microbiota actively interact with the epithelium barrier to regulate intestinal permeability and protection against infiltration by pathogens. For example, *Bifidobacterium infantis* stabilizes tight junction protein expression and promotes intestinal barrier function in mice.[31] Bacteriocins secreted by *Lactobacillus plantarum* were also found to interact with the intestinal epithelium and enhance the production of tight junction protein ZO-1.[32] Below the epithelial barrier is the GVB, which regulates translocation of bacteria into portal circulation and liver. Diet-induced dysbiosis is associated with disrupted GVB, resulting in bacterial translocation into the blood and nonalcoholic steatohepatitis development.[33]

In addition to the physical barriers, antimicrobial compounds are produced to combat pathogens. Despite containing the microbiota at the mucosal layer, the immune system detects and responds to the presence of intestinal bacteria. Paneth cells secrete antimicrobial peptides (AMP) which play an important role in the small intestine where the mucus layer is a single layer that is loosely attached. AMP usually mediate killing through targeting the bacterial cell wall structure and its production has been shown to be induced and regulated by the gut microbiota. For instance, antibacterial lectin RegIIIγ expression is suppressed in antibiotic-treated or germfree mice, while microbiota from conventional mice helped restore the expression.[34] While a healthy microbiota is necessary for AMP production, studies discovered that specific species including *B. thetaiotaomicron* and *Lactobacillus innocua* are inducers of the production.[35,36] Apart from AMP, immunoglobulin A (IgA) secreted from plasma cells in the gut binds to bacteria to avoid overgrowth, or conversely to promote bacterial colonization. Germ-free animals have reduced IgA levels, which are restored by microbial colonization.[37] Gut microbiota also enhance other immune responses against pathogens, including inflammasome activation and cytokines expression (Fig. 54.2).[38]

54.3 Dietary risk factor for dysbiosis and strategy for healthy gut microbiome and food safety

54.3.1 Dietary components as risk factor for dysbiosis

Gut microbiota not only influence xenobiotic metabolism, but also mediate the effect of diet through changing microbial ecology and function. Food components, ranging from macronutrient composition to specific food additives or toxins, shape the GI microbiota community. While beneficial compounds shift the microbiome to a more desirable community composition, harmful foods may cause deleterious effects that are associated with dysbiosis. Dietary modulation of gut microbiota composition also governs favorable and adverse effects on host health and physiology. Consequently, the diet-microbiota interaction plays a critical role in determining the impact of dietary factors on food safety.

54.3.1.1 Dietary imbalance

Western diet is characterized by high fat and refined sugar, low fiber content and containing a large proportion of processed food. This diet is strongly linked to various western diseases including obesity, diabetes, and cardiovascular risk. Considerable evidence shows dysbiosis is associated with dietary imbalance and harm to host health, but its role in disease onset is not clearly understood since detrimental as well as compensatory responses may be enacted. Expansion of *Firmicutes* and contraction of *Bacteroidetes* is regularly reported with western diet consumption.[39,40] The increase in *Firmicutes: Bacteroidetes* ratio is often associated with enhanced energy harvesting and obesity.[41,42] In support of this notion, western diet-induced increased adiposity is

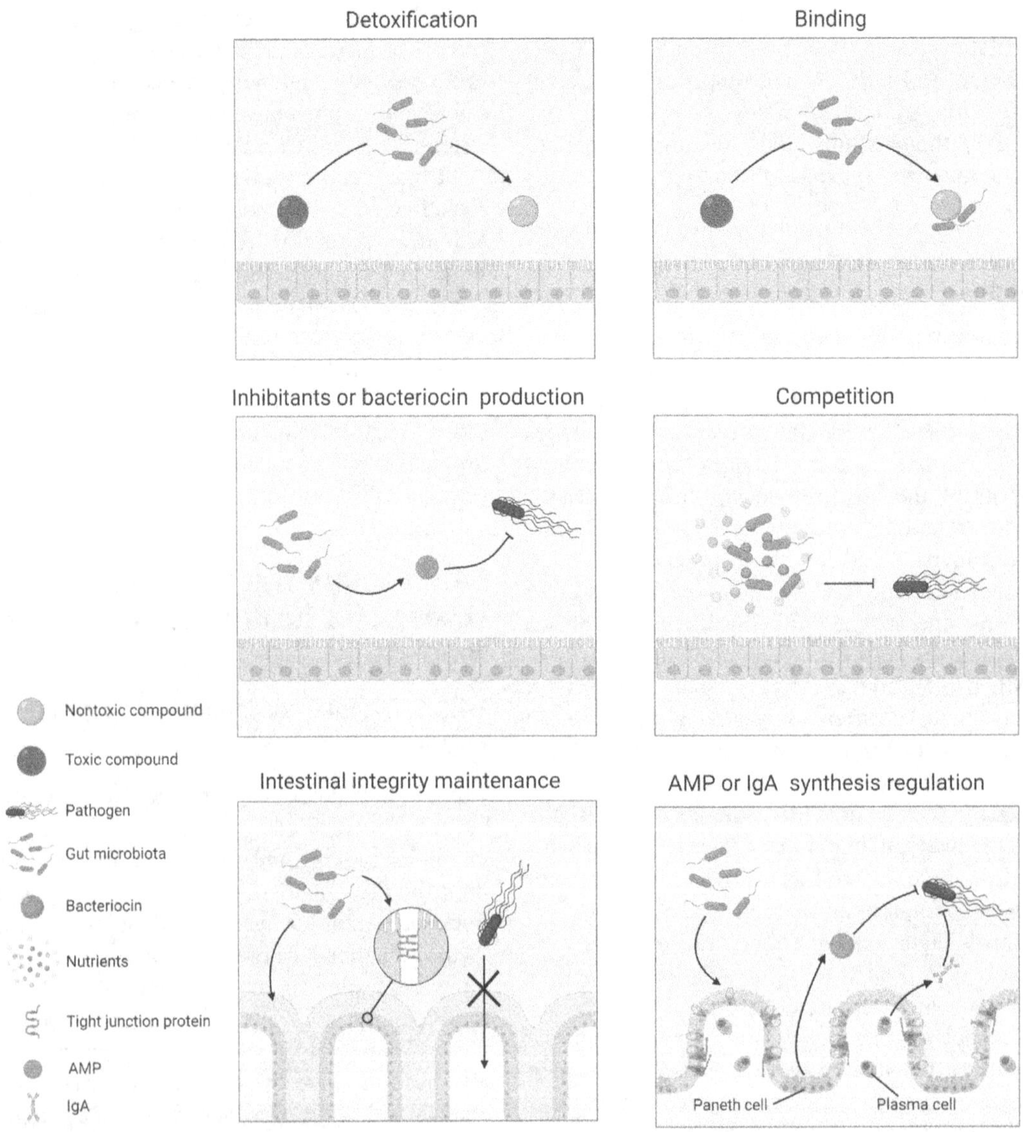

FIGURE 54.2 Mechanisms of gut microbiota protect against toxins or pathogens.

transmitted by transfer of an obese but not lean human gut microbiota community into recipient gnotobiotic mice, implying causation in mediating the effects of western diet on metabolic phenotype.[39]

One of the major characteristics of a western diet is high fat content. The effect of fat consumption on gut microbiota community composition has been extensively studied. High-fat diet (HFD) consumption leads to dramatic shifts in microbiota community structure, which can contribute to chronic inflammation and metabolic disorders. In animals, HFD causes dysbiosis that is positively associated with weight gain, insulin resistance, inflammation and increased gut permeability.[43–47] Short-term studies revealed that the HFD-induced dysbiosis preceded onset of obesity, indicating that gut microbiota may be involved in early pathophysiological changes rather than reflecting an altered metabolic milieu.[48] HFD-induced dysbiosis is also observed in humans. In healthy young adults, consumption of a HFD for 6 months caused an increase in fecal *Alistipes* and *Bacteroides*, with a decrease in *Faecalibacterium*.[49] In the same study, high-fat consumption increased metabolites associated with metabolic disorder and inflammation. In addition to the amount of fat consumed, fatty acid composition also influences gut microbiota. Saturated fat, n-6 polyunsaturated fat (PUFAs) and trans-fat are abundant in the western diet[50] and consumption is associated with dysbiosis linked to enhanced inflammation.[51–55] The western diet is also low in n-3 polyunsaturated fat, which are considered as beneficial in reversing dysbiosis.[52,56]

High refined sugar content is another feature of the western diet. Although sugars are believed to be absorbed in the upper GI tract and are unavailable for microbiota metabolism in the distal gut, evidence shows that sugar consumption modulates gut microbiota composition. Sucrose, glucose, and fructose are commonly found in modern diets. Fructose and glucose are capable of blocking the synthesis of protein required for colonization by a gut bacterium associated with lean and healthy individuals.[57] High-fructose or high-glucose diets also reduce GI microbiota diversity and composition, as well as metabolite profiles.[58–60] While most studies combine high-sucrose and high-fat to study pathophysiological effects of a western diet, one study evaluated the impact of high-sucrose content alone and reported reduced microbial diversity with dysbiosis linked to increased adiposity.[61]

Western diet is also characterized by its low fiber content. Dietary fiber is composed of a variety of monosaccharides polymerized into carbohydrate polymers and oligomers. It is nondigestible by the host and reaches the distal gut where it is processed by the gut microbiota. Specifically, these carbohydrates are metabolized by the gut bacteria and are defined as "microbiota-accessible carbohydrate (MAC)."[62] This serves as important energy and carbon sources for microbiota and is crucial in shaping the gut microbiota community structure and microbial activities. Supplementation of MAC enhances growth of beneficial gut bacteria, with concomitant SCFAs production that promotes host health.[63–65] In a *meta*-analysis, dietary fiber, particularly fructans and galacto-oligosaccharides, increased the abundance of beneficial microbiota, including *Bifidobacterium* spp. and *Lactobacillus* spp.[66] Conversely, low MAC intake reduces microbial diversity and SCFAs production.[62] Furthermore, a diet lacking fiber leads to expansion of mucin-degrading bacteria, which causes erosion of intestinal unstirred layer and promotes pathogen susceptibility.[67] Although alteration is reversible in a single generation, consumption of a low-MAC diet results in loss of gut microbial diversity in offspring and this loss was not recoverable over several generations in mice.[68]

54.3.1.2 Maillard reaction products

During thermal processing of food, chemical reactions such as Maillard reaction may occur. Maillard reaction is known as a complex network of nonenzymatic browning reactions that involves several steps. First, it starts with condensation of amino groups with reducing sugars, followed by various reactions forming different intermediate products such as advanced glycation end products (AGEs), HCAs, and 5-Hydroxymethylfurfural (HMF). The process ends with condensation of amino compounds and sugar fragments into polymerized melanoidins. A wide range of Maillard reaction products (MRPs) are formed during this process and are commonly found in Western diets. While some products are beneficial, some are potentially harmful to gut microbiota structure and human health.

AGE-mediated protein cross-linking during the Maillard reaction reduces digestibility. MRPs subsequently escape digestion and enter the lower GI tract.[69,70] Furthermore, gut microbiota are capable of metabolizing MRPs, for example, *N*-ε-fructosyllysine (FL), *N*-ε-carboxymethyllysine (CML), pyrraline (PYR) which are formed during intermediate stages of degradation by colonic microbiota.[71] Consequently, dietary intake of MRPs may modulate gut microbiota composition. Early in vitro studies observed that MRPs have species-dependent effects on the gut microbiota, that is, enhanced growth of *lactobacilli* but not *E. coli*.[72] Conversely, another study showed consumption of bread crust which is a major source of MRPs resulted in decreases in *Lactobacilli* and *Bifidobacteria*, compared with increases in *Escherichia/Shigella*.[73]

Later studies investigated the effect of specific MRPs that modulate gut microbiota composition. Melanoidins, the product of the final Maillard reaction stage, caused a nonspecific expansion of anaerobic bacteria in fecal bacteria culture.[74] AGEs treatment reduced intestinal microbial diversity and richness, as well as SCFAs-producing bacteria.[75] A human study of peritoneal dialysis patients showed dietary AGE restriction modulated gut microbiota composition, that is, reduction of *Prevotella copri* and *Bifidobacterium animalis* and caused an expansion of *Alistipes indistinctus*, *Clostridium hathewayi*, *Clostridium citroniae*, and *Ruminococcus gauvreauii*. In healthy mice, consumption of CML, one of the AGEs, caused expansion of several *Bacteroidetes* families and *Desulfovibrionaceae*, and reduced the abundance of *Lachnospiraceae* and *Sutterella*.[76] However, CML did not influence three strains of *E. coli* isolated from piglet and human feces.[77] Intake of Amadori compounds, HMF and CML was negatively correlated to total fecal bacteria and *lactobacilli* abundance, but did not correlate with *bifidobacteria* in rats.[78] In human adolescents, HMF and CML are negatively associated with *lactobacilli* numbers while Amadori compounds are negatively associated with *bifidobacteria* abundance.[78] In the early 2000s, acrylamide was discovered as a potential carcinogen formed during the Maillard reaction.[79] Recent in vitro studies have shown that high concentrations of acrylamide reduces the viability of lactic acid bacteria and influences the morphology of *L. plantarum*.[80,81]

The huge variety of MRPs and study models, as well as variations in experimental conditions have added complexity and difficulty when comparing and summarizing different studies. While some studies suggest MRPs exert a desirable effect on gut microbial communities,[76,82,83] some show opposite outcomes.[78,84] Nevertheless, the effect of MRPs on the gut microbiota should not be overlooked and needs to be evaluated as a potential safety concern associated with food products.

54.3.1.3 Food additives

Food additives are naturally occurring or synthetic ingredients added into processed food to improve the flavor, texture, nutritional value and safety of products. Currently, there are over 3000 additives approved by the Food and Drug Administration (FDA). However, with advances in evaluating gut microbiota communities and their interaction with the host, mounting evidence suggests that seemingly inert additives may modulate gut microbiota composition and cause undesirable effects. Food additives are classified into different groups based on their functions. One of those is artificial sweetener substitutes for sugar. Although food-use-approved sweeteners are generally recognized as safe and well tolerated, recent reports indicate an effect on glucose tolerance and alteration to gut microbiota composition. Using genetically modified bioluminescent *E. coli*, researchers suggested that several FDA-approved artificial sweeteners are toxic towards gut microbiota.[85] Commonly used sweeteners, including saccharin, sucralose, and aspartame, were reported to enhance glucose intolerance through inducing dysbiosis.[86,87] Specifically, several of the bacterial taxa that were affected by the sweeteners, for example, increases in *Bacteroides* and decreases in *Clostridiales*, were closely related to type 2 diabetes. Alterations in gut microbiota induced by sucralose are also associated with increased risk of tissue inflammation.[88] Additionally, Splenda, a commercial formulation of sucralose, reduces the abundance of beneficial fecal microflora in rats.[89] Apart from the nonnutritive artificial sweeteners, low-calorie sweeteners such as polyols are used as a substitution of sugar. Excessive consumption of polyols induces GI discomfort or provides a laxative effect, which could possibly be associated with altered gut microbiota composition. For instance, xylitol reduces the abundance of *Bacteroidetes* phylum and *Barnesiella* genus in mice.[90] Furthermore, the fecal microbiome composition shifts from gram-negative to gram-positive bacteria by xylitol in both humans and rodents.[91] Despite these concerns of potential undesirable effects of polyols, other studies report no effect or beneficial shifts in gut microbiome composition;[92] thus, further studies are needed to determine their impact on human and animal health.

Apart from artificial sweeteners, dietary emulsifiers also alter the gut microbial community. There are natural emulsifiers such as gum arabic, carrageenan, as well as synthetic emulsifiers such as carboxylmethylcellulose (CMC) and polysorbate 80 (P80). Emulsifiers are amphiphilic molecules which possess both hydrophobic and hydrophilic groups. They reduce the surface tension between water and oil to maintain a stable and homogenous mixture. Due to their detergent-like properties, dietary emulsifiers cause bacterial encroachment into intestinal mucus layers, promote bacterial translocation across the intestinal barrier and affect gut microbiota composition.[93–95] The gut mucosal barrier is important for innate immunity by covering and protecting intestinal epithelial cells from direct contact with pathogens. These disturbances are suggested to lead to chronic inflammatory disease including inflammatory bowel disease and metabolic syndrome. For instance, CMC and P80 altered the microbial community structure, including increasing the abundance of mucolytic bacteria and reducing levels of *Bacteroidales* in mice. These mechanisms are proposed to mediate dietary emulsifier-induced metabolic syndrome and inflammation.[95] Additionally, CMC and P80 induce sex-specific alterations to gut microbiota which drives sex-dependent changes in anxiety-related and social behaviors in mice.[96] Using an ex vivo approach, it was also found that CMC and P80 directly affect human gut microbiota by enhancing proinflammatory responses as reflected by elevated levels of bioactive flagellin.[97]

Another class of commonly consumed food additive is dietary preservatives or antimicrobial agents. These slow food spoilage and lengthen product shelf-life. As preservatives work mainly through preventing microbial growth, their potential effect on intestinal bacteria is of concern as well. Researchers showed a mixture of commonly used food preservatives caused overgrowth of *Proteobacteria* and a decrease in *Clostridiales* in a human-microbiota-associated mouse model.[98] Sulfite is a widely-used food preservative for controlling microbial growth, yet it may trigger adverse responses including abdominal pain and diarrhea. In relation to that, sodium bisulfite and sodium sulfite inhibits growth of beneficial bacterial species in in vitro settings.[99] Another dietary antimicrobial agent, ε-polylysine, also induced a transient alteration of gut microbiota composition and their predicted functions.[100]

54.3.1.4 Food toxins and pathogens

Apart from the aforementioned components of the western diet, consumption of toxin- or pathogen-contaminated food are also harmful to the gut microbiota. Such adverse effects may aggravate toxicity of the compounds and should be taken into account when evaluating tolerable levels and related regulations. Consumption of toxic metals such as cadmium (Cd), copper (Cu), and lead (Pb) causes damage to various organs and represent a significant threat to human health. In addition to the extensively studied effects on tissue organs, metal exposure may result in dysbiosis.[101–104] For instance, exposure to Cd reduces gut microbiome diversity and alters the microbiome and metabolome related to metabolic health.[105] The undesirable effects are metal-specific and time-dependent.[106] Apart from contamination with metals, concerns are also raised towards the extensive use of pesticides due to the emerging evidence of their toxicity on nontarget organisms. Pesticides, for example, glyphosate herbicide, permethrin and chlorpyrifos inhibited growth of gut bacteria, and particularly beneficial bacteria in "in vitro" settings.[107–109] Regarding their in vivo effect, a study reported that the shift of gut microbiota structure and metabolic profile induced by chlorpyrifos subsequently led to intestinal inflammation and abnormal intestinal permeability in mice.[110] Furthermore, chlorpyrifos induced a pro-obesity phenotype in rats and altered the gut microbiota including bacteria that are associated with obesity and diabetes.[111] Researchers also demonstrated that propamocarb, a commonly used fungicide, could disturb metabolism through altering gut microbiota and microbial metabolites profile in mice.[112] Other toxic contaminants found in food may also lead to dysbiosis. For instance, bisphenol A (BPA), a structural component of food containers, alters the abundance of bacteria associated with various disorders.[113]

In addition to metals and chemicals, foodborne pathogens also cause dysbiosis. Norovirus, one of the leading causes of foodborne illness, causes vomiting and abdominal discomfort. Although the illness duration is usually short, disruption of the gut microbiota in infected patients suggests an elevated risk of long-term health complications.[114] Apart from norovirus, infection of *Salmonella enterica Serovar Typhimurium* altered microbiome community structure and function, with an increased abundance of *Enterobacteriaceae* and reduced biosynthetic gene cluster potential.[115]

Pathogens may harm human health in different ways. Natural microbial toxins in foods are produced by living microorganisms as a tactic to favor their growth through gaining advantage when competing with other microbes or manipulating host cell function. These toxins are not harmful to the producing organisms themselves, but may possess deleterious effects on human health and intestinal microbiota after consumption. Mycotoxins are produced by fungi and are potentially toxic to humans and animals. For instance, deoxynivalenol (DON, also known as vomitoxin), is a mycotoxin commonly found in cereal crops and causes vomiting, as well as gastroenteritis with nausea and diarrhea. Researchers found that a 4-week treatment of DON increased fecal Bacteroides/Prevotella and decreased *E. coli* in a human microbiota-associated rat model.[116] Additionally, *in vivo* and *in vitro* studies demonstrated that DON exposure increases genotoxicity of *E. coli* strains.[117] Apart from DON, evidence shows that Ochratoxin A (OTA), a mycotoxin commonly found in coffee, also affects the gut microbiome. A study using bioreactors revealed that OTA reduced the abundance of beneficial species such as *Lactobacillus reuteri*, despite a desirable microbial conversion of OTA into less toxic metabolites.[118]

54.3.2 Probiotics as a strategy to maintain healthy gut microbiome and improve food safety practices

Probiotics are defined as "live microorganisms which when administered in adequate amounts confer a health benefit on the host" by the Food and Agriculture Organization of the United Nations (FAO) and the World Health Organization (WHO) in 2001.[119] There are several commonly studied and used probiotics strains, particularly members of the *Lactobacillus* and *Bifidobacterium* genera, for example, *Lactobacillus acidophilus*, *L. casei*, *L. rhamnosus* and *Bifidobacterium bifidum*. Probiotics are added into food products such as yogurt but are also available as dietary supplements in capsules, powders, and tablets form.

As mentioned in the previous section, the gut microbiota plays a significant role in protection against food toxins and foodborne illnesses. Consumption of probiotics therefore helps restore desirable gut microbiota composition and reduce susceptibility to food poisoning in humans. Furthermore, probiotics also bind to toxins such as mycotoxins and reduce their bioavailability and toxicity.[120,121]

Probiotics are also commonly used in agriculture and aquacultures. Considering the rise of antibiotic resistance and multidrug-resistant organisms, use of antibiotics in healthy livestock for growth promotion and disease prevention has been prohibited. In view of the health benefits and relatively few side effects associated with probiotics use, substitution for antibiotics in enhancing animal health and growth has gained popularity. Numerous evidence are available on the beneficial effects of probiotics on animal production, in terms of growth performance, disease prevention and immunity.[122,123] In relation to food safety, the supplementation of probiotics reduces the use of chemotherapy and levels of pathogens in animal production, thus avoiding foodborne infections in humans. Taking the poultry industry as an example, probiotics treatment improves growth performance of broilers, which could possibly be due to enhanced enzyme activity and increased capacity to ferment complex polysaccharides.[124] Probiotics treatment in poultries also enhances intestinal immunity against subclinical necrotic enteritis, which was previously prevented by antibiotics.[125] In addition, contaminated egg is a major source of *S. enterica* serovar Enteritidis infection in humans. Treatment with

Lactobacilli strains prevents *S. enterica* serovar Enteritidis colonization in chicks.[126] Treatment with microbiota may also provide desirable effects on animal production without benefiting the host. For instance, although carriage of *E. coli* O157 does not harm cattle, humans may be infected due to contact with infected animals or their feces, or consumption of contaminated water or food. Direct-fed microbiota treatment, particularly combination of *L. acidophilus* (NP 51) and *Propionibacterium freudenreichii* (NP 24), is effective in reducing prevalence of fecal *E. coli* O157 shedding in cattle thus minimizing the chance of human infection.[127]

Apart from being used as probiotics in preharvest production, bacteria and their products are also added to extend shelf life and inhibit pathogen growth in food products. Fermented food products such as kimchi, fermented cabbage, and yogurt contain microbial species with antimicrobial function. Bio-preservation generally includes inoculation of protective culture, which are effective against spoilage or pathogenic bacteria; or addition of microbial metabolites or products such as bacteriocin.[128] Although selected protective culture and bacteriocin should be safe for consumption, able to survive food production process and do not cause detrimental effects on the target food products, further safety studies are required since emerging data indicates that bacteriocins can also signal to regulate, for example, host intestinal barrier function. Many lactic acid producing bacteria (LAB), which are commonly used as protective cultures, are considered as "generally regarded as safe" (GRAS) by the FDA and granted with the Qualified Presumption of Safety by EFSA.[129,130] They produce lactic acid, hydrogen peroxide, and bacteriocins which inhibit growth of food spoilage and pathogenic bacteria.[131] Apart from fermented food, LAB are also applied to nonfermented food such as chicken, beef, smoked salmon, and apples.[128] Furthermore, several bacteriocins produced by LAB are isolated and applied as bio-preservatives in dairy, vegetable or meat product. For example, nisin, a FDA-approved bacteriocin produced by *L. lactis* subsp. *lactis*, is added in cheese or other food products as food preservative. It was first used for inhibition of *Clostridium botulinum* in cheese, but is also effective against other pathogenic bacteria including *Listeria monocytogenes* and *Salmonella* spp, as well as heat resistant spores of pathogens in food production.[132] In addition to prevention of food spoilage, microorganism help detoxification in foods. For instance, fungal pathogens produce mycotoxins in crops, which may enter into the food chain and cause adverse health outcome in human and animal health. Unfortunately, contamination may happen postharvest and preharvest measures do not entirely eliminate the risk. Microbial detoxification is therefore suggested as one of the strategies to reduce mycotoxins contamination.[133] The function has a long history, since the detoxification of aflatoxin by *Flavobacterium aurantiacum* was discovered in 1966.[134] Accumulating evidence also shows different strains are capable of converting other mycotoxins, such as the detoxification of DON by soil-originating microorganism.[135]

Despite the numerous advantages of probiotics, several challenges need to be overcome in the field and further research has to be done on various aspects. Consensus is needed on selection of novel strains and regulations. There are certain prerequisites to be fulfilled for microorganisms as food cultures or animal feed additives. The large scale production of probiotics and protective culture is one of the major challenges in incorporating them into food production. Additionally, probiotics have to be viable and effective beyond food processing procedures and storage period. There are also increasing concerns regarding the long-term safety of probiotics consumption. For example, the possibility of antibiotic resistance of dietary probiotics transferred to pathogens is recently being addressed.[136] Furthermore, genetic stability, pathogenicity and metabolic effect of probiotic strains have to be reviewed as well.[137] Finally, there is potential for significant socio-economical harm, as purchasing ineffective and unproven probiotic formulations can leave the family income at significant odds with perceived health claims (Fig. 54.3).

54.4 Technical aspects to evaluate the role of gut microbiota in food safety studies

Emerging evidence on the association between gut microbiota and food safety urges the inclusion of gut microbiota in risk assessment and food safety evaluation. Advances in experimental systems and analytic tools allow the investigation of microbiota–microbiota interactions, microbial metabolism of food components, effect of food components on microbial community, as well as the interaction between host and gut microbiota. This section describes current methods for studying the influence and modulation of the gut microbiota, as well as current tools for evaluating gut microbiota composition.

54.4.1 Experimental models to assess gut microbiota influence and changes

In vitro experimental systems are useful for screening purposes prior to in vivo studies. The systems offer platform to study different microbial processes and reaction, such as bioconversion and change in microbial community in response to xenobiotics exposure. In vitro systems can generally be classified into batch and continuous cultures. Batch cultures is one of the long-established, simple and common models for studying gut microbiota. It is conducted in a closed system, for example, batch

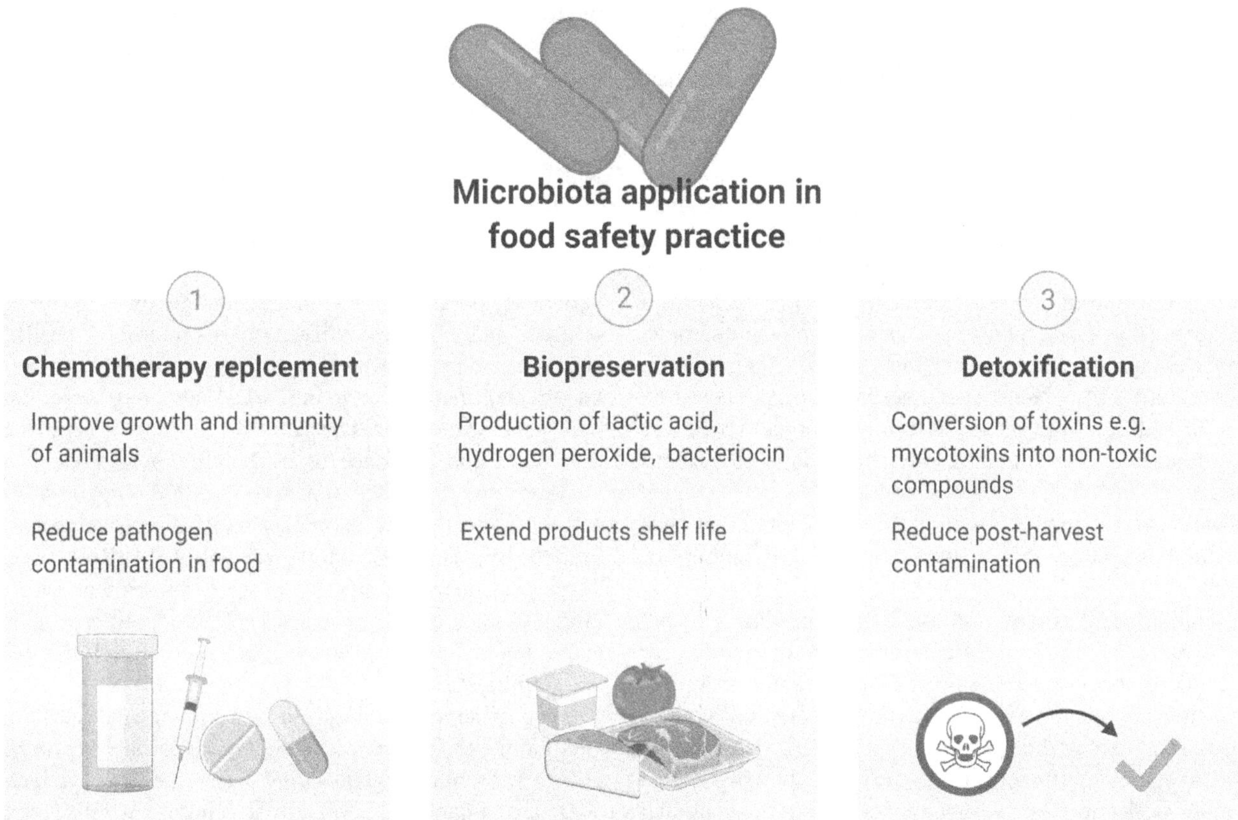

FIGURE 54.3 Summary of microbiota application in food safety practice.

reactors, test tubes and well plates, with components for microbial growth such as nutrient broth included at the beginning of experiments. In contrast to batch cultures, medium flows for nutrients supply and waste removal to maintain microbial growth in continuous cultures. The continuous model has an advantage of enabling extended study period while experimental conditions are under control. One of the well-developed continuous culture systems is the Simulated Human Intestinal Microbial Ecosystem (SHIME), which consists of multiple compartments and simulates progressive digestive process of the entire GI tract, including stomach, small intestine, and colon. The system has been used for studying effect of food components, for example, dietary polyphenols,[138] as well as toxins, for example, insecticide[109] on gut microbiota. Due to its high flexibility, it can be modified to study digestive conditions of interest. Its modified model mucosal SHIME (M-SHIME) incorporates mucin-covered microcosms and simulates mucosal microbial colonization.[139] Another example of continuous culture is the minibioreactor array (MBRAs), which consists of replicate bioreactors and peristaltic pumps for continuous flow of medium. The small size and simple design is advantageous in reducing cost and time for higher-throughput analysis and efficient cultivation of reproducible microbial communities.[140] It has been applied in the study of competition of *C. difficile* ribotypes in the presence of complex fecal microbiota,[141] and identification of simplified microbial communities that inhibit *C. difficile* invasion.[142] In relation to food safety, the model was also used in investigation of effect of dietary disaccharide trehalose on virulence of epidemic *C. difficile*.[143] In vitro studies have several advantages including the high output and reproducibility, as well as the availability of pure isolated cultures, etc. However, the lack of microbiota–host interaction is a common drawback of in vitro models. New technologies such as microfluid and microfabrication can be integrated for development of novel experimental models.[144] Gut-microbiome-on-a-chip, a recently reported in vitro model, takes advantage of the microfluidic gut-on-a-chip setup and enables study of microbial–human interaction within the gut.[145] It consists of a lower layer of endothelial cells, and an upper layer of epithelial cells which directly contact with the microbiota. An oxygen gradient is established across the layers, and a complex human gut microbiome is cocultured with endothelial and epithelial cells for extended time. Yet, systemic components beyond the gut are still not taken into account, thus physiological relevance is limited.

Animal models, mainly rodents, are extensively used in study of gut microbiota due to the easier control of experimental conditions compared to human studies, while providing higher physiological relevance compared to in vitro models. However, the differences between human and animals in gut microbiota composition and host–microbe interaction limit the extrapolation to human system. To overcome this pitfall, humanized microbiota mice were developed by introducing human microbiota into germ-free mice. The humanized mice contain a majority of genus-level taxa detected in the donor sample, and was applied in characterizing gut microbial changes by western diet.[39] Nonetheless, several aspects should be considered carefully when performing animal studies of gut microbiota to minimize variability and other confounding factors. For instance, how animals are cocaged, as well as the standardization of gut microbiota in animals or randomization of animals in the beginning of studies.[146]

Human studies are restrained by sampling method. Fecal samples are the most commonly used specimen for gut microbiota, as other samples may require relatively invasive procedure. This limits the investigation on the location of events happening within the gut. Despite the ethical issues and practical limitations in human studies, human is potentially the best model for studying human gut microbiota due to the physiological relevance. Studies have reported that the human gut microbiome is influenced by sex, age, region, and dietary habits. Therefore researchers have to be cautious in selection of experimental participants and control group. Baseline microbiota can be considered as inclusion or exclusion criteria of participants selection in intervention studies.[147] The use of longitudinal cross-over designs, where each participant receive both control and experimental treatment in different time period, may increase power and help minimize interindividual variations. Efforts should also be done to assess or control dietary differences, for example, by stabilizing or standardizing their diet, or by conducting food frequency questionnaires or 24-h dietary recalls. However, the current dietary assessment are prone to reporting error and have limited ability in capturing dietary details in relation to gut microbiota.[148] Hence, there is a need for development of improved dietary assessment methods, while experimental designs and data analysis have to be considered carefully in the meantime (Fig. 54.4).

54.4.2 Tools for evaluation of gut microbiome

Advancement in DNA sequencing and computational methods facilitates the study of the gut microbiome. Targeted sequencing, or gene amplicon sequencing, is a popular and affordable approach for characterization of microbial diversity. It relies on DNA specific binding and makes use of one or several marker genes which are highly conserved yet vary among bacterial species to identify known bacteria taxa. For example, 16S rRNA gene is commonly targeted as phylogenetic marker and widely recognized as the "gold standard" for bacterial identification. It encodes small subunit ribosomal RNA molecules and plays significant role in cell survival. It consists of highly conserved regions, as well as the hypervariable regions (V1–V9) that reflect genome divergence of taxa and allow identification of microbial profiles. However, analysis using the targeted method is limited to known taxa. Furthermore, individual taxa may share identical gene sequence resulting in difficulties in identification of unique sequence or differentiation of taxa.[149] In addition, this method is sensitive to rRNA copy numbers and the resolution to taxon especially species or strain is limited by relatively short size of 16S rRNA gene. Targeted sequencing are also prone to biases that arise in different steps of the analysis, such as variation in DNA extraction efficiency from different species and preferential amplification.[150]

In comparison to targeted sequencing approach, the genome-wide shotgun metagenomics approach, or untargeted metagenomics sequencing, target the entire genomic content and capture all microbial genomes within a sample. Using this approach, all DNA is fragmented and sequenced independently. It is advantageous in providing high resolution taxonomic information and potential functional dynamics of the gut microbiome.[149] Despite the complexity of data sets and high demand of computational capacity and cost, the reducing price of sequencing and advancement in computational method are going to enhance the popularity of shotgun metagenomics method. Nevertheless, current metagenomics methods still have limitations. For instance, limited information is provided on state and activity of microbes. Furthermore, it is highly sensitive to contamination and loss of DNA.

Current targeted sequencing and metagenomics method provide valuable information regarding microbiota composition, yet strategies for obtaining functional details with minimal biases are needed. Recent *meta*-omics methods including metatranscriptomics and metaproteomics aid analysis of activity of pathways and enhance function understanding of the microbiome beyond the genome level. Metatransciptomics measures RNA expression and provide higher sensitivity, linearity, and reproducibility compared to metagenomics. However, there are several challenges, for example, low stability of RNA, contamination of host RNA, and low relevance with actual microbial activity. In particular, the transcript level does not necessarily reflect protein expression and activity. Metaproteomics focuses on protein expression of the microbiome and is able to identify active pathways

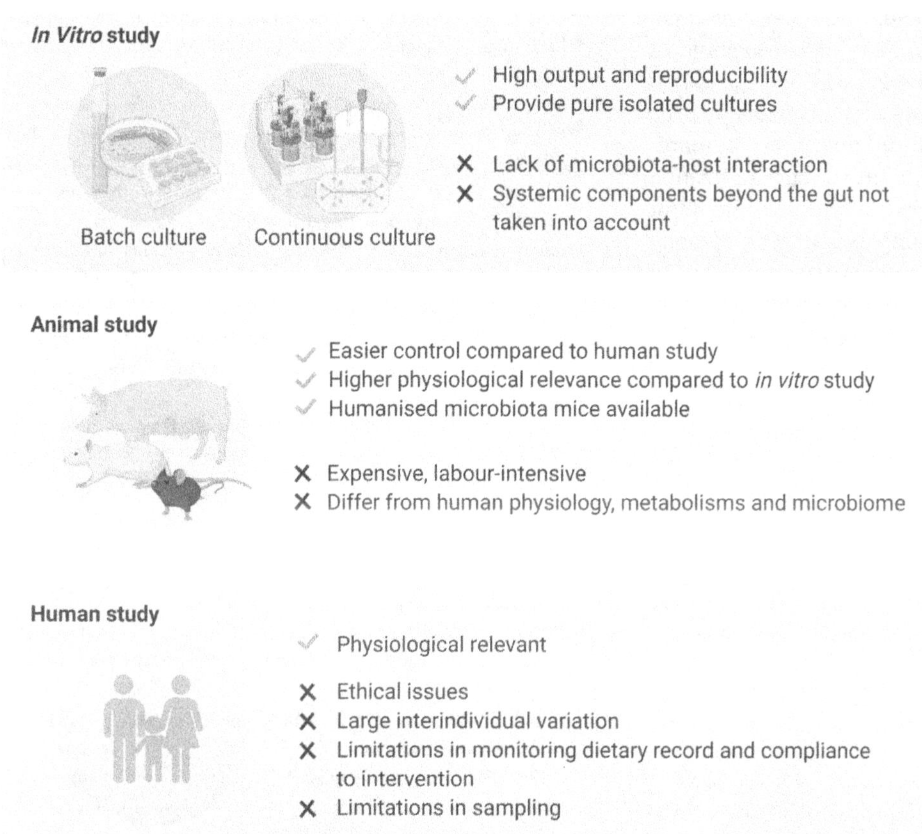

FIGURE 54.4 Pros and cons of experimental setups in gut microbiota studies.

and analyze posttranslation modifications of proteins. It is considered as a method which provides more valuable information regarding taxonomy, function and pathways of the gut microbiome compared to metagenomics. Yet, metaproteomics is still constrained by several limitations such as low protein yield, inability in measuring low-abundance protein and bioinformatic challenges. In particular, peptide identification using database search method restricts the identity to available reference while de novo sequencing is prone to errors.[149] Metaproteogenomics, an integrated approach based on the combined analysis of genomic and proteomic data, promote protein identification through a matched metagenome database. It has gained interest in recent years to overcome limitations of both methods yet still requires further improvement.[151] Other *meta*-omics approaches may also be integrated to facilitate the study of gut microbiome and to provide additional insight, for example, the integration of metagenomics and metatranscriptomics in analyzing transcript ratio and expression level of the microbiome.[152]

Last but not least, metabolomics focuses the metabolite profile and provide information on the biochemical events and host-microbiota interaction. It can be carried out as untargeted approach which analyses the global metabolite profile, or the targeted approach which measures specific metabolites. Metabolomics is useful in assessing the state and function of the microbiome, as well as providing valuable information on the host-microbiome interaction and the influence of diet. However, one of the major challenges is to identify whether the compounds are derived from the host or the microbiome.

54.5 Research gap and future perspectives

This chapter has illustrated the significance of gut microbiota in food safety. It has become exceedingly clear that gut microbiota play an important role in human health, while considerable evidence links them to food safety. This pushes us to change our perspectives towards food safety, and act by taking account of gut microbiota in food regulations. Current standards or tolerable limits for food chemicals have to be re-evaluated. Meanwhile, the reciprocal interaction between food components and intestinal microbial community has to be further characterized. As microbial composition varies among individuals, there is a need to evaluate the interaction in different groups and identify those who are more vulnerable to adverse outcomes. These tasks will assist in providing stronger basis for re-evaluation of regulations. Furthermore, the application of probiotics and protective cultures in food safety practices can be encouraged. Yet, more work is needed to examine their interaction with host or pathogens. Further research on the safety of food cultures and implementation of related safety regulations are also required.

Nevertheless, there are several key challenges to be addressed. Firstly, interindividual difference of gut microbiota composition increases difficulty in standardization and summarization of findings. Secondly, huge amount of effort is needed to unravel the complex interaction among host, gut microbiota and dietary components, as well as to consider whether a mixture of food components could interfere the interaction. Last but not least, a reproducible, highly physiological, and functional relevant experimental model is needed for more comprehensive and powerful studies in characterizing the role of human microbiome.

Acknowledgment

Figures of the chapter are created with BioRender.com. This publication was supported by the National Institutes of Health grants P30-DK56338, PO-AI152999, and U01-AI24290.

References

1. Claus SP, Guillou H, Ellero-Simatos S. The gut microbiota: a major player in the toxicity of environmental pollutants? *NPJ Biofilms Microbiomes*. 2016;2:16003.
2. Zheng X, Zhao A, Xie G, et al. Melamine-induced renal toxicity is mediated by the gut microbiota. *Sci Transl Med*. 2013;5 (172):172ra22. ra22.
3. Van de Wiele T, Vanhaecke L, Boeckaert C, et al. Human colon microbiota transform polycyclic aromatic hydrocarbons to estrogenic metabolites. *Environ Health Perspect*. 2005;113(1):6–10.
4. Xu H, Heinze TM, Chen S, Cerniglia CE, Chen H. Anaerobic metabolism of 1-amino-2-naphthol-based azo dyes (Sudan dyes) by human intestinal microflora. *Appl Environ Microbiol*. 2007;73 (23):7759–7762.
5. Feng J, Cerniglia CE, Chen H. Toxicological significance of azo dye metabolism by human intestinal microbiota. *Front Biosci (Elite Ed)*. 2012;4:568–586.
6. Bickel MH, Burkard B, Meier-strasser E, Van Den Broek-Boot M. Entero-bacterial formation of cyclohexylamine in rats ingesting cyclamate. *Xenobiotica*. 1974;4(7):425–439.
7. Hirayama K, Baranczewski P, Åkerlund J-E, Midtvedt T, Möller L, Rafter J. Effects of human intestinal flora on mutagenicity of and DNA adduct formation from food and environmental mutagens. *Carcinogenesis*. 2000;21(11):2105–2111.
8. Humblot C, Murkovic M, Rigottier-Gois L, et al. β-Glucuronidase in human intestinal microbiota is necessary for the colonic genotoxicity of the food-borne carcinogen 2-amino-3-methylimidazo [4,5- f]quinoline in rats. *Carcinogenesis*. 2007;28(11):2419–2425.
9. Bakke J, Gustafsson J, Gustafsson B. Metabolism of propachlor by the germfree rat. *Science*. 1980;210(4468):433–435.
10. Björkholm B, Bok CM, Lundin A, Rafter J, Hibberd ML, Pettersson S. Intestinal microbiota regulate xenobiotic metabolism in the liver. *PLoS One*. 2009;4(9):e6958.
11. Selwyn FP, Cui JY, Klaassen CD. RNA-Seq quantification of hepatic drug processing genes in germ-free mice. *Drug Metab Dispos*. 2015;43(10):1572–1580.
12. Toda T, Saito N, Ikarashi N, et al. Intestinal flora induces the expression of Cyp3a in the mouse liver. *Xenobiotica*. 2009;39 (4):323–334.
13. Clayton TA, Baker D, Lindon JC, Everett JR, Nicholson JK. Pharmacometabonomic identification of a significant host-microbiome metabolic interaction affecting human drug metabolism. *Proc Natl Acad Sci U S A*. 2009;106(34):14728–14733.
14. Zhang J, Lacroix C, Wortmann E, et al. Gut microbial beta-glucuronidase and glycerol/diol dehydratase activity contribute to dietary heterocyclic amine biotransformation. *BMC Microbiol*. 2019;19(1):99.
15. Stidl R, Sontag G, Koller V, Knasmüller S. Binding of heterocyclic aromatic amines by lactic acid bacteria: results of a comprehensive screening trial. *Mol Nutr Food Res*. 2008;52 (3):322–329.
16. Orrhage K, Sillerström E, Gustafsson JÅ, Nord CE, Rafter J. Binding of mutagenic heterocyclic amines by intestinal and lactic acid bacteria. *Mutat Res*. 1994;311(2):239–248.
17. Breton J, Daniel C, Dewulf J, et al. Gut microbiota limits heavy metals burden caused by chronic oral exposure. *Toxicol Lett*. 2013;222(2):132–138.
18. Assefa S, Köhler G. Intestinal microbiome and metal toxicity. *Curr Opin Toxicol*. 2020;19:21–27.
19. Pickard JM, Zeng MY, Caruso R, Núñez G. Gut microbiota: role in pathogen colonization, immune responses, and inflammatory disease. *Immunol Rev*. 2017;279(1):70–89.
20. Rea MC, Sit CS, Clayton E, et al. Thuricin CD, a posttranslationally modified bacteriocin with a narrow spectrum of activity against *Clostridium difficile*. *Proc Natl Acad Sci U S A*. 2010;107 (20):9352–9357.
21. Aguirre AM, Yalcinkaya N, Wu Q, et al. Bile acid-independent protection against Clostridioides difficile infection, *PLoS Pathog* 2021;17(10):e1010015. Available from https://doi.org/10.1371/journal.ppat.1010015.
22. Jacobson A, Lam L, Rajendram M, et al. A gut commensal-produced metabolite mediates colonization resistance to *Salmonella* infection. *Cell Host Microbe*. 2018;24(2):296–307.e7.
23. Piewngam P, Zheng Y, Nguyen TH, et al. Pathogen elimination by probiotic *Bacillus* via signalling interference. *Nature*. 2018;562 (7728):532–537.
24. Pilmis B, Le Monnier A, Zahar J-R. Gut microbiota, antibiotic therapy and antimicrobial resistance: a narrative review. *Microorganisms*. 2020;8(2):269.
25. Kamada N, Kim Y-G, Sham HP, et al. Regulated virulence controls the ability of a pathogen to compete with the gut microbiota. *Science (NY)*. 2012;336(6086):1325–1329.
26. Maltby R, Leatham-Jensen MP, Gibson T, Cohen PS, Conway T. Nutritional basis for colonization resistance by human commensal *Escherichia coli* strains HS and Nissle 1917 against *E. coli* O157: H7 in the mouse intestine. *PLoS One*. 2013;8(1):e53957.
27. Momose Y, Hirayama K, Itoh K. Competition for proline between indigenous *Escherichia coli* and *E. coli* O157:H7 in gnotobiotic mice associated with infant intestinal microbiota and its contribution to the colonization resistance against *E. coli* O157:H7. *Antonie van Leeuwenhoek*. 2008;94(2):165–171.

28. Deriu E, Liu JZ, Pezeshki M, et al. Probiotic bacteria reduce *Salmonella typhimurium* intestinal colonization by competing for iron. *Cell Host Microbe*. 2013;14(1):26–37.
29. Johansson MEV, Jakobsson HE, Holmén-Larsson J, et al. Normalization of host intestinal mucus layers requires long-term microbial colonization. *Cell Host Microbe*. 2015;18(5):582–592.
30. Petersson J, Schreiber O, Hansson GC, et al. Importance and regulation of the colonic mucus barrier in a mouse model of colitis. *Am J Physiol-Gastrointestinal Liver Physiol*. 2010;300(2):G327–G333.
31. Bergmann KR, Liu SXL, Tian R, et al. Bifidobacteria stabilize claudins at tight junctions and prevent intestinal barrier dysfunction in mouse necrotizing enterocolitis. *Am J Pathol*. 2013;182 (5):1595–1606.
32. Heeney DD, Zhai Z, Bendiks Z, et al. *Lactobacillus plantarum* bacteriocin is associated with intestinal and systemic improvements in diet-induced obese mice and maintains epithelial barrier integrity in vitro. *Gut Microbes*. 2019;10(3):382–397.
33. Mouries J, Brescia P, Silvestri A, et al. Microbiota-driven gut vascular barrier disruption is a prerequisite for non-alcoholic steatohepatitis development. *J Hepatol*. 2019;71(6):1216–1228.
34. Ismail AS, Severson KM, Vaishnava S, et al. Gammadelta intraepithelial lymphocytes are essential mediators of host-microbial homeostasis at the intestinal mucosal surface. *Proc Natl Acad Sci U S A*. 2011;108(21):8743–8748.
35. Hooper LV, Stappenbeck TS, Hong CV, Gordon JI. Angiogenins: a new class of microbicidal proteins involved in innate immunity. *Nat Immunol*. 2003;4(3):269–273.
36. Cash HL, Whitham CV, Behrendt CL, Hooper LV. Symbiotic bacteria direct expression of an intestinal bactericidal lectin. *Science (NY)*. 2006;313(5790):1126–1130.
37. Macpherson AJ, Hunziker L, McCoy K, Lamarre A. IgA responses in the intestinal mucosa against pathogenic and non-pathogenic microorganisms. *Microbes Infect*. 2001;3(12):1021–1035.
38. Cheng H-Y, Ning M-X, Chen D-K, Ma W-T. Interactions between the gut microbiota and the host innate immune response against pathogens. *Front Immunol*. 2019;10:607.
39. Turnbaugh PJ, Ridaura VK, Faith JJ, Rey FE, Knight R, Gordon JI. The effect of diet on the human gut microbiome: a metagenomic analysis in humanized gnotobiotic mice. *Sci Transl Med*. 2009;1 (6):6ra14. 6ra.
40. Turnbaugh PJ, Bäckhed F, Fulton L, Gordon JI. Diet-induced obesity is linked to marked but reversible alterations in the mouse distal gut microbiome. *Cell Host Microbe*. 2008;3(4):213–223.
41. Riva A, Borgo F, Lassandro C, et al. Pediatric obesity is associated with an altered gut microbiota and discordant shifts in Firmicutes populations. *Environ Microbiol*. 2017;19(1):95–105.
42. Koliada A, Syzenko G, Moseiko V, et al. Association between body mass index and Firmicutes/Bacteroidetes ratio in an adult Ukrainian population. *BMC Microbiol*. 2017;17(1):120.
43. Kim SJ, Kim S-E, Kim AR, Kang S, Park M-Y, Sung M-K. Dietary fat intake and age modulate the composition of the gut microbiota and colonic inflammation in C57BL/6J mice. *BMC Microbiol*. 2019;19(1):193.
44. Serino M, Luche E, Gres S, et al. Metabolic adaptation to a high-fat diet is associated with a change in the gut microbiota. *Gut*. 2012;61(4):543–553.
45. Cani PD, Bibiloni R, Knauf C, et al. Changes in gut microbiota control metabolic endotoxemia-induced inflammation in high-fat diet–induced obesity and diabetes in mice. *Diabetes*. 2008;57 (6):1470–1481.
46. Shen W, Wolf PG, Carbonero F, et al. Intestinal and systemic inflammatory responses are positively associated with sulfidogenic bacteria abundance in high-fat–fed male C57BL/6J mice. *J Nutr*. 2014;144(8):1181–1187.
47. Daniel H, Gholami AM, Berry D, et al. High-fat diet alters gut microbiota physiology in mice. *ISME J*. 2014;8(2):295–308.
48. Araújo JR, Tomas J, Brenner C, Sansonetti PJ. Impact of high-fat diet on the intestinal microbiota and small intestinal physiology before and after the onset of obesity. *Biochimie*. 2017;141:97–106.
49. Wan Y, Wang F, Yuan J, et al. Effects of dietary fat on gut microbiota and faecal metabolites, and their relationship with cardiometabolic risk factors: a 6-month randomised controlled-feeding trial. *Gut*. 2019;68(8):1417–1429.
50. Cordain L, Eaton SB, Sebastian A, et al. Origins and evolution of the Western diet: health implications for the 21st century. *Am J Clin Nutr*. 2005;81(2):341–354.
51. Miao Z-L, Zheng J-S, Chen Y-M. Erythrocyte n-6 polyunsaturated fatty acids, gut microbiota and incident type 2 diabetes: a prospective cohort study. *Curr Dev Nutr*. 2020;4(Suppl 2):1452.
52. Ghosh S, Molcan E, Decoffe D, Dai B, Gibson D. Diets rich in n-6 PUFA induce intestinal microbial dysbiosis in aged mice. *Br J Nutr*. 2013;110:1–9.
53. Caesar R, Tremaroli V, Kovatcheva-Datchary P, Cani Patrice D, Bäckhed F. Crosstalk between gut microbiota and dietary lipids aggravates wat inflammation through tlr signaling. *Cell Metab*. 2015;22(4):658–668.
54. Abulizi N, Quin C, Brown K, Chan YK, Gill SK, Gibson DL. Gut mucosal proteins and bacteriome are shaped by the saturation index of dietary lipids. *Nutrients*. 2019;11(2):418.
55. Ge Y, Liu W, Tao H, et al. Effect of industrial trans-fatty acids-enriched diet on gut microbiota of C57BL/6 mice. *Eur J Nutr*. 2019;58(7):2625–2638.
56. Costantini L, Molinari R, Farinon B, Merendino N. Impact of omega-3 fatty acids on the gut microbiota. *Int J Mol Sci*. 2017;18 (12):2645.
57. Townsend GE, Han W, Schwalm ND, et al. Dietary sugar silences a colonization factor in a mammalian gut symbiont. *Proc Natl Acad Sci U S A*. 2019;116(1):233–238.
58. Do MH, Lee E, Oh M-J, Kim Y, Park H-Y. High-glucose or -fructose diet cause changes of the gut microbiota and metabolic disorders in mice without body weight change. *Nutrients*. 2018;10(6):761.
59. Silva JCP, Mota M, Martins FO, et al. Intestinal microbial and metabolic profiling of mice fed with high-glucose and high-fructose diets. *J Proteome Res*. 2018;17(8):2880–2891.
60. Li J-M, Yu R, Zhang L-P, et al. Dietary fructose-induced gut dysbiosis promotes mouse hippocampal neuroinflammation: a benefit of short-chain fatty acids. *Microbiome*. 2019;7(1):98.
61. Sen T, Cawthon CR, Ihde BT, et al. Diet-driven microbiota dysbiosis is associated with vagal remodeling and obesity. *Physiol Behav*. 2017;173:305–317.
62. Sonnenburg Erica D, Sonnenburg Justin L. Starving our microbial self: the deleterious consequences of a diet deficient in microbiota-accessible carbohydrates. *Cell Metab*. 2014;20(5):779–786.
63. Lin D, Peters BA, Friedlander C, et al. Association of dietary fibre intake and gut microbiota in adults. *Br J Nutr*. 2018;120 (9):1014–1022.

64. Myhrstad MCW, Tunsjø H, Charnock C, Telle-Hansen VH. Dietary fiber, gut microbiota, and metabolic regulation-current status in human randomized trials. *Nutrients*. 2020;12(3):859.
65. Makki K, Deehan EC, Walter J, Bäckhed F. The impact of dietary fiber on gut microbiota in host health and disease. *Cell Host Microbe*. 2018;23(6):705–715.
66. So D, Whelan K, Rossi M, et al. Dietary fiber intervention on gut microbiota composition in healthy adults: a systematic review and *meta*-analysis. *Am J Clin Nutr*. 2018;107(6):965–983.
67. Desai MS, Seekatz AM, Koropatkin NM, et al. A dietary fiber-deprived gut microbiota degrades the colonic mucus barrier and enhances pathogen susceptibility. *Cell*. 2016;167(5):1339–1353.e21.
68. Sonnenburg ED, Smits SA, Tikhonov M, Higginbottom SK, Wingreen NS, Sonnenburg JL. Diet-induced extinctions in the gut microbiota compound over generations. *Nature*. 2016;529 (7585):212–215.
69. Delgado-Andrade C, Tessier FJ, Niquet-Leridon C, Seiquer I, Pilar, Navarro M. Study of the urinary and faecal excretion of Nε-carboxymethyllysine in young human volunteers. *Amino Acids*. 2012;43 (2):595–602.
70. Tuohy KM, Hinton DJ, Davies SJ, Crabbe MJ, Gibson GR, Ames JM. Metabolism of Maillard reaction products by the human gut microbiota–implications for health. *Mol Nutr Food Res*. 2006;50 (9):847–857.
71. Hellwig M, Bunzel D, Huch M, Franz CMAP, Kulling SE, Henle T. Stability of individual maillard reaction products in the presence of the human colonic microbiota. *J Agric Food Chem*. 2015;63 (30):6723–6730.
72. Jemmali M. Influence of the Maillard reaction products on some bacteria of the intestinal flora. *J Appl Bacteriol*. 1969;32 (2):151–155.
73. Delgado-Andrade C, Pastoriza de la Cueva S, Peinado MJ, Rufián-Henares JÁ, Navarro MP, Rubio LA. Modifications in bacterial groups and short chain fatty acid production in the gut of healthy adult rats after long-term consumption of dietary Maillard reaction products. *Food Res Int*. 2017;100:134–142.
74. Ames JM, Wynne A, Hofmann A, Plos S, Gibson GR. The effect of a model melanoidin mixture on faecal bacterial populations in vitro. *Br J Nutr*. 1999;82(6):489–495.
75. Qu W, Yuan X, Zhao J, et al. Dietary advanced glycation end products modify gut microbial composition and partially increase colon permeability in rats. *Mol Nutr Food Res*. 2017;61 (10):1700118.
76. Aljahdali N, Gadonna-Widehem P, Delayre-Orthez C, et al. Repeated oral exposure to nε-carboxymethyllysine, a Maillard reaction product, alleviates gut microbiota dysbiosis in colitic mice. *Digestive Dis Sci*. 2017;62(12):3370–3384.
77. Helou C, Marier D, Jacolot P, et al. Microorganisms and Maillard reaction products: a review of the literature and recent findings. *Amino Acids*. 2014;46(2):267–277.
78. Seiquer I, Rubio LA, Peinado MJ, Delgado-Andrade C, Navarro MP. Maillard reaction products modulate gut microbiota composition in adolescents. *Mol Nutr Food Res*. 2014;58(7):1552–1560.
79. Mottram DS, Wedzicha BL, Dodson AT. Acrylamide is formed in the Maillard reaction. *Nature*. 2002;419(6906):448–449.
80. Rivas-Jimenez L, Ramírez-Ortiz K, González-Córdova AF, Vallejo-Cordoba B, Garcia HS, Hernandez-Mendoza A. Evaluation of acrylamide-removing properties of two *Lactobacillus* strains under simulated gastrointestinal conditions using a dynamic system. *Microbiol Res*. 2016;190:19–26.
81. Petka K, Tarko T, Duda-Chodak A. Is acrylamide as harmful as we think? A new look at the impact of acrylamide on the viability of beneficial intestinal bacteria of the genus *Lactobacillus*. *Nutrients*. 2020;12:1157.
82. Borrelli RC, Fogliano V. Bread crust melanoidins as potential prebiotic ingredients. *Mol Nutr Food Res*. 2005;49(7):673–678.
83. Dominika Ś, Arjan N, Karyn RP, Henryk K. The study on the impact of glycated pea proteins on human intestinal bacteria. *Int J Food Microbiol*. 2011;145(1):267–272.
84. Mills DJS, Tuohy KM, Booth J, et al. Dietary glycated protein modulates the colonic microbiota towards a more detrimental composition in ulcerative colitis patients and non-ulcerative colitis subjects. *J Appl Microbiol*. 2008;105(3):706–714.
85. Harpaz D, Yeo LP, Cecchini F, et al. Measuring artificial sweeteners toxicity using a bioluminescent bacterial panel. *Molecules*. 2018;23 (10):2454.
86. Suez J, Korem T, Zeevi D, et al. Artificial sweeteners induce glucose intolerance by altering the gut microbiota. *Nature*. 2014;514 (7521):181–186.
87. Palmnäs MSA, Cowan TE, Bomhof MR, et al. Low-dose aspartame consumption differentially affects gut microbiota-host metabolic interactions in the diet-induced obese rat. *PLoS One*. 2014;9(10): e109841.
88. Bian X, Chi L, Gao B, Tu P, Ru H, Lu K. Gut microbiome response to sucralose and its potential role in inducing liver inflammation in mice. *Front Physiol*. 2017;8:487.
89. Abou-Donia MB, El-Masry EM, Abdel-Rahman AA, McLendon RE, Schiffman SS. Splenda alters gut microflora and increases intestinal P-glycoprotein and cytochrome P-450 in male rats. *J Toxicol Environ Health A*. 2008;71(21):1415–1429.
90. Uebanso T, Kano S, Yoshimoto A, et al. Effects of consuming xylitol on gut microbiota and lipid metabolism in mice. *Nutrients*. 2017;9(7):756.
91. Salminen S, Salminen E, Koivistoinen P, Bridges J, Marks V. Gut microflora interactions with xylitol in the mouse, rat and man. *Food Chem Toxicol*. 1985;23(11):985–990.
92. Ruiz-Ojeda FJ, Plaza-Díaz J, Sáez-Lara MJ, Gil A. Effects of sweeteners on the gut microbiota: a review of experimental studies and clinical trials. *Adv Nutr*. 2019;10(Suppl_1):S31–S48.
93. Swidsinski A, Ung V, Sydora BC, et al. Bacterial overgrowth and inflammation of small intestine after carboxymethylcellulose ingestion in genetically susceptible mice. *Inflamm Bowel Dis*. 2009;15 (3):359–364.
94. Roberts CL, Keita ÅV, Duncan SH, et al. Translocation of Crohn's disease *Escherichia coli* across M-cells: contrasting effects of soluble plant fibres and emulsifiers. *Gut*. 2010;59(10):1331–1339.
95. Chassaing B, Koren O, Goodrich JK, et al. Dietary emulsifiers impact the mouse gut microbiota promoting colitis and metabolic syndrome. *Nature*. 2015;519(7541):92–96.
96. Holder MK, Peters NV, Whylings J, et al. Dietary emulsifiers consumption alters anxiety-like and social-related behaviors in mice in a sex-dependent manner. *Sci Rep*. 2019;9(1):172.
97. Chassaing B, Van de Wiele T, De Bodt J, Marzorati M, Gewirtz AT. Dietary emulsifiers directly alter human microbiota composition and gene expression ex vivo potentiating intestinal inflammation. *Gut*. 2017;66(8):1414–1427.

98. Hrncirova L, Machova V, Trckova E, Krejsek J, Hrncir T. Food preservatives induce proteobacteria dysbiosis in human-microbiota associated Nod2-deficient mice. *Microorganisms.* 2019;7(10):383.
99. Irwin SV, Fisher P, Graham E, Malek A, Robidoux A. Sulfites inhibit the growth of four species of beneficial gut bacteria at concentrations regarded as safe for food. *PLoS One.* 2017;12(10): e0186629.
100. You X, Einson JE, Lopez-Pena CL, et al. Food-grade cationic antimicrobial ε-polylysine transiently alters the gut microbial community and predicted metagenome function in CD-1 mice. *NPJ Sci Food.* 2017;1(1):8.
101. Namkung H, Gong J, Yu H, de Lange CFM. Effect of pharmacological intakes of zinc and copper on growth performance, circulating cytokines and gut microbiota of newly weaned piglets challenged with coliform lipopolysaccharides. *Can J Anim Sci.* 2006;86(4):511–522.
102. Sadykov R, Digel I, Artmann A, uuml LT, Porst D, et al. Oral lead exposure induces dysbacteriosis in rats. *J Occup Health.* 2009;51(1):64–73.
103. Fazeli M, Hassanzadeh P, Alaei S. Cadmium chloride exhibits a profound toxic effect on bacterial microflora of the mice gastrointestinal tract. *Hum Exp Toxicol.* 2011;30(2):152–159.
104. Liu Y, Li Y, Liu K, Shen J. Exposing to cadmium stress cause profound toxic effect on microbiota of the mice intestinal tract. *PLoS One.* 2014;9(2):e85323.
105. Li X, Brejnrod AD, Ernst M, et al. Heavy metal exposure causes changes in the metabolic health-associated gut microbiome and metabolites. *Environ Int.* 2019;126:454–467.
106. Zhai Q, Li T, Yu L, et al. Effects of subchronic oral toxic metal exposure on the intestinal microbiota of mice. *Sci Bull.* 2017;62 (12):831–840.
107. Kittle RP, McDermid KJ, Muehlstein L, Balazs GH. Effects of glyphosate herbicide on the gastrointestinal microflora of Hawaiian green turtles (*Chelonia mydas*) Linnaeus. *Mar Pollut Bull.* 2018;127:170–174.
108. Nasuti C, Coman MM, Olek RA, et al. Changes on fecal microbiota in rats exposed to permethrin during postnatal development. *Environ Sci Pollut Res.* 2016;23(11):10930–10937.
109. Joly C, Gay-Quéheillard J, Léké A, et al. Impact of chronic exposure to low doses of chlorpyrifos on the intestinal microbiota in the simulator of the human intestinal microbial ecosystem (SHIME®) and in the rat. *Environ Sci Pollut Res.* 2013;20 (5):2726–2734.
110. Zhao Y, Zhang Y, Wang G, Han R, Xie X. Effects of chlorpyrifos on the gut microbiome and urine metabolome in mouse (*Mus musculus*). *Chemosphere.* 2016;153:287–293.
111. Fang B, Li JW, Zhang M, Ren FZ, Pang GF. Chronic chlorpyrifos exposure elicits diet-specific effects on metabolism and the gut microbiome in rats. *Food Chem Toxicol.* 2018;111:144–152.
112. Wu S, Jin C, Wang Y, Fu Z, Jin Y. Exposure to the fungicide propamocarb causes gut microbiota dysbiosis and metabolic disorder in mice. *Environ Pollut.* 2018;237:775–783.
113. Javurek AB, Spollen WG, Johnson SA, et al. Effects of exposure to bisphenol A and ethinyl estradiol on the gut microbiota of parents and their offspring in a rodent model. *Gut Microbes.* 2016;7(6):471–485.
114. Nelson AM, Walk ST, Taube S, et al. Disruption of the human gut microbiota following Norovirus infection. *PLoS One.* 2012;7 (10):e48224.
115. Bratburd JR, Keller C, Vivas E, et al. Gut microbial and metabolic responses to *Salmonella enterica, Serovar Typhimurium* and *Candida albicans. mBio.* 2018;9(6):e02032–18.
116. Saint-Cyr MJ, Perrin-Guyomard A, Houée P, Rolland J-G, Laurentie M. Evaluation of an oral subchronic exposure of deoxynivalenol on the composition of human gut microbiota in a model of human microbiota-associated rats. *PLoS One.* 2013;8(11): e80578.
117. Payros D, Dobrindt U, Martin P, et al. The food contaminant deoxynivalenol exacerbates the genotoxicity of gut microbiota. *mBio.* 2017;8(2):e00007–e00017.
118. Ouethrani M, Van de Wiele T, Verbeke E, et al. Metabolic fate of ochratoxin A as a coffee contaminant in a dynamic simulator of the human colon. *Food Chem.* 2013;141(4):3291–3300.
119. FAO/WHO. Probiotics in food. Health and nutritional properties and guidelines for evaluation. Report of a joint FAO/WHO expert consultation on evaluation of health and nutritional properties of probiotics in food including powder milk with live lactic acid bacteria. Cordoba, Argentina; 2001.
120. Turner PC, Wu QK, Piekkola S, Gratz S, Mykkänen H, El-Nezami H. Lactobacillus rhamnosus strain GG restores alkaline phosphatase activity in differentiating CaCO-2 cells dosed with the potent mycotoxin deoxynivalenol. *Food Chem Toxicol.* 2008;46(6):2118–2123.
121. El-Nezami HS, Chrevatidis A, Auriola S, Salminen S, Mykkänen H. Removal of common Fusarium toxins in vitro by strains of *Lactobacillus* and Propionibacterium. *Food Addit Contam.* 2002;19(7):680–686.
122. Park YH, Hamidon F, Rajangan C, et al. Application of probiotics for the production of safe and high-quality poultry meat. *Korean J Food Sci Anim Resour.* 2016;36(5):567–576.
123. Yirga H. The use of probiotics in animal nutrition. *J Probiotics Health.* 2015;03.
124. Wang Y, Gu Q. Effect of probiotic on growth performance and digestive enzyme activity of Arbor Acres broilers. *Res Vet Sci.* 2010;89(2):163–167.
125. Wang H, Ni X, Qing X, et al. Probiotic enhanced intestinal immunity in broilers against subclinical necrotic Enteritis. *Front Immunol.* 2017;8:1592.
126. Van Coillie E, Goris J, Cleenwerck I, et al. Identification of lactobacilli isolated from the cloaca and vagina of laying hens and characterization for potential use as probiotics to control *Salmonella Enteritidis. J Appl Microbiol.* 2007;102 (4):1095–1106.
127. Wisener LV, Sargeant JM, O'Connor AM, Faires MC, Glass-Kaastra SK. The use of direct-fed microbials to reduce shedding of escherichia coli o157 in beef cattle: a systematic review and *meta*-analysis. *Zoonoses Public Health.* 2015;62(2):75–89.
128. Gaggia F, Di Gioia D, Baffoni L, Biavati B. The role of protective and probiotic cultures in food and feed and their impact in food safety. *Trends Food Sci Technol.* 2011;22:S58–S66.
129. EFSA. Scientific committee. introduction of a qualified presumption of safety (QPS) approach for assessment of selected microorganisms referred to EFSA1. Opinion of the Scientific Committee (Question No EFSA-Q-2005-293). *EFSA J.* 2007;587:1–16.
130. Silva CCG, Silva SPM, Ribeiro SC. Application of bacteriocins and protective cultures in dairy food preservation. *Front Microbiol.* 2018;9(594).

131. Mokoena MP. Lactic acid bacteria and their bacteriocins: classification, biosynthesis and applications against uropathogens: a mini-review. *Molecules.* 2017;22(8):1255.
132. Gharsallaoui A, Oulahal N, Joly C, Degraeve P. Nisin as a food preservative: part 1: physicochemical properties, antimicrobial activity, and main uses. *Crit Rev Food Sci Nutr.* 2016;56(8):1262–1274.
133. Karlovsky P, Suman M, Berthiller F, et al. Impact of food processing and detoxification treatments on mycotoxin contamination. *Mycotoxin Res.* 2016;32(4):179–205.
134. Ciegler A, Lillehoj EB, Peterson RE, Hall HH. Microbial detoxification of aflatoxin. *Appl Microbiol.* 1966;14(6):934–939.
135. Islam R, Zhou T, Christopher Young J, Goodwin PH, Peter, Pauls K. Aerobic and anaerobic de-epoxydation of mycotoxin deoxynivalenol by bacteria originating from agricultural soil. *World J Microbiol Biotechnol.* 2012;28(1):7–13.
136. Zheng M, Zhang R, Tian X, Zhou X, Pan X, Wong A. Assessing the risk of probiotic dietary supplements in the context of antibiotic resistance. *Front Microbiol.* 2017;8(908).
137. Sanders ME, Akkermans LMA, Haller D, et al. Safety assessment of probiotics for human use. *Gut Microbes.* 2010;1(3):164–185.
138. Boever PD, Deplancke B, Verstraete W. Fermentation by gut microbiota cultured in a simulator of the human intestinal microbial ecosystem is improved by supplementing a soygerm powder. *J Nutr.* 2000;130(10):2599–2606.
139. Van den Abbeele P, Roos S, Eeckhaut V, et al. Incorporating a mucosal environment in a dynamic gut model results in a more representative colonization by Lactobacilli. *Microb Biotechnol.* 2012;5(1):106–115.
140. Auchtung JM, Robinson CD, Britton RA. Cultivation of stable, reproducible microbial communities from different fecal donors using minibioreactor arrays (MBRAs). *Microbiome.* 2015;3(1):42.
141. Robinson CD, Auchtung JM, Collins J, Britton RA. Epidemic <span class = "named-content genus-species" id = "named-content-1" > *Clostridium difficile* < /span> strains demonstrate increased competitive fitness compared to nonepidemic isolates. *Infect Immun.* 2014;82(7):2815–2825.
142. Auchtung JM, Preisner EC, Collins J, Lerma AI, Britton RA. Identification of simplified microbial communities that inhibit *Clostridioides difficile* infection through dilution/extinction. *BioRxiv.* 2020.
143. Collins J, Robinson C, Danhof H, et al. Dietary trehalose enhances virulence of epidemic *Clostridium difficile. Nature.* 2018;553(7688):291–294.
144. Ashammakhi N, Nasiri R, Barros NRd, et al. Gut-on-a-chip: current progress and future opportunities. *Biomaterials.* 2020;255:120196.
145. Jalili-Firoozinezhad S, Gazzaniga FS, Calamari EL, et al. A complex human gut microbiome cultured in an anaerobic intestine-on-a-chip. *Nat Biomed Eng.* 2019;3(7):520–531.
146. Licht TR, Bahl MI. Impact of the gut microbiota on chemical risk assessment. *Curr OpToxicol.* 2019;15:109–113.
147. Swann JR, Rajilic-Stojanovic M, Salonen A, et al. Considerations for the design and conduct of human gut microbiota intervention studies relating to foods. *Eur J Nutr.* 2020.
148. Johnson AJ, Zheng JJ, Kang JW, Saboe A, Knights D, Zivkovic AM. A guide to diet-microbiome study design. *Front Nutr.* 2020;7(79).
149. Wu Q, Chen T, El-Nezami H, Savidge T. Food ingredients in human health: ecological and metabolic perspectives implicating gut microbiota function. *Trends Food Sci Technol.* 2020;100.
150. McLaren MR, Willis AD, Callahan BJ. Consistent and correctable bias in metagenomic sequencing experiments. *Elife.* 2019;8:e46923.
151. Schiebenhoefer H, Van Den Bossche T, Fuchs S, Renard BY, Muth T, Martens L. Challenges and promise at the interface of metaproteomics and genomics: an overview of recent progress in metaproteogenomic data analysis. *Expert Rev Proteom.* 2019;16 (5):375–390.
152. Zhang X, Li L, Butcher J, Stintzi A, Figeys D. Advancing functional and translational microbiome research using *meta*-omics approaches. *Microbiome.* 2019;7(1):154.

Chapter 55

Bacterial cell-to-cell communication and its relevance to food safety

Felipe Alves de Almeida[1], Leonardo Luiz de Freitas[2], Deisy Guimarães Carneiro[2] and Maria Cristina Dantas Vanetti[2]

[1]*Department of Nutrition, Federal University of Juiz de Fora (UFJF), Governador Valadares, Brazil,* [2]*Department of Microbiology, Federal University of Viçosa (UFV), Viçosa, Brazil*

Abstract

Bacteria can interact and regulate, in a coordinated manner, gene expression in response to population density through a mechanism of cellular communication known as quorum sensing (QS). This communication has been described in Gram-positive and Gram-negative bacteria; it is based on population density and includes production, excretion, and response to a signal molecule called autoinducer. Relevant phenotypes associated with virulence, resistance to stress conditions, enzyme production, sporulation, and antimicrobial resistance are regulated by QS, which impact the action of bacteria in food. Knowledge of this mechanism of gene regulation and its possible effects on food microbiology is essential to understand bacterial activity and develop strategies to combat undesirable microorganisms. The inhibition of QS, called quorum quenching, is an attractive strategy for bacterial control since blocking cell communication inhibits the expression of certain phenotypes. This chapter focuses on the design of microbial communication networks and their disruption to ensure food safety.

Keywords: Autoinducer; cellular communication; foodborne pathogen; quorum quenching; quorum sensing

55.1 Introduction

The presence and activity of microorganisms in food is an exciting study area as they are involved in various activities including production, preservation, spoilage, and safety. The ability of pathogenic and spoilage microorganisms to overcome the stress conditions faced in the natural environment of food and during processing is concerning. Understanding the strategies they use to establish themselves in food and food-processing environments can be useful in designing approaches for food preservation, to prevent spoilage and to enhance food safety. Bacteria are highly interactive and have an extraordinary ability to communicate and modulate cell decisions to adopt necessary measures for fitness, facilitating collective survival. Many bacterial species have complex inter- and intracellular mechanisms that allow them to communicate with neighboring cells of the same species, different species, and even from different kingdoms, in addition to interacting with their environment and acting as a cooperative population in a process known as quorum sensing (QS).[1] The discovery of QS has been one of the most significant developments in the field of microbiology in the past 30 years. Fuqua et al.[1] have coined the term "quorum sensing" for a microbial cell-to-cell communication system, but the phenomenon had already been observed in *Vibrio fischeri*, now *Aliivibrio fischeri*, by Nealson et al.[2] These authors described it as a "cell density-dependent autoinducer (AI)" behavior after observing luminescence in this marine symbiont bacterium that inhabits light organs of squid *Euprymna scolopes*, produced at high cell densities.

QS is a chemical process of cell-to-cell communication dependent on population density and based on the production, detection, and response to diffuse or transport extracellular signal molecules called AIs. AIs produced by bacterial cells accumulate in the environment and, upon reaching a threshold concentration, bind to cellular receptors and regulate target gene expression. QS allows groups of bacteria present in the surrounding medium to synchronously alter their behavior in response to changes in population density and act as a multicellular organism. Bacteria also establish efficient chemical communication with other

Present Knowledge in Food Safety. DOI: https://doi.org/10.1016/B978-0-12-819470-6.00025-1

kinds of bacteria, where two species must exist in microspatial proximity of each other (~ <70 μM), use the same signals, and activate similar or complementary genes that influence subsequent coordinated activities.[3,4] The capacity to behave collectively as a group has obvious advantages that include the ability to migrate to a more suitable environment or to a better nutrient supply and to adopt new modes of growth, such as biofilm formation, entry into a dormancy state (spores), which may afford protection from deleterious environments in addition to regulating other important phenotypes such as antimicrobial resistance, bioluminescence, and competence, among others.[5]

The development of chemical communication between two species in culture has been widely observed and the probability of the phenomenon occurring in natural environments should be assessed. The importance of AI gradients in mediating effective communication between distant cells should be considered and it is likely that cell-to-cell communication occurs not only within dense populations, but also in small groups of cells. Therefore, this cellular activity is more common and effective than hitherto envisaged. Cell-to-cell communication is believed to be governed more by the spatial proximity of cells within AI gradients than by the need for a high-density quorum group.

55.2 Cell-to-cell communication mechanisms in bacteria

Bacterial language is chemical in nature and numerous signaling molecules or AIs have been integrated into bacterial communication by QS. Currently, there are four well-defined classes of AIs: (1) *N*-acyl homoserine lactones (AHLs), which are fatty acid derivatives generically called autoinducer-1 (AI-1), produced and used by Gram-negative bacteria; (2) a furanosyl borate diester, which is derived from the recycling of *S*-adenosyl-homocysteine to homocysteine and known as autoinducer-2 (AI-2), produced by both Gram-positive and Gram-negative bacteria; (3) autoinducer-3 (AI-3), belonging to the pyrazinone family and serving as a QS signal for Enterohemorrhagic *Escherichia coli* (EHEC) and *Salmonella*, in addition to cross-talking with mammalian epinephrine and norepinephrine host cell signaling systems; and (4) autoinducing peptides (AIPs), which are produced and used by Gram-positive bacteria. Each signaling molecule class contains several members differing in minor molecular details, such as the length and type of molecular side chains attached to the same general molecular scaffold.[6] Other molecules similar to those in QS systems have also been described and include indole, 2-heptyl-3-hydroxy-4-quinolone, 2-(2-hydroxyphenyl)-thiazole-4-carbaldehyde, and diketopiperazines (cyclic dipeptides).[7,8]

Besides AIs, other fundamental elements in the QS circuit are signal synthase, signal transporter, signal receptor, signal response regulator, and regulated genes. During the initial stage of bacterial growth, the signal molecules occur at low concentrations in the surrounding environment, which increase with an increase in bacterial density. When the concentration of AIs attains a threshold level, they are sensed by the receptors present inside the bacterial cytoplasm or on the cell membrane.

The most studied QS signaling molecules are the AHLs, also known as AI-1, that comprise neutral lipid molecules, generally produced by LuxI or homologous proteins, from the lactone fraction of *S*-adenosyl methionine (SAM), mainly by Gram-negative bacteria. In most cases, the acyl chain is obtained from intermediates of the fatty acid biosynthesis pathway.[7] The acyl chain length can range from 4 to 18 carbons and may or may not have a 3-oxo or 3-hydroxy function.[9] Short side-chain AHLs are directly released from the cell upon synthesis, whereas long side-chain AHLs are actively secreted to the environment.[10] The size of the chain affects the stability of the molecule and may provide a mechanism for the processing of temporal information by the microbial community.[11] At high concentrations, this diversity of AHLs is recognized by the cognate LuxR-type protein, which binds to a specific Lux-boxes promoter sequence, affecting the expression of QS target genes, including genes associated with AI-1 synthesis (Fig. 55.1A). The autoinduction loop apparently endorses synchrony in the population and brings about phenotypic effects by QS-regulating gene expression.

In some bacteria of the *Enterobacteriaceae* family, such as *E. coli* and *Salmonella*, the LuxI/R system is incomplete since there is no gene in the genome that encodes the synthase; therefore AHLs are not synthesized. However, they are able to detect and alter their gene expression in response to AHLs produced by other species, since they encode a protein called SdiA, with a sequence similar to that of LuxR type transcriptional activators,[12] as shown in Fig. 55.1B. It is believed that a deletion event removed the *luxI* counterpart after the divergence of the genera *Pantoea* and *Erwinia*, leaving only the LuxR.[13] A systematic survey of LuxR domains in sequenced bacterial genomes, included in the InterPro database, identified that in 40%–70% of cases, there is a complete QS system, depending on the taxa, whilst the other species have only orphaned LuxR.[14]

The AI-2, a furanosyl borate diester, is derived from 4,5-dihydroxy-2,3-pentanedione (DPD) and identified in Gram-positive and Gram-negative bacterial species; it is recognized as a universal signaling molecule and used in the intra- and interspecies communication of bacteria.[15] The AI-2 is produced in three enzymatic steps from an *S*-ribosilhomocysteine (SRH), a product of the SAM

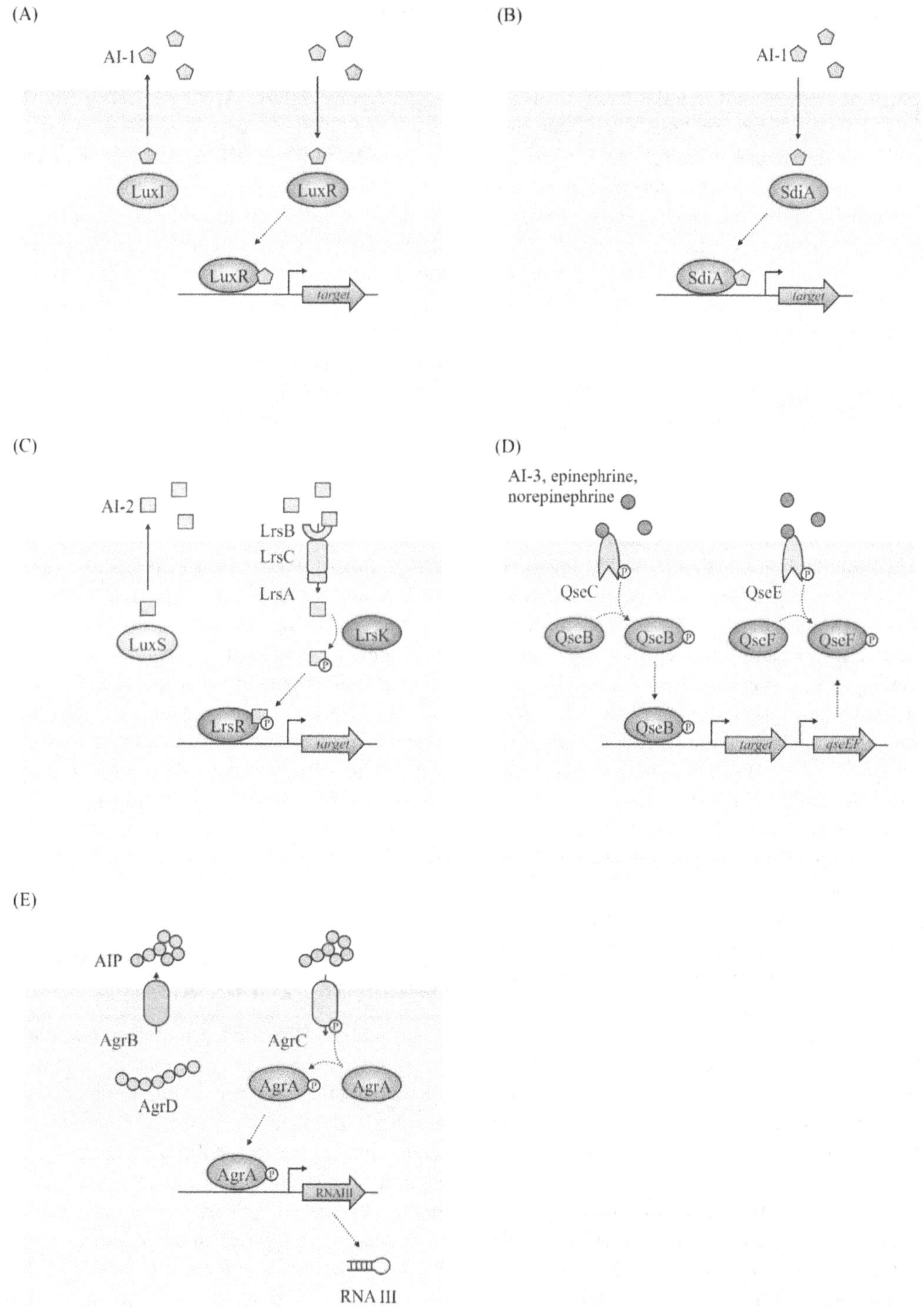

FIGURE 55.1 Quorum sensing (QS) systems: (A) autoinducer-1 (AI-1) by LuxR protein, (B) AI-1 by SdiA protein, (C) autoinducer-2 (AI-2), (D) autoinducer-3 (AI-3), and (E) autoinducing peptides (AIPs).

pathway, which is cleaved by the LuxS protein to form homocysteine (HC) and the precursor DPD.[15,16] In the model system in *Vibrio harveyi*, the AI-2 unleashes an integrated response of two distinct QS systems, LuxMN and CqsAS through histidine kinase sensors linked to the membrane. In mechanisms involving AI-2, the receptor protein is submitted to a cascade of phosphorylation, and the phosphorylated protein activates gene expression. Initially, AI-2 is detected by LuxP, a periplasmic protein. The LuxP-AI-2 complex interacts with LuxQ, a histidine kinase sensor, which acts as phosphatase, removing the phosphate group from the receptor proteins, LuxU and LuxO. Dephosphorylated LuxO is inactive and therefore there is no expression of small regulatory RNAs that destabilize the LuxR regulatory protein, which activates the expression of the luciferase operon.[17] In *E. coli* and *Salmonella*, AI-2 is recognized by the periplasmic protein LrsB and is internalized by the ATP binding cassette (ABC) transporter, composed of LsrC and LsrA. Once internalized, AI-2 is phosphorylated by LsrK and interacts with the transcriptional repressor LsrR to relieve the repression of the *lsrACDBFGE* operon,[15] as shown in Fig. 55.1C.

The AI-3 is an aromatic amino compound produced by bacteria from the intestinal microbiota and by some enteric pathogens such as *E. coli* and *Salmonella*.[18,19] Kim et al.[20] identified the structure of AI-3 as molecules that belong to the pyrazinone family. Using ^{13}C-labeled amino acids, the most significant potent inducer has been shown to be 3,6-dimethylpyrazin-2-one. Additional ^{13}C-labeled amino acid feeding experiments and subsequent structural analyses revealed that AI-3 is formed from two molecules of threonine. In addition, AI-3 analogs can be formed by reacting tRNA synthetase products with aminoacetone or 1-amino-3-methylbutan-2-one to form dipeptide ketones, which can undergo cyclizations and oxidations.[20] The AI-3 detection system has been well described for *E. coli* O157: H7 (EHEC) (Fig. 55.1D). The AI-3 and the molecules produced by the host cells, such as epinephrine and norepinephrine, are recognized by the same receptor, a sensor kinase, QseC. Upon detecting the molecules, QseC phosphorylates the QseB response regulator, which activates its own expression and that of the target genes. It also activates the transcription of a two-component QseEF system (Fig. 55.1D), which may also be involved in the detection of host hormones.[18,21] Homologs of the *E. coli* QseC/QseB and QseE/QseF systems have already been identified in different commensal and pathogenic Gram-negative bacteria, including foodborne pathogens such as *Salmonella*, *Shigella*, *Yersinia*, and *Coxiella*.[19–21]

Gram-positive bacteria have their own language, and AIPs are used for communication. They are small molecules ribosomally synthesized, varying from 5 to 26 amino acid residues and sometimes undergo posttranslational modifications to increase functionality and stability.[16] Peptides are generally transported via an ABC transporter to the extracellular environment, as they cannot permeate bacterial cell membranes. When the peptide signal's extracellular concentration accumulates to the minimal level, a protein histidine sensor kinase detects it. The QS of *Staphylococcus aureus* is one of the most studied systems among the Gram-positive bacteria (Fig. 55.1E) and in this pathogen, the AIP is encoded by the *agrD* gene. Subsequently, AgrB processes the precursor peptide for the active mature AIP by adding a thiolactone ring and transports the AIP out of the cell, which upon accumulation, is detected by a cognate sensor kinase ArgC. Upon binding, ArgC transfers a phosphate to ArgA, which upregulates its own promoter transcription and actives the regulatory RNA (RNA III), which in turn leads to the expression of target genes.[22]

Besides these recognized autoinducers, some bacterial metabolites that play important roles in host metabolism and modulate the immune response, also act in communication. Among these metabolites, indole, produced by a variety of Gram-positive and Gram-negative bacteria, has received considerable attention. The first evidence that indole can act as an extracellular signaling molecule was found in *E. coli*. Indole is produced through the degradation of tryptophan by the enzyme tryptophanase (TnaA), transported to the extracellular medium through membrane proteins, such as AcrEF, and absorbed, mainly, through Mtr permease.[23,24] However, there is evidence that indole does not require a carrier and freely crosses the membrane. Gene regulation does not occur through binding to receptor proteins but through the activation of genes or the actuation in regulatory proteins.[24] Several environmental factors such as cell population, carbon sources, temperature, and pH can affect the accumulation of extracellular indole.[25] Interestingly, the recognition of metabolites as QS signals demonstrates the process of bacterial adaptation to the environment to survive, whilst the classic QS, mediated by AIs, is much more related to the evolutionary ability of bacteria to form social communities.[8]

55.3 Quorum sensing in foodborne pathogenic bacteria

A large body of evidence indicates that pathogenic bacteria share common strategies to modulate virulence, and QS is one such strategy adapted not only to modify their metabolic demands but also to regulate virulence factor production. In some foodborne pathogens, the QS mechanism regulates numerous phenotypes, which can contribute to survival in adverse conditions and assist in host colonization. A deeper understanding of when and how cell-to-cell communication is involved in the virulence of bacteria is therefore useful and will allow designing approaches for the specific blocking of these communication systems, reducing or inhibiting pathogen virulence.

Bacterial pathogens are faced with stressful conditions in food and food industry environments, in the passage through the gastrointestinal tract, and within phagocytic cells. Some pathogens have developed mechanisms to survive in those environments, and QS is critical to the success of these adaptations. The adhesion of different foodborne pathogenic bacteria, including *Salmonella*,

Listeria monocytogenes, and *S. aureus*, and with subsequent biofilm formation on food-processing surfaces, can be associated with food spoilage and/or foodborne diseases. The biofilm, an agglomerate of surface-associated microbial cells in a complex three-dimensional structure surrounded by extracellular polymeric substance, protecting the cells against harmful factors, is directly regulated by QS. The AHL-mediated QS increases the biofilm formation by *Salmonella enterica* serovar Enteritidis in specific conditions.[26,27] In this pathogen, AHL-mediated QS affects the expression of genes that encode important factors for adhesion and biofilm formation.[26] However, this cell-to-cell communication system downregulates biofilm formation in *Yersinia pseudotuberculosis*, *Campylobacter jejuni*, and *E. coli* strains.[28–30] This difference in the role of AHL-mediated QS in the regulation of biofilm formation is intriguing and seems to be specific for each group of microorganisms. Moreover, the LuxS/AI-2 QS system also regulates the adhesion of *C. jejuni* on polystyrene surfaces,[31] as well as the biofilm formation of *E. coli* BW30044[32] and *Vibrio parahaemolyticus*.[33] In *Vibrio cholerae*, an etiological agent of the disease cholera, the cholera AI-1 (CAI-1; (*S*)-3-hydroxytridecan-4-one) and the AI-2 are involved in aggregation, biofilm formation and dispersal, demonstrating that both QS pathways are necessary to control these phenotypes and for the colonization of this pathogen in other niches.[34]

The biofilm phenotype is regulated by AIPs in some Gram-positive pathogens. The *agr* operon, responsible for the synthesis of AIP, directly regulates biofilm formation at different stages in *S. aureus*. Mutants with inactivation in *agr* operon genes form more biofilms than wild-type strains. However, activation results in the detachment of the biofilm due to upregulation of extracellular enzymes that disrupt the biofilm matrix.[35,36] This explains the constant isolation of QS-dysfunctional *S. aureus* strains from infections associated with biofilm.[37] Similar observations have shown that the AIP-mediated QS system controls biofilm formation in other foodborne pathogens such as *L. monocytogenes* and *Clostridium perfringens*.[38,39] Zetzmann et al.[40] have observed that the *agrD* of *L. monocytogenes* controls the biosynthesis, structure, and function of the cell envelope by regulating several factors, including genes for internalins, peptidoglycan-associated proteins, penicillin-binding proteins, and proteins with wall-hydrolyzing activity. This regulatory profile shows that *agrD* participates in adhesion and interaction with the abiotic surface, neighboring bacteria and/or the biofilm matrix.[40] Further, *L. monocytogenes* isolates from food and forming biofilms have an increased expression of the *agr* system genes, whereas isolates that do not form biofilms have a low expression of these genes,[41] which confirms the importance of QS in biofilm regulation in this foodborne pathogen.

The role of QS in stress resistance has been described as an important factor for the maintenance of pathogens in the environment and the host. The protein SdiA of *E. coli* is required to survive in an acidic condition by regulating the expression of specific genes.[42] Interestingly, although they do not produce AI-1, *E. coli* and *Salmonella* show increased acid tolerance when exposed to exogenous AHL.[43,44] Thus the AHL-regulated phenotype suggests that the detection of these autoinducer molecules by pathogens promotes resistance to acidic stress and possibly contributes to survival during passage through the stomach or within phagocytic cells. In addition, *Salmonella* was more resistant to nisin, a cationic peptide, when cultivated with AHL and this behavior is related to alterations in the fatty acid composition as well as in the increase in *phoPQ* and *pmrAB* expression.[44] The PhoPQ and PmrAB are directly involved in cationic antimicrobial peptide and polymyxin B resistance in some Gram-negative pathogens.[45] The presence of exogenous AHLs increased the transition rate to a viable but nonculturable (VBNC) state in strains of *C. jejuni*.[29] The VBNC cells, usually stress-induced, do not grow in traditional culture media but can retain certain features of viable cells, such as cellular integrity, metabolic activity, and virulence.[46]

The AI-2 also participates in the regulation of resistance phenotypes to different stresses. For example, *C. jejuni luxS*-deficient mutant, a nonproducer of AI-2, is more sensitive to oxidative stress, and its survival in chicken meat juice stored at low temperature is affected.[47,48] In EHEC *luxS*-deficient mutant, the growth ability in an acidic condition was reduced and the tolerance to osmotic stress was increased when compared to the wild-type strain.[49] Also, the role of QS in the survival of Gram-positive foodborne pathogens under stress has been reported, especially in the presence of antibiotics. The mutation of the *luxS* gene in *S. aureus* increased the expression of *vraRS* genes. These genes encode the VraSR two-component system, which is responsible for the regulation of cell wall biosynthesis pathways. These modifications caused by the LuxS/AI-2 QS system resulted in resistance to antibiotics such as vancomycin as well as decreased autolysis; they can also affect the survival rate of this pathogen in human blood and macrophages.[50,51]

Furthermore, the virulence of many foodborne pathogens is directly regulated by QS. This system controls phenotypes related to virulence in *C. jejuni*, *Y. pseudotuberculosis*, *E. coli*, *Shigella flexneri*, and *Salmonella*.[26,29,52] In *Salmonella* serotypes, the presence of exogenous AHLs increased adhesion and invasion in eukaryotic cells[52] as well as virulence in *Galleria mellonella* larvae.[53] The mutation in the *luxS* gene, which results in no production of AI-2, affects the virulence of some pathogens.

The *C. jejuni luxS*-deficient mutant inoculated orally failed completely to colonize the gastrointestinal tract of guinea pigs and chickens.[54] In addition, this mutant has its motility and invasion of INT407 cells reduced as well as a reduction in the expression of genes that encode toxins.[31,55] In *S. flexneri*, the LuxS/AI-2 QS system is not required for virulence in L2 fibroblasts but controls the expression of the *virB* gene, a transcriptional factor involved in virulence.[56]

The role of QS in controlling virulence and persistence of *V. cholerae* in the intestinal environment is intriguing. The QS activates or represses specific genes that contribute to the control of virulence factors, which allows the perception of the presence or absence of oxygen, the production of enzymes important for invasion in the mucus barrier of the gastrointestinal epithelium, the colonization of mouse intestines, and the prevention of signal interference within the host as well as cholera enterotoxin and toxin-coregulated-pilus synthesis.[57,58]

Although poorly understood, interkingdom communication controls several virulence factors. The AI-3-mediated QS system or epinephrine and norepinephrine can regulate the virulence of EHEC by controlling the locus of enterocyte effacement, a pathogenicity island.[59] In addition, the epinephrine acts in EHEC-regulating virulence gene expression and the colonization of HeLa cells.[60] The compound, 3,4-dihydroxymandelic acid (DHMA), a metabolite of norepinephrine, also induces the expression of genes related to pathogenicity and increases attachment to intestinal epithelial cells in a QseC-dependent manner in EHEC.[61] In *S. enterica* serovar Typhimurium, adrenergic hormones or the QseCB system cause changes in antimicrobial peptide resistance, flagellar motility, invasion of epithelial cells, intramacrophage replication, and systemic infection in mice.[19,62,63]

Similarly, in Gram-positive foodborne pathogens, such as *S. aureus*, *L. monocytogenes*, *Clostridium*, and *Bacillus* the AIP-mediated QS is also involved in virulence. For example, in *S. aureus*, the *agrBDCA* operon, which encodes a set of proteins that will produce and detect an AIP, controls the expression of several virulence factors, including lipases, toxic shock syndrome toxins, alpha- and beta-hemolysin, protein A, exfoliative toxin A, and staphylococcal serine protease.[64,65] In addition, this system is also required for infection in vivo. The *S. aureus* strains with *agr* mutations reduce the ability to cause infections such as skin infection, pneumonia, endocarditis, and osteomyelitis in different animal models.[65] *S. aureus* AK23, a piezotolerant isolate less invasive in Caco-2 cells when compared to the wild-type strain, presents part of the genes belonging to the *agr* system downregulated, which possibly impairs its virulence characteristics.[66] The mutation in the *agrD* gene in *L. monocytogenes* affects the transcription of more than 650 genes and impairs the invasion in Caco-2 cells, in addition to dissemination and virulence in affected mice.[67] This significant reduction in virulence clearly indicates the contribution of the AIP to controlling gene expression and, consequently, to pathogenicity. Also, the *agrA* gene is not necessary for invasion and multiplication of *L. monocytogenes* in cells in vitro, but is required for virulence in mice, which reinforces the QS role in the mortality of mammalian models.[68]

The *agr*-like QS system is important for the pathogenicity of members of the genus *Clostridium*. Orthologs of *agrB* and *agrD* have been identified in the *C. perfringens* genome, which positively control the production of several toxins, including alpha-toxin, beta-toxin, perfringolysin-O, epsilon-toxin, and enterotoxin.[69] In *Clostridioides difficile*, previously named *Clostridium difficile*, which causes severe gastrointestinal illness, the AIP produced by the *agr* system regulates multiple functions, including motility, sporulation, and toxin production.[70] In *Clostridium botulinum*, the *agr* operon is important in sporulation and neurotoxin production.[71]

Therefore the meticulous regulatory control promoted by QS allows pathogens to adjust cellular processes and metabolism mediated by signaling molecules in response to environmental cues, which possibly contributes to adaptability and pathogenicity. Despite the role QS plays in virulence during animal and plant laboratory-engineered infections, QS mutants are frequently isolated from natural infections, demonstrating that the function of QS during infection and its role in pathogenesis remain poorly understood and are fruitful areas for future research.[72] Thus the role of QS in regulating multiple systems in bacteria needs to be understood in more detail and the characterization and understanding of these regulation mechanisms are crucial for the development of control strategies for many foodborne pathogens.

55.4 Detection of quorum sensing signals in foods

QS signaling is an important component of bacterial metabolism and, therefore, it is reasonable to assume that it also plays a significant role in food ecology and spoilage activity. Signaling molecules such as AI-1 and AI-2, present in different food systems, are associated with their deterioration. These molecules have been detected in a variety of deteriorating foods, such as cold-smoked salmon[73] and vacuum-packed meat,[74] as well as in frozen fish samples, tomato, cantaloupe, carrots, tofu, milk samples,[75] and in minced beef.[76] However, the role of QS in food spoilage and in the survival and virulence of foodborne pathogens has only recently been addressed, and available data are scarce. It is relevant to consider that many factors influence the critical concentration of QS signals needed by microorganisms to recognize the quorum and alter their gene expression profiles. The spatial distribution of contaminating microbiota attached in solid food products and the production, diffusion, and chemical degradation of the signals in the dynamic abiotic conditions of the food product affect QS signaling. Therefore, these variables to be considered for evaluating the effect of AIs produced by microbiota in food are complex but necessary to understand the mechanisms of signaling and regulation of virulence of pathogenic bacteria present in food.

The AHLs and AI-2 are potential biomarkers for the detection of pathogen and spoilage bacteria in food and consequently, represent an alternative strategy for conventional microbiological analysis methods. This may provide an opportunity to enhance the fight against food contamination and bacterial pathogens.[77] The most used method for detecting these signal molecules or producing bacteria is the use of biosensors. These strains are genetically modified to not produce AHL but can recognize these signaling molecules from cell-free supernatants, extracts of food samples, spent culture supernatants of bacteria isolated from food products or from the bacteria themselves. In general, biosensors contain a functional LuxR-family protein cloned together with a target promoter, which positively controls a phenotype (e.g., bioluminescence, β-galactosidase activity, green-fluorescent protein expression, and violacein pigment production). Also, thin-layer chromatography (TLC) is constantly associated with biosensors to identify AHLs by comparing migration between the target sample and standard AHLs.[78,79] However, more sophisticated methods have been applied in this area such as high-performance liquid chromatography (HPLC), ultra-performance liquid chromatography (UPLC), mass spectrometry (MS), liquid chromatography-MS (LC-MS), nuclear magnetic resonance spectroscopy (NMR), surface-enhanced Raman spectroscopy, or surface-enhanced Raman scattering (SERS), among other instrumental techniques.[80–83] The new technologies have advantages in detecting low concentrations of signaling molecules as well as in elucidating the molecular structure.

55.5 Quorum quenching in food safety

Because of the phenotypes regulated by the different mechanisms of QS in foodborne pathogens and consequently their importance in food safety, the inhibition of QS has become the target of studies with the aim to inhibit or alter the transcription of virulence genes. The mechanism of QS inhibition is called quorum quenching (QQ) and can occur by different strategies leading to changes in gene regulation, but without interfering with cell growth. QQ occurs naturally in some organisms to recycle or discard their AIs or even to eliminate those molecules produced by other organisms in a competitive relationship.[84,85]

Interestingly, in the literature, enzymes that inactivate AIs are called QQ enzymes, whilst compounds that interrupt QS pathways are called QS inhibitors.[85] However, in this chapter, we standardize all enzymes, antibodies, and compounds with QQ activity as quorum quenchers (QQer).

Different QQ strategies are known and vary in nature, such as the use of enzymes, antibodies and compounds; the mode of action, such as cleavage of AIs, and competitive inhibition, among others; targets of the QS system, such as synthesis, diffusion, accumulation, and perception of the AI. Physical parameters such as temperature and pH can also affect the half-life of AIs. Thus an overview of the QQ strategies is shown in Fig. 55.2.

The AI antagonism is the most studied strategy, followed by the degradation of AI through enzymes, since compounds and enzymes can be found easily in several sources, including food. In addition, they can be used for various pathogens, are applied easily, and do not depend on sophisticated technologies.[85,86]

Different QQer screening and identification strategies are used, including in silico, in vitro, and in situ methods. Virtual or in silico screenings allow the quick and economical selection of promising QQer from vast libraries of molecules, such as drugs already approved by official agencies that are likely endowed with low cytotoxicity and favorable pharmacological properties, as well as compounds from different sources, such as algae, marine sponges, plants, food, bacteria, and fungi. Thus the time and cost requirements for searching for QQer are lower than those for conventional in vitro processes, since only promising compounds will be validated through these experiments.[87,88] Molecular docking is the most widely used screening strategy for QQer in silico and can be performed in conjunction with molecular dynamics, as it allows predicting the mode of binding between the compound and the target, providing a molecular basis for its optimization in terms of binding affinity.[89] Another in silico analysis used is the search for genes potentially involved in QQ, such as genes that encode the enzymes lactonases, acylase, hydrolase, and oxidoreductase, in the genome of a single organism or in the metagenomic library.[90]

The strategies for the validation of the results in silico as well as for in vitro screening of QQer are numerous. These involve the use of the AI biosensor or reporter strain; quantification of AIs by TLC, HPLC, UPLC, MS, LC-MS, NMR, and SERS, among other instrumental techniques; evaluation of the interaction between QQer and the receptor protein of AIs by calorimetry and SERS; and qualitative and quantitative systems of phenotypes

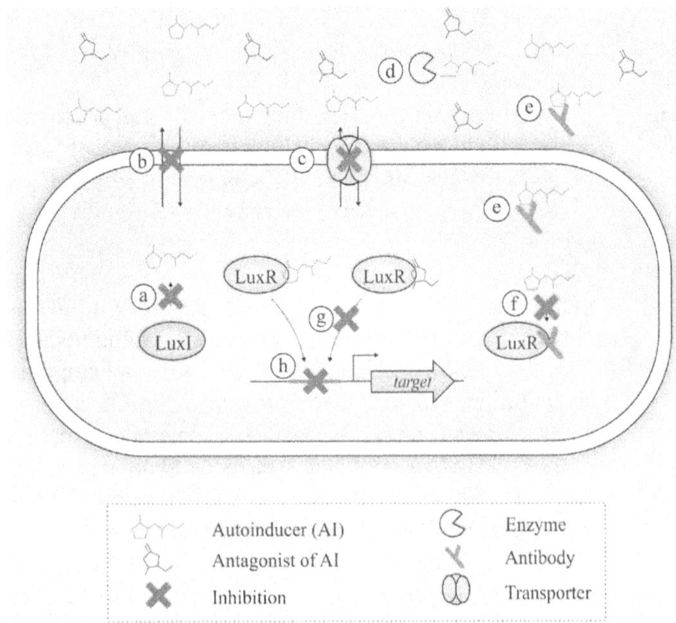

FIGURE 55.2 Quorum quenching (QQ) strategies: (a) inhibition of autoinducers (AIs) synthesis; (b and c) inhibition of AI secretion, transport, and internalization; (d) degradation of AIs using either catalytic antibodies, such as abzymes or enzymes, such as lactonases, acylase, hydrolase, and oxidoreductase; (e) sequestration of AIs using, for example, antibodies against AIs; (f) antibodies that "cover" and therefore block AI receptors; (g) antagonist of AIs, such as compounds; (h) inhibition of targets downstream of the binding of the AI to the receptor.

regulated by the QS. Examples of the latter are motility, violacein production, bioluminescence, elastase, exoproteases, siderophores, exotoxins, rhamnolipid, pyocyanin, and pyoverdin, among other phenotypes. The strategy for identifying and quantifying the phenotypes regulated by the QS is used most often because it is fast, cheap, and reliable.[80,84,90,91] It is worth mentioning that for the identification of QQer by in vitro strategies, it must be below the minimal inhibitory concentration, without altering the final cell density and growth kinetics of the evaluated microorganism.[92] The SERS can also be used to study QS signaling by releasing pyocyanin in situ, as in biofilms and QQer can be detected by modifying substrates due to its presence.[80]

QQ has become an important tool to inhibit virulence factors of pathogenic bacteria, mainly due to the increase in the number of strains resistant to antibiotics. QQ strategies can decrease the risk of developing resistance and tolerance to antibiotics and sanitizer products, prevent the production of virulence factors, toxins, and enzymes, and can be used as an adjuvant therapy for the treatment of infections. In the food industry, QQ could help to reduce the colonization of food surfaces, thereby contributing to food safety, integrity, and quality. Thus the search for QQer against bacteria in vitro can occur by investigating numerous sources, which can be evaluated in the form of extracts, essential oils, compounds, and enzymes, as well as through the application of nanotechnology strategies.[85,93–97] Some examples are shown in Table 55.1.[27,87,90,91,98–112]

The first QQer studied were the halogenated furanones produced by the Australian red algae, *Delisea pulchra*, which are antagonists of AIs. These compounds lead to a reduced expression of virulence factors, but their cytotoxicity and chemically unstable nature are undesirable characteristics.[113,114] Thus the toxicity and allergenicity of QQer identified through in silico and/or in vitro strategies must be evaluated for use as adjuvant therapy for the treatment of infections and for applications in food, since they will be in direct and/or indirect contact with food. Pharmacological properties are also essential to assess the solubility, lipophilicity, cell membrane permeability, and other characteristics of the QQer under study, which may interfere with its effectiveness.[87]

In silico tools and databases allow prior assessment of toxicity and pharmacological properties, such as OpenVirtualToxLab,[115] SwissADME,[116] and PubChem database,[117] among others available. However, these QQer must be validated by in vitro and in vivo experiments to identify the limits of acceptable daily intake and the level of adverse effects not observed, among other parameters. A good strategy is to use molecules with properties already known or approved by official agencies, as they probably have a low toxicity and favorable pharmacological properties.[87,88] However, in recent years, the demand for more natural products often present in food, plants, and other natural sources has increased, but to a large extent, their activities and properties are unknown. Bio-preservatives are an option, given the growing number of strains of multidrug-resistant food pathogens.[94,97]

The identified QQer that has ideal and favorable properties can be applied and evaluated by direct and/or indirect incorporation in food, packaging, cleaning, and sanitizing products or as adjuvant therapy for the treatment of infections, as shown in Fig. 55.3. However, these

TABLE 55.1 Examples of QQer identified in different sources and forms as well as their applications in food.

Source	Specific source	Form	Application	Target bacteria	Evaluated phenotype	Reference
Algae	*Sarcodiotheca gaudichaudii*; *Chondrus crispus*	Aqueous extract	Culture medium; *Caenorhabditis elegans*	*Salmonella* Enteritidis	Growth; biofilm formation; motility; expression of genes; survival	Kulshreshtha et al.[98]
Marine sponges	*Siphonochalina siphonella*	Isolated compound: siphonocholin; structure	Culture medium; in silico	*Acinetobacter baumannii* ATCC BAA747; *Chromobacterium violaceum* ATCC 12472; *Pseudomonas aeruginosa* PAO1; Methicillin-resistant *Staphylococcus aureus* ATCC 43300	Growth; pellicle and biofilm formation; swarming motility; production of violacein, elastase, protease, pyocyanin, chitinase, and exopolysaccharide; molecular docking	Alam et al.[99]
Plants	Essential oils of tea tree [*Melaleuca alternifolia* (Maiden & Betche) Cheel] and rosemary (*Rosmarinus officinalis* L.); extract of propolis; bee pollen; pomegranate dried extract	Dissolved in dimethyl sulfoxide (DMSO)	Culture medium	*C. violaceum* ATCC 12472; *Escherichia coli* O157:H7 ATCC 25158; *Listeria monocytogenes*	Growth; production of violacein	Alvarez et al.[100]
	Oregano (*Lippia graveolens*)	Essential oil	Culture medium; pectin film in medium, coating shrimp (*Litopenaeus vannamei*) and cucumber (*Cucumis sativus* L.)	*C. violaceum* ATCC 12472; *E. coli* O157:H7 ATCC 43890; *L. monocytogenes* ATCC 7644; *Salmonella* Choleraesuis ATCC 7001; *S. aureus* ATCC 6538	Growth; production of violacein	Alvarez et al.[101]
	Peppermint (*Mentha piperita*)	Essential oil	Culture medium; *C. elegans*	*Aeromonas hydrophila* WAF38; *C. violaceum* CV026; *E. coli* pEAL08-2 and MG4/pKDT17; *P. aeruginosa* PAO1	Growth; biofilm formation; swarming motility; production of violacein, elastase, protease, pyocyanin, chitinase, and exopolysaccharide; bioluminescence; survival	Husain et al.[102]
	Star anise (*Illicium verum* Hook. f.)	Extract	Culture medium; pasteurized milk	*C. violaceum ATCC 12472; P. aeruginosa ATCC 9027; Salmonella Typhimurium ATCC 50013; S. aureus ATCC 6538*	Growth; biofilm formation; swarming motility; production of violacein and exopolysaccharide; acidity test; total plate counts	Rahman et al.[103]

(*Continued*)

TABLE 55.1 (Continued)

Source	Specific source	Form	Application	Target bacteria	Evaluated phenotype	Reference
Foods	Rio red and Marsh white grapefruits	Supernatant juice; isolated compounds: dihydroxybergamottin and bergamottin	Culture medium	*E. coli* O157:H7; *P. aeruginosa*; *Salmonella* Typhimurium; *Vibrio harveyi* BB886, BB170, and BB120	Growth; biofilm formation; bioluminescence	Girennavar et al.[104]
	Pulp and seed of jambolan [*Syzygium cumini* (L.) Skeels]	Ethanolic fraction dissolved in water	Culture medium; active film using cellulose acetate	*A. hydrophila* IOC/FDA 110-36; *C. violaceum* ATCC 12472; *E. coli* ATCC 10536; *L. monocytogenes* ATCC 7644; *P. aeruginosa* ATCC 15442; *Pseudomonas fluorescens* NCTC 10038; *Salmonella* Typhimurium ATCC 14028; *Serratia marcescens* RM1; *S. aureus* ATCC 6538P	Antioxidant activity; growth; biofilm formation; swarming motility; production of violacein	Santos et al.[105]
Bacteria	*Bacillus licheniformis* DAHB1; *Bacillus subtilis* DAHB2; *Bacillus pumilus* DAHB3; *Bacillus thuringiensis* DAHB4	Bacterium; supernatant; isolated enzyme: AHL-lactonase (AiiA)	Culture medium; shrimps (*Fenneropenaeus indicus*)	*C. violaceum* CV026; *Vibrio parahaemolyticus* DAHP1	Growth; biofilm formation; production of violacein; virulence	Vinoj et al.[106]
	B. subtilis KATMIRA1933	Isolated compound: subtilosin	Culture medium	*C. violaceum* ATCC 12472; *E. coli* O157:H7; *Gardnerella vaginalis* ATCC 14018; *L. monocytogenes* ScottA; *P. aeruginosa* ATCC 14213	Growth; biofilm formation; production of violacein and AI-2	Algburi et al.[107]
	Lactic acid bacteria (LAB) from raw milk cheese and cheese processing environments	Sequencing of 9216 recombinant clones; clones of LAB	In silico; Culture medium	Metagenomic library; *C. violaceum* DSMZ 30191; *V. harveyi* DSMZ 19623	Functional screening; production of violacein; bioluminescence	Alexa (Oniciuc) et al.[90]
Fungi	*Penicillium chrysogenum* DXY-1	Isolated compound: tyrosol; structure	Culture medium; in silico	*C. violaceum* CV026; *P. aeruginosa* PAO1	Growth; biofilm formation; production of violacein, pyocyanin, elastase, and protease; molecular docking	Chang et al.[108]
Compounds	Resveratrol	Dissolved in DMSO	Culture medium	*C. violaceum* ATCC 12472; *E. coli* O157:H7 ATCC 25158; *L. monocytogenes*	Growth; production of violacein	Alvarez et al.[100]
	Menthol	Structure	Culture medium; *C. elegans;* in silico	*A. hydrophila* WAF38; *C. violaceum* CV026; *E. coli* pEAL08-2 and MG4/pKDT17; *P. aeruginosa* PAO1	Growth; biofilm formation; swarming motility; production of violacein, elastase, protease, pyocyanin, chitinase, and exopolysaccharide; bioluminescence; survival; molecular docking	Husain et al.[102]

	3-Methyl2(5H)-furanone; 2-methyltetrahydro-3-furanone; 2(5H)-furanone; 2,2-dimethyl-3(2H)-furanone	Mixture of four furanones dissolved in acetonitrile; structure	Culture medium; in silico	*Salmonella* Enteritidis PT4 578	Planktonic growth; swarming and twitching motility; adhesion and biofilm formation; molecular docking	Almeida et al.[27]
	Acetic acid; citric acid; lactic acid	-	Culture medium; cucumber	*C. violaceum* CV026 and CV 2656; *E. coli* MTCC 727; *Salmonella* Typhimurium ATCC 14028; Eight isolates of *E. coli*; Four isolates of *Salmonella* sp.	Growth; biofilm formation; swimming and swarming motility; production of violacein and exopolysaccharide	Amrutha et al.[109]
	107 plant compounds; 73 nonsteroidal antiinflammatory drugs; 5 furanones	Structure	In silico	*Salmonella* Enteritidis PT4 578	Biofilm formation; molecular docking; absorption; solubility; permeability	Almeida et al.[87]
	Curcumin	-	Culture medium	*A. hydrophila* ATCC 7966; Three isolates of *A. hydrophila*	Growth; biofilm formation; swimming and swarming motility; production of protease and hemolysin; expression of genes	Mangoudehi et al.[110]
	L-Ascorbic acid (vitamin C)	Dissolved in medium	Culture medium; Indian cottage cheese (Paneer)	*E. coli* EMC17	Growth; survival; killing; cell damage; reactive oxygen species; biofilm formation; production of AHL and exopolysaccharide; expression of genes; sensory analysis	Shivaprasad et al.[111]
Nanotechnology strategies	Essential oils from cumin (*Cuminum cyminum*); pepper (*Piper nigrum*); fennel (*Foeniculum vulgare*)	Nanoemulsion	Culture medium	*C. violaceum* MTCC 2656 and CV026; *E. coli* MTCC 727; *Klebsiella pneumoniae* MTCC 12202; *Salmonella* Typhimurium ATCC 14028	Growth; killing; biofilm formation; production of violacein and exopolysaccharide	Venkadesaperumal et al.[112]
	Nigella sativa seed extract	ZnO nanoparticles synthesized with extract	Culture medium; beef extract model media; lettuce leaf model media	*C. violaceum* ATCC 12472 and CV026; *E. coli*; *L. monocytogenes*; *P. aeruginosa* PAO1	Growth; biofilm formation; swarming motility; production of violacein, elastase, protease, pyocyanin, alginate, and exopolysaccharide; expression of genes	Al-Shabib et al.[91]

AHL, *N*-acyl homoserine lactones.

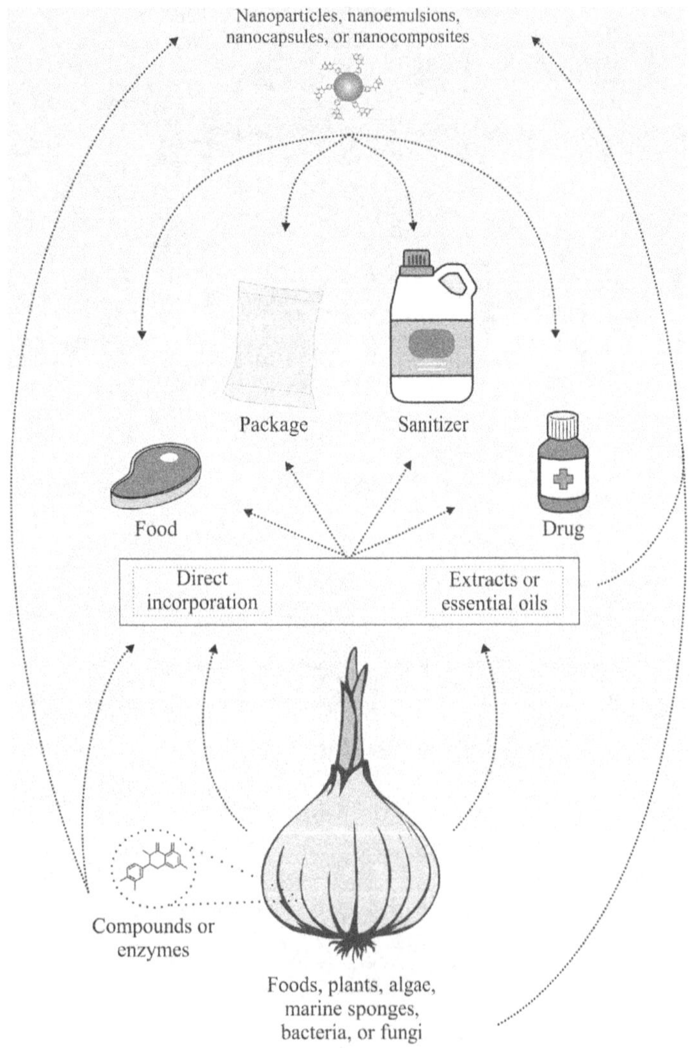

FIGURE 55.3 Direct and/or indirect incorporation of QQer in food, packaging, cleaning, and sanitizing products or as adjuvant therapy for the treatment of infections in its direct form or in extracts, essential oils, compounds, and enzymes, or using nanotechnological and pharmaceutical strategies.

studies are scarce (Table 55.1), but fundamental because of the different QS systems that can coexist synergistically or interfere with each other in a dynamic system. Food components can also inhibit some QS systems and improve others, just as they can inhibit added QQer and their effects. The microarchitecture of food as well as biotic and abiotic factors can drastically influence cell-to-cell communication and consequently, the QQ mechanism.[16,91,118] The direct incorporation of QQer into foods can also be a worrying factor, especially in the case of essential oils, as they can alter the sensory and rheological properties of foods.[97,119]

In addition to all the desirable properties of the QQer mentioned so far, their cost is also a crucial point for their application in food, as their value will be added to that of the product. The costs of synthesis, purification, and commercialization of QQer must be considered, as well as the costs of recovery of enzymes with QQ activity for their reuse. The cost–benefit ratio is an excellent parameter because it relates the cost of a QQer with its beneficial effect on the safety and useful life of the food; however, this ratio will depend on the type of food and the cost of the finished product. The added value is another important parameter, especially for QQer of natural origin, as there may be an appeal as bio-preservers of food.[97,120]

In this sense, QQer can be used as food additives or drugs with a QQ function to increase food safety and shelf life or in adjuvant therapy for the treatment of infections, respectively. However, for food, they must have QQ activity in situ in food or in vivo, a "Generally Recognized as Safe" status, and must be regulated by some official agency, such as the Food and Drug Administration (FDA) and the European Commission (EC) among other agencies depending on the country, or the Food and Agriculture Organization (FAO) and/or the World Health Organization (WHO) of the United Nations, at international level. In fact, some drugs, food additives and ingredients approved by these official agencies as well as other compounds naturally present in foods, have already been evaluated in silico, in vitro, in vivo, and/or in foods, showing that they have QQ activity,[94,97] as shown in Table 55.1. However, to date, none of these agencies has regulated any enzymes or compounds with QQ activity as a QQer for use in food and health fields.

55.6 Final considerations and perspectives

As shown in this chapter, knowing the QS mechanism of foodborne pathogens is extremely important to understand its role in cell physiology, in regulating biofilm formation, motility, enzyme production, and several other virulence factors of concern for food safety. Thus it is becoming increasingly necessary to develop AI detection and/or quantification techniques directly in food to understand AI correlation with food safety and spoilage of the product. In addition, the search for QQer from different sources against pathogens has shown promising results, but so far, no enzyme or compound with QQ activity has been regulated as QQer for use in food and health fields.

References

1. Fuqua WC, Winans SC, Greenberg EP. Quorum sensing in bacteria: the LuxR-LuxI family of cell density-responsive transcriptional regulators. *J Bacteriol.* 1994;176(2):269–275. Available from: https://doi.org/10.1128/jb.176.2.269-275.1994.
2. Nealson KH, Platt T, Hastings JW. Cellular control of the synthesis and activity of the bacterial luminescent system. *J Bacteriol.* 1970;104(1):313–322. Available from: https://doi.org/10.1128/JB.104.1.313-322.1970.
3. Gantner S, Schmid M, Dürr C, et al. *In situ* quantitation of the spatial scale of calling distances and population density-independent *N*-acylhomoserine lactone-mediated communication by rhizobacteria colonized on plant roots. *FEMS Microbiol Ecol.* 2006;56(2):188–194. Available from: https://doi.org/10.1111/j.1574-6941.2005.00037.x.
4. Prescott RD, Decho AW. Flexibility and adaptability of quorum sensing in nature. *Trends Microbiol.* 2020;28(6):436–444. Available from: https://doi.org/10.1016/j.tim.2019.12.004.
5. Vanetti MCD, Carneiro DG, Almeida FA, et al. *Autoinducer-1 quorum sensing communication mechanism in Gram-negative bacteria.* Trends in Quorum Sensing and Quorum Quenching. New Perspectives and Applications. CRC Press; 2020:9–29. Available from: http://doi.org/10.1201/9780429274817-2.
6. János J, Pongor S, Ligeti B. *Toward a systematic genomic survey of bacterial quorum sensing genes.* Trends in Quorum Sensing and Quorum Quenching. New Perspectives and Applications. CRC Press; 2020:31–45. Available from: http://doi.org/10.1201/9780429274817-3.
7. Papenfort K, Bassler BL. Quorum sensing signal–response systems in Gram-negative bacteria. *Nat Rev Microbiol.* 2016;14(9):576–588. Available from: https://doi.org/10.1038/nrmicro.2016.89.
8. Wu L, Luo Y. Bacterial quorum-sensing systems and their role in intestinal bacteria-host crosstalk. *Front Microbiol.* 2021;12:611413. Available from: https://doi.org/10.3389/fmicb.2021.611413.
9. Churchill MEA, Chen L. Structural basis of acyl-homoserine lactone-dependent signaling. *Chem Rev.* 2011;111(1):68–85. Available from: https://doi.org/10.1021/cr1000817.
10. Liu J, Fu K, Wu C, Qin K, Li F, Zhou L. "In-group" communication in marine *Vibrio*: a review of *N*-acyl homoserine lactones-driven quorum sensing. *Front Cell Infect Microbiol.* 2018;8:139. Available from: https://doi.org/10.3389/fcimb.2018.00139.
11. Von Bodman SB, Willey JM, Diggle SP. Cell-cell communication in bacteria: united we stand. *J Bacteriol.* 2008;190(13):4377–4391. Available from: https://doi.org/10.1128/JB.00486-08.
12. Soares JA, Ahmer BMM. Detection of acyl-homoserine lactones by *Escherichia* and *Salmonella*. *Curr Opin Microbiol.* 2011;14(2):188–193. Available from: https://doi.org/10.1016/j.mib.2011.01.006.
13. Sabag-Daigle A, Ahmer BMM. ExpI and PhzI are descendants of the long lost cognate signal synthase for SdiA. *PLoS One.* 2012;7(10):e47720. Available from: https://doi.org/10.1371/journal.pone.0047720.
14. Subramoni S, Salcedo DVF, Suarez-Moreno ZR. A bioinformatic survey of distribution, conservation, and probable functions of LuxR solo regulators in bacteria. *Front Cell Infect Microbiol.* 2015;5:16. Available from: https://doi.org/10.3389/fcimb.2015.00016.
15. Pereira CS, Thompson JA, Xavier KB. AI-2-mediated signalling in bacteria. *FEMS Microbiol Rev.* 2013;37(2):156–181. Available from: https://doi.org/10.1111/j.1574-6976.2012.00345.x.
16. Skandamis PN, Nychas G-JE. Quorum sensing in the context of food microbiology. *Appl Environ Microbiol.* 2012;78(16):5473–5482. Available from: https://doi.org/10.1128/AEM.00468-12.
17. Ng W-L, Bassler BL. Bacterial quorum-sensing network architectures. *Annu Rev Genet.* 2009;43:197–222. Available from: https://doi.org/10.1146/annurev-genet-102108-134304.
18. Sperandio V, Torres AG, Jarvis B, Nataro JP, Kaper JB. Bacteria host communication: the language of hormones. *Proc Natl Acad Sci U S A.* 2003;100(15):8951–8956. Available from: https://doi.org/10.1073/pnas.1537100100.
19. Moreira CG, Weinshenker D, Sperandio V. QseC mediates *Salmonella enterica* serovar Typhimurium virulence *in vitro* and *in vivo*. *Infect Immun.* 2010;78(3):914–926. Available from: https://doi.org/10.1128/IAI.01038-09.
20. Kim CS, Gatsios A, Cuesta S, et al. Characterization of autoinducer-3 structure and biosynthesis in *E. coli*. *ACS Cent Sci.* 2020;6(2):197–206. Available from: https://doi.org/10.1021/acscentsci.9b01076.
21. Hughes DT, Clarke MB, Yamamoto K, Rasko DA, Sperandio V. The QseC adrenergic signaling cascade in Enterohemorrhagic *E. coli* (EHEC). *PLoS Pathog.* 2009;5(8):e1000553. Available from: https://doi.org/10.1371/journal.ppat.1000553.
22. Thoendel M, Kavanaugh JS, Flack CE, Horswill AR. Peptide signaling in the staphylococci. *Chem Rev.* 2011;111(1):117–151. Available from: https://doi.org/10.1021/cr100370n.
23. Wang D, Ding X, Rather PN. Indole can act as an extracellular signal in *Escherichia coli*. *J Bacteriol.* 2001;183(14):4210–4216. Available from: https://doi.org/10.1128/JB.183.14.4210-4216.2001.
24. Zarkan A, Liu J, Matuszewska M, Gaimster H, Summers DK. Local and universal action: the paradoxes of indole signalling in bacteria. *Trends Microbiol.* 2020;28(7):566–577. Available from: https://doi.org/10.1016/j.tim.2020.02.007.

25. Lee J-H, Lee J. Indole as an intercellular signal in microbial communities. *FEMS Microbiol Rev.* 2010;34(4):426–444. Available from: https://doi.org/10.1111/j.1574-6976.2009.00204.x.
26. Campos-Galvão MEM, Ribon AOB, Araújo EF, Vanetti MCD. Changes in the *Salmonella enterica* Enteritidis phenotypes in presence of acyl homoserine lactone quorum sensing signals. *J Basic Microbiol.* 2016;56(5):493–501. Available from: https://doi.org/10.1002/jobm.201500471.
27. Almeida FA, Pimentel-Filho NJ, Pinto UM, Mantovani HC, Oliveira LL, Vanetti MCD. Acyl homoserine lactone-based quorum sensing stimulates biofilm formation by *Salmonella* Enteritidis in anaerobic conditions. *Arch Microbiol.* 2017;199(3):475–486. Available from: https://doi.org/10.1007/s00203-016-1313-6.
28. Atkinson S, Goldstone RJ, Joshua GWP, et al. Biofilm development on *Caenorhabditis elegans* by *Yersinia* is facilitated by quorum sensing-dependent repression of type III secretion. *PLoS Pathog.* 2011;7(1):e1001250. Available from: https://doi.org/10.1371/journal.ppat.1001250.
29. Moorhead SM, Griffiths MW. Expression and characterization of cell-signalling molecules in *Campylobacter jejuni. J Appl Microbiol.* 2011;110(3):786–800. Available from: https://doi.org/10.1111/j.1365-2672.2010.04934.x.
30. Culler HF, Couto SCF, Higa JS, et al. Role of SdiA on biofilm formation by atypical Enteropathogenic *Escherichia coli. Genes (Basel).* 2018;9(5):253. Available from: https://doi.org/10.3390/genes9050253.
31. Šimunović K, Ramić D, Xu C, Smole Možina S. Modulation of *Campylobacter jejuni* motility, adhesion to polystyrene surfaces, and invasion of INT407 cells by quorum-sensing inhibition. *Microorganisms.* 2020;8(1):104. Available from: https://doi.org/10.3390/microorganisms8010104.
32. Kaur A, Capalash N, Sharma P. Expression of *Meiothermus ruber luxS* in *E. coli* alters the antibiotic susceptibility and biofilm formation. *Appl Microbiol Biotechnol.* 2020;104(10):4457–4469. Available from: https://doi.org/10.1007/s00253-020-10480-8.
33. Guo M, Fang Z, Sun L, et al. Regulation of thermostable direct hemolysin and biofilm formation of *Vibrio parahaemolyticus* by quorum-sensing genes *luxM* and *luxS. Curr Microbiol.* 2018;75(9):1190–1197. Available from: https://doi.org/10.1007/s00284-018-1508-y.
34. Bridges AA, Bassler BL. The intragenus and interspecies quorum-sensing autoinducers exert distinct control over *Vibrio cholerae* biofilm formation and dispersal. *PLoS Biol.* 2019;17(11):e3000429. Available from: https://doi.org/10.1371/journal.pbio.3000429.
35. Boles BR, Horswill AR. *agr*-mediated dispersal of *Staphylococcus aureus* biofilms. *PLoS Pathog.* 2008;4(4):e1000052. Available from: https://doi.org/10.1371/journal.ppat.1000052.
36. Grande R, Nistico L, Sambanthamoorthy K, et al. Temporal expression of *agrB*, *cidA*, and *alsS* in the early development of *Staphylococcus aureus* UAMS-1 biofilm formation and the structural role of extracellular DNA and carbohydrates. *Pathog Dis.* 2014;70(3):414–422. Available from: https://doi.org/10.1111/2049-632X.12158.
37. He L, Le KY, Khan BA, et al. Resistance to leukocytes ties benefits of quorum sensing dysfunctionality to biofilm infection. *Nat Microbiol.* 2019;4(7):1114–1119. Available from: https://doi.org/10.1038/s41564-019-0413-x.
38. Vidal JE, Shak JR, Canizalez-Roman A. The CpAL quorum sensing system regulates production of hemolysins CPA and PFO to build *Clostridium perfringens* biofilms. *Infect Immun.* 2015;83(6):2430–2442. Available from: https://doi.org/10.1128/IAI.00240-15.
39. Lee Y, Wang C. Links between S-adenosylmethionine and Agr-based quorum sensing for biofilm development in *Listeria monocytogenes* EGD-e. *Microbiologyopen.* 2020;9(5). Available from: https://doi.org/10.1002/mbo3.1015.
40. Zetzmann M, Bucur FI, Crauwels P, et al. Characterization of the biofilm phenotype of a *Listeria monocytogenes* mutant deficient in *agr* peptide sensing. *Microbiologyopen.* 2019;8(9). Available from: https://doi.org/10.1002/mbo3.826.
41. Gandra TKV, Volcan D, Kroning IS, et al. Expression levels of the *agr* locus and *prfA* gene during biofilm formation by *Listeria monocytogenes* on stainless steel and polystyrene during 8 to 48 h of incubation 10 to 37°C. *Int J Food Microbiol.* 2019;300:1–7. Available from: https://doi.org/10.1016/j.ijfoodmicro.2019.03.021.
42. Ma X, Zhang S, Xu Z, et al. SdiA improves the acid tolerance of *E. coli* by regulating GadW and GadY expression. *Front Microbiol.* 2020;11:1078. Available from: https://doi.org/10.3389/fmicb.2020.01078.
43. Van Houdt R, Aertsen A, Moons P, Vanoirbeek K, Michiels CW. *N*-acyl-L-homoserine lactone signal interception by *Escherichia coli. FEMS Microbiol Lett.* 2006;256(1):83–89. Available from: https://doi.org/10.1111/j.1574-6968.2006.00103.x.
44. Freitas LL, Santos CIA, Carneiro DG, Vanetti MCD. Nisin and acid resistance in *Salmonella* is enhanced by *N*-dodecanoyl-homoserine lactone. *Microb Pathog.* 2020;147:104320. Available from: https://doi.org/10.1016/j.micpath.2020.104320.
45. Richards SM, Strandberg KL, Conroy M, Gunn JS. Cationic antimicrobial peptides serve as activation signals for the *Salmonella* Typhimurium PhoPQ and PmrAB regulons *in vitro* and *in vivo. Front Cell Infect Microbiol.* 2012;2. Available from: https://doi.org/10.3389/fcimb.2012.00102.
46. Ramamurthy T, Ghosh A, Pazhani GP, Shinoda S. Current perspectives on viable but non-culturable (VBNC) pathogenic bacteria. *Front Public Health.* 2014;2:103. Available from: https://doi.org/10.3389/fpubh.2014.00103.
47. He Y, Frye JG, Strobaugh TP, Chen C-Y. Analysis of AI-2/LuxS-dependent transcription in *Campylobacter jejuni* strain 81-176. *Foodborne Pathog Dis.* 2008;5(4):399–415. Available from: https://doi.org/10.1089/fpd.2008.0106.
48. Ligowska M, Cohn MT, Stabler RA, Wren BW, Brøndsted L. Effect of chicken meat environment on gene expression of *Campylobacter jejuni* and its relevance to survival in food. *Int J Food Microbiol.* 2011;145(suppl 1:):S111–S115. Available from: https://doi.org/10.1016/j.ijfoodmicro.2010.08.027.
49. Park H, Lee K, Yeo S, Shin H, Holzapfel WH. Autoinducer-2 quorum sensing influences viability of *Escherichia coli* O157:H7 under osmotic and *in vitro* gastrointestinal stress conditions. *Front Microbiol.* 2017;8:1077. Available from: https://doi.org/10.3389/fmicb.2017.01077.
50. Zhao L, Xue T, Shang F, Sun H, Sun B. *Staphylococcus aureus* AI-2 quorum sensing associates with the KdpDE two-component system to regulate capsular polysaccharide synthesis and virulence. *Infect Immun.* 2010;78(8):3506–3515. Available from: https://doi.org/10.1128/IAI.00131-10.
51. Xue T, Zhao L, Sun B. LuxS/AI-2 system is involved in antibiotic susceptibility and autolysis in *Staphylococcus aureus* NCTC 8325.

Int J Antimicrob Agents. 2013;41(1):85–89. Available from: https://doi.org/10.1016/j.ijantimicag.2012.08.016.
52. Nesse LL, Berg K, Vestby LK, Olsaker I, Djønne B. *Salmonella* Typhimurium invasion of HEp-2 epithelial cells *in vitro* is increased by *N*-acylhomoserine lactone quorum sensing signals. *Acta Vet Scand*. 2011;53(1):44. Available from: https://doi.org/10.1186/1751-0147-53-44.
53. Freitas LL, Silva FP, Fernandes KM, et al. The virulence of *Salmonella* Enteritidis in *Galleria mellonella* is improved by *N*-dodecanoyl-homoserine lactone. *Microb Pathog*. 2021;152:104730. Available from: https://doi.org/10.1016/j.micpath.2021.104730.
54. Plummer P, Sahin O, Burrough E, et al. Critical role of LuxS in the virulence of *Campylobacter jejuni* in a guinea pig model of abortion. *Infect Immun*. 2012;80(2):585–593. Available from: https://doi.org/10.1128/IAI.05766-11.
55. Jeon B, Itoh K, Ryu S. Promoter analysis of cytolethal distending toxin genes (*cdtA, B*, and *C*) and effect of a *luxS* mutation on CDT production in *Campylobacter jejuni*. *Microbiol Immunol*. 2005;49(7):599–603. Available from: https://doi.org/10.1111/j.1348-0421.2005.tb03651.x.
56. Day WAJ, Maurelli AT. *Shigella flexneri* LuxS quorum-sensing system modulates *virB* expression but is not essential for virulence. *Infect Immun*. 2001;69(1):15–23. Available from: https://doi.org/10.1128/IAI.69.1.15-23.2001.
57. Mashruwala AA, Bassler BL. The *Vibrio cholerae* quorum-sensing protein VqmA integrates cell density, environmental, and host-derived cues into the control of virulence. *mBio*. 2020;11(4). Available from: https://doi.org/10.1128/mBio.01572-20.
58. Watve S, Barrasso K, Jung SA, et al. Parallel quorum-sensing system in *Vibrio cholerae* prevents signal interference inside the host. *PLoS Pathog*. 2020;16(2):e1008313. Available from: https://doi.org/10.1371/journal.ppat.1008313.
59. Walters M, Sperandio V. Autoinducer 3 and epinephrine signaling in the kinetics of locus of enterocyte effacement gene expression in Enterohemorrhagic *Escherichia coli*. *Infect Immun*. 2006;74(10):5445–5455. Available from: https://doi.org/10.1128/IAI.00099-06.
60. Bansal T, Englert D, Lee J, Hegde M, Wood TK, Jayaraman A. Differential effects of epinephrine, norepinephrine, and indole on *Escherichia coli* O157:H7 chemotaxis, colonization, and gene expression. *Infect Immun*. 2007;75(9):4597–4607. Available from: https://doi.org/10.1128/IAI.00630-07.
61. Sule N, Pasupuleti S, Kohli N, et al. The norepinephrine metabolite 3,4-dihydroxymandelic acid is produced by the commensal microbiota and promotes chemotaxis and virulence gene expression in Enterohemorrhagic *Escherichia coli*. *Infect Immun*. 2017;85(10). Available from: https://doi.org/10.1128/IAI.00431-17.
62. Karavolos MH, Spencer H, Bulmer DM, et al. Adrenaline modulates the global transcriptional profile of *Salmonella* revealing a role in the antimicrobial peptide and oxidative stress resistance responses. *BMC Genomics*. 2008;9:458. Available from: https://doi.org/10.1186/1471-2164-9-458.
63. Moreira CG, Sperandio V. Interplay between the QseC and QseE bacterial adrenergic sensor kinases in *Salmonella enterica* serovar Typhimurium pathogenesis. *Infect Immun*. 2012;80(12):4344–4353. Available from: https://doi.org/10.1128/IAI.00803-12.
64. Le KY, Otto M. Quorum-sensing regulation in staphylococci – an overview. *Front Microbiol*. 2015;6. Available from: https://doi.org/10.3389/fmicb.2015.01174.
65. Jenul C, Horswill AR. Regulation of *Staphylococcus aureus* virulence. *Microbiol Spectr*. 2019;7(2). Available from: https://doi.org/10.1128/microbiolspec.GPP3-0031-2018.
66. Karatzas KAG, Lemmens-den Toom NA, Tassou CC, Leeuwen W, Belkum A. Molecular characterization of piezotolerant and stress-resistant mutants of *Staphylococcus aureus*. *J Appl Microbiol*. 2021;130(3):901–912. Available from: https://doi.org/10.1111/jam.14832.
67. Riedel CU, Monk IR, Casey PG, Waidmann MS, Gahan CGM, Hill C. AgrD-dependent quorum sensing affects biofilm formation, invasion, virulence and global gene expression profiles in *Listeria monocytogenes*. *Mol Microbiol*. 2009;71(5):1177–1189. Available from: https://doi.org/10.1111/j.1365-2958.2008.06589.x.
68. Autret N, Raynaud C, Dubail I, Berche P, Charbit A. Identification of the *agr* locus of *Listeria monocytogenes*: role in bacterial virulence. *Infect Immun*. 2003;71(8):4463–4471. Available from: https://doi.org/10.1128/iai.71.8.4463-4471.2003.
69. Ohtani K, Shimizu T. Regulation of toxin production in *Clostridium perfringens*. *Toxins (Basel)*. 2016;8(7):207. Available from: https://doi.org/10.3390/toxins8070207.
70. Ahmed UKB, Shadid TM, Larabee JL, Ballard JD. Combined and distinct roles of Agr proteins in *Clostridioides difficile* 630 sporulation, motility, and toxin production. *mBio*. 2020;11(6). Available from: https://doi.org/10.1128/mBio.03190-20.
71. Cooksley CM, Davis IJ, Winzer K, Chan WC, Peck MW, Minton NP. Regulation of neurotoxin production and sporulation by a putative *agrBD* signaling system in proteolytic *Clostridium botulinum*. *Appl Environ Microbiol*. 2010;76(13):4448–4460. Available from: https://doi.org/10.1128/AEM.03038-09.
72. Azimi S, Klementiev AD, Whiteley M, Diggle SP. Bacterial quorum sensing during infection. *Annu Rev Microbiol*. 2020;74(1):201–219. Available from: https://doi.org/10.1146/annurev-micro-032020-093845.
73. Gram L, Christensen AB, Ravn L, Molin S, Givskov M. Production of acylated homoserine lactones by psychrotrophic members of the Enterobacteriaceae isolated from foods. *Appl Environ Microbiol*. 1999;65(8):3458–3463. Available from: https://doi.org/10.1128/AEM.65.8.3458-3463.1999.
74. Bruhn JB, Christensen AB, Flodgaard LR, et al. Presence of acylated homoserine lactones (AHLs) and AHL-producing bacteria in meat and potential role of AHL in spoilage of meat. *Appl Environ Microbiol*. 2004;70(7):4293–4302. Available from: https://doi.org/10.1128/AEM.70.7.4293-4302.2004.
75. Lu L, Hume ME, Pillai SD. Autoinducer-2-like activity associated with foods and its interaction with food additives. *J Food Prot*. 2004;67(7):1457–1462. Available from: https://doi.org/10.4315/0362-028X-67.7.1457.
76. Blana VA, Nychas G-JE. Presence of quorum sensing signal molecules in minced beef stored under various temperature and packaging conditions. *Int J Food Microbiol*. 2014;173:1–8. Available from: https://doi.org/10.1016/j.ijfoodmicro.2013.11.028.
77. Özcan SS, Dieser M, Parker AE, Balasubramanian N, Foreman CM. Quorum sensing inhibition as a promising method to control biofilm growth in metalworking fluids. *J Ind Microbiol Biotechnol*. 2019;46(8):1103–1111. Available from: https://doi.org/10.1007/s10295-019-02181-7.
78. Pinto UM, Viana ES, Martins ML, Vanetti MCD. Detection of acylated homoserine lactones in gram-negative proteolytic

psychrotrophic bacteria isolated from cooled raw milk. *Food Control*. 2007;18(10):1322–1327. Available from: https://doi.org/10.1016/j.foodcont.2006.09.005.

79. Steindler L, Venturi V. Detection of quorum-sensing *N*-acyl homoserine lactone signal molecules by bacterial biosensors. *FEMS Microbiol Lett*. 2007;266(1):1–9. Available from: https://doi.org/10.1111/j.1574-6968.2006.00501.x.
80. Bodelón G, Montes-García V, López-Puente V, et al. Detection and imaging of quorum sensing in *Pseudomonas aeruginosa* biofilm communities by surface-enhanced resonance Raman scattering. *Nat Mater*. 2016;15(11):1203–1211. Available from: https://doi.org/10.1038/nmat4720.
81. Lépine F, Milot S, Groleau M-C, Déziel E. Liquid chromatography/mass spectrometry (LC/MS) for the detection and quantification of *N*-acyl-L-homoserine lactones (AHLs) and 4-hydroxy-2-alkylquinolines (HAQs). *Methods Mol Biol*. 2018;1673:49–59. Available from: https://doi.org/10.1007/978-1-4939-7309-5_4.
82. Rothballer M, Uhl J, Kunze J, Schmitt-Kopplin P, Hartmann A. Detection of the bacterial quorum-sensing signaling molecules *N*-acyl-homoserine lactones (HSL) and *N*-acyl-homoserine (HS) with an enzyme-linked immunosorbent assay (ELISA) and via ultrahigh-performance liquid chromatography coupled to mass spectrometry (UHPLC-MS). *Methods Mol Biol*. 2018;1673:61–72. Available from: https://doi.org/10.1007/978-1-4939-7309-5_5.
83. Cutignano A. Analytical approaches for the identification of quorum sensing molecules. In: Tommonaro G, ed. *Quorum Sensing – Molecular Mechanism and Biotechnological Application*. Academic Press; 2019:29–53. Available from: http://doi.org/10.1016/B978-0-12-814905-8.00002-2.
84. Adak S, Upadrasta L, Kumar S, Soni R, Banerjee R. Quorum quenching – an alternative antimicrobial therapeutics. In: Méndez-Vilas A, ed. *Science Against Microbial Pathogens: Communicating Current Research and Technological Advances*. Formatex Research Center; 2011:586–593.
85. Grandclément C, Tannières M, Moréra S, Dessaux Y, Faure D. Quorum quenching: role in nature and applied developments. *FEMS Microbiol Rev*. 2016;40(1):86–116. Available from: https://doi.org/10.1093/femsre/fuv038.
86. Zhang J, Feng T, Wang J, Wang Y, Zhang X-H. The mechanisms and applications of quorum sensing (QS) and quorum quenching (QQ). *J Ocean Univ China*. 2019;18(6):1427–1442. Available from: https://doi.org/10.1007/s11802-019-4073-5.
87. Almeida FA, Vargas ELG, Carneiro DG, Pinto UM, Vanetti MCD. Virtual screening of plant compounds and nonsteroidal anti-inflammatory drugs for inhibition of quorum sensing and biofilm formation in *Salmonella*. *Microb Pathog*. 2018;121:369–388. Available from: https://doi.org/10.1016/j.micpath.2018.05.014.
88. Mellini M, Di Muzio E, D'Angelo F, et al. *In silico* selection and experimental validation of FDA-approved drugs as anti-quorum sensing agents. *Front Microbiol*. 2019;10:2355. Available from: https://doi.org/10.3389/fmicb.2019.02355.
89. Reuter K, Steinbach A, Helms V. Interfering with bacterial quorum sensing. *Perspect Med Chem*. 2016;8:1–15. Available from: https://doi.org/10.4137/PMC.S13209.
90. Alexa (Oniciuc) EA, Walsh CJ, Coughlan LM, et al. Dairy products and dairy-processing environments as a reservoir of antibiotic resistance and quorum-quenching determinants as revealed through functional metagenomics. *mSystems*. 2020;5(1). Available from: https://doi.org/10.1128/mSystems.00723-19. e00723-19.
91. Al-Shabib NA, Husain FM, Ahmed F, et al. Biogenic synthesis of zinc oxide nanostructures from *Nigella sativa* seed: prospective role as food packaging material inhibiting broad-spectrum quorum sensing and biofilm. *Sci Rep*. 2016;6(1):36761. Available from: https://doi.org/10.1038/srep36761.
92. Defoirdt T, Brackman G, Coenye T. Quorum sensing inhibitors: how strong is the evidence? *Trends Microbiol*. 2013;21(12):619–624. Available from: https://doi.org/10.1016/j.tim.2013.09.006.
93. Suga H, Smith K. Molecular mechanisms of bacterial quorum sensing as a new drug target. *Curr Opin Chem Biol*. 2003;7(5):586–591. Available from: https://doi.org/10.1016/j.cbpa.2003.08.001.
94. Bai AJ, Rai VR. Bacterial quorum sensing and food industry. *Compr Rev Food Sci Food Saf*. 2011;10(3):183–193. Available from: https://doi.org/10.1111/j.1541-4337.2011.00150.x.
95. Silvestre C, Duraccio D, Cimmino S. Food packaging based on polymer nanomaterials. *Prog Polym Sci*. 2011;36(12):1766–1782. Available from: https://doi.org/10.1016/j.progpolymsci.2011.02.003.
96. Kalia VC. Quorum sensing inhibitors: an overview. *Biotechnol Adv*. 2013;31(2):224–245. Available from: https://doi.org/10.1016/j.biotechadv.2012.10.004.
97. Barberis S, Quiroga HG, Barcia C, Talia JM, Debattista N. Natural food preservatives against microorganisms. In: Grumezescu AM, Holban AM, eds. *Food Safety and Preservation*. Elsevier; 2018:621–658. Available from: http://doi.org/10.1016/B978-0-12-814956-0.00020-2.
98. Kulshreshtha G, Borza T, Rathgeber B, et al. Red seaweeds *Sarcodiotheca gaudichaudii* and *Chondrus crispus* down regulate virulence factors of *Salmonella* Enteritidis and induce immune responses in *Caenorhabditis elegans*. *Front Microbiol*. 2016;7:421. Available from: https://doi.org/10.3389/fmicb.2016.00421.
99. Alam P, Alqahtani AS,#Mabood Husain F, et al. Siphonocholin isolated from red sea sponge *Siphonochalina siphonella* attenuates quorum sensing controlled virulence and biofilm formation. *Saudi Pharm J*. 2020;28(11):1383–1391. Available from: https://doi.org/10.1016/j.jsps.2020.09.002.
100. Alvarez MV, Moreira MR, Ponce A. Antiquorum sensing and antimicrobial activity of natural agents with potential use in food. *J Food Saf*. 2012;32(3):379–387. Available from: https://doi.org/10.1111/j.1745-4565.2012.00390.x.
101. Alvarez MV, Ortega-Ramirez LA, Gutierrez-Pacheco MM, et al. Oregano essential oil-pectin edible films as anti-quorum sensing and food antimicrobial agents. *Front Microbiol*. 2014;5:699. Available from: https://doi.org/10.3389/fmicb.2014.00699.
102. Husain FM, Ahmad I, Khan MS, et al. Sub-MICs of *Mentha piperita* essential oil and menthol inhibits AHL mediated quorum sensing and biofilm of Gram-negative bacteria. *Front Microbiol*. 2015;6:420. Available from: https://doi.org/10.3389/fmicb.2015.00420.
103. Rahman MRT, Lou Z, Zhang J, et al. Star Anise (*Illicium verum* Hook. f.) as quorum sensing and biofilm formation inhibitor on foodborne bacteria: study in milk. *J Food Prot*. 2017;80(4):645–653. Available from: https://doi.org/10.4315/0362-028X.JFP-16-294.
104. Girennavar B, Cepeda ML, Soni KA, et al. Grapefruit juice and its furocoumarins inhibits autoinducer signaling and biofilm formation in bacteria. *Int J Food Microbiol*. 2008;125(2):204–208. Available from: https://doi.org/10.1016/j.ijfoodmicro.2008.03.028.

105. Santos CA, Almeida FA, Quecán BXV, et al. Bioactive properties of *Syzygium cumini* (L.) Skeels pulp and seed phenolic extracts. *Front Microbiol*. 2020;11:990. Available from: https://doi.org/10.3389/fmicb.2020.00990.
106. Vinoj G, Vaseeharan B, Thomas S, Spiers AJ, Shanthi S. Quorum-quenching activity of the AHL-lactonase from *Bacillus licheniformis* DAHB1 inhibits *Vibrio* biofilm formation *in vitro* and reduces shrimp intestinal colonisation and mortality. *Mar Biotechnol (NY)*. 2014;16(6):707–715. Available from: https://doi.org/10.1007/s10126-014-9585-9.
107. Algburi A, Zehm S, Netrebov V, Bren AB, Chistyakov V, Chikindas ML. Subtilosin prevents biofilm formation by inhibiting bacterial quorum sensing. *Probiotics Antimicrob Proteins*. 2017;9(1):81–90. Available from: https://doi.org/10.1007/s12602-016-9242-x.
108. Chang A, Sun S, Li L, et al. Tyrosol from marine fungi, a novel quorum sensing inhibitor against *Chromobacterium violaceum* and *Pseudomonas aeruginosa*. *Bioorg Chem*. 2019;91:103140. Available from: https://doi.org/10.1016/j.bioorg.2019.103140.
109. Amrutha B, Sundar K, Shetty PH. Effect of organic acids on biofilm formation and quorum signaling of pathogens from fresh fruits and vegetables. *Microb Pathog*. 2017;111:156–162. Available from: https://doi.org/10.1016/j.micpath.2017.08.042.
110. Mangoudehi HT, Zamani H, Shahangian SS, Mirzanejad L. Effect of curcumin on the expression of *ahyI/R* quorum sensing genes and some associated phenotypes in pathogenic *Aeromonas hydrophila* fish isolates. *World J Microbiol Biotechnol*. 2020;36(5):70. Available from: https://doi.org/10.1007/s11274-020-02846-x.
111. Shivaprasad DP, Taneja NK, Lakra A, Sachdev D. *In vitro* and *in situ* abrogation of biofilm formation in *E. coli* by vitamin C through ROS generation, disruption of quorum sensing and exopolysaccharide production. *Food Chem*. 2021;341(Pt 1):128171. Available from: https://doi.org/10.1016/j.foodchem.2020.128171.
112. Venkadesaperumal G, Rucha S, Sundar K, Shetty PH. Anti-quorum sensing activity of spice oil nanoemulsions against food borne pathogens. *LWT Food Sci Technol*. 2016;66:225–231. Available from: https://doi.org/10.1016/j.lwt.2015.10.044.
113. Givskov M, de Nys R, Manefield M, et al. Eukaryotic interference with homoserine lactone-mediated prokaryotic signalling. *J Bacteriol*. 1996;178(22):6618–6622. Available from: https://doi.org/10.1128/jb.178.22.6618-6622.1996.
114. Hentzer M, Riedel K, Rasmussen TB, et al. Inhibition of quorum sensing in *Pseudomonas aeruginosa* biofilm bacteria by a halogenated furanone compound. *Microbiology*. 2002;148(Pt 1):87–102. Available from: https://doi.org/10.1099/00221287-148-1-87.
115. Vedani A, Dobler M, Hu Z, Smieško M. OpenVirtualToxLab—a platform for generating and exchanging *in silico* toxicity data. *Toxicol Lett*. 2015;232(2):519–532. Available from: https://doi.org/10.1016/j.toxlet.2014.09.004.
116. Daina A, Michielin O, Zoete V. SwissADME: a free web tool to evaluate pharmacokinetics, drug-likeness and medicinal chemistry friendliness of small molecules. *Sci Rep*. 2017;7(1):42717. Available from: https://doi.org/10.1038/srep42717.
117. Kim S, Chen J, Cheng T, et al. PubChem in 2021: new data content and improved web interfaces. *Nucleic Acids Res*. 2021;49(D1):D1388–D1395. Available from: https://doi.org/10.1093/nar/gkaa971.
118. Galié S, García-Gutiérrez C, Miguélez EM, Villar CJ, Lombó F. Biofilms in the food industry: health aspects and control methods. *Front Microbiol*. 2018;9:898. Available from: https://doi.org/10.3389/fmicb.2018.00898.
119. Bai AJ, Vittal RR. Quorum sensing inhibitory and anti-biofilm activity of essential oils and their *in vivo* efficacy in food systems. *Food Biotechnol*. 2014;28(3):269–292. Available from: https://doi.org/10.1080/08905436.2014.932287.
120. David JRD, Steenson LR, Davidson PM. Expectations and applications of natural antimicrobials to foods: a guidance document for users, suppliers, research and development, and regulatory agencies. *Food Prot Trends*. 2013;33:238–247.

Chapter 56

Significance of identifying microbial DNA in foods and raw materials without concomitant detection of respective viable populations

Luca Cocolin

Department of Agriculture, Forest and Food Sciences, University of Turin, Grugliasco, Italy

Abstract

The advent of molecular biology–based methods in food microbiology has revolutionized the way detection and quantification of foodborne pathogens are carried out. We may not rely anymore on the capability of the microbial cell to grow on synthetic media, as we search for nucleic acids belonging to the target microorganism to assess its presence or absence. The stability of DNA, though, introduces some challenges in the interpretation of the results obtained, especially when PCR is employed to amplify the target. In this chapter we will describe the strategies to use and to correctly interpret the results of a food safety analysis. As it will be indicated a hybrid approach, based on a preenrichment period, followed by PCR amplification should guarantee the robustness of the result, based on which the food business operator can take the appropriate decisions with the final goal of protecting public health.

Keywords: Nucleic acids stability; viable not culturable state; molecular methods; culture-dependent methods; culture-independent methods

56.1 Introduction

Food safety is an aspect food business operators (FBOs) must address on a daily basis. According to the food legislation, FBO have to guarantee the absence of hazards that could harm the consumers, thereby protecting public health. If those safety criteria are not respected, food cannot be commercialized.

Nowadays, there a number of approaches that allow FBOs to move safely in this context and the implementation of risk analysis, including hazard analysis critical control points, is one of the most effective strategies, that has been introduced since the beginning of the 2000s with the entering into force of the Regulation 178/2002.[1]

When it comes to microbiological food safety, the FBO has to compromise between the need for fast results on the presence, absence, and quantification of specific pathogenic bacteria and the slowness of traditional culturing methods, which need several days to obtain the needed result. Especially in a context of globalization, where foodstuffs are moved around the globe, and due to the fact that shelf-life has become a challenge, because consumers' desire is to access foods that are as less as possible processed and retaining the characteristics of fresh produce, thereby food processing should be as mild as possible, FBOs have to find suitable solutions to properly address the food safety objectives and be absolutely sure that foods that are exiting from their plants are free of foodborne pathogens.

This aspect becomes even more relevant if we consider the fact that the microbiological methods recognized as official, are all based on cultivation (e.g., ISO (International Organization for Standardisation) methods) and if other analytical approaches are used, they have to be validated by following international guidelines [e.g., Food and Drug Administration (FDA), Guidelines for the Validation of Microbiological Methods for the FDA Foods Program, Third Edition] and have to meet the satisfaction of the food safety authority inspector.

In the last 50 years, we have assisted to a revolution in the way microbiological analysis can be executed, changing paradigms such as the need to cultivate microorganisms in

Present Knowledge in Food Safety. DOI: https://doi.org/10.1016/B978-0-12-819470-6.00020-2

order to detect them. Instead of promoting their growth in synthetic media and in laboratory conditions, often very far away from the real situation in which microorganisms are found in food, we have learnt to look at other ways to understand if they are present or not in a given sample. These alternative ways of detecting microbes have been promoted essentially by the significant advancements in the field of molecular biology. The possibility to search for microorganisms, without the need to cultivate them, let the differentiation between culture-dependent methods and culture-independent methods.[2] To note that the differentiation is not based on the use of molecular methods, in fact PCR applied to identify microbial isolates from a given ecosystem, is culture based.

56.2 The molecular biology area

As indicated above, the differentiation between culture-dependent and culture-independent methods is the use or omission of cultivation, respectively, to detect microorganisms. In culture-dependent methods we exploit the ability of microbes to grow in synthetic media, both solid and liquid, and after an isolation in pure culture, microorganisms are identified by using phenotypic and genotypic tests. In culture-independent methods, the cultivation is by-passed and the detection takes place by targeting microbial macromolecules, such as DNA, RNA, and proteins. With the use of culture-dependent methods we are able to detect alive microbial populations, while with culture-dependent methods we analyze the total microbial populations and, most of the times, it is not possible to assess if those are alive or dead. This circumstance has important implications when addressing food safety. In fact, only foods containing alive populations of pathogens should be considered at risk if consumed. What is the significance, then, of having positive results from DNA without knowing if the target foodborne pathogen is alive or not?

The accuracy of the culture-dependent methods to assess the safety of foodstuffs has been criticized mainly because:

- injured and stressed cells are not always recovered due to the fact that in selective media, usually supplemented with antibiotics and other selective agents, they are not able to grow and as a consequence false-negative results can be obtained;
- low numbers of pathogenic microorganisms are complicated to recover, especially when they are hard to handle in laboratory[3] or when they do not show competitive power and they grow slow.[4] Sometimes they may even be impossible to cultivate.[5]

Lastly, as already mentioned above, the traditional methods require long time to obtain the results.

In the field of molecular biology, polymerase chain reaction (PCR) is undoubtedly the most revolutionary invention,[6] which allowed for the design of new approaches in microbiological examination. By PCR it is indeed possible to detect and quantify specific microorganisms by targeting their DNA and/or RNA. From its first introduction in the field of food safety,[7] PCR has become an essential tool for researchers working with foodborne microorganisms (including pathogenic bacteria) and an impressive number of papers are still published nowadays. PCR has enormous potential in modern food diagnostics; however, some disadvantages are still playing against its wide application in the food sector. In Fig. 56.1,[8] the advantages and disadvantages of PCR in the diagnostics of foodborne pathogens are summarized.

PCR is able to detect the target microorganism independently of its physiological state, thereby stressed or injured cells are picked up by the method, avoiding the false-negative results described above for the traditional microbiological methods. Moreover, the time required for the analysis is much shorter if compared to the cultural methods. This last aspect is very relevant for the food industry. PCR results can be obtained in a minimum of 3 h to a maximum of 24 h, if an enrichment step is included in the analysis, which is necessary for the detection of small numbers of pathogenic microorganisms. The initial investment for the PCR equipment, even if the market has seen a significant decrease in the prices of the instruments, and the requirement for trained personnel, still remain hurdles for the implementation of PCR methods in industrial settings.

Apart from PCR, other amplification methods are available to detect foodborne pathogens in foods.

Nucleic acid sequence-based amplification and the loop-mediated isothermal amplification have the great advantage to be carried out at a constant temperature, thereby avoiding the necessity to purchase expensive equipment for the thermal cycling, classical in PCR amplification. However, they suffer from the same disadvantages PCR has, mainly due to the characteristics of the target molecule, which is often represented by DNA.[9]

Following the advancements in optics technology, PCR has become quantitative by the end of the 1990s. This technique called quantitative PCR (qPCR) revolutionized the molecular approaches in food microbiology. Not only it is possible to quantify one specific microorganism in food, but is also possible to study its behavior as a consequence of the influence of the environment (i.e., food composition, temperature, pH, oxygen, etc.). Moreover, there is no need for postamplification treatment, such as gel electrophoresis, saving time, and simplifying the qPCR application.[10]

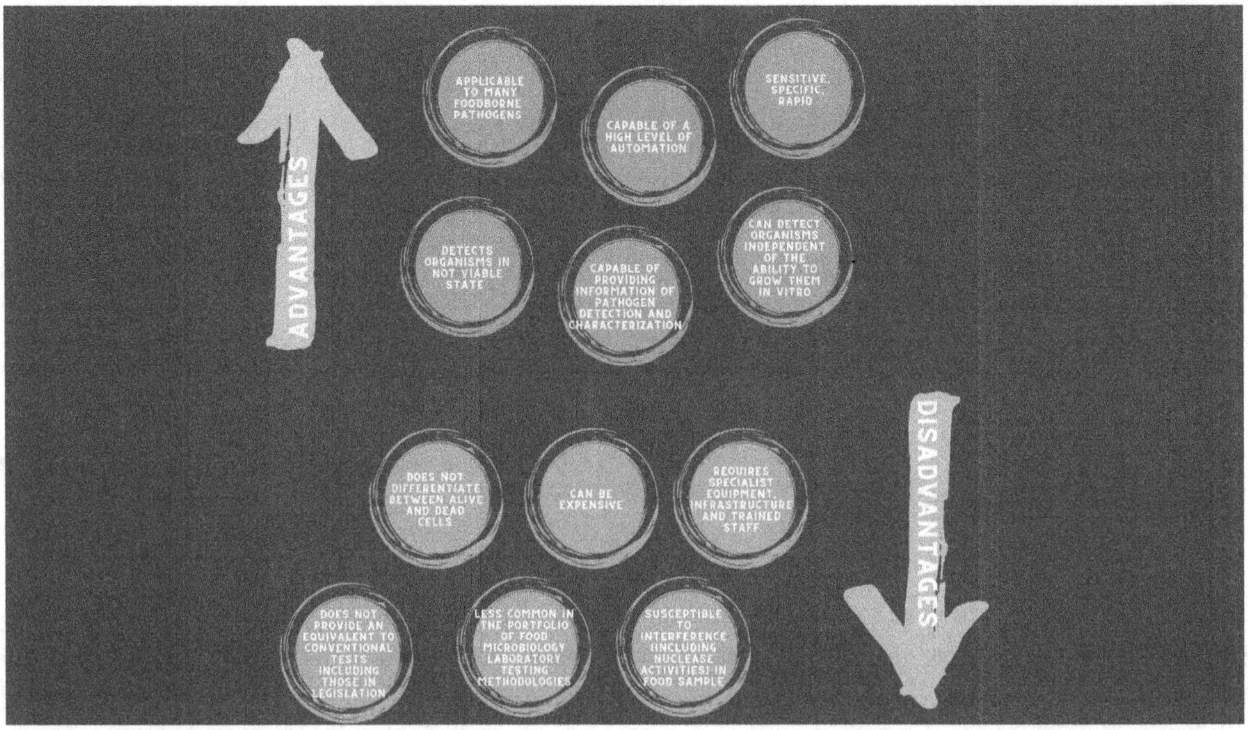

FIGURE 56.1 Advantages and disadvantages of sequence-based amplification of foodborne pathogens. *Adapted from Cocolin L, Donaghy J, Renault P, Ross P, Van Ranst M. Safety implications of the presence of nucleic acids of inactivated microorganisms. ILSI Europe Report Series. <https://ilsi.eu/publication/safety-implications-of-the-presence-of-nucleic-acids-of-inactivated-microorganisms-in-foods/>; 2013.*[8]

PCR is still the method of choice to detect nucleic acid in food, although due to its high specificity, it could only allow detection of well-defined targets, the sequence of which is used as a basis to define primers. In case there is an interest in understanding the overall ecology of a food ecosystem, understanding the context in which pathogens live in, high-throughput sequencing (HTS) methods are better suited. However, the same limitations explained for the PCR method apply also here. The fact that only microorganisms that are at a significant level in the food can be detected by HTS is a great concern for food safety. Last, they still cost too much for a routine application in food industry.

56.3 Impact of processing technologies on the stability of nucleic acids

Food processing is characterized by a number of procedures with well define objectives, which aim to make raw materials edible, improve their safety and organoleptic profile, and protect foods from decay, thereby prolonging their shelf-life. With regards to their impact on nucleic acids stability, the thermal treatments, and specifically those exploiting high temperatures, efficiently used to control the development of microorganisms, both pathogenic and spoilage, but with side effects on the nutritional content and the sensory profiles, are able to determine their fragmentation and denaturation. Mechanical procedures, such as milling and cutting, have less impact on nucleic acid integrity, although also those can determine shredding of the nucleic acid molecules and rupture of the microbial cell, which release DNA and RNA in the food matrix.

Free nucleic acids are degraded either spontaneously or by enzymatic action (see the following section); however, their stability depends on the initial concentration of the microorganisms, and as a consequence the concentration of nucleic acids, the type of inactivation, and the food matrix. Moreover, depending on the processing technique, microorganisms can die but maintain their structure, thereby the nucleic acids are not released in the external environment. In this context, the validation of a processing step to reduce or eliminate foodborne pathogens should be planned and performed correctly to avoid misleading results. Specifically, the microbiological analysis cannot rely completely on the results of molecular methods (i.e., PCR amplification) due to the presence of DNA either free or contained in dead cells. From this point of view, it is necessary to combine the molecular methods with a preenrichment step, in a way that only cells that are alive, can multiply and increase in numbers, and as a consequence be detected by the molecular method. In case of positive signals, it is also advisable to proceed with the confirmation of the pathogen presence by culturing. The effect of different processing techniques on the persistence of free nucleic acids (DNA and RNA) has been reviewed in great detailed in Ceuppens et al. (2014).

An important element that should be considered, when using molecular methods, and more specifically PCR amplification, to detect foodborne pathogens in processed foods, is the length of the target region. Short PCR products have more possibilities to be amplified long after the treatment, due to the fact that nucleic acids, even if partially degraded, will generate small fragments which will be detected by the amplification process. If longer pieces are looked at, then there is more probability that they will disappear after the inactivation of the microorganism, resulting in (true) negative PCR results.

56.4 The viable but not culturable state and its significance for the food industry

Foods are complex microbial ecosystems in which a great microbial diversity can be encountered, in terms of species, growth requirements, and physiological states. Particularly relevant for the food industry is the viable but not culturable (VBNC) state. Cells in VBNC state are metabolically active, but incapable of undergoing the cellular division required for growth in or on a medium normally supporting growth of that cell.[11] VBNC state may be considered as survival strategy and response to adverse environmental conditions (i.e., starvation, acid stress, etc.).[12] The implementation of the hurdle technology,[13] where mild processing conditions are used to avoid big changes in the organoleptic characteristics of foods, thereby responding to the consumers demand of processed food which maintain sensory profiles resembling freshness, there is a high-probability VBNC state can emerge.

VBNC states have been described for several foodborne pathogens.[14] Cells in VBNC state represent a great risk for the food industry; in fact it cannot be excluded that such cells will exit from this state when entering the human body. When interpreting the results of the PCR amplification of DNA, it will not be possible to discriminate dead or VNBC cells, while RNA will give additional information about the presence of alive cells of the target organism, although it will not be possible to identify its VNBC state. Only if the results will be integrated by a culture-dependent approach, such as cultivation in standard broths or agar media, the evidence of microorganisms in VBNC state will be highlighted.

56.5 DNA versus RNA detection and the interpretation of the results

Nucleic acids undergo spontaneously hydrolytic degradation in solution. RNA is particularly susceptible due to the fact that its phosphodiester bond is less stable than that of DNA.[15] However, DNA is more susceptible to depurination (loss of the bases adenine and guanine) and to a lesser extent to depyrimidination (loss of the bases cytosine and thymine). Moreover, hydrolytic deamination, oxidation, and alkylation can damage DNA creating aberrant base derivatives, and ultimately decomposition of DNA. DNA and RNA can also be degraded by extracellular (microbial) DNases and RNases.[16]

The persistence of DNA from inactivated microorganisms in food depends on the temperature, the food matrix, and the presence of other microorganisms during storage after inactivation. Moreover, it is also highly dependent on the initial concentration of the microorganism. Similarly, the degradation of RNA in microorganisms after lethal treatments depends on several factors such as the type of transcript, its stability and its abundance, the type and the severity of the inactivation treatment, the type of microorganism and its physiological condition prior to inactivation, and the subsequent holding conditions.[17] Ribosomal RNAs (rRNAs) are among the most persistent transcripts, but the decay of different messenger RNAs (mRNAs) after bacterial death is not generally predictable (Ceuppens et al., 2014).

There is a profound difference in the significance of the results obtained when, by molecular methods, DNA or RNA is detected. DNA is a molecule that shows a great stability in the environment and this is supported by the studies of recovery of DNA from archeological and paleontological sites. DNA from specimens thousands of years old have been successfully amplified by PCR.[18] In the field of food safety, the detection of DNA should be carefully interpreted. Positive amplifications by PCR of DNA from pathogenic microorganism do not necessarily imply the presence of alive populations of such pathogen in the tested food. This relates to the concepts expressed above and mainly to the stability of fragments of DNA in the environment (in this case represented by foodstuffs). Detection of RNA in reverse-transcription PCR (RT-PCR), as well as exclusion of dead cells on the basis of their permeable membrane to intercalating dyes, such as ethidium monoazide, in, for example, EMA-PCR (Ethidium Monoazide Bromide) format, are alternatives to DNA amplification for the detection of solely live cells. In the case of the EMA-PCR, the dye penetrates the dead cell, because of the lost functionality of the cell wall and membrane, and binds to the DNA preventing its amplification. It is important to underline the fact that this approach, though, was never considered completely and always successful due to its complexity and susceptibility to several factors, such as food matrix and type of dye.[19]

RNA should be considered as a more representative target to assess bacterial viability, due to the fact that mRNA molecules persist for only short periods of time in actively growing bacteria cells with an average half-life of minutes.[20] mRNA-based approaches have proved difficult to exploit mainly because of the experimental complexity such as the extraction of detectable levels of intact mRNA from small numbers of bacteria and a lack of basic information about the significance of detecting mRNA in stressed or injured cells.[21] Another RNA molecule which can be exploited in molecular detection is the rRNA, since the number of intact ribosomes can reflect the rate of protein synthesis and for this reason can be used as a marker for general metabolic activity.[22] rRNA has a higher level of protection when compared to mRNA and this should be taken into account when interpreting results from its detection and amplification.

RT-PCR, where RNA is first retro-transcribed in complementary DNA (cDNA) and then amplified by PCR, is the common method to detect RNA molecules. It can become a quantitative assay if coupled with qPCR. In terms of food safety, the detection of RNA in a processed food should underline the presence of viable population of a specific foodborne pathogen, although it should be recognized that rRNA may still be intact long after the inactivation of the foodborne pathogen.[23]

How to interpret then the results of nucleic acids amplification when compared to classical cultivation? In Fig. 56.2, the different combinations of the positive and negative results, together with some guidance on how to evaluate the results, are displayed. As already indicated above, when the molecular method used for pathogen detection is PCR, it is extremely relevant to always have in mind that longer amplification products correlate better to the presence of live populations, with respect to small PCR products. On the other hand, the longer the sequence to amplify the lower the efficiency of amplification, thereby there is a risk to have false-negative results due to technical pitfalls and not because of the absence of the target organism.

When both methodologies give back negative results, the food should be considered free of the microbial contaminant and can be commercialized, because it will not represent any health risk, situation that is instead found when both culture-dependent and PCR methods produce positive results. In this last case, foodborne pathogens are viable in the sampled product and they may pose important risks for the consumers. Apart from those two straightforward scenarios, also two intermediate situations, where results of the two approaches are not in agreement, can be observed. The case of positive cultivation-based methodology and negative

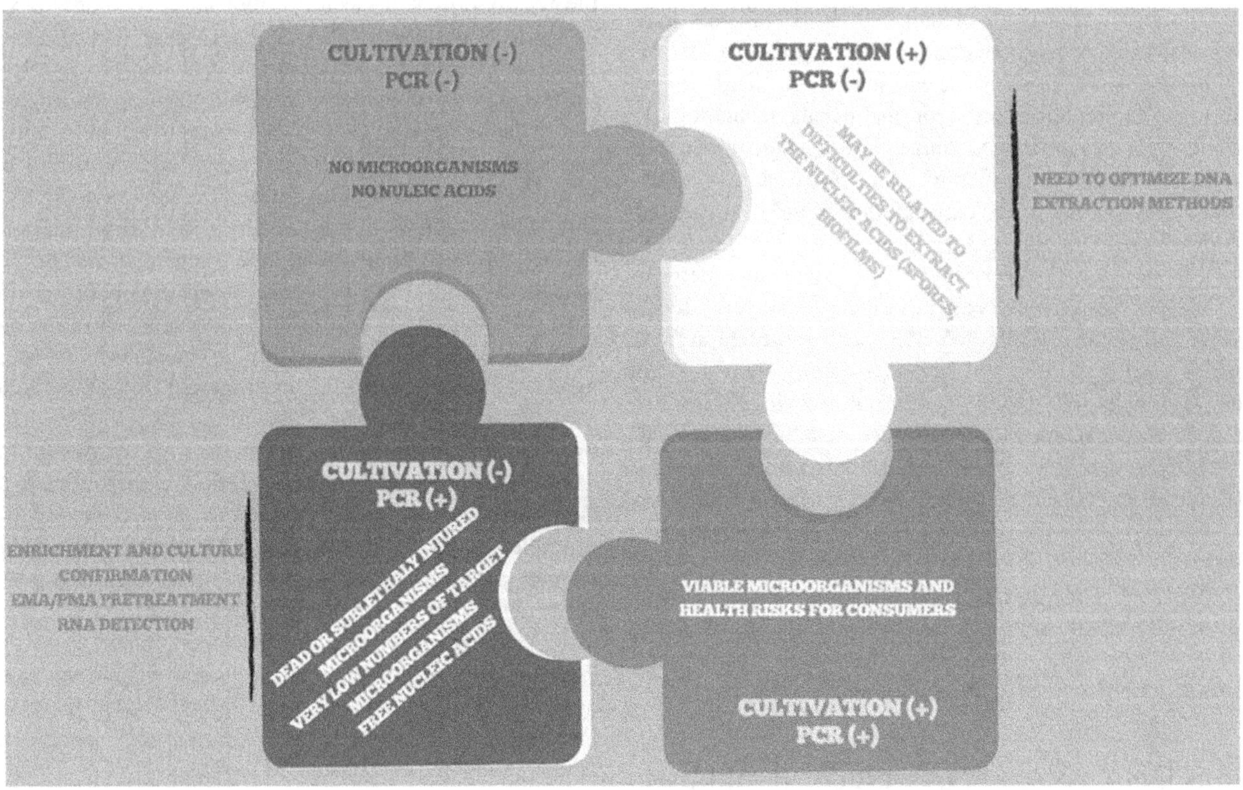

FIGURE 56.2 The interpretation of the polymerase chain reaction amplification results in comparison with the classical microbiological methods. *Modified from Siele Ceuppens, Dan Li, Mieke Uyttendaele, Pierre Renault, Paul Ross, Marc Van Ranst, Luca Cocolin, John Donaghy, Molecular Methods in Food Safety Microbiology: Interpretation and Implications of Nucleic Acid Detection, Comprehensive Reviews in Food Science and Food Safety, 2014, 13, 4, 551-577.*

PCR results highlights some technical problems mainly related to nucleic acids extraction. Possible causes for negative PCR results may be related to microorganisms present as spores, embedded in biofilms and internalized in tissues, such as in plants, situations which makes DNA and RNA extractions more complicated and special pretreatments, such as mechanical solicitations, should be used. Negative amplification results may also be related to inhibitory substances extracted together with the nucleic acids, which halts the DNA polymerase in its activity. There are a number of compounds in foods which have been already identified as inhibitory for PCR, such as polyphenols, carbohydrates, fats, and blood.[24] Also in this case, the extraction protocol should be equipped with steps able to remove those compounds, by separation or absorption, in a way that they do not accompany the nucleic acids and inhibit the PCR reaction. In both cases, the optimization of the extraction phase is essential in order to avoid to incur into false-negative results by molecular methods.

In case of negative results by cultivation and positive results by PCR, the explanation for such a deviation is more complicated and it considers a number of different possibilities related mainly but not only to the physiological state of the target cells. A simple explanation of this inconsistency may be the different sensitivity limit of the two methodologies. It is known that theoretically, PCR is able to amplify one single copy of the target DNA, thereby the single cell that would not be detected by the culture-based methods can contain the necessary quantity of nucleic acids needed to allow PCR amplification. However, more often this difference in the result is really due to the presence of dead target cells, or even free target DNA. As underlined above, this is one of the major drawbacks of the molecular methods when targeting the DNA, in fact, without other confirmation, it will never be possible to understand if the cells are alive or dead. This case is also possible when cells are sublethally injured, situation that happens often in the food production processes, where, for example, high and low temperatures are used, or in presence of preservatives. Cells if are not given the possibility to recover in a proper medium, if cultured in selective media (as it is the case for the detection of pathogenic bacteria in food), instead of growing, they will dye. The nonagreement of the results in this case can be solved if a recovery is carried out. This step will allow the recovery of stressed and injured cells, and at the same time diluting the effect of the inhibitory substances on the microbial growth, thereby they will be able to grow and become detectable by culture-dependent methods; moreover, the enrichment will solve the issue of the low number of target cells, since they will increase during the incubation. The enigma of the dead or alive cells can also be addressed by using pretreatments with EMA and propidium monoazide, allowing the exclusion of dead cells from the amplification, or by targeting the RNA, which may be a better indication for viability as discussed above.

56.6 Modern metagenomic approaches: can they help in the detection of foodborne pathogens in processed foods?

In the last 20 years we have experienced a big advancement in the nucleic acids sequencing techniques. From the Sanger method, which did not allow the sequencing of more than one DNA molecule at a time and it was a rather low-throughput method, we have nowadays the possibility to sequence DNA mixtures in short time and with a great deepness. The next-generation sequencing techniques are in fact able to generate millions of DNA (or cDNA) sequences in a few hours and from complex microbial ecosystems, allowing not only the description of the ecological set up, but also their functional make up. More precisely, with metataxonomics (or amplicon sequencing or metagenetics) we are able to understand the taxonomic composition of the ecosystem and the technique allows for the sequencing of a mixture of PCR products, derived from the 16S rRNA gene, or other conserved genes. With metagenomics, the total DNA (or cDNA), extracted from a sample, is directly sequenced, without any prior amplification, and in this case the approach makes it possible to understand not only the diversity (by analyzing the ribosomal genes) but also the functions that are present and that are characterizing the ecosystem.[25] While with metataxonomics we are able to create taxonomic maps, with metagenomics we can study the putative metabolic activities by constructing pathways from the sequencing libraries produced. Metataxonomics are probably most suitable to use when interested in detection of foodborne pathogens, with respect to metagenomics. While in the first case, the sequencing of fragments amplified starting from the DNA of a pathogenic microorganism is a strong evidence of its presence, retrieving sequences from metagenomic libraries aligning with pathogenic microorganism genomes makes very difficult the interpretation of the outcomes. In addition, the lack of quantitative significance of the data, especially in the case of metataxonomics due to the amplification process prior to sequencing, poses important challenges in the correct interpretation of the results. To that end, only the presence or absence of the pathogenic microorganism nucleic acids can be determined, as it can be done by using a conventional PCR methodology.

The potential of metagenomics, and in general of omics techniques, has been addressed in detail in volume 287 of the International Journal of Food Microbiology, introduced by Cocolin et al.[26] collecting articles from experts from the academia and industry entitled “Omics in MRA – the integration of omics in microbiological risk assessment."

Undoubtedly, metaomics approaches can help industry to produce safer food; however, we are still in a phase where more efforts are needed in order to fully understand how to translate physiological evidences (e.g., stress response to processing techniques) and ecological insights into foodborne pathogen behavior and presence/absence in foods, respectively.

Unfortunately, all the aspects described in this chapter related to nucleic acids significance and persistence are also valid for these more sophisticated techniques. Moreover, the cost for the analysis, especially in the case of metagenomics, is still too high to consider it suitable for routine analysis in food industries.

56.7 Conclusions

Since the target for the amplification is mainly represented by DNA, molecule characterized by high stability also after cell death, a positive result by PCR does not necessarily indicate the presence of alive pathogenic microorganisms in foods. This evidence is extremely important for processed foods, that is, thermally processed, where the production includes a step, in which foodborne pathogens are eliminated. This pitfall of the PCR has been addressed in different ways by the researchers and it is generally accepted that if positive results are obtained after an enrichment step this implies the presence of viable populations that were able to multiply and their DNA was subsequently amplified by PCR.[27] Nonetheless, even the mere presence of dead cells indicates that somewhere along the food production line there has been a breach of food safety measures (initial contamination of raw materials in the best case), which puts an additional "fail-safe" pressure on the intervention measure located at a downstream critical control point.

In conclusion, the detection and quantification of residual DNA from processed foods by molecular methods such as conventional or quantitative PCR do not necessarily indicate the presence of a safety risk for the consumer in terms of direct pathogenesis of the detected pathogens. RNA is the most suitable target to assess microbial viability, thereby its testing is more accurate in order to guarantee the safety of processed foods.

References

1. Anonymous. Regulation (EC) No 178/2002 of the European Parliament and of the Council of 28 January 2002 laying down the general principles and requirements of food law, establishing the European Food Safety Authority and laying down procedures in matters of food safety; 2002.
2. Cocolin L, Alessandria V, Dolci P, Gorra R, Rantsiou K. Culture independent methods to assess the diversity and dynamics of microbiota during food fermentation. *Int J Food Microbiol.* 2013;167:29–43.
3. García-Sánchez L, Melero B, Rovira J. *Campylobacter* in the food chain. *Adv Food Nutr Res.* 2018;86:215–252.
4. Bannantine JP, Barletta RG, Stabel JR, Paustian ML, Kapur V. Application of the genome sequence to address concerns that *Mycobacterium avium* subspecies *paratuberculosis* might be a foodborne pathogen. *Foodborne Pathog Dis.* 2004;1(1):3–15.
5. Ramírez-Castillo FY, Loera-Muro A, Jacques M, et al. Waterborne pathogens: detection methods and challenges. *Pathogens.* 2015;4 (2):307–334.
6. Saiki RK, Gelfand DH, Stoffel S, et al. Primer-directed enzymatic amplification of DNA with a thermostable DNA polymerase. *Science.* 1988;239(4839):487–491.
7. Wernars K, Delfogou E, Soentoro PS, Notermans S. Successful approach for the detection of low numbers of enterotoxigenic *Escherichia coli* in minced meat by using the polymerase chain reaction. *Appl Environ Microbiol.* 1991;57:1793–1798.
8. Cocolin L, Donaghy J, Renault P, Ross P, Van Ranst M. Safety implications of the presence of nucleic acids of inactivated microorganisms. ILSI Europe Report Series.<https://ilsi.eu/publication/safety-implications-of-the-presence-of-nucleic-acids-of-inactivated-microorganisms-in-foods/>; 2013.
9. Ceuppens S, Li S, Uyttendaele M, et al., Molecular Methods in Food Safety Microbiology: Interpretation and Implications of Nucleic Acid Detection, Comprehensive Reviews in Food Science and Food Safety, 2014, 13, 4, 551–577
10. Cocolin L, Rajkovic A, Rantsiou K, Uyttendaele M. The challenge of merging food safety diagnostic needs with quantitative PCR platforms. *Trends Food Sci Technol.* 2011;22:S30–S38.
11. Ayrapetyan M, Oliver JD. The viable but non-culturable state and its relevance in food safety. *Curr Opin Food Sci.* 2016;8:127–133.
12. Rowan NJ. Viable but non-culturable forms of food ad waterborne bacteria: Quo Vadis. *Trends Food Sci Technol.* 2004;15:462–467.
13. Leistner L. Principles and applications of hurdle technology. In: Gould GW, ed. *New Methods of Food Preservation.* Glasgow: Blackie Academic and Professional; 1995:1–21.
14. Gao R, Liao X, Zhao X, Liu D, Ding T. The diagnostic tools for viable but nonculturable pathogens in the food industry: current status and future prospects. *Compr Rev Food Sci Food Saf.* 2021;20(2):2146–2175.
15. Lindahl T. Instability and decay of the primary structure of DNA. *Nature.* 1993;362(6422):709–715.
16. Palchevskiy V, Finkel SE. A role for single-stranded exonucleases in the use of DNA as a nutrient. *J Bacteriol.* 2009;191 (11):3712–3716.
17. Cenciarini C, Courtois S, Raoult D, La Scola B. Influence of long time storage in mineral water on RNA stability of *Pseudomonas aeruginosa* and *Escherichia coli* after heat inactivation. *PLoS One.* 2008;3(10):e3443.
18. Landweber L. Something old for something new: the future of ancient DNA in conservation biology. In: Landweber L, Dobson AP, eds. *Genetics and Extinction of Species: DNA and the Conservation of Biodiversity.* Princeton: Princeton University Press; 1999:163–186.

19. Nogva H, Dromtorp SM, Nissen H, Rudi K. Ethidium monoazide for DNA-based differentiation of viable and dead bacteria by 5'-nuclease PCR. *Biotechniques*. 2003;34:804–813.
20. Arraiano CM, Yancey SD, Kushner SR. Stabilization of discrete mRNA breakdown products in *ams, pnp* and *rnb* multiple mutants of *Escherichia coli* K-12. *J Bacteriol*. 1988;170:4625–4633.
21. Sheridan GEC, Masters CI, Shallcross JA, Mackey BM. Detection of mRNA by reverse transcription-PCR as an indicator of viability in *Escherichia coli* cells. *Appl Environ Microbiol*. 1998;64: 1313–1318.
22. Gosalbes MJ, Durban A, Pignatelli M, et al. Metatranscriptomic approach to analyze the functional human gut microbiota. *PLoS One*. 2011;6:e17447.
23. Blazewicz SJ, Barnard RL, Daly RA, Firestone MK. Evaluating rRNA as an indicator of microbial activity in environmental communities: limitations and uses. *ISME J*. 2013;7 (11):2061–2068.
24. Sajali N, Wong SC, Hanapi UK, Abu Bakar Jamaluddin S, Tasrip NA, Mohd Desa MN. The challenges of DNA extraction in different assorted food matrices: a review. *J Food Sci*. 2018;83 (10):2409–2414.
25. Berg G, Rybakova D, Fischer D, et al. Microbiome definition re-visited: old concepts and new challenges. *Microbiome*. 2020;8 (1):103.
26. Cocolin L, Membré J-M, Zwietering MZ. Editorial: Integration of omics into MRA. *Int J Food Microbiol*. 2018;287:1–2.
27. Rossen L, Holstrom K, Olsen JE, Rasmussen OF. A rapid polymerase chain reaction (PCR)-based assay for the identification of *Listeria monocytogenes* in food samples. *Int J Food Microbiol*. 1991;14:135–145.

Chapter 57

Whole-genome sequencing for food safety

Nigel French

New Zealand Food Safety Science and Research Centre, School of Veterinary Science, Massey University, Palmerston North, New Zealand

Abstract

Next-generation sequencing (NGS) technologies are increasingly being embraced and adopted by public health agencies and the food industry for the control of foodborne pathogens. This chapter describes the application of these technologies for whole-genome sequencing (WGS) of bacterial pathogens in the food chain. Examples are provided showing how WGS has been used for different applications, from global to local and factory-scale. Applications include outbreak investigation, source attribution and genomic epidemiology, processing plant investigations of contamination, and understanding pathogen evolution. Despite the promise and potential of WGS and NGS technology, there remain concerns regarding access to the technology, particularly in low- and middle-income settings, and issues relating to speed and cost, data governance, and the implications of sharing data. Advances in bioinformatics and visualization, and a strong focus on collaboration, standardization, and harmonization, will help to ensure the tools and technologies are adopted and used effectively for food safety decision-making.

Keywords: Food safety; whole-genome sequencing; next generation sequencing; outbreak investigation; genomic epidemiology; microbial hazard management

Chapter points

- Advances in whole-genome sequencing (WGS) technology provide unprecedented opportunities for improving food safety.
- There are many applications of WGS for improving public health and managing microbial hazards in the food industry.
- The technology needs to be applied in an interdisciplinary context, allowing sequencing data to be appropriately interpreted, in context, to improve decision making.
- Applications at a *global scale* include identifying the source of outbreaks, and the use of phylogeographic methods to describe how foodborne pathogens have been transmitted between countries over time.
- Applications at a *country scale* include using sequencing and modeling to understand how foodborne pathogens are transmitted in primary production, between farms, and for the detection of national outbreaks and sources of sporadic cases.
- Applications at a *plant scale* include determining the relatedness and potential links between isolates from different food production facilities, and 'micro-mapping' to determine pathogen entry and control points.
- When combined with phenotypic testing, genome sequencing can be used to determine antimicrobial resistance, virulence, and other traits to inform and optimize control strategies.
- Data governance and sharing of genome sequencing data remain an important concern, with many ethical, commercial, and legal considerations.
- Future advances are likely to include non-culture-based methods that can be applied in near real-time to inform decision-making.

57.1 Introduction

Foodborne pathogens continue to be an important cause of illness and mortality worldwide.[1] Although recent trends show a decline in the overall incidence of foodborne illness, the costs of compliance and the number of recalls are increasing.[2,3] New technologies have emerged in recent years that provide novel approaches to improving hazard and risk management within the food industry and improving public health. One such advance is the advent of next-generation or high throughput DNA/RNA sequencing (NGS). This has revolutionized our approach to the detection, characterization, and management of foodborne pathogens, and has spawned a plethora of novel approaches to data analysis and presentation, making it more accessible and beneficial for decision

Present Knowledge in Food Safety. DOI: https://doi.org/10.1016/B978-0-12-819470-6.00065-2

making. This chapter focuses on the application of NGS technology for whole-genome sequencing (WGS) of foodborne pathogens that have been isolated by culture methods. The application of NGS to non-culture-based methods, including metabarcoding and shotgun metagenomics, is briefly discussed but is not the focus of this chapter.[4]

Food safety has already benefitted from the application of WGS. Advances in recent years have been characterized by transformational improvements in sequencing technology (hardware and software), enabling higher sample throughput and increased speed of turnaround from sample to sequence. At the same time, the cost per sample has fallen, allowing the technology to be applied more widely and readily in public health and food industry settings. Open data platforms have transformed the way WGS data is stored, shared, and analyzed, greatly enhancing the utility of this technology for multiple applications in many fields. For food safety these include (with example references):

- Identifying the source of outbreaks and sporadic cases of foodborne disease.[5,6]
- Foodborne pathogen surveillance.[7,8]
- Understanding how foodborne pathogens are transmitted, both locally and globally.[9,10]
- Determining the source of contamination in food processing facilities.[11]
- Identifying and characterizing strains resident in food production facilities.[11]
- Pathogen risk profiling.[12]
- Screening probiotic strains.[13]
- Understanding how foodborne pathogens are evolving.[14,15]

One of the most striking early applications of WGS to inform food safety was during the large-scale, severe outbreaks of STEC O104 in Europe in 2011.[16] Two outbreaks occurred concurrently, one with a focus in Germany involving ~4000 cases of bloody diarrhea, 850 cases of hemolytic uremic syndrome (HUS) and 50 deaths. The other was a much smaller outbreak in France. Both outbreaks were epidemiologically linked to fenugreek seeds used to produce beansprouts. Using conventional molecular tools such as pulsed field gel electrophoresis and 7-gene multilocus sequence typing (MLST) the isolates from the outbreak were indistinguishable. With WGS, a much higher resolution was achieved, allowing inferences on the likely origin and evolution of this newly emerged lineage to be made.[15] The successful application of this technology, which involved the rapid, early sharing of sequence data with the global community, was a major stimulus for the wider adoption of WGS for surveillance of foodborne and other pathogens.

This chapter describes the application of second and third-generation sequencing technology for sequencing the genomes of isolates of foodborne pathogens. This is a rapidly moving field; at the time of writing there has been an explosion of publications that have described the use of WGS technology for food safety (in broad terms). This review includes many examples of studies that have been published in the last 2 years, along with earlier examples demonstrating novel applications of relevance to food safety today. Other more comprehensive reviews of the application of WGS for food safety are highly recommended.[17,18] The chapter outlines the need and value of high-resolution genotyping, allowing the tracking of important pathogen lineages and the emergence and spread of antimicrobial and virulence genes. It will underline the value of the technology for hazard and risk assessment, describe trends in the development of NGS technology, modeling, and visualization tools, and give examples of applications at varying scales; from global to food factory scale.

57.2 Main text

57.2.1 Advances in genome sequencing technologies and analytical tools

Next-generation sequencing (NGS) or High Throughput Sequencing technologies emerged around 2008 and have advanced rapidly over the last 15 years.[19,20] The major advances in NGS compared to earlier technologies include:

- Higher resolution.
- Greater speed – NGS instruments sequence many billions of base pairs per day compared to 1–2 million with lower-throughput, earlier technology
- Reduced size and greater portability – small benchtop and hand-held devices are now commonplace.
- Reduced cost.

The National Human Genome Research Institute has regularly updated graphs of the cost of sequencing per megabase of sequence. Fig. 57.1 shows the trend in cost per megabase illustrating the dramatic decline in cost between 2007 and 2015 followed by a slower decline by 2020.[a] Moore's law is plotted as a benchmark trend.[b]

57.2.1.1 Next-generation sequencing technologies

There are several basic NGS technologies.[20,21] These include 'shotgun' methods whereby genome fragmentation is followed by parallelization and template generation. The outputs are raw 'reads' that are multiple overlapping stretches of DNA (or RNA) that are compiled by statistical algorithms into longer contiguous sequences (contigs). The different technologies can be broadly categorized by the length of reads into short and long-read technologies. Although many technologies and instruments have been

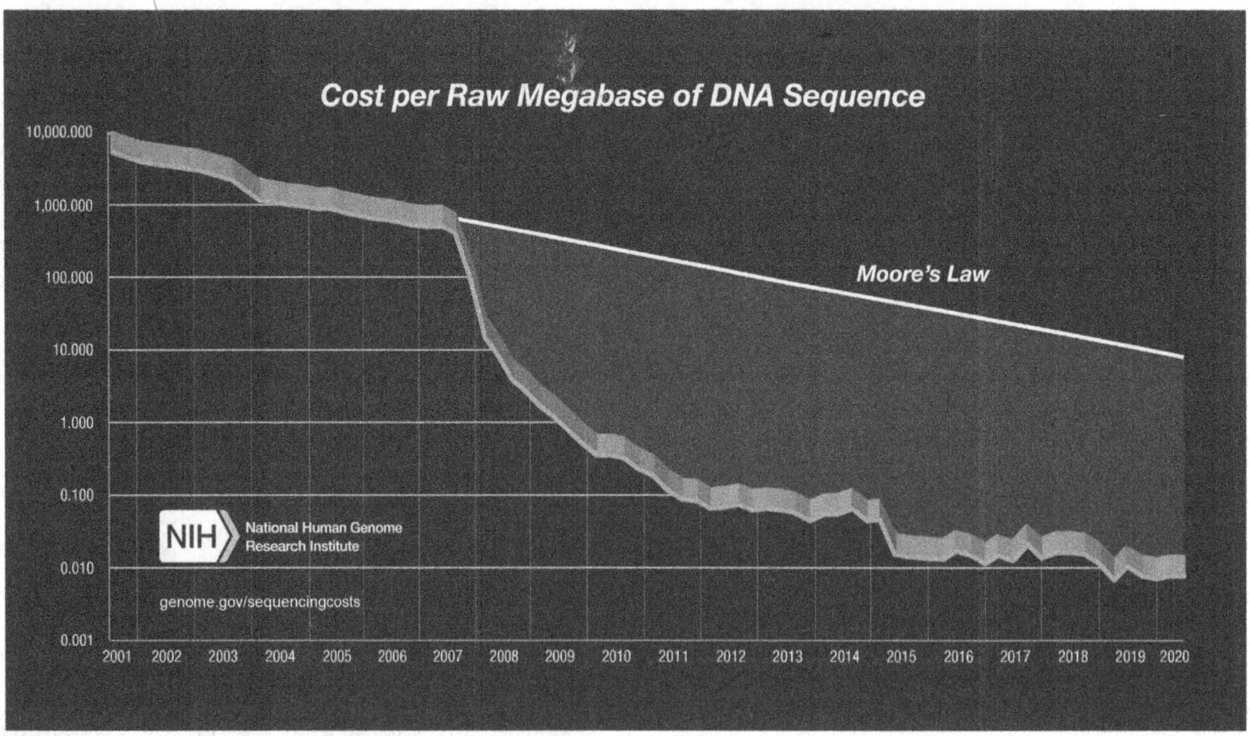

FIGURE 57.1 Trend in cost of sequencing per megabase of DNA sequence, taken from the National Human Genome Research Institute (NHGRI).[g] Data from 2001 to October 2007 represent the costs of generating DNA sequence using Sanger sequencing and capillary-based instruments. From 2008, the data represent the costs of generating DNA sequence using NGS.

developed, a small number are more commonly used for food safety and public health applications including:

- Illumina dye sequencing (short read)
- Pacific Biosciences (PacBio) single-molecule real-time sequencing (long read)
- Oxford Nanopore sequencing (long read)
- Ion Torrent semiconductor sequencing (short read)
- Beijing Genomics Institute Combinatorial probe anchor synthesis with DNA nano ball sequencing (short read).

Short-read sequencing is generally less expensive per isolate and the high throughput short read instruments can generate extremely large numbers of replicate reads at the same time in a single run, giving a greater coverage depth. There are disadvantages of short-read sequencing, including the loss of observed genetic variation resulting from gaps between assembled regions, difficulty in assembling genomes due to repetitive regions, and the PCR steps introducing errors into the DNA sequence.

Long-read sequencing tends to have a consistent level of coverage across the genome, and better detection of genetic variation. However, the higher cost of long-read sequencing still presents a significant barrier to use in food safety and public health settings, and earlier applications of the technology were associated with lower sequence read accuracy compared to short-read sequencing. Long-read sequencing is often combined with short-read sequencing using 'hybrid assemblies' to generate complete reference genomes that can be used as scaffolds for larger collections of isolates sequenced using short-read technology.

NGS machines used for food safety applications vary considerably in terms of factors such as their speed, portability, throughput, read length, data management, and error rates. As an example, two contrasting technologies used for food safety applications include Illumina Dye's short-read sequencing and Oxford Nanopore's long-read sequencing. Benchtop Illumina instruments currently available are the iSeq and MiniSeq, suitable for a relatively small number of samples, and the MiSeq and NextSeq, suitable for higher throughput. Standalone high throughput Illumina machines are the HiSeq and NovaSeq. Oxford Nanopore machines include the portable hand-held MinION and even smaller SmigION; both can be used in field applications for generating sequence data in real-time. Higher throughput Oxford Nanopore desktop devices include the GridION and the larger PromethION.

57.2.2 Reads, assemblies, and contigs

As indicated earlier, genome sequencing technologies produce millions of overlapping 'raw' reads, comprising stretches of

DNA or RNA sequence that are 100 s (e.g., for Illumina short-read technology) to 1000 s of bases long (e.g., for PacBio or Nanopore technology). These raw overlapping reads are used to generate assembled "contigs" that comprise long stretches of a sequence determined by computational algorithms[22,23] to be the most likely sequence of nucleotides within the chromosome or extra-chromosomal elements (e.g., plasmids) of the target organism – in the case of food safety applications described in this chapter these are isolates of bacterial foodborne pathogens. Generally, better genome assemblies are achieved with higher read coverage (depth), longer reads, and good read quality. Successful application of long-read sequencing, often combined with short-read sequencing, can produce large circular contigs, comprising the complete genome of the host's chromosome and mobile genetic elements (e.g., plasmids). These can then be annotated, using bioinformatics tools such as PROKKA,[24] to provide well-characterized reference genomes.

57.2.3 From pangenome to core genome and multilocus sequence typing

For populations of organisms, such as bacteria, the entire complement of genes across the target population is called the pangenome. The target population may be the entire global population of all sequenced isolates from a particular bacterial species, or a sample from, for example, a particular country at a particular time point. A subset of these genes may be in all members of the population, and this is called the core genome. Those genes that are in some, but not all, of the target population, comprise the accessory or variable genome, and therefore the core plus the accessory genome comprise the pangenome. There are subtle variations to this simplified description; for example, genes that are in all or the vast majority of a population may be called the hardcore genome, whereas the genes that are in most, as defined by a threshold, may be called the softcore genome. When typing bacterial populations, a subset of loci (sequences of interest) from genes common to most of the entire population of sequenced isolates from a particular species may be used to define a core genome multilocus genotyping scheme (cgMLST). Examples include the *Campylobacter jejuni* and *Campylobacter coli* cgMLST scheme used in PubMLST,[25] comprising over 1300 loci. Alternatively, samples of genomes can be compared by examining all genes common to most or all the subset of genomes represented by the sample. This is usually a larger set of loci than those used in cgMLST schemes derived from comprehensive global datasets and are used for whole-genome MLST (wgMLST) comparisons. wgMLST profiles can be compared using predetermined schemes, or ad hoc schema development methods.[26,27]

For some analyses, further subsets of genes/loci may be analyzed from WGS data. Commonly used examples are ribosomal MLST (rMLST), which uses the ~50 genes encoding the bacterial ribosome protein subunits[28] and seven gene housekeeping schemes.[29] The latter was initially developed for use with Sanger sequencing, but 7-gene MLST allele profiles and sequence types (STs) may also be derived from WGS data to indicate lower-resolution ST groupings of isolates compatible with earlier schemes.

57.2.4 Analysis of whole-genome sequencing data for food safety – in silico typing, alleles, single nucleotide polymorphisms, trees, and 'zip-codes'

There are several ways WGS data can be analyzed, and the approach taken will depend on the food safety question(s) being addressed. This may include confirmation of a bacterial species; low to high resolution genotyping for source attribution; identification of genes associated with virulence or antimicrobial resistance; and pairwise comparisons of genetic relatedness to determine transmission pathways or membership of an outbreak cluster.

57.2.4.1 In silico species determination and low-resolution genotyping

Examination of raw or processed WGS reads and assembled contigs can be used to identify or confirm the species of the organism in question. For example, species can be determined by examination of the 16S genes and comparison with annotated databases of 16S sequences such as Greengenes[30] and RDP.[31] Other approaches to inferring species include k-mer[c]-based methods[32] and 7-gene MLST. 7-gene MLST and other relatively low-resolution 'traditional' genotyping schemes can be determined from WGS data. For example, assembled contigs can be uploaded to the PubMLST database to determine the 7-gene ST and clonal complex of an isolate.[33] This can be valuable for determining which broad lineage a set of isolates belong to, allowing backward comparison with low-resolution data generated, for example, by Sanger sequencing. It's often valuable to link the whole genome sequenced isolates to data held in traditional, lower-resolution typing databases; this enables the isolate to be placed in a broader historical context and can assist with, for example, outbreak investigations. Large, curated databases of isolates typed by lower resolution methods such as a 7-gene MLST contain valuable information, and the ability to extract comparative data, in silico, from low- and high-resolution methods, can greatly enhance food safety investigations. For example, the PubMLST

C. jejuni/coli database has a genome collection of over 50,000 isolates, whereas the lower resolution 7-gene MLST collection contains information on ~100,000 isolates.

57.2.4.2 In silico phenotype prediction – antimicrobial resistance, virulence, and serotype

WGS data can be used to determine the complement of genes associated with serotype, virulence traits, and antimicrobial resistance. Tools and databases publicly available for predicting the antimicrobial resistance and virulence status of certain bacterial species include the Center for Genomic Epidemiology ResFinder,[34] the CARD database,[35] and VirulenceFinder.[36] The ability of these to detect particular phenotypes will improve as more WGS data and accompanying phenotypic data become available.[37]

WGS data can also be used to predict serotypes for certain species, such as *Escherichia coli*[38] and *Salmonella enterica*,[39] by searching for genes associated with serotypes, or by extrapolating from an isolate's location within the overall population structure. This is an example of backward compatibility with earlier typing schemes that enable isolates to be placed in a broader historical context. Freely available online tools, such as SerotypeFinder[38] and SISTR[39] are examples of web-based interactive databases that enable serotypes to be inferred from WGS data.

57.2.4.3 Methods to determine relatedness and the 'genetic unit' of interest

A key component of any analysis of WGS data is determining the 'relatedness' of isolates from different samples. The more closely related two isolates are, the more likely they are to share a recent common ancestor. This is important because the more likely they are to share a common ancestor, the more likely they are to be linked to some event; such as transmission from a food product to a person causing foodborne illness, or from an ingredient source to a final product.

Determining relatedness requires pairwise comparisons of the genetic data provided by sequencing, and WGS provides the highest resolution available for fine-scale linking of isolates. A sample of genomes can be characterized by comparing them all with a standard reference genome (usually a fully annotated, publicly available genome) or one of the isolates within the sample (usually the one with the fewest contigs and highest N50 value[d]). Alternatively, they can be compared with each other without the use of a reference genome, also called 'alignment-free' methods.

Comparisons can be made using different features of the genome[40] or 'genetic units'. These include:

- Single nucleotide polymorphisms (SNPs). These are single base changes that can occur anywhere in the genome and arise because of 'errors' during replication. They may be analyzed across the entire genome or subsets of the genome, such as the core genome. They are often referred to as high-quality SNPs (hqSNPs) if the sequence data provide a sufficient level of confidence that they are true SNPs and not the result of sequencing error (see below).[e]
- Alleles or gene-by-gene-based methods. Alleles are unique sequences of full-length genes or parts of genes (loci). Particular gene/locus sets are used as standard sets for typing schemes applied to many pathogens, for example, the core genome MLST set[25]; the ~50 ribosomal rMLST set[28]; or seven housekeeping gene set used for 7-gene MLST[29]).
- K-mers. These are substrings of nucleotides of a particular length, k. The creation of k-mers from raw sequence data is an essential step in the assembling of raw reads into longer contigs. However, they are also used for assessing the relatedness of pairs of isolates. In one approach, genome sequences are converted into datasets of k-mers of a specific size, called sketches. The distributions of the most frequent sketches are compared to provide pairwise comparisons of isolates.[41]

There are advantages and disadvantages to each approach. For example, SNP analyses can provide higher resolution than allele-based analyses because a single allele difference between a pair of isolates can result from single or multiple SNPs within the same locus. However, evolutionary relationships can be distorted by recombination events, whereby a single introduction of a recombinant fragment can introduce multiple SNPs. If this is not accounted for it may be concluded that two isolates are distantly related based on the number of SNPs, whereas they are separated by a single evolutionary event. For organisms that frequently undergo homologous recombination through mechanisms such as the uptake of naked DNA (i.e. natural transformation in panmictic organisms such as *C. jejuni*), allele-based approaches may provide a better indication of the true evolutionary relationships between isolates.

SNP and allele-based analyses are frequently used in food safety applications, including the use of SNPs for outbreak investigation, understanding transmission in production facilities, and the presence of resident strains.[11] Allele-based approaches have been central to the development of schemes and databases for multiple species and include whole genome or core-genome MLST schemas available in databases such as pubMLST for multiple pathogens including *C. jejuni/coli*,[33] Institut Pasteur MLST for *Listeria*[42] and Enterobase for *E. coli*, *S. enterica* and *Yersinia* spp.[43]

Rapid visual assessment of relatedness between pairs of isolates can be achieved through the construction of phylogenetic trees, multivariate visualization methods, or the assignment of 'zip-codes'. There are many ways of representing phylogenetic trees including rooted, unrooted, circular/radial, and minimum spanning trees, but the underlying principle is the same – isolates that are more closely connected through the branches of the tree are more similar to each other than isolates that are separated by longer branches (Fig. 57.2).

Alternative ways of visualizing pairwise differences between isolates include multivariate methods, such as discriminant analysis of principal components, that provide two-dimensional maps summarizing genetic distances[49,50] and the assignment of allele codes[51] or SNP addresses to individual isolates.[52] These are analogous to Zip codes used for identifying the local physical addresses. For example, allele codes used in PulseNet[51] include the organism identifier and version of the code script used for naming, followed by a string of up to six numbers representing the genetic similarity of the isolate at different allelic thresholds compared with other isolates in the database. Thresholds of 5, 10, 25, 50, 100, and 250 allelic differences are commonly used (see Fig. 57.3 for an example). The codes are optimized for individual bacterial species using allelic thresholds demonstrated to be the most stable for each species.[42]

57.2.5 Data sharing – underlining the need for quality control, standardization, harmonization, and accreditation

The utility of WGS for food safety has been greatly enhanced by the development of NGS technology, enabling genomic DNA to become standard data for surveillance, providing high-resolution information and discrimination between isolates, and enabling pathogens to be stored, readily shared, and analyzed.[53] Storing and sharing genomic pathogen data and related surveillance metadata analyses as "open data" has transformed global pathogen surveillance.[54] Examples of the success of this model, including GenomeTrakr and PulseNet, come from the United States,[51,55,56] partnered with countries such as the United Kingdom[57] and Australia.[58]

The value of WGS data is greatly enhanced through the development of open data platforms and databanks that store raw reads, aligned sequences, and metadata. Examples include the following:

- National Center for Biotechnology Information
- GenomeTrakr Network[59]
- Global Microbial Identifier (GMI)[60]

To make valid and useful comparisons from WGS data it is essential to understand how repeatable, accurate and reliable the data are. This is important when comparing data from different sites and at different time points within the same site. With the advent of widespread sharing of data from different laboratories, the ability to make meaningful comparisons becomes particularly important for dealing with, for example, outbreaks that are inter-jurisdictional or cross-border.

Data generated by NGS technology will undergo initial quality checks before further bioinformatic analyses. Inter and intra laboratory variation in WGS data can occur for a variety of reasons including the following:

- Differences in the NGS technology and its application – different platforms have different sequencing error rates, and data may be generated with different read lengths, sequencing depth, and coverage.
- Differences in bioinformatics platforms and settings – different pipelines may use different analytical approaches and bioinformaticians may apply different parameters, thresholds, or settings which can result in differences in, for example, SNP calling.
- SNPs were generated in vitro during the culture of the primary sample.

A summary of the many reasons for false positive and false negative SNP calling is provided in the paper by Croucher et al.[61]

The above underlines the importance of quality control, and the standardization and harmonization of approaches, and is the impetus for schemes and accreditation programs being developed around the world for different pathogens. Examples include standardization of *Listeria monocytogenes* typing using WGS.[62] In general allele based methods, such as extended MLST schemes (e.g., cgMLST and wgMLST) provide greater opportunities for developing a stable, internationally standardized nomenclature, compared to SNP-based methods.[63]

Harmonization of data for sharing, both genomic and associated metadata, is crucial.[18] Data need to be sufficiently standardized to be comparable between sites, well-curated and FAIR: findable, accessible, interoperable, and reusable.[64] Many efforts to date have attempted to harmonize approaches to generating and combining genomic and clinical data, for example using standardized classification systems and protocols (e.g., the PhenX toolkit for standardized collection of clinical data[65] and ARTIC protocols for genome sequencing).[66] Similarly, the Genomic Epidemiology Ontology project seeks a global standard for the contextual information (metadata) that is associated with WGS data.[67] There is a clear need for globally harmonized guidelines for the interpretation of WGS data; this is essential when sharing information, particularly during multi-

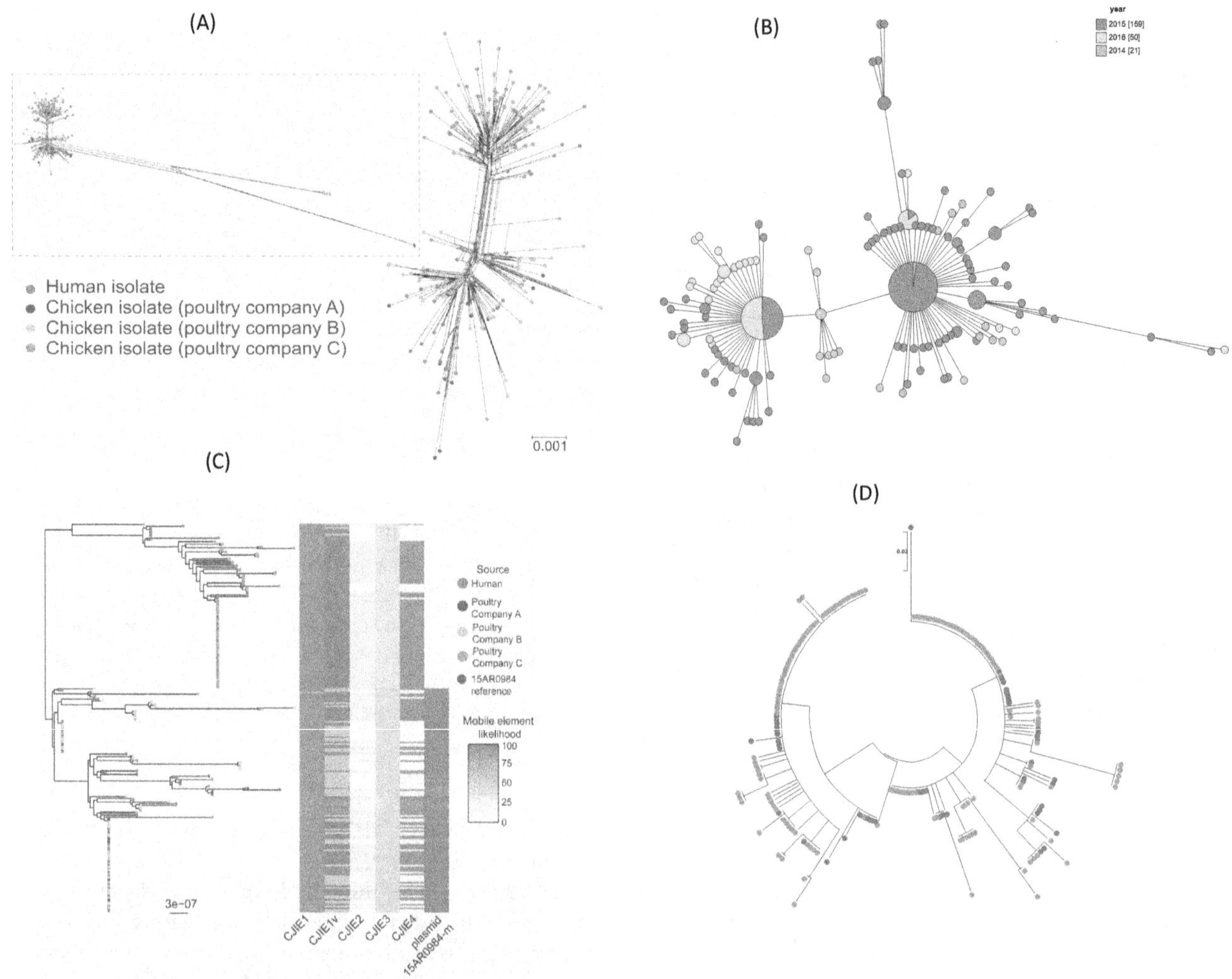

FIGURE 57.2 Different representations of phylogenetic relatedness using trees. All trees were produced using WGS data from the same set of isolates of *Campylobacter jejuni* ST6964 from humans and different poultry companies in New Zealand.[44] (A) is a non-rooted phylogenetic network produced using the programme Splitstree.[45] The genetic distance is the difference in the whole genome allele profile between pairs of isolates generated by the programme Fast-Gep[26] and is represented by the length of the branches connecting the nodes. Uncertainty in the shape of the tree is captured by the net-like structures. (B) is a minimum spanning tree representation of the difference between pairs of isolates based on pairwise comparisons of core genome MLST allele profiles generated using PubMLST,[25] and visualised using GrapeTree.[46] (C) shows the genetic relatedness of the isolates based on the difference in core genome SNPs identified using Snippy version 4.3.5 (https://github.com/tseemann/snippy). This is a rooted maximum likelihood tree, generated using IQ-Tree[47] and visualized using the program ggtree in R (https://www.r-project.org), and includes a plot of the presence and absence of mobile genetic elements as a heatmap to the right of the tree. (D) is a circular dendrogram generated from a k-mer based distance matrix produced using Mashtree[41] and displayed using the Interactive Tree of Life.[48]

jurisdictional events, but there is still much to do to improve global uptake and utility of these initiatives.

57.2.6 Visualization and web-based interactive tools

Following in the wake of recent advances in standardization and data sharing, are new initiatives aimed at improving the visualization and presentation of genome sequencing and related metadata. Examples of such platforms include interactive web-based platforms such as Nextstrain[68] and Microreact.[69] These provide accessible tools for analyzing genomic data that are scalable, from the global transmission of pathogens to source tracking in processing plants, and can accommodate public and private data. Both Nextstrain and Microreact have multiple examples that are readily accessible from their websites (https://nextstrain.org/ and https://microreact.org/) and provide open-source software for end-users to develop their applications. Although there are few examples of foodborne pathogens currently available on public sites, food companies in countries such as New Zealand have used Microreact to develop interactive dashboards, combining plant-scale maps with phylogenetic trees based on WGS and metadata.

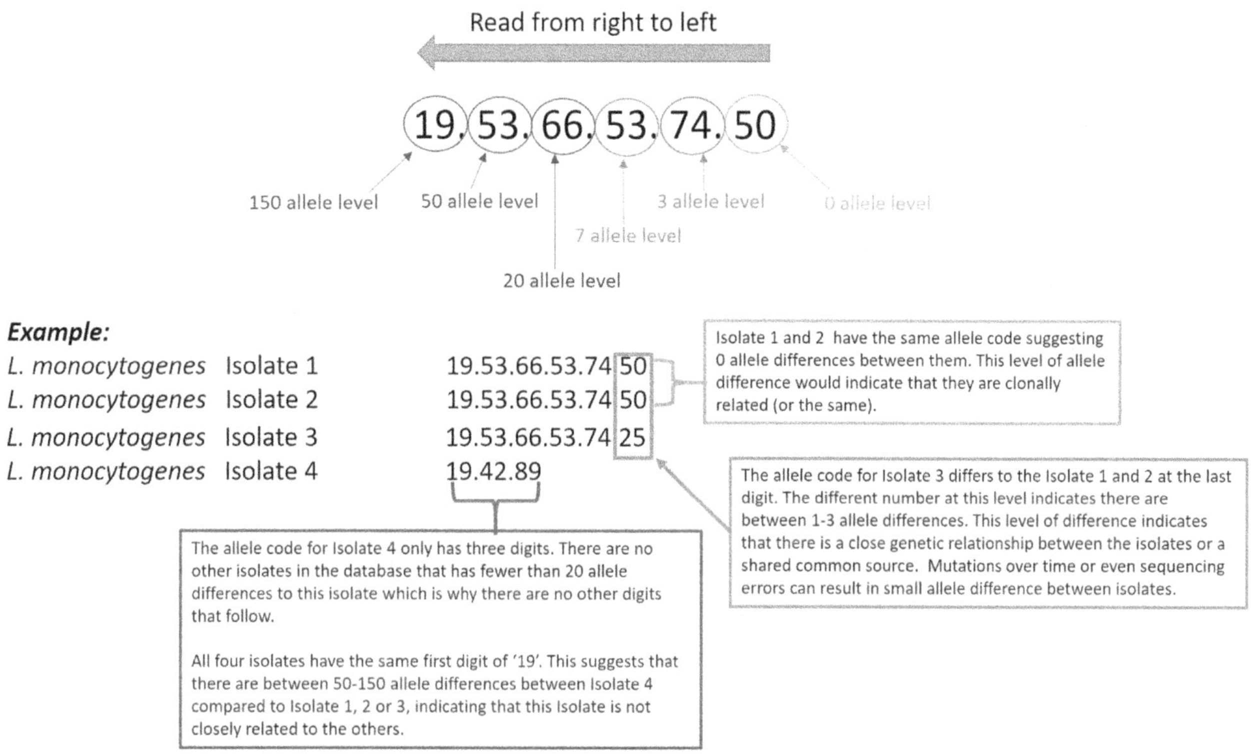

FIGURE 57.3 A 'Zip-code' scheme for *Listeria monocytogenes* (courtesy of Drs Brent Gilpin and Lucia Rivas).

The global pandemic of COVID-19 also saw the emergence of other web-based platforms that combined epidemiological data with genome sequence information to provide easy to interpret, interactive websites that are designed to aid decision making. The website https://outbreak.info/ is one such site that was developed to display epidemiological information and the emergence of genetic variants in near real-time. Again, although this was not developed for a foodborne pathogen, the technology could readily be applied to address the emergence and spread of any pathogen.

57.2.7 Whole-genome sequencing in low-resource countries

Although the cost of WGS has declined markedly in recent years, there remain significant challenges to the adoption of this powerful technology for food safety management in low to middle-income countries.[70] While there are examples of funded research studies examining the transmission of foodborne pathogens in low-resource countries, for example, the transmission of Non-Typhoidal Salmonella in Africa,[71,72] there are relatively few examples of the routine adoption of this technology for regulatory purposes, outbreak management or day-to-day food safety management in the food industry.[73] There are many reasons for the relatively low adoption of WGS in low to middle-income countries and these include[17,18,70]:

- Relatively limited awareness of the utility of WGS for regulatory food safety activities at the level of national or regional government.
- Relatively low investment in the hardware and other laboratory resources needed to collect and analyze WGS data.
- A lack of bioinformaticians and computational biologists with the experience to carry out the analyses needed to inform decision making, and to train others in these skills.

The gap between high and low- and middle-income countries in the adoption of WGS technology, particularly for regulatory purposes, is likely to result in inequality in the international food trade. This underlines the importance of international organizations, and those countries with well-developed systems, to help with training and resourcing less developed nations, enabling them to take full advantage of the technology and resources available.

The FAO recommended a step-by-step approach for the implementation of WGS in low- and middle-income countries, in recognition of the lack of minimum equipment and other resources required for the implementation of the technology in routine, national food safety management, and the fact that each country is likely to have its own unique set of challenges when implementing this technology.[17] They recommend a set of key actions in four phases which can be summarized:

- Phase 1: Before considering WGS, raise awareness with policymakers on global trends in the application of WGS in food safety management, considering benefits and limitations. Assess the level and suitability of current and planned infrastructure, including laboratory resources, and examine existing links with relevant regional and international organizations.

- Phase 2: If infrastructure for WGS adoption is deemed not yet suitable for WGS adoption, strengthen the country's food safety system, including enhancing and strengthening the monitoring and testing of food, the human health surveillance system for targeted foodborne pathogens, and food safety and public health laboratories.
- Phase 3: Once the infrastructure for WGS adoption is deemed suitable, develop tools to guide decision-makers critical for the adoption of WGS at a national level. Provide training to build capability through, for example, online courses or placements in organizations with advanced skills in the use of WGS in food safety.
- Phase 4: Transition to WGS by involving key experts and stakeholders from research providers, including universities and research institutes, government agencies, and other international organizations. Establish a mechanism to coordinate WGS activities at the national level, including surveillance and monitoring systems, data management, enhanced communication systems, a sustainable and ongoing program of training in relevant skills, and harmonization of techniques (e.g., standardized SOPs and reference standards) and stakeholder engagement. Developing links and partnering with other countries, international organizations, and/or international networks and consortia will help with adoption; for example, with PulseNet International and/or GMI. Ongoing financial support is essential to ensure a sustainable program of adoption of WGS technology for food safety management.

57.2.8 Examples of the application of whole-genome sequencing for food safety and the control of foodborne pathogens

In this section, a variety of applications of WGS for food safety are presented, focusing on recent publications. Examples are provided that illustrate a range of pathogens and applications, at varying spatial and temporal scales; from global to local and from long-term to short-term. For further examples of food safety applications see Anon.[17]

57.2.8.1 The global spread of foodborne pathogens

The sharing of sequence data between researchers in different parts of the world, combined with advances in evolutionary modeling[74] has provided the basis for many studies examining the spatial and temporal spread of a variety of viral and bacterial pathogens, with the most recent examples being the transmission of SARS-CoV-2.[75,76] Understanding how pathogens are transmitted around the world is important for the development of mitigation measures aimed at both preventing the emergence of new pathogens and their subsequent widespread dissemination. This approach has also been used to examine the global spread of foodborne pathogens such as Shiga toxin-producing *E. coli* (STEC).[10,77]

Franz et al.[10] used WGS data on STEC serotype O157 from 17 countries on 4 continents to explore the historical movement of this pathogen. They used methods that reconstruct the ancestral history, based on the dates of isolation, their location, and genome sequences. They estimated the date of the common ancestor of the isolates examined was likely to have been around the end of the 19th century, with the most likely location in Northern Europe. The authors conclude that emergence was followed by multiple local and long-range intercontinental movements, most likely associated with the trade-in live animals, particularly cattle and sheep, around the world (Fig. 57.4). A similar approach was taken by Browne et al.[77] who examined the global spread of STEC serotype O26. This showed a consistent pattern of emergence and dissemination and, as with O157, was most likely attributable to the global trade in live animals.

57.2.8.2 The evolution and persistence of pathogens in food processing and along the production chain

Detailed genomic analysis of populations of pathogens in processing environments and along production chains can help to understand how strains adapt, survive, and persist to become foodborne hazards. This can lead to novel approaches to mitigate the risk associated with pathogens such as *L. monocytogenes*[78] and *Campylobacter* spp.[79] An analysis of multiple *L. monocytogenes* contamination events in processing plants showed that WGS could not only demonstrate diversity and sub-populations associated with different time points and different locations/production lines in the same plant, but also revealed specific microevolution events that occurred in processing environments.[78] Similarly, a genome-wide association study of *C. jejuni/coli* isolated from various stages of the poultry processing chain, revealed a selection of lineages with specific genetic elements associated with survival and virulence.[79]

WGS can indicate the presence of genetic traits that may be associated with persistence in processing environments, such as resistance to heat or biocides and the ability to form biofilms. To inform control strategies, it is valuable to assess not only gene content but also phenotypic behavior. A recent study of *L. monocytogenes* isolates from a meat processing plant in Switzerland combined low and high-resolution genotyping with

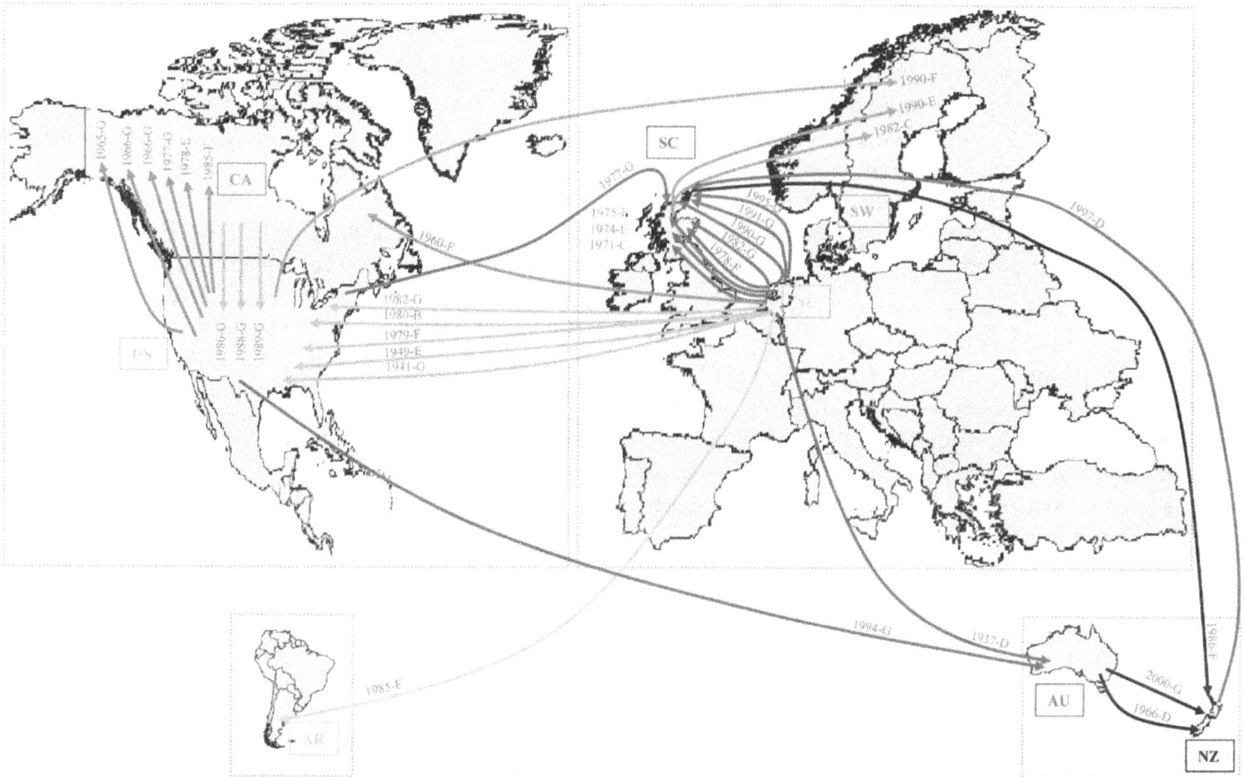

FIGURE 57.4 The estimated 'phylogeography' of STEC serotype O157 determined by Franz et al.,[10] indicating the likely dates and sources of introduction of the pathogen into different locations around the globe.

phenotyping experiments to explore their ability to form biofilms and resistance to biocides benzalkonium chloride and peracetic acid.[80] Genotyping revealed evidence of persistence of several clonal populations for at least four years. All strains showed high biofilm-forming capacity. Genes encoding for efflux pumps for benzalkonium chloride were present in several strains with high minimal inhibitory concentrations (MICs) for this biocide, while other strains showed very low MICs. Further evidence of high MICs for peracetic acid indicated that this biocide might also be ineffective at controlling *L. monocytogenes* in the meat processing facility. Together, information from WGS, lower resolution typing, phenotyping assays, and an understanding of the cleaning procedures used in the plant, can help inform strategies to eliminate persistent strains.

57.2.8.3 Source attribution

Effective control of foodborne pathogens with multiple animal reservoirs, such as *S. enterica* and *C. jejuni*, requires an understanding of the likely 'source' of human infection. 'Source' can be defined broadly as the animal reservoir or maintenance host (e.g., poultry, cattle, or sheep) or, more precisely, the consumption of a particular food product.[81] The various tools and techniques devised for 'Source Attribution' include low technology solutions, such as the elicitation of expert opinion, to quantitative hazard and risk modeling and molecular techniques. There are many approaches to source attribution using molecular tools, including many model-based methods using a subset of the genome[82] or the whole genome.[6,71,83] Source attribution based on the subset of 7 housekeeping genes used for the *C. jejuni/coli* MLST scheme[29] has been used to infer the source of campylobacteriosis in many countries.[84–87]

Although there are many technical issues concerning the use of high-resolution WGS data for modeling source attribution, there are recent examples of publications applying new techniques for attributing campylobacteriosis[88–90] and salmonellosis[83] to animal reservoirs, using WGS. Recent innovations include the development and application of new models that are well-validated, for example, they can perform well in self-attribution of isolates from known sources.[82]

57.2.8.4 Outbreak investigation

WGS is contributing to a more rapid resolution of outbreaks of foodborne disease. In the United States, a collaboration between multiple agencies began performing real-time WGS on all *L. monocytogenes* isolates from human clinical cases, food, and the environment, and data were posted in a public repository. When contemporary comparisons were made with the year before implementation, it was evident that WGS, working alongside epidemiological and product trace-back data, detected more listeriosis clusters and solved more outbreaks post-implementation compared to pre-implementation. [91]

There are many other well-documented examples of the application of WGS for outbreak investigation. Recent examples include the following:

Listeriosis in South Africa[73]

WGS was used to investigate the source of a large outbreak of listeriosis in South Africa in 2017, in which 937 human cases were identified, of which at least 193 died. A case-control study identified the consumption of polony, a ready-to-eat processed meat, as a risk factor. Analysis of 609 human clinical isolates identified one particular 7 gene MLST type of *L. monocytogenes*, ST6, in 93% of cases. The same ST was also identified in polony samples. Higher-resolution cgMLST showed the isolates from the patients and the polony belonged to the same cluster, separated by 4 or fewer allelic differences. WGS confirmed polony produced at a single food production facility to be the source of the outbreak, leading to a large-scale recall of ready-to-eat processed meat products from this facility. This was followed by a rapid decline in the number of human cases of listeriosis associated with *L. monocytogenes* ST6 infections.

STEC O157 in the UK[92]

WGS of isolates from an outbreak of STEC O157:H7 in England in 2017 indicated cases arose from a common source. Of twelve outbreak cases, eight were hospitalized and four developed HUS. This led to several plausible hypotheses that were tested in a case-case study using focused questionnaires and shopping history, as determined by 'loyalty card' data. Frozen beef burgers from a national retailer were identified as the putative cause of the outbreak, and this was confirmed by follow-up testing of burger samples obtained from the freezers of two of the cases from different households, and a sample retained from the production facility – all were found to be positive for the outbreak strain. This led to a voluntary recall by the retailer which likely prevented further cases. WGS played an important role in linking the cases to the same cluster and identifying the vehicle responsible for the outbreak.

Salmonella *Kottbus in Germany*[93]

In June 2017, an outbreak of *Salmonella* Kottbus infection was suspected in Germany. The outbreak was investigated with WGS and the implementation of a case-control study. Forty-six isolates from 69 cases were subtyped and three distinct WGS clusters were identified. Compared to the control population, cluster 1 cases were associated with the consumption of raw smoked ham bought at a particular supermarket chain, whereas cluster 2 cases interviewed were associated with the consumption of quail eggs. Timely WGS of this relatively rare *Salmonella* serotype was useful for distinguishing concurrent outbreaks with different etiologies.

Listeriosis in Germany[94]

In Germany, routine WGS, cgMLST, and SNP-based typing are used for subtyping *L. monocytogenes* isolates from human cases of listeriosis and suspected foods. An unusually large cluster of *L. monocytogenes* isolates was identified in 2018/2019. WGS confirmed the presence of 134 highly clonal, benzalkonium-resistant ST6 isolates collected from 112 notified listeriosis cases. Epidemiological and WGS-based molecular investigations identified blood sausage contaminated with *L. monocytogenes* strains that were highly related to the clinical isolates to be the likely source, and removal of the product from the market ended the outbreak. This investigation demonstrated the value of WGS of isolates from food and clinical samples, combined with epidemiological investigations of food isolates, to identify the source of one of the largest reported outbreaks of listeriosis in Europe over the previous 25 years.

Salmonella *Enteritidis in China*[95]

In July 2018 an outbreak of 10 cases of *S. enterica* serovar Enteritidis infection occurred in Shenzhen, China. An outbreak investigation was augmented by WGS and traced the source to food ordered online. The investigation was one of the first to highlight the emergence of online food delivery platforms as a mode of foodborne disease transmission.

57.2.8.5 Safety evaluation of probiotic strains

Probiotics are used widely in the food industry and guidelines produced by the Food and Agriculture Organization/World Health Organization (FAO/WHO) recommend certain criteria and methodological approaches for the evaluation of their safety.[96] In addition, to standard phenotypic assays, probiotic bacteria are increasingly sequenced using NGS technology to determine their complement of potential virulence and antimicrobial resistance genes. Recent examples of the application of WGS for probiotic safety evaluation include assessing genomes of *Lactobacillus plantarum*[97] and *Bacillus coagulans*[98] for the presence of genes associated with virulence and antimicrobial resistance.

57.2.8.6 Determining the genetic basis of antimicrobial resistance

WGS can be used to identify genes and alleles associated with antimicrobial resistance in foodborne pathogens, such as *Campylobacter* spp.,[44,99] *Listeria* spp.[80] and *S. enterica*.[9] This includes the presence of genes as well as variants of genes (i.e. alleles) known to encode for resistance to specific antibiotics used to treat human clinical cases, as well as biocides and sanitizers used in the food chain to prevent contamination of food products.

57.2.8.7 Understanding transmission in food supply chains

57.2.8.7.1 Transmission from primary production to consumption

A study by Yang et al.[100] describes the population structure and spread of *Vibrio parahaemolyticus* by analyzing genomes from 383 food-associated isolates from six provinces of China in 2014. The isolates were sampled from different sources along the food chain from primary production to circulation and consumption. The study revealed the genetic diversity to be similar across different geographical locations, sample types, and sources, and along the food chain, with some evidence of the spread of lineages along the production chain. Of interest was the lack of distinct boundaries in genetic diversity between isolates from inland and coastal regions or fresh and seawater products. Further, virulence genes and genomic islands were relatively rare, indicating the disease risk from these strains was relatively low. The authors highlight the utility and limitations of using WGS to track *V. parahaemolyticus* from farm-to-table.

WGS was used to examine the transmission of *S. enterica* in the poultry production chain in Hebei Province in China and characterize the isolates in terms of their population structure and antimicrobial resistance gene profile.[101] The authors isolated 148 *S. enterica* from a breeder flock, a hatchery, and a commercial chicken farm, of which all but one were *Salmonella* Enteritidis. WGS revealed that all 147 *Salmonella* Enteritidis strains belonged to ST11 and could be further divided into 4 different ribosomal MLSTs and 64 core genome MLSTs. Using SNP-based analysis they provided evidence for vertical transmission of *Salmonella* Enteritidis from the breeder flock to the commercial chicken farm. Genes associated with antimicrobial resistance and virulence were identified on three plasmids including one blaCTX-M-14-carrying plasmid and two virulence-resistance plasmids. They concluded that routine surveillance in breeding chicken farms is valuable for the control of *Salmonella* Enteritidis along the production chain.

57.2.8.7.2 Transmission from one food processing company to another

Pightling et al.[11] describe a study of the transmission of *L. monocytogenes* from an ingredient supplier to an ice-cream producer. In 2016, the pathogen was detected in finished ice cream products. Investigations by the Regulator identified the source of contamination was likely to be an ingredient provided by another company. Samples were collected from finished products and environmental samples from the ingredient supplier facility. *L. monocytogenes* was isolated from both sets of samples and, using an SNP-based analysis, WGS helped to confirm that the contamination in the ingredient arose from a reservoir population in the ingredient supplier's facility. The investigators compared the populations of *L. monocytogenes* from the final product in 2016 with those from historical samples from the producer and isolates from the ingredient supplier's facility. The pairwise SNP distances revealed a relatively genetically diverse reservoir population, but phylogenetic analysis showed that the finished ice cream isolates from the producer and the environmental isolates from the ingredient supplier formed a 'monophyletic group'; defined as a single cluster of isolates on a phylogenetic tree that is descended from a common ancestor containing only isolates from the populations of interest – in this case, the final product and the ingredient supplier. A bootstrap analysis provided strong support for this branch on the phylogenetic tree, adding further evidence for a direct ancestral link between the isolates. The investigators did not rely on WGS alone - traceback investigations were carried out that revealed that the ice cream producer sourced ingredients from the ingredient supplier to produce ice cream products. The authors concluded that this example shows that WGS can be used to provide further support for identifying sources of contamination in the food chain, and can be used by food safety regulators to identify sources of pathogen contamination both quickly and efficiently. They also caution that WGS data alone is not sufficient, and this must be supported by other evidence, such as traceback data.

57.2.8.7.3 Between farm transmission

A study by Greening et al.[102] used WGS of an antimicrobial-resistant strain of *C. jejuni* (ST 6964) to explore the transmission pathways linking poultry farms in New Zealand. Pathways included local spread indicated by geographical and road distances between farms, and the networks of suppliers of feed, hatching eggs, live birds, and waste litter removal. Genetic relatedness between isolates ($N = 167$ from 30 farms) was determined by wgMLST allele profiles and this was formally compared with the pairwise differences between farms in terms of road distance and shared services (Fig. 57.5). Multivariate analysis and distance-based linear models identified significant associations between the genetic relatedness of the *C. jejuni* isolates and the parent company, road distance, and network distance of transporting feed vehicles. This

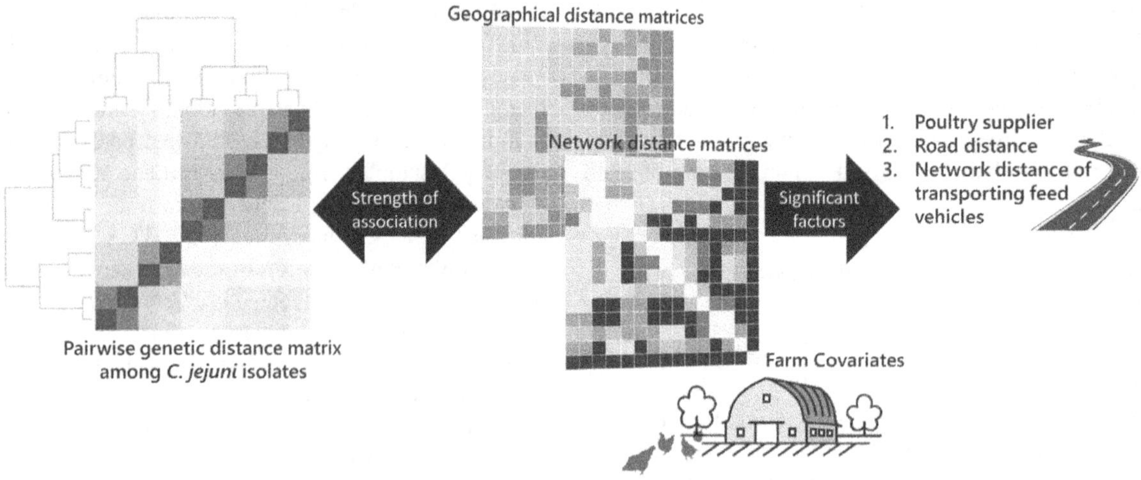

FIGURE 57.5 The application of WGS to understand the local drivers of transmission of *Campylobacter jejuni* between poultry flocks described in Greening et al.[102]

highlighted the importance of within-company spread and mechanisms of the local spread between flocks, leading to recommendations to the industry to improve biosecurity and hygiene barriers between flocks.

57.2.9 Research gaps and future directions

WGS is a tool that is being increasingly used by the food industry and public health agencies to inform decision-making and to reduce the risk to consumers. It can be viewed as one of a number of tools generating 'big' data for 'precision food safety' and 'precision public health'.[103] Applications are many and varied, from understanding global patterns of transmission of food-borne pathogens to source attribution and plant scale micro-mapping. While it is undoubtedly a powerful tool, there remain many concerns about data governance and sharing of sequence data and metadata, with wide-ranging implications for sensitive issues such as patient confidentiality and commercial liability.

Sequencing technologies will likely become more accessible, portable, cheaper, and accurate, and this will make them of greater value to public health agencies for outbreak investigations and determining the source of sporadic cases of foodborne illness, and for the food industry for in-house management of food safety hazards. A recent study has indicated that judicious use of WGS in public health settings "... provides a level of additional information that more than balances the additional costs if used effectively".[104] Similar cost-benefit analyses are needed for the food industry.

The utility of WGS will be further enhanced with the advent of more refined data management and visualization tools. Although there are few published examples, the combination of WGS with phylogenetic trees and mapping of sampling locations has been developed for healthcare settings (https://haiviz.beatsonlab.com/). A similar approach using Microreact (https://microreact.org/) as the interactive visualization tool has been applied for farm and factory-scale micro-mapping for several commercial food companies in New Zealand, by the New Zealand Food Safety Science and Research Centre (https://www.nzfssrc.org.nz/).

A major limitation of the applications of WGS technology described in this chapter, is the need to culture organisms from samples. This adds cost and time to the process. Non-culture-based approaches, therefore offer an exciting new frontier for the application of NGS technologies in food safety. Large food companies are collaborating and applying shotgun metagenomics approaches to genomic characterization of food components[105] and the food chain microbiome, to manage food security and food safety risks.[f] In healthcare settings, affordable, bedside, real-time sequencing applications using Oxford Nanopore technology are being developed to inform clinical decision-making. Protocols developed for real-time genomic epidemiology and outbreak response are increasingly sophisticated and publicly available, such as the Read Assignment, Mapping, and Phylogenetic Analysis in Real-Time (RAMPART) tool (https://artic.network/rampart) developed through the ARTIC network (https://artic.network/). Such tools are likely to see a greater application for public health responses to food safety incidents and for managing microbial hazards in the food chain.

Endnotes

[a]Note the y-axis is logged.

[b]Moore's Law is a benchmark often used to indicate the expected rate of technological progress against the cost of the technology – originally a perception that the number of transistors on a microchip doubles every two years, though the cost of computers is halved.

[c]A kmer is a nucleotide stretch of length k. These are also used for pairwise comparisons to determine relatedness as described below.

[d]This is a measure of the quality of an isolate's sequence. For a set of contigs compiled in descending order according to their size (i.e. sequence length), the N50 is the length of the shortest contig at 50% of the total genome length, i.e. 50% of the whole genome assembly is contained in contigs equal to or larger than this value.

[e]Rapid bacterial SNP identification can be carried out quickly from raw reads, using a suitable reference genome, in the software Snippy (https://github.com/tseemann/snippy). This is implemented in Nullarbor, a pipeline containing multiple bioinformatics tools for generating reports from sequenced isolates (https://github.com/tseemann/nullarbor).

[f]Sequencing the Food Supply Chain Consortium (SFSCC) https://www.research.ibm.com/client-programs/foodsafety/

[g]Wetterstrand KA. DNA Sequencing Costs: Data from the NHGRI Genome Sequencing Program (GSP) Available at: www.genome.gov/sequencingcostsdata. Accessed 4/6/2021. Costs include labour, administration, management, utilities, reagents, and consumables, sequencing instruments and other large equipment (including depreciation), informatics directly related to sequence production and submission of data to a public database.

References

1. Havelaar AH, Kirk MD, Torgerson PR, et al. World health organization global estimates and regional comparisons of the burden of foodborne disease in 2010. *PLoS Med.* 2015;12(12):e1001923. Available from: https://doi.org/10.1371/journal.pmed.1001923.
2. Song H, Chen K. Trade effects and compliance costs of food safety regulations: the case of China. *Agr Agr Sci Proc.* 2010;1:429–438.
3. Ducharme J. You're not imagining it: food recalls are getting more common. Here's why. *Time.* 2019.
4. Townsend A, Li S, Mann DA, Deng X. A quasimetagenomics method for concerted detection and subtyping of *Salmonella enterica* and *E. coli* O157:H7 from romaine lettuce. *Food Microbiol.* 2020;92:103575. Available from: https://doi.org/10.1016/j.fm.2020.103575.
5. Jenkins C, Dallman TJ, Grant KA. Impact of whole genome sequencing on the investigation of food-borne outbreaks of Shiga toxin-producing *Escherichia coli* serogroup O157:H7, England, 2013 to 2017. *Euro Surveill.* 2019;24(4). Available from: https://doi.org/10.2807/1560-7917.Es.2019.24.4.1800346.
6. Mather AE, Vaughan TG, French NP. Molecular approaches to understanding transmission and source attribution in Nontyphoidal *Salmonella* and their application in Africa. *Clin Infect Dis.* 2015;61(Suppl 4):S259–S265. Available from: https://doi.org/10.1093/cid/civ727.
7. Dallman TJ, Byrne L, Ashton PM, et al. Whole-genome sequencing for national surveillance of Shiga toxin-producing *Escherichia coli* O157. *Clin Infect Dis.* 2015;61(3):305–312. Available from: https://doi.org/10.1093/cid/civ318.
8. Moura A, Tourdjman M, Leclercq A, et al. Real-time whole-genome sequencing for surveillance of *Listeria monocytogenes*, France. *Emerg Infect Dis.* 2017;23(9):1462–1470. Available from: https://doi.org/10.3201/eid2309.170336.
9. Mather AE, Reid SW, Maskell DJ, et al. Distinguishable epidemics of multidrug-resistant *Salmonella* Typhimurium DT104 in different hosts. *Science.* 2013;341(6153):1514–1517. Available from: https://doi.org/10.1126/science.1240578.
10. Franz E, Rotariu O, Lopes B, et al. Phylogeographic analysis reveals multiple international transmission events have driven the global emergence of *Escherichia coli* O157:H7. *Clin Infect Dis.* 2019;29(5146342).
11. Pightling AW, Pettengill JB, Luo Y, Baugher JD, Rand H, Strain E. Interpreting whole-genome sequence analyses of foodborne bacteria for regulatory applications and outbreak investigations. *Front Microbiol.* 2018;9:1482. Available from: https://doi.org/10.3389/fmicb.2018.01482.
12. Lupolova N, Dallman TJ, Matthews L, Bono JL, Gally DL. Support vector machine applied to predict the zoonotic potential of *E. coli* O157 cattle isolates. *Proc Natl Acad Sci U S A.* 2016;113(40):11312–11317. Available from: https://doi.org/10.1073/pnas.1606567113.
13. Li B, Zhan M, Evivie SE, et al. Evaluating the safety of potential probiotic *Enterococcus durans* KLDS6.0930 using whole genome sequencing and oral toxicity study. *Front Microbiol.* 2018;9:1943. Available from: https://doi.org/10.3389/fmicb.2018.01943.
14. Zamudio R, Haigh RD, Ralph JD, et al. Lineage-specific evolution and gene flow in *Listeria monocytogenes* are independent of bacteriophages. *Environ Microbiol.* 2020;22(12):5058–5072. Available from: https://doi.org/10.1111/1462-2920.15111.
15. Rasko DA, Webster DR, Sahl JW, et al. Origins of the *E. coli* strain causing an outbreak of hemolytic-uremic syndrome in Germany. *N Engl J Med.* 2011;365(8):709–717. Available from: https://doi.org/10.1056/NEJMoa1106920.
16. Grad YH, Lipsitch M, Feldgarden M, et al. Genomic epidemiology of the *Escherichia coli* O104:H4 outbreaks in Europe, 2011. *Proc Natl Acad Sci U S A.* 2012;109(8):3065–3070. Available from: https://doi.org/10.1073/pnas.1121491109.
17. Anon. *Applications of Whole Genome Sequencing in Food Safety Management.* Food and Agriculture Organization of the United Nations in collaboration with the World Health Organization; 2016.
18. Anon. Whole genome sequencing for foodborne disease surveillance: landscape paper. Geneva: World Health Organization. Licence: CC BY-NC-SA 3.0 IGO. 2018. 9241513861.
19. Heather JM, Chain B. The sequence of sequencers: the history of sequencing DNA. *Genomics.* 2016;107(1):1–8. Available from: https://doi.org/10.1016/j.ygeno.2015.11.003.
20. Goodwin S, McPherson JD, McCombie WR. Coming of age: ten years of next-generation sequencing technologies. *Nat Rev Genet.* 2016;17(6):333–351. Available from: https://doi.org/10.1038/nrg.2016.49.
21. Quail MA, Smith M, Coupland P, et al. A tale of three next generation sequencing platforms: comparison of Ion Torrent, Pacific Biosciences and Illumina MiSeq sequencers. *BMC Genomics.* 2012;13:341. Available from: https://doi.org/10.1186/1471-2164-13-341.
22. Souvorov A, Agarwala R, Lipman DJ. SKESA: strategic k-mer extension for scrupulous assemblies. *Genome Biol.* 2018;19(1):153. Available from: https://doi.org/10.1186/s13059-018-1540-z.
23. Bankevich A, Nurk S, Antipov D, et al. SPAdes: a new genome assembly algorithm and its applications to single-cell sequencing. *J Comput Biol.* 2012;19(5):455–477. Available from: https://doi.org/10.1089/cmb.2012.0021.
24. Seemann T. Prokka: rapid prokaryotic genome annotation. *Bioinformatics.* 2014;30(14):2068–2069. Available from: https://doi.org/10.1093/bioinformatics/btu153.

25. Cody AJ, Bray JE, Jolley KA, McCarthy ND, Maiden MCJ. Core genome multilocus sequence typing scheme for stable, comparative analyses of *Campylobacter jejuni* and C. coli human disease isolates. *J Clin Microbiol.* 2017;55(7):2086–2097. Available from: https://doi.org/10.1128/jcm.00080-17.
26. Zhang J, Xiong Y, Rogers L, Carter GP, French N. Genome-by-genome approach for fast bacterial genealogical relationship evaluation. *Bioinformatics.* 2018;34(17):3025–3027. Available from: https://doi.org/10.1093/bioinformatics/bty195.
27. Silva M, Machado MP, Silva DN, et al. chewBBACA: a complete suite for gene-by-gene schema creation and strain identification. *Microb Genom.* 2018;4(3). Available from: https://doi.org/10.1099/mgen.0.000166.
28. Jolley KA, Bliss CM, Bennett JS, et al. Ribosomal multilocus sequence typing: universal characterization of bacteria from domain to strain. *Microbiol (Read).* 2012;158(Pt 4):1005–1015. Available from: https://doi.org/10.1099/mic.0.055459-0.
29. Dingle KE, Colles FM, Falush D, Maiden MC. Sequence typing and comparison of population biology of *Campylobacter coli* and *Campylobacter jejuni. J Clin Microbiol.* 2005;43(1):340–347. Available from: https://doi.org/10.1128/jcm.43.1.340-347.2005.
30. DeSantis TZ, Hugenholtz P, Larsen N, et al. Greengenes, a chimera-checked 16S rRNA gene database and workbench compatible with ARB. *Appl Env Microbiol.* 2006;72(7):5069–5072. Available from: https://doi.org/10.1128/aem.03006-05.
31. Cole JR, Wang Q, Fish JA, et al. Ribosomal database project: data and tools for high throughput rRNA analysis. *Nucleic Acids Res.* 2014;42(D1):D633–D642.
32. Wood DE, Salzberg SL. Kraken: ultrafast metagenomic sequence classification using exact alignments. *Genome Biol.* 2014;15(3):R46. Available from: https://doi.org/10.1186/gb-2014-15-3-r46.
33. Jolley KA, Bray JE, Maiden MCJ. Open-access bacterial population genomics: BIGSdb software, the PubMLST.org website and their applications. *Wellcome Open Res.* 2018;3:124. Available from: https://doi.org/10.12688/wellcomeopenres.14826.1.
34. Zankari E, Hasman H, Cosentino S, et al. Identification of acquired antimicrobial resistance genes. *J Antimicrob Chemother.* 2012;67(11):2640–2644. Available from: https://doi.org/10.1093/jac/dks261.
35. Jia B, Raphenya AR, Alcock B, et al. CARD 2017: expansion and model-centric curation of the comprehensive antibiotic resistance database. *Nucleic Acids Res.* 2017;45(D1):D566–D573. Available from: https://doi.org/10.1093/nar/gkw1004.
36. Kleinheinz KA, Joensen KG, Larsen MV. Applying the ResFinder and VirulenceFinder web-services for easy identification of acquired antibiotic resistance and *E. coli* virulence genes in bacteriophage and prophage nucleotide sequences. *Bacteriophage.* 2014;4(1):e27943. Available from: https://doi.org/10.4161/bact.27943.
37. McDermott PF, Tyson GH, Kabera C, et al. Whole-genome sequencing for detecting antimicrobial resistance in nontyphoidal *Salmonella. Antimicrob Agents Chemother.* 2016;60(9):5515–5520. Available from: https://doi.org/10.1128/aac.01030-16.
38. Joensen KG, Tetzschner AM, Iguchi A, Aarestrup FM, Scheutz F. Rapid and easy in silico serotyping of *Escherichia coli* isolates by use of whole-genome sequencing data. *J Clin Microbiol.* 2015;53(8):2410–2426. Available from: https://doi.org/10.1128/jcm.00008-15.
39. Yoshida CE, Kruczkiewicz P, Laing CR, et al. The *Salmonella In Silico* Typing Resource (SISTR): an open web-accessible tool for rapidly typing and subtyping draft *Salmonella* genome assemblies. *PLoS One.* 2016;11(1):e0147101. Available from: https://doi.org/10.1371/journal.pone.0147101.
40. Henri C, Leekitcharoenphon P, Carleton HA, et al. An assessment of different genomic approaches for inferring phylogeny of *Listeria monocytogenes. Front Microbiol.* 2017;8:2351. Available from: https://doi.org/10.3389/fmicb.2017.02351.
41. Katz LS, Griswold T, Morrison SS, et al. Mashtree: a rapid comparison of whole genome sequence files. *J Open Source Softw.* 2019;4(44):1762.
42. Moura A, Criscuolo A, Pouseele H, et al. Whole genome-based population biology and epidemiological surveillance of *Listeria monocytogenes. Nat Microbiol.* 2016;2:16185. Available from: https://doi.org/10.1038/nmicrobiol.2016.185.
43. Zhou Z, Alikhan NF, Mohamed K, Fan Y, Achtman M. The EnteroBase user's guide, with case studies on *Salmonella* transmissions, *Yersinia pestis* phylogeny, and *Escherichia* core genomic diversity. *Genome Res.* 2020;30(1):138–152. Available from: https://doi.org/10.1101/gr.251678.119.
44. French NP, Zhang J, Carter GP, et al. Genomic analysis of fluoroquinolone- and tetracycline-resistant *Campylobacter jejuni* sequence type 6964 in humans and poultry, New Zealand, 2014-2016. *Emerg Infect Dis.* 2019;25(12):2226–2234. Available from: https://doi.org/10.3201/eid2512.190267.
45. Huson DH. Application of phylogenetic networks in evolutionary studies. *Mol Biol Evol.* 2006;23(2):254–267. Available from: https://doi.org/10.1093/molbev/msj030.
46. Zhou Z, Alikhan NF, Sergeant MJ, et al. GrapeTree: visualization of core genomic relationships among 100,000 bacterial pathogens. *Genome Res.* 2018;28(9):1395–1404. Available from: https://doi.org/10.1101/gr.232397.117.
47. Nguyen LT, Schmidt HA, von Haeseler A, Minh BQ. IQ-TREE: a fast and effective stochastic algorithm for estimating maximum-likelihood phylogenies. *Mol Biol Evol.* 2015;32(1):268–274. Available from: https://doi.org/10.1093/molbev/msu300.
48. Letunic I, Bork P. Interactive Tree Of Life (iTOL) v4: recent updates and new developments. *Nucleic Acids Res.* 2019;47(W1):W256–W259. Available from: https://doi.org/10.1093/nar/gkz239.
49. Jombart T, Devillard S, Balloux F. Discriminant analysis of principal components: a new method for the analysis of genetically structured populations. *BMC Genet.* 2010;11:94. Available from: https://doi.org/10.1186/1471-2156-11-94.
50. Williamson DA, Baines SL, Carter GP, et al. Genomic insights into a sustained national outbreak of *Yersinia pseudotuberculosis. Genome Biol Evol.* 2016;8(12):3806–3814. Available from: https://doi.org/10.1093/gbe/evw285.
51. Tolar B, Joseph LA, Schroeder MN, et al. An overview of PulseNet USA databases. *Foodborne Pathog Dis.* 2019;16(7):457–462. Available from: https://doi.org/10.1089/fpd.2019.2637.
52. Inns T, Ashton PM, Herrera-Leon S, et al. Prospective use of whole genome sequencing (WGS) detected a multi-country outbreak of *Salmonella* Enteritidis. *Epidemiol Infect.* 2017;145(2):289–298. Available from: https://doi.org/10.1017/s0950268816001941.
53. Timme RE, Wolfgang WJ, Balkey M, et al. Optimizing open data to support one health: best practices to ensure interoperability of genomic

data from bacterial pathogens. *One Health Outlook*. 2020;2(1):20. Available from: https://doi.org/10.1186/s42522-020-00026-3.

54. Timme RE, Strain E, Baugher JD, et al. Phylogenomic pipeline validation for foodborne pathogen disease surveillance. *J Clin Microbiol*. 2019;57(5). Available from: https://doi.org/10.1128/jcm.01816-18.
55. Allard MW, Bell R, Ferreira CM, et al. Genomics of foodborne pathogens for microbial food safety. *Curr Opin Biotechnol*. 2018;49:224–229. Available from: https://doi.org/10.1016/j.copbio.2017.11.002.
56. Allard MW, Strain E, Rand H, et al. Whole genome sequencing uses for foodborne contamination and compliance: discovery of an emerging contamination event in an ice cream facility using whole genome sequencing. *Infect Genet Evol*. 2019;73:214–220. Available from: https://doi.org/10.1016/j.meegid.2019.04.026.
57. Ashton PM, Nair S, Peters TM, et al. Identification of *Salmonella* for public health surveillance using whole genome sequencing. *PeerJ*. 2016;4:e1752. Available from: https://doi.org/10.7717/peerj.1752.
58. Ford L, Carter GP, Wang Q, et al. Incorporating whole-genome sequencing into public health surveillance: lessons from prospective sequencing of *Salmonella* Typhimurium in Australia. *Foodborne Pathog Dis*. Mar 2018;15(3):161–167. Available from: https://doi.org/10.1089/fpd.2017.2352.
59. Timme RE, Rand H, Sanchez Leon M, et al. GenomeTrakr proficiency testing for foodborne pathogen surveillance: an exercise from 2015. *Microb Genom*. 2018;4(7). Available from: https://doi.org/10.1099/mgen.0.000185.
60. Moran-Gilad J, Sintchenko V, Pedersen SK, et al. Proficiency testing for bacterial whole genome sequencing: an end-user survey of current capabilities, requirements and priorities. *BMC Infect Dis*. 2015;15:174. Available from: https://doi.org/10.1186/s12879-015-0902-3.
61. Croucher NJ, Harris SR, Grad YH, Hanage WP. Bacterial genomes in epidemiology--present and future. *Philos Trans R Soc Lond B Biol Sci*. 2013;368(1614):20120202. Available from: https://doi.org/10.1098/rstb.2012.0202.
62. ECDC. European Centre for Disease Prevention and Control. *Fifth external quality assessment scheme for Listeria monocytogenes typing*. Stockholm: ECDC; 2018.
63. Nadon C, Van Walle I, Gerner-Smidt P, et al. PulseNet international: vision for the implementation of whole genome sequencing (WGS) for global food-borne disease surveillance. *Euro Surveill*. 2017;22(23). Available from: https://doi.org/10.2807/1560-7917.Es.2017.22.23.30544.
64. Wilkinson MD, Dumontier M, Aalbersberg IJ, et al. The FAIR guiding principles for scientific data management and stewardship. *Sci Data*. 2016;3:160018. Available from: https://doi.org/10.1038/sdata.2016.18.
65. Hendershot T, Pan H, Haines J, et al. Using the PhenX toolkit to add standard measures to a study. *Curr Protoc Hum Genet*. 2015;86:1.21.1–1.21.17. Available from: https://doi.org/10.1002/0471142905.hg0121s86.
66. Li J, Wang H, Mao L, et al. Rapid genomic characterization of SARS-CoV-2 viruses from clinical specimens using nanopore sequencing. *Sci Rep*. 2020;10(1):17492. Available from: https://doi.org/10.1038/s41598-020-74656-y.
67. Griffiths E, Dooley D, Graham M, Van Domselaar G, Brinkman FSL, Hsiao WWL. Context is everything: harmonization of critical food microbiology descriptors and metadata for improved food safety and surveillance. *Front Microbiol*. 2017;8:1068. Available from: https://doi.org/10.3389/fmicb.2017.01068.
68. Hadfield J, Megill C, Bell SM, et al. Nextstrain: real-time tracking of pathogen evolution. *Bioinformatics*. 2018;34(23):4121–4123. Available from: https://doi.org/10.1093/bioinformatics/bty407.
69. Argimón S, Abudahab K, Goater RJE, et al. Microreact: visualizing and sharing data for genomic epidemiology and phylogeography. *Microb Genom*. 2016;2(11):e000093. Available from: https://doi.org/10.1099/mgen.0.000093.
70. Apruzzese I, Song E, Bonah E, et al. Investing in food safety for developing countries: opportunities and challenges in applying whole-genome sequencing for food safety management. *Foodborne Pathog Dis*. 2019;16(7):463–473. Available from: https://doi.org/10.1089/fpd.2018.2599.
71. Crump JA, Thomas KM, Benschop J, et al. Investigating the meat pathway as a source of human nontyphoidal *Salmonella* bloodstream infections and diarrhea in East Africa. *Clin Infect Dis*. 2020;. Available from: https://doi.org/10.1093/cid/ciaa1153.
72. Kagambèga A, Lienemann T, Frye JG, Barro N, Haukka K. Whole genome sequencing of multidrug-resistant *Salmonella enterica* serovar Typhimurium isolated from humans and poultry in Burkina Faso. *Trop Med Health*. 2018;46:4. Available from: https://doi.org/10.1186/s41182-018-0086-9.
73. Thomas J, Govender N, McCarthy KM, et al. Outbreak of listeriosis in South Africa associated with processed meat. *N Engl J Med*. 2020;382(7):632–643. Available from: https://doi.org/10.1056/NEJMoa1907462.
74. Kühnert D, Stadler T, Vaughan TG, Drummond AJ. Phylodynamics with migration: a computational framework to quantify population structure from genomic data. *Mol Biol Evol*. 2016;33(8):2102–2116. Available from: https://doi.org/10.1093/molbev/msw064.
75. Geoghegan JL, Ren X, Storey M, et al. Genomic epidemiology reveals transmission patterns and dynamics of SARS-CoV-2 in Aotearoa New Zealand. *Nat Commun*. 2020;11(1):6351. Available from: https://doi.org/10.1038/s41467-020-20235-8.
76. du Plessis L, McCrone JT, Zarebski AE, et al. Establishment and lineage dynamics of the SARS-CoV-2 epidemic in the UK. *Science*. 2021;371(6530):708–712. Available from: https://doi.org/10.1126/science.abf2946.
77. Browne AS, Biggs PJ, Wilkinson DA, et al. Use of genomics to investigate historical importation of Shiga toxin-producing *Escherichia coli* Serogroup O26 and nontoxigenic variants into New Zealand. *Emerg Infect Dis*. 2019;25(3):489–500. Available from: https://doi.org/10.3201/eid2503.180899.
78. Yang H, Hoffmann M, Allard MW, Brown EW, Chen Y. Microevolution and gain or loss of mobile genetic elements of outbreak-related *Listeria monocytogenes* in food processing environments identified by whole genome sequencing analysis. *Front Microbiol*. 2020;11:866. Available from: https://doi.org/10.3389/fmicb.2020.00866.
79. Yahara K, Méric G, Taylor AJ, et al. Genome-wide association of functional traits linked with *Campylobacter jejuni* survival from farm to fork. *Environ Microbiol*. 2017;19(1):361–380. Available from: https://doi.org/10.1111/1462-2920.13628.
80. Stoller A, Stevens MJA, Stephan R, Guldimann C. Characteristics of *Listeria monocytogenes* strains persisting in a meat processing facility over a 4-year period. *Pathogens*. 2019;8(1). Available from: https://doi.org/10.3390/pathogens8010032.

81. Wagenaar JA, French NP, Havelaar AH. Preventing *Campylobacter* at the source-why is it so difficult? *Clin Infect Dis.* 2013;57(11):1600–1606.
82. Cody AJ, Maiden MC, Strachan NJ, McCarthy ND. A systematic review of source attribution of human campylobacteriosis using multilocus sequence typing. *Euro Surveill.* 2019;24(43). Available from: https://doi.org/10.2807/1560-7917.Es.2019.24.43.1800696.
83. Munck N, Njage PMK, Leekitcharoenphon P, Litrup E, Hald T. Application of whole-genome sequences and machine learning in source attribution of *Salmonella* Typhimurium. *Risk Anal.* 2020;40(9):1693–1705. Available from: https://doi.org/10.1111/risa.13510.
84. Boysen L, Rosenquist H, Larsson JT, et al. Source attribution of human campylobacteriosis in Denmark. *Epidemiol Infect.* 2014;142(8):1599–1608. Available from: https://doi.org/10.1017/s0950268813002719.
85. Mughini Gras L, Smid JH, Wagenaar JA, et al. Risk factors for campylobacteriosis of chicken, ruminant, and environmental origin: a combined case-control and source attribution analysis. *PLoS One.* 2012;7(8):e42599. Available from: https://doi.org/10.1371/journal.pone.0042599.
86. Nohra A, Grinberg A, Marshall JC, Midwinter AC, Collins-Emerson JM, French NP. Shifts in the molecular epidemiology of *Campylobacter jejuni* infections in a sentinel region of New Zealand following implementation of food safety interventions by the poultry industry. *Appl Environ Microbiol.* 2020;86(5). Available from: https://doi.org/10.1128/aem.01753-19.
87. Sheppard SK, Dallas JF, Strachan NJ, et al. *Campylobacter* genotyping to determine the source of human infection. *Clin Infect Dis.* 2009;48(8):1072–1078. Available from: https://doi.org/10.1086/597402.
88. Jehanne Q, Pascoe B, Bénéjat L, et al. Genome-wide identification of host-segregating SNPs for source attribution of clinical *Campylobacter coli* isolates. *Appl Environ Microbiol.* 2020;. Available from: https://doi.org/10.1128/aem.01787-20.
89. Thépault A, Rose V, Quesne S, et al. Ruminant and chicken: important sources of campylobacteriosis in France despite a variation of source attribution in 2009 and 2015. *Sci Rep.* 2018;8(1):9305. Available from: https://doi.org/10.1038/s41598-018-27558-z.
90. Lake RJ, Campbell DM, Hathaway SC, et al. Source attributed case-control study of campylobacteriosis in New Zealand. *Int J Infect Dis.* 2021;103:268–277. Available from: https://doi.org/10.1016/j.ijid.2020.11.167.
91. Jackson BR, Tarr C, Strain E, et al. Implementation of nationwide real-time whole-genome sequencing to enhance listeriosis outbreak detection and investigation. *Clin Infect Dis.* 2016;63(3):380–386. Available from: https://doi.org/10.1093/cid/ciw242.
92. Byrne L, Kaindama L, Bentley M, et al. Investigation into a national outbreak of STEC O157:H7 associated with frozen beef burgers, UK, 2017. *Epidemiol Infect.* 2020;148:e215. Available from: https://doi.org/10.1017/s0950268820001582.
93. Enkelmann J, von Laer A, Simon S, et al. Disentangling outbreaks using whole-genome sequencing: concurrent multistate outbreaks of *Salmonella* Kottbus in Germany, 2017. *Epidemiol Infect.* 2020;148:e51. Available from: https://doi.org/10.1017/s0950268820000394.
94. Halbedel S, Wilking H, Holzer A, et al. Large nationwide outbreak of invasive listeriosis associated with blood sausage, Germany, 2018-2019. *Emerg Infect Dis.* 2020;26(7):1456–1464. Available from: https://doi.org/10.3201/eid2607.200225.
95. Jiang M, Zhu F, Yang C, et al. Whole-genome analysis of *Salmonella enterica* serovar Enteritidis isolates in outbreak linked to online food delivery, Shenzhen, China, 2018. *Emerg Infect Dis.* 2020;26(4):789–792. Available from: https://doi.org/10.3201/eid2604.191446.
96. Anon. Probiotics in food: health and nutritional properties and guidelines for evaluation: report of a Joint FAO/WHO Expert Consultation on Evaluation of Health and Nutritional Properties of Probiotics in Food including Powder Milk with Live Lactic Acid Bacteria, Cordoba, Argentina, 1-4 October 2001 [and] Report of a Joint FAO/WHO Working Group on Drafting Guidelines for the Evaluation of Probiotics in Food, London, Ontario, Canada, 30 April–1 May 2002. FAO food and nutrition paper, 0254-4725; 85. Food and Agriculture Organization of the United Nations, World Health Organization; 2006.
97. Arellano K, Vazquez J, Park H, et al. Safety evaluation and whole-genome annotation of *Lactobacillus plantarum* strains from different sources with special focus on isolates from green tea. *Probiotics Antimicrob Proteins.* 2020;12(3):1057–1070. Available from: https://doi.org/10.1007/s12602-019-09620-y.
98. Saroj DB, Gupta AK. Genome based safety assessment for *Bacillus coagulans* strain LBSC (DSM 17654) for probiotic application. *Int J Food Microbiol.* 2020;318:108523. Available from: https://doi.org/10.1016/j.ijfoodmicro.2020.108523.
99. Wallace RL, Bulach D, McLure A, et al. Antimicrobial resistance of *Campylobacter* spp. causing human infection in Australia: an international comparison. *Microb Drug Resist.* 2020;. Available from: https://doi.org/10.1089/mdr.2020.0082.
100. Yang C, Zhang X, Fan H, et al. Genetic diversity, virulence factors and farm-to-table spread pattern of *Vibrio parahaemolyticus* food-associated isolates. *Food Microbiol.* 2019;84:103270. Available from: https://doi.org/10.1016/j.fm.2019.103270.
101. Lei CW, Zhang Y, Kang ZZ, et al. Vertical transmission of *Salmonella* Enteritidis with heterogeneous antimicrobial resistance from breeding chickens to commercial chickens in China. *Vet Microbiol.* 2020;240:108538. Available from: https://doi.org/10.1016/j.vetmic.2019.108538.
102. Greening SS, Zhang J, Midwinter AC, et al. Transmission dynamics of an antimicrobial resistant *Campylobacter jejuni* lineage in New Zealand's commercial poultry network. *Epidemics.* 2021;37:100521. Available from: https://doi.org/10.1016/j.epidem.2021.100521.
103. Donaghy JA, Danyluk M, Ross T, Krishna B, Farber J. Big data impacting dynamic food safety risk management in the food chain. *Front Microbiol.* 2021;12:952.
104. Alleweldt F, Kara Ş, Best K, et al. Economic evaluation of whole genome sequencing for pathogen identification and surveillance-results of case studies in Europe and the Americas 2016 to 2019. *Euro Surveill.* 2021;26(9). Available from: https://doi.org/10.2807/1560-7917.Es.2021.26.9.1900606.
105. Haiminen N, Edlund S, Chambliss D, et al. Food authentication from shotgun sequencing reads with an application on high protein powders. *NPJ Sci Food.* 2019;3(1):24. Available from: https://doi.org/10.1038/s41538-019-0056-6.

Chapter 58

Drug-resistant bacteria from "farm to fork": impact of antibiotic use in animal production

Michaela van den Honert[1] and Louwrens Hoffman[2]

[1]Centre for Food Safety, Department of Food Science, University of Stellenbosch, Matieland, South Africa, [2]Centre for Nutrition and Food Sciences, Queensland Alliance for Agriculture and Food Innovation, The University of Queensland, Gatton, QLD, Australia

Abstract

Antibiotic resistance of zoonotic foodborne pathogens is now considered by the World Health Organization to be one of this century's leading global health challenges. Unfortunately, we are currently in danger of entering a "post-antimicrobial era," where the efficacy of antimicrobials may be significantly compromised by the emergence of antimicrobial resistant microorganisms. The farming industry has come under scrutiny over recent years for being considered a major contributor to the emergence of antibiotic resistance worldwide. There are various practices that can be implemented to help reverse or slow down the development of antibiotic resistance in animal production. In an attempt to better control and contain antibiotic resistance, the World Health Organization and Food and Agriculture Organization have published an action plan on antimicrobial resistance. The World Health Organization suggested that every country should develop an antimicrobial resistance action plan in line with their Global Action Plan.

Keywords: Horizontal gene transfer; prophylaxis; One Health; foodborne illness; pathogens; animal production systems; agriculture

58.1 Introduction

Antimicrobial agents are considered one of modern medicine's greatest discoveries, saving millions of lives annually.[1] Antimicrobial resistance is the ability of a microorganism to resist the action of an antimicrobial agent that has been designed to kill it through targeting different parts of the microorganism's cell, which are essential for growth and survival.[2] The antimicrobial resistant microorganism is thus able to survive and grow, despite the presence of an antimicrobial agent. The development of antimicrobial resistance is inherent and unavoidable and can be described as a Darwinian process—that is, selection of the fittest.[3]

Unfortunately, we are currently in danger of entering a "post-antimicrobial era," where the efficacy of most antimicrobials may be significantly compromised by the emergence of antimicrobial resistant microorganisms.[4,5] This would pose a major global threat to human health. Increased treatment failures, increased infection severity, and increased occurrence of infections that would not otherwise have occurred in both animals and humans, will become prevalent.[3]

Antimicrobial resistance of bacterial origin, known as antibiotic resistance (ABR), of zoonotic foodborne pathogens, is now considered by the World Health Organization (WHO) to be one of this century's leading global health challenges due to bacteria's inherent ability to rapidly and easily multiply.[6–8] This has brought about increased public concerns and scientific interest over the last decade.[9,10] The One Health initiative aims to improve future human, animal, and environmental health through interdisciplinary collaborations and communications.[11] The WHO, the Food and Agriculture Organization (FAO), and the World Organization for Animal Health have collaborated to take collective action to minimize the emergence and spread of antimicrobial resistance.

This phenomenon emerges largely as a result of a selective pressure created in a bacterial community, which creates a "survival of the fittest" evolutionary change.[12] The antibiotic agent exerted onto the bacterial population creates a stressed environment where all the susceptible bacteria are killed and the few resilient bacteria are able to survive and resist the antibiotic action.[3,13] The resistant bacteria that survived the treatment then go

Present Knowledge in Food Safety. DOI: https://doi.org/10.1016/B978-0-12-819470-6.00011-1

on to replicate and, over time, produce a larger resistant population.[3]

The misuse, overuse, and inappropriate use of antimicrobials in human medicine and animal medicine and husbandry create an enormous selection pressure toward developing ABR.[1] This increases and accelerates the likelihood that bacteria will adapt and multiply to produce a more resistant population. The epidemic of ABR was initially bound to hospital environments but has since emerged into community-acquired and livestock-acquired resistant bacteria. For example, methicillin-resistant *Staphylococcus aureus* (MRSA) was once only detected in hospitals but is now evident in livestock, wildlife, and the community since the past two decades.[1,14] Since the mid-2000s, livestock have become a primary reservoir of MRSA strains. A new variant, CC398, first noted in European countries, has recently been found in animals, especially intensively reared production animals like pigs, cattle, and poultry.[15]

It is not just resistant pathogens which are a concern but also the resistant nonpathogenic commensal bacteria. This is because resistant commensals can create a large resistance gene pool where resistant traits can be readily transferred, even to pathogenic bacteria.[16]

The farming industry has come under scrutiny over recent years for being considered a major contributor to the emergence of ABR worldwide, followed closely by the human medicine industry.[4,17] This arises in part because antibiotics are used to a greater extent in the agricultural industry than in human medicine, as the former relies heavily on antibiotics to improve animal health and productivity, especially in intensively reared species.[18,19] It is time to review agricultural practices in this regard.

Although there is still no consensus on the degree to which antibiotic usage in food-producing animals contributes to the development and spread of ABR in humans, experimental evidence exists that suggests a relationship between antimicrobial use and ABR development in animals and the spread to humans, especially via the food chain.[20]

The potential for transmission of zoonotic pathogenic and commensal bacteria to humans, either by direct contact with animals or through indirect contact via the food chain, presents a major challenge to the future of human health.[8]

TABLE 58.1 Mechanisms of action of the main antibiotic classes.[21,22]

Antibiotic mechanism of action	Antibiotic class
Disruption or inhibition of cell wall synthesis	Beta-lactams and subclasses, bactitracin polypeptides, glycopeptides
Alteration or interference of cell membrane	Polymyxins, lipopeptides
Disruption or inhibition of protein synthesis	Tetracyclines, aminoglycosides, macrolides, streptogramins, lincosamides, oxazolidinones, amphenicols, pleuromutilins
Inhibition of nucleic acid synthesis/metabolism	Sulfonamides, quinolones, rifamycins, trimethoprim

58.2 Development and transfer of antibiotic resistance

The discovery and production of antibiotics in the early 1900s contributed to a significant increase in the human lifespan.[5] Antibiotics kill bacteria by targeting various parts or processes of the bacterial cell. Table 58.1 lists the mechanism of action of various antibiotic classes. Antibiotic resistant bacteria have developed various mechanisms to counteract the action of antibiotics.

The first antibiotic, penicillin, was discovered in 1928. Back then, it was believed that ABR development would be minor, based on the assumption that the emergence of antibiotic resistant mutants would be negligible.[5] The ability of bacteria to interchange genes through a process of horizontal gene transfer (HGT) was largely unforeseen. Likewise, a microorganism's ability to adapt to environmental conditions was greatly overlooked and underestimated.

Bacteria exhibit a number of ABR mechanisms, including (1) efflux pumps which actively pump out the antibiotic from the bacterial cell and thus decrease the intracellular antibiotic concentration, (2) enzyme modification of the antibiotic which renders it ineffective, (3) degradation of the antimicrobial compound, (4) the use of alternative metabolic pathways to those inhibited by the antibiotic, (5) overproduction of the target enzyme, (6) modification of antibiotic targets, and lastly, (7) alteration of cell wall permeability, which stops the antimicrobial agent entering the cell and reaching the target sites.[23]

In nature, a harmonious balance exists between antibiotic levels produced by antibiotic-producing bacteria and antibiotic resistant bacteria in an ecological population.[24] Antibiotics produced by organisms in the natural environment serve the purpose of cell-to-cell signaling networks and homeostasis of bacterial communities, over and above, that is, the use of antibiotics to increase the chances of survival in a compromised or competitive environment.[24,25] What's more is that some antibiotic resistant mechanisms have existed in nature even before the use of antibiotics began by humans. For example, efflux pumps originally served the purpose of signal trafficking and for removing toxic substances.[26] Some of the most commonly used antibiotics are of natural origin. For example, the well-known penicillin antibiotic is produced by the *Penicillium* fungus; streptomycin, chloramphenicol, and tetracycline are produced by *Streptomyces* bacteria and vancomycin is made by *Amycolatopsis* bacteria.[25]

A microorganism may even be resistant to antimicrobials to which it has never been exposed. This is either due to intrinsic resistance or as a result of cross-resistance or coresistance.[27] Intrinsic resistance is naturally occurring and is related to physiological attributes, such as the complexity of the cell wall, as in Gram-negative bacteria.[27] Gram-negative bacteria usually have a higher level of intrinsic ABR than Gram-positive bacteria, owing to their impermeable double membrane in the cell wall, making them innately resistant to antibiotics such as penicillin, which cannot enter their cell wall.[27] Another characteristic of intrinsic resistance is the ability of some microorganisms to form a biofilm which protects the microbial cells through secretion of exopolysaccharides, creating a physical barrier between the antibiotic and the bacterial cell.[27]

Intrinsic resistance is shown in various studies where ABR was detected in environments in which antibiotics have never been used before.[28] For example, a microbiome in an isolated cave in New Mexico exhibited ABR to several commercially available antibiotics, suggesting that ABR is prehistoric and occurs naturally in order to increase the chance of survival of microorganisms in a compromised environment.[23] One of the first antibiotic resistant bacteria studied in wildlife was found in wild pigeons around 1975, when strains of *Escherichia coli* were found to be resistant to various antibiotics.[29] However, this naturally existing ABR gene pool is not a major threat to human and animal health as it contributes to a minute portion of ABR in populated environments.[30]

Cross-resistance can develop to structurally related antibiotics, either to antibiotics within the same class or across different classes, either due to overlapping drug targets or if the efflux pump is capable of removing different classes of antibiotics from the bacterial cell, known as "multidrug efflux pumps."[31] For example, resistance genes to the antibiotics vancomycin and avoparcin from the glycopeptide antibiotic class are located on the same resistance gene cluster and thus resistance can be selected for both antibiotics, as the resistance genes are not located on a mobile genetic element.[32]

Coresistance or cotransfer is the development of resistance to structurally unrelated antibiotics. This generally occurs if the resistance genes are located on the same mobile genetic elements, such as a plasmid. Therefore antibiotic resistant determinants which are located on the bacterial chromosome, such as is the case for quinolone resistance, are not likely to be coselected by use of other antibiotics.[33]

Research has also shown that biocides, such as disinfectants and preservatives, as well as heavy metals can coselect ABR.[25] For example, copper, zinc, and mercury have been correlated with the *sul*A and *sul*III ABR genes. This generally happens if a mobile genetic element contains resistance genes and also heavy metal resistance genes. This is because the mechanisms of resistance toward heavy metals are similar to those for ABR. Like antibiotics, heavy metals exert a stress on bacteria. It is also common to find ABR genes and heavy metal resistance genes located on the same mobile genetic element. For example, studies have found links between using zinc in animal feeds and the occurrence of MRSA, where a zinc resistance gene, *czr*C is located on the same mobile genetic element "SCC*mec*," which encodes for methicillin resistance too.[32] The link between biocide and ABR is less well known and is still controversial. However, it is thought that some biocides increase the risk of ABR development.[34] For example, it was reported that exposure of quaternary ammonium compounds, a disinfectant, to *E. coli* resulted in the development of resistance to various antibiotics such as beta-lactams, tetracycline, and fluoroquinolones.[34] This association is likely due to the development of increased efflux activity and improved biofilm capability.[34]

Of greater concern over intrinsic resistance is the ability of bacteria to *acquire* resistance, which is widely considered the most important form of ABR development. Acquired resistance occurs either through genetic mutations or horizontal transfer of genetic material via mobile genetic elements from other resistant microorganisms.[3,35]

Transfer of antibiotic resistant genetic material through HGT is of greater concern than random genetic mutations because it can occur more often with a more specific outcome. In addition, HGT can occur between bacterial strains, species, and even between genera that share the same ecological niche, and, more worryingly, from nonpathogenic to pathogenic bacterial strains.[3] This genetic transfer can occur almost anywhere, such as in food-producing animals or in the environment, for example, the soil.[3,35]

There are various ways in which HGT can take place, namely, conjugation, transduction, and transformation.[3]

58.2.1 Conjugation

The conjugational pathway, illustrated in Fig. 58.1, constitutes a direct cell-to-cell exchange of genetic material through enzyme activities involving a donor and a recipient cell.[36] The transfer of genetic material between the two cells can occur within species or between species.[36] Exchange of genetic material occurs via a specific hair-like temporary attachment called a "pilus" on the surface of the donor cell which creates a bridge between the two

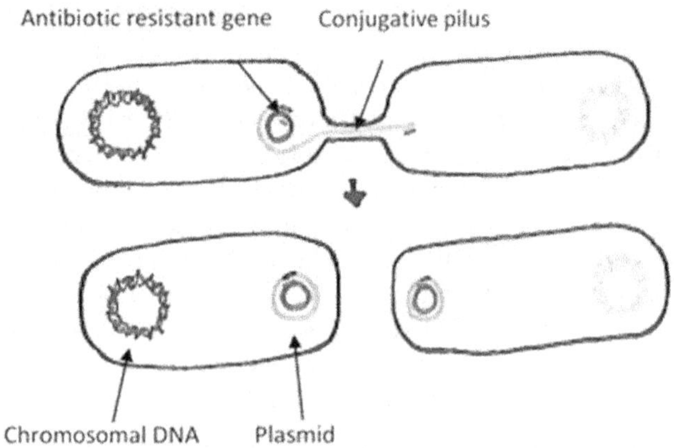

FIGURE 58.1 The exchange of conjugative plasmids. *Adapted from von Wintersdorff CJH, Penders J, Van Niekerk JM, et al. Dissemination of antimicrobial resistance in microbial ecosystems through horizontal gene transfer.* Front Microbiol. *2016;7:1–10.*

cells.[3] Enzymes then initiate the transportation of a single DNA strand to the recipient, which synthesizes a double DNA strand to create a copy of the antibiotic resistant gene.[36] Not only can chromosomal DNA be transferred to other hosts but so can plasmids, transposons, integrons, and insertion sequences which all bear one or more genes from the donor cell.[13] The exchange of conjugative plasmids is the most efficient and common form of genetic transfer. This is because of independent replication in the host cell. This can therefore be considered as the most likely way in which ABR is acquired.[30,36]

58.2.2 Transduction

Transduction involves injection of genetic material into a host cell by making use of a "vector."[3] Genetic material can be passed onto a suitable bacterial host by a bacteriophage that has previously replicated in another bacterium and contains random DNA fragments, such as insertion elements, plasmids, and chromosome fragments.

Transduction appears to play a key part in bacterial evolution due to the transfer of virulence and antibiotic resistant genes to new bacterial hosts by bacteriophages that are highly abundant in nature.[37] Transduction has been considered a rare event in the past but due to the abundance of phages and hosts in many environments and due to the additional fact that phages have excellent survival capabilities, genetic transfer via transduction has been postulated to contribute significantly to ABR in microbial communities.[37] However, gene transfer via transduction is still at this stage considered a minor mechanism compared to other genetic transfer routes such as conjugation and transformation. Fig. 58.2 demonstrates the transfer of DNA between bacteria via phages.[38]

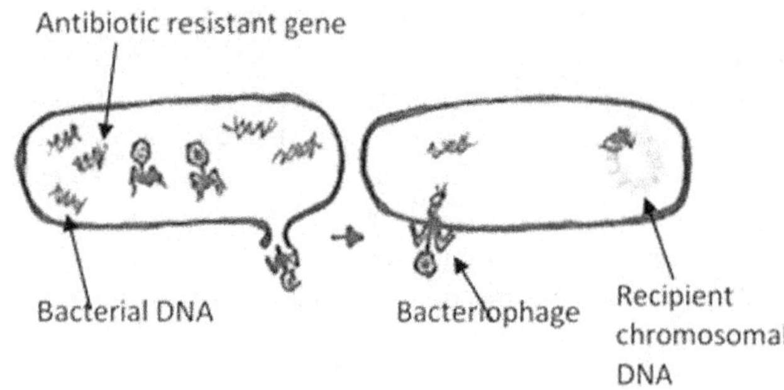

FIGURE 58.2 The transfer of DNA between bacteria via phages, known as transduction. *Adapted from Balcazar JL. Bacteriophages as vehicles for antibiotic resistance genes in the environment. PLOS Pathog. 2014;10:1–4.*

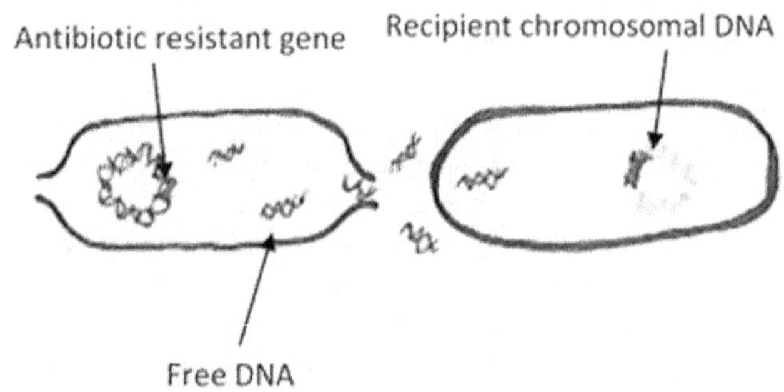

FIGURE 58.3 The uptake of free DNA from a nearby bacterium cell, known as transformation. *Adapted from Fronzes R, Christie PJ, Waksman G. The structural biology of type IV secretion systems.* Nat Rev Microbiol. *2009;7:703–714.*

58.2.3 Transformation

The third type of transmission mechanism of bacterial genetic material in addition to conjugation and transduction is transformation, shown in Fig. 58.3.[39] This occurs via the uptake of free DNA from a bacterial cell close to a donor cell.[13] The donor cell in such a scenario, is usually dead and releases its plasmids or short fragments of DNA into the environment, allowing its genetic material to be acquired directly by a healthy bacterial cell through its cell wall.[3] This type of genetic transfer has limitations and can only effectively occur in certain bacteria and in those that have the genetic capacity to absorb the loose DNA.[36] Additionally, the DNA must be compatible with the recipient.[36]

The rise in antibiotic resistant bacterial species is a result of a complex mix of factors. Some factors are unavoidable and inherent in nature, such as those mentioned above, where bacteria have the ability to adapt rapidly to changing environmental conditions because of their short generation time and some are intrinsically resistant to certain antibiotics.[40] But some variables are man-made, such as the extensive use of antibiotics as growth promoters in the farming industry.[1,41]

58.3 Epidemiology of antibiotic resistance

ABR in the environment occurs in many sectors, from aquaculture, food processing, and healthcare to wildlife, companion animals, and food animals.[16,42] The activities of these sectors often result in a constant release of low-level antibiotic concentrations, which has shown to encourage ABR development and can make its way into water sources and soil through wastewater treatment plant effluents, sewage, agricultural waste and bio-solid application to fields, among others.[25,43] Mobile vectors can assist in transferring ABR between these different sectors and include elements such as the wind, crops, and flies.[44,45] Fig. 58.4 displays a schematic of pathways, transfer vectors, and practices which are all involved in the dissemination of ABR throughout the environment and demonstrate that each sector is indeed interconnected one way or another.

There are various stages and interactions in the food production chain where antibiotic resistant bacteria and antibiotic residues can enter. A concern with regards to antibiotic dissemination into the environment is that antibiotics remain largely unchanged after metabolism.[46] On the farm environment, the most obvious source of direct antibiotic contamination and antibiotic resistant bacteria is the application of antibiotics in animal feed for livestock and aquaculture food production. Antibiotic resistant bacteria can spread directly between animals that are in close proximity to each other, as well as between farmers and their animals.[16] Other animals such as birds and small rodents have also shown to be carriers of antibiotic resistant bacteria by releasing fecal matter over vast areas during movement and migration.

More indirect sources of antibiotic resistant bacteria and antibiotic residues can enter the farm environment from human waste, animal waste, and industrial waste, and can make its way into other environments via soil, water, and manure.[46] This can happen during soil fertilization with raw animal manure, contamination of water sources such as rivers from human, animal, or industrial waste runoff or discharge, seeping of animal manure into the surface and groundwater, irrigation with contaminated water or untreated wastewater, or contamination of water sources from antibiotic use in aquaculture. Farming activities such as cograzing with livestock and wildlife on the same farm can cause a bidirectional transfer of antibiotic resistant bacteria at the interface.[47]

During food production, there are processing steps such as farming activities, slaughtering practices, and

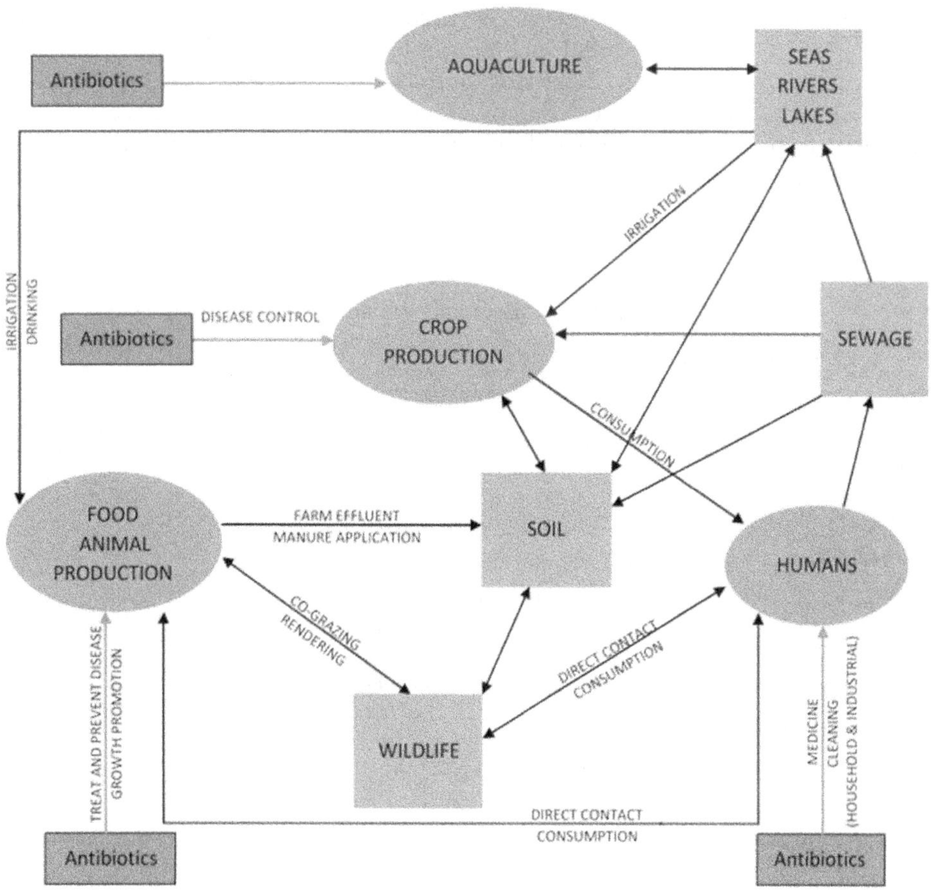

FIGURE 58.4 The epidemiology of antimicrobial resistance. *Adapted from Landers TF, Cohen B, Wittum TE, Larson EL. A review of antibiotic use in food animals: perspective, policy, and potential. Public Health Rep. 2012;127:4–22. and Anonymous. Antimicrobial resistance: implications for the food system. Compr Rev Food Sci Food Saf. 2006;5:71–137.*

meat processing activities which could possibly introduce resistant bacteria into the food chain. During slaughter, contamination of the meat with fecal matter or contaminated water, or by personal contact can transfer antibiotic resistant bacteria onto the meat. Contaminated meat processing equipment and food handlers can cause further contamination of the meat. Residual antibiotics in raw meat could result in the development of antibiotic resistant bacteria in the human gut.[48]

The food products through which antibiotic resistant bacteria may be present include meat, fish, milk, and eggs. However, plant-based foods can also contain antibiotic resistant bacteria which could have originated either via contaminated irrigation water or improper handling.

58.4 Existing antibiotic resistant microorganisms

The potential danger of the development of antibiotic resistant bacteria was first noted by Sir Alexander Fleming in the early 1900s. He predicted that if penicillin were to be misused following its introduction, then *S. aureus* mutants could develop that would build resistance to the antimicrobial compound.[3] Quite correctly, only a few years later, a significant amount of *S. aureus* strains were resistant to the treatment of penicillin due to the development of resistant strains.[30]

The WHO published a list of the highest priority antibiotic resistant pathogens where there is urgent need to develop new antibiotics to fight against these emerging resistant pathogens, which pose a major threat to human health; they are listed in Table 58.2.

Acinetobacter baumannii is a Gram-negative nosocomial pathogen which has shown increased ABR worldwide in hospitals, especially in intensive care units.[50] *A. baumannii* have become resistant to a wide range of antibiotics, owing to their ability to easily exchange genetic material.[50] Currently only carbapenems are still effective in treating *A. baumannii* infections but resistance to this class of antibiotic is also rising.[51] Although *Acinetobacter* is not a classical foodborne pathogen, multidrug resistant (MDR) *Acinetobacter* has been detected in raw milk and raw meat, suggesting that food of animal origin could serve as vectors of MDR *Acinetobacter* into the community and hospital settings.[52] MDR *Acinetobacter* could also contaminate fruits and vegetables from contaminated irrigation water.[52]

Pseudomonas aeruginosa is a Gram-negative pathogen which can colonize a wide range of environments, including hospitals, animals, and aquatic environments.[53] It is the pathogen which is most commonly responsible for community or hospital-acquired pneumonia. *P. aeruginosa* has unique intrinsic antibiotic resistant mechanisms and metabolic versatility over other Gram-negative pathogens, which has resulted in the emergence of multidrug resistant strains.[54] The transfer of antibiotic resistant *Pseudomonas* to humans has predominantly been implicated in drinking water and via person-to-person contact.[46]

Selection of resistant mutants and the uptake of antibiotic resistant genes from the environment have led to the recent development of extended spectrum beta-lactamase

TABLE 58.2 The top pathogens of concern with regards to antibiotic resistance as listed by WHO.[49]

Priority category	Pathogen	Antibiotic resistance of concern
Critical	*Acinetobacter baumannii*	Carbapenem-resistant
	Pseudomonas aeruginosa	Carbapenem-resistant
	Enterobacteriaceae spp.	Third-generation cephalosporin-resistant
High	*Enterococcus faecium*	Vancomycin-resistant
	Staphylococcus aureus	Methicillin-resistant, vancomycin intermediate and resistant
	Helicobacter pylori	Clarithromycin-resistant
	Campylobacter	Fluoroquinolone-resistant
	Salmonella spp.	Fluoroquinolone-resistant
	Neisseria gonorrhoeae	Third-generation cephalosporin-resistant and Fluoroquinolone-resistant
Medium	*Streptococcus pneumoniae*	Penicillin-nonsusceptible
	Haemophilus influenzae	Ampicillin-resistant
	Shigella spp.	Fluoroquinolone-resistant

WHO, World Health Organization.

(ESBL)-producing Enterobacteriaceae, frequently found in *E. coli* and *Klebsiella pneumoniae*.[55] They have caused many infections, for example urinary tract infections.[55] They are antibiotic resistant bacteria that produce beta-lactamase enzymes that can hydrolyze beta-lactam antibiotics such as penicillin and third-generation cephalosporin antibiotics, thus rendering them resistant.[56] ESBLs are often located on plasmids which are easily transferred via HGT to other bacteria.[57] The prevalence of ESBL-producing Enterobacteriaceae has been increasing since the 1980s and has been found in healthy food animals and even in wild animals.[58] It is thought that the emergence of resistance caused by ESBL-producing Enterobacteriacae is related to the spread from animal reservoirs via the environment and food.[59]

Another antibiotic resistant pathogen of concern is vancomycin-resistant *Enterococcus faecium*, which was first documented in the 1980s.[60] Over the past two decades, enterococci have emerged as common causes of hospital-acquired infections, notably due to their ability to exchange genetic material.[61] Enterococci predominantly inhabit the gastrointestinal tract of humans and animals and thus can serve as a hygiene indicator for food production.[62] Enterococci also occur in the soil, water, and on plants. Thus they can colonize raw foods such as milk, cheese, and meat.[46,62] Glycopeptide-resistant *E. faecium* has been identified in animal husbandry, largely due to the use of the antibiotic avoparcin as a feed additive.[46] But enterococci isolated from foods have been found to be resistant to many other antibiotics. Of concern to human health is the ability of antibiotic resistant enterococci to survive the gastric passage and result in intestinal colonization.[46]

Nowadays, penicillin-resistant *S. aureus* is common, and the increase of MRSA strains is of great concern, not just in hospital settings but also in livestock and the community. MRSA has been found to be associated with domestic animals, food-producing animals, and various food items such as meat, street food, vegetables, and milk, mainly due to contamination by infected humans.[46,63] *S. aureus* produces enterotoxins in food which cause gastroenteritis.

Helicobacter pylori is a Gram-negative pathogen that causes diseases of the upper gastrointestinal tract in humans.[64] Multiantibiotic therapies are employed to fight *H. pylori* infections.[65] However, resistance to these currently utilized antibiotics is becoming an emerging problem in the treatment of *H. pylori* infections.[66] *H. pylori* may occur in food and water due to fecal contamination, where it can then enter the stomach and cause an infection.[67] Thus *H. pylori* foodborne infections are more common in areas where there are poor hygienic conditions.[67] Milk has been implicated as a food commodity which may play a more significant role in the transmission of *H. pylori* infection than other foods. This is due to the bacteria's ability to survive in acidic pH and in the presence of urea.[67]

Campylobacter species cause Campylobacteriosis which is a foodborne infection causing gastroenteritis, particularly from food of animal origin, where poultry and pigs are a major source after being contaminated with fecal matter.[68] Campylobacteriosis, as well as salmonellosis, are the leading causes of bacterial foodborne infection in the European Union (EU) and United States over the last decade.[69,70] *Campylobacter coli* and *Campylobacter jejuni* are the most common species associated with enteric disease in humans.[7] *Campylobacter* species have shown increased resistance to fluoroquinolones and macrolides.

Salmonella enterica subsp. *enterica* is the leading cause of foodborne salmonellosis and causes gastroenteritis.[71] Isolates resistant to first-line treatment antibiotics have been recorded since the 1980s and today, third-generation cephalosporins and azithromycin are used to treat resistant infections.[72] Antibiotic resistant *Salmonella* species have been found in various food products such as meat and eggs, dairy, drinking water, and vegetables.[46]

Shigella is responsible for the foodborne illness shigellosis, which is an infection of the colon causing bloody diarrhea.[73] This pathogen has been labeled by the Center for Diseases Control and Prevention (CDC) as the third most common bacterial pathogen which causes foodborne disease.[73] *Shigella* finds its way most commonly into the food chain via poor hygiene practices of an infected food handler or via contaminated water.[73] Currently, ceftriaxone and azithromycin are used to treat shigellosis but isolates resistant to these antibiotics have already been reported.[74]

The four key bacterial pathogens of concern to human health with regards to the spread of ABR from animals to humans are *E. coli*, *Enterococcus*, *Campylobacter*, and *Salmonella*.[32] These bacteria are enteric bacteria and are considered to be the most frequently transmitted from animals to humans in the food chain.

58.5 Use of antibiotics in animal farming

The human population is rapidly growing and is forecasted by some demographic experts, to reach 8 billion by 2030. This has been accompanied by a parallel increase in the global demand for food. Food demand on this scale has required industrial scale production of food to meet the global population's requirements for protein and energy. However, with industrialization and intensification of food production systems comes increased risks of contamination of food with pathogens.[75] Various approaches have been used to combat these foodborne pathogens such as Good Manufacturing Practices, Hazard Analysis Critical Control Points (HACCP) and Good

Agricultural Practices (GAP).[75] To keep up with the enormous scale of global food production and limited resources, food producers have applied new technologies and alternative production methods to industrialize food production[75]—these technologies and production methods are continuously evolving at a rapid rate.

The use of antibiotics in food animal production has been one of the means in which farmers have been able to keep up with large-scale production. The uses of antibiotics in the food animal industry include treatment of bacterial infections, prevention of infections, and growth promotion.[8,24] The application of mass medication and the use of broad-spectrum antibiotics in animal husbandry is common, because it is often impractical to treat animals individually.[3]

The benefits of growth promotants was first discovered in the 1940s when chickens were observed to grow faster when they were fed by-products of tetracycline fermentation.[76] The use of antibiotics as growth promotants is predominantly in monogastric animals such as pigs, chickens, and turkeys, farmed fish/aquaculture, and less in ruminants. The mechanisms of growth promoters are still largely unknown, but it is hypothesized that they work by altering the micro-intestinal flora, which results in more efficient digestion and metabolism, resulting in increased weight gain and milk supply, reduced feed requirements, as well as disease and pathogen suppression, which all result in potential increased profitability, depending on the extent of these effects and the cost of the antibiotics themselves.[32,76] More specifically, growth promotion is achieved through four main mechanisms: (1) enhancement of protein metabolism which improves digestion, (2) stabilization of the gut microflora by suppressing pathogens, (3) increased vitamin production by gastrointestinal microorganisms, and (4) increased feed efficiency by increasing intestinal absorption of nutrients by reducing the numbers of intestinal bacteria that would divert nutrition away from the animal.[36]

It is also argued that there are environmental benefits of using growth promotants, especially in intensive farming, as increased feed efficiency can lead to reduced manure, nitrogen, and methane output.[32]

The classes of antibiotics most commonly used in food animal production globally are tetracyclines, penicillins, and trimethoprim/sulfonamides.[77–80] However, polypeptides, macrolides, quinolones, aminoglycosides, and polymyxin are also commonly used.[77–80] Table 58.3 lists the

TABLE 58.3 The applications of the most commonly used antibiotic classes.[76,81–84]

Antibiotic	Human medicine	Veterinary medicine (food animals)	Comments
Aminoglycosides	Yes	Yes	
Babermycins	No	Yes	Used solely for growth promotion in food animals.
Carbapenems	Yes	No	Usually reserved for known or suspected MDR bacterial infections.
Cephalosporins	Yes	Yes	
Glycopeptides	Yes	Yes	Avoparcin is banned for use as a growth promoter in the EU.
Ionophores	No	Yes	
Lincosamides	Yes	Yes	
Macrolides	Yes	Yes	Also used in aquaculture. Spiramycin and tylosin are banned for use as a growth promoter in the EU.
Monobactams	Yes	No	
Penicillins	Yes	Yes	
Phenicols	Yes	No	Chloramphenicol is banned for use in food animals by the FDA, EU and most other countries. Florfenicol is typically only used in veterinary medicine; it is also used in aquaculture.
Pleuromutilins	No	Yes	
Polypeptides	Yes	Yes	Bacitracin is banned for use as a growth promoter in the EU.
Streptogramins	Yes	Yes	Virginiamycin is banned for use as a growth promoter in the EU.
Sulfonamides and trimethoprim combos	Yes	Yes	Also used in aquaculture.

(Continued)

TABLE 58.3 (Continued)

Antibiotic	Human medicine	Veterinary medicine (food animals)	Comments
Tetracyclines	Yes	Yes	Also used in aquaculture.
Quinolones	Yes	Yes	Also used in aquaculture.
Quinoxalines	No	Yes	Carbadox is used exclusively for veterinary medicine.

EU, European Union; *FDA*, Food and Drug Administration; *MDR*, multidrug resistant.

TABLE 58.4 Various antibiotics which are permitted for growth promotion for food animals.

Antibiotic class	Antibiotic	Food animal species	Country
Arsenicals	3-Nitro-arsonic acid	Pigs, poultry	United States/Australia
Beta-lactams	Penicillin	Pigs	United States
Glycopeptides	Avoparcin	Pigs, poultry, cattle	Australia
Lincosamides	Lincomycin	Pigs	United States
Macrolides	Erythromycin Tylosin Kitasamycin Oleandomycin	Pigs, cattle, poultry	United States Canada/Australia/South Africa Australia/South Africa Australia
Pleuromutilins	Tiamulin	Pigs	United States
Ionophores	Lasalocid Monensin Salinomycin	Cattle Pigs	Canada/Australia/South Africa United States/EU/Canada/Australia/South Africa EU/Canada/Australia/South Africa
Oligosaccharides	Avilamycin	Pigs, poultry	EU/South Africa
Polypeptides	Bacitracin	Pigs, poultry, cattle	United States/Canada/Australia/South Africa
Quinoxalines	Carbadox Olaquindox	Pigs, poultry	United States/Canada South Africa Australia/South Africa
Streptogramins	Virginiamycin	Pigs, poultry, cattle	United States/Canada/Australia/South Africa
Tetracyclines	Tetracycline	Pigs, poultry, cattle	United States/South Africa

EU, European Union.
Adapted from Joint Expert Advisory Committee on Antibiotic Resistance. *The Use of Antibiotics in Food-producing Animals: Antibiotic Resistant Bacteria in Animals and Humans*. Canberra: Commonwealth of Australia; 1999 and Eagar H, Swan G, van Vurren M. A survey of antimicrobial usage in animals in South Africa with specific reference to food animals. J S Afr Vet Assoc. 2012;1(83):1–8.

most common antibiotic classes that are used in veterinary and or human medicine.

The volume of antimicrobial use in the food animal production industry is comparable with that of medicine.[85] The Centre for Disease Dynamics, Economics and Policy estimated that 80% of antibiotics used in the United States are used in the feed of food animals during production.[86] Worryingly, many antimicrobials that are regarded as important to human health are used in animal food production.[16] Antibiotics used for growth promotion such as bambermycins and ionophores, have little or no application in human medicine, whereas some antibiotics commonly used therapeutically and for prophylaxis in livestock are closely related to those used in human medicine and pose a threat to efficacy of human medicine. These include the penicillins, sulfonamides, tetracyclines, macrolides, glycopeptides, quinolones, streptogramins, and lincosamides.[76] Antibiotics considered important to human health are restricted for use in veterinary medicine in most countries.[19,87] Table 58.4 lists the antibiotics registered in various countries for use as growth promotants in food animals. It should be noted that antibiotics are not commonly used for growth promotion in aquaculture farming.[88]

58.6 Antibiotic resistance in food animals

The use of antibiotics in food animal production is usually seen as important for ensuring a consistent supply of healthy and sizeable animals, leading to greater profitability and efficient production.[3] However, this application of antibiotics at low concentrations over extended time periods favors the emergence of ABR. This is due to accelerated HGT and mutation, where the high density of animals involved in intensive production facilitates its spread.[89]

The use of antibiotics in the agricultural industry has increasingly come under scrutiny due to their overall impact on human health.[18,87] Food animals have been considered an important source of antimicrobial resistant bacteria that can affect humans.[76] As pointed out earlier, the misuse, overuse, and inappropriate use of antimicrobials in human medicine and animal husbandry create an enormous selection pressure, which causes bacteria to adapt in response to the selective pressure, resulting in a more resistant population. This is therefore a key factor that drives the development of ABR.[8,89] Consequently, the farming industry has been established as an ABR reservoir "hotspot."[36]

One of the first consequences of the misuse of antimicrobials in the agricultural industry was documented in 1963 when an increased level of resistance in *S. enterica* ser. Typhimurium was observed in several feedlots in the United Kingdom and several resistant isolates were identified.[90] Numerous other studies have shown that the use of antibiotics in intensive food-producing animals, especially for nontherapeutic use, is linked to resistance seen in people on farms and even in the general population via the food chain.[6] Although the topic is still controversial, recent studies have demonstrated that intensive food animal farming results in higher ABR as well as increased virulence genes, compared to free-range or organic farming.[91–93] There is also concern with respect to the spread of antibiotic resistant bacteria from the farms into nearby environments via groundwater contamination or run-off and via small insects and rodents. For example, Graham et al. found that enterococci and staphylococci isolates from flies near poultry farms carried similar antibiotic susceptibility patterns to the isolates from poultry litter on the farms.[94]

Due to the fact that many foodborne illnesses in humans are commonly associated with animal species and the surrounding environment, food-producing animals are of particular relevance to the emergence and transfer of antimicrobial resistance (AMR) to humans via the food chain.[8,95] The potential threat to human health from the misuse of antibiotics in food animals is significant. Its impact has not been fully comprehended because of inadequate research and documentation;[16] this is particularly relevant in developing countries in Africa and Asia.

According to the Centre for Science in the Public Interest (CSPI) in the United States, from 1973 to 2011, most antibiotic resistant outbreaks from food were due to dairy products, ground beef and poultry.[96] The most commonly identified foodborne pathogens that have been associated with bacterial resistance in humans and farm animals include MRSA, *E. coli*, *Campylobacter*, *Salmonella*, and *Enterococcus* species.[6,76] Antibiotic resistant outbreaks have been recorded since the 1970s but the majority have occurred from the 2000s onward; however, data on foodborne illness outbreaks caused by antibiotic resistant bacteria is limited.[96] Some of these outbreaks are listed in Table 58.5.

As a result of the findings summarized in Table 58.5, it is clear that the foodborne route is one of the major

TABLE 58.5 Studies of antibiotic resistant microorganisms detected in food animals and in food products and humans.

Study author, year, location	Study findings
Holmberg et al., 1984, United States	Resistant plasmid from *Salmonella* detected in hamburger meat from beef cattle fed subtherapeutic chlortetracycline and patients infected with Salmonellosis.
van den Bogaard et al., 1997, the Netherlands	Vancomycin-resistant enterococci (VRE) isolated from 50% of the turkey samples, 39% of farmers, and 20% of turkey slaughterers. VRE more prevalent among turkeys fed avoparcin.
van den Bogaard et al., 2002, the Netherlands	Resistant traits from enterococci in chickens were transferred to enterococci in humans. Resistant enterococci more prevalent among broiler chickens and their farmers than among laying hens and their farmers.
Cui et al., 2005, United States	Resistant *Campylobacter* and *Salmonella* more prevalent among conventional reared chicken than organic reared chicken isolates.
Gundogan et al., 2005, Turkey	Resistant *Staphylococcus aureus* isolates were recovered from retail calf, lamb, and chicken products.

(Continued)

TABLE 58.5 (Continued)

Study author, year, location	Study findings
Ramchandani et al., 2005, United States	Resistant *Escherichia coli* isolates from humans of a multistate outbreak of urinary tract infections suggested to originate from food animals and acquired through the food chain.
Johnson et al., 2007, United States	Source of infection of bacteremic hospital patients linked to resistant *E. coli* in slaughtered chickens from the same area.
Angulo et al., 2004, United Kingdom	The use of fluoroquinolones in dairy cows in the United Kingdom was linked to an infection outbreak in humans caused by nalidixic acid-resistant *Salmonella enterica* ser. Typhimurium.

Adapted from Marshall BM, Levy SB. Food Animals and antimicrobials: impacts on human health. Clin Microbiol Rev. 2011;24:718–733 and Landers TF, Cohen B, Wittum TE, Larson EL. A review of antibiotic use in food animals: perspective, policy, and potential. Public Health Rep. 2012;127:4–22.

transfer vectors of antibiotic resistant bacteria, as well as pathogenic bacteria, from animals to humans. Some examples of current antibiotic resistant foodborne pathogens include ESBL-producing *Salmonella* and *E. coli*, quinolone-resistant *Salmonella* and *E. coli* and also livestock-acquired MRSA.[42] Most cases of antibiotic resistant foodborne infections are due to the use of antibiotics in food animal production and thus the use of antibiotics in food-producing animals is becoming a risk to human health and consequently needs to be much more strictly controlled.[42]

58.7 Consequences of reducing the use of antibiotics in food animal farming

The ABR problem we face today due to the extensive use and misuse of antibiotics, is not likely to disappear immediately after reducing antibiotic use.[97] Typically, mutations conferring ABR to microorganisms impose a large fitness cost, thereby reducing the microorganisms' ability to replicate and survive in a competitive environment in the absence of the antibiotic because these mutations target mechanisms which are required for proper functioning of the cell. This allows sensitive microorganisms that do not have to pay the cost of resistance, to replicate faster and eventually replace the resistant microorganisms, in the absence of a selection pressure.[98] However, research suggests that this is not always the case, as some studies have shown that resistant bacteria have remained abundant or even increased in a population despite the absence of an antibiotic.[98] Furthermore, the reduction of antibiotic use has rarely shown to eliminate resistant strains completely. The persistence of resistance has been explained by three hypotheses: first, different resistant mutations are more costly than others, while some do not have a fitness cost associated with it. Secondly, second-site mutations may occur which helps to increase fitness without compromising resistance. Thirdly, resistance genes may be coselected with other mutations and will not get eliminated in the absence of the antibiotic.[98]

In general, the prevalence and persistence of ABR is a result of a complex interaction between the microorganisms, antimicrobials, the host, and the surrounding environment.[87] It has been found that after removal of an antimicrobial agent and thus the selection pressure in a given environment, the resistance persists for different periods of time depending on the type of antimicrobial agent and type of microorganism involved, among other factors.[87,98] For example, Gram-positive bacteria generally have a higher fitness cost associated with resistant mutations than Gram-negative bacteria due to their thicker cell wall. Melnyk et al. determined that, for example, the antibiotic trimethoprim has a relatively low fitness cost, but rifampicin has a relatively high fitness cost.[98]

Even longer periods of persistence can occur if the resistant bacteria obtain a selective growth advantage over the susceptible bacteria and thus continue to thrive in the environment. This selective growth advantage is often linked with genes that encode for survival, virulence, and multiplication characteristics, for example, biocide resistance.[87] This relationship between virulence and antibiotic resistant genes has been demonstrated in some studies in which strains of enterotoxigenic *Escherichia coli* (ETEC) have higher resistance levels than non-ETEC strains.[87]

There have been recommendations by global health authorities to ban the use of nontherapeutic antibiotics in food animals. However, this has been difficult to implement in many countries, although the EU has adopted this policy since 2006.[18,30,76] Others suggest that reduced antimicrobial consumption that is more strictly controlled would be more effective than a complete ban of antimicrobial usage in food animal production, as this can potentially cause negative repercussions on animal health, productivity, and thus also on food prices.[19,30]

One of the major consequences of decreasing the total consumption of antibiotics for nontherapeutic purposes in animal husbandry is the subsequent increase in usage of antibiotics for therapeutic uses, especially during the first stages of production.[3] This is the period when animal infections are most likely to occur, leading to a decline in production, reduced weight gain, and an increase in mortality rates which the Joint Expert Advisory Committee on Antibiotic Resistance (JETACAR) in Australia has estimated to be at about 1%–2%.[3,32] These adverse effects were observed following the ban of growth promoters in Denmark in 1994.[3] This subject is still being debated in the EU, as other countries have only reported a small increased consumption of therapeutic antibiotics, which tends to decline after two or three years following removal of growth-promoting antibiotics.[3]

Despite the increase in antibiotic use for therapeutic use, some countries have reported a decline in antibiotic resistant bacteria after the ban. To demonstrate, the banning of avoparcin and virginiamycin, chemically similar to vancomycin, as a growth promoter in animal feed in Europe, has resulted in a decrease in vancomycin-resistant enterococci in Danish broilers from 80% to 3%.[3,19] In Sweden, growth-promoting antibiotics have been banned for use in food animals since 1986, and production has been able to continue (although a 1.5% loss in production has been noted) due to stricter hygiene measures and improvements in feed formulations.[30] Since the ban, total consumption of antibiotics has dropped by 50% in food animal production in Sweden.

Another more indirect consequence of banning antibiotic growth promoters is the increased prevalence of pathogenic microorganisms, such as *Salmonella* and *Campylobacter*, due to the fact that farm animals not given growth promoters tend to have larger variations in size at slaughter, leading to more frequent rupture of the gastrointestinal tract during slaughter and consequent contamination of the carcass with pathogens which greatly comprises food safety.[3] The animal species most affected by the ban of antibiotic growth promoters are chickens and weaner pigs. In chickens, necrotic enteritis is the main problem and in weaner pigs, postweaning diarrhea; a 1.5% increase in mortality and time to reach slaughter weight increased by 5–6 days were the main issues faced. Various measures can be applied to reduce the occurrence of these negative consequences, such as improved housing and hygiene, production of pigs using the same pen from birth to slaughter and the addition of various ingredients in animal feed.[32] However, the application of these are sometimes costly and will only become the norm when the producers will see an increase in profitability.

Doyle et al. suggest that at least five years are needed after a ban of growth-promoting antibiotics to reduce resistance levels in food animals by significant amounts.[99] In order to improve animal welfare and reduce the risk of mortalities following a ban of growth promoters, it is important to improve farm hygiene and to implement good farming practices and production conditions in order to lessen infections from occurring and spreading.[3] Some examples of farm hygiene and good farming practices are: (1) having a planned herd health program such as vaccinations and parasite control, (2) frequent inspection of animal health status, (3) regular cleaning of animal housing areas, (4) keeping records of animal medications and feeds, (5) keeping an appropriately-sized herd, and (6) ensuring clean, uncontaminated water supplies.[100] If these steps are actively followed, it has been forecasted that comparatively good production can be obtained without the use of growth promoters in animal feed.[3]

58.8 Consequences of antibiotic resistance in food animals on human health

One of the first fears about ABR in humans was recorded in Denmark in 1994 due to the development of vancomycin-resistant *E. faecium* in humans. This occurrence was associated with the use of avoparcin, a chemically related antimicrobial agent to vancomycin, which was used as a growth-promoting agent in food animals such as pigs and poultry.[8]

The presence of antibiotic resistant bacteria in humans could affect the future of human health adversely as certain infections would become more difficult to treat.[36,101] ABR can also create complications to medical procedures such as organ transplants or prosthesis implants.[3] This, in turn, creates a burden on the public health system since more people require hospitalization and the likelihood of rising mortality rates increases.[104]

The main threat of ABR to human health is the transfer of resistant bacteria between animals and humans. The main transmission route is via the food chain. Antibiotic resistant bacteria, as well as pathogens, can be transferred to humans through consumption of contaminated meat or other animal products that are improperly cooked and/or inappropriately handled during food preparation.[36,89] Consumption of contaminated fresh produce can also be a source of antibiotic resistant bacteria but is less common than animal products.

A concern of the transfer of antibiotic resistance to humans is the subsequent colonization of the human intestine.[36,101] To demonstrate, the CDC reported that the foodborne pathogens *Salmonella* and *Campylobacter*, cause an estimated 410,000 antibiotic resistant infections in the United States alone each year. In the EU and European Economic Area, more than 25,000 people a year die from infections caused by antibiotic resistant bacteria.[8]

The same safety and hygiene procedures that are used to prevent and control the spread of pathogens and unwanted microorganisms via food in the food industry will help to control the spread of antibiotic resistant bacteria in the food chain.[3]

Another transmission pathway which antibiotic resistant bacteria can transfer from animals to humans is via direct or close contact. There are many documented cases where there has been a direct spread of ABR from animals, namely livestock, to nearby humans, such as farm workers or residents living nearby (Table 58.5). This type of situation was first described where tetracycline-resistant *E. coli* strains present in chickens that were fed tetracycline in their feed were also present in the workers on the chicken farm.[102]

An additional concern to human health is the presence of antibiotic residues in the muscles or organs of food animals, which can have toxic or allergenic properties if present in high amounts.[103] The antibiotic residues may exert a selective pressure on the intestinal flora, encouraging the growth of resistant microorganisms and could also alter the enzyme activity of the microbial flora.[103] Some researchers have suggested that antibiotic residues in animal products do not pose a big health risk to humans as the heat applied during food processing and cooking significantly reduces the concentration of residues and most antibiotics administered to food animals are also approved for human use.[103,105]

Of greater importance than the presence of antibiotic residues in animal tissues is the concentration it is present in. The WHO and the FAO of the United Nations has stipulated in the Codex Alimentarius, a list of maximum residue limits (MRL) for residues of veterinary drugs, which includes antibiotics, for various food animal tissues, as well as the acceptable daily intake.[106] These are in place to encourage farmers to adhere to the correct dosages of antibiotics used during animal production and also to adhere to the withdrawal periods prior to slaughter so that the drug residue concentrations in the animal products stays below the MRL.

58.9 Curbing the spread of antibiotic resistance in food agriculture

Various practices can be implemented to help reverse or slow down the development of ABR in various environments, including agriculture, which has largely been caused by the misuse of antibiotics.[8,90]

On the farm, mass administration of antibiotics in animal husbandry should be avoided or reduced wherever possible, especially those used in human medicine, as this creates unnecessary selection of antibiotic resistant bacteria in the environment.[107] Additionally, antibiotic use needs to be used correctly and responsibly. This involves maximizing the therapeutic effect of antibiotics, while *minimizing* the potential for resistant bacteria to develop.[107] Elimination or a reduction in the use of antibiotics as growth promoters is one of the most effective ways to reduce the development of antibiotic resistant bacteria. It should be noted that there are various indirect sources of antibiotics and antibiotic resistant bacteria which are sometimes added into animal feed and these can include bone meal, carcass meal, and poultry manure.[108] These feed sources should also be avoided in animal feed.

Restriction on the critically important antibiotics for human health would help to conserve the effectiveness of these drugs for when they are truly needed.[99] Furthermore, increasing hygiene and good herd management in livestock farming could reduce the need for antibiotics to treat diseases. This could be further improved by reducing animal density on farms, which helps to prevent the spread of diseases, as well as ABR,[27] although producers argue that they need high density/intensive systems to meet the projected food demand.

Vaccines, too, can reduce the need for antibiotics by preventing diseases from occurring. Various studies, as listed by Hoelzer et al.,[109] have demonstrated this, for example, the implementation of a vaccine against *Aeromonas salmonicida* in the farmed salmon industry led to a significant decrease in antibiotic use. Immune enhancers can also be administered to further prevent illnesses from occurring.[26] Furthermore, inclusion of probiotic and beneficial bacteria in livestock feed can potentially reduce the occurrence of pathogenic bacteria in the gut by competitive exclusion, thereby reducing the chances of development and spread of pathogens.[107] The use of enzymes as alternative to antibiotics in animal feed has shown to improve digestion of various chemical components which would either be poorly digested or undigested.[32] Other animal feed ingredients, such as organic salts, fiber and plant extracts, have also shown to reduce the dependence on antibiotics.[32]

Antimicrobial peptides have shown to be attractive candidates as alternative antimicrobial agents and as a potential for use in feed additives in livestock production, because of the low risk of developing bacterial resistance.[110,111] Unlike conventional antibiotics which function through a specific target mechanism, antimicrobial peptides exert multiple antimicrobial activities, resulting in a broad spectrum of activity against microorganisms.[110] Their main mechanism of action is membrane disruption via the attraction of its positive charge to the negatively charged bacterial membrane.[110,111] There are many other modes of actions of antimicrobial peptides, including interactions involved with the host's immune system.[110]

In addition to their antimicrobial effect, peptides also play a role in the maintenance of gut health, enhanced immunity, and reduced inflammatory response.[110] There are, however, several issues facing commercialization and continuous use of peptides, including product degradation during storage, product stability under physiological conditions, reducing host cell toxicity, and potential developments of resistance mechanisms such as reduction of cell membrane surface charge, among others.[111,112]

Additionally, due to the fact that 70%–90% of an antibiotic which is administered to animals remains unchanged in their feces or urine, treatment of raw animal manure before application onto fields or crops can significantly reduce the spread of antimicrobial resistant bacteria and genes throughout the environment.[113] Treatment options include composting and anaerobic digestion.

In food production, efforts should focus on minimizing the transmission of foodborne pathogens via the food chain, despite their antibiotic susceptibility profile, by adopting good hygiene practices at all stages of food production, including food marketing and food preparation by the consumer.

To better control and contain ABR, the WHO and FAO have published an action plan on antimicrobial resistance. The WHO suggests that every country should develop an action plan in line with their Global Action Plan. One of the key strategies is to implement a surveillance program to monitor and report on antibiotic usage and antimicrobial resistance development.[46,114]

According to WHO, strategies aimed at reducing exposure to antibiotics and strict control of existing antibiotics should have the greatest effect at curbing the emergence of resistance.[114,115] JETACAR's ABR management program has five key elements which are considered critical for any ABR management program to be successful and include (1) implementing or tightening regulatory controls over the registration, import and use of antibiotics for both human and animal use to minimize the use of antibiotics and to ban the use of animal in-feed antibiotics which are critical to human and animal health; (2) standardized monitoring and surveillance of the prevalence of antibiotic resistant bacteria in human, animal, environmental, and food-chain organisms (including molecular studies of resistance genes) and on antibiotic use patterns; (3) implementing hygienic measures and infection prevention strategies on the farm and throughout the food chain; (4) education of the stakeholders involved in the use of antibiotics for veterinary and human medicine so that they can understand the rationale behind these strategies and education of the general public about safe food handling, infections, and the hazards and risks involved; (5) further research on clinical and veterinary problems of ABR and on possible solutions.[32] The conclusions and efforts of the management program should be communicated to stakeholders, regulatory bodies, and the general public. Various countries across the globe have implemented antimicrobial resistance surveillance programs and/or policies. Some of these initiatives are listed in Table 58.6. There are also various global initiatives currently in place, such as the Global Antibiotic

TABLE 58.6 Current antimicrobial resistance surveillance programs and/or policies which have been implemented by various countries.[101,116,117]

Program or policy	Year implemented	Country
The Japanese Veterinary Antimicrobial Resistance Monitoring System in the Field of Animal Hygiene (JVARM)	2013	Japan
Danish Integrated Antimicrobial Resistance Monitoring and Research Programme (DANMAP)	2014	Denmark
Norwegian Surveillance System for Antimicrobial Drug Resistance (NORM/NORM-VET)	2015	Norway
Deutsche Antibiotika-Resistenzstrategie (DART)	2015	Germany
National Antimicrobial Resistance Monitoring System (NARMS)	2014	United States
Monitoring of Antimicrobial Resistance and Antibiotic Usage in Animals in the Netherlands (MARAN)	2015	Netherlands
Swedish Veterinary Antimicrobial Resistance Monitoring (SVARM)	2015	Sweden
European Surveillance of Antimicrobial Consumption Network (ESAC-Net) and European Antimicrobial Resistance Surveillance Network (EARS-Net)	2014–2015	Europe
Central Asian and Eastern European Surveillance of Antimicrobial Resistance (CAESAR)	2012	Asian and eastern Europe
The Finnish Veterinary Antimicrobial Resistance Monitoring and Consumption of Antimicrobial Agents report (FINRES-VET)	2007	Finland

(Continued)

TABLE 58.6 (Continued)

Program or policy	Year implemented	Country
Canadian Integrated Program for Antimicrobial Resistance Surveillance (CIPARS)	2014	Canada
L'Observatoire National de l'Epidémiologie de la Résistance Bactérienne aux Antibiotiques (ONERBA)	2015	France
Pilot Surveillance Program for Antimicrobial Resistance in Bacteria of Animal Origin and the National Antimicrobial Resistance Strategy for 2015–2019	2007 and 2015	Australia
The New Zealand Antimicrobial Resistance Action Plan	2017	New Zealand
Africa CDC Framework for Antimicrobial resistance, 2018–23	2018	Africa
National guidelines for antibiotic use	2013	India
National Action Plan to Contain AMR for 2016–20	2016	China
Antibiotic Resistance Containment Program for 2012–16	2012	Thailand
National Framework of Antimicrobial Resistance for 2014–24	2014	South Africa
Colombian Integrated Program for Antimicrobial Resistance Surveillance (COIPARS)	2011	Columbia
Kor-GLASS surveillance program	2016	South Korea

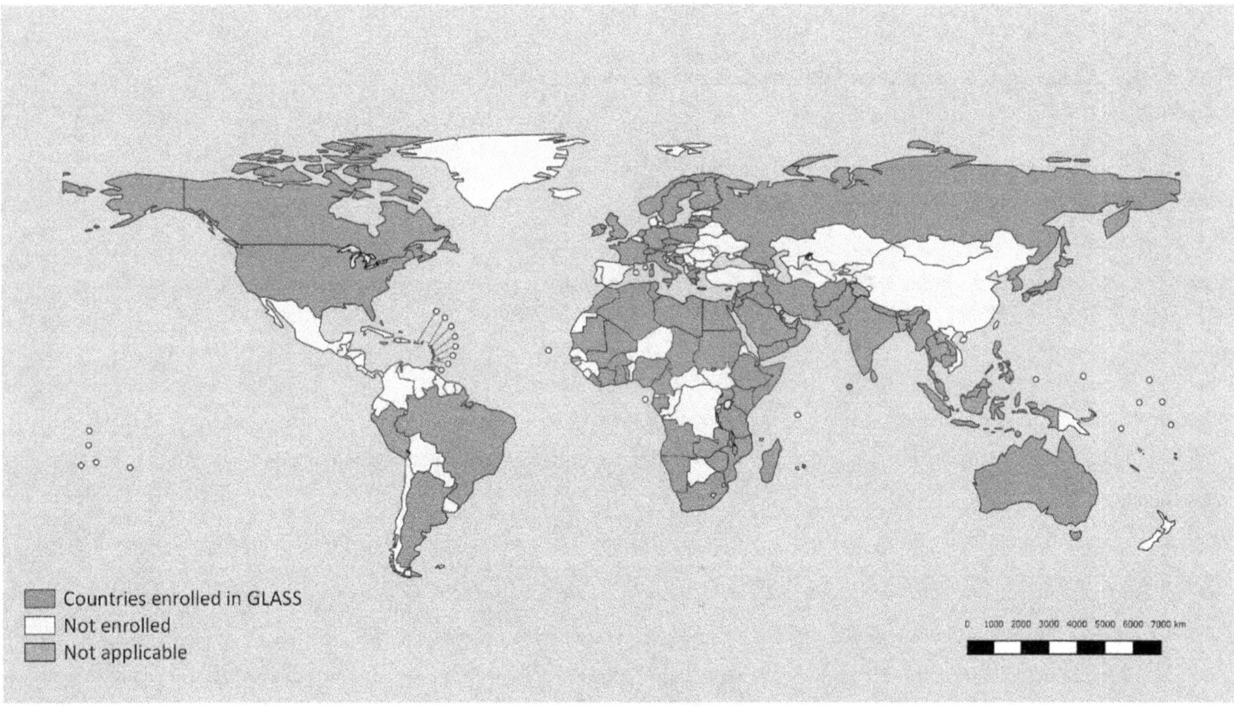

FIGURE 58.5 Countries which have enrolled in the Global Antimicrobial Resistance Surveillance System (GLASS) program, as of December 2020. *Adapted from World Health Organization. Global antimicrobial resistance surveillance system (GLASS). Country participation. https://www.who.int/glass/country-participation/en/; Accessed 03.11.20.*

Resistance Partnership, Global Research on Antimicrobial Resistance, and the Global Antimicrobial Resistance Surveillance System (GLASS). Currently as of December 2020, 99 countries have enrolled in the GLASS program, consisting of developed and developing countries, as depicted in Fig. 58.5.[118] The challenge faced by these global initiatives is to get more countries to actively participate.

58.10 Detection of antibiotic resistant microorganisms

There are two types of testing methods that can be used to assess a bacterium's ABR profile, namely, phenotypic and genotypic methods (see Table 58.7). Phenotypic testing determines the observed level of susceptibility a bacterium has toward an antibiotic. Genotypic testing, on the other hand, determines the presence of mutations that are known to confer ABR expression.[119] However, the presence of a resistance gene does not always result in phenotypic resistance and hence treatment failure, because phenotypic resistance is also dependent on the mode and level of expression of the resistant genes.[122] There are advantages and disadvantages to using phenotypic and genotypic methods to assess the ABR profile of bacteria.

Due to limitations of both methods, it has been recommended to use a combination of phenotypic and genotypic methods to obtain a reliable and accurate result. Usually this would involve the use of phenotypic methods to screen for ABR, followed by confirmation of resistance and determination of resistance mechanisms using genotypic methods.[120]

58.10.1 Phenotypic methods for determining antibiotic resistance

The most commonly used phenotypic susceptibility testing methods are either based on diffusion of the antimicrobial agent in agar (Stokes method and Kirby–Bauer method), dilution in broth or agar [minimum inhibitory concentration (MIC) method] or a combination (E-test method).

Automated instrumental techniques are also based on variations of diffusion and/or dilution. They can produce results in shorter time periods and are more sensitive than manual readings because of optical detection systems capable of detecting subtle changes in bacterial growth.[123] Examples of such automated systems include Vitek AST cards, Autobac, Microscan, and the Abbott Ms-2 system.[124]

The two most commonly used international antimicrobial susceptibility phenotypic testing methods and standards are the European Committee on Antimicrobial Susceptibility Testing (EUCAST) and Clinical and Laboratory Standards Institute (CLSI).[125,126] These standards categorize the results based on breakpoints, which determine whether a bacterium is considered resistant or

TABLE 58.7 Advantages and disadvantages of phenotypic versus genotypic methods for detection of antibiotic resistant bacteria.[119–121]

Advantages	Disadvantages
Phenotypic tests	
Can detect degree of susceptibility	Labor-intensive
Can detect resistance to an antibiotic without prior knowledge of resistant mechanisms	More time-consuming (a pure culture first needs to be obtained and then grown in the presence of an antibiotic)
Relatively inexpensive	Classification of resistance is dependent on what drug concentration is considered significant according to standards
Testing methods are generally simple to perform	Difficult to test low-level resistance
	In vitro selective pressures which may result in biases or variations in results
Genotypic tests	
Rapid (testing can be conducted directly on the specimen)	Cannot detect degree of susceptibility, only presence or absence of resistance gene (although some WGS models have tried to predict the MIC and RT-PCR is quantitative)
The resistance mechanism can be determined	Often more expensive than phenotypic methods
Minority resistant populations can be detected	Only known resistance genes can be detected (except when using DNA sequencing)
Difficult to culture or slow-growing microorganisms can be sequenced	False-negative results due to detection of incorrect gene(s) as phenotypic resistance can be a result of numerous mutations (although some WGS models have shown high sensitivity and specificity for phenotypes)
	False-positive results due to contamination or sequencing errors
	Requires more advanced technical knowledge to perform tests

MIC, Minimum inhibitory concentration; *RT-PCR*, real-time polymerase chain reaction; *WGS*, whole genome sequencing.

susceptible to the antibiotic. These breakpoints are set by international agencies and are regularly revised. The EUCAST breakpoints are based on epidemiological MIC cutoffs and pharmacokinetic-pharmacodynamic (PK-PD) properties. The CLSI breakpoints are based on MIC distributions, PK-PD properties, and mechanisms of resistance.[127] Additional differences in the two standards include different breakpoint values, incubation times, conditions and media.

58.10.1.1 Dilution

Dilution methods are used to determine what the minimum concentration of an antimicrobial is which will inhibit or kill the microorganism. This is important to know in diagnosing treatment of serious clinical infections. They are commonly used in Dutch, Danish, and Norwegian AMR monitoring systems.[8,123]

Dilution methods yield quantitative results via interpretation of the MIC, which is determined as the lowest antibiotic concentration inhibiting the growth of the organism, as judged by the lack of turbidity (growth) in the test tube. The broth dilution method is used to test a small number of bacterial isolates in a simple manner. A standard bacterial suspension is inoculated into prepared stock dilutions of antibiotic at varying concentrations.[123] This method is tedious and time-consuming, and some authors have found that higher MIC values are obtained in broth than in solid media due to stronger expression of resistance in liquid media.[126] Studies have revealed an excellent correlation between the values obtained from disk diffusion and dilution methods.[8]

58.10.1.2 Disk diffusion

The Kirby–Bauer disk diffusion method and adaptions thereof are the most prevalent AST methods used in laboratories today. It is an affordable, simple, well- standardized method and is recommended by the CLSI and EUCAST.[8,126] The method is performed by applying a standardized bacterial suspension to a Mueller–Hinton agar plate and then applying paper antibiotic disks that contain a fixed concentration of antibiotic.[123] The diameter of the zone of inhibition, which is the area around the disk where no growth occurred, is measured. The results classify the zone of inhibition into categories of susceptibility according to criteria published by the CLSI and EUCAST.[123] The CLSI is approved by the Food and Drug Administration (USA) and is recommended by the WHO. The results are qualitative but can be converted into MIC breakpoint values using standard curves.[8,123] This method is the least-expensive phenotypic method and offers simplicity and flexibility, allowing the categorical results to be easily interpreted by members of the public.[123] The disk diffusion method also gives insight into the heterogeneity of the cell population of the bacterial isolate.[123] For these reasons, the disk diffusion method is seen as the most practical method that yields clinically relevant results.

58.10.1.3 E-test

The epsilometer (E-test) is a testing method that uses a combination of dilution and diffusion of the antibiotic into the medium, creating an exponential gradient.[123] The method uses a thin test strip impregnated with a predefined antimicrobial gradient which is applied onto an inoculated agar plate. The intersection of the ellipse shaped inhibitory zone edge with the test strip indicates the MIC value. This allows testing over a wide concentration range. This method is generally used in particular instances such as when organisms require a special incubation atmosphere, as this is a more expensive method. It can sometimes result in systematic biases with certain antibiotic–organism combinations.[123]

58.10.2 Genotypic methods for determining antibiotic resistance

There are various molecular techniques which are currently being used to detect antibiotic resistant genes, namely, polymerase chain reaction (PCR), probe technology, and DNA sequencing.[123,128] Detection of resistance genes in bacterial isolates is useful to confirm phenotypic ABR, as well as to better understand the mechanism of resistance the bacterial isolate harbors as resistant genes encode for specific resistant mechanisms.

58.10.2.1 Polymerase chain reaction

PCR is one of the most commonly used methods in laboratories today to detect resistant genes as it is a reliable and quick detection method for genes whose sequence is known. Its popularity as a method is also due to its ease of use and its cost.[129] This method amplifies a specific DNA sequence, which is known to encode for a resistant gene, in a DNA sample. The PCR product is then run on a gel via electrophoresis and if the gene is present in the DNA sample, it can be visualized on the gel at the specific base pair length. Multiplex PCR can be performed, which amplifies multiple genes in one PCR run.

Real-time PCR (RT-PCR) has more recently been used to detect resistant genes and to quantify them. This method is based on a comparison of the number of DNA copies obtained when bacteria are cultivated in breakpoint-equivalent concentration of antibiotics after, and before, incubation and the control, that is, those grown without the presence of the antibiotic.[77] If a resistant bacterium is present, the number of DNA copies would increase in a similar fashion to the control. Conversely, if the bacteria are susceptible to the antibiotic, then the number of DNA copies would remain similar to those before incubation in the presence of the antibiotic.[77] Other techniques utilizing RT-PCR include quantification of gene copy number and gene expression analysis.

58.10.2.2 DNA hybridization

DNA hybridization involves using a probe with a known DNA sequence that can pair up with open DNA from a sample. If hybridization occurs (the resistant gene of interest is present in the sample) then a detectable signal will occur.[122] DNA arrays and DNA chips are based on the principle of DNA hybridization. These are devices that can detect a large number of DNA sequences at once.[122]

58.10.2.3 DNA sequencing

DNA sequencing can detect the presence of antibiotic resistant genes within the genome sequence of an isolate by comparing the sequence against known gene sequences using an ABR reference gene database.[121] Therefore specific primers are not needed, and this enables a much more comprehensive detection of ABR genes. This technique also enables the discovery of any novel antibiotic resistant genes which may be present if the target sequence is incomplete or has low similarity to existing antibiotic resistant genes in a database but still confers phenotypic ABR patterns.[130]

Whole genome sequencing (WGS) has gained recent interest in antimicrobial resistance surveillance.[131] WGS covers the entire genome so that hundreds of resistance genes are detected and not just a select few as with PCR.[132]

58.11 Research gaps and future directions

Antibiotic resistant cases in the farming industry are commonly documented in intensive animal production systems, such as broiler chickens and feedlot cattle and pigs, where the use of antibiotics is evident and regularly employed.[17,76] However, research on extensively produced food animals, such as free-range livestock and game species, is narrowly documented.[12] This scarcity of research in these environments may be due to low, or negligible, expectations of intrinsic and acquired resistance patterns in these natural environments; but microbial ecosystems in nature are never isolated and thus extensive gene exchange occurs in nature, usually via mobile genetic elements.[19]

Despite the perception of a low risk of ABR developing in natural environments, studies[132] have shown that ABR among wild animals is a growing public health issue, due to increased wildlife contact between humans, livestock and domestic animals, as well as increased cohabitation with other animals, among others.[47,133,134] In addition, there is a rising trend of consumption of game meat with meat known as a source of bacteria.[43,47,133] Furthermore, biodiversity in the natural, more remote environments could be threatened by ABR pollution.[45,47] It is not just a human health issue—it is a one-health issue.

Clinical laboratories still employ culture-based antimicrobial susceptible testing as its primary method, although WGS is gaining popularity in antimicrobial resistance research as it becomes more efficient and affordable. WGS is a powerful tool which has many applications in ABR research, from assisting in developing novel antibiotics to detecting the various factors which are involved in emergence and persistence of ABR. WGS makes it possible to compare ABR across different reservoirs, which encourages research using the "One Health" approach.[135]

The use of WGS for routine use in laboratories is currently limited due to the process being too slow and expensive and requires high-throughput machines and bioinformaticians for data processing.[129] Nevertheless, continual improvements and advancements in this technology are paving the way to allow WGS to be used as the primary tool for routine use in antimicrobial resistance diagnostics and research. This would require the development of user-friendly software to process data, standardization of software and data storage and public sharing of databases, among others.[135,136]

JETACAR have listed various topics which should be focused on in future research on ABR and include (1) alternatives to antibiotic growth promotants in animal production, (2) alternatives to antibiotics to prevent and treat infections in human and animal medicine such as vaccines, (3) the epidemiology of ABR which includes molecular research, (4) what the effects are of intervention programs which reduce the use of antibiotics, (5) development of rapid diagnostic tests, and (6) clinical efficacy studies.[32]

The fight against antimicrobial resistance requires a One Health approach. Antimicrobial resistance is a complex, multisectoral problem, and it requires integration of environmental, animal, and human sectors in order to combat this worldwide problem we face.

References

1. Ventola CL. The antibiotic resistance crisis. *Pharm Therap.* 2015;40:277–283.
2. Munita JM, Arias CA. Mechanisms of antibiotic resistance. *Microbiol Spectr.* 2016;4(2):1–36.
3. Capita R, Alonso-calleja C, Capita R, Alonso-calleja C. Antibiotic-resistant bacteria: a challenge for the food industry antibiotic-resistant bacteria. *Crit Rev Food Sci Nutr.* 2016;53:11–48.

4. Morley PS, Apley MD, Besser TE, et al. Antimicrobial drug use in veterinary medicine. *J Vet Intern Med.* 2005;19:617–629.
5. Van Hoek AHAM, van Mevius D, Guerra B, Mullany P, Roberts AP, Aarts HJM. Acquired antibiotic resistance genes: an overview. *Front Microbiol.* 2011;2:1–27.
6. Marshall BM, Levy SB. Food Animals and antimicrobials: impacts on human health. *Clin Microbiol Rev.* 2011;24:718–733.
7. Nyenje ME, Ndip RN. The challenges of food-borne pathogens and antimicrobial chemotherapy: a global perspective. *Afr J Microbiol Res.* 2013;7:1158–1172.
8. Mc Nulty K, Soon JM, Wallace CA, Nastasijevic I. Antimicrobial resistance monitoring and surveillance in the meat chain: a report from five countries in the European Union and European Economic Area. *Trends Food Sci Technol.* 2016;58:1–13.
9. Wellington EMH, Boxal ABA, Cross P, et al. The role of the natural environment in the emergence of antibiotic resistance in gram-negative bacteria. *Lancet Infect Dis.* 2013;13:155–165.
10. Fair RJ, Tor Y. Antibiotics and bacterial resistance in the 21st century. *Perspect Med Chem.* 2014;6:25–64.
11. Anonymous. One Health initiative. <http://www.onehealthinitiative.com/index.php>; Updated 2017 Accessed 09.09.17.
12. Szmolka A, Nagy B. Multidrug resistant commensal *Escherichia coli* in animals and its impact for public health. *Front Microbiol.* 2013;4:1–13.
13. Levy SB. The challenge of antibiotic resistance. *Sci Am.* 1998;3:46–53.
14. Van den Honert MS, Gouws PA, Hoffman LC. A preliminary study: antibiotic resistance of *Escherichia coli* and *Staphylococcus aureus* from the meat and faeces of various South African wildlife species. *Food Sci Anim Resour.* 2021;41:135–144.
15. Salmenlinna S, Lyytikäinen O, Vainio A, et al. Human cases of methicillin-resistant *Staphylococcus aureus* CC398 infection, Finland. *Emerg Infect Dis.* 2010;16:1626–1629.
16. Landers TF, Cohen B, Wittum TE, Larson EL. A review of antibiotic use in food animals: perspective, policy, and potential. *Public Health Rep.* 2012;127:4–22.
17. Gilchrist MJ, Greko C, Wllinga DB, Beran GW, Riley DG, Thorne PS. The potential roles of concentrated animal feeding operations in infectious disease epidemics and antibiotic resistance. *Environ Health Perspect.* 2007;115:313–316.
18. Moyane JN, Jideani AIO, Aiyegoro OA. Antibiotics usage in food-producing animals in South Africa and impact on human: antibiotic resistance. *Afr J Microbiol Res.* 2013;7:2990–2997.
19. Woolhouse M, Ward M, van Bunnik B, Farrar J. Antimicrobial resistance in humans, livestock and the wider environment. *Philos Trans R Soc B.* 2015;370:1–7.
20. Van Vurren M. Antibiotic resistance, with special reference to poultry production. *OIE Conf.* 2001;53:135–146.
21. Kapoor G, Saigal S, Elongavan A. Action and resistance mechanisms of antibiotics: a guide for clinicians. *J Anaesthesiol Clin Pharmacol.* 2017;33(3):300–305.
22. Carlson-Banning KM, Zechiedrich L. Antibiotic classes and mechanisms of resistance. In: Nelson K, ed. *Encyclopedia of Metagenomics.* New York: Springer; 2013:1–13.
23. Bhullar K, Waglechner N, Pawlowski A, et al. Antibiotic resistance is prevalent in an isolated cave microbiome. *PLoS One.* 2012;7:1–12.
24. Rolain J. Food and human gut as reservoirs of transferable antibiotic resistance encoding genes. *Front Microbiol.* 2013;4:1–10.
25. Ramey AM, Ahlstrom CA. Antibiotic resistant bacteria in wildlife: perspectives on trends, acquisition and dissemination, data gaps, and future directions. *J Wildl Dis.* 2019;56(1):1–15.
26. Martínez JL. Antibiotics and antibiotic resistance genes in natural environments. *Sci Mag.* 2008;21:365–367.
27. Anonymous. Antimicrobial resistance: implications for the food system. *Compr Rev Food Sci Food Saf.* 2006;5:71–137.
28. Jeters RT, Rivera AJ, Boucek LM, Stumpf RM, Leigh SR, Salyers AA. Antibiotic resistance genes in the vaginal microbiota of primates not normally exposed to antibiotics. *J Bacteriol.* 2009;191: 6374–6382.
29. Bonnedahl J, Järhult JD. Antibiotic resistance in wild birds. *Upsala J Med Sci.* 2016;119:113–116.
30. Davies J, Davies D. Origins and evolution of antibiotic resistance. *Microbiol Mol Biol Rev.* 2010;74:417–433.
31. Wales AD, Davies RH. Co-selection of resistance to antibiotics, biocides and heavy metals, and its relevance to foodborne pathogens. *Antibiotics.* 2015;4:567–604.
32. Joint Expert Advisory Committee on Antibiotic Resistance. *The Use of Antibiotics in Food-producing Animals: Antibiotic Resistant Bacteria in Animals and Humans.* Canberra: Commonwealth of Australia; 1999.
33. Harada K, Asai T. Role of antimicrobial selective pressure and secondary factors on antimicrobial resistance prevalence in *Escherichia coli* from food-producing animals in Japan. *J Biomed Biotechnol.* 2010;1–12.
34. Cheng G, Ning J, Ahmed S, et al. Selection and dissemination of antimicrobial resistance in Agri-food production. *Antimicrob Resist Infect Control.* 2019;8(158):1–13.
35. von Wintersdorff CJH, Penders J, Van Niekerk JM, et al. Dissemination of antimicrobial resistance in microbial ecosystems through horizontal gene transfer. *Front Microbiol.* 2016;7:1–10.
36. Essack SY, Bester L. Antibiotic resistance via the food chain: fact or fiction? *S Afr J Sci.* 2010;106:1–5.
37. Muniesa M, Colomer-Lluch M, Jofre J. Potential impact of environmental bacteriophages in spreading antibiotic resistance genes. *Future Microbiol.* 2013;8:739–751.
38. Balcazar JL. Bacteriophages as vehicles for antibiotic resistance genes in the environment. *PLoS Pathog.* 2014;10:1–4.
39. Fronzes R, Christie PJ, Waksman G. The structural biology of type IV secretion systems. *Nat Rev Microbiol.* 2009;7:703–714.
40. Laxminarayan R, Duse A, Wattal C, et al. Antibiotic resistance – the need for global solutions. *Lancet Infect Dis.* 2013;13: 1057–1098.
41. Lowy F. Antimicrobial resistance: the example of *Staphylococcus aureus.* *J Clin Investig.* 2003;111:1265–1273.
42. Wegner HC. *Antibiotic resistance-linking human and animal health. Improving Food Safety Through a One Health Approach.* Washington, DC: The National Academies Press; 2012:331–347.
43. Dias D, Torres RT, Kronvall G, Fonseca C, Mendo S, Caetano T. Assessment of antibiotic resistance of *Escherichia coli* isolates and screening of *Salmonella* spp. in wild ungulates from Portugal. *Res Microbiol.* 2015;166:584–593.
44. Heuer H, Schmitt H, Smalla K. Antibiotic resistance gene spread due to manure application on agricultural fields. *Curr Opin Microbiol.* 2011;14:236–243.
45. Mercat M, Clermont O, Massot M, Ruppe E, Garine-wichatitsky M, Miguel E. *Escherichia coli* population structure and antibiotic

resistance at a buffalo/cattle interface in Southern Africa. *Appl Environ Microbiol.* 2016;82:1459–1467.

46. Manyi-Loh C, Mamphweli S, Meyer E, Okoh A. Antibiotic use in agriculture and its consequential resistance in environmental sources: potential public health implications. *Molecules.* 2018;23 (795):1–48.
47. Van den Honert MS, Gouws PA, Hoffman LC. Importance and implications of antibiotic resistance development in livestock and wildlife farming in South Africa. *S Afr J Anim Sci.* 2018;48: 401–412.
48. Kjeldgaard J, Cohn MT, Casey PG, Hill C, Ingmer H. Residual antibiotics disrupt meat fermentation and increase risk of infection. *mBio.* 2012;3:1–4.
49. World Health Organization. WHO publishes list of bacteria for which new antibiotics are urgently needed. <http://www.who.int/en/news-room/detail/27-02-2017-who-publishes-list-of-bacteria-for-which-new-antibiotics-are-urgently-needed>; Updated 2017 Accessed 10.05.18.
50. Perez F, Hujer AM, Hujer KM, Decker BK, Rather PN, Bonomo RA. Global challenge of multidrug-resistant *Acinetobacter baumannii. Antimicrob Agents Chemother.* 2007;51:3471–3484.
51. Chen L-K, Kuo S-C, Chang K-C, et al. Clinical antibiotic-resistant *Acinebacter baumannii* strains with higher susceptibility to environmental phages than antibiotic-sensitive strains. *Nat Sci Rep.* 2017;7:1–10.
52. De Amorim AM, Nascimento JDS. *Acinetobacter*: an underrated foodborne pathogen? *J Infect Dev Ctries.* 2017;11(2):111–114.
53. Yayan J, Ghebremedhin B, Rasche K. Antibiotic resistance of *Pseudomonas aeruginosa* in pneumonia at a single university hospital center in Germany over a 10-year period. *PLoS One.* 2015;10:1–20.
54. Cabot G, Zamorano L, Moyà B, et al. Evolution of *Pseudomonas aeruginosa* antimicrobial resistance and fitness under low and high mutation rates. *Antimicrob Agents Chemother.* 2016;60:1767–1778.
55. Hawkey PM. Molecular epidemiology of clinically significant antibiotics resistance genes. *Br J Pharmacol.* 2008;153:S406–S413.
56. Rupp ME, Fey PD. Extended spectrum beta-lactamase (ESBL)-producing *Enterobacteriaceae*: considerations for diagnosis, prevention and drug treatment. *Drugs.* 2003;63:353–365.
57. Reinthaler FF, Feierl G, Galler H, et al. ESBL-producing *E. coli* in Austrian sewage sludge. *Water Res.* 2010;44:1981–1985.
58. Poeta P, Radhouani H, Gonçalves A, et al. Genetic characterisation of antibiotic resistance in enteropathogenic *Escherichia coli* carrying extended-spectrum β-lactamases recovered from diarrhoeic rabbits. *Zoonoses Public Health.* 2009;57:162–170.
59. Anonymous. Scientific opinion on the public health risks of bacterial strains producing extended spectrum β-lactamases and/or AmpC β-lactamases in food and food-producing animals. *EFSA J.* 2011;9:2322.
60. Cetinkaya Y, Falk P, Mayhall CG. Vancomycin-resistant *Enterococci. Clin Microbiol Rev.* 2013;13:686–707.
61. Miller WR, Munita JM, Arias CA. Mechanisms of antibiotic resistance in enterococci. *Expert Rev Anti Infect Ther.* 2014;12: 1221–1236.
62. Giraffa G. Enterococci from foods. *FEMS Microbiol Rev.* 2002;26:163–171.
63. Porrero MC, Mentaberre G, Sánchez S, et al. Carriage of *Staphylococcus aureus* by free-living wild animals in Spain. *Appl Environ Microbiol.* 2014;80:4865–4870.
64. Thung I, Aramin H, Vavinskaya V, et al. Review article: the global emergence of *Helicobacter pylori* antibiotic resistance. *Aliment Pharmacol Ther.* 2015;43:514–533.
65. Alba C, Blanco A, Alarcón T. Antibiotic resistance in *Helicobacter pylori. Curr Opin Infect Dis.* 2017;30:489–497.
66. Mégraud F. *H pylori* antibiotic resistance: prevalence, importance, and advances in testing. *Gut.* 2004;53:1374–1384.
67. Quaglia NC, Dambrosio A. *Helicobacter pylori*: a foodborne pathogen? *World J Gastroenterol.* 2018;24(31):3472–3487.
68. Butzler JP, Oosterom J. *Campylobacter*: pathogenicity and significance in foods. *Int J Food Microbiol.* 1991;12(1):1–8.
69. The World Health Organization. *The Burden of Foodborne Diseases in the WHO European Region.* WHO; 2017: 1–47.
70. Centers for Disease Control and Prevention. Foodborne Diseases Active Surveillance Network (FoodNet). <https://www.cdc.gov/foodnet/reports/prelim-data-intro-2019.html>; Accessed 19.10.20.
71. DiMarzio M, Shariat N, Kariyawasam S, Barrangou R, Dudley EG. Antibiotic resistance in *Salmonella enterica* serovar Typhimurium assocaites with CRISPR sequence type. *Antimicrob Agents Chemother.* 2013;57:4282–4289.
72. Klemm EJ, Shakoor S, Page AJ, et al. Emergence of an extensively drug-resistant *Salmonella enterica* serovar Typhi clone harbouring a promiscuous plasmid encoding resistance to fluoroquinolones and third-generation cephalosporins. *mBio.* 2018;9:1–10.
73. Warren BR, Parish ME, Schneider KR. *Shigella* as a foodborne pathogen and current methods for detection in food. *Crit Rev Food Sci Nutr.* 2007;46:551–567.
74. Puzari M, Sharma M, Chetia P. Emergence of antibiotic resistant *Shigella* species: a matter of concern. *J Infect Public Health.* 2017;11:451–454.
75. Koluman A, Dikici A. Antimicrobial resistance of emerging foodborne pathogens: status quo and global trends. *Crit Rev Microbiol.* 2013;39:57–69.
76. Phillips I, Casewell M, Cox T, et al. Does the use of antibiotics in food animals pose a risk to human health? A critical review of published data. *J Antimicrob Chemother.* 2004;53:28–52.
77. Rolain JM, Mallet MN, Fournier PE, Raoult D. Real-time PCR for universal antibiotic susceptibility testing. *J Antimicrob Chemother.* 2004;54:538–541.
78. De Briyne N, Atkinson J, Pokludová L, Borriello SP. Antibiotics used most commonly to treat animals in Europe. *Vet Rec.* 2014;175:1–8.
79. Dorado-Garcia A, Mevius DJ, Jacobs JJH, et al. Quantitative assessment of antimicrobial resistance in livestock during the course of a nationwide antimicrobial use reduction in the Netherlands. *J Antimicrob Chemother.* 2016;71:3067–3619.
80. Kimera ZI, Mshana SE, Rweyemamu MM, Mboera LEG, Matee MIN. Antimicrobial use and resistance in food-producing animals and the environment: an African perspective. *Antimicrob Resist Infect Control.* 2020;9(37):1–12.
81. Barton M. Antibiotic use in animal feed and its impact on human health. *Nutr Res Rev.* 2001;13:279–299.
82. Casewell M, Friss C, Marco E, McMullin P, Phillips I. The European ban on growth-promoting antibiotics and emerging consequences for human and animal health. *J Antimicrob Chemother.* 2003;52:159–161.
83. Moulin G, Cavalié P, Pellanne I, et al. A comparison of antimicrobial usage in human and veterinary medicine in France from 1999 to 2005. *J Antimicrob Chemother.* 2008;62:617–625.

84. OIE. *OIE List of Antimicrobials of Veterinary Importance*. Paris: OIE; 2007.
85. Anonymous. Antimicrobials in agriculture and the environment: reducing unnecessary use and waste. Review on Antimicrobial Resistance. <https://ec.europa.eu/health/amr/sites/amr/files/amr_-studies_2015_am-in-agri-and-env.pdf>; Updated 2015 Accessed 10.01.18.
86. Nelson DW, Moore JE, Rao JR. Antimicrobial resistance (AMR): significance to food quality and safety. *Food Qual Saf.* 2019;3:15–22.
87. Catry B, Laevens H, Devriese LA, Opsomer G, De Kruif A. Antimicrobial resistance in livestock. *J Vet Pharmacol Ther.* 2003;26:81–93.
88. Ibrahim M, Ahmad F, Yaqub B, et al. *Current trends of antimicrobials used in food animals and aquaculture. Antibiotics and Antimicrobial Resistance Genes in the Environment.* Elsevier; 2020:39–69.
89. Lerma LL, Benomar N, Casado C, Gálvez A, Abriouel H. Antibiotic multiresistance analysis of mesophilic and psychrotrophic *Pseudomonas* spp. isolated from goat and lamb slaughterhouse surfaces throughout the meat production process. *Appl Environ Microbiol.* 2014;80:6792–6806.
90. Khachatourians GG. Agricultural use of antibiotics and the evolution and transfer of antibiotic-resistant bacteria. *Can Med Assoc J.* 1998;159:1129–1136.
91. Luangtongkum T, Morishita TY, Ison AJ, Huang S, McDermott PF, Zhang Q. Effect of conventional and organic practices on the prevalence and antimicrobial resistance of *Campylobacter* spp. in poultry. *Appl Environ Microbiol.* 2006;72:3600–3607.
92. Millman JM, Waits K, Grande H, et al. Prevalence of antibiotic-resistant *E. coli* in retail chicken: comparing conventional, organic, kosher, and raised without antibiotics. *F1000 Res.* 2014;2:1–14.
93. Koga VL, Scandorieiro S, Vespero EC, et al. Comparison of antibiotic resistance and virulence factors among *Escherichia coli* isolated from conventional and free-range poultry. *BioMed Res Int.* 2015;1–8.
94. Graham JP, Price LB, Evans SL, Graczyk TK, Silbergeld EK. Antibiotic resistant enterococci and staphylococci isolated from flies collected near confined poultry feeding operations. *Sci Total Environ.* 2009;407:2701–2710.
95. Karesh WB, Loh E, Machalaba C. *Food safety: a view from the wild side. Improving Food Safety Through a One Health Approach.* Washington, DC: The National Academies Press; 2012:207–211.
96. Center for Science in the Public Interest. *Antibiotic Resistance in Foodborne Pathogens*. Washington, DC: Center for Science in the Public Interest; 2013.
97. Anderson AC, Jonas D, Huber I, et al. *Enterococcus faecalis* from food, clinical specimens, and oral sites: prevalence of virulence factors in association with biofilm formation. *Front Microbiol.* 2016;6:1–14.
98. Melnyk AH, Wong A, Kassen R. The fitness costs of antibiotic resistance mutations. *Evol Appl.* 2014;8:273–283.
99. Doyle MP, Loneragan GH, Scott HM, Singer RS. Antimicrobial resistance: challenges and perspectives. *Compr Rev Food Sci Food Saf.* 2013;12:234–248.
100. Anonymous. Animal welfare guidelines for beef farmers. <https://www.teagasc.ie/media/website/animals/beef/dairybeef/AnimalWelfareGuidelinesforBeefFarmers2003--Dept-of-Agr.pdf>; Updated 2003 Accessed 03.02.19.
101. Founou LL, Founou RC, Essack SY. Antibiotic resistance in the food chain: a developing country-perspective. *Front Microbiol.* 2016;7:1–19.
102. Levy SB, FitzGerald GB, Macone AB. Spread of antibiotic resistant plasmids from chicken to chicken and from chicken to man. *Nature.* 1976;260:40–42.
103. Serrano PH. Responsible use of antibiotics in aquaculture. In: *FAO Fisheries Technical paper 469.* Rome: FAO; 2005.
104. Angulo FJ, Nargund VN, Chiller TC. Evidence of an association between use of anti-microbial agents in food animals and antimicrobial resistance among bacteria isolated from humans and the human health consequences of such resistance. *J Vet Med.* 2004;51:374–379.
105. Vivienne EE, Josephine O-KO, Anaelom NJ. Effect of temperature (cooking and freezing) on the concentration of the oxytetracycline residue in experimentally induced birds. *Vet World.* 2018;11:167–171.
106. Codex Alimentarius International Food Standards. Maximum residue limits (MRLs) and risk management recommendations (RMRs) for the residues of veterinary drugs in foods. 2018, 1–46.
107. McEwen SA, Fedorka-Cray PJ. Antimicrobial use and resistance in animals. *Clin Infect Dis.* 2002;34:93–106.
108. Van den Honert MS, Gouws PA, Hoffman LC. A preliminary study: antibiotic resistance patterns of *Escherichia coli* and *Enterococcus* species from wildlife species subjected to supplementary feeding on various South African farms. *Animals.* 2020;10(396):1–20.
109. Hoelzer K, Bielke L, Blake DP, et al. Vaccines as alternatives to antibiotics for food producing animals. Part 1: challenges and needs. *Vet Res.* 2018;49(64):1–10.
110. Wang S, Zeng X, Yang Q, Qiao S. Antimicrobial peptides as potential alternatives to antibiotics in food animal industry. *Int J Mol Sci.* 2016;17(5):603.
111. Mejía-Argueta EL, Santillán-Benítez JG, Ortiz-Reynoso M. Antimicrobial peptides, an alternative to combat bacterial resistance. *Acta Biol Colomb.* 2020;25(2):294–302.
112. Roněevic T, Puizina J, Tossi A. Antimicrobial peptides as anti-infective agents in pre-post-antibiotic era? *Int J Mol Sci.* 2019; 20:1–32.
113. Massé DI, Saady NM, Gilbert Y. Potential of biological processes to eliminate antibiotics in livestock manure: an overview. *Animals.* 2014;4:146–163.
114. Wallmann J. Monitoring of antimicrobial resistance in pathogenic bacteria from livestock animals. *Int J Med Microbiol.* 2006;296: 81–86.
115. Sandora TJ, Goldmann DA. Preventing lethal hospital outbreaks of antibiotic-resistant bacteria. *N Engl J Med.* 2012;367: 2168–2170.
116. Simonsen GS. Antimicrobial resistance surveillance in Europe and beyond. *Euro Surveill.* 2018;23(42):1–3.
117. Schall J, Rajkhowa A, Ikua K, Rao P, Moore CE. Surviellance and monitoring of antimicrobial resistance: limitation and lessons from the GRAM project. *BMC Med.* 2019;17(176):1–3.
118. World Health Organization. Global antimicrobial resistance surveillance system (GLASS). Country participation. <https://www.who.int/glass/country-participation/en/>; Accessed 03.11.20.

119. Hanna GJ, D'Aquila RT. Clinical use of genotypic and phenotypic drug resistance testing to monitor antiretroviral chemotherapy. *HIV/AIDS*. 2001;32:774–782.
120. Georgios M, Egki T, Effrosyni S. Phenotypic and molecular methods for the detection of antibiotic resistance mechanisms in gram negative nosocomial pathogens. *Trends Infect Dis*. 2014;2014: 139–162.
121. Anjum MF. Screening methods for the detection of antimicrobial resistance genes present in bacterial isolates and the microbiota. *Future Microbiol*. 2015;10:317–320.
122. Fluit AC, Visser MR, Schmitz F-J. Molecular detection of antimicrobial resistance. *Clin Microbiol Rev*. 2001;14:836–871.
123. Jorgensen JH, Ferraro MJ. Antimicrobial susceptibility testing: a review of general principles and contemporary practices. *Clin Infect Dis*. 2009;49:1749–1755.
124. Kelly MT, Latimer JM, Balfour LC. Comparison of three automated systems for antimicrobial susceptibility testing of gram-negative bacilli. *J Clin Microbiol*. 1982;15:902–905.
125. Silley P. Susceptibility testing methods, resistance and breakpoints: what do these terms really mean? *Rev Sci Tech*. 2012; 31:33–41.
126. Kassim A, Omuse G, Premji Z, Revathi G. Comparison of Clinical Laboratory Standards Institute and European Committee on Antimicrobial Susceptibility Testing guidelines for the interpretation of antibiotic susceptibility at a University teaching hospital in Nairobi, Kenya: a cross-sectional study. *Ann Clin Microbiol Antimicrob*. 2016;15:1–7.
127. Schlegelova J, Rysïânek D, Sïedivâ I, Babâk V. Comparison of methods for the determination of antimicrobial resistance in *Staphylococcus aureus* from bovine mastitis. *J Vet Med*. 2001; 48:21–29.
128. Healy M, Huong J, Bittner T, et al. Microbial DNA typing by automated repetitive sequence based PCR. *J Clin Microbiol*. 2005;43:199–207.
129. Gorski L, Csordas A. *Molecular detection: principles and methods. Molecular Detection of Foodbourne Pathogens*. Boca Raton, FL: CRC Press; 2010:3–10.
130. Gupta SK, Padmanabhan BR, Diene SM, et al. ARG-ANNOT, a new bioinformatic tool to discover antibiotic resistance genes in bacterial genomes. *Antimicrob Agents Chemother*. 2014;58:212–220.
131. Oniciuc EA, Likotrafiti E, Alvarez-Molina A, Prieto M, Santos JA, Alvarez-Ordóñez A. The present and future of whole genome sequencing (WGS) and whole metagenome sequencing (WMS) for surveillance of antimicrobial resistant microorganisms and antimicrobial resistance genes across the food chain. *Genes*. 2018;9:1–28.
132. Tyson GH, McDermott PF, Li C, et al. WGS accurately predicts antimicrobial resistance in *Escherichia coli*. *J Antimicrob Chemother*. 2015;70:2763–2769.
133. Vittecoq M, Godreuil S, Prugnolle F, et al. Antimicrobial resistance in wildlife. *J Appl Ecol*. 2016;53:519–529.
134. Sousa M, Silva N, Igrejas G, et al. Antimicrobial resistance determinants in *Staphylococcus* spp. recovered from birds of prey in Portugal. *Vet Microbiol*. 2014;171:436–440.
135. Hendriksen RS, Bortolaia V, Tate H, Tyson GH, Aarestrup FM, McDermott PF. Using genomics to track global antimicrobial resistance. *Front Public Health*. 2019;7(242):1–17.
136. Su M, Satola SW, Read TD. Genome-based prediction of bacterial antibiotic resistance. *J Clin Microbiol*. 2019;57(3):1–15.

Chapter 59

Quick detection and confirmation of microbes in food and water

Ricardo Franco-Duarte[1], Snehal Kadam[2], Karishma S. Kaushik[2], Sakshi Painuli[3], Prabhakar Semwal[3], Natália Cruz-Martins[4,5,6] and Célia Fortuna Rodrigues[6,7]

[1]*Centre of Molecular and Environmental Biology (CBMA), Department of Biology, University of Minho, Braga, Portugal,* [2]*Institute of Bioinformatics and Biotechnology, Savitribai Phule Pune University, Pune, India,* [3]*Department of Biotechnology, Graphic Era University, Dehradun, India,* [4]*Faculty of Medicine, University of Porto, Porto, Portugal,* [5]*Institute for Research and Innovation in Health (i3S), University of Porto, Porto, Portugal,* [6]*TOXRUN - Toxicology Research Unit, University Institute of Health Sciences, Polytechnic and University Cooperative (CESPU), Gandra, Portugal,* [7]*LEPABE – Laboratory for Process Engineering, Environment, Biotechnology and Energy, ALiCE-Associate Laboratory in Chemical Engineering - Faculty of Engineering, University of Porto, Porto, Portugal*

Abstract

The ingestion of contaminated food or water is a great threat to public health. In fact, food and water contamination can result in serious infections, and are associated with high morbidity and mortality. The food and water supply chain need to guarantee the safety and quality of all food products; however, this can be laborious, since it depends on several segments, starting from food sample handling, storage, sample processing, transport, and retail. Essentially, for food and waterborne pathogen detection, cell culture methods continue to be the "gold standard" (low-cost, sensitive and microorganism specific), but traditional methods do have several drawbacks: high time spent for sample preparation, large volumes of reagents needed, and prerequisite of qualified personnel. In order to surpass these issues, rapid, sensitive, on-site, and reliable methods have been developed and implemented in modern food production systems. This chapter will recapitulate available methods, and discuss them in the context of their applications, and possible use as alternatives to gold-standard methods.

Keywords: Cell culture; foodborne pathogen; waterborne pathogen food safety; immunoassay; molecular biology method; MALDI-TOF; microfluidics

59.1 Introduction

Food and water contamination by toxins and microorganisms is a major public health problem. Indeed, infections derived from food and waterborne pathogens are responsible for high morbidity, mortality, and treatment costs. The World Health Organization (WHO) considers foodborne diseases as a serious public health challenge, given that more than 200 diseases can be spread through food alone.[1,2] Globally, approximately 1 in 10 persons (~600 million) fall ill every year from contaminated food and, among them, 420,000 die.[2] Between 1980 and 2015, about 1.3 million global deaths originated from diarrheal infections.[3] Particularly in the United States, these infections increased from 2000 to 2014, resulting in 0.41–2.41 deaths/100,000 individuals.[4] The European Centre for Disease Prevention and Control (ECDC) has reported an average of 100 food and waterborne outbreaks per week in 2017, in several countries (total: 5079). With the need of an increase in quantity and safer food, a new era in food safety is rapidly approaching, where the global food safety testing market is expected to grow more than 21.5 billion by 2023.[5]

Pathogens responsible for food contaminations—foodborne pathogens—can be grouped as bacteria, fungi, parasites, and viruses. The most common are *Salmonella enterica*, *Clostridium* spp., *Campylobacter* spp., *Shigella* spp., *Escherichia coli*, *Vibrio* spp., *Penicillium* spp., *Aspergillus* spp., *Cladosporium* spp., *Giardia lamblia*, *Trichinella spiralis*, *Cryptosporidium* spp., *Taenia* spp., Hepatitis A, Norwalk virus, and calicivirus.[6,7] Among the ECDC reported outbreaks, *Salmonella* sp. were the most common cause of foodborne outbreaks, and the rising trend of listeriosis continued to cause deaths in vulnerable groups. Furthermore, after several years of decline, the downward trend of European Union (EU) salmonellosis that started in 2008 has now stalled and cases have flattened out. *Cronobacter* spp. has also been

Present Knowledge in Food Safety. DOI: https://doi.org/10.1016/B978-0-12-819470-6.00030-5

described as a relevant pathogen, particularly to infant infections associated with powdered infant formula. This genus has a high mortality rate (40%–80%),[2] causing serious diseases both in children and adults, for example, necrotizing enterocolitis, meningitis, brain abscesses, kidney and liver failure, brain and neural disorders, reactive arthritis, cancer, septicemia, and several sequelae, as quadriplegia.[2] The Czech Republic recently revealed in a study that 31% of the several samples tested, were positive to *Cronobacter* spp.[2] *Campylobacter* spp. was the most commonly reported gastrointestinal bacterial pathogen in humans in the EU and has been so since 2005.[2] Notably, *Campylobacter* spp. was the third most common cause of mortality among the pathogens considered.[2] In 2010, WHO reports suggested that 600 million incidences of ailments were triggered by 31 different foodborne threats[6] (Table 59.1).

There are various other factors that are also relevant to the rise of foodborne infections. According to the ECDC, climatic factors impact the growth and survival of pathogens and transmission routes. Global warming affects the replication cycles of foodborne pathogens, and prolonged seasons might increase the chances of food-handling mistakes. Notably, in 32% of investigated foodborne outbreaks in Europe, "temperature misuse" was indicated as a contributing factor.[8] Furthermore, as a result of economic growth, lifestyle, and globalization, the demand and availability of different type of foods (e.g., fully cooked, raw, or undercooked) has also augmented. Therefore it is important to understand how the preparation and cooking conditions impact foodborne pathogen survival in different foods.[9]

The statistics clearly corroborate the urgent need for implementation of quality monitoring systems in food production processes. These systems already exist, and started to be employed in the early 1960s, in the United States.[10] It was firstly applied in slaughterhouses and meat processing firms, in order to avoid food contamination at the source (e.g., site construction, hygiene practices, animal access, slaughtering procedure, appropriate detergents, and other key points). The goal was to stop contamination and the dissemination of pathogenic microorganisms in the meat. This was, in fact, the first Hazard Analysis and Critical Control Point (HACCP) standard system for the elimination of pathogens from food goods. The system relies on the conduction of hazard analysis, critical control points/critical limits, procedure-monitoring, corrective actions, and verification and documentation processes.[11] After initial positive results, HACCP was applied across the food industry and restructured with the commitment of putting wide-ranging guidelines of hygiene for foodstuffs and procedures for certification. In Europe, HACCP was applied for food industry in 1993. HACCP established the basic rules for food business operators, who are obliged to follow specific regulations, to ensure the quality and safety of food products.[11]

As obvious, there is no doubt that food and waterborne infections are a substantial cause of human illness and urgently need to be reduced. European Food Safety Authority's recommendations are to enhance efforts, to push down the figures further. In a global perspective, these infections threaten the achievement of several of the United Nations (UN)' sustainable-development-goals (SDGs), in particular the third SDG: *Good Health and Well-Being*.

With reference to microbiological methods used for food microbial control, culture methods continue to be the "gold standard" approach. These techniques are low-cost, sensitive, and specific. Nonetheless, these methods have many drawbacks, such as time required for sample preparation, the demand for large reagent volumes, and necessity of qualified personnel.[12,13] In order to surpass these issues, rapid, sensitive, on-site, and reliable methods have been developed and implemented in modern food

TABLE 59.1 Main incidences of foodborne diseases in the period of 2007–15, according to WHO.[6]

Foodborne threat	Incidence
Norovirus	124,000,000
Campylobacter spp.	95,000,000
Enterotoxigenic *Escherichia coli*	86,000,000
Giardia spp., *Entamoeba histolytica*, and *Cryptosporidium* spp.	68,000,000
Shigella spp.	51,000,000
Salmonella Typhi	7,000,000
Nontyphoidal *Salmonella enterica*	59,000

production chains. This includes various tests using immunoassays (e.g., ELISA), molecular microbiology techniques [e.g., polymerase chain reaction (PCR), matrix-assisted laser desorption ionization time-of-flight (MALDI-TOF)], fluorescent-based methods [e.g., fluorescence in situ hybridization (FISH)], improved classical methods [e.g., most probable number (MPN)], or biosensors [e.g., bioluminescence, Fourier transform infrared spectroscopy (FT-IR)]. This chapter summarizes past and current novel methods to detect foodborne pathogens (Fig. 59.1).

59.2 Methods for microbial testing in food and water

59.2.1 Culture-based rapid approaches: an overview

59.2.1.1 Modifications to the standard colony count method

Traditional methods to detect microorganisms in food and water have relied on standard colony counts using the "plate count" method.[14] Briefly, in this approach, the

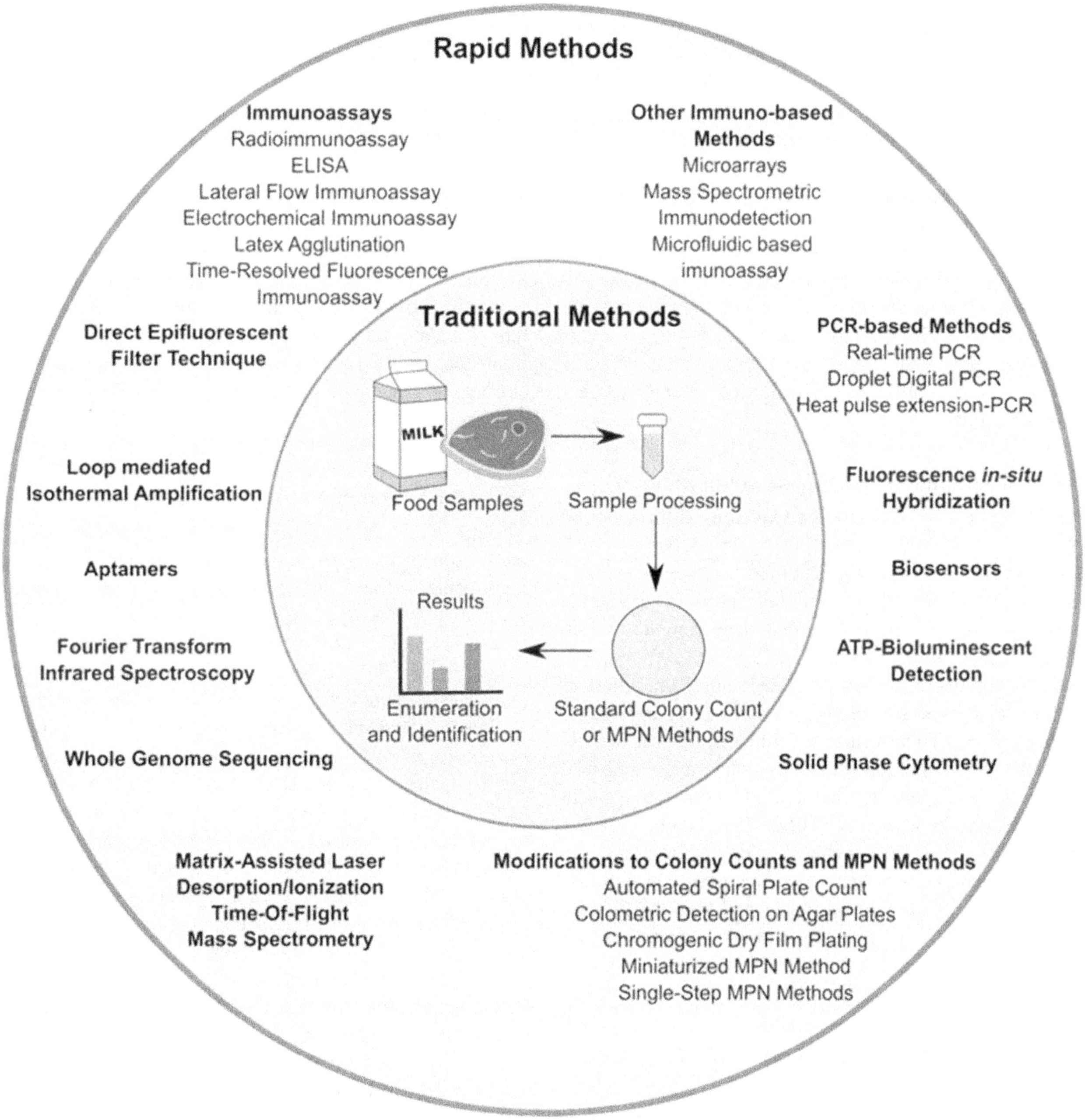

FIGURE 59.1 Current methods for microbial detection in food and water.

food or water sample is homogenized and diluted in sterile medium (often phosphate buffer saline). Dilutions are plated on a solid nutrient medium by the spread plate or pour plate method, following which plates are typically incubated at 37°C for 24–48 h. Microorganisms, if present in the food or water sample, grow to form visible colonies (colony-forming units, CFUs) on the plate, which can be counted. Dilutions with 30–300 colonies are counted, given that less than 30 colonies (in some cases, less than 10) is considered statistically unreliable, and it is impossible to count individual colonies at counts greater than 300 (error). While this has been standard practice for several years in food and water microbiology, a major limitation is the turn-around-time (TAT) of the results. For detection with the naked eye, the colonies on the plate need to be incubated overnight (at least 16–18 h), following which they can be counted. Furthermore, if plated on nonselective media, colonies will have to be suitably identified with biochemical tests (traditional or rapid testing methods). Together, this means that results can be reported, at the earliest possible, 2–3 days after the food or water sample has been brought to the laboratory. In addition, while the materials needed for the standard colony count method are routinely found in microbiology laboratories, and the techniques associated with the assay are well-documented, the standard colony count method does involve a significant utilization of laboratory manpower and time.

59.2.1.1.1 Automated spiral plate count method

There have been several modified versions of the standard colony count method, with the aim to accelerate the TAT of the method and automate segments of the assay. The spiral plate count method is widely used to enumerate microorganisms present in food and water samples.[15,16] In this method, an automated machine deposits a known volume of a homogenized food or water sample on a plate in the form of concentric spirals, in successively decreasing concentrations. This results in dilution of the sample across the concentric spirals, and by counting an appropriate area on the plate, the number of microorganisms in the sample can be estimated. The major advantage of this method over the manual standard colony count method is the need for minimal training, less recourse consumption (several dilutions on a single plate), and high throughput. The detection of microbial colonies still requires overnight incubation, and enumeration requires a special counting grid.

59.2.1.1.2 Colorimetric detection of microorganisms on agar plates

Following overnight growth, protocols in food and water microbiology require the identification and typing of microbial colonies. In standard microbiology practice, this is done via biochemical tests, often with rapid identification test kits. However, although these composite detection systems have reduced laboratory time and manpower, they require the addition of a pure microbial culture. To overcome this, a range of rapid detection methods based on direct plating of homogenized and enriched food and water samples on chromogenic agar plates, and subsequent colorimetric detection of microorganisms.[17–19] Widely known as CHROMagar, these media have been adapted to detect a wide range of foodborne bacteria/fungi, particularly Gram-negative pathogens, such as *Salmonella* spp., *Listeria* spp., *Proteus* spp., and coliforms. The agar plates contain synthetic chromogenic substrates that via a specific biochemical reaction, impart a color to the select pathogen. The presence of combinations of chemical inhibitors prevents the overgrowth of Gram-positive organisms. Therefore they possess the advantage of being both selective and differential, but also enable the detection of pathogens with high specificity. The major consideration with the use of chromogenic agar media is the need for laboratory time and manpower, as well as the requirement of overnight incubation. Notwithstanding, this method enables detection faster than standard microbiology practices, and has the additional advantage of obtaining the bacteria/fungi in pure culture for susceptibility testing (as opposed to molecular approaches).

59.2.1.1.3 Chromogenic dry film plating methods

Variations in chromogenic detection methods include ready-to-use dry nutrient beds (CompactDry) on which homogenized food, and water samples, can be directly applied.[17,20] The system typically consists of a special spread sheet with culture medium containing nutrients, a gelling agent, and a color indicator, enclosed in a disposable plastic container. The food or water solution is applied to the center of the dry spread sheet, following which it spreads through the medium. Following overnight incubation, the chromogenic substrates in the medium enable simultaneous detection and identification of pathogenic bacteria. While the system requires overnight incubation, it does serve to lessen manual components of laboratory work such as preparing plates, quality check of media, spreading of the sample, and subsequent biochemical analysis of the pathogens.

Another modification of this approach is the 3M Petrifilm Rapid Aerobic Count Plates (3M Petrifilm Coliform; 3M Petrifilm Anaerobic) with variations to detect only *E. coli*/coliforms and Enterobacteriaceae. The Rapid Coliform Count Plate is a dry film plating method which uses Violet Red Bile Lactose agar, and contains nutrients, a gelling agent, a pH indicator, and tetrazolium indicator. The food or water sample is place directly on the surface of the bottom film, following which the sample-containing gel is incubated overnight. Plates can be counted with a standard colony counter to enumerate colony numbers. Prior to overnight enumeration of colonies, the system accelerates the detection of coliforms by the appearance of yellow acid zones (which can appear as early as 6 h), and appearance of gas bubbles around the edge of early colonies.

59.2.1.2 Modifications to the most probable number method

The MPN technique is a well-known method for quantitative estimations of bacteria in food and water samples.[21] Briefly, replicate portions of the food or water samples are serially diluted in tubes, followed by incubation and enumeration of growth in the tubes. The presence of even a single viable bacterium in the tube will result in visible changes, observed as turbidity. Based on Poisson distribution, the dilutions and replicates employed can be used to estimate the bacterial density of the original sample. Guide tables are used to define the most probable number of bacteria (MPN index) and contain upper and lower confidence limits. Widely used in food and water microbiology to estimate fecal contamination with coliforms, the coliform MPN test employs three steps—presumptive estimation with lactose broth tubes (gas production by coliforms), the MPN confirmation procedure with brilliant green lactose broth (gas production of total and fecal coliforms, incubated at different temperatures), and completed tests with eosin methylene blue agar plates.

While an established standard, the traditional MPN method requires several sets of media, incubation at different temperatures, and up to 72 h for results. Given this, several modifications to the technique have been developed, to reduce laboratory manpower and time, and speed up the acquisition of results.

59.2.1.2.1 Miniaturized most probable number method

Several studies have reported the use of microplates to reduce the labor and reagent costs that limit the standard MPN method.[22,23] In these modifications, the wells of microplates (24 or 96) are used as "miniature" tubes, so constituting the miniaturized MPN method. The major modification, in addition to the smaller volumes of the microplate format, is the use of enrichment media or semisolid media (often modified semisolid Rappaport-Vassiliadis) to facilitate the recovery of coliforms and enteric pathogens from small volumes. In most modifications, incubation for 24–48 h was sufficient for detection and enumeration of colonies.

59.2.1.2.2 Single-step most probable number methods

Several single-step MPN procedures have been developed, particularly for the selection and identification of fecal coliforms. In one procedure, the media was modified to eliminate agar, mannitol, and dyes from the standard MPN procedure media, and instead modified media containing nutrients was used, and pH was adjusted to 7.3.[24] These modifications conferred selectivity toward fecal coliforms in the samples, given its lactose-based composition, presence of surfactants, and increased incubation temperature (44.5°C). The modified approach proved to be simple and rapid, providing results overnight, and comparable with the standard MPN assay.

59.2.2 Nonculture-based rapid approaches

59.2.2.1 Direct epifluorescent filter technique

One of the earliest rapid methods for pathogen detection in food and water samples, the direct epifluorescent filter technique (DEFT), uses the principles of membrane filtration and epifluorescence microscopy to directly visualize the presence of bacteria.[25–29] The standard protocol employs a 0.22 μm pore-sized membrane filter and staining with acridine orange. Visualized bacteria can be counted with automated techniques, since viable bacteria appear orange. Given the need for filtration, DEFT is typically suited for liquid samples of food such as milk, beverages, and water, but has also been modified for solid foods, with suitable homogenization and prefiltration modifications.[30] In one study, prefiltration of the homogenized sample through nylon filters (pore size 5 μm) was observed to get rid of most of the solid food debris, while minimally affecting bacterial counts.[30]

While the DEFT technique is certainly rapid (the procedure takes less than 30 min), allowing estimation of bacteria from samples within hours, it has certain limitations. Firstly, it does not enable the identification of bacterial species; this is particularly important given the association of certain pathogenic bacteria with food and waterborne infections. To overcome this, a modification of the DEFT technique employs a Gram staining procedure prior to staining with acridine orange.[31] In doing so, it could at least differentiate all Gram-positive bacteria, and viable Gram-negative bacteria, albeit not at species level.

A modified DEFT technique for the detection of yeasts in food samples[32] employed the use of an enrichment protocol, followed by prefiltration and use of the stain Viablue 1. A similar approach was used for the detection of *E. coli* O157:H7 in beef samples, with enrichment prior to DEFT, followed by visualization with anti-O157 fluorescent antibody (Ab-DEFT). The use of the antibody made the assay specific for the detection of O157:H7, a common pathogen found in meat and meat products. More recent DEFT modifications employ live-dead staining techniques, such as the BacLight bacterial viability assay,[33,34] thereby allowing the detection of total and viable bacterial counts.

While DEFT serves as an excellent screening method even today, it does not result in isolation of a pure bacterial culture, which is needed for species-level identification and antimicrobial susceptibility.

59.2.2.2 Biosensors

Biosensor-based approaches allow for the detection of microbes using a biology-based sensing function and have been investigated for their ability to detect microbes in food and water.[35–41] The typical design of a biosensor is a detection component, usually an antibody (but also nucleic acids, receptors, peptides, enzymes), and a transducing component that converts the recognized entity into a detectable signal. The type of detection system used to detect a particular molecule can highly influence the sensitivity and selectivity of the biosensor. Different types of transducers and their working principles have been discussed in detail elsewhere.[35,36,40,42] Briefly, biosensors can have optical, electrochemical or mass-based transducers.[36,38,40,42–44] Optical biosensors involve an optical readout of the detected microbial signal in the form of fluorescence, quantum dots, surface plasmon resonance (SPR), and other spectrophotometric methods. Surface SPR–based biosensors have bioactive molecules that facilitate the detection (via antigen/antibody, enzyme/substrate interactions). This detection component is immobilized on the surface of a conducting film on a metal surface, and when light passes through this, it interacts with the electrons on the metal surface at a specific angle. A binding event is detected by a change in this angle (and subsequent change in reflectance). Another type of optical biosensor is based on quantum dots. These are more advantageous than normal fluorescence dyes as they are brighter and have improved resistance to photobleaching. Electrochemical biosensors make use of redox-based chemical reactions involving transfer of electrons, leading to a change in the signal (current, resistance, voltage, impedance) measured. A typical electrochemical biosensor consists of electrodes, with the detection component coated or immobilized onto the electrode surface (silver, gold, platinum, copper, carbon electrodes). The binding event leads to an electrochemical change, which is then measured by the biosensor. Mass-based biosensors measure a change in mass due to the detection event. Most mass-based biosensors make use of piezoelectric crystals to detect small changes in mass. The detecting agent, such as antibodies, is coated onto the crystal surface. A binding event leads to a very minor, but detectable change in crystal mass sensed by the biosensor.

The type of biosensor used also determines the sample preparation required. For example, in a colorimetric based biosensor that detected protease activity,[45] *L. monocytogenes*-specific peptide substrates were conjugated on magnetic nanoparticles and deposited on a gold-plated self-adhesive sheet mounted on a plastic strip as its sensing surface. To test spiked milk and minced meat samples, minimal sample preparation was required. The samples were centrifuged, and the supernatants were filtered and added onto the sensor surface to determine bacterial load visualized as a color change. Some biosensors are designed to require minimal sample pretreatments; however, those that use small volumes of sample require preenrichment processes to concentrate the sample.[42,46] The combination of the recognition and transducing components, along with the pathogen being detected, determines the efficiency and detection limits of the biosensor. Biosensors can provide low detection limits (some as low as <10 CFU/mL) with quick detection times (most biosensors requiring less than 2 h).[42]

An electrochemical impedance spectroscopy–based biosensor using species-specific aptamers coated on gold nanoparticle–deposited electrodes was able to detect *S. Typhimurium* in spiked samples of egg and water with a sensitivity of 10^1 CFU/mL.[47] Another electrochemical-based biosensor used antibodies attached to the carbon electrodes to detect *S. Typhimurium* in lychee and orange juice with a limit of detection of $\sim 10^1$ CFU/mL.[48] Multiple other electrochemical biosensors have been explored to detect microbes in food and water.[44,49] Biosensors of single-walled carbon nanotubes with immobilized antibodies for *Y. enterocolitica* were able to detect the bacteria in kimchi with a 10^4 CFU/mL detection limit.[50] A magnetoelastic biosensor with a filamentous E2 phage coating was able to detect *S. Typhimurium* directly from spiked tomato surfaces.[51] Commercial biosensors such as Spreeta, a SPR–based biosensor, has been tested for its ability to detect *E. coli* O157:H7 in spiked apple juice, milk, and ground beef.[52] While biosensors have various advantages like high sensitivity and selectivity, and quick detection times, some challenges associated with biosensors can be the equipment required, background noise due to sample, and the detection of multiple bacterial species within one sensor simultaneously. In the food and water industry, biosensors are used to analyze safety.[53,54] This is tested at different stages of the process, right from the freshly acquired produce to the final finished product. Some products, such as BactoBox from SBT Instruments, are specific to testing of water (and limited liquid samples).[55]

59.2.2.3 Fourier transform infrared spectroscopy

The FT-IR approach makes use of radiation emitted from an IR source (between the visible and microwave regions of the electromagnetic spectrum), passed through an interferometer and its absorbance by the sample to detect microbial presence.[56–58] Different chemical groups have different IR bands associated with them, determined by the way they absorb radiation and vibrate.[56] Each bacterial/fungal species thus leads to a different IR spectral molecular fingerprint, due to differences in the absorbance of radiation by molecules in cells, such as DNA, RNA, and several proteins and small molecules, and thus can be uniquely identified.[59–61] The sample preparation procedure varies with the sampling method used and the kind of sample being analyzed. Solid foods can be powdered, and liquid samples may need further processing (such as filtration or immunomagnetic separation to capture the microorganism) depending on the type of FT-IR being used (attenuated total reflectance, specular reflectance, transmission, photo-acoustic and others). Some FT-IR techniques also require drying of the sample into a film. In a study that used FT-IR combined with either filtration or immunomagnetic separation to detect *E. coli* O157:H7 in spike ground beef, the sample processing was different based on the separation technique.[62] Filtered liquid from the stomached spiked ground beef was used as the starting material. Using a 0.45 μm pore size filter, bacteria were collected on the filter surface and their spectra were acquired. In comparison, to separate bacteria by immunomagnetic separation, Dynabeads coated with antibodies against *E. coli* O157:H7 were used with the filtered inoculated beef samples. The beads were coated on a gold-coated glass slide and air-dried before the spectra were acquired with FT-IR. However, in a study using horizontal attenuated total reflectance FT-IR to detect microbial spoilage of chicken meat,[63] excised fragments from the comminuted chicken meat were placed in direct contact with the ZnSe crystal and spectra were recorded. In the presence of multiple microorganisms within a sample, a separation step may also be required to better visualize the IR spectra.[58] The detection limit varies between 10^3 and 10^6 CFU/mL. The major advantages associated with FT-IR-based microbial detection are its speed, sensitivity, ability to process solid and liquid samples, detection of multiple species, and quantitative analysis.

Other previous studies have also detected microbes in food and water using FT-IR approaches.[58,63,64] In the study that separated *E. coli* O157:H7 from ground beef using filtration and immunomagnetic separation techniques, a detection limit of 10^5 CFU/g was observed.[62] Another study was able to detect and differentiate between eight bacterial species in spike apple juice at the lowest concentration tested of 10^3 CFU/mL.[65] Using individual cultures of eight bacterial species, six dilutions per species were made in sterile apple juice and these different spiked apple juice samples were analyzed using attenuated total reflectance FT-IR. The spectra were acquired from 80 μL of the sample loaded directly onto the ZnSe crystal. Using a two-step approach in canonical variate analysis of the first derivative of the spectra measured, the eight species were distinguishable. However, it should be noted that a multispecies-inoculated apple juice sample was not tested.

This method requires a FT-IR spectrophotometer. The costs for these instruments can go up with the addition of multiple modes of spectral acquisition, additional software analysis tools, improvements in signal-to-noise ratio, and more. However, FT-IR instruments are becoming popular in the food industry to determine food and beverage quality and test adulteration.[66,67] Hence, these can also be adapted to help detect microbial contaminants through the food and water industry.

59.2.2.4 Solid-phase cytometry

Solid-phase cytometry (SPC) detects microbial presence in samples via fluorescent labeling.[68–70] Samples are passed through a black polycarbonate or polyester filter with the appropriate pore size to retain microbes on the surface of the filter. Since this method is dependent on filtration, it is used largely for the analysis of water and other liquids, which are then labeled with fluorescent probes. The probes can be labeled antibodies, labeled species-specific nucleic acid probes, markers of certain enzyme activities, or nonfluorescent substrates that fluoresce only when they are taken up by the cells and cleaved.[70] Depending on the probes, the detection can be nonspecific or species/strain-specific, and can detect both viable and dead cells (most common), or only viable cells. Once the sample is filtered, the entire filter surface is scanned with a solid-phase cytometer, a laser-scanning device that capture microbes on a solid surface (the filter), to determine fluorescent signals from the microbial cells. An advantage of this method is that it requires approximately 3 min for a 25 mm filter to be scanned, and hence is a rapid method of detection. Since the whole filter is scanned, it has a detection limit as low as 1 cell per filter. This method allows one to enumerate the cells in the sample directly based on the fluorescence. The use of viability stains allows this method to detect microbial cells that would have been difficult to culture using traditional culture-based methods.[68] The filtration process involved make this a preferred method for microbial detection in water.[68,69,71–73] In a study to test SPC-based methods for detection of *C. jejuni* in spiked tap water (presterilized to remove other contaminants) incubated over 85 days, an aliquot from the water was passed through a 0.4 μm pore size black polyester membrane filter.[68] After a brief incubation period, the filter was exposed to a dye and further incubated and then scanned by an automated software to identify microbial cells within 3 min. The requirement of filterability limits the type of samples that can be analyzed using SPC. Since food samples are not filterable, studies that use SPC to detect microbes in food are scarce. This method is used as a sterility test to check for contaminants in water. is a commercial SPC-based system, that has been evaluated for its sterility testing (SCANRDI, bioMerieux).[74,75]

59.2.2.5 ATP-bioluminescent detection

This detection method uses the well-studied luciferin-luciferase system. Based on the detection of microbial ATP in the sample, the luciferase mediated ATP-dependent oxidative decarboxylation of luciferin proceeds to give luminescence as the output. Standard curves assist in converting luminescence detected into ATP (which is then converted into number of microbial cells). This assay is widely used in the food and beverage industry to evaluate sterility and hygiene at various processing stages.[76] For example, the Celsis Innovate ATP-bioluminescence based system uses this method of detection with applications in beverage and diary product sterility. While their system uses the standard ATP-bioluminescence assay, they provide proprietary reagents for a pretreatment step that helps reduce ATP background (from nonmicrobial sources in the sample). The Milliflex Rapid Detection system by Millipore also makes use of this detection method.[77] While this assay is rapid, it lacks the specificity with which different bacterial species can be detected by other methods.

59.2.2.6 Immunoassays

The presence of microbial pathogens in food and water can be detected by different immunological methods.[78] Briefly defined as immunoassays, they comprise bioanalytical techniques in which the analytes detection is based on the interaction between the antigen and the antibody. In 1917, while investigating the antigenicity of small molecules, Karl Landsteiner provided the framework for developing immuno-based assays capable of detecting low molecular–weight compounds.[78] In the period between 1995 and 2017, many advanced immuno-based assays were developed, allowing the quantitative, semi-quantitative, or qualitative identification of analytes.[79] Immunological assays are generally based on competitive binding reaction occurring between a specific amount of labeled analyte and an unspecified amount of unlabeled sample for a fixed amount of receptor binding sites available on a specific antianalyte antibody. As a result of this reaction, the analyte binds to the antibody to form an immune complex. The resulting immune complexes can be separated from the unbound reagent by chemical or physical separation methods for further analysis. Finally, the analysis is performed by assessing the labeled analyte activity through several detection techniques, like radiation, fluorescent, calorimetric, or enzymatic assays, where their sensitivity and specificity depend on the antibody characteristics. Nowadays, various methods have been used for the detection of multiple pathogens, including radioimmunoassay (RIA), enzyme-linked immunoassay [enzyme-linked immunosorbent assay (ELISA), ELFA], lateral flow immunoassay (LFIA), latex agglutination and reverse passive latex agglutination, time-resolved fluorescence immunoassay (TRFIA), chemiluminescent immunoassay (CLIA), and others. Due to high sensitivity and accuracy of immunochemical techniques, they became promising methods for detecting microorganisms and their toxins in water and food items. Some immunoassays, like ELISA, RIA, latex agglutination, among others, can be directly used for the determination of food and water contaminants (like microorganisms or substances, toxins, proteins, glycoproteins, among others, they produce) without a prior step of isolation.[12,80] In this section we will discuss several important methods used for detecting microorganism in food and water.

59.2.2.6.1 Radioimmunoassay

RIA is an old technique that is still used for the detection of unknown quantities of clinically and biologically important components. This is a highly sensitive and precise technique and uses radioactive compounds for quantitative and qualitative analysis of antigens present in samples. In late 1950s, Rosalyn Yalow and Solomon Berson developed this technique to detect plasma insulin levels and received the Nobel Prize for their work in 1977.[81] In the food industry, the technique has been used for the detection of *Staphylococcal enterotoxins* (A, B, C, D, E) in food items, such as milk, cheese, nonfat dry milk, hamburger, and boiled egg.[82–86] RIA technique was also used to determine the enterotoxin produced by *Clostridium perfringens* and other mycotoxins that can contaminate food, wheat, peanut butter, and maize.[87,88] This technique works on the principle of competitive binding, where an antigen labeled with radioactive compound, also known as "tracer," competes with nonlabeled antigens for a limited amount of antibody (receptor binding sites). When the nonlabeled antigens in a sample have a higher concentration than the labeled antigens, a competitive reaction occurs between the two types of antigens for the antibody binding site, resulting in the displacement of radiolabeled antigen and binding of nonlabeled antigen to the receptor binding site. The antigen–antibody complex so formed, will emit different radioactivity than before, and further, this radio emission of the antigen–antibody complex is measured and a binding curve is produced to determine the amount of analyte or unlabeled antigen in a sample.[89] By using antibodies with high affinity (Kd = 10^{-8}–10^{-11} M) it is possible to analyze even a few picograms of an analyte. Although this technique is very useful for the determination of microbial cells and toxins, it has some limitations including the high costs of reagents and equipment, in comparison to other techniques, and shorter shelf-life of radiolabeled compounds, among others. Presently, this method has been replaced by calorimetry and florescence-based methods (enzyme-based methods).

59.2.2.6.2 Enzyme-linked immunosorbent assay

ELISA or enzyme immunoassay (EIA) is a widely used immunological assay designed for qualitative and quantitative analysis of antigens, hormones, antibodies, glycoproteins, and proteins in biological samples. It was first conceptualized by the two research teams, Engvall and Perlmann and Van Weemen and Schuurs, in 1971.[90,91] ELISA is extensively used for detecting *Salmonella* in food items.[87,92–94] Other foodborne microorganisms, like *L. monocytogenes*, *E. coli* O157:H, *Alicyclobacillus* spp., and *Bacillus cereus* can also be detected by the ELISA technique, from meat, complex material, apple juice, and even other food products.[95–98] There are a few commercially available ELISA kits for identification of microbiological pathogens or microbial toxins in food.[94] The list comprises various ELISA kits for the detection of foodborne pathogens or microbial toxins, like *B. cereus* diarrheal enterotoxin, *Clostridium botulinum* neurotoxin, *Salmonella*, Shiga toxin, under the trade name *Bacillus* diarrheal enterotoxin, BoNT, *Salmonella*-TeK, *Salmonella* VIA, and Premier EHEC.[99] These ELISA kits are suitable for high-throughput screening with minimal manual handling, and most of them are based on sandwich ELISA. Basically, ELISA uses an enzyme for detecting the binding between a specific antigen and an antibody. Generally, the antigen or target molecule is stabilized on a solid surface (such as microtiter plate wells) and the enzyme-linked antibody is allowed to react with it. If the antigen and antibody are compatible with each other, they form a complex and the linked reporter enzyme triggers a colorimetric change in the solution after the addition of an appropriate substrate. This colorimetric change can be easily detected by several detectors and the concentration of the analyte can be determined by plotting a standard curve. On the basis of antigen–antibody combination, there are different types of ELISA methods—direct ELISA, indirect ELISA, competitive ELISA, and sandwich ELISA. The major advantages of ELISA are its specificity and simplicity along with low-cost, safety, and speed of operation.

59.2.2.6.3 Lateral flow immunoassay

LFIA, also known as immunochromatographic assay, has been effectively used for more than 50 years in detection of numerous diseases and conditions. This method is well known for its rapid ability to detect analytes or molecular ligands in complex mixtures. Due to its multifaceted properties, LFIA is immensely utilized in many other industrial sectors, for environmental testing, pharma sector, food testing, plant and crop health, and animal health. LFIA is a simple diagnostic technique with a paper-based platform, and methods based on LFIA like immunochromatography, dipstick, and immune-filtration are gaining interest in pathogen and mycotoxin detection in the food industry.[100] LFIA-based dipstick method was established for the rapid detection of aflatoxin B in pig feed[101] and contaminated samples of peanut, hazelnut, pistachio, and almonds.[102] Luo et al.[103] reported important commercial lateral flow assay kits for the diagnosis of microbiological pathogens in food items. Among others, such kits were capable of detecting foodborne pathogen, including *E. coli* O157, *Salmonella*, *Listeria*, *Campylobacter*, *B. cereus*, *Shigella*, *Vibrio cholerae*, and *Vibrio parahaemolyticus* from food samples, like raw beef, meat products, vegetables, fish, and sea food.[103]

In LFIA, mainly liquid samples are used for analysis; however, solid samples are homogenized and pretreated before analysis. The solid sample pretreatment method depends on the nature of matrix.[104] The liquid sample containing the target analyte moves on a polymeric strip by capillary action, and the analyte interacts with specific immobilized biological components on the strip.[105] The polymeric strip is composed of a sample pad, a conjugate release pad, a membrane having immobilized antibody, and an adsorbent pad. The liquid sample is deposited on the sample pad and it moves toward the conjugate release pad. Here, specific antibodies conjugated to fluorescent particles (colloidal gold or latex microsphere) interact with the analyte, and the complex moves to the detection zone. The interaction between the analyte and the immobilized biological component in the detection zone results in the appearance of a test line, while a control line indicates the proper flow of liquid sample on the strip. The appearing of the test line on the strip can be observed by a naked eye, or by a dedicated reader, and the results appear within 5–30 min.

59.2.2.6.4 Electrochemical immunoassay

In last few years electrochemical immunoassays have been developed and have become promising alternatives for current immunochemical assays. This assay is based on the assessment of few parameters, like interfacial capacitance, electrode potential, redox current, or impedance, whose measurement depends on the interfacial behavior of the oxidation reaction or electrode surface, or of the intrinsic reduction of a target analyte molecule, being, as seen in impedance, potential capacitance, and amperometry immunoassays.[106] Electrochemical immunoassays have several benefits, including speed, sensitivity, and accuracy of the method. For example, sandwich electrochemical immunoassay based on immobilized thiolated antibodies has been successfully used for the detection of *Staphylococcal enterotoxin* B,[107] whereas nonenzymatic sandwich electrochemical immunoassay has been developed for quantitative detection of *E. coli* with ATCC no. 25922 and *E. coli* O157:H7 in pork and milk samples.[108,109]

59.2.2.6.5 Latex agglutination and reverse passive agglutination assay

Latex agglutination test (LAT) was first developed in 1980s for the detection of toxin A and was later used for the detection of glutamate hydrogenase in toxigenic and nontoxigenic *Clostridium difficile* isolates.[110] It is a very common technique used for detection of microbial pathogens. According to the LAT principle, antigen and antibody molecules get bound, in a random arrangement, to the surface of latex or polystyrene beads.[111] The large amount of antibody or antigen molecules bound to the latex bead results in a high number of binding sites. Antibodies or antigen in the sample binds to the binding sites of the corresponding antibody/antigen, resulting in the formation of cross-linked aggregates of the latex particle and the sample antibody/antigen. These large-sized particles of latex enable the visualization of the antigen and antibody reaction. However, reverse passive agglutination test is a unique kind of particle agglutination assay in which the antigen or analyte in the sample are detected by the carrier molecules coated with antibodies. These agglutination assays are being continuously developed for the detection of a wide range of foodborne pathogens and toxins, like *C. difficile* toxin A and B, *E. coli* O157:H7, *Staphylococcus aureus*, and *Staphylococcal enterotoxins* from raw milk, meat, dairy products, and sausages.[112–116]

59.2.2.6.6 Time-resolved fluorescence immunoassay

TRFIA is an analytical technique which involves the use of rare earth metals or nonisotopes for detection of target analytes. The technique is based on the estimation of the fluorescence produced by rare earth metals (especially when the metal is present in complexes with suitable organic chelators).[117] Briefly, TRFIA utilizes a spectroscopic approach to investigate dynamic procedures in materials or chemical components. This technique can be used to detect any procedure which can cause variations in the material properties. In TRFIA, the fluorescence of the analyte or sample is observed as a function of time after the excited state by the flash.[118] The technique uses a specific fluorescent molecule, that is lanthanide. Lanthanide possess the rare property of emitting fluorescence for a long time period (estimated in milliseconds) after excitation, whereas other prominently used fluorescent dyes have an emitting period of only few nanoseconds. This TRFIA technique was used to detect *E. coli* O157:H7 in apple cider.[119] Multicolor time-resolved fluorescence assay was fabricated for the simultaneous detection of *S. aureus* and *S. typhimurium*.[120,121] After positive result, the method was validated by analyzing these two strains (of *S. aureus* and *S. typhimurium*) in milk sample.[121] TRFIA is very useful and sensitive compared to other commercial EIAs.[122]

59.2.2.6.7 Chemiluminescent immunoassay

CLIA is consistently gaining attention as a detection method due to its high specificity, sensitivity, simple equipment, wide linear range, and wide range of applications, in the field of clinical diagnostics, life sciences, pharmaceutical sector, food safety, and environmental monitoring.[123] This technique is used to detect the concentration of a sample or analyte based on the intensity of chemiluminescence that is emitted during a chemical reaction. CLIA is a joint result of chemiluminescence and immunoreactions.[124] In CLIA some of the target reagents are chemiluminescent-labeled, and following the addition of chemiluminescent substrates, the reaction results in luminescence, the intensity of which is based on the sample concentration that is detected. Commonly used chemiluminescence substrates are isoluminol, luminol, and their derivatives, alkaline phosphatase, peroxidase, and acridine ester derivative, and the most popular labeling enzymes are alkaline phosphatase and horseradish peroxidase.[123] Briefly, a buffer containing magnetic beads coated with specific antigen is added to a prediluted sample and incubated for 10 min. Incubation is followed by a washing step, and then the tracer (antibodies labeled with chemiluminescent) is added to the mixture. The mixture is incubated again for 10 min and washed to remove impurities. Chemiluminescence is measured with the help of a luminometer. CLIA technique is also capable of detecting microbes in a sample of low abundance, and has wide applications in different fields of biological sciences.[123] Rapid multiplexed CLIA has been developed for diagnosis of *Y. enterocolitica*, *E. coli* O157:H7, *L. monocytogenes*, and *S. typhimurium*.[125] A gold nanoparticle–based chemiluminescence immunosensor was developed for the detection of *Staphylococcal enterotoxin B* from mushroom, Gerber's meat, baby food, and tomato.[126] Another study shows the rapid and successful detection of *Salmonella* from different samples of milk and chicken by combination of immunomagnetic separation technique with chemiluminescence microparticle immunoassay.[127] Xu et al. developed a chemiluminescence EIA for the histamine detection (a biogenic amine responsible for food poisoning and allergies) from food samples, like shrimp, fish ball, carp, and soy sauce.[128]

59.2.2.7 Other immunoassay-based methods

59.2.2.7.1 Protein/antibody microarrays

Protein microarrays, also known as protein chips, is a high-throughput technique used to identify proteins interactions and activities, and also their function at a large scale.[129] The major benefit of using this technique is that it can track large quantity of proteins simultaneously. The proteins are immobilized on a surface or chip of support surface, like a nitrocellulose membrane, glass slide, and microtiter plate or bead.[130] In this technique, the probe molecules added to the array are labeled with a fluorescent dye. The interaction between the probe molecule and captured protein results in the emission of fluorescent signals and these signals are measured by a laser scanner. Protein microarrays require less amounts of samples and reagents and are known to be automated, cost-effective, highly sensitive, and rapid.[131] Antibody microarray is a specific type of protein microarray where antibodies are immobilized on a chip, and the probe molecules, composed by proteins or target molecules, are allowed to react with antibodies. The reaction produces fluorescence which is measured by the scanners and further data analysis is done for accurate results.[132] Antibody microarrays are one of the most promising approaches in future among multiplexed immunoassay technologies. Huelseweh and colleagues developed an antibody microarray for the detection of several foodborne and waterborne pathogens, including *Francisella tularensis*, *Brucella melitensis*, and *Burkholderia mallei*, by using sandwich immunoassays.[133]

59.2.2.7.2 Mass spectrometric immunodetection

Mass spectrometric immunodetection or immunoassay (MSIA) is a rapid technique for detection and quantification of antigens or antibody analytes in biological samples. MSIA has been increasingly used for the detection of *S. aureus* from raw milk.[134] The method is based on analyte affinity extraction (either by antibodies or antigens) to isolate the target analytes.[135–137] The method is highly sensitive and allows the detection of multiple analytes (either antigens or antibodies) in a single assay. This technique also has the ability to identify the point mutations in proteins.[136,138] Each analyte is detected precisely according to their specific molecular mass. For instance, Schlosser and colleagues detected *Staphylococcal enterotoxin B* from milk sample by combining immunomagnetic separation method with MALDI-ToF-mass spectroscopy (Ms),[134] while Jadhav et al. revealed the ability of MALDI-TOF-Ms for detecting *L. monocytogenes*, *E. coli* O157:H7, and *S. enterica* in red meat samples.[139]

59.2.2.7.3 Microfluidic immunoassay

A microfluidic immunoassay is a combination of two techniques, microfluidics and immunoassays, and in recent years, is gaining an increasing interest from researchers in the clinical, pharmaceutical, and environmental sectors. Generally, microfluidic systems are known as a "micro-total-analysis-system," "biochips," or a "lab-on-a-chip" system. In this method, the miniaturized systems perform each step of the protocol. The system carries out sample pretreatment, sample transport, mixing, interaction, detection, and even product collection.[140] The microfluidic immunoassay (based on lateral flow) have been used for the detection of different types of microbial pathogens, including *L. monocytogenes* (pork samples),[141] *E. coli* O157:H7 (bread, milk, jelly),[142] and *Staphylococcal enterotoxins* (milk, apple juice, cheese, rice).[143] The microfluidic immunoassay has a number of advantages, like less sample consumption, reduced risk of contamination, high sensitivity, functionality, and reliability.[144] In spite of these advantages, there are also few limitations, like bubble formation and dead volume microdevices which can result in poor performance.

Few examples of microbial pathogens detection in food and water samples by using different immune-based assays are presented in Table 59.2.

59.2.3 Polymerase chain reaction–based methods

PCR is a technique commonly used in many fields of science, consisting of the synthesis of multiple copies of a template DNA, using a set of short single-stranded DNA sequences called primers, and a heat-stable DNA-polymerase enzyme, usually *Taq* polymerase. Since its discovery in 1985 by Kary Mullis, this technique was applied broadly, from the diagnosis of genetic diseases to the field of criminology. In pathogen detection, PCR revealed to be precise and effective, using as DNA template a very specific region of the microbial genome, often a virulence gene. In the last years, with the technical and scientific advances, new approaches have been developed, based on the PCR technique, that allowed an increase in sensitivity and, most important, in reaction time.

TABLE 59.2 Detection of microbial pathogens in food and water samples using different immune-based assays.

Name of immunoassay	Detected microbial pathogen	Analyzed samples	References
Chemiluminescence assay	*Escherichia coli* O157:H7	Spring water, apple juice, milk	Zhang et al.[145]
Immunochromatography assay	*Campylobacter jejuni*	Food, water	Xu et al.[146]
Immunoassay strip assay	Food allergen glycinin	Powdered milk	Wang et al.[147]
Enzyme-based colorimetric assay	*E. coli* O157:H7	Milk	Park et al.[148]
ELISA	*Salmonella typhimurium*	Low fat milk	Chattopadhyay et al.[92]
ELISA	*Listeria monocytogenes*	Meat	Shim et al.[96]
ELISA	*Escherichia coli* O157:H7	Complex material	Pappert et al.[95]
ELISA	*Alicyclobacillus* spp.	Apple juice	Wang et al.[97]
Fluorescence immunochromatographic assay	*L. monocytogenes*	Sausage, pork, milk	Li et al.[149]
Fluorescence immunoassay	*Escherichia coli* O157:H7	Water	Zhu et al.[150]
Immunochromatographic assay	*Escherichia coli* O157:H7	Beef, milk, water	Li et al.[127]
Immunoassay	*Aeromonas* spp.	Water, fish	Wang et al.[151]
ELISA	*Bacillus cereus*	Food	Zhu et al.[98]
ELISA	*Salmonella typhimurium*	Milk	Wang et al.[94]
ELISA	*Salmonella* spp.	Milk powder	Mansfield and Forsythe[93]
Lateral flow immunoassays	*E. coli* O157:H7	Water, milk, purple cabbage	Wang et al.[152]
Lateral flow immunoassays	*Cronobacter* spp.	Dairy products	Akineden et al.[153]
Lateral flow fluorescent immunoassay	*Salmonella* spp.	Meat	Zhuang et al.[154]
Latex agglutination assays	*E. coli*	Food	Medina et al.[114]
Latex agglutination assays	*Staphylococcus aureus*	Bovine raw milk	Mansour et al.[112]
Reverse passive latex agglutination	*Staphylococcal enterotoxins*	Dairy products	Rose et al.[115]
Reverse passive latex agglutination	*S. aureus*	Meat, dairy products	Mathenge et al.[113]
Time-resolved fluoro-immunoassay	*E. coli* O157:H7	Apple cider	Yu et al.[119]
Time-resolved fluoro-immunoassay	*Salmonella* spp.	Food material	Hagren et al.[120]
Chemiluminescent immunoassay	*E. coli, Salmonella typhimurium*	Food material	Magliulo et al.[125]
Capillary immunoassay	*Salmonella typhimurium*	Meat product	Kim et al.[155]
Electrochemical immunoassay	*Staphylococcal enterotoxin*	Food products	Tang et al.[156]
Electrochemical immunoassay	*Pseudomonas aeruginosa*	Water	Krithiga et al.[157]
Electrochemical immunoassay	*E. coli*	Dairy products	Zhang et al.[158]
Mass spectrometric immunoassay	*S. aureus*	Raw milk	Schlosser et al.[134]

59.2.3.1 Real-time polymerase chain reaction

Real-time PCR, also known as quantitative PCR (qPCR), is a sophisticated technique that allows real-time and continuous identification of amplified DNA fragments. This technique combines the amplification procedure of PCR, performed by automated temperature cycling, with product analysis, usually performed using double-stranded DNA-specific fluorescent dyes, which allows the continuous monitoring of fluorescence during amplification.[159] Several dyes are available nowadays, being the most common SYBR Green I,[160] and by associating its fluorescence to the reaction temperature, in each cycle one can determine the amount of DNA being amplified, increasing the fluorescence signal with the number of PCR molecules generated, in direct proportion. Real-time PCR softwares allow the plotting, in real time, of the fluorescence signal against the reaction cycle number, allowing the user to analyze the accumulation of product over the reaction time. The main advantages of this technique are its precision, allowing the measurement of the starting DNA material in a particular sample, and the capacity to monitor in real time the progress of the reaction.

Real-time PCR have been widely used lately in many areas of applied microbiology (reviewed in Filion M, 2012),[161] with great predominance in food safety, food spoilage, and in assessment of water quality, in which it is already routinely used in many laboratories to analyze pathogens. RT-PCR has been used with success to detect microbial contamination in several food products, especially the ones involving microbial fermentation. One example relates with dairy products, in which a rapid, precise, and simple technique is needed to detect a wide range of organisms that usually are responsible for spoilage of the product. Agrimonti et al.[162] reviewed the main applications of real-time PCR to analyze dairy products, compiling information from more than 50 food analyses, considering products varying from yogurt, milk, and cheese, to milk powder, infant formula, and ice-cream, in which this molecular technique allowed to detect several foodborne pathogens. Other food products have also been successfully tested using RT-PCR, sustaining its routine use: (1) detection of mayonnaise spoilage yeast *Pichia kudriavzevii*[163]; (2) detection of spoilage yeast *Brettanomyces bruxellensis* in wine[164–166]; (3) detection of *Vibrio* contamination in shellfish and in water[167]; (4) detection of lactic acid bacteria in sourdough[168]; (5) detection of *L. monocytogenes* in food[169,170]; (6) detection of human enteric viruses in food samples.[171]

59.2.3.2 Droplet digital PCR

Droplet digital PCR (ddPCR) is a third generation of PCR reactions. This technique aims at the exact quantification of a DNA or RNA amplicon within a sample, with higher accuracy and sensitivity than real-time PCR. This technique consists in the use of a water-oil emulsion droplet system that leads to the formation of particular droplets in which template DNA molecules will be partitioned. In brief, these droplets will mimic the division of the reaction in different wells, occurring in each one a miniaturized version of a reaction, repeated massively.[172] The main advantage of this technique is the measurement of thousands of independent amplifications in a single reaction.

ddPCR has been applied in the past with great success, although mainly in the clinical field, to detect pathogens of infectious diseases,[173] to monitor tumoral DNA,[174] in tuberculosis research[175] and in oncology.[176] However, great advances have been achieved by the use of this methodology to detect microbial contamination of food and water. This fact is mainly due to the advantages that highlight this method as an alternative to real-time PCR: (1) it is not so sensitive to PCR inhibitors; (2) allows absolute quantification of DNA or RNA, without the need of standard curves; (3) shows higher sensitivity allowing detection of targets present in low copy numbers.[172,177,178] Several examples allow to sustain the successful use of this technique to detect mainly food adulteration and feed contamination. Already in 2013, Morisset et al.[179] applied ddPCR for routine analysis of food and feed samples, detecting the presence of genetically modified organisms. Ren et al.[180] used ddPCR to quantify the presence of chicken in sheep and goat meat products, confirming the potential of the method to accurately confirm the presence or absence of adulterants in meat. Many other examples are available considering application of ddPCR in food genomics, detecting contamination or adulteration of food products, mainly applied to meat[181,182] or to the detection of genetically modified organisms.[178] However, this technique was also already applied to water quality assessment, in particular, ddPCR was revealed as a successful technique to quantify general and human-associated fecal indicators in water.[183] In this work, *Enterococcus* spp. and the human fecal-associated HF183 marker were quantified in 131 fecal and water samples with higher precision and reproducibility. This high-precision molecular procedure allowed also to quantify human adenovirus and norovirus in river waters,[184,185] enteric pathogens in surface water samples in California,[186] and even zoonotic bacterial pathogens in poultry processing water samples.[187]

59.2.3.3 Heat pulse extension-polymerase chain reaction

In certain scenarios, conventional PCR protocols cannot be used to amplify certain DNA templates, especially considering extremely GC-rich and/or long sequences. Several optimizations have been attempted in order to modify PCR procedure and reagents to be able to address these kinds of DNA templates (reviewed in Orpana et al.[188]). However, this type of sequences was still a challenge until the development of the technique of heat pulse extension-PCR. With this method, the extension step of the PCR is altered to improve amplification efficiency over difficult target sequences with higher GC-content.[188] With the help of heat pulses, secondary structures that require usually high melting temperatures, and that are considered as the main obstacle to primers annealing, will temporarily be weakened, improving extension step and, consequently, increasing efficiency and specificity of the reaction. This technique is still new and less explored until now, and no report of its use in food or water pathogens detection was found. However, due to its particularities, we consider it to have a good potential to be explored, serving as alternative to detect pathogens with long DNA chains, large CTG base repeats and/or a high content of GC.

59.2.4 Aptamers

The use of aptamers constitutes an alternative method used nowadays in different scientific fields, mainly for the detection of microorganisms. This method consists in the use of oligonucleotides or peptide molecules—aptamers—that bind to specific target molecules, such as proteins, peptides, or carbohydrates. Aptamers can assume a wide range of shapes due to their tendency to form helices and single-stranded loops, binding to targets with high specificity and selectivity. The selection of a certain aptamer to have affinity with a particular target is done using a large oligonucleotide library through a process called systematic evolution of ligands by exponential enrichment (SELEX). As reviewed by Schmitz et al.[189], this process involves an incubation of oligonucleotides library, the separation, the amplification by PCR, and finally the purification of the products.

Despite its wide use in medicine, aptamer-based nanostructures have been used also in the last decade to detect food contamination and ensure food safety, mainly screening samples for the presence of *Salmonella* spp. in pasteurized milk, shrimp, and chicken breasts,[190,191] and in pork.[192] This method was also recently able to detect, as target, the presence of *Streptococcus pyogenes* in cooked chicken,[193] and several species of *Staphylococcus aureus* in milk, fresh fish, and pork meat.[194–196] Some adaptations were also performed using aptamers, as for example the use of gold nanoparticles to be conjugated with aptamers and with a colorimetric detection method, which already allowed the high sensible detection of *S. enterica* and other microbial pathogens.[197] Also, in terms of environment monitoring, aptamers have been extensively used to minimize environmental pollutants and their effects, in particular to detect antibiotics used in farm animals such as chloramphenicol[198] and tetracycline.[199] In water samples, especially unclean ones, *S. aureus* was also detected using aptamers approaches.[200]

59.2.5 Whole genome sequencing

The decrease in costs and the increase of accessibility of next-generation sequencing technologies have revolutionize the field of genomics applied to almost all fields of life sciences. Especially in microbiology, an exponential increase occurred in the last decade allowing fast and simple whole genome sequencing (WGS) of several organisms, becoming already a routine procedure in many laboratories. In comparison with other methods, WGS allows an unparallel analysis of the entire genome of a particular organism, dissecting base-by-base comparisons and allowing to understand secondary parameters such as virulence, resistance, and evolutive marks. Foodborne pathogens of genera *Salmonella*, *Listeria*, *Campylobacter*, *Escherichia*, and *Vibrio* was already sequenced in many works using WGS (reviewed by Brown et al.[201]), and in association with the field of phylogenetics, it was possible to provide useful insights into past foodborne outbreak investigations.[202–211]

59.2.6 Fluorescence in situ hybridization

FISH technique was described in 1980[212] for the detection of specific DNA sequences in animal cells, using a single fluorescent probe. This technique involves the use of phylogenetic dyes (15–25 base pairs) which are fluorescent oligonucleotides, whose base sequences are complementary to the ribosomal RNA sequences, and that will penetrate into the cell. The great advantage of this technique is the use of specific dyes, that react with only one species or, in some cases, with species of a particular phylogenetic group.

For microbial detection, FISH has been described as being advantageous especially in terms of time-saving. This technique promotes a short time-to-result (full procedure usually takes between 60 and 100 min), saving also the time for microbial culturing, which allows a great spectrum of applications for the detection of pathogenic microorganisms.[213] However, and when comparing with other techniques such as real-time PCR, the sensitivity of FISH has been revealed as being smaller.

Although not yet used routinely, FISH showed already promising results in food and water microbial analysis. In 2003, Fang et al.[214] used a FISH approach for the detection and identification of *Salmonella* species in food, using two species-specific 23S rRNA-targeted oligonucleotide probes. Results showed a positive result for the 51 tested *Salmonella* strains, obtaining no cross-reactions with other strains of the family Enterobacteriaceae. Even though the majority of FISH studies sleuthing foodborne pathogens have focused in the detection of the bacteria *Salmonella*, identification of the other genera showed already promising results, especially considering

Campylobacter and *Listeria*.[215–223] Bisha and Brehm-Stecher[216,217] applied also FISH to the detection of *E. coli* in food products, in particular in beef, milk, and vegetables, but also in beverages (juice, beer, wine, tea). One last example of success is the works of Moreno et al.[224] and Schmid et al.[221] which detected the presence of *Campylobacter* spp. in chicken products using FISH, and 16S and DNA probes.

59.2.7 Loop-mediated isothermal amplification

In order to surpass many disadvantages of other molecular techniques used routinely (such as the need for trained personnel, expensive equipment, and fancy reagents), in 2000, a new isothermal nucleic acid amplification method was developed[225]—loop-mediated isothermal amplification (LAMP). Since its first publication, LAMP has been widely used for microbial identification, mainly due to its high specificity, efficiency, and easiness of operation.

The principle of the technique is based in the use of a set of four to six primers that bind to 6–8 regions on the target gene, which makes the process highly specific.[226] The main particularity of the technique is the use of outer and inner primers, and also loop primers, both forward and backward (reviewed in Wong et al.[227]). Several microbial pathogens have been identified successfully using LAMP in food products and wastewaters, as for example the following genera: *Campylobacter*,[228–230] *Listeria*,[231–238] *Entamoeba*,[239–243] *Helicobacter*,[244,245] *Pseudomonas* and *Actinetobacter*,[246] *Toxolasma*,[239] *Vibrio*,[247–249] *Escherichia*,[250–253] and *Staphylococcus*.[254–257]

59.2.8 Matrix-assisted laser desorption/ ionization time-of-flight mass spectrometry

The necessity to identify rapidly, accurately, and in a cost-efficient way microbials associated with food spoilage and contamination, demanded the appearance of new methods, especially the ones with high sensibility. MALDI-TOF method was developed to go in line with these requirements, to detect nucleic acids, peptides, proteins, sugars and small molecules, generating fingerprints and correlating results with spectra available in databases. The principle of the technique is based on the ionization of a neutral molecule and then in the determination of the resulting primary ions and their decay products in high vacuum.[258]

MALDI-TOF has been routinely used in laboratories performing microbial identifications, but the major spectra of applicability relate with their use to identify yeasts, bacteria, and filamentous fungi in clinical samples.[259] In food microbiology, MALDI-TOF showed good results analyzing meat,[260,261] kimchi,[262] poultry carcasses,[263] yoghurt,[264] and cheese.[265–267] In particular for filamentous fungi, one of the groups of organisms mainly responsible for food spoilage and contamination, MALDI-TOF showed 90% of accurate identification in experiments testing 619 strains of fungi belonging to 136 species.[268] The comprehensive database resulting from this work will allow the correct identification of a wide array of food spoilage fungi in the future. One additional advantage of MALDI-TOF is the potential ability to differentiate between different strains, already assessed with success for some species of yeasts and bacteria.[269,270]

59.3 Future remarks

Food and water safety and quality are critical factors for prevention of food/water-related illnesses, and a frequent microbiological food/water examination along the production process, is crucial to reduce the risk of poisoning outbreaks.

Advances in manufacturing combined with greater understanding of the complexity of food/waterborne diseases, as well as the remarkable availability of increasingly powerful computing technologies, have made it possible to decrease food and water contaminations, and to rapidly treat patients with intoxications/infections. To minimize the loss of production and occurrence of food and waterborne outbreaks, the classical culture techniques are still widely used for microbial identification, but these procedures take too long to provide a conclusive result. However, culture techniques are being replaced by other faster and very sensible methods that can be easily integrated into food and water processing, such as MALDI-TOF, PCR, the use of biosensors, or immunoassays.

Acknowledgments

R.F.-D. acknowledges the strategic programs UID/BIA/04050/2013 (PO-CI-01-0145-FEDER-007569) and UID/BIA/04050/2019 funded by national funds through the FCT, I.P., and by the ERDF through the COMPETE2020—Programa Operacional Competitividade e Internacionalização (POCI) and Sistema de Apoio à Investigação Científica e Tecnológica (SAICT). The academic appointments of KSK and SK are funded by the Ramalingaswami Re-entry Fellowship, Department of Biotechnology, Government of India (BT/HRD/35/02/2006).

Contributions

KSK and SK contributed to the section on culture-based rapid approaches, and in nonculture-based rapid approaches to the sections on DEFT, biosensors, FT-IT, SPC, and ATP-bioluminescent detection. RFD contributed to the conceptualization of the chapter and the section on PCR-based methods. SP, PS, and NC-M prepared the immunoassays section. CFR contributed with chapter conceptualization, abstract, introduction, future remarks, reviewed and analyzed the data.

Conflicts of interest

The authors declare no conflicts of interest.

References

1. WHO. Ten threats to global health in 2019. <https://www.who.int/news-room/feature-stories/ten-threats-to-global-health-in-2019>. Accessed 02.03.20.
2. Boelaert F, Van der Stede Y, Stoicescu A, et al. The European Union summary report on trends and sources of zoonoses, zoonotic agents and food-borne outbreaks in 2017. 2018.
3. Wang H, Naghavi M, Allen C, et al. Global, regional, and national life expectancy, all-cause mortality, and cause-specific mortality for 249 causes of death, 1980–2015: a systematic analysis for the Global Burden of Disease Study 2015. *Lancet*. 2016;388:1459–1544. Available from: https://doi.org/10.1016/S0140-6736(16)31012-1.
4. El Bcheraoui C, Mokdad AH, Dwyer-Lindgren L, et al. Trends and patterns of differences in infectious disease mortality among US counties, 1980–2014. *JAMA*. 2018;319:1248–1260. Available from: https://doi.org/10.1001/jama.2018.2089.
5. Liu Y, Cao Y, Wang T, et al. Detection of 12 common food-borne bacterial pathogens by TaqMan real-time PCR using a single set of reaction conditions. *Front Microbiol*. 2019;10:222. Available from: https://doi.org/10.3389/fmicb.2019.00222.
6. WHO. WHO estimates of the global burden of foodborne diseases. <https://www.who.int/foodsafety/publications/foodborne_disease/fergreport/en/3M Petrifilm e 3MTM PetrifilmTM Rapid Coliform Count Plate Interpretation Guide 3M Petrifilm Rapid Aerobic Count Plates | 3M Food Safety | 3M United States>; 2015.
7. FDA. Foodborne pathogens. <https://www.fda.gov/food/outbreaks-foodborne-illness/foodborne-pathogens>; 2019. Accessed 05.01.21.
8. MarketsandMarkets. Global food safety testing market anticipated growing at a 7.7% CAGR. <https://www.globenewswire.com/news-release/2019/11/04/1940425/0/en/Global-Food-Safety-Testing-Market-Anticipated-Growing-at-a-7-7-CAGR.html>; Accessed 05.01.21.
9. Horn B, Hewitt J, Withers H, et al. Review of microbial pathogen inactivation relevant to Sous Vide cooking at temperatures below 55°C prepared for MPI. 2016.
10. Wadhams EHC. Hygiene in abattoirs and meat processing plants. *R Soc Health J*. 1961;81:268–276. Available from: https://doi.org/10.1177/146642406108100553.
11. Machado Nardi VA, Auler DP, Teixeira R. Food safety in global supply chains: a literature review. *J Food Sci*. 2020;85:883–891. Available from: https://doi.org/10.1111/1750-3841.14999.
12. Law JWF, Mutalib NSA, Chan KG, Lee LH. Rapid methods for the detection of foodborne bacterial pathogens: principles, applications, advantages and limitations. *Front Microbiol*. 2014;5:770. Available from: https://doi.org/10.3389/fmicb.2014.00770.
13. Velusamy V, Arshak K, Korostynska O, et al. An overview of foodborne pathogen detection: in the perspective of biosensors. *Biotechnol Adv*. 2010;28:232–254. Available from: https://doi.org/10.1016/j.biotechadv.2009.12.004.
14. Brackett RE. *Microbial quality. Postharvest Handling*. Elsevier; 1993:125–148.
15. Gilchrist JE, Campbell JE, Donnelly CB, et al. Spiral plate method for bacterial determination. *Appl Microbiol*. 1973;25:244–252. Available from: https://doi.org/10.1128/aem.25.2.244-252.1973.
16. Jarvis B, Lach VH, Wood JM. Evaluation of the spiral plate maker for the enumeration of micro-organisms in foods. *J Appl Bacteriol*. 1977;43:149–157. Available from: https://doi.org/10.1111/j.1365-2672.1977.tb00734.x.
17. Mizuochi S, Kodaka H. Evaluation of dry sheet medium culture plate (Compactdry TC) method for determining numbers of bacteria in food-samples. *J Food Prot*. 2000;63:665–667. Available from: https://doi.org/10.4315/0362-028X-63.5.665.
18. Perry JD. A decade of development of chromogenic culture media for clinical microbiology in an era of molecular diagnostics. *Clin Microbiol Rev*. 2017. Available from: https://doi.org/10.1128/CMR.00097-16.
19. Fallon D, Ackland G, Andrews N, et al. A comparison of the performance of commercially available chromogenic agars for the isolation and presumptive identification of organisms from urine. *J Clin Pathol*. 2003;56:608–612. Available from: https://doi.org/10.1136/jcp.56.8.608.
20. R-Biopharm. Microbiology: detection of microbiological contamination.
21. de Man JC. The probability of most probable numbers. *Eur J Appl Microbiol*. 1975;1:67–78. Available from: https://doi.org/10.1007/BF01880621.
22. Colla FL, Mion L, Parizotto L, et al. Miniaturized most probable number for the enumeration of *Salmonella* sp in artificially contaminated chicken meat. *Rev Bras Cienc Avic*. 2014;16:45–48. Available from: https://doi.org/10.1590/S1516-635X2014000100006.
23. Kuai L, Nair AA, Polz MF. Rapid and simple method for the most-probable-number estimation of arsenic-reducing bacteria. *Appl Environ Microbiol*. 2001;67:3168–3173. Available from: https://doi.org/10.1128/AEM.67.7.3168-3173.2001.
24. Munoz EF, Silverman MP. Rapid, single-step most-probable-number method for enumerating fecal coliforms in effluents from sewage treatment plants. 1979.
25. O'Connor F. Rapid methods for estimating microbial quality of foods. *Irish J Food Sci Technol*. 1983;7:61–67.
26. Pettipher GL. *Status and future of the direct epifluorescent filter technique. Rapid Methods and Automation in Microbiology and Immunology*. Berlin, Heidelberg: Springer; 1985:629–637.
27. Qvist SH, Jakobsen M. Application of the direct epifluorescent filter technique as a rapid method in microbiological quality assurance in the meat industry. *Int J Food Microbiol*. 1985;2:139–144. Available from: https://doi.org/10.1016/0168-1605(85)90032-7.
28. Pettipher GL. Review: the direct epifluorescent filter technique. *Int J Food Sci Technol*. 1986;21:535–546. Available from: https://doi.org/10.1111/j.1365-2621.1986.tb00392.x.
29. Mesa MM, Macías M, Cantero D, Barja F. Use of the direct epifluorescent filter technique for the enumeration of viable and total acetic acid bacteria from vinegar fermentation. *J Fluoresc*. 2003;13:261–265. Available from: https://doi.org/10.1023/A:1025094017265.

30. Pettipher GL, Rodrigues UM. Rapid enumeration of microorganisms in foods by the direct epifluorescent filter technique. 1982.
31. Rodrigues UM, Kroll RG. The direct epifluorescent filter technique (DEFT): increased selectivity, sensitivity and rapidity. *J Appl Bacteriol.* 1985;59:493–499. Available from: https://doi.org/10.1111/j.1365-2672.1985.tb03351.x.
32. Rowe MT, McCann GJ. A modified direct epifluorescent filter technique for the detection and enumeration of yeast in yoghurt. *Lett Appl Microbiol.* 1990;11:282–285. Available from: https://doi.org/10.1111/j.1472-765X.1990.tb00182.x.
33. Rodrigues UM, Kroll RG. Use of the direct epifluorescent filter technique for the enumeration of yeasts. *J Appl Bacteriol.* 1986;61:139–144. Available from: https://doi.org/10.1111/j.1365-2672.1986.tb04267.x.
34. Boulos L, Prévost M, Barbeau B, et al. LIVE/DEAD(®) BacLight (TM): application of a new rapid staining method for direct enumeration of viable and total bacteria in drinking water. *J Microbiol Methods.* 1999;37:77–86. Available from: https://doi.org/10.1016/S0167-7012(99)00048-2.
35. Oluwaseun AC, Phazang P, Sarin NB. *Biosensors: a fast-growing technology for pathogen detection in agriculture and food sector. Biosensing Technologies for the Detection of Pathogens – A Prospective Way for Rapid Analysis.* IntechOpen; 2018.
36. Poltronieri P, Mezzolla V, Primiceri E, Maruccio G. Biosensors for the detection of food pathogens. *Foods.* 2014;3:511–526. Available from: https://doi.org/10.3390/foods3030511.
37. Rainbow J, Sedlackova E, Jiang S, et al. Integrated electrochemical biosensors for detection of waterborne pathogens in low-resource settings. *Biosensors.* 2020;10:36.
38. Choudhary U. Biosensors for detection of foodborne pathogens. *Pharma Innov J.* 2019;8:386–396.
39. Esfandiari L, Wang S, Wang S, et al. PCR-independent detection of bacterial species-specific 16S rRNA at 10 fM by a pore-blockage sensor. *Biosensors.* 2016;6. Available from: https://doi.org/10.3390/bios6030037.
40. Ali AA, Altemimi AB, Alhelfi N, Ibrahim SA. Application of biosensors for detection of pathogenic food bacteria: a review. *Biosensors.* 2020;10:58.
41. Kumar H, Bhardwaj K, Kaur T, et al. Detection of bacterial pathogens and antibiotic residues in chicken meat: a review. *Foods.* 2020;9. Available from: https://doi.org/10.3390/foods9101504.
42. Sentürk E, Aktop S, Sanlibaba P, Tezel BU. Biosensors: a novel approach to detect food-borne pathogens. 2018. Available from: https://doi.org/10.4172/2471-9315.1000151.
43. Mungroo NA, Neethirajan S. *Optical biosensors for the detection of food borne pathogens. Nanobiosensors for Personalized and Onsite Biomedical Diagnosis.* Institution of Engineering and Technology; 2016:181–208.
44. Riu J, Giussani B. Electrochemical biosensors for the detection of pathogenic bacteria in food. *TrAC Trends Anal Chem.* 2020;126:115863.
45. Alhogail S, Suaifan GARY, Zourob M. Rapid colorimetric sensing platform for the detection of *Listeria monocytogenes* foodborne pathogen. *Biosens Bioelectron.* 2016;86:1061–1066. Available from: https://doi.org/10.1016/j.bios.2016.07.043.
46. Leonard P, Hearty S, Brennan J, et al. Advances in biosensors for detection of pathogens in food and water. *Enzyme Microb Technol.* 2003;32:3–13.
47. Pathania P, Sharma A, Kumar B, et al. Selective identification of specific aptamers for the detection of non-typhoidal salmonellosis in an apta-impedimetric sensing format. *Microchim Acta.* 2017;184:1499–1508. Available from: https://doi.org/10.1007/s00604-017-2098-2.
48. Mutreja R, Jariyal M, Pathania P, et al. Novel surface antigen based impedimetric immunosensor for detection of *Salmonella typhimurium* in water and juice samples. *Biosens Bioelectron.* 2016;85:707–713. Available from: https://doi.org/10.1016/j.bios.2016.05.079.
49. Vizzini P, Braidot M, Vidic J, Manzano M. Electrochemical and optical biosensors for the detection of *Campylobacter* and *Listeria*: an update look. *Micromachines.* 2019;10:500.
50. Sobhan A, Lee J, Park MK, Oh JH. Rapid detection of *Yersinia enterocolitica* using a single-walled carbon nanotube-based biosensor for Kimchi product. *LWT Food Sci Technol.* 2019;108:48–54. Available from: https://doi.org/10.1016/j.lwt.2019.03.037.
51. Li S, Li Y, Chen H, et al. Direct detection of *Salmonella typhimurium* on fresh produce using phage-based magnetoelastic biosensors. *Biosens Bioelectron.* 2010;26:1313–1319. Available from: https://doi.org/10.1016/j.bios.2010.07.029.
52. Waswa J, Irudayaraj J, DebRoy C. Direct detection of *E. coli* O157:H7 in selected food systems by a surface plasmon resonance biosensor. *LWT Food Sci Technol.* 2007;40:187–192.
53. Mehrotra P. Biosensors and their applications – a review. *J Oral Biol Craniofacial Res.* 2016;6:153–159.
54. Bunney J, Williamson S, Atkin D, et al. The use of electrochemical biosensors in food analysis. *Curr Res Nutr Food Sci.* 2017;5:183–195. Available from: https://doi.org/10.12944/CRNFSJ.5.3.02.
55. SBT. Bactobox®.
56. Alvarez-Ordóñez A, Prieto M. *Technical and Methodological Aspects of Fourier Transform Infrared Spectroscopy in Food Microbiology Research.* Springer; 2012: 1–18.
57. Rodriguez-Saona LE, Khambaty FM, Fry FS, Calvey EM. Rapid detection and identification of bacterial strains by Fourier transform near-infrared spectroscopy. *J Agric Food Chem.* 2001;49:574–579. Available from: https://doi.org/10.1021/jf000776j.
58. Davis R, Davis R, Mauer LJ. Fourier transform infrared (FT-IR) spectroscopy: a rapid tool for detection and analysis of foodborne pathogenic bacteria.
59. Al-Masoud N, Muhamadali H, Chisanga M, et al. Discrimination of bacteria using whole organism fingerprinting: the utility of modern physicochemical techniques for bacterial typing. *Analyst.* 2021;. Available from: https://doi.org/10.1039/d0an01482f.
60. Quintelas C, Ferreira EC, Lopes JA, Sousa C. An overview of the evolution of infrared spectroscopy applied to bacterial typing. *Biotechnol J.* 2018;13:1700449. Available from: https://doi.org/10.1002/biot.201700449.
61. Wenning M, Scherer S. Identification of microorganisms by FTIR spectroscopy: perspectives and limitations of the method. *Appl Microbiol Biotechnol.* 2013;97:7111–7120. Available from: https://doi.org/10.1007/s00253-013-5087-3.
62. Davis R, Irudayaraj J, Reuhs BL, Mauer LJ. Detection of *E. coli* O157:H7 from ground beef using Fourier transform infrared (FT-IR) spectroscopy and chemometrics. *J Food Sci.* 2010;75. Available from: https://doi.org/10.1111/j.1750-3841.2010.01686.x.

63. Ellis DI, Broadhurst D, Kell DB, et al. Rapid and quantitative detection of the microbial spoilage of meat by Fourier transform infrared spectroscopy and machine learning. *Appl Environ Microbiol.* 2002;68:2822–2828. Available from: https://doi.org/10.1128/AEM.68.6.2822-2828.2002.
64. Al-Qadiri HM, Al-Holy MA, Lin M, et al. Rapid detection and identification of *Pseudomonas aeruginosa* and *Escherichia coli* as pure and mixed cultures in bottled drinking water using Fourier transform infrared spectroscopy and multivariate analysis. *J Agric Food Chem.* 2006;54:5749–5754. Available from: https://doi.org/10.1021/jf0609734.
65. Yu C, Irudayaraj J, Debroy C, et al. Spectroscopic differentiation and quantification of microorganisms in apple juice. *J Food Sci.* 2006;69:268–272. Available from: https://doi.org/10.1111/j.1365-2621.2004.tb13627.x.
66. Rodriguez-Saona LE, Allendorf ME. Use of FTIR for rapid authentication and detection of adulteration of food. *Annu Rev Food Sci Technol.* 2011;2:467–483.
67. Franca AS, Oliveira LS. Potential uses of Fourier transform infrared spectroscopy (FTIR) in food processing and engineering. *Food Eng.* 2011;.
68. Cools I, D'Haese E, Uyttendaele M, et al. Solid phase cytometry as a tool to detect viable but non-culturable cells of *Campylobacter jejuni. J Microbiol Methods.* 2005;63:107–114. Available from: https://doi.org/10.1016/j.mimet.2005.02.023.
69. Lisle JT, Hamilton MA, Willse AR, McFeters GA. Comparison of fluorescence microscopy and solid-phase cytometry methods for counting bacteria in water. *Appl Environ Microbiol.* 2004;70:5343–5348. Available from: https://doi.org/10.1128/AEM.70.9.5343-5348.2004.
70. Vanhee LM, D'Haese E, Cools I, et al. Detection and quantification of bacteria and fungi using solid-phase cytometry. 2010: 25–41.
71. Clark SA, Thompson KC, Keevil CW, Smith MS, eds. *Rapid Detection Assays for Food and Water.* Cambridge: Royal Society of Chemistry; 2001.
72. Rompré A, Servais P, Baudart J, et al. Detection and enumeration of coliforms in drinking water: current methods and emerging approaches.
73. Van Poucke SO, Nelis HJ. A 210-min solid phase cytometry test for the enumeration of Escherichia coli in drinking water. *J Appl Microbiol.* 2000;89:390–396. Available from: https://doi.org/10.1046/j.1365-2672.2000.01125.x.
74. SCANRDI® rapid and sensitive detection. bioMérieux Industrial Microbiology.
75. Shintani H. Validation study of rapid assays of bioburden, endotoxins and other contamination. 2016.
76. Dostálek P, Brányik T. Prospects for rapid bioluminescent detection methods in the food industry – a review. *Czech J Food Sci.* 2005.
77. Milliflex® rapid microbiology detection and enumeration system. Milliflex Rapid Testing.
78. Picó Y. *Food Toxicants Analysis: Techniques, Strategies and Developments.* Elsevier B.V.; 2007.
79. Vashist SK, Luong JHT. Chapter 1 – Immunoassays: an overview. In: Vashist SK, Luong JH, eds. *Handbook of Immunoassay Technologies: Approaches, Performances, and Applications.* Academic Press; 2018:1–18.
80. Notermans S, Wernars K. Immunological methods for detection of foodborne pathogens and their toxins. *Int J Food Microbiol.* 1991;12:91–102. Available from: https://doi.org/10.1016/0168-1605(91)90050-Y.
81. Goldsmith SJ. Radioimmunoassay: review of basic principles. *Semin Nucl Med.* 1975;5:125–152. Available from: https://doi.org/10.1016/S0001-2998(75)80028-6.
82. Collins WS, Johnson AD, Metzger JF, Bennett RW. Rapid solid-phase radioimmunoassay for Staphylococcal enterotoxin A. *Appl Microbiol.* 1973;25:774–777.
83. Johnson HM, Bukovic JA, Kauffman PE, Peeler JT. Staphylococcal enterotoxin B: solid-phase radioimmunoassay. *Appl Microbiol.* 1971;22:837–841.
84. Nedelkov D, Nelson RW. Detection of *Staphylococcal enterotoxin* B via biomolecular interaction analysis mass spectrometry. *Appl Environ Microbiol.* 2003;69:5212–5215. Available from: https://doi.org/10.1128/aem.69.9.5212-5215.2003.
85. Niyomvit N, Stevenson K, McFeeters R. Detection of *Staphylococcal enterotoxin* B by affinity radioimmunoassay. *J Food Sci.* 1978;43:735–739. Available from: https://doi.org/10.1111/j.1365-2621.1978.tb02405.x.
86. Su Y-C, Wong ACL. Current perspectives on detection of *Staphylococcal enterotoxins. J Food Prot.* 1997;60:195–202. Available from: https://doi.org/10.4315/0362-028X-60.2.195.
87. Candlish AAG. Immunological methods in food microbiology. *Food Microbiol.* 1991;8:1–14. Available from: https://doi.org/10.1016/0740-0020(91)90012-Q.
88. Stelma GN, Crawford RG, Spaulding PL, Twedt RM. Evidence that *Clostridium perfringens* produces only one enterotoxin. *J Food Prot.* 1985;48:232–233. Available from: https://doi.org/10.4315/0362-028X-48.3.232.
89. Madigan MT, Bender KS, Buckley DH, et al. 15th ed. *Brock Biology of Microorganisms.* vol. 15. Pearson; 2018.
90. Engvall E, Perlmann P. Enzyme-linked immunosorbent assay (ELISA) quantitative assay of immunoglobulin G. *Immunochemistry.* 1971;8:871–874. Available from: https://doi.org/10.1016/0019-2791(71)90454-X.
91. Van Weemen BK, Schuurs AHWM. Immunoassay using antigen–enzyme conjugates. *FEBS Lett.* 1971;15:232–236. Available from: https://doi.org/10.1016/0014-5793(71)80319-8.
92. Chattopadhyay S, Kaur A, Jain S, et al. Functionalized polymeric magnetic nanoconstructs for selective capturing and sensitive detection of *Salmonella typhimurium. Anal Chim Acta.* 2016;937:127–135. Available from: https://doi.org/10.1016/j.aca.2016.07.014.
93. Mansfield LP, Forsythe SJ. The detection of *Salmonella* using a combined immunomagnetic separation and ELISA end-detection procedure. *Lett Appl Microbiol.* 2000;31:279–283. Available from: https://doi.org/10.1046/j.1472-765x.2000.00811.x.
94. Wang W, Liu L, Song S, et al. A highly sensitive ELISA and immunochromatographic strip for the detection of *Salmonella typhimurium* in milk samples. *Sensors (Basel).* 2015;15:5281–5292. Available from: https://doi.org/10.3390/s150305281.
95. Pappert G, Rieger M, Niessner R, Seidel M. Immunomagnetic nanoparticle-based sandwich chemiluminescence-ELISA for the enrichment and quantification of *E. coli. Microchim Acta.* 2010;168:1–8.

96. Shim W-B, Choi J-G, Kim J-Y, et al. Enhanced rapidity for qualitative detection of *Listeria monocytogenes* using an enzyme-linked immunosorbent assay and immunochromatography strip test combined with immunomagnetic bead separation. *J Food Prot*. 2008;71:781–789. Available from: https://doi.org/10.4315/0362-028x-71.4.781.
97. Wang Z, Yue T, Yuan Y, et al. Development and evaluation of an immunomagnetic separation–ELISA for the detection of *Alicyclobacillus* spp. in apple juice. *Int J Food Microbiol*. 2013;166:28–33. Available from: https://doi.org/10.1016/j.ijfoodmicro.2013.06.015.
98. Zhu L, He J, Cao X, et al. Development of a double-antibody sandwich ELISA for rapid detection of *Bacillus cereus* in food. *Sci Rep*. 2016;6:16092. Available from: https://doi.org/10.1038/srep16092.
99. Mccarthy J, Colworth U. *Immunological Techniques: ELISA*. Elsevier Science; 2003.
100. Zhao X, Lin C-W, Wang J. Advances in rapid detection methods for foodborne pathogens. *J Microbiol Biotechnol*. 2014;24:297–312. Available from: https://doi.org/10.4014/jmb.1310.10013.
101. Delmulle BS, De Saeger SMDG, Sibanda L, et al. Development of an immunoassay-based lateral flow dipstick for the rapid detection of aflatoxin B1 in pig feed. *J Agric Food Chem*. 2005;53:3364–3368. Available from: https://doi.org/10.1021/jf0404804.
102. Tang D, Sauceda JC, Lin Z, et al. Magnetic nanogold microspheres-based lateral-flow immunodipstick for rapid detection of aflatoxin B2 in food. *Biosens Bioelectron*. 2009;25:514–518.
103. Luo K, Kim H-Y, Oh M-H, Kim Y-R. Paper-based lateral flow strip assay for the detection of foodborne pathogens: principles, applications, technological challenges and opportunities. *Crit Rev Food Sci Nutr*. 2020;60:157–170. Available from: https://doi.org/10.1080/10408398.2018.1516623.
104. Sajid M, Kawde A-N, Daud M. Designs, formats and applications of lateral flow assay: a literature review. *J Saudi Chem Soc*. 2015;19:689–705.
105. Koczula KM, Gallotta A. Lateral flow assays. *Essays Biochem*. 2016;60:111–120. Available from: https://doi.org/10.1042/EBC20150012.
106. Pawliszyn J. *Sampling theory and methodology. Comprehensive Sampling and Sample Preparation: Analytical Techniques for Scientists*. Academic Press; 2012. 3200 p.
107. Chatrathi MP, Wang J, Collins GE. Sandwich electrochemical immunoassay for the detection of Staphylococcal enterotoxin B based on immobilized thiolated antibodies. *Biosens Bioelectron*. 2007;22:2932–2938. Available from: https://doi.org/10.1016/j.bios.2006.12.013.
108. Kozitsina A, Svalova T, Malysheva N, et al. A new enzyme-free electrochemical immunoassay for *Escherichia coli* detection using magnetic nanoparticles. *Anal Lett*. 2016;49:245–257. Available from: https://doi.org/10.1080/00032719.2015.1072824.
109. Zhu F, Zhao G, Dou W. A non-enzymatic electrochemical immunoassay for quantitative detection of *Escherichia coli* O157:H7 using Au@Pt and graphene. *Anal Biochem*. 2018;559:34–43. Available from: https://doi.org/10.1016/j.ab.2018.08.016.
110. Bennett JE, Dolin R, Blaser MJ. *Mandell, Douglas, and Bennett's Principles and Practice of Infectious Diseases*. vol. 2. Elsevier B. V.; 2014.
111. Trovero AC, Mazza M, Rogé A, et al. Production of a latex agglutination reagent for the rapid diagnosis of cryptococcal meningitis. *Rev Argent Microbiol*. 2020;52:169–175. Available from: https://doi.org/10.1016/j.ram.2019.06.002.
112. Mansour AS, Wagih GE-S, Morgan SD, et al. Detection of *Staphylococcus aureus* enterotoxigenic strains in bovine raw milk by reversed passive latex agglutination and multiplex polymerase chain reaction. *Vet World*. 2017;10:843–847. Available from: https://doi.org/10.14202/vetworld.2017.843-847.
113. Mathenge JM, Okemo P, Ng'ang'a P, et al. Identification of enterotoxigenic *Staphylococcus aureus* strains from meat and dairy products by multiplex PCR and reverse passive latex agglutination test in Nairobi, Kenya. 2015.
114. Medina MB, Shelver WL, Fratamico PM, et al. Latex agglutination assays for detection of non-O157 Shiga toxin–producing *Escherichia coli* serogroups O26, O45, O103, O111, O121, and O145. *J Food Prot*. 2012;75:819–826. Available from: https://doi.org/10.4315/0362-028X.JFP-11-430.
115. Rose SA, Bankes P, Stringer MF. Detection of staphylococcal enterotoxins in dairy products by the reversed passive latex agglutination (SET-RPLA) kit. *Int J Food Microbiol*. 1989;8:65–72. Available from: https://doi.org/10.1016/0168-1605(89)90081-0.
116. Favier GI, Lucero Estrada C, Cortiñas TI, Escudero ME. Detection and characterization of Shiga toxin producing *Escherichia coli*, *Salmonella* spp., and *Yersinia* strains from human, animal, and food samples in San Luis, Argentina. *Int J Microbiol*. 2014;2014:284649. Available from: https://doi.org/10.1155/2014/284649.
117. Papanastasiou-Diamandis A, Bhayana V, Diamandis EP. A simple time-resolved fluoroimmunoassay of total thyroxine in serum. *Ann Clin Biochem*. 1989;26:238–243. Available from: https://doi.org/10.1177/000456328902600305.
118. Boreham A, Brodwolf R, Walker K, et al. Time-resolved fluorescence spectroscopy and fluorescence lifetime imaging microscopy for characterization of dendritic polymer nanoparticles and applications in nanomedicine. *Molecules*. 2016;22:17. Available from: https://doi.org/10.3390/molecules22010017.
119. Yu LSL, Reed SA, Golden MH. Time-resolved fluorescence immunoassay (TRFIA) for the detection of *Escherichia coli* O157:H7 in apple cider. *J Microbiol Methods*. 2002;49:63–68. Available from: https://doi.org/10.1016/S0167-7012(01)00352-9.
120. Hagren V, von Lode P, Syrjälä A, et al. An 8-hour system for *Salmonella* detection with immunomagnetic separation and homogeneous time-resolved fluorescence PCR. *Int J Food Microbiol*. 2008;125:158–161. Available from: https://doi.org/10.1016/j.ijfoodmicro.2008.03.037.
121. Wang X, Huang Y, Wu S, et al. Simultaneous detection of *Staphylococcus aureus* and *Salmonella typhimurium* using multi-color time-resolved fluorescence nanoparticles as labels. *Int J Food Microbiol*. 2016;237:172–179. Available from: https://doi.org/10.1016/j.ijfoodmicro.2016.08.028.
122. McDonald SLR, Maple PAC, Andrews N, et al. Evaluation of the time resolved fluorescence immunoassay (TRFIA) for the detection of varicella zoster virus (VZV) antibodies following vaccination of healthcare workers. *J Virol Methods*. 2011;172:60–65. Available from: https://doi.org/10.1016/j.jviromet.2010.12.021.
123. Cinquanta L, Fontana DE, Bizzaro N. Chemiluminescent immunoassay technology: what does it change in autoantibody

detection? *Auto Immun Highlights*. 2017;8:9. Available from: https://doi.org/10.1007/s13317-017-0097-2.

124. Wang C, Wu J, Zong C, et al. Chemiluminescent immunoassay and its applications. *Chin J Anal Chem*. 2012;40:3–10. Available from: https://doi.org/10.1016/S1872-2040(11)60518-5.

125. Magliulo M, Simoni P, Guardigli M, et al. A rapid multiplexed chemiluminescent immunoassay for the detection of *Escherichia coli* O157:H7, *Yersinia enterocolitica*, *Salmonella typhimurium*, and *Listeria monocytogenes* pathogen bacteria. *J Agric Food Chem*. 2007;55:4933–4939. Available from: https://doi.org/10.1021/jf063600b.

126. Yang M, Kostov Y, Bruck HA, Rasooly A. Gold nanoparticle-based enhanced chemiluminescence immunosensor for detection of Staphylococcal enterotoxin B (SEB) in food. *Int J Food Microbiol*. 2009;133:265–271.

127. Li Q, Yang Y, Hu F, et al. Rapid detection of *Escherichia coli* O157:H7 by a fluorescent microsphere-based immunochromatographic assay and immunomagnetic separation. *Anal Biochem*. 2019;564–565:32–39. Available from: https://doi.org/10.1016/j.ab.2018.10.009.

128. Xu L, Zhou J, Eremin S, Dias ACP, Zhang X. Development of ELISA and chemiluminescence enzyme immunoassay for quantification of histamine in drug products and food samples. *Anal Bioanal Chem*. 2020;412:4739–4747.

129. Melton L. Proteomics in multiplex. *Nature*. 2004;429:105–107. Available from: https://doi.org/10.1038/429101a.

130. Renault NK, Gaddipati SR, Wulfert F, et al. Multiple protein extract microarray for profiling human food-specific immunoglobulins A, M, G and E. *J Immunol Methods*. 2011;364:21–32. Available from: https://doi.org/10.1016/j.jim.2010.10.004.

131. Lee BH, Nagamune T. Protein microarrays and their applications. *Biotechnol Bioprocess Eng*. 2004;9:69–75. Available from: https://doi.org/10.1007/BF02932987.

132. Chen Z, Dodig-Crnković T, Schwenk JM, Tao S-C. Current applications of antibody microarrays. *Clin Proteom*. 2018;15:7. Available from: https://doi.org/10.1186/s12014-018-9184-2.

133. Huelseweh B, Ehricht R, Marschall HJ. A simple and rapid protein array based method for the simultaneous detection of biowarfare agents. *Proteomics*. 2006;6:2972–2981.

134. Schlosser G, Kacer P, Kuzma M, et al. Coupling immunomagnetic separation on magnetic beads with matrix-assisted laser desorption ionization-time of flight mass spectrometry for detection of staphylococcal enterotoxin B. *Appl Environ Microbiol*. 2007;73:6945–6952. Available from: https://doi.org/10.1128/AEM.01136-07.

135. Niederkofler EE, Tubbs KA, Gruber K, et al. Determination of β-2 microglobulin levels in plasma using a high-throughput mass spectrometric immunoassay system. *Anal Chem*. 2001;73:3294–3299. Available from: https://doi.org/10.1021/ac010143j.

136. Niederkofler EE, Tubbs KA, Kiernan UA, et al. Novel mass spectrometric immunoassays for the rapid structural characterization of plasma apolipoproteins. *J Lipid Res*. 2003;44:630–639. Available from: https://doi.org/10.1194/jlr.D200034-JLR200.

137. Krastins B, Prakash A, Sarracino DA, et al. Rapid development of sensitive, high-throughput, quantitative and highly selective mass spectrometric targeted immunoassays for clinically important proteins in human plasma and serum. *Clin Biochem*. 2013;46:399–410. Available from: https://doi.org/10.1016/j.clinbiochem.2012.12.019.

138. Tubbs KA, Nedelkov D, Nelson RW. Detection and quantification of beta-2-microglobulin using mass spectrometric immunoassay. *Anal Biochem*. 2001;289:26–35. Available from: https://doi.org/10.1006/abio.2000.4921.

139. Jadhav SR, Shah RM, Karpe AV, et al. Detection of foodborne pathogens using proteomics and metabolomics-based approaches. *Front Microbiol*. 2018;9:3132.

140. Lin C-C, Wang J-H, Wu H-W, Lee G-B. Microfluidic immunoassays. *J Assoc Lab Autom*. 2010;15:253–274. Available from: https://doi.org/10.1016/j.jala.2010.01.013.

141. Wang Y, Li H, Wang Y, et al. Development of multiple cross displacement amplification label-based gold nanoparticles lateral flow biosensor for detection of *Listeria monocytogenes*. *Int J Nanomed*. 2017;12:473–486.

142. Song C, Liu J, Li J, Liu Q. Dual FITC lateral flow immunoassay for sensitive detection of *Escherichia coli* O157:H7 in food samples. *Biosens Bioelectron*. 2016;85:734–739.

143. Kant K, Shahbazi MA, Dave VP, et al. Microfluidic devices for sample preparation and rapid detection of foodborne pathogens. *Biotechnol Adv*. 2018;36:1003–1024.

144. Lin Q, Wen D, Wu J, et al. Microfluidic immunoassays for sensitive and simultaneous detection of IgG/IgM/antigen of SARS-CoV-2 within 15 min. *Anal Chem*. 2020;92:9454–9458. Available from: https://doi.org/10.1021/acs.analchem.0c01635.

145. Zhang Y, Tan C, Fei R, et al. Sensitive chemiluminescence immunoassay for *E. coli* O157:H7 detection with signal dual-amplification using glucose oxidase and laccase. *Anal Chem*. 2014;86:1115–1122. Available from: https://doi.org/10.1021/ac4028774.

146. Xu F, Di X, Ming X, et al. Quantum dot-based immunochromatography test strip for rapid detection of *Campylobacter jejuni*. *J Nanosci Nanotechnol*. 2013;13:4552–4559.

147. Wang Y, Deng R, Zhang G, et al. Rapid and sensitive detection of the food allergen glycinin in powdered milk using a lateral flow colloidal gold immunoassay strip test. *J Agric Food Chem*. 2015;63:2172–2178. Available from: https://doi.org/10.1021/jf5052128.

148. Park JY, Park K, Ok G, et al. Detection of *Escherichia coli* O157:H7 using automated immunomagnetic separation and enzyme-based colorimetric assay. *Sensors (Basel)*. 2020;20:1395. Available from: https://doi.org/10.3390/s20051395.

149. Li Q, Zhang S, Cai Y, et al. Rapid detection of *Listeria monocytogenes* using fluorescence immunochromatographic assay combined with immunomagnetic separation technique. *Int J Food Sci Technol*. 2017;52:1559–1566. Available from: https://doi.org/10.1111/ijfs.13428.

150. Zhu P, Shelton DR, Li S, et al. Detection of *E. coli* O157:H7 by immunomagnetic separation coupled with fluorescence immunoassay. *Biosens Bioelectron*. 2011;30:337–341. Available from: https://doi.org/10.1016/j.bios.2011.09.029.

151. Wang W, Liu D, Gao Y, et al. Identification of twelve *Aeromonas* spp. species with monoclonal antibody-based immunoassay in water and fish samples. *Aquaculture*. 2020;516:734646. Available from: https://doi.org/10.1016/j.aquaculture.2019.734646.

152. Wang Z, Yao X, Zhang Y, et al. Functional nanozyme mediated multi-readout and label-free lateral flow immunoassay for rapid detection of Escherichia coli O157:H7. *Food Chem*. 2020;329:127224. Available from: https://doi.org/10.1016/j.foodchem.2020.127224.

153. Akineden Ö, Wittwer T, Geister K, et al. Nucleic acid lateral flow immunoassay (NALFIA) with integrated DNA probe degradation for the rapid detection of *Cronobacter sakazakii* and *Cronobacter malonaticus* in powdered infant formula. *Food Control*. 2020;109:106952. Available from: https://doi.org/10.1016/j.foodcont.2019.106952.
154. Zhuang L, Gong J, Ji Y, et al. Lateral flow fluorescent immunoassay based on isothermal amplification for rapid quantitative detection of *Salmonella* spp. *Analyst*. 2020;145:2367–2377. Available from: https://doi.org/10.1039/C9AN02011J.
155. Kim B, Su X-L, Li Y. Evaluation of a capillary immunoassay system for detection of *Salmonella* Typhimurium in poultry products. *J Food Prot*. 2005;68:1799–1803. Available from: https://doi.org/10.4315/0362-028X-68.9.1799.
156. Tang D, Tang J, Su B, Chen G. Ultrasensitive electrochemical immunoassay of Staphylococcal enterotoxin B in food using enzyme-nanosilica-doped carbon nanotubes for signal amplification. *J Agric Food Chem*. 2010;58:10824–10830. Available from: https://doi.org/10.1021/jf102326m.
157. Krithiga N, Viswanath KB, Vasantha VS, Jayachitra A. Specific and selective electrochemical immunoassay for *Pseudomonas aeruginosa* based on pectin–gold nanocomposite. *Biosens Bioelectron*. 2016;79:121–129. Available from: https://doi.org/10.1016/j.bios.2015.12.006.
158. Zhang X, Zhang F, Zhang H, et al. Functionalized gold nanorod-based labels for amplified electrochemical immunoassay of *E. coli* as indicator bacteria relevant to the quality of dairy product. *Talanta*. 2015;132:600–605. Available from: https://doi.org/10.1016/j.talanta.2014.10.013.
159. Ririe KM, Rasmussen RP, Wittwer CT. Product differentiation by analysis of DNA melting curves during the polymerase chain reaction. *Anal Biochem*. 1997;245:154–160.
160. Wittwer CT, Herrmann MG, Moss AA, et al. BioFeature continuous fluorescence monitoring of rapid cycle DNA amplification. *BioTechniques*. 1997;22:130–138.
161. Filion M. *Quantitative Real-Time PCR in Applied Microbiology*. Norfolk: Caister Academic Press; 2012.
162. Agrimonti C, Bottari B, Sardaro MLS, et al. Application of real-time PCR (qPCR) for characterization of microbial populations and type of milk in dairy food products. *Crit Rev Food Sci Nutr*. 2017;59:423–442.
163. Syromyatnikov MY, Kiryanova Sv, Popov VN. Development and validation of a TaqMan RT-PCR method for identification of mayonnaise spoilage yeast *Pichia kudriavzevii*. *AMB Express*. 2018;8. Available from: https://doi.org/10.1186/s13568-018-0716-y.
164. Garijo P, González-Arenzana L, López-Alfaro I, et al. Analysis of grapes and the first stages of the vinification process in wine contamination with *Brettanomyces bruxellensis*. *Eur Food Res Technol*. 2014;240:525–532.
165. Tubia I, Prasad K, Pérez-Lorenzo E, et al. Beverage spoilage yeast detection methods and control technologies: a review of *Brettanomyces*. *Int J Food Microbiol*. 2018;283:65–76.
166. Willenburg E, Divol B. Quantitative PCR: an appropriate tool to detect viable but not culturable *Brettanomyces bruxellensis* in wine. *Int J Food Microbiol*. 2012;160:131–136.
167. Panicker G, Myers ML, Bej AK. Rapid detection of *Vibrio vulnificus* in shellfish and Gulf of Mexico water by real-time PCR. *Appl Environ Microbiol*. 2004;70:498–507.
168. de Vuyst L, Vancanneyt M. Biodiversity and identification of sourdough lactic acid bacteria. *Food Microbiol*. 2007;24:120–127.
169. Yan B, Jiang Y-J, Qu Y-Y, et al. Detection of viable *Listeria monocytogenes* in milk by real time RT-PCR. *Food Sci*. 2008;.
170. Ye K, Zhang Q, Jiang Y, et al. Rapid detection of viable *Listeria monocytogenes* in chilled pork by real-time reverse-transcriptase PCR. *Food Control*. 2012;25:117–124.
171. Sair AI, D'Souza DH, Moe CL, et al. Improved detection of human enteric viruses in foods by RT-PCR. *J Virol Methods*. 2002;100:57–69.
172. Morley AA. Digital PCR: a brief history. *Biomol Detect Quantif*. 2014;1:1–2.
173. Li H, Bai R, Zhao Z, et al. Application of droplet digital PCR to detect the pathogens of infectious diseases. *Biosci Rep*. 2018;38:1–8.
174. Postel M, Roosen A, Laurent-Puig P, et al. Droplet-based digital PCR and next generation sequencing for monitoring circulating tumor DNA: a cancer diagnostic perspective. *Expert Rev Mol Diagn*. 2018;18:7–17.
175. Nyaruaba R, Mwaliko C, Kering KK, et al. Droplet digital PCR applications in the tuberculosis world. *Tuberculosis*. 2019;117:85–92.
176. Olmedillas-López S, García-Arranz M, García-Olmo D. Current and emerging applications of droplet digital PCR in oncology. *Mol Diagn Ther*. 2017;21:493–510.
177. Mayer W, Schuller M, Viehauser MC, et al. Quantification of the allergen soy (*Glycine max*) in food using digital droplet PCR (ddPCR). *Eur Food Res Technol*. 2019;245:499–509.
178. Iwobi A, Gerdes L, Busch U, et al. Droplet digital PCR for routine analysis of genetically modified foods (GMO) – a comparison with real-time quantitative PCR. *Food Control*. 2016;69:205–213.
179. Morisset D, Štebih D, Milavec M, et al. Quantitative analysis of food and feed samples with droplet digital PCR. *PLoS One*. 2013;8. Available from: https://doi.org/10.1371/journal.pone.0062583.
180. Ren J, Deng T, Huang W, et al. A digital PCR method for identifying and quantifying adulteration of meat species in raw and processed food. *PLoS One*. 2017;12:1–17.
181. Naaum AM, Shehata HR, Chen S, et al. Complementary molecular methods detect undeclared species in sausage products at retail markets in Canada. *Food Control*. 2018;84:339–344.
182. Floren C, Wiedemann I, Brenig B, et al. Species identification and quantification in meat and meat products using droplet digital PCR (ddPCR). *Food Chem*. 2015;173:1054–1058.
183. Cao Y, Raith MR, Griffith JF. Droplet digital PCR for simultaneous quantification of general and human-associated fecal indicators for water quality assessment. *Water Res*. 2015;70:337–349.
184. Jahne MA, Brinkman NE, Keely SP, et al. Droplet digital PCR quantification of norovirus and adenovirus in decentralized wastewater and graywater collections: implications for onsite reuse. *Water Res*. 2020;169. Available from: https://doi.org/10.1016/j.watres.2019.115213.
185. Sedji MI, Varbanov M, Meo M, et al. Quantification of human adenovirus and norovirus in river water in the north-east of France. *Environ Sci Pollut Res*. 2018;25:30497–30507.

186. Cooley MB, Carychao D, Gorski L. Optimized co-extraction and quantification of DNA from enteric pathogens in surface water samples near produce fields in California. *Front Microbiol.* 2018;9:1–9.
187. Rothrock MJ, Hiett KL, Kiepper BH, et al. Quantification of zoonotic bacterial pathogens within commercial poultry processing water samples using droplet digital PCR. *Adv Microbiol.* 2013;03:403–411.
188. Orpana AK, Ho TH, Stenman J. Multiple heat pulses during PCR extension enabling amplification of GC-rich sequences and reducing amplification bias. *Anal Chem.* 2012;84:2081–2087.
189. Schmitz FRW, Valério A, de Oliveira D, et al. An overview and future prospects on aptamers for food safety. *Appl Microbiol Biotechnol.* 2020;104:6929–6939.
190. Duan N, Wu S, Ma X, et al. A universal fluorescent aptasensor based on AccuBlue dye for the detection of pathogenic bacteria. *Anal Biochem.* 2014;454:1–6.
191. Duan YF, Ning Y, Song Y, et al. Fluorescent aptasensor for the determination of *Salmonella* typhimurium based on a graphene oxide platform. *Microchim Acta.* 2014;181:647–653.
192. Ma X, Jiang Y, Jia F, et al. An aptamer-based electrochemical biosensor for the detection of *Salmonella*. *J Microbiol Methods.* 2014;98:94–98.
193. Huang Y, Wang X, Duan N, et al. Selection and characterization, application of a DNA aptamer targeted to *Streptococcus pyogenes* in cooked chicken. *Anal Biochem.* 2018;551:37–42.
194. Hao L, Gu H, Duan N, et al. An enhanced chemiluminescence resonance energy transfer aptasensor based on rolling circle amplification and WS2 nanosheet for *Staphylococcus aureus* detection. *Anal Chim Acta.* 2017;959:83–90.
195. Jia F, Duan N, Wu S, et al. Impedimetric aptasensor for *Staphylococcus aureus* based on nanocomposite prepared from reduced graphene oxide and gold nanoparticles. *Microchim Acta.* 2014;181:967–974.
196. Yuan J, Wu S, Duan N, et al. A sensitive gold nanoparticle-based colorimetric aptasensor for *Staphylococcus aureus*. *Talanta.* 2014;127:163–168.
197. Lavu PSR, Mondal B, Ramlal S, et al. Selection and characterization of aptamers using a modified whole cell bacterium SELEX for the detection of *Salmonella enterica* serovar Typhimurium. *ACS Comb Sci.* 2016;18:292–301.
198. Burke DH, Hoffman DC, Pardi A, et al. RNA aptamers to the peptidyl transferase inhibitor chloramphenicol. *Chem Biol.* 1997;4:833–843.
199. Kim YJ, Kim YS, Niazi JH, et al. Electrochemical aptasensor for tetracycline detection. *Bioprocess Biosyst Eng.* 2010;33:31–37.
200. Zelada-Guillén GA, Sebastián-Avila JL, Blondeau P, et al. Label-free detection of *Staphylococcus aureus* in skin using real-time potentiometric biosensors based on carbon nanotubes and aptamers. *Biosens Bioelectron.* 2012;31:226–232.
201. Brown E, Dessai U, Mcgarry S, et al. Use of whole-genome sequencing for food safety and public health in the United States. *Foodborne Pathog Dis.* 2019;16:441–450.
202. Ashton PM, Peters T, Ameh L, et al. Whole genome sequencing for the retrospective investigation of an outbreak of *Salmonella* Typhimurium DT 8. *PLoS Curr.* 2015;7. Available from: https://doi.org/10.1371/currents.outbreaks.2c05a47d292f376afc5a6fcdd8a7a3b6.
203. Chen Y, Luo Y, Curry P, et al. Assessing the genome level diversity of *Listeria monocytogenes* from contaminated ice cream and environmental samples linked to a listeriosis outbreak in the United States. *PLoS One.* 2017;12:1–19.
204. Haendiges J, Jones J, Myers RA, et al. A nonautochthonous U.S. strain of *Vibrio parahaemolyticus* isolated from Chesapeake Bay oysters caused the outbreak in Maryland in 2010. *Appl Environ Microbiol.* 2016;82:3208–3216.
205. Hoffmann M, Luo Y, Monday SR, et al. Tracing origins of the *Salmonella* Bareilly strain causing a food-borne outbreak in the United States. *J Infect Dis.* 2016;213:502–508.
206. Hoffmann M, Zhao S, Pettengill J, et al. Comparative genomic analysis and virulence differences in closely related *Salmonella enterica* serotype Heidelberg isolates from humans, retail meats, and animals. *Genome Biol Evol.* 2014;6:1046–1068.
207. Kozyreva VK, Truong CH, Greninger A, Crandall J, Mukhopadhyay RC. Validation and Implementation of Clinical Laboratory Improvements Act-compliant whole-genome sequencing in the public health microbiology. *J Clin Microbiol.* 2017;55:2502–2520.
208. Nichols M, Conrad A, Whitlock L, et al. Short communication: multistate outbreak of *Listeria monocytogenes* infections retrospectively linked to unpasteurized milk using whole-genome sequencing. *J Dairy Sci.* 2020;103:176–178.
209. Nouws S, Bogaerts B, Verhaegen B, et al. The benefits of whole genome sequencing for foodborne outbreak investigation from the perspective of a national reference laboratory in a smaller country. *Foods.* 2020;9. Available from: https://doi.org/10.3390/foods9081030.
210. Type SS, Fruit CS, Chen Y, et al. crossm monocytogenes Associated with Three Multistate Outbreaks Linked to. 2017;55:931–941.
211. Yang H, Hoffmann M, Allard MW, et al. Microevolution and gain or loss of mobile genetic elements of outbreak-related *Listeria monocytogenes* in food processing environments identified by whole genome sequencing analysis. *Front Microbiol.* 2020;11:1–29.
212. Bauman JGJ, Wiegant J, Borst P, et al. A new method for fluorescence microscopical localization of specific DNA sequences by in situ hybridization of fluorochrome-labelled RNA. *Exp Cell Res.* 1980;128:485–490.
213. Frickmann H, Zautner AE, Moter A, et al. Fluorescence in situ hybridization (FISH) in the microbiological diagnostic routine laboratory: a review. *Crit Rev Microbiol.* 2017;43:263–293.
214. Fang Q, Brockmann S, Botzenhart K, et al. Improved detection of *Salmonella* spp. in foods by fluorescent in situ hybridization with 23S rRNA probes: a comparison with conventional culture methods. *J Food Prot.* 2003;66:723–731.
215. Almeida C, Azevedo NF, Fernandes RM, et al. Fluorescence in situ hybridization method using a peptide nucleic acid probe for identification of *Salmonella* spp. in a broad spectrum of samples. *Appl Environ Microbiol.* 2010;76:4476–4485.
216. Bisha B, Brehm-Stecher BF. Combination of adhesive-tape-based sampling and fluorescence in situ hybridization for rapid detection of Salmonella on fresh produce. *J Vis Exp.* 2010;. Available from: https://doi.org/10.3791/2308.
217. Bisha B, Brehm-Stecher BF. Simple adhesive-tape-based sampling of tomato surfaces combined with rapid fluorescence in situ hybridization for *Salmonella* detection. *Appl Environ Microbiol.* 2009;75:1450–1455.

218. Fuchizawa I, Shimizu S, Ootsubo M, et al. Specific and rapid quantification of viable *Listeria monocytogenes* using fluorescence in situ hybridization in combination with filter cultivation. *Microbes Environ.* 2009;24:273–275.
219. Kljujev I, Raicevic V, Vujovic B, et al. *Salmonella* as an endophytic colonizer of plants – a risk for health safety vegetable production. *Microb Pathog.* 2018;115:199–207.
220. Oliveira M, Vieira-Pinto M, Martins da Costa P, et al. Occurrence of *Salmonella* spp. in samples from pigs slaughtered for consumption: a comparison between ISO 6579:2002 and 23S rRNA Fluorescent In Situ Hybridization method. *Food Res Int.* 2012;45:984–988.
221. Schmid MW, Lehner A, Stephan R, et al. Development and application of oligonucleotide probes for in situ detection of thermotolerant *Campylobacter* in chicken faecal and liver samples. *Int J Food Microbiol.* 2005;105:245–255.
222. Vieira-Pinto M, Oliveira M, Bernardo F, et al. Evaluation of fluorescent in situ hybridization (fish) as a rapid screening method for detection of *Salmonella* in tonsils of slaughtered pigs for consumption: a comparison with conventional culture method. *J Food Saf.* 2005;25:109–119.
223. Vieira-Pinto M, Oliveira M, Bernardo F, et al. Rapid detection of *Salmonella* sp. in pork samples using fluorescent in situ hybridization: a comparison with VIDAS®-SLM system and ISO 6579 cultural method. *Arq Bras Med Vet Zootec.* 2007;59:1388–1393.
224. Moreno Y, Hernández M, Ferrús MA, et al. Direct detection of thermotolerant Campylobacters in chicken products by PCR and in situ hybridization. *Res Microbiol.* 2001;152:577–582.
225. Iwamoto T, Sonobe T, Hayashi K. Loop-mediated isothermal amplification for direct detection of *Mycobacterium tuberculosis* complex, *M. avium*, and *M. intracellulare* in sputum samples. *J Clin Microbiol.* 2003;41:2616–2622.
226. Notomi T, Okayama H, Masubuchi H, et al. Loop-mediated isothermal amplification of DNA. *Nucleic Acids Res.* 2000;28:e63.
227. Wong YP, Othman S, Lau YL, et al. Loop-mediated isothermal amplification (LAMP): a versatile technique for detection of micro-organisms. *J Appl Microbiol.* 2018;124:626–643.
228. Pham NTK, Trinh QD, Khamrin P, et al. Loop-mediated isothermal amplification (LAMP) for detection of *Campylobacter jejuni* and *C. coli* in Thai children with diarrhea. *Jpn J Infect Dis.* 2015;68:432–433.
229. Romero MR, Cook N. A rapid lamp-based method for screening poultry samples for *Campylobacter* without enrichment. *Front Microbiol.* 2018;9:1–8.
230. Yamazaki W, Taguchi M, Ishibashi M, et al. Development and evaluation of a loop-mediated isothermal amplification assay for rapid and simple detection of *Campylobacter jejuni* and *Campylobacter coli*. *J Med Microbiol.* 2008;57:444–451.
231. Birmpa A, Kalogeropoulos K, Kokkinos P, et al. Evaluation of two loop-mediated isothermal amplification methods for the detection of *Salmonella* Enteritidis and *Listeria monocytogenes* in artificially contaminated ready-to-eat fresh products. *Ital J Food Saf.* 2015;4. Available from: https://doi.org/10.4081/ijfs.2015.5383.
232. Shan X, Zhang Y, Zhang Z, et al. Rapid detection of food-borne *Listeria monocytogenes* by real-time quantitative loop-mediated isothermal amplification. *Food Sci Biotechnol.* 2012;21:101–106.
233. Tang MJ, Zhou S, Zhang XY, et al. Rapid and sensitive detection of *Listeria monocytogenes* by loop-mediated isothermal amplification. *Curr Microbiol.* 2011;63:511–516.
234. Wachiralurpan S, Sriyapai T, Areekit S, et al. Development of a rapid screening test for *Listeria monocytogenes* in raw chicken meat using loop-mediated isothermal amplification (LAMP) and lateral flow dipstick (LFD). *Food Anal Methods.* 2017;10:3763–3772.
235. Wachiralurpan S, Sriyapai T, Areekit S, et al. Rapid colorimetric assay for detection of *Listeria monocytogenes* in food samples using LAMP formation of DNA concatemers and gold nanoparticle-DNA probe complex. *Front Chem.* 2018;6:1–9.
236. Wang L, Li Y, Chu J, et al. Development and application of a simple loop-mediated isothermal amplification method on rapid detection of *Listeria monocytogenes* strains. *Mol Biol Rep.* 2012;39:445–449.
237. Wang Y, Wang Y, Ma A, et al. The novel multiple inner primers-loop-mediated isothermal amplification (MIP-LAMP) for rapid detection and differentiation of *Listeria monocytogenes*. *Molecules.* 2015;20:21515–21531.
238. Ye L, Li Y, Zhao J, et al. Development of a real-time loop-mediated isothermal amplification assay for the sensitive and rapid detection of *Listeria monocytogenes*. *Lett Appl Microbiol.* 2015;61:85–90.
239. Ajonina C, Buzie C, Möller J, et al. The detection of *Entamoeba histolytica* and *Toxoplasma gondii* in wastewater. *J Toxicol Environ Health.* 2018;81:1–5.
240. Foo PC, Chan YY, Mohamed M, et al. Development of a thermostabilised triplex LAMP assay with dry-reagent four target lateral flow dipstick for detection of *Entamoeba histolytica* and non-pathogenic *Entamoeba* spp. *Anal Chim Acta.* 2017;966:71–80.
241. Mwendwa F, Mbae CK, Kinyua J, et al. Stem loop-mediated isothermal amplification test: comparative analysis with classical LAMP and PCR in detection of *Entamoeba histolytica* in Kenya. *BMC Res Notes.* 2017;10:1–9.
242. Rivera WL, Ong VA. Development of loop-mediated isothermal amplification for rapid detection of *Entamoeba histolytica*. *Asian Pac J Tropical Med.* 2013;6:457–461.
243. Singh P, Mirdha BR, Ahuja V, et al. Loop-mediated isothermal amplification (LAMP) assay for rapid detection of *Entamoeba histolytica* in amoebic liver abscess. *World J Microbiol Biotechnol.* 2013;29:27–32.
244. Bakhtiari S, Alvandi A, Pajavand H, et al. Development and diagnostic evaluation of loop-mediated isothermal amplification using a new gene target for rapid detection of helicobacter pylori. *Jundishapur J Microbiol.* 2016;9. Available from: https://doi.org/10.5812/jjm.28831.
245. Yari F, Abiri R, Aryan E, et al. Loop-mediated isothermal amplification as a fast noninvasive method of *Helicobacter pylori* diagnosis. *J Clin Lab Anal.* 2016;30:464–470.
246. Kim HJ, Kim HS, Lee JM, et al. Rapid detection of *Pseudomonas aeruginosa* and *Acinetobacter baumannii* harboring blaVIM-2, blaIMP-1 and blaOXA-23 genes by using loop-mediated isothermal amplification methods. *Ann Lab Med.* 2016;36:15–22.
247. Lee JE, Mun H, Kim SR, et al. A colorimetric loop-mediated isothermal amplification (LAMP) assay based on HRP-mimicking molecular beacon for the rapid detection of *Vibrio parahaemolyticus*. *Biosens Bioelectron.* 2020;151. Available from: https://doi.org/10.1016/j.bios.2019.111968.
248. Li W, Lin L, Yamasaki S, et al. Rapid detection of *Vibrio parahaemolyticus* by loop-mediated isothermal amplification method. *Food Sci.* 2008;7:382–385.

249. Surasilp T, Longyant S, Rukpratanporn S, et al. Rapid and sensitive detection of *Vibrio vulnificus* by loop-mediated isothermal amplification combined with lateral flow dipstick targeted to rpoS gene. *Mol Cell Probes*. 2011;25:158–163.
250. Hara-Kudo Y, Konishi N, Ohtsuka K, et al. Detection of verotoxigenic *Escherichia coli* O157 and O26 in food by plating methods and LAMP method: a collaborative study. *Int J Food Microbiol*. 2008;122:156–161.
251. Hara-Kudo Y, Nemoto J, Ohtsuka K, et al. Sensitive and rapid detection of Vero toxin-producing *Escherichia coli* using loop-mediated isothermal amplification. *J Med Microbiol*. 2007;56:398–406.
252. Liu JS, Wang Q, Zhang JB, et al. Construction and functional activity of a recombinant vector expressing rat glutamic acid decarboxylase 65. *Neurosci Bull*. 2011;27:430–435.
253. Wang D, He B, Li F, et al. The influence of injection processing on the shrinkage variation and dimensional stability of wax pattern in investment casting. *Adv Mater Res*. 2012;538–541:1217–1221.
254. Goto M, Hayashidani H, Takatori K, et al. Rapid detection of enterotoxigenic *Staphylococcus aureus* harbouring genes for four classical enterotoxins, SEA, SEB, SEC and SED, by loop-mediated isothermal amplification assay. *Lett Appl Microbiol*. 2007;45:100–107.
255. Suwanampai T, Pattaragulvanit K, Pattanamahakul P, et al. Evaluation of loop-mediated isothermal amplification method for detecting enterotoxin a gene of *Staphylococcus aureus* in pork. *Southeast Asian J Trop Med Public Health*. 2011;42:1489–1497.
256. Wang D, Liu F, Huo G, et al. Development and evaluation of a loop-mediated isothermal amplification method for detecting *Escherichia coli* o157 in raw milk. *J Rapid Methods Autom Microbiol*. 2009;17:55–66.
257. Yang H, Ma X, Zhang X, et al. Development and evaluation of a loop-mediated isothermal amplification assay for the rapid detection of *Staphylococcus aureus* in food. *Eur Food Res Technol*. 2011;232:769–776.
258. Pavlovic M, Huber I, Konrad R, et al. Application of MALDI-TOF MS for the identification of food borne bacteria. *Open Microbiol J*. 2013;7:135–141.
259. Welker M, van Belkum A, Girard V, et al. An update on the routine application of MALDI-TOF MS in clinical microbiology. *Expert Rev Proteomics*. 2019;16:695–710.
260. Doan NTL, van Hoorde K, Cnockaert M, et al. Validation of MALDI-TOF MS for rapid classification and identification of lactic acid bacteria, with a focus on isolates from traditional fermented foods in Northern Vietnam. *Lett Appl Microbiol*. 2012;55:265–273.
261. Höll L, Behr J, Vogel RF. Identification and growth dynamics of meat spoilage microorganisms in modified atmosphere packaged poultry meat by MALDI-TOF MS. *Food Microbiol*. 2016;60:84–91.
262. Kim E, Cho EJ, Yang SM, et al. Novel approaches for the identification of microbial communities in Kimchi: MALDI-TOF MS analysis and high-throughput sequencing. *Food Microbiol*. 2021;94. Available from: https://doi.org/10.1016/j.fm.2020.103641.
263. Yu Z, Peruzy MF, Dumolin C, et al. Assessment of food microbiological indicators applied on poultry carcasses by culture combined MALDI-TOF MS identification and 16S rRNA amplicon sequencing. *Food Microbiol*. 2019;82:53–61.
264. Angelakis E, Million M, Henry M, et al. Rapid and accurate bacterial identification in probiotics and yoghurts by MALDI-TOF mass spectrometry. *J Food Sci*. 2011;76:568–572.
265. Nacef M, Chevalier M, Chollet S, et al. MALDI-TOF mass spectrometry for the identification of lactic acid bacteria isolated from a French cheese: the Maroilles. *Int J Food Microbiol*. 2017;247:2–8.
266. Rau J, Korte N, Dyk M, et al. Rapid animal species identification of feta and mozzarella cheese using MALDI-TOF mass-spectrometry. *Food Control*. 2020;117. Available from: https://doi.org/10.1016/j.foodcont.2020.107349.
267. Kačániová M, Kunová S, Nagyová L, et al. Application of MALDI-TOF mass spectrometry for identification of bacteria isolated from traditional Slovak cheese "Parenica.". *J Microbiol Biotechnol Food Sci*. 2019;8:1294–1297.
268. Quéro L, Girard V, Pawtowski A, et al. Development and application of MALDI-TOF MS for identification of food spoilage fungi. *Food Microbiol*. 2019;81:76–88.
269. Dieckmann R, Helmuth R, Erhard M, et al. Rapid classification and identification of Salmonellae at the species and subspecies levels by whole-cell matrix-assisted laser desorption ionization-time of flight mass spectrometry. *Appl Environ Microbiol*. 2008;74:7767–7778.
270. Stübiger G, Wuczkowski M, Mancera L, et al. Characterization of yeasts and filamentous fungi using MALDI lipid phenotyping. *J Microbiol Methods*. 2016;130:27–37.

Section X

Safety assessment of genetically modified organisms and other biological alterations

Chapter 60

New genetic modification techniques: challenges and prospects

Graham Head[1] and George T. Tzotzos[2]
[1]Bayer Crop Science, Chesterfield, MO, United States, [2]Bioinformatics researcher, Vienna, Austria

Abstract

Several new genetic modification (nGM) techniques have emerged in the last few years through rapid advancements in plant molecular biology and genomic research. The technical underpinnings of these techniques are diverse, and so are their potential outcomes. Some nGMs are intended to introduce heritable genomic modifications, while others aim to induce transient changes in gene expression patterns without the insertion of foreign DNA. This chapter presents an overview of the technical features of each of these techniques, as well as their similarities and differences compared to *recombinant DNA* and plant breeding technologies. The chapter also deals with the perceived safety issues associated with the application of nGMs. It gives due consideration to the suitability of genetically modified organism regulations to deal with the products of these technologies. It concludes that the diversity of nGM products may require risk assessment procedures that are flexible and proportional to anticipated risks.

Keywords: New plant breeding techniques (NBPT); genome editing; ZFNs; TALENs; CRISPR/Cas; synthetic biology; risk assessment

60.1 Introduction

New genetic modification techniques (nGMs) are emerging as powerful tools in plant research and crop improvement. They have some similarities to conventional plant breeding and recombinant DNA (rDNA) techniques, but they are much more versatile and efficient. nGMs employ diverse methodologies (Table 60.1). The resulting end-products may or may not contain *exogenous* DNA sequences, and in some cases, may be indistinguishable from those resulting from conventional breeding. In this chapter, Sections 60.2–60.7 describe the scientific underpinnings of nGMs, indicative applications of the techniques, and their comparative advantages and disadvantages. Although synthetic biology (SynBio) is not an nGM technology, its inclusion in Section 60.8 is based on its potential for breakthrough innovations in the near future. Sections 60.9 and 60.10 describe the safety issues and the analytical methods available to detect and characterize unintended effects related to the application of nGMs. Section 60.11 concludes this chapter.

60.2 Genome editing

Plant breeders have traditionally relied on spontaneous natural mutations to broaden the genetic diversity of genotypes. With the advent of rapid and cheap sequencing technologies, numerous mutagenesis methods coupled with tissue culture and molecular-based trait selection have been incorporated into breeding programs.[1] The advent of genetic engineering (GE) broadened the pool of agriculturally useful traits by allowing the transfer of genes between distantly related, or even unrelated, organisms. However, the random integration of exogenous DNA into the recipient plant genome is a significant limitation of GE, henceforth referred to as conventional GE or cGE. More recently, genome editing techniques have emerged as the tools of choice for the GM of plants. This is because of the efficacy and efficiency with which these techniques generate precise changes in targeted loci in the recipient plant genome with or without exogenous DNA integration. In nature, nuclease enzymes effect the single or double-stranded break (DSB) of target DNA, and they are essential components of the DNA repair machinery.

Genome editing relies on engineered site-directed nucleases (SDNs) that are tailor-made to induce DSBs with great specificity. Engineered SDNs function in a complex with short oligonucleotides or RNA sequences, guiding the complex to the targeted genomic locus where they catalyze a DNA double-strand break (DSB). Highly efficient genome editing in plants has been achieved with zinc-finger nucleases (ZFNs), transcription activator-like effector nucleases (TALENs), and the clustered regularly

Present Knowledge in Food Safety. DOI: https://doi.org/10.1016/B978-0-12-819470-6.00017-2

TABLE 60.1 New genetic modification (GM) techniques: objectives and product outcomes.

	Objective of the technique	GM in the final product
Genome editing	Targeted knockout and knock-in mutations Transgene insertions are possible	Present and heritable
Oligonucleotide-directed mutagenesis	Targeted single nucleotide polymorphisms	Present and heritable
Cis- and transgenesis	Insertion of cis-genes or intra-genes	Present and heritable
Transgrafting	Production of chimeric plants	May be absent
Agroinfiltration	Modification of somatic tissues	May be absent
RNA-dependent DNA methylation	Modification of gene expression	Absent but epigenetic modifications may be passed on to progeny for some generations
Reverse breeding	Enable or speed up breeding programs	Absent

interspaced short palindromic repeats (CRISPR)-associated nuclease (CRISPR/Cas system). Another technology, namely, oligonucleotide-directed mutagenesis (ODM), has also been demonstrated to be effective in providing custom-made single nucleotide polymorphisms (SNPs).

60.2.1 Engineered nucleases and oligonucleotides

60.2.1.1 Zinc finger nucleases

Zinc fingers (ZFs) are zinc ion–regulated small structural motifs in proteins. In ZFNs, ZF domains, usually but not exclusively three ZF repeats, have been synthesized to recognize nearly all 64 nucleotide codons.[2,3] Thus a ZF domain comprising three ZF modules can recognize 9 bp sequences in the target DNA. ZF domains are typically fused to a non-specific DNA cleavage domain from the *FokI* endonuclease through a linker oligopeptide sequence forming a ZF-nuclease complex (ZFN). Endonuclease activity requires the dimerization of the *FokI* domain, and therefore two ZFN complexes are needed to recognize and bind to opposite strands of the target DNA (Fig. 60.1A).

60.2.1.2 Transcription activator-like effector nucleases

Like ZFNs, TALENs comprise two *FokI* domains, each of which is linked to a TAL effector that serves as a guide to DNA recognition and binding. TAL effectors (TALEs) are proteins secreted by *Xanthomonas* bacteria after infection of appropriate plant hosts. Most TALEs consist of 12–27 nearly identical repeat units, each of which comprises a highly conserved 33–34 amino acid sequences. The amino acids at positions 12 and 13 of each unit are highly variable and can recognize specific nucleotide bases. They are referred to as the repeat variable diresidue (RVD) and have a one-to-one relationship to DNA nucleotides. This allows the engineering of tailored DNA-binding domains by combining repeat units with the appropriate RVDs[3] (Fig. 60.1B).

60.2.1.3 Clustered regularly interspaced short palindromic repeats-Cas editing

The CRISPR-Cas editing system is a synthetic construct that works similarly to a genome editing system naturally found in bacteria in response to viral transfection. Bacteria integrate segments of DNA formed by small fragments of viral DNA. These segments, known as CRISPR arrays, allow bacteria to produce RNA sequences that are able to recruit Cas9 or a similar nuclease. The CRISPR-Cas9 complex acts as "scissors" cutting the DNA of the invading virus and, as such, plays a vital role in the antiviral defense system of prokaryotes.

Synthetic CRISPR-Cas systems consist of two key molecules, namely a nuclease enzyme (Cas, usually but not exclusively Cas9) and an RNA sequence predesigned to match the target DNA sequence. The latter, known as single-guide RNA (sgRNA), binds to the target DNA where Cas9 mediates its cleavage. The target specificity of the CRISPR/Cas9 system is mainly determined by the sgRNA sequence matching genomic loci within 10–12 bp upstream of a required 5′-NGG protospacer adjacent motif (PAM)[4] (Fig. 60.1C). Whereas the 5'-NGG protospacer adjacent motif comprises any nucleobase ("N") followed by two guanine nucleobases ("GG"),[5] an enormous variety of Cas protein families recognize distinct PAM motifs, and different protein engineering approaches aim to construct designer PAM-interaction domains.[6] Some variants of the CRISPR/Cas system utilize a catalytically impaired nuclease fused to a single-stranded DNA deaminase enzyme. These variants, known as base editors, do not

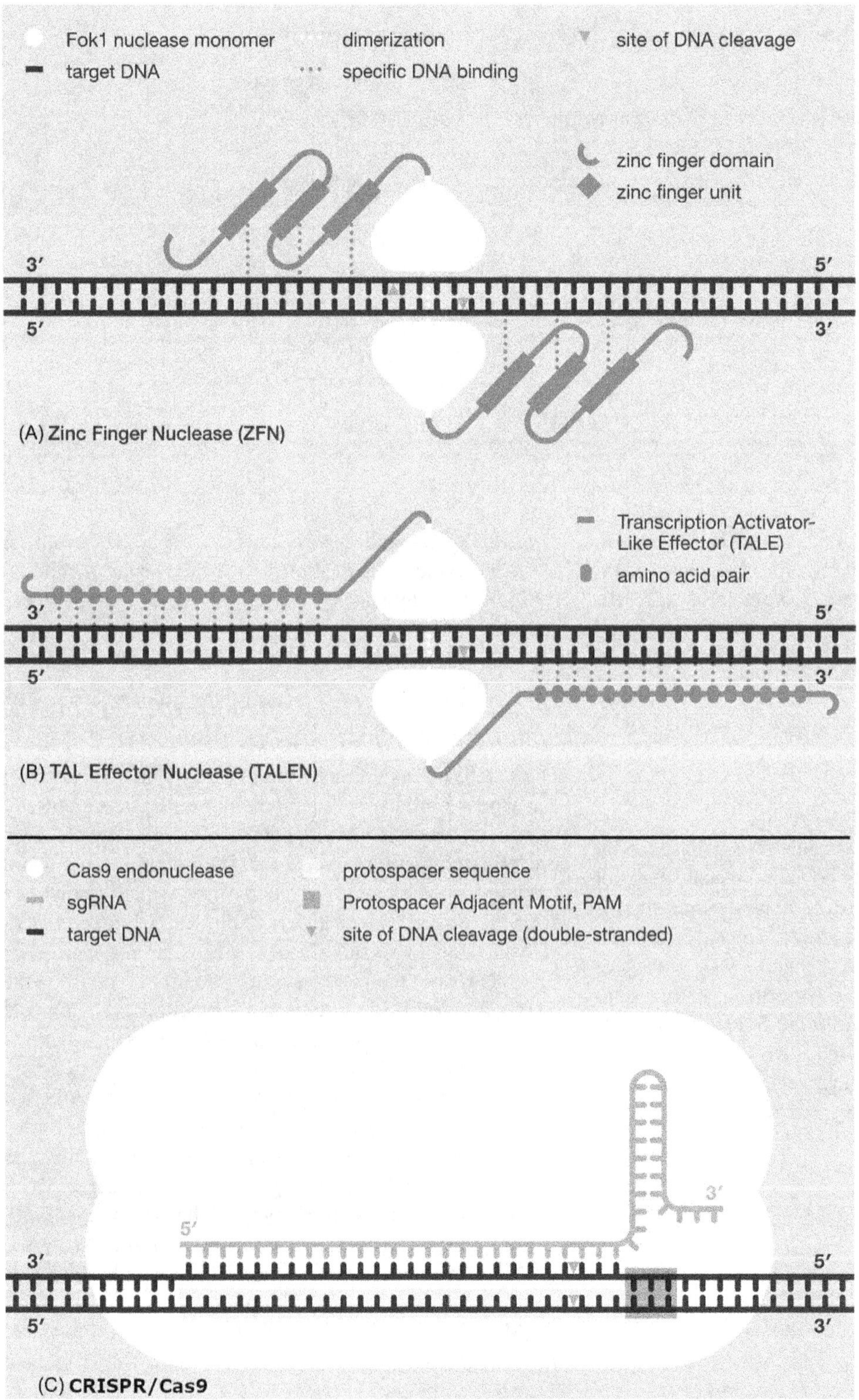

FIGURE 60.1 Schematic depiction of site directed nucleases used in genome editing.

require DSBs or donor templates and do not rely on homologous recombination (HR). These editors may convert C-G base pairs to T-A base pairs (cytosine editors) or A-T base pairs to G-C base pairs (adenine editors). Prime editors are different variants of the CRISPR/Cas system. They are fusion proteins consisting of a Cas9 nickase domain and an engineered reverse transcriptase domain that can induce all six base-pair conversions.[7]

60.2.1.4 Meganucleases

Meganucleases (MNs), also known as homing endonucleases, are naturally occurring enzymes in many microorganisms, yeast, algae, and some plants. They are encoded by mobile introns, and despite their name, they are considerably smaller (~165 amino acids) than the corresponding proteins of the ZFNs, TALENs, and CRISPR/Cas9 systems. MNs recognize large DNA target sequences ranging from 12 to 40 bp. The action of MNs causes DSBs in alleles that lack MN coding introns. The ensuing DNA repair involves intron harboring alleles acting like repair templates copying the MN coding sequence into the target DNA site.[8,9] One of the problems limiting the usability of MNs in genome editing is the difficulty in engineering tailor-made DNA sequence specificity. Unlike editing with the other SDN systems described above, in MN editing, the cleavage and DNA-binding domains overlap. As a result, changes intended to alter the specificity of binding of MNs to the target DNA may compromise their catalytic activity.[10]

60.2.1.5 Oligonucleotide-directed mutagenesis

ODM is a nontransgenic genome editing platform using chemically synthesized oligonucleotides, approximately 20–100 nucleotides in length. Depending on the type of plant cells, polyethylene glycol (PEG)-mediated transfection of protoplast or biolistics can be used to deliver the oligonucleotides. The oligonucleotides are synthesized to be homologous to a target sequence, albeit containing one or a few nucleotides that are not complementary to the target DNA. Highly specific mutations are obtained following the annealing of oligonucleotides with their target DNA sequences and the induction of the cellular mismatch repair mechanism.[1] Cellular enzymes degrade the oligonucleotides, and the induced mutations are stable and heritable. The method's success has been demonstrated in relatively few plants (*Arabidopsis*, tobacco, rice, oilseed rape, maize) with modest conversion rates regardless of the delivery method. The efficiency of transformation depends on various factors, including the target plant's cell biology, the length and concentration of the oligonucleotides used, and the targeted strand (coding or noncoding).[11]

60.2.2 Comparative advantages and disadvantages of site-directed nucleases

Each SDN platform has comparative advantages and disadvantages relating to their respective activity, specificity, and deliverability, as well as the ease and costs of engineering them (Table 60.2). The CRISPR/Cas system was

TABLE 60.2 Features of different site-directed nuclease platforms.

	ZFNs	TALENs	CRISPR/Cas
Recognition site	Zn-finger protein	RVD tandem repeat of TALE protein	Single-strand RNA
Target sequence size	18–36 bp per ZFN pair	28–40 bp per TALEN pair	~20 bp guide sequence plus PAM sequence
Mechanism of target recognition	DNA–protein interaction	DNA–protein interactions	DNA–RNA interaction via Watson–Crick base pairing
Specificity	Tolerate a small number of positional mismatches	Tolerate a small number of positional mismatches	Tolerate multiple consecutive mismatches
Design and cloning	Available Zn-finger motifs with predefined target specificity. Challenging design. Zn-finger motifs assembled in arrays can affect the specificity of neighboring Zn-finger motifs. Requires engineering linkages between Zn-finger motifs	Easy design. TALE motifs with target specificities are well-defined. Complex molecular cloning methods. It can be done using Golden Gate assembly	Easy design based on complementarity with the target DNA. Standard cloning procedures and oligo synthesis. Numerous expression *vectors* for Cas9 are available
Delivery	Relatively easy due to the small size of ZFN expression elements	Difficult because of the large size of the functional components	The size of the Cas9 can be a problem. It can be delivered as a DNA expression vector or directly as an RNA molecule or preloaded Cas9-RNA complex

CRISPR, Clustered regularly interspaced short palindromic repeats; *TALENs*, transcription activator-like effector nucleases; *RVD*, repeat variable di-residue; *ZFN*, zinc-finger nucleases.

first used to edit mammalian genomes in 2013. It was used in plant genome editing shortly after and became the editing platform of choice. It has been used to edit an enormous variety of plant species and commercial crops.[12] However, this does not mean the CRISPR/Cas system has totally eclipsed the other editing platforms. Considerable progress has been made in the redesign of protein-DNA specificity of the other nuclease systems.[13] However, the limited scope of genome editing with MNs and the difficulty and costs of engineering and cloning of ZFNs and TALENs partially prevent their large-scale adoption by academic laboratories.[14]

Gene editing with ZFNs is less specific than editing with TALENs, and in general, causes high frequencies of off-target edits and higher levels of cytotoxicity. Also, for some applications, the use of TALENs is not without problems. For example, DNA methylation is a significant factor in the adaptation of plants to stress, and TALENs, unlike CRISPR/Cas9, cannot target methylated DNA. As a result, TALENs has limited value for the development of stress-tolerant plants.[12]

60.2.3 Mechanisms and outcomes of genome editing

Cells repair DNA damage by either HR or nonhomologous end-joining (NHEJ). NHEJ is the predominant DNA repair mechanism in higher plants, but the nuclease action can also stimulate HR to repair DSBs.[13] Delivery of the engineered nucleases is intended to generate targeted DSBs, followed by appropriate genomic changes. The type of GM outcome depends not only on the intrinsic activity of SDNs but also on their ability to steer DNA repair by either the HR or the NHEJ pathways. Delivery of the SDN to the target plant cells with or without an exogenous DNA template determines which pathway is recruited to repair the DSB. User-supplied templates can be DNA sequences homologous to the target DNA locus and contain one or a few nucleotide substitutions, longer sequences, and even one or more *transgenes*. The NHEJ and HR pathways of DNA repair are described in detail in recent papers.[13,14]

Genome editing applications can lead to diverse end products, some of which can be devoid of exogenous DNA sequences or include modifications of a few nucleotides in targeted genomic loci, or even contain integrated DNA elements of heterologous origin. To enable the comparison of products of such a diverse range of genotypic and phenotypic traits, the European Food Safety Authority (EFSA) Panel on Genetically Modified Organisms (GMOs) proposed a scheme grouping them by the type of SDN-meditated modification. The scheme allows a direct comparison of genome-edited products with those developed by conventional breeding programs or transgenesis. Three broad categories of SDN modifications have been defined, namely, SDN-1, SDN-2, and SDN-3.[15,16]

SDN-1 includes edits generated by SDNs in the absence of donor DNA or a repair template, and thus the outcome of the nuclease action depends on NHEJ as this is the predominant DSB repair pathway. Further subdivision of this category includes events with small indels (SDN-1a), larger deletions caused by tandemly arranged SDNs (SDN-1b), inversions (SDN-1c), and translocations (SDN-1d).[17] SDN-1-type modifications usually result in loss-of-function mutations (gene knockouts) (Fig. 60.2A).

SDN-2 includes edits generated by an SDN supplied together with an additional donor DNA template designed to possess the required modifications. The DNA template sequences include regions that are homologous with the sequences flanking the cut site. The template acts as the substrate for HR repair following the induction of one or two adjacent DSBs. Modifications up to 20 nucleotides are indistinguishable from genomic changes of similar size occurring naturally. ODM-induced modifications are deemed to be comparable to SDN-2.[17] Gain-of-function mutations (knock-ins) are the usual outcome of SDN-2 modifications (Fig. 60.2B, top).

SDN-3 includes edits following the introduction of an SDN together with long stretches of DNA (e.g., transgenes) targeting DNA insertion at a predefined genomic locus. The process relies on HR-mediated DSB repair. Mechanistically, the process is like SDN-2, differing from the latter, mainly in the size of the inserted sequence.[17] SDN-3 modifications result in gain-of-function insertions equivalent to transgenesis (Fig. 60.2B, bottom). Mechanistically, the SDN-2 and SDN-3 processes are similar and the discrimination between the two processes is arbitrary based on the size of the inserted sequences.

60.2.4 Targeted knockout mutations in plants

Engineered nuclease NHEJ-induced mutations are the simplest and most frequently implemented type of genome editing. The editing is precise for the targeted site but not for the resulting type of mutation. NHEJ is the predominant DNA-repair pathway when SDNs are delivered without an exogenous DNA template. NHEJ is not entirely error-free and introduces small localized indels or localized substitutions of a few base pairs in the rejoined DNA. Indels occurring in open reading frames cause frameshifts and premature stop of translation, leading to gene knockouts. SDN targeting of promoter regions can thus modulate gene expression.

In terms of applications, the ability to induce recessive mutations in all alleles of a targeted locus is of particular importance in dealing with polyploids, and this is a major advantage of SDN-1 editing compared to mutation breeding.[18] Another important application is multiplexing, that

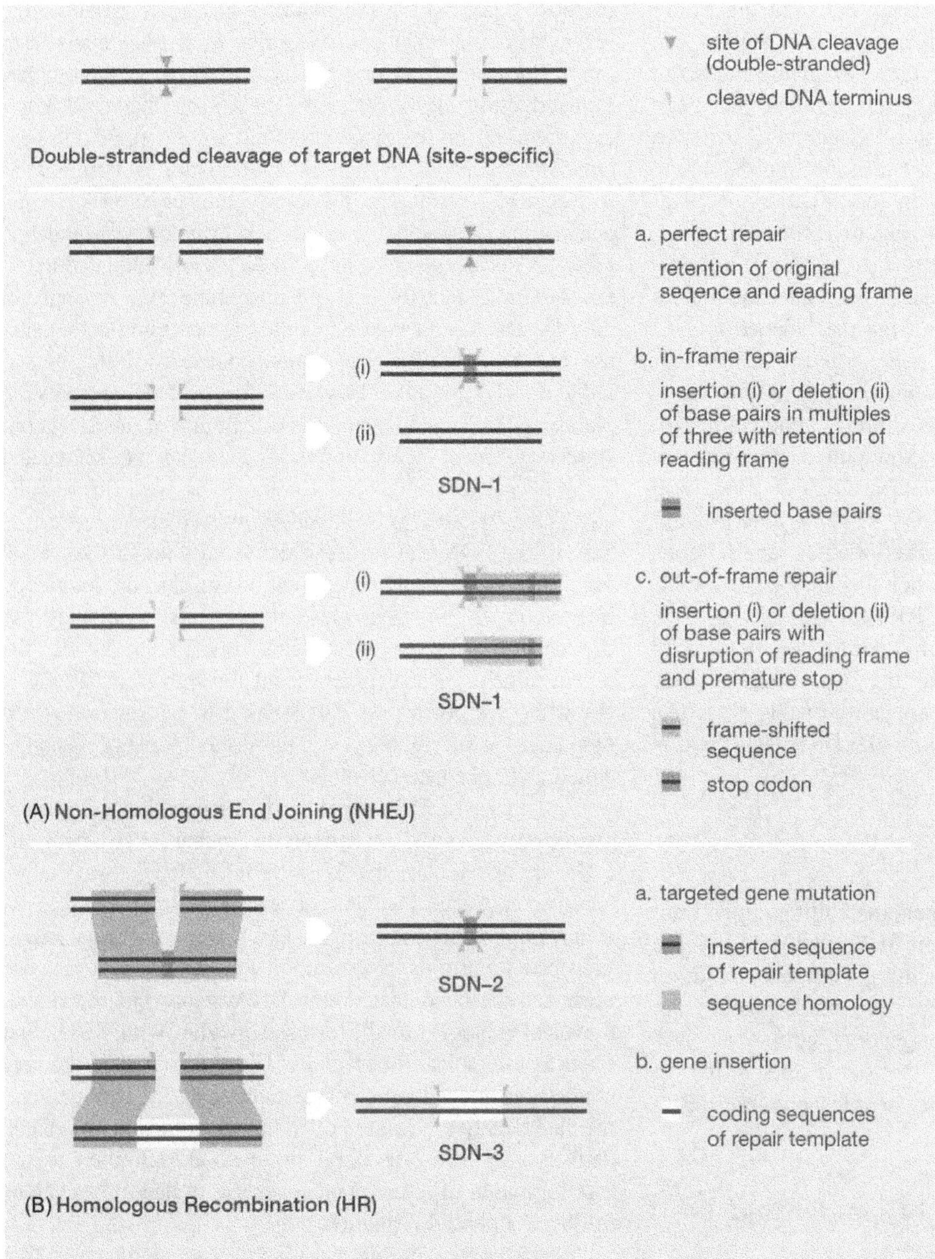

FIGURE 60.2 Genome editing with site-specific nucleases. (A) DNA cleavage by site-specific nucleases is repaired by nonhomologous end-joining (NHEJ), or homologous recombination (HR) (B, top) to yield edited or novel gene sequences (B, bottom).

is the ability to mutate several functional genes in a single step. Multiplexing is likely to find many applications in improving food quality, storage, and processing. For example, multiplexing was used to knockout 35 different alpha-gliadin genes in a wild-type wheat line resulting in the development of low gluten wheat.[19]

60.2.5 Targeted knock-in mutations in plants

Knock-in mutations are generated by site-specific DNA integration of exogenous DNA sequence templates. These can be DNA sequences of a few base pairs or more extensive DNA sequences, including entire genes or even sets of genes. Unlike knockout mutations that usually result in loss of function, knock-in mutations are intended to gain or modify gene function. As mentioned earlier, in this type of applications, the SDN system is delivered together with a user-supplied exogenous DNA repair template that is homologous to the targeted area and the regions flanking the DSB site. The repair template can contain sequence modifications ranging from a single nucleotide to one or more transgenes.

Subject to the type of the target cell and the donor DNA template's architecture, the repair mechanism can involve NHEJ or be HR-driven.[20] Nuclease-mediated NHEJ-directed editing via a supplied template has been used to introduce a single amino acid change of a native gene (*acetohydroxyacid synthase*) in allohexaploid bread wheat.[21] However, the controlled modification of plant genomes by HR is still challenging to achieve because, even in the presence of an extrachromosomal template, the balance between HR and NHEJ lies predominantly in favor of the latter. Therefore shifting the balance toward HR is a significant challenge in gene targeting (GT).[22]

It is beyond the scope of this chapter to provide a comprehensive list of genome editing applications in research and commercial crop development. A recent literature search of bibliographic databases shows over 1300 SDN genome editing applications in 68 different plant species, of which 99 were market-oriented applications focused on 28 crops. The overwhelming majority of studies were conducted using the CRISPR/Cas platform.[23] A commercially available herbicide-tolerant canola cultivar was edited using ODM-based editing. A soybean cultivar with modified oil composition was edited using TALENs technology, while field trials with the first CRISPR/Cas edited canola are underway.[24]

60.2.6 Delivery systems

The efficacy and efficiency of genome editing depend not only on the high specificity of SDNs but also on the methods used to deliver the editing components, often referred to as effectors, and regenerate whole plants from transformed cells. In general, genome editing is performed using three strategies: the stable integration of SDNs, transient SDN expression, or transgene-free delivery of SDNs.

60.2.6.1 Stable integration of site-directed nucleases

Where stable integration of the editing components is required, the most commonly used delivery methods are *PEG-* or *Agrobacterium-mediated* transformation and particle bombardment (biolistics). PEG-mediated delivery of SDNs has been successfully performed in protoplasts of several crop species with high frequency. The efficiency of protoplast transformation depends on the tissue from which the cells were harvested, the plant species, or even the cultivar. In those cases where plants can be regenerated from protoplasts, SDNs are not integrated into the plant genome as they are expressed transiently and are degraded through the action of cellular enzymes.[1] For many important crops, the main drawback of the method is the difficulty to regenerate whole plants from the transformed protoplasts.[22] However, in those cases where regeneration has been possible, the regenerated plants inherit mutations in a Mendelian fashion.[25] Because of the drawbacks associated with protoplast transformation, *Agrobacterium-* or biolistic-mediated delivery of editors are the most commonly used methods. In general, *Agrobacterium*-mediated transformation is preferable as it frequently results in low-copy number insertions and enables the integration of transgenes at unlinked Mendelian loci.[26] A disadvantage of the *Agrobacterium*-mediated delivery system is that the host plant genome may contain not only the DNA sequences encoding the programmable nuclease but also marker genes and sequences of the tumor-inducing (Ti) plasmid. However, for sexually reproducing plants, as DSB and the site(s) of integration of the SDN constructs are most likely unlinked, they can be segregated away by backcrossing.[1] SDN delivery by biolistics has the advantage, relative to *Agrobacterium*-mediated transformation, of the SDN editors being delivered without the exogenous DNA material. The method results in multicopy integration of transgene(s), and also, its successful use depends on the type of explants used. For example, the regeneration of whole plants from the transformed calli is not without problems, as callus-based transformation methods often result in chimeric tissues comprising genome-edited and nonedited cells.[25]

In the case of SDN-2 and SDN-3 applications, the nuclease construct must be delivered simultaneously with the DNA repair template that is to be integrated into the target chromosomal site. Delivery of the repair templates can be achieved through incoming T-DNA from A. tumefaciens, transfected plasmids, biolistics, or viral replicons. It has also been demonstrated that donor DNA stably integrated into the plant genome can be excised in vivo with SDNs and serve as a template for *in planta* GT.[27] Other SDN delivery methods include floral-dip (see Section 60.7), nanoparticle-mediated delivery and pollen magnetofection–mediated delivery. To date, the floral-dip method is limited to the transformation of a few plant species only due to limitations in flower and seed formation.[28]

However, the problem with template delivery is that the frequencies of successful integration into the target locus are extremely low as NHEJ is the predominant pathway for transgene integration. Several strategies have been employed to tilt the balance between NHEJ and HR in favor of the latter. These include repression of NHEJ factors, the application of geminivirus replicons as GT vectors for HR,[29] and biolistics to deliver high amounts of repair template.[22]

60.2.6.2 Transient gene expression of nuclease editors

It is possible to deliver the SDN components into the plant cells by transfecting protoplasts with plasmids carrying the

DNA coding sequences of these components, thus avoiding the integration of exogenous DNA into the recipient genome. Alternatively, the transient expression can be achieved by vacuum infiltration[5] (see Section 60.7). The method is not flawless, and unintended insertions of exogenous DNA have been observed in the cut site.[30] Nonintegrating plasmids have also been used as vehicles for nuclease delivery. However, these plasmids are degraded by endogenous nucleases, and the resulting small DNA fragments can be inserted into the host cells.[31]

60.2.6.3 Transgene-free genome editing

ODM is an example of a transgene-free process as no stable or transient expression system is needed to deliver the oligonucleotide into the recipient plant cell. For SDN applications, the introduction of nuclease-containing vectors into the host plant genome greatly increases the risk of off-target effects, making phenotypic stability a concern. Several strategies have been adopted to remove foreign DNA insertions from the recipient plant genome. As mentioned earlier, SDN-1 applications in sexually propagated plants, even in the cases where SDN constructs and marker genes are integrated into chromosomes, are unlinked to the site of DSB and, therefore, can be segregated by backcrossing.[32]

Another strategy to obtain transgene-free plants is to deliver the components of the editing systems as purified protein or mRNA.[33] Transgene-free plants have been obtained in this way in proof-of-concept studies. Protoplast fusion, electroporation, and in a few cases biolistics, were used to deliver the purified SDNs.[34] An example of a strategy to generate transgene-free plants involves using a pair of suicide transgenes that effectively kill all of the nuclease-containing pollen and embryos produced by T0 plants. This strategy virtually eliminates the nuclease transgenes in all the T1 plants and reduces drastically the time needed to identify transgene-free plants having the targeted mutations generated from the action of the nuclease.[35] An *in planta* GT technology provides another promising way to remove exogenous DNA. It relies on a stably integrated T-DNA harboring a site-specific nuclease and a GT repair template that could be inserted into the plant genome via its homologous regions. Expression of the nuclease induces the simultaneous excision of the GT repair template from the donor molecule and the activation of the target site for somatic HR. As GT events occur during the whole life cycle of the plant, these eventually enter the germline and can be harvested as seeds in the next generation. Another advantage of this *in planta* technology is that it is, in principle, amenable even for crops that are recalcitrant to efficient transformation and regeneration.[22,36]

60.3 *Cis*-genesis and *intra*-genesis

In *cis*-genesis, a plant is transformed with a coding DNA sequence (CDS), including its promoter and terminator regions, derived from the same plant species or closely related species capable of sexual hybridization. In *intra*-genesis, the transformation may involve new gene combinations generated by in vitro rearrangements of functional elements originating from the recipient plant species or sexually compatible species.[37] The DNA sequences comprising *cis*-genes and *intra*-genes originate from the traditional plant breeders' gene pool.

These techniques offer significant advantages over conventional plant breeding. For example, while it took almost 50 years to introgress a single late blight resistance (R) gene into potato cultivars employing conventional breeding, *cis*-genic potato varieties with broad-spectrum resistance to the late blight fungus *Phytophthora infestans* were obtained in less than 10 years.[38]

60.4 Transgrafting

Grafting is a common technique used in horticulture and fruit-bearing trees. It is commonly used to improve fruit quality and resistance to biological stressors. It involves the joining of two severed plant segments together, usually a scion and a rootstock. Healing of the wound produces a chimeric plant. The scion and the stock need to be compatible, and grafts of different species within the same genus can form viable chimaeras. Root-scion interactions, mediated by hormonal signaling, influence the grafted plant's phenotype and may alter physiological and morphological features. It was shown that in grafting sexually incompatible species, complete chloroplast genomes could translocate short distances across the graft site from one species into another, suggesting that grafting may lead to asexual speciation.[39] Heritable phenotypic variation may result as a consequence of grafting through epigenetic modifications. Other graft transmissible sequences include miRNAs that have been shown to silence the expression of one or more genes, as well as protein-coding mRNAs, which may also play an essential role in cell signaling.[40]

Recently, the technique has been applied to graft a non-GM wild-type scion onto a grapevine GM-rootstock resistant to an insect-transmitted bacterial disease caused by *Xylella fastidiosa (Xf)* (Pierce's disease). While the DNA in the fruit is unchanged, it is resistant to Pierce's disease.[41] The acquired protection is derived through the production of proteins in the scion adjusted by the rootstock.

60.5 RNA-directed DNA Methylation (RdDM)

RdDM can be used to improve a wide variety of plant traits such as tolerance to biotic and abiotic stresses, nutritional quality, or longer shelf life without altering the plant's genetic material. In plants, RdDM is the primary small RNA–mediated pathway regulating several transcriptional processes, leading to transgenerational epigenetic effects on gene expression and phenotype.[42,43] In plant breeding, the technique relies on introducing short double-stranded RNA molecules (dsRNA) that are homologous to the target chromosomal site of the plant genome. The dsRNA molecules are recognized by the plant's natural defense system, which recruits a ribonuclease III enzyme (Dicer) that processes dsRNA into small interfering RNAs (siRNAs). The latter induce epigenetic changes at the target site through DNA methylation resulting in transcriptional gene silencing. The production of dsRNA into the plant is achieved either through transfection with a plant virus engineered to produce a particular dsRNA or by introducing a transgene coding for it. In the case of virus-induced gene silencing (VIGS), the virus's genetic material containing the sequences for the production of dsRNA is lost during meiosis. If dsRNA is introduced using a transgene, the latter is removed by backcrossing. The methylation pattern, and thus the desired trait, can be maintained for several generations following the elimination of the inserted genes. The duration of the induced epigenetic changes cannot be predicted as these may gradually be lost.

60.6 Reverse breeding

In conventional plant breeding, elite hybrids are obtained by crossing homozygous parental lines (forward breeding). The hybrid (F1) progeny are usually more robust or vigorous than their homozygous parents due to a phenomenon known as hybrid vigor or heterosis. The exploitation of heterosis in crop plants is considered one of the landmark innovations in modern agriculture and is of outstanding economic importance. The degree of heterosis is calculated as the difference in the phenotypic performance of a trait between a hybrid and the average of its two distinct parents. Despite the importance of heterosis in modern agriculture, the poor understanding of the underlying driving mechanisms confounds the optimization of breeding programs. Despite the introduction of new tools to assist the development of elite hybrids, the process is laborious and time-consuming as it is difficult to predict which parental lines will give the best progeny.

Furthermore, classical heterozygous hybrids cannot be stably maintained due to meiotic recombination. Therefore one of the most significant challenges in plant breeding is developing methods to preserve heterozygous genotypes. Reverse breeding provides an alternative strategy intended to generate populations with high levels of heterozygosity and random variation and enable homozygous parental lines from any heterozygous plant. When mated, these parental homozygous lines can perfectly reconstitute the selected heterozygous plant and can thus be propagated indefinitely.[44] The underlying process of reverse breeding is depicted in Fig. 60.3. The first stage of the process involves integrating an RNA interference construct into one of the chromosomes of a chosen elite plant. This suppresses the genes involved in the meiotic recombination process (achiasmatic meiosis).[44] The intermediate transgenic plants are backcrossed to generate plants free of transgenic sequences, known as null segregants. This stage is followed by the regeneration of the plants from the transformed cells. Doubled haploid plants can be obtained from unfertilized ovules (gynecogenesis) or microspore and anther cultures (androgenesis) resulting from achiasmatic meiosis. The diploid microspores can develop into embryos and subsequently into homozygous plants. The latter constitute the homozygous parental lines. Doubled haploids can then be crossed to obtain nontransgenic heterozygous plants. Marker-assisted selection can be used to speed up the overall RB process.

60.7 Agroinfiltration

Agroinfiltration allows the delivery of exogenous DNA into the intercellular space of plant tissue, usually the leaf, using different application-specific protocols. The main ones are discussed below.

Syringe agroinfiltration. This is the most popular method as it does not require specialized equipment and is flexible enough to allow the infiltration into different areas of the leaf of one target T-DNA construct or several. As the name implies, a syringe is used to inject the infiltration medium into a small nick in the epidermis on the leaf's underside. The transient expression of the exogenous DNA results in high levels of recombinant proteins, which can be recovered from the plant tissue within 1–2 weeks after the infiltration. The technique is amenable for a broad range of applications, including plant interactions with biotic and abiotic stressors, gene expression assays, and protein localization and function.[45]

Vacuum agroinfiltration. In this variant of the method, a vacuum chamber is used containing the plant leaves and the infiltration medium of the *Agrobacterium* strain that harbors the target T-DNA. A negative atmospheric pressure applied to the vacuum chamber draws air from the submerged leaves' interstitial spaces. Releasing the vacuum allows *Agrobacterium* to infiltrate the empty interstitial space. Although relatively demanding in technical terms, the technique is much more scalable and allows

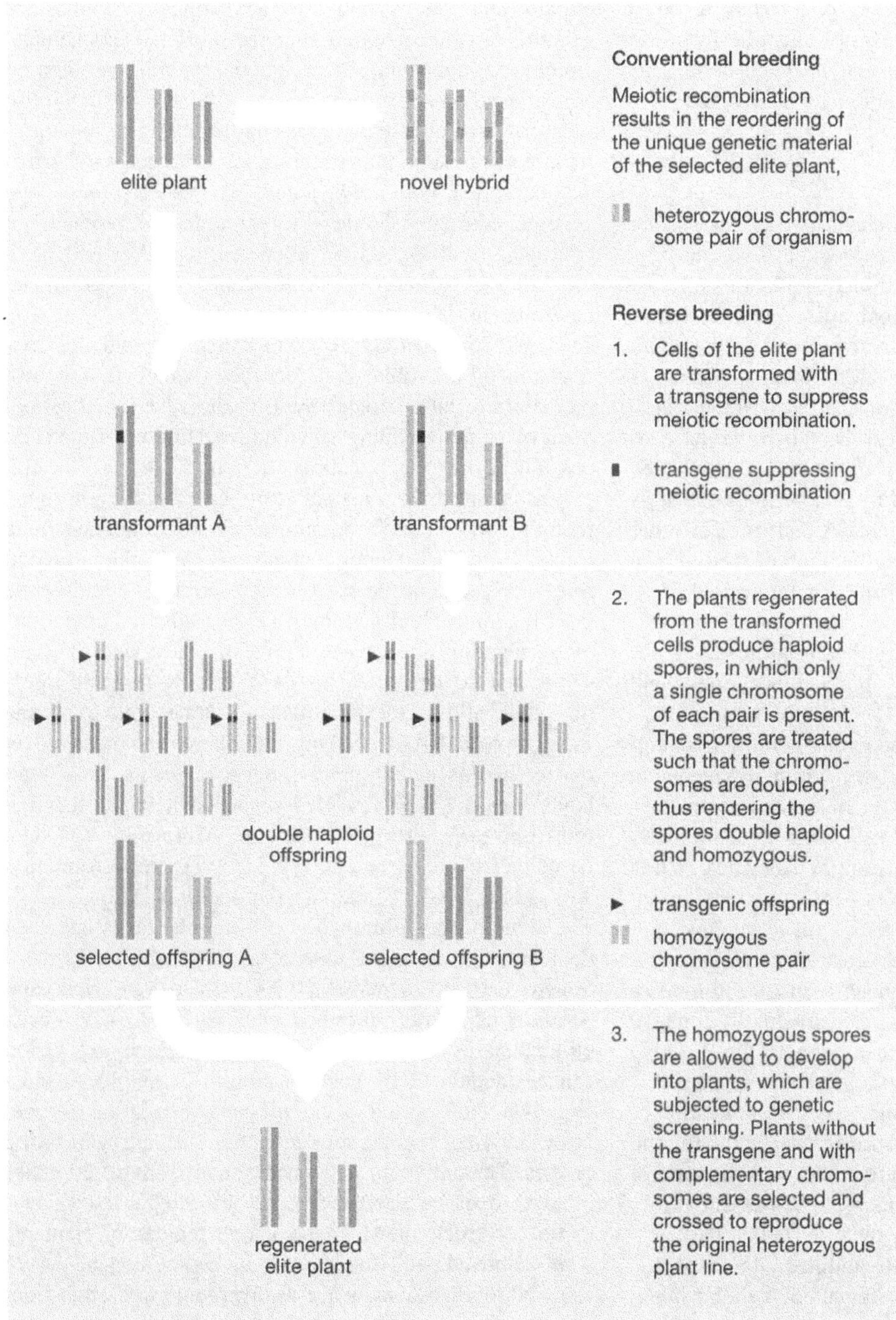

FIGURE 60.3 Schematic representation of the reverse breeding procedure.

functional analysis of genes of plant species that are not amenable to syringe infiltration. For example, RNA virus–based vectors providing RNA interference capability of regulating gene expression via the VIGS technology have been used to introduce desired traits into grapevine without heritable modifications to the genome.[46]

Floral dip. Unlike the other infiltration methods, floral dip results in heritable changes in the plant genome. Limited initially to the transformation of plants of the Brassicaceae family, the method has been demonstrated to work for a small number of other plants.[47] In this method, germline tissues, typically flowers or inflorescences, are immersed in the infiltration medium containing the *Agrobacterium* carrying the target DNA. Transformed embryos are selected at the germination state and grown into mature plants. The method appears to apply to those plants that allow *Agrobacterium* to colonize the interior of developing ovaries and transform the female gametophyte cell lineages. As no plant tissue culture is required, somaclonal variation can be avoided.[48]

60.8 Synthetic biology

Since ancient times, the yeast *Saccharomyces cerevisiae* has been used as a cell factory to produce food and beverages. Apart from these traditional applications, yeast has been used in biofuels and biochemicals and the heterologous expression of proteins. Another cell factory with a long track record in research and industry is *Escherichia coli*. Other production platforms for biotechnological processes have emerged. They involve the evolutionary optimization or random mutagenesis of selected microbial species based on performance criteria, such as yield and response to environmental stressors. Yet other approaches have relied on the modification of well-known species such that they are optimized to meet desired product and bioprocess conditions. In most cases, species-specific constraints hinder further optimization of microbial hosts from meeting productivity and yield objectives.[49]

The recent advances in the so-called "omics" technologies, systems biology, next-generation sequencing (NGS), and genome editing have rekindled interest in designing and assembling novel cell factories using metabolic engineering and synthetic biology (SynBio). While metabolic engineering involves the redirection or enhancement of cellular metabolism, SynBio applies engineering principles to design and construct biological systems. Metabolic engineering can be seen as a top-down approach to retrofitting cellular metabolism. In contrast, SynBio is a bottom-up approach aiming at the de novo assembly of individual parts into a synthetic living cell.[50] A more formal definition of SynBio is "the application of science, technology and engineering to facilitate and accelerate the design, manufacture and/or modification of genetic materials in viable organisms."[51] An essential prerequisite for tailor-made cellular factories is that they possess engineered functions streamlined for specific applications. These differently "formatted" cellular hosts, or "chassis," can be defined as "the physical, metabolic and regulatory containment for plugging-in and plugging-out dedicated genetic circuits and regulatory devices."[52] The construction and engineering of the chassis may follow a top-down approach involving a combination of computational systems analysis, experimental data, and models regarding metabolic, regulatory, and signal networks to identify genes that are essential for cellular life. The chassis is then constructed by removing nonessential genes. Alternatively, a bottom-up strategy may be followed. Such an approach involves the in silico design of circuits and the assembly of a chemically synthesized genome capable of expressing the designed biochemical circuitry components. The synthetic genome can then be transplanted into an appropriate cellular host.[53] SynBio relies on several research areas and enabling technologies such as (1) genetic part libraries, (2) *protocells* and artificial cells, (3) *xenobiology*, and (4) DNA synthesis and genome editing.[54] Some early commercial products of microbial SynBio include artemisin, vanillin, and algal oil, all of which were developed in a contained environment.[55]

Applications of SynBio can extend beyond the construction of microbial cell factories. Although it is still premature to talk of plant SynBio, the advent and refinement of genome editing techniques enable us to envision possible SynBio applications in plants. Indeed, several projects point this way, such as projects targeting nitrogen fixation in cereals[56] or improving the photosynthetic capacity of rice.[57] Genome engineering can play a pivotal role in SynBio projects by engineering (1) multigenic insertions into plant genomes, (2) genomic manipulations by elimination or reprogramming of genes, and (3) transcriptional control of metabolic fluxes. Multigenic insertions that allow "mix-and-match," on-demand transgene integration and trait stacking have been demonstrated in maize. In this technique, a sequence serving as a "trait landing pad" (TLP) is added such that it flanks the first transgene targeted by the nuclease. More traits can then be delivered precisely into the TLP via cotransformation with donor DNAs containing the additional transgenes.[58] The simultaneous elimination of multiple genes has been demonstrated, as in the case of alpha-gliadin genes mentioned earlier (Section 60.2.4). Also, in rice and *Arabidopsis*, large chromosomal segments have been eliminated by multiplex technology.[59] Gene expression can be modulated by genome editing of multigene clusters, as in the example of the *nif* genes regulating nitrogenase activity which are essential in nitrogen-fixing cereals. The native *nif* gene cluster consisting of 20 genes in seven operons was "refactored" by using a totally synthetic construct, in which all native regulatory elements were removed, and the codons of essential genes were changed to a DNA sequence as divergent as possible from the wild-type gene.[56] A comprehensive review of potential applications of genome editing for plant SynBio is given in Baltes et al.[60]

60.9 Safety assessment considerations

60.9.1 Genome editing applications

Consideration of the safety of SDN-derived products should take into account (1) the presence or absence of exogenous DNA sequences and (2) the novelty of the resulting phenotype. Based on the operational definition of SDN (Section 60.2.3), SDN-3 is intended to introduce functional genes much like *cis*- and *intra*-genesis or transgenesis. In this regard, it is logical to expect that the premarket safety assessment of SDN-3 derived products will follow the procedures described in Chapter 62. However, it is recognized that because the inserted DNA sequences are directed to a predefined region in the host plant's chromosome, hazards associated with the disruption of genes, and/or regulatory elements in the host plant genome will be minimized in relation to those caused by cGE.[1,8,61]

SDN-1 and SDN-2 applications result, respectively, in random or predicted mutations at targeted genomic loci. Site-directed mutagenesis can be achieved by (1) the stable integration of the nuclease into the plant genome in tandem with a selectable marker to facilitate the identification of transformants, (2) the transient expression of the nuclease, and (3) DNA-free methods. ODM, much like SDN-2, results in targeted modifications at specific loci, but unlike SDN-2, it is delivered to the host plant without any stable or transient expression system. In those events where exogenous DNA is stably integrated into the plant genome, unwanted DNA sequences may be segregated away during backcrossing. Although this is possible for sexually reproducing plants, it may not be possible in perennial and vegetatively propagated plants.[62] In such cases, the edited plant may be considered to be transgenic, and its safety assessment may be conducted according to the procedures described in Chapter 62. SDN-1 and SDN-2 modifications effected through transient expression or DNA-free nuclease delivery methods may also result in the unintended integration of exogenous DNA sequences. Molecular characterization conducted as part of the risk assessment process can identify potential hazards from the unintentional integration of exogenous DNA sequences (Chapter 62, Section 2).

It is too early to anticipate or even consider risks associated with SynBio. This is because risks related to a particular application may not be relevant for another application with different design objectives. However, in terms of SynBio-derived products, toxicity and allergenicity will remain the focus of risk assessment, and consequently, the established risk assessment methods are adequate.[63]

The possibility of unintended off-target genomic modifications has been brought into the focus of the risk assessment of SDN products. Significant research effort has been dedicated to assessing the frequency of occurrence of such events.[23] Different types of unintended effects associated with genome editing are reviewed in recent literature.[64,65] Off-target mutations occur because SDN modifications are not entirely precise and can result in unintended genomic changes. Cleavage at off-target sites followed by indel formation with NHEJ may result in gene inactivation or mutation. Chromosomal rearrangements (chromosomal deletion and inversion or chromosomal translocation) are also known to occur due to multiple concomitant cleavages. All of the above are also known to occur as a result of natural recombination processes, conventional breeding, and mutagenesis programs, and therefore "unintended" does not necessarily mean "harmful." Factors that affect off-target changes include[66]:

1. The presence of homologous sequences at genomic sites other than the targeted one. Such off-target sequences can be identified with available bioinformatics tools.
2. The levels of nuclease expression increase the probability of off-target DSBs. Nuclease expression can be downregulated by reducing the input of the nuclease expression vector.
3. Duration of exposure to the nuclease. Transient gene expression of the nuclease or DNA-free delivery decreases the time of exposure.
4. Target site accessibility. The epigenetic status of off-target loci affects the accessibility to nuclease cleavage.

Several biased and unbiased methods are available for the identification of off-target sites. Biased methods depend predominantly on bioinformatics tools, whereas the unbiased methods follow in vitro off-target site screening. Some biased methods relying on bioinformatics tools are described in recent publications.[67,68] The precision of biased methods is compromised by the inability to predict the effects of single mismatches and the dependence of the cleavage frequency on genomic and epigenomic factors. Consequently, these methods have to be complemented with unbiased ones.[67] These are described in Martin et al.[67] and Yee[66] and references therein and are summarized in Table 60.3.

Mitigation of unintended effects can be achieved with a variety of methods. For example, as the specificity of the CRISPR/Cas system depends on the availability of appropriate PAM motifs, alterations of either the PAM motif or length of the sgRNA have a dramatic effect on the system's ability to generate DSBs. There are numerous CRISPR design tools enabling selecting appropriate functionalities to minimize off-target effects.[12] Likewise, off-target effects can be reduced by orders of magnitude using truncated sgRNAs or in combination with mutated nickase Cas9.[75] Reducing the duration of exposure to the nuclease and, thus, the possibility of unintended effects can be achieved by delivering preassembled Cas9 protein-sgRNA ribonucleoproteins or controlling the transgene copy numbers to moderate concentration of sgRNA.[12] Another strategy to reduce the frequency of off-target

TABLE 60.3 Unbiased strategies for off-target site detection.

Strategy	Underlying methods
Integration defective lentiviral vector (IDLV)	Uses IDLV to mark DSBs, which are then mapped by nonrestrictive linear amplification–mediated PCR (nrLAM-PCR)[69]
Genome-wide, unbiased identification of DSBs enabled by sequencing (GUIDE-seq)	Based on NHEJ-mediated capture of double-stranded oligodeoxynucleotides (dsODNs) by DSBs. The dsODNs and their flanking sequences are amplified by PCR and subjected to high-throughput sequencing[70]
Chromatin mmunoprecipitation sequencing (ChIP-seq)	Chromatin immunoprecipitation and high-throughput genome sequencing (ChIP-seq) can identify well-defined regions for target and off-target binding[71]
High-throughput genome-wide translocation sequencing (HTGTS)	HTGTS relies on chromosomal translocations between DSBs at on- and off-target sites, which are then captured by LAM-PCR[72]
Breaks labeling, enrichment on streptavidin and next-generation sequencing (BLESS)	Direct in situ BLESS involves the direct ligation of a biotin-labeled proximal linker to DSBs generated during genomic DNA extraction[73]
Digenome-seq	Digested whole-genome sequencing is based on identifying indels formed in vitro at off-target sites employing nuclease digestion of the purified genomic DNA[74]

DSB, Double-stranded break; *NHEJ*, nonhomologous end-joining; *PCR*, polymerase chain reaction.

mutations is the directed insertion of the nuclease *cassette* into predetermined plant genomic safe harbors (GSHs).[76] GSHs are chromosomal regions in which transgenes can be inserted without disruption of the host organism genome. The insertion of a carotenoid biosynthesis cassette in two GSHs of marker-free rice plants has been achieved without detectable penalty in morphology or yield. Whole-genome sequencing (WGS) has confirmed the absence of off-target mutations.[77]

NGS has shown that plant species populations carry millions of SNPs and many copy and structural variants. The rate of spontaneous mutations has been estimated to be $\sim 10^{-8}$ to 10^{-9} per site per generation. Much higher mutation rates occur due to physical or chemical mutagenesis.[78] In genome editing technologies, off-target changes are of the same type and occur with less frequency than those produced by recombinant DNA (rDNA) techniques.[63,79]

60.9.2 Other new genetic modification applications

Biosafety issues related to plants and products derived using the other nGM technologies are summarized below.

60.9.2.1 *Cis*-genesis and *intra*-genesis

In terms of safety assessment of *cis*- and *intra*-genic plants and products, the methodology presented in Chapter 62 is applicable. A scientific opinion of the EFSA Panel on GMOs concluded that the potential hazards associated with conventional breeding and *cis*-genesis are similar. At the same time, *intra*-genesis may give rise to novel hazards due to new combinations of genetic elements. In terms of potential unintended effects, conventional breeding, *cis*- and *intra*-genesis were deemed likely to give rise to effects of variable frequency and severity. While the methodology described in Chapter 62 is appropriate for the safety assessment of *cis*- and *intra*-genic plants and products, they should be assessed case-by-case.[61]

60.9.2.2 Transgrafting

Two distinct outcomes are possible depending on whether (1) a GM scion is grafted onto a non-GM rootstock or (2) a non-GM scion is grafted onto a GM rootstock. Although it has been argued that both outcomes result in GM plants, there is no scientific consensus on this point. In the EU, while the chimeric plant resulting from the grafting of a non-GM scion onto a GM rootstock is captured under the regulations of GMOs, the products of this grafting process are considered to be GMO-free. Issues that may be relevant for risk assessment relate to unintended effects on the scion physiology or nontarget organisms resulting from the movement of gene products through the graft union.

60.9.2.3 RNA-directed DNA methylation (RdDM)

The regulatory status of RdDM-derived plants may depend on the following factors. Insertion of a gene template encoding dsRNA by direct or vector-mediated techniques that is stably integrated and inherited in the next generation could result in plants considered to be GMOs. However, if gene expression within the cell occurs transiently (a few days, at most) and the template is degraded, the changed methylation pattern is transmitted to progeny even if the transgene that induced the methylation is deleted or segregated out. The only factor determining whether an RdDM-derived plant is transgenic or not is the possible genomic integration of RNA or vector sequences by reverse transcription.[80] For such plants, the regulatory status of RdDM plants would depend on whether the GMO definition applies to the intermediate organisms or the final product. In some cases, the introduction of rDNA molecules can be avoided altogether by spraying purified siRNA molecules on plant leaves.

60.9.2.4 Reverse breeding

The breeding outcomes of this technique are the same as those obtained from conventional breeding. Although the intermediate plants contain transgenic sequences used to suppress meiosis, these are backcrossed out to generate null segregants. The resulting homozygous parental cell lines and their offspring are non-GM.

60.9.2.5 Agroinfiltration

The offspring of plants produced by syringe and vacuum agroinfection are free of foreign DNA and, therefore, may not be subject to regulations that require "a stable integration event" be detected, as is the case of the EU Directive 2001/18/EC. As the progeny of these plants are free of transgenes and vector sequences, they cannot be considered to be GMOs. Furthermore, the infiltration area and any inserted T-DNA are likely to be lost through natural senescence. However, due to the presence of recombinant bacterial or viral vectors in the plant tissues, these plants may be considered to be "containers" of GM microorganisms and, therefore, fall under the purview of relevant regulations [e.g., EU Directive 2009/41/EC (Annex I, Part A)]. The floral dip method may give rise to transgenic plants, in which case GMO regulations would apply.

60.9.3 The regulatory context

To date, very few nGM products have obtained market or field-testing approvals (Table 60.4). To an extent, this reflects the lack of competency of current safety regulations to deal with such products. In many countries, regulatory authorities are faced with the conundrum of applying GMO regulations to assess the safety of products developed by means of nGMs. For example, the *Cartagena Protocol* defines *LMOs* as organisms deemed to possess novel combinations of genetic material. Similarly, in EU regulations, a GMO is defined as an organism whose "genetic material has been altered in a way that does not occur naturally by mating and/or natural recombination." In the case of plants developed by SDN-1, SDN-2, ODM, and RB applications, it is not apparent what types of combinations of genetic material these plants must possess in order to be considered "genetically novel." Point mutations occur spontaneously and, together with natural selection, are vital drivers of evolution. Crop domestication has been driven by combinations of many different types of mutagenic events, including not only point mutations but also gene rearrangements, DNA deletions, and transposon insertions, to name but a few. Many of these events could not have occurred without human intervention.

Furthermore, "omics" techniques have shown that species barriers are permeable and horizontal gene transfer has been shown to occur in nature, even between kingdoms. nGM plant products that lack exogenous DNA represent genotypes and phenotypes that are indistinguishable from plant variation that arises from natural or conventional breeding processes. At a practical level, this raises the question of whether the available detection and identification methods have the appropriate resolution to distinguish nGM products from counterparts developed using rDNA or conventional breeding technologies (see Section 60.10).

The shortcomings of GMO regulations to deal with nGM-derived products have prompted several countries to update their legal interpretation of GMO regulations. For example, Latin American countries, including Argentina, Brazil, Chile, and Colombia, have passed normative resolutions which allow regulatory authorities to assess nGM products on a case-by-case basis.[34] Other countries have adopted or are in the process of adopting different approaches. In Canada, providing that a given plant-trait combination has a history of safe use, it is exempted from regulation. In the United States, no planting permits are required for plants that are shown to be devoid of potential risk factors, such as exogenous DNA from plant pathogens. In Japan, SDN-1 and SDN-2 derived plants are regulated in the same manner as conventionally bred varieties. Some other countries consider the deregulation of plants developed by SDN-1 and SDN-2 applications.[82] India's planned legislation proposes a tiered approach grouping products based on risk. Low-risk products would include SDN-1 and SDN-2 plants, whereas high-risk plants would be those whose genomes contain large DNA insertions or exogenous DNA. However, according to the proposal, even low-risk products would require a compositional assessment and complete molecular and phenotypic characterization, agronomic equivalence, and, potentially, environmental safety assessments.[82] A point to be made is that excessive data requirements for the safety assessment of genome-edited products can

TABLE 60.4 Regulatory status of food crop varieties developed by nGM techniques.[81]

nGM	Developer	Crop	Trait	Status (year). Regulator
Transgrafting	National Institute for Agricultural Research (INRA), France	Grapevine	Resistance to grapevine fanleaf virus	Field-trial approval (2010). French Ministry of Agriculture, Biomolecular Engineering Commission
*Cis-, intra-*genesis	University of Florida	Grapevine	Red color in seed berries	Nonregulated. Nonplant pest (2012). USDA APHIS
Cis-genesis	Wageningen University	Apple	Scab resistance	May be regulated. Plant pest vector used (2012). USDA APHIS
ODM	Cibus Canada	Canola	Imidazolinone and sulfonylurea herbicide tolerance	Approved for food and feed use. Confined release (2013). Health Canada, Canadian Food Inspection Agency
ZFN	Dow AgroSciences	Maise	Reduced phytate production	Nonregulated. Nonplant pest. Null segregant (2012). USDA APHIS
TALEN	Cellectis Plant Sciences	Soybean[a]	High oleic acid	Nonregulated. Nonplant, nonnoxious weed. Null segregant (2015). USDA APHIS
TALEN	Cellectis Plant Sciences	Soybean[b]	High oleic acid	Nonregulated. Nonplant, nonnoxious weed. Null segregant (2015). USDA APHIS
TALEN	Iowa State University	Rice	Disease resistance	Nonregulated. Nonplant, nonnoxious weed. Null segregant (2015). USDA APHIS
TALEN	Calyxt	Wheat	Powdery mildew resistance	Nonregulated. Nonplant, nonnoxious weed. Null segregant (2016). USDA APHIS

nGM, New genetic modification; *NHEJ*, nonhomologous end-joining; *ODM*, oligonucleotide-directed mutagenesis; *TALEN*, transcription activator-like effector nuclease; *USDA APHIS*, US Department of Agriculture Animal and Plant Health Inspection Service; *ZFN*, zinc-finger nucleases.
[a]*FAD2-1A and FAD2-1B knockouts via NHEJ.*
[b]*FAD3 knockout via NHEJ.*

be as discouraging as overly restrictive regulations. Furthermore, regulatory requirements for excessive safety assessment tests impose a cost burden that discourages all but the larger agri-food companies from being involved in the forefront of agricultural innovations.[83]

In summary, country regulations cover a spectrum that extends from the deregulation of SDN-1 and SDN-2 to partial deregulation based on case-by-case assessment to regulation of genome-edited plants as GMOs. Furthermore, unless there is some harmonization concerning the diverse legal definitions and interpretations for genome-edited plants, trade barriers to agri-food commodities will be unavoidable.[34]

60.10 Detection and identification

Detection refers to analytical techniques used to investigate the differences between the original and modified plants. The most amenable techniques for analyzing the targeted chromosomal locus are based on DNA amplification and DNA sequencing. Other techniques such as hybridization assays and protein and metabolite analysis methods can also be used, but their applicability is limited. Identification refers to techniques that ascertain whether an end product is the outcome of an nGM or conventional breeding process.

60.10.1 DNA amplification

The most common detection method is PCR. An absolute prerequisite for applying PCR is knowledge of the exact DNA sequence at the chromosomal site that is being investigated. This is because PCR uses primers made of oligonucleotides complementary to the target sequence and a polymerase for DNA amplification. Short sequence changes resulting from the SDN-1, SDN-2, and ODN processes are detectable by using specific probes for real-time or digital PCR.[84] For point mutations, such as SNPs, genotypic approaches can be used subject to the availability of an appropriate reference sequence.[85]

60.10.2 DNA sequencing

WGS methods have been used for GMO detection and can be extended to genome-edited plants. WGS does not require prior information on the target sequence and can be applied to detect unknown genomic changes. Very large genomes and the presence of many repetitive sequences, as in the case of allopolyploid plants, render WGS impractical in many cases. NGS is well suited for GMO analysis and appropriately adapted may be used for genome-edited plants. Unlike WGS, which is used for untargeted detection, NGS is targeted to specific genomic sites and therefore relies on the availability of a reference sequence from the parental plant.

60.10.3 Other analysis methods

Southern blots and DNA microarrays may be appropriate for detecting transgenes and integrated exogenous DNA, but they are unsuitable for changes induced by SDN-1, SDN-2, and ODN.[86] ELISA immunoassays and mass spectrometry have been used to detect GMOs and could potentially be applied for SDN-3 modifications but not SDN-1, SDN-2, and ODN. Metabolic profiling of genome-edited plants by mass spectrometry or NMR is possible but of limited value. This is because the detected difference in metabolic profiles is determined by environmental conditions and the type of matrix from which the analytes were extracted. Generally, detection techniques based on RNA, protein, and metabolic content show significant variance in concentrations depending on the respective tissue (embryo, meristem, endosperm) of the plant under consideration.[87]

60.10.4 Identification of the process

Detection techniques allow the comparison of analytes against a reference standard. The limitation of this is that these techniques can only detect what is being looked for. If the genes coding for the gene-editing components are transiently expressed or absent, as in the case of DNA-free plants, it is challenging, if not impossible, to identify the GM process. Using bioinformatics methods to detect SDN-1 and SDN-2 mutations is confounded because such mutations are indistinguishable from those occurring naturally. The same applies to longer indels because chromosomal, segmental substitutions or additions can also result from natural recombination processes. WGS can detect transgenes inserted by means of SDN-3. Even so, WGS genotyping does not allow the identification of individual genotypes in cases of heterogeneous samples. In such cases, WGS has to be conducted separately for several plants.[87] This makes the identification of specific genotypes in commodities demanding, particularly in the light of the ever-increasing number of transgenic events and the types of the introduced structural elements.

60.11 Conclusion and prospects

This chapter has reviewed techniques that are diverse, not only in terms of how they induce genetic variation but also in terms of product characteristics. Grouping nGMs together may not be cogent because the technological implications of the individual technologies vary significantly. Regardless of this, nGMs will broaden the potential of plant breeding programs and lead to significant innovations in the agri-food sector. Genome editing, in particular, is expected to have profound impacts both in research and commercial crop applications. Inevitably, attention has fallen on the safety of nGM products and, mainly, on unintended effects due to the application of these technologies.

However, focusing the risk assessment of nGM products on potential unintended effects may be counterproductive or even futile. Unintended effects are also known to arise from conventional breeding methods (*pleiotropic* or *epistatic* effects, *linkage drag*), from random mutagenesis, or transgenesis (insertional mutations). Equally important, not all unintended effects are harmful. Any biological intervention has unintended consequences, and it is counterproductive to attempt to predict all of them. This is because the focus on unintended effects shifts the attention from evaluating the trait characteristics of a product to the method by which it was produced. Molecular profiling to characterize the presence of foreign DNA in modified plants in conjunction with molecular techniques that increase the precision of genome editing hold the prospect of mitigating undesired outcomes (see Section 60.9). There is little point in basing the risk assessment process on "unintended" mutations when little or nothing is known about their biological relevance.[88] Instead, the emphasis should be on identifying the possible risk sources and biologically meaningful variables (endpoints) that can be measured as a test of a given risk hypothesis. Therefore the data requirements for risk assessment should be matched to the nature and level of the anticipated risks. This requires a paradigm shift toward more flexible safety evaluation procedures. In a case-by-case assessment and depending on the product under evaluation, only a subset of the data required for GMOs may be needed. In other words, the information requirements for risk assessment should be scaled in accordance with the expected risks.[89] Failure to do so may negatively impact innovations that are much needed to improve agricultural productivity, and more importantly, meet the challenges of achieving food security globally.

Glossary

AHAS	Acetohydroxyacid synthase.
Cartagena Protocol	The *Cartagena Protocol on Biosafety to the Convention on Biological Diversity* is an international agreement which aims to ensure the safe handling, transport, and use of living modified organisms (LMOs) resulting from modern biotechnology that may have adverse effects on biological diversity, taking also into account risks to human health. It was adopted on January 29, 2000 and entered into force on September 11, 2003.
Cassette	Usually, an expression cassette. See definition on vector below.
Epistatic	Epistasis is the interaction of nonallelic genes. In particular, the dependence of a gene mutation effect on the presence or absence of mutations in one or more nonallelic genes, known as modifier genes.
Exogenous	DNA or RNA originating outside the plant species that is being modified.
Linkage drag	Genetic linkage describes how two closely associated genes on the same chromosome are frequently inherited together. In plant breeding, "breaking" the linkage drag refers to the separation of a desirable gene affecting trait X from a linked gene that has an undesirable effect on a different trait (Y).
LMO	Living modified organisms.
Null segregant	These are genetically modified organism (GMO)-derived plants that have lost the transgenic event due to segregation during generations of crosses with non-GMO plants (see section on reverse breeding). As a result, null segregants do not contain detectable sequences of the original transgenic event and are therefore indistinguishable from plants obtained through conventional breeding.
PEG	Polyethylene glycol.
Pleiotropic	Refers to the situation in which a particular gene has an effect on several different traits.
Protocell	Refers to the aggregation of self-organizing molecular components, an RNA replicase and lipids forming a fatty acid membrane. They are considered to be the precursors of modern living cells.
rDNA	Recombinant DNA (rDNA) is a technology that uses enzymes to splice together DNA sequences of interest.
Transgene	One or more DNA sequences from species A introduced into species B.
Vector	Vehicles that ferry rDNA into a host cell where it can be copied or expressed. An expression cassette consists of one or more transgenes and the sequences that control their expression.
Xenobiology	Refers to the engineering of biological systems that do not exist in nature, as for example, the synthesis of artificial chromosomes using xeno nucleic acids (XNA). XNA is different from its natural counterparts in a variety of tailor-made structural and chemical changes.

References

1. Songstad DD, Petolino JF, Voytas DF, Reichert NA. Genome editing of plants. *Crit Rev Plant Sci.* 2017;36(1):1–23. Available from: https://doi.org/10.1080/07352689.2017.1281663.
2. Gaj T, Gersbach CA, Barbas 3rd CF, ZFN, TALEN, and CRISPR/Cas-based methods for genome engineering. Trends Biotechnol. 31 (7):397–405. doi:10.1016/j.tibtech.2013.04.004.
3. Weeks DP, Spalding MH, Yang B. Use of designer nucleases for targeted gene and genome editing in plants. *Plant Biotechnol J.* 2016;14(2):483–495. Available from: https://doi.org/10.1111/pbi.12448.
4. Hsu PD, Scott DA, Weinstein JA, et al. DNA targeting specificity of RNA-guided Cas9 nucleases. Nat Biotechnol. 31(9):827–832. doi:10.1038/nbt.2647.
5. Ma X, Zhu Q, Chen Y, Liu YG. CRISPR/Cas9 platforms for genome editing in plants: developments and applications. *Mol Plant.* 2016;9(7):961–974. Available from: https://doi.org/10.1016/j.molp.2016.04.009.
6. Gleditzsch D, Pausch P, Muller-Esparza H, et al. PAM identification by CRISPR-Cas effector complexes: diversified mechanisms and structures. *RNA Biol.* 2019;16(4):504–517. Available from: https://doi.org/10.1080/15476286.2018.1504546.
7. Anzalone AV, Koblan LW, Liu DR. Genome editing with CRISPR-Cas nucleases, base editors, transposases and prime editors. *Nat Biotechnol.* 2020;38(7):824–844. Available from: https://doi.org/10.1038/s41587-020-0561-9.
8. Stoddard BL. Homing endonucleases: from microbial genetic invaders to reagents for targeted DNA modification. *Structure.* 2011;19(1):7–15. Available from: https://doi.org/10.1016/j.str.2010.12.003.
9. Voytas DF. Plant genome engineering with sequence-specific nucleases. *Annu Rev Plant Biol.* 2013;64:327–350. Available from: https://doi.org/10.1146/annurev-arplant-042811-105552.
10. Smith J, Grizot S, Arnould S, et al. A combinatorial approach to create artificial homing endonucleases cleaving chosen sequences. *Nucleic Acids Res.* 2006;34(22):e149. Available from: https://doi.org/10.1093/nar/gkl720.
11. Sauer NJ, Mozoruk J, Miller RB, et al. Oligonucleotide-directed mutagenesis for precision gene editing. *Plant Biotechnol J.* 2016;14(2):496–502. Available from: https://doi.org/10.1111/pbi.12496.
12. Zhao H, Wolt JD. Risk associated with off-target plant genome editing and methods for its limitation. *Emerg Top Life Sci.* 2017;1 (2):231–240. Available from: https://doi.org/10.1042/ETLS20170037.

13. Huang TK, Puchta H. CRISPR/Cas-mediated gene targeting in plants: finally a turn for the better for homologous recombination. *Plant Cell Rep.* 2019;38(4):443–453. Available from: https://doi.org/10.1007/s00299-019-02379-0.
14. Knoll A, Fauser F, Puchta H. DNA recombination in somatic plant cells: mechanisms and evolutionary consequences. *Chromosome Res.* 2014;22(2):191–201. Available from: https://doi.org/10.1007/s10577-014-9415-y.
15. EFSA. Scientific opinion addressing the safety assessment of plants developed using Zinc Finger Nuclease 3 and other Site-Directed Nucleases with similar function. *EFSA J.* 2012;10(10):31.
16. Podevin N, Davies HV, Hartung F, Nogue F, Casacuberta JM. Site-directed nucleases: a paradigm shift in predictable, knowledge-based plant breeding. *Trends Biotechnol.* 2013;31(6):375–383. Available from: https://doi.org/10.1016/j.tibtech.2013.03.004.
17. Pacher M, Puchta H. From classical mutagenesis to nuclease-based breeding – directing natural DNA repair for a natural end-product. *Plant J.* 2017;90(4):819–833. Available from: https://doi.org/10.1111/tpj.13469.
18. van de Wiel CCM, Schaart JG, Lotz LAP, Smulders MJM. New traits in crops produced by genome editing techniques based on deletions. *Plant Biotechnol Rep.* 2017;11(1):1–8. Available from: https://doi.org/10.1007/s11816-017-0425-z.
19. Sanchez-Leon S, Gil-Humanes J, Ozuna CV, et al. Low-gluten, nontransgenic wheat engineered with CRISPR/Cas9. *Plant Biotechnol J.* 2018;16(4):902–910. Available from: https://doi.org/10.1111/pbi.12837.
20. Petolino JF, Kumar S. Transgenic trait deployment using designed nucleases. *Plant Biotechnol J.* 2016;14(2):503–509. Available from: https://doi.org/10.1111/pbi.12457.
21. Ran Y, Patron N, Kay P, et al. Zinc finger nuclease-mediated precision genome editing of an endogenous gene in hexaploid bread wheat (*Triticum aestivum*) using a DNA repair template. *Plant Biotechnol J.* 2018;16(12):2088–2101. Available from: https://doi.org/10.1111/pbi.12941.
22. Wolter F, Puchta H. In planta gene targeting can be enhanced by the use of CRISPR/Cas12a. *Plant J.* 2019;100(5):1083–1094. Available from: https://doi.org/10.1111/tpj.14488.
23. Modrzejewski D, Hartung F, Sprink T, Krause D, Kohl C, Wilhelm R. What is the available evidence for the range of applications of genome-editing as a new tool for plant trait modification and the potential occurrence of associated off-target effects: a systematic map. *Environ Evid.* 2019;8(1):27. Available from: https://doi.org/10.1186/s13750-019-0171-5.
24. Menz J, Modrzejewski D, Hartung F, Wilhelm R, Sprink T. Genome edited crops touch the market: a view on the global development and regulatory environment. *Front Plant Sci.* 2020;11:586027. Available from: https://doi.org/10.3389/fpls.2020.586027.
25. Park J, Choe S. DNA-free genome editing with preassembled CRISPR/Cas9 ribonucleoproteins in plants. *Transgenic Res.* 2019;28(suppl 2):61–64. Available from: https://doi.org/10.1007/s11248-019-00136-3.
26. Vain P. Thirty years of plant transformation technology development. *Plant Biotechnol J.* 2007;5(2):221–229. Available from: https://doi.org/10.1111/j.1467-7652.2006.00225.x.
27. Fauser F, Roth N, Pacher M, et al. In planta gene targeting. *Proc Natl Acad Sci U S A.* 2012;109(19):7535–7540. Available from: https://doi.org/10.1073/pnas.1202191109.
28. Sandhya D, Jogam P, Allini VR, Abbagani S, Alok A. The present and potential future methods for delivering CRISPR/Cas9 components in plants. *J Genet Eng Biotechnol.* 2020;18(1):25. Available from: https://doi.org/10.1186/s43141-020-00036-8.
29. Baltes NJ, Gil-Humanes J, Cermak T, Atkins PA, Voytas DF. DNA replicons for plant genome engineering. *Plant Cell.* 2014;26(1):151–163. Available from: https://doi.org/10.1105/tpc.113.119792.
30. Andersson M, Turesson H, Olsson N, et al. Genome editing in potato via CRISPR-Cas9 ribonucleoprotein delivery. *Physiol Plant.* 2018;164(4):378–384. Available from: https://doi.org/10.1111/ppl.12731.
31. Woo JW, Kim J, Kwon SI, et al. DNA-free genome editing in plants with preassembled CRISPR-Cas9 ribonucleoproteins. *Nat Biotechnol.* 2015;33(11):1162–1164. Available from: https://doi.org/10.1038/nbt.3389.
32. Voytas DF, Gao C. Precision genome engineering and agriculture: opportunities and regulatory challenges. *PLoS Biol.* 2014;12(6):e1001877. Available from: https://doi.org/10.1371/journal.pbio.1001877.
33. Stoddard TJ, Clasen BM, Baltes NJ, et al. Targeted mutagenesis in plant cells through transformation of sequence-specific nuclease mRNA. *PLoS One.* 2016;11(5):e0154634. Available from: https://doi.org/10.1371/journal.pone.0154634.
34. Metje-Sprink J, Menz J, Modrzejewski D, Sprink T. DNA-free genome editing: past, present and future. *Front Plant Sci.* 2018;9:1957. Available from: https://doi.org/10.3389/fpls.2018.01957.
35. He Y, Zhu M, Wang L, et al. Programmed self-elimination of the CRISPR/Cas9 construct greatly accelerates the isolation of edited and transgene-free rice plants. *Mol Plant.* 2018;11(9):1210–1213. Available from: https://doi.org/10.1016/j.molp.2018.05.005.
36. Schiml S, Fauser F, Puchta H. The CRISPR/Cas system can be used as nuclease for in planta gene targeting and as paired nickases for directed mutagenesis in *Arabidopsis* resulting in heritable progeny. *Plant J.* 2014;80(6):1139–1150. Available from: https://doi.org/10.1111/tpj.12704.
37. Schaart JG, van de Wiel CCM, Lotz LAP, Smulders MJM. Opportunities for products of new plant breeding techniques. *Trends Plant Sci.* 2016;21(5):438–449. Available from: https://doi.org/10.1016/j.tplants.2015.11.006.
38. Haverkort AJ, Boonekamp PM, Hutten R, et al. Durable late blight resistance in potato through dynamic varieties obtained by cisgenesis: scientific and societal advances in the DuRPh project. *Potato Res.* 2016;59(1):35–66. Available from: https://doi.org/10.1007/s11540-015-9312-6.
39. Stegemann S, Keuthe M, Greiner S, Bock R. Horizontal transfer of chloroplast genomes between plant species. *Proc Natl Acad Sci U S A.* 2012;109(7):2434–2438. Available from: https://doi.org/10.1073/pnas.1114076109.
40. Wang J, Jiang L, Wu R. Plant grafting: how genetic exchange promotes vascular reconnection. *N Phytol.* 2017;214(1):56–65. Available from: https://doi.org/10.1111/nph.14383.
41. Dandekar AM, Jacobson A, Ibáñez AM, et al. Trans-graft protection against Pierce's disease mediated by transgenic grapevine rootstocks. *Front Plant Sci.* 2019;10:84. Available from: https://doi.org/10.3389/fpls.2019.00084.
42. Matzke MA, Mosher RA. RNA-directed DNA methylation: an epigenetic pathway of increasing complexity. *Nat Rev Genet.* 2014;15(6):394–408. Available from: https://doi.org/10.1038/nrg3683.

43. Erdmann RM, Picard CL. RNA-directed DNA methylation. *PLoS Genet.* 2020;16(10):e1009034. Available from: https://doi.org/10.1371/journal.pgen.1009034.
44. Dirks R, van Dun K, de Snoo CB, et al. Reverse breeding: a novel breeding approach based on engineered meiosis. *Plant Biotechnol J.* 2009;7(9):837–845. Available from: https://doi.org/10.1111/j.1467-7652.2009.00450.x.
45. Chen Q, Lai H, Hurtado J, Stahnke J, Leuzinger K, Dent M. Agroinfiltration as an effective and scalable strategy of gene delivery for production of pharmaceutical proteins. *Adv Tech Biol Med.* 2013;1(1). Available from: https://doi.org/10.4172/atbm.1000103.
46. Kurth EG, Peremyslov VV, Prokhnevsky AI, et al. Virus-derived gene expression and RNA interference vector for grapevine. *J Virol.* 2012;86(11):6002–6009. Available from: https://doi.org/10.1128/JVI.00436-12.
47. Hu D, Bent AF, Hou X, Li Y. Agrobacterium-mediated vacuum infiltration and floral dip transformation of rapid-cycling *Brassica rapa*. *BMC Plant Biol.* 2019;19(1):246. Available from: https://doi.org/10.1186/s12870-019-1843-6.
48. Bent A. *Arabidopsis thaliana* floral dip transformation method. *Methods Mol Biol.* 2006;343:87–103. Available from: https://doi.org/10.1385/1-59745-130-4:87.
49. Kavscek M, Strazar M, Curk T, Natter K, Petrovic U. Yeast as a cell factory: current state and perspectives. *Microb Cell Fact.* 2015;14:94. Available from: https://doi.org/10.1186/s12934-015-0281-x.
50. Jullesson D, David F, Pfleger B, Nielsen J. Impact of synthetic biology and metabolic engineering on industrial production of fine chemicals. *Biotechnol Adv.* 2015;33(7):1395–1402. Available from: https://doi.org/10.1016/j.biotechadv.2015.02.011.
51. EFSA Scientific Committee. Evaluation of existing guidelines for their adequacy for the microbial characterisation and environmental risk assessment of microorganisms obtained through synthetic biology. *EFSA J.* 2020;18(10):50. Available from: https://doi.org/10.2903/j.efsa.2020.6263.
52. Calero P, Nikel PI. Chasing bacterial chassis for metabolic engineering: a perspective review from classical to non-traditional microorganisms. *Microb Biotechnol.* 2019;12(1):98–124. Available from: https://doi.org/10.1111/1751-7915.13292.
53. Chi H, Wang X, Shao Y, et al. Engineering and modification of microbial chassis for systems and synthetic biology. *Synth Syst Biotechnol.* 2019;4(1):25–33. Available from: https://doi.org/10.1016/j.synbio.2018.12.001.
54. Epstein MM, Vermeire T. Scientific opinion on risk assessment of synthetic biology. *Trends Biotechnol.* 2016;34(8):601–603. Available from: https://doi.org/10.1016/j.tibtech.2016.04.013.
55. Robaey Z, Spruit SL, van de Poel I. The food warden: an exploration of issues in distributing responsibilities for safe-by-design synthetic biology applications. *Sci Eng Ethics.* 2018;24(6):1673–1696. Available from: https://doi.org/10.1007/s11948-017-9969-0.
56. Temme K, Zhao D, Voigt CA. Refactoring the nitrogen fixation gene cluster from *Klebsiella oxytoca*. *Proc Natl Acad Sci U S A.* 2012;109(18):7085–7090. Available from: https://doi.org/10.1073/pnas.1120788109.
57. Zhou H, Liu B, Weeks DP, Spalding MH, Yang B. Large chromosomal deletions and heritable small genetic changes induced by CRISPR/Cas9 in rice. *Nucleic Acids Res.* 2014;42(17):10903–10914. Available from: https://doi.org/10.1093/nar/gku806.
58. Ainley WM, Sastry-Dent L, Welter ME, et al. Trait stacking via targeted genome editing. *Plant Biotechnol J.* 2013;11(9):1126–1134. Available from: https://doi.org/10.1111/pbi.12107.
59. Malzahn A, Lowder L, Qi Y. Plant genome editing with TALEN and CRISPR. *Cell Biosci.* 2017;7:21. Available from: https://doi.org/10.1186/s13578-017-0148-4.
60. Baltes NJ, Voytas DF. Enabling plant synthetic biology through genome engineering. *Trends Biotechnol.* 2015;33(2):120–131. Available from: https://doi.org/10.1016/j.tibtech.2014.11.008.
61. EFSA Panel on Genetically Modified Organisms (GMO). Scientific opinion addressing the safety assessment of plants developed through cisgenesis and intragenesis. *EFSA J.* 2012;10(2):33. Available from: https://doi.org/10.2903/j.efsa.2012.2561.
62. Zhang Y, Liang Z, Zong Y, et al. Efficient and transgene-free genome editing in wheat through transient expression of CRISPR/Cas9 DNA or RNA. *Nat Commun.* 2016;7:12617. Available from: https://doi.org/10.1038/ncomms12617.
63. SAM. New techniques in agricultural biotechnology. Explanatory Note of the High Level Group of Scientific Advisors; 2017.
64. Kawall K, Cotter J, Then C. Broadening the GMO risk assessment in the EU for genome editing technologies in agriculture. *Environ Sci Eur.* 2020;32(1):106. Available from: https://doi.org/10.1186/s12302-020-00361-2.
65. Eckerstorfer MF, Dolezel M, Heissenberger A, et al. Corrigendum: an EU perspective on biosafety considerations for plants developed by genome editing and other new genetic modification techniques (nGMs). *Front Bioeng Biotechnol.* 2019;7:90. Available from: https://doi.org/10.3389/fbioe.2019.00090.
66. Yee JK. Off-target effects of engineered nucleases. *FEBS J.* 2016;283(17):3239–3248. Available from: https://doi.org/10.1111/febs.13760.
67. Martin F, Sanchez-Hernandez S, Gutierrez-Guerrero A, Pinedo-Gomez J, Benabdellah K. Biased and unbiased methods for the detection of off-target cleavage by CRISPR/Cas9: an overview. *Int J Mol Sci.* 2016;17(9). Available from: https://doi.org/10.3390/ijms17091507.
68. Hahn F, Nekrasov V. CRISPR/Cas precision: do we need to worry about off-targeting in plants? *Plant Cell Rep.* 2019;38(4):437–441. Available from: https://doi.org/10.1007/s00299-018-2355-9.
69. Wang X, Wang Y, Wu X, et al. Unbiased detection of off-target cleavage by CRISPR-Cas9 and TALENs using integrase-defective lentiviral vectors. *Nat Biotechnol.* 2015;33(2):175–178. Available from: https://doi.org/10.1038/nbt.3127.
70. Tsai SQ, Zheng Z, Nguyen NT, et al. GUIDE-seq enables genome-wide profiling of off-target cleavage by CRISPR-Cas nucleases. *Nat Biotechnol.* 2015;33(2):187–197. Available from: https://doi.org/10.1038/nbt.3117.
71. Muhammad II, Kong SL, Akmar Abdullah SN, Munusamy U. RNA-seq and ChIP-seq as complementary approaches for comprehension of plant transcriptional regulatory mechanism. *Int J Mol Sci.* 2019;21(1). Available from: https://doi.org/10.3390/ijms21010167.
72. Frock RL, Hu J, Meyers RM, Ho YJ, Kii E, Alt FW. Genome-wide detection of DNA double-stranded breaks induced by engineered nucleases. *Nat Biotechnol.* 2015;33(2):179–186. Available from: https://doi.org/10.1038/nbt.3101.
73. Crosetto N, Mitra A, Silva MJ, et al. Nucleotide-resolution DNA double-strand break mapping by next-generation sequencing. *Nat Methods.* 2013;10(4):361–365. Available from: https://doi.org/10.1038/nmeth.2408.

74. Kim D, Bae S, Park J, et al. Digenome-seq: genome-wide profiling of CRISPR-Cas9 off-target effects in human cells. *Nat Methods.* 12 (3):237–243, 1 p following 243. Available from: https://doi.org/10.1038/nmeth.3284.
75. Lozano-Juste J, Cutler SR. Plant genome engineering in full bloom. *Trends Plant Sci.* 2014;19(5):284–287. Available from: https://doi.org/10.1016/j.tplants.2014.02.014.
76. Papapetrou EP, Schambach A. Gene insertion into genomic safe harbors for human gene therapy. *Mol Ther.* 2016;24(4):678–684. Available from: https://doi.org/10.1038/mt.2016.38.
77. Dong OX, Yu S, Jain R, et al. Marker-free carotenoid-enriched rice generated through targeted gene insertion using CRISPR-Cas9. *Nat Commun.* 2020;11(1):1178. Available from: https://doi.org/10.1038/s41467-020-14981-y.
78. Graham N, Patil GB, Bubeck DM, et al. Plant genome editing and the relevance of off-target changes. *Plant Physiol.* 2020;183(4):1453–1471. Available from: https://doi.org/10.1104/pp.19.01194.
79. EFSA GMO Panel. Applicability of the EFSA Opinion on site-directed nucleases type 3 for the safety assessment of plants developed using site-directed nucleases type 1 and 2 and oligonucleotide-directed mutagenesis. *EFSA J.* 2020;18(11): e06299. Available from: https://doi.org/10.2903/j.efsa.2020.6299.
80. Hartung F, Schiemann J. Precise plant breeding using new genome editing techniques: opportunities, safety and regulation in the EU. *Plant J.* 2014;78(5):742–752. Available from: https://doi.org/10.1111/tpj.12413.
81. Ishii T, Araki M. Consumer acceptance of food crops developed by genome editing. *Plant Cell Rep.* 2016;35(7):1507–1518. Available from: https://doi.org/10.1007/s00299-016-1974-2.
82. Schmidt SM, Belisle M, Frommer WB. The evolving landscape around genome editing in agriculture: many countries have exempted or move to exempt forms of genome editing from GMO regulation of crop plants. *EMBO Rep.* 2020;21(6):e50680. Available from: https://doi.org/10.15252/embr.202050680.
83. Whelan AI, Gutti P, Lema MA. Gene editing regulation and innovation economics. *Front Bioeng Biotechnol.* 2020;8:303. Available from: https://doi.org/10.3389/fbioe.2020.00303.
84. Stevanato P, Biscarini F. Digital PCR as New Approach to SNP Genotyping in Sugar Beet. *Sugar Tech* 2016;18(4):429–432. Available from: https://doi.org/10.1007/s12355-015-0408-82, https://doi.org/10.1007/s12355-015-0408-8C.
85. Broccanello C, Chiodi C, Funk A, McGrath JM, Panella L, Stevanato P. Comparison of three PCR-based assays for SNP genotyping in plants. *Plant Methods.* 2018;14:28. Accession Number: 29610576, PMCID: PMC5872507. Available from: https://doi.org/10.1186/s13007-018-0295-6, https://www.ncbi.nlm.nih.gov/pubmed/29610576.
86. Lusser M, Parisi C, Plan D, Rodriguez-Cerezo E. Deployment of new biotechnologies in plant breeding. *Nat Biotechnol* 2012;30 (3):231–239. Accession Number: 22398616. Available from: https://doi.org/10.1038/nbt.2142, https://www.ncbi.nlm.nih.gov/pubmed/22398616.
87. Grohmann L, Keilwagen J, Duensing N, et al. Detection and identification of genome editing in plants: challenges and opportunities. *Front Plant Sci.* 2019;10:236. Available from: https://doi.org/10.3389/fpls.2019.00236.
88. Raybould A. Problem formulation and phenotypic characterisation for the development of novel crops. *Transgenic Res.* 2019;28(suppl 2):135–145. Available from: https://doi.org/10.1007/s11248-019-00147-0.
89. Kleter GA, Kuiper HA, Kok EJ. Gene-edited crops: towards a harmonized safety assessment. *Trends Biotechnol.* 2019;37 (5):443–447. Available from: https://doi.org/10.1016/j.tibtech.2018.11.014.

Chapter 61

Safety assessment of food and feed derived from genetically modified plants

Hanspeter Naegeli
Institute of Veterinary Pharmacology and Toxicology, University of Zurich, Zurich, Switzerland

Abstract
Genetic engineering inserts or modifies DNA sequences to generate genetically modified (GM) plants that display constituents novel to the recipient species or altered in quantity. These changes involve nutrients like proteins, carbohydrates, or fatty acids, and other dietary ingredients that, if consumed in appropriate amounts, do not cause adverse effects. The safety evaluation is, therefore, focused on possible new hazards arising from the engineered plants in comparison to non-GM comparators. This comparative approach considers effects intended by the genetic modification as well as unintended effects. The consequences of any lack of equivalence between the engineered plant and its comparators, apart from intentional changes, will be assessed to ensure that GM products are as safe and nutritious as conventional food and feed. A sustainable agriculture covering the growing needs of the world's population should take advantage of scientific advances that simplify, without lowering safety, the regulatory approval of GM crops.

Keywords: Allergen; GMO; newly expressed protein; stacks; transformation

Chapter points

- The safety assessment of genetically modified (GM) food and feed considers information on the recipient and donor organisms and analyzes the effects of the genetic modification.
- The molecular characterization describes the transformation process, the introduced DNA sequences, the potential for horizontal gene transfer, the biological function and activity of newly expressed proteins, and, if applicable, an evaluation of RNA interference.
- The comparative assessment involves an analysis of phenotypic characteristics and agronomic performance as well as an evaluation of the nutrient, antinutrient, and toxin content of raw commodities and relevant products.
- A weight-of-evidence approach evaluates the safety of newly expressed proteins and the potential allergenicity of the GM food and feed.
- On a case-by-case basis, this thorough assessment provides assurance that the GM food and feed is as safe and nutritious as non-GM counterparts.

61.1 Introduction

This chapter describes the principles of the premarket risk assessment of genetically modified (GM) plants. The majority of GM crops currently commercialized have been designed to express heterologous proteins, so-called newly expressed proteins (NEPs), which confer a desired phenotype like herbicide tolerance or pest protection. Other traits of GM crops include increased yield, drought resistance, or changes in nutrient composition. Due their so far scarce market approval,[1] the risk assessment of food and feed derived from GM animals is not included, but the interested reader is referred to existing guidance documents.[2] Table 61.1 presents a glossary of recurrent technical terms and abbreviations.

The widely approved health-based analysis with risk = hazard × exposure, consisting of hazard identification, hazard characterization, exposure assessment, and risk characterization, is also applicable to GM plants. Commission Regulation 503/2013, which constitutes vinculating law in the European Union (EU) for the risk assessment of GM food and feed, lays down the following definitions[3]:

- Hazard identification describes "the identification of biological, chemical and physical agents capable of causing adverse health effects which may be present in a particular food and feed."

Present Knowledge in Food Safety. DOI: https://doi.org/10.1016/B978-0-12-819470-6.00033-0

TABLE 61.1 Glossary of technical terms and abbreviations.

Term	Abbreviation (if applicable)	Definition
Acceptable daily intake	ADI	Amount of a substance that can be ingested orally on a daily basis over a lifetime without a health risk
Adequate intake	AI	The recommended average daily intake of a nutrient that is assumed to be adequate
Allergenicity	–	The potential of a material to cause sensitization and elicit allergic reactions
Codex Alimentarius Commission	–	Internationally recognized committee that establishes standards, codes of practice, and guidelines relating to food production and safety
Comparator	–	Any non-GM plant (conventional counterpart or non-GM commercial variety) that is included as a baseline reference for the comparative analysis
Conventional counterpart	–	A comparator line with a genetic background that is closely related to that of the GM plant
Dietary reference value	DRV	Amount of a nutrient that must be consumed on a regular basis to maintain health
European Food Safety Authority	EFSA	Agency of the European Union that provides independent scientific advice on food safety
European Union	EU	Political and economic union of member states located in Europe
Event	–	Stable outcome of a genetic transformation process including inserted DNA elements and flanking genomic sequences
Genetically modified organism	GMO	An organism in which the genetic material has been changed in a way that does not occur naturally
Genetically modified plant	GM plant	A plant in which the genetic material has been changed in a way that does not occur naturally
Genome editing	–	Alterations in the genome achieved with high precision and efficiency
Horizontal gene transfer	HTG	The movement of genetic material across boundaries independently of reproduction
Newly expressed protein	NEP	Proteins that are expressed in the GM plant but not in non-GM comparators
Non-GM commercial varieties	–	Conventional comparators for which safety has been established based on their common use as a source of food and feed
No observable adverse effect	NOAEL	The highest dose of a substance where no adverse treatment-related findings are observed
Organization for Economic Cooperation and Development	OECD	International organization to stimulate economic progress and world trade
Open reading frames	ORFs	Any nucleotide sequence between two stop codons in the same reading frame
RNA interference	RNAi	A sequence homology-dependent process of gene silencing
Site-directed nuclease	SDN	A nuclease guided to a specific DNA sequence target for cleavage
Small interfering RNA	siRNA	A noncoding RNA molecule of 20–25 nucleotides in length that interferes with the expression of genes with complementary nucleotide sequences
Stacked events	–	Combination of transformation events by conventional plant breeding
Synthetic biology	SynBio	The application of science, technology, and engineering to facilitate and accelerate the design, manufacture, or modification of genetic materials in living organisms
Trait	–	Any observable characteristic, in the context of this chapter, conferred by a genetic modification

(Continued)

TABLE 61.1 (Continued)

Term	Abbreviation (if applicable)	Definition
Transformation	–	Transfer of DNA followed by stable integration into the chromosome(s) or organelle genome(s) of the recipient organism
Upper intake level	UL	Maximum dietary daily intake of a nutrient (over a lifetime and from all sources) judged to be unlikely to pose a risk of adverse health effects

Please see Table 61.2 for the nomenclature of proteins.

- Hazard characterization is "the qualitative and/or quantitative evaluation of the nature of the adverse health effects associated with biological, chemical and physical agents."
- Risk characterization involves a "qualitative and/or quantitative estimation, including attendant uncertainties, of the probability of occurrence and severity of known or potential adverse health effects."

After giving basic principles in Section 61.1, this chapter describes in Sections 61.2–61.7 the tests and trials needed for the identification and characterization of hazards related to GM plants, whereas Section 61.8 deals with exposure assessment and risk characterization. Risk management considerations (Section 61.9) are followed by a conclusion and future perspectives (Section 61.10). Represented is the view of the author based on his experience as a member (since 2012) and as the chair (from 2015 to 2021) of the Panel on Genetically Modified Organisms (GMO Panel) at the European Food Safety Authority (EFSA), without necessarily reflecting the opinion of other Panel members or of the EFSA.

61.1.1 Risk assessment strategy

For the safety assessment of GM plants, internationally recognized bodies like the Organization for Economic Cooperation and Development (OECD), the Codex Alimentarius Commission, and the EFSA converge on a robust scheme based on the concept of substantial equivalence.[4–10] A comparative analysis constitutes the centerpiece of this approach, implying that, rather than an absolute assessment of safety, genetically transformed plants are evaluated relative to non-GM comparators usually obtained from thousands of years of conventional breeding. An important consequence of this approach is that the risk analysis is only applicable to traits introduced in plant species with a history of safe consumption, or which have at least gained familiarity as a source of food and feed. In practice, the comparative approach is dependent on the existence of an appropriate conventional counterpart, which is genetically closely related to the GM plant under scrutiny, as well as the availability of non-GM varieties that are being commercialized. Various procedures aim at identifying differences between the GM crop and its non-GM comparators and the follow-up evaluation serves to assess the safety of intended and, if present, unintended differences induced by the genetic transformation. Of note, such a rigorous analysis is unique to GM organisms, whereas, traditionally, new plant varieties are evaluated by breeders for morphologic characteristics and agronomic performance but are not subjected to any safety assessment prior to marketing (with the exception of toxic alkaloid contents in some legislations).

61.1.2 Scope of market authorization

GM plants are usually employed for the same purpose as their conventional counterparts, generally for the production of food and feed. It should be noted that, on a global biomass basis, most GM crops are currently used in farms as animal feed.[11] A full market scope nevertheless implies that the risk assessment will be performed under the assumption of a theoretically possible 100% replacement of conventional food and feed with the GM plant under evaluation. This assumption is not applicable if the introduced trait changes drastically the nutrient or safety profile and, hence, does not comply with the principle of substantial equivalence. An example is GM maize expressing a heat-tolerant α-amylase from microbial origin known as AMY797E protein.[12] This maize was developed for ethanol production, whereby the starch contained in grains is hydrolyzed into glucose, which is subsequently converted to ethanol by fermentation. The protein- and lipid-rich residue remaining after fermentation and ethanol extraction is employed as animal feed. However, maize expressing AMY797E should not enter the regular food chain because the newly expressed α-amylase, by breaking down starch, changes fundamentally the texture, composition, safety and nutritional property of processed products as compared to those obtained from conventional maize.[13] This case exemplifies why the risk assessment of GM plants should consider specific methods of manufacturing triggered by the nature of the genetic modification and phenotypic trait, possibly leading to food and feed with novel characteristics.

61.1.3 Background information on the recipient plant

The assessment of GM plants starts with a description of the recipient including its name, family name, genus, species, subspecies, cultivar, and breeding scheme. Transformation events (defined as newly inserted DNA sequences together with genomic flanking sequences) are usually tested in a particular host genetic background although, after market authorization, these same events may be crossed into other varieties by conventional breeding to optimize agronomic performances. A documentation of the safety record of the recipient should include where and how the plant is typically cultivated, which parts of the plant are used as food and feed (grains, seeds, forage, etc.), with what nutrients the plant contributes to the human and animal diet, and whether processing is required to render its products safe for consumption. Known antinutrients as well as inherent toxic or allergenic constituents of the recipient should be listed. An adverse attribute of plants, although used safely as food and feed since thousands of years, is illustrated by soy and other legumes because the ingestion of their raw beans may cause gastrointestinal disorders (abdominal discomfort, nausea, vomiting, diarrhea, and malabsorption). These manifestations are caused by protease inhibitors, which interfere with the digestive enzymes trypsin and chymotrypsin, and by lectins, which damage the gut mucosa by binding to the carbohydrate moiety of cell surface glycoproteins. A range of industrial and home processing practices (soaking, fermentation, cooking, toasting, etc.) are employed to reduce the content and biological activity of these antinutrients.[14,15]

61.2 Molecular characterization

The risk assessment further includes an appraisal of the donor organisms, transformation method, inserted DNA sequences and their functionality, as well as modifications of genomic flanking regions. Where this molecular characterization identifies potential hazards, the risk assessment should outline what follow-up analyses described in Sections 61.3–61.7 contribute to the safety evaluation.

61.2.1 Genetic modification

The characterization of the DNA vector used to deliver genetic material to the recipient plant comprises a description of the biological function of its components, including gene regulatory motifs, as well as the size, sequence, location, and orientation of all elements in the construct. A map of the vector with restriction sites and positions of hybridization primers, used in polymerase chain reactions, and probes for Southern blotting should be indicated for the interpretation of molecular tests. The vector region intended for insertion should be defined. It is necessary to provide a synopsis of how the vector has been constructed and which intermediate hosts were used. Equally important is information on the donor organisms of newly inserted DNA sequences. Of relevance is whether these donor organisms possess a history of safe consumption or use in food or feed production or, alternatively, whether they exhibit characteristics of pathogenicity, toxin production or allergenicity, or have other adverse traits. In the latter case, information should be provided to ensure that genes coding for known toxins, antinutrients, or allergens present in the donor organisms are not transferred to the GM plant. Any modification of the original sequence of genetic elements, as they occur in donor organisms, is to be notified. The method employed for the DNA transfer (e.g., *Agrobacterium*-mediated transformation or microprojectile bombardment) should be documented and helper plasmids or carrier nucleic acids, if used for transformation, should be described. If applicable, enzymes and recognition sequences exploited for site-directed integration into the recipient genome should be listed. Marker genes facilitate the selection and identification of successfully transformed cells. In view of the bacterial resistance crisis, the choice of an antibiotic resistance as the selection strategy is viewed skeptically because of the possibility of horizontal gene transfer (HGT). It is acknowledged that, with preexisting high levels of spontaneously occurring bacteria that have already lost susceptibility to a given antibiotic, the likelihood of a resistance transfer from these bacteria will be orders of magnitude higher than the likelihood of a transfer from GM plants (see Section 61.2.3 for considerations related to HGT). Nevertheless, antibiotic resistance genes for selection should be avoided.

61.2.2 Molecular description of the new trait

To understand the biological implications of a genetic transformation process, it is indispensable to characterize the resulting transformation event, which in turn allows for the evaluation of any newly expressed RNA or protein. This molecular characterization of the event includes the following information:

- confirmation of a single insertion site or, alternatively, identification of the number of insertion sites in the host genome;

- size, organization, orientation, and complete sequence of each insert and regions surrounding the insertion locus;
- any evidence indicating that endogenous genes or regulatory sequences in the host plant have been interrupted or deleted by the insertion of foreign DNA sequences;
- subcellular location of inserts, which might be in the nucleus, chloroplasts, or mitochondria;
- demonstration of the stability of the transgenic locus over multiple (e.g., five) generations and description of its inheritance pattern;
- identification of open reading frames (ORFs) within the inserted sequences and newly created by the insertion within the contiguous host DNA.

The molecular characterization will also confirm that the genetic material used for the insertion is conserved, that is, that no mutations, deletions, rearrangements, or addition of extra sequences have occurred during the procedure. It should be avoided that, by genetic engineering, toxins or allergens are transferred from one organism to another or that genetic engineering "creates" new toxins or allergens. Therefore the molecular characterization next proceeds with information on newly expressed substances in the GM plant, including:

- the description of any NEP or untranslated RNA product;
- the biological function of these expression products;
- a prediction of changes in the morphologic and agronomic characteristics of the GM plant, relative to non-GM comparators, resulting from the newly introduced trait;
- a prediction of altered composition of the GM plant, focusing on the edible parts, particularly if the function of expressed sequences is to alter the nutritional profile.

Sequence comparisons should be carried out against appropriate databases (see Sections 61.1 and 61.1) to rule out that ORFs display any similarity to known toxins or allergens. The molecular characterization will reveal the presence of promoters near ORFs driving their expression and the existence of genetic elements supporting their translation. Depending on the outcome, additional tests like transcription or translation analyses of ORF sequences may be required. When complex genetic modifications are produced, for example, by transfer of multiple elements with a single vector or retransformation of a preexisting GM line, it is important to consider known or expected interactions between the newly expressed RNA, NEPs, or other new constituents. Such interactions may exert synergistic or antagonistic phenotypic effects.

61.2.3 Potential for horizontal gene transfer

The inherently dynamic nature of genes may lead to their horizontal movement to humans, animals, and microorganisms, primarily to gut bacteria, potentially conferring new properties. HGT occurs by multiple routes among bacteria, but the only mechanism known to facilitate the transfer of chromosomal DNA segments from plants to the genome of microorganisms is by homologous recombination. This process requires the presence of DNA sequences that are similar between the insert and potential recipients. Practical guidance on how to identify sequence stretches with sufficient identity to promote homologous recombination can be found in an EFSA explanatory note.[16] In addition to homology-based recombination, illegitimate recombination by nonhomologous end joining or microhomology-mediated end joining may theoretically take place.[17] However, the expected transformation rates for illegitimate recombination are many orders of magnitude lower than for homologous recombination. To summarize, the occurrence of HGT from plants (or their products) is considered a rare possibility because of the complex molecular reactions that would need to be deployed.[18,19] A horizontal transfer of recombinant genes from plants to bacteria has never been demonstrated under field conditions with GM plants used in agriculture. The safety impact of gene movements depends in any case on the selection pressure as such transfers are only relevant if the introduced DNA conveys a selective advantage to the recipient microorganisms.

61.2.4 Characterization of newly expressed proteins

An overview of NEPs assessed so far by the EFSA GMO Panel shows that the most popular traits mediate herbicide tolerance and insect resistance (Table 61.2).

The characterization of these NEPs involves the following:

- description of their biological function;
- determination of their amino acid sequence, molecular mass, degree of glycosylation, or other known post-translational modifications;
- for newly expressed enzymes, information on the specific activity, reaction conditions (temperature, pH), substrate specificity, and enzymatic products.

The molecular characterization of GM plants also involves a measurement of the concentration of NEPs in edible parts (grains, seeds, forage, and, if appropriate, pollen) obtained from field trials. Expression in other parts of the plant might be relevant if tissue-specific promoters are in place that might raise safety concerns, for example,

TABLE 61.2 List of NEPs that have been evaluated by the EFSA GMO Panel between 2005 and 2022.

Trait	NEPs
Selection of transformed cells by:	
Hygromycin B resistance	Aminoglycoside phosphotransferase (APH)
Neomycin resistance	Neomycin phosphotransferase (NPT)
Utilization of mannose as carbon source	Phosphomannose isomerase (PMI)
Visualization of successful insertion	β-Glucuronidase (GUS)
Tolerance to the following herbicides:	
Dicamba	Dicamba monooxygenase (DMO)
Glufosinate ammonium	Phosphinothricin acetyltransferase (PAT)
Glyphosate	5-Enolpyruvylshikimate-3-phosphate synthase (EPSPS), glyphosate acetyltransferase (GAT), glyphosate oxidoreductase (GOX)
Imidazolinones, sulfonylureas	Acetohydroxy acid synthase (AHAS), also known as acetolactate synthase (ALS), *Glycine max* herbicide-resistant acetolactate synthase (GM-HRA)
Mesotrione	4-Hydroxyphenylpyruvate dioxygenase (HPPD)
Phenoxy herbicides like 2,4-dichlorophenoxyacetic acid, quizalofop	Aryloxyalkanoate dioxygenase (AAD), FT_T dioxygenase
Protection from insect pests:	
Coleoptera-specific	Cry3A, Cry3Bb1, Cry34Ab1, Cry35Ab1, eCry3.1Ab, IPD072Aa[a], IPD079Ea[b]
Lepidoptera-specific	Cry1A.105, Cry1Ab, Cry1Ac, Cry1F, Cry2Ab2, Cry2Ae, Vip3Aa, Vip3Aa19, Vip3Aa20
Protection from nematode pests:	Cry14Ab1
Improved agronomic performance by:	
Drought tolerance	Cold shock protein B (CSPB)
Increased biomass	Transcription factors AtHB17Δ113 and ZMM28[c]
Male sterility/fertility restorer system[c]	Barnase (an RNase)/Barstar (RNase inhibitor)[d]
Altered composition of plant products:	
High omega-3 stearidonic acid (C18:4n-3) soybean	Desaturases PjΔ6D and NcΔ15D
High omega-3 long-chain polyunsaturated fatty acid (including C20:5n-3 and C22:6n-3) oilseed rape	Biochemical pathway catalyzed by desaturases Pavsa-Δ5D, Micpu-Δ6D, Lackl-Δ12D, Picpa-ω3D, and elongases Pyrco-Δ6E and Pyrco-Δ5E; biochemical pathway catalyzed by Δ4D(Pl), Δ4D(Tc), Δ5D(Tc), Δ6D(Ot), Δ12D(Ps), ω3D(Pi), ω3D(Pir), Δ5E(Ot), Δ6E(Tp), and Δ6E(Pp)
Conversion of starch to oligosaccharides	Thermostable α-amylase (AMY797E)
Meat-like taste	Soy leghemoglobin

Crystal (Cry) insecticidal proteins and vegetative insecticidal proteins from the soil bacterium *Bacillus thuringiensis* are toxic to different insect orders, as indicated. *EFSA*, European Food Safety Authority; *GMO*, genetically modified organism; *NEPs*, newly expressed proteins.
[a]*(refers to IPD072Aa): Selective insecticidal protein from* Pseudomonas chlororaphis.
[b]*(refers to IPD079Ea): Selective insecticidal protein from* Ophidoglossum pendulum.
[c]*(refers to ZMM28): Extended and increased expression of maize ZMM28 protein.*
[d]*(refers to to male sterility/fertility restorer system): For hybrid production in Brassica crops.*

because of leakiness. To be representative, expression values should be determined from multiple growing sites or over several seasons. More advice on how to measure NEP levels can be found in an EFSA explanatory note.[20]

61.2.5 Evaluation of RNA interference

The newly inserted DNA may serve to express RNA sequences that, instead of being translated to proteins, mediate gene silencing. By exploiting natural gene regulation mechanisms, RNA interference (RNAi) is used to modulate morphologic, agricultural, and compositional characteristics. In RNAi plants, inserted DNA sequences lead to the expression of double-stranded RNA subsequently processed to small interfering RNA (siRNA) of 20–30 nucleotides in length, which silence genes at the posttranscriptional level. In most cases, RNAi targets plant genes, implying that the effector siRNA consists of fragments of endogenous sequences that by themselves hold a record of safe consumption. In other cases, RNAi is deployed against pathogens (viruses, nematodes, insects) by the expression of new RNA sequences not related to any endogenous plant gene.[21–23] To combat the western corn rootworm (*Diabrotica virgifera*), for example, DNA constructs have been inserted in maize that drive the expression, in an inverted repeat configuration, of complementary sequences of parasite genes coding for essential proteins.[24] Unlike vertebrates, *D. virgifera* is endowed with mechanisms for RNA uptake and systemic spread[25] such that, when the larvae feed on the RNAi maize, silencing of the essential target leads to insect lethality and, hence, protection from root damage (see Section 61.5.1 for the food and feed safety assessment of RNAi sequences).

Effector siRNA molecules are designed to lack ORFs and translation initiation signals for protein synthesis and, therefore, the risk assessment is focused on the gene silencing machinery. In the EU, Regulation 503/2013 requests an in silico bioinformatic screen to search for potential "off-target" genes in the plant host that might be unintentionally down regulated. Such a prognostic analysis is supported by the fact that silencing RNA sequences in plants are perfectly or nearly perfectly complementary to their target transcripts.[26,27] Thus bioinformatic studies retrieving transcripts that match the newly expressed siRNA sequences could potentially indicate off-targets, but the genome of typical crops are only partially sequenced and known reference genomes do not take into account sequence differences between cultivars.[28] While acknowledging the limitations of bioinformatic searches, the EFSA GMO Panel issued practical recommendations[29] whereby a set of parameters allows for the detection of potential RNAi off-targets in plants, whereas in vertebrate animals and humans the complementarity between the siRNA molecules and their targets is more flexible, thus preventing reliable predictions.[30] The proposed procedure covers all 21-nucleotide siRNA sequences that derive from a given RNA precursor, with the degree and position of base pairing between siRNA and the target mRNA being primary factors determining the efficiency of silencing. The safety assessment of potential off-targets in the plant should consider the abundance and number of siRNAs showing relevant similarity to the same transcript, as the likelihood for silencing increases with multiple siRNA sequences that bind to the same mRNA molecule. Depending on the nature and function of potential off-targets, the assessment may require the measurement of additional phenotypic/agronomic or compositional endpoints over the standard comparative analysis outlined in Section 61.3.

61.2.6 Breeding stacks and subcombinations

Upon market approval, GM lines are combined by conventional breeding to generate "stacked" transformation events. The typical case is a maize stack containing five events, which in combination impart herbicide tolerance (by expression of EPSPS), insect resistance (by expression of Cry1A.105, Cry2Ab2 and Vip3Aa20), as well as drought tolerance mediated by CSPB[31] (see Table 61.2 for protein abbreviations). Plants with stacked events need to be evaluated for potential synergistic or antagonistic interactions occurring between the different DNA inserts, and supplementary analyses might be prompted if such interactions are anticipated from the biological function of each single event. Relevant cross-talks between events may occur, for example, if the genetic modifications affect metabolic pathways with a combinatorial impact on composition.[32]

In the EU, the evaluation of stacked GM plants requires not only the prior analysis of each single event, but also by default a complete assessment of the breeding stack including field trials for comparative analyses and determination of NEP levels. However, the incremental experience gained from the examination of breeding stacks shows that, in practice, interactions between events are a rare phenomenon and, even if present, generally have no consequences for food and feed safety. One foreseeable possibility is that the combined expression of different Cry, vegetative insecticidal proteins, or other insecticidal proteins may mutually potentiate their action against target pests and nontarget insects or nematodes,[33,34] but without raising concerns in view of their concomitant presence in food and feed. It is, therefore, questionable whether a full risk analysis of stacked GM plants including field trials provides any additional safety benefit.[35]

In the situation of stacked GM crops grown as hybrids, each harvest results in grain or seed progeny containing various subcombinations of events segregating by Mendelian rules. The aforementioned five-event stack maize generates grains comprising 25 different subcombinations of events[31] whereas, for example, a four-event stack rapeseed generates seeds with 10 distinct subcombinations. The problem is that current control methods do not allow distinguishing the origin of such subcombinations as they may also have been generated by conventional crossing of just a subset of single events. Therefore Regulation

503/2013 stipulates that, in the EU, applications for the approval of segregating stacks must provide sufficient data to cover all subcombinations that have not yet been authorized. The EFSA GMO Panel devised a strategy by which subcombinations of the stacks can be evaluated on the basis of the outcome of the assessment of the corresponding single events and of the highest stack. This strategy builds on the principle that, if the assessment of the single events and/or stack identifies unintended effects linked to any event, the risk raised by combinations of these events can be predicted without the need for additional experimental data.[36]

61.3 Comparative analysis

A detailed comparative assessment is the key cornerstone for the evaluation of GM plants. The goal is to exclude differences between the GM plant and its comparators that might pose safety concerns. A straightforward protocol for this comparative analysis includes a statistical test of difference combined with a statistical test of equivalence.[37,38] The first compares the GM plant with the conventional counterpart and, by the analysis of many variables, this test will almost always identify significant differences. To account for baseline fluctuations at the location of the field trial, therefore, these differences are related to the natural variation by the test of equivalence involving an additional comparison with a range of non-GM commercial cultivars with a history of safe use.

61.3.1 Choice of the conventional counterpart and other nongenetically modified comparators

The GM crop is compared with a genetically close counterpart, ideally a near isogenic parental line. In practice, this may not be feasible at all times, in which case a line genetically as close as possible should be chosen.[39] When no appropriate conventional counterpart is identified, a comparative safety analysis cannot be carried out and the risk assessment will remain incomplete. Non-GM commercial varieties should be included in the experimental design in sufficient number to ensure a reliable estimate of natural variability. These non-GM commercial comparators are selected on the basis of the particular growth conditions and customary agronomic practices at each test location and, hence, may vary between individual sites of the field trial.

61.3.2 Controlled field trial for the comparative analysis

Levels of nutrients, antinutrients, and other constituents may change depending on soil characteristics, climate, humidity, parasite damage, or weed profile. The location of trial sites should, consequently, be representative of the conditions under which the GM plant is expected to be grown for commercial purposes. The number of trial sites should be sufficient to allow for an assessment of the plants' attributes over the range of conditions met in the field. To minimize environmental effects and account for natural variability, each trial site should be replicated. In the EU, Regulation 503/2013 requires that the field trial is carried out at a minimum of eight representative sites with at least four replicates at each site, which is a scheme derived from practicability considerations[40] rather than purely statistical criteria. A thorough description of the field trial includes, in particular, information on management of the field before sowing, soil type, pesticide use, metereologic and other environmental conditions during growth, pathogen or weed pressure, as well as conditions during harvest and postharvest storage.[41] For herbicide-tolerant GM plants, the following test materials should be grown:

- the conventional counterpart and commercial non-GM comparators treated with standard agrochemicals,
- the GM plant treated with the same standard agrochemicals as above,
- the GM plant exposed to the intended herbicide in addition to standard agrochemicals.

This comparison with the GM plant grown under its foreseen agronomic management (sprayed with the intended herbicide in addition to maintenance pesticides) is thought to test whether agricultural practices influence the measured endpoints by exerting herbicide-induced stress. Plants need to be sampled in adequate amounts and the methods of analysis should be sufficiently sensitive and specific to detect variations in the measured endpoints. The biological relevance of any observed difference (determined by the test of difference) between the GM plant and its conventional counterpart should be judged in the context of the natural variation of that same parameter in non-GM reference varieties grown simultaneously (determined by the test of equivalence).

61.3.3 Comparative analysis of phenotypic characteristics and agronomic performance

Morphologic and agronomic features (e.g., stand count, plant height, flowering duration, seed weight, and yield) are typically monitored in selecting new varieties for commercialization. For the assessment of GM plants, phenotypic and agronomic endpoints should be compared with those of the conventional counterpart and non-GM reference varieties grown and harvested under identical conditions (Section 61.3.2). The goal of this phenotypic/agronomic branch of the comparative analysis is to determine whether there are new characteristics of the GM plant that need further investigations.[41] This analysis may confirm desired traits that are intended to improve plant growth, grain yield, or pest protection. Considerations should also be given to the potential impact on human or animal health, as substantial changes of phenotypic/agronomic characteristics might be indicative of compositional shifts in the GM plant compared to non-GM comparators.

61.3.4 Comparative analysis of composition

The raw agricultural commodity for compositional analysis (grains/seeds and forage for most crops) is selected taking into account the prospective uses as food and feed. Besides the proximates (ash, moisture, proteins, fat, carbohydrates, fiber), quantitative analyses entail macronutrients (e.g., amino acids, fatty acids), micro-nutrients (vitamins, minerals), antinutrients (like lectins in soybean), toxins (e.g., gossypol in cotton), and allergens, which are characteristic for the crop species and are listed in consensus documents developed under the OECD patronage (see for instance the list of compositional variables for maize[42]). Selected vitamins and minerals should be those that are present at relevant levels, that is, that make nutritionally important contributions to the diet in the amounts at which the plant is consumed. The concentrations of nutrients/antinutrients, toxins, and allergens of the GM plant are compared to those of the conventional counterpart and non-GM references grown, harvested, and stored under the same conditions (Section 61.3.2).

Food and feed analyses address both beneficial and harmful components. The goal of this compositional part of the comparative analysis is to determine whether there are ingredients of the GM plant that, when compared to non-GM comparators, need investigation.[43] The risk associated with such compounds would to be assessed with usual procedures for establishing safety or nutritional impact. In general, a large proportion of statistically significant differences in composition are spurious in magnitude. Only rarely, biologically relevant changes in composition between a GM plant and its comparators have been identified. An example of such a difference—large enough to justify a more thorough examination—was an up to 36% increased concentration of lectins observed in GM soybean expressing AAD and PAT enzymes for herbicide tolerance (see Table 61.2 for protein abbreviations). Lectin activity was significantly higher in GM soybean seeds than in the conventional counterpart for two of the four field trial conditions and fell outside of the equivalence limits determined by non-GM reference varieties (Table 61.3[14]). The follow-up assessment took into account that:

- The toxicity of lectins in soybean is low compared to other commonly consumed legumes.
- The observed increase is not relevant in the context of the high natural variability reported for lectin content and/or activity in raw soybean.[44–46]
- The safe use of soybean as food and feed depends on industrial and home processing practices that considerably reduce lectin content and/or activity.

Based on these considerations it was concluded that the observed increase of lectin activity in the GM soybean seeds relative to the conventional counterpart is unlikely to raise additional concerns compared to non-GM soybean varieties.[14]

The detailed characterization of the introduced trait may allow for the anticipation of specific compositional changes and, thereby, trigger the analyses of extra compounds in addition to the standard repertoire of endpoints. These effects might be intended as it is the case when the aim of the genetic transformation is to alter the nutrient profile of the plant (see Section 61.7). An example of unintended effect emerged from the characterization of the GAT protein (see Table 61.2 for protein abbreviations), which is used to confer glyphosate tolerance by virtue of its capacity to inactivate this herbicide by acetylation. In vitro assays revealed that the GAT enzyme also acetylates amino acids and, consequently, *N*-acetylated amino acids were found in higher concentrations in grains of the GM crop compared to the conventional counterpart. In particular, the level of *N*-acetyl-aspartic acid (NAA) was in one instance >500-fold higher in GM maize grains (Table 61.4[47]). The evaluation of this enhanced NAA content relied on a previously published 90-day feeding study in rats, where the daily oral NAA intake at 500 mg/kg led to an increased incidence of hypertrophy of mucus-secreting cells in salivary glands.[48] In view of this

TABLE 61.3 Lectin levels measured in an herbicide-tolerant GM soybean and its non-GM comparators.

	Conventional counterpart	GM soybean treatment				Equivalence limits from non-GM varieties
		None	2,4-D	Glufosinate	2,4-D and glufosinate	
Lectin activity	48.2	53.7	65.8*	53.5	56.0*	21.0–52.8

Lectin activity was determined as hemagglutinin units per milligram protein. Asterisk indicates statistically significant differences between the GM soybean and its conventional counterpart. *GM*, genetically modified.

TABLE 61.4 Mean levels of acetylated amino acids (mg/kg) in the grains of maize expressing the GAT protein.

Analyte	Year	Conventional counterpart	GM maize	Fold change
N-acetyl-L-aspartic acid (NAA)	2006	0.90	403	448
	2007	4.03	292	72
	2008	1.01	542	537
N-acetyl-L-glutamate (NAG)	2006	0.50	79.0	158
	2007	0.21	84.0	400
	2008	0.05	13.0	260
N-acetylglycine (NAGly)	2006	0.07	0.23	3
	2007	0.06	0.12	2
	2008	0.06	0.12	2
N-acetylserine (NAS)	2006	0.90	1.97	2
	2007	0.86	1.49	2
	2008	1.16	2.03	2
N-acetylthreonine (NAT)	2006	0.18	2.99	17
	2007	0.16	1.97	12
	2008	0.18	1.42	8

Samples from field trials carried out during different years were analyzed side-by-side as indicated. GM, genetically modified.

potentially harmful response to NAA administration, which was not observed in rats administered nonacetylated aspartic acid, the highest dose level with no observable adverse effect (NOAEL) was 250 mg/kg body weight. Based on human consumption data, it was then concluded that there is a sufficient margin, that is, factors of 250–2500 between the amounts of NAA consumed in the worst-case scenario of a 100% replacement of conventional maize with the GM maize of Table 61.4 (at the 95th percentile of exposure) and the NOAEL of 250 mg/kg/day derived from the 90-day study.[47] More problematic are the lower margins for farm animals fed with this particular GM maize.

61.3.5 Effect of food or feed processing

Considerations on the effect of food and feed processing may be required on a case-by-case basis for two reasons. On the one hand, it is likely that preservation procedures, industrial food processing or home preparations, influence the level of a substance that has been identified as a hazard by deactivating, degrading, or eliminating antinutrients, toxicants, or allergens. The nature of the product for consumption determines the types of processing which would be applied and its effects on the presence of any particular substance in the final products. This applies for example to the evaluation of rapeseed expressing the GOX protein (see Table 61.2 for protein abbreviations). An assessment concluding on the safety of this GM rapeseed recognized that the GOX protein is absent in the oil used for human consumption and is present only in trace amounts in the toasted meal used for animal feeding. However, this conclusion does not extend to new formulations consisting of extracted proteins (protein isolates) from rapeseed. As GOX has the potential to be concentrated in such protein isolates, human and animal exposure would be substantially higher and, therefore, toxicologic studies were needed to extend the risk assessment to all rapeseed products.[49,50]

On the other hand, the example of a heat-tolerant α-amylase presented in Section 61.1.2 illustrates how NEPs can influence the final composition of plant products.[13] Therefore a description of the processing used for the manufacture of food, feed, and ingredients (like, e.g., vegetable oil) is needed. This aspect is particularly important if a GM plant is processed differently than non-GM comparators, in which case-specific products should be analyzed as appropriate.

61.3.6 What about unexpected unintended effects?

In imparting a specific trait, which constitutes the intended effect of inserted DNA sequences, extra attributes of the plant could, in theory, be acquired and existing characteristics could be modified or lost. Such unintended effects are subdivided into two groups, that is, those that are expected and those that are unexpected.

Many unintended effects are predictable based on the molecular characterization of the inserted event (Section 61.2). Conversely, unexpected changes can result from the random insertion of DNA sequences into the plant genome, thus resulting in the disruption, silencing, or activation of endogenous genes. Also, newly expressed RNA or NEPs may regulate gene activity in an unexpected manner or elicit unanticipated biochemical reactions, for example, due to a promiscuous substrate specificity in the case of enzymes.[47,51] These effects may change the nutrient, antinutrient, and, in certain crops, the toxin and allergen content of edible parts. However, unintentional effects are an inherent phenomenon in plant breeding and do not necessarily influence safety. Moreover, unintended effects, as they might originate from the insertion of new sequences at a single genomic location, or at few locations, are likely to be less severe in magnitude than those occurring during conventional breeding relying on genome-wide mutagenesis by treatment with uncontrollable genotoxic agents.[52,53] Physicochemical mutagenesis, which uses radiation or DNA-damaging substances to alter the genetic code, has been practiced since the 1950s. Notably, recent advances in biotechnology allow for targeted integrations without the accidental disruption of regulatory or coding sequences in the host genome and, hence, further diminish the probability of unintended effects. For example, site-specific meganucleases can be employed to introduce, by homologous recombination, a landing pad at defined genomic locations for the subsequent insertion, by a second recombination reaction, of the desired expression cassette.[54]

Once the new trait is stably introduced by genetic transformation, the next step is to ascertain that essential attributes of the recipient plant are not distorted in a way that cannot be balanced out by backcrossing or by spontaneous genomic or metabolic adjustments. This assessment takes into account phenotypic and agronomic characteristics (Section 61.3.3) that provide a screen for unusual properties. Despite the natural variability in nutrient/antinutrient contents, the compositional analysis (Section 61.3.4) provides another indicator of potential unintended effects. For the risk assessment, it is necessary to evaluate the relevance of possible unintended effects, which might be neutral, beneficial, or deleterious with respect to the safety of food and feed. By and large, unintended effects identified or assumed to occur in GM crops exert no adverse effects on human and animal health.

61.4 Assessment of newly expressed proteins

The canonical principles of toxicologic risk assessment involving oral administration studies in rodents have been developed to evaluate small-molecule substances (additives, contaminants, pesticide or veterinary drug residues). For the assessment of NEPs, rodent studies are frequently not necessary and, in other instances, not or only partially feasible, such that a more adaptable weight-of-evidence approach is used for their evaluation.

61.4.1 Weight-of-evidence evaluation of NEP safety

The studies for assessment of the NEP safety are selected on a case-by-case basis depending on the available knowledge with regard to:

- the source of the protein,
- its biological function,
- the history of consumption of the protein by humans and animals,
- its heat stability,
- its digestibility,
- the in silico analysis of its amino acid sequence.

The relevance of protein source, biological function, and history of consumption is exemplified by the assessment of an HPPD protein conferring herbicide tolerance to soybean (see Table 61.2 for protein abbreviations). HPPD proteins are evolutionary conserved, ubiquitously present in aerobic organisms, and widely expressed in plants, where they participate in the synthesis of carotenoids and tocopherols. Sequence comparisons showed a high degree of identity between the transgenic HPPD and natural HPPDs in food and feed plants, including oat, wheat, barley, rice, maize, and potato. On the basis of this information, it was concluded that, even assuming a 100% replacement, the intake of HPPD from the GM soybean is in the same range as the consumption of highly similar proteins naturally present in different crops, thus documenting a robust record of use that provides assurance as to the safety of the NEP under evaluation.[55]

Another part of the weight-of-evidence evaluation of NEPs involves their susceptibility to heat treatment, which provides information on their inactivation during food or feed processing. The susceptibility of NEPs to in vitro degradation by the digestive proteolytic enzyme pepsin indicates whether they are likely to reach the intestinal mucosa as intact proteins (or as fragments containing biologically active domains) with the potential to cause adversity. NEP breakdown products are also evaluated with regard to their allergenic potential (Section 61.6.1). The assessment of NEPs proceeds by appropriate algorithms to test for amino acid sequence similarities to toxins, antinutrients, or any other protein linked directly or indirectly to toxicity.[56] The query sequences also comprise those that are hypothetically formed from unintentional ORFs in the insert or crossing its borders with the surrounding host genome (Section 61.2.2). Unfortunately, primary amino acid sequences are notoriously poor predictors as the secondary/tertiary structure of proteins with a common biological function shows more similarity than their primary sequence.[57,58] Therefore it would be useful to identify sequence alerts by the comparison with folding motifs that determine the three-dimensional structure of toxins or other pathogenic proteins. Much progress has been made in using artificial intelligence to predict protein structures from primary amino acid sequences. Machine learning techniques, for example, exploit the evolutionary covariation of sequences to identify physically interacting amino acid residues that are responsible for building the structure of proteins.[59] Validation of artificial intelligence tools may allow to screen NEPs for specific sequence elements that build hazardous three-dimensional shapes.

In the case that the above weight of evidence is well documented, toxicity studies with laboratory animals are not required. Conversely, remaining uncertainties as to the safety of NEPs are currently addressed by in vivo assays in rodents. Such studies may be carried out, for example, if the NEP is not sufficiently similar to proteins that are being consumed safely in food and feed. Internationally agreed protocols are recommended and, for the initial hazard identification, subacute (28-day) repeated dose studies according to OECD Guidelines[60] provide the most appropriate approach to evaluate a continued intake. In this assay, the NEP in purified form is orally administered daily to groups of male and female rodents for a period of 28 days. The preferred species is the rat. The use of mice as a smaller species is possible, but may result in an increased variability due to technical challenges in the administration of the test substance, dissection of organs, or the analysis of small sample volumes. The test protein is administered via the diet or by gavage. In principle, a control group and at least three test groups with incremental doses should be used to allow for an indication of the dose–response relationship and determination of the NOAEL. Except for the treatment with the test substance, control animals should be handled in an identical manner. If a vehicle is used in administering the test substance, the control group should receive this vehicle in the highest volume employed. For NEPs, frequently no low-dose effects are expected and, consequently, a so-called limit dose assay at 1000 mg/kg body weight per day may be performed. During the 28-day study period, the animals are observed for signs of toxicity. Body weight as well as food and water consumption are monitored. At the end of the study, samples are taken for hematology, clinical biochemistry analyses, and coagulation tests. The animals are sacrificed and subjected to gross necropsy and histopathology examinations. Adverse effects detected in the 28-day study may indicate the need for additional tests.

61.4.2 Material for newly expressed protein safety assessment

Test proteins should correspond to the NEPs as they appear in the GM plant. However, their isolation directly from plants is difficult because NEPs tend to represent a very minor biomass fraction. A practical alternative is their production by a prokaryotic expression system (usually *Escherichia coli*), but the resulting substitute should be structurally and functionally equivalent to the protein expressed in the GM plant. Attention should be given to posttranslational modifications occurring in distinct hosts (eukaryotic vs prokaryotic), which may have an impact on the toxic and allergic potential. Some proteins have properties that make them extremely difficult or impossible to express, purify, and concentrate in a native and functional form.[61] Membrane-associated NEPs belong to such recalcitrant proteins because, in their native folding, they are inserted into lipid bilayers. Such proteins may be produced in bacteria in an insoluble form as inclusion bodies that become soluble only in the presence of a strong denaturant. More advanced expression systems for membrane proteins are available, but eventually their solubilization requires disruption of the lipid bilayer by means of detergents exhibiting an inherent oral toxicity. It is challenging to identify detergents that maintain the solubility and native folding of isolated membrane proteins, yet without confounding the results of animal toxicity studies.

61.5 Safety of new constituents other than newly expressed proteins

Constituents other than NEPs include, besides RNA (see below), novel metabolites generated by newly expressed enzymes. An example is acetyl-aminoadipate, which has never been found before as an endogenous plant metabolite but detected in GM plants expressing the bialaphos resistance protein, an acetyltransferase from *Streptomyces hygroscopicus*.[51] As of yet, there is no information on this acetylated compound that would suggest a hazard hypothesis justifying further studies. Generally, the safety evaluation of new constituents would take into account the chemical nature and biological activity of the novel substance. Determination of its concentration in edible parts of the GM plant is needed to anticipate dietary exposure levels and predict possible effects upon ingestion by humans and animals. This risk assessment may require appropriate toxicologic testing including, as appropriate, genotoxicity/carcinogenicity, and reproductive toxicity assays.

61.5.1 Newly expressed RNA

The use of RNAi as a biocidal agent (Section 61.2.5) raises the question of whether siRNAs that are lethal to invertebrates could harm humans, domestic animals, or other vertebrates. It has been noted that noncoding RNA sequences found in plants may display similarity or even identity to genomic regions of humans and animals.[62,63] This observation opens the possibility that dietary siRNA, of natural occurrence or inserted into RNAi plants, may elicit effects upon consumption. However, the mammalian digestive tract provides an efficient barrier to the uptake of exogenous RNA, which is inherently unstable.[64] The degradation of ingested RNA begins in saliva, which is a rich source of ribonucleases.[65] Next, the milieu in the stomach with low pH promotes RNA depurination and hydrolytic fragmentation. Even pepsin, which is commonly thought to be a protease only, has been shown to digest nucleic acids including RNA.[66] Pancreatic enzymes (nucleases, phosphodiesterases and nucleoside phosphorylases) are secreted into the intestinal lumen and further degrade ingested RNA.[67,68] Finally, the intestinal epithelium—deploying tight junctions—is a physical barrier to nucleic acids and any RNA that may bypass cellular membranes by endocytosis will be sequestered into lysosomes and degraded by lysosomal enzymes.[69] In summary, the systemic absorption of orally ingested RNA is negligible in vertebrates and, in fact, reports of microRNA (miRNA) of plant sources appearing in the bloodstream of humans and rodents were due to misidentification or technical artifacts.[70–72] Trace amounts of dietary RNA that might be absorbed into the blood are anyway subjected to rapid degradation and hepatic or renal clearance[73,74] and few remaining RNA molecules would not be able to exert any activity in cells.[75–78] Oral toxicity studies on RNA sequences are, therefore, not necessary.[24,79]

61.5.2 The disputed 90-day feeding test

Rodent studies cannot readily be applied to the testing of whole food and feed, which are extremely complex mixtures of substances, often characterized by a wide variation in composition and nutritional value, thus dampening the sensitivity of the assay. One problem is that the dose of individual ingredients of whole food/feed is too low to identify potential hazards in the unlikely case that unintended effects may remain undetected in the extensive analyses of Sections 61.2–61.4. Also, whole feed cannot be given to rodents at multiples of the amount that might be present in the diet of some farm animals (the inclusion rate of test materials in the rodent feed ranges from 10% for cottonseed meal to 50% for maize grains). Another aspect to consider in conducting rodent feeding studies is the nutritional balance of the diet, in order to avoid adverse effects induced by alimentary deficiencies not related to the genetic transformation. Finally, in view of the natural variability of clinical and pathological endpoints, any attempt to relate the expected small effects in feeding studies conclusively to the tested GM food/feed is problematic. It is, therefore, highly questionable whether whole food/feed testing helps to detect potential adverse effects of GM plants.[80,81]

In its guidance, the GMO panel at EFSA indicated that, notwithstanding the above limitations, a 90-day feeding study in rodents with whole food/feed may help to clarify uncertainties resulting from the comparative assessment.[8] This is applicable to complex genetic modifications that change fundamentally the nutritional properties of the GM crop, although the level of uncertainty, which would trigger the need for such a rodent study, has not been defined. Some competent authorities defend the principle that the 90-day feeding study should be performed in the context of all applications for the authorization of single transformation events, even when the comparative assessment fails to identify any hypothesis for an adverse effect. Thus the EU still imposes a 90-day feeding study for the risk assessment of single events,[3] but it was planned to review this decision in light of the outcome of research carried out within the 7th Framework Program.[82–84] It is in any case not appropriate to subject experimental animals to a study that, given its insensitivity and problematic interpretation, is unable to yield meaningful data for the risk assessment.

61.6 Allergenicity assessment

The purpose is to demonstrate that the GM plant does not deploy a higher allergenic potential than the conventional counterpart and non-GM reference varieties.

61.6.1 Weight-of-evidence allergenicity evaluation of newly expressed proteins

Immunoglobulin E (IgE)-mediated reactions, which affect the skin as well as the gastrointestinal, respiratory, and cardiovascular systems, represent the main form of food allergy that may manifest with severe symptoms including life-threatening anaphylaxis. The paradigm of GM soybean expressing a methionine-rich 2S albumin from the Brazil nut (*Bertholletia excelsa*) highlights the hazard that could arise in sensitized subjects when an allergen is transferred by genetic transformation.[85,86] This experimental GM crop was never advanced to the market but illustrates why NEPs that could be present in final products should be analyzed for their potential to cause allergic reactions. The questions are whether a NEP is one to which certain individuals may already be sensitive and whether a protein new to the food supply is likely to induce novel allergic reactions by de novo sensitization. It is advisable to avoid the transfer of gene sequences from commonly allergenic foods (e.g., peanuts, soybean, tree nuts) and from cereals known to elicit gluten-sensitive enteropathy (Section 61.6.4), unless it can be demonstrated that the transferred sequence is innocuous.

Food allergy is a pathologic deviation of the immune system in a subset of the population (2%–4% of adults, 5%–8% of children) and, hence, is not a property of proteins that can be reliably evidenced experimentally.[87,88] As there is no single test to predict allergic responses, a weight-of-evidence procedure is taken to assess the possible allergenicity of NEPs.[8,89] This approach entails several elements:

- the allergenic status of the organism from which the NEP originates, that is, whether the source of the NEP has been recognized as an oral, respiratory, or contact allergen;
- any relevant similarity between the amino acid sequence of the NEP and that of known allergens recorded in databases;
- protein properties including, but not limited to, the susceptibility to heat treatment and enzymatic degradation.

The search for epitopes by amino acid sequence analysis serves to identify potential IgE cross-reactivities between the NEP and known allergens. The value of very short amino acid sequence matches for the prediction of allergenicity has been dismissed.[90] Therefore the most commonly used method compares the sequence of the NEP under scrutiny with that of proven allergens by a contiguous search over a sliding window of 80 amino acids. The threshold of concern is set at >35% sequence identity using alignment algorithms developed to recognize domain homologies, whereby inserted gaps are treated as mismatches.[91,92] This screen generates false positives due to the inability to distinguish between true homologies between proteins and irrelevant sequence similarities. Another caveat is that many NEPs are present in crops at low concentrations that may be insufficient to cause symptoms of allergy.

A resistance to pepsin digestion had been linked previously to allergenicity.[93] Consequently, degradation tests with pepsin or simulated gastric fluid were thought to indicate if further analyses should be conducted to determine the likelihood of the NEP being allergenic. However, protein stability is poorly associated with an allergenic potential as digestive activities may abolish, decrease, have no effect, or even augment the allergenicity of proteins.[94–98] Because of this lack of a clear readout, it has been proposed to remove digestion tests from the allergenicity assessment scheme.[99]

For NEPs that originate from a source known to be allergenic, or have sequence homology with a known allergen, immunological tests should be performed. Specifically, sera from sensitized individuals with a clinically validated allergy to the source of the protein, or to a potentially cross-reacting antigen, are used to test for the presence of IgE antibodies recognizing the NEP under assessment. A critical limitation is the availability of human sera from a sufficient number of individuals, but negative results from eight relevant sera confer a 99% certainty that the new protein is not an allergen.[91] Auxiliary allergenicity testing using *in vitro* cell–based assays or in vivo bioassays in animal models have not yet been validated for regulatory purposes in the food sector.

61.6.2 Allergenicity of the whole genetically modified plant

When the recipient plant is known to be allergenic, the EU regulation requests that the comparative analysis described in Section 61.3.4 should include a repertoire of documented allergens of that plant. The goal is to ascertain that the genetic transformation does not unintentionally increase the expression of allergens above the upper equivalence limit defined in the field trial by the non-GM reference varieties. To date, this requirement applies only to endogenous allergens found in soybean[100,101] as listed in the relevant OECD consensus document.[45] This additional data is not requested by competent authorities outside the EU.

61.6.3 Adjuvanticity

Immuno-adjuvants are substances that, when coadministered with an antigen, stimulate immune responses and may thereby enhance an allergic reaction. Sequence similarities to a known adjuvant protein (e.g., cholera toxin subunit B) may indicate a possible adjuvant activity of NEPs. Such an evaluation is requested in the EU but, so far, none of the NEPs assessed and listed in Table 61.2 display characteristics that may confer the ability to act as an adjuvant by the oral route.[102,103]

61.6.4 Gluten-sensitive enteropathy

Celiac disease (also known as gluten-sensitive enteropathy) is an autoimmune disorder of the intestinal villi. This enteropathy is triggered by dietary gluten or gluten-like proteins (storage proteins of wheat, barley, rye, and possibly oat) in genetically predisposed individuals that possess the DQ2 or DQ8 haplotype of human leukocyte antigen (HLA). An involvement of the immune system is demonstrated by the recruitment—to the intestinal mucosa—of T lymphocytes specific for gluten-derived peptides bound to HLA-DQ2 or HLA-DQ8 complexes. Although the disease penetrance in individuals with one or both of these haplotypes is incomplete,[104–106] NEPs should be evaluated for a sequence similarity with HLA-DQ2- or HLA-DQ8-restricted epitopes known to elicit celiac disease. The Codex Alimentarius states that this assessment is needed if the introduced genetic material derives from cereals associated with celiac disease.[7] In the EU, there is a broader requirement to screen the amino acid sequence of NEPs whenever there is no history of safe consumption of the protein among subjects with celiac disease. A dedicated guidance provides bioinformatic methods to rule out the presence of nine-amino acid peptides matching with known celiac-causing epitopes.[107,108] In the case that a partial match is found, the guidance describes three-dimensional modeling to determine whether the peptides would be able to bind to HLA-DQ2 or HLA-DQ8 in a way that this could lead to activation of T cell receptors. Depending on the outcome of these in silico studies, in vitro experiments like HLA-DQ binding or T cell activation tests should be considered.[109]

61.7 Nutritional assessment

The purpose is to demonstrate that the genetic transformation does not generate products that are nutritionally disadvantageous as compared to the food and feed that it is intended to replace. This assessment considers the consequences of any change in composition, beyond background fluctuations, observed in the GM plant relative to its comparators, and is important if the particular crop is known to be a relevant source of the specific nutrient with altered concentration. It should be estimated to what extent the measured change will affect the intake of that nutrient by humans and animals. The first step is to determine the level of the substance in question in the parts of the plant intended for food and feed uses. The concentrations from the compositional analysis (Section 61.3.4) need to be combined with the anticipated intake of the crop and derived products using regional or national consumption data (e.g., the EFSA Food Consumption Database for EU populations). Implications of an altered nutrient concentration should be predicted both at average and maximal levels of consumption, also considering variations in food preferences and vulnerable population groups such as infants, children and the elderly. Dietary reference values, adequate intake (AI), upper intake levels, or acceptable daily intake levels, as appropriate, might support the assessment. When no such guidance values exist, consideration may be given to the record of safe use of nutrients consumed as part of the diet. Similarly, animal nutrient requirements and nutrition guidelines serve as the reference to assess possible consequences of changes in feed composition. Supporting feeding studies with rapidly growing farm animals such as broiler chicks (as a monogastric model), lambs (as a ruminant model), or fish (as an aquatic species) may be presented in this context. Control diets in such studies should include the conventional counterpart and, if available, additional comparators. In the case of a herbicide tolerance trait, the test material should come from GM plants exposed to the intended herbicide.

If GM plants have undergone modifications to intentionally alter their nutritional profile, the assessment should include the possibility that the overall intake of particular nutrients is affected by the market introduction of the novel food and feed. A paradigmatic example is oil from soybean with an increased content of monounsaturated fatty acids. The purpose of this GM soybean with reduced omega-6 fatty acid desaturase activity (through siRNA-mediated silencing) is to obtain oil with a higher proportion of heat-stable oleic acid (C18:1) mainly at the expense of heat-labile polyunsaturated fatty acids (C18:2 and C18:3) prone to oxidation (Table 61.5[110]). This oil tends to become less rancid and is more suited for frying and bakery without the need for chemical stabilization by hydrogenation. In view of this favorable feature, oil from GM soybean with reduced omega-6 fatty acid desaturase might potentially replace other oils in addition to the conventional soybean counterpart. As a consequence, the change of fatty acid composition was assessed in a broad human exposure scenario where not only soybean oil but all conventional vegetable oils are replaced with oil from the GM soybean, taking into account that consumers need to attain AIs of polyunsaturated fatty acids. Despite this total replacement scenario, which is far beyond the actually intended use of the new product, the calculated reduction in the dietary omega-6 fatty acid availability did not raise health concerns.

61.8 Exposure assessment and risk characterization

Follow-up steps of the risk assessment are usually minimized by the recognition that, for many GM plants, a thorough hazard identification, as described in Sections 61.2–61.7, reveal no concerns needing further assessment. An exception is for example the surge of acetylated amino acids in GM maize expressing the GAT enzyme (Section 61.3.4). Most regulatory authorities nevertheless request a *pro forma* full risk assessment regardless of the case-specific attributes of the GM plant under scrutiny, that is, even in the absence of any evidence of hazards or a plausible hypothesis warranting exposure estimates or risk characterization.

TABLE 61.5 Fatty acid composition of the seeds of a herbicide-tolerant, nutritionally altered GM soybean and its non-GM comparator.

Analyte	Conventional counterpart	GM soybean	
		Untreated	Sulfonylurea herbicide
Mono-unsaturated fatty acids			
Heptadecenoic acid (C17:1)	0.06	1.26	1.26
Oleic acid (C18:1)	19.2	73.7	72.7
Nonadecenoic acid (C19:1)	0.04	0.31	0.32
Eicosenoic acid (C20:1)	0.17	0.35	0.35
Polyunsaturated fatty acids			
Linoleic acid (C18:2)	54.9	4.26	4.48
Linolenic acid (C18:3)	8.28	4.84	4.72

The GM soybean was either untreated or exposed to the intended sulfonylurea herbicide. Fatty acid proportions are indicated as the percentages of total fatty acids. *GM*, genetically modified.

61.8.1 Anticipated extent of use

Production and import quantities as well as realistic levels of use of the GM food and feed are difficult to predict. For an estimate of the expected intake (or "exposure"), the risk assessment is, therefore, carried out by assuming that the GM plant will replace the respective conventional food and feed by 100%. On the basis of representative consumption data for products obtained from the corresponding conventional plant, it is then possible to estimate anticipated average and maximum intakes of the GM food and feed. To complete the risk assessment, it is also possible to calculate the expected intake of constituents of which the levels have been altered as a result of the genetic transformation (based on compositional analyses, Section 61.3.4), the expected intake of new plant constituents (based on their concentration in edible parts of the plant, Section 61.5), and the expected intake of NEPs (based on the protein expression levels, Section 61.2.4). These estimates may take into account the effects of treatment of the food and feed in question, for example, a potential accumulation or reduction during processing (Section 61.3.5).

61.8.2 Risk characterization

An integrated assessment of GM food and feed is based on the data obtained from hazard identification and hazard characterization (Sections 61.2–61.7) and the anticipated intake levels (Section 61.8.1). In the vast majority of cases, this risk characterization is of qualitative nature by addressing whether the GM food and feed is as safe and nutritious as the corresponding non-GM comparators under similar processing practices and consumption patterns. This risk characterization process also comprises a qualitative evaluation of the remaining uncertainties and an appraisal on whether the overall uncertainty is acceptable or if, on the other hand, the uncertainty reaches a degree that might conceal a health risk for humans or animals. Market authorization is rejected if potentially disadvantageous characteristics of the GM plant relative to non-GM comparators translate to any predictable risk.

61.9 Risk management

Following completion of the safety assessment, the GM crop might be subjected to special risk management measures that accompany its commercial distribution. To ensure scientific integrity and full transparency, there should always be a functional separation of risk assessment and risk management. However, special considerations as the ones outlined below may necessitate a closer dialog between risk assessors and risk managers.

61.9.1 Postmarket monitoring

Monitoring of marketed food and feed derived from GM crops can be requested if, once the safety of GM food and feed has been demonstrated, it is appropriate to confirm the anticipated consumption levels. Particular attention should be paid in this respect to those GM plants that are aimed at changing nutritional profiles of foods and feeds. In these cases, postmarket monitoring might be useful to detect changes in the dietary intake pattern and to confirm that such changes would not result in adverse effects.

61.9.2 Pesticide residues

Some GM plants exhibit traits (most prominently herbicide tolerance) which could result in the accumulation of pesticide residues or novel pesticide metabolites. Procedures for establishing the safety of such residues and validated methods for their detection should be in place.[111] It must be ensured, in particular, that the herbicide is authorized and that the maximum residue levels established for the commodity and its products also include metabolites formed in herbicide-tolerant plants.

61.9.3 Low-level presence

Traces of GM plants that have passed the safety assessment in one or more countries may appear in importing countries, where the relevant GM food and feed has not been authorized. Two distinct exposure scenarios are possible[7]:

- Commodities like grains, beans, or seeds, in which the GM food or feed would be diluted to low-level amounts at any time. Because these commodities are sourced from multiple farms and commingled during harvest, storage, shipment, import, and processing, any inadvertent GM material would be present only at minute levels in final products.
- Foods that are commonly consumed whole and undiluted, such as fruits and vegetables like potatoes, tomatoes, and papaya. While the likelihood of consuming material from an unauthorized GM variety and the likelihood of repeated intake would be low, any such consumption might be of an entire unauthorized fruit or vegetable.

For the first, more common case of low-level presence, upon request by the European Commission the EFSA GMO Panel issued guidance for the evaluation of GM crops intended for markets other than in the EU.[112] In this context, the presence at low level has been defined at a maximum of 0.9% GM plant material per ingredient. In view of this low exposure, only certain parts of the risk assessment will be relevant. In principle, the molecular characterization of the transformation event and its intended effects should be performed, whereas studies aiming at identifying unintended effects are not necessary in this low-level scenario.

61.10 Conclusion and perspectives

The above case-by-case analysis provides assurance that the GM plant under assessment does not cause harm to humans and farm/domestic animals when harvested, processed, and consumed according to its foreseen purposes. Each risk assessment will conclude whether the GM products are as safe and nutritious as non-GM comparators with a documented record of use. If applicable, the assessment should inform risk managers on any postmarket monitoring or restrictions that might be needed to mitigate uncertainties. Conversely, an incomplete hazard identification and characterization will lead to an inconclusive assessment. Unfortunately, it can be observed that the implementation of these principles of a comparative assessment tends to solicit many regulatory authorities to overscrutinize GM plants by requesting an increasingly complex set of studies with costs and timelines that are inconsistent with identifiable risks.[52,53]

The aim of crop breeding is to introduce advantageous heritable traits while minimizing adverse unintended effects. To that end, tremendous progress is being made in developing new methods to add, remove, or alter nucleotide sequences in the plants' genome. With such genome-editing tools, specific changes to the DNA can now be made at particular locations with very high precision.[113–115] The resulting genome-edited plants are in most cases indistinguishable from spontaneously occurring variants as the same alterations could also result from natural mutations. By exploiting such advanced breeding tools, it will hopefully be possible to cover the growing demand of the world's population for high-quality and sustainable food supplies. In the agriculture of the future, high-precision plant breeding could for example adapt the plants to the deterioration of arable land (resulting from erosion or increased salinity), to the changing climate (associated with heat waves, droughts, and flooding), and to an increasing pathogen stress, thus reducing crop losses and diminishing the need for fertilizers and pesticides.[116]

Competent authorities in the United States, Australia, and other countries decided not to regulate such high-precision genome-editing technologies in plants if they do not introduce foreign sequences. This includes, for example, the use of site-directed nucleases (SDNs) or other site-specific DNA modifiers, as long as the recipient cell is allowed to restore the double helix integrity by natural means, that is, without foreign templates for repair synthesis. By contrast, the Court of Justice of the EU ruled that organisms obtained by genome editing, for example using SDNs, are to be categorized as GM and, consequently, bound to the regulatory obligations described in this chapter.[9] It is true that the comparative risk assessment is also applicable in part (with substantial derogations) to plants altered by modern genome-modifying techniques. Nevertheless, imposing the onerous regulatory framework designed for GM organisms to the market approval of genome-edited plants will dampen entrepreneurship in the European food and feed industry. One reason for this negative impact on innovation is that the financial resources (entailing scientists and patent lawyers) necessary to bring a GM product to the market will remain outside the reach of small and medium-sized enterprises. To foster advances in this vital economic sector, therefore, the existing regulation will hopefully be deescalated while preserving the elements needed to guarantee the safety of gene-edited food and feed, but with the aim of rolling out superfluous data requirements for which there is no scientific justification and that confer no added value for the safety evaluation.

Some more challenging traits, like enhanced photosynthesis, disease resistance, or vitamin fortification, will depend on the practical application of advances in the fast-evolving synthetic biology (SynBio) research field. The introduction of multifactorial traits by SynBio will, presumably, be achieved through multiplex genome modifications using various genetic engineering techniques. For a fit-to-purpose evaluation of emerging and, potentially, very valuable plants created by SynBio assembly, it will eventually be unavoidable to switch from the current technology-driven risk perception to a more trait-based appraisal irrespective of the underlying technology.[52,117] The familiarity gained during the last decades in the assessment of GM plants justifies this future change of paradigm, as benefits and risks posed by foods and feeds are entirely determined by their nutritional characteristic and safety profile, not by the processes employed for their production.

Acknowledgments

The author wishes to thank all GMO Panel members over four terms (2012–2024) for their contributions to the risk assessment of GM plants. Of outstanding value was the support from my very friendly colleagues Josep Casacuberta, Andrew Chesson, Huw Jones, Gijs Kleter, Harry Kuiper, Fabien Nogué, Nils Rostoks and Jeremy Sweet. Also acknowledged is the pleasant collaboration with all scientific officers of the GMO Unit at EFSA. The author wishes to thank particularly Elisabeth Waigmann, Anna Lanzoni and Michele Ardizzone for many interesting discussions.

References

1. Ledford H. Creators of gene-edited animals bypass US market. *Nature*. 2016;566:433–434.
2. EFSA GMO and AHAW Panels. Scientific opinion on the guidance on the risk assessment of food and feed from genetically modified animals and animal health and welfare. *EFSA J*. 2012;10:2501. Available from: https://doi.org/10.2903/j.efsa.2012.2501.
3. European Commission. Regulation No 503/2013 of 3 April 2013 on applications for authorisation of genetically modified food and feed. <https://eur-lex.europa.eu/legal-content/EN/TXT/HTML/?uri = CELEX:32013R0503&from = EN>; Accessed 31.12.20.
4. Organization for Economic Co-operation and Development. *Safety Evaluation of Foods Derived by Modern Biotechnology, Concepts and Principles*. Paris, France; 1993.
5. Organization for Economic Co-operation and Development. *Genetically Modified Foods: Widening the Debate on Health and Safety*. Paris, France; 2000.
6. Codex Alimentarius Commission. *Guideline for the Conduct of Food Safety Assessment of Foods Derived from Recombinant-DNA Plants*. FAO and WHO; 2003.
7. Codex Alimentarius Commission. *Foods Derived from Modern Biotechnology*. FAO and WHO; 2009.
8. EFSA GMO Panel. Scientific opinion on guidance for risk assessment of food and feed from genetically modified plants. *EFSA J*. 2011;9:2150. Available from: https://doi.org/10.2903/j.efsa.2011.2150.
9. Bruetschy C. The EU regulatory framework on genetically modified organisms (GMOs). *Transgenic Res*. 2019;28:169–174.
10. Schiemann J, Dietz-Pfeilstetter A, Hartung F, et al. Risk assessment and regulation of plants modified by modern biotechniques: current status and future challenges. *Annu Rev Plant Biol*. 2019;70:699–726.
11. Giraldo PA, Shinozuka H, Spangenberg GC, et al. Safety assessment of genetically modified feed: is there any difference from food? *Front Plant Sci*. 2019;10:1592. Available from: https://doi.org/10.3389/fpls.2019.01592.
12. EFSA GMO Panel. Scientific opinion on application (EFSA-GMO-UK-2006-34) for the placing on the market of genetically modified maize 3272 with a thermotolerant alpha-amylase, for food and feed uses, import and processing under Regulation (EC) No 1829/2003 from Syngenta Crop Protection AG. *EFSA J*. 2013;11:3252. Available from: https://doi.org/10.2903/j.efsa.2013.3252.
13. EFSA GMO Panel. Statement complementing the EFSA Scientific Opinion on application (EFSA-GMO-UK-2006-34) for authorisation of food and feed containing, consisting of and produced from genetically modified maize 3272. *EFSA J*. 2019;17:5844. Available from: https://doi.org/10.2903/j.efsa.2019.5844.
14. EFSA GMO Panel. Scientific opinion on an application by Dow AgroSciences LLC (EFSA-GMO-NL-2011-91) for the placing on the market of genetically modified herbicide-tolerant soybean DAS-68416-4 for food and feed uses, import and processing under Regulation (EC) No 1829/2003. *EFSA J*. 2017;15:4719. Available from: https://doi.org/10.2903/j.efsa.2017.4719.
15. Lee TC, Edrington TC, Bell E, et al. Effect of common processing of soybeans on the enzymatic activity and detectability of the protein, Dicamba Mono-Oxygenase (DMO), introduced into dicamba-tolerant MON 87708. *Regul Toxicol Pharmacol*. 2019;102:98–107.
16. EFSA. Explanatory note on DNA sequences similarity searches in the context of the assessment of horizontal gene transfer from plants to microorganisms. *EFSA Support Publ*. 2017;EN-1273. Available from: https://doi.org/10.2903/sp.efsa.2017.EN-1273.
17. Brigulla M, Wackernagel W. Molecular aspects of gene transfer and foreign DNA acquisition in prokaryotes with regard to safety issues. *Appl Microbiol Biotechnol*. 2010;86:1027–1041.

18. Kleter GA, Peijnenburg AC, Aarts HJ. Health considerations regarding horizontal gene transfer of microbial transgenes present in genetically modified crops. *J Biomed Biotechnol.* 2005;4: 326–352.
19. Rizzi A, Raddadi N, Sorlini C, et al. The stability and degradation of dietary DNA in the gastrointestinal tract of mammals – implications for horizontal gene transfer and the biosafety of GMOs. *Crit Rev Food Sci Nutr.* 2012;52:142–161.
20. EFSA. Explanatory note on the determination of newly expressed protein levels in the context of genetically modified plant applications for EU market authorization. *EFSA Support Publ.* 2010;EN-1466. Available from: https://doi.org/10.2903/sp.efsa.2018.EN-1466.
21. Baum JA, Bogaert T, Clinton W, et al. Control of coleopteran insect pests through RNA interference. *Nat Biotechnol.* 2007; 25:1322–1326.
22. Gordon KH, Waterhouse PM. RNAi for insect-proof plants. *Nat Biotechnol.* 2007;25:1231–1232.
23. Mao YB, Cai WJ, Wang JW, et al. Silencing a cotton bollworm P450 monooxygenase gene by plant-mediated RNAi impairs larval tolerance of gossypol. *Nat Biotechnol.* 2007;25:1307–1313.
24. EFSA GMO Panel. Assessment of genetically modified maize MON 87411 for food and feed uses, import and processing, under Regulation (EC) No 1829/2003 (application EFSA-GMO-NL-2015-124). *EFSA J.* 2018;16:5310. Available from: https://doi.org/10.2903/j.efsa.2018.5310.
25. Huvenne H, Smagghe G. Mechanisms of dsRNA uptake in insects and potential of RNAi for pest control: a review. *J Insect Physiol.* 2010;56:227–235.
26. Senthil-Kumar M, Mysore KS. Caveat of RNAi in plants: the off-target effect. *Methods Mol Biol.* 2011;744:13–25.
27. Paces J, Nic M, Novotny T, Svoboda P. Literature review of baseline information to support the risk assessment of RNAi-based GM plants. *EFSA Support Publ.* 2017;EN-1246. Available from: https://doi.org/10.2903/sp.efsa-2017.EN-1246.
28. Casacuberta JM, Devos Y, du Jardin P, et al. Biotechnological uses of RNAi in plants: risk assessment consideration. *Trends Biotechnol.* 2015;33:145–147.
29. EFSA GMO Panel. Annex II of the minutes of the 118th Plenary Meeting. <https://www.efsa.europa.eu/sites/default/files/event/171025-m.pdf>; 2017 Accessed 31.12.20.
30. Pinzón N, Li B, Martinez L, et al. MicroRNA target prediction programs predict many false positives. *Genome Res.* 2017;27: 234–245.
31. EFSA GMO Panel. Assessment of genetically modified maize MON 87427 x MON 87460 × MON 89034 × MIR162 × NK603 and subcombinations, for food and feed uses, under Regulation (EC) No 1829/2003 (application EFSA-GMO-NL-2016-134). *EFSA J.* 2019;17:57–74. Available from: https://doi.org/10.2903/j.efsa.2019.5774.
32. Kramer C, Brune P, McDonald J, et al. Evolution of risk assessment strategies for food and feed uses of stacked GM events. *Plant Biotechnol J.* 2016;14:1899–1913.
33. De Schrijver A, De Clercq P, De Maagd RA, et al. Relevance of Bt toxin interaction studies for environmental risk assessment of genetically modified crops. *Plant Biotechnol J.* 2015;13:1221–1223.
34. Baranek J, Konecka E, Kaznowski A. Interaction between toxin crystals and vegetative insecticidal proteins of *Bacillus thuringiensis* in lepidopteran larvae. *BioControl.* 2017;62:649.
35. Kok EJ, Pedersen J, Onori R, et al. Plants with stacked genetically modified events: to assess or not to assess? *Trends Biotechnol.* 2014;32:70–73.
36. EFSA GMO Panel. Annex I of the minutes of the 115th Plenary Meeting. <https://www.efsa.europa.eu/sites/default/files/event/170517-m.pdf>; 2017 Accessed 31.12.20.
37. van der Voet H, Perry JN, Amzal B, et al. A statistical assessment of differences and equivalences between genetically modified and reference plant varieties. *BMC Biotechnol.* 2011;11:15. Available from: https://doi.org/10.1186/1472-6750-11-15.
38. van der Voet H, Paoletti C. Equivalence testing approaches in genetically modified organism risk assessment. *J Agric Food Chem.* 2019;67:13506–13508.
39. EFSA GMO Panel. Guidance on selection of comparators for the risk assessment of genetically modified plants and derived food and feed. *EFSA J.* 2011;9:2149. Available from: https://doi.org/10.2903/j.efsa.2011.2149.
40. EFSA GMO Panel. Statistical considerations for the safety evaluation of GMOs. *EFSA J.* 2010;8:1250. Available from: https://doi.org/10.2903/j.efsa.2010.1250.
41. EFSA GMO Panel. Guidance on the agronomic and phenotypic characterisation of genetically modified plants. *EFSA J.* 2015;13:4128. Available from: https://doi.org/10.2903/j.efsa.2015.4128.
42. Organization for Economic Co-operation and Development. *Consensus Document on Compositional Considerations for New Varieties of Maize (Zea mays): Key Food and Feed Nutrients, Anti-nutrients and Secondary Plant Metabolites.* Paris, France; 2002.
43. Paoletti C, Favilla S, Leo A, et al. Variability of crops' compositional characteristics: what do experimental data show? *J Agric Food Chem.* 2018;66:9507–9515.
44. Becker-Ritt AB, Mulinari F, Vasconcelos IM, et al. Antinutritional and/or toxic factors in soybean (*Glycine max* (L.) Merril) seeds: comparison of different cultivars adapted to the southern region of Brazil. *J Sci Food Agric.* 2004;84:263–270.
45. Organization for Economic Co-operation and Development. *Revised Consensus Document on Compositional Considerations for New 452 Varieties of Soybean [Glycine max (L.) Merr.]: Key Food and Feed Nutrients, 453 Antinutrients, Toxicants and Allergens.* Paris, France; 2012.
46. Maria John KM, Khan F, Luthria DL, et al. Proteomic analysis of anti-nutritional factors (ANF's) in soybean seeds as affected by environmental and genetic factors. *Food Chem.* 2017;218:321–329.
47. EFSA GMO Panel. Scientific opinion on application (EFSA-GMO-UK-2008-53) for the placing on the market of herbicide tolerant genetically modified maize 98140 for food and feed uses, import and processing under Regulation (EC) No 1829/2003 from Pioneer Overseas Corporation. *EFSA J.* 2013;11:3139. Available from: https://doi.org/10.2903/j.efsa.2013.3139.
48. Karaman S, Barnett J, Sykes GP, et al. Subchronic oral toxicity assessment of N-acetyl-L-aspartic acid in rats. *Food Chem Toxicol.* 2011;49:3192–3205.
49. EFSA GMO Panel. Scientific Opinion on application (EFSA-GMO-NL-2010-87) for the placing on the market of genetically modified herbicide tolerant oilseed rape GT73 for food containing or consisting of, and food produced from or containing ingredients produced from, oilseed rape GT73 (with the exception of refined oil and food additives) under Regulation (EC) No 1829/2003 from Monsanto. *EFSA J.* 2013;11:3079. Available from: https://doi.org/10.2903/j.efsa.2013.3079.

50. EFSA GMO Panel. Assessment of genetically modified oilseed rape GT73 for renewal authorization under Regulation (EC) No 1829/2003 (application EFSA-GMO-RX-002). *EFSA J.* 2020;18:6199. Available from: https://doi.org/10.2903/j.efsa.2020.6199.
51. Christ B, Hochstrasser R, Guyer L, et al. Non-specific activities of the major herbicide-resistance gene BAR. *Nat Plants.* 2017;3:937–945.
52. Tagliabue G. Product, not process! Explaining a basic concept in agricultural biotechnologies and food safety. *Life Sci Soc Policy.* 2017;13:3.
53. Wolt JD. Current risk assessment approaches for environmental and food and feed safety assessment. *Transgenic Res.* 2019;28:111–117.
54. Christensen HM, Crane V, Hu X, et al. Maize event DP-023211-2 and methods for detection thereof. International Patent C12N 15/82 (2006.01). <https://patentimages.storage.googleapis.com/ee/ff/f8/90f1f2112adabe/WO2019209700A1.pdf>; 2019 Accessed 31.12.20.
55. EFSA GMO Panel. Assessment of genetically modified soybean SYHT0H2 for food and feed uses, import and processing, under Regulation (EC) No 1829/2003 (application EFSA-GMO-DE-2012-111). *EFSA J.* 2020;18:5946. Available from: https://doi.org/10.2903/j.efsa.2020.5946.
56. Franceschi N, Paraskevopoulos K, Waigmann E, et al. Predictive protein toxicity and its use in risk assessment. *Trends Biotechnol.* 2017;35:483–486.
57. Hoang TX, Marsella L, Trovato A, et al. Common attributes of native-state structures of proteins, disordered proteins, and amyloid. *Proc Natl Acad Sci U S A.* 2006;103:6883–6888.
58. Fieldhouse RJ, Merrill AR. Needle in the haystack: structure-specific toxin discovery. *Trends Biochem Sci.* 2008;33:546–556.
59. Senior AW, Evans R, Jumper J, et al. Improved protein structure prediction using potentials from deep learning. *Nature.* 2020;577:706–710.
60. Organization for Economic Co-operation and Development. *Test No. 407: Repeated Dose 28-Day Oral Toxicity Study in Rodents.* Paris, France; 2008.
61. Bushey DF, Bannon GA, Delaney BF, et al. Characterization and safety assessment of intractable proteins in genetically modified crops. *Regul Toxicol Pharmacol.* 2014;69:154–170.
62. Heisel SE, Zhang Y, Allen E, et al. Characterization of unique small RNA populations from rice grains. *PLoS One.* 2008;3:e2871. Available from: https://doi.org/10.1371/journal.pone.0002871.
63. Ivashuta SI, Petrick JS, Heisel SE, et al. Endogenous small RNAs in grain: semi-quantification and sequence homology to human and animal genes. *Food Chem Toxicol.* 2009;47:353–360.
64. Dàvalos A, Henriques R, Latasa MJ, et al. Literature review of baseline information on non-coding (ncRNA) to support the risk assessment of ncRNA-based genetically modified plants for food and feed. *EFSA Support Publ.* 2019; EN-1688. Available from: https://doi.org/10.2903/sp.efsa.2019.EN-1688.
65. Park NJ, Li Y, Yu T, et al. Characterization of RNA in saliva. *Clin Chem.* 2007;52:988–994.
66. Liu Y, Zhang Y, Dong P, et al. Digestion of nucleic acids starts in the stomach. *Sci Rep.* 2015;5:11936. Available from: https://doi.org/10.1038/srep11936.
67. Jain KK. Stability and delivery of RNA via the gastrointestinal tract. *Curr Drug Deliv.* 2008;5:27–31.
68. O'Neill MJ, Bourre L, Melgar S, et al. Intestinal delivery of non-viral gene therapeutics: physiological barriers and preclinical models. *Drug Discov Today.* 2011;16:203–218.
69. Gilmore IR, Fox SP, Hollins AJ, et al. The design and exogenous delivery of siRNA for post-transcriptional gene silencing. *J Drug Target.* 2004;12:315–340.
70. Tosar JP, Rovira C, Naya H, et al. Mining of public sequencing databases supports a non-dietary origin for putative foreign miRNAs: underestimated effects of contamination in NGS. *RNA.* 2014;20:754–757.
71. Kang W, Bang-Berthelsen CH, Holm A, et al. Survey of 800+ data sets from human tissue and body fluid reveals xenomRs are likely artifacts. *RNA.* 2017;23:433–445.
72. Witwer KW. Alternative miRNAs? Human sequences misidentified as plant miRNAs in plant studies and in human plasma. *F1000Res.* 2018;7:244. Available from: https://doi.org/10.12688/f1000research.14060.1.
73. Vaishnaw AK, Gollob J, Gamba-Vitalo C, et al. A status report on RNAi therapeutics. *Silence.* 2010;1:14. Available from: https://doi.org/10.1186/1758-907X-1-14.
74. Christensen J, Litherland K, Faller T, et al. Metabolism studies of unformulated internally 3H-labeled short interfering RNAs in mice. *Drug Metab Dispos.* 2013;41:1211–1219.
75. Sioud M. On the delivery of small interfering RNAs into mammalian cells. *Expert Opin Drug Deliv.* 2005;2:639–651.
76. Dickinson B, Zhang Y, Petrick JS, et al. Lack of detectable oral bioavailability of plant microRNA after feeding in mice. *Nat Biotechnol.* 2013;31:965–967.
77. Petrick JS, Brower-Toland B, Jackson AL, et al. Safety assessment of food and feed from biotechnology-derived crops employing RNA-mediated gene regulation to achieve desired traits: a scientific review. *Regul Toxicol Pharmacol.* 2013;66:167–176.
78. Rodrigues TB, Petrick JS. Safety considerations for humans and other vertebrates regarding agricultural uses of externally applied RNA molecules. *Front Plant Sci.* 2020;11:407. Available from: https://doi.org/10.3389/fpls.2020.00407.
79. Papadopoulou N, Devos Y, Alvarez-Alfageme F, et al. Risk assessment considerations for genetically modified RNAi plants: EFSA's activities and perspective. *Front Plant Sci.* 2020;11:445. Available from: https://doi.org/10.3389/fpls.2020.00445.
80. Kuiper HA, Kok EJ, Davies HV. New EU legislation for risk assessment of GM food: no scientific justification for mandatory animal feeding trials. *Plant Biotechnol J.* 2013;11:781–784.
81. Devos Y, Naegeli H, Perry JN, et al. 90-day rodent feeding studies on whole GM food/feed: is the mandatory EU requirement for 90-day rodent feeding studies on whole GM food/feed fit for purpose and consistent with animal welfare ethics? *EMBO Rep.* 2016;17:942–945.
82. Zeljenková D, Ambrušová K, Bartušová M, et al. Ninety-day oral toxicity studies on two genetically modified maize MON810 varieties in Wistar Han RCC rats (EU 7th Framework Programme project GRACE). *Arch Toxicol.* 2014;88:2289–2314.
83. Steinberg P, van der Voet H, Goedhart PW, et al. Lack of adverse effects in subchronic and chronic toxicity/carcinogenicity studies on the glyphosate-resistant genetically modified maize NK603 in Wistar Han RCC rats. *Arch Toxicol.* 2019;93:1095–1139.
84. G-TwYST. Final Report Summary. <https://cordis.europa.eu/project/id/632165/reporting/de>; 2018 Accessed 31.12.20.

85. Nordlee JA, Taylor SL, Townsend JA, et al. Identification of a Brazil-nut allergen in transgenic soybeans. *N Engl J Med.* 1996;334:688–692.
86. Moreno FJ, Clemente A. 2S Albumin storage proteins: what makes them food allergens? *Open Biochem J.* 2008;2:16–18.
87. Castan L, Bogh KL, Maryniak NZ, et al. Overview of in vivo and ex vivo endpoints in murine food allergy models: suitable for evaluation of the sensitizing capacity of novel proteins? *Allergy.* 2019;75:289–301.
88. Costa J, Bavaro SL, Benedé S, et al. Are physicochemical properties shaping the allergenic potency of plant allergens? *Clin Rev Allergy Immunol.* 2020;. Available from: https://doi.org/10.1007/s12016-020-08810-9. online ahead of print.
89. EFSA GMO Panel. Scientific opinion on the assessment of allergenicity of GM plants and microorganisms and derived food and feed. *EFSA J.* 2010;8:1700. Available from: https://doi.org/10.2903/j.efsa.2010.1700.
90. Silvanovich A, Nemeth MA, Song P, et al. The value of short amino acid sequence matches for prediction of protein allergenicity. *Toxicol Sci.* 2006;90:252–258.
91. Food and Agriculture Organization of the United Nations, *Evaluation of Allergenicity of Genetically Modified Foods.* Rome, Italy; 2001.
92. Song P, Herman R, Kumpatla S. 1:1 FASTA update: using the power of E-values in FASTA to detect potential allergen cross-reactivity. *Toxicol Rep.* 2015;2:1145–1148.
93. Astwood JD, Leach JN, Fuchs RL. Stability of food allergens to digestion in vitro. *Nat Biotechnol.* 2010;14:1269–1273.
94. Bogh KL, Madsen CB. Food allergens: is there a correlation between stability to digestion and allergenicity? *Crit Rev Food Sci Nutr.* 2016;56:1545–1567.
95. Mackie A, Dupont D, Torcello-Gomez A, et al. Report on EFSA project OC/EFSA/GMO/2017/01 "In vitro protein digestibility" (Allergestion). *EFSA Support Publ.* 2019;EN-1765. Available from: https://doi.org/10.2903/sp.efsa.2019.EN-1765.
96. Wang R, Wang Y, Edrington TC, et al. Presence of small resistant peptides from new in vitro digestion assays detected by liquid chromatography tandem mass spectrometry: an implication of allergenicity prediction of novel proteins? *PLoS One.* 2020;15:e0233745. Available from: https://doi.org/10.1371/journal.pone.0233745.
97. Herman RA, Roper JM, Zhang JXQ. Evidence runs contrary to digestive stability predicting protein allergenicity. *Transgenic Res.* 2020;29:105–107.
98. EFSA GMO Panel. Statement on in vitro protein digestibility tests in allergenicity and protein safety assessment of GM plants. *EFSA J.* 2021;19:6350.
99. Verhoeckx K, Bogh KL, Dupont D, et al. The relevance of a digestibility evaluation in the allergenicity risk assessment of novel proteins. Opinion of a joint initiative of COST action ImpARAS and COST action INFOGEST. *Food Chem Toxicol.* 2019;129:405–423.
100. Fernandez A, Mills EN, Lovik M, et al. Endogenous allergens and compositional analysis in the allergenicity assessment of genetically modified plants. *Food Chem Toxicol.* 2013;62:1–6.
101. Selb R, Wal JM, Moreno FJ, et al. Assessment of endogenous allergenicity of genetically modified plants exemplified by soybean – where do we stand? *Food Chem Toxicol.* 2017;101:139–148.
102. Joshi SS, Barnett B, Doerrer NG, et al. Assessment of potential adjuvanticity of Cry proteins. *Regul Toxicol Pharmacol.* 2016;79:149–155.
103. Parenti MD, Santoro A, Del Rio A, et al. Literature review in support of adjuvanticity/immunogenicity assessment of proteins. *EFSA Support Publ.* 2019;EN-1551. Available from: https://doi.org/10.2903/sp.efsa.2019.EN-1551.
104. Plenge RM. Unlocking the pathogenesis of celiac disease. *Nat Genet.* 2010;42:281–282.
105. DeGeorge KC, Fry JW, Stein KM, et al. Celiac disease and gluten sensitivity. *Prim Care.* 2017;44:693–707.
106. Tye-Din JA, Galipeau HJ, Agardh D. Celiac disease: a review of current concepts in pathogenesis, prevention, and novel therapies. *Front Pediatr.* 2018;6:350. Available from: https://doi.org/10.3389/fped.2018.00350.
107. EFSA GMO Panel. Guidance on allergenicity assessment of genetically modified plants. *EFSA J.* 2017;15:4862. Available from: https://doi.org/10.2903/j.efsa.2017.4862.
108. Sollid LM, Tye-Din JA, Qiao SW, et al. Update 2020: nomenclature and listing of celiac disease-relevant gluten epitopes recognized by CD4 + T cells. *Immunogenetics.* 2020;72:85–88.
109. Fernandez A, Mills EN, Koning F, et al. Safety assessment of immune-mediated adverse reactions to novel food proteins. *Trends Biotechnol.* 2019;37:796–800.
110. EFSA GMO Panel. Scientific opinion on application EFSA-GMO-NL-2007-45 for the placing on the market of herbicide-tolerant, high-oleic acid, genetically modified soybean 305423 for food and feed uses, import and processing under Regulation (EC) No 1829/2003 from Pioneer. *EFSA J.* 2013;11:3499. Available from: https://doi.org/10.2903/j.efsa.2013.3499.
111. Kleter GA, Unsworth JB, Harris CA. The impact of altered herbicide residues in transgenic herbicide-resistant crops on standard setting for herbicide residues. *Pest Manag Sci.* 2011;67:1193–1210.
112. EFSA GMO Panel. Guidance for the risk assessment of the presence at low level of genetically modified plant material in imported food and feed under Regulation (EC) No 1829/2003. *EFSA J.* 2017;15:5048. Available from: https://doi.org/10.2903/j.efsa.2017.5048.
113. Kleter GA, Kuiper HA, Kok EJ. Gene-edited crops: towards a harmonized safety assessment. *Trends Biotechnol.* 2019;37:443–447.
114. Chen KL, Wang YP, Zhang R, et al. CRISPR/Cas genome editing and precision plant breeding in agriculture. *Annu Rev Plant Biol.* 2019;70:667–697.
115. Nogué F, Vergne P, Chèvre A-M, et al. Crop plants with improved culture and quality traits for food, feed and other uses. *Transgenic Res.* 2019;28:65–73.
116. Bailey-Serres J, Parker JE, Ainsworth EA, et al. Genetic strategies for improving crop yields. *Nature.* 2019;575:109–118.
117. Eriksson D. Recovering the original intentions of risk assessment and management of genetically modified organisms in the European Union. *Front Bioeng Biotechnol.* 2018;6:52. Available from: https://doi.org/10.3389/fbioe.2018.00052.

Section XI

Food safety: risk perception and communicating with the public

Chapter 62

Consumer attitudes about the use of new technologies in agrifood industries

Roger Clemens[1], Peter Pressman[2,3] and A. Wallace Hayes[4]

[1]*Department of Regulatory and Quality Science, School of Pharmacy, University of Southern California, Los Angeles, CA, United States,* [2]*Saba University School of Medicine, Saba, Dutch Caribbean,* [3]*Polyscience Consulting, Chatsworth, CA, United States,* [4]*College of Public Health, University of South Florida, Tampa, FL, United States*

Abstract

Providing the global consumer with safe foods is the priority of professionals in agriculture, food technology, nutrition, and regulatory agencies. The pioneering and initially criticized food safety efforts by German Chemist Friedrich Christian Accum (1769–1838) in London and Harvey Wiley (1844–1930) in the United States triggered significant advances to reduce dangerous substances in foods, and the promulgation of critical regulations that focused on safe foods and safe food production working conditions.

Since those early days of food processing and food safety regulations, a myriad of technologies and an array of food additives have increased the safety of food products, improved the nutritional value of foods, and extended the shelf-life of a range of foods. Some of those technologies include, but are not limited to, pasteurization, aseptic processing, nonthermal processing, flash-pasteurization, edible and smart packaging, biofortification, clustered regularly interspaced short palindromic repeats (CRISPR) and biotechnology. Several of these technologies and food additives as a food ingredient category and ingredient sourcing have triggered consumer concerns, stimulated international debates, and prompted numerous reactionary food regulations and restrictions that have impacted global food trade, product availability, and consumer misunderstandings.

Meaningful protection against real hazards is everyone's business, but the challenges inherent in implementing and disseminating food safety seem complicated by consumer perceptions equating food processing and food technologies in general with health risks and poor product quality. Moreover, while seemingly privileged western food activists often focus on the availability of high-quality artisanal and locally produced organic foods, the United Nations estimates that 1 billion people live with chronic hunger and malnutrition. Communication with, and education of consumers have emerged as an overarching mandate for industry and government alike.

Keywords: Food safety; food regulations; agriculture technology; consumer attitudes

62.1 Introduction

From a cursory overview of food regulations promulgated since 1906, particularly the Pure Food and Drug Act and the Federal Meat Inspection Act of that year, one quickly observes that all of the legislative actions in the United States, except the Food Safety and Modernization Act of 2011,[1] were triggered by a spectrum of adverse events (see Fig. 62.1). This Act was a major proactive reformation to provide additional safety of the food supply through the implementation of five key elements. Those elements are prevention, inspection, imported food, partnerships, and cooperation. Jointly, these regulations were developed to impart to consumers that measures taken by regulatory agencies and food manufacturers assure the safety of food by initiating critical steps in quality assurance and effective and nonmisleading communications.

A series of food and health surveys conducted in the United States since 2010 indicate consumers have changed their attitudes and behaviors toward foods and food ingredients, beliefs about food production and food technologies, and pursuit of plant-based foods and related dietary patterns. Interestingly, the primary sources of food safety information stem from food labels and websites, whereas television, magazines, and newspapers have little impact on informing consumers about food safety. During the past decade, consumers have become more aware of dietary components that may affect their health, such as dietary fats and sodium, while at the same time, paying more attention to their health, including weight management and noncommunicable diseases and their associated health risks while continuing to demand for foods that are safer and more nutritious. Unfortunately, much of this information fails to provide consumers and even scientists with the critical essence of much of the original research

Present Knowledge in Food Safety. DOI: https://doi.org/10.1016/B978-0-12-819470-6.00034-2

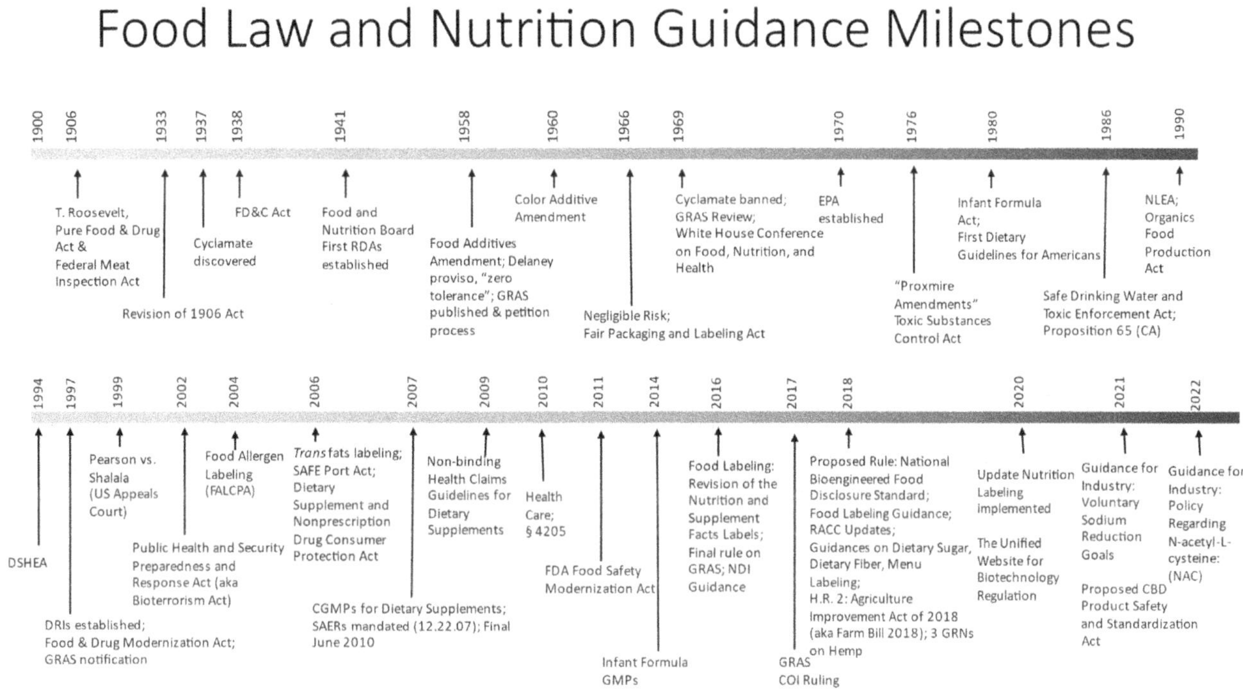

FIGURE 62.1 Food law and nutrition guidance milestones within the United States since 1906.

on these and other nutrition and health topics. The traditional systematic reviews and metaanalyses often are fraught with statistical model errors and incomplete coverage of the topics as evidenced by the prejudiced inclusion and exclusion criteria applied to peer-reviewed publications.[2,3]

The Centers for Disease Control and Prevention (CDC) monitor the incidence and prevalence of foodborne illnesses.[4] According to the CDC, more than 48 million people get sick from 31 pathogens that contribute to foodborne illness, 128,000 are hospitalized, and 3000 succumb annually. The primary vectors of foodborne illnesses appear to be an array of bacteria, viruses, and parasites, as well as harmful toxins and chemicals that can also contaminate foods. Recent estimates suggest the cost burden of foodborne illnesses may exceed \$2000 (USD) per case or between \$34.2 and \$161.8 billion as estimated using an array of models at the upper 90% of the estimate.[5] According to the World Bank, the global costs associated with foodborne illnesses are about \$110 billion (USD) annually in low and middle-income countries.[6] These costs are spread through at least three sectors, namely households, the food industry, and public health.[7]

The globalization of the food supply chain and changes in technologies applied to agricultural practices and food product production, the lack of international harmonization on food policies, including the foundations of food safety, and the inconsistent risk communications pertinent to food quality, and food and ingredient sourcing have impacted consumer perceptions of food safety and food-related hazards.[8]

The consumer perceptions of risk resulting from the globalization of the food supply chain transposes differently in differing settings, including time, restaurants, and culture. The subjective nature of food quality and food safety, at least in the minds of most consumers, makes it difficult for consumers to understand the need for both food quality and safety. For example, more than two decades ago, some investigators noted an interesting hierarchical value map for fresh fish that included terms such as happiness and well-being, good health and a long life, good and nourishing as well as factors influencing costs and preparation, but not food quality or safety.[9]

Restaurant operations within the United States are obliged to adhere to food safety standards as outlined, for example, in the ServeSafe program sponsored by the National Restaurant Association. The ServSafe program offers various personnel training programs for food handlers and management guidelines, such as sanitation practices to avoid contamination with food allergens and microbes, and a spectrum of system approaches to assure food safety. (https://www.servsafe.com/). Interestingly, a recent assessment by the CDC indicated restaurants with food safety training management programs tended to have fewer foodborne outbreaks, such as those caused by norovirus and *Clostridium perfringens*.10 Consumer reports on restaurant-based foodborne outbreaks indicated consumers are concerned with food safety practices among personnel, which, in turn, influenced their choice of dining locations. Consumers were particularly anxious about cleanliness and handling of ready-to-eat foods in these facilities, regardless of ethnic cuisines.[11–13]

Consumers continue to voice concerns over food service among the airlines and cruise ships. In a Turkish's study, more than 80% of passengers did not have high expectations for quality of foods and beverages served during flights.[14] In this setting, food safety remained an on-going concern, and was described as an essential compounded of food security within the transportation industry. However, an earlier study out of Spain suggested food safety was not a concern among those experiencing catering services at airports.[15]

A 2020 consumer survey among 1000 adults (>18 years old) intended to represent the diverse population within the United States indicated nearly half of the respondents were concerned about food safety when preparing foods at home, while voicing traditional concerns regarding food contaminants, safe cooking techniques, clean cutting boards, and food allergens.[16,17] Meanwhile, the survey participants indicated preferences of avoiding foods and beverages that included sugar, salt, fat, meat, and food additives since their perceptions of these ingredients were unsafe and unhealthful.

62.2 Genetically modified organisms

Three US regulatory agencies regulate most genetically modified foods (GMOs): the US Food and Drug Administration (FDA), the US Environmental Protection Agency (EPA), and the US Department of Agriculture (USDA). GMOs or genetically engineered foods, or bioengineered foods are produced from organisms that have had changes introduced into their DNA using the methods of genetic engineering.

The FDA regulates most human and animal food, including GMO foods. GMO foods or GMO ingredients must meet the same safety standards as all other foods. The EPA regulates the safety of substances that protect GMO plants, referred to as plant-incorporated protectants that are in some GMO plants to make them resistant to pests and diseases. The USDA Animal and Plant Health Inspection Service sets regulations to make sure GMO plants are not harmful to other plants, and the USDA Biotechnology Regulatory Services implements these regulations.

The 1992 FDA guidance to industry policy applied to all foods derived from new plant varieties, including varieties produced through traditional plant breeding as well as those developed using recombinant deoxyribonucleic acid (DNA) technology.[18–20] In 2017 the FDA published a notice titled "Genome Editing in New Plant Varieties Used for Foods" seeking public input to help inform its regulatory approach to human and animal foods derived from plants produced using genome editing.[21] This request was in response to the development of new techniques to modify the DNA sequences of plants and to characterize such modifications. In addition, new GMOs with compositional differences that make them materially different from their traditional counterpart, require labeling that identifies such differences.

In 2016 Congress passed the National Bioengineered (BE) Food Disclosure Standard Law, directing the USDA Agricultural Marketing Service to establish a national mandatory standard for disclosing bioengineered foods. The Standard defines bioengineered foods as those that contain detectable genetic material that has been modified through certain laboratory techniques and cannot be created through conventional breeding or found in nature.[22] This standard is in sharp contrast to the European Union (EU) regulations, namely 1829/2003 and 1830/2003, that acknowledge and accept GMOs in a proportion no higher than 0.9% or lower thresholds without mandated product labeling.[23,24]

A 2021 survey among more than 420 consumers indicated only 8% sought foods without GMO ingredients.[16,17] Fourteen years of International Food Information Council (IFIC)-sponsored food and health surveys indicate that less than 10%of respondents indicated any negative perspectives on GMO foods or ingredients.

62.3 Cultured meat products

Cultured meat products are beginning to supplement traditional nonmeat alternatives to beef and chicken products. Vegetarian burgers and chicken nugget-type products have been available for some time. However, advances in molecular and cellular biology have resulted in the development of cell-based, cultured meat. In many cases, there is a need to modify the biology of the donor cells to enhance output. These modifications are made using current genetic engineering techniques resulting in cells that will reproduce and remain healthy while being kept alive outside of the normal biological state.

Within the United States, the USDA is responsible for the safety of meat products as well as fruits and vegetables, whereas the FDA is fundamentally responsible for other food products and their ingredients. Thus, as the cultured meat market within this country, there is an array regulatory challenges, including the term "meat." One is reminded that the term "meat" refers to the flesh of animals (including fishes and birds) used as food, that can be part of a healthful diet. Clearly, cultured or plant-based meat, and cultured alternative protein products are not meat as defined by the USDA, even though many of the cultured meat products are derived in vitro cultivation of animal tissue. Importantly, meat is a major source of key nutrients, such as high-quality protein, iron, and B vitamins for many people. The nutritional value of tradition meat is often lost in discussions that include "clean label" that refers to products made with as few ingredients, and terms that consumers are likely to recognize and think of as wholesome. Clean label does not have any statutory definition within the Unites States.

A recent study among about 700 Germans indicated concerns with cultured meat indicated three issues.[25] Those concerns focused on ethics, emotions, and globalization. At this point, the panel indicated that Germans are moderately prepared to accept cultured meat. A small survey among approximately 500 Italians revealed that younger, highly educated, and those somewhat familiar with cultured meat, meat consumers, and willing to reduce meat consumption were more likely to accept these kinds of products.[26] Similar surveys among more than 2000 meat eater and nonmeat consumers in Croatia, Greece, and Spain perceived cultured meat as kind to animals, unnatural, healthy and environmentally-friendly, disgusting, and possibly tasty.[27] An earlier study among nearly 500 consumers who associated themselves at omnivores, pescatarians, vegetarians, or vegans in the United States differed in their perspectives on the cultured meat concept based on their attitudes and beliefs.[28] When the participants identified word associations with cultured meat, the top categories were artificial (e.g., fake, unnatural), science (e.g., science, laboratory chemicals), and positive (e.g., good, awesome, super). Less than 2%of the word association responses were categorized as uncertain, environment, special diet, and cost.

62.4 Alternative protein sources

Among the many trends within the food industry is the expansion of the alternative proteins market, even though plant-based "meat" only represents 2%of all packaged meat sales.[29] Unfortunately, the complexities of dietary proteins and the health implications of these proteins across diverse, and often underserved, populations are not addressed. While the food industry explores the future of food across basic issues, such as environmental footprint, agriculture inclusivity, shifting demographics, food technology innovations, and nutrition and health,[30] sustainability of alternative protein sources remains a priority among European consumers, particularly among older adults (>65 years old).[31] However, alternative protein sources, including plants, insects, single-cell, microalgae, and an array of microorganisms represent numerous challenges, which include, but not limited to, safety, quality, bioavailability, analytical assessment, and regulatory standardization.

Insects, which represent a significant and diverse biomass, are consumed by more than 80% of the world's population. However, the quality of insect proteins, such as those provided by crickets, reflects limits in essential amino acids, including methionine and cysteine, tryptophan, histidine, and leucine. In addition, these insects may represent a zoonotic spillover due to Cordyceps fungi and densoviruses. As a result, in 2015, the European Food Safety Authority (EFSA) Scientific Committee noted concerns for both biological and chemical hazards associated with insect production.[32] Other viruses innate to insects include Poxviruses, Iridoviruses, Parvoviruses, Dicistroviruses, Iflaviruses, and Reoviruses.[33] Meanwhile, the typical microbiological assessments of insect-based proteins do not include any form of virology. Importantly, data on the potential pathogenicity of these viruses from insects are limited, and little is known about the prions and viruses innate to crickets.

A recent study among consumers in the Unites States, Mexico, and Spain evaluated their perception on the use of insect powder as an ingredient in chocolate chip cookies.[34] Cookies with 15% insect power (replaced all-purpose flour) were similar to control products as deemed by consumers in the Unites States, whereas consumers in Mexico and Spain liked this sample over the control and the cookie with 30% insect powder. However, participants preferred the control over the product with the highest level of insect powder.

An earlier review on global entomophagy suggest that insects may be important sources of quality protein for an expanding population, while emphasizing the importance of increased consumer studies on the psychological and cultural barriers to eating insects.[35] Interestingly, this review did not address potential protein quality challenges or food safety issues associated with insect consumption, especially with apparent reluctances in Western culture. It was also noted that an increasing consumer demand and acceptance are vital for globalized entomophagy.

Perhaps one of several precautions that should be considered is the consumption of plant-based dairy products fed to children. A recent evaluation of these products emphasized that plant-based beverages should not be substituted for cow's milk for children less than 24 months of age based in their nutrient profile and potential allergenicity.[36] These authors also noted that while some of the plant-based products may be favorable to adult perceptions of healthfulness due to less sugars and fats, the quality and quantities of nutrients, such as calcium and vitamin B_{12}, are often lacking or of poor bioavailability, and the protein quality is markedly lower than the casein and whey innate to mammalian milks. Rice-based beverages typically contain lower levels of lipids, especially the omega-3 fatty acids, lower protein quality, and inadequate levels of vitamin A and D, which are critical for children growth and development. Similar analyses of coconut-based and oat-based beverages indicate significant nutritional inadequacies for children. These nutritional inadequacies may be critical for other vulnerable populations, such as pregnant and lactating women, and older adults.

Consumer perceptions of plant-based beverages often reflect their health concerns associated with traditional dairy products and their sustainability.[37] It appears that consumer continue to perceive the natural sugar (lactose-free is "in") in fluid milk and its fat content to be inconsistent with their "healthy" lifestyle.[38] The sustainability and packaging messages with plant-based beverages are more favorable in today's market. Very few of the surveys reviewed included consumer comments on the safety and different nutritional contributions of these kinds of products relative to traditional fluid milk. One recent survey posed the question regarding the perceived safety of plant-based products as perceived by 1000 consumers.[39] The third greatest concern focused on plant-based beverages. In fact, the Kerry-sponsored study revealed that more than 60%of consumers read a product's ingredient statement and nutritional panel. These plant-based products have a longer ingredient declaration than traditional fluid milk products that have a standard of identity, and include many "no-no" components as perceived by the participants.

62.5 Cellular agriculture

Cellular agriculture includes cells from animals, plants, and microbes.[40] Products from these sources include food proteins and an array of flavor components, and materials, such as proteins that are silk and leather-like. While the concept of cellular agriculture is somewhat unfamiliar among consumers, a 2021 qualitative study out of the Netherlands indicated consumers are quite concerned with process and products associated with cultured agriculture that includes cultured meat.[41] These investigators emphasized the importance of the food chain and legal framework associated with cultured meat in the EU. The survey noted that the primary concern among stakeholders and consumers is the safety of the end products of this technology. Interestingly, these experts observed that the classic food chains for these kinds of products have yet to be established, which raises concerns among those involved in consumer protection and consumer education. Perhaps some of these concerns may be mitigated through transparent communications and future consumer acceptance of the critical balance of risks and hazards characterized by cultured agriculture and other food-related technologies.

A 2018 report out of Australia addresses emerging technologies in agriculture from the consumers' perspective.[42] This team reported an array of consumer drivers and concerns that impact the developing trends in agriculture technologies. Some of those technologies include blockchain, artificial intelligence, robotics, nanomaterials, genetic editing, synthetic biology, 3D printing, satellites, and drones. For example, consumers perceive these technologies may improve product quality, increase health benefits, and demonstrate social responsibility. On the other hand, consumers expressed concerns about sustainability and environmental impact of such technologies, animal welfare, and "industrial" or corporate agriculture instead of embracing smaller scale farming that is recognized as more "natural."

A 2017 FAO report addresses significant trends and challenges in agriculture, particularly as the organization continues to focus on global hunger and malnutrition.[43] Importantly, and within this context, FAO emphasizes food safety as the key element that must be the priority as agriculture is challenged with sustainable productivity and natural resources.

62.6 Food additives

62.6.1 Background

There are more than 30 classifications of food additives according to the Code of Federal Regulations. Those classifications include, but not limited to, preservatives, flavors, leavening agents, humectants, emulsifiers, drying agents, nonnutritive sweeteners, antimicrobial agents, pH control agents, and dough strengtheners. The substances in these classifications may be used directly or indirectly as a food component that affects the characteristics of any food, such as nutritional value, stability, and sensory qualities. Many food additives/ingredients have received *prior sanction* status from the FDA since they had a long history of use without adverse events. Examples of these food additives include preservatives that function as antimicrobials, such as ascorbic acid (vitamin C), potassium sorbate, and potassium bisulfite.

Food additives do not include pesticides, food colors *per se*, or substances that have been reviewed as Generally Recognized As Safe (GRAS). GRAS is a US FDA designation that a chemical or substance added to food is considered safe by experts. An ingredient with a GRAS designation is exempted from the usual Federal Food, Drug, and Cosmetic Act food additive tolerance requirements. It is important to note that as of September 1, 2021, more than 1000 new food ingredients have been reviewed or are pending review by the FDA via the GRAS petition process. These ingredients have been examined by experts through the GRAS affirmation process that was initiated in 1972 for which the FDA has not been notified. The safety standards for GRAS determinations were finalized in 2016. Another critical component of food ingredient safety is the 1958 Delaney Clause, which prohibits the addition of any chemical to the food supply that causes cancer in humans or animals.[44]

Food colorants, both exempt and certified, are reviewed by experts under the provisions presented in the 1960 Color Additives amendment (21 U.S.C. 301). As of 2015 there are nine certified and 27 color additives exempt from batch certification for food applications as stated in the Federal regulations, such as 21 CFR 74 and 21 CFR 73, respectively. (https://www.fda.gov/industry/color-additive-inventories/summary-color-additives-use-united-states-foods-drugs-cosmetics-and-medical-devices#table1A; Accessed 01.09.21).

62.6.2 Consumer perceptions

Concerning consumer attitudes on artificial food additives, a study in Switzerland indicated an understanding of risk versus benefits impacts on their acceptance or rejection of these substances.[45] This understanding includes consumer awareness of and trust in the regulatory environment, and consumer exposure to actual risk communication.[46]

In an era of social media communications, rapid communications are the norm. Such communications, such as blogs, podcasts, Twitter, and other social media platforms, often convey information without facts check and typically without an understanding of the spectrum of scientific data, regardless of study methods, scientific models, or public health implications. Thus consumers frequently receive inaccurate information, which is misleading, yet may reinforce the consumers' vested interests, while affecting their behaviors that may have a negative impact on public and individual health.[47]

Even in South Korea, consumers have voiced concerns about food additives, such as preservatives, food colors, artificial sweeteners, curing agents, and antioxidants.[48] While the study participants were aware of an array of food additives, the study demonstrated that better education on the safety and functional properties of food additives tended to improve consumers' value of these substances and permitted them to make better food choices, regardless of the nature of processed foods. A similar study among consumers in China reinforced the importance of accurate risk communications, such that improved knowledge about food additives tended to reduce negative perceptions on food safety issues pertinent to these substances.[49]

Within the United States, a 2018 survey indicated the America public was closely divided on the health risks associated with food additives and GMOs.[50] According to this survey sponsored by the PEW Research Center, about 70%of respondents believed that science has had a mostly positive effect on the quality of food in the United States. Yet, slightly more than half of the people indicated they would face a serious health risk from food additives over their lifetime. The primary areas of concern included meat from animals given antibiotics or hormones, fruits and vegetables grown with pesticides, food and drinks with artificial preservatives, and food and drinks with artificial coloring. At the same time, about the same percentage of participants indicated that GMO-derived foods increase one's health risks, despite the extensive publicly available evidence to the contrary.

Interestingly, using a recombinant DNA procedure for medications, such as human insulin (Humulin) produced using a strain of *Escherichia coli* or *Saccharomyces cerevisiae*, or human growth hormone as a product of Chinese Hamster ovary cells or plasmids of *E. coli* (Protropin), consumers, in general, have yet to voice concerns. There are some exceptions relative to other recombinant medications approved by the FDA. Such was the Zohydro case where the public evidence suggested that the safety, efficacy, and medical necessity of this pharmaceutical was not adequately demonstrated.[51]

62.7 Food colors

Within the United States, food colors are regulated by the FDA through the Color Additives Amendment of 1960. This amendment to the Food, Drug and Cosmetic Act outlined the general provisions to assess the safety and usage of pigments in the food supply. Basically, there are two classifications of food colors: those that are water-soluble, known as dyes, and those that are fat-soluble, known as lakes. From a statutory perspective, the United States does not have natural colors, even though many colors in the food supply originate from natural sources. There are certified colors (each batch of color is certified through extensive analytical analyses) and exempt colors. Consumers often consider exempt—exempt from certification—colors as natural, since they are derived from natural sources.

The initial food color and health controversy emerged in the 1970s. The Feingold hypothesis suggested that artificial food additives and colors were linked to hyperkinesis and learning disabilities among children.[52] A controversy ensued among consumers and the medical community, which culminated in a regulation based on public pressure, not scientific evidence. That regulation stipulates that those foods and pharmaceuticals with the yellow-color tartrazine must contain a label with a warning statement. That statement notes the "...product contains FD&C Yellow No. 5 (tartrazine) which may cause allergic-type reactions (including bronchial asthma) in certain susceptible persons. Although the overall incidence of FD&C Yellow No. 5 (tartrazine) sensitivity in the general population is low, it is frequently seen in patients who also have aspirin hypersensitivity."[19,20]

The public's reaction to the tartrazine issue prompted concerns within the medical community. The subsequent clinical evidence did suggest that those children who presented allergy-related atopic dermatitis tended to be more sensitive to the consumption of foods with this colorant.[53] This condition, a common inflammatory skin disorder, affects about 13%of children.[54]

Consumer negative reactions to food colors were heightened following the 2007 publication of the South Hampton study. This study suggested that the consumption of artificial food color additives (5 mg sunset yellow, 2.5 mg carmoisine, 7.5 mg tartrazine, and 5 mg ponceau 4R) by children altered their behavior patterns and contributed to their hyperactivity.[55] Despite this study being rejected by the EFSA due to some inconsistencies in the data and conclusions,[56] several organizations and parents called for the banning of artificial colors.[57] Since the acceptance of 15 certified colors in 1931, some colors, such as Orange No. 2 and Red Dye No. 2, were banned by the FDA. Today, seven of these colors meet the safety standards under the 1960 Colors Additives Amendment, and only six of these remain in usage in foods and pharmaceuticals. As consumers call for a reduction of these colors, they also call for the use of "natural" or exempt colors. Technical issues aside, the color industry continues to conduct research in alternative color sources, such as those found in mineral deposits, plants, fungi, insects, microorganisms, and algae that are safe for human consumption, and are stable when exposed to a variety of food processing environments, such as heat, light, and pH.

Meanwhile, in light of the virtual absence of untoward effects of food colors, there is a "free-from" movement across the consuming public in the United States. Consumers are driving this "free-from" market, thus the appearance of "gluten-free," "lactose-free," "preservative-free," and similar statements on food packages and presented in social media outlets. In 2018 the USDA chimed in by stating that natural refers to products "containing no artificial ingredient or added color and only minimally processed. Minimal processing means that the product was processed in a manner that does not fundamentally alter the product."[58] However, the FDA has yet to finalize the rulemaking to establish a formal definition for the term "natural," even though there was call for public input in 2016. Remarkably, the "free-from" movement has sparked numerous consumer-initiated litigations or class-action suits against the food industry that claim "natural" or "all natural" on their products or declared ingredients.

62.8 Carrageenan

From Carrageenan County, Ireland emerges a red algae extract called carrageenan that has been used in a spectrum of foods and medications for many centuries. The FDA, EFSA, and World Health Organization support the safety of food-grade carrageenan for its intended use, including in infant formula and follow-on products, at levels consistent with good manufacturing practices. Some of those approved uses leverage an array of functional properties, such as thickener, gelling and stabilizing agent, and emulsifier in a variety of foods and household products, and as an excipient in and production aid for pharmaceutical products, including some antibiotics.[59–61]

Carrageenan is an alkaline aqueous extract from various members of red seaweeds (Rhodophyceae).[62] Importantly, this extraction process avoids the production of low molecular – weight polymers ($<5\%$), which are the focus of scrutiny and continued controversy. The most common forms of carrageenan in the food supply are kappa-, iota- and lambda. These forms vary in their degree of sulfation (20%–40%) and linkage of highly flexible hexose units of galactose and anhydrogalactose. The molecular weight of food-grade carrageenan typically ranges between 200 and 800kDa with average >100 kDa, although a molecular weight range is not stipulated in any food regulations.[63]

Poligeenan, formerly known as "degraded carrageenan," is the product of acid hydrolysis (pH: 0.9–1.3) conducted at high temperatures ($>80°C$) for extended periods of time. This product has a molecular weight of approximately 10–30 kDa. Importantly, poligeenan is not a food additive or found in the food supply. Current evidence indicates dietary carrageenan is not absorbed, hydrolyzed, or converted to poligeenan following ingestion by rodents, dogs, and nonhuman primates, or by intestinal microflora[59,64]

The absence of intestinal degradation of carrageenan is supported by the lack of endogenous enzymes, such as carrageenases and galactosidases that recognize the unique structure of carrageenan.[61,65] However, it should be noted that some species of marine organisms, not components of human microflora, produce κ-carrageenase.[66]

The degradation of carrageenan to poligeenan has not been demonstrated in in vivo studies. A review of animal studies with poligeenan, a surrogate of carrageenan exposure, indicate this product can elicit inflammatory responses in the small bowel and in in vitro studies with various human cell lines.[67] As noted by EFSA, these findings did not present additional data for its 2018 comprehensive review on carrageenan.[68]

Another assessment of inflammatory potential of carrageenan demonstrated when injected into the footpad of rats.[69] On the other hand, topical administration of carrageenan suggested this polysaccharide may function as a microbicide by inhibiting Herpes Simplex Virus, Human Papillomavirus, and Human Immunodeficiency Virus[70,71]. These findings emphasize and clearly indicate the route of administration is a critical and fundamental variable in assessing the potential toxicity and safety of any substance, whether that substance is a possible food ingredient or prospective component in a pharmaceutical mixture.

Several early studies assessed the potential carcinogenicity of carrageenan when fed to rodents. These studies, following the subcutaneous injection of three different colon tumor initiators and coadministration of diets containing 6% or 15% of various forms of carrageenan, indicated an increase in colon cancer based on tumor burden.[72,73] Upon careful examination of these studies indicates the diets were nutritionally insufficient and high carrageenan concentration (>5%) are inappropriate to assess safety based on contemporary research (e.g., International Conference on Harmonization (ICH) and Organisation for Economic Cooperation and Development (OECD)) protocols. Follow-up studies on the possible genotoxicity of carrageenan indicated this food additive was not mutagenic.[74,75]

A comprehensive review on the potential impact of food-grade carrageenan on the immune system indicated the absence of any adverse effect.[64] As suggested by other investigators, poligeenan does exhibit toxicological properties at high doses (>10%), levels of which do not occur in the food supply.

Clearly, the physical and toxicological properties of carrageenan and poligeenan differ considerably. From a practical perspective, evidence indicates poligeenan does not have any functional properties in aqueous food matrices, whereas carrageenan is typically used at concentrations of 0.01% or less.

Despite the compelling evidence on the safety of carrageenan, the controversy among consumers, the scientific community, and healthcare professionals continues. A 2018 assessment suggests there remain at least significant information gaps germane to the safety of this polysaccharide.[76] For example, these authors claim that there is insufficient information regarding current levels of public exposure to carrageenan, the potential association of the physicochemical properties of carrageenan and its impact on digestive proteolysis, as well as its impact on the colon microbiome and possible gut inflammatory events, such as those experienced among the elderly and those presenting inflammatory bowel disease. An earlier study also advances the position that carrageenan and carboxymethylcellulose contribute to the development of gut inflammatory episodes as reflected in possible modulation of the immune system and a possible gut dysbiosis.[77] It is important to note that these kinds of outcomes are not components to assess the safety of food additives directed to foods for the healthy, general public. The primary criteria for safety assessment of direct food additives and principles for GRAS determinations for intended populations are clearly presented within the respective framework.[78,79] (FDA, 2009; FDA, 2016). These criteria for safety must provide reasonable certainty of no harm under their intended conditions of use before they can be intentionally added to food.

The spectrum of scientific literature over more than three decades of research and food applications indicates carrageenan is a food additive that is safe for consumers of all ages, and that it has broad applications in the food industry. However, social media and medical news letters continue to communicate possible negative health effects allegedly related to carrageenan consumption without any qualification pertinent to studies reviewed by the international community of regulatory agencies and scientific organizations.

62.9 The sociology of consumer activism

The sociological convention holds that consumerism emphasizes a consumer's right for protection against adulterated, deficient, or unsafe products and services. Specifically, social marketing states that consumerism is attempting to tell industry something their research has not found, or that management has rejected or ignored.[80] Kotler[81] defines consumerism as "a social movement seeking to augment the rights and powers of buyers in relation to sellers." According to Kotler, consumerism ought to be ultimately beneficial for both consumers and businesses. Ideally, consumerism mobilizes the energies of consumers, industry, and government leaders to seek solutions and advance society, and ensures short-term and long-term values for consumers.

In any discussion of consumer attitudes, it is valuable to consider the sociological underpinnings of why it may be that consumers are vocally and even legally opposing global brands and expressing grave and strident concerns about corporate products and practices. Consumer activism is either grassroots collective organization of consumption or its withdrawal.[82]

Consumer activism, also known as "ethical shopping, ethical purchase behavior, ethical consumption, political consumption, political consumerism, and critical consumerism,"[83] generally relates to the choices a consumer makes in the marketplace. Such choices are influenced by a myriad of forces and factors. Among other things, the consumer activist intends to give the purchase an ethical and/or moral impact beyond the purchase involved,[83] and this belief and associated action is ostensibly driven by a perception of evidence that demonstrates that the purchase or product in question is not beneficial and may present a health hazard.

Common sense and sociological convention hold that consumerism emphasizes a consumer's right for protection against adulterated, deficient, or unsafe products and services. Traditionally, social marketing states that consumerism is attempting to tell industry something their research has not found, or that management has rejected or ignored.[80] Kotler[81] notes that consumerism ought to be ultimately beneficial for both consumers and businesses. Ideally, consumerism mobilizes the energies of consumers, industry, and government leaders to seek solutions and advance society, and ensures short-term and long-term values for consumers. Yet, Johnston[84] observed that a condition has arisen which idealizes markets and consumers as primary guardians of the public good, and "occludes the importance" of nonmarket measures and democratically and scientifically accountable entities to provide for the safety and guide citizen efforts in an evidence-based fashion to "protect and preserve the commons."

Hollenbeck and Zinkhan[85] studied the "anti-brand movement." They concluded that this growing movement has reinforced negativity toward the brand and influences a member's attitude and/or decision to take action against a corporation. Their research suggests the relevancy of the role online communities play in present social action endeavors and, with internet capabilities, these communities are more powerful (e.g., number of participants) and progressive (e.g., technology-driven action strategies) than earlier social movements.

More recently, Cardello[86] observed that the power to shape consumer tastes and behavior has been hijacked to a large degree by new influencers—celebrity nutritionists, politicians, food bloggers—who have their own agendas and can influence public sentiment as never before. Their megaphone is sympathetic media, especially online: social media, consumer websites, and an exploding number of alternative news outlets. Yet again, the sociological impact of the internet is felt.

Cardello goes on to cite national, well-organized campaigns for restrictions such as taxes on large-sized sugary drinks, and forced labeling of products containing putative GMOs. He notes excoriating films like *Fed Up* and polemics like Michael Moss' book *Salt, Sugar, Fat* that paint the food industry as indifferent to consumer health and focused only on profit. Finally, he calls into question organizations such as the Center for Science in the Public Interest, which targets big-name brands, from Coke to Oreos to the Trix rabbit with dubious and cherry-picked assertions. A concluding summary is worth quoting verbatim:

> *Outside influencers, both well-meaning experts and articulate novices, are scrambling corporate communications and often spreading their own uninformed interpretations about food ingredients, working conditions, fair trade, and other concerns. Using social media to amplify and spread those messages quickly, activists, lawmakers, and others have captured the public's attention, even when the charges are reckless.*

Thus what may have begun as a means to satisfy ethical and moral imperatives, to induce corporations to harmonize policies with well-founded consumer activist desires, has evolved to a significant degree into strident, litigious, and financially destructive behavior that does not necessarily promote superior products or public health. It appears that consumer awareness may be increasingly impaired and thus activism is no longer simply about the moral identity of the consumer, but an unintentional and often profound mis-perception and misunderstanding of food safety as practiced commercially and as overseen by regulators.

62.10 Conclusion

The era of COVID-19 has elevated consumer perceptions of food safety. A 2020 survey among consumers indicated about 50%of consumers are doing less in-person grocery shopping, eating more home-cooked meals, and are more attentive to handwashing and minimizing contact with surfaces while in-person shopping.[87] Importantly, nearly 80% of the survey respondents indicated they were confident or somewhat confident that the foods they purchased were safe for consumption.

Food safety is the primary focus by regulatory agencies, the food industry, among restaurants, public transportation networks, and consumer food-handling practices. Understanding food safety measures and criteria that connote food and ingredient safety is critical for all consumers. A key element of that understanding is the establishment of trust and reliability of information sources—sources that are unbiased and complete and that are truthful and not misleading.

References

1. FDA. Public law 111−353—JAN. 4, 2011. Food Safety Modernization Act 2011. <https://www.govinfo.gov/content/pkg/PLAW-111publ353/pdf/PLAW-111publ353.pdf>; 2011.
2. Ioannidis J. The challenge of reforming nutritional epidemiological research. *JAMA*. 2018;320:969−970. Available from: https://doi.org/10.1001/jama.2018.11025.
3. Page M, Altman D, McKenzie J, et al. Flaws in the application and interpretation of statistical analyses in systematic reviews of therapeutic interventions were common: a cross-sectional analysis. *J Clin Epidemiol*. 2018;95:7−18. Available from: https://doi.org/10.1016/j.jclinepi.2017.11.022.
4. CDC. Centers for Disease Control and Prevention. <https://www.cdc.gov/foodsafety/foodborne-germs.html>; March 2020.
5. Scharff R. The economic burden of foodborne illness in the United States. In: Scharff RL, ed. *Food Safety Economics, Food*

Microbiology and Food Safety Book Series. Springer International Publishing AG; 2018:123–142. Available from: http://doi.org/10.1007/978-3-319-92138-9_8.

6. Jaffee S, Henson S, Unnevehr L, Grace D, Cassou E. *The Safe Food Imperative: Accelerating Progress in Low- and Middle-Income Countries*. Washington, DC: World Bank Group; 2019. Available from: http://doi.org/10.1596/978-1-4648-1345-0.
7. Devlesschauwer B, Scharff R, Kowalcyk B, Havelaar A. Burden and risk assessment of foodborne disease. In: En RT, ed. *Food Safety Economics, Food Microbiology and Food Safety Book Series*. Springer International Publishing AG; 2018:83–106. Available from: http://doi.org/10.1007/978-3-319-92138-9_6.
8. Frewer L, de Jonge J, van Kleef E. Consumer perceptions of food safety. In: Mansourian EB, Wojtczak A, Sayers B, eds. *Encyclopedia of Life Support Systems*. Oxford: EOLSS Publishers Co. Ltd; 2009:86–109.
9. Nelson N, Sørensen E, Grunert K. Consumer motives for buying fresh or frozen plaice: a means end chain approach. In: Luter EJ, Borresen T, eds. *Seafood from Producer to Consumer: Integrated Approach to Quality*. Amsterdam: Elsevier; 1997:31–43.
10. CDC. Environmental Health Services; 2019. https://www.cdc.nceh/ehs/ehsnet/plain_language/how-eh-specialists-investigate-outbreaks.htm.
11. Knight A, Worosz M, Todd E. Dining for safety: consumer perceptions of food safety and eating out. *J Hosp Tour Res*. 2009;33:471–486. Available from: https://doi.org/10.1177/1096348009344211.
12. Lee L, Niode O, Simonne A, Bruhn C. Consumer perceptions on food safety in Asian and Mexican restaurants. *Food Control*. 2012;26:531–538. Available from: https://doi.org/10.1016/j.foodcont.2012.02.010.
13. Liu P, Lee Y. An investigation of consumers' perception of food safety in restaurants. *Int J Hosp Manag*. 2018;73:29–35. Available from: https://doi.org/10.1016/j.ijhm.2018.01.018.
14. Dolekoglu C, Veziroglu P, Keiyinci S. Analysing passenger behavior towards on perception in-flight food safety and quality. *N Trends Issues Proc Humanit Soc Sci*. 2017;4:417–425.
15. Castillo-Manzano J, López-Valpuesta L. Analysing passenger behaviour towards the catering industry: implications for airport management. *Int J Hosp Manag*. 2013;35:258–260. Available from: https://doi.org/10.1016/j.ijhm.2013.06.010.
16. IFIC. From "Chemical-sounding" to "Clean": consumer perspectives on food ingredients. <https://foodinsight.org/wp-content/uploads/2021/06/Food-Ingredients-LSI-Survey.May-2021.pdf>; 2021a.
17. IFIC. Consumer survey: trends, habits and attitudes related to food safety. Food & Health Survey. <https://foodinsight.org/2021-food-health-survey/>; 2021b.
18. FDA. FDA's Voluntary Plant Biotechnology Consultation Program eases pathway to marketplace. <https://www.fda.gov/news-events/fda-voices/fdas-voluntary-plant-biotechnology-consultation-program-eases-pathway-marketplace>; 2019.
19. FDA. Consultation Programs on Food from New Plant Varieties. <https://www.fda.gov/food/food-new-plant-varieties/consultation-programs-food-new-plant-varieties> 2020a.
20. FDA. 21 CFR 74.1705: FD&C Yellow No. 5. En FDA, *Code of Federal Regulations*; 2020b.
21. FDAHHS. Federal Register/Vol. 82, No. 12/Thursday, January 19, 2017. Genome Editing in New Plant Varieties. <https://www.govinfo.gov/content/pkg/FR-2017-01-19/pdf/2017-00840.pdf>; 2017.
22. USDA. What is a bioengineered food? USDA, Agriculture Marketing Service: https://www.ams.usda.gov/sites/default/files/media/BE_Consumer.pdf>; 2016.
23. EU. Regulation (EC) No 1829/2003 of the European Parliament and of the Council. *Off J Eur Union*. <https://eur-lex.europa.eu/legal-content/EN/TXT/PDF/?uri = CELEX:32003R1829>; 2003a.
24. EU. Regulation (EC) No 1830/2003 of the European Parliament and of the Council. *Off J Eur Union*. <https://eur-lex.europa.eu/legal-content/EN/TXT/PDF/?uri = CELEX:32003R1830&from = EN>; 2003b.
25. Weinrich R, Strack M, Neugebauer F. Consumer acceptance of cultured meat in Germany. *Meat Sci*. 2020;162:107924. Available from: https://doi.org/10.1016/j.meatsci.2019.107924.
26. Mancini M, Antonioli F. Exploring consumers' attitude towards cultured meat in Italy. *Meat Sci*. 2019;150:101–110. Available from: https://doi.org/10.1016/j.meatsci.2018.12.014.
27. Franceković P, García-Torralba L, Sakoulogeorga E, Vučković T, Perez-Cueto F. How do consumers perceive cultured meat in Croatia, Greece, and Spain? *Nutrients*. 2021;13:1284. Available from: https://doi.org/10.3390/nu13041284.
28. Bryant C, Dillard C. The impact of framing on acceptance of cultured meat. *Front Nutr*. 2019;6:103. Available from: https://doi.org/10.3389/fnut.2019.00103.
29. Good Food Institute. U.S. retail market data for the plant-based industry. <https://gfi.org/marketresearch/>; 2021.
30. Global Market Insights. Top 8 challenges of food and beverage industry to watch out for. <https://www.gminsights.com/blogs/challenges-in-food-and-beverage-industry>; 2020.
31. Grasso A, Hung Y, Olthof M, Verbeke W, Brouwer I. Older consumers' readiness to accept alternative, more sustainable protein sources in the European Union. *Nutrients*. 2019;11:1904. Available from: https://doi.org/10.3390/nu11081904.
32. EFSA Scientific Committee. Risk profile related to production and consumption of insects as food and feed. *EFSA J*. 2015;13:4257. Available from: https://doi.org/10.2903/j.efsa.2015.4257.
33. King A, Lefkowitz E, Adams M, Carstens E, eds, *Virus Taxonomy: Ninth Report of the International Committee on Taxonomy of Viruses*. Elsevier Academic Press; 2012.
34. Delgado M, Carbonell-Barrachina A, Artiaga L, Quintanar R, Hernandez A. Consumer acceptability in the USA, Mexico, and Spain of chocolate chip cookies made with partial insect powder replacement. *J Food Sci*. 2020;85:1621–1628. Available from: https://doi.org/10.1111/1750-341.15175.
35. Sun-Waterhouse D, Waterhouse G, You L, et al. Transforming insect biomass into consumer wellness foods: a review. *Food Res Int*. 2016;89:129–151. Available from: https://doi.org/10.1016/j.foodres.2016.10.001.
36. Verduci E, D'Elios S, Cerrato L, et al. Cow's milk substitutes for children: nutritional aspects of milk from different mammalian species, special formula and plant-based beverages. *Nutrients*. 2019;11:1739. Available from: https://doi.org/10.3390/nu11081739.
37. Schiano A, Harwood W, Gerard P, Drake M. Consumer perception of the sustainability of dairy products and plant-based dairy alternatives. *J Dairy Sci*. 2020;103:11228–11243. Available from: https://doi.org/10.3168/jds.2020-18406.

38. McCarthy K, Parker M, Ameerally A, Drake S, Drake M. Drivers of choice for fluid milk vs plant-based beverages: what are consumer perceptions of fluid milk? *J Dairy Sci.* 2017;100:6125–6138. Available from: https://doi.org/10.3168/jds.2016-12519.
39. de Vegt B. Conquering food safety challenges for plant-based ingredients. Food Safety Magazine (August/September). <https://www.food-safety.com/articles/7300-conquering-food-safety-challenges-for-plant-based-ingredients>; 2021.
40. Rischer H, Szilvay G, Oksman-Caldentey K. Cellular agriculture–industrial biotechnology for food and materials. *Curr Opin Biotechnol.* 2020;61:128–134. Available from: https://doi.org/10.1016/j.copbio.2019.12.003.
41. Ketelings L, Kremers S, de Boer A. The barriers and driers of a safe market introduction of cultured meat: a qualitative study. *Food Control.* 2021;130:108299. Available from: https://doi.org/10.1016/j.foodcont.2021.108299.
42. GHD, AgThentic. Emerging agricultural technologies: consumer perceptions around emerging agtech. AgriFutures – National Rural Issues. <https://www.agrifutures.com.au/wp-content/uploads/2019/01/18-048.pdf>; 2018.
43. FAO. *The Future of Food and Agriculture – Trends and Challenges.* Rome: FAO. <http://www.fao.org/3/i6583e/i6583e.pdf>; 2017.
44. Merrill R. Food safety regulation: reforming the Delaney Clause. *Annu Rev Public Health.* 1997;18:313–340. Available from: https://doi.org/10.1146/annurev.publhealth.18.1.313.
45. Bearth A, Cousin M-E, Siegrist M. The consumer's perception of artificial food additives: influences on acceptance, risk and benefit perceptions. *Food Qual Prefer.* 2014;38:14–23. Available from: https://doi.org/10.1016/j.foodqual.2014.05.008.
46. Rutsaert P, Regan A, Pieniak Z, et al. The use of social media in food risk and benefit communication. *Trends Food Sci Technol.* 2013;30:84–91. Available from: https://doi.org/10.1016/j.tifs.2012.10.006.
47. Suarez-Lledo V, Alvarez-Galvez J. Prevalence of health misinformation on social media: systematic review. *J Med Internet Res.* 2021;23:e17187. Available from: https://doi.org/10.2196/17187.
48. Shim S-M, Seo S, Lee Y, Moon G-I, Kim M-S, Park J-H. Consumers' knowledge and safety perceptions of food additives: evaluation on the effectiveness on transmitting information on preservatives. *Food Control.* 2011;22:1054–1060. Available from: https://doi.org/10.1016/j.foodcont.2011.01.001.
49. Miao P, Chen S, Li J, Xie X. Decreasing consumers' risk perception of food additives by knowledge enhancement in China. *Food Qual Pref.* 2020;79:103781. Available from: https://doi.org/10.1016/j.foodqual.2019.103781.
50. Funk C, Kennedy B, Hefferon M. Public perspectives on food risks. Pew Research Center. <http://www.pewresearch.org>; 2018.
51. Manchikanti L, Atluri S, Candido K, et al. Zohydro approval by Food and Drug Administration: controversial or frightening? *Pain Physician.* 2014;17:E437–E450.
52. Feingold B. Hyperkinesis and learning disabilities linked to artificial food flavors and colors. *Am J Nurs.* 1975;75:797–803.
53. Feketea G, Tsabouri S. Common food colorants and allergic reactions in children: myth or reality? *Food Chem.* 2017;230:578–588. Available from: https://doi.org/10.1016/j.foodchem.2017.03.043.
54. NEA. Atopic dermatitis in children. National Eczema Association. <https://nationaleczema.org/eczema/children/atopic-dermatitis>; 2021.
55. McCann D, Barrett A, A. C, et al. Food additives and hyperactive behaviour in 3-year-old and 8/9-year old children in the community: a randomised, double-blinded, placebo-controlled trial. *Lancet.* 2007;370:1560–1567. Available from: https://doi.org/10.1016/S0140-6736(07)61306-3.
56. EFSA. Scientific opinion of the Panel on Food Additives, Flavourings, Processing Aids and Food Contact Materials (AFC) on a request from the commission on the results of the study by McCann et al. (2007) on the effect of some colours and sodium benzoate on chil. *EFSA J.*. 2008;660:1–54. Available from: https://doi.org/10.2903/j.efsa.2008.660.
57. Potera C. The artificial food day blues. *Environ Health Perspect.* 2010;118:A428. Available from: https://doi.org/10.1289/ehp.118-a428.
58. USDA. What does natural meat and poultry mean? <https://ask.usda.gov/s/article/What-does-natural-meat-and-poultry-mean>; 2019.
59. McKim J. Food additive carrageenan: part I: a critical review of carrageenan in vitro studies, potential pitfalls, and implications for human health and safety. *Crit Rev Toxicol.* 2014;44:211–243. Available from: https://doi.org/10.3109/10408444.2013.861797.
60. Necas J, Bartosikova L. Carrageenan: a review. *Vet Med.* 2013;58:187–205. Available from: https://doi.org/10.17221/6758-VETMED.
61. Weiner M. Food additive carrageenan: part II: a critical review of carrageenan in vivo safety studies. *Crit Rev Toxicol.* 2014;1–26. Available from: https://doi.org/10.3109/10408444.2013.861798.
62. Shukla P, Borza T, Critchley A, Prithiviraj B. Carrageenans from red seaweeds as promoters of growth and elicitors of defense response in plants. *Front Mar Sci.* 2016;3:1–9. Available from: https://doi.org/10.3389/fmars.2016.00081.
63. Campo V, Kawano D, da Silva D, Carvalho I. Carrageenans: biological properties, chemical modifications and structural analysis – a review. *Carbohydr Polym.* 2009;77:167–180. Available from: https://doi.org/10.1016/j.carbpol.2009.01.020.
64. Cohen S, Ito N. A critical review of the toxicological effects of carrageenan and processed eucheuma seaweed on the gastrointestinal tract. *Crit Rev Toxicol.* 2002;35:413–444. Available from: https://doi.org/10.1080/20024091064282.
65. Lecacheux D, P R, Brigand G, Martin G. Molecular weight distribution of carrageenans by size exclusion chromatography and low angle laser light scattering. *Carbohydr Polym.* 1985;5:423–440. Available from: https://doi.org/10.1016/0144-8617(85)90003-7.
66. Potin P, Sanseau A, Le Gall Y, Rochas C, Kloareg B. Purification and characterization of a new K-carrageenase from a marine *Cytophaga*-like bacterium. *Eur J Biochem.* 1991;201:241–247. Available from: https://doi.org/10.1111/j.1432-1033.1991.tb16280.x.
67. Tobacman J. Review of harmful gastrointestinal effects of carrageenan in animal experiments. *Environ Health Perspect.* 2001;109:983–994. Available from: https://doi.org/10.1289/ehp.01109983.
68. EFSA. Scientific opinion on the re-evaluation of carrageenan (E407) and processed Eucheuma seaweed (E 407a) as food additives. *EFSA J.* 2018;16:5238. Available from: https://doi.org/10.2903/j.efsa.2018.5238.

69. Harmuth-Hoene A, Schwerdtfeger E. Effect of indigestible polysaccharides on protein digestibility and nitrogen retention in growing rats. *Nutr Metab.* 1979;23:399–407. Available from: https://doi.org/10.1159/000176285.
70. Marais S, Pepper DJ, Marais BJ, Török ME. HIV-associated tuberculous meningitis–diagnostic and therapeutic challenges. *Tuberculosis (Edinb).* 2010;90(6):367–74. Available from: https://doi.org/10.1016/j.tube.2010.08.006.
71. Marais S, Pepper DJ, Schutz C, Wilkinson RJ, Meintjes G. Presentation and outcome of tuberculous meningitis in a high HIV prevalence setting. *PLoS One.* 2011;6(5):e20077. Available from: https://doi.org/10.1371/journal.pone.0020077.
72. Arawawa S, Okumura M, Yamada S, Ito M, Tejima S. Enhancing effect of carrageenan on the induction of rat colonic tumors by 1,2-dimethyhydrazine and its relation to beta-glucuronidase activities in feces and other tissues. *J Nutr Sci Vitaminol (Tokyo).* 1986;32:481–485. Available from: https://doi.org/10.3177/jnsv.32.481.
73. Watanabe K, Reddy B, Wong C, Weisburger J. Effect of dietary undegraded carrageenan on colon carcinogenesis in F344 rats treated with azoxymethane or methylnitrosourea. *Cancer Res.* 1978;4427–4430.
74. IARC. *IARC Monographs on the Evaluation of the Carcinogenic Risk of Chemicals to Humans.* 31. International Agency for Research on Cancer; 1983.
75. JECFA. *Safety Evaluation of Certain Food Additives.* Geneva: World Health Organization; 1999.
76. Shlomit D, Levi C, Fahoum L, Ungar Y. Revisiting the carrageenan controversy: do we really understand the digestive fate and safety of carrageenan in our foods? *Food Funct.* 2018;9:1344. Available from: https://doi.org/10.1039/c7fo01721a.
77. Martino J, Van Limbergen J, Cahill L. The role of carrageenan and carboxymethylcellulose in the development of intestinal inflammation. *Front Pediatr.* 2017;5:96. Available from: https://doi.org/10.3389/fped.2017.00096.
78. FDA, 2009. "Guidance for Industry: Recommendations for Submission of Chemical and Technological Data for Direct Food Additive Petitions," (Available from: http://www.fda.gov/Food/GuidanceRegulation/GuidanceDocumentsRegulatoryInformation/ucm124917.htm).
79. FDA, 2016. Federal Register / Vol. 81, No. 159 / August 17, 2016 / Pages 54960-55055. (Available from: https://govinfo.gov/content/pkg/FR-2016-08-117/pdf/2016-19164.pdf.
80. Buskirk R, Rothe J. Consumerism—an interpretation. *J Mark.* 1970;34:61–65. Available from: https://doi.org/10.1177/002224297003400410.
81. Kotler P. What consumerism means to marketers. *Harv Bus Rev.* 1972;50:48–57.
82. Glickman L. *Buying Power: A History of Consumer Activism in America.* Chicago: The University of Chicago Press; 2009. Available from: http://doi.org/10.1177/14695405100020601.
83. Jacobsen E, Dulsrud A. Will consumers save the world? The framing of political consumerism. *J Agric Environ Ethics.* 2007;20:469–482. Available from: https://doi.org/10.1007/s10806-007-9043-z.
84. Johnston J. The citizen-consumer hybrid: ideological tensions and the case of Whole Foods Market. *Theory Soc.* 2008;229–270. Available from: https://doi.org/10.1007/s11186-007-9058-5.
85. Hollenbeck C, Zinkhan G. Consumer activism on the Internet: the role of anti-brand communities. In: Pechmann EC, Price L, eds. *NA – Advances in Consumer Research.* vol. 33. Association for Consumer Research; 2006:479–485. Available from: http://www.acrwebsite.org/volumes/12299/volumes/v33/NA-33.
86. Cardello H. Message to food companies: food activists are your new brand managers. Forbes Online. <https://www.forbes.com/sites/forbesleadershipforum/2016/08/18/message-to-food-companies-food-activists-are-your-new-brand-managers/>; August 18, 2016.
87. IFIC. *COVID-19: Impact on Food Purchasing, Eating Behaviors, and Perceptions of Food Safety.* Washington, DC: International Food Information Council; 2020. Available from: http://www.foodinsight.org.

Chapter 63

Microbiological risks versus putative chemical risks based on hazard rather than exposure: can it be rationalized for public understanding?

John O'Brien

The Food Observatory, UK and Nutrition Innovation Centre for Food and Health, School of Biomedical Sciences, Ulster University, Coleraine, United Kingdom

Abstract

Both hazard- and risk-based approaches are used to manage the safety of foods. Each approach has merits. However, the different methodologies and terminology used can lead to challenges for public understanding and for risk communication. The widespread application of hazard analysis and critical control point (now evolving as hazard analysis and risk-based preventive controls) supported by chemical and microbial risk assessment is part of a modern food system that delivers very safe food. Nonetheless, many consumers are worried about food safety and there are professional differences about the best ways of protecting public health. Several approaches have been proposed for the better classification of chemical hazards. In addition, frameworks are evolving that can support better regulation based on hazards and risks. This has the potential to improve priority setting and public understanding. Risk assessment has been in the public spotlight during the COVID-19 pandemic and new scientific tools have been deployed (e.g., wastewater surveillance) that have the potential to improve food microbial risk assessment and consumer understanding. Finally, data triangulation from multiple methods may support better hazard identification and risk assessment with the potential to improve public confidence in food safety.

Keywords: Hazard; food safety; labeling; risk assessment; consumer perception; regulation; risk management; risk communication; foodborne illness

63.1 Introduction

The golden rule in risk analysis is to design actions and messages that are proportionate to the risks. The coincidence of different classes of risk can be especially challenging to manage, especially when data are limited. When miscalculations occur in the risk analysis process, the consequences can be truly disastrous. The significance of such errors was highlighted by a large cholera outbreak in Lima, Peru in 1991.[1] The outbreak had its origins in raw seafood. Once in the human population, the bacteria contaminated drinking water supplies. Water treatment should have prevented such contamination. Indeed, it appeared that water filtration facilities were satisfactory. However, the backstory to the outbreak was the interpretation of research published by the US EPA on carcinogenicity of disinfection by-products (in this case the trihalomethanes).[2] Local authorities, acting upon US EPA studies decided to stop chlorination of many of Lima's water supplies. Removing the disinfection step and the safeguard of residual chlorine in the distribution network removed a vital protection against contaminated water reaching the consumer. The epidemic reportedly caused 3516 deaths and more than 300,000 cases of illness. The main lessons learned from the incident, and which are relevant to the theme of this chapter, can be summarized as follows:

1. Not to lose sight of the larger risks that need to be managed (in this case the prevention of waterborne infections).
2. It is necessary to place risk assessment (and risk communication) in its larger context (i.e., the practical constraints and options for dealing with risks of different magnitudes).
3. Importance of better communication of uncertainties and limitations of risk assessment (in this case, the risk of a waterborne infection was very real, whereas the risk of cancer was theoretical, based on extrapolation from high-dose rodent feeding studies).

Present Knowledge in Food Safety. DOI: https://doi.org/10.1016/B978-0-12-819470-6.00003-2

The important lessons from the Lima outbreak need to be placed in the larger context of the mastering of risk analysis in a complex and dynamic environment. Food is a good example of both a complex and dynamic risk environment. There is increasing recognition that the optimal approach to many of the more complex food challenges is to adopt a systems approach, that is, food at the intersection of multiple interacting systems. This is not an argument to ignore smaller carcinogenic risks. Such cases demand an ALARA approach (as low as reasonably achievable) whereby current best practices are applied to minimize risk.

Discussions around hazards are often seductively simple. Humans are hard-wired to identify rapidly, and react to, known hazards. Little thinking or effort is required and action is swift.[a] Errors of judgment occur, but throughout human history, the cost of errors was generally low: "better safe than sorry!" Such simple, binary, thinking is no longer useful in confronting the risks in modern life. Of particular relevance to an evaluation of the pitfalls of hazard- versus risk-based approaches is the observation by Kahneman,[3] "it is easier to construct a coherent story when you know little, when there are fewer pieces to fit into the puzzle." Thus "can cause cancer" is much easier to process than "nongenotoxic rodent carcinogen at maximum tolerated dose."

BOX 63.1 Simple definitions of health risk and hazard.[a]

Health risk	Hazard
• A probability	• A property or characteristic of a material, substance, or organism
• Depends on a specified level of exposure	• Depends on method of measurement
• Refers to a specific adverse health effect	• Makes no inference about scale of risk
• Applies to a specific group of people	• Makes no inference about scale of exposure

Caveats
- Hazard≠risk
- Hazard in medium A (e.g., air)≠hazard in medium B (e.g., food)
- Risk assessment≠risk of occurrence of a hazard
- Risk assessment≠risk analysis

[a]Further reading, Paustenbach.[4]

63.2 Terminology, definitions, and challenges of communication

The correct definition of risk and hazard is fundamental in underpinning their correct application (Box 63.1). Therefore well-constructed statements on risk should be qualified and context specific. Statements on hazards, on the other hand, make no such assumptions and only depend on the methodology to identify the hazard.

The assessment and management of microbial and chemical risks in foods have developed through different pathways,[5] with the consequence that different terminology is used (Table 63.1). Until recently, the management of microbial food safety was overwhelmingly hazard based,[8] whereas the management of chemicals in food used a risk-based approach largely informed by data from animal studies.[5] As will be seen below, there are examples where the definition and communication of hazards are highly standardized; the fact that the processes are different does not devalue the outputs. Such distinctions are not always clear in published narratives on hazard and risk. Even expert authorities have been observed to conflate risk concepts such as evidence of association with evidence of causation.[13] Different terminologies and approaches sometimes lead to confusion and difficulty to translate easily from one paradigm to another. Frequently, risk and hazard are used interchangeably leading to confusion. Furedi[14] observed that the phrase "at risk" in UK newspapers had grown almost 10-fold during the 1990s. This was not due to an increase in risks per se but to a journalistic trend. He concluded, "our obsessions with so-called theoretical risks actually distract society from dealing with those old-fashioned dangers that have always threatened our lives."[14] This observation is truer today than ever.

The word risk is itself relative. Slovic[15] observed, "Human beings have invented the concept *risk* to help them understand and cope with the dangers and uncertainties of life. Although these dangers are real, there is no such thing as 'real risk' or 'objective risk'." Absolute risk as measured objectively may be very different from perceived risk. Most consumers apply the word "risk" in an everyday sense but may use the term inconsistently or have no understanding of the scientific definition of risk.

Each hazard has a unique profile of perceived qualities.[16] The perception of "controversial" hazards can differ markedly between experts and laypersons. The perception of hazards differs significantly across categories and between experts and consumers.[17] Cultural, social, political, and historical factors can have a huge impact.[18] Thus hazards that are of little concern in one country can make front-page news in another. In the case of crop protection, consumers tend to be less accepting of chemical pesticides compared with biotechnology provided when the latter is seen as natural.[19] This means that different groups would rank hazards differently, based on different criteria. Consumers generally express more concern about chemical risks in food than microbial risks.[20] This is part of the great challenge of food risk communication: experts rank sources of health risks in foods associated with pathogenic microorganisms and nutritional

TABLE 63.1 Comparison of terms used in microbial and chemical food safety.[a]

Microbial food safety		Chemical food safety	
Abbreviation	**Description**	**Abbreviation**	**Description**
HACCP	Hazard analysis and critical control point.	HBGV	Health-based guidance value (e.g., ADI and TDI). Daily dose (e.g., mg/kg body weight) acceptable or tolerable over a lifetime exposure.
HARPC	Hazard analysis and risk-based preventive controls (terminology derived from US FSMA Act).	ADI	Acceptable daily intake (HBGV applied to, e.g., food additives and pesticides).
GHP	Good hygienic practices.	TDI	Tolerable daily intake (HBGV applied to, e.g., environmental chemical contaminants).
ALOP	Appropriate level of (consumer) protection. Level of protection, expressed as disease incidence, deemed tolerable by a public health authority. Used to set the FSO.	MRL	Maximum residue level (EU). Maximum residue limit (Codex Alimentarius). Applied to pesticide and veterinary residues in food.
Microbiological criteria	Rules defining limits of microbial contamination for specific microbe–food combinations. May be private specifications, regulatory standards, or guidelines.	ML	Maximum level. Term generally used for regulatory limits of natural and environmental contaminants.
FSO	Food safety objective. Risk-based approach to microbial safety. An expression of the maximum level of microbiological hazard in food that would be tolerable (e.g., <100 CFU/g *Listeria monocytogenes*).	NOAEL	No observed adverse effect level (dose used as a basis to set ADI/TDI for threshold toxicants following application of an uncertainty factor).
PC	Performance criterion. An outcome of control measure(s), e.g., 12D reduction[b] of *Clostridium botulinum* in retort processing.	LOAEL	Lowest observed adverse effect level (dose).
PO	Performance objective. Maximum frequency/ concentration of a microbial hazard in a food at a specific step in the food chain.	BMD	Benchmark Dose. Mathematically derived value for a dose giving a specific response (e.g., 1%, 10%) in a dose–response curve.

[a]*From Paustenbach,[4] Whiting,[6] US FDA,[7] IFST,[8] Lanzoni et al.,[9] IFST,[10] FAO,[11] FAO/WHO.[12]*
[b]*Decimal reduction time expressed in log_{10} units.*

imbalances as greater than the toxicological risks from natural toxicants, environmental contaminants, food additives, and pesticides residues.[21] Big gaps between expert and public understanding are an acknowledged challenge for regulatory systems because regulatory action out of line with citizen expectations can lead to erosion of trust.[22]

The emotional attitude to hazards drives belief about their benefits and risks. This is called the affect heuristic[23] whereby people's likes and dislikes determine their beliefs about the world. Media coverage can also skew the judgments of causes of injury and death. This is the so-called availability heuristic—the process of judging the frequency of an event by the ease with which instances come to mind.[23] This is especially important in the field of food safety if food risks receive media attention that is out of proportion to the real statistical risks. The phenomenon of the social amplification of risk has been known for many years.[24] Ruzza et al.[25] analyzed media coverage of the 2017 Fipronil alert and egg product recall and concluded that, while the online information correctly communicated the risks to consumers as low, the alert was amplified because the general news media could represent it as a political scandal. Kahneman[3] describes how our predilection for causal thinking leads to a bias toward confidence over doubt. When a story is compelling, we tend to focus on the story rather than assessing the reliability of the result. Certainty is easier than doubt and we pay more attention to the content of messages rather than attempting to analyze their reliability.

As mentioned above, there are multiple conceptions of risk and risk is multidimensional.[15] In the context of food safety the use of risk assessment will generally be interpreted as applying to health risk. However, "risk" is often used to denote risk of exposure or risk of contamination as opposed to health risk. "Risk assessment" is also applied to the evaluation of risks of food fraud, for example, in the application of supply chain vulnerability risk assessment.[8] The outcome of such assessments does not necessarily imply a health risk.

63.3 Microbial hazards in foods

Microbial hazards in foods are classified into a small number of broad classes: parasites, fungi, bacteria, viruses, and prions.[26] Within these groups of hazards, some may produce toxins that lead to food contamination (e.g., toxigenic fungi such as *Aspergillus* or bacteria such as *Clostridium botulinum*) and some have the potential to cause infections in humans and animals (e.g., *Salmonella* spp., norovirus, *Cryptosporidium parvum*). The bacteria may be spore formers or nonspore formers, which will determine the type of process required for destruction. The parasites include protozoa (e.g., *Cryptosporidium* spp. and *Toxoplasma* spp.), tapeworms (e.g., *Echinococcus* spp.), and nematode worms (e.g., *Trichinella* spp.).[27,28] The list of hazards is changing over time. For example, listeria was unknown as a foodborne pathogen before the early 1980s.[29] Recently, attention has focused on new or changing biohazards in foods (such as *Clostridium difficile*),[30] hepatitis E virus,[31] and the microbial safety of fresh produce.[32] In addition, attention has shifted back to foodborne parasites.[27]

In the case of microbial hazards, four main factors influence the risk to consumers:

- The microorganism (e.g., infectious dose, virulence factors, and disease severity).
- The food matrix. Some matrices permit microbial growth and some do not. High-fat content can protect bacteria from the effects of stomach acid and bile. Indigenous flora may outcompete or destroy contaminating pathogens.
- The consumer (host factors include age, immune status, pregnancy, medication such as antacids, status of the gut microbiome).
- Consumption factors (level of contamination and food intake).

In addition to the above, manufacturers need to consider the process and storage conditions: some food processes have the potential to successfully eliminate a hazard and some do not; some storage conditions permit microbial growth and some do not.

63.4 Chemical hazards in foods

There is much more diversity in chemical hazards compared with microbial hazards. As an illustration, the European Food Safety Authority (EFSA) has compiled a chemical hazards database based on >5500 substances evaluated in more than 2000 scientific opinions since its inception.[33] Toxicological data are lacking for many of the 85,000 plus chemicals in commercial use.[34] In addition, natural food constituents bring the potential number of chemical substances in food to at least 100,000. Many hazards reflect many different chemical substances and many different modes of toxic action. Historically, chemical hazard identification and characterization were heavily dependent on animal bioassays. In recent years, animal assays have gradually been replaced or augmented by in silico predictive methods [(Q)SARS, biokinetic modeling], data read across, thresholds of toxicological concern, and in vitro assays.[35] Such changes are driven by scientific developments, ethical standards, and by legislation (see, e.g., EC/1907[36] and US House of Representatives).[37]

Carcinogen hazards have been a focus of concern since the 1950s. The Delaney Clause of the US Food Drug and Cosmetic Act (1958) prohibited the use in foods of substances shown to induce cancer in humans or animals.[5] If a substance has been shown to cause cancer in an animal study, knowledge of the mechanism of carcinogenicity is necessary to assess the risk for humans. In addition, it is necessary to determine if the substance acts via a genotoxic or nongenotoxic mode of action. Generally, genotoxic carcinogens are assumed to have no identifiable threshold of toxicity, whereas nongenotoxic carcinogens may have a threshold below which no adverse effects can be seen. Substances that are genotoxic are usually not added deliberately to foods and would be screened out during premarket assessment.[38] Contaminants (natural and environmental) that are genotoxic generally have maximum levels in food set to levels that are ALARA.[39] The methods used to determine genotoxicity for regulatory purposes are clearly defined (e.g., EFSA).[40] In addition, the application of ALARA may be highly dependent on the contaminant, food commodity, and agriculture system. It is particularly challenging for policy makers, and public understanding, when a substance is shown to be positive in one assay for genotoxicity and negative in another. There is an ongoing challenge of defining what "genotoxic," "nongenotoxic," and "carcinogenic" mean in regulatory toxicology.[41]

More recently, a lot of attention has focused on endocrine disruption. This was typified by concern about bisphenol A (BPA) from food contact materials and other sources.[42] A large number of substances have been identified as possessing endocrine activity. The number of structures is diverse due to

1. The number of endocrine organs and responsive tissues and the many potential modes of action.
2. In the case of the estrogen (ER) receptor, the ability to accommodate a diverse array of chemical structures, what chemists sometimes call "receptor promiscuity."[43]

This creates a challenge for researchers, regulators, industry risk managers, and for consumer understanding. The absence of agreed working definitions and consensus on test systems has led to a large number of endocrine disruptors described according to hazard. While ~800 chemicals have been reported to have the potential to interact with endocrine receptors, or affect hormone synthesis or conversion, only a small fraction of these have been investigated in intact organisms.[44] It is time consuming, expensive, and inappropriate to conduct risk assessments of thousands of chemicals. While chemicals such as BPA and diethylstilbestrol have a huge amount of toxicity data, many hundreds of compounds have little information beyond the presence of the endocrine activity hazard. La Merrill et al.[45] used a pragmatic approach inspired by hazard identification of carcinogens to propose 10 key characteristics (KCs) with which to classify endocrine disrupters, and assays that could be used to identify them and provide mechanistic data. The proposed KCs are clearly defined and biologically based: for example, KC1: interacts with or activates hormone receptors; KC3: alters hormone receptor expression; KC4: alters signal transduction in hormone-responsive cells; KC9: alters hormone metabolism or clearance.

63.5 The case for hazard-based approaches

A complete risk assessment is not necessary to take appropriate risk management action. In food microbiology, hazard-based approaches to food safety management have served the world well for 60 years since the food safety demands of space travel led to the development of HACCP (hazard analysis and critical control point) thinking for food manufacturing.[8] Hazard identification is easier and more rapid than a risk assessment (Table 63.2). While HACCP is based on hazards rather than risks, it depends on the reasonable likelihood of a given hazard being present in a given raw material or processing environment.[8] For many operations, the protection offered by classical HACCP and increasingly HARPC (hazard analysis and risk-based preventive controls) approaches, offers a high level of consumer protection without the need for full risk assessment. While this paper advocates more attention to underpinning food regulatory decisions by scientific risk assessment, more risk assessment is not a remedy for all food safety challenges. Better, more consistent, and more targeted application of existing tools is also needed.

Epidemiology can highlight the biohazard-food combinations leading to disease in humans.[6] These data are useful and can inform hazard-based approaches for microbial food safety management. However, there are limitations. First, the quality and coverage of epidemiology data vary throughout the world (including in developed countries). In all countries, only a fraction of all foodborne diseases is reported. Furthermore, there are limitations in statistical power. Ebel and Williams[46] applied a Bayesian model to baseline US FoodNet Salmonella data and concluded that the power to detect a 10% reduction in salmonellosis incidence over a 1-year hypothetical period could be as low as 0.04 (4% confidence). In addition, epidemiology depends on imperfect data and a wide variety of evidence is generally necessary to imply a causal relationship between exposure and disease.[47]

Approaches to determine likelihood and severity can be qualitative (as in a basic HACCP approach), semiquantitative, or fully quantitative (in a quantitative microbial risk assessment).[5] Even qualitative approaches emphasize the value of knowledge and good quality information in the choice and ranking of hazards to include in a food safety plan. Thus the selection of hazards is rational, practical, and selective, taking into account factors such as

TABLE 63.2 Comparison of hazard- and risk-based approaches to risk management.

Parameter	Hazard based	Risk based
Time	Rapid	Slow
Data	Data light	Data intense
Expertise	Requires less expertise	High level of expertise
Complexity	Simple	Complex
Cost	Cheap	Expensive
Risk–benefit comparison	No	Yes
Risk ranking	None or simple classes	Yes
Facilitate cost–benefit	No	Yes
Evaluation of mixtures	Limited	Possible

historical data about known hazards in raw materials and ingredients, current guidelines and codes of practice, legislation and microbiological criteria, customer requirements, target consumers, and the latest scientific research. The selected hazards should be realistic and reasonably expected to occur.[8] Identified hazards should

1. be directly or indirectly associated with the food chain AND/OR
2. have the potential to become food chain hazards (even if they are not currently considered as such).

This ensures targeted risk management.

There is sometimes a general perception that microbial risk assessment is not as developed as chemical risk assessment. It can, however, more easily avail of data from human epidemiology to inform the hazard identification and hazard characterization steps. This is greatly assisted by the recent advent of next-generation sequencing in outbreak investigations.[48] The value of epidemiological investigations in the setting of standards in food safety microbiology was illustrated by a recent outbreak of listeriosis associated with ice cream consumption. The outbreak had a number of features that led to an improved hazard characterization of *Listeria monocytogenes* in ice cream.[49] First, the outbreak was well investigated and benefitted from both pulse-field gel electrophoresis and whole-genome sequencing data which linked human cases with consumption of products. Second, a large amount of product analytical data was generated. Third, *L. monocytogenes* is stable over time and does not grow in frozen ice cream meaning that good estimates of human exposures were possible; it was reasonable to expect that analytical data from the finished product reflected levels that were in the product at the time of consumption.

Hazard-based food safety management such as HACCP is flexible enough and simple enough to be applicable at many levels in food production: for example, at farm level, water treatment, fisheries, manufacturing, retail, and food service.[50] Millions of workers contribute to successful hazard-based management in food and other industries.

Microbiological criteria for foods are used extensively in risk management by food businesses. The criteria, with expert guidance, link specific food commodities with given pathogenic hazards and an acceptable public health level of protection.[10] The concept of appropriate level of protection (ALOP) was introduced to complement the HACCP concept with a risk context derived from population disease incidence[6] (Table 63.1). The ALOPs and food safety objectives are linked via the dose–response relationship of an organism in a specific setting. Microbial dose–response data have become more abundant and avails of data from the following sources: foodborne disease data (observational); characteristics of the population at risk (e.g., demographics; data on vulnerability); animal and in vitro studies (experimental data); human volunteer trials (experimental data).

In the case of chemicals, EFSA[51] is considering a combined approach whereby a hazard-driven process is used to group chemicals in mixtures based on toxicity data. The combinations of chemicals can then be prioritized based on exposure alone or risk (combining exposure assessment and hazard characterization).

Rapid hazard screening assays can be efficient tools in product safety by design. The relatively low-cost, high-throughput nature of such assays can support the prioritization of constituents of food contact materials for risk assessment when combined with chemical analysis. Koster et al.[52] reviewed the application of genotoxicity, endocrine activity, and cytotoxicity bioassays in vitro for nonintentionally added substances in food contact materials. Such an approach, in combination with other tools, can provide direction and insights when complex chemical mixtures need to be characterized and when toxicity data are lacking. The range of potential assays available is extensive and includes in vitro assays targeting a variety of endocrine receptors: ER, androgen, glucocorticoid, progesterone, and thyroid.[53] A large number of in vitro assays are available for the detection of genotoxicity via different modes of action (e.g., Ames *Salmonella* mutagenicity tests; refer Koster et al.[52] and Van Bossuyt et al.).[54] While such assays are not mandated by regulations for food contact materials, the application of an integrated testing approach has the potential to increase regulatory compliance of finished products increasing consumer confidence.[53]

63.5.1 Disadvantages

Because human judgment is required to respond to hazards in an appropriate way, one of the errors associated with HACCP is the misperception of the risks associated with the hazard.[55] Hazard-based approaches can result in black and white answers and a lack of flexibility.[38,56] This may lead to inconsistency in the approach used in food chemical risk management or lack of proportionality in risk regulation due to under or overly conservative risk assessments. Both consequences conflict with the principles of good regulatory practice. To support consumer trust and to facilitate innovation and legitimate business activities, consistent, transparent, proportional, and targeted approaches are needed.

The risk of overregulation has been suggested to be lower for risk-based compared with hazard-based approaches.[56] This may be an oversimplistic representation of the challenge of evaluating hazard- versus risk-based options. Risk assessments incorporating high levels of uncertainty or applying unrealistically high exposure assumptions may also lead to disproportionate regulatory action. However, the risk-assessment process is in principle more transparent and can lead to constructive dialog between different stakeholders.

Hazard detection without risk information, unfortunately, is amenable to political intervention whereby food safety risk may be overlooked in favor of some other goal.

63.6 The case for risk assessment

The WHO/FAO risk analysis paradigm is applicable to the assessment, management, and communication of all foodborne risks (Fig. 63.1).[38,57] In risk assessment, hazard identification, hazard characterization, exposure assessment, and risk characterization are applicable to both chemical and microbial risk assessment.

Whether dealing with chemical or microbial hazards, the important metrics of safety are not measured exposure to the hazard but the health outcomes in terms of disease incidence. Ultimately, the health outcomes should shed light on the specific cases, in specific groups exposed to specific foods per head of population per year. Pragmatic approaches to risk analysis start with an evaluation of exposure. Thus in principle,

Hazard $\times$ zero exposure = zero risk
High hazard $\times$ zero exposure = zero risk

In practice, there is no such thing as zero risk as there are always theoretical possibilities coupled with uncertainties which together make the statement of zero risk impossible. However, if the conclusion of negligible risk is robust and based on an acceptable analysis, then there is no case for specific management action and the public can be given appropriate unambiguous advice and reassurance. There is a caveat, however. Risk is always a specific and bounded concept (Box 63.1). It must always be used to indicate a probability of a specific adverse health outcome, in a specific individual (or group), under specified conditions of exposure. If any of these conditions change, the risk changes. Therefore considerations of nonexposure must take into account not just the hazardous agent, but also the possible pathways to exposure as well as those exposed.

Risk assessments conducted to protect consumer health are, by design, conservative and have a built-in level of precaution. Inherent to such precaution is a set of assumptions. In the past, some such assumptions deviated significantly from what would be considered normal food consumption or food use. The data used to define high intakes should ideally be based on evidence and sense-checked against what a diet based on an extreme scenario would look like.[58] Scenarios and assumptions used in the process should be evidence-led where possible. Would such a scenario be plausible in practice? Would such an exposure scenario engender health risks unrelated to the risk assessment being conducted (e.g., high fat, calories, protein, or other nutritional imbalance)?

The science of risk assessment is constantly evolving and this brings with it more complexity. Deluyker[59] paraphrased Karl Popper in describing the process as not concluding that a microorganism or chemical is safe but defining the context under which they do *not* constitute a risk (my emphasis). This underlines the conditional or context-specific nature of risk assessment. Hazard on the other hand, as a property, is easy to grasp and tends to be fixed (guided by definitions, e.g., what is flammable, toxic, and carcinogenic). Deluyker[59] went further and compared scientific risk assessment with an experimental approach in

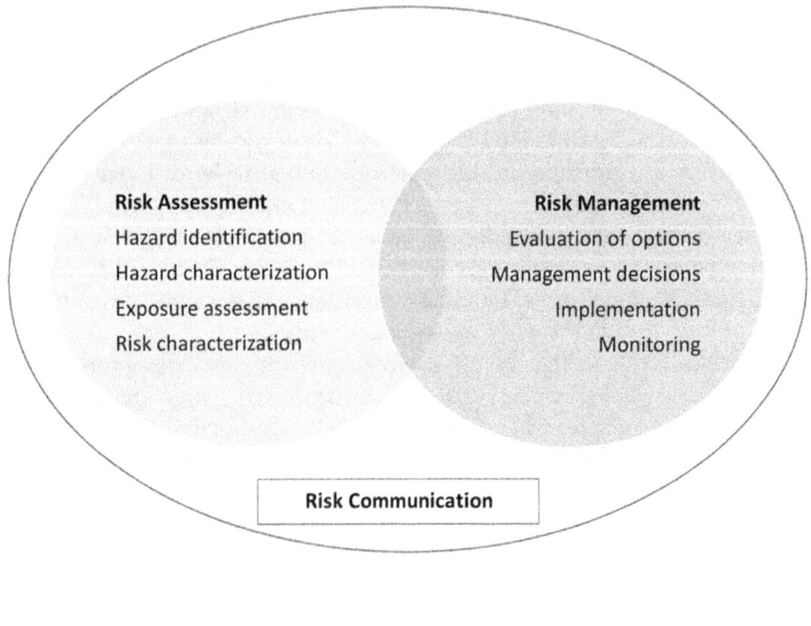

FIGURE 63.1 The risk analysis process. *After FAO/WHO, 2006.* Food Safety Risk Analysis. A Guide for National Food Safety Authorities. Paper 87. *Rome: Food and Agriculture Organisation of the United Nations.*

that it is step-wise and hypothesis driven. Not everyone agrees that risk assessment can be compared with hypothesis testing. They have parallels in that both require careful formulation of the (research) question, objectivity, and a disciplined generation of data. However, MacGillivray[60] pointed out that risk assessment operates within a broader context than research involving a range of interest groups, societal considerations, and many disciplines ranging from philosophy to statistics. While null hypothesis testing can contribute to the process, the inferential part of risk assessment is much broader involving such tasks as weighing evidence, uncertainty, model selection, and estimating the consequences of action and inaction.[60]

63.6.1 Disadvantages

As outlined above (Table 63.2), risk assessment is time consuming and expensive and requires far more data than hazard identification. The methodology may be challenging to communicate. Some hazards such as genotoxic carcinogens present special challenges compared with toxicants for which thresholds are identifiable. A risk of risk assessment is the risk of miscommunication or misunderstanding of the limits and assumptions inherent in the assessment. A further danger is the assumption that a risk assessment in one setting (e.g., high-dose respiratory or dermal occupational exposure) can be extrapolated to another (e.g., ingestion of low levels in the diet or drinking water). Such data may be useful. However, extrapolation is only valid if the mode of toxic action via different routes of exposure is the same.

Awareness of hazards, especially those that receive much media attention, can lead to recall bias in case-control epidemiology studies.[61] This is difficult to control for and it is not possible to obtain objective and precise exposure data from such studies.

The application of epidemiology in chemical risk assessment is more challenging than that for food microbiology, but new developments point to more opportunities in this area. Classical epidemiology based on statistical association between exposures and disease were fraught with uncertainties due to the fact that disease processes for noncommunicable diseases spanned years and decades and were confounded by other factors, including genetics, that influenced disease development.[62] There has been rapid progress in recent years in the use of biomarkers of toxicity, genome-wide association studies, and epigenetic markers to improve the integration of in vitro, experimental animal and human data.[63]

63.7 Balancing and reconciling different risks

Food is a special case as there are three major classes of risk to be managed: microbiological, chemical, and nutritional. Frequently, there is an interplay between these risks; if one is modified, it frequently leads to a change in another. For example, removal of the chemical risk associated with a preservative agent could lead to a large increase in microbial risk if no mitigating measures were taken.[21] Comparison of different risks and comparison of risks and benefits is not possible using hazard-based approaches alone and generally requires a risk-based methodology and outcome measures that can be compared.[64]

Risk assessment rather than hazard-based approaches is generally applied to whole foods and natural toxicants in foods.[38] This reflects the chemical complexity of whole foods, the need to consider the nutritional and economic implications, the complexity of formulating appropriate dietary guidelines, and the history of food use. The following case studies explore recent challenges in risk analysis associated with a whole foods (red and processed meats), presence of a disinfection by-product from biocidal control of microbial risks (chlorate), and acrylamide, a cooking/processing by-product.

63.7.1 Whole food example: meat and cancer risk

In 2015 the International Agency for Research on Cancer (IARC) published a summary of the conclusions of a working group on meat consumption and cancer.[65] The Agency assigned the consumption of processed meat to Group 1 of the IARC Carcinogenic Hazard Classification (carcinogenic to humans) and red meat to Group 2a (probably carcinogenic to humans). Much controversy ensued as to the methodology used to inform the IARC classification and to explain why the opinion of different expert bodies may be different. The monograph published in 2018 clarified that the IARC monographs evaluate hazards despite the use of the word "risk" in the titles.[66] Thus the terminology is nuanced to indicate "capable of causing cancer" rather than "carcinogen."[66] The challenge with identifying meat as a cancer hazard is that it is not possible to treat meat as one could a carcinogenic industrial chemical such as 2-naphthylamine (IARC Group 1, carcinogenic to humans). Therefore authorities need to respond to such research through the formulation of dietary guidelines taking into account many factors such as cancer risk, nutrition benefit and risk, microbial risk, and consumer choice and preferences.

Observational epidemiology studies have consistently revealed an association between red and processed meat consumption and colorectal cancer.[67] Many animal, cell culture, and analytical studies have addressed potential mechanisms by which meat could increase colorectal cancer risk. There has been much commentary in the scientific literature on the presence of carcinogens in red and processed meat, especially those produced during cooking.[68] Even when all the evidence is assembled, there remains uncertainty and disagreement, in particular for the following reasons:

1. Observational studies on diets are not perfect tools, alone, with which to pinpoint the causes of diseases such as cancer.
2. Many dietary and lifestyle factors may be involved in colorectal carcinogenesis: gut microbiota,[69] energy intake, dietary fat, fruit, vegetable, and dairy consumption.[70,71]
3. Many of the animal studies have used levels of meat consumption and diets that are not reflective of normal human diets.[72,73]
4. While several mutagenic heterocyclic amines (e.g., PhIP and MEIQ) may be present in cooked meat, they do not appear to be associated with colorectal cancer in epidemiology studies.[68]

The use of biomonitoring data looks promising as a means of integrating experimental data with observational human epidemiology data.[74] However, while adduct formation can be related mechanistically with carcinogenesis for DNA-reactive carcinogens, it is difficult to relate the presence of adducts directly to risk of cancer due to a number of factors, including DNA repair, adducts that do not lead to mutations, mutations that do not lead to cancers, background adduct formation, and cellular apoptosis.[75]

63.7.2 Chlorate, a by-product of disinfection: balancing microbial and chemical risks

The toxicity of biocides has been the subject of much attention in recent years, including concerns about some applications in food preparation, environmental, and household applications. Disinfectants are used in food manufacturing to manage microbial contamination. Microorganisms are ubiquitous and microbial food safety depends on multiple independent measures, including disinfection, to deliver a safe product. However, disinfection is not a panacea and prevention of contamination is always preferable to decontamination. As highlighted in Section 63.1, disinfectant residues and their derivatives may give rise to the presence of a chemical hazard. Therefore risk management requires a balance between chemical and microbial risks. This is achieved by identifying the optimal best sanitary practices which may vary from region to region and depends on the raw material, type of process, and finished product specification.

Chlorate is an anionic by-product of disinfection of water with chlorine-based agents. Its use in the EU as a pesticide was discontinued in 2008, and a default maximum residue limit (MRL) of 0.01 ppm is applicable to all foods under EU law.[76] Therefore products with levels in excess of the limit are technically in breach of regulations. This presented a challenge for authorities in 2016 when analytical data revealed widespread contamination of products with chlorate.[77] Chlorine is still probably the most widespread disinfectant for water and food production equipment; strict application of low MRLs could remove or reduce the use of an important biocide, with potential microbial safety implications. Strict one-sided risk management is not appropriate under such circumstances.[78,79] This was summed up succinctly by an ACMSF[78] opinion: "Complexity (competition) associated with coincident chemical and microbial hazards ensures that one-sided minimization is not explicitly a precautionary approach." A number of solutions were proposed to deal with the challenge:

1. Defining best sanitation practices.
2. Application of the WHO guideline for drinking water of 0.7 ppm chlorate.

This is a good illustrative case study as it highlights the challenge of comparison of a chemical risk by extrapolation from toxicology studies with the potential for presence of microbial hazards due to removal of a risk-based preventive control.

63.7.3 Thermal processing and cooking contaminant: acrylamide

From a regulatory perspective, neither risk assessment nor classical epidemiology has the power to detect directly an increase in risk of less than one in a thousand (let alone the one in a million risk deemed to be acceptable by some authorities).[62] Therefore extrapolation is required from finite numbers of animals treated at high doses (for statistical power) or by combining several sources of evidence to increase confidence in epidemiology observations. Both approaches have uncertainties.

Since its discovery in 2002,[80] thousands of papers have been published on acrylamide in food. Due to the mechanism of formation via a pathway of the Maillard reaction, it is very difficult to avoid during cooking or thermal processing. Acrylamide is widely used as a man-made industrial chemical, but its formation via natural chemical pathways was a surprise and a challenge. Of particular concern to toxicologists was the evidence that (1) acrylamide is classified as a probable human carcinogen (Group 2A). (2) The calculated margins of exposure (MOEs) for acrylamide (based on $BMDL_{10}$ modeling of carcinogenicity dose–response in B6C3F mice) were 425–89 for mean exposure estimates and as 283–50 for

95th percentile exposure estimates. EFSA[81] uses a "cut-off" MOE of >10,000 to signify a low level of concern (based on $BMDL_{10}$ modeling of rodent dose–response data for substances that are both carcinogenic and genotoxic). Thus risk-assessment data for acrylamide give cause for concern across all age groups.

The challenges presented for consumer understanding were highlighted by the media commentary on a UK Food Standards Agency campaign to help consumers to reduce acrylamide exposure via home-cooked food[82]; the above media article drew attention to the complexity of the available evidence including the impossibility of assigning a precise risk to acrylamide in food. The rationale for the campaign, derived from risk assessment, was well founded. There has been limited success in reducing levels of acrylamide in manufactured foods over the past two decades.[83] MOEs for dietary acrylamide remain of concern and steps can be taken to minimize acrylamide formation in home-cooked foods. However, the translation of risk-assessment science into consumer action is far more limited (especially in the context of the many public health messages consumers receive) compared with industrial manufacturing. This argues for different approaches and outcomes for interventions at the consumer level compared with food businesses, whether dealing with chemical or microbiological hazards.

Thermal processing of food is a special case where a purely hazard-based approach does not resolve the challenge of the simultaneous elimination of microbial hazards and achieving culinary acceptability while limiting the potentially harmful consequences of cooking: nutrient destruction and generation of chemical process contaminants (e.g., acrylamide and furan). Reassuringly, epidemiology studies have not indicated that acrylamide in food increases the risk of cancers in humans.

63.8 Hazard and risk ranking

As discussed above, one of the challenges arising from identifying hazards is the development of measures to respond to them. Various approaches have been proposed for the comparison and ranking of hazards. These are divided into either "top-down" surveillance-based methods (e.g., disease data, biomarker data, pathogen prevalence in foods) or bottom-up predictive approaches (e.g., using experimental data on toxicity or virulence).[84] Epidemiological data have clear advantages over extrapolation from experimental data. However, epidemiology data are not abundant and may not be available in some regions. Hazard ranking has the potential to be of value to risk assessors, policy makers, risk managers, and possibly in risk communication with consumers. However, all approaches have their limitations.

A simple worst case risk scenario for pesticides was proposed by Low et al.[85]:

$$\text{Risk} = \text{Exposure/ADI (acceptable daily intake)}$$

where exposure = food consumption × highest concentration detected in food.

While such an approach has the attraction of simplicity, its use for exposures below the ADI is not valid as a means of risk ranking (at best, it would be a form of safety ranking), while exceeding the ADI does not necessarily imply a risk. It is also challenging to compare compounds using such an approach as there will be different modes of action, adverse outcomes, and dose–response curves. In effect, it would amount to comparing different hazards without accounting for the nature of those hazards—in layman's terms, comparing apples and oranges.

More recently, Langerholc et al.[86] proposed a hazard ranking for chemical hazards termed a severity-adjusted MOE approach. The approach used a ratio of a reference point [e.g., benchmark dose (BMD), LOAEL, or NOEAL] divided by the product of (exposure) × (a severity factor) × (an adjustment factor) (using a default of 100 for intra and interspecies variability). The severity factor used a scale of 1–100 for mild effects (e.g., changes in biomarkers) to severe effects (e.g., cancer). The approach was applied to compare hazards with very different modes of action such as acrylamide, methyl mercury and sunset yellow.

Lindqvist et al.[87] advocated the use of health-adjusted life years to compare across hazard classes. This approach is also fraught with difficulty as input data for such an exercise are always incomplete and agreement is needed on default scenarios. When attempting to compare chemical and microbial hazards, there are challenges associated with the methods used in risk assessment, the need to deal with both acute and chronic health end-points, and the different types of data used to identify and characterize the hazards (e.g., in silico, in vitro, in vivo animal studies, and human epidemiology). A possible solution is to use separate approaches for the two classes of hazard.

The so-called human exposure-rodent potency of Ames et al.[88] was an early attempt to rank carcinogenic hazards based on a point estimate of human exposure divided by an estimate of TD50 (daily dose over a lifespan of a species resulting in tumors in 50% of test animals) derived from the Carcinogenic Potency Database. The approach was heavily criticized[89] not least for the fact that the TD50 relied on using one point on the dose–response curve. The currently accepted approach of deriving a BMD (usually $BMDL_{10}$; lower-bound estimate of the dose resulting in a 10% response using the most appropriate cancer endpoint) from appropriate mathematical models gives a more sound basis for comparison,[90] assuming that enough data are available to build the model. Using the $BMDL_{10}$ as a point of departure for a ratio of potency to exposure is the basis for the MOE approach. In this case, conservative assumptions are also used to produce an exposure estimate at the higher end of the expected range (generally the 95th percentile or higher).[91] The approach is useful for assigning levels of concern to genotoxic carcinogens, where the identification of biological thresholds is not possible.[91] However, the MOE approach can be applied across a range of hazards in foods and other systems. While the MOE is not a measure of risk *per se*, it is possible to state that high MOEs (lower potency and/or lower exposure) represent lower risk than low MOEs. In the case of genotoxic carcinogens, the EFSA has concluded that a MOE of $>10,000$ can be interpreted as of low concern.[81] This is a useful communication and standardization tool.

The use of the MOE to assign priorities to food chemicals is a robust way of applying BMD methodology to ensure optimal analysis of dose–response data. However, the current BMD methodology is evolving rapidly.[92] As the BMD is not a fixed number in time, neither is the MOE. Nonetheless, comparisons of MOEs derived using the same methodology will remain of value.

63.9 Hazard warning labels on foods

Hazard warning labels on chemical agents are commonplace for the protection of worker and consumer safety. The methods for hazard identification and classification and the communication of the hazards in the form of pictograms are highly standardized[93,94] (Fig. 63.2). Consistent guidance is generally provided on appropriate application of such labels and recommended protective measures. Professionals handling chemical and biological hazards will generally have training in the interpretation of hazard labels. Information provided to users in the form of such hazard labels or in Material Safety Data Sheets do not constitute a risk assessment. The information is provided to inform their own risk assessments and/or risk management measures as necessary. In the case of foods a number of hazard warning labels are in use. In some cases the information offers valuable protection to consumers. However, the value in other cases is questionable or unknown.

63.9.1 Allergens

Allergen labeling is a good example of a hazard warning label. There are at least 170 foods that have been identified as potentially allergenic.[95] Major allergens are required by law to be labeled in most countries. In the EU, 14 allergens must be highlighted in product labels when present[96]: cereals containing gluten, crustaceans, eggs, fish, peanuts, soybeans, milk and products (including lactose), nuts (almonds, hazelnuts, walnuts, cashews, pecans, Brazil nuts, pistachio nuts, macadamia nuts), celery, mustard, sesame seeds, sulfur dioxide and sulfites, lupin, and molluscs. The incidence of food allergy differs in different parts of the world. This is reflected in the rules for mandatory labeling. For example, in Japan mandatory labeling covers 7 allergens, while there is a recommendation to label an additional 20 ingredients.[97] Japan also specifies that labels apply if the concentration allergen protein is >10 mg/kg. In the United States, eight allergens are subject to mandatory labeling[98]: milk, eggs, wheat, tree nuts, peanuts, fish, shellfish, and soybeans;

Pictogram	Hazard description	Meaning/Application
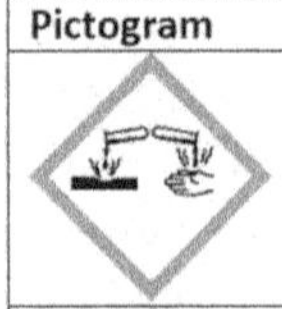	Corrosive	May corrode metals, cause severe skin burns and eye damage/drain cleaner, acids, bases
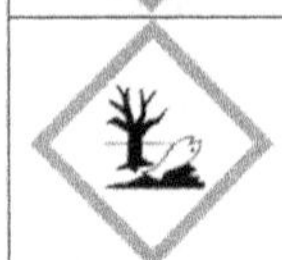	Environmental hazard	Toxic to aquatic life/herbicides, turpentine, gasoline, varnish
	Health hazard	Harmful if swallowed or inhaled, harmful to the environment/washing detergents, toilet cleaner, cleaning fluid
	Skull and crossbones (acute toxicity)	Can harm or kill if swallowed, inhaled or in contact with skin/insecticides, nicotine refills for e-cigarettes

FIGURE 63.2 Examples of chemical hazard pictographs employed worldwide in the UN Globally Harmonized System of Classification and Labelling of Chemicals (GHS) to ensure consistent communication of chemical hazards. *From US Occupational Safety and Health Administration. https://www.osha.gov/hazcom/pictograms; https://echa.europa.eu/regulations/clp/clp-pictograms.*

sesame will be added from 2023. The labels are based on the presence of the allergen hazard, which means that if a sensitive method detects the presence of the protein, it has to be labeled. An additional challenge in allergen management is how to determine if public health concern is important enough to warrant regulation of an existing or new food allergen. Food allergy prevalence data are often sparse or of poor quality. Consumers may benefit from more information on food production practices, but this may not, in itself, be easy to translate into risk. A risk-based framework for food allergens has been proposed based on elicitation potency (ED50 in human trials).[95]

While hazard-based labeling has worked well to inform consumers of allergenic risk of food ingredients, it has not been a great success in informing consumers about the possible incidental contamination. In Australia and New Zealand, a risk-based labeling system is in place the Voluntary Incidental Trace Allergen Labelling (VITAL) program. VITAL labeling is based upon reference doses (ED01, ED05, or both) derived from dose-distribution models.[99] The approach is yet to be adopted outside of Australia and New Zealand. Precautionary allergen labeling (PAL) is a form of hazard warning to support decision making by allergic consumers. The wording of such labels varies. One such format is "may contain X," where "X" is a major allergen; however, many phrases are in current use to signify the possible unintended presence of an allergen hazard. The lack of standardization of PAL phrasing leads to confusion among consumers. In a US study, Marchisotto et al.[100] reported that 37% of consumers believed the label signaled the amount of allergen present. There is also concern about the high use of PAL labels by businesses and the fact that some allergic consumers ignore PAL labels.[101] Pele et al.[102] reported that while the presence of a PAL led to a higher frequency of positive analytical results, 75% of cookie products bearing a PAL label did not contain detectable traces of allergen. A risk-based system of labeling for incidental contamination could help protect consumers while avoiding unnecessary food avoidance and food waste.

63.9.2 Proposition 65

In the area of food safety, one of the best known (and most controversial) hazard-based warning systems is that of the State of California Proposition 65 of the Safe Drinking Water and Toxic Enforcement Act (1986). Proposition 65 mandates warnings for >900 different chemicals (not all of which are foodborne) identified as carcinogens or reproductive toxicants.[103] The act is sometimes described by regulators as a "right to know law."[104] However, there is no discrimination between the risks posed by exposure to such chemicals, which varies by several orders of magnitude. Equally, there is no discrimination between different chemicals based on the quality of the hazard identification data. Naturally occurring carcinogens, such as aflatoxin, are usually exempt from the labeling rules. However, acrylamide, present as a cooking by-product in many foods, is not. This means that the regulation covers whole foods in addition to food additives, pesticides, and anthropogenic contaminants. In the context of food, warnings are used both on product labels and in restaurants (Fig. 63.3). An example of a product label would be "Warning: This product contains a chemical known in the state of California to cause cancer."[105] In addition to enforcement of the act by state and local authorities, private citizens have the right to bring suits under the act.[106] This leads to a large amount of litigation under the law.

The challenge of providing a large volume of information as a regulatory strategy is ensuring consumers can process the information and be empowered to take action to protect their health.[104] With an increasing complexity and volume of information, there is a danger when hazard warnings become so widespread that individuals will ignore the information or become unduly concerned by small risks while potentially ignoring large ones. One research study suggested that a majority of consumers interpreted a Proposition 65 warning on cereal labels as equivalent to a cigarette packet warning.[107]

It has been suggested that cancer epidemiology data provide little evidence that Proposition 65 has had an influence on cancer incidences in California.[106] However, in the absence of additional supporting evidence (e.g., biomarker data, exposure data), the ability of epidemiology alone to "see" changes in cancer incidence attributable to the law is very limited.

63.9.3 Artificial food colors

Based on a double-blind placebo-controlled randomized trial, McCann et al.[108] concluded that mixtures of artificial food colors or a sodium benzoate preservative (or both) in the diet resulted in increased hyperactivity in children in the general population. The EFSA concluded that evidence did not constitute a causal link between individual food colors and behavior in children.[109] The potential effects of artificial food colors on behavior in children were given a great deal of attention by the UK news media and the case highlights the importance of different risk perceptions among different nations. The use of the six colors concerned (sunset yellow FCF, quinoline yellow, carmoisine, allura red, tartrazine, and ponceau 4R) is still permitted in foods. However, the UK applied the "right to know" regulatory approach and mandated the label "May have an adverse effect on activity and attention in children." The

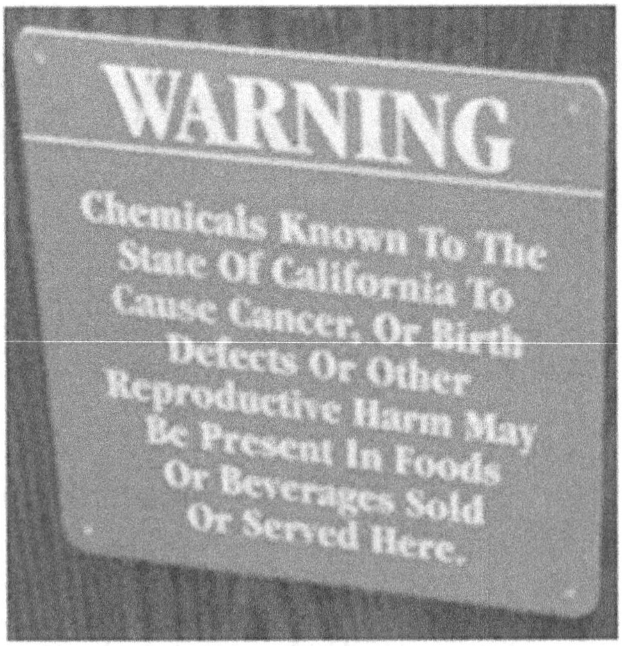
WARNING
Chemicals Known To The State Of California To Cause Cancer, Or Birth Defects Or Other Reproductive Harm May Be Present In Foods Or Beverages Sold Or Served Here.

FIGURE 63.3 Example of a restaurant warning sign complying with the state of California Proposition 65 rules.

labels led to the reformulation of many products to avoid the labeling requirement and stimulated ongoing innovation to achieve "cleaner" labels. The pressure on artificial food additives reflects consumer preference for products that are perceived to be natural.[110] However, experts frequently underline that "natural" does not necessarily mean safe.[111] Specifications for natural food colors can be very challenging. It is also worth recalling that artificial colors were introduced because many natural colors are unstable during food processing and storage.[112] Food businesses have been encouraged to avoid negative claims and to better communicate the choices available in food formulation.[113]

63.9.4 Other hazard labels

Many food safety hazards are routinely managed using labels to inform consumers and food businesses. A number of additional mandatory hazard warning labels are used to protect vulnerable consumers (Table 63.3). In addition, there are many precautionary hazard labels in use. These include labels to alert consumers to the possible presence of pieces in bone in fillets of fish or stones in fruit. They may be used to alert consumers, when necessary, to the presence of raw meat or fish requiring cooking. In some countries, a voluntary label is used to advise consumers not to give honey to infants under the age of 1 year. This precautionary label is designed to protect against infant botulism, a rare but serious condition, that may be caused by *C. botulinum* spores in honey.[116] In recent years, policy makers in several countries have employed front-of-pack warning labels to highlight "unhealthy" nutrient profiles. An example was the introduction of the black and white "stop sign" label in Chile in 2016.[117] While impacts on consumption of target products have been reported, it remains to be seen if such dietary changes will endure or wear off over time.

In summary warning labels on foods based on hazard, may in limited circumstances offer useful guidance to consumers. They can offer a simple, low-cost approach, in principle enabling consumers to make decisions for themselves.[104] In the case of allergic consumers, they can provide information directly to those at risk. However, as a minimum, such labels should

1. be used sparingly as abundant use can lead to their being ignored,
2. be designed to enable consumers to discriminate between large and minor risks and enable simple decisions about whether to use the product, and
3. be subject to periodic reviews of efficacy to verify intended public health protection and value for money.

63.10 Learning from the COVID-19 pandemic

Despite the notable scientific successes in the areas of diagnostics, sequencing, modeling, and vaccine development, risk analysis had little experience or preparation for dealing with a global viral pandemic. Concerns were expressed early during the COVID-19 pandemic about the lack of attention to non-COVID-19 risks (e.g., healthcare, economics, and education). Risk communication, while intensive, was often inconsistent.[118] This is against a backdrop of previous evidence[119] pointing to the possibility of a global viral pandemic. Many of the learnings for risk analysis arising from the COVID-19 pandemic will also be applicable to food hazards and risks.

Wastewater pathogen surveillance for SAR-CoV2 received widespread use during the pandemic.[120,121] Wastewater analysis can form the basis for a useful easy to explain early warning system.[122] The approach is also being applied to surveillance for other pathogens including foodborne microorganisms.[123] Wastewater data can point to which organisms are causing infections in specific areas and indicate whether rates are increasing or decreasing. Wastewater epidemiology can also be used to explore chemical and food exposures.[124] Such observational data can be a valuable complement to experimental and clinical data in underpinning risk management decisions and in supporting public understanding of the basis of such decisions.

Several expert committees concluded early in the COVID-19 outbreak that there was little, if any, risk of transmission via food.[125–127] Publication of hazard data

TABLE 63.3 Selected food hazard warning labels for the protection of vulnerable consumers.[a]

Ingredient	Target consumer	Wording
Aspartame	Consumers with phenylketonuria	"Contains a source of phenylalanine"
Caffeine (>150 m/L)	Children, pregnant women, those sensitive to caffeine	"Not suitable for children, pregnant women and persons sensitive to caffeine"
Licorice	All; consumers with hypertension	"Contains licorice"
Polyols (>10%)	All	"Excess consumption may cause a laxative effect"
Raw milk	All	"This milk has not been heat-treated and may therefore contain organisms harmful to health"
Skimmed milk	Infants	Wording not fixed but must state that the product is not suitable for infant feeding

[a]*From FSAI*[114]*; FSA.*[115]

from the results of polymerase chain reaction monitoring of viral RNA led to concerns about foodborne transmission and of transmission via contaminated food packaging.[128] As the worldwide number of cases continued to grow, China imposed additional controls in September 2020 on imported food, mandating PCR testing of swabs of imported food packaging[129] The United States shared its concerns with the World Trade Organisation in November 2020, asserting that such measures were unjustified and lacking scientific support.[130] Such food control challenges highlight the dangers of using hazard-based safety management alone during an international health crisis. Hazard-based approaches are easy to perform and implement but can lead to unjustified (nontariff) barriers to trade, generate avoidable food waste, and ultimately may have no impact on public health. Testing for the presence of hazards (e.g., presence of viral RNA) may be of great value but needs to be informed by information on risk.[131] The principles of HACCP/HARPC emphasize the importance of not relying on finished product testing to protect public health, but of ensuring the operation of validated preventive measures providing assurance that those measures continue to work. The FAO/WHO[132] guide on dealing with food safety emergencies highlights the value of applying the same risk analysis process in emergencies and in routine operations, the value of having suitable procedures in place in advance, and, when hazards are not fully identified, the value of using scientifically guided surrogate hazard data.

63.11 Future challenges and opportunities

In highlighting the limitations of hazard-based approaches in risk communication, it is easy to assume that the solution is to provide more quantitative risk data. Generally, the public response to risk communication is improved when communicated visually and when it is personalized. The role of social media in risk communication is predicted to grow.[133] This has been clearly illustrated during the COVID-19 pandemic. While news and social media play a role in informing populations about risks to human health, they can also have a numbing or desensitizing effect.[134] People now tend to have a limited understanding of complex issues and lean heavily on their community of knowledge as a basis for their beliefs. To be successful, attempts to improve science literacy must instill change in the community of knowledge or associate the learner with a different community.[135] Science and risk literacy is a social as well as an educational process. The pandemic has helped the public to understand that science is constantly evolving and is always associated with uncertainty.[136] There is a case to reexplore the recommendations of the UK Bodmer Report[137] in the light of the science and antiscience response to the COVID-19 pandemic. Food risk analysis will need to respond strongly as society faces the challenges of creating safer, more sustainable more healthy food systems.

Culture and language are important considerations in tackling the challenge of public understanding. Scientists are quite comfortable bringing uncertainty into discussions. It underlines the nature of scientific thinking after Karl Popper that science is always ready to evolve to a better explanation of the natural world when new data emerge. However, to the nonscientist, uncertainty can constitute a reason to dismiss scientific opinion or an argument to wait for more clarity. The challenge of public distrust has been widely discussed in the context of risk analysis. There is an opportunity to better understand the origins of public distrust and develop novel ways of addressing mismatches between expert opinion and public expectations.[138]

There are particular challenges associated with the risk assessment and public understanding of the risks associated with chemical mixtures.[139] As mentioned above, various tools are being developed to combine hazard- and risk-based approaches to deal with mixtures. As food is a complex mixture, such approaches should be compatible with the safety assessment of whole foods. There is an opportunity to combine experimental toxicity data with epidemiology data.[140]

Ord[141] advocated a portfolio approach for dealing with existential risks highlighting the challenge of managing multiple concurrent risks with limited resources. Though not as high on the risk scale, food risks would benefit from more portfolio thinking whereby limited resources necessitate trade-offs between the value of addressing a risk, the tractability of the problem (a measure of how easy it is to solve the problem), and the degree to which so-called "neglectedness" of a topic (the degree to which resources have been spent on a problem; the idea being that after a while marginal resources would be better spent on a different risk). The ideal global portfolio allocates resources to each risk in proportion to its contribution to the total risk. This notion is applicable to many food-related risks.

The pandemic has led to calls for more horizon scanning and foresight analysis to enable better preparation for possible high-impact events.[119] Horizon scanning applied to food systems can support better planning for dealing with new hazards in foods or new evidence or changing exposure to known hazards.[142]

Risk assessment generally does not analyze the risks associated with managerial or organizational performance in the risk analysis process. As human behavior and organizational factors play an important role in risk management, there is a strong case to incorporate an analysis of such factors as part of risk assessment.[138]

63.12 Conclusions and recommendations

Can the differences in hazard-based approaches for microbiological risk and putative chemical risks based on risk assessment be rationalized for public understanding? The answer is that better public understanding is both possible and necessary. The following prerequisites and steps may support that goal:

1. Transparency and consistency of guidelines, assessments, and data will continue to be a prerequisite without which there can be no public trust regardless of the level of public understanding.
2. The lessons learnt during the pandemic in many countries underscore the urgency of progress in the area of public understanding of science and risk literacy. Measures to improve understanding should ideally start at primary school level and continue through the entire education system.
3. The communication of allergen hazards could be improved if consensus were achieved on appropriate risk-based thresholds for labeling nonintentional (incidental) allergen presence in association with appropriate hazard management standards.
4. Infectious disease surveillance has advanced recently in all regions of the world. Better use of surveillance data in the identification of food microbiology hazards will support better targeting of hazards, better risk assessments and regulatory limits, and better public understanding/acceptance of regulatory measures.
5. Hazard identification and characterization tools are proliferating. There is a need for better standards and guidance for hazard identification and tools and guidance for comparing risks and hazards in foods. More work is needed to support the use of (Q)SAR models in regulatory decision making.
6. It is challenging to use inference from one data source alone to construct a basis for risk management. When several methodologies are combined, it can improve the quality of the risk assessment and also improve public understanding and confidence, especially when a complex methodology is employed. Guidance on combining different approaches (including method and evidence triangulation) would support scientifically valid and consistent ways of working.
7. There is an opportunity to harmonize genotoxic and carcinogenic hazard identification and definition (to better define what positive and negative results mean). This would improve regulatory consistency and support public understanding of expert opinions.
8. An ALARA approach is used for many contaminants. It would help regulators and support public understanding and acceptance if better technical guidance were available on the application of ALARA.

Endnotes

[a]Kahneman[3] described two modes of thinking, labeled System 1 and System 2. System 1 refers to automatic, rapid thinking with little effort or mental cost. System 2, on the other hand, describes processes demanding considerable mental effort and complex computations. By definition, it has a mental cost and is not instantaneous or automatic. Of particular relevance to the present discussion is the observation from many psychology studies that people who are simultaneously challenged by a demanding cognitive problem and the temptation to accept a simple heuristic tend to yield to the latter. Of more importance is that the division of labor between the two systems is highly efficient. System 2 can help if the cognitive challenge becomes too great for System 1. However, System 2 may also erroneously accept the "intuitive" conclusion of System 1. This is critical since when people believe a conclusion to be true, they are also likely to believe the arguments supporting it. We can thus be blind to our blindness. Jumping to conclusions saves time and mental energy.[3]

References

1. Anderson C. Cholera epidemic traced to risk miscalculation. *Nature.* 1991;354:255. Available from: https://doi.org/10.1038/354255a0.
2. Pendygraft GW, Schlegel FE, Huston MJ. Organics in drinking water: a health perspective. *J Am Water Works Assoc.* 1979;71:118–126. Available from: https://www.jstor.org/stable/41269698.
3. Kahneman D. *Thinking Fast and Slow.* London: Penguin Random House; 2012.
4. Human and ecological risk assessment. In: Paustenbach DJ, ed. *Theory and Practice.* New York: Wiley; 2002.
5. Wu F, Rodricks JV. Forty years of food safety risk assessment: a history and analysis. *Risk Anal.* 2020;40:2218–2230. Available from: https://doi.org/10.1111/risa.13624.
6. Whiting RC. What risk assessments can tell us about setting criteria. *Food Control.* 2011;22:1525–1528. Available from: https://doi.org/10.1016/j.foodcont.2010.07.011.
7. US FDA. Current good manufacturing practice, hazard analysis, and risk-based preventive controls for human. *Food Fed Reg.* 2015;80:55907–56168.
8. IFST (Institute of Food Science and Technology). *Food & Drink Good Manufacturing Practice. A Guide to Its Responsible Management.* 7th ed. Chichester: Wiley; 2018.
9. Lanzoni A, Castoldi AF, Kass GEN, et al. Advancing human health risk assessment. *EFSA J.* 2019;17:1–21. Available from: https://doi.org/10.2903/j.efsa.2019.e170712.
10. IFST (Institute of Food Science and Technology). *Handbook of Microbiological Criteria for Foods.* London: Institute of Food Science & Technology; 2020.
11. FAO. *Understanding Codex.* 5th ed. Rome: Food & Agriculture Organisation of the United Nations; 2018. Available from: http://www.fao.org/3/CA1176EN/ca1176en.pdf.
12. FAO/WHO. Microbiological Risk Assessment. Guidance for Food. In: *Microbiological Risk Assessment Series 36.* Rome: Food and Agriculture Organisation of the United Nations; 2021.
13. Cox T, Lowrie K. From the Editors. *Risk Anal.* 2020;40:657–659. Available from: https://doi.org/10.1111/risa.13490.
14. Furedi F. *Culture of Fear.* London: Continuum Books; 2002.
15. Slovic P. Trust, emotion, sex, politics, and science: surveying the risk-assessment battlefield. *Risk Anal.* 1999;19:689–700.
16. Slovic P. Risk perception and risk analysis in a hyperpartisan and virtuously violent world. *Risk Anal.* 2020;40:2231–2239.
17. Hartmann C, Hübner P, Siegrist M. A risk perception gap? Comparing expert, producer and consumer prioritization of food hazard controls. *Food Chem Toxicol.* 2018;116:100–107. Available from: https://doi.org/10.1016/j.fct.2018.04.006.
18. Lofstedt R. Risk communication and the FSA: the food colourings case. *J Risk Res.* 2009;12:537–557. Available from: https://doi.org/10.1080/13669870903132695.
19. Saleh R, Bearth A, Siegrist M. How chemophobia affects public acceptance of pesticide use and biotechnology in agriculture. *Food Qual Prefer.* 2021;91:104197. Available from: https://doi.org/10.1016/j.foodqual.2021.104197.
20. Meagher KD. Public perceptions of food-related risks: a cross-national investigation of individual and contextual influences. *J Risk Res.* 2019;22:919–935. Available from: https://doi.org/10.1080/13669877.2017.1422789.
21. Bidlack WR, Birt D, Borzelleca J, et al. Expert report: making decisions about the risks of chemicals in foods with limited scientific information: an IFT expert report funded by the IFT foundation. *Compr Rev Food Sci Food Saf.* 2009;8:269–303. Available from: https://doi.org/10.1111/j.1541-4337.2009.00081.x.
22. Lloyds Register Foundation. Foresight review of the future of regulatory systems. Regulating in a disruptive world. <http://www.lrfoundation.org.uk>; 2021.
23. Slovic P, Finucane ML, Peters E, MacGregor DG. Risk as analysis and risk as feelings: some thoughts about affect, reason, risk, and rationality. *Risk Anal.* 2004;24:311–322.
24. Renn O, Siovic P, Burns WJ, Kasperson JX, Kasperson RE. Social amplification theory: theoretical foundations and empirical applications. *J Soc Issues.* 1992;48:127–160.
25. Ruzza M, Tiozzo B, Rizzoli V, Giaretta M, D'Este L, Ravarotto L. Food risks on the web: analysis of the 2017 Fipronil alert in the Italian online information sources. *Risk Anal.* 2020;40:2071–2092.
26. Shaw IC. *Food safety. The Science of Keeping Food Safe.* 2nd ed. Chichester: Wiley-Blackwell; 2018.
27. EFSA BIOHAZ Panel. (EFSA Panel on Biological Hazards), scientific opinion on the public health risks associated with food-borne parasites. *EFSA J.* 2018;16(12):5495, 113 pp. Available from: https://doi.org/10.2903/j.efsa.2018.5495.
28. Gajadhar AA, Pozio E, Ray Gamble H, et al. Trichinella diagnostics and control: mandatory and best practices for ensuring food safety. *Vet Parasitol.* 2009;159:197–205. Available from: https://doi.org/10.1016/j.vetpar.2008.10.063.
29. Schlech WF, Lavigne PM, Bortolussi RA, et al. Epidemic listeriosis—evidence for transmission by food. *N Engl J Med.* 1983;308:203–206.
30. Candel-Pérez C, Ros-Berruezo G, Martínez-Graciá C. A review of *Clostridioides [Clostridium] difficile* occurrence through the food chain. *Food Microbiol.* 2019;77:118–129. Available from: https://doi.org/10.1016/j.fm.2018.08.012.
31. EFSA BIOHAZ Panel. (EFSA Panel on Biological Hazards), scientific opinion on the public health risks associated with hepatitis E virus (HEV) as a food-borne pathogen. *EFSA J.* 2017;15(7):4886. Available from: https://doi.org/10.2903/j.efsa.2017.4886. 89 pp.
32. Bennett SD, Sodha SV, Ayers TL, Lynch MF, Gould LH, Tauxe RV. Produce-associated foodborne disease outbreaks, USA, 1998–2013. *Epidemiol Infect.* 2018;146:1397–1406. Available from: https://doi.org/10.1017/S0950268818001620.
33. Kovarich S, Ceriani L, Ciacci A, et al. *OpenFoodTox: EFSA's Chemical Hazards Database (Version 3) [Data set].* Zenodo; 2020. https://doi.org/10.5281/zenodo.3693783.
34. Gross L, Birnbaum LS. Regulating toxic chemicals for public and environmental health. *PLoS Biol.* 2017;15:2–4. Available from: https://doi.org/10.1371/journal.pbio.2004814.
35. US National Academy of Sciences. *Using 21st Century Science to Improve Risk-Related Evaluations.* Washington, DC: The National Academies Press; 2017. Available from: http://nap.edu/24635.
36. EC Regulation 1907/2006 of the European Parliament and of the Council of 18 December 2006 concerning the Registration, Evaluation, Authorisation and Restriction of Chemicals (REACH),

establishing a European Chemicals Agency, amending Directive 1999/45/EC and repealing Council Regulation (EEC) No 793/93 and Commission Regulation (EC) No 1488/94 as well as Council Directive 76/769/EEC and Commission Directives 91/155/EEC, 93/67/EEC, 93/105/EC and 2000/21/EC.

37. US House of Representatives. Frank R. Lautenberg chemical safety for the 21st century act, <https://www.congress.gov/114/plaws/publ182/PLAW-114publ182.pdf>; 2016.

38. Barlow SM, Boobis AR, Bridges J, et al. The role of hazard- and risk-based approaches in ensuring food safety. *Trends Food Sci Technol.* 2015;46:176–188. Available from: https://doi.org/10.1016/j.tifs.2015.10.007.

39. EC/1881. *Commission Regulation Setting Maximum Levels for Certain Contaminants in Foodstuffs*; 2006.

40. EFSA. Scientific opinion on genotoxicity testing strategies applicable to food and feed safety assessment. *EFSA J.* 2011;9(9):2379. Available from: https://doi.org/10.2903/j.efsa.2011.2379.

41. Schrenk DS. What is the meaning of 'A compound is carcinogenic'? *Toxicol Rep.* 2018;5:504–511. Available from: https://doi.org/10.1016/j.toxrep.2018.04.002.

42. Beausoleil C, Pasquier E, Rousselle C, Michel C. Editorial. Special issue: is BPA an ED? *Mol Cell Endocrinol.* 2018;475:4–9.

43. Baker ME, Lathe R. The promiscuous estrogen receptor: evolution of physiological estrogens and response to phytochemicals and endocrine disruptors. *J Steroid Biochem Mol Biol.* 2018;184:29–37. Available from: https://doi.org/10.1016/j.jsbmb.2018.07.001.

44. Bergman A, Jobling S, Heindel JJ, Kidd K, Zoeller RT, eds. *State-of-the-Science of Endocrine Disrupting Chemicals 2012*. United Nations Environment Programme; 2012.

45. La Merrill MA, Vandenberg LN, Smith MT, et al. Consensus on the key characteristics of endocrine-disrupting chemicals as a basis for hazard identification. *Nat Rev Endocrinol.* 2020;16:45–57. Available from: https://doi.org/10.1038/s41574-019-0273-8.

46. Ebel ED, Williams MS. When are qualitative testing results sufficient to predict a reduction in illnesses in a microbiological food safety risk assessment? *J Food Prot.* 2015;78:1451–1460. Available from: https://doi.org/10.4315/0362-028X.JFP-15-042.

47. Pearce N, Vandenbroucke JP, Lawlor DA. Causal inference in environmental epidemiology: old and new approaches. *Epidemiology.* 2019;30:311–316.

48. Gerner-Smidt P, Besser J, Concepción-Acevedo J, et al. Whole genome sequencing: bridging one-health surveillance of foodborne diseases. *Front Public Heal.* 2019;7:1–11. Available from: https://doi.org/10.3389/fpubh.2019.00172.

49. Chen Y, Burall LS, Macarisin D, et al. Prevalence and level of *Listeria monocytogenes* in ice cream linked to a listeriosis outbreak in the United States. *J Food Prot.* 2016;79:1828–1832. Available from: https://doi.org/10.4315/0362-028X.JFP-16-208.

50. Manning L, Luning PA, Wallace CA. The evolution and cultural framing of food safety management systems—where from and where next? *Compr Rev Food Sci Food Saf.* 2019;18:1770–1792. Available from: https://doi.org/10.1111/1541-4337.12484.

51. EFSA. Draft guidance document on scientific criteria for grouping chemicals into assessment groups for human risk assessment of combined exposure to multiple chemicals. <https://connect.efsa.europa.eu/RM/s/publicconsultation/a0c1v00000HnXIB/pc0014>; 2021.

52. Koster S, Bani-Estivals MH, Bonuomo M, et al. *Guidance of Best Practices on the Risk Assessment of NIAS in Food Contact Materials and Articles*. ILSI Europe; 2015.

53. Severin I, Souton E, Dahbi L, Chagnon MC. Use of bioassays to assess hazard of food contact material extracts: state of the art. *Food Chem Toxicol.* 2017;105:429–447. Available from: https://doi.org/10.1016/j.fct.2017.04.046.

54. Van Bossuyt M, Van Hoeck E, Vanhaecke T, Rogiers V, Mertens B. Prioritizing substances of genotoxic concern for in-depth safety evaluation using non-animal approaches: the example of food contact materials. *ALTEX—Altern Anim Exp.* 2019;36(2):215–230. Available from: https://doi.org/10.14573/altex.1810011.

55. Motarjemi Y. Human factors in food safety management. In: Motarjemi Y, Lelieveld H, eds. *Food Safety Management. A Practical Guide for the Food Industry*. London: Academic Press; 2014:975–986.

56. de Boer A. Scientific assessments in European food law: making it future-proof. *Regul Toxicol Pharmacol.* 2019;108. Available from: https://doi.org/10.1016/j.yrtph.2019.104437.

57. FAO/WHO. *Food Safety Risk Analysis. A Guide for National Food Safety Authorities. Paper 87.* Rome: Food and Agriculture Organisation of the United Nations; 2006.

58. Tennant DR, Bruyninckx C. The potential application of European market research data in dietary exposure modelling of food additives. *Food Addit Contam.* 2017;35:412–424. Available from: https://doi.org/10.1080/19440049.2017.1400187.

59. Deluyker H. Is scientific assessment a scientific discipline? *EFSA J.* 2017;15. Available from: https://doi.org/10.2903/j.efsa.2017.e15111.

60. MacGillivray BH. Null hypothesis testing ≠ scientific inference: a critique of the shaky premise at the heart of the science and values debate, and a defense of value-neutral risk assessment. *Risk Anal.* 2019;39:1520–1532. Available from: https://doi.org/10.1111/risa.13284.

61. Crump K. The potential effect of recall bias and selection bias on the epidemiological evidence for the carcinogenicity of glyphosate. *Risk Anal.* 2020;40:696–704.

62. Calderon RL. Measuring risks in humans: the promise and practice of epidemiology. *Food Chem Toxicol.* 2000;38:59–63. Available from: https://doi.org/10.1016/s0278-6915(99)00134-9.

63. Blaauboer BJ, Boekelheide K, Clewell HJ, et al. The use of biomarkers of toxicity for integrating in vitro hazard estimates into risk assessment for humans. *ALTEX.* 2012;29:411–425. Available from: https://doi.org/10.14573/altex.2012.4.411.

64. Vidry S, Hoekstra J, Hart A, et al. Benefit-risk analysis for foods (BRAFO) – executive project summary. *Eur J Nutr Food Saf.* 2013;3:146–153.

65. Bouvard V, Loomis D, Guyton KZ, Grosse Y, El Ghissassi F, et al. Carcinogenicity of consumption of red and processed meat. *Lancet Oncol.* 2015;16(16):599–1600. Available from: https://doi.org/10.1016/S1470-2045(15)00444-1.

66. IARC (International Agency for Research on Cancer). *Red Meat and Processed Meat, IARC Monographs*. Lyons: IARC; 2018.

67. Knuppel A, Papier K, Fensom GK, et al. Meat intake and cancer risk: prospective analyses in UK Biobank. *Int J Epidemiol.* 2020;49:1540–1552. Available from: https://doi.org/10.1093/ije/dyaa142.

68. Le NT, Silva Michels FA, Song M, et al. A prospective analysis of meat mutagens and colorectal cancer in the Nurses' Health Study

and Health Professionals Follow-up Study. *Environ Health Perspect*. 2016;124:1529–1536. Available from: https://doi.org/10.1289/EHP238.

69. Abu-Ghazaleh N, Chua WJ, Gopalan V. Intestinal microbiota and its association with colon cancer and red/processed meat consumption. *J Gastroenterol Hepatol*. 2021;36:75–88. Available from: https://doi.org/10.1111/jgh.15042.
70. Sneyd MJ, Cox B. Do low-fat foods alter risk of colorectal cancer from processed meat? *Public Health*. 2020;183:138–145. Available from: https://doi.org/10.1016/j.puhe.2020.03.026.
71. Hur SJ, Yoon Y, Jo C, Jeong JY, Lee KT. Effect of dietary red meat on colorectal cancer risk—a review. *Compr Rev Food Sci Food Saf*. 2019;18:1812–1824. Available from: https://doi.org/10.1111/1541-4337.12501.
72. Turner ND, Lloyd SK. Association between red meat consumption and colon cancer: a systematic review of experimental results. *Exp Biol Med*. 2017;242:813–839. Available from: https://doi.org/10.1177/1535370217693117.
73. Kruger C, Zhou Y. Red meat and colon cancer: a review of mechanistic evidence for heme in the context of risk assessment methodology. *Food Chem Toxicol*. 2018;118:131–153. Available from: https://doi.org/10.1016/j.fct.2018.04.048.
74. Aloisi CMN, Sandell ES, Sturla SJ. A chemical link between meat consumption and colorectal cancer development? *Chem Res Toxicol*. 2021;34:12–23. Available from: https://doi.org/10.1021/acs.chemrestox.0c00395.
75. Kobets T, Iatropoulos MJ, Williams GM. Mechanisms of DNA-reactive and epigenetic chemical carcinogens: applications to carcinogenicity testing and risk assessment. *Toxicol Res*. 2019;8:123–145.
76. EC/865. *Commission Decision of 10 November 2008 Concerning the Non-Inclusion of Chlorate in Annex I to Council Directive 91/414/EEC and the Withdrawal of Authorisations for Plant Protection Products Containing That Substance*; 2008.
77. Panseri S, Nobile M, Arioli F, Biolatti C, Pavlovic R, Chiesa LM. Occurrence of perchlorate, chlorate and polar herbicides in different baby food commodities. *Food Chem*. 2020;330:127205. Available from: https://doi.org/10.1016/j.foodchem.2020.127205.
78. ACMSF (Advisory Committee on the Microbial Safety of Food). *Food Safety-Maximum Safety Levels of Chlorate in Foods*. Food Standards Agency, UK; 2019. https://acmsf.food.gov.uk/sites/default/files/acm-1306-mrls-for-chlorate-in-food_0.pdf.
79. EFSA CONTAM Panel. (EFSA Panel on Contaminants in the Food Chain), scientific opinion on risks for public health related to the presence of chlorate in food. *EFSA J*. 2015;13(6):4135. Available from: https://doi.org/10.2903/j.efsa.2015.4135. 103 pp.
80. Tareke E, Rydberg P, Karlsson P, Eriksson S, Törnqvist M. Analysis of acrylamide, a carcinogen formed in heated foodstuffs. *J Agric Food Chem*. 2002;50:4998–5006. Available from: https://doi.org/10.1021/jf020302f.
81. EFSA. Scientific opinion on the applicability of the margin of exposure approach for the safety assessment of impurities which are both genotoxic and carcinogenic in substances added to food/feed. *EFSA J*. 2012;10:2578. Available from: https://doi.org/10.2903/j.efsa.2012.2578.
82. Devlin, H. How burnt toast and roast potatoes became linked to cancer. *The Guardian*. January 27, 2017. https://amp.theguardian.com/science/2017/jan/27/how-burnt-toast-became-linked-to-cancer-acrylamide.
83. Powers SJ, Mottram DS, Curtis A, Halford NG. Progress on reducing acrylamide levels in potato crisps in Europe, 2002 to 2019. *Food Addit Contam – Part A Chem Anal Control Expo Risk Assess*. 2021;. Available from: https://doi.org/10.1080/19440049.2020.1871083.
84. Newsome R, Tran N, Paoli GM, et al. Development of a risk-ranking framework to evaluate potential high-threat microorganisms, toxins, and chemicals in food. *J Food Sci*. 2009;74. Available from: https://doi.org/10.1111/j.1750-3841.2008.01042.x.
85. Low F, Lin H-M, Gerrard JA, Cressey PJ, Shaw IC. Ranking the risk of pesticide dietary intake. *Pest Manag Sci*. 2004;60:842–848.
86. Langerholc T, Lindqvist R, Sand S. Risk ranking of chemical and microbiological hazards in food. *EFSA J*. 2018;16:1–9. Available from: https://doi.org/10.2903/j.efsa.2018.e160813.
87. Lindqvist R, Langerholc T, Ranta J, Hirvonen T, Sand S. A common approach for ranking of microbiological and chemical hazards in foods based on risk assessment – useful but is it possible? *Crit Rev Food Sci Nutr*. 2020;60:3461–3474. Available from: https://doi.org/10.1080/10408398.2019.1693957.
88. Ames BN, Magaw R, Gold LS. Ranking possible carcinogenic hazards. *Science*. 1987;236:271–280.
89. Tomatis L, Melnick RL, Haseman J, Barrett JC, Huff J. Alleged 'misconceptions' distort perceptions of environmental cancer risks. *FASEB J*. 2001;15:195–203.
90. Slob W. Benchmark dose and the three Rs. Part I. Getting more information from the same number of animals. *Crit Rev Toxicol*. 2014;44:557–567. Available from: https://doi.org/10.3109/10408444.2014.925423.
91. O'Brien J, Renwick AG, Constable A, et al. Approaches to the risk assessment of genotoxic carcinogens in food: a critical appraisal. *Food Chem Toxicol*. 2006;44:1613–1635. Available from: https://doi.org/10.1016/j.fct.2006.07.004.
92. Jensen SM, Kluxen FM, Ritz C. A review of recent advances in benchmark dose methodology. *Risk Anal*. 2019;39:2295–2315. Available from: https://doi.org/10.1111/risa.13324.
93. United Nations. Globally harmonized system of classification and labelling of chemicals (GHS). <https://doi.org/10.14927/reeps.10.2_60>; 2017.
94. EC Regulation 1272/2008 of the European Parliament and of the Council of 16 December 2008 on classification, labelling and packaging of substances and mixtures, amending and repealing Directives 67/548/EEC and 1999/45/EC, and amending Regulation (EC) No 1907/2006.
95. Houben G, Burney P, Chan CH, et al. Prioritisation of allergenic foods with respect to public health relevance. Report from an ILSI Europe Food Allergy Task Force Expert Group. *Food Chem Toxicol*. 2016;89:8–18. Available from: https://doi.org/10.1016/j.fct.2015.12.028.
96. EU Regulation 1169/2011 of the European Parliament and of the Council of 25 October 2011 on the provision of food information to consumers, amending Regulations (EC) No 1924/2006 and (EC) No 1925/2006 of the European Parliament and of the Council, and

repealing Commission Directive 87/250/EEC, Council Directive 90/496/EEC, Commission Directive 1999/10/EC, Directive 2000/13/EC of the European Parliament and of the Council, Commission Directives 2002/67/EC and 2008/5/EC and Commission Regulation (EC) No 608/2004.

97. Shoji M, Adachi R, Akiyama H. Japanese food allergen labeling regulation: An update. *J AOAC Int.* 2018;101:8–13. Available from: https://doi.org/10.5740/jaoacint.17-0389.

98. US House of Representatives. Food Allergen Labelling and Consumer Protection Act of 2004, <https://www.fda.gov/media/77570/download>; 2004

99. Taylor SL, Baumert JL, Kruizinga AG, et al. Establishment of reference doses for residues of allergenic foods: report of the VITAL Expert Panel. *Food Chem Toxicol.* 2014;63:9–17. Available from: https://doi.org/10.1016/j.fct.2013.10.032.

100. Marchisotto MJ, Harada L, Kamdar O, et al. Food allergen labeling and purchasing habits in the United States and Canada. *J Allergy Clin Immunol Pract.* 2017;5:345–351.

101. Remington BC, Baumert JL, Blom WM, Houben GF, Taylor SL, Kruizinga AG. Unintended allergens in precautionary labelled and unlabelled products pose significant risks to UK allergic consumers. *Allergy Eur J Allergy Clin Immunol.* 2015;70:813–819. Available from: https://doi.org/10.1111/all.12625.

102. Pele M, Brohée M, Anklam E, Van Hengel AJ. Peanut and hazelnut traces in cookies and chocolates: relationship between analytical results and declaration of food allergens on product labels. *Food Addit Contam.* 2007;24:1334–1344. Available from: https://doi.org/10.1080/02652030701458113.

103. State of California. The Proposition 65 list. <https://oehha.ca.gov/proposition-65/proposition-65-list/>; 2021.

104. Robinson LA, Viscusi WK, Zeckhauser R. Efficient warnings, not "wolf" or "puppy" warnings. In: Kunreuther H, Meyer RJ, Michel-Kerjan EO, eds. *The Future of Risk Management.* University of Pennsylvania Press; 2019:227–248.

105. Linnekin BJ. The "California Effect" and the future of American food: how California's growing crackdown on food and agriculture harms the state and the nation. *Chapman Law Rev.* 2010;13(2):357–389.

106. Marlow ML. Too much questionable information?. *Regulation. Winter* 2013–2014. 2013;20–28.

107. Viscusi WK. Predicting the effects of food cancer risk warnings on consumers. *Food Drug Cosmetic Law J.* 1988;43(2):283–307.

108. McCann D, Barrett A, Cooper A, et al. Food additives and hyperactive behaviour in 3-year-old and 8/9-year-old children in the community: a randomised, double-blinded, placebo-controlled trial. *Lancet.* 2007;370:1560–1567.

109. EFSA. EFSA updates safety advice on six food colours. <https://www.efsa.europa.eu/en/press/news/091112>; 2009.

110. Bearth A, Cousin ME, Siegrist M. The consumer's perception of artificial food additives: influences on acceptance, risk and benefit perceptions. *Food Qual Prefer.* 2014;38:14–23. Available from: https://doi.org/10.1016/j.foodqual.2014.05.008.

111. Scotter MJ. Emerging and persistent issues with artificial food colours: natural colour additives as alternatives to synthetic colours in food and drink. *Qual Assur Saf Crops Food.* 2011;3:28–39.

112. Lehtoa S, Buchweitzb M, Klimmb A, Straßburgerb R, Bechtolda C, Ulbertha F. Comparison of food colour regulations in the EU and the US: a review of current provisions. *Food Addit Contam, A.* 2017;34:335–355.

113. Van Gunst A, Roodenburg AJC. Consumer distrust about E-numbers: a qualitative study among food experts. *Foods.* 2019;. Available from: https://doi.org/10.3390/foods8050178.

114. FSAI. Food information on pre-packed foods. <https://www.fsai.ie/publications_labelling_FIC/>; 2014.

115. FSA. Food labelling: giving food information to consumers. <https://www.gov.uk/guidance/food-labelling-giving-food-information-to-consumers#tell-the-consumer-about-certain-ingredients>; 2017.

116. Aureli P, Franciosa G, Fenicia L. Infant botulism and honey in Europe: a commentary. *Pediatr Inf Dis J.* 2002;21:866–868.

117. Reyes M, Garmendia ML, Olivares S, Aqueveque C, Zacarías I, Corvalán C. Development of the Chilean front-of-package food warning label. *BMC Public Health.* 2019;19:1–11. Available from: https://doi.org/10.1186/s12889-019-7118-1.

118. Haas C. Coronavirus and risk analysis. *Risk Anal.* 2020;40:660–661. Available from: https://doi.org/10.1111/risa.13481.

119. Collins A, Florin MV, Renn O. COVID-19 risk governance: drivers, responses and lessons to be learned. *J Risk Res.* 2020;23:1073–1082. Available from: https://doi.org/10.1080/13669877.2020.1760332.

120. Randazzo W, Cuevas-Ferrando E, Sanjuán R, Domingo-Calap P, Sánchez G. Metropolitan wastewater analysis for COVID-19 epidemiological surveillance. *Int J Hyg Environ Health.* 2020;. Available from: https://doi.org/10.1016/j.ijheh.2020.113621.

121. Westhaus S, Weber FA, Schiwy S, et al. Detection of SARS-CoV-2 in raw and treated wastewater in Germany – suitability for COVID-19 surveillance and potential transmission risks. *Sci Total Environ.* 2021;751:141750. Available from: https://doi.org/10.1016/j.scitotenv.2020.141750.

122. Lapolla P, Lee R, Mingoli A. Wastewater as a red flag in Covid-19 spread. *Public Health.* 2020;185:26.

123. Yanagimoto K, Yamagami T, Uematsu K, Haramoto E. Characterization of *Salmonella* isolates from wastewater treatment plant influents to estimate unreported cases and infection sources of salmonellosis. *Pathogens.* 2020;. Available from: https://doi.org/10.3390/pathogens9010052.

124. Choi PM, Tscharke B, Samanipour S, et al. Social, demographic, and economic correlates of food and chemical consumption measured by wastewater-based epidemiology. *Proc Natl Acad Sci USA.* 2019;116:21864–21873. Available from: https://doi.org/10.1073/pnas.1910242116.

125. FSA. Qualitative risk assessment: what is the risk of food or food contact materials and surfaces being a source or transmission route of SARS-CoV-2 for UK consumers?. <https://www.food.gov.uk/sites/default/files/media/document/qualitative-risk-assessment-covid-19-v.2.2.pdf>; 2020.

126. ICMSF. ICMSF opinion on SARS-CoV-2 and its relationship to food safety. <https://www.icmsf.org/wp-content/uploads/2020/09/ICMSF2020-Letterhead-COVID-19-opinion-final-03-Sept-2020.BF_.pdf>; 2020.

127. Lacombe A, Quintela I, Liao Yt, Wu VCH. Food safety lessons learned from the COVID-19 pandemic. *J Food Saf.* 2020;41. Available from: https://doi.org/10.1111/jfs.12878.

128. Pang X, Ren L, Wu S, et al. Cold-chain food contamination as the possible origin of COVID-19 resurgence in Beijing. *Natl Sci Rev.* 2020;7:1861–1864.

129. WTO. Committee on sanitary and phytosanitary measures, document G/SPS/N/CHN/1173, 21 September 2020, notification of emergency

measures. <https://docs.wto.org/dol2fe/Pages/SS/directdoc.aspx?filename = q:/G/SPS/NCHN1173.pdf&Open = True>; 2020a.

130. WTO. Committee on sanitary and phytosanitary measures, document G/SPS/GEN/1863, 18 November 2020, China's Covid-19 related trade actions against food and agricultural products – new specific trade concern, Submission by the United States of America. <http://www.wto.org>; 2020b.

131. Dyani L. *COVID-19 rarely spreads through surfaces. So why are we still deep cleaning? Nature.* 590. 202126–28.

132. FAO/WHO. *FAO/WHO Guide for Application of Risk Analysis Principles and Procedures During Food Safety Emergencies.* Rome: FAO; 2011.

133. UK Parliament. POSTnote 564. Communicating risk. <https://post.parliament.uk/research-briefings/post-pn-0564/>; 2017.

134. Bhatia S, Walasek L, Slovic P, Kinreuther H. The more who die, the less we care: evidence from natural language analysis of online news articles and social media posts. *Risk Anal.* 2021;41:179–203.

135. Sloman S, Fernabch P. *The knowledge illusion. Why We Never Think Alone.* New York: Riverhead Books; 2017.

136. Anon. How epidemiology has shaped the COVID pandemic. *Nature.* 2021;589:491–492. Available from: https://doi.org/10.1038/d41586-021-00183-z.

137. Royal Society. *The Public Understanding of Science.* London: The Royal Society; 1985. Available from: https://royalsociety.org/topics-policy/publications/1985/public-understanding-science/.

138. Goble R. Through a glass darkly: how natural science and technical communities looked at social science advances in understanding risk. *Risk Anal.* 2021;41:414–428.

139. Hernández AF, Tsatsakis AM. Human exposure to chemical mixtures: challenges for the integration of toxicology with epidemiology data in risk assessment. *Food Chem Toxicol.* 2017;103:188–193. Available from: https://doi.org/10.1016/j.fct.2017.03.012.

140. Bornehag CG, Kitraki E, Stamatakis A, et al. A novel approach to chemical mixture risk assessment—linking data from population-based epidemiology and experimental animal tests. *Risk Anal.* 2019;39:2259–2271. Available from: https://doi.org/10.1111/risa.13323.

141. Ord T. *The Precipice. Existential Risk and the Future of Humanity.* London: Bloomsbury Publishing; 2020.

142. IFST. *Horizon Scanning Report.* London: IFST; 2021. Available from: https://www.ifst.org/resources-policy/horizon-scanning-report.

Chapter 64

Communicating about risk in relation to food with the public and countering media alarmism

Katherine Rich[1] **and Gary Bowering**[2]

[1]New Zealand Food & Grocery Council, Wellington, New Zealand, [2]Independent Science Communicator, Wellington, New Zealand

Abstract

Trained food safety experts have a science-based understanding of the concepts of hazard, risk, and mitigation. Those same three words, however, are strongly emotion-based for most other people. It is this gulf that is used by news media, campaigners, and other interest groups to generate fear and outrage, whether well-meaning or otherwise. We examine the reasons for this difference and propose techniques and processes that food safety risk communicators can use to move audience and stakeholder publics towards mutual understanding and ideally into agreement. We present the "HOT" (honest, open, transparent) communications approach and underpin this with the "4Rs" (rapid, reliable, relevant, repeated) principles and look at how communicators can embrace effective storytelling in order to deliver desired health protection outcomes, whether they be preventing or limiting consumption to mitigate a hazard; or encouraging people to consume more of certain food groups so as to lower risk of poor health outcomes.

Keywords: Risk communication; risk perception; media reporting; journalism; food; misinformation

64.1 Introduction—"Everything's a risky hazard"

Everything appears to be killing us these days—from broccoli to burning incense, tannins in tea leaves to traveling on an airplane, wearing a bra and deodorant to having punk-style hair or sprinkling talcum powder. Sometimes we are just bombarded with so many of these Doomsday stories that it seems miraculous that any of us are still alive.

There is an increasing tendency for activists and columnists to argue there is a risk associated with a common object, then use that risk to create significant public concern and demand political change on the basis that people are worried. At a fundamental level, there is nothing wrong with this. Freedom to share one's views is a vital principle in a civilized society. Raising concerns is the cycle we followed when we rightly stopped using lead-based make-up and, more recently, asbestos insulation. Smoking tobacco is another, although one that is still an issue.

In these cases, science and public opinion were in agreement. However, in many other modern examples the science is misrepresented, misused, or ignored, to create anxiety. The level of risk is not put into any meaningful context and the dangers are exaggerated or even invented. The existence of a hazard and the perceived risk it poses are often poles apart.

When food health risks are being discussed, it is vital to be very precise. The correct use of science, statistics, and language is critical. Too often, discussions in the media and online fail even the simplest tests.

One of the most high-profile examples of this situation is Bisphenol A (BPA), a compound which was commonly used in plastic food packaging and utensils. We use the past tense because BPA has been phased out in most developed nations, including New Zealand.

BPA was widely used, with plenty of solid science saying it was safe. Then one report indicated it was a compound (usually pejoratively referred to as a "toxic chemical") which had the potential to increase the chance of cancer later in life. That story went right around the world and New Zealand got caught up in it.

Food Standards Australia New Zealand (FSANZ) attempted to dampen concerns by releasing its own dietary modeling. This showed that a 5 kg baby would have to drink around 80 bottles of formula a day every day for

Present Knowledge in Food Safety. DOI: https://doi.org/10.1016/B978-0-12-819470-6.00038-X

a lifetime before even approaching the safety limit. That is between 15 and 20 times more than a baby consumes each day. The infant would have to keep up this consumption for many years (into adulthood!) to have any measurable risk of cancer from BPA. It simply could not happen. Even if it could, the massive over-consumption of food would cause far more harm, far more quickly, than the tiny quantity of BPA that might be in it.

FSANZ concluded that BPA "does not pose a risk to public health for any age group," a position affirmed by additional research findings since. But that did not seem to matter in the slightest. Media reports continued to refer to "baby bottles with the potential to cause cancer." One of this chapter's authors, as a mother, knows that no parent will pay any attention to the word "potential" in that phrase. Companies will support the science to a point, before responding to the will of consumers as they start to shift their spending to goods that proclaim to be "free" of the chemical du jour.

What the media and activists failed to do with BPA was to explain the level of risk, which was minute. By creating and growing unfounded fear and anxiety, governments in Canada and several US states were pressured by campaigners into banning BPA even though their own food safety and health experts were adamant it was safe. Those bans were then used by activists in other countries, New Zealand included, to call for their governments to follow suit. The same reporters who helped create the initial story could then legitimately return to the story in light of these developments, claiming the status of consumer advocate. It is a circle, but hardly a virtuous one.

The irony is that BPA was phased out and replaced by plastics which had not been tested nearly as rigorously. In addition, the considerable supply chain costs of disposing of unwanted product and introducing new products and packaging were eventually recouped from consumers, whether through price increases, lower returns for shareholding investors, or other mechanisms.

Several experts also said the "cancer scare" took attention away from the much more important issues of informing parents and caregivers about the hygienic preparation of infant formula, correct care and storage of children's bottles, and feeding practices.

Those critical lessons, about more clear and present food safety hazards, risks and issues, were lost in the maelstrom.

Life is fundamentally a series of hazards with their associated risk. Everything we ever do as human beings has a certain element of risk involved. It could be argued that being alive is the single most dangerous activity in the world, and death is guaranteed. We all intuitively know this but seem to be more and more likely to suspend this mindset when confronted with the next food safety horror story, whether it is the breathless revelation of extremely low levels of arsenic in most of the drinking water; another celebrity swearing off deodorant because she believes it to cause cancer; or someone getting into "vampire facials" to promote skin renewal.

These stories and many others point to the real or perceived existence of a hazard while downplaying or even concealing the often extremely low level of the risk. Such an approach makes us more worried than we need be, often shifting focus and resource away from real issues. Disseminating such misinformation is rarely done by lying; more often by omitting key facts and context or framing the available science in a particular way.

The internet can be a useful tool. We use it extensively to communicate with friends and colleagues, and to gather information from around the world. It can also amplify groundless concerns and facilitate scaremongering, which generate genuine anxiety and fear for the public. The critical point is when science and public opinion diverge. Most people now do their research on the internet using Google's search engine, but Google Search measures a page's popularity—not its accuracy, and ranks results on that basis. With the readership of newspapers in decline over the last few decades, many younger citizens do not even search for news, relying instead on information which appears on their social media feeds be it Facebook, TikTok, Instagram or other channels.

When it comes to health hazards and risk, the science, statistics, and language are of paramount importance. Hazard and risk must be put into context. If the risks are significant, they need to be addressed. If the risks are negligible, we should put our efforts into other areas which might make a difference. This could include the ones that are known to delay the inevitable: promoting a healthy balanced lifestyle of hygienically prepared moderate diet; and getting enough exercise.

Time is a finite commodity. We should spend it on the risks that matter. In this chapter, we aim to provide concepts and tools to assist people involved with food safety issues to help their publics and consumers to do just that.

64.2 Risk communication

"Risk communication" is a phrase that is widely used. Unfortunately, it can be—and is—also interpreted broadly, leading to confusion, misperception, and abuse. This is especially so when it comes to communicating risk about food, particularly with public and nonexpert media and audiences. Here it is subject to, or can lead to, confusion of the terms hazard, risk and mitigation. Risk communication is also at the mercy of a general misunderstanding of concepts such as uncertainty and weight of robust science-based evidence.

The act of communication is itself subject to cognitive and belief factors that need special consideration. Although these apply to all communication, food is an area where these principles often assume most significance. Food has the obvious biological necessity for a healthy existence and, especially in countries where famine or extreme poverty remains, a worrying part of many peoples' daily lives. For those fortunate to have an adequate supply of food, cultural, societal, or religious factors often come into play when food assumes a ceremonial, cultural or other meaningful role. And all this is before mainstream and social media has entered the picture with their overriding goal of producing content that gathers eyeballs and/or generates clicks.

These issues, and more, are why the seemingly simple subject of "risk communication" often becomes complex while the communication process itself remains, as we will show, relatively uncomplicated.

For our purposes, the first step in navigating the complexity of food risk communication is defining what it is. The FAO/WHO's 2016 definition is useful:

Risk communication is the exchange of information and opinions concerning risk and risk-related factors among risk assessors, risk managers, consumers and other interested parties.[1]

This is a broad definition, especially with the inclusion of "risk-related factors" and "other interested parties," both of which can mean many things to many people. This does, however, allow for recognition of the importance of an individual's perceptions and biases, and the phenomenon of outrage, which we will address.

A key word in the FAO/WHO definition is "exchange." Risk communication is rarely effective without some understanding of existing perception, knowledge, beliefs, and motivations within society. It also requires feedback during and after the communication process to adjust and tailor messaging and measure effectiveness. This generally requires some form of active and ongoing dialog (hence the use of "exchange" in the definition), with the term covering a spectrum from, for example, consumer research to face-to-face meetings.

The FAO/WHO handbook (pp. 57–58) lists questions that are useful to have answered to guide food safety risk communication. A point we add to those made in the handbook is that having answers to these, and being able to explain how the answers were obtained, will assist with any media alarmism and provide a counterpoint to claims made by activists or other groups that it is only they that "understand" or "represent" the public or consumer. The questions are:

- What do the target audiences understand about this food safety risk?
- What misconceptions do they have?
- What do the target audiences want to know about this food safety risk?
- Do the target audiences consider the risk to be high or low?
- What are the target audiences' specific concerns and perceptions? For example, who do they perceive to be most vulnerable to the hazard?
- How do the target audiences prefer to receive information about food safety risks? Is it through scientists, NGOs, the media, or from an authoritative government official or spokesperson?
- What sources of information do the target audiences trust? Is it the media, scientists, food safety risk managers and communicators, or NGOs?
- Are the planned information sources and channels accessible to the target audiences?
- Who are the opinion leaders that are likely to influence the target audiences?

We would add to these an extra question that helps the risk communicator to understand the individual's or group's motivations:

- Why do they have the knowledge, beliefs, or concerns that they do?

In some cases, the answer to this extra question might be inferred from data gained from the FAO/WHO handbook questions listed earlier, much is likely to be conjecture. The link between risk perception and protection motivation is well known.[2] However, for the purposes of risk communication we usually need to create that perception in the first place or change an existing perception. Therefore it is important to know what may motivate a person or audience to form or change a risk perception of a hazard. Unfortunately, this is rarely straightforward.

In psychology there are many theories of motivation. These include Maslow's commonly quoted (and often overstated) 1943 Hierarchy of Needs[3] and a wide range of more modern models that cover drive, goal, emotion, personality, change, and happiness. This subject is beyond this chapter's scope. We mention it here to note that this is one area that helps create complexity noted at the outset. It also means that, while we recommend asking questions that will help you gain insight into motivation, we are unable to provide specific questions themselves – they need to be tailored to the context, time, place, and situation. For example, for an issue that affects manufactured baby food, the motivational questions you might explore are likely to be different to those for an issue that involves unpackaged fresh meat or produce consumed by adults.

Information about the audience(s) you are communicating with is just as important as information about the food safety hazard, risk, and mitigation itself. If you do not understand the person or people you are communicating with, and their motivations, you are less likely to communicate successfully or effectively, meaning that even the most well-constructed and delivered message may not reach its target effectively.

64.3 Hazard; real and perceived risk; mitigation; outrage

The FAO/WHO handbook (p. 13) touches on the problem of outrage in its definition of hazard, risk, and risk perception, where it is referred to as "judgement":

Hazard: a biological, chemical or physical agent in, or condition of, food with the potential to cause an adverse health effect.

Risk: a function of the probability of an adverse effect resulting from a hazard in food and the severity of that effect.

Risk perception: the judgement that people make about the characteristics, likelihood, and severity of a specific risk.

"Judgement" is directly linked to the level of a person's outrage about an event or situation. For example, a person's degree of unhappiness about having to dispose of food because of a contamination event will likely be the same whether they were notified of this in a timely manner or not. However, they will be more outraged if, for example, they perceive that the notification of the recall was not timely. If harm has been caused, outrage will be even greater no matter how timely the recall (and especially high if there is actual harm and a perception of delay).

Outrage may also vary in degree, from low to high, if an individual believes that the cause of the contamination was an act of God (natural causes), an accident, or as a result of negligence. A person may have the same escalation, but higher levels at each stage—if the contamination was affecting a population they consider vulnerable (e.g., a contamination of baby food rather than a food for adult consumption). Further, levels of outrage will also vary if the individual is directly affected (generally higher) or merely aware of the issue (generally lower).

Outrage introduces further complexity into the communication of risk and impacts the management and mitigation of that risk for the decision-makers tasked with determining an appropriate response. There are many factors that both generate outrage and affect its level. Box 1.4 (p. 13) of the FAO/WHO handbook lists these as:

Factor	Increase perceived risk	Decrease perceived risk
Perceived naturalness	Unnatural/human-made	Natural hazard
Perceived controllability	Uncontrollable	Personal controllability
Scientific knowledge	Risks are unknown to science	Risks are known to science
Familiarity	New risk	Familiar risk
Voluntariness of exposure	Involuntary exposure	Choice about exposure
Perceived catastrophic potential	Many people are affected at the same time	People are affected over a greater period of time
Severity of consequences	Severe consequence (regardless of likelihood of occurrence)	Consequences not severe
Immediacy of consequences	Consequences are immediate	Consequences are delayed
Who is affected	Vulnerable people (e.g., children, infants, and pregnant women)	Not vulnerable people
Perceived distribution of risks and benefits	Unequal distribution of risks and benefits	Equal distribution of risks and benefits
Ethical and moral concerns	Risk is seen as ethically or morally wrong (e.g., fraudulent acts)	No ethical or moral concerns

These perceived risk factors create risk communication complexity and drive consumer, interest group, and activist outrage. Food science and industry professionals generally understand hazard, risk, mitigation, and uncertainty. Risk perception is often given less consideration yet is almost always the most important factor for consumers, who often make personal purchase and consumption choices with limited information. It is this gulf that leads to outrage and its attendant media coverage or political intervention consequences, as a 2015 paper in *Journalism & Mass Communication Quarterly* confirmed. In this study of 200 Korean journalists, outrage factors perceived by the reporters were influential in determining the degree of newsworthiness, with "catastrophic potential" the most salient.[4]

The study was based on the pioneering work of Dr. Peter M. Sandman, who developed the "risk = hazard + outrage" formula.* He notes:

The most important fact about risk communication is the incredibly low correlation between a risk's "hazard" (how much harm it's likely to do) and its "outrage" (how upset it's likely to make people). If you know a risk is dangerous, that tells you almost nothing about whether it's upsetting. If you know it's upsetting, that tells you almost nothing about whether it's dangerous.[5]

*Australian science communicator, Dr Craig Cormick, has a similar view: "Many of the problems relating to risk communication stem from the fact that scientific definitions of risk can be very different from community attitudes to risk. I sum this up as the scientific formula for risk as: 'Risk = probability × impact' while the public view is: 'Risk = OMG × WTF.'" http://www.asc.asn.au/blog/2017/12/06/presidents-update-32/comment-page-1/. Accessed January 8, 2021.

Sandman uses this insight to categorize risk communication into four tasks:

- When hazard is high and outrage is low, the task is "precaution advocacy"—alerting insufficiently upset people to serious risks. "Watch out!"
- When hazard is low and outrage is high, the task is "outrage management"—reassuring excessively upset people about small risks. "Calm down."
- When hazard is high and outrage is also high, the task is "crisis communication"—helping appropriately upset people cope with serious risks. "We'll get through this together."
- When hazard and outrage are both intermediate, you're in the "sweet spot"—dialoguing with interested people about a significant but not urgent risk. "And what do you think?"

This is not complicated. But it is, as with other aspects of food safety risk communication, complex. Just a few influencing or confounding factors include: individuals have different levels of knowledge, understanding and perception; people vary in their personal tolerance to risk and also often have a different tolerance when loved ones are considered; beliefs for costs versus benefits span a wide range; and multiple potential sources of information (and misinformation). In addition, these factors often change with time, and some individuals, groups or audiences will be in different states of outrage. It is possible that one event or issue may require communicators to work on two or more outrage tasks at once. For example, a higher-than-expected prevalence of a foodborne pathogen on fresh poultry may be a "sweet spot" task for the food preparation professionals in hospitality (who are likely, if properly trained, to have some understanding of the hazard, risk, and mitigation) but a "precaution advocacy" task for consumers. Of course, for the latter it might also be (or become) an "outrage management" task if, for example, media have raised more alarm than is justified.

It can be argued that food producers and manufacturers have not done themselves any favors by making blanket promises of health and safety when all food inherently carries some risk. Things might well be different if, instead of an escalation of statements of "safe," the conversation had been one of "becoming safer." A parallel can be drawn here with the common experience of road transport, in which consumers accept that driving has hazards, have some understanding of risk and perceptions of that risk, and some knowledge of the mitigations that have been or can be made—whether by the roading authorities, vehicle manufacturers or themselves as drivers or passengers. Tellingly, only one major car brand (Volvo) has made "safe" a key ownership proposition.

Yet, the opposite is true for food producers, manufacturers and even regulators. Almost all tout "their" food as "safe" or even "the safest." This is likely to be one of the reasons that road accidents and incidents, although vastly more common than those relating to food, generate far less day-to-day concern and outrage. This is especially so when it is realized that "safe," to the general consumer, has a hugely variable meaning: some will see any food produced using "chemicals" as unsafe; others will be fearful of allergens or specific ingredients (based on a medical diagnosis or self-perception); certain groups will have influencer-based views of carbohydrate, sugar, fats and other food components, whether it's Sarah Wilson's "I Quit Sugar" advocacy, celebrity chef Pete Evans' promotion of the paleo diet; or 'Food Babe' Vana Hari's marketing of her Truvani range of foods.

It is here, too, that communication of mitigation can run into problems. When "safety" is touted as a key benefit of a food or a food system, it is natural for consumers to sheet home the unlimited responsibility for safety to those making that claim. This is the same mindset that applies in, for example, advertising where an explicit claim that is shown or proven to be untrue generates far more emotional response (outrage) than an implicit claim, or one that expressly notes any consumer responsibilities (such as safe and proper use, storage, etc.). In such cases, the mitigation messages often need to be different, or expressed in a different way, because individuals will react and be motivated differently depending on whether they feel they should share any blame.

Sandman's "risk = hazard + outrage" is important and must be recognized and applied. Early consideration of which one(s) of the four tasks need to be achieved is also likely to assist in gaining an insight into possible motivations because it can help communicators "put themselves in their audience's shoes".

Two Examples

Eating 10 kg of Raspberry Lamington... every day

A lifestyle columnist for a large New Zealand daily newspaper "reviewed" a packaged commercial bakery product. They found many supposed issues with the product, including that it "can sit on a supermarket shelf for a month." They failed to mention, however, anything about modified atmospheric packaging, instead referring to "a vast cocktail of preservatives, humectants, thickeners, stabilizers, emulsifiers, and antioxidants."

The columnist also attempted to terrify readers by stating that Azorubine is "not approved for use in the United States" and amaranth (E123), a purple color has "been banned in the United States since 1976." While these statements are true as they stand, it is more correct to say that both substances are approved for use in Australia and New Zealand, and that the amounts of each in the product were well within acceptable levels. Indeed,

(Continued)

(Continued)

conservative calculations by FSANZ showed that, for amaranth, a 60 kg person would need to eat 33 packets of the product (about 10 kg) every day to reach the Acceptable Daily Intake (ADI). For Azorubine the figure to reach the ADI was over 9000 packets. That's 2970 kg of Lamington consumed every day.

Serial killer sweets

Another example, from 2009, generated international coverage, including in New Zealand. The headline ran: "Sweets Can Turn Your Kids Into Serial Killers."

In the story the claim was made that researchers[6] had found that "letting your kids eat sweets could turn them into serial killers." The story went on to quote one of the researchers as saying that sweets "may nurture a taste for sweetened food," asserting that this would, in later life, lead to exposure to additives, "the consumption of which may also contribute toward adult aggression."

At the time, one of the authors of this chapter, having become progressively more frustrated with stories of this nature, took the unusual step of writing directly to the scientist whose research was being quoted as the basis of the claim. He was absolutely horrified that was how it was being reported.

He said they had found no causal relationship between sweets and serial killing, and that they had been very careful to stress this when presenting the findings. Even the scientist noted that it was entirely likely there were no serial killers in his sample survey, so he could not possibly have reached that conclusion. That is probably scant consolation to kids around the world who did not get a lolly because Dad was worried about them turning into Hannibal Lector.

However, the chapter did have this unfortunate line in its abstract: "Children who ate confectionery daily at the age of 10 years were significantly more likely to have been convicted for violence at the age of 34 years, a relationship that was robust when controlling for ecological and individual factors." It can be seen how even a conscientious journalist could misinterpret and overstate this statement in a story or attention-seeking headline.

Valid criticism[7] of the chapter, in 2010, received, as far as we can tell, no mainstream media coverage at all, despite it being pointed out that "there are serious methodological concerns, which make the overall findings questionable," and "as the authors recognise, the number of violent people in their cohort is very low." It was also noted that "only about 33 participants were violent (0.47% of 6942) and of these, only 23 (69% of the 33 violent individuals) had eaten confectionery excessively. With such numbers, it is highly discouraged in the biostatistical literature to model the probability of being violent using as many parameters (8) as the authors did, since the fit is essentially driven by the number of cases and not by the entire sample size."

(Continued)

(Continued)

While we did earlier concede that even a conscientious journalist could misinterpret and overstate the conclusions of Original chapter, we find it difficult to see how the news that the original news wasn't actually news, cannot be new news (if you follow).

Indeed, today, the University of Florida, in its "CRIM CCJ 4700 Research Methods" course, uses the chapter as a classic example of the difference between causation and correlation.

In both cases (lamingtons and sweets), despite the relevant science-based information being supplied to the relevant media, they took no action and their audiences remained ill-informed. We acknowledge that some media outlets will sometimes respond appropriately. However, almost always, the damage is done and cannot be fully corrected. The media will have created its sensational fodder for eyes and ears, and the level of public outrage will have grown. While this is not a new complaint and dates back centuries, (with one of the earliest observations being Jonathan Swift who noted in 1710: "Falsehood flies, and the truth comes limping after it"), some 300 years later with the dramatic digital and social media connectivity across the world, it's obvious that falsehoods can fly at even faster speeds than at any other time in human history.

64.4 Storyteller importance

Human communication is strongly based around stories. We have greater emotional reactions when we hear about people than when we are told facts. For many people, that also generates a greater trust in the person telling the story ("they understand people") than in a person explaining facts. As Sundin, Andersson & Watt note:

> *Storytelling is a two-way interaction, written or oral, between someone telling a story and one or more listeners. It is a well-known and powerful means of communicating messages and engaging audiences... Using storytelling to explain complex research has, in the past, not been considered a rigorous method of communicating science. But an increasing number of studies are showing how narratives can be useful for developing trust with an audience and increasing knowledge retention as well as the ability and willingness by audiences to learn and take action. Being easily digested by the human brain, stories help bridging between our logos and pathos; when an audience becomes emotionally receptive of facts, chances increase that they will respond and act on the knowledge.*[8]

Who is telling the story is one reason why what are, to experts, minor concerns or even non-issues can quickly become anxieties in the public and political domains. Examples are numerous and include GMOs, BPA, sweeteners, nitrates, colorings, preservatives, pesticide residues,

MSG, and modified atmosphere packaging. Even entire food groups have been demonized: wheat, meat, vegetables, milk, and corn are examples that spring to mind.

Many of these are direct results of strong storytelling, usually involving cherry-picking of data, loose interpretation of results or simply pure anecdote. Interest group organizations and activists have driven much of the anti-GMO narrative, with cherry-picking and ignoring the weight of evidence being common. Loose data interpretation has led to other issues, particularly the antichemical ones such as MSG, residues, and BPA getting traction. Anecdotal storytelling has been especially strong in preservatives, colorings, and sweeteners, likely because many people perceive these as "unnecessary" and therefore apply conspiracy theory thinking and question the "real reason" they are in food products.

Food safety communicators can also use storytelling to counteract these. Three current examples include popular nonfiction authors and commentators: McGill University Professor of chemistry Dr. Joe Schwarcz; "Angry Chef" Anthony Warner; and James Madison University Associate Professor of religious studies Alan Levinovitz. Each of these commentators use a friendly, reasoned, and reasonable, human (as opposed to "scientist") voice, tone, and manner. They include, where appropriate, humor or light-hearted phrasing and avoid it where it is not appropriate. They use personal anecdote or the stories of other individuals to illustrate points that back up the evidence or uncertainty they cite. This is communication that uses storytelling well and is an especially effective approach. It may not be appropriate for all situations, and not possible in others, but it is recommended for consideration, especially where longer written pieces can be used, or in face-to-face situations such as meetings and some media interactions.

There are usually two main differences when storytelling is used, depending upon whether its purpose is science-based risk communication or to promote a belief-based view and/or sell products. These are:

1. the use of weight of evidence backed with illustrative anecdote versus the use of anecdote connected to cherry-picked data
2. acknowledgment of risk uncertainty and the context in which it applies versus promotion of uncertainty as the risk itself.

In both cases, the science-based communicator needs to carefully consider the issues and many factors (as outlined above, and later in this chapter). This includes whether a storytelling approach will be, in each case, more or less effective than a comparatively bland fact-based one.

Once again, this is complex, and space here does not allow an exploration of all that is involved. The main consideration for storytelling is, by its very human nature, that it introduces emotion and personality, and these may not be appropriate in some situations, times, or places. Two such examples are the 2008 global melamine in milk powder food safety issue which affected several thousand infants (among others), and the 1980s–1990s UK BSE outbreak. Many food safety and risk communicators will be familiar with the example of UK Agriculture Minister John Gummer, who, in May 1990, staged a media event in which he was filmed and photographed eating a beef burger with his 4-year-old daughter. The incident is so notorious that it is still referenced in media stories on other health issues, including COVID-19.[9]

If using a storytelling approach, or elements of storytelling, in food safety risk communications it will often be important to find a way for the audience to understand the relevance of the concept of "weight of evidence." To use a little storytelling ourselves, a humorous take on weight of evidence occurred in an episode of the 1986 BBC television comedy "Blackadder II." In the scene (set in the year 1582), aboard a chartered ship lost at sea, title character Edmund Blackadder discusses the problem with the vessel's Captain Rum:

> ***Edmund****: Look, there's no need to panic. Someone in the crew will know how to steer this thing.*
>
> ***Rum****: The crew, milord?*
>
> ***Edmund****: Yes, the crew.*
>
> ***Rum****: What crew?*
>
> ***Edmund****: I was under the impression that it was common maritime practice for a ship to have a crew.*
>
> ***Rum****: Opinion is divided on the subject.*
>
> ***Edmund****: Oh, really?*
>
> ***Rum****: Yahs. All the other captains say it is; I say it isn't.*[10]

For some people, and perhaps most, this will give them a better insight into the concept of "weight of evidence", and its value, than even the most plain-language definition. As noted, however, such an approach will only sometimes be appropriate.

The other aspect that is common with most food safety storytellers on both sides of most issues: they address uncertainty. As noted, the difference is generally that those creating alarm (when alarm is not considered justified) use uncertainty to create fear, whereas those taking a balanced and realistic approach address uncertainty, and add context, to inform.

Science-based risk communicators can struggle with the uncertainty that comes from not having answers to the many and varied media and citizen questions posed, both at the time they must begin their communication process, and as the situation develops. This is understandable and reasonable because humans vary greatly in their intolerance of uncertainty.[11] People who are more anxious find ambiguity and the lack of absolute or categorical assurances unsettling and distressing, leading them to greater worry and often more likely to accept at face value either purported concerns or solutions.

Food safety risk communication, especially messaging that uses strong and vibrant storytelling, is often used to highlight uncertainty in such a way as to increase fear to generate outrage. Because of its importance to individuals, groups and cultures, food is even used to focus attention on broader issues. For example, with COVID-19, suggestions of virus contamination led the safety of food itself to be questioned, and fears about supply led to unnecessary panic buying. Another recent example: in early 2021, UK politicians used fears of "substandard food imports" to make political points about post-Brexit trade deals and its perceived threats to British farming. Yet, many UK citizens travel extensively in Europe and presumably eat local food while they're there!

In situations where food is less-peripherally connected, such as biological, chemical, or physical agents, the relationship between uncertainty and fear is often seemingly more apparent and more urgent. This can be used by activist and single-interest groups and actors[†] to generate outrage for their cause, usually to get consumer and political attention and media coverage, or to sell more of their own product. We cannot, of course, blame them for this—they are often doing what they think is right. The point is that, in this process, they are simply showing how Sandman's outrage equation works.

The challenge is to address and communicate uncertainty in a way that does not increase fear and, if possible, reduces it. Adhering to the key principles of risk communication will help achieve success, although this is rarely easy because countering fearmongering requires the introduction of the concept of mitigation, and associated costs and benefits, in the face of what are usually calls for outright bans or prohibitions.

64.5 Approach and principles for food safety risk communication

We consider that good food safety risk communicators, both individuals and organizations, require an approach that is honest, open and transparent (the acronym **HOT** may assist recall) and adherence to four communication principles: rapid, reliable, relevant, repeated (the **4Rs**)[‡].

This approach and these principles will greatly assist risk communicators to move people along the risk communications pathway from (1) misunderstanding and disagreement, through (2) understanding but disagreement, to (3) understanding and agreement. Note that these three stages are the ideal—in many cases, people may come to understand the risk or hazard but remain in disagreement with the assessment or mitigation (or decision not to mitigate) just as, in some cases, certain individuals will continue to misunderstand and disagree despite the risk communications.

64.5.1 HOT risk communications approach

64.5.1.1 Honest

This is, essentially, about respecting each of the audiences regardless of whether there is agreement or disagreement on the issues. It is vital that what you say is accurate, truthful, and complete. It is important to avoid hyperbole and language that can be interpreted as an attempt to "sell" a situation or obfuscate. For example, if a pesticide residue testing regime is changed and fewer samples are tested or analyses are made, the message should not be that "it is better," especially if the motivation for the change is cost reduction. You need to be honest because this puts you in a stronger position to then explain why the changes have been made. Even if the "why" has no upside for some audiences, you must be honest, or you will lose trust. If this happens, you will not be able to move the conversation to a point of mutual understanding but disagreement, let alone mutual understanding and agreement.

64.5.1.2 Open

There are two parts to an open approach. The first is about being open to engaging with all food safety stakeholders (once again, whether there is agreement or disagreement on the issues), including those at risk as well as those responsible for the hazard and that associated risk. The second part is openness of information, ensuring that, wherever possible, all information is available to your audiences. For example, carefully consider the use of embargoes. This is because it will add even more complexity to the risk communications as some audiences will be suspicious of the need for one (some people will see it as a delaying tactic). If you do embargo, you will

†. We include in this term those food producers, manufacturers and sellers using fear or demonization to differentiate or promote their own products.

‡. The 4Rs risk communication principles are different from, but related to, the emergency management "four Rs" (reduction, readiness, response, recovery). Indeed, good emergency management communications must embed the risk communication 4Rs principles throughout the emergency management process. In this sense, the communications 4Rs can be considered more widely as "the 4Rs communication principles."

need to be honest, open, and transparent about why an embargo was necessary. Embargoes are best avoided if you can, so you don't confuse or sidetrack some audiences.

64.5.1.3 Transparent

The concept of transparency to some extent underlies honesty and openness. It can be difficult to define, but the FAO/WHO handbook (p. 25) has a useful outline:

> *Transparency implies a set of policies, practices, and procedures that enable stakeholders and the interested public to understand how decisions on risk assessment, management, and communication have been made. This means that information on which decisions are made, and documentation about the decision-making process, should be made accessible to stakeholders and the public.*

It is clear from this definition how adopting a transparent approach can assist communicators to build trust and minimize emotion-based fears and objections. If reports and meeting minutes are readily and completely available, one of the most common issues that impact risk communications effectiveness—belief that something is being hidden, is easier to avoid.

Transparency does mean that communicators, as well as administrators and politicians, must understand and prepare for potential downsides that can include (but are not limited to) internal dissent or differing views becoming public and creating media stories themselves; economic, reputational, or other damage to organizations, regions or countries; and concerns about confidentiality, proprietary rights, and intellectual property.

The HOT risk communications approach is not complicated, but its intricacies should not be underestimated.

64.5.2 4Rs risk communications principles

Each of the 4Rs risk communication principles (rapid, reliable, relevant, repeated) are equally important. This should be kept in mind as we discuss each in turn.

64.5.2.1 Rapid

Messages must reach their target audiences as soon as those people need and can use the information. In practice, of course, immediacy is not achievable and there will be a delay between the discovery of any issue or the occurrence of an event and communication of the hazard and its risk. The key is to minimize that delay. This is neither new nor surprising. It should, indeed, be common sense to any good risk communicator who often must initiate the communication process well before s/he is in receipt of all necessary facts.

This is, however, when communications professionals can come into conflict within their organizations in cases where others insist on taking time to consider scientific, legal, or political aspects. This can be a serious problem. The solution is strong leaders who understand that quick approvals of communications and messages is vital for protecting health and minimizing harm. There also needs to be acceptance that mistakes are bound to happen, highlighting the need for a process in place that will deliver continuous improvements without blame. It is our experience that, in many cases, food safety risk communication rarely leaves all parties happy. In most instances, however, applying the "front page of the newspaper test" will help decision-making around when communications should start: if criticism can be successfully countered by saying "if we'd waited then things would have been worse," then the decision not to wait was the correct one.

Note here that the "rapid" principle does not advocate applying a precautionary approach to the situation in question. That is a philosophical matter outside the scope of this chapter. Suffice to say that it is our experience that being precautionary often leads to other problems or consequences, as the earlier example of BPA shows.

64.5.2.2 Reliable

This principle is another that has two equally important facets. The first refers to ensuring that the message content and advice on action is accurate, substantiated, and as complete as it can be at the time: the person receiving the message can rely on it to act appropriately and in a timely manner to reduce the risk.

The other facet of "reliable" is an organizational one and refers to the trust in the storyteller, as noted earlier in this chapter. It is what makes "reliable" the most complex of the 4Rs: your messages can be perfect and entirely reliable, but it is the perception of the reliability of who is delivering them that matters. In the last few decades, as communication channels have multiplied through social media and web-based outlets, establishing reliability has become more fraught and difficult since it relies heavily on perception of reputation, something that almost always is built slowly and over the long-term.

The importance of reputation is often underestimated. This is understandable—it is human nature to believe that you and your organization are doing good work and are seen externally to be so. Many communicators naturally assume that everyone else feels the same as they do. However, lessons from the world of marketing are relevant here. Advertising expert and author Bob Hoffman states[12]:

> *If you're a marketer and you believe people care about your brand just because they buy it, you're headed for*

trouble. What we blithely call 'brand loyalty' is mostly just habit, convenience, mild satisfaction or easy availability.

While it is unlikely that many people care about your brand as much as you imagine they do (which, in the case of government and regulatory organizations, is usually your department's name) they are likely to have a perception of your reputation, and that will have a strong and direct bearing on how much they believe and trust your communications and message content. For the receiver of your message to perceive it as reliable they must trust the messenger. The best-case scenario is that you are known as being trustworthy; if people haven't heard of you, you may be given the benefit of the doubt.

Establishing and maintaining trust and reputation—let alone rebuilding from a negative view, is a subject for an entire book. All organizations involved with food safety risk communications should have in place a properly resourced trust and reputation program. This will involve robust research to determine what each audience or public thinks of you and why they hold that view; a willingness to address any issues identified; and a process to do so, including ongoing research to measure success and identify new or evolving problems.

If you cannot deliver on the "reliable" principle, then it will matter little if you are "rapid" or not. We temper this by noting, of course, that most organizations will be viewed as highly reliable and reputable by some people, while others will hold the opposite view. The challenge is always to move the individuals in the latter group into, or closer to, the former. For example, messaging about the dangers of drinking raw milk, delivered by a respected food safety agency or individual expert, will be perceived by many as solid advice and may well enhance their view of the reputation and credibility of the messenger. Other people may not know the organization brand or individual's name but, should the message seem credible, are likely to give it some credence and consideration and move towards a view of good reputation. The group of staunch raw milk advocates will dismiss the information, likely label it as "typical" propaganda, and have an already negative reputational view reinforced. C'est la vie!

64.5.2.3 Relevant

The third of the 4Rs is much more straightforward. Relevance simply refers to ensuring that the receiver of the communications or message will, within the first few seconds, recognize the WIIFM ("what's in it for me?") message requirement for the receiver of the message. Good risk communications should grab the attention of individuals in the target audience yet avoid overstatement or sensationalizing (which would lower credibility to the detriment of the "reliable" principle).

Relevance also covers the communications art of using just enough words (or images) to allow the recipient to get the correct clear message, assign it the appropriate degree of attention, and then act or behave as required to minimize risk and harm. Ideally, this means tailoring communications to every segment of the target population or public. In practice, it needs care to ensure that the dissemination of the message is not slowed ("rapid") and confusion is avoided, since individuals are likely to use more than one channel for information, and see messages targeted at segments other than themselves.

For example, a recall for a snack food that is consumed widely may need messages that warn children not to eat it and other messages tailored to parents. Many or all of these messages may also need to be translated into different languages, disseminated across a range of different paid and unpaid media channels, as well as directly to consumers and retailers. Relevant communications for each is likely to involve different wording and calls to action.

Communicators should also beware instances where a simple, but accurate, message could be perceived as having information withheld when seen alongside a more detailed message, particularly where this has the potential to derail the public or media conversation from the food safety issue to a debate about the communication of it.

This is where good storytelling techniques come into play and the same, or more, consideration that you give to what you say must be given to **how** you say it.

64.5.2.4 Repeated

This is related to the "relevant" 4Rs above. It is the principle of having the same message or content in more than one place (different channels) multiple times. Lessons can again be taken from the world of advertising. As we note above, consumers generally care less about brands than we often imagine as communicators or marketers. Similarly, people don't care about messages per se; they only care once the content of the message has cut through the noise of the sum total of communications that we are all exposed to throughout each day of our lives and judge that the message is of some relevance to them. Even then, landing a message with the appropriate target can and does take time. One study, a *meta*-analysis conducted in 2015[13] found that, in an experimental setting, maximum attitude (response to an advertisement) is reached at approximately 10 exposures, while recall increases linearly and does not level off before the eighth exposure.

As with our earlier discussion of reputation, it is easy for risk communicators and their organizations to fall into the trap of thinking that their food safety messaging is especially important and so automatically attract notice and enough attention to induce risk-minimization behaviors. In some cases, where the issue becomes headline news, this might be true. Consider, however, estimates that the average US consumer was exposed to 500 advertisements a day in the 1970s, rising to between 6,000 and 10,000 daily today. Include news items and general "life" messages (emails, phone calls, conversations, etc.) and the noise is obviously considerable.

Repeating risk communication messages and content can assist with cutting through this noise. It can also help build credibility and relevance (the "truth effect"[14]) if repetition is judicious: too much repetition may lead to negative credibility. Communicators should be mindful that the quality of the message remains of the utmost importance: no amount of repetition will rescue a poorly crafted message nor inadequate content.

64.6 COVID-19 food safety communications

Accepted science is clear: the SARS-CoV-2 virus does not pose a food safety hazard. This was an early unknown which was widely covered by mainstream news media in the first few months of 2020 and has now largely subsided. From time-to-time, however, the discovery of the virus on food or food packaging (especially in laboratory settings) is reported, despite the presence not indicating any public health risk. While such reporting does help keep the seriousness of the COVID-19 risk in the public mind, it can raise unfounded public fear and political reaction.

An example of this, which has received global media attention, has been the actions of China, which has implemented technical barriers to trade many times based on the reported detection of SARS-CoV-2 on frozen food packaging, with more than 20 countries affected to date.

Chinese authorities have been able to use this to reject or delay imported food shipments. While this will have some cost to their local importing businesses and consumers, it may also advantage some local Chinese producers. A few examples (from many) of the products that have been affected are Argentinian beef, German pork, Indian cuttlefish, New Zealand mussels, Indonesian fishery products, Brazilian chicken, Ecuadorian prawns, and Saudi shrimp.

Requirements on imports, such as disinfecting and testing before release onto the market, impose additional costs that are borne by the foreign exporter and/or domestic importer, depending on specific business agreements. Cold-chain logistics, with international multistage workflows, make it unreasonable to blame the country of origin when products test positive. However, hazard and risk misinformation make it easier for unreasonable actions to be taken.

We are seeing this in the case of China with SARS-CoV-2/COVID-19. We have seen it with food colors, BPA, and a myriad more.

Food safety professionals and risk communicators must work together with the goal of making unreasonable action itself unreasonable and return the focus to making a real difference by addressing real hazards that have real risks and public health consequences.

64.7 Ban the avocado!

We all have a vested interest in ensuring high standards of food safety. This requires government regulation that is fit for purpose and appropriate individual and family knowledge about preparation and consumption. Good regulation, knowledge, and behaviors also apply to those involved in food production, manufacture, transport, storage, sale, supply, and service as well.

If bread is the staff of life, then food safety risk communications is the bread bin that keeps it safe and suitable. Just like a bread bin, good risk communication is generally not a complicated process. There are simple things to do and steps to take. However, unlike the humble bread bin, those steps involve individuals, their level of knowledge and understanding, and their (often ever-changing) perceptions. And that is where something that it not in essence complicated can become multifaceted and complex.

We leave you with an example, and a call to ban the sale of fresh avocado[§].

In New Zealand, during 2019, 428 people were injured by food, at a cost of more than $800,000 ($1869 each, on average). In 2020 researchers at Emory University in the United States described "an epidemic" with the same food estimated to have injured 50,413 people between 1998 and 2017, with over half happening in the last decade[15]... and that's not counting those who did not seek medical attention.

This food presents a clear and obvious hazard that has a high risk of harm. An obvious hazard requires an obvious action: fresh avocados should be banned from sale, with the only option being a processed form. We make this (tongue-in-cheek) call because, over many years of risk communication, people are still cutting themselves when they try to remove the stone from an avocado.

Or, do we use this example to remind us that all food is an hazard to some people some of the time? Do we remember that context, perspective, and common sense are sometimes over-looked when food and food safety issues become emotional? Do we acknowledge that perception and outrage play a big (the biggest?) part on food safety risk communication?

§. We think that, in concluding, a little humor is appropriate!

Our call to ban the avocado—while evidence-based, is bound to fail because, despite an hazard with a high and real risk, outrage is low. Why? Because cutting your hand when preparing an avocado is not the fault of the avocado grower (or the knife-maker), nor the fault of the greengrocer (or knife-seller). When there is no one to blame but yourself, there is no outrage—just some (in most cases) small annoyance, pain, a bit of blood and a mental note to be more careful next time.

Sadly, far less important food hazards, with far less risk of harm, can cause food safety communicators their own fair share of annoyance and pain—but hopefully no blood!. And, if you follow good risk communications principles and practice from the start, no need to make a note to take more care next time.

References

1. World Health Organization. Risk communication applied to food safety: handbook. (Food safety and quality series, 2) <http://www.fao.org/3/a-i5863e.pdf>; 2016. Accessed 08.01.2021.
2. Ferrer RA, Klein WMP, Avishai A, Jones K, Villegas M, Sheeran P. When does risk perception predict protection motivation for health threats? A person-by-situation analysis. *PLoS One*. 2018;13(3): e0191994. Available from: https://doi.org/10.1371/journal.pone.0191994.
3. Maslow AH. A theory of human motivation. *Psychol Rev*. 1943;50 (4):370–396. Available from: https://doi.org/10.1037/h0054346.
4. You M, Ju Y. The influence of outrage factors on journalists' gatekeeping of health risks. *J Mass Commun Q (JMCQ)*. 2015;92 (4):959–969.
5. Sandman PM. Introduction to risk communication and orientation to this website. The Peter M. Sandman risk communication website. <https://www.psandman.com/index-intro.htm> Accessed 08.01.2021.
6. Moore SC, Carter LM, van Goozen S. Confectionery consumption in childhood and adult violence. *Br J Psychiatry*. 2009;195(4): 366–367. Available from: https://doi.org/10.1192/bjp.bp.108.061820.
7. Gregori D. Confectionery consumption and violence. *Br J Psychiatry*. 2010;196(3):245. Available from: https://doi.org/10.1192/bjp.196.3.245.
8. Sundin A, Andersson K, Watt R. Rethinking communication: integrating storytelling for increased stakeholder engagement in environmental evidence synthesis. *Environ Evid*. 2018;7:6. Available from: https://doi.org/10.1186/s13750-018-0116-4.
9. Financial Times website. The battle at the heart of British science over coronavirus. <https://www.ft.com/content/1e390ac6-7e2c-11ea-8fdb-7ec06edeef84>; Accessed 09.01.2021.
10. Blackadder Quotes website. Blackadder Series 2 Episode 3—Potato full script. <https://blackadderquotes.com/blackadder-series-2-episode-3-potato-full-script>; Accessed 09.01.2021.
11. Carleton RN. The intolerance of uncertainty construct in the context of anxiety disorders: theoretical and practical perspectives. *Expert Rev Neurother*. 2012;12(8):937–947. Available from: https://doi.org/10.1586/ern.12.82.
12. The Ad Contrarian website. Nobody gives a flying shit about your brand. <http://adcontrarian.blogspot.com/2015/05/nobody-gives-flying-shit-about-your.html>; Accessed 21.02.2021.
13. Eisend M, Schmidt S. Advertising repetition: a *meta*-analysis on effective frequency in advertising. *J Advert*. 2015;44:415–428. Available from: https://doi.org/10.1080/00913367.2015.1018460.
14. Fazio LK, Brashier NM, Payne BK, Marsh EJ. Knowledge does not protect against illusory truth. *J Exper Psychol General*. 2015;144(5):993–1002.
15. Farley KX, Aizpuru M, Boden SH, Wagner ER, Gottschalk MB, Daly CA. Avocado-related knife injuries: describing an epidemic of hand injury. *Am J Emerg Med*. 2020;38(5):864–868. Available from: https://doi.org/10.1016/j.ajem.2019.06.051.

Chapter 65

Consumer attitudes toward novel agrifood technologies: a critical review on genetic modification and synthetic biology

Shan Jin[1,2], Wenjing Li[1,3], Francis Z. Naab[1], David Coles[1] and Lynn J. Frewer[1]

[1]School of Natural and Environmental Sciences, Newcastle University, Newcastle upon Tyne, United Kingdom, [2]Faculty of Business and Law, University of Portsmouth, Portsmouth, United Kingdom, [3]School of Economics and Management, Huazhong Agricultural University, Wuhan, P.R. China

Abstract

Consumer acceptance is an important driver of success in the process of commercializing novel agrifood technologies and their applications. It needs to be measured and considered throughout the whole process of technological innovations. Here, genetically modification (GM) and synthetic biology (SB) are considered as two cases which can be employed as lenses to assess consumers' responses to novel agrifood technologies. Risk and benefit perceptions are considered to be important determinants of acceptance. Application attributes, affect heuristic, ethical concerns, individual characteristics, and social contexts are also discussed. However, some inconsistent findings in relation to factors impacting on consumers' attitudes were mainly about the role of information provision, prior knowledge, and social trust. The European Union and US regulations of GM and SB applied to food production were also compared. Based on the above findings, an explanatory framework for understanding consumer attitudes towards novel agrifood technologies in general, and specific GM- and SB-based applications in particular, has been proposed. Limitations in existing research and implications for future studies are presented.

Keywords: Genetically modified food; synthetic biology; consumer acceptance; risk and benefit perception

65.1 Introduction

Developing and implementing novel technologies, including genetic modification (GM) and synthetic biology (SB), within the agrifood sector is considered a promising way of closing the yield and nutrition gaps, and simultaneously reducing the use of natural resources and synthetic agricultural chemicals, to bring benefits to the environment and society.[1,2] However, social responses to different technologies might differ, with some being easily accepted and others essentially rejected by the public. This in turn may affect the development and commercialization trajectories of these technologies and relevant products.[3] Previous research has shown that some technologies are more accepted by consumers than others. For example, in the case of food preservation techniques, high-pressure and pulsed electric field processing of food were more acceptable to consumers, while food irradiation was associated with more negative public views.[4] Nanotechnology is another potentially controversial area in terms of public acceptance of its applications. Consumers showed a relatively positive attitude towards nanotechnology in food production, although food applications were less accepted than other areas of application.[4] GM technology was perceived to be riskier and less beneficial than nanotechnology, representing a prominent example associated with societal negativity in many parts of the world, in particular in Europe.[5] A variety of determinants shaping public attitudes towards GM food have been identified by previous studies, mainly conducted after social opposition to GM products had occurred, suggesting those determinants were better predictors of people's rejection rather than acceptance.[4] In contrast, SB is a rather new area associated with very limited research investigating social responses including those in relation to the agrifood applications, which should be initiated prior to the commercialization process and in turn refine the commercialization trajectory if relevant.[6]

Despite SB currently being under the legal definition of GM in the European Union (EU) Directive No 2001/18/EC,[a]

Present Knowledge in Food Safety. DOI: https://doi.org/10.1016/B978-0-12-819470-6.00035-4

there exist some technical differences between GM and SB. GM mainly involves the transfer of DNA from one organism to a different organism,[7] while SB integrates science and engineering principles to synthesize and assemble artificial and/or natural components for producing novel living systems, which are more predictable, efficient and "off-the-shelf" compared with traditional GM technology, and can be transferred to different organisms for producing expected products.[8,9] There has been a variety of SB-based applications delivering different benefits to the agrifood sector, for example, crops with increased resistance to abiotic (e.g., drought) and biotic stress (e.g., pests and diseases),[10] crops with improved nutritional values,[11] and novel food and food ingredient production based on modified microbes.[12]

However, different risks linked to health, environmental, economic and social aspects could also emerge, associated with specific applications. Food or food ingredients based on GM and SB technologies, for example, may be associated with (perceived) uncertainty about the long-term human health impacts.[13] As has been the case with other novel foods, the increased allergenicity resulting from the new substance produced in certain GM products could be a problem, especially when the allergens do not exist in the corresponding natural products and are not accurately labeled.[14] The ecological risk relates to the release of modified organisms into the environment, in particular plants and microbes, which might threaten natural species and harm human health if, for example, ecosystems are disrupted and food security is compromized.[15] SB is particularly associated with the risk of release of biological agents by people within or outside research institutes, not least because of open-sourcing platforms, which in turn might increase risks to the environment and human health.[15] Also, if unbalanced adoption of novel applications (e.g., excessive cultivation of modified energy crops) occurs among farmers, there may be negative impacts on farmer livelihoods.[16] Novel food applications with tangible benefits may sometimes negatively impact existing industries as well as lead to potential financial losses among certain stakeholders.

Given that novel food technologies potentially bring both benefits and risks to society, it is important to understand public perceptions of these so as to develop better risk-benefit communication strategies and optimize commercialization trajectories of applications. As such, the present study selects GM and SB as two cases for investigating consumer responses to food technologies and their applications through a critical review. The findings contribute to the development of a conceptual framework for better understanding consumer decision-making regarding the application of technologies to food production. On the other hand, it provides information for helping align relevant product development and policy-making in line with public preferences.

65.2 Public attitudes towards genetic modification and synthetic biology

Numerous studies have investigated public attitudes towards GM technology applied to food production and its specific applications, in different countries and regions.[17,18,19,20] Overall, the research suggested that consumers prefer conventionally produced foods to those made using GM technology. European consumers were generally reluctant to accept GM food on the basis of their perceived risks. The results of a systematic review has indicated that Europeans hold more negative attitudes, but lower ethical concerns, compared with North American and Asian study participants.[5] Against this, very limited research has been undertaken in relation to societal responses to SB applied to food production. At the time of publication, the media portrayal of SB has been relatively positive,[21,22] implying that, unlike GM foods, social amplification of perceived risks has not occurred and an "inherent societal aversion" to SB as an enabling technology has not resulted.[23,24] In addition, research into GM food and SB indicated that there are certain applications potentially more accepted by the public, such as food products with enhanced nutrition via the technological innovation process.[6,25] This indicates there is a need to investigate public priorities and preferences regarding specific food applications of technological innovation in different social contexts.

65.3 Public perceptions of benefits and risks

Public perceptions of benefits and risks as well as ethical issues in relation to GM and specific agrifood applications were considered to largely determine public attitudes.[26–28] While environmentalists paid much attention to, such as super weeds and biodiversity, the public were more concerned about potential adverse and uncertain health effects in the long term due to consuming GM foods.[29] Interestingly, some benefits certain GM food claims to deliver, such as increased food supply, price discounts and extended shelf-life, also generated negative attitudes.[25] People's reliance on different perceptions in the decision-making of the technology and specific applications might also differ due to, for instance, demographic, cultural, geographical, and policy contexts.[30,31]

65.3.1 Prior attitudes and application types

Prior attitudes towards GM technology applied to food production might be largely shaped by how the technology or its first product was initially introduced to a society and also affected by the social context (e.g., relevant policies and media portrayal) and personal attributes. Its influence on one's product-specific attitude can be strong in particular in the absence of actual GM food experience.[32,33] However, most studies into public attitudes focused on GM food in general rather than specific types of application, which can be regarded as people's prior attitudes. As was mentioned, before investigating in what way GM food should be introduced into society so it can receive more public support, strong social opposition had already emerged in Europe.[4] Thus, future research that explores public responses to a novel food technology should be conducted at an early stage so as to avoid such opposition.

In the research into the influence of information presented on consumers' attitudes towards specific GM products in Denmark, Germany, Italy, and the UK, prior attitudes appeared to "over-ride" any external information that was given.[34] Bredahl[33] suggested public attitudes towards GM food on a case-by-case basis might emerge as more products are available on the market. Some subsequent studies have identified attitudinal differences across different types of GM applications. For instance, consumers tend to accept GM food with enhanced nutrition and health benefits, but are more resistant to GM applications with increased production, reduced price and extended shelf lives.[25,35] More negative attitudes were associated with animal-based GM applications, in particular in relation to food production, compared with the plant-based applications.[36]

65.3.2 Influence of affect heuristic

A negative relationship between risk and benefit perceptions of GM food has often been identified in different studies, despite the inconsistent strengths reported.[30,37,38] Slovic and Peters[39] studied people's instinctive and intuitive reactions to a technology, in this case, nuclear power. They found that positive feelings increased benefit perceptions and negative feelings increased risk perceptions. The influence of this "affect" heuristic on the negative relationship was also identified in relation to nanotechnology-derived food products.[40] Here, affect heuristic represents a stimuli-evoked image which has been marked to varying degrees of affect, either positive or negative, in one's affect pool.[41] Other studies, however, associated the effect with the discounting effect of risks respondents perceived on their benefit perceptions, in which trade-offs between these perceived benefits and risks were made during consumers' decision-making associated with GM food.[42] As the actual strength of negative relationship to some degree implies the possibility of reducing risk perceptions by increasing benefit perceptions or vice versa, more research into the mechanism is required in the context of both GM and SB applied to food production.

65.3.3 Effects of information and knowledge

The effects of information and knowledge on consumer attitudes towards novel food technologies and specific applications have also been studied. Scholderer and Frewer[34] found no systemic change in participants' attitudes towards applying GM technology to produce food products after being presented balanced information about GM technology or information about specific products (i.e., beer produced by means of GM yeast and fat-free yoghurt produced with GM starter culture). Participants' choice probability of GM food products with related information was lower than those without extra information. Zhu and Xie[43] reported no effect of benefit information on participants' attitudes, whereas balanced information and risk information decreased participants' acceptance of GM applied in food production. In contrast, a positive influence of benefit information on participants' acceptance of a chocolate chip cookie made with GM ingredients was identified in the United States and the United Kingdom but not in France, and the effect of benefit types (i.e., environmental, health and world benefits) on participants' attitudes differed across regions.[44] It was also found that consumers with negative prior attitudes were less affected by benefit information in comparison to those with more positive prior attitudes, again showing the importance of prior attitudes in shaping acceptance of specific applications.[44] Some research has attributed the unstable effects of benefit information to the confirmatory bias, where participants with clear positive or negative attitudes tended to favor information that supported their prior attitudes, and explained the negative influence of risk information by a negativity bias, where participants with intermediate attitudes could be more affected by negative information than positive information.[45]

Besides information provision, the importance of knowledge in shaping public attitudes has been a topic of research.[25,26,46] The knowledge includes objective and subjective knowledge, of which the former is tested using questions in relation to technical or product attributes of GM, and the latter represents the extent to which people perceive themselves knowledgeable about GM. House et al.[47] found a positive correlation only between subjective but not objective knowledge and consumer attitudes. Christoph et al.[48] found no clear relationship between participants' knowledge of genetics and biotechnology and their acceptance of GM applied in food production. Connor and Siegrist[49] tested objective knowledge from three aspects including knowledge about basic biology, GM technology and relevant regulation, which showed no significant effect on participants' risk and benefit perceptions of, and no effect on attitudes towards, GM food applications. In contrast, some studies have identified the effect of objective knowledge in reducing consumers' risk perceptions regarding GM applied in food production.[43,50–52] Connor and Siegrist[53] argued people with more knowledge about basic biology and genetics were more likely to base their attitudes on cognitive judgements of relevant risks and benefits. Another alternative explanation, however, related to people's education in particular in science, which may result in people being more pro-technology. Zhu and Xie[43] tested participants' benefit and risk knowledge about GM food, showing positive and negative impacts respectively on participants' acceptance of GM applied in food production. However, it might be difficult to distinguish whether benefit and risk knowledge should be assigned to participants' objective knowledge or predictors of their overall risk and benefit perceptions of GM food. At present, there is no solid conclusion about how to properly test objective knowledge of GM as well as the actual effects of both objective and subjective knowledge on consumer attitudes.

65.3.4 Social trust in institutions and information sources

Some studies showed that trust in institutions, such as official bodies, experts, industry and NGOs, plays an important role in shaping people's perceptions of, and prior attitudes towards, GM applied to food production as well as specific applications, in particular when people had a lack of knowledge.[50,49,54,55] The effects on public responses, however, might differ across types of trusted institutions due to their distinct attitudes towards GM affecting the public.[56] For instance, NGOs in Europe often had more negative attitudes, and therefore increased people's risk perceptions and rejection of relevant applications.[54] In contrast, some researchers found that social trust in institutions might reflect people's prior attitudes towards GM applied in food production, which was named the "associationist" view of trust.[57] Poortinga and Pidgeon[58] found social trust was largely expression of general attitudes, while it still contributed to people's acceptance of GM food, despite its very low level of correlation. The influence of trust in institutions on people's risk and benefit perceptions and acceptance of specific GM applications was also identified.[49] Unfortunately, Connor and Siegrist did not include people's prior attitudes towards GM applied in food production in the study, which therefore could not test whether the influence of trust was mediated by prior attitudes.

Trust in information sources about technologies may also be influential. There was research showing that Chinese consumers most frequently use television, the internet and personal communication as information channels to obtain information about food safety including that in relation to GM food, while they tended to trust more medical doctors, personal experience and research institutes, despite medical doctors being not professional in food issues.[59] However, Frewer et al.[32] argued that trust in information sources appeared to be more driven by people's prior attitudes to GM food, rather than trust affecting people's reactions to different types of information.

65.3.5 Individual attributes and social contexts

Research into people's perceptions of, and attitudes towards, GM/SB and its food applications has observed differences across certain socio-demographic attributes, for example, gender, education, age, and income.[48,60,61] Women in the United States perceived higher risks in relation to SB as compared to men.[62] Such gender difference has also been reported in other technologies (e.g., food irradiation), which was attributed to men perceiving themselves to be more involved in controlling and benefiting from technologies than women.[63] The influence of educational level and gender on public attitudes, however, was sometimes found insignificant in quantitative studies in both SB- and GM-related studies.[64–67] For example, when participants were presented GM food products with tangible benefits, the attitudinal difference across gender disappeared.[66]

Food neophobia, food technology neophobia and food disgust sensitivity also predicted attitudes towards GM foods,[17,33,68] as do attitudes towards environment and nature,[33,69] religion affiliation[70] and personality traits (e.g., openness and conscientiousness as predictors of consumer acceptance of GM animal products).[71] In addition, the potential effect of social contexts on public responses to GM food was studied, such as press media reporting, interpersonal networks, cultural values, and the regulatory framework being employed,[30,72–75] which aligns with the theoretical framework of social amplification and attenuation of risks.[76]

65.4 Ethical concerns

There has been much discussion about ethical consideration with respect to novel agrifood technologies generally, and GM- and SB-based foods in particular. A number of scholars have debated whether SB constitutes a "special case" for ethical consideration. If yes, this suggests the necessity of establishing distinct ethics to discuss SB. The consensus that has been reached suggested that a subfield for ethics of SB is unnecessary, and the normal ethical analysis approach (i.e., four prima facie principles) of autonomy (self-determination), beneficence (do good), nonmaleficence (to do no bad), and justice (equal and equitable) can still be effectively employed to SB.[77–81] Based on this, an Ethical Matrix was utilized to facilitate the analysis of ethical issues in relation to some agrifood technologies (e.g., GM, genomic technologies and nanotechnology) and specific applications (e.g., GM salmon) in consideration of different stakeholder groups.[79,82,83] This body of research suggested that sufficient information (focused on both risks and benefits) about the technologies and products should be provided by producers and distributors to enable consumers' informed choice-making. Products derived from different technologies should have minimal risks to human health and the environment and deliver benefits which are appreciated by consumers. Besides the technical risks, socio-economic risks that relate to justice (e.g., equity of access to the technology, and technological benefits) should also be included, and a clear, consistent and transparent regulatory framework should be developed to provide assurance of compliance throughout the food chain.[82] This might relate to scientists' or product developers' research process, in which public preferences should be considered and applicable regulation must be followed. This calls for the development of consensus regarding how to estimate, evaluate and manage risks, due consideration was applied to any scientific uncertainty where this exists, and ideally on a case-by-case basis; and also raises the requirement for better engagement of stakeholders, such as scientists, product developers, the public, manufacturers and distributors, risk researchers and government representatives.[84] Research has also suggested a framework based on a specific technology in the area of SB (i.e., gene drive), which includes six domains for comprehensive ethics assessment: standard research ethics, risk identification and interpretation, fiduciary responsibility, democratizing technology, epistemology and power, and procedural ethics. The framework focused on the final product and the whole research process.[85] The framework, as well as the Ethical Matrix, can represent useful tools for identifying potential ethical issues of different agrifood technologies and specific products at the early stage and provide policy-makers with more information.

Moral and ethical issues associated with GM and SB from a laypersons' perspective have also been investigated, as well as the influence on people's attitudes towards these technologies and applications. The most frequently discussed concerns related to the "unnaturalness" of the GM and SB *per se* as well as their derived products, which were particularly linked to animal-based applications. Consumers' resistance to unnatural products they perceived has been demonstrated by previous research.[83,86] The notion that using GM or SB is "playing god" or "tampering with nature" informed ethical concerns. The bottom-up approach of SB that intends to synthesize cells from scratch may represent a further step to artificial life and might be more ethically controversial than GM, for example, the total synthesis of *Escherichia coli* with a recoded genome.[87–90] Dragojlovic and Einsiedel[91] reported that people with a stronger belief in God are less supportive of SB due to their use of value-based considerations as heuristics. This indicated that some people's negative attitudes could be largely determined by their moral or ethical objections. Other ethical issues in relation to SB and GM were studied, such as biosafety (i.e., unintended risk events) and biosecurity (i.e., deliberate misuse of SB for nefarious purposes), patent and benefit distribution, research integrity, and regulations.[80,92,93] Pino and other coauthors (2016) argued that perceptions of producers' higher corporate social responsibility could improve their acceptance of relevant GM food products. This suggested that producers' moral and ethical considerations linked to the process of commercializing GM food may *positively* impact consumer attitudes and purchase intentions. However, some researchers argued that moral and ethical issues have limited influence on consumers' attitude formation.[94] Despite so, it is still important to investigate consumers' attitudes towards different ethical issues in relation to different stakeholders and activities throughout the agrifood chain, as trust is much easier to destroy than to create,[45] and ethically developed and commercialized products derived from GM and SB might be more acceptable in the long term.

65.5 Regulations of genetic modification and synthetic biology

Currently, there are no specific regulations on SB-based applications in the agrifood sector in Europe or elsewhere. They commonly fall under the existent regulations of biotechnology (e.g., GM technology), while the regulation targets differ between the US and EU. The US regulation is "trait-based" and is focused on new traits linked to final products. The EU applies precautionary principles, and thus regulates the initial application of genetic engineering in specific organisms to its release into the environment.[95] In the EU, SB and GM are both covered by The Contained Use Directive (2009/41/EC)[b] and The Deliberate Release Directive (2001/18/EC), while, as more novel SB-based applications are being developed, ambiguities in regulation may emerge. For instance, a synthetic bacterium contained in a secure casing has been developed for sensing arsenic, while the developers' application for exemption from The Contained Use Directive (2009/41/EC) and The Deliberate Release Directive (2001/18/EC) was not approved in the EU. This was because, despite this application being technically "contained," it was applied outside the laboratory, which results in it being considered "uncontained."[96] In contrast, the US regulation is relatively favorable to the development of GM food products, mainly focusing on the nature of the end products, according to health, safety, and environmental legislation governing conventional products, rather than how they were produced.[97]

Another regulatory issue is the labeling of GM feeds and foods, which also relates to the ethical consideration of providing both risk and benefit information about the technologies and products to enable consumers' informed choice-making. In the EU, feed and food products that contain or consist of, as well as those which are produced from or contain ingredients from, GM organisms (GMOs) must be labeled, covered by Regulation (EC) No. 1829/2003.[c] The requirement, however, excludes food products with no higher than 0.9% GM ingredients and those with adventitious or technically unavoidable presence of GM ingredients during cultivation, harvest, or transport. In the United States, some labeling legislation has been implemented in certain states (e.g., mandatory labeling for certain GM products implemented in 2016 in Vermont). The National Bioengineered Food Disclosure Law was implemented on 1 January 2020, with requirement for mandatory compliance initiating from 1 January 2021.[98] However, this Standard defines bioengineered foods as those, containing genetic material that has been modified using in vitro recombinant DNA techniques, and that cannot be created through conventional breeding or found in nature, for human consumption. In other words, GM foods obtained through biotechnologies (e.g., SB and gene-editing) without detectable in vitro recombinant DNA and possibly gained through conventional breeding or in nature as well as GM feed is not regulated by this Standard. Also, food served in a restaurant or similar retail food establishment, food produced and sold by very small manufacturers, animals fed with bioengineered feed and their products (e.g., eggs, meat, and milk), refined foods without detectable in vitro recombinant DNA, and food with inadvertent or technically unavoidable presence of bioengineered substances of up to 5% for each ingredient have been exemplified.[98]

Overall, the EU legislation associated with GM and SB tends to be more conservative and stricter than the US legislation. This may limit European researchers' innovations in experiments, which has resulted in researchers' demands for upgrading the existing regulatory framework.[84] There has been limited research into consumers' attitudes towards government regulations of GM food. European consumers were relatively uninformed about GM food regulations, and the majority of them considered the regulations not enough to protect people from risks in relation to GM.[30] The impacts of labeling on consumer attitudes towards GM foods were not consistent in the existing studies, with some research showing discounted consumer willingness to purchase food products after being labeled,[99] while some indicating the implemented labeling policy that led to reduction of opposition to GM food.[100] Some research suggested mandatory labeling policies as being more in line with consumer preferences than voluntary labeling policies,[101] while some gave opposite conclusions.[102] Nonetheless, more research is needed to study public attitudes in the context of different regulatory frameworks, thereby avoiding public controversy during the policy-making of novel agrifood technologies.

65.6 Implications for future research and strategy-making

There are different frameworks which have been established for explaining consumer acceptance of agrifood technology-based innovations (e.g., GM and nanotechnology). However, these tend to focus on technologies in themselves and neglected specific contexts, such as the type of applications derived from these technologies and how they interact with social contexts. Here, we have proposed an explanatory framework for understanding consumer attitudes towards novel agrifood technologies generally and specific GM- and SB-based applications in particular (Fig. 65.1). This provides some insights into future strategy-making for improving public acceptance of GM and SB applied to food production. First, it might be a bit upsetting that building or rebuilding social trust and disseminating information about technologies may not be able to directly resolve risk controversies surrounding certain agrifood technologies, in particular when prior negative attitudes have been formed. However, it does not mean these actions have little value in risk communication. For instance, this could be effective in relation to targeting the groups with less negative prior attitudes or insufficient self-assessed knowledge about the technologies.[103] Given the moderate but significant relationship between social trust and risk perceptions after controlling for prior attitudes, building or rebuilding social trust might still impact on consumer attitudes and behaviors especially in the long term.[58] In terms of novel food technologies that have not raised strong societal concerns, it is valuable to further explore how one technology or its first product is developed, described, and introduced to a specific society, can shape a more positive attitude, which could benefit future commercialization of other products. Second, as consumer preferences for applications with tangible benefits have been identified,[104] it is important to further investigate the application attributes consumers are enthusiastic about by involving the consumers in the product design. This helps avoid potential societal rejection of the application or even other products based on this technology. Nonetheless, consumers' concerns surrounding these applications with tangible benefits should also be considered, based on which strategies could be

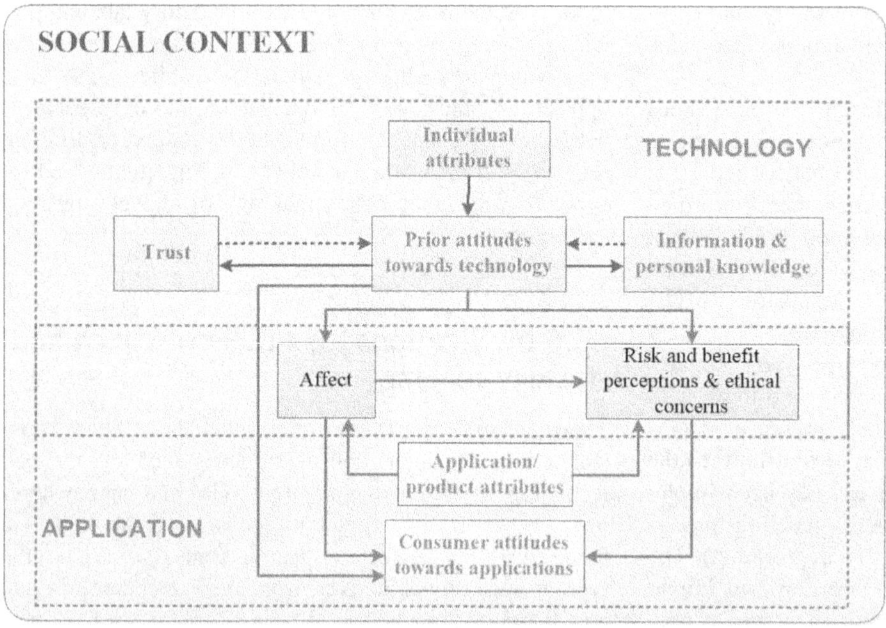

FIGURE 65.1 Conceptual framework of consumer attitudes towards novel agrifood technologies.

made to attenuate or reduce their risk perceptions.[105] Third, consumers' emotional responses to applications may need to be more considered in risk communication as it largely shapes consumer attitudes.[106] Notably, the specific attributes of products and other factors that evoke negative or positive affect should be investigated, which can help reduce consumers' perceived risk and increase their perceived benefit, thereby improving acceptability. Finally, in terms of information design for risk communication, the heterogeneity of consumers should be further researched, such as the responses to distinct information types, and the preferred media channels and trusted stakeholders for obtaining information among different segments of consumers. While it has often called for a balanced introduction to both benefit and risk information about certain GM food, there was evidence showing that consumers also want to get information about the adopted risk control mechanism as well as what is being done to reduce the relevant risk in a transparent manner.[25,107] Moreover, increased stakeholder engagement, which includes the public and applies a multiway approach (e.g., dialog and deliberation), will enable coproduction of effective risk communication.[108] This would be particularly important in a society with low social trust as ignorance of public needs and concerns could further destroy the public trust in regulatory authorities.[109]

Some problems might need to be addressed in future studies. First, the calibration of testing certain constructs may be needed. For example, questions that test objective knowledge about GM food were highly differentiated, and sometimes mixed with questions focused on basic biological knowledge, GM technology in general and specific products, and relevant regulations. This has made it difficult to define the impacts of objective knowledge clearly and needs to be more standardized. In addition, some questions might reflect on consumer attitudes or behaviors rather than objective knowledge, such as using "Have you eaten foods made from GM crops?" to test consumers' knowledge.[52] McPhetres et al.[52] emphasized, in their research, a focus on knowledge about GM technology rather than about benefits or risks in relation to GM food in other studies.[32,43] However, questions or statements used in their survey, such as "What are the current benefits of having foods made from GM crops?" and "GMOs cause more damage to the environment because of the chemicals involved." should be assigned to the measurement of benefit perceptions of the current commercialized GM food and risk perceptions associated with GMOs, respectively, rather than the knowledge about GM technology *per se*. This might partially explain why objective knowledge was such a strong predictor of consumer attitudes towards GM applied in food production in that study. This was also the case for a study investigating the influence of benefit and risk knowledge about GM food, which could be reflections on participants' perceived benefits and risks rather than actual knowledge.[43] Second, the methods used for data collection may create biases and inequalities. At present, the survey is still the dominant method for investigating consumer acceptance of novel agrifood technologies, which sometimes might limit in-depth exploration of key issues, or understanding of causal relationships. Other methods, such as experiments, can be used to complement survey-based studies. Sample representativeness also needs to be considered when trying to generalize findings as subjects in some studies were university students-dominant.[43,52] Third, more inclusive engagement with broader agrifood supply chain stakeholders rather than only consumers should be conducted to investigate diverse perceptions, viewpoints and potential consensus. These must be measured and considered throughout the whole process of technological innovations so as to codevelop more ethically and socially acceptable food technologies and applications.

Endnotes

[a]https://eur-lex.europa.eu/legal-content/EN/TXT/?uri = celex%3A32001L0018 (Accessed 01.07.2022).

[b]https://eur-lex.europa.eu/legal-content/EN/TXT/?uri = celex%3A32009L0041 (Accessed 01.07.2022).

[c]https://eur-lex.europa.eu/legal-content/EN/ALL/?uri = CELEX%3A32003R1830 (Accessed 01.07.2022).

References

1. Brookes G, Barfoot P. Environmental impacts of genetically modified (GM) crop use 1996–2015: impacts on pesticide use and carbon emissions. *GM Crops Food.* 2017;8(2):117–147. Available from: https://doi.org/10.1080/21645698.2017.1309490.
2. Pretty J, Benton TG, Bharucha ZP, et al. Global assessment of agricultural system redesign for sustainable intensification. *Nat Sustain.* 2018;1:441–446. Available from: https://doi.org/10.1038/s41893-018-0114-0.
3. Cardello AV. Consumer concerns and expectations about novel food processing technologies: effects on product liking. *Appetite.* 2003;40(3):217–233. Available from: https://doi.org/10.1016/S0195-6663(03)00008-4.
4. Frewer LJ, Bergmann K, Brennan M, et al. Consumer response to novel agri-food technologies: implications for predicting consumer acceptance of emerging food technologies. *Trends Food Sci Technol.* 2011;22(8):442–456. Available from: https://doi.org/10.1016/j.tifs.2011.05.005.
5. Frewer LJ, van der Lans IA, Fischer ARH, et al. Public perceptions of agri-food applications of genetic modification—a systematic review and *meta*-analysis. *Trends Food Sci Technol.* 2013;30(2):142–152. Available from: https://doi.org/10.1016/j.tifs.2013.01.003.
6. Jin S, Clark B, Kuznesof S, Lin X, Frewer LJ. Synthetic biology applied in the agrifood sector: public perceptions, attitudes and implications for future studies. *Trends Food Sci Technol.* 2019;91:454–466. Available from: https://doi.org/10.1016/j.tifs.2019.07.025.
7. Colwell RK, Norse EA, Pimentel D, Sharples FE, Simberloff D. Genetic engineering in agriculture. *Science.* 1985;229(4709):111–112. Available from: https://doi.org/10.1126/science.229.4709.111.
8. Canton B, Labno A, Endy D. Refinement and standardization of synthetic biological parts and devices. *Nat Biotechnol.* 2008;26:787–793. Available from: https://doi.org/10.1038/nbt1413.
9. European Commission. Synthetic biology applying engineering to biology. Brussels. Retrieved from <https://haseloff.plantsci.cam.ac.uk/resources/SynBio_reports/NEST_syntheticbiology_2005.pdf>; 2005
10. Park S, Peterson FC, Mosquna A, Yao J, Volkman BF, Cutler SR. Agrochemical control of plantwater use using engineered abscisic acid receptors. *Nature.* 2015;520:545–548. Available from: https://doi.org/10.1038/nature14123.
11. Fraser PD, Enfissi EMA, Bramley PM. Genetic engineering of carotenoid formation in tomato fruit and the potential application of systems and synthetic biology approaches. *Arch Biochem Biophysics.* 2009;483(2):196–204. Available from: https://doi.org/10.1016/j.abb.2008.10.009.
12. Nigam PS, Luke JS. Food additives: production of microbial pigments and their antioxidant properties. *Curr OpFood Sci.* 2016;7:93–100. Available from: https://doi.org/10.1016/j.cofs.2016.02.004.
13. Bawa AS, Anilakumar KR. Genetically modified foods: safety, risks and public concerns—a review. *J Food Sci Technol.* 2013;. Available from: https://doi.org/10.1007/s13197-012-0899-1.
14. van Putten MC, Frewer LJ, Gilissen LJWJ, Gremmen B, Peijnenburg AACM, Wichers HJ. Novel foods and food allergies: a review of the issues. *Trends Food Sci Technol.* 2006;17(6):289–299. Available from: https://doi.org/10.1016/j.tifs.2005.11.010.
15. Polizzi, K, Stanbrough, L, Heap, J. A new lease of life, understanding the risks of synthetic biology. London, UK. Retrieved from <https://www.lloyds.com/news-and-risk-insight/risk-reports/library/understanding-risk/a-new-lease-of-life>; 2018.
16. Harvey M, Pilgrim S. The new competition for land: food, energy, and climate change. *Food Policy.* 2011;36(Supplement 1):40–51. Available from: https://doi.org/10.1016/j.foodpol.2010.11.009.
17. Egolf A, Hartmann C, Siegrist M. When evolution works against the future: disgust's contributions to the acceptance of new food technologies. *Risk Anal.* 2019;39(7):1546–1559. Available from: https://doi.org/10.1111/risa.13279.
18. Larson RB. Examining consumer attitudes toward genetically modified and organic foods. *Br Food J.* 2018;120(5):999–1014. Available from: https://doi.org/10.1108/BFJ-09-2017-0502.
19. Pino G, Amatulli C, De Angelis M, Peluso AM. The influence of corporate social responsibility on consumers' attitudes and intentions toward genetically modified foods: evidence from Italy. *J Clean Prod.* 2016;112(4):2861–2869. Available from: https://doi.org/10.1016/j.jclepro.2015.10.008.
20. Popek S, Halagarda M. Genetically modified foods: consumer awareness, opinions and attitudes in selected EU countries. *Int J Consum Stud.* 2017;41(3):325–332. Available from: https://doi.org/10.1111/ijcs.12345.
21. Ancillotti M, Holmberg N, Lindfelt M, Eriksson S. Uncritical and unbalanced coverage of synthetic biology in the Nordic press. *Public Underst Sci.* 2017;26(2):235–250. Available from: https://doi.org/10.1177/0963662515609834.
22. Pauwels E, Lovell A, Rouge E. *Trends in American & European Press Coverage of Synthetic Biology:Tracking the Years 2008–2011.* Washington, D.C: *Woodrow Wilson International Center for Scholars*; 2012, Retrieved from. Available from: http://www.synbioproject.org/publications/why_scientists_should_care/.
23. Betten AW, Broerse JEW, Kupper F. Dynamics of problem setting and framing in citizen discussions on synthetic biology. *Public*

Underst Sci. 2018;27(3):294–309. Available from: https://doi.org/10.1177/0963662517712207.

24. Pauwels E. Review of quantitative and qualitative studies on U.S. public perceptions of synthetic biology. *Syst Synth Biol*. 2009;. Available from: https://doi.org/10.1007/s11693-009-9035-6.
25. Hess S, Lagerkvist CJ, Redekop W, Pakseresht A. Consumers' evaluation of biotechnologically modified food products: new evidence from a *meta*-survey. *Eur Rev Agric Econ*. 2016;43(5):703–736. Available from: https://doi.org/10.1093/erae/jbw011.
26. Costa-Font M, Gil JM, Traill WB. Consumer acceptance, valuation of and attitudes towards genetically modified food: review and implications for food policy. *Food Policy*. 2008;33(2):99–111. Available from: https://doi.org/10.1016/j.foodpol.2007.07.002.
27. Dabrock P. Playing god? Synthetic biology as a theological and ethical challenge. *Syst Synth Biol*. 2009;3(1–4):47–54. Available from: https://doi.org/10.1007/s11693-009-9028-5.
28. Frewer LJ, Howard C, Shepherd R. Public concerns in the united kingdom about general and specific applications of genetic engineering: risk, benefit, and ethics. *Sci Technol Hum Values*. 1997;. Available from: https://doi.org/10.1177/016224399702200105.
29. Gaskell G, Allum N, Wagner W, et al. GM foods and the misperception of risk perception. *Risk Anal*. 2004;24(1):185–194. Available from: https://doi.org/10.1111/j.0272-4332.2004.00421.x.
30. Costa-Font M, Gil JM. Structural equation modelling of consumer acceptance of genetically modified (GM) food in the Mediterranean Europe: a cross country study. *Food Qual Preference*. 2009;20(6):399–409. Available from: https://doi.org/10.1016/j.foodqual.2009.02.011.
31. Bearth A, Siegrist M. Are risk or benefit perceptions more important for public acceptance of innovative food technologies: a *meta*-analysis. *Trends Food Sci Technol*. 2016;49(March):14–23. Available from: https://doi.org/10.1016/j.tifs.2016.01.003.
32. Frewer LJ, Scholderer J, Bredahl L. Communicating about the risks and benefits of genetically modified foods: the mediating role of trust. *Risk Anal*. 2003;23(6):1117–1133. Available from: https://doi.org/10.1111/j.0272-4332.2003.00385.x.
33. Bredahl L. Determinants of consumer attitudes and purchase intentions with regard to genetically modified foods–results of a cross-national survey. *J Consum Policy*. 2001;24:23–61. Available from: https://doi.org/10.1023/A:1010950406128.
34. Scholderer J, Frewer LJ. The biotechnology communication paradox: experimental evidence and the need for a new strategy. *J Consum Policy*. 2003;26(2):125–157. Available from: https://doi.org/10.1023/a:1023695519981.
35. Mucci A, Hough G. Perceptions of genetically modified foods by consumers in Argentina. *Food Qual Preference*. 2004;15(1):43–51. Available from: https://doi.org/10.1016/S0950-3293(03)00021-1.
36. Frewer LJ, Coles D, Houdebine L-M, Kleter GA. Attitudes towards genetically modified animals in food production. *Br Food J*. 2014;116(8):1291–1313. Available from: https://doi.org/10.1108/BFJ-08-2013-0211.
37. Traill WB, Yee WMS, Lusk JL, et al. Perceptions of the risks and benefits of genetically-modified foods and their influence on willingness to consume. *Food Econ - Acta Agric Scand, Sect C*. 2006;3:12–19. Available from: https://doi.org/10.1080/16507540600733900.
38. Zhang Y, Jing L, Bai Q, et al. Application of an integrated framework to examine Chinese consumers' purchase intention toward genetically modified food. *Food Qual Preference*. 2018;65:118–128. Available from: https://doi.org/10.1016/j.foodqual.2017.11.001.
39. Slovic P, Peters E. Risk perception and affect. *Curr Direct Psychol Sci*. 2006;15(6):322–325. Available from: https://doi.org/10.1111/j.1467-8721.2006.00461.x.
40. Siegrist M, Cousin ME, Kastenholz H, Wiek A. Public acceptance of nanotechnology foods and food packaging: the influence of affect and trust. *Appetite*. 2007;49:459–466. Available from: https://doi.org/10.1016/j.appet.2007.03.002.
41. Slovic P, Finucane ML, Peters E, MacGregor DG. Risk as analysis and risk as feelings: some thoughts about affect, reason, risk, and rationality. *Risk Anal*. 2004;24(2):311–321. Available from: https://doi.org/10.1111/j.0272-4332.2004.00433.x.
42. Hu W, Hünnemeyer A, Veeman M, Adamowicz W, Srivastava L. Trading off health, environmental and genetic modification attributes in food. *Eur Rev Agric Econ*. 2004;31(3):389–408. Available from: https://doi.org/10.1093/erae/31.3.389.
43. Zhu X, Xie X. Effects of knowledge on attitude formation and change toward genetically modified foods. *Risk Anal*. 2015;35(5):790–810. Available from: https://doi.org/10.1111/risa.12319.
44. Lusk JL, House LO, Valli C, et al. Effect of information about benefits of biotechnology on consumer acceptance of genetically modified food: evidence from experimental auctions in the United States, England, and France. *Eur Rev Agric Econ*. 2004;31(2):179–204. Available from: https://doi.org/10.1093/erae/31.2.179.
45. Poortinga W, Pidgeon NF. Trust, the asymmetry principle, and the role of prior beliefs. *Risk Anal*. 2004;24(6):1475–1486. Available from: https://doi.org/10.1111/j.0272-4332.2004.00543.x.
46. Savadori L, Savio S, Nicotra E, Rumiati R, Finucane M, Slovic P. Expert and public perception of risk from biotechnology. *Risk Anal*. 2004;24(5):1289–1299. Available from: https://doi.org/10.1111/j.0272-4332.2004.00526.x.
47. House L, Lusk JH, Jaeger S, et al. Objective and subjective knowledge: impacts on consumer demand for genetically modified foods in the United States and the European Union. *Ag Bio Forum*. 2004;7(3):113–123. Available from: http://www.agbioforum.org/.
48. Christoph IB, Bruhn M, Roosen J. Knowledge, attitudes towards and acceptability of genetic modification in Germany. *Appetite*. 2008;51(1):58–68. Available from: https://doi.org/10.1016/j.appet.2007.12.001.
49. Connor M, Siegrist M. Factors influencing people's acceptance of gene technology: the role of knowledge, health expectations, naturalness, and social trust. *Sci Commun*. 2010;32(4):514–538. Available from: https://doi.org/10.1177/1075547009358919.
50. Chen MF, Li HL. The consumer's attitude toward genetically modified foods in Taiwan. *Food Qual Preference*. 2007;18(4):662–674. Available from: https://doi.org/10.1016/j.foodqual.2006.10.002.
51. Klerck D, Sweeney JC. The effect of knowledge types on consumer-perceived risk and adoption of genetically modified foods. *Psychol Mark*. 2007;24(2):171–193. Available from: https://doi.org/10.1002/mar.20157.
52. McPhetres J, Rutjens BT, Weinstein N, Brisson JA. Modifying attitudes about modified foods: increased knowledge leads to more positive attitudes. *J Environ Psychol*. 2019;64:21–29. Available from: https://doi.org/10.1016/j.jenvp.2019.04.012.

53. Mielby H, Sandøe P, Lassen J. The role of scientific knowledge in shaping public attitudes to GM technologies. *Public Underst Sci.* 2013;22(2):155–168. Available from: https://doi.org/10.1177/0963662511430577.
54. Olofsson A, Öhman S, Rashid S. Attitudes to gene technology: the significance of trust in institutions. *Eur Societies.* 2006;8(4): 601–624. Available from: https://doi.org/10.1080/14616690601002707.
55. Siegrist M. The influence of trust and perceptions of risks and benefits on the acceptance of gene technology. *Risk Anal.* 2000;20(2): 195–204. Available from: https://doi.org/10.1111/0272-4332.202020.
56. Marques MD, Critchley CR, Walshe J. Attitudes to genetically modified food over time: how trust in organizations and the media cycle predict support. *Public Underst Sci.* 2015;24(5):601–618. Available from: https://doi.org/10.1177/0963662514542372.
57. Eiser JR, Miles S, Frewer LJ. Trust, perceived risk, and attitudes toward food technologies. *J Appl Soc Psychol.* 2002;32(11): 2423–2433. Available from: https://doi.org/10.1111/j.1559-1816.2002.tb01871.x.
58. Poortinga W, Pidgeon NF. Trust in risk regulation: cause or consequence of the acceptability of GM food? *Risk Anal.* 2005;25 (1):199–209. Available from: https://doi.org/10.1111/j.0272-4332.2005.00579.x.
59. Liu R, Pieniak Z, Verbeke W. Food-related hazards in China: consumers' perceptions of risk and trust in information sources. *Food Control.* 2014;46:291–298. Available from: https://doi.org/10.1016/j.foodcont.2014.05.033.
60. Ganiere P, Chern WS, Hahn D. A continuum of consumer attitudes toward genetically modified foods in the United States. *J Agric Resour Econ.* 2006;31(1):129–149. Available from: https://doi.org/10.2307/40987310.
61. Kimenju SC, De Groote H. Consumer willingness to pay for genetically modified food in Kenya. *Agric Econ.* 2008;38(1):35–46. Available from: https://doi.org/10.1111/j.1574-0862.2007.00279.x.
62. Braman D, Mandel GN, Kahan DM. Cultural cognition and synthetic biology risk perceptions: a preliminary analysis. *GW Law Faculty Publ Other Work.* 2008;282. Available from: https://doi.org/10.2139/ssrn.1264804.
63. Finucane ML, Slovic P, Mertz CK, Flynn J, Satterfield TA. Gender, race, and perceived risk: the 'white male' effect. *Health Risk Soc.* 2000;2(2):159–172. Available from: https://doi.org/10.1080/713670162.
64. Akin H, Rose KM, Scheufele DA, et al. Mapping the landscape of public attitudes on synthetic biology. *BioScience.* 2017;67 (3):290–300. Available from: https://doi.org/10.1093/biosci/biw171.
65. Verdurme A, Viaene J. Consumer beliefs and attitude towards genetically modified food: basis for segmentation and implications for communication. *Agribusiness.* 2003;19(1):91–113. Available from: https://doi.org/10.1002/agr.10045.
66. Frewer LJ, Howard C, Shepherd R. Effective communication about genetic engineering and food. *Br Food J.* 1996;98(4/5):48–52. Available from: https://doi.org/10.1108/00070709610119883.
67. Kahan DM, Braman D, Mandel GN. Risk and culture: is synthetic biology different? Harvard Law School Program on Risk Regulation Research Paper No. 09-2; Yale Law School, Public Law Working Paper No. 190. <https://doi.org/10.2139/ssrn.1347165>; 2009.
68. Vidigal MCTR, Minim VPR, Simiqueli AA, Souza PHP, Balbino DF, Minim LA. Food technology neophobia and consumer attitudes toward foods produced by new and conventional technologies: a case study in Brazil. *LWT - Food Sci Technol.* 2015;60(2):832–840. Available from: https://doi.org/10.1016/j.lwt.2014.10.058.
69. Siegrist M. Belief in gene technology: the influence of environmental attitudes and gender. *Personal Individ Differ.* 1998;24 (6):861–866. Available from: https://doi.org/10.1016/S0191-8869(98)00021-X.
70. Costa-Font J, Mossialos E, Rudisill C. Are feelings of genetically modified food politically driven? *Risk Manag.* 2008;10:218–234. Available from: https://doi.org/10.1057/rm.2008.5.
71. Lin W, Ortega DL, Caputo V, Lusk JL. Personality traits and consumer acceptance of controversial food technology: a cross-country investigation of genetically modified animal products. *Food Qual Preference.* 2019;76:10–19. Available from: https://doi.org/10.1016/j.foodqual.2019.03.007.
72. Vilella-Vila M, Costa-Font J. Press media reporting effects on risk perceptions and attitudes towards genetically modified (GM) food. *J Socio-Econ.* 2008;37(5):2095–2106. Available from: https://doi.org/10.1016/j.socec.2008.04.006.
73. Brosig S, Bavorova M. Association of attitudes towards genetically modified food among young adults and their referent persons. *PLoS One.* 2019;14(2):e0211879. Available from: https://doi.org/10.1371/journal.pone.0211879.
74. Finucane ML, Holup JL. Psychosocial and cultural factors affecting the perceived risk of genetically modified food: an overview of the literature. *Soc Sci Med.* 2005;60(7):1603–1612. Available from: https://doi.org/10.1016/j.socscimed.2004.08.007.
75. Frewer LJ, Miles S, Marsh R. The media and genetically modified foods: evidence in support of social amplification of risk. *Risk Anal.* 2002;22(4):701–711. Available from: https://doi.org/10.1111/0272-4332.00062.
76. Kasperson RE, Renn O, Slovic P, et al. The social amplification of risk: a conceptual framework. *Risk Anal.* 1988;8(2):177–187. Available from: https://doi.org/10.1111/j.1539-6924.1988.tb01168.x.
77. Gillon R. Medical ethics: four principles plus attetion to scope. *Br Med J.* 1994;309(6948):184–188. Retrieved from https://search.proquest.com/docview/1777514508/fulltextPDF/72E6BD468A674508PQ/1?accountid = 14620%0Ahttp://www.jstor.org.login.ezproxy.library.ualberta.ca/stable/pdf/29724194.pdf?refreqid = excelsior%3Aa520b0d86c2f17d1825f7eaf62b05c30.
78. Kaiser M, Millar K, Thorstensen E, Tomkins S. Developing the Ethical Matrix as a decision support framework: GM fish as a case study. *J Agric Environ Ethics.* 2007;20(1):65–80. Available from: https://doi.org/10.1007/s10806-006-9023-8.
79. Mepham B. A framework for the ethical analysis of novel foods: the ethical matrix. *J Agric Environ Ethics.* 2000;12(2):165–176. Available from: https://doi.org/10.1023/A:1009542714497.
80. Newson A. Synthetic biology: ethics, exeptionalism and expectations. *Macquarie Law J.* 2015;15:45–58, Retrieved from. Available from: http://content.ebscohost.com/ContentServer.asp?T = P&P = AN&K = 108715935&S = R&D = ofs&EbscoContent = dGJyMNLe80SeprM4zdnyOLCmr0%2BeqK9Sr664Sa%2BWxWXS&ContentCustomer = dGJyMPGpt02xr65LuePfgeyx43zx.
81. Parens E, Johnston J, Moses J. Do we need 'synthetic bioethics'? *Science.* 2008. Available from: https://doi.org/10.1126/science.1163821.

82. Coles D, Frewer LJ. Nanotechnology applied to European food production—a review of ethical and regulatory issues. *Trends Food Sci Technol*. 2013;34(1):32–43. Available from: https://doi.org/10.1016/j.tifs.2013.08.006.
83. Coles D, Frewer LJ, Goddard E. Ethical Issues and potential stakeholder priorities associated with the application of genomic technologies applied to animal production systems. *J Agric Environ Ethics*. 2015;28:231–253. Available from: https://doi.org/10.1007/s10806-015-9529-z.
84. Jin S, Clark B, Li W, Kuznesof S, Frewer LJ. Social dimensions of synthetic biology in the agrifood sector: the perspective of Chinese and EU scientists. *British Food Journal*. 2021;123 (12):4135–4154. Available from: https://doi.org/10.1108/BFJ-12-2020-1142.
85. Thompson PB. The roles of ethics in gene drive research and governance. *J Responsible Innov*. 2018;5(51):S159–S179. Available from: https://doi.org/10.1080/23299460.2017.1415587.
86. Tenbült P, De Vries NK, Dreezens E, Martijn C. Perceived naturalness and acceptance of genetically modified food. *Appetite*. 2005; 45(1):47–50. Available from: https://doi.org/10.1016/j.appet.2005.03.004.
87. Chen Y, Yin Z, Shao Z, Xie Q. The defence of artificial life by synthetic biology from ethical and social aspects. *J Coll Physicians Surg Pak*. 2015;25(7):519–524, Retrieved from. Available from: http://www.scopus.com/inward/record.url?eid = 2-s2.0-84938083514&partnerID = 40&md5 = ade46820b271b2e1a7706e5cc90c1d68.
88. Fredens J, Wang K, de la Torre D, et al. Total synthesis of *Escherichia coli* with a recoded genome. *Nature*. 2019;569:514–518. Available from: https://doi.org/10.1038/s41586-019-1192-5.
89. Häyry M. Synthetic biology and ethics: past, present, and future. *Camb Q Healthc Ethics*. 2017;26(2):186–205. Available from: https://doi.org/10.1017/S0963180116000803.
90. Heavey P. Synthetic biology: the response of the commission of the (Catholic) bishops' conferences of the European community. *Camb Q Healthc Ethics*. 2017;26(2):257–266. Available from: https://doi.org/10.1017/S0963180116000852.
91. Dragojlovic N, Einsiedel E. Playing God or just unnatural? Religious beliefs and approval of synthetic biology. *Public Underst Sci*. 2012;22(7):869–885. Available from: https://doi.org/10.1177/0963662512445011.
92. Miles S, Frewer LJ. Investigating specific concerns about different food hazards. *Food Qual Preference*. 2001;12(1):47–61. Available from: https://doi.org/10.1016/S0950-3293(00)00029-X.
93. Rogers W. Ethical issues in synthetic biology: a commentary. *MacQuire Law J*. 2011;2011–2016, Retrieved from. Available from: https://www.mq.edu.au/__data/assets/pdf_file/0020/213761/mlj_2015_rogers.pdf.
94. Vilella-Vila M, Costa-Font J, Mossialos E. Consumer involvement and acceptance of biotechnology in the European Union: a specific focus on Spain and the UK. *Int J Consum Stud*. 2005;29 (2):108–118. Available from: https://doi.org/10.1111/j.1470-6431.2004.00425.x.
95. Breeman G, Giest S, Rimkutė D. Food security and the sustainability of GMOs in the United States and the European Union. *Adv Food Security Sust*. 2017;2:165–193. Available from: https://doi.org/10.1016/bs.af2s.2017.09.005.
96. European Food Safety Authority. Risk assessment of the genetically modified microorganism 'Arsenic Biosensor', a derivative of *Bacillus subtilis* 168 trpC2, for the purpose of its inclusion in Part C Annex II of Council Directive. Retrieved from <https://www.efsa.europa.eu/en/supporting/pub/en-917>; 2015.
97. Library of Congress. Restrictions on genetically modified organisms, United States. Retrieved from <https://www.loc.gov/law/help/restrictions-on-gmos/usa.php#_ftn1>; 2014.
98. USDA. National bioengineered food disclosure standard. Retrieved from <https://www.federalregister.gov/documents/2018/12/21/2018-27283/national-bioengineered-food-disclosure-standard>; 2018.
99. Huffman WE, Shogren JF, Rousu M, Tegene A. Consumer willingness to pay for genetically modified food labels in a market with diverse information: evidence from experimental auctions. *J Agric Resour Econ*. 2003;28(3):481–502. Available from: https://doi.org/10.2307/40987963.
100. Kolodinsky J, Lusk JL. Mandatory labels can improve attitudes toward genetically engineered food. *Sci Adv*. 2018;4(6):eaaq1413. Available from: https://doi.org/10.1126/sciadv.aaq1413.
101. Hu W, Veeman MM, Adamowicz WL. Labelling genetically modified food: heterogeneous consumer preferences and the value of information. *Can J Agric Econ*. 2005;53(1):83–102. Available from: https://doi.org/10.1111/j.1744-7976.2005.04004.x.
102. Zhao L, Gu H, Yue C, Ahlstrom D. Consumer welfare and GM food labeling: a simulation using an adjusted Kumaraswamy distribution. *Food Policy*. 2013;42:58–70. Available from: https://doi.org/10.1016/j.foodpol.2013.06.006.
103. Siegrist M, Cvetkovich G. Perception of hazards: the role of social trust and knowledge. *Risk Anal*. 2000;20(5):713–719. Available from: https://doi.org/10.1111/0272-4332.205064.
104. Magnusson MK, Koivisto Hursti U-K. Consumer attitudes towards genetically modified foods. *Appetite*. 2002;39(1):9–24. Available from: https://doi.org/10.1006/appe.2002.0486.
105. Frewer LJ. Societal issues and public attitudes towards genetically modified foods. *Trends Food Sci Technol*. 2003;14(5–8): 319–332. Available from: https://doi.org/10.1016/S0924-2244(03)00064-5.
106. Fischer ARH, Frewer LJ. Consumer familiarity with foods and the perception of risks and benefits. *Food Qual Preference*. 2009;20(8):576–585. Available from: https://doi.org/10.1016/j.foodqual.2009.06.008.
107. Frewer LJ, Miles S, Brennan M, Kuznesof S, Ness M, Ritson C. Public preferences for informed choice under conditions of risk uncertainty. *Public Underst Sci*. 2002;11(4):363–372. Available from: https://doi.org/10.1088/0963-6625/11/4/304.
108. Pidgeon N. Engaging publics about environmental and technology risks: frames, values and deliberation. *J Risk Res*. 2020;1–19. Available from: https://doi.org/10.1080/13669877.2020.1749118.
109. Bier VM. On the state of the art: risk communication to the public. *Reliab Eng Syst Saf*. 2001;71:139–150. Available from: https://doi.org/10.1016/S0951-8320(00)00090-9.

Section XII

New and emerging foods and technologies

Chapter 66

Safety, nutrition and sustainability of plant-based meat alternatives

Jane M. Caldwell[1] and E.N. Clare Mills[2]

[1]*Caldwell Food Safety LLC, Springfield, MO, United States,* [2]*Division of Immunity, Infection and Respiratory Medicine, School of Biological Sciences, Manchester Academic Health Sciences Centre, Manchester Institute of Biotechnology, Manchester, United Kingdom*

Abstract

Plant-based meat alternatives (PBMA) are a rapidly growing and much publicized segment of the processed food industry due to affluent consumer's desire for sustainable nonmeat choices to help reduce the carbon emissions, animal welfare concerns, and land usage required by traditional meat and poultry production. Formulations of PBMA are complex and require the use of many ingredients, further processing, and occasionally, genetically engineered components. The end goal is to emulate animal meat in organoleptic properties and nutritional content at a similar price point. Challenges for development include antinutrients, off-flavors, sensory attributes, novel allergens, bioavailability of nutrients, and identifying necessary microbial and chemical testing. Long-term effects of a diet based on PBMA will need to be evaluated. PBMA have the potential to disrupt traditional protein sources by supplying products which are more environmentally friendly, cause no harm to animals, and are cost-effective.

Keywords: Plant-based meat alternatives; ultra-processed foods; protein isolates; bioavailability; allergens; sustainability; GMOs; antinutrients; extrusion; formulations

66.1 Introduction

Plant-based meat alternatives (PBMA) are targeting vegetarians and flexitarians who want to eliminate or reduce their consumption of meat but still crave the texture, mouthfeel, and feeling of satiety provided by the consumption of animal-derived foods. Many startups and traditional meat producers are entering the market which is predicted to reach over US$21 billion globally by 2025.[1] These novel foods are attracting significant investment and media attention as they are marketed as healthier and more sustainable than animal meat. Beyond Meat, Gardein, and Impossible Foods are three of the most visible new manufacturers. Tyson, Smithfield, Perdue Farms, Hormel Foods, and Maple Leaf are traditional meat and poultry producers who have also entered this burgeoning market.[2] This chapter will cover PBMA only, excluding in vitro or laboratory cultured meats and older technologies which use commercially grown fungi mycelia such as Quorn.[3]

66.2 Formulation

PBMA have complicated formulations and are "ultra-processed" according to the NOVA food classification system.[4] Ultra-processed foods are those manufactured with little or no whole foods.[5] They contain processed ingredients such as protein isolates, hydrogenated oils and fats, flours, starches, sugar variants, refined carbohydrates, and other value-added ingredients.[6] PBMA buck the current trend in North America where consumers will pay a premium for minimally processed foods with few ingredients.[5] Sha and Xiong[2] detailed the ingredients used in some formulations. This section summarizes their article.

To achieve the desired sensory characteristics of meat, PBMA formulations combine plant protein sources with binders and additives. Soy protein, pea protein, and wheat gluten are the most commonly used plant protein alternatives. However, other plant proteins are utilized to provide structural and nutritional properties. Prepared by aqueous alcohol washing, the widely used textured vegetable protein is comprised most commonly of soy protein concentrate. Wheat gluten is often used to create meat-like chewiness. Potato, mung bean, and rice proteins may also be incorporated to enhance and alter texture. These plant protein sources add amino acids complementary to those in legumes, to create a nutritionally balanced amino acid profile. The ultimate formulation goal is to combine plant proteins which bind together to simulate the interstitial spaces between meat muscle myofilaments. These myofilaments

Present Knowledge in Food Safety. DOI: https://doi.org/10.1016/B978-0-12-819470-6.00063-9

trap and retain water, which is released during chewing to create the sensation of juiciness.

Oils and fats are also used to create mouthfeel and faux marbling similar to animal fat. Plant fats, such as those extracted from coconut and cocoa beans, are solid at room temperature. They are often blended with oils which are liquid at room temperature, such as sunflower, canola, sesame, and avocado oils for nutritional as well as flavor purposes. To further bind water and reduce syneresis, carbohydrate polymers are added. These include crude fibers from wheat, oat, apple, digestible starch, and purified polysaccharides.

Many additives are used in PBMA, and their labels may contain more than 20 listed ingredients. These products contain more ingredients and additives for flavoring, coloring, and binding agents than meats.[5] Leghemoglobin, a heme and pigment-containing protein expressed in soybean root nodules, has been genetically engineered for production in yeast cultures. Leghemoglobin may be used at a level of up to 0.8% of a product's final weight to simulate the bloody appearance of meat. Red and orange pigments from red beets, red cabbage, berries, paprika, and carrots are also used. A United States generally recognized as safe (GRAS) colorant, titanium dioxide, is used in plant-based chicken as a whitener and brightener. This ingredient will need to be reexamined as the European Food Safety Authority (EFSA) has updated its safety assessment on titanium dioxide and no longer considers it safe as a food additive.[7] To compensate for lack of flavor, yeast extracts, nucleotides, sugars, and spices are added. They may also be used to mask undesirable beany off-flavors. Vitamins and minerals are added to fortify and make up for the deficiencies in plant matrices as compared with meat. Antioxidants are added to reduce the oxidation and rancidity caused by high-temperature processing. Organic acids and phosphate compounds are added to improve microbial stability and shelf-life. Consumers desiring clean labels or short ingredient lists may object to PBMA due to the many additives on the labels or the inclusion of a genetically modified (GM) protein.

66.3 Processing

Most PBMA are processed using extrusion, a high-temperature and high-pressure method which creates the desired form and texture while simultaneously reducing the microbial load. Extrusion is considered a time-temperature treatment and a critical control point which promotes the safety and shelf-life of the product. Other processing methods such as shear cells and spinning are used to create meat-like fibrous structures.[8] Shear cell technology, like extrusion, also uses high heat to form fibrous structures to mimic meat. There are two types of spinning processes, wet spinning and electrospinning.[8] In wet spinning a viscous solution is pushed through a spinneret, a cap or plate containing small holes, producing stretched and aligned fibers.[8] The fibers are then solidified in a coagulation bath containing salts, acids or alkali solutions. This creates a large waste stream for manufacturers, so electrospinning is the more attractive option.[8] In electrospinning, high voltage produces the fibers from the viscous solution. Electrospraying is another form of electrospinning in which the polymer solution is sprayed from a nozzle.[8] Extrusion is still the preferred method since soy proteins have complex secondary and tertiary structures which are difficult to electrospin without carriers such as plastics or animal-based ingredients such as gelatin.[8]

Carcinogens produced by high temperature processing have not been studied in PBMA. Carcinogenic compounds such as polycyclic aromatic hydrocarbons, nitrosamines, and heterocyclic aromatic amines, found in meats cooked at high temperature, may also occur in PBMA.[9]

66.4 Microbial Safety and Testing

Published research concerning safety, shelf-life, and long-term nutritional and health effects of PBMA is limited. Companies developing these products and organizations promoting them have funded much of the available research so it is not always in the public domain.[10] With a few exceptions, PBMA are based on food ingredients that are GRAS for human consumption. PBMA are high-moisture foods and include ready-to-eat and raw products.[2] Therefore microbial safety, storage conditions, shelf-life, and lipid oxidation should be studied with an eye to postprocessing handling.[2]

PBMA have near-neutral pH, relatively low salt and high protein moisture content making them susceptible to microbial growth.[11] In a study assessing microbial communities in vegetarian, vegan, and insect imitations of meat products, bacterial counts were relatively low but wide-ranging (<2.0–8.7 log CFU/g).[12] In the same study, 426 bacterial isolates were identified using radiolabeled oligonucleotide $(GTG)_5$-polymerase chain reaction (PCR) fingerprinting. The isolates from the vegetarian and vegan meat substitutes consisted primarily of *Lactobacillus sakei*, *Enterococcus faecium*, and *Carnobacterium divergens*. The insect-derived products contained not only *E. faecium*, but *Macrococcus caseolyticus* and *Cronobacter sakazakii*. The authors concluded that the relatively high levels of enterococci indicated that food safety was a concern for these products due to potential virulence factors, possible infections, antibiotic resistance, and gene transfer associated with *E. faecium*.[12]

Wild et al.[11] evaluated the microbial load of a PBMA. Products which were exposed to the high temperatures of the extrusion process averaged less than 100 CFU/g total microbial load (methods and specific microorganisms were not cited). However, the researchers felt the products were susceptible to postprocessing contamination. Therefore they recommended that further thermal treatments and refrigerated storage be instituted postextrusion to increase the safety and shelf-life of the products. They also stated that: "The storage and handling of these products should mimic that of raw meats." While not evaluated in the study, they suggested that endospores such as *Bacillus* spp. and *Clostridium* spp. may survive the extrusion process. Risks with high bioburdens of raw materials have been reported in retort processing of meat analogs containing textured soy protein and wheat gluten[13] and a procedure to quantify spore destruction in extruded plant foods is not available.[14] Unfortunately, spores can be reactivated in other posttreatment steps for PBMA.[8] Postprocessing contamination can occur during packaging in a nonaseptic environment and with the addition of nonsterilized flavor ingredients such as spices, herbs, and marinades.[8,15]

Diagnostic tests for screening of pathogens must be validated by kit manufacturers and organizations such as AOAC International. Erin Crowley, president of AOAC International, stated: "Matrix extension of current claims as well as verification of these new products should be analyzed to hasten the determination of fit for purpose methods in the evaluation of plant-based meat alternatives. This is a great opportunity for AOAC to identify unmet needs in the food industry." She said lessons learned from evaluation of cannabis products should be applied to develop guidance for other novel food commodities, such as PBMA. Kit manufacturers for food and pet food molecular screening tests have begun extending matrices for verification. The Hygiena Company recently demonstrated that the BAX systems for detection of *Salmonella* and *Listeria monocytogenes* in PBMA are equivalent to the Food and Drug Administration Bacteriological Analytical Manual (FDA BAM) method.[16] Third-party analytical laboratories can also verify and extend matrices but these data are considered the intellectual property of those organizations and are not publicly shared.

One academic study noted that the appearance of PBMA in the marketplace was ahead of US FDA matrix extension verification procedure (Section 5.1.1) for *Salmonella* BAM.[17] To remedy this, the efficacy of three preenrichment broths (lactose, universal preenrichment and buffered peptone water) were evaluated for the detection of *Salmonella* in five plant-based burger (PBB) products.[17] Each product type was spiked with either *Salmonella enteritidis* or *Salmonella agona* with <30 CFU per 25 g sample. Additionally, seven negative control replicates were tested with all broths. Pathogen recovery was evaluated with *Salmonella* BAM Chapter 5 or quantitative PCR molecular methods. Final results found no significant difference between the effectiveness of each broth. However, the greatest level of detection was found with lactose broth at 95.7%.[17] The study demonstrated that lactose broth, the current BAM recommended preenrichment broth, was effective for the detection of *Salmonella* in PBMA. At the time of publication, this was the only academic peer-reviewed article found extending pathogen testing to PBMA matrices. With new companies entering the market almost on a daily basis, more disinterested third-party testing needs to occur to guarantee the safety of novel PBMA.

66.5 Allergens

Soybean and wheat are two of the "big eight" allergenic foods identified and codified by the US FDA. Wheat is associated with gluten sensitivities in the form of celiac disease in <1% of the US population. Allergenicity has been associated with legume crops such as chickpeas and peas.[18] AllergenOnline[19] is an interactive website that provides allergen lists and a searchable database for the identification of potential allergens in novel proteins or food varieties. Because many PBMA contain concentrated protein isolates, consumers may receive much higher doses of potential allergens. Dr. Goodman, Research Professor at the University of Nebraska – Lincoln, cautions that with more than 2000 proteins recognized as allergens, it is hard to predict the effects of regular consumption of higher protein concentrations, new processing methods which may alter and combine proteins, and the consumption of proteins from novel sources. Consumers with known allergies should read the labels and pay attention to the source of the plant proteins. Many consumers avoid gluten and seek products which are gluten-free. Research studies using zein, a nongluten protein from maize, are underway to replace wheat gluten in formulations.[20]

66.6 Allergenicity risk assessment of alternative proteins

The need to assess the allergenicity of novel foods has emerged in 1990s as the application of transgenesis for crop improvement emerged and expression of a Brazil nut allergen in soybean to improve its nutritional value was found to pose a risk of causing allergic reactions in individuals with IgE (immunoglobulin E)-allergies to Brazil nut.[21] This leads to the development of an internationally recognized approach for assessing the allergenic risks posed by GM crops using transgenesis which was also applied to novel foods.[22] Although initially a decision tree approach was suggested risk assessments are now generally undertaken in an integrative manner drawing on data on a number of different aspects (Fig. 66.1). An early example of a novel food protein allergenicity risk assessment is that of the ice-structuring protein (ISP) identified in ocean pout (*Macrozoarces americanus*) and can be

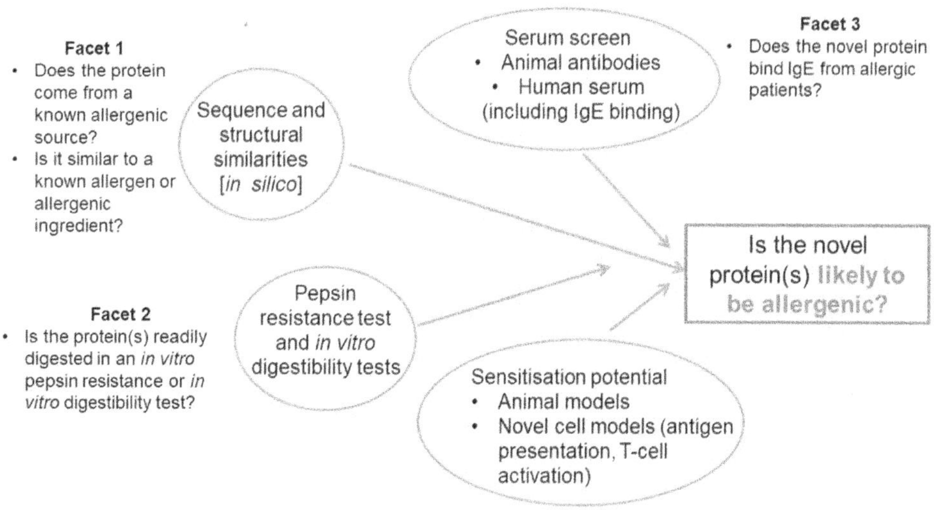

FIGURE 66.1 A weight-of-evidence integrative approach to allergenicity risk assessment.

used to illustrate the approach in practice. The protein binds to ice and structures ice crystal formation, a property which led to its being developed as a processing aid in ice cream manufacture. The different facets of the risk assessment process for the ISP can be summarized as follows:

Facet 1: Does the protein or ingredient come from a known allergenic source? Is it similar to a known allergen or allergenic ingredient? Since the protein originated from a food source that was already considered to be allergenic an initial assessment was performed by comparing the sequence of the protein with known allergens using both a global and local alignment approach. This is done on the basis that if part of the amino acid sequence of a novel protein resembled that of a known allergen and was long enough to contain either B-cell or T-cell epitopes there is an increase likelihood that it would be recognized by the immune system of an allergic individual. The global alignment identified a short region of 10 amino acid residues (i.e., long enough to contain a T-cell epitope) in ISP which had 63% sequence similarity with 10 amino acid regions showing in a superoxide dismutase allergen from *Aspergillus fumigatus*, Asp f6. However, no similarity across the entire protein sequence was identified.[23]

Facet 2: Is it readily digested in an in vitro pepsin resistance test? Subsequently the resistance of the protein to digestion to pepsin, an approach which had been developed for allergenicity risk assessment of GM crops.[24] Using a combination of gel-based methods and mass spectrometry the ISP and a recombinant version of the protein produced in yeast were shown to be rapidly digested with a half-life of less than 6 min, further indicating a lower likelihood of causing an allergic reaction in a sensitized individual.[23,25]

Facet 3: Does the novel protein bind IgE from allergic patients? An investigation of serum IgE-binding using a panel of fish allergic individuals confirmed the lack of IgE-reactivity by the ISP.[25]

Based on such data ISP has GRAS status in the United States and in Europe the EFSA stated in 2008 that ISP was unlikely to cause an allergic reaction in the fish allergic population.[26] Since that time the EFSA allergenicity risk assessment guidance has been further elaborated and addresses both the risk of sensitization and risk posed to the existing allergic population.[27] It has also been broadened to include aspects relating to non-IgE-mediated food allergies.[28,29] More recent novel foods applications relate to complex food ingredients comprising a mixture of proteins, such as oil seed rape powder and meal worm flour, which means some of the methodology developed for single protein molecules needs to be adapted. This is especially true of the bioinformatic assessment since although a host of informatic tools have been developed to support allergenicity prediction,[30,31] they have been designed for assessing allergenic potential of a single type of protein. Their application to whole food ingredients is complex since there are gaps in data on the genome and proteome of the new ingredients.[32] Furthermore in silico methods rely on having access to well-curated sequences of allergens and nonallergenic proteins to train algorithms but there are well-defined deficiencies in many of these databases which are often unfunded academic initiatives.[33] In silico tools are imperfect and consequently other tools and methods, including IgE binding studies, are still required as part of the integrative risk assessment process. This extends to in vitro digestibility tests and it will be important to benchmark those used for allergenicity risk assessment designed for use with purified proteins molecules[34,35] against those developed for analysis of whole foods which are also used to assess nutritional quality.[36–38] The lack of an effective animal model for food allergy also hampers assessment of de novo sensitization and a range of cell-based models are being developed although this work is also hampered by a lack of consensus as to what allergenic comparators should be used, making this part of the risk assessment process uncertain.[39] Thus much remains to be done to improve the quality of the allergenicity risk assessment process.[40]

For example, the seeds of oilseed rape (*Brassica napus*) have previously been shown to be allergenic[41] with a high level of sequence similarity to the European priority food allergen mustard (*Brassica sinapis*, *Brassica nigra*).[42] Consequently, although EFSA considered two oil seed rape ingredients to be safe to consume, the issues of allergies were highlighted and that it was likely to cause reactions in mustard allergic subjects.[43,44] This was consequently addressed by requiring a precautionary label to be used on foods using oil seed rape powder in the European Union: "this ingredient may cause allergic reaction to consumers who are allergic to mustard and products thereof." However, such precautionary allergen labeling has not been well received by the clinical community as the view is that the cross-reactivity between oils seed rape and mustard allergies is not proven and that such "type II" precautionary allergen labeling should be avoided.[45] It is evident that insect proteins pose a similar issue, with meal worm flour having been shown to cause allergic reaction during oral food challenge in shrimp-allergic subjects[46] reflecting the high levels of relatedness between crustacean shellfish allergens and those in insects.[47,48] A recent EFSA opinion on mealworm flour also acknowledged its likelihood of causing de novo sensitization but nevertheless concluded it was generally safe to consume.[49] Given such uncertainties over the allergenicity risk assessment process there is an urgent need to address the need for effective postmarket surveillance which would demonstrate the effectiveness or the allergenicity risk assessment process and any management decisions that results, such as the use of advisory labels.[50]

Despite such difficulties and challenges the risk assessment processes do provide some levels of assurance and it is notable that novel proteins, such as ISP, have not caused allergenicity risks after being introduced into the market. Similarly other, more complex novel ingredients, such as the widely consumed fungal protein source *Fusarium venenatum* used in the manufacture of Quorn, have only one case report of allergy in the literature to date[51] (Fig. 66.1).

66.7 Contaminants, chemicals, and GMOs

Contaminants of concern that have not been widely studied in PBMA are heavy metals, pesticides,[9] and aflatoxins. Concerning occupational health, the chemicals hexane or ethanol are used in processing soy protein isolates. Consumer advocacy groups are concerned about the use of hexane as it is a neurotoxin, highly explosive, and an air pollutant.[10] Although evaluated for safety and unlikely to cause adverse reactions, some PBMA contain the genetically engineered protein, leghemoglobin, which certain consumers may wish to avoid. A study conducted by Impossible Foods, a PBMA manufacturer, evaluated soy leghemoglobin protein, which is used for coloration, flavoring, and bloody exudate-appearance in PBMA and found no toxicological issues.[52] Systemic toxicity was assessed in a 28-day dietary study in male and female Sprague Dawley rats fed leghemoglobin levels 100 times greater than the 90th percentile estimated daily intake. There were no mortalities observed, no effects on male reproduction, nor adverse clinical findings related to leghemoglobin consumption. A potential estrous cycle distribution effect in female rats warranted a second dietary study, which found that leghemoglobin-fed female reproductive parameters were comparable to controls. Studies with heme iron from soybean root nodules, leghemoglobin, have shown iron bioavailability similar to bovine hemoglobin using an in vitro Caco-2 cell culture model.[53]

66.8 Antinutrients and off-flavors

Legume seeds contain protein inhibitors which are antinutritional in effect when consumed. These include inhibitors of alpha-amylase and trypsin, enzymes which hasten carbohydrate and protein digestion in mammals.[18] Trypsin inhibitors in soy protein isolates could be lowered through ultra-high-temperature pretreatment at 143°C–154°C.[54] Phytic acids, also present in these plant seeds, can reduce the bioavailability of minerals through the formation of indigestible salts. This can cause mineral deficiency in humans.[18] Antinutrients such as phytic acid could be treated with phytase to reduce the content as much as 800-fold.[55] Iron absorption from soy protein isolates was increased four- to fivefold when phytic acid was reduced enzymatically. However, iron absorption was still only half that of the egg white control. Therefore other factors must contribute to the poor iron availability in soy protein isolates.[55] High calcium may reduce iron absorption when consumed from the same food and high sodium and potassium levels may increase mineral loss through urination.[56,57] The use of lower salt marinades has been suggested as a means of enhancing the water-holding capacity of PBMA while reducing the sodium content.[58]

Strong off-flavors are produced during processing of plant materials and include grassy and beany flavors from soybeans due to endogenous lipoxygenases. There are also bitter and astringent flavors from saponins and isoflavones, which are both antinutritional and anticarcinogenic.[18] PBMA formulations are created to mask and reduce the potency of these off-flavors. Fermentations with *Lactobacillus*, *Lactococcus*, and *Streptococcus* bacteria species, yeasts, and fungi such as *Aspergillus* and *Rhizopus* should be a future strategy, not only to remove or mask off-flavors but to produce meaty aromas and flavors.[59]

66.9 Nutritional comparisons

PBMA have been formulated to mimic meat both in sensory and nutritional characteristics. Naturally present and supplemental nutrients which are heat sensitive can be destroyed or reduced due to vigorous processing methods such as high temperature extrusion. This raises the question of whether they are equal nutritionally to animal meat and can be used as replacements, especially concerning at-risk groups such as pregnant women, children, the elderly, and those with metabolic impairments. In 2021 several peer-reviewed articles compared the nutritional components of animals meats versus PBMA. In a metabolomic study, 4 oz patties of grass-fed beef ($n = 18$) and PBMA ($n = 18$) were cooked in a nonstick skillet, core samples obtained then stored at $-80°C$ until analysis.[60] Metabolites were characterized by gas chromatograph-mass spectrophotometry analysis.[60] Despite very similar Nutrition Facts panels (Fig. 66.2A)[60] and being matched for serving size (4 oz)

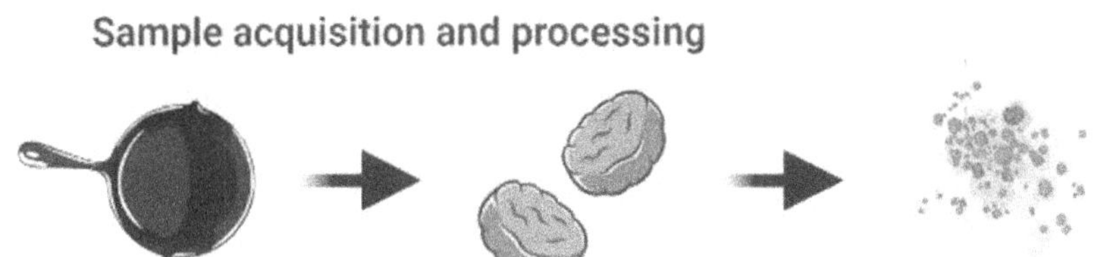

Ground Beef

Nutrition Facts

Serving size	(113g)
Amount Per Serving **Calories**	**220**
	% Daily Value*
Total Fat 14g	**18%**
Saturated Fat 5g	**25%**
Trans Fat 0g	
Cholesterol 60mg	**20%**
Sodium 70mg	**3%**
Total Carbohydrate 0g	**0%**
Dietary Fiber 0g	**0%**
Total Sugars 0g	
Includes 0g Added Sugars	**0%**
Protein 23g	**46%**
Vitamin D 0.1mcg	0%
Calcium 12mg	0%
Iron 2mg	10%
Potassium 289mg	6%
Thiamin 0.05mg	4%
Riboflavin 0.2mg	15%
Niacin 4.8mg	30%
Vitamin B6 0.4mg	25%
Folate 6mcg	2%
Vitamin B12 2mcg	80%
Phosphorus 175mg	15%
Zinc 4.6mg	40%

*The % Daily Value (DV) tells you how much a nutrient in a serving of food contributes to a daily diet. 2,000 calories a day is used for general nutrition advice.

Plant Alternative

Nutrition Facts

Serving size	(113g)
Amount Per Serving **Calories**	**250**
	% Daily Value*
Total Fat 14g	**18%**
Saturated Fat 8g	**40%**
Trans Fat 0g	
Cholesterol 0mg	**0%**
Sodium 370mg	**16%**
Total Carbohydrate 9g	**3%**
Dietary Fiber 3g	**11%**
Total Sugars 0g	
Includes 0g Added Sugars	**0%**
Protein 19g	**38%**
Vitamin D 0mcg	0%
Calcium 180mg	15%
Iron 4.2mg	25%
Potassium 610mg	15%
Thiamin 28.2mg	2350%
Riboflavin 0.4mg	30%
Niacin 4.8mg	30%
Vitamin B6 0.4mg	25%
Folate 115mcg	30%
Vitamin B12 3mcg	120%
Phosphorus 180mg	15%
Zinc 5.5mg	50%

*The % Daily Value (DV) tells you how much a nutrient in a serving of food contributes to a daily diet. 2,000 calories a day is used for general nutrition advice.

FIGURE 66.2 Nutrition facts panels of grass-fed ground beef and the plant-based meat alternative. Source*: Reproduced and modified with permission from, Vman Vliet S, Bain JR, Muehlbauer MJ, et al. A metabolomics comparison of plant-based meat and grass-fed meat indicated large nutritional differences despite comparable Nutrition Facts panels.* Sci Rep. *2021;11:13828. https://doi.org/10.1038/s41598-021-93100-3.*

and fat content (14 g), the metabolite abundances between PBMA and ground beef differed by 90% (171 out of 190 profiled metabolites) (Fig. 66.3).[60] Twenty-two metabolites were found only in beef and included docosahexaenoic acid, vitamin B3, glucosamine, hydroxyproline, and the antioxidants allantoin, anserine, cysteamine, spermine, and squalene. Vitamin C, phytosterols, and phenolic antioxidants such as loganin, sulfurol, syringic acid, tyrosol, and vanillic acid were found exclusively in PBMA. Large differences in metabolites from nutrient classes such as amino acids, dipeptides, vitamins phenols, tocopherols, and fatty acids led to the conclusion that these two product types were not truly interchangeable, but perhaps could be described as complementary in the nutrients provided.[60] These data based on comparisons of deep metabolomics profiles could not determine which source may be healthier to consumer.[60]

Another study compared the nutritional composition of raw meat-based burgers (MBB) and raw PBB assessing color, pH, carbohydrates, fiber, moisture, cooking loss,

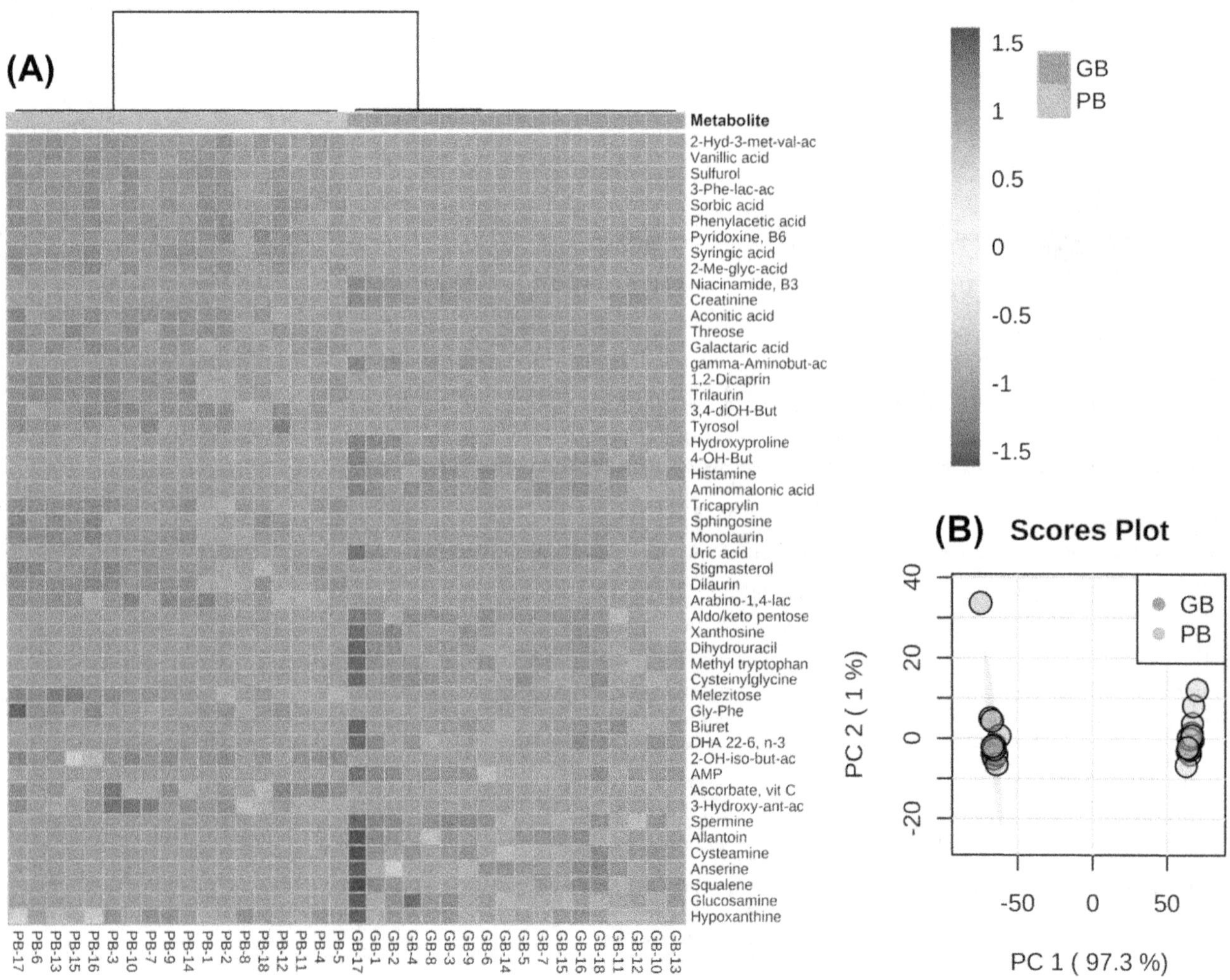

FIGURE 66.3 Metabolomics revealed distinct differences in metabolite profiles between grass-fed ground beef (GB) and the plant-based meat alternative (PB). (A) Heatmap of the top 50 metabolites, ranked by *P* values (lowest to highest), that were significantly different ($P < .05$) between beef and the plant-based meat alternative. Red (intensity ranges from 0 to 1.5) means higher abundance of the corresponding metabolite, whereas blue means lower abundance (intensity ranges from −0 to −1.5). The numbers below the heatmap represent individual samples (GB-1 to 18 and PB-1 to 18, respectively; $n = 18$ for each group). Metabolites in beef and the plant-based meat alternative were compared by the Wilcoxon rank sum test with Benjamini−Hochberg adjusted *P* values at 5% ($P < .05$). (B) Principal component analysis (PCA) analysis of beef and plant-based meat revealed a distinct difference in metabolite composition between the grass-fed GB and the plant-based meat, with 97.3% of the variance explained within the first principal component (PC1)—which illustrates that large differences exist between beef and the plant-based meat alternative. Red and green colors above the heatmap (A) and the PCA plot (B) represent the GB and the plant-based meat, respectively. The 95% confidence interval of the groups is depicted in their respective color. A full list of potential bioactivities and health effects of each individual metabolite is reported in Table 66.1. Figure was created with MetaboAnalyst 4.0 (http://www.metaboanalyst.ca). Source*: Reproduced and modified with permission from, Van Vliet S, Bain JR, Muehlbauer MJ, et al. A metabolomics comparison of plant-based meat and grass-fed meat indicated large nutritional differences despite comparable Nutrition Facts panels.* Sci Rep. *2021;11:13828. https://doi.org/10.1038/s41598-021-93100-3.*

TABLE 66.1 Gross composition (of the raw product) and gross energy (of the raw product and in DM, dry matter).

Item	Meat-based burger		Plant-based burger		*P*-value
	Median	95% $CI_{50\%}$	Median	95% $CI_{50\%}$	
Moisture (%)	65.91	61.51–69.60	60.91	52.81–64.01	.037
Ashes (%)	1.79	1.77–1.82	2.52	1.87–3.47	.003
Protein (%)	17.96	15.89–18.75	18.01	13.30–18.43	.514
• Collagen[b] (%)	2.49	1.37–2.83	—	—	—
Fat (%)	12.51	7.98–20.33	11.10	8.76–19.08	.631
• Cholesterol (mg/100 g of the raw product)	50.60	48.81–54.26	3.98	3.88–4.55	.003
Carbohydrates (%)	2.09	2.00–2.76	8.37	7.62–10.03	.003
• Starch (%)	0.93	0.86–1.14	0.31	0.10–1.21	.161
• Fructose (%)	0.022	0.019–0.055	0.013	0.010–0.056	.571
• Total dietary fiber (%)	0.74	0.48–0.98	4.27	2.90–5.02	.003
Gross energy (MJ/kg DM)	28.42	26.11–30.26	24.86	23.98–28.61	.031
Gross energy (MJ/kg of the raw product)	9.69	7.94–12.19	9.41	8.92–13.50	1.00

Results are reported as median and 95% $CI_{50\%}$.[a]
[a]*95% $CI_{50\%}$: median 95% confidence interval.*
[b]*Collagen percentage was calculated as (hydroxyproline × 8)/10^3.*

TABLE 66.2 Cooking loss (%), volume loss (%), and shear force (N) of cooked burgers in water bath or in plate.

Trait	Meat-based burger		Plant-based burger		*P*-value
	Median	95% $CI_{50\%}$	Median	95% $CI_{50\%}$	
Cooking loss[b] (%)	25.67	24.15–32.47	16.01	8.55–20.41	.004
Volume loss[b] (%)	26.01	17.89–34.41	20.23	13.50–25.02	.094
Shear force[b] (N)	12.85	10.70–16.89	6.34	5.92–6.67	.004
Cooking loss[c] (%)	23.06	21.15–26.16	21.04	18.79–26.11	.071
Volume loss[c] (%)	27.96	25.32–48.13	21.84	14.24–35.12	.246
Shear force[c] (N)	13.70	10.57–18.27	10.10	8.78–15.01	.086

Results are reported as median and 95% $CI_{50\%}$.[a]
[a]*95% $CI_{50\%}$: median 95% confidence interval.*
[b]*Using the water bath method.*
[c]*Using the cooking plate methods.*
Source: Taken from De Marchi M, Costa A, Pozza M, Goi A, Manuelian CL. Detailed characterization of plant-based burgers. *Sci Rep.* 2021;11:2049. https://doi.org/10.1038/s41598-021-81684-9

mineral, protein, and fatty acid profiles (Table 66.1).[61] The raw PBB had a slightly higher and more variable pH (median 5.81, range 5.58–7.29) than the raw MBB (median 5.48, range 5.28–5.70) due to the greater alkalinity and diversity of ingredients.[61] While both product types had the same lightness (L*), MBB had greater green-red (a*) and blue-yellow (b*) color components than PBB, probably due to the hemoglobin content in the former. PBB had greater content in both carbohydrates (median, 8.37%) and total dietary fiber (median, 4.27%) compared to MBB (medians, 2.04% and 0.74%, respectively). Using the water bath method, PBB had lower cooking loss (median, 16.01%) compared to MBB (median, 25.67%; Table 66.2).[61]

The greater moisture content of raw MBB (median, 65.91%) compared to raw PBB (median, 60.91%), plus the lower fiber content could explain the greater cooking loss in MBB. The PBB exhibited a lower shear force (6.34 N) when compared to MBB (12.85 N) when cooked using the water bath method (Table 66.2).[61] They concluded that increased dietary fiber could be obtained by consuming more PBB compared to MBB and that pH values near neutral put PBMA in danger of microbial growth including spores.

In both PBB and MBB, the most abundant minerals were calcium, potassium, magnesium, sodium, phosphate, and sulfur. Sodium, sulfur, and silicon content was similar in both (Table 66.3).[61] Zinc was less abundant in PBB than in MBB. Ash content was greater in raw PBB (median, 2.52%) than raw MBB (median, 1.79%). Heavy metals such as lead, arsenic, and mercury were not detected in either group. One of the PBB brands had cadmium and lithium in all four samples, while only one MBB sample contained lithium. This would be a safety concern because higher levels of cadmium are potentially toxic. Boron and molybdenum were only present in PBB.[61] Iron was found to be two times higher in PBB (26.51 mg/kg raw product vs 13.05 mg/kg in MBB) than MBB. However, heme-iron was not evaluated. This is an

TABLE 66.3 Mineral composition (mg/kg of the raw product).

Mineral	Meat-based burger		Plant-based burger		*P*-value
	Median	95% $CI_{50\%}$	Median	95% $CI_{50\%}$	
Major minerals					
Na	4267.44	4214.72–4445.18	4284.66	3653.16–7152.97	1.000
K	2717.57	2524.12–2959.74	3457.13	3279.45–5448.62	.003
P	1270.13	1191.41–1415.95	2098.92	1558.16–3647.59	.003
S	1325.11	1297.02–1537.88	1442.76	1113.35–1692.15	.460
Mg	159.42	151.84–174.21	614.94	181.17–1404.44	.003
Ca	85.62	79.72–141.48	715.39	176.82–853.47	.003
Trace minerals					
Zn	30.69	27.61–36.33	21.38	8.35–25.11	.003
Si	20.89	19.26–23.61	20.43	16.21–98.81	.965
Fe	13.05	11.62–14.14	26.51	23.93–33.09	.003
Cu	1.52	0.80–4.28	3.52	2.62–9.12	.009
Sr	0.50	0.46–0.53	2.76	0.61–3.03	.007
Mn	0.18	0.17–0.27	10.52	2.96–11.30	.003
Li[b]	0.10	-	0.28	0.26–0.38	-
Cr	0.08	0.07–0.11	0.18	0.15–0.31	.003
Ba	0.07	0.06–0.26	0.53	0.14–2.36	.005
Ni	0.06	0.06–0.10	0.22	0.19–0.33	.003
Ti	0.05	0.04–0.07	0.17	0.11–0.81	.003
B[c]	—	—	0.79	0.15–4.14	—
Mo	—	—	0.22	0.10–0.88	—
Heavy metals					
Cd[d]	—	—	0.14	0.14–0.15	—

Results are reported as median and 95% $CI_{50\%}$.[a]
[a]*95% CI50%: median 95% confidence interval.*
[b]*Li was only detected in one sample of meat-based burgers, and in four samples of the same plant-based burgers brand.*
[c]*B was only detected in nine samples of plant-based burgers.*
[d]*Cd was only detected in four samples of plant-based burgers of the same brand.*
Source: Taken from De Marchi M, Costa A, Pozza M, Goi A, Manuelian CL. Detailed characterization of plant-based burgers. *Sci Rep*. 2021;11:2049. https://doi.org/10.1038/s41598-021-81684-9

important omission because heme-iron is much more bioavailable than the nonheme sources usually found in plants. Phytates, which can affect the absorption of minerals and vitamins in a food were not quantified.

Although total protein content was similar between the categories (raw PBB, median 18.01% and raw MBB, median 17.96%), 5 out of 18 amino acids in the detailed protein profile were significantly different (Table 66.4).[61] Like the van Vliet study, hydroxyproline was only found in MBB samples. Therefore one could employ infrared spectroscopy to detect hydroxyproline for rapid detection and authentication of meat products. Alanine, glycine, and especially methionine (21 times lower) were less abundant in PBB when compared to MBB. One of the nine essential amino acids in human nutrition, methionine has been known as the limiting amino acid in legumes and pulses such as soy and pea for over 70 years.[62] However, amino acids, cysteine and glutamic acid were more abundant in PBB. With methionine as the exception, PBMA provided a relatively complete protein profile. Protein digestibility–corrected amino acid scores, the preferred method for the measurement of protein values in human nutrition,[63] have shown that plant sources such as soy protein isolate and pea protein concentrate have similar digestibilities to animal protein sources.[64]

No differences were found between the total fat content in the burger categories (raw PBB, median, 11.10% and raw MBB, median, 12.51%). However, raw PBB had much lower cholesterol content (median, 3.98 mg/100 g) than raw MBB (median, 50.60 mg/100 g). PBB had a comparable saturated fat content when compared to MBB due to the inclusion of coconut oil.[61]

In a third peer-reviewed study, proximate analysis of PBMA, ground pork (GP) and data from the USDA-ARS Food Data Center nutrient database for ground beef (GB) indicated that crude protein and crude fat content did not

TABLE 66.4 Amino acids composition (mg/100 g of the raw product).

Amino acid	Meat-based burger		Plant-based burger		*P*-value
	Median	95% $CI_{50\%}$	Median	95% $CI_{50\%}$	
Alanine	1096.24	815.93–1214.69	686.97	605.63–818.55	.007
Arginine	1085.62	912.53–1489.29	1060.73	930.21–1478.36	.965
Aspartic acid	1581.08	1232.11–1885.85	1925.04	1549.21–2502.18	.062
Cysteine	154.13	141.88–187.69	251.91	174.84–308.23	.012
Glycine	1305.27	949.08–1910.00	689.43	640.20–761.76	.003
Glutamic acid	30.27.17	2275.92–3515.55	4351.61	4017.72–5805.17	.003
Hydroxyproline	310.93	171.16–354.14	—	—	—
Isoleucine[b]	554.97	463.71–749.81	507.7	472.27–618.83	.631
Histidine[b]	582	498.67–773.87	591.48	417.03–869.42	.965
Leucine[b]	1164.39	962.76–1496.66	1214.58	872.24–1500.31	.965
Lysine[b]	1391.19	1046.08–1836.15	927.82	707.09–1604.09	.138
Methionine[b]	300.11	243.62–392.31	13.76	9.64–51.06	.003
Phenylalanine[b]	661.94	613.06–891.79	899.28	630.23–1066.58	.101
Proline	855.61	696.31–1047.03	774.66	534.19–1159.60	.631
Serine	672.63	535.50–884.56	902.61	593.11–1038.95	.215
Tyrosine	481.56	436.45–642.64	591.16	365.79–675.24	.760
Threonine[b]	686.22	579.13–927.21	572.28	468.41–647.78	.062
Tryptophan[b]	102.51	93.19–133.41	108.28	87.09–128.34	.965
Valine[b]	612.10	575.45–825.46	559.02	516.81–671.49	.215

Results are reported as median and 95% $CI_{50\%}$.[a]
[a]*95% $CI_{50\%}$: median 95% confidence interval.*
[b]*Essential amino acids.*
Source: Taken from De Marchi M, Costa A, Pozza M, Goi A, Manuelian CL. Detailed characterization of plant-based burgers. *Sci Rep*. 2021;11:2049. https://doi.org/10.1038/s41598-021-81684-9

differ statistically for each PBMA tested and GP in either raw or cooked states.[65] Calcium and sodium were significantly greater in PBMA compared to GP. Iron and zinc were greater for most PBMA tested than in GP. However, zinc content was numerically greater in GB when compared to PBMA and GP.[65] Vitamin E content in both raw and cooked PBMA was significantly greater than in raw and cooked GP. Total saturated fat was numerically greater in PBMA when compared to GP. Total essential amino acid content was greater in some PBMA compared to GP but methionine and lysine were statistically greater in GP.[65] While PBMA had many nutrient parameters comparable to animal meats, empirical trials should be performed to assess their bioavailability in humans before making recommendations to young, old, pregnant, and individuals with metabolic disorders.

66.10 Health benefits

Because they are recent additions to Western diets, there are no long-term studies on the effects of consuming PBMA. There are limited scientific data on safety and conflicting reports on the health benefits. In a review article penned by the Johns Hopkins Bloomberg School of Public Health, the authors outlined some of the differing perspectives.[10] Some professionals assert that replacing meat with PBMA does not guarantee a healthier dietary lifestyle.[66] Increased consumption of ultra-processed foods may reduce the consumption of whole foods which can cause excess calorie intake, weight gain, and may produce unknown and unintended consequences.[67] Many PBMA contain comparable amounts of calories, protein, and iron compared with meat.[5] Some products contain coconut oil which has saturated fat levels comparable to or higher than poultry and pork.[10] In contrast, diets rich in legumes, whole grains, vegetables, and nuts have been associated with reduced risk for adverse health outcomes.[68] However, it is not known if plant protein isolates offer similar nutritional benefits as their whole legume counterparts.[66] Because soy isolates are highly processed, they lack some of the beneficial nutritional components found in whole soybeans.[69] Inconsistent research findings with soy proteins and their effect on heart disease have caused the FDA to revoke an authorized health claim granted to the products in 1999.[70] Despite the fact that gut microbiomes are more diverse with plant-based diets, it is uncertain how PBMA might affect microbiomes.[66] In one study, a lower muscle protein synthetic response occurred when plant-based proteins from soy and wheat were compared with several animal-based proteins.[64] The lower skeletal muscle anabolic response was attributed to the lower digestibility, greater splanchnic extraction, amino acids taken up by the gut and liver, and urea synthesis of plant protein-derived amino acids.[64] In addition to nutritional comparisons, both chemical and empirical, future research should concentrate on the long-term health effects of diets rich in PBMA, especially for the elderly who exhibit increased splanchnic extraction as they age.[71]

66.11 Sustainability

In a Beyond Meat-commissioned study conducted by the University of Michigan, researchers compared the Beyond Burger production system with that of an existing life cycle assessment of US beef production commissioned by the National Cattleman's Beef Association.[72] They concluded that "... Beyond Burger generates 90% less greenhouse gas emissions, requires 46% less energy, and has $>$ 99% less impact on water scarcity, and 93% less impact on land use than a quarter pound of U.S. beef." Other studies have shown that a diet containing limited amounts of meat can be environmentally beneficial when animals are fed on marginal lands or with products inedible to humans: land use is most efficient when humans derive 12% of their dietary protein from animals, especially in the form of milk.[73,74] While there are many studies with whole plant foods, there are few studies on the environmental impacts of plant proteins derived from these whole foods. Some studies indicate that legumes and their concentrates are environmentally friendly as protein sources.[75] Plant proteins such as peas and beans have the lowest land use per kilogram of protein.[76] In contrast, the production of 1 kg of meat protein requires an input of up to 10 kg of plant proteins.[77]

Studies with whole plant foods suggest, and PBMA stakeholders insist, that PBMA have less environmental impact than meats. The fourth estate is parroting the environmental and sustainability halos claimed by makers and marketers of PBMA. Here is a typical quote from the media: "Alternative meats, in general, reduce land use and deforestation, protect biodiversity, produce less air and water pollution..."[78] Does increasing use of plant proteins in products such as PBMA really reduce deforestation and protect diversity as stated in PBMA marketing releases and popular media? Most of the PBMA on the market are derived from environmental questionable resources such as soy.[79] Soybean production has been associated with monocultures, deforestation, and nitrate run-off in watersheds. Row crop production has accelerated social and environmental change especially in developing nations. The deforestation of the South American Chaco region was driven by the increasing global demand for soybean[80]; the Chaco being the largest continuous stretch of tropical dry forest in South America. Other researchers observing global land use policies have concluded that cattle ranching and the large-scale expansion of soybean production in the early 2000s were the main drivers in deforestation.[81] Brazilian deforestation, in particular, was driven by land speculation, where the speculators would deforest an area, sell off the timber, convert the land to pasture, and then quickly sell the land to a soy producer at a much greater price.[82] This caused Brazil to initiate the Soy Moratorium: a commitment by the world's largest traders to halt soybean purchases from areas which were deforested after July 2006. This moratorium was largely successful. It was noted that from 2006 to 2010 deforestation of the Mato Grosso in the Amazon frontier was reduced by 30%.[83] Declining deforestation also coincided with a collapse of commodity markets. Therefore scientists caution that policies alone may not be enough to slow deforestation if future markets spur global demands for soy production.[83] In Brazil soybeans are much more damaging than other crops because they justify massive transportation infrastructure projects to facilitate export.[84] When compared to pastureland, soybean cropland expansion showed a significantly higher precipitation decrease due to the high albedo of the plants[85]; the albedo being the measurement of surface reflectivity of solar energy.

In the US Midwest region, corn and soybean production combined with decreased crop diversity has been correlated to greater levels of nitrates leaching into nearby aquatic systems[86] and hypoxia or dead zones in the Gulf of Mexico.[87] Most of the soybean produced in the US Midwest go to animal feeds. Will PBMA cause this balance to shift to food ingredients? Despite new innovations and calls for sustainability, demand for meat from animal sources remains strong not only in the North America and Europe but worldwide. Globally, we are expected to consume more meat in 2021 than any previous year. The United Nations Food and Agriculture Organization projects that meat consumption will increase by 1% this year.[78] The fastest growth is occurring where incomes are rising such as in low- and middle-income nations.[78] This points to a continued expansion of land needed for soybean production, both for livestock feed and direct human consumption of products such as PBMA.

Instead of producing more soybeans for PBMA, another approach is to side stream or waste stream plant proteins from products already in use, such as cereals and legumes used in oil production or animal feeds, or from plants which grow in diverse agricultural regions. Rapeseed meal is currently used as animal feed and seldom consumed as a food ingredient.[88] Rapeseed meal can be washed with aqueous ethanol, as is done with soybean meal, to create rapeseed protein concentrate. This would be an upcycled by-product of rapeseed (canola) oil and a contender for a sustainable meat analog ingredient.[88] When compared to soybeans from Brazil, rapeseed from Germany had lower fuel, electricity, fertilizer, and pesticides inputs but lower yields.[75] The environmental impact of cultivation was therefore slightly lower for soybean then rapeseed, 7.06 versus 7.65. However, deforestation would not be an issue when using a waste stream from an already extant crop.

Faba bean seeds are grown in many climatic zones from Europe and Asia to Africa and are rich in proteins, vitamins, and dietary fiber.[76] Faba beans can be side streamed and further processed to obtain a protein-rich faction.[76] Other interesting alternatives are light-yellow microalgae, *Auxenochlorella protothecoides*, which have lower land use needs. When combined with soy concentrates the microalgae improved the extrudates' nutritional profile by adding vitamins B and E and increased the tenderness when compared to pure soy extrudates.[79] *A. protothecoides* also enhanced lutein and zeaxanthin, carotenoids with protective effects against eye diseases. These nutritional factors' elevated levels were retained even after high-pressure and high-temperature extrusion.[79]

The discovery of food technology by Silicon Valley and libertarian venture capitalists has driven the creation of ambitious meat alternatives and spurred great media attention.[89] In the rush to embrace technology, we sometimes disregard simple solutions or ignore what we already have. Recently, sociologists collaborated with food scientists to create an approach to compare new food innovations with behavioral or low technological alternatives. In order to examine and compare meat alternatives they developed the Reflexive Integrative Comparative Heuristics.[89] They compared the plausibility and desirability of alternative options for meats in the immediate and long-term future.[89] They concluded that "... [PBMA's] potential sustainability benefits may turn out to be disappointing, due to the extensive processing that is required, which takes energy and leads to losses during the transformation from raw materials into final products." They also cited the relative neglect of existing alternatives such as eating less meat and the consumption of pulses which would produce immediate and significant sustainability gains. Western diets already contain an excess of protein. Based on an average need of 50 g of daily protein per adult, meat intake in the industrial world could be reduced by up to one-third without a negative impact on human health and without the need for a replacement.[89] Supported by food activists, local producers, and the United Nations, the consumption of pulses in whole form offers the largest potential sustainability gain as they need very little processing and have lower environmental impacts than animal proteins.[89]

66.12 Research gaps and future directions

Animal meat has advantages over plant protein sources due to the completeness of its amino acid profile, and the density and availability of its vitamins and minerals. Also, meat provides sensory satisfaction: flavors, mouthfeel, and satiety that are hard to mimic with plant ingredients without the use of extensive additives and processing. PBMA endeavor to replace or reduce meat consumption in order to meet growing population demands for protein and reduce the environmental impact of animal agriculture. However, the environmental costs of quality protein are high, regardless of the source. PBMA developers and manufacturers should consider waste streams from extant products and other underutilized protein-rich by-products. They should move away from soy and utilize more diverse protein sources in the legume and cereal families and nontraditional alternatives such as microalgae and insects. Older technologies such as fungi should be reexamined.[3] Manufacturers and food scientists should optimize technologies which reduce the nutrient degradation and energy consumption caused by ultra-processing. Additionally, PBMA formulations should move toward reduced sodium and saturated fat levels to improve their health halo. Nutritionists need to study the long-term effects of PBMA consumption, especially by young, pregnant, elderly, and metabolically challenged individuals. Empirical data from clinical trials are needed to ensure that vitamin and mineral fortifications and amino acid profiles of PBMA are nutritionally equivalent to animal meat, if they wish to completely replace the latter option. Research gaps such as the formation of potential carcinogenic compounds during processing, environmental contaminants such as aflatoxins, heavy metals, pesticides, and industrial chemicals from extractions need to be explored and quantified to conform to the respective regulations of the country in which the PBMA are manufactured.

Ultra-processed foods such as PBMA are here to stay due to their sensory attributes, convenience, and longer shelf-lives. PBMA fulfill certain consumers' needs to explore new products which more closely align with their beliefs, their political and social agendas. They are not the only choice for food sustainability and security but one of many intriguing lifestyle options for consumers to consider.

Acknowledgments

Some of this material was originally published as "How Safe are Plant-Based Meat Alternatives?" by Jane M. Caldwell for the February 2021 issue of IFT Food Technology magazine (http://www.ift.org).

References

1. Zion Market Research. Global plant-based meat market will reach USD 21.23 billion by 2025. <https://www.zionmarketresearch.com/news/plant-based-meat-market>; 2019.
2. Sha L, Xiong YL. Plant protein-based alternatives of reconstructed meat: science, technology, and challenges. *Trends Food Sci Technol.* 2020;102:51–61. Available from: https://doi.org/10.1016/j.tifs.2020.05.022.
3. Reynolds M. Watch out, Beyond Burgers, the Fungi Renaissance is here. Wired UK. <https://www.wired.com/story/fungi-renaissance-is-here/>; August 8, 2021.
4. Anonymous. The NOVA food classification system. <https://edu-change.com/wp-content/uploads/2018/09/NOVA-Classification-Reference-Sheet.pdf>; 2018.
5. Boher BM. An investigation of the formulation and nutritional composition of modern meat analogue products. *Food Sci Hum Wellness.* 2019;8:320–329.
6. Monteiro CA, Cannon G, Moubarac JC, et al. The UN decade of nutrition, the NOVA food classification and the trouble with ultra-processing. *Public Health Nutr.* 2018;21:5–17. Available from: https://doi.org/10.1017/S1368980017000234.
7. Gelski J. European panel finds titanium dioxide no longer safe in food. Food Business News. <https://www.foodbusinessnews.net/articles/18597-european-panel-finds-titanium-dioxide-no-longer-safe-in-food>; May 12, 2021.
8. Kyriakopoulou K, Dekkers B, van der Goot AJ. Chapter 6: Plant-based meat analogues. In: *Sustainable Meat Production and Processing*. Academic Press; 2019. <https://doi.org/10.1016/B978-0-12-814874-7.00006-7>.
9. He J, Evans NM, Liu H, et al. A review of research on plant-based meat alternatives: driving forces, history, manufacturing, and consumer attitudes. *Compr Rev Food Sci Food Saf.* 2020;19:2639–2656.
10. Santo RE, Kim BF, Goldman SE, et al. Considering plant-based meat substitutes and cell-based meats: a public health and food systems perspective. *Front Sustain Food Syst.* 2020;4:1–23.
11. Wild F, Czerny M, Janssen AM, et al. The evolution of a plant-based alternative to meat. *Agro Food Ind Hi-Tech.* 2014;25:45–49.
12. Geeraerts W, Vuyst LD, Leroy F. Ready-to-eat meat alternatives, a study of their associated bacterial communities. *Food Biosci.* 2020;37:100681. Available from: https://doi.org/10.1016/j.fbio.2020.100681.
13. Filho GCS, Vessoni Penna TC, Schaffner DW. Microbiological quality of vegetable proteins during the preparation of a meat anlog. *Ital J Food Sci.* 2005;17:269–283.
14. Mwangi R. Inactivation of wild-type Bacillus spores in soy meat analog model by extrusion cooking [Master's thesis]. ProQuest Dissertations and Theses, 181. <https://mospace.umsystem.edu/xmlui/bitstream/handle/10355/5763/research.pdf?sequence = 3>; 2008.
15. Sagoo SK, Little CL, Greenwood M, et al. Assessment of the microbiological safety of dried spices and herbs from production and retail premises in the United Kingdom. *Food Microbiol.* 2009;26:39–43.
16. Weller J, Kuhnel V, Likanchuk A, et al. *Evaluation of the Hygiena BAX® system for the detection of* Salmonella *and* L. monocytogenes *in plant-based meat substitutes. IAFP Poster Session.* 2021.
17. Sampson GL. Assessing the efficacy of Bacteriological Analytical Manual (BAM) enrichment broths for detection of *Salmonella* spp. in meat analogs [Master's thesis, Chapman University]. <https://doi.org/10.36837/chapman.000292>; 2021.
18. Joshi VK, Kumar S. Meat analogues: plant-based alternatives to meat products – a review. *Int J Food Ferment Technol.* 2015;5:107–119.
19. University of Nebraska – Lincoln Food Allergy Research and Resource Program. AllergenOnline. <http://www.allergenonline.org/>; 2019.

20. Mattice KD, Marangoni AG. Evaluating the use of zein in structuring plant-based products. *Curr Res Food Sci.* 2020;3:59–66.
21. Nordlee JA, Taylor SL, Townsend JA, Thomas LA, Bush RK. Identification of a Brazil-nut allergen in transgenic soybeans. *N Engl J Med.* 1996;334:688–692.
22. Poulsen LK. Allergy assessment of foods or ingredients derived from biotechnology, gene-modified organisms, or novel foods. *Mol Nutr Food Res.* 2004;48:413–423.
23. Baderschneider B, Crevel RW, Earl LK, Lalljie A, Sanders DJ, Sanders IJ. Sequence analysis and resistance to pepsin hydrolysis as part of an assessment of the potential allergenicity of ice structuring protein type III HPLC 12. *Food Chem Toxicol.* 2002;40:965–978.
24. Astwood JD, Leach JN, Fuchs RL. Stability of food allergens to digestion in vitro. *Nat Biotechnol.* 1996;14:1269–1273.
25. Bindslev-Jensen C, Sten E, Earl LK, et al. *Assessment of the potential allergenicity of ice structuring protein type III HPLC 12 using the FAO/WHO 2001 decision tree for novel foods. Food Chem Toxicol.* 41. 200381–87.
26. European Food Safety Authority. Safety of 'Ice Structuring Protein (ISP) – Scientific Opinion of the Panel on Dietetic Products, Nutrition and Allergies and of the Panel on Genetically Modified Organisms. *EFSA J.* 2008;6:768.
27. EFSA Panel on Dietetic Products NaA, Turck D, Bresson J-L, Burlingame B, Dean T, Fairweather-Tait S, et al. Guidance on the preparation and presentation of an application for authorisation of a novel food in the context of Regulation (EU) 2015/2283. *EFSA J.* 2016;14:e04594.
28. Fernandez A, Mills ENC, Koning F, Moreno FJ. Safety assessment of immune-mediated adverse reactions to novel food proteins. *Trends Biotechnol.* 2019;37:796–800.
29. EFSA Panel on Genetically Modified Organisms, Naegeli H, Birch AN, et al. Guidance on allergenicity assessment of genetically modified plants. *EFSA J.* 2017;15:e04862.
30. Maurer-Stroh S, Krutz NL, Kern PS, et al. AllerCatPro-prediction of protein allergenicity potential from the protein sequence. *Bioinformatics.* 2019;35:3020–3027.
31. Westerhout J, Krone T, Snippe A, et al. Allergenicity prediction of novel and modified proteins: not a mission impossible! Development of a Random Forest allergenicity prediction model. *Regul Toxicol Pharmacol.* 2019;107:104422.
32. Abdelmoteleb M, Zhang C, Furey B, et al. Evaluating potential risks of food allergy of novel food sources based on comparison of proteins predicted from genomes and compared to http://www.AllergenOnline.org. *Food Chem Toxicol.* 2021;147:111888.
33. Radauer C, Breiteneder H. Allergen databases – a critical evaluation. *Allergy.* 2019;74:2057–2060.
34. Thomas K, Aalbers M, Bannon GA, et al. A multi-laboratory evaluation of a common in vitro pepsin digestion assay protocol used in assessing the safety of novel proteins. *Regul Toxicol Pharmacol.* 2004;39:87–98.
35. Mandalari G, Adel-Patient K, Barkholt V, et al. In vitro digestibility of beta-casein and beta-lactoglobulin under simulated human gastric and duodenal conditions: a multi-laboratory evaluation. *Regul Toxicol Pharmacol.* 2009;55:372–381.
36. Brodkorb A, Egger L, Alminger M, et al. INFOGEST static in vitro simulation of gastrointestinal food digestion. *Nat Protoc.* 2019;14:991–1014.
37. Torcello-Gomez A, Dupont D, Jardin J, et al. Human gastrointestinal conditions affect in vitro digestibility of peanut and bread proteins. *Food Funct.* 2020;11:6921–6932.
38. Torcello-Gómez A, Dupont D, Jardin J, et al. Human gastrointestinal conditions affect in vitro digestibility of peanut and bread proteins. *Food Funct.* 2020;11:6921–6932.
39. Lozano-Ojalvo D, Benedé S, Antunes CM, et al. Applying the adverse outcome pathway (AOP) for food sensitization to support in vitro testing strategies. *Trends Food Sci Technol.* 2019;85:307–319.
40. Fernandez A, Mills ENC, Koning F, Moreno FJ. Allergenicity assessment of novel food proteins: what should be improved? *Trends Biotechnol.* 2021;39:4–8.
41. Puumalainen TJ, Poikonen S, Kotovuori A, et al. Napins, 2S albumins, are major allergens in oilseed rape and turnip rape. *J Allergy Clin Immunol.* 2006;117:426–432.
42. Rahman M, Baten A, Mauleon R, King GJ, Liu L, Barkla BJ. Identification, characterization and epitope mapping of proteins encoded by putative allergenic napin genes from *Brassica rapa. Clin Exp Allergy.* 2020;50:848–868.
43. EFSA Panel on Nutrition, Novel Foods and Food Allergens, Turck D, Castenmiller J, et al. Safety of rapeseed powder from *Brassica rapa* L. and *Brassica napus* L. as a Novel food pursuant to Regulation (EU) 2015/2283. *EFSA J.* 2020;18:e06197.
44. EFSA Panel on Dietetic Products NaA. Scientific opinion on the safety of "rapeseed protein isolate" as a novel food ingredient. *EFSA J.* 2013;11:3420.
45. Fiocchi A, Dahdah L, Riccardi C, Mazzina O, Fierro V. Preacutionary labelling of cross-reactive foods: the case of rapeseed. *Asthma Res Pract.* 2016;2:13.
46. Broekman H, Verhoeckx KC, den Hartog Jager CF, et al. Majority of shrimp-allergic patients are allergic to mealworm. *J Allergy Clin Immunol.* 2016;137:1261–1263.
47. Barre A, Pichereaux C, Velazquez E, et al. Insights into the allergenic potential of the edible yellow mealworm (*Tenebrio molitor*). *Foods.* 2019;8.
48. Verhoeckx KC, van Broekhoven S, den Hartog-Jager CF, et al. House dust mite (Der p 10) and crustacean allergic patients may react to food containing Yellow mealworm proteins. *Food Chem Toxicol.* 2014;65:364–373.
49. EFSA Panel on Nutrition, Novel Foods and Food Allergens, Turck D, Castenmiller J, et al. Safety of dried yellow mealworm (*Tenebrio molitor* larva) as a novel food pursuant to Regulation (EU) 2015/2283. *EFSA J.* 2021;19:e06343.
50. Hepburn P, Howlett J, Boeing H, et al. The application of post-market monitoring to novel foods. *Food Chem Toxicol.* 2008;46:9–33.
51. Hoff M, Trueb RM, Ballmer-Weber BK, Vieths S, Wuethrich B. Immediate-type hypersensitivity reaction to ingestion of mycoprotein (Quorn) in a patient allergic to molds caused by acidic ribosomal protein P2. *J Allergy Clin Immunol.* 2003;111:1106–1110.
52. Fraser RZ, Shitut M, Agrawal P, et al. Safety evaluation of soy leghemoglobin protein preparation derived from *Pichia pastoris*, intended for use as a flavor catalyst in plant-based meat. *Int J Toxicol.* 2018;37:241–262.
53. Proulx AK, Reddy MB. Iron bioavailability of hemoglobin from soy root nodules using a Caco-2 cell culture model. *J Agric Food Chem.* 2006;54:1518–1522.

54. Kwok KC, Qin WH, Tsang JC. Heat inactivation of trypsin inhibitors in soymilk at ultra-high temperatures. *J Food Sci.* 1993;58:859–862. Available from: https://doi.org/10.1111/j.1365-2621.1993.tb09377.x.
55. Hurrell RF, Juillerat MA, Reddy MB, et al. Soy protein, phytate, and iron absorption in humans. *Am J Clin Nutr.* 1992;56:573–578. Available from: https://doi.org/10.10093/ajcn/56.3.573.
56. Lynch SR. The effect of calcium on iron absorption. *Nutr Res Rev.* 2000;13:141–158.
57. Matkovic V, Ilich JZ, Andon MB, Hsieh LC, Tzagournis MA, et al. Urinary calcium, sodium, and bone mass of young females. *Am J Clin Nutr.* 1995;62:417–425.
58. Cornet SHV, Snel SJE, Lesschen J. Enhancing the water holding capacity of model meat analogues through marinade composition. *J Food Eng.* 2021;290:110283.
59. Flores M, Piornos JA. Fermented meat sausages and the challenge of their plant-based alternatives: a comparative review on aroma-related aspects. *Meat Sci.* 2021;. Available from: https://doi.org/10.1016/j.meatsci.2021.108636Get_rights_and_content.
60. Van Vliet S, Bain JR, Muehlbauer MJ, et al. A metabolomics comparison of plant-based meat and grass-fed meat indicated large nutritional differences despite comparable Nutrition Facts panels. *Sci Rep.* 2021;11:13828. Available from: https://doi.org/10.1038/s41598-021-93100-3.
61. De Marchi M, Costa A, Pozza M, Goi A, Manuelian CL. Detailed characterization of plant-based burgers. *Sci Rep.* 2021;11:2049. Available from: https://doi.org/10.1038/s41598-021-81684-9.
62. Jaffe WG. Limiting essential amino acids of some legume seeds. *Exp Biol Med.* 1949;. Available from: https://doi.org/10.3181/00379727-71-17203. Available from: https://journals.sagepub.com/doi/abs/10.3181/00379727-71-17203.
63. Schaafsma G. The protein digestibility-corrected amino acid score. *J Nutr.* 2000;130(7):1865S–1867S. Available from: https://doi.org/10.1093/jn/130.7.1865S. Available from: https://pubmed.ncbi.nlm.nih.gov/10867064/.
64. van Vliet S, Burd NA, van Loon LJC. The skeletal muscle anabolic response to plant- vs animal-based protein consumption. *J Nutr Crit Rev.* 2015;145:1981–1991. Available from: https://pubmed.ncbi.nlm.nih.gov/26224750/.
65. Swing CJ, Thompson TW, Guimaraes O, Geornaras I, Engle TE, Belk KE, et al. Nutritional composition of novel plant-based meat alternatives and traditional animal-based meats. *J Food Sci Nutr.* 2021;7:2.
66. Hu FB, Otis BO, McCarthy G. Can plant-based meat alternatives be part of a healthy and sustainable diet? *J Am Med Assoc.* 2019;322:1547–1548.
67. Hall KD, Ayuketah A, Brychta R, et al. Ultra-processed diets cause excess calorie intake and weight gain: an inpatient randomized controlled trial of *ad libitum* food intake. *Cell Metab.* 2019;30:67–77. Available from: https://doi.org/10.1016/j.cmet.2019.05.008.
68. Nelson ME, Hamm MW. Alignment of healthy dietary patterns and environmental sustainability: a systematic review. *Adv Nutr.* 2016;7:1005–1025.
69. Messina M, Messina V. The role of soy in vegetarian diets. *Nutrients.* 2010;2:855–888.
70. Statement from Susan Mayne, Ph.D., on proposal to revoke health claim that soy protein reduces risk of heart disease. 2017. <https://www.fda.gov/news-events/press-announcements/statement-susan-mayne-phd-proposal-revoke-health-claim-soy-protein-reduces-risk-heart-disease>.
71. Jourdan M, Deutz NEP, Cynober L, Aussel C. Features, causes and consequences of splanchnic sequestration of amino acid in old rats. *PLoS One.* 2011;6:e27002. Available from: https://www.ncbi.nlm.nih.gov/pmc/articles/PMC3210777/pdf/pone.0027002.pdf.
72. Heller MC, Keoleian GA. Beyond Meat's Beyond Burger life cycle assessment: a detailed comparison between a plant-based and an animal-based protein source. CSS Report, Publication No. CSS18-10. University of Michigan, Ann Arbor, MI. <http://css.umich.edu/publication/beyond-meats-beyond-burger-life-cycle-assessment-detailed-comparison-between-plant-based>; 2018.
73. Van Kernebeek HRJ, Oosting SJ, Van Ittersum MK, Bikker P, De Boer IJM. Saving land to feed a growing population: consequences for consumption of crop and livestock products. *Int J Life Cycle Assess.* 2016;21:677–687.
74. Van Zanten HHE, Mollenhorst H, Klootwijk CW, van Middelaar CE, De Boer IJM. Global food supply land use efficiency of livestock systems. *Int J Life Cycle Assess.* 2016;21:747–758.
75. Blonk Consultants. Agri-footprint. Part 2 – Description of data. p. 101. Version 5.0, Gouda, The Netherlands. <https://simapro.com/wp-content/uploads/2020/10/Agri-Footprint-5.0-Part-2-Description-of-data.pdf>; 2020.
76. Heusala H, Sinkko T, Sozer N, Hytonen E, Mogensen L, Knudsen MT. Carbon footprint and land use of oat and faba bean protein concentrates using a life cycle assessment approach. *J Clean Prod.* 2020;242:118376. Available from: https://doi.org/10.1016/j.jclepro.2019.118376.
77. Reijinders L, Soret S. Quantification of the environmental impact of different dietary protein choices. *Am J Clin Nutr.* 2003;78:6645–6685.
78. Blaustein-Rejto D, Smith A. We're on track to set a new record for global meat consumption. *MIT Technol Rev.* April 26, 2021;. Available from: https://www.technologyreview.com/2021/04/26/1023636/sustainable-meat-livestock-production-climate-change/.
79. Caporgno MP, Bocker L, Mussner C, et al. Extruded meat analogues based on yellow, heterotrophically cultivated *Auxenochlorella protothecoides* microalgae. *Innov. Food Sci Emerg Technol.* 2020;59:102275. Available from: https://doi.org/10.1016/j.ifset.2019.102275.
80. Fehlenberg V, Baumann M, Gasparri NI, et al. The role of soybean production as an underlying driver of deforestation in the South American Chaco. *Global Environ Change.* 2017;45:24–34.
81. Gollnow F, Hissa LDV, Rufin P, Lakes T. Property-level direct and indirect deforestation for soybean production in the Amazon region of Mato Grosse, Brazil. *Land Use Policy.* 2018;78:377–385.
82. Prager A. Brazil's key deforestation drivers: pasture, cropland, land speculation. Mongabay. <https://news.mongabay.com/2019/03/brazils-key-deforestation-drivers-pasture-cropland-land-speculation/>; March 19, 2019.
83. Macedo MN, DeFries RS, Morton DC, et al. Decoupling of deforestation and soy production in the southern Amazon during the late 2000s. *Proc Natl Acad Sci U S A.* 2012;109:1341–1346.
84. Fearnside PM. Soybean cultivation as a threat to the environment in Brazil. *Environ Conserv.* 2001;28:23–38.
85. Costa MH, Yanagi SNM, Souza PJOP, et al. Climate change in Amazonia caused by soybean cropland expansion as compared to caused by pastureland expansion. *Geophys Res Lett.* 2007;34:L07706.

86. Burke MWV, Shahabi M, Xu Y, Zheng H, Zhang X, VanLooy J. Identifying the driving factors of water quality in a sub-watershed of the Republican River basin, Kansas USA. *Int J Environ Res Public Health.* 2018;15:1041. Available from: https://doi.org/10.3390/ijerph15051041.
87. Jones CS, Nielsen JK, Schilling KE, Weber LJ. Iowa stream nitrate and the Gulf of Mexico. *PLoS One*. 2018. Available from: https://doi.org/10.1371/journal.pone.0195930.
88. Jia W, Curubeto N, Rodriguez-Alonzo E, Keppler JK, van der Goot AJ. Rapeseed protein concentrate as a potential ingredient for meat analogues. *Innov Food Sci Emerg Technol.* 2021;72:102758. Available from: https://doi.org/10.1016/j.ifset.2021.102758.
89. Van der Weele C, Feindt P, van der Goot AJ, et al. Meat alternatives: an integrative comparison. *Trends Food Sci Technol.* 2019;88:505–512.

Chapter 67

The role of Big Data and Artificial Intelligence in food risk assessment and prediction

Giannis Stoitsis, Mihalis Papakonstantinou, Manos Karvounis and Nikos Manouselis
Agroknow, Maroussi, Greece

Abstract
Risk assessment is one of the most important tools to prevent recalls. The assessment and management of risk is challenging as it needs to take into account all the stages of the supply chain and to use the data that is produced at each stage, namely production, incoming ingredients, processing & manufacturing, storage, distribution, and services. This chapter focuses on the role of Big Data and Artificial Intelligence technologies in risk assessment and prediction. Available systems and tools are reviewed and their role in the different steps of risk assessment is analyzed. A methodology for the risk assessment and prediction using global food safety data, Big Data and Artificial Intelligence technologies is presented. The proposed assessment and prediction approach was applied on fruits and vegetables and the results are presented. Food risk predictions could be generated so that Food Safety and Quality Assurance teams can be prepared to handle the situation before a major product recall happens and causes financial expenditures and, most importantly, damages the brand's trust and reputation.

Keywords: Big Data; Artificial Intelligence; food safety; food recall prevention; food risk prediction

67.1 Introduction

Today, although we have good food safety standards, food safety systems, certifications and risk assessment strategies, recalls and border rejections are increasing: the number of recalls and border rejections reported by Authorities in 2019 was doubled compared to 2014 (Fig. 67.1).

To this we need to add the COVID-19 situation, which created a bottleneck to the food industry.[1] Under this new situation, industry has to deal with a disturbed supply chain, companies need to immediately change suppliers, because when they are looking for shorter supply chains, less budget is available and due to the travel restrictions experts cannot conduct audits. This situation is moving us to exploring the possibilities for new risk assessment approaches that can utilize all the available data in the supply chain.

The Global Food Safety Initiative (GFSI) standards and regulations like Food Safety Modernization Act (FSMA) require detailed risk assessment of hazards for ingredients, finished products, processes and suppliers. According to the GFSI standards and FSMA, generic risk assessment for product categories and suppliers is no longer sufficient. The standards and new regulation require assessing risk for suppliers, for facilities, and for all the materials used in each facility.

In addition to that, **consumers** trends for less processing and new ingredients and the increased complexity and globalization of the supply chain calls for a risk assessment approach that

- is using accurate data about reported issues in the global and company's supply chain
- is not static and is updated frequently because microbial, chemical, allergen and fraud risks are continuously evolving
- applies predictive models of pathogens growth, toxins and chemicals contaminants
- takes into account consumption and population data
- takes into account the processing steps applied to materials (cooking, partitioning, packaging, storing)
- concludes to recommendations on how to mitigate risks

Risk assessment is one of the most important tools to prevent recalls. However, today risk assessment is too

Present Knowledge in Food Safety. DOI: https://doi.org/10.1016/B978-0-12-819470-6.00041-X

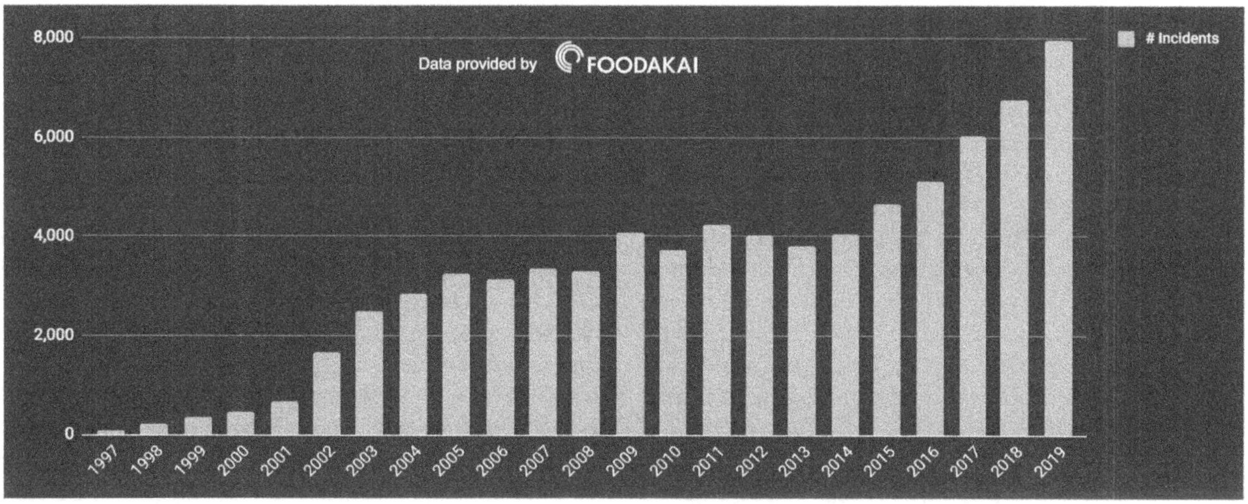

FIGURE 67.1 Number of recalls and border rejections reported by National Authorities. *FOODAKAI platform https://www.foodakai.com/*

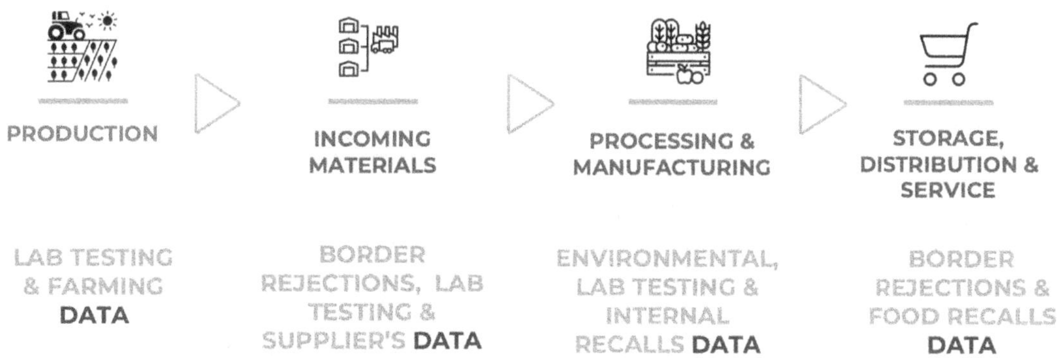

FIGURE 67.2 Stages of the supply chain and corresponding data that can be used for risk assessment.

often approached as a checklist compliance task. Not utilizing appropriate technology, data and good strategies to the fullest extent is poor risk management practice. It causes resources to be misdirected towards redundant activities or towards addressing events that are unlikely to occur. The risk assessment approaches followed in the industry are based on historical incidents and cannot really help experts to identify emerging and increasing risks.

The assessment and management of risk is challenging as it needs to take into account all the stages of the supply chain and to use the data that is produced at each stage, namely production, incoming ingredients, processing and manufacturing, storage, distribution and services (Fig. 67.2).

At the production level, laboratory testing data of the harvested agricultural products and farming data (cultivation practices, soil type, fertilizers, plant protection products applied) are generated and can be very helpful for the risk assessment in order to identify at an early stage the exceedances of chemicals and high levels of toxins. At the incoming materials level, data about border rejections, laboratory testing results and supplier's information including certificates, audits results, are generated. Data from this level is very helpful to identify risks for the ingredients and materials before getting them in the plant. At the processing level we have a lot of data including laboratory test results, environmental data and internal recalls data. At the storage, distribution, and service level we have data about border rejections, controls on the market and recalls. We should also add to the picture data that is highly relevant for all the stages such as commodity pricing data, country risk indicators and foodborne disease outbreaks.

From all these stages of the supply chain, a wealth of data and knowledge is generated about risks in foods due to better monitoring systems, testing technologies and research advances.[2] An important challenge is how to integrate all this data in order to use it to assess and predict risk. The data is highly scattered, heterogenous, multilingual, and disconnected. To integrate all this data a significant amount of time and specialized effort is needed.

Food industry needs to understand and predict food safety risk in order to switch from reaction to prevention. This requires combining new analytical tools, new methods and food safety data to enable a timely and proactive risk assessment approach. The current chapter focuses on how the challenge of assessing and predicting risk using all the available supply chain data can be addressed with efficient data processing and prediction workflows that include steps for collecting, processing, translating, mining and semantic annotation. The role of the Big Data and Artificial Intelligence (AI) technologies for addressing this challenge is described along with relevant workflows, systems and tools that can be used to achieve a timely risk assessment and risk prediction.

67.2 Available systems and tools for risk assessment

Nowadays we have systems, tools and platforms that can help us in performing risk assessment for any ingredient, material and finished product. The main types of such tools and systems are:

- online systems that can be used to access accurate and timely data about reported incidents in the global supply chain
- web-based systems designed to analyze data concerning microbial and chemical hazards in food and return an estimate of the resulting health burden on a population level
- online tools that can predict the behavior of a specific microorganism under a variety of conditions
- compliance management software systems that conduct Risk Assessment based on international best practices.
- systems that collect and process environmental data in plants. Data can be collected using sensors, environmental swabs, product testing, sanitation conformance, compliance measures, and many other data elements.

The list of the systems and tools presented here is a subset of the available systems that can help in food risk assessment and management. Starting from the accurate and timely data that food safety experts need to have at hand about reported incidents in the global supply chain, one can use online systems like HorizonScan[3] and FOODAKAI.[4]

HorizonScan[3] is a web-based information service with a suite of proprietary Risk Assessment and Supplier Check tools tracking current and historical global food fraud and contamination issues in near real time. The HorizonScan ingredient risk assessment system monitors safety & fraud alerts worldwide, collecting data daily from over 110 food safety agencies and other reliable sources to deliver timely alerts on emerging food safety issues affecting the global supply chain. The risk assessment is based on the occurrences of the hazards in specific materials.

FOODAKAI[4] is a software enterprise platform that generates tailor-made insights about the food supply chain from global food safety data. It helps food businesses to monitor food safety hazards (micro, chemical, physical, contact material) and food fraud issues in different food materials. The platform collects, translates and enriches more than **100 million food safety records** for food recalls, import refusals and laboratory testing analysis results that are published by National Authorities. The platform identifies **risk level for each hazard type** implementing a computational model that classifies risk to high, medium, or low based on the number of recalls and severity of the hazard that occurred in specific food materials.

Moving to the estimation of the health burden of microbial and chemical hazards, experts can use **FDA-iRisk**.[5] FDA-iRISK is a web-based system designed to analyze data concerning microbial and chemical hazards in food and return an estimate of the resulting health burden on a population level. It uses second-order Monte Carlo simulation to combine the impact of variability from all user inputs into the final estimates of risk. It also provides the option of specifying quantitative descriptions of uncertainty, the so-called Second-order Monte Carlo simulation, to the majority of model parameters.

When food safety experts need to predict the behavior of a specific microorganism under a variety of conditions, you may use **ComBase**[6] and **CB Premium**.[7] ComBase is an online tool for quantitative food microbiology. The focus of ComBase is describing and predicting how microorganisms survive and grow under a variety of primarily food-related conditions. It provides access to over 60,000 records, describing how food environments, such as temperature, pH, and water activity, as well as other factors (e.g., preservatives and atmosphere) affect the growth of bacteria.

CB Premium[7] is a web portal of predictive models and risk management tools to help enhance the safety and quality of food. What differentiates CB Premium from ComBase is it's sole focus on predictive models that have been developed for and validated in real commercial foods. CB Premium models focus on how microorganisms grow and die in commercial foods. It provides predictive models for microbial hazards. It is connected to ComBase models. Bibliographic reference to each predictive model is available.

When it comes to assessing the risk for your supply chain taking into account processes and international rules, you can use a software like **Safefood360**.[8] This is a compliance management software that conducts Risk Assessment based on international best practices. The software allows users to build custom Risk Assessment models and to apply them in workflows for HACCP, Management Processes, PRPs, and Monitoring programs. Using SafeFood360 a food business can build risk assessment models for different supplier and material types.

A comparison of these tools and systems using the important dimensions that we analyzed is presented in the following table (Table 67.1).

Several critical steps are involved in the process of risk assessment. The following table summarizes the main steps for a technology enhanced risk assessment and maps to the corresponding tool and system that can be used to implement each step (Table 67.2).

It's critical to take into account that risk assessment is not a one off task or a task that can be performed once or twice in a year. Our supply chain is complex, global and affected by situations like the COVID-19 but also environmental and social economical factors. Food industry needs to monitor new hazards that may increase risk in your supply chain and to follow new scientific and technological advancements that may improve the risk assessment process.

TABLE 67.1 Comparison of systems and tools that can be used to perform risk assessment.

System	Global data about reported hazards in foods	Supported types of hazards	Predictive models support	Supplier risk assessment support	Risk estimation for commercial food products
HorizonScan	Yes	All	No	No	No
FOODAKAI	Yes	All	Yes	Yes	Yes
FDA-iRisk	No	Microbiological, chemical	Yes	No	Yes
SafeFood360	No	All	No	Yes	Yes
ComBase	No	Microbiological	Yes	No	No
CP Premium	No	Microbiological	Yes	No	Yes

TABLE 67.2 Steps of a technology enhanced risk assessment.

Risk assessment step	System or tool that can be used to support the step
1. Hazards monitoringxx	HorizonScan
Collect the right data for incidents reported in the global supply chain about new hazards that may affect your products, ingredients, raw materials, facilities	FOODAKAI
2. Data management	
Manage the verification processes and the corresponding food safety records of your company (e.g., testing results, audit results)	SafeFood360
3. Hazard identification	HorizonScan
For each ingredient perform a hazard analysis to identify known and foreseeable hazards	FOODAKAI
4. Hazard characterization	FDA-iRisk
For each hazard estimate the chemical and micro risk based on the conditions and processing steps	ComBase
	CB Premium
5. Risk characterization	FOODAKAI
Characterize and rank the risk based on the hazard's probability and severity	HorizonScan
	SafeFood360
6. Risk updates	FOODAKAI
Continuously monitor risk changes to identify increasing and emerging risks.	

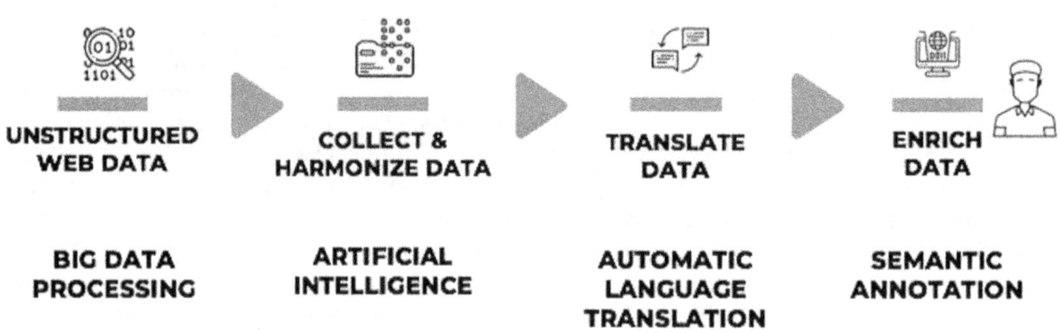

FIGURE 67.3 Data processing workflow of the Big Data platform.

67.3 Applying Big Data and Artificial Intelligence for food risk assessment and prediction

67.3.1 Workflow for Big Data processing

The first and very important step towards a technology enhanced risk assessment is the collection and processing of all the scattered and heterogeneous data that are generated every single minute in our supply chain. To address this challenge we have developed a Big Data processing workflow. The main goal of Big Data processing workflow is to take advantage of the computers' power in dealing with Big Data and combine it with the knowledge and experience of the food safety experts.[9] The development of the Big Data Platform for the food safety sector focused at targeting the needs of the food safety industry using Big Data processing, text mining, semantic and AI technologies (Fig. 67.3). The platform is responsible for collecting, processing, indexing and publishing heterogeneous food and agriculture data from a large variety of data sources. The platform was designed using microservice architecture,[10] with different technology components handling different aspects of the data lifecycle. Automatically processed and enriched data are reviewed by the experts to enable high quality and harmonized data.

The data platform stores and processes millions of food safety data records that can be used for risk assessment and prediction. The data types that can be used for risk assessment and prediction are presented in the following table (Table 67.3).

TABLE 67.3 Data types stored and processed by the Big Data platform.

Data type	Number of records (as of March 2021)
Food recalls	78,466
Border rejections	381,842
Inspections	228,306
Laboratory testing results	108,169,332
Suppliers	702,578
Prices	415,670
Country risk and corruption indicators	3519
News items	68,971
Maximum residue level limit	141,594
Product brands	28,081
Sensor data	12,437,743

67.3.2 Risk assessment

For the implementation of the Risk Estimation we used a mathematical model that is based on the frequency of the incidents and the severity of the identified hazards in the incidents. The risk is estimated for all the possible product (ingredient, raw material) hazard pairs as suggested in guidelines for risk assessment published.[11] Considering that the data platform includes more than 12,000 products (ingredients and materials) and more than 4300 hazards, the risk estimation should be conducted for a large number of pairs.

More specifically, the following risk estimation formula was used for the estimation of the risk based on global food safety incidents data that are collected and processed by the data platform.

$$\text{Risk} = \text{Incident Severity} \times \text{Hazard Severity} \times \text{Probability}$$

where

Incident Severity: is the severity based on the type of the incident (e.g., food recall, food alert, border rejection). A table with the severity classification values mapped to incident types is presented later in this document.

Hazard Severity: is the severity of the hazard based on the health impact. The hazard severity is classified as: 1, 2, 3 and follows the classification defined by organizations such as FDA (e.g., listeria spp = 3, pesticide = 2).

TABLE 67.4 Classification used for the incident severity factor.

Incident severity	Value
Food alert/recall	5
Border rejection	4
Information	3
Information for attention	2
Information for follow up	1

Detailed values for the hazard severity are presented later in this document.

Probability: is the probability of the specific hazard to occur for the specific ingredient. The estimation of the probability is based on the frequency of the incidents that a big data system such as FOODAKAI collects and processes everyday.

In the following table, we present the classification used for the incident severity. The classification of incidents are based on the types of incidents used in official data sources such as the Rapid Alert for Food and Feed (Table 67.4).[12]

For the estimation of the incident severity for each specific ingredient in a category we are using the mean value. For instance if for aflatoxin and for pistachio there are 100 alerts, 120 border rejections and 10 information for attention the Severity $= (100 \times 5 + 120 \times 4 + 10 \times 2)/230 = 4.34$ (the closest integer is used, i.e., 4).

In the following table we present the classification of the hazard severity for the most important hazard categories. It should be pointed out that in some cases there are hazards that have different classification values than their category. For instance in a category like Biological there are hazards such as coliforms and molds that have a classification of 2 due to the fact that the health impact is lower. On the other hand there may be cases that a specific hazard may have higher classification value than its category (Table 67.5).

The classification that is used in FOODAKAI is based on the FDA's classification of hazards depicted in the following table (Table 67.6).[13]

The probability can be estimated using two different approaches.

Approach 1: The **first approach** is estimated as the fraction of the number of incidents for the specific ingredient and hazard to the total number of incidents for the specific ingredient.

$$P = \frac{\text{Number of incidents of a hazard for the specific ingredient}}{\text{Total number of incidents for the specific ingredient}}$$

TABLE 67.5 Classification value for the severity factor for the major hazards categories.

Hazard category	Value
Allergens	3
Biological	3
Chemical	2
Foreign bodies	2
Organoleptic	1
Fraud	2
Food contact materials	2

TABLE 67.6 Classification used for the hazard severity factor.

Hazard severity classification	
3	This is a health hazard situation where there is a reasonable probability that the use of the product will cause serious, adverse health consequences or death.
2	This is a health hazard situation where there is a remote probability of adverse health consequences from the use of the product.
1	This is a situation where the use of the product will not cause adverse health consequences.

Approach 2: The **second approach** focuses on the probability a hazard for a specific ingredient to occur in the ingredient category that the ingredient belongs (e.g., a hazard to occur for okra that belongs to fruits and vegetables). It is estimated as the fraction of the # incidents for the specific ingredient and hazard to the total number of the incidents for the specific category of the ingredient and the specific hazard.

$$P = \frac{\text{Number of incidents of a hazard for the specific ingredient}}{\text{Total number of incidents of hazard for the specific ingredient category}}$$

The ranking of the probability is done based on the values in the following table (Table 67.7).

The estimated risk can be classified as Low, Medium, and High as follows:

- 15 = I—Low
- 16–24 = II—Low
- 25–48 = III—Medium
- 49–75 = IV—High

The potential values of the risk for the risk dimensions, namely hazard severity, incident severity and probability, are presented in the following matrix for a specific slice in which Hazard Severity equals to 3 (Fig. 67.4).

67.3.3 Identifying emerging risks

According to European Food Safety Agency, an emerging risk is: "a risk resulting from a newly identified hazard to which a significant exposure may occur, or from an unexpected new or increased significant exposure and/or susceptibility to a known hazard".

Using the analyzed risk estimation approach and the live data stream of the global food safety incidents, it is possible to identify emerging risks by monitoring the tendency of the risk and if there are new unknown hazards that are reported for the first time by the National Authorities. New risks (for a specific hazard and ingredient) are the ones that came up for the first time within the last 12 months and was not identified before in the incidents within the reference period (36 months or 60 months).

Regarding the risk tendency, we can identify increasing and decreasing trends of the estimated risk by comparing the risk of the last 12 months (1 year) with the historical risk for the specific ingredient–hazard pair. More specifically, for the case of the 3 years Risk, the system estimates the Risk of the last 12 months (current date−1 year) and compares it to the Risk of 2 years before the last year.

The formula for the estimation of the tendency is:

$$\text{Tendency}(\%) = \frac{\text{Risk for the period of the last 12 months} - \text{Risk for the period of } N - 12 \text{ months}}{\text{Risk for the period of last } N - 12 \text{ months}}$$

where N is the period of historical incidents that we would like to use for the risk estimation.

If the tendency is negative then we have a decrease and if the tendency is positive we have an increase of the risk. The tendency of the risk is presented in percentage format (%).

TABLE 67.7 Ranking of the probability factor used in the risk assessment.

Probability	Rank	
>75%	5	Frequent
75%–50%	4	Possible
50%–25%	3	Occasional
10%–25%	2	Small possibility
<10%	1	Unlikely

67.3.4 Risk prediction

A robust methodology is needed to generate predictions that are tailor made to the supply chain of a company that is using a specific set of ingredients. The first step of such methodology (Fig. 67.5) is to prepare the datasets that include data specific for a sector and not generic. The second step is to select the AI algorithm that can be applied to this data and fit well to the problem. Different parameters for the AI model need to be explored in terms of performance. The variations of the model need to be trained and tested. Several AI algorithms may be applied to the data of food recalls and border rejections, both machine learning and deep learning algorithms. In this study we selected an algorithm that can work well in a time series prediction problem.

More specifically, food incident data of the last 30 years is used to train a prediction model to predict food

Hazard Severity=3					
	Probability				
Incident Severity	(1) Unlikely	(2) Small possibility	(3) Occasional	(4) Possible	(5) Frequent
I (Low)	I (3)	I (6)	I (9)	I (12)	I (15)
II	I (6)	I (12)	II (18)	II (24)	III (30)
III	I (9)	II (18)	III (27)	III (36)	III (45)
IV	I (12)	II (24)	III (36)	III (48)	IV (60)
V (High)	I (15)	III (30)	III (45)	IV (60)	IV (75)

FIGURE 67.4 Example of a risk matrix.

incidents in the future. The incidents' dataset becomes available through the Data API of the data platform. To that direction, a request to the Data API of the workflow presented in Section 67.3.1 is sent with the product (ingredient or material) for which we want to predict the incidents of the next 12 months. We can build prediction models for specific hazards and specific regions by filtering the result set with the country of interest and the hazard.

For the implementation of the prediction models that are based on the historical food safety incidents Prophet is used.[14] Prophet is a procedure for forecasting time series data based on an additive model where nonlinear trends are fit with yearly, weekly, and daily seasonality, plus holiday effects. It works best with time series that have strong seasonal effects and several seasons of historical data. Prophet is robust to missing data and shifts in the trend, and typically handles outliers well.

The validation of a forecasting model like the one that was used in this study, can be achieved by holding some data back from the model, such as the last 12 months. Then, fitting the model on the first portion of the data, using it to make predictions on the held-pack portion, and calculating an error measure, such as the mean absolute error across the forecasts (e.g., a simulated out-of-sample forecast). The score gives an estimate of how well we might expect the model to perform on average when making an out-of-sample forecast. This can be done with the samples data by creating a new dataset for training with the last 12 months removed.

67.3.5 Setting up a live and automated risk assessment and prediction

Here we would like to focus on how the available data, new innovative digital solutions and the systems that a company already has, can be combined to enable a live and automated risk assessment (Fig. 67.6).

To set up a live risk assessment, we need to feed our risk assessment module with data from different stages of the supply chain such as global data about recalls and lab tests, company internal data about lab tests, non conformities and environmental conditions. This is live data that we continuously collect from public sources and company's data sources. All this data needs to be harmonized and linked so it can be used in the risk assessment steps. The interconnection of this data is achieved using the data workflows that we analyzed earlier in this article.

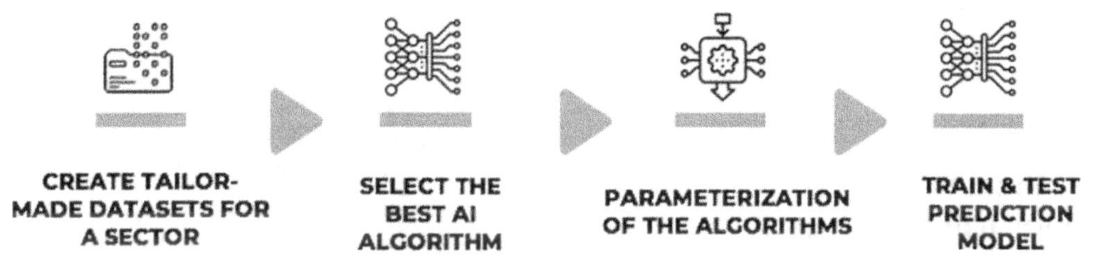

FIGURE 67.5 Risk prediction methodology.

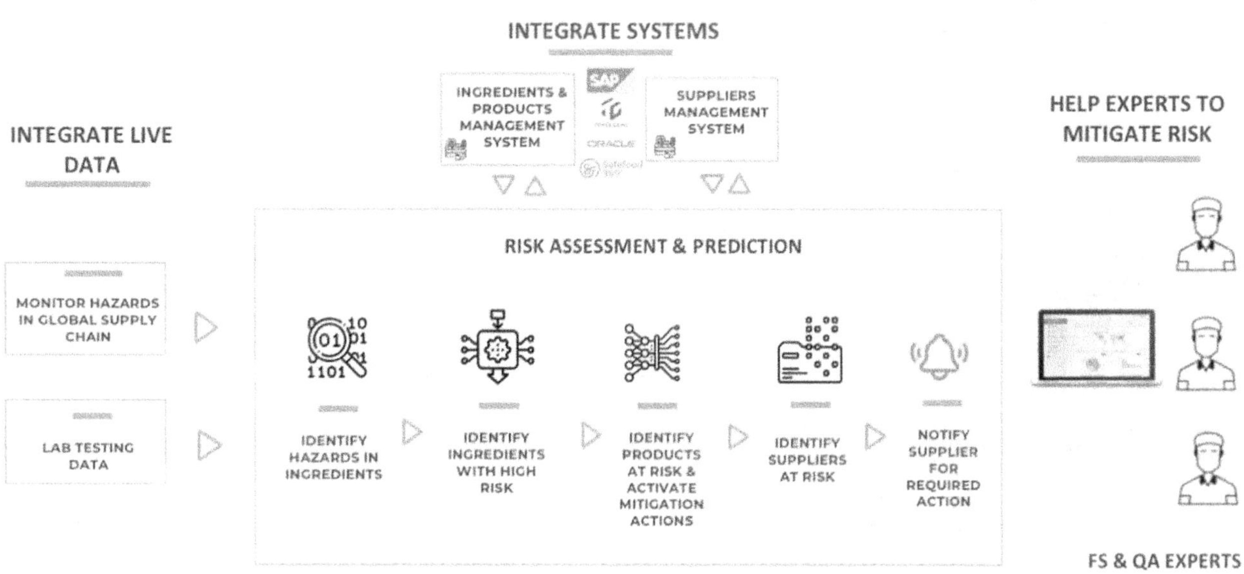

FIGURE 67.6 Automated and integrated risk assessment setup.

The harmonized live data can be then used to monitor hazards in ingredients and to identify ingredients at high risk. Using the information of the ingredients and products management system that the company has, we can identify the products that will be affected and this will help the experts to define the internal mitigation actions. By using the information of the company's suppliers management system, we can notify the suppliers at risk for the required actions, for example, to do extra lab tests, to add a processing control step.

As already analyzed previously in this chapter, today we have both the data and technologies to establish a robust risk assessment strategy that is dynamic and automated. The main points of such strategy are:

- Take advantage of all the available data from different stages of the supply chain
- Combine different tools and software systems that can estimate risk at different stages of the supply chain
- Do not rely on static risk estimations but continuously update the risk
- Automate the approach by connecting risk systems with company's internal systems

Implementing these points, we can help food industry to move away from dealing risk assessment as a manual task based on scattered spreadsheets to a more dynamic, automated, and proactive approach able to identify increasing and emerging risks.

67.4 Case study: risk assessment and prediction for fruits and vegetables

In this section we are focusing on the application of the proposed risk assessment and prediction methodology for fruits and vegetables, a category connected to numerous other products, including dairy and beverages, to unravel how interconnected, enriched and curated food safety data can assist in preventing future product recalls, by generating reliable predictions and useful insights, invaluable to critical business decisions and strategic pivots.

In this use case we created a specific dataset using 78,466 food recalls and 333,842 border rejections. According to historical data from FOODAKAI, fruits and vegetables have the highest percentage (27%) of all incidents in the last 10 years (Fig. 67.7).

Over the years the incidents in this category have increased with the highest peak in 2019. As in most categories in 2020 there was a decreasing tendency, likely due to Covid-19 since less official inspections and tests were taking place (Fig. 67.8).

Top hazards over the last decade in fruits and vegetables were chemical, followed by biological incidents. Together they account for more than 95% of all reported incidents.

In order to generate predictions for this specific category, first we used 20 years of historical data from official, international, and trusted sources. Then, we created a training dataset with the relevant incidents for fruits and vegetables and followed our systematic method to test, measure, and select the right AI algorithms to generate the most accurate and reliable predictions (Fig. 67.9).

According to the prediction model, in the next 12 months we expect a 46% increase in food safety incidents in fruits and vegetables.

To identify specific hazards that are likely to increase for the category of fruits and vegetables, the prediction models were applied for all the potential hazards in this food category. The results of the prediction for hazards are presented in Table 67.8 (Fig. 67.10).

The predictions models were also applied to identify potential new hazards that will emerge in fruits and

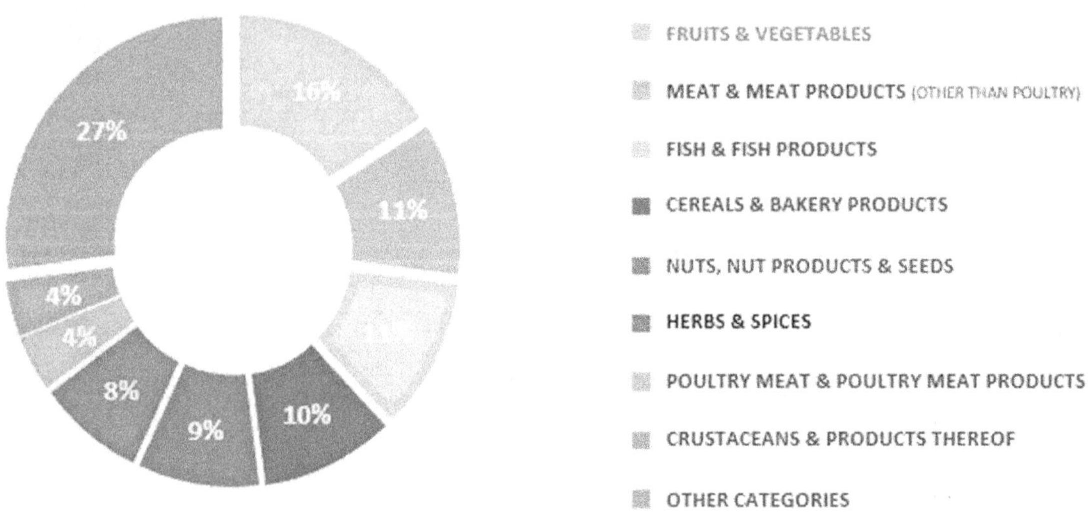

FIGURE 67.7 Distribution of the food safety incidents per product category.

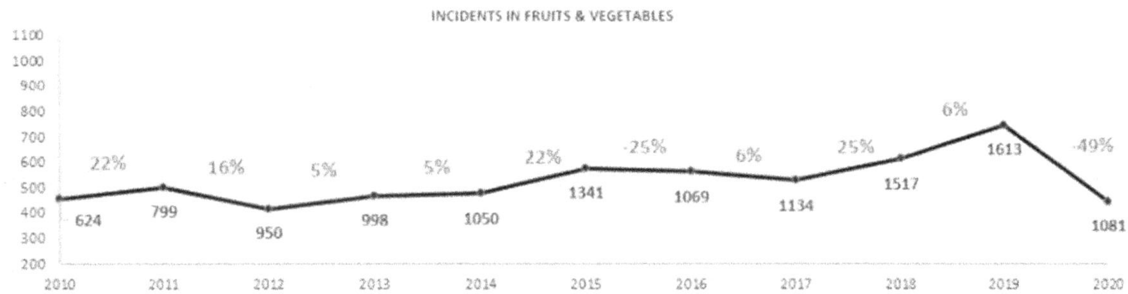

FIGURE 67.8 Trend of the food safety incidents for fruits and vegetables.

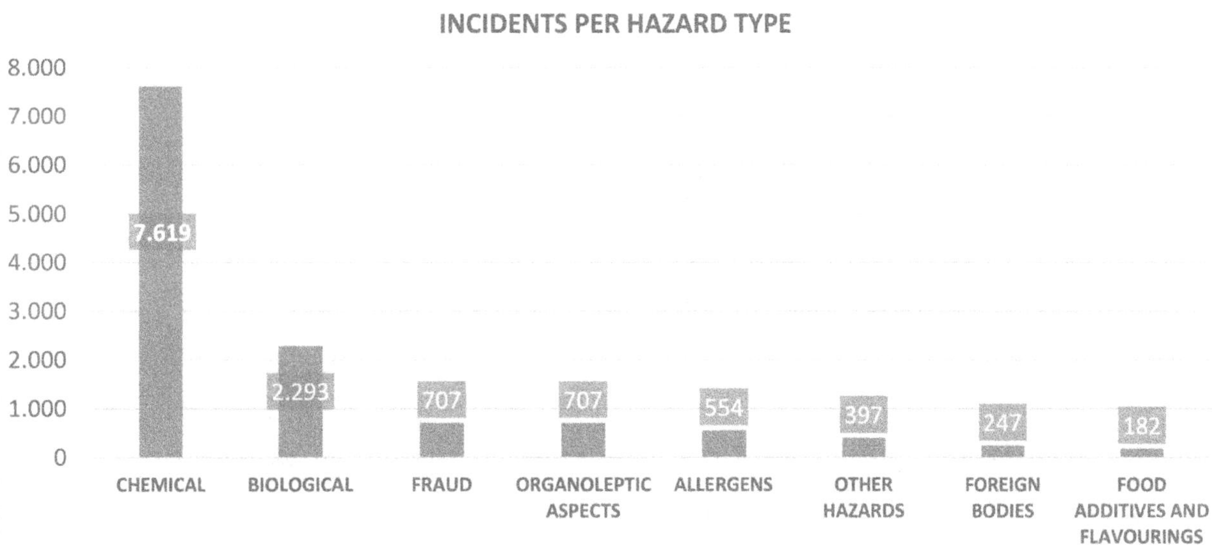

FIGURE 67.9 Distribution of the food safety incidents for fruits and vegetables per hazard category.

TABLE 67.8 Hazards likely to increase for fruit and vegetables.

Hazard	Last 12 months' incidents	Next 12 months' incidents	Tendency (%)
Pesticides	736	1077	46
Chlorpyrifos	115	119	3
Aflatoxin	91	111	22
Chlorpyriphos	4	104	2500
Listeria monocytogenes	48	156	225
Salmonella	89	152	71

vegetables within the next few months. The following hazards were identified:

- chlorinated hydrocarbon
- dieldrin
- nondioxin-like polychlorobifenyls
- paraffin coating

Using the predicted trend for the hazards, we can apply the risk assessment model presented earlier in this chapter in order to predict the trend for the risks in fruits and vegetables. The heatmap of the risk for each hazard and the level of the risk is visualized in the following heatmap (Fig. 67.11). As one can see, the highest predicted risk is for pesticides.

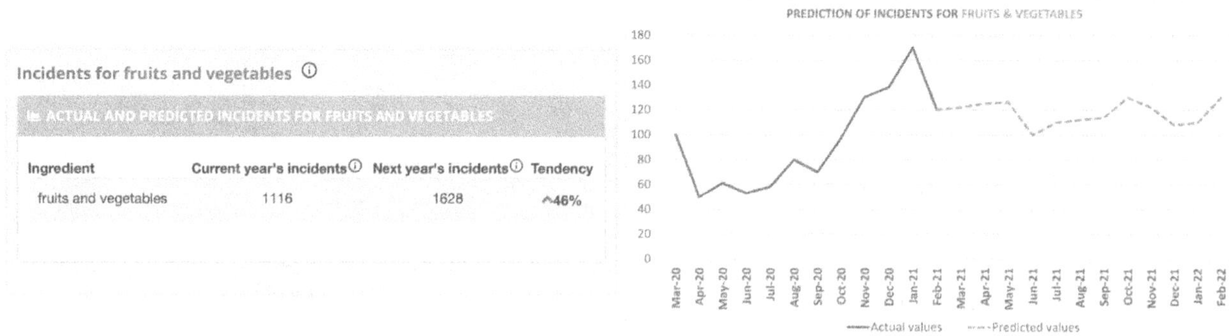

FIGURE 67.10 Prediction of incidents for fruits and vegetables.

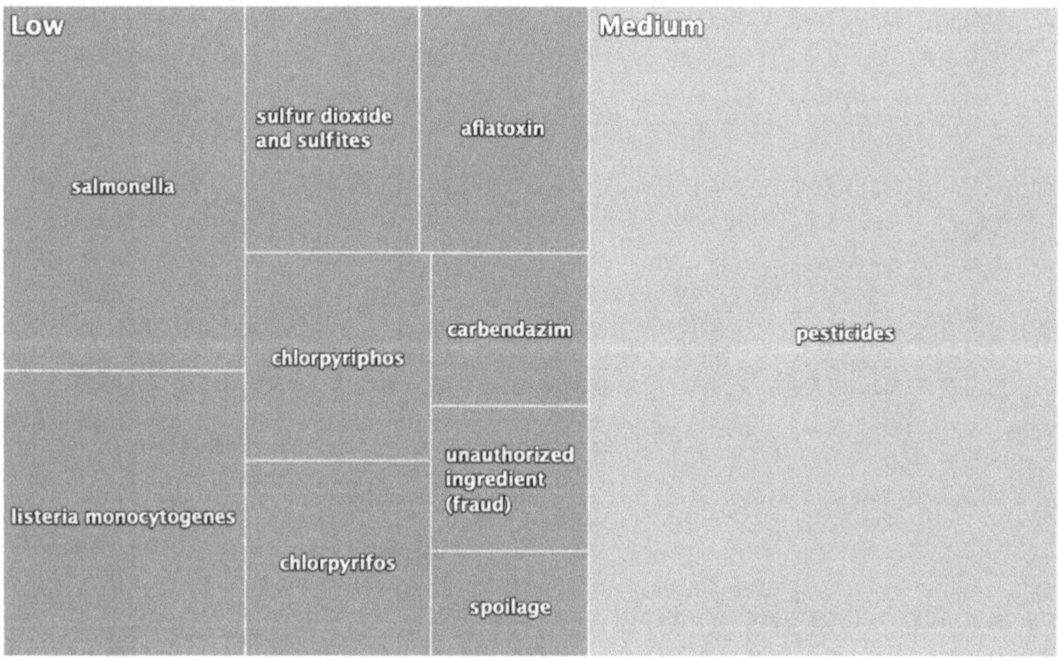

FIGURE 67.11 Heatmap for the predicted risks in fruits and vegetables.

Predictions models can be applied to predict how the risk of a specific hazard in fruits and vegetables will evolve in the next months. As one can see in Fig. 67.12, the risk of pesticides in fruits and vegetables had a significant peak in 2016 and based on the prediction models will increase by 4% within the next 12 months.

By having access to reliable incident predictions for food safety, risks and emerging hazards in the international food supply chain and being able to perform risk assessment for company's key ingredients and suppliers, food safety experts can establish the backbone of a smarter food safety strategy that mitigates food recalls, maintains brand loyalty, and most importantly, protects consumers.

67.5 Research gaps and future perspectives

When it comes to food safety, adopting a proactive strategy to prevent risks from appearing in the food supply chain is currently the most essential shift that the leaders of the largest food manufacturers around the globe are considering. Damage control after a product recall becomes a more outdated practice everyday. Predictive analytics, which have been a hot topic in the food industry for many years, may be an important tool to strengthen the risk assessment approaches.

Today, we are able to predict food safety incidents and identify emerging risks in numerous product categories,

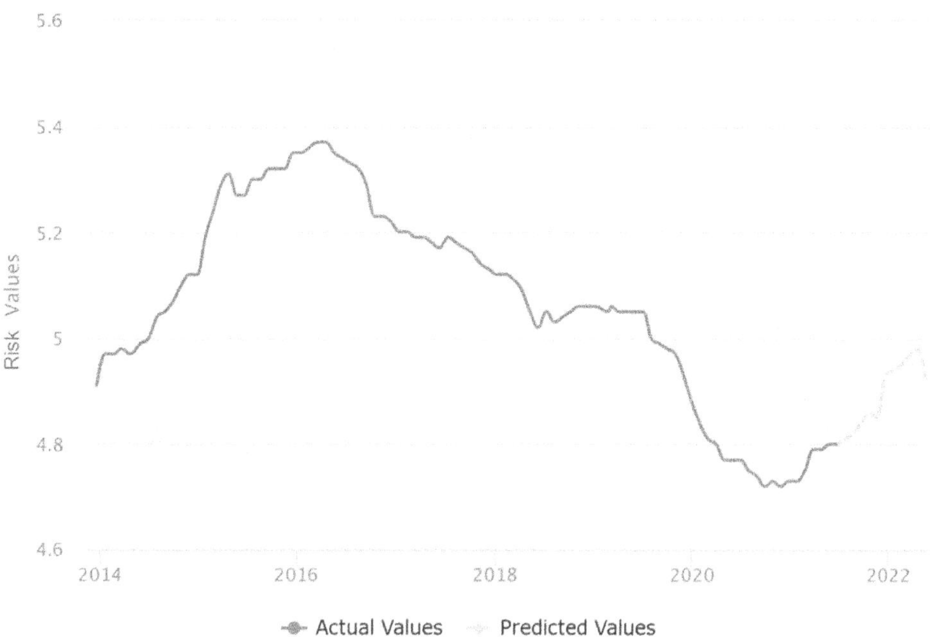

FIGURE 67.12 Risk estimation and prediction for pesticides in fruits and vegetables.

ingredients and international suppliers by harnessing the power of Big Data and AI. Food risk predictions could be generated so that Food Safety and Quality Assurance teams can be prepared to handle the situation before a major product recall happens and causes financial expenditures and, most importantly, damages the brand's trust and reputation. However, mere application of such technologies will not lead to the development of prediction models that will model the complexity of the supply chain. The experience and the knowledge of experts will be needed to develop meaningful and accurate prediction models. Thus it is critical for such prediction models to be developed in close collaboration between scientists, technology experts and food safety experts.

Food industry needs both short term predictions and long term predictions. On the one hand, short term predictions can help in adjusting the laboratory test plan and to optimize it so it can prevent risks. The short term predictions can be like weather forecasts that are used everyday by farmers to plan their farming activities of the next few hours and days. On the other hand, long term risk predictions may help in designing the risk mitigation strategy of the company for the next few years. An example is to use predictive analytics in order to decide the region from which a company will source ingredients in order to minimize the risk of chemical contaminants.

It's important for the risk assessment and prediction approaches to take into consideration all the parameters that may affect the increase of the risk. Previous works have demonstrated the value of applying prediction models to predict fraud.[15] Experts can be involved in the process of selecting which are the risk drivers using interviews and online questionnaires.[16] For each risk driver identified the next step is to find the corresponding data sources that will be used for building the prediction models.

The integration of the latest results from the scientific work that is conducted in the area of food safety and food fraud, into the prediction models can highly contribute to the development of accurate prediction models. A large number of publications and scientific opinions is published and is challenging for the experts to monitor all the research advances and findings. AI can be used to automatically identify these findings by analyzing thousands of publications and reports.[17]

In this study we focused on presenting a method for short term risk prediction. Future perspectives of the current study including the utilization of more parameters in the risk estimation model such as consumption data, manufacturing processes contamination probability, growth potential and cost of illnesses. In addition to that, we plan to test and validate more prediction algorithms that will exploit parameters that are early indicators of emerging risks such as climate change, social data, production data, price data and others that will be indicated by food safety experts. This will enable long term risk predictions in the global food supply chain.

In this chapter we presented how the Big Data and AI technologies can be utilized to assess and predict the risks in foods. The challenges that the food industry is facing and tools that can be used for risk assessment were analyzed. It was concluded that short term risk predictions can help in activating early mitigation actions and that food safety leaders need long term predictions to design the mitigation strategy that will help in reducing the number of food recalls.

Acknowledgment

This work is funded with the support by European Commission, and more specifically project TheFSM "The Food Safety Market: an SME-powered industrial data platform to boost the competitiveness of European food certification" (Grant No. 871703) (https://foodsafetymarket.eu/), which is funded by the schema "Innovation Actions (IA)" under the work programme topic "H2020-EU.2.1.1. – INDUSTRIAL LEADERSHIP – Leadership in enabling and industrial technologies - Information and Communication Technologies (ICT)". This publication reflects the views only of the authors, and the Commission cannot be held responsible for any use, which may be made of the information contained therein.

References

1. Rizou M, Galanakis I, Aldawoud T, Galanakis C. Safety of foods, food supply chain and environment within the COVID-19 pandemic. *Trends Food Sci Technol.* 2020;102:293–299.
2. Cangyu Jin, Bouzembrak Y, Zhou J, et al. Big Data in food safety: a review. *Curr OpFood Sci.* 2020;36:24–32.
3. FERA, HorizonScan. <https://horizon-scan.fera.co.uk/>.
4. Polychronou I, Katsivelis P, Papakonstantinou M, Stoitsis G, Manouselis N. Machine learning algorithms for food intelligence: towards a method for more accurate predictions. In: *International Symposium on Environmental Software Systems*; 2020:165–172.
5. Chen Y, Dennis S, Hartnett E, et al. FDA-iRISK—a comparative risk assessment system for evaluating and ranking food-hazard pairs: case studies on microbial hazards. *J Food Prot.* 2013;76(3):376–385. Available from: https://doi.org/10.4315/0362-028X.JFP-12-372.
6. Baranyi J, Tamplin M. ComBase: a common database on microbial responses to food environments. *J Food Prot.* 2004;67(9):1967–1971. Available from: https://doi.org/10.4315/0362-028X-67.9.1967.
7. University of Tasmania. CB Premium. <https://www.cbpremium.org>.
8. Safefood360. <https://safefood360.com/>.
9. Polychronou I, Stoitsis G, Papakonstantinou M, Manouselis N. Stress-testing big data platform to extract smart and interoperable food safety analytics. *Int J Metadata Semant Ontol.* 2020;14(4).
10. Indrasiri K, Siriwardena P. Microservices for the Enterprise: Designing, Developing, and Deploying, *Berkeley*. Springer; 2018.
11. Center for Food Safety and Applied Nutrition Food and Drug Administration, U.S. Department of Health and Human Services, Methodological Approach to Developing a Risk-Ranking Model for Food Tracing FSMA Section 204 (21 U.S. Code Section 2223). https://www.fda.gov/media/142247/download; 2020.
12. European Food Safety Agency, RASFF—the Rapid Alert System for Food and Feed. <https://ec.europa.eu/food/safety/rasff_en>.
13. United States Department of Agriculture, Food Safety and Inspection Service, Food Recalls Classification. <https://www.fsis.usda.gov/wps/portal/fsis/topics/food-safety-education/get-answers/food-safety-fact-sheets/production-and-inspection/fsis-food-recalls/fsis-food-recalls>.
14. Taylor SJ, Letham B. Forecasting at scale. *Am Statistician.* 2018;72(1):37–45.
15. Marvin H, Bouzembrak Y, Janssen E, Van der Fels- Klerx HJ, Van Asselt E, Kleter G. A holistic approach to food safety risks: food fraud as an example. *Food Res Int.* 2016;89(1):463–470.
16. Marvin H, Esther van Asselt, Kleter G, et al. Expert-driven methodology to assess and predict the effects of drivers of change on vulnerabilities in a food supply chain: aquaculture of Atlantic salmon in Norway as a showcase. *Trends Food Sci Technol.* 2020;103:49–56.
17. Gavai A, Bouzembrak Y, van den Bulk LM, et al. Artificial intelligence to detect unknown stimulants from scientific literature and media reports. *Food Control.* 2021;130:108360.

Chapter 68

Blockchain: an enabler for safe food in global supply networks

John G. Keogh[1], Abderahman Rejeb[2], Nida Khan[3] and Khaldoon Zaid-Kaylani[4]

[1]*Henley Business School, University of Reading, Henley-on-Thames, United Kingdom,* [2]*University of Rome Tor Vergata, Rome, Italy,* [3]*Nash FintechX, Esch-sur-Alzette, Luxembourg,* [4]*InCube Mobility Solutions, Oakville, ON, Canada*

Abstract

Recurring food safety and food fraud incidents have negatively impacted the food industry's credibility and consumer confidence. As a result, food safety management and food fraud risk have garnered significant attention. Food business operators are aware of the need to respond to consumer concerns regarding product quality and safety and shape consumer attitudes regarding food. In parallel, businesses with local, regional, or global food supply chains (FSCs) are continually evaluating the use of advanced technologies to improve supply chain efficiency and flexibility and reduce risk. In this regard, scholars have examined food safety issues and proposed blockchain technology. Blockchain is a foundational innovation that has the potential to radically transform FSCs and support the efficient management and operations of food industry stakeholders. In this chapter, we aim to expand the academic understanding of the full potential of the technology and the impediments to its adoption in the food industry by providing a comprehensive review and understanding of the literature's most prominent topics. As the chapter's primary sources of information, two blockchain use cases were selected, summarised, and analysed to highlight the practical relevance of adopting the technology in the FSC. The chapter's findings indicate that blockchain can improve FSC traceability, transparency and trust, collaboration and trade, and contributes to food safety management. However, the technology's benefits cannot be realised until technical, organisational, and regulatory issues are resolved.

Keywords: Blockchain; food; supply chains; traceability; transparency; trust; food integrity

68.1 Introduction

Globalization has increased the complexity of the agrifood sector, which now includes numerous interconnected ecosystems ranging from primary production to foodservice and retail.[1] Food is both a fundamental human right and an integral part of the economy of every nation.[2] Additionally, access to safe, nutritious, and affordable food is critical for an economy's health, well-being, productivity, and sustainable development.[3,4] Consumers in developed and developing economies can now access foods once considered seasonal or exotic, but several factors affect their availability and safety for consumption. Among these factors are food quality and perishability, food safety and the risk of food fraud. Food fraud is a complicated issue that encompasses everything from documentation fraud (e.g., fake food safety test results, fabricating organic or halal certification, and fabricating country of origin) to product dilution, substitution, concealment, unapproved enhancements, and mislabeling.[5]

On a global scale, developing nations may face a shortage of skilled labor, inadequate infrastructural (e.g., roads, refrigeration, warehousing), and technological deficiencies on farms and in information and communications technologies (ICT).[6] As a result, designing global food supply chains (FSCs) is a complicated task due to the intrinsic focus and governance required of the food product, and the extrinsic focus needed to build and maintain FSCs that ensure the integrity of food in transit.[7]

Furthermore, institutional investors are concerned about the environmental, social, and corporate governance (ESG) implications of FSCs and the lack of transparency surrounding them. For instance, in November 2020, the CEOs of Canada's top eight pension funds with a combined $1.6 trillion in assets under management stated that they would be demanding increased transparency from the companies in which they invest and that ESG factors would play a role in their investment decisions.[8]

FSCs encompass a diverse range of interconnected ecosystems, and a breakdown or disruption in the FSC can cause panic if supply is disrupted.[2] According to

Present Knowledge in Food Safety. DOI: https://doi.org/10.1016/B978-0-12-819470-6.00008-1

Maloni and Brown,[9] agrifood is one of the few sectors that receives significant public attention due to well-documented vulnerabilities (e.g., food safety, food quality, food fraud) and the concerns over the rising cost of food products. As a result, management of the FSC requires a strategic approach to governance and risk mitigation associated with improper or unauthorized practices.[7] Failure to mitigate risk can result in a variety of food frauds or low quality and unsafe products being placed on the market with potentially severe consequences such as foodborne illness and deaths and resulting in a costly product safety recall. Ensuring FSC efficiency while understanding and mitigating consumer risks is of paramount importance. Blockchain technology may be a useful tool for reducing uncertainties and friction between exchange parties in FSCs.

According to Treiblmaier[10] (p. 547), blockchain is a *digital, decentralized, and distributed ledger in which transactions are logged and added in chronological order with the goal of creating permanent and tamperproof records*. Blockchain can also be conceptualized as a combination of multiple technologies, tools, and methods that are configured to address a particular problem or business use case.[11] A blockchain eliminates the need for third-party intermediaries in the transaction process, allowing users to directly exchange value and resources.[12] The decentralized ledger of records and transactions is distributed across the different computers that form the entire system. Data is saved in blocks distributed on a peer-to-peer basis in the blockchain system, with changes being made via a consensus mechanism.[13] Blockchain participants are involved in an iterative process[14] in which each computing node contributes to the authentication of transactions[13] and the security of the entire system is maintained across a high number of untrusted nodes.[15] Consensus mechanisms are a core component of blockchain as they provide a fault-tolerant mechanism for how data entries are accepted and validated onto a blockchain-based distributed ledger.[16] Its high-security characterizes blockchain technology's data structure due to cryptographic methods such as hashing and encryption.[14,15,17–19] Moreover, the chaining of blocks allows users to trace the whole chain of valid network transactions back to the first block initiated in the blockchain. Apart from eliminating intermediaries and reducing transaction costs, blockchain's unique features include data provenance and transparency, immutability, enhanced security, increased reliability, and auditability that have served as the main drivers for its application in different sectors of the economy.

Blockchain is viewed as a potential game changer in the agrifood sector, with the potential to reshape numerous activities and (digital) business processes.[20] The technology enables FSC stakeholders to enhance critical functions such as end-to-end traceability and the ability to conduct rapid product safety recalls.[21] Additionally, blockchain has the potential to ameliorate friction between FSC stakeholders by providing a reliable, auditable, and accessible record of food products' entire life cycle from primary production to retail.[22] The recurrence of incidents involving food quality, food safety, and food fraud is alarming and undermines consumer trust. Subsequently, food organizations are constantly evaluating advanced technologies such as blockchain, IoT-based sensor devices, Artificial Intelligence (AI), and other tools to improve the traceability of food products, permit predictive analytics, and enhance the overall performance and integrity of their global FSCs.

Organizations can use blockchain technology to assuage mounting public anxiety about the lack of transparency and low trust in globalized food ecosystems. Concerns about recurring ethical, moral, and social license violations such as forced labor, child labor, deforestation, product cross-contamination and food safety recalls. Blockchain technology enables organizations to improve data transparency, verifiability, security, and trust in the FSC.[23] The blockchain is a cutting-edge technology that can be used as part of a food safety management program because it creates a permanent, unfalsifiable record for every transaction between FSC stakeholders.[24,25] While not covered in this chapter, organizations can layer Internet of Things (IoT) sensor devices like real-time temperature monitoring and AI on top of blockchain to gain real-time and predictive capabilities.

According to the literature, developing blockchain-based FSCs can aid in assuring the provenance and safety of food products,[26] improve relationships between FSC stakeholders and reduce friction,[27] and support transactional security and privacy.[28] It is critical to note here that both peer-reviewed research papers and marketing literature frequently conflate *data provenance* or when data was entered into the blockchain, with *scientific provenance*[a] of food, as determined by analytical science methods such as stable isotope analysis or trace element analysis. In this regard, data provenance could be providing *false provenance* of the food.

Additionally, numerous studies demonstrate that blockchain is not a silver bullet for achieving efficient, sustainable, and safe FSCs.[29–31] For example, several technical issues surrounding blockchain continue to be unresolved, including scalability, redundancies, and privacy. Due to the technical immaturity of blockchain technology and its potential novel applications in the food industry, questions are raised about the availability of technical experts with the necessary in-depth knowledge and skills to deploy the technology.[32] For these reasons, blockchain deployment in FSCs is likely to be a long and arduous process.[33] Moreover, Iansiti and Lakhani[33] argued that blockchain should not be viewed as *disruptive*. Instead, blockchain should be considered a *foundational* technology that will take time to implement and eventually deliver significant societal benefits.

While the literature continues to debate the benefits and limitations of blockchain in supply chain management, additional research is needed to elucidate the technology's specific role(s) in FSCs and to broaden academic and practitioners' knowledge and empirical evidence. A more comprehensive assessment of the full potentials and limitations of blockchain technology in relation to FSCs is required. As such, we aim to partially fill this void by conducting a review of the academic literature to determine how blockchain technology can make FSCs safer. Throughout the chapter, we will examine several research questions related to the integration of blockchain in the food industry, including:

68.1.1 Research question: what are the benefits and limitations of blockchain in global food supply chains?

We add to the existing body of knowledge by synthesizing blockchain research in the FSC. Additionally, we concur with Yiannas[34] that blockchain is deserving attention due to the technology's inherent characteristics and implications when applied to FSCs. This includes the significant structural changes that this entails, the potential societal consequences, and the barriers to the development of blockchain-based food ecosystems.

The chapter is organized as follows. Following the introduction, we describe the methodology we used to compile the pertinent academic contributions to blockchain and the FSC. Section 68.3 contains the review's descriptive statistics. The following section discusses the study's findings based on keyword coding. Section 68.5 provides a technical overview of blockchain technology, followed by Section 68.6, which illustrates the technology's value in the FSC through two case studies. Finally, the chapter concludes with a summary.

68.2 Methodology

To address our research questions, we conducted a systematic review of the literature (SLR) in the manner described by Tranfield et al.[35] SLR is a well-established and rigorous scientific method that has been widely used in numerous supply chain management and logistics-related studies.[29,36,37] SLRs are distinct from traditional and narrative reviews of the literature in that they require specific planning and methodical processes. The steps in conducting a systematic review are as follows: (1) formulation of research questions, (2) literature search, (3) evaluation and selection of pertinent studies, (4) analysis and synthesis of results, and (5) reporting of review findings.[35] The research questions for this chapter are determined by our research objectives, which are to investigate blockchain as a potential enabler of secure FSCs. The search for related literature began with an assessment of the state of current research in the respective field through the collection and identification of all pertinent studies. In October 2020, one of the research team's authors conducted an extensive search of the Scopus database to locate and select relevant studies. The initial investigation discovered a dearth of recent publications on the nexus between blockchain and the FSC. In comparison to other scientific databases, Scopus is well-known for its effectiveness[38] and comprehensive coverage of the literature in a variety of fields including science, social sciences, technology, medical sciences, and the art and humanities.[39] The following keywords were used in the title, abstract, and keywords fields to compile relevant studies for this review:

68.2.1 Blockchain and food

To ensure the materials high-quality, we considered only peer-reviewed journal articles. Given the widespread interest in blockchain among academics working in a variety of fields of study, no subject areas were used to group the publications. Additionally, there was no time constraints applied, as this could result in unsatisfactory search results. To begin, the search query returned 117 publications that had their titles and abstracts screened for relevance. Second, a spreadsheet was used to organize and facilitate the systematic review of the publications. After the initial screening, we identified 100 publications that were relevant to the scope of our chapter. Although the majority of the excluded articles contained the keywords *"blockchain"* and *"food"* in their abstracts, they were either technical in nature or lacked an explicit focus on blockchain applications in the food industry (e.g.,[40,41]). During the second screening, we read the entirety of each publication and determined whether to include or exclude the documents based on our research objectives. As a result, we ended up with a final dataset of 92 articles for review and analysis. The search process used in this chapter is depicted in Fig. 68.1.

68.3 Descriptive results

68.3.1 Year-wise distribution of publications

The annual distribution of the reviewed literature is depicted in Fig. 68.2. The distribution of publications by year demonstrates an exponential growth in the number of journal articles discussing blockchain applications in the food industry. The first article on this topic was published in 2017, proposing a new blockchain consensus algorithm for transactions related to the IoT data and food history.[42]

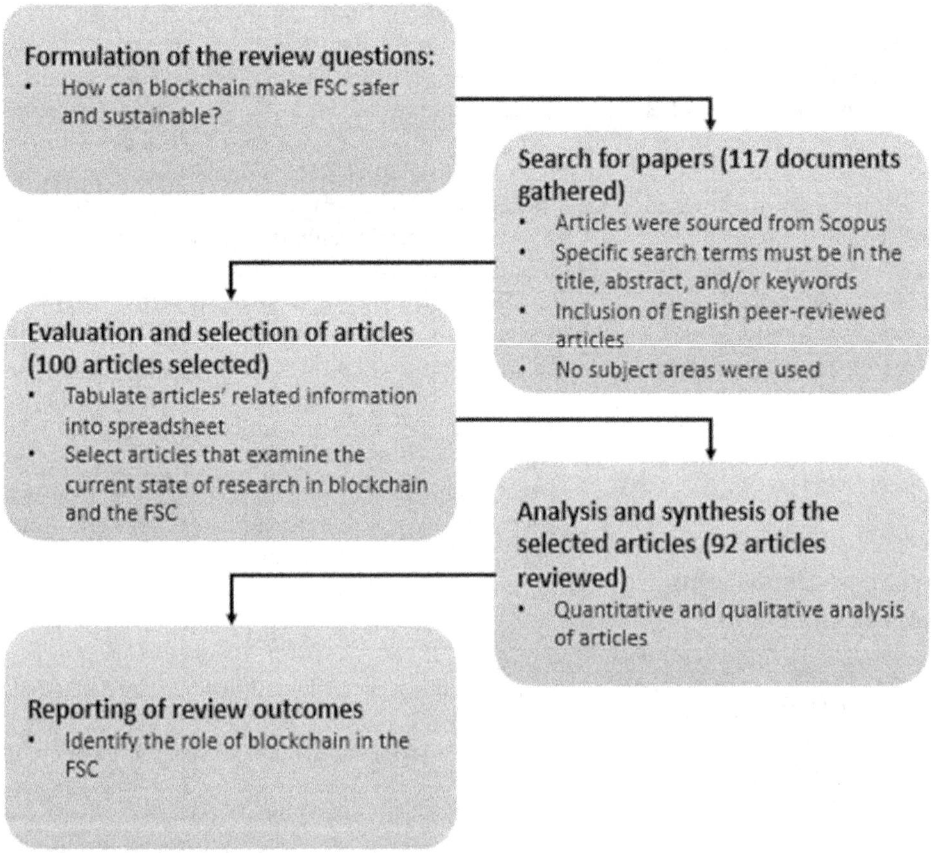

FIGURE 68.1 Schematic presentation of the review protocol.

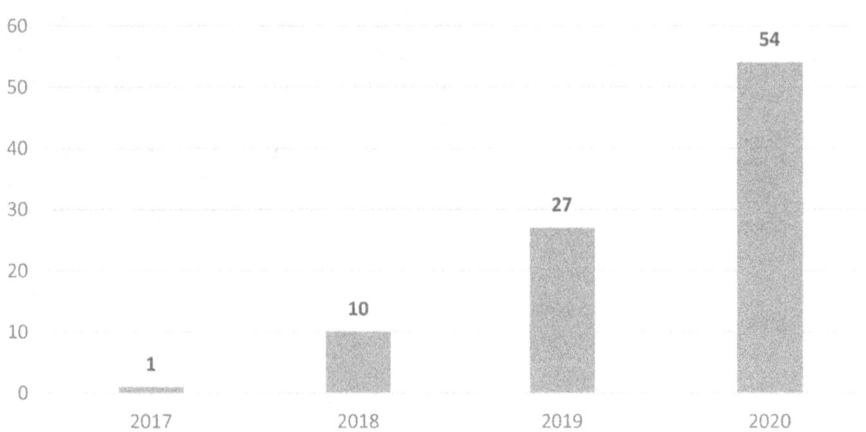

FIGURE 68.2 Annual distribution of selected articles.

Since 2018, the number of articles published has increased significantly, reflecting a widespread interest in blockchain. The growing scholarly and practitioner interest in blockchain technology is expected to increase, resulting in a continued growth of future publications.

68.3.2 Journal-wise distribution of publications

Table 68.1 presents the classification of articles according to academic journals. Overall, the 92 articles were published in 65 academic journals. *IEEE Access* stands out from the rest of the journals, publishing the highest number of articles. To a lesser extent, the *Journal of Cleaner Production* published five articles. *International Journal of Information Management* and *Trends in Food Science and Technology* published three articles each. Ten journals published two articles each, and the remaining journals on the list published only one article on blockchain and the FSC. The analysis of the articles, according to the sources, reflects the topical richness of blockchain research from the FSC perspective, which appeals to various academic communities, including those that focus on

TABLE 68.1 Distribution of articles according to journals.

Source title	Number of publications
IEEE Access	10
Journal of Cleaner Production	5
International Journal of Information Management	3
Trends in Food Science and Technology	3
Computers in Industry	2
Food Control	2
International Journal of Advanced Computer Science and Applications	2
International Journal of Environmental Research and Public Health	2
International Journal of Production Economics	2
IT Professional	2
Production Planning and Control	2
Sensors	2
Supply Chain Management	2
Sustainability	2
Others (One article per journal)	51

computer science, engineering, production operations, business and management, and food sciences.

68.3.3 Content analysis

Identifying the topics discussed in the literature often requires a subjective content analysis of the selected publications manually, reading the full text of the publications, or using dedicated software. To identify the prevailing research themes on blockchain technology in the context of FSCs, we used author-supplied keywords, following the procedure suggested by Ferreira[43] and Furrer et al.[44] We coded the keywords into key themes of categories. The author-supplied keywords indicate each publication's content since authors choose the keywords that best convey their publication content to potential readers and serve indexing purposes.

Of the 92 journal articles, 244 author-supplied keywords were treated. The coding process was necessary to obtain interpretable results. One coder categorized each keyword into eight key themes: (1) traceability, (2) combination of blockchain with other technologies (IoT, smart contracts, Big Data, AI, (3) food safety, (4) trust and transparency, (5) sustainability, (6) data management and security, (7) food trade, and (8) barriers to blockchain adoption. Table 68.2 presents the classification of the reviewed literature into the major themes based on author-supplied keywords. We obtained a clear overview

TABLE 68.2 Content analysis of the reviewed literature.

Themes	Example of supporting literature
(1) Traceability	Antonucci et al.,[45] Astill et al.,[46] Barge et al.,[47] Behnke & Janssen,[48] Casino et al.,[49] Chan et al.,[50] Creydt & Fischer,[51] Demestichas et al.,[52] dos Santos et al.,[53] Feng et al.,[54] Galvez et al.,[55] George et al.,[21] Gopi et al.,[56] Grecuccio et al.,[57] Guido et al.,[58] Hao et al.,[59] Hao et al.,[60] He et al.,[61] Hew et al.,[62] Kamble et al.,[63] Kayikci et al.,[64] Khan et al.,[65] Khanna et al.,[66] Kim & Laskowski,[67] Lin et al.,[68] Lin et al.,[69] Longo et al.,[70] Patelli & Mandrioli,[71] Prashar et al.,[72] Qian et al.,[73] Qian et al.,[74] Qian et al.,[75] Rao et al.,[76] Salah et al.,[77] Samal & Pradhan,[78] Scuderi et al.,[27] Shahid et al.,[79] Stranieri et al.,[80] Surasak et al.,[81] Tan et al.,[82] Torky & Hassanein,[83] Tripoli & Schmidhuber,[84] Tsang et al.,[85] Tsolakis et al.,[86] Wallace & Manning[87]
(2) Combination of blockchain with other technologies (IoT, smart contracts, Big Data, Artificial Intelligence)	*IoT*: Alonso et al.,[88] Antonucci et al.,[45] Astill et al.,[46] Barge et al.,[47] Cho et al.,[42] Feng et al.,[54] Grecuccio et al.,[57] Khan et al.,[65] Klerkx et al.,[89] Lezoche et al.,[90] Mondal et al.,[91] Surasak et al.,[81] Torky & Hassanein,[83] Tsang et al.,[85] Violino et al.,[92] Zhao et al.[30] *Smart contracts*: Casino et al.,[49] dos Santos et al.,[53] Khanna et al.,[66] Kim & Laskowski,[67] Lin et al.,[68] Prashar et al.,[72] Qian et al.,[73] Salah et al.,[77] Tan et al.,[82] Tao et al.,[93] Yu et al.,[94] Zhang et al.,[95] *Big Data*: Astill et al.,[46] Lezoche et al.,[90] Liu et al.[96] *AI*: Antonucci et al.,[45] Lezoche et al.,[90] Qian et al.[73]
(3) Food safety and security	Bumblauskas et al.,[97] Dinesh Kumar et al.,[24] Dinesh Kumar et al.,[25] Guido et al.,[58] Hao et al.,[60] Hew et al.,[62] Kayikci et al.,[64] Lin et al.,[68] Longo et al.,[70] Qian et al.,[73] Rogerson & Parry,[23] Salah et al.,[77] Tao et al.,[93] Tripoli & Schmidhuber,[84] Violino et al.,[92] Zhang et al.[95]
(4) Trust and transparency	Astill et al.,[46] Chan et al.,[50] Feng et al.,[54] Hao et al.,[60] Kamble,[98] Kamble,[63] Kittipanya-ngam & Tan,[100]; Prashar et al.,[72] Rogerson & Parry,[23] Shahid et al.,[79] Tsolakis et al.[86]
(5) Sustainability	Astill et al.,[46] Davies & Garrett,[100] Feng et al.,[54] Kamble et al.,[63] Klerkx & Rose,[101] Kouhizadeh et al.,[102] Mao et al.,[103] Tiscini et al.,[104] Tsolakis et al.[86]

(*Continued*)

TABLE 68.2 (Continued)

Themes	Example of supporting literature
(6) Data management and security	Feng et al.,[54] Galvez et al.,[55] Hao et al.,[60] He et al.,[61] Kumar et al.,[26] Lin et al.,[69] Scuderi et al.,[27] Shivaanivarsha & Santhoshkumar,[105] Steinwandter & Herwig,[106] Surasak et al.[81]
(7) Food trade	Hao et al.,[60] Mao et al.,[103] Qian et al.,[73] Tripoli & Schmidhuber[84]
(8) Barriers to blockchain adoption	Kouhizadeh et al.,[102] Rao et al.,[76] Yadav et al.[107]

of the topics covered and discussed in the selected articles in applying this procedure. Although prior studies categorized each article into one category (e.g.[44]), we allowed articles to be in more than one category to recognize the research's multidimensional nature. As such, an article may be categorized into the theme "Traceability" and "Transparency" based on the author-supplied keywords.

68.4 Findings

This section elaborates on the main themes identified from the coding procedure applied to author-supplied keywords. It should be noted that some themes (e.g., a combination of blockchain with other technologies) are highly diffused, overlapping the content of the different themes (e.g., traceability, trust, and transparency), and therefore are not separately analyzed.

68.4.1 Traceability

Aung and Chang[108] define food traceability as the:

> part of logistics management that capture, store, and transmit adequate information about a food, feed, food-producing animal or substance at all stages in the food supply chain so that the product can be checked for safety and quality control, traced upward, and tracked downward at any time required. *(p. 35)*

Traceability is viewed as a strategic tool that can be used to improve food safety systems including the management of raw materials and finished goods, product safety recalls and can enhance competitive advantage for businesses.[49,108] While food producing organizations require traceability for regulatory compliance, it is critical for building consumer trust and upholding food quality and food safety standards.[109] Implementing traceability remains difficult and costly when food products contain multiple ingredients from different countries.[110] Prior research has established that tracking and tracing (collectively traceability) of food is a difficult and complicated task in conventional supply chain that are geographically dispersed, scattered, and disconnected.[63] According to Prashar et al.[72] implementing traceability is costly and challenging. And the consequences of failing to implement the necessary traceability systems may be severe for food organizations in the form of costly recalls, litigation, and reputation damage. Thus to address the numerous issues associated with traditional FSC traceability approaches, blockchain technology represents a potentially transformative tool that can enable interoperability between exchange partners and can enhance transparency and trust from primary production to the end consumer.[49] Blockchain technology can be used to improve the trace back to a foods geographic origin (food provenance) through the design of origin chains that are secure, visible, and adaptable to accommodate regulatory changes in compliance.[109] In their recent study, Bumblauskas et al.[97] note that blockchain could be used to supplement food traceability in new and current supply chains because it is a solution to siloed FSC activities and can be integrated into existing systems and technologies without requiring significant process or behavioral changes on the part of the FSC stakeholders. The integrity of food products in global FSCs can be further enhanced when food safety, authenticity, claims verification, and provenance data from analytical laboratory testing are stored in chronological order and protected against manipulation. In this regard, Galvez et al.[55] noted that blockchain technology enhances analytical processes, data acquisition, and management, thereby (digitally) assuring the quality and safety of food products.

There is a plethora of academic literature on the role of blockchain technology in facilitating food traceability, with several scholars proposing FSC designs based on the technology.[111] For example, Tsang et al.[85] present a blockchain and IoT-based food traceability system (BIFTS) that integrates blockchain, IoT technology, and fuzzy logic into a fully traceable shelf-life management system for managing and monitoring perishable food products. The proposed traceability system is compatible with the requirements of today's FSC environment and enables reliable and intelligent monitoring, food tracking, and quality assurance. He et al.[61] propose a decentralized and irreversible traceability system based on blockchain technology for storing commodity data. Through the analysis of traceability data, such a system would enable users to determine whether a commodity is potentially a counterfeit. Hao et al.[59] created a traceability system for agricultural products using an Interplanetary File System

(IPFS), blockchain, and IoT. If users have doubts about the product's origin, data can be verified using blockchain (i.e., to validate the data provenance whereas analytical science is needed to validate the true or scientific geographic origin of the food). dos Santos et al.[53] investigated the traceability requirements for recipe-based foods and proposed a substitute for full-chain traceability. Apart from facilitating the traceability of food ingredients, the proposed system establishes a framework for food certification that ensures the confidentiality of business-sensitive data for foods derived from comingling operations.

Similarly, Lin et al.[68] developed a food safety traceability system based on blockchain and the joint GS1 and ISO interoperability standard called EPCIS. The system aims to provide a management architecture for on-chain and off-chain data where the traceability system can overcome potential data explosion issues of the blockchain for IoT. Overall, the common point between these systems is that data collected in blockchain-based food traceability systems constitutes an effective tool since blockchain provides more granular information about food products. The integration of blockchain helps to minimize the production and distribution of unsafe and unsatisfactory food products. Moreover, it can also accelerate recalling a particular lot or batch of hazardous food products rather than recalling all products in the FSC. According to George et al.,[21] the speed of detecting certain food frauds can be instantaneous instead of a centralized food traceability system. The authors further note that blockchain features can be used as a beneficial marketing tool to strengthen consumer loyalty. The assurance that blockchain gives on food traceability enhances customer value, increases their willingness to pay for traceable food products, and improves awareness regarding the certified, safe, and sustainable origin of food products.[104]

68.4.2 Trust and transparency

Trust is defined in the business-to-business (B2B) context as the willingness to rely on a trading partner in whom one has confidence. It refers to the degree to which trading partners (i.e., buyers and suppliers) regard one another as credible, reliable, and benevolent.[112–114] Trust between trading partners facilitates the establishment of long-term relationships.[115,116] Numerous studies emphasize the critical nature of developing trusting relationships within FSCs.[117,118]

Consumer trust is critical in a business-to-consumer (B2C) context for the continued existence of a market for food products with credence claims (e.g., organic, grass-fed, wild-caught) that command premium prices.[119] Transparency is a prerequisite for increasing consumer trust in food products, as it eliminates uncertainties and increases information visibility throughout the entire FSC processes.[120] Due to the growing emphasis on environmental, social, and governance (ESG) issues and rising consumer expectations, transparency is a critical property for FSCs and a management priority.[121,122]

Transparency is defined in the FSC context as the breath of coverage from upstream to downstream FSC stakeholders and the degree to which information is visible to downstream members.[123] Because FSC operations are frequently fast-paced, climate-sensitive, and involve perishable products, trust and transparency are strategic management concerns.[124] While enhancing trust and transparency in FSCs is acknowledged to be difficult, advanced technologies such as blockchain can be used to increase the transparency of food production systems.[46]

Due to the distributed nature of blockchain technology, it aligns with FSC transparency requirements (i.e., improving the visibility and flow of information) and may mitigate the weaknesses inherent in centralized supply chain management solutions.[50] When implemented properly, blockchain enables "gap-less transparency" between the FSCs exchange parties. Moreover, the blockchain is structured to increase transparency and trust, which reduces friction between exchange parties and helps to improving relationships.[109] According to Kayikci et al.[64] a blockchain consortium is the most widely accepted and suitable business model because it has the potential to bring like-minded organizations together in the FSC and provides a new level of trust and transparency based on a single view of the truth. For instance, Walmart, IBM, and Beijing Tsinghua University collaborated to develop a model for food traceability, supply chain transparency, and audibility using blockchain technology.[55] Further, food waste can be reduced when blockchain is combined with IoT-based sensors that perform data capture and sharing of temperature information during storage and distribution.[86] According to Kamble et al.[63] blockchain adoption in the FSC increases information visibility and transparency, and ameliorates trust-related issues. By utilizing blockchain technology to increase FSC transparency, food organizations can reduce the risks related to product safety recalls, while boosting consumer confidence in FSC processes, and increasing consumer satisfaction.[80]

The increased transparency enabled by blockchain technology has the potential to improve coordination and process synchronization, as well as to reduce friction and drive down the transaction costs associated with an FSC.[99] Additionally, the transparency enabled by blockchain technology is critical for food organizations to ensure data and information authenticity, maintain food integrity along the value chain, and retain consumer trust. Tan et al.,[82] for example, note that public permissionless or private permissionless blockchains are appropriate for promoting information transparency and integrity and for strengthening halal FSCs. According to the authors, blockchain technology can be used in conjunction with smart contracts to achieve complete FSC transparency, as QR codes can be validated by smart contracts that require each process to adhere to specific guidelines (e.g., halal).

Historically, FSC transparency has been lacking, and consumers have been forced to search for information to make informed decisions.[125,126] Consumers can now access expanded information about the product's source, type of ingredients, cultivation and processing methods, as well as other information about the social conditions of workers, thanks to blockchain-enabled FSCs.[48] Agrifood organizations can also leverage blockchain's transparency features to increase trust in the FSC, provide real-time transparency,[65] and increase control over FSC processes.[53] Thus blockchain technology serves as a critical driver and tool for FSC compliance and, when combined with IoT sensors, enables real-time monitoring of product quality.

68.4.3 Data management and security

FSCs are being pushed by new technologies towards a data-driven digital supply ecosystem.[98] Numerous challenges arise as a result of the increasing availability of data and information about food preparation through point-of-sale and delivery to final consumers. For instance, insufficient and ineffective management of information systems may result in food loss in the preconsumption stages (i.e., before food is ready for human consumption) and food waste in production, distribution, retail and foodservice.[127] The adoption of novel technologies such as IoT-based sensors results in the generation of massive amounts of data, which may jeopardize agrifood organizations' ability to manage and effectively use the data collected by IoT sensors deployed throughout the FSC. As a result, FSC systems integration, interoperability, and data governance are critical components of today's business ecosystems.[128] To improve the management and security of FSC data, blockchain has emerged as a promising technology for operational efficiency, data management, responsiveness, and smart contract management.[109] Due to the technical characteristics of blockchain technology, it improves data management by enabling faster and more secure access to FSC data.[71,109,111] While centralized and nonblockchain-based technologies can improve data management and FSC efficiency, blockchain remains an irreplaceable solution for FSC processes that require a high level of trust among stakeholders.[129] This is because blockchain-based data management systems in FSCs have the potential to significantly boost the food industry's ability to manage disparate applications such as farmland and land usage records, purchase details and usage information for farm equipment, seeds, agrochemicals and labor inputs, as well as traceability and financial transactions across the entire FSC.[63]

Additionally, blockchain technology can be used to securely connect all exchange parties along the entire FSC, reducing the risk of food adulteration and enhancing food safety management.[109] Chen et al.[130] argue that blockchain technology can provide greater data security because it increasingly employs encryption technology combinations, such as hash functions, asymmetric encryption algorithms and digital signatures. The blockchain design structure makes it ideal for data sharing between FSC stakeholders and regulatory authorities. Dutta et al.[109] recognize this point when developing intelligent logistics systems for operational efficiency and data security using blockchain and big data technology. Similarly, Feng et al.[28] demonstrate that a blockchain-based multisensors (WSN) monitoring system can be used to achieve real-time control of shellfish quality while also increasing data security and reliability. The relevance of blockchain technology in FSCs is further attributed to its collaborative capabilities. As such, blockchain technology has the potential to facilitate and enhance data sharing among actors in the FSC and to foster more integrated, frictionless, and cooperative business processes.[131] Blockchain technology enables smart contracts, which can be used to automate business rules, simplify data sharing, and facilitate continuous process improvement among FSC participants.[28] Given that data quality is a prerequisite for effective information sharing,[132] blockchain technology can be used to address the FSCs historical poor data quality problem[109] in demand forecasting by making immutable product-process links smarter and more accessible to data and market information.[90] As a result, data sharing between FSC actors facilitates increased visibility, traceability, and monitoring of food quality and safety. Additionally, the combination of blockchain and IoT is a promising technological enabler for effective communication and data quality, providing a slew of data management and analytics benefits.[49]

Additionally, the FSC benefits from the fusion of blockchain and big data analytics, including robust data security, privacy, and transparency.[96,109] Blockchain technology is critical in developing a secure and transparent ledger for all data generated throughout the FSC.[30] According to Chen et al.,[130] blockchain technology improves FSC interoperability by standardization of data and streamlining supply chain data management in complex FSCs. Nonetheless, the technology's potential may be limited if it compromises data privacy and precludes error corrections due to nonreversible mechanisms (e.g., immutability). As a result, mutable and self-editing blockchains can be explored to overcome these issues.[96]

68.4.4 Food trade

Globalization has been instrumental in facilitating global trade in agricultural products.[88] For example, the international agriculture trade is worth more than two trillion dollars and employs more than a billion people worldwide.[133] While transnational food trade increased food choice and availability regardless of season,[134,135] several obstacles remained. For instance, the complexities of the FSC and the information asymmetry between traders have complicated regulators' efforts to collect reliable and authentic information necessary for supervising and managing traders and trade flows.[136] Additionally, growing segments of consumers are becoming more informed and are expressing concern with supply chain transparency and the safety of their food.[137] As a result of these growing concerns, agrifood organizations can leverage blockchain technology to meet the rising consumer expectations for transparency, high-quality, and safe products. Additionally, the technology can help reduce information asymmetry between exchange partners and consumers, while also increasing FSC efficiencies.[45,109] By ensuring secure ownership transfer, intercountry trades, and information sharing without the need for intermediaries, the use of blockchain and smart contracts can help coordinate strategic partnerships in international food trade.[109] Blockchain technology, as a decentralized economic infrastructure, increases transparency in food trade processes, fosters honest relationships among the FSC stakeholders and democratizes supply chain processes. In light of these points, Dutta et al.[109] argue that blockchain technology enables a secure, accurate, and real-time cost-effective supply chain that will promote fair trade of coffee products. According to Hao et al.[60] blockchain's robustness, decentralization, and end-to-end credibility make it a viable alternative to traditional food trading platforms. Furthermore, the authors propose a novel food trading platform based on consortium blockchain technology to increase trust and security and to enable food trading in decentralized, transparent, and secure market environments.

Similarly, Mao et al.[103] develop a blockchain-based credit evaluation system to improve the effectiveness of FSC supervision and management. By implementing this system, traders can be held accountable for their actions during the transaction and credit evaluation process; at the same time, regulators will collect more reliable, authentic, and sufficient data on traders. Additionally, blockchain significantly improves trade settlement, as trading parties in the FSC no longer have to worry about payment failures or trade settlement delays.[63] Furthermore, the economic benefits of blockchain in the food trade include the facilitation of faster transactions, and the prevention of price coercion and retroactive payments.[64] As such, blockchain enables the establishment of an authoritative record for trade data and information, enabling food organizations to reconcile invoices automatically, thereby increasing accountability and transactional efficiency.[63]

Kayikci et al.[64] cite the Louis Dreyfus Company as an example of a firm that used blockchain technology to trade 60,000 tonnes of American soybeans with China. In this scenario, blockchain enables increased transactional food trade and significantly reduces overall logistics time by 80 percent. According to Qian et al.,[74] blockchain technology can help build trust in international food trade by enabling tamper-proof data recording and decentralized management, as well as enhancing collaboration and interoperability under multilateral trade rules. Tsolakis et al.[86] support this argument, claiming that blockchain technology has the potential to reshape seafood trade and logistics in developing countries by establishing direct connections between processors and consumers. Kittipanya-ngam and Tan[99] note that blockchain technology can ensure the validity and efficiency of information gathered from various traders and authorities in the international fish supply chains, thus increasing governance and compliance to environmental and sustainable standards. As a result, blockchain technology is expected to facilitate international food trade by upholding the necessary sanitary and phytosanitary standards, promoting sustainability compliance, and helping to mitigate food-related contamination and safety concerns.[63]

68.4.5 Barriers to adoption

Despite its enormous potential for the FSC, several technical issues must be resolved before the full potential of blockchain in the food industry can be realized.[23,30,64,80,102] For example, blockchain implementation introduces a slew of complications related to the processing of large numbers of transactions and the storage of blocks that are growing in size.[102] Scalability of contemporary blockchain-based systems is still limited,[138] as is transaction speed.[107] According to Dutta et al.,[109] as the number of users increases, blockchain scalability issues arise, resulting in large block sizes, slow response times, and prohibitively high fees. While blockchain's transaction processing performance is currently inferior to that of established payment systems such as Visa, blockchain may be more adaptable.[139] While private blockchains may offer more scalability, they are less sustainable, wasting an enormous amount of energy in the process.[139] Access to FSC data is required for management[46] which blockchain may not guarantee or provide. To illustrate, the IBM Food Trust case demonstrates how private blockchains are unable to provide data access to all stakeholders across the entire FSC, resulting in data asynchrony.[129] Another technical requirement for blockchain integration in the FSC is data and information security.[28] Blockchain technology is not impervious to security threats, as attackers can compromise the system when they gain control over the blockchain protocol.[138] In this regard, Torky and Hassanein[83] identify a number of security risks associated with blockchain-based IoT systems in agriculture, including denial of services (DoS) attacks, Sybil attacks, Eclipse attacks, and routing attacks. Shahid et al.[79] detail the decentralized autonomous organization (DAO) hack, which resulted in a USD 70 million loss, highlighting the vulnerabilities of smart contracts-based blockchain systems such as bugs, call stack attacks, and time dependency. As a result, blockchain security is a critical priority that must be addressed in order to minimize vulnerabilities and increase the resilience of blockchain against hacking attacks, system failures, and data corruption.

In the FSC, privacy represents one of the critical concerns to consider in the use of blockchain. Food organizations need to maintain their business confidentiality among their competitors.[107] Although blockchain can ensure higher transactional privacy, possibilities of privacy intrusion are likely to occur even with permission management.[30] For public blockchains, Torky and Hassanein[83] further add that anonymity is not ensured because blockchain transactions are shared publicly, increasing the chance for attackers to analyze transactions and infer users' real identities. As a result, food organizations would be skeptical about engaging in blockchain and sharing their information across organizational boundaries.[102] Privacy concerns continue to occur when FSC stakeholders feel that blockchain is too invasive and that their ability to remain anonymous can be eroded.

The potential value of blockchain deployment in the FSC is diminished by a number of impediments to widespread adoption in the agrifood industry. Among these are apprehensions about adopting the technology due to its perceived immaturity.[23,26,64,102,131,140] Apart from posing operational and technical challenges such as limited scalability, usability, and interoperability,[23] blockchain's immaturity increases managers' uncertainty and has a detrimental effect on their commitment and support of blockchain for their FSCs.[102] Blockchain technology is still in its infancy, requiring significant effort to reach maturity and widespread adoption.[131] To realize its full potential, blockchain technology must rise above the hype by emphasizing its capacity to enable stronger forms of collaboration in order to manage global FSCs more effectively.[55] Businesses view blockchain adoption as a difficult task that requires additional knowledge and education about the technology and its integration into the FSC.[70]

Klerkx and Rose[101] argue that digital technologies have an impact on FSC operations and require FSC actors to acquire different knowledge, skills, and methods of labor management. Digitalization (e.g., business process and role automation) through the use of blockchain technology requires a long-term commitment and vision with compelling business value propositions, competencies, and availability of resources.[125] Additionally, the adoption and use of blockchain in the FSC may result in additional costs for agrifood organizations. For instance, Dutta et al.[109] argue that the nontrivial operations cost and implementation associated with blockchain should not be underestimated. Additionally, the maintenance costs of FSC-based blockchain systems' should be adequately controlled[68] in order to achieve competitive advantage.[26] To justify the necessary resources, blockchain applications for food traceability must demonstrate a positive return on investment to justify the necessary resources.[141] As such, blockchain-based food traceability systems may be unaffordable to small organizations with limited budgets and resources, as digital systems can be costly to implement and expensive to maintain.[64] In contrast to the latter statements, the growth of blockchain-enabled traceability solutions-as-a-service with a low monthly fee provides a significant opportunity for micro, small, and medium-sized businesses to improve their FSCs and position themselves as an attractive supplier to larger firms and end consumers seeking increased transparency and trust.

While government support for information and communication technology (ICT) is critical for the development of technology-driven FSCs,[142] regulations are sovereign to a nation and generally not harmonized (exceptions exist such as within the European Union framework). While numerous governments are experimenting with blockchain technology, regulations supporting or mandating blockchain are almost certainly being considered but currently don't exist due to its novelty and often controversial nature.[102] There is a general dearth of standards and governance mechanisms for blockchain implementation in areas such as FSC sustainability.[23,55,90,102] Numerous scholars have documented the negative consequences of the absence of standards and government policies to promote widespread adoption of blockchain in the FSC. For instance, Kayikci et al.[64] argue that the lack of uniform technology standards makes widespread adoption of blockchain a pipe dream. Yadav et al.[107] identify regulatory uncertainty as a significant barrier to blockchain adoption in the Indian agriculture supply chain (ASC). Kamble et al.[63] warn that the ability for blockchain to circumvent government surveillance and control may result in legal restrictions that limit the value the technology can provide in the agrifood sector.

Summarizing, Fig. 68.3 presents the main topics discussed in the nexus of blockchain and the FSC.

68.5 Blockchain as an enabler of food supply chains

This section discusses blockchain technology, highlighting the fundamentals and the different kinds of blockchain

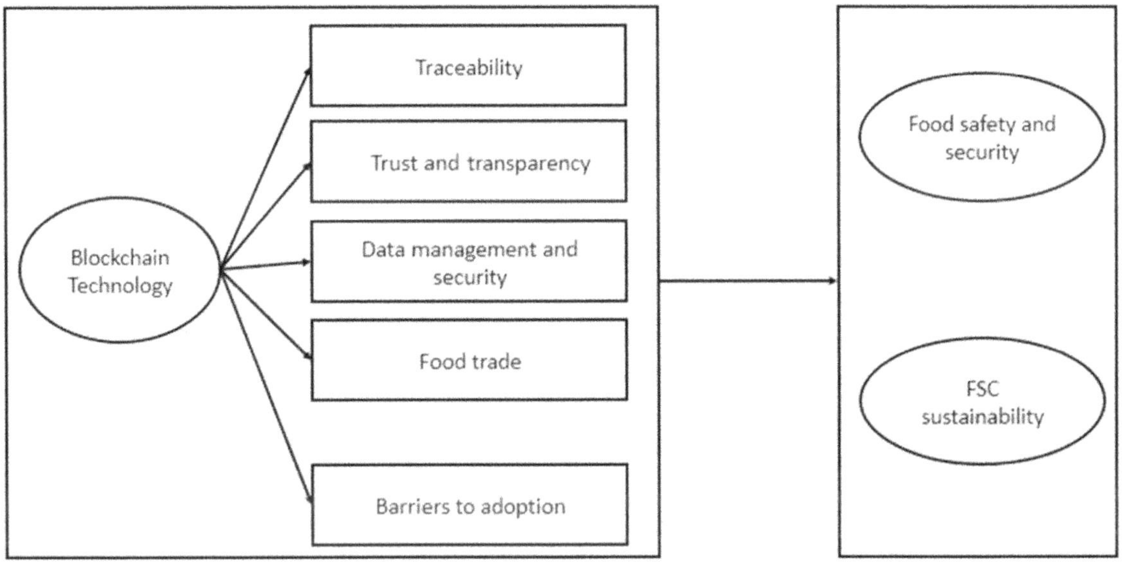

FIGURE 68.3 The topics at the blockchain–food supply chain nexus.

platforms available, focusing on the FSC. The section also elaborates on alternative solutions that can be used in place of blockchain. The section will provide insights, giving the relevant background, on the reasons behind blockchain usage as a technological enabler for FSCs.

68.5.1 Technical overview

Blockchain was invented by an unknown person or persons with the introduction of Bitcoin in 2008 by the pseudonymous Satoshi Nakamoto.[143] It consists of a decentralized, distributed database operating in a peer-to-peer network. In a public blockchain, any user can read and add data to the blockchain. Since the right to update the database is distributed, there is a necessity for a mutual agreement to decide which user will update the data in a particular instance of time. This mutual agreement is termed as consensus and is algorithmically imposed using different consensus mechanisms like proof of work in Bitcoin and Ethereum. The users who update the database are called validators (miners in proof of work blockchains) and are given a monetary reward for their contribution. The database is a chain of blocks that are cryptographically linked to each other, rendering traceability a default characteristic. Each block is timestamped and contains data/transactions added in a certain cycle of updating the blockchain database. Manipulating the data implies changing the entire chain of blocks, or else the cryptographic linkage would be broken to reveal the tampering.

Fig. 68.4 shows the process of mining in the Ethereum blockchain. Two miners compete to add their data to the blockchain. Each user maintains a local copy of the blockchain database, and all transactions are broadcasted to all users. Miners add the transactions to their local block. The winning miner, who gets to add his local block as the next block in the blockchain, is the one who can solve a complex cryptographic puzzle by finding a random number, referred to as a Nonce. In return for his services to the network, the miner gains Ether, the cryptocurrency of Ethereum. Ethereum is presently working on a proof of stake consensus mechanism to ensure scalability.[144,145]

Smart contracts are viewed as one of the most important applications of blockchains. However, all blockchain platforms do not support smart contracts, which might be an essential requirement in certain use cases like monitoring the cold chain parameters of food items in transit and automatically executing payments if the agreed parameters (e.g., temperature during transit) are met.[146] Smart contracts operate in the blockchain network, ensuring their immutability and transparency. They are used to formalize relationships and agreements in a network and are analogous to legal agreements in the physical world. A blockchain that is chosen to function in an FSC should be reviewed and adapted based on the particular use case requirements, and such considerations like whether the blockchain offers smart contracts or not is an important criterion for determining the choice.

68.5.2 Types of blockchain platforms

Blockchain platforms can be broadly categorized into the following two types, based on the permissibility to be a validator as being open or subject to restrictions by authorizing entities.

1. *Permissionless*: Public blockchain platforms like Bitcoin and Ethereum are permissionless. No entity

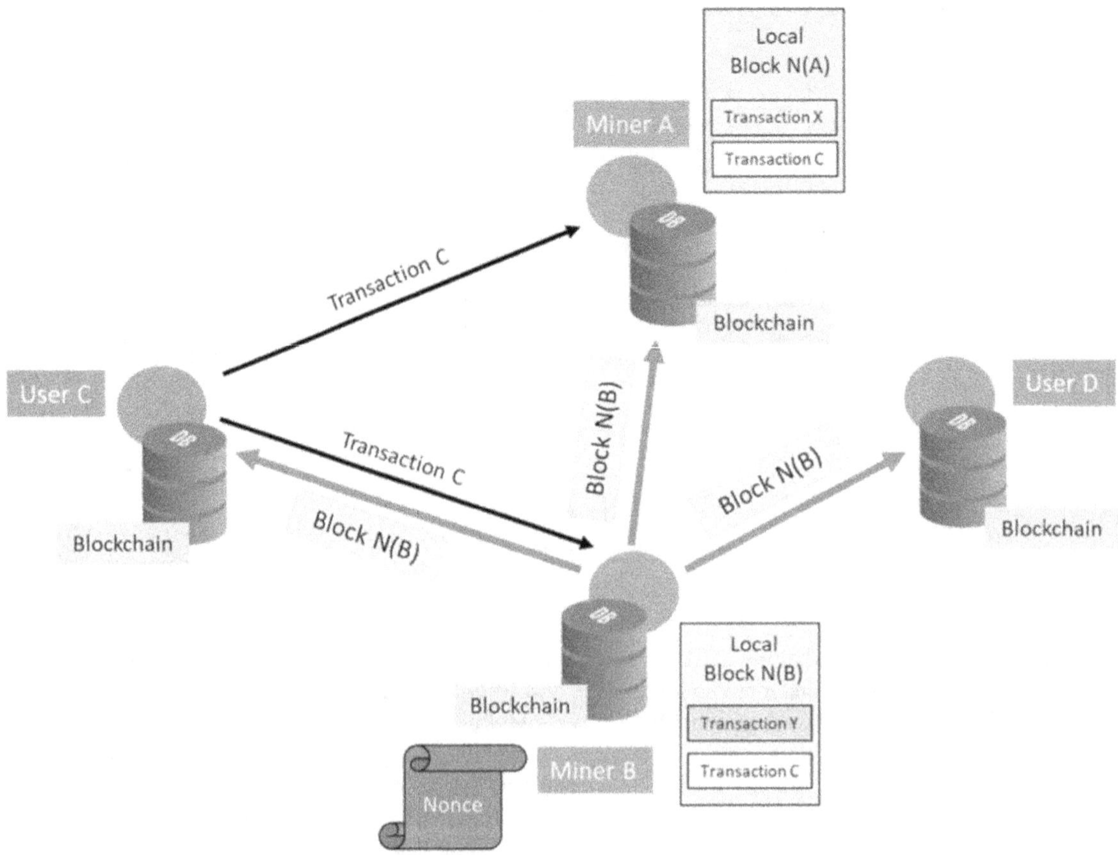

FIGURE 68.4 Mining. *Data from Khan N. Blockchain-enabled traceability and immutability for financial applications. University of Luxembourg, Luxembourg.<https://orbilu.uni.lu/handle/10993/43941>; 2020.*

controls these blockchain platforms, and the right to validate transactions is open to anybody. The right to read data from the blockchain platform is also open to all. The blockchain platforms are highly transparent but exhibit low performance. These open systems exhibit poor scalability,[147] and research is ongoing to make blockchains scalable.

2. *Permissioned*: Private and consortium blockchain platforms like R3 Corda and Hyperledger belong to this category. These blockchain platforms can be owned and controlled by a single/group of entities. The controlling entities confer the right to read data as well as the right to validate transactions. Transparency is less with an increase in performance and scalability. However, scalability is still restricted.[147]

There are several ways to evaluate the efficacy of the different kinds of blockchain platforms. Table 68.3 outlines the evaluation parameters for permissioned or permissionless blockchain.

Like Monero, Zcash, and Enigma, privacy-preserving blockchain platforms have emerged but remained vulnerable to privacy breaches,[148] together with an increase in complexity. A permissioned blockchain platform can be customized to ensure data privacy to manage read-write access to the blockchain data. On the other hand, a permissionless blockchain cannot be made compliant with privacy-related regulatory requirements like the European Union's General Data Protection Regulation.[149]

In the context of immutability, since a permissionless blockchain has a presumably higher number of validators than a permissioned blockchain, it is comparatively more difficult to corrupt the distributed database, where the ledger is stored with innumerable validating entities. A permissionless blockchain is less secure than a permissioned one as permissioned blockchains can have an access layer, regulating the users allowed to interact with the blockchain platform. Governance in both kinds of blockchain platforms can be off-chain or on-chain. Still, a permissioned blockchain platform can be governed more easily than a permissionless one, where more incentives would be needed to ensure that all users comply with the blockchain platform's overall objectives. Governance in a permissioned blockchain would be similar to the scenario of governing a technology company,[150] whereas a permissionless in the absence of an administrative body would be more challenging.

The factors mentioned in Table 68.3 can help stakeholders and business organizations choose the most appropriate

TABLE 68.3 Permissionless versus permissioned blockchains.

Evaluation parameter	Permissionless	Permissioned
Owner	Nobody	Single/group of entities
Validators	Anybody	Restricted
Performance	Low throughput	Higher throughput
Scalability	Poor	Comparatively more
Privacy	Public	Privacy achievable
Security	Less	High
Governance	Off-chain/on-chain	Off-chain/on-chain
Transaction cost	Yes	Depends on the owner/free
Database	Decentralized and distributed	Centralized/decentralized and distributed
Transparency	Yes	Not guaranteed
Immutability	Yes	Not ensured
Examples	Ethereum, Bitcoin, Algorand	Hyperledger, R3 Corda, Quorum

blockchain platform for their particular use case. For example, a business solution where traceability is of paramount importance can choose either of the two categories of blockchain platforms depending upon other requirements like data privacy, security, and compliance to the operating region's regulatory environment. Organizations that focus on preventing and eliminating recalls can utilize a permissionless blockchain platform, proven to be more resilient to manipulating the data and ensuring data immutability and integrity. However, if trusted entities, even the government, back the permissioned blockchain platform, then a permissioned blockchain will ensure compliance with regulations and immutability.

68.5.3 Blockchain alternatives and competitors

Blockchain is characterized by a distributed database in a peer-to-peer network. Alternative solutions exist that can also provide data storage mechanisms. We will discuss the alternative solutions, focusing on the points that make the blockchain as the database of choice for a FSC, as the advantages offered by the alternative solutions are well documented and known.

1. *Centralized databases*: A centralized database is owned and managed by a central authority as depicted in Fig. 68.5. The central authority confers the management rights to the database administrator. Each organization maintains its own database to record the details of its clients. The database administrator manages access to the database, including read and write access. In the depicted figure, only the central authority has the right to update the data in the database. This contrasts with the distributed database, which is a characteristic of a blockchain. In a distributed database, multiple users can read and write to the database. Fig. 68.5 depicts the distributed database of public Ethereum blockchain,[151] where the users who can add data to the database are the miners. All the users in a distributed database maintain a local copy of the entire database and hence corrupting or tampering with the data is extremely difficult. In a light client of the blockchain, the users, excluding the miners, need not store a local copy of the entire database to reduce the high storage requirements that accompany using a blockchain platform.

   Consider the case of a FSC utilizing a centralized database. In case of an issue with a food item, the seller can tamper with its own database to indicate the desired attributes in the concerned food item. The database maintained by an intermediary in the FSC might show a different record for the same food item and there is no way to resolve this conflict. If a single database is maintained by all the parties in the FSC, even then a seller/some company can manipulate the database administrator to alter records. However, this is not factually possible in a distributed database maintained by a blockchain.

2. *Cloud databases*: Cloud databases ease the work of the database administrator, permitting organizations to utilize the benefits of traditional databases with the advantages of cloud computing.[152] Cloud databases facilitate hosting a database in the cloud without purchasing and maintaining the required hardware resources for it. The cloud provider provides the database as a service with a cloud architect setting up the

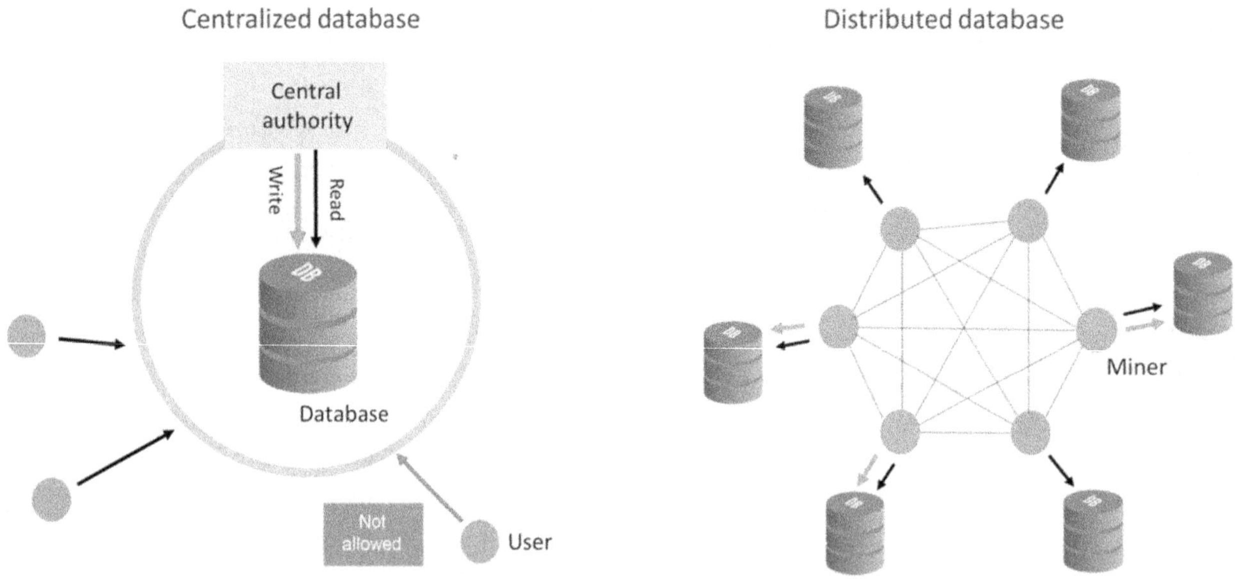

FIGURE 68.5 Centralized versus distributed database. *Khan N. Blockchain-enabled traceability and immutability for financial applications. University of Luxembourg, Luxembourg. <https://orbilu.uni.lu/handle/10993/43941>; 2020. Durham University. Blockchain, cryptocurrency and ethical projects. Durham University. https://www.dur.ac.uk/business/research/accounting-and-finance/ethical-finance/events/?id = 38144&eventno = 38144; 2020.*

database and thereafter assigning the work of management to the database administrator. These roles can be combined or if equipped with the necessary skills, one can take the role of another. Here the possibility of data tampering exists in accessing the database by the organizational users and hence the connection needs to be secured. Additionally, the cloud architect/database administrator can also tamper with the records. In order to prevent this Microsoft Azure has introduced immutable *blob storage*, whereby the data adheres to WORM (Write Once, Read Many) state.[153] Utilizing an immutable blob would be like a permissioned blockchain platform in the context of immutability and preserving data integrity.

3. *Distributed ledgers*: A distributed ledger is the parent technology of blockchain. It implies a decentralized database that is distributed among different computers or nodes.[154] There is no central point of failure as in a centralized database. However, in a distributed ledger, there is no defined structure in which the database should be organized so we have both blockchain and DAG (directed acyclic graph) technology being categorized under distributed ledgers. Blockchain has a data structure, where the data is organized into blocks. The blocks are timestamped and cryptographically linked to the previous block. In a DAG, transactions are organized as nodes in a graph, which are joined to each other by directed links.[144] Research is ongoing in DAGs to explore the potential applications.[155] DAGs seem to overcome the bottlenecks faced by blockchains in scalability, speed, and efficiency, but they are still in the stage of initial research compared to blockchains, which have been around for more than 10 years now. DAGs witness loss of decentralization, leading to a somewhat centralized network relying on a trusted coordinator to validate transactions as seen in IOTA, an implementation of DAG technology. There are ongoing efforts to mitigate this.[156] DAGs are seen as an enabler for blockchain, but it needs more robust testing and large-scale use to be usable for practical deployments.

68.6 Case studies

We did not apply any exclusive criteria for the selection of use cases because the anticipated number of cases was small. As a result, random sampling is not typically a viable approach.[157] As primary informants of this chapter, two cases were selected, summarized, and analyzed to identify the importance of blockchain in the FSC. The use cases were derived as a follow-on to the lead author's series[b] "2020 Future of Food 10 × 10 Blockchain Series." In this series, the lead author interviewed ten executives from ten blockchain firms for ten minutes. The series concluded with an academic panel discussion.

68.6.1 Case study 1: connecting food

Connecting Food (CF) is a technology provider based in Paris, France with numerous household brands as clients. CF operates as a food tech and blockchain platform aimed at enhancing transparency and trust in food chains. CF has developed a reliable and scalable blockchain-based

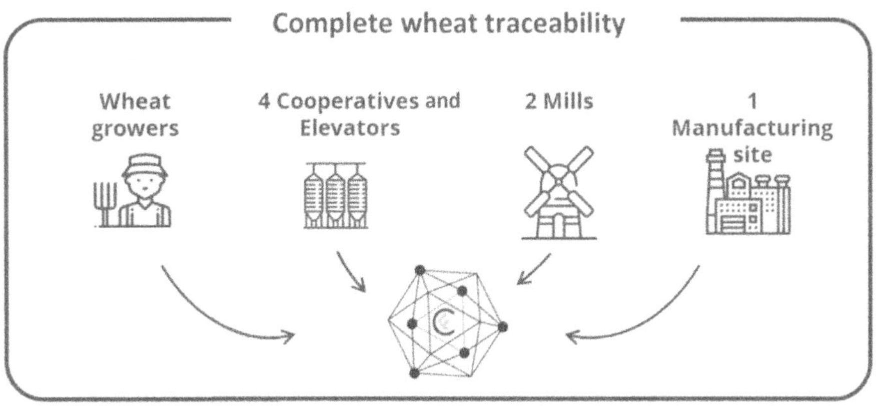

FIGURE 68.6 Complete wheat traceability. *Connecting Food.*

traceability solution to enable its customer, an international food company behind a famous biscuit brand, to improve traceability and quality control information and enhance transparency and trust. By implementing the CF's blockchain platform, the food brand aimed to promote its strong commitment to a strict quality charter and share it with its consumers, thereby reinforcing consumer trust. Moreover, the company's goals include developing high integrity levels in data exchanged between the farms and factories. Furthermore, the solution helps to reconnect consumers with farmers by increasing their knowledge through authentic stories. Moreover, the brand aimed at showing consumers the geographic proximity and short distribution lines between farms and factories.

The deployment of a permission-based blockchain has facilitated secure information sharing among the involved cooperatives, millers, and processing plants (see Fig. 68.6). To enhance the integrity of the supply ecosystem, CF created a unique LiveAudit module, which performs a real-time audit of the integrity of information and ensures that each product is compliant with the quality charter. As a result, the brand can mitigate the risk of "garbage in-garbage out" and enhance efficiencies in quality management and reduce noncompliance. Utilizing blockchain, consumers can track their food products' whole journey through a simple scan of an on-pack QR code with their smartphones, thereby increasing consumer trust in product claims. Overall, blockchain, coupled with CFs LiveAudit module, enabled the brand to move from the marketing of claims towards real-time and specific marketing of proof. Further benefits include improving product quality compliance, maximizing supply ecosystem efficiencies, enhancing consumer trust and transparency.

68.6.2 Case study 2: Origin Chain Networks: universal farm compliance

Origin Chain Networks is an Irish technology provider of software solutions in the agrifood sector focused on cocreating a secure, stable, and transparent food value-chain. Their distributed ledger technology *Agritrust* is a mobile farming solution that incentivizes and facilitates *digitization* (analog to digital) of farm data and *digitalization* (business process and role automation) for farm management and compliance purposes. Through on-chain and off-chain data flow analyses, Origin Chain Networks modeled stakeholder data in the decentralized system. The system view described in Fig. 68.7 utilizes a data flow analysis based on ISO TS23257 Blockchain and DLT: Reference Architecture.

According to Origin Chain Networks, farm compliance processes form the basis of transparency and trust and are ready for transformation across several areas including audit checking, antifraud measures and deadlines. For many farmers, online and digital means intermittent or sparse internet access which are compounded by low technical skill levels and worries around data privacy and data ownership.

The Origin Chain Agritrust mobile farming solution provides a mobile and edge computing solution. It reduces friction, enables smart data entry and decentralized data governance. The system uses access permission which is an important *farmer-first* data ownership model that safeguards access to potential new revenue streams for farmers using the system.

Accelerated adoption of foundational technologies including blockchain and DLT is central to the European Union's Digital Strategy. It is envisaged that digital reform across the public and private sectors will enhance cohesion and reduce friction in trade across the single digital marketplace. The Origin Chain Networks universal farm compliance/Agritrust mobile farming solution exemplifies how, in the distributed governance context of agriculture compliance, a decentralized approach can resolve barriers to cooperation and regulatory oversight.

The solution leverages infrastructure and resources available through Connecting Europe Facility (CEF) and EU Blockchain Service Infrastructure (EBSI v1.0 Infrastructure Specification). Furthermore, the platform

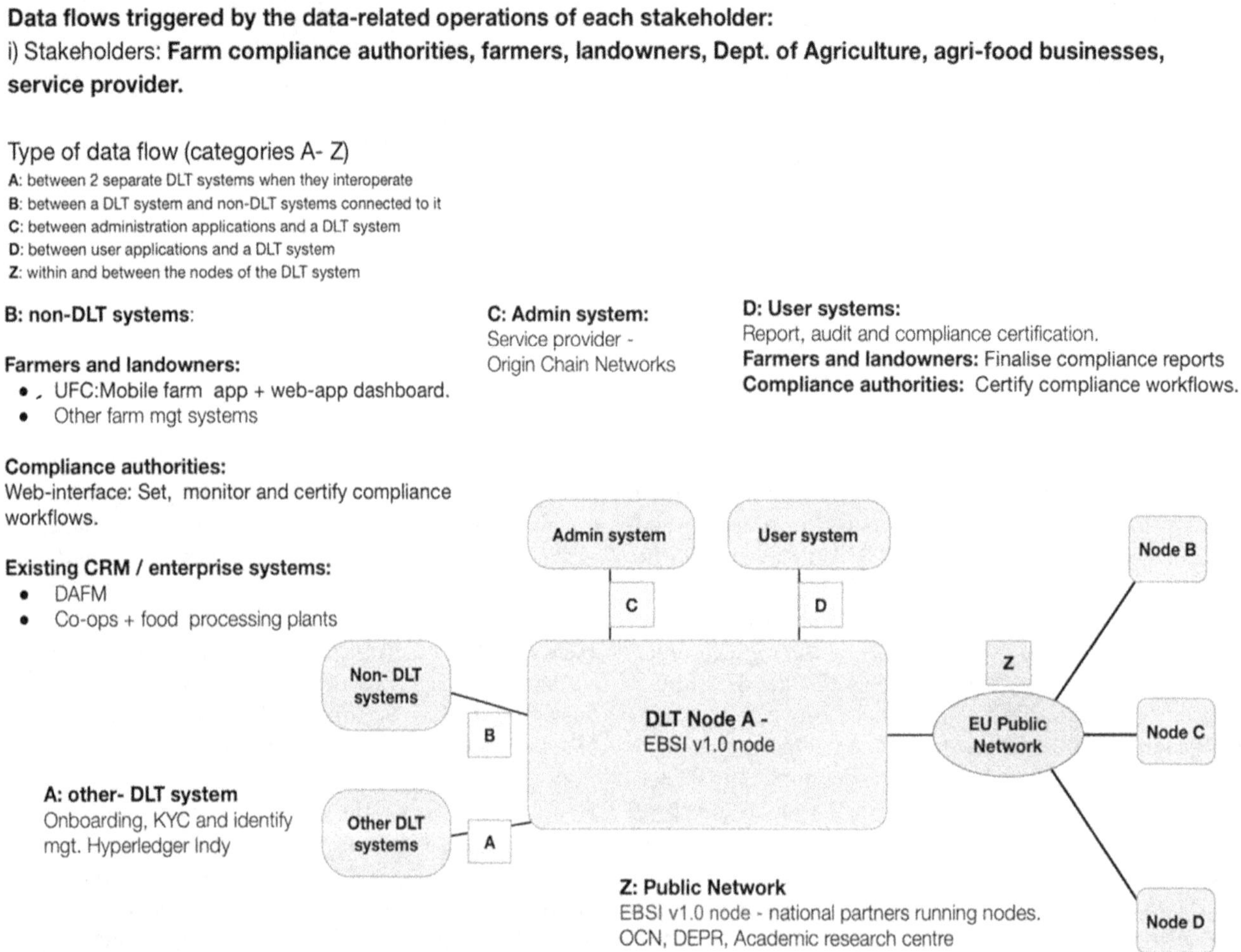

FIGURE 68.7 Universal Farm Compliance/Agritrust mobile farming. Origin Chain Networks (2021). Data flow analysis. *ISO TR3242:2021. Blockchain and DLT use cases. Reproduced with permission from Origin Chain Networks.*

redesigns the interface between public sector and farming communities, forges new models of engagement and brings the benefits of emerging technologies to farming data and efficiencies in farm compliance processes.

68.7 Conclusion

Food safety has become an increasingly critical issue. As a result, traceability requirements have increased to mitigate the risks related to perishability and food fraud vulnerability. This is occurring in agrifood environments that are under increasing pressure to enhance operational performance and competitive advantage. Food products' quality and freshness can be maintained and managed more efficiently with highly coordinated and interoperable FSCs. Tighter supply chain integration can significantly assist organizations in lowering their overall supply chain risks and transaction costs. Food industry stakeholders can enhance food safety, establish efficient risk management, and ensure food quality from farm to retail with the help of blockchain technology. We have demonstrated in this chapter that blockchain technology has the potential to significantly benefit the food industry. Through increased fine-grained data capture and data sharing processes, food organizations can leverage the technology to develop more efficient food traceability systems.

The implementation of blockchain technology enables FSC stakeholders to reduce friction, increase trust, enhance transparency, and more securely and efficiently manage information flows. Additionally, the adoption of blockchain technology in the food industry has the potential to improve food trade, promote ethical and fair-trading practices, and optimize transactional efficiency (e.g., by reducing transactional and relational friction). However, realizing blockchains transformative potential in the food industry is complicated by the technology's technical limitations, the organizational complexity of food companies, and the absence of supporting regulatory frameworks. Without addressing these issues, FSC stakeholders will fall short of ensuring food quality and safety and increasing consumer trust in food integrity and compliance with food standards. Given blockchain's growing popularity in a variety of FSC use cases, it is expected that the technology will be a game changer in future FSCs spanning transnational food supply ecosystems. We hope that practitioners and scholars can use blockchain technology to address more specific FSC vulnerabilities. Additional awareness campaigns must be developed to promote the technology's effective integration into the food industry and encourage widespread adoption by the FSC.

The UK Food Standards Agency (FSA) released a report called "Insights and learnings from the Food Standards Agency (FSA) exploring the use of Blockchains." We recommend practitioner access and review the findings in this report.

The report can be accessed here:

https://www.food.gov.uk/sites/default/files/media/document/fsa-blockchain-first-steps-to-next-steps.pdf

Wageningen University and UNFAO released a joint Whitepaper on the use of Blockchain called "Applying blockchain for climate action in agriculture: state of play and outlook." This paper notes that "blockchain can help improve transparency and accountability of climate change activities and impacts in a wide range of verticals in agriculture."

The report can be found here http://www.fao.org/3/cb3495en/cb3495en.pdf.

Endnotes

[a]The Future of Food mini-series with scientists on food provenance. https://www.youtube.com/watch?v = 91cAyNWPfRw&list = PLtx-MnDXwDwUB87AjHOioy3l4_Xd_3Xuf.

[b]https://www.youtube.com/watch?v = 7y2CAsci8BA&list = PLtx-MnDXwDwWUvchdJQpNzwKm5PMAJzQP.

References

1. Wee HM, Budiman SD, Su LC, Chang M, Chen R. Responsible supply chain management—an analysis of Taiwanese gutter oil scandal using the theory of constraint. *Int J Logist Res Appl*. 2016;19(5):380–394. Available from: https://doi.org/10.1080/13675567.2015.1090964.
2. Azmat F, Ha H. Corporate social responsibility, customer trust, and loyalty—perspectives from a developing country. *Thunderbird Int Bus Rev*. 2013;55(3):253–270. Available from: https://doi.org/10.1002/tie.21542.
3. Munoz A, Clements MD. Disruptions in information flow. A revenue costing supply chain dilemma. *J Theor Appl Electron Commer Res*. 2008;3(1):30–40.
4. Campoy-Muñoz P, Cardenete MA, Delgado MC. Economic impact assessment of food waste reduction on European countries through social accounting matrices. *Resour, Conserv Recycling*. 2017;122: 202–209. Available from: https://doi.org/10.1016/j.resconrec.2017.02.010.
5. Pink J, Bedard B, Keogh J, Moyer DC, Scimeca J, Vasan A. International survey of food fraud and related terminology: preliminary results and discussion. *J Food Sci*. 2019;84:2705–2718.
6. Kamble SS, Raut RD. Evaluating the factors considered for procurement of raw material in food supply chain using Delphi-AHP methodology—a case study of potato chips processing company in India. *Int J Product Qual Manag*. 2019;26(2):176–189. Available from: https://doi.org/10.1504/IJPQM.2019.097765.
7. Ting SL, Tse YK, Ho GTS, Chung SH, Pang G. Mining logistics data to assure the quality in a sustainable food supply chain: a case in the red wine industry. *Int J Prod Econ*. 2014;152:200–209. Available from: https://doi.org/10.1016/j.ijpe.2013.12.010.
8. BCIMC (2020) article https://www.prnewswire.co.uk/news-releases/ceos-of-eight-leading-canadian-pension-plan-investment-managers-call-on-companies-and-investors-to-help-drive-sustainable-and-inclusive-economic-growth-895852223.html.
9. Maloni MJ, Brown ME. Corporate social responsibility in the supply chain: an application in the food industry. *J Bus Ethics*. 2006;68(1):35–52. Available from: https://doi.org/10.1007/s10551-006-9038-0.
10. Treiblmaier H. The impact of the blockchain on the supply chain: a theory-based research framework and a call for action. *Supply Chain Manage An Int J*. 2018;23(6):545–559. Available from: https://doi.org/10.1108/SCM-01-2018-0029.
11. Rejeb A, Sűle E, Keogh JG. Exploring new technologies in procurement. *Transp Logist Int J*. 2018;18(45):76–86.
12. Alammary A, Alhazmi S, Almasri M, Gillani S. Blockchain-based applications in education: a systematic review. *Appl Sci (Switz)*. 2019;9(12). Available from: https://doi.org/10.3390/app9122400.
13. Pence HE. Blockchain: will better data security change chemical education? *J Chem Educ*. 2019;97:1847–1854. Available from: https://doi.org/10.1021/acs.jchemed.9b00560.
14. Swan M. (2018). Blockchain for business: next-generation enterprise artificial intelligence systems. (Raj, P. and Deka, G.C., Ed.) Blockchain Technology: Platforms, Tools and Use Cases. San Diego: Elsevier Academic Press Inc. <https://doi.org/10.1016/bs.adcom.2018.03.013>.
15. Guo R, Shi H, Zheng D, Jing C, Zhuang C, Wang Z. Flexible and efficient blockchain-based ABE scheme with multi-authority for medical on demand in telemedicine system. *IEEE Access*. 2019;. Available from: https://doi.org/10.1109/ACCESS.2019.2925625.
16. Hasselgren A, Kralevska K, Gligoroski D, Pedersen SA, Faxvaag A. Blockchain in healthcare and health sciences-a scoping review. *Int J Med Inform*. 2020;. Available from: https://doi.org/10.1016/j.ijmedinf.2019.104040.
17. Radanović I, Likić R. Opportunities for use of blockchain technology in medicine. *Appl Health Econ Health Policy*. 2018;16(5):583–590. Available from: https://doi.org/10.1007/s40258-018-0412-8.
18. Rejeb A, Keogh JG, Treiblmaier H. Leveraging the Internet of Things and blockchain technology in supply chain management. *Future Internet*. 2019;11(7):161. Available from: https://doi.org/10.3390/fi11070161.
19. Turkanović M, Hölbl M, Košič K, Heričko M, Kamišalić A. EduCTX: a blockchain-based higher education credit platform. *IEEE Access*. 2018;6:5112–5127. Available from: https://doi.org/10.1109/ACCESS.2018.2789929.

20. Woodside JM, Augustine Jr. FK, Giberson W. Blockchain technology adoption status and strategies. *J Int Technol Inf Manag.* 2017;26(2):65–93.
21. George RV, Harsh HO, Ray P, Babu AK. Food quality traceability prototype for restaurants using blockchain and food quality data index. *J Clean Prod.* 2019;240. Available from: https://doi.org/10.1016/j.jclepro.2019.118021.
22. Babich V, Hilary G. Blockchain and other distributed ledger technologies in operations. *Found Trends Technol, Inf Oper Manag.* 2019;12(2–3):152–172.
23. Rogerson M, Parry GC. Blockchain: case studies in food supply chain visibility. *Supply Chain Manag.* 2020;25(5):601–614. Available from: https://doi.org/10.1108/SCM-08-2019-0300.
24. Dinesh Kumar K, Manoj Kumar DS, Anandh R. Blockchain technology in food supply chain security. *Int J Sci Technol Res.* 2020;9(1):3446–3450.
25. Dinesh Kumar K, Senthil P, Manoj Kumar DS. Educational certificate verification system using blockchain. *Int J Sci Technol Res.* 2020;9(3):82–85.
26. Kumar A, Liu R, Shan Z. Is blockchain a silver bullet for supply chain management? Technical challenges and research opportunities. *Decis Sci.* 2019;1–30. Available from: https://doi.org/10.1111/deci.12396.
27. Scuderi A, Foti VT, Timpanaro G. The supply chain value of pod and pgi food products through the application of blockchain. *Quality-Access Success.* 2019;20(S2):580–587.
28. Feng H, Wang X, Duan Y, Zhang J, Zhang X. Applying blockchain technology to improve agri-food traceability: a review of development methods, benefits and challenges. *J Clean Prod.* 2020;260. Available from: https://doi.org/10.1016/j.jclepro.2020.121031.
29. Rejeb A, Keogh JG, Zailani S, Treiblmaier H, Rejeb K. Blockchain technology in the food industry: a review of potentials, challenges and future research directions. *Logistics.* 2020;4(4):27. Available from: https://doi.org/10.3390/logistics4040027.
30. Zhao G, Liu S, Lopez C, et al. Blockchain technology in agri-food value chain management: a synthesis of applications, challenges and future research directions. *Comput Ind.* 2019;109:83–99. Available from: https://doi.org/10.1016/j.compind.2019.04.002.
31. Keogh JG, Rejeb A, Khan N, Dean K, Hand KJ. Blockchain and GS1 standards in the food chain: a review of the possibilities and challenges. In: Detwiler D, ed. *Building the Future of Food Safety Technology.* 1st Ed London: Elsevier; 2020.
32. Atlam HF, Alenezi A, Alassafi MO, Wills G. Blockchain with Internet of Things: Benefits, challenges, and future directions. *Int J Intell Syst Appl.* 2018;10(6):40–48.
33. Iansiti M, Lakhani KR. (2017) The Truth About Blockchain. Harvard Business Review. https://hbr.org/2017/01/the-truth-about-blockchain.
34. Yiannas F. A new era of food transparency powered by blockchain. *Innov Technol, Gov Global.* 2018;12(1–2):46–56. Available from: https://doi.org/10.1162/inov_a_00266.
35. Tranfield D, Denyer D, Smart P. Towards a methodology for developing evidence-informed management knowledge by means of systematic review. *Br J Manag.* 2003;14(3):207–222. Available from: https://doi.org/10.1111/1467-8551.00375.
36. Queiroz MM, Telles R, Bonilla SH. Blockchain and supply chain management integration: a systematic review of the literature. *Supply Chain Manage Int J.* 2019;25(2):241–252. Available from: https://doi.org/10.1108/SCM-03-2018-0143.
37. Strozzi F, Colicchia C, Creazza A, Noè C. Literature review on the 'Smart Factory' concept using bibliometric tools. *Int J Prod Res.* 2017;55(22):6572–6591. Available from: https://doi.org/10.1080/00207543.2017.1326643.
38. Tober M. PubMed, ScienceDirect, Scopus or Google Scholar—Which is the best search engine for an effective literature research in laser medicine? *Med Laser Appl.* 2011;26(3):139–144. Available from: https://doi.org/10.1016/j.mla.2011.05.006.
39. Jacsó P. The h-index, h-core citation rate and the bibliometric profile of the Scopus database. *Online Inf Rev.* 2011;35(3):492–501. Available from: https://doi.org/10.1108/14684521111151487.
40. Khatoon A. A blockchain-based smart contract system for healthcare management. *Electronics.* 2020;9(1):94. Available from: https://doi.org/10.3390/electronics9010094.
41. Low KFK, Mik E. Pause the blockchain legal revolution. *Int Comp Law Q.* 2019;. Available from: https://doi.org/10.1017/S0020589319000502.
42. Cho SH, Park SY, Lee SR. Blockchain consensus rule based dynamic blind voting for non-dependency transaction. *Int J Grid Distrib Comput.* 2017;10(12):93–106. Available from: https://doi.org/10.14257/ijgdc.2017.10.12.09.
43. Ferreira MP. A bibliometric study on Ghoshal's managing across borders. *Multinatl Bus Rev.* 2011;19(4):357.
44. Furrer O, Thomas H, Goussevskaia A. The structure and evolution of the strategic management field: a content analysis of 26 years of strategic management research. *Int J Manag Rev.* 2008;10(1):1–23. Available from: https://doi.org/10.1111/j.1468-2370.2007.00217.x.
45. Antonucci F, Figorilli S, Costa C, Pallottino F, Raso L, Menesatti P. A review on blockchain applications in the agri-food sector. *J Sci Food Agric.* 2019;99(14):6129–6138. Available from: https://doi.org/10.1002/jsfa.9912.
46. Astill J, Dara RA, Campbell M, et al. Transparency in food supply chains: a review of enabling technology solutions. *Trends Food Sci Technol.* 2019;91:240–247. Available from: https://doi.org/10.1016/j.tifs.2019.07.024.
47. Barge P, Biglia A, Comba L, Aimonino DR, Tortia C, Gay P. Radio frequency identification for meat supply-chain digitalisation. *Sens (Switz).* 2020;20(17):1–17. Available from: https://doi.org/10.3390/s20174957.
48. Behnke K, Janssen MFWHA. Boundary conditions for traceability in food supply chains using blockchain technology. *Int J Inf Manag.* 2019;101969. Available from: https://doi.org/10.1016/j.ijinfomgt.2019.05.025.
49. Casino, F., Kanakaris, V., Dasaklis, T.K., Moschuris, S., & Rachaniotis, N.P. (2019). Modeling food supply chain traceability based on blockchain technology. In Ivanov D., Dolgui A, Yalaoui F (Ed.), IFAC-PapersOnLine (Vol. 52, pp. 2728–2733). Elsevier B.V. <https://doi.org/10.1016/j.ifacol.2019.11.620>.
50. Chan KY, Abdullah J, Khan AS. A framework for traceable and transparent supply chain management for agri-food sector in malaysia using blockchain technology. *Int J Adv Comput Sci Appl.* 2019;10(11):149–156. Available from: https://doi.org/10.14569/IJACSA.2019.0101120.
51. Creydt M, Fischer M. Blockchain and more—algorithm driven food traceability. *Food Control.* 2019;105:45–51. Available from: https://doi.org/10.1016/j.foodcont.2019.05.019.
52. Demestichas K, Peppes N, Alexakis T, Adamopoulou E. Blockchain in agriculture traceability systems: a review. *Appl Sci*

(Switz). 2020;10(12):1–22. Available from: https://doi.org/10.3390/APP10124113.

53. dos Santos RB, Torrisi NM, Yamada ERK, Pantoni RP. IGR token-raw material and ingredient certification of recipe based foods using smart contracts. *Informatics*. 2019;6(1):11. Available from: https://doi.org/10.3390/informatics6010011.
54. Feng H, Wang W, Chen B, Zhang X. Evaluation on frozen shellfish quality by blockchain based multi-sensors monitoring and SVM algorithm during cold storage. *IEEE Access*. 2020;8:54361–54370. Available from: https://doi.org/10.1109/ACCESS.2020.2977723.
55. Galvez JF, Mejuto JC, Simal-Gandara J. Future challenges on the use of blockchain for food traceability analysis. *Trends Anal Chem*. 2018;107:222–232. Available from: https://doi.org/10.1016/j.trac.2018.08.011.
56. Gopi K, Mazumder D, Sammut J, Saintilan N. Determining the provenance and authenticity of seafood: a review of current methodologies. *Trends Food Sci Technol*. 2019;91:294–304. Available from: https://doi.org/10.1016/j.tifs.2019.07.010.
57. Grecuccio J, Giusto E, Fiori F, Rebaudengo M. Combining blockchain and IoT: food-chain traceability and beyond. *Energies*. 2020;13(15). Available from: https://doi.org/10.3390/en13153820.
58. Guido R, Mirabelli G, Palermo E, Solina V. A framework for food traceability: case study-Italian extra-virgin olive oil supply chain. *Int J Ind Eng Manag*. 2020;11(1). Available from: https://www.scopus.com/inward/record.uri?eid = 2-s2.0-85083581451&partnerID = 40&md5 = 04379d8beb25ccf5491f74d92167d88d.
59. Hao J, Sun Y, Luo H. A safe and efficient storage scheme based on blockchain and IPFs for agricultural products tracking. *J Comput (Taiwan)*. 2018;29(6):158–167. Available from: https://doi.org/10.3966/199115992018122906015.
60. Hao Z, Mao D, Zhang B, Zuo M, Zhao Z. A novel visual analysis method of food safety risk traceability based on blockchain. *Int J Environ Res Public Health*. 2020;17(7). Available from: https://doi.org/10.3390/ijerph17072300.
61. He X, Chen X, Li K. A decentralized and non-reversible traceability system for storing commodity data. *KSII Trans Internet Inf Syst*. 2018;13(2):619–634. Available from: https://doi.org/10.3837/tiis.2019.02.008.
62. Hew J-J, Wong L-W, Tan GW-H, Ooi K-B, Lin B. The blockchain-based Halal traceability systems: a hype or reality? *Supply Chain Manag*. 2020;25(6):863–879. Available from: https://doi.org/10.1108/SCM-01-2020-0044.
63. Kamble SS, Gunasekaran A, Sharma R. Modeling the blockchain enabled traceability in agriculture supply chain. *Int J Inf Manag*. 2019;52. Available from: https://doi.org/10.1016/j.ijinfomgt.2019.05.023.
64. Kayikci Y, Subramanian N, Dora M, Bhatia MS. Food supply chain in the era of Industry 4.0: blockchain technology implementation opportunities and impediments from the perspective of people, process, performance, and technology. *Prod Plan Control*. 2020;. Available from: https://doi.org/10.1080/09537287.2020.1810757.
65. Khan PW, Byun Y-C, Park N. IoT-blockchain enabled optimized provenance system for food industry 4.0 using advanced deep learning. *Sens (Switz)*. 2020;20(10). Available from: https://doi.org/10.3390/s20102990.
66. Khanna T, Nand P, Bali V. Permissioned blockchain model for end-to-end trackability in supply chain management. *Int J e-Collab*. 2020;16(1):45–58. Available from: https://doi.org/10.4018/IJeC.2020010104.
67. Kim HM, Laskowski M. Toward an ontology-driven blockchain design for supply-chain provenance. *Intell Syst Accounting, Financ Manag*. 2018;25(1):18–27. Available from: https://doi.org/10.1002/isaf.1424.
68. Lin Q, Wang H, Pei X, Wang J. Food safety traceability system based on blockchain and EPCIS. *IEEE Access*. 2019;7:20698–20707. Available from: https://doi.org/10.1109/ACCESS.2019.2897792.
69. Lin W, Huang X, Fang H, et al. Blockchain technology in current agricultural systems: from techniques to applications. *IEEE Access*. 2020;8:143920–143937. Available from: https://doi.org/10.1109/ACCESS.2020.3014522.
70. Longo F, Nicoletti L, Padovano A. Estimating the impact of blockchain adoption in the food processing industry and supply chain. *Int J Food Eng*. 2020;16(5–6). Available from: https://doi.org/10.1515/ijfe-2019-0109.
71. Patelli N, Mandrioli M. Blockchain technology and traceability in the agrifood industry. *J Food Sci*. 2020;. Available from: https://doi.org/10.1111/1750-3841.15477.
72. Prashar D, Jha N, Jha S, Lee Y, Joshi GP. Blockchain-based traceability and visibility for agricultural products: a decentralizedway of ensuring food safety in India. *Sustainability (Switz)*. 2020;12(8). Available from: https://doi.org/10.3390/SU12083497.
73. Qian J, Dai B, Wang B, Zha Y, Song Q. Traceability in food processing: problems, methods, and performance evaluations—a review. *Crit Rev Food Sci Nutr*. 2020;. Available from: https://doi.org/10.1080/10408398.2020.1825925.
74. Qian J, Ruiz-Garcia L, Fan B, et al. Food traceability system from governmental, corporate, and consumer perspectives in the European Union and China: a comparative review. *Trends Food Sci Technol*. 2020;99:402–412. Available from: https://doi.org/10.1016/j.tifs.2020.03.025.
75. Qian J, Wu W, Yu Q, et al. Filling the trust gap of food safety in food trade between the EU and China: an interconnected conceptual traceability framework based on blockchain. *Food Energy Security*. 2020;. Available from: https://doi.org/10.1002/fes3.249.
76. Rao MS, Chakraborty G, Murthy KS. Market drivers and discovering technologies in meat species identification. *Food Anal Methods*. 2019;12(11):2416–2429. Available from: https://doi.org/10.1007/s12161-019-01591-8.
77. Salah K, Nizamuddin N, Jayaraman R, Omar M. Blockchain-based soybean traceability in agricultural supply chain. *IEEE Access*. 2019;7:73295–73305, Presented at the IEEE Access. Available from: https://doi.org/10.1109/ACCESS.2019.2918000.
78. Samal A, Pradhan BB. Boundary traceability conditions in food supply chains using block chain technology. *Int J Psychosoc Rehabil*. 2019;23(6):121–126. Available from: https://doi.org/10.37200/IJPR/V23I6/PR190745.
79. Shahid A, Almogren A, Javaid N, Al-Zahrani FA, Zuair M, Alam M. Blockchain-based agri-food supply chain: a complete solution. *IEEE Access*. 2020;8:69230–69243. Available from: https://doi.org/10.1109/ACCESS.2020.2986257.
80. Stranieri S, Riccardi F, Meuwissen MPM, Soregaroli C. Exploring the impact of blockchain on the performance of agri-food supply chains. *Food Control*. 2021;119. Available from: https://doi.org/10.1016/j.foodcont.2020.107495.

81. Surasak T, Wattanavichean N, Preuksakarn C, Huang SC-H. Thai agriculture products traceability system using blockchain and Internet of Things. *Int J Adv Comput Sci Appl.* 2019;10(9):578–583.
82. Tan A, Gligor D, Ngah A. Applying blockchain for halal food traceability. *Int J Logist Res Appl.* 2020;. Available from: https://doi.org/10.1080/13675567.2020.1825653.
83. Torky M, Hassanein AE. Integrating blockchain and the internet of things in precision agriculture: analysis, opportunities, and challenges. *Comput Electron Agric.* 2020;. Available from: https://doi.org/10.1016/j.compag.2020.105476.
84. Tripoli M, Schmidhuber J. Optimising traceability in trade for live animals and animal products with digital technologies. *Rev Sci Tech (Int Office Epizootics).* 2020;39(1):235–244. Available from: https://doi.org/10.20506/rst.39.1.3076.
85. Tsang YP, Choy KL, Wu CH, Ho GTS, Lam HY. Blockchain-driven IoT for food traceability with an integrated consensus mechanism. *IEEE Access.* 2019;7:129000–129017. Available from: https://doi.org/10.1109/ACCESS.2019.2940227.
86. Tsolakis N, Niedenzu D, Simonetto M, Dora M, Kumar M. Supply network design to address United Nations sustainable development goals: a case study of blockchain implementation in Thai fish industry. *J Bus Res.* 2020;. Available from: https://doi.org/10.1016/j.jbusres.2020.08.003.
87. Wallace CA, Manning L. Food provenance: assuring product integrity and identity. *CAB Rev Perspect Agric Vet Sci Nutr Nat Resour.* 2020;15(32). Available from: https://doi.org/10.1079/PAVSNNR202015032.
88. Alonso RS, Sittón-Candanedo I, García Ó, Prieto J, Rodríguez-González S. An intelligent Edge-IoT platform for monitoring livestock and crops in a dairy farming scenario. *Ad Hoc Netw.* 2020;98. Available from: https://doi.org/10.1016/j.adhoc.2019.102047.
89. Klerkx L, Jakku E, Labarthe P. A review of social science on digital agriculture, smart farming and agriculture 4.0: new contributions and a future research agenda. *NJAS—Wageningen J Life Sci.* 2019;100315. Available from: https://doi.org/10.1016/j.njas.2019.100315.
90. Lezoche M, Panetto H, Kacprzyk J, Hernandez JE, Alemany Díaz MME. Agri-food 4.0: a survey of the supply chains and technologies for the future agriculture. *Comput Ind.* 2020;117. Available from: https://doi.org/10.1016/j.compind.2020.103187.
91. Mondal S, Wijewardena KP, Karuppuswami S, Kriti N, Kumar D, Chahal P. Blockchain inspired RFID-based information architecture for food supply chain. *IEEE Internet Things J.* 2019;6(3):5803–5813. Available from: https://doi.org/10.1109/JIOT.2019.2907658.
92. Violino S, Pallottino F, Sperandio G, et al. Are the innovative electronic labels for extra virgin olive oil sustainable, traceable, and accepted by consumers? *Foods.* 2019;8(11). Available from: https://doi.org/10.3390/foods8110529.
93. Tao Q, Cui X, Huang X, Leigh AM, Gu H. Food safety supervision system based on hierarchical multi-domain blockchain network. *IEEE Access.* 2019;7:51817–51826. Available from: https://doi.org/10.1109/ACCESS.2019.2911265.
94. Yu B, Zhan P, Lei M, Zhou F, Wang P. Food quality monitoring system based on smart contracts and evaluation models. *IEEE Access.* 2020;8:12479–12490. Available from: https://doi.org/10.1109/ACCESS.2020.2966020.
95. Zhang X, Sun P, Xu J, et al. Blockchain-based safety management system for the grain supply chain. *IEEE Access.* 2020;8:36398–36410. Available from: https://doi.org/10.1109/ACCESS.2020.2975415.
96. Liu P, Long Y, Song H-C, He Y-D. Investment decision and coordination of green agri-food supply chain considering information service based on blockchain and big data. *J Clean Prod.* 2020;277. Available from: https://doi.org/10.1016/j.jclepro.2020.123646.
97. Bumblauskas D, Mann A, Dugan B, Rittmer J. A blockchain use case in food distribution: do you know where your food has been? *Int J Inf Manag.* 2020;52. Available from: https://doi.org/10.1016/j.ijinfomgt.2019.09.004.
98. Kamble SS, Gunasekaran A, Gawankar SA. Achieving sustainable performance in a data-driven agriculture supply chain: a review for research and applications. *Int J Prod Econ.* 2019;219:179–194. Available from: https://doi.org/10.1016/j.ijpe.2019.05.022.
99. Kittipanya-ngam P, Tan KH. A framework for food supply chain digitalization: lessons from Thailand. *Prod Plan Control.* 2020;31(2–3):158–172. Available from: https://doi.org/10.1080/09537287.2019.1631462.
100. Davies FT, Garrett B. Technology for sustainable urban food ecosystems in the developing world: strengthening the nexus of food–water–energy–nutrition. *Front SustaFood Syst.* 2018;2. Available from: https://doi.org/10.3389/fsufs.2018.00084.
101. Klerkx L, Rose D. Dealing with the game-changing technologies of Agriculture 4.0: how do we manage diversity and responsibility in food system transition pathways? *Glob Food Security.* 2020;24. Available from: https://doi.org/10.1016/j.gfs.2019.100347.
102. Kouhizadeh M, Saberi S, Sarkis J. Blockchain technology and the sustainable supply chain: theoretically exploring adoption barriers. *Int J Prod Econ.* 2021;231:107831. Available from: https://doi.org/10.1016/j.ijpe.2020.107831.
103. Mao D, Hao Z, Wang F, Li H. Innovative blockchain-based approach for sustainable and credible environment in food trade: a case study in Shandong Province, China. *Sustainability (Switz).* 2018;10(9). Available from: https://doi.org/10.3390/su10093149.
104. Tiscini R, Testarmata S, Ciaburri M, Ferrari E. The blockchain as a sustainable business model innovation. *Manag Decision.* 2020;(Ahead-of-print). Available from: https://doi.org/10.1108/MD-09-2019-1281.
105. Shivaanivarsha N, Santhoshkumar DR. Secured food delivery and monitoring using blockchain algorithm. *Test Eng Manag.* 2020;82:14343–14349.
106. Steinwandter V, Herwig C. Provable data integrity in the pharmaceutical industry based on version control systems and the blockchain. *PDA J Pharm Sci Technol.* 2019;73(4):373–390. Available from: https://doi.org/10.5731/pdajpst.2018.009407.
107. Yadav VS, Singh AR, Raut RD, Govindarajan UH. Blockchain technology adoption barriers in the Indian agricultural supply chain: an integrated approach. *Res Conserv Recycling.* 2020;161. Available from: https://doi.org/10.1016/j.resconrec.2020.104877.
108. Aung MM, Chang YS. Traceability in a food supply chain: safety and quality perspectives. *Food Control.* 2014;39:172–184. Available from: https://doi.org/10.1016/j.foodcont.2013.11.007.
109. Dutta P, Choi T-M, Somani S, Butala R. Blockchain technology in supply chain operations: applications, challenges and research

opportunities. *Transport Res Part E: Logist Transport Rev*. 2020;142. Available from: https://doi.org/10.1016/j.tre.2020.102067.

110. Swaffield SR, Corry RC, Opdam P, McWilliam W, Primdahl J. Connecting business with the agricultural landscape: business strategies for sustainable rural development. *Bus Strat Environ*. 2019;28(7):1357–1369. Available from: https://doi.org/10.1002/bse.2320.

111. Casino F, Kanakaris V, Dasaklis TK, et al. Blockchain-based food supply chain traceability: a case study in the dairy sector. *Int J Prod Res*. 2020;1–13. Available from: https://doi.org/10.1080/00207543.2020.1789238.

112. Doney PM, Cannon JP. An examination of the nature of trust in buyer–seller relationships. *J Mark*. 1997;61(2):35–51. Available from: https://doi.org/10.1177/002224299706100203.

113. Ganesan S. Determinants of long-term orientation in buyer-seller relationships. *J Mark*. 1994;58(2):1–19. Available from: https://doi.org/10.1177/002224299405800201.

114. Kumar N, Scheer LK, Steenkamp J-BEM. The effects of supplier fairness on vulnerable resellers. *J Mark Res*. 1995;32(1):54–65. Available from: https://doi.org/10.1177/002224379503200107.

115. Carolan MS. Social change and the adoption and adaptation of knowledge claims: whose truth do you trust in regard to sustainable agriculture? *Agric Hum Values*. 2006;23(3):325–339. Available from: https://doi.org/10.1007/s10460-006-9006-4.

116. DuPuis EM, Gillon S. Alternative modes of governance: organic as civic engagement. *Agric Hum Values*. 2009;26(1):43–56. Available from: https://doi.org/10.1007/s10460-008-9180-7.

117. Smithers J, Lamarche J, Joseph AE. Unpacking the terms of engagement with local food at the farmers' market: insights from Ontario. *J Rural Stud*. 2008;24(3):337–350. Available from: https://doi.org/10.1016/j.jrurstud.2007.12.009.

118. Moore O. Understanding postorganic fresh fruit and vegetable consumers at participatory farmers' markets in Ireland: reflexivity, trust and social movements. *Int J Consum Stud*. 2006;30(5):416–426. Available from: https://doi.org/10.1111/j.1470-6431.2006.00537.x.

119. Insch A, Cuthbert R. Why country of origin still matters in food retailing: implications for promotion management research. *J Promotion Manag*. 2018;24(3):363–375. Available from: https://doi.org/10.1080/10496491.2018.1378304.

120. Ab Rashid N, Bojei J. The relationship between halal traceability system adoption and environmental factors on halal food supply chain integrity in Malaysia. *J Islamic Mark*. 2019;11(1):117–142. Available from: https://doi.org/10.1108/JIMA-01-2018-0016.

121. Faisal MN. A study of inhibitors to transparency in red meat supply chains in Gulf cooperation council (GCC) countries. *Bus Process Manag J*. 2015;21(6):1299–1318. Available from: https://doi.org/10.1108/BPMJ-11-2014-0107.

122. Foscht T, Lin Y, Eisingerich AB. Blinds up or down? The influence of transparency, future orientation, and CSR on sustainable and responsible behavior. *Eur J Market*. 2018;52(3/4):476–498. Available from: https://doi.org/10.1108/EJM-10-2016-0576.

123. Sporleder TL, Goldsmith PD. Network embeddedness in the food supply chain and firm strategy on signaling quality. *Paradoxes Food Chains Netw*. 2002;720–728.

124. Opara LU. Traceability in agriculture and food supply chain: a review of basic concepts, technological implications, and future prospects. <https://agris.fao.org/agris-search/search.do?recordID=FI2016100260>; 2003 Accessed 05.11.20.

125. Bastian J, Zentes J. Supply chain transparency as a key prerequisite for sustainable agri-food supply chain management. *Int Rev Retail Distrib Consum Res*. 2013;23(5):553–570. Available from: https://doi.org/10.1080/09593969.2013.834836.

126. Curtis D, Hill A, Wilcock A, Charlebois S. Foodborne and waterborne pathogenic bacteria in selected organisation for economic cooperation and development (OECD) countries. *J Food Sci*. 2014;79(10):R1871–R1876. Available from: https://doi.org/10.1111/1750-3841.12646.

127. Zhong DRY, Tan PK, Bhaskaran PG. Data-driven food supply chain management and systems. *Ind Manag Data Syst*. 2017;117(9):1779–1781. Available from: https://doi.org/10.1108/IMDS-06-2017-0269.

128. Gessner DGH, Volonino DL, Fish LA. One-up, one-back ERM in the food supply chain. *Inf Syst Manag*. 2007;24(3):213–222. Available from: https://doi.org/10.1080/10580530701404561ff.

129. Köhler S, Pizzol M. Technology assessment of blockchain-based technologies in the food supply chain. *J Clean Prod*. 2020;269. Available from: https://doi.org/10.1016/j.jclepro.2020.122193.

130. Chen Y, Li Y, Li C. Electronic agriculture, blockchain and digital agricultural democratization: origin, theory and application. *J Clean Prod*. 2020;268. Available from: https://doi.org/10.1016/j.jclepro.2020.122071.

131. Astarita V, Giofre VP, Mirabelli G, Solina V. A review of blockchain-based systems in transportation. *Information*. 2020;. Available from: https://doi.org/10.3390/info11010021.

132. Moberg CR, Cutler BD, Gross A, Speh TW. Identifying antecedents of information exchange within supply chains. *Int J Phys Distrib Logist Manag*. 2002;32(9):755–770. Available from: https://doi.org/10.1108/09600030210452431.

133. Harshavardhan Reddy B, Aravind Reddy Y, Sashi Rekha K. Blockchain: to improvise economic efficiency and supply chain management in agriculture. *Int J Innov Technol Explor Eng*. 2019;8(12):4999–5004. Available from: https://doi.org/10.35940/ijitee.L3749.1081219.

134. Weber CL, Matthews HS. Food-miles and the relative climate impacts of food choices in the United States. *Environ Sci Technol*. 2008;42(10):3508–3513. Available from: https://doi.org/10.1021/es702969f.

135. Weber CL, Matthews HS. Quantifying the global and distributional aspects of American household carbon footprint. *Ecol Econ*. 2008;66(2):379–391. Available from: https://doi.org/10.1016/j.ecolecon.2007.09.021.

136. Mao D, Wang F, Hao Z, Li H. Credit evaluation system based on blockchain for multiple stakeholders in the food supply chain. *Int J Environ Res Public Health*. 2018;15(8). Available from: https://doi.org/10.3390/ijerph15081627.

137. Meyerding SGH, Trajer N, Lehberger M. What is local food? The case of consumer preferences for local food labeling of tomatoes in Germany. *J Clean Prod*. 2019;207:30–43. Available from: https://doi.org/10.1016/j.jclepro.2018.09.224.

138. Gopalakrishnan PK, Ananth V, Lewis K, Behdad S. A decision-making framework for blockchain technology selection. *Smart Sustain Manuf Syst*. 2019;3(2):148–168. Available from: https://doi.org/10.1520/SSMS20190021.

139. Perboli G, Musso S, Rosano M. Blockchain in logistics and supply chain: a lean approach for designing real-world use cases.

IEEE Access. 2018;1. Available from: https://doi.org/10.1109/ACCESS.2018.2875782.

140. Rejeb A, Rejeb K. Blockchain and supply chain sustainability. *Logforum*. 2020;16(3):363–372. Available from: https://doi.org/10.17270/J.LOG.2020.467.
141. Chen S, Liu X, Yan J, Hu G, Shi Y. Processes, benefits, and challenges for adoption of blockchain technologies in food supply chains: a thematic analysis. *Inf Syst e-Business Manag*. 2020;. Available from: https://doi.org/10.1007/s10257-020-00467-3.
142. Tan MII, Razali RN, Husny ZJ. Adoption Halal Transportations Technol Halal Logist Serv Providers Malays. 2012;6(3):8.
143. Nakamoto S. Bitcoin: a peer-to-peer electronic cash system. <http://Www.Bitcoin.Org>; 2008:9. https://doi.org/10.1007/s10838-008-9062-0
144. Khan N. Blockchain-enabled traceability and immutability for financial applications. University of Luxembourg, Luxembourg. https://orbilu.uni.lu/handle/10993/43941; 2020.
145. EthHub. Ethereum proof of stake—EthHub. <https://docs.ethhub.io/ethereum-roadmap/ethereum-2.0/proof-of-stake/>; 2020 Accessed 08.02.20.
146. Law A. Smart contracts and their application in supply chain management (Thesis). Massachusetts Institute of Technology. <https://dspace.mit.edu/handle/1721.1/114082>; 2017.
147. Dinh TTA, Wang J, Chen G, Liu R, Ooi BC, Tan K-L. BLOCKBENCH: a framework for analyzing private blockchains. In: *Proceedings of the 2017 ACM International Conference on Management of Data*. New York: Association for Computing Machinery; 2017:1085–1100. <https://doi.org/10.1145/3035918.3064033>.
148. Khan N, Nassar M. A look into privacy-preserving blockchains. In: Proceedings of the IEEE/ACS Sixteenth International Conference on Computer Systems and Applications (AICCSA); 2019. <https://doi.org/10.1109/AICCSA47632.2019.9035235>
149. Khan N, Lahmadi A, Kraussl Z, State R. Management plane for differential privacy preservation through smart contracts. In: Proceedings of the IEEE/ACS Seventeenth International Conference on Computer Systems and Applications (AICCSA). Antalya; 2020.
150. Khan N, Ahmad T, Patel A, State R. Blockchain governance: an overview and prediction of optimal strategies using nash equilibrium. *arXiv:2003.09241 [cs]*. <http://arxiv.org/abs/2003.09241>; 2020 Accessed 06.11.20.
151. Durham University. Blockchain, cryptocurrency and ethical projects. Durham University. https://www.dur.ac.uk/business/research/accounting-and-finance/ethical-finance/events/?id = 38144&eventno = 38144; 2020 Accessed 06.11.20.
152. Al Shehri W. Cloud database. Database as a service. *Int J Database Manag Syst*. 2013;5(2):1.
153. Microsoft docs. Store business-critical blob data with immutable storage. <https://docs.microsoft.com/en-us/azure/storage/blobs/storage-blob-immutable-storage>; 2019. Accessed 06.11.20.
154. Maull R, Godsiff P, Mulligan C, Brown A, Kewell B. Distributed ledger technology: applications and implications. *Strategic Change*. 2017;26(5):481–489. Available from: https://doi.org/10.1002/jsc.2148.
155. Li Y, Cao B, Peng M, et al. Direct acyclic graph-based ledger for internet of things: performance and security analysis. *IEEE/ACM Trans Netw*. 2020;28(4):1643–1656, Presented at the IEEE/ACM Transactions on Networking. Available from: https://doi.org/10.1109/TNET.2020.2991994.
156. Simmons J IOTA publishes updated whitepaper on Coordicide. *Crypto News Flash*. <https://www.crypto-news-flash.com/iota-foundation-publishes-updated-whitepaper-on-coordicide/>; 2020 Accessed 06.11.20.
157. Seawright J, Gerring J. Case selection techniques in case study research: a menu of qualitative and quantitative options. *Pol Res Q*. 2008;61(2):294–308. Available from: https://doi.org/10.1177/1065912907313077.

Further reading

Chen A 1 in 10 people around the world gets sick from food every year. *NPR.org*. <https://www.npr.org/sections/thesalt/2015/12/16/459971675/1-in-10-people-around-the-world-get-sick-from-food-every-year>; 2015 Accessed 05.11.20.

DeLind LB, Howard PH. Safe at any scale? Food scares, food regulation, and scaled alternatives. *Agric Hum Values*. 2008;25(3):301–317. Available from: https://doi.org/10.1007/s10460-007-9112-y.

Hollands T, Martindale W, Swainson M, Keogh JG. Blockchain or bust for the food industry? *Food Sci Technol*. 2018;33(4). Available from: https://www.fstjournal.org/features/32-4/blockchain.

Stevenson M, Spring M. Flexibility from a supply chain perspective: definition and review. *Int J Oper Prod Manag*. 2007;27(7):685–713. Available from: https://doi.org/10.1108/01443570710756956.

van der Vorst JGAG, Tromp S-O, van der Zee D-J. Simulation modelling for food supply chain redesign; integrated decision making on product quality, sustainability and logistics. *Int J Prod Res*. 2009;47(23):6611–6631.

Section XIII

Hazard versus risk-based approaches to food safety regulations

Chapter 69

Pros and cons of hazard- versus risk-based approaches to food safety regulation

Jyotigna M. Mehta[1] and Ivonne M.C.M. Rietjens[2]

[1]*ADAMA Agricultural Solutions, Reading, United Kingdom,* [2]*Division of Toxicology, Wageningen University, Wageningen, The Netherlands*

Abstract

Legislation and regulations around the globe currently use a mixture of hazard- and risk-based approaches for ensuring the safety of food. This chapter focusses on the pros and cons of hazard- versus risk-based approaches to food safety regulation providing examples to illustrate the concepts and arguments provided. Hazard-based approaches only perform the first of the four steps that are part of risk assessment including hazard identification, hazard characterization, exposure assessment, and risk assessment. Hazard-based approaches are, for example, common practice in the field of allergenicity or genotoxicity, and also show a tendency to be increasingly applied as a result of the need for the replacement, reduction, and refinement (3Rs) of animal testing, resulting in use of a wide range of in vitro assays elucidating hazards but not risks. Recent developments, however, indicate a need for risk-based approaches even in the field of genotoxicity testing and allergenicity, while physiologically-based kinetic modeling is able to translate in vitro data to the in vivo situation enabling a risk rather than a hazard-based approach. Risk management and risk communication based on hazard assessment lead to unnecessary risk mitigation actions and consumer fear. Risk perception and the impact of globalization are key considerations for the future.

It is concluded that future developments should be directed at moving away from hazard- toward risk-based evaluations and educating the risk assessors, risk managers, and the public on the fact that a hazard does not translate into a risk at certain levels of exposure, even for genotoxic carcinogens or allergens.

Keywords: Food safety; risk assessment; hazard-based; risk management; risk communication

69.1 Introduction

Legislation and regulations around the globe currently use a mixture of hazard- and risk-based approaches for ensuring the safety of food. In hazard-based approaches (focused on inherent properties), the mere presence of a compound can form the basis of a regulatory decision without taking the level of exposure, and thus the actual potential for an adverse effect to occur, into account. In contrast, risk-based approaches (focused on likelihood of adverse effects occurring) combine exposure assessment with the hazard assessment to conclude on the risk for human health as a basis for regulatory decisions. Many of the regulatory systems in the world use a risk-based approach for evaluating concerns arising from exposure to chemicals, although there are some countries and/or regulations that still focus on hazard data as the critical data for safety decisions. These different approaches result in inconsistencies in evaluation strategies and testing needs. A focus on hazard not only limits the acceptance of new innovative products but is also not scientifically justified nor sustainable. Hazard only or hazard first strategies may require the use of large numbers of animals and the performance of redundant and often costly studies that provide little value in informing human or environmental risk decisions. Alternatively, hazards may be derived from in vitro assays without taking the consequences of in vivo kinetics, including absorption, distribution, metabolism, and excretion of the compound under study, into account, which may also result in inadequate conclusions on safety. Another outcome of hazard only assessments is the elimination of the use of substances or products without considering risk management practices, which can successfully mitigate exposure. Examples of hazard-based approaches are the regulations related to so-called carcinogenic, mutagenic, and reproductive (CMR) substances. Their classification is based on evidence supporting that they present a hazard to human health because of CMR effects. This implies that the evidence can theoretically be derived from

Present Knowledge in Food Safety. DOI: https://doi.org/10.1016/B978-0-12-819470-6.00024-X

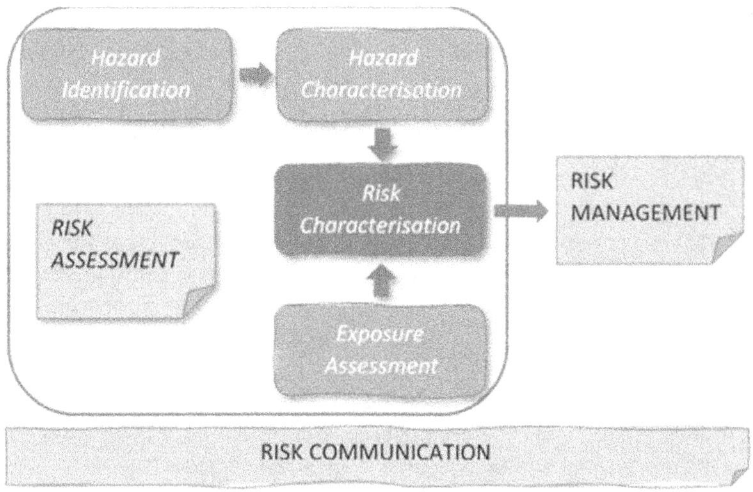

FIGURE 69.1 The process of risk assessment, consisting of four steps: hazard identification, hazard characterization, exposure assessment, and risk characterization; these guide risk management decisions and risk communication.

in vitro bioassays, without taking in vivo kinetics and/or actual exposure levels into account. Examples of compounds regulated by a risk-based approach are food additives and veterinary drug residues in animal-based foods, for which, based on a risk assessment including evaluation of exposure versus proposed health-based guidance values (HBGV) such as acceptable daily intakes (ADIs), regulations underlying their safety in use can be put in place.

The process of risk assessment is generally accepted to consist of four essential steps (as shown in Fig. 69.1) including hazard identification, hazard characterization, exposure assessment, and risk characterization.[1] In a hazard-based approach only, the step of hazard identification is required, and hazard characterization, in which dose–response curves and HBGV are defined, is not needed. It is also of interest to note that the process of risk management and risk communication is not part of the process of risk assessment but is based on the outcomes of the risk assessment and sector-specific regulations. Differences have evolved in safety assessment approaches for food chemicals (occurring either as contaminants, residues, or deliberately added), food allergens, whole foods and ingredients, including novel and genetically modified foods, and pathogenic microorganisms in food. This is due mainly to inherent differences in their nature.

This chapter focusses on the pros and cons of hazard- versus risk-based approaches to food safety regulation providing examples to illustrate the different aspects across these various food chain components.

69.2 The concept of hazard in the 21st century

69.2.1 General principles

A hazard can be defined as something that has the potential to cause harm. A hazard does not include any information of whether the hazard will actually result in this harm. This explains why a hazard-based evaluation assessment consists of only the hazard identification step and does not include the other three steps of risk assessment. At a societal level, some hazards are accepted (e.g., consumption of caffeine and alcoholic drinks) whereas others are not (e.g., food allergen or microbial contaminant), some being of more acute concern while others are more chronic in nature. The basis for this acceptance by consumers is debatable and could provide an interesting risk-benefit analysis, which is often missing (and not the focus of this chapter). As defined by OECD, food safety means having "a reasonable certainty that no harm will result from intended uses under the anticipated conditions of consumption."[2] Obviously, a hazard-based approach does not comply with this definition.

For non-food industrial chemicals, a hazard-based regulation has been in use for decades (e.g., for flammable, explosive, and corrosive hazards) and has been extended to cover certain toxicological hazards. In the EU, hazard-based regulation was covered in the past by the Dangerous Substances Directive (DSD) and the Dangerous Preparations Directive (DPD),[3,4] which have been replaced by the EU REACH and CLP Regulations.[5] As an example of foodborne chemicals, other regions around the world utilized the WHO hazard classification system for pesticides (WHO Chronicle, 22, 397–401 (1975)), or other similar national systems, based essentially on acute toxicity hazard endpoints. The CLP Regulation takes into account the Global Harmonization System (GHS) on classification and labeling (C&L) that has been developed (originally mandated in 1992) and implemented internationally as a non-legally binding agreement.[6] These types of legislation and agreement aim to ensure that knowledge about hazards is more widely available, that criteria for hazard classification and communication of hazard information are more uniform internationally, and that information on hazards is passed to users so that chemicals can be transported, used, and disposed safely. For example, internationally recognizable pictograms and hazard statements (formerly called risk phrases under the DSD and DPD) have been introduced to enable quick identification of hazards on containers of chemicals or environmental signage.

While regulations for C&L have evolved, the changing societal environment for requiring C&L has not been factored in. Basic intrinsic properties of substances are only considered, which may have been suitable >50 years ago. Today, our knowledge of chemicals and their utility has hugely advanced, manufacturing technology provides adequate mitigation and control to protect workers, and exposure science has developed to help understand situations of concern. Therefore the question arises whether these hazard-based systems are still fit-for-purpose.

69.2.2 Hazard-based approaches in food safety regulation

Use of hazard-based approaches in ensuring the safety of food has been applied when evaluating so-called avoidable regulated chemicals. For such avoidable compounds, a full risk assessment is performed but when in the initial step of this risk assessment a genotoxic hazard is identified, this identified hazard triggers a zero tolerance approach and prevents such compounds from entering the market or being present in food items. Since more than 10 years in the EU, this concept has been extended to what are called CMR substances. Classification of a substance as a CMR substance automatically implies legislative restrictions on its approval, manufacture, market entrance and use, without opportunity for a risk assessment being conducted, depending on the sector-specific regulations[7]. In this way, for example, within the framework of the EU REACH and CLP Regulations, risk management may be based on hazard identification alone. Also, although criteria for determination of endocrine disrupting properties have not yet been agreed upon in the EU for harmonized classification, substances that test positive in bioassays for endocrine activity may be treated in the same way[7]. Under the specific Plant Protection Products Regulation (EC) 1107/2009, substances showing endocrine disrupting properties are currently not permitted to be approved on the EU market unless negligible exposure can be demonstrated (even though harmonized classification criteria for such effects are not established in the EU). Based on analytical tools available today, detection limits can be very low and "negligible" exposure is not easy to demonstrate. For more than a decade, a zero-residue concept has also been suggested for fresh produce or commodities due to pressures from secondary legislation (i.e., food suppliers or supermarkets within the food chain creating their own conditions of sale). This "zero-residue" is difficult to define, depends on limits of detection based on analytical methods used, and often gets confused with no residue being present at all. Thus, within the REACH and CLP Regulations on classification, labeling and packaging, substances, and mixtures may be evaluated by ECHA (European Chemicals Agency) based on hazard, while the evaluation of their residues in food upon use (as defined under regulations for different food safety sectors) may be evaluated based on risk by EU Member States and the European Food Safety Authority (EFSA). These contradictions add to debate and confusion, especially at a global food safety level, impacting trade, and import of food commodities, and raise uncertainty, mistrust, or concerns among consumers and other stakeholders.

An example of an area that has evolved is the field of food allergens, which may trigger adverse reactions at relatively low exposures in sensitive individuals. Since the thresholds for elicitation of allergic reactions can be extremely low and it is difficult to establish the thresholds for each allergen that may be of importance, traditionally, a hazard-based approach has been taken, for instance in communicating possible unintended allergen presence due to cross-contact contamination. Given that the hazard also relates to only a small percentage of the whole population, allergenicity has also not been used as a critical effect to define HBVGs. Food safety in this field has thus been approached by indicating the (possible) presence of an allergen by labeling so that those who are susceptible can avoid that food item. However, such precautionary labeling ("may contain...") can restrict food choice unnecessarily due to its excessive and indiscriminate use. Hence, a risk-based approach has been developed (the VITAL project, see http://www.eu-vital.org/en/home.html), based on the establishment of reference doses elaborated from a safety objective or accepted risk level agreed upon by stakeholders.[8] Bindslev-Jensen et al.[9] showed that threshold data could be modeled statistically, with a view to predicting the proportions of the at-risk population that would be likely to react to specified doses. They illustrated the use of this approach with data from human beings, that is, the species of interest, in contrast to most other types of toxicological safety data. Dose-distribution modeling became the preferred method for characterizing allergen hazard and was adopted for subsequent major projects. ILSI Europe's considerations included the criteria to be applied to identify allergens of public health concern through methodologies to determine the relationship between dose and the proportion of allergic individuals reacting, as well as the nature of the observed responses.[10–13] They also promoted the application of novel, probabilistic risk assessment methods to better delineate the impact of benchmarks, such as reference doses, and actively participated in major European food allergy projects, such as EUROPREVALL ("The prevalence, cost and basis of food allergy across Europe"; http://cordis.europa.eu/result/rcn/51771_en.html) and iFAAM ("Integrated approaches to food allergen and allergy risk management"; http://research.bmh.manchester.ac.uk/iFAAM), both being EU-funded projects. The evaluation includes a review of analytical methods and how different ones can best be deployed given their strengths and limitations as a basis for reliable exposure data and development of a framework for stakeholders to achieve consensus on acceptable risk.

A more complex situation exists for the risk assessment of pathogenic microorganisms in food, which has to take into account the fact that microorganisms can grow (multiply) during food processing and storage, that they are often inactivated during processing and preparation (e.g., sterilization, pasteurization), and that cross contamination may occur. Exposure to the microorganisms can only be assessed making use of processing data and predictive models, and based on prevalence and concentration data in the raw material or the food product, some time prior to consumption. A single living cell may—in theory—result in illness because microorganisms may multiply in the gut. These features have a large impact on the methods applied for both exposure assessment and hazard characterization and, therefore, for the terminology used in microbiological risk assessment, challenging what constitutes the actual hazard. For example, in microbiological risk assessment, the agent itself (microorganism) is considered a hazard and a hazard-based approach is generally based only on hazard assessment, excluding consideration of exposure characterization. Control of exposure to the microorganism is called "hazard-based" when it is known to decrease prevalence and/or concentrations of the specific hazard of concern, but the impact on human health risk is still unknown. However, it is called "risk-based" when risk assessment is applied to assess impact on the incidence of human illness.[14,15]

Some chemicals are regarded as so inherently hazardous to human health or the environment that they have triggered internationally agreed moves to ban or severely restrict their import, export, and use. This includes a number of persistent chemicals with adverse effects on the environment and/or human health, such a DDT, aldrin, lindane, polychlorinated biphenyls, and perfluorinated compounds.[16] It also includes pesticides with very high acute toxicity, such as paraquat, and certain cholinesterase inhibiting compounds, which have not only caused deaths from suicide, but also many accidental deaths among exposed workers, particularly in developing countries, and, less commonly, deaths from food contamination.[17–19] This history has led to a renewed call from the Food and Agricultural Organization of the United Nations (FAO), World Health Organization (WHO), and the World Bank that highly hazardous pesticide products should not be available to small-scale farmers who lack knowledge and the proper sprayers, protective gear, and storage facilities to manage such products appropriately.[20] Particular examples are some organophosphates that have been listed under the 1998 Rotterdam Convention as severely hazardous pesticide formulations and are subject to the agreed prior informed consent procedure on import and export.[16] As a result, several such pesticides have been banned or severely restricted in many countries, but not necessarily worldwide. Even for substances with very high acute toxicity, different advisory bodies may reach differing conclusions with respect to hazard and risk and, consequently, legislative jurisdictions may take different decisions on whether it is necessary to ban their use dependent on the local situation or to define appropriate risk mitigation measures. This is where risk benefit and risk management need to be considered and well communicated.

69.3 Risk-based approaches in safety assessment

Risk assessment–based approaches in safety assessment of chemicals and products used or found in foodstuff have been adopted in different ways across different food sectors and global regions. A mechanism is needed for the food industry and associated regulatory agencies to have a globally harmonized way to focus evaluation efforts for risk management of chemicals to better incorporate innovation and ensure societal needs are met.

A globally harmonized, risk assessment–based regulatory decision-making process, achieved by the application of advances in science via integration of new methods and traditional data to create tailored exposure-driven risk assessments, would help to resolve inconsistencies in regulatory practice. Using a risk-based evaluation strategy increases the ability to use alternative approaches and new technologies to inform risk assessment, better characterize risk, and improve management decisions. These new, more scientifically robust methods are more human relevant and also frequently decrease the number of animals needed to determine human health risk. Recently, the US EPA has published a directive to greatly diminish the use of mammalian laboratory animals for the testing of chemicals, including agrochemicals.[21] Good exposure estimates and knowledge of their uncertainties are a prerequisite for reliable risk characterization.

As an example, to advance innovation more rapidly and efficiently within the agricultural chemistry community, a globally coordinated effort bringing together regulatory authorities and the regulated industries to discuss scientific and technical aspects of data requirements and registration was sought.[22] Such an evaluation process would emulate the goals of the International Conference of Harmonization (ICH) of Technical Requirements for Pharmaceuticals for Human Use (http://www.ich.org/home.html) or the Veterinary ICH (https://www.vichsec.org/en/). An important consideration for achieving success for such endeavors is the encouragement of direct communication between the regulatory community and the regulated industry, which will enable a more rapid evaluation and incorporation of new technologies and scientific advances into the regulatory process and lead to the elimination of outmoded practices that no longer serve their intended purpose. Broader implementation of such approaches across all food sectors will increase the speed, efficiency, and accuracy of regulatory decision-making for food safety. This approach also recognizes the global aspect of the food sector industries and encourages uniformity and best practices for data generation and evaluation to support approval of safe uses for products with scientifically defensible human health risk assessments.

69.3.1 General principle

The basic principle behind risk-based approaches in safety assessment was first coined by Paracelsus more than 500 years ago (1493–1541):

> *All substances are poisons; there is none which is not a poison. The right dose differentiates a poison and a remedy.*

This quotation has been undermined by misleading interpretation of, for example, the Precautionary Principle (Article 191 of the Treaty of the Functioning of the European Union https://eur-lex.europa.eu/LexUriServ/LexUriServ.do?uri = CELEX:12008E191:EN:HTML; WTO Uruguay Round Agreement on the Application of Sanitary and Phytosanitary (SPS) Measures, Article 5 https://www.wto.org/english/tratop_e/sps_e/spsagr_e.htm[23]; EU Commission, 2000 http://eur-lex.europa.eu/legal-content/EN/TXT/?uri = LEGISSUM:l32042; Science for Environment Policy[24]), which shall be informed by *three specific principles*:

- the fullest possible scientific evaluation, the determination, as far as possible, of the degree of scientific uncertainty;
- a risk evaluation and an evaluation of the potential consequences of inaction;
- the participation of all interested parties in the study of precautionary measures, once the results of the scientific evaluation and/or the risk evaluation are available.

In addition, the *general principles* of risk management remain applicable when the Precautionary Principle is invoked. These are the following five principles:

- proportionality between the measures taken and the chosen level of protection;
- non-discrimination in application of the measures;
- consistency of the measures with similar measures already taken in similar situations or using similar approaches;
- examination of the benefits and costs of action or lack of action;
- review of the measures in the light of scientific developments.

These principles reflect the use of best science and innovation to provide relevant risk assessments and safety evaluation for decision-making, incorporating all available knowledge and data, and state that the appropriate use of mitigation, where necessary, should be uniformly applied.

For chemicals in foods, the risks to health mostly depend on the duration, frequency, and level of exposure. Low-level exposures are often of no or negligible risk, with the likelihood of risk increasing as exposure increases and/or when eventually thresholds for triggering of toxicological effects are exceeded. Hence, risk-based approaches are more commonly used to guide appropriate risk management decisions.

69.3.2 The data-rich versus the data-poor

Robust risk assessments require various data generated from a variety of well-designed and analyzed studies, including exposure data, understanding use scenarios, representative toxicological data, and much more. However, an "ideal" dataset is rarely available in the real world. Suboptimal study design, bioanalytical limitations, lack of investment in data generation, and differing regulatory requirements between jurisdictions can result in data "gaps," which impede the risk assessment process. Across the different food regulation sectors, there are variable degrees of data available in support of the hazard or risk assessments, some areas being data-rich and others being data-poor. For this reason, and to avoid unnecessary animal testing, many alternative approaches [recently referred to as new approach methodologies (NAMs)] have been developed to provide reasonable solutions to demonstrate safety. It is also not practical to generate data for all substances as this is a resource issue for both society (high costs and limited facilities with required capabilities) and risk assessment bodies (with conflicting prioritization tasks).

For example, the REACH regulation (2008) for chemicals adopts a tonnage-driven tiered approach to hazard data generation (a form of exposure-based approach). This has further been reviewed by an ECETOC taskforce to consider exposure-based adaptations and a new transformational program to move away from the current "tonnage-based testing annex"–driven assessment to an exposure-led chemical safety assessment, integrating different sources of information, including NAMs, in an objective way to provide sufficient weight of evidence (WoE) using a tiered approach to conduct risk assessments with confidence (ECETOC Workshop Report No. 37; ECETOC Technical Report No. 137).

One of the more data-rich areas relates to pesticides, where globally, the data requirements have been the most comprehensive for decades, driven by the need to understand the intrinsic hazard properties of the substances, irrespective of the volume of manufacture or exposure scenarios. During these last 15–20 years, many multistakeholder evaluations have been conducted for agrochemicals to review the data requirements to elucidate the critical studies and species for testing considering the types of risk assessment needed.[25–27] An advancement of this latter effort is a new Health and Environmental Sciences Institute (HESI) initiative to transform evaluation of agrochemicals, making it fit-for-purpose and applicable to the changing global (and regional) needs for regulatory decisions that incorporate relevant evolving science inputs (https://hesiglobal.org/transforming-the-evaluation-of-agrochemicals-tea/).

69.3.3 Case example review: threshold of toxicological concern

For situations where human exposure is expected to be low or data are limited for a substance, the concept of the threshold of toxicological concern (TTC) was developed as a pragmatic solution. This estimates the probability of no adverse effects occurring for a substance of unknown toxicity at a specified daily intake level. It is not intended to be applied to regulated chemicals for which specific requirements exist for their hazard and risk assessment,[28] though the latter may not be considered a scientific justification for exclusion. The TTC concept is currently used for the following areas:

- food flavoring substances (EFSA & JECFA);
- food additives, for example, impurities, metabolites, and degradation products present in food additives (EFSA);
- food contact materials (FDA);
- recycled plastics—safety of recycling processes—criteria for mechanical processes to produce recycled polyethylene terephthalate (PET) for materials and articles in contact with food (EFSA);
- contaminants, for example, pharmacologically active substances in food of animal origin (EFSA);
- pesticide metabolites in groundwater in the EU; metabolites and degradation products of plant protection products relevant to residue definition for risk assessment (EFSA);
- flavoring additives in feed—"Maximum acceptable feed concentrations" from default values for feed consumption (EFSA);
- genotoxic impurities in pharmaceuticals (EMEA);
- genotoxic constituents in herbal substances and preparations (EMEA);
- micropollutants and impurities in drinking water (AUS).

Notably, there is potential for its broader utility as a first screening step, even for regulated chemicals.

The TTC approach is a resource-effective, de minimis method for the safety assessment of chemicals, based on a distributional analysis of the results of numerous toxicological studies.[28,29] It is being increasingly used to screen and prioritize substances with low exposure for which there is little or no toxicological information, provided the chemical structure of the compound is known and that it does not belong to one of the so-called excluded classes.[30,31] The first step in the approach is the identification of substances that may be DNA-reactive genotoxins, to which the lowest TTC value is applied. This TTC value was originally based on the analysis of the cancer potency database and involved several assumptions that no longer reflect the state-of-the-science and some of which were not as transparent as they could have been. Hence, the database has been reviewed using inclusion and exclusion criteria reflecting current knowledge. A strategy was defined to select appropriate substances for TTC determination based on consideration of WoE for genotoxicity and carcinogenicity. Differentiation between substances that are carcinogenic by DNA-reactive genotoxic modes of action and those that act by nongenotoxic modes of action will enable the protectiveness to be determined of both the TTC for DNA-reactive genotoxicity and that applied by default to substances that may be carcinogenic but are unlikely to be DNA-reactive genotoxins (i.e., for Cramer class I–III compounds). Critical to the application of the TTC approach to substances that are likely to be DNA-reactive genotoxins is the reliability of the software tools used to identify such compounds.

Thresholds have been in consideration for decades. Frawley first introduced this principle in 1967 following analysis of a large dataset of 220 two-year chronic toxicity studies on food additives, industrial, and consumer chemicals and pesticides.[32] This review serves as an interesting insight as to how concepts develop and evolve over time.

Most chemicals (180/220) had NOELs greater than 100 mg/kg of diet (100 ppm), 19 had NOELs below 10 mg/kg of diet (10 ppm) but all of these were pesticides or heavy metals, and 5 chemicals had NOELs below 1 mg/kg of diet (1 ppm) but these were pesticides with known toxicity (either they accumulated or affected the nervous system at low doses). It is of interest to note that at this time NOAELs were expressed in mg/kg diet whereas in more recent approaches levels in the diet are generally converted to mg/kg bw. Frawley thus suggested a level of 10 mg/kg of diet for food packaging materials and applying an additional safety factor of 100 which gave a level of 0.1 mg/kg in the human diet or 100 parts-per-billion (ppb) as a dietary concentration threshold.

In 1969, the FDA proposed a threshold of 50 ppb for levels of migrants into food or food-simulating solvents.[33] Finally, in 1977, following petitioning, the FDA modified its regulations so that uses of substances that resulted in levels of migration into foods at levels ≤ 50 ppb would be exempt from food-additive regulation unless they raised safety concerns.

In later establishing a Threshold of Regulation (TOR), the FDA had to determine a level and establish a review framework that would meet this "reasonable certainty of no harm" standard, including the prohibition against FDA authorization of known carcinogens under the Delaney Clause [Section 409(c)(3)(A) of the Act]. The FDA had to choose a TOR low enough to ensure that the public health would be protected even if an exempted substance was later found to be a carcinogen. Rulis conducted a further analysis using the FDA's Priority Based Assessment of Food Additives (PAFA) database containing 159 compounds with subchronic and chronic studies, and determined that an intake of between 1 and 10 μg/kg bw/day of various chemicals might not pose a risk to humans.[34]

In 1986, the FDA proposed a probabilistic approach to the TOR to address overall safety and concerns about potential carcinogenicity of untested additives. In 1987, scientists outside of the FDA considered factors that suggested a practical threshold between 1 part per trillion (ppt) and 5 ppb in the diet. In 1990, the Canadian Center for Toxicology proposed a dietary concentration of 1 ppb as the TOR for components of food-contact articles for which no toxicology data had been developed, expressing a clear confidence in the concept of regulating based on thresholds.

In 1995, the FDA finally adopted the TOR for food contact substances,[35] that would result in minimal migration into food, but which would be exempted from regulation as food additives. The threshold was set at 0.5 ppb or less, that is, an intake of 1.5 μg/person/day (0.025 μg/kg bw/day). Below this level, FDA required no specific toxicity testing and performed an abbreviated safety assessment mainly focused on intake (exposure) assessment. The value of 0.5 ppb was derived from a distribution plot of chronic dose rates based on the dose descriptor TD_{50}, the daily dose rate required to induce a calculated 50% tumor incidence based on analysis of the Cancer Potency Database (CPDB) and linear extrapolation. However, several conditions had to be met, such as the substance must not have been shown to be carcinogenic, the structure of the substance does not provide reason to suspect it might be carcinogenic, and the substance is free of carcinogenic impurities of specified potency.

Further work by the FDA[36] has provided support for the use of higher thresholds, though this tiered approach was not adopted, based on Ames negative data and a lack of structural alerts. Efforts to derive structural-based TTCs on endpoints other than carcinogenicity have typically made use of the structural decision rules defined by Cramer et al.[37] Munro et al.[38] explored the relationship between structure and toxicity by compiling a large database of over 600 substances that had been tested for a variety of noncancer endpoints by the oral route. The resulting database contained 2941 NOELs for a total of 613 organic substances, which were then assigned to one of three structural classes that revealed to have a bearing on toxicity, based on Cramer's rules,[37] that is, Class I (simple structures efficiently metabolized to innocuous products; anticipated low order of oral toxicity); Class II (intermediate structures, less innocuous than substances in Class I, but no positive indication of toxic potential); Class III (complex structures; metabolism to reactive products suggestive of potential toxicity).

For each of the distributions of NOELs, the lower 5th percentile was estimated (the point on the distribution where 5% of the chemicals had lower NOELs and 95% had higher NOELs) and divided by a traditional 100-fold safety factor. This defined three human exposure thresholds, that is, TTC values, which have since been further supplemented.[31] Recommended exclusions to this decision tree include those chemical classes underrepresented in the database or outside of the application domain (such as metals, organometallics, organosilicon chemicals, nanomaterials, radioactive substances, and proteins) or those with special properties (such as substances with a potential for bioaccumulation, steroids, and high-potency carcinogens) or mixtures of substances containing unknown chemical structures.

Later, the ICH M7 guidance proposed a TTC for pharmaceutical impurities, in which an intake level below 1.5 μg/person/day does not increase excess lifetime cancer risk more than over 10^{-5} (1:100,000), even when there is a concern that the impurity may have DNA-reactive genotoxicity (https://www.pmda.go.jp/files/000208234.pdf); however, the guidance indicates that highly potent DNA-reactive carcinogens (e.g., aflatoxin-like, azoxy-, or *N*-nitroso-carcinogens) are outside of the application of the TTC approach, and are sometimes called the "cohort of concern" (COC).[39] Both the US FDA and ICH adopt the same value of 1.5 μg/person/day as the TOR and TTC, respectively. However, the former excludes DNA-reactive genotoxic chemicals while the latter includes them. The policy differences may depend on the usage of the chemicals, and associated risk-benefit analysis. Food contact materials do not necessarily provide health benefits to consumers, and therefore the policy for an acceptable level of risk is more conservative or strict, whereas pharmaceuticals may be needed to maintain or improve health conditions of patients, even if the drugs contain some DNA-reactive impurities, thus forming a basis for risk-benefit analysis.

EFSA/WHO[30] later proposed a level 10 times lower, that is, 0.15 μg/person/day or 0.0025 μg/kg bw/day (which reflects a risk level of 1:1,000,000), than that proposed by ICH as a sufficiently protective TTC for DNA-reactive genotoxic chemicals.[31,39]

TTCs have been proposed for specific chemical classes such as organophosphates and carbamates, and also for other endpoints such as prenatal developmental toxicity[40] and skin sensitization[41] where TTC values are derived based on systemic toxicity endpoints by the oral route. Other routes of exposure such as inhalation have also been considered[42,43] and the EU COSMOS project (http://www.cosmostox.eu) explored oral to dermal extrapolation.

TTC assumes a lifetime exposure but staged TTC were proposed by Muller et al.[44] to consider if higher TTC values could be proposed when exposure duration is likely to be shorter term, <1 year. This might allow accommodation of the risk/benefit of a particular pharmaceutical substance, for example, presence of genotoxic impurities. Higher TTC values were proposed when accounting for occupational versus consumer exposures also.

Efforts have been made to integrate TTC with high-throughput exposure data.[45,46] Ranking and prioritization of 7968 chemicals with respect to the upper 95th percentile predicted exposure (mg/kg/day) for the US population and children 6–11 years showed that less than 5% of the 95th percentile values for any chemical in any demographic group were above the Cramer Class 3 TTC value.

The value gained in exploring larger (ever increasing) datasets to set thresholds confidently is clear. These efforts provide significant progress in assessing risk in the absence of substance-specific toxicity data, thus providing a confident tool to minimizing the use of animals in several contexts.

For the use of veterinary drugs in food-producing animals, which may lead to residues in animal-derived foodstuffs, potentially posing a risk to human safety, the process of residue risk assessment continues to evolve as new data emerge. A recurring challenge is when suboptimal or incomplete data are provided with the expectation of supporting a robust risk assessment. The Joint FAO/WHO Expert Committee on Food Additives (JECFA) is comprised of international experts who routinely deal with such data challenges when performing veterinary drug residue evaluations. Recent developments in veterinary drug residue risk assessment include specific consequences of suboptimal data during the risk assessment process. Case examples from recent JECFA evaluations help to quantify and illustrate the concepts and facilitate the generation of improved quality data, enabling more timely and robust risk assessments.[47] In some situations, hazard characterization challenges can be mitigated through a variety of strategies to facilitate HBGV derivation and continue the residue assessment. Such strategies may include using more conservative uncertainty (i.e., safety) factors, or using surrogate values based on TTCs or quantitative structure–activity relationship models enabling read-across. However, because JECFA closely integrates the hazard characterization and residue assessment processes, strategies to address hazard characterization deficiencies may impact the residue assessment (e.g., leading to derivation of more conservative maximum residue levels (MRLs) than necessary had a complete toxicological/microbiological dataset been available).[48]

A potential limitation for the TTC approach is that it uses toxicological data from oral doses administered to experimental animals to estimate an equivalent human external exposure. A refinement of the TTC approach would be to take into consideration the internal exposure (e.g., plasma concentrations quantified for example via physiologically based pharmacokinetic modeling), converting the chemical-specific external NOAELs (in mg/kg/day) in the TTC database to this estimated internal exposure, and linking it to the internal concentration at the target leading to the occurrence of adversity and/or even to the human situation. The use of an internal TTC (iTTC) has been proposed by several researchers[49–51] and, if successful, this development could provide a more precise way of assessing various sources of uncertainty associated with the TTC. However, the prediction of an internal exposure for chemicals with no or very limited data may prove challenging. Once distribution of internal exposures exists, approaches to determine and apply appropriate toxicokinetic and toxicodynamic uncertainty factors may be evaluated and then applied to the 5th percentile threshold level to derive the final iTTC values.[49] These efforts continue to progress exposure science to allow relevant tiered risk assessments to be conducted without the need for extensive in vivo toxicity testing.

Although improvements to an approach should always be sought, it is clear from this TTC development example that these thresholds are robustly derived from large datasets and should thus provide confidence as a first tier approach to risk assessment in the absence of substance-specific data.

When the TTC approach is applied, one of the practical challenges remains the accurate calculation of relevant exposure scenarios against which these thresholds are compared. Two factors that need to be addressed are the consideration of all possible sources of exposure (aggregate) for one chemical (e.g., environmental background, biocidal uses, veterinary medicinal products and in some cases even endogenous sources from internal biochemical pathways) and the combined exposure to multiple chemicals (cumulative) with similar toxicological impact on human health. These two issues in many cases hinder the application and acceptance of the TTC approach for regulatory purposes in some areas, and thus would benefit from further work.[28]

69.3.4 Weight of evidence based on science

WoE is a term used frequently, but often mis-represented. As a concept, it refers to situations where several pieces of evidence are used to reach a conclusion. As a procedure, it refers to the process of assembling, weighing (reliability, relevance, consistency), and evaluating evidence to integrate into a scientifically defensible conclusion.[52] The WoE approach is used when scientific questions can only be answered by using several different pieces of evidence. Using intelligent science approaches to provide a WoE based on available or new data (which were developed using good scientific practices, such as adherence to GLP) within the context of the use and exposure scenario for any chemical or product is essential. This is theoretically captured well by Suter et al.[53] who compared systematic evidence and WoE and illustrated how assessors should follow scientific standards of transparency concerning the reasons for choosing and implementing their methods. By focusing on the needs of the assessment, thus defining the problem formulation rather than traditional practices (e.g., hazard identification by a preordained list), one can defensibly support evidence-based decision-making.

69.3.5 Clarity and consistency

Those involved in testing to meet regulatory requirements would be able to work more efficiently if there was only one global standard or requirement to meet. Preservation of risk assessment as the operating principle for regulatory decision-making is essential to product stewardship. The conduct of risk assessments may differ, and the underlying data may vary depending upon the populations and their practices or exposure scenarios. However, how these data are used and how decisions are made should be more uniform. Harmonization attempts (e.g., OECD, NAFTA, EU) with uniform data requirements and mutual recognition (work-sharing) have tried to tackle this, but do not go far enough to transform our risk assessment and management sciences to be globally aligned or accepted. Hazard and exposure have a global definition. However, their utility is too fragmented (e.g., as experienced with adoption of GHS), often takes a long time and sometimes becomes too politicized. How can scientists attempt to follow the 3R's Principles when they are required to conduct additional studies beyond core data packages to meet unrealistic needs or aims of specific nations (leading to redundant or irrelevant testing)? How can society then have confidence in the generated data (which regulators evaluate) if they see different requirements in different countries with, more importantly, different interpretations? How would scientists explain themselves to Paracelsus, 500 years on? More can certainly be done to achieve consistency in scientific understanding and interpretation of data, and the application of this knowledge in various contexts. This education often needs to begin at an early stage in the scientist's development. Alongside accumulating the knowledge is a need for appropriately communicating the science and data interpretation. Global efforts to create more harmonization (e.g., WHO, OECD) need to be more widely adopted at national level to bring greater clarity about food safety for the consumer.

An example of developing consistency is the pathology terminology used. Since 2006, the European Society of Toxicological Pathologists (ESTP) is involved in the INHAND project, with the target to standardize the nomenclature and diagnostic criteria for rats and mice in toxicologic pathology. INHAND is a global collaboration project of the major Toxicological Pathology societies (e.g., ESTP, STP, BSTP and JSTP; https://www.eurotox-path.org/nomenclature/index.php). This type of initiative then helps with consistent interpretation of findings, enabling better comparison between studies (especially if conducted at different laboratories).

69.3.6 Compounds with and without thresholds

With the notable exception of genotoxic carcinogens,[54] most chemicals are generally assumed to have thresholds. In practice, however, the same types of (sigmoidal) dose−response models are used descriptively for all groups of chemicals as part of the hazard characterization and derivation of the point of departure.[15] Chemical risk assessment differs between compounds with respect to what is done after derivation of the reference point. Dose−response modeling in microbial risk assessment generally uses non-threshold models (a single pathogen can cause infection) for infectious microorganisms and threshold or probability of toxin production for toxin-producing microorganisms (e.g., *C. botulinum*). Microbial dose−response modeling has been reviewed.[55] In contrast to chemicals, assessment factors are generally not employed in microbial risk assessment even when models are based on animal data or on specific population subgroups but are considered as a source of uncertainty (e.g., FDA/FSIS[56]).

Recent developments also include approaches to account for variability in pathogen virulence and susceptibility of different human populations and how it can be characterized in terms of the r-parameter (reproduction parameter)[57]. This approach has been used in recent years to consider the influenza outbreaks[58] and the recent Covid 19 pandemic.[59,60]

69.4 Examples of hazard-based food safety regulation

69.4.1 Genotoxicity

Genotoxicity is a hazard that is frequently used as a basis for safety regulations or risk management decisions in the field of food safety. Especially when one considers so-called avoidable chemicals, for example, food additives, food flavors, pesticides, food contact materials, or food packaging materials, a compound or mixture that tests positive for genotoxicity is generally not allowed to enter the market. The in vitro bioassays used to detect this hazard may take bioactivation into account but do not take further in vivo ADME (absorption, distribution, metabolism and excretion) characteristics into account. This implies that positive outcomes in an in vitro bioassay may be overruled by negative data from in vivo genotoxicity testing. These kinds of regulatory testing guidelines acknowledge that in vivo kinetics may affect internal exposure and thus the actual in vivo hazard. However, when the compound tests positive in vivo, that hazard is not easily overruled, not even by negative data on carcinogenicity since regulators or risk assessors may argue that also germ cells could be mutated so carcinogenicity is not the only endpoint of concern for a genotoxic compound. Recent scientific developments in the field, however, provide data and arguments that question the concept of a non-threshold approach for genotoxic chemicals.[61] This is based on the consideration that DNA damage may also induce repair instead of leading to a mutation and that genotoxicity will only be observed when that repair is overwhelmed or saturated. Thus, at low concentrations or dose levels, generally relevant for intake via the human diet, actual concentration response curves or dose–response curves for DNA damage and/or genotoxicity may be sublinear pointing at an apparent threshold.[62,63]

69.4.2 Endocrine disruption

Should endocrine disruptors (EDs) be considered or assessed in any different way to any other toxicological endpoint? Within the European Union, various legislative acts contain specific provisions on endocrine disruption, requiring the regulation of substances with endocrine disrupting properties via a hazard-based approach, thus minimizing exposure. Presumably this is due to an assumed lack of thresholds for the adverse effects of such substances. Conversely, in other jurisdictions, such as the United States, Canada, Australia, and Japan, EDs are regulated using a risk-based approach and focus more on estrogenic compounds. This has led to increasing controversy on whether thresholds can be inferred for endocrine-mediated effects. There is concern that the endocrine system is too complex to allow estimation of safe levels of exposure to such chemicals. Based on an evaluation of the available scientific evidence in this area, Brescia[64] presents a sound and robust conclusion that there is nothing special or unique about endocrine disruption and that there are no greater uncertainties in its assessment compared to other non-genotoxic forms of toxicity that would justify adopting a non-threshold approach by default. Biology predicts that thresholds of adversity exist and are the rule for all endpoints, including those arising from endocrine disruption (and as observed for directly acting genotoxic agents). A threshold approach to the risk assessment of endocrine disrupting chemicals is scientifically justified.[64]

Importantly, both synthetic EDs (S-EDCs) and natural (exogenous and endogenous) EDs (N-EDCs) can interact with endocrine receptors and disturb hormonal balance. However, compared to endogenous hormones, S-EDCs are only weak partial agonists with receptor affinities several orders of magnitude lower than N-EDCs. Thus, to elicit observable, adverse effects, S-EDCs require considerably higher concentrations to attain sufficient receptor occupancy or to displace natural hormones and other endogenous ligands. Significant exposures to exogenous N-EDCs may result from ingestion of foods such as soy-based diets, green tea, and sweet mustard. While their potencies are lower as compared to natural endogenous hormones, they usually are considerably more potent than S-EDCs. Effects of exogenous N-EDCs on the endocrine system are observed at high dietary intakes. A causal relation between their mechanism of action and these effects is often established and biologically plausible. In contrast, the assumption that the much lower human exposures to S-EDCs may induce observable endocrine effects is not plausible. Hence, it is not surprising that epidemiological studies searching for an association between S-EDC exposure and health effects have failed to find causal links. Regarding testing for potential endocrine effects, Autrup et al.[65] suggested that a scientifically justified screen should use in vitro tests to compare potencies of S-EDCs with those of reference N-EDCs. When the potency of the S-EDC is similar or smaller than that of the N-EDC, further testing in laboratory animals and regulatory consequences would then not be warranted. An example of the contradictory effects of natural substances is shown in a comprehensive review of phytoestrogens,[66] discussing the prevalence of these different plant-derived dietary compounds, their supposed mode(s) of action and recent evidence on their supposed beneficial effects as compared with their potential (anti)estrogenic properties, which may cause endocrine disruption. This clearly demonstrates that further assessment is needed to understand risks and benefits at relevant exposure levels.

EDs substantially cost society as a result of increases in disease and disability but—unlike other toxicant classes such as carcinogens—have yet to be codified into regulations as a hazard category, though this is currently being considered by ECHA. The economic, regulatory, and policy approaches to limit human ED exposures and potential improvements are evolving areas.[67] Minimization of human exposure is unlikely without a clear overarching definition for EDs, a better understanding of realistic exposure and implementation of relevant testing requirements to better assess any risks posed.

69.5 Disadvantages and limitations of hazard-based safety regulation

Use of a hazard-based approach to make food safety decisions clearly has advantages. It is simple and can be based on in vitro bioassays only, thus being more cost effective and less resource intensive. It will also not need animal or human data that facilitate definition of HBGVs. Additionally, provided the bioassay includes adequate systems for bioactivation, it will also detect compounds for which the metabolites raise a concern. The approach is also conservative in terms of safety, since a hazard detected will result in regulatory action and risk management directed at limiting or preventing exposure. However, there are also disadvantages. The major disadvantage is that a hazard-based system is over-protective and raises unnecessary concerns. It may also result in regulations that would result in bans or limitations for economically or nutritionally essential food items[7]. For example, foods that naturally contain toxic constituents, such as herbs like basil or products thereof like pesto or vegetables like fennel that contain the alkenylbenzenes estragole and/or methyleugenol, potatoes that contain solanine, wheat and thus bread containing mycotoxins like deoxynivalenol or nuts containing aflatoxin B1, would all face risk management actions independent of the level of the respective constituents and consumption of the respective food item. The same holds for products in which compounds that are genotoxic and carcinogenic such as acrylamide, polycyclic aromatic hydrocarbons, aromatic heterocyclic amines, and furans are introduced as a result of food processing methods such as frying or roasting. This would affect French fries, chips, fried hamburgers, barbequed meat, and coffee, to name but a few. It could also hold for wine that contains alcohol known to be a genotoxic carcinogen. Clearly, the approach toward such compounds and products has to be risk-based and not hazard-based to come to adequate conclusions on the risk management actions needed for society. Without a risk assessment, it is uncertain if adequate conclusions would emerge from the hazard-based approach for these and other chemicals.

There are, however, also situations where a hazard-based approach can be of help. This is especially the case when adequate exposure and full risk assessment appear not feasible, because of time limitations or inadequate data. Here, information on the hazard can be of initial help. However, whenever possible, taking exposure into account will always be more informative and relevant. Even for compounds that test positive for genotoxicity, performing a risk assessment using the so-called margin of exposure (MOE) assessment (indicating a safety margin between the exposure level and the dose causing the adverse effects or preferably using the $BMDL_{10}$ for tumor induction) is informative and results in a more balanced risk management approach than what would be initiated based on hazard identification alone. This can be illustrated by the example of calculating the MOE resulting from exposure to genotoxic polycyclic aromatic hydrocarbons via food as reported by EFSA.[68] In their opinion, the CONTAM Panel of EFSA estimated the margins of exposure based on the estimated exposure of the European population and concluded that the MOEs for average consumers were 17,900 for benzo[a]pyrene, 15,900 for PAH2, 17,500 for PAH4, and 17,000 for PAH8. Based on these values that were above the cut-off value of 10,000, it was concluded that these MOEs indicate a low concern for consumer health at the average estimated dietary exposures. For high-level consumers, the respective MOEs were 10,800, 9500, 9900, and 9600 and thus close to or less than 10,000, indicating a potential concern for consumer health and a possible need for specific risk management action.

A similar risk assessment for acrylamide,[69] however, resulted in MOE values that were all substantially lower than the value of 10,000, identifying a concern for human health. This comparison further illustrates the importance of risk assessment instead of only hazard evaluation to set priorities for risk management mitigation and regulation.

69.5.1 Relevance of kinetics

As stated earlier, a major disadvantage with a hazard-based system is that it is over-protective, raising unnecessary concerns, and/or results in defining the wrong priorities. A further example of this would be the fact that electron donating molecules, including antioxidants like flavonoids (e.g., quercetin), vitamin C, and the amino acid cysteine, will test positive for inhibition of thyroid peroxidase (TPO) in the so-called NCCT-TPO-AUR-dn assay[70] and other assays for TPO activity.[71–73] This implies that in a hazard-based approach, vitamin C, the amino acid cysteine, and the tea flavonoid quercetin would be classified as EDs. This example illustrates that hazard-based approaches may classify compounds as a potential food safety issue while, in reality, they are not.

Discrepancy between what is detected in an in vitro assay and in vivo may often originate from the fact that, in vivo, so-called ADME characteristics may play an important role. This may result in limited bioavailability of the compound of interest in vivo at the target site, due to limited absorption, distribution preventing delivery at the target site, efficient metabolism, and/or efficient excretion. These aspects are generally not accounted for in hazard-based approaches.

69.6 Implications for risk management

For all stakeholders, there is a need to understand risks in context as this can influence views on the levels of risk that are considered to be acceptable. For example, the risks posed by one substance or product that may no longer be permitted/available need to be compared with those of potential replacements, or with other chemicals used in the same sector, or with natural chemicals that can produce the same effect of concern. Food risks also need to be seen alongside benefits in order to make a balanced decision. Environmental and human health challenges are multifaceted[74] and a good example of this complexity is exposure to ethanol via both exogenous sources and endogenous formation.[75]

A difficulty with the use of hazard-based approaches in the food safety arena is that it is not possible to undertake any meaningful comparison with benefit. Benefit encompasses not only the area of nutritional benefit, which can be weighed against known or potential toxicological risks in risk-benefit analyses of individual foods,[76] but also encompasses food security, which includes physical availability of food, agricultural demand or environmental/climate pressure, economic and physical access to food, utilization of food, and stability of the food supply.[77]

Often, benefit considerations have been narrowly focused on nutritional aspects or have not been considered at all. This has the potential to lead to bias in the overall conclusions of regulators and risk managers, who may not have been presented with the benefits or importance of particular foods. The aim of food legislation should be to ensure the achievement of the right balance between minimizing potential risks to human health and the environment and maximizing the benefits to society (as per OECD[2]). A risk-based assessment allows for this by incorporating any relevant impacting factors.

69.6.1 Risk perception and risk acceptance

Perception and acceptance of risk are where the current paradigm has the most limitations and contradictions. For example, most regions globally operate a dual scheme for the registration of agrochemicals whereby risk assessment and hazard-based classification sit side by side. Although the risk assessment methodology and approaches may differ between regions, they are basically consistent. Where the biggest contradiction and discrepancy in risk management occur are with the regional variation in the consequences of hazard-based classification. Typically, CMR classifications attract the most regulatory attention and concern. In some regions (notably the United States and Canada), classification based on these outcomes leads to approaches such as the use of additional uncertainly factors (such as the FQPA—Food Quality Protection Act—safety factor) or health protective statistical approaches (such as Q* methodology). In other regions (mainly the EU), a classification as a CMR (Category 1a and 1b) means that the active ingredient cannot be registered or re-registered regardless of risk assessments that may demonstrate safe uses (the so called "Cut-Off" approach). This fundamental regional dichotomy illustrates the lack of a global approach to safety and leads to a high degree of unpredictability and uncertainly for registrants and within the food chain.

Because of the impact of classification on registrability, registrants must devote considerable resources (often involving generation of extensive additional animal data) in understanding mode of action (MoA) and relevance to humans of the outcome leading to classification. For example, to set aside a classification outcome in the EU, the competent authority requires extensive MoA data and human relevance assessments on a case-by-case basis, for each substance and even for "common" modes of actions such as nuclear hormone interaction leading to high dose–level liver tumors in rodents. Read-across between the same MoA and/or chemical groups is not easily accepted and the inability of some regulators to understand and accept any degree of uncertainty makes this approach ever more difficult and unpredictable. As more examples of these cases are developed, and understanding into AOPs grows, more of this uncertainty will eventually be addressed. However, even if the MoA is unknown, due to adverse findings having a threshold dose, a risk assessment can still be conducted.

On a slightly more positive note, some regulators (mainly in the United States and Canada) are more open to scientific advances to the extent that certain study types can be waived if scientific information is provided that can reasonably be expected to predict the outcome of the current standard animal study. However, even one region regulating on hazard alone means that for global registrability of that substance, the studies that are conducted and the way in which they are specified will remain rooted in hazard-based thinking without any advantage in protecting human health.

The approach and data needed for a risk assessment are dependent on the risk management question(s) and the reason for doing an assessment (problem formulation). For example, the assessments considered fit for purpose for chemicals and microbiological agents are fundamentally different. In chemical risk assessment, if exposure assessment is lower or higher than the corresponding HBGV, the situation related to the chemical substances are considered to be of no concern or of potential concern, respectively. For compounds that are both genotoxic and carcinogenic, EFSA recommends using an MOE of 10,000 or higher to be protective. Thus, for chemicals, the estimated exposure is usually compared, in one way or another, with a HBGV, reference dose or point of departure (e.g., PoD). Therefore chemical risk assessment relates in most cases to safety assessments rather than risk assessments, since a margin between the current exposure and some guideline value intends to ensure the absence of adverse effects rather than an estimate of the probability or degree of response under the current exposure. In contrast, in risk-based approaches for microbiological agents, it is not necessarily that human exposure is estimated (or measured) but the prevalence and concentration of the microorganism within the food chain should be determined, from which the magnitude of the potential risk can be assessed to judge whether it is acceptable or not. The aim is to calculate the probability of illness based on the current exposure and estimate the consequences in terms of the selected endpoint of the dose–response model with any biases associated with the data, assumptions, and models.[15]

69.6.2 Uncertainties put into context

How uncertainties vary in their type and impact for risk assessment approaches and their interpretation should be transparently and clearly explained to all stakeholders. A better understanding of uncertainties is needed but also a better communication of these uncertainties and what they mean for the consumer. Quantification of uncertainties in both hazard and risk assessment gives some direction toward where further work or research may be needed or could be focused. It may not be possible to fully eliminate uncertainty, but clarity will help to derive better risk management decisions and consumer confidence. In the absence of clarity or understanding, it is easier to embrace a hazard-based approach.

It was highlighted in EFSA's third Scientific Conference[78] that there is a need to advance forms of risk assessment that are more contextual and socially sound and accountable, while remaining scientifically robust. A fit-for-purpose risk assessment needs to begin with a clear articulation of policy to provide context and boundaries for the risk assessment and help guide risk managers to make decisions that align with the societal goals. This allows the risk assessment to include contextual relevance and reflects reality. A hazard-based approach does not do this. In the absence of clarity, risk assessors are left to make a series of small policy decisions with varying degrees of success. While policy shapes the objectives of the risk assessment, science informs the process, which ensures the outcomes of the risk assessment are robust, repeatable, and defensible. Improving the science used for risk assessment alone is not enough, as it is also necessary to ensure that the risk assessment is consistent with the objectives of the guiding policy. Modern analytical methods can produce prodigious amounts of data that can lead risk assessors down unproductive avenues with the mistaken impression that more data will inevitably yield a more precise outcome. In this context, a risk assessment to determine whether an activity is acceptable becomes a loop of data generation and scientific inquiry where the original problem formulation becomes lost and the risk manager is left to reach a decision without guidance. They often default to a hazard-based approach as it seems easier on the surface for decision-making.

There is a need to manage value-laden judgments in risk assessment through efforts that promote reflection, openness, and engagement. Likewise, it is essential to acknowledge and communicate risks and unavoidable scientific uncertainty in a transparent and trustworthy way, relevant to the societal context. Early empirical research suggests that if uncertainty can be communicated with confidence, preferably as a range, then trust in the source is not diminished. It was noted that intelligent transparency requires the information to be accessible, intelligible, useable, and assessable due to ever-increasing complexities. Communication requires professional input, listening to audiences, addressing misunderstandings, and testing all outputs for comprehension and usefulness. Only in doing so can risk assessment meet the demands of the public to generate and communicate knowledge that safeguards society.[79]

Another example where there is a tendency to place more trust in a hazard-based system instead of a risk-based approach is the field of mixture toxicity. Over the last 20 years or more, many efforts have been made to better understand mixture toxicity and cumulative risk assessment by researchers and regulators, with huge programs of funding, innovation, and collaboration (e.g., EU Horizon 2020 EuroMix; OECD combined exposure guidance development; US EPA cumulative risk assessment, EFSA development of methods for cumulative risk assessment).

An overview of different approaches has been recently compiled in an OECD document (https://www.oecd.org/chemicalsafety/risk-assessment/considerations-for-assessing-the-risks-of-combined-exposure-to-multiple-chemicals.pdf). Several international frameworks and guidance documents are available for the assessment of chemical mixtures, for example, from WHO/IPCS (https://www.sciencedirect.com/science/article/pii/S0273230011000638?via%3Dihub), OECD (https://www.oecd.org/chemicalsafety/risk-assessment/considerations-for-assessing-the-risks-of-combined-exposure-to-multiple-chemicals.pdf), or EFSA (https://www.efsa.europa.eu/en/efsajournal/pub/5634).

One of the issues with these various programs is the regionally diverse approaches undertaken to address what are in fact common concerns. Many start from a hazard identification perspective across multiple chemicals and due to the perceived better understanding of the toxicity profiles, it can be misconstrued that the uncertainties in the hazard assessment are far fewer than those in the ultimate risk assessments because we have less data or poorer understanding of the exposure scenarios required for the latter. More recent recommendations are to begin with problem formulation (e.g., the OECD approach), and to start with a better understanding of the scope of the mixture of concern in relation to vulnerable populations (using food consumption and residue monitoring data such as NHANEs Database in the United States, EFSA monitoring reports; EU total food diets). Many activities are also looking at aggregate exposure or more holistic views to environmental exposure (EC platform IPCHEM; CARES, EUROMix). The missing point is the global context to the concerns and having a unified risk-based approach to provide consistent, comparable risk assessments which better communicate the safety to consumers.[80]

69.7 Communication along the food chain

In terms of the pros and cons of hazard- versus risk-based assessments, communication of safety along the food chain is critical to reassure consumers. Communication should be based on risk assessments and not purely on hazard criteria, because the former incorporates the relevant factors for ensuring safety following a more insightful understanding of the exposure situation. Due to a diverse mix of stakeholders, tailored risk communication strategies are needed to convey the complexities of different levels of certainty and uncertainty in the risk assessment process depending on the knowledge-base of the various audiences. Key actors in the food chain include decision-makers such as risk managers, national food safety agencies, European and international scientific advisory bodies, academia, industry, and non-governmental and consumer organizations. Key European agencies dealing with chemical risk assessment include the EFSA, the ECHA within the REACH directive, and the European Medicines Agency (EMA) for pharmaceuticals. Key national and international scientific advisory bodies include the FAO/WHO Joint Expert Committees on Food Additives (JECFA) and the Joint Meeting on Pesticide Residues (JMPR), the US Environmental Protection Agency (US-EPA), the US Food and Drug Administration (FDA), the Food Safety Commission of Japan and the Organisation for Economic Cooperation and Development (OECD), to cite but a few. Over the past 60 years, these international and national bodies have performed risk assessment for thousands of substances in food, water, air, or consumer products.

Appropriate communication, education, and training will ensure that there is increasing awareness among regulators, manufacturers, and the general public of the consequences of any uncertainty for risk-based conclusions on food safety, which can never be absolute. Characterization of the uncertainty will lead to refined data gap analysis and improved mitigation opportunities for managing the risks. An interesting example of the impact along the food chain is given by a fipronil contamination incident in the EU.

69.7.1 Fipronil eggs

Fipronil, a broad spectrum phenylpyrazole pesticide, is used to prevent insects such as fleas and ticks from plaguing cats and dogs as well as repelling a variety of pests from crops and homes. It is not approved for use in any food animal species in any country.[81] A recent event in 2017/2018 involved a cleaning agent for sanitizing hen houses laced with fipronil as an illegal treatment against red lice. Due to the application of the fipronil-containing cleaning agent mainly in the Netherlands and Belgium (who issued the first EU-wide alert), but also in a limited number of farms in Germany, laying hens were exposed to fipronil via contaminated feed, dermal contact or by preening (grooming) their feathers, leading to absorption, accumulation in tissues, and excretion via eggs and excreta. Many articles appeared in the media (e.g., Deutsche Welle, Science: https://p.dw.com/p/2hgNS) adding fuel to the incident. Hundreds of farms were affected and tons of produce destroyed ($>$39 million dollars financial damage). Ultimately, more than 16 EU countries, China and Switzerland were impacted.

A Dutch company, Chickfriend, had used fipronil at poultry farms to combat red mite. Fipronil is not allowed for the purpose of controlling pests. The NVWA

(Netherlands Food and Consumer Safety Authority) took the precautionary measure of blocking nearly 200 farms and required them to withdraw their eggs after the determination was made that these eggs contained residues of fipronil above the standards permitted, which might be harmful for the health of children if ingested daily. This hazard-based decision meant that not just the eggs, but also chickens and manure were not allowed to leave the yard. The sales of table eggs declined dramatically, impacting Germany where a large part of the eggs produced in the Netherlands is sold. In this way, major financial consequences for poultry farms and other companies within the egg production/distribution chain were observed.

The comprehensive contamination of table eggs with fipronil and the response of the authorities caused agitation in the food industry and uncertainty among consumers. This incident questioned the food safety protocols in place and whether sufficient endeavors were made by the food producers to ensure safety. A number of concerns were highlighted by both the Netherlands and Belgian authorities during their investigation of the incident.

The most important (and simple) management measure is to prevent the use and/or the placing on the market of contaminated eggs, egg products, and poultry meat. This hazard-based approach does not account for which produce was actually contaminated, and at what level or how much exposure would result and thus no actual risk characterization was made. Operators must usually ensure that their eggs, egg products, and poultry meat that are placed on the market or used as a raw material/ingredient in the production of foodstuffs comply with the MRL for fipronil.

In the context of using fipronil as a pesticide for plants, MRLs have been fixed not only in plant products but also in animal products since food-producing animals might be exposed to fipronil residues in feed. A risk assessment conducted by the German Federal Institute for Risk Assessment came to the conclusion that for this particular fipronil egg contamination event, only up to 7.8% of the ADI would be reached for various European consumer groups (based on German and European egg consumption data) indicating no concern. This placed the initial hazard into relevant context. This contamination event had also shown the need for finer quantitative predictions of fipronil transfer, including uncertainty estimations and better predictions of the depuration phase. A toxicokinetic model calibrated specifically with fipronil and laying hens could be useful for the assessment and management of human health risks as a consequence of feed and egg contamination. Because of its predictive power, this modeling can potentially be used to set thresholds and maximum levels that are coherent between feed and food.[82] Having reliable data to ensure the safety of consumers is critical in these situations to provide appropriate communication based on consideration of all relevant information and to then implement pertinent risk management measures. The food chain stakeholders are then better able to manage such contamination issues with more dependable and less drastic outcomes.

69.7.2 Residues on food items

Many reports are seen in media about exposure to pesticide residues and their potential harmful effects and even attempts to link them to disease prevalence. However, these media reports are often an example of hazard- instead of risk-based communication. Not many robust epidemiological data are available to define cause and effect, though good epidemiological practices to support such research has been better defined in recent years.[83] Often due to this press, pesticides generically receive a bad name leading to unnecessarily conservative risk assessments, and hence impractical risk mitigation measures. Secondary legislation became popular, which allowed, for example, supermarkets to further restrict presence of pesticide residues on produce sold driven by such pressures. The farmers are expected to comply with these hazard-driven market needs, otherwise their crops would not be sold. Other forms of crop protection such as organics have become populist due to their perceived safer profiles (e.g., less synthetic chemical use). Now, biopesticides and GMOs are being approved for use as pesticides, often used in combination with conventional products as part of the integrated pest management programs. There is a perception that these products are less hazardous than conventional chemical or synthetic products. As these tools for the farmer develop alongside changes in spraying technology and increasing climatic demands, new innovative products (both naturally derived and synthetically derived) will continue to come to the market. The consumer though has little concept as to their benefits and how they interact with crops to improve yields, with the pressures of ever-decreasing land availability, to improve the food available globally. If hazard-based approaches are used to regulate these products, there would be insufficient tools available for farmers to grow healthy high-yield crops. Life expectancy has grown over the century, a key factor contributing to this is the improved quality of raw commodity used for food production and improved hygiene. It is essential to have a risk-based approach to consider both the exposure scenarios and the consequent risk profile to demonstrate safe use of products to better inform farmer and consumer choice. Mixed messages along the food chain regarding safety (even scare-mongering) can deter consumers from making healthy food choices. Thus it is incumbent upon all stakeholders to have a consensus around the approaches used for risk assessment in food safety and its unbiased communication. Unfortunately, the anxiety caused leads to more strict regulations without a clear scientific basis and overly conservative risk assessments, which move further away from real-life exposure and risk profiles.

69.7.3 Public perception

The public does not generally differentiate between hazard and risk. The public is overwhelmed by contradictory messages on the hazard or risk for a variety of food-related issues and, understandably, there is difficulty in knowing whom to trust.[84] This in turn complicates efforts to communicate effectively the distinction between hazard and risk, and their actual implications. It is clear that the terms hazard and risk are perceived and used very differently in risk communication depending very much on the perspective and knowledge base of the stakeholders, including among so-called experts and across different global regions.[85] Public attitudes are complex and influenced by many factors.

Different types of potential food hazards are classified according to whether or not they have been deliberately or accidentally introduced into the food chain, or are naturally occurring, and whether they represent acute or chronic risks. It is critical to ensure an effective flow and/or exchange of information between consumers and other stakeholders in the area of food safety (e.g., risk assessors, regulators, and the food industry) and to focus on risk-based assessment outcomes.[86]

For those individuals who are generally more risk averse with respect to exposure to chemicals, they may view chemicals as being "not natural" (as observed in the organic and GMO foods debate), as being of benefit to industry rather than to consumers ("Big Business" concept), and that chemicals are over-used and mis-used, resulting in human disease and environmental pollution. Consequently, exposure to chemicals is seen as involuntary and of concern.[87,88] Consumer tolerance of risks is significantly influenced by awareness of the risk. For example, individuals with allergies have high awareness and are more likely to accept some risk. On the other hand, the sporadic nature of microbial food poisoning results in low awareness of its risks, while most people are not even aware whether chemical risks are important or not.

69.7.4 Impact of globalization

Globalization has led to greater awareness and (faster) access to information. Differences in approaches to food safety evaluation have become more obvious. For the global citizen, the One Health paradigm (https://www.onehealthcommission.org/en/why_one_health/what_is_one_health/) is more relevant with its collaborative approach to recognizing the interconnections between people, animals, plants, and their shared environment. Having different approaches for assessing the same one chemical entity in different regions (e.g., using the hazard-based vs. risk-based approaches) does not benefit the consumer or provide any added protection, thus a safety assessment approach needs to reflect this.

The sharing of advances in consistently applied risk-based methodologies will facilitate harmonization and consistency across food sectors, across regions, and across other chemical sectors. Further advances in the science of exposure assessment will benefit all sectors as a key component of any risk assessment providing regional/local relevance. Regional exposure data are needed to ensure relevant assessments are performed, adequate to the nature of exposure and mitigation options available to the local population. These should be the driver for conducting any risk assessment to direct resources to real safety concerns. Risk assessments need to be transparent, of high quality and address uncertainties. Better clarity, consistency, and communication of findings by risk assessors and risk communicators and the use of opportunities, such as stakeholder forums and the teaching of risk assessment and especially the difference between hazard and risk in school and university curricula, will facilitate wider understanding of the issues and improve public trust in the outcomes of risk assessment.

Scientific aspects are an important component of a common language for all the stakeholders. Adoption of science-based risk assessment approaches provides a way of applying common principles and approaches consistently for all stakeholders, based on objective evidence and its inherent uncertainties. Communication and the use of appropriate language is one of the challenges.

69.8 Future perspectives

The review by Barlow et al.[7] already clearly described that, with the current state-of-the-art, the regulation of chemicals in the field of food safety, and also in other fields, is a mix of both hazard- as well as risk-based approaches. It has to be recognized, however, that a basic rule in modern safety science is the concept introduced by Paracelsus that the dose makes the poison. Regulatory actions and risk management decisions based on hazard identification alone are not in line with this basic concept. Although there can be several practical arguments to decide on a hazard-based approach including, for example, the possibility to use in vitro bioassays and replace animal testing, from a scientific point of view it does not seem the way forward. A hazard-based approach does not enable the definition of risk management priorities, and it also does not provide insight in the risks for different (sub)groups within the population. In the long run, the major disadvantages of a risk-based approach, including the fact that it requires more data, the inaccuracy of the exposure assessments, and the introduction of uncertainty, should rather be seen as future challenges to work on. For example, in cases where one wants to keep the advances of in vitro bioassays for hazard identification, the (future) combination of the outcomes of in vitro testing with physiologically based kinetic (PBK) modeling to enable translation of effective in vitro concentrations into actual in vivo effect levels seems an essential way forward. Currently, within the TOX21 program these approaches are adopted and they provide a way to take kinetics into account. These PBK model-based reverse dosimetry approaches for quantitative in vitro to in vivo extrapolation also allow the combination of human data on kinetics and in vitro toxicity data from relevant human in vitro cell models, to allow prediction of dose−response curves for human, thereby providing the opportunity of moving away from animal-based in vitro or in vivo models.[89,90]

Another field where future progress may argue in favor of risk-based instead of hazard-based evaluations is the development in the field of genotoxicity. More sensitive detection methods seem to reveal sublinear concentration response curves for DNA damage and genotoxicity pointing at potential practical thresholds at low concentrations that are relevant at realistic low-dose human exposure.[63]

This illustrates the need for future consideration of a risk-based instead of a hazard-based approach toward even the endpoint of genotoxicity. The MOE approach introduced in the risk assessment of genotoxic carcinogens actually already takes exposure into account to come to a prioritization of risk and, in some cases, even to the conclusion that the exposure to a genotoxic compound is of low-safety concern. Although with the present state of the art, this approach is only applied for unavoidable chemicals or for unavoidable contaminants in avoidable food constituents, future developments may define possibilities to extend this approach. When further developing the MOE approach for the risk assessment of genotoxic carcinogens attention should also be devoted to defining how to evaluate exposure during less than a lifetime duration such as exposure to a supplement that is likely to be only used by consumers during short periods of time instead of life-long.

Furthermore, in a risk-based instead of hazard-based approach, it can be taken into account that for some genotoxic carcinogens to which we may be exposed via food, also endogenous sources add to the overall exposure. In a risk-based assessment, the external exposure could be compared to this endogenous formation of the chemical informing on whether the external exposure would substantially add to the risk or not. An example of this approach can already be found in the various risk assessments for ethanol, which has been subject of many human safety evaluations.[91] Endogenous formation of ethanol resulting from microbial fermentation by the gut microbiota, or from its formation in pathways endogenous to host metabolism, may substantially add to the overall exposure. In a risk-based assessment, the external exposure may be evaluated against this endogenous exposure. For example, the exposure to ethanol resulting from use of ethyl esters as flavor constituents was concluded to not raise a safety concern because it would not add substantially to the overall exposure. This importance of endogenous formation to the overall exposure has recently been discussed in more detail.[92,93]

It is important to recognize that the global aspect of food safety and therefore uniformity in assessment requirements should be encouraged. To accomplish this, having established best practices for data generation and evaluation to demonstrate safe uses and scientifically defensible human health and food safety assessments is imperative. Such an effort would transcend the traditional mutual acceptance of data to a mutually accepted approach of risk assessment through a globally accepted framework for knowledge generation and evaluation. New technologies offer the opportunity to improve testing paradigms and will provide better solutions for evaluating risk while decreasing the need for animal testing. Better targeting of resources to understanding exposure will provide a more relevant basis for risk management. Implementing a globally harmonized risk assessment−based approach for regulatory decision-making of products will increase the speed, efficiency, and accuracy of regulatory decision-making for protection, while increasing the efficiency of getting safe and effective innovative products into the food chain. This will provide a more consistent and understandable basis for risk communication to the global consumer.

It is concluded that future developments should be directed at moving away from hazard- to risk-based evaluations and educating the risk assessors, risk managers, and the public on the fact that a hazard does not translate into a risk at certain levels of exposure, even for genotoxic carcinogens or allergens.

References

1. CODEX. *Working Principles for Risk Analysis for Food Safety for Application by Governments. CAC/GL62−2007.* Rome: Communication Division Electronic Publishing Policy and Support Branch, FAO; 2007.
2. OECD. *Safety Evaluation of Foods Produced by Modern Biotechnology e Concepts and Principles.* Paris: OECD; 1993. Available at. Available from: http://dbtbiosafety.nic.in/guideline/OACD/Concepts_and_Principles_1993.pdf.
3. EC. Directive C. Council Directive 67/548/EEC of 27 June 1967 on the approximation of laws, regulations and administrative provisions relating to the classification, packaging and labelling of dangerous substances. *Off J Eur Commun.* 1967;196(16.8):1. Available at:. Available from: https://op.europa.eu/en/publication-detail/-/publication/8e12a450-cb71-4356-bd3b-8a9f980208a0.

4. EC. Directive 1999/45/EC of the European parliament and of the council of 31 May 1999 concerning the approximation of the laws, regulations and administrative provisions of the member states relating to the classification, packaging and labelling of dangerous preparations. Offic J Eur Commun. L 200/234e256, 30.7.1999. Available at: https://eur-lex.europa.eu/legal-content/EN/TXT/?uri = CELEX%3A01999L0045-20150601.
5. EC. Regulation (EC) No 1272/2008 of the European Parliament and of the Council of 16 December 2008 on classification, labelling and packaging of substances and mixtures, amending and repealing Directives 67/548/EEC and 1999/45/EC, and amending Regulation (EC) No 1907/2006. Official Journal of the European Union. L 353/1–1355, 31.12.2008. Available at: http://eur-lex.europa.eu/LexUriServ/LexUriServ.do?uri = OJ:L:2008:353:0001:1355:EN:PDF.
6. UN. Globally Harmonized system of classification and labelling (GHS) (Fourth Revised Edition). ST/SG/AC.10/30/Rev.4. United Nations, New York and Geneva. 2011. Available at: http://www.unece.org/fileadmin/DAM/trans/danger/publi/ghs/ghs_rev04/English/ST-SG-AC10-30-Rev4e.pdf.
7. Barlow SM, Boobis AR, Bridges J, et al. The role of hazard- and risk-based approaches in ensuring food safety. *Trends Food Sci Technol.* 2015;46:176–188. Available from: https://doi.org/10.1016/j.tifs.2015.10.007.
8. Allen KJ, Remington BC, Baumert JL, et al. Allergen reference doses for precautionary labeling (VITAL 2.0): clinical implications. *J Allergy Clin Immunol.* 2014;133(1):156–164.
9. Bindslev-Jensen C, Briggs D, Osterballe M. Can we determine a threshold level for allergenic foods by statistical analysis of published data in the literature? *Allergy.* 2002;57(8):741–746. Available from: https://doi.org/10.1034/j.1398-9995.2002.23797.x.
10. Crevel RW, Baumert JL, Baka A, et al. Development and evolution of risk assessment for food allergens. *Food Chem Toxicol.* 2014;67:262–276.
11. Crevel RW, Baumert JL, Luccioli S, et al. Translating reference doses into allergen management practice: challenges for stakeholders. *Food Chem Toxicol.* 2014;67:277–287.
12. Crevel RR, Ronsmans S, Marsaux CF, Bánáti D. ILSI Europe's Food Allergy Task Force: from defining the hazard to assessing the risk from food allergens. *J AOAC Int.* 2018;101(1):91–95. Available from: https://doi.org/10.5740/jaoacint.17-0397.
13. Hattersley S, Ward R, Baka A, Crevel RW. Advances in the risk management of unintended presence of allergenic foods in manufactured food products–an overview. *Food Chem Toxicol.* 2014;67:255–261.
14. Alimentarius C. *Guidelines for the Control of Campylobacter and Salmonella in Chicken Meat [CAC/GL 78/2011].* Rome: FAO; 2011. Available at. Available from: http://www.codexalimentarius.org/input/download/standards/11780/CXG_078e.pdf.
15. Lindqvist R, Langerholc T, Ranta J, Hirvonen T, Sand S. A common approach for ranking of microbiological and chemical hazards in foods based on risk assessment-useful but is it possible? *Crit Rev Food Sci Nutr.* 2020;60(20):3461–3474. Available from: https://doi.org/10.1080/10408398.2019.1693957.
16. UNEP. Rotterdam convention on the prior informed consent procedure for certain hazardous chemicals and pesticides in international trade (Revised in 2013). In Rotterdam Convention Secretariat, United Nations Environmental Programme, Geneva, Switzerland. 2013. Available at: http://www.pic.int/TheConvention/Overview/TextoftheConvention/tabid/1048/language/en-US/Default.aspx.
17. Idrovo AJ. Food poisoned with pesticide in Bihar, India: new disaster, same story. *Occup Environ Med.* 2014;71(3):228.
18. IFCS. Acutely toxic pesticides initial input on extent of problem and guidance for risk management. International Forum on Chemical Safety. IFCS/FORUM-IV/10w. *Original Engl.* 2003;, 23 April 2003. Available at:. Available from: http://www.who.int/ifcs/documents/forums/forum4/en/10w_f4_en.pdf?ua = 1.
19. Kishi M. IFCS: acutely toxic pesticides. InInternational forum on chemical safety. 2002 Jun 6. Available at: http://www.who.int/heli/risks/toxics/bibliographyikishi.pdf.
20. FAO. Highly hazardous pesticides should be phased out in developing countries. *Food Agric Organ.* 2013;. Available at. Available from: http://www.fao.org/news/story/en/item/180968/icode/.
21. US EPA Directive to prioritize efforts to reduce animal testing. 2019. Available: https://www.epa.gov/research/administrator-memo-prioritizing-efforts-reduce-animal-testing-september-10-2019.
22. Wolf DC, Aggarwal M, Battalora M, et al. Implementing a globally harmonized risk assessment-based approach for regulatory decision-making of crop protection products. *Pest Manag Sci.* 2020;76(10):3311–3315.
23. WTO. The WTO agreement on the application of sanitary and phytosanitary measures (SPS agreement). 2015. Available at: https://www.wto.org/english/docs_e/legal_e/15-sps.pdf.
24. Science for Environment Policy. The Precautionary Priniple: decision making under uncertainty. Future Brief 18. Produced for the European Commission DG Environment by the Science Communication Unit, UWE, Bristol. 2017. Available at: http://ec.europa.eu/science-environment-policy.
25. Doe JE, Boobis AR, Blacker A, et al. A tiered approach to systemic toxicity testing for agricultural chemical safety assessment. *Crit Rev Toxicol.* 2006;36(1):37–68. Available from: https://doi.org/10.1080/10408440500534370.
26. Carmichael NG, Barton HA, Boobis AR, et al. Agricultural chemical safety assessment: a multisector approach to the modernization of human safety requirements. *Crit Rev Toxicol.* 2006;36(1):1–7. Available from: https://doi.org/10.1080/10408440500534354.
27. Parsons P, Freeman E, Weidling R, et al. Using existing knowledge for the risk evaluation of crop protection products in order to guide exposure driven data generation strategies and minimise unnecessary animal testing. *Crit Rev Toxicol.* 2021;51(7):600–621. Available from: https://doi.org/10.1080/10408444.2021.1987384.
28. Serafimova R, Coja T, Kass GE. Application of the threshold of toxicological concern (TTC) in food safety: challenges and opportunities. *Front Toxicol.* 2021;3:655951. Available from: https://doi.org/10.3389/ftox.
29. Boobis A, Brown P, Cronin MT, et al. Origin of the TTC values for compounds that are genotoxic and/or carcinogenic and an approach for their re-evaluation. *Crit Rev Toxicol.* 2017;47(8):10–732. Available from: https://doi.org/10.1080/10408444.2017.1318822.
30. EFSA and WHO. Review of the Threshold of Toxicological Concern (TTC) approach and development of new TTC decision tree. *EFSA Support Public.* 2016;13(3):1006E.
31. EFSA. Guidance on the use of the Threshold of Toxicological Concern approach in food safety assessment. *EFSA J.* 2019;17(6):17. Available from: https://doi.org/10.2903/j.efsa.2019.5708.5708.

32. Frawley JP. Scientific evidence and common sense as a basis for food-packaging regulations. *Food Cosmet Toxicol.* 1967;5(3):293–308.
33. Ramsey LL. The food additive problem of plastics used in food packaging. In National Technical Conference of the Society of Plastics Engineers (USA)(4–6 November 1969) 1969. Commonly referred to as the Ramsey Proposal.
34. Rulis A. De minimis and the threshold of regulation. In: Felix CW, ed. *Food Protection Technology*. Chelsea, MI: Lewis; 1986:29–37.
35. FDA. TOR process outlined in Title 21 of the Code of Federal Regulations (CFR) part 170.39, Threshold of Regulation for substances used in food-contact articles. Food and Drug Administration. Food Additives: Threshold of regulation of substances used in food-contact articles: Final Rule. *Fed Register.* 1995;60:36582–36596.
36. Cheeseman MA, Machuga EJ, Bailey AB. A tiered approach to threshold of regulation. *Food Chem Toxicol.* 1999;37(4):387–412.
37. Cramer GM, Ford RA, Hall RL. Estimation of toxic hazard—a decision tree approach. *Food Cosmet Toxicol.* 1976;16(3):255–276.
38. Munro IC, Ford RA, Kennepohl E, Sprenger JG. Correlation of structural class with no-observed-effect levels: a proposal for establishing a threshold of concern. *Food Chem Toxicol.* 1996;34(9):829–867.
39. Kroes R, Renwick AG, Cheeseman M, et al. Structure-based thresholds of toxicological concern (TTC): guidance for application to substances present at low levels in the diet. *Food Chem Toxicol.* 2004;42(1):65–83.
40. Van Ravenzwaay B, Dammann M, Buesen R, Schneider S. The threshold of toxicological concern for prenatal developmental toxicity. *Regulat Toxicol Pharmacol.* 2011;59(1):81–90. Available from: https://doi.org/10.1016/j.yrtph.2010.09.009.
41. Safford RJ. The Dermal Sensitisation Threshold—a TTC approach for allergic contact dermatitis. *Regulat Toxicol Pharmacol.* 2008; 51(2):195–200.
42. Carthew P, Clapp C, Gutsell S. Exposure based waiving: the application of the toxicological threshold of concern (TTC) to inhalation exposure for aerosol ingredients in consumer products. *Food Chem Toxicol.* 2009;47(6):1287–1295. Available from: https://doi.org/10.1016/j.fct.2009.02.024.
43. Nelms MD, Patlewicz G. Derivation of new Threshold of Toxicological Concern values for exposure via inhalation for environmentally-relevant chemicals. *Front Toxicol.* 2020;2:5. Available from: https://doi.org/10.3389/ftox.2020.580347.
44. Müller L, Mauthe RJ, Riley CM, et al. A rationale for determining, testing, and controlling specific impurities in pharmaceuticals that possess potential for genotoxicity. *Regul Toxicol Pharmacol.* 2006;44:198–211.
45. Patlewicz G, Wambaugh JF, Felter SP, Simon TW, Becker RA. Utilizing Threshold of Toxicological Concern (TTC) with high throughput exposure predictions (HTE) as a risk-based prioritization approach for thousands of chemicals. *Comput Toxicol.* 2018;7:58–67.
46. Wambaugh JF, Wang A, Dionisio KL, et al. High throughput heuristics for prioritizing human exposure to environmental chemicals. *Environ Sci Technol.* 2014;48(21):12760–12767. Available from: https://doi.org/10.1021/es503583j.
47. Chicoine A, Erdely H, Fattori V, et al. Assessment of veterinary drug residues in food: considerations when dealing with sub-optimal data. *Regulat Toxicol Pharmacol.* 2020;104806. Available from: https://doi.org/10.1016/j.yrtph.2020.104806.
48. Boobis A, Cerniglia C, Chicoine A, et al. Characterizing chronic and acute health risks of residues of veterinary drugs in food: latest methodological developments by the joint FAO/WHO expert committee on food additives. *Crit Rev Toxicol.* 2017;47(10):889–903.
49. Ellison CA, Api AM, Becker RA, et al. Internal threshold of toxicological concern (iTTC): where we are today and what is possible in the near future. *Front Toxicol.* 2021;2:621541. Available from: https://doi.org/10.3389/ftox.2020.621541.
50. Blackburn KL, Carr G, Rose JL, Selman BG. An interim internal Threshold of Toxicologic Concern (iTTC) for chemicals in consumer products, with support from an automated assessment of ToxCast™ dose response data. *Regulat Toxicol Pharmacol.* 2020;114:104656.
51. Partosch F, Mielke H, Stahlmann R, Kleuser B, Barlow S, Gundert-Remy U. Internal threshold of toxicological concern values: enabling route-to-route extrapolation. *Arch Toxicol.* 2015;89(6):941–948. Available from: https://doi.org/10.1007/s00204-014-1287-6.
52. EFSA. 2017. Scientific Opinion on the guidance on the use of the weight of evidence approach in scientific assessments. *EFSA J.* 2017;15(8):69. Available from: https://doi.org/10.2903/j.efsa.2017.4971. 4971.
53. Suter G, Nichols J, Lavoie E, Cormier S. Systematic review and weight of evidence are integral to ecological and human health assessments: they need an integrated framework. *Integr Environ Assess Manag.* 2020;16(5):718–728. Available from: https://doi.org/10.1002/iea.
54. Nohmi T. Thresholds of genotoxic and non-genotoxic carcinogens. *Toxicol Res.* 2018;34(4):281–290. Available from: https://doi.org/10.5487/TR.2018.34.4.281.
55. WHO/FAO. *Hazard Characterization for Pathogens in Food and Water, Guidelines, Microbiological Risk Assessment Series: Food Safety Department.* Geneva: World Health Organization; 2003.
56. FDA/FSIS.Quantitative assessment of relative risk to public health from foodborne listeria monocytogenes among selected categories of ready-to-eat foods. Food and Drug Administration Center for Food Safety and Applied Nutrition, U.S. Department of Health and Human Services, Food Safety and Inspection Service, U.S. Department of Agriculture. 2003. https://www.foodsafety.gov/~dms/lmr2-toc.html. 2003 Dec 4.
57. Pouillot* R, Hoelzer K, Chen Y, Dennis SB. Listeria monocytogenes dose response revisited—incorporating adjustments for variability in strain virulence and host susceptibility. *Risk Anal.* 2015;35(1):90–108. Available from: https://doi.org/10.1111/risa.12235.
58. Ridenhour, et al. Unraveling R_0: considerations for public health applications. *Syst Rev Am J Public Health.* 2014;104(2). Available from: https://doi.org/10.2105/AJPH.2013.301704.
59. Kucharski AJ, Russell TW, Diamond C, et al. Early dynamics of transmission and control of COVID-19: a mathematical modelling study. *Lancet Infect Dis.* 2020;20(5):553–558. Available from: https://doi.org/10.1016/S1473-3099(20)30144-4.
60. The Royal Society. *Number R. and Growth Rate (r) of the COVID-19 Epidemic in the UK: Methods of Estimation, Data Sources, Causes of Heterogeneity, and Use as a Guide in Policy Formulation.* 2020. London: The Royal Society; 2020:1–86.

61. Hartwig A, Arand M, Epe B, et al. Mode of action-based risk assessment of genotoxic carcinogens. *Arch Toxicol.* 2020;94(6):1787–1877. Available from: https://doi.org/10.1007/s00204-020-02733-2.
62. Kobets T, Williams GM. Review of the evidence for thresholds for DNA-reactive and epigenetic experimental chemical carcinogens. *Chem-Biol Interact.* 2019;301:88–111.
63. Schulte-Hubbert R, Küpper JH, Thomas AD, Schrenk D. Estragole: DNA adduct formation in primary rat hepatocytes and genotoxic potential in HepG2-CYP1A2 cells. *Toxicology.* 2020;444:152566. Available from: https://doi.org/10.1016/j.tox.2020.152566.
64. Brescia S. Thresholds of adversity and their applicability to endocrine disrupting chemicals. *Crit Rev Toxicol.* 2020;50(3):213–218. Available from: https://doi.org/10.1080/10408444.2020.1740973.
65. Autrup H, Barile FA, Berry SC, et al. Human exposure to synthetic endocrine disrupting chemicals (S-EDCs) is generally negligible as compared to natural compounds with higher or comparable endocrine activity: how to evaluate the risk of the S-EDCs? *Arch Toxicol.* 2020;94:2549–2557. Available from: https://doi.org/10.1016/j.tiv.2020.104861.
66. Rietjens IMCM, Louisse J, Beekmann K. The potential health effects of dietary phytoestrogens. *Br J Pharmacol.* 2017;174(11):1263–1280.
67. Kassotis CD, Vandenberg LN, Demeneix BA, Porta M, Slama R, Trasande L. Endocrine-disrupting chemicals: economic, regulatory, and policy implications. *Lancet Diabet Endocrinol.* 2020;8(8):719–730. Available from: https://doi.org/10.1016/S2213-8587(20)30128-5.
68. EFSA. Polycyclic aromatic hydrocarbons in food-scientific opinion of the panel on contaminants in the food chain. *EFSA J.* 2008;6(8):724. Available from: https://doi.org/10.2903/j.efsa.2008.724.
69. EFSA. CONTAM E. Scientific opinion on acrylamide in food. EFSA CONTAM Panel (EFSA Panel on Contaminants in the Food Chain). *EFSA J.* 2015;13(6):4104–4425. Available from: https://efsa.onlinelibrary.wiley.com/doi/epdf/10.2903/j.efsa.2015.4104.
70. Paul KB, Hedge JM, Rotroff DM, Hornung MW, Crofton KM, Simmons SO. Development of a thyroperoxidase inhibition assay for high-throughput screening. *Chem Res Toxicol.* 2014;27(3):387–399. Available from: https://doi.org/10.1021/tx400310w.
71. Carvalho DP, Ferreira AC, Coelho SM, Moraes JM, Camacho MA, Rosenthal D. Thyroid peroxidase activity is inhibited by amino acids. *Braz J Med Biol Res.* 2000;33(3):355–361. Available from: https://doi.org/10.1590/s0100-879x2000000300015.
72. Jomaa B, de Haan LH, Peijnenburg AA, Bovee TF, Aarts JM, Rietjens IMCM. Simple and rapid in vitro assay for detecting human thyroid peroxidase disruption. *ALTEX-Alternat Anim Experim.* 2015;32(3):191–200.
73. White-Stevens RH. Interference by ascorbic acid in test systems involving peroxidase. I. Reversible indicators and the effects of copper, iron, and mercury. *Clin Chem.* 1982;28(4):578–588.
74. Worth AP. Computational modelling for the sustainable management of chemicals. *Comput Toxicol.* 2020;14:100122.
75. Farland WH, Lynch A, Erraguntla NK, Pottenger LH. Improving risk assessment approaches for chemicals with both endogenous and exogenous exposures. *Regulat Toxicol Pharmacol.* 2019;103:210–215. Available from: https://doi.org/10.1016/j.yrtph.2019.01.029.
76. Vidry S, Boobis A, Hoekstra J, Watzl B, Verhagen H. Benefit risk analysis for foods (BRAFO): qualitative and quantitative comparison of human health risks and benefits of foods and food components. *Food Chem Toxicol.* 2012;50.
77. FAO. An introduction to the basic concepts of food security food security information for action. *Food Agric Organ.* 2008;2008:1–3. Available from: http://www.fao.org/docrep/013/al936e/al936e00.pdf.
78. EFSA. Conducting fit-for-purpose food safety risk assessments. *EFSA J.* 2019;17(S1):e170707. 2019.
79. EFSA. Guidance on communication of uncertainty in scientific assessments. *EFSA J.* 2019;17(1):5520.
80. Kumar V, Boobies AR, Moreto A. Test and risk assessment strategies for combined exposure to multiple chemicals. *Food Chem Toxicol.* 2020;144. ISSN: 0278-6915.
81. Stafford EG, Tell LA, Lin Z, et al. Consequences of fipronil exposure in egg-laying hens. *J Am Veter Med Assoc.* 2018;253(1):57–60. Available from: https://doi.org/10.2460/javma.253.1.57.
82. Gerletti P, Von Kleist M, Mielke H, et al. Transfer kinetics of fipronil into chicken (*Gallus gallus domesticus*) eggs. *Comput Toxicol.* 2020;15:100131. Available from: https://doi.org/10.1016/j.comtox.2020.100131.
83. Goodman JE, Prueitt RL, Boffetta P, Halsall C, Sweetman A. "Good epidemiology practice" guidelines for pesticide exposure assessment. *Int J Environ Res Public Health.* 2020;17(14):5114. Available from: https://doi.org/10.3390/ijerph17145114.
84. Scheer D, Benighaus C, Benighaus L, et al. The distinction between risk and hazard: understanding and use in stakeholder communication. *Risk Anal.* 2014;34(7):1270–1285.
85. IPCS. *World Health Organization, Inter-Organization Programme for the Sound Management of Chemicals. IPCS Risk Assessment Terminology.* World Health Organization; 2004, 2004. Available at:. Available from: http://www.who.int/ipcs/methods/harmonization/areas/ipcsterminologyparts1and2.pdf?ua = 1.
86. Frewer LJ, Fischer AR, Brennan M, et al. Risk/benefit communication about food—a systematic review of the literature. *Crit Rev Food Sci Nutr.* 2016;56(10):1728–1745. Available from: https://doi.org/10.1080/10408398.2013.801337.
87. Rembischevski P, Caldas (ED). Risk perception related to food. *Food Sci Technol.* 2020;40:779–785.
88. Saleh R, Bearth A, Siegrist M. Addressing chemophobia: informational vs affect-based approaches. *Food Chem Toxicol.* 2020;140:111390.
89. Louisse J, Beekmann K, Rietjens IMCM. Use of physiologically based kinetic modeling-based reverse dosimetry to predict in vivo toxicity from in vitro data. *Chem Res Toxicol.* 2017;30(1):114–125.
90. Punt A, Firman J, Boobis A, et al. Potential of ToxCast data in the safety assessment of food chemicals. *Toxicol Sci.* 2020;174(2):326–340. Available from: https://doi.org/10.1093/toxsci/kfaa008.
91. IARC. *Consum Alcoholic Beverag.* 2018;110.
92. Jecfa JF. *WHO Expert Committee on Food Additives. Toxicological Evaluation of Some Extraction Solvents and Certain Other Substances.* World Health Organization; 1970. Available from: http://www.inchem.org/documents/jecfa/jecmono/v48aje01.htm.
93. Rietjens IMCM, Michael A, Hermann MB, et al. The role of endogenous versus exogenous sources in the exposome of putative genotoxins and consequences for risk assessment. *Arch Toxicol.* 2022;96:1297–1352.

Section XIV

Impact of food safety on global trade

Chapter 70

Global Food Safety Initiative (GFSI): underpinning the safety of the global food chain, facilitating regulatory compliance, trade, and consumer trust

Anne Gerardi

GFSI at the Consumer Goods Forum, Paris, France

Abstract

In the past 22 years, Global Food Safety Initiative (GFSI) has grown into a vast, global multi-stakeholder movement that brings together key actors of the food industry to collaboratively drive continuous improvement in food safety management systems (FSMS) and practices around the world. With a vision of Safe food for consumers everywhere, food industry leaders created GFSI in 2000 to find collaborative solutions to collective concerns, notably to reduce food safety risks, and audit duplication and costs while building trust throughout the supply chain.

This article explains how the role and scope of influence of GFSI have evolved in global food systems underpinning the paramount necessity of safe food and its associated challenges linked to the Sustainable Development Goals (SGD) and strengthening market access for fairest trade and the new digital and big data revolution. It also explains how GFSI has evolved from a benchmarking organization of recognized certification programs made for retailers and manufacturers dedicated to harmonization food safety audits of food safety management systems and practices to an organization delivering strategic outcomes on regulatory affairs and capability building by facilitating regulatory compliance for food business operators, creating dialogue for the shared objective of improving the understanding and application of CODEX standards and creating more access to capacities within food safety supply chains for safe food for consumers everywhere.

Keywords: Food safety; consumers trust; regulatory compliance; international trade; capability building; food systems; benchmarking; global food supply chains; food safety management systems; sustainable development goals; digital technologies

70.1 Introduction

70.1.1 Global Food Safety Initiative history: "once recognized, certified everywhere"

GFSI is a 22-year-old initiative based on collaboration and on a historical scientific risk-based approach initiative[a] from retailers and manufacturers to improve food safety in the food chain for safe food for consumers everywhere

Over the past several decades, the world has seen numerous food safety crises in the headlines, eroding consumers' trust in the safety of the food they buy, the brands they love, and even the food industry at large. During the 90s, there had been a series of high-profile international food safety crises including BSE, dioxin, and listeria. Within the food industry, there was growing audit fatigue as retailers and brand manufacturers audited factories against their countless in-house standards, each developed in isolation and with no consideration of convergence. The results showed no consistency. Consumer and food industry confidence was low. The CEOs of the world's food retailers, working through their independent network CIES – The Food Business Forum, now the Consumer Goods Forum (CGF), agreed to take collaborative action. The Global Food Safety Initiative (GFSI) was created in May 2000 to help address those global challenges with the vision of safe food for consumers everywhere by providing continuous improvement in food safety management systems and practices to ensure confidence in the delivery of safe food to consumers worldwide. It is a landmark initiative of the CGF, a consumer goods industry CEO platform working to support Better Lives Through Better Business. GFSI aims to build consumers'

Present Knowledge in Food Safety. DOI: https://doi.org/10.1016/B978-0-12-819470-6.00058-5

trust in the food they buy – no matter where their food has come from, nor where in the world they live.

In the past 22 years, GFSI has grown into a vast, global multi-stakeholder movement that brings together key actors of the food industry to collaboratively drive continuous improvement in food safety management systems and practices around the world. With a vision of Safe food for everyone, food industry leaders created GFSI in 2000 to find collaborative solutions to collective concerns, notably to reduce food safety risks, audit duplication, and costs while building trust throughout the supply chain. The GFSI community works on a volunteer basis and is composed of the world's leading food safety experts from retail, manufacturing, food service companies, primary producers, including upstream suppliers, as well as international governmental organizations (IGOs), governments, academia, and services providers to the global food industry.

The main goal was laid out at the very beginning of GFSI and remains a compelling message: once certified, recognized everywhere. GFSI chose the benchmarking approach as there were existing foundations. The British Retail Consortium had already published its first BRC food safety standard in 1998. The German and French retailers were starting to work together on the International Food Standard and the Food Marketing Institute, the Trade Association for the North American retailers, was developing their Safe Quality Food Standard. The benchmarking model would credibly determine equivalency between food safety certification programs, whilst leaving flexibility and choice in the marketplace with the following objectives:

- Reduce food safety risks by delivering equivalence and convergence between effective food safety management systems
- Manage cost in the global food system by eliminating redundancy and improving operational efficiency
- Develop competencies and capacity building in food safety to create consistent and effective global food systems
- Provide a unique international stakeholder platform for collaboration, knowledge exchange, and networking.

GFSI was born with a unique role that has to specify the recognition of food safety certification programs to defined requirements in its Benchmarking Requirements, bring together food safety experts within a global network, and drive global change through multi-stakeholder projects on strategic issues (e.g., auditors' requirements, regulatory affairs, and food safety management systems for small suppliers). GFSI's role is very clear and its intention is not to take a role in making policy for retailers, manufacturers, any food business operators (FBOs) or food safety certification program owners (CPOs), nor undertake any accreditation or certification activities, own any food safety schemes or standards, undertake training programs, or to have any involvement outside of the scope of food safety, such as animal welfare or sustainability issues.

70.1.2 Global Food Safety Initiative in the past decade: "safe food for consumers everywhere"

Over the past 20 years, GFSI has grown into a vast, global multi-stakeholder community. We enable the extensive collaboration that is so critical to ensuring a safe global food system, involving both the private and public sectors.

GFSI has presided over a community that delivers food safety assurance through benchmarking and the harmonization of food safety programs that are recognized as meeting the GFSI Benchmarking Requirements. The GFSI eco-system relies on multiple actors playing multiple parts in delivering food safety audits and certification upon which the global food industry relies.

GFSI has developed to become more than a benchmarking organization, and has based all its work on three strategic priorities since 2017:

- benchmarking and harmonization
- Public-private partnerships (PPPs)
- Capability building.

Those strategic priorities have evolved in the last three years into three strategic outcomes for which GFSI operates and that can be defined as such:

1. **Harmonization:**
   GFSI recognizes, accredited, 3rd party certification guarantees an FSMS which provides essential elements for the provision of safe food to consumers everywhere
2. **Public-private partnerships**
   Food safety regulators trust that GFSI certification can be used for risk-based resource allocation
3. **Capability building:**
   Enabling improvements in the FSMS of non GFSI certified FBOs such that they can achieve GFSI certification and/or regulatory compliance resulting in safer food for consumers everywhere.

70.1.3 Global Food Safety Initiative today: "safe food for all": towards a more trusted ecosystem for safer food systems for all

The original genesis of GFSI focused on setting requirements for food safety globally in a non-competitive way. The *GFSI Benchmarking Requirements* provide a high-level framework against which individual food safety certification programs can be assessed. In short, GFSI is responsible for the food safety "*what*" not the food safety "*how.*", hence its key relationships with its stakeholders as GFSI relies on the industry and the extended community serving the industy to implement its strategic framework.

Over the past few years, trust and confidence in third-party certification to deliver food safety assurance has been challenged. The quality of the outputs of some audits leading to certification to a GFSI-recognized Certification Program has been questioned. There has been understandable concerns about the efficacy of audits and more specifically the competence of some food safety auditors themselves.

Consulting with strategic stakeholders, GFSI has recognized in 2019 that the issues lie not just with the auditors but with the entire ecosystem and its mechanisms leading to certifications to a GFSI-recognized Certification Program, and overseen by the Certification Programme Owners, the Certification Bodies (CBs), and the Accreditation Bodies (ABs). GFSI Board convened to discuss the ongoing challenges which they felt were inherent in the quality of GFSI certificates. They shared industry data that highlighted stark contrasts between the quality of GFSI third party audits and their own second party food safety audits. The GFSI Board concluded that despite best efforts to improve aspects of the GFSI ecosystem, trust and confidence in GFSI certificates were at an all-time low and something radical had to be done and at pace, to address the inherent audit outputs.

GFSI committed to developing and delivering a bold new vision designed to shape what was termed "The Race to The Top" (RTTT) approved unanimously in Seattle, US in February 2020 as an initial suite of measures specifically designed to improve the sphere of influence that GFSI had over its entire food safety certification and assurance system.

The RTTT is the sum of multiple work streams and projects designed to ensure that there is a fundamental shift in culture from "compliance being enough", to a new era and demands for "continuous improvement" at all touchpoints within the GFSI sphere of influence – Certification Programme Owners, Certification Bodies, auditors and the Food Business Operators themselves by building and enhancing trust and confidence in GFSI certificates by all stakeholders. The conceptual framework of GFSI's modernization combines to deliver a bold vision and enable the RTTT. In broad terms, GFSI is moving to assume explicit oversight for what good looks like in all aspects of the GFSI ecosystem.

The conceptual framework includes two phases with the following elements for each. Four fundamental features of the RTTT phase I framework were shaped with the support of stakeholders, comprising representatives from ABs, CBs, CPOs, members, and the broader industry who provided significant inputs between the October 2019 and February 2020 GFSI Board Meetings. Phase II of the Race to the Top will be entirely dedicated to GFSI future capability building framework, boldly reshaping the outdated GFSI Global Markets Programme to support food business operators in a more inclusive, harmonized, protected, sustainable and educative manner to build capabilities in their food safety management systems.

70.1.3.1 Phase I – Race to the top: building more trust in the existing ecosystem

1. Developing a new benchmarking activity: harmonization and benchmarking requirements for providers of food safety auditor training and ongoing Continuing Professional Development.
2. Moving to deliver a process of ongoing assessment and continuous alignment to the GFSI requirements for CPOs.
3. Developing a collaborative approach to the management of Certification Bodies between Certification Program Owners, Accreditation Bodies, and GFSI.
4. Developing a online GFSI certificate platform – enabling access to certificate data and status of all FBOs certified to a GFSI-recognized Program.

The vision depends upon breaking down the current silos where performance information is held. It requires an information infrastructure where information is input once, then made available to relevant stakeholders on a "need to know" basis. Centralization of the information facilitates effective governance and protection of the information, whilst enabling GFSI to oversee and exercise control over all the factors which impact the integrity of the GFSI benchmarking process. The RTTT framework proposes the enhancement of oversight of the GFSI ecosystem intending to improve trust, transparency, and confidence in GFSI-recognized certification and audit outcomes. Additionally, GFSI is seeking to stay true to its core purpose as a benchmarking and harmonization organization responsible for the "what" – not the "how" – of food safety.

GFSI intends to move away from a checklist compliance model to a more risk-based, data-driven, continuous improvement mindset and approach through its tools and deliver outcomes linked to its strategic objectives. It will also describe how GFSI intends to place more emphasis on science (HACCP, risk assessment, root cause analysis, etc.) and new technologies in the near future.

70.1.3.2 Phase 2 – Race to the top: enhancing a new ecosystem to serve capacities for safe food for all

70.1.3.2.1 Global Food Safety Initiative Global Markets Program

With the development and evolution of the GFSI Benchmarking Requirements came the need to create by GFSI members, 14 years ago, a dynamic and systematic route to third-party certification for small and developing businesses that had aspirations to be certified but who lacked the internal resource and food safety management system expertise to achieve it. GFSI developed the GFSI Global Markets Program (GMaP) capability tool in 2008 to support small or less developed Food Business Operators to achieve certification to GFSI-recognized food safety programs and to improve market access.

The aim was to help target companies develop effective food safety management systems through a systematic continuous improvement process through the following specific objectives:

- To provide a route for small and less developed businesses to achieve GFSI accredited certification.
- To support capability-building efforts and improve market access opportunities for small suppliers operating locally.

The GMaP was a voluntary program, with a toolkit that contains a food safety checklist and a protocol to drive continuous improvement. Companies may choose to use the GMaP, or they may decide to implement the program as part of business development activities in manufacturing sites and/or primary production. It is a free access tool and voluntary program that businesses can use to implement according to their needs and strategic objectives, available on GFSI website. The documents guide the food businesses, service providers, and stakeholders in the form of a toolkit. The GMaP was originally designed as an introductory three-step program toward full GFSI-certification. During the last 12 years, various pilot programs have used the GMaP checklists to introduce food safety management systems into smaller and less developed businesses around the world. Pioneer countries include Ukraine, China, Japan, Russia, Chile, Malaysia, the USA, and Zambia amongst many others. Businesses participating include retailers and brand manufacturers in partnership with international organizations and universities that have funded training and mentoring programs to raise awareness and build capability.

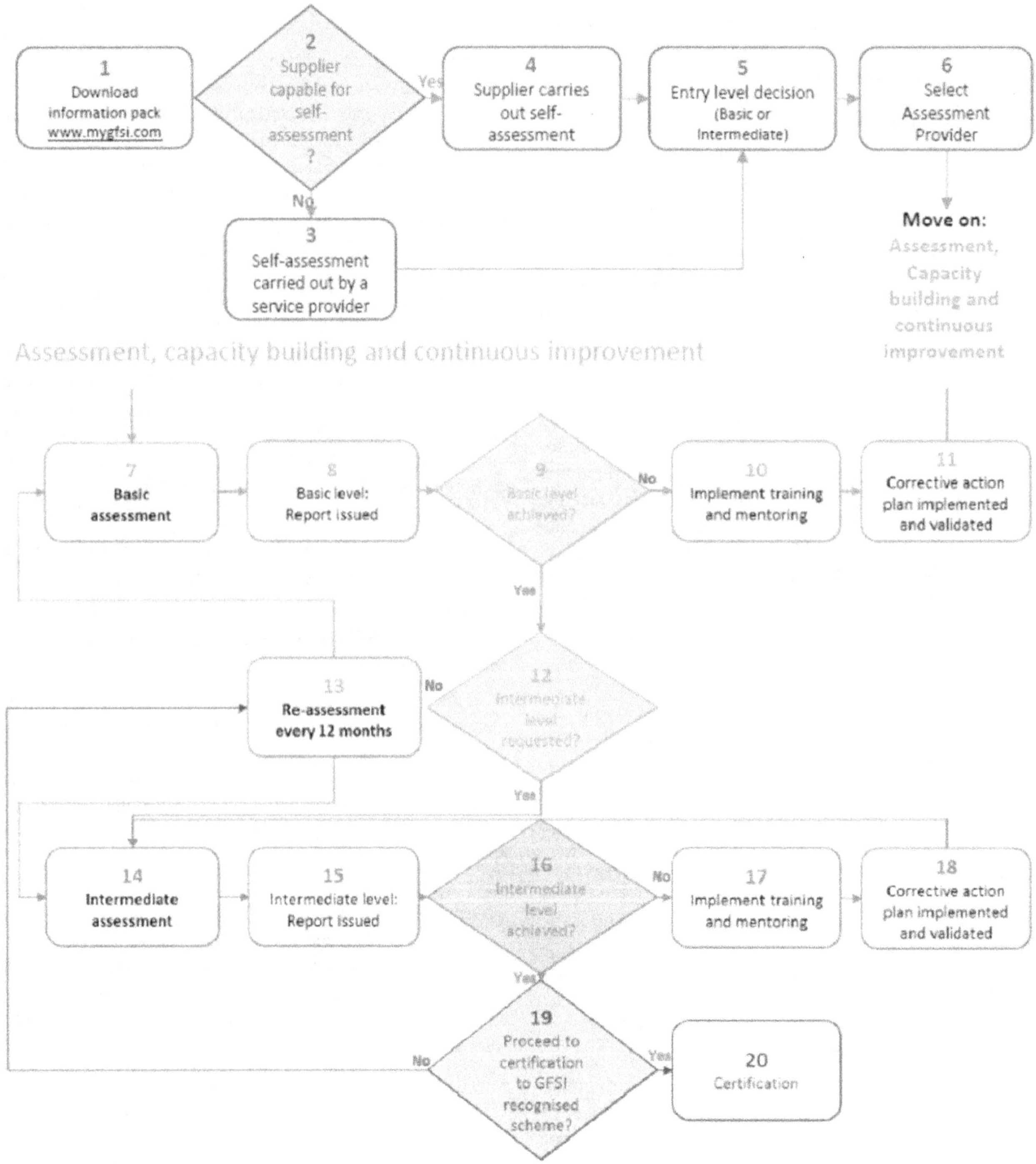
1 Download information pack www.mygfsi.com
2 Supplier capable for self-assessment?
Yes
No
3 Self-assessment carried out by a service provider
4 Supplier carries out self-assessment
5 Entry level decision (Basic or Intermediate)
6 Select Assessment Provider
Move on: Assessment, Capacity building and continuous improvement
Assessment, capacity building and continuous improvement
7 Basic assessment
8 Basic level: Report issued
9 Basic level achieved?
No
10 Implement training and mentoring
11 Corrective action plan implemented and validated
Yes
12 Intermediate level requested?
No
13 Re-assessment every 12 months
Yes
14 Intermediate assessment
15 Intermediate level: Report issued
16 Intermediate level achieved?
No
17 Implement training and mentoring
18 Corrective action plan implemented and validated
Yes
19 Proceed to certification to GFSI recognised scheme?
No
Yes
20 Certification

It was never intended to be a fully stand-alone program, which unintentionally could devalue full certification. The end destination was always full certification after a three-year process. With the development of this program, without proper oversight from GFSI, the program has lost its initial objective and purpose,[b] has become an additional cost for some FBOs to improve their food safety management systems, and has proven to be a risk in jeopardizing GFSI certification. Despite GFSI's success in driving improvements in food safety capabilities through the GMaP, there is no room for complacency.

This framework was shared for formal stakeholder consultation in the Spring of 2020. When responses to the RTTT consultation were reviewed, GFSI noted a significant number of concerns from stakeholders specifically relating to the efficacy and integrity of the GMaP. Given the fact that no strategic review of the GMaP had been undertaken since its launch in 2010 it seemed timely to consider a review of the GMaP during the second phase of the RTTT. In September 2020 GFSI launched a strategic review of the GMaP of which this consultation is a critical part. Along with a public consultation on its GFSI website from February to March 2021 GFSI convened a Uited Nations Food Systems Summit independent dialogue on March 9, 2021 to engage stakeholders' views on how to strategically review its capability-building tool. This multi-stakeholder global dialogue brought together businesses, international organizations, academics, and governments from UN member states responsible for, or with an interest in, food safety. It gathered 120 participants from 45 governments[c] (mainly ministries of health, agriculture and trade) and 35 companies (mainly manufacturers and retailers, along with less sophisticated food producers).

This dialogue was the culmination of three preparatory discussions that took place with participants from Asia, Africa, and Central and South America from January to March 2021 and included 186 participants from more than 25 countries on those three continents.

With the following ideas/outcomes were generated from the dialogue:

- the future capability-building framework shall benefits to food business operators first, and to support regulators and food safety IGOs to design and finance easily capability building programs in emerging markets to strengthen supply chains and facilitate trade
- the future framework should ensure safe food for all including food banks, informal markets, micro-enterprises customers, humanitarian beneficiaries, and consumers everywhere with no distinction on the safety of the food between exports and domestic consumption (to avoid a two-speed system)
- the future framework should help develop leaders and champions in small and very small enterprises and MSMEs by empowering them with appropriate food safety managements systems tools and supporting them to strengthen food safety culture in their companies, cities, regions, and countries via the following:
- Ensure women are empowered as they are key contributors to healthier lifestyles and more sustainable food systems
- use innovative ways to educate and spread awareness should be used such as ancestral communication techniques, and internet-based solutions, to educate easily with non-literary tools about good hygiene practices
- People who are lacking literacy need to be targeted with the fit for purpose innovative solutions to empower them via education and training programs
- the new program needs to encourage sustainable and nutritious food systems production and equitable livelihoods, in rural communities at a very small scale and should ensure that it develops harmonized food safety management systems aligned with the SDGs linked to trade, food safety, and food security (especially 2, 3, 6, 12, 17)
- Small is the answer to making the change with the future framework: a renewed focus should be applied to involve MSMEs, informal markets, new small disruptive players in the food industry, and small restaurants.
- Training and education are paramount! The value of training was underscored repeatedly, and there was broad agreement that there is a genuine thirst for knowledge of food safety. GFSI must be engaged in providing a training and educational pathway framework not only for businesses but also for food inspectors, where regulators wish to collaborate. Some regulators also noted that some regulators in developing countries at the local level could also benefit from training. Regulators would also benefit from GFSI to create a Global markets checklist for inspectors in jurisdictions where public resources are scare
- The development of a community of FBOs focused on food safety via a future framework can provide mutual support and encourage the sharing of best practices while understanding shared local challenges and culture. Development of mentorship programs may also be of value.

The principal conclusion from all participants was that efforts towards capacity building for small and very small FBOs were fundamental to providing access to safe food for all, and to increase access to markets. Stakeholders agreed that given the size and complexity of the task, GFSI private-public partnerships forum offers the most promising opportunities to make a difference, and increased collaboration could help to avoid duplication and better leverage efforts of businesses and governments. It was clear that if the objective was to ensure that "no one is left behind" and that safe food should be for all, then the scope of capacity-building programming and tools should extend to all food businesses to be more inclusive and agents and GFSI could make a great impact there. Regulators noted that investments in capacity building can also contribute to greater regulatory compliance.

70.2 Global Food Safety Initiative's new capability building approach: enhancing more inclusive trade via food safety capacities

70.2.1 A new paradigm for food systems: the shift of focus towards lower- and middle-income countries and the opportunities and challenges linked to the SDGs[d]

According to FAO and OECD,[e] low- and middle-income countries are the source of most demand food and drive most of the global production growth of food from 2021 to 2030.

> *It is also projected by FAO and OECD*[f] *that production growth in agriculture will be predominantly located in emerging economies and low-income countries and will be driven by productivity-increasing investments in agricultural infrastructure and research and development, wider access to agricultural inputs, and improved management skills in these regions.*

The world has been organized by gigantic modern supply chains in the western world for the past 30 years. As the world faces one of its most important challenges linked to food systems by needing to include greater resilience and inclusivity in food systems to address major drivers such as conflict, climate variability, and climate change extremes, economic crisis, provide more affordable, healthier, sustainable, and inclusive food while ending hunger, food insecurity and malnutrition in all its forms, the production and consumption of food are shifting towards lower- and middle-income countries. Food Safety is front and center of food systems, and those challenges and drivers, as *if it is not safe, is not food*, it is vital to produce safe food for everyone and food safety is vital for achieving the Sustainable Development Goals by 2030, as *The Safe Food Imperative: accelerating progress in low and income countries' report*[g] *states*: *Food safety is linked in direct and indirect ways to achieving many of the Sustainable Development Goals, especially those on ending hunger and poverty, and promoting good health and well-being. Food and nutritional security are realized only when the essential elements of a healthy diet are safe to eat, and when consumers recognize this. The safety of food is vital for the growth and transformation of agriculture, which are needed to feed a growing and more prosperous world population, for the modernization of national food systems, and for a country's efficient integration into regional and international markets.*

As all those enduring drivers will impact food safety and food systems via all supply chains and all its traditional and new stakeholders, GFSI has a role to play as a convening forum and network and as a historical player in providing tools for more Food Business Operators from various sizes, sophistication levels and regions to improve their food safety management systems to share and enhance food safety capacities to support FBOs from all over the world with this new paradigm and the challenges linked to attaining the SDGs.

70.2.2 The revolution of digital technologies and big data in the food system

Digital technologies linked to big data have a very high potential for further development of the agricultural sector, by reshaping food supply chains. They also have the potential to contribute toward more efficient, resilient, and transparent food systems and specific supply chains. They also should support more and better inclusion of small farmers and small FBOs from all over the world but especially in low- and middle-income countries' supply chains says Đuric'[1] and Baragwanath[2]. Those digital technologies should if used the right way and given access in a fair way, enable more efficient and more inclusive local and global agricultural markets. The benefits could be tremendous, such as reducing the gap in information asymmetries and giving opportunities to reduce transaction costs for smaller agribusiness players hence increasing market access. Also with the right mechanisms, they could be providing financial inclusion to all the smaller stakeholders by supporting them to tackle a lot of the challenges linked to attaining the SDGs.

70.2.3 The challenge of climate change on food systems and food safety

Climate change represents an unprecedented challenge to the biosphere and the world[3]. Therefore, it also represents a unique challenge for plant health and therefore food safety, FAO[h] writes *the evidence assessed strongly indicates that climate change has already expanded some pests' host range and geographical distribution and may further increase the risk of pest introduction to new areas.*

The impacts of climate change on the environment are well known (unprecedented damage to our ecosystem with increasing temperatures, ocean warming and acidification, severe and repeated weather events, and crisis such as droughts, wildfires, altered precipitation patterns, melting glaciers, rising sea levels) and therefore has implications on food security and food safety[i] as FAO describes in *Climate change: Unpacking the burden on food safety*. This report identifies and attempts to quantify some current and anticipated food safety issues that are associated with climate change, food safety hazards considered in the publication are foodborne pathogens and parasites, harmful algal blooms, pesticides, mycotoxins, and heavy metals with emphasis on methylmercury.

70.2.4 Global Food Safety Initiative future capability building approach: a unique opportunity to cooperate

Acknowledging that smaller and better-informed food systems are the future, GFSI is designing a new food safety capability building framework that intends to bring solutions for FBOs from everywhere to all those challenges in one new trusted food safety ecosystem. This new capability building framework will consist of a holistic approach, barrier-free but managed model to become a full operational capability building framework within 2–3 years, creating a full architecture to support building capacities, linking players of goodwill and all means in all the food safety systems aspects for safe food for all everywhere. The overall value proposition is to facilitate market access for all FBOs by giving access to a trusted ecosystem for FBOs to find techincal, educational, financial, resources to strenghten food safety capacities by coordinating efforts of the exisitng food safety community in one place.

GFSI's new role and objective with its new capability building strategic framework will be to support every stakeholder in building or supports building food safety capacities in more decentralized food systems with better access to intelligence and education on food safety management in a digital environment while integrating with various components of the SDGs impacting safe food.

70.3 Public-private partnership: a cornerstone of Global Food Safety Initiative strategy to seek recognition from regulators of Global Food Safety Initiative certification as a risk-based tool in national food control systems

70.3.1 Global Food Safety Initiative's role and objective in the public-private partnership context is to facilitate trade: collaboration between the public and private sectors for better dialogue and partnerships

As our food network becomes more globalized and interconnected, we have seen a shift towards greater transparency and integrity as consumers are awakened to issues of food safety and traceability. National and international public partners cannot build a safer and more efficient food supply chain without the support of the industry. One of GFSI's strategic priorities, on PPP, consists in creating the right environment to create trust, engage dialogue and create scaled-up impact so that accredited third-party certification against one of the 12 GFSI recognized CPOs is understood and trusted by public authorities so that they can use it in their national food control systems for risk-based resource allocation tool.

GFSI believes that by utilizing our collective resources, industry stakeholders and governments can work more effectively together to ensure that there are tools in place along the entire value chain, from origination to the end consumer to ensure safe food for people everywhere. With this understanding that we can't do it alone, GFSI has made it a priority to foster PPPs between private companies, government food safety regulators, and intergovernmental organizations (IGOs) to harmonize global food safety regulations and reduce trade barriers. By stimulating dialogue and joint programs between public and private sectors, GFSI is working to advance food safety worldwide while building consumer trust and increasing industry efficiency, this is why one of GFSI's three strategic outcomes is to strengthen PPPs so that food safety regulators trust that GFSI certification can be used for risk-based resource allocation.

70.3.2 Debunking the myths around third party certification to strengthen efforts on food safety

GFSI believes developed collaboration as an enhancing and necessary tool for public-private action to enhance trade via better understanding. There is a need for public actors to fully support the use of all available food safety management tools for FBOs and to overcome the myths around accredited third-party certification. GFSI believes that national food control systems are the foundation in support of consumer safety.

Therefore, GFSI intends to play only a complementary role as a benchmarking organization with its recognized accredited third-party certification programs to be used as a risk-based indicator for national food control systems to have more informed and risk-based resource allocation of their inspections activities in the context of good regulatory practices. This is the overall strategic outcome sought by GFSI for one of its three strategic priorities (on PPP). GFSI recognized accredited certification programs can- and should be considered – as an effective tool in assisting relevant regulatory authorities in meeting their NFCS objectives: knowledge regarding a FBO's certification status and scope can be valuable input in helping to decide where regulatory resources should be spent.

The GFSI benchmarking requirements are intended to transcend borders and build food safety into all aspects of a company, from management commitment to processes and procedures. FBOs across the globe have demonstrated their commitment to safe food for people everywhere by undertaking a voluntary accredited third-party certification in a GFSI recognized program, often with a significant investment in resources. FBOs who are certified may represent a diminished risk in the food landscape since regimented rules and procedures are in place to grant the certification and to maintain ongoing certification, including onsite audits.

70.3.3 A complementary role for Global Food Safety Initiative in the global food safety systems governance

GFSI voluntary third-party assurance programs (vTPA) are designed to support FBOs with a total view of food safety and serve as a complementary program to a country's National Food Control System (NFCS). As such, the programs are not intended to mirror any country's food laws but are intended to serve as the cornerstone for effective food safety and quality management systems. GFSI believes that national food control systems are the foundation in support of consumer safety.

GFSI's benchmarking requirements are built through the consensus of experts and are based on internationally recognized standards Codex Alimentarius, IPPC and OIE. These standards form a widely accepted understanding of what constitutes a robust food safety certification program. Additionally, GFSI takes proactive measures in establishing new criteria based on scientific evidence and stakeholder expertise. These criteria help to ensure that the programs continue to deliver on GFSI's vision, often ahead of discussions that may be happening within an NFCS.

GFSI believes it can play a complementary role as a benchmarking organization with its recognized accredited third-party certification programs to be used as a risk-based indicator for national food control systems to have more informed and risk-based resource allocation of their inspections activities in the context of good regulatory practices. GFSI recognized accredited certification programs can- and should be considered – as an effective tool in assisting relevant regulatory authorities in meeting their NFCS objectives: knowledge regarding a FBO's certification status and scope can be valuable input in helping to decide where regulatory resources should be spent. GFSI and its members believe in robust national food control systems and regulatory oversight. The first criteria required for each FBO audited against one of the GFSI recognized CPOs is to be compliant with the applying regulatory framework in which the FBO operates. The benchmarking requirements are intended to transcend borders and build food safety into all aspects of a company, from management commitment to processes and procedures with concrete tools that can be evident during an audit while reducing the audit burden and duplication in a supplier, but neither to duplicate national, regional, or international regulatory control system and standard nor to replace any regulatory oversight.

FBOs who are certified against a GFSI-recognized CPO represent a diminished risk in the food landscape since regimented rules and procedures are in place to grant the certification and to maintain ongoing certification, including onsite audits. Those efforts should be encouraged and incentivized by regulators and UN agencies such as WHO and FAO; as FBOs using voluntary accredited third-party certification are the first supporters of safer food for their customers and people everywhere. FBOs across the globe have demonstrated their commitment to food safety by undertaking a voluntary accredited third-party certification in a GFSI recognized program, always with a significant investment in resources (people's expertise, processes, machines....). GFSI believes that the immensity of the challenges linked to food safety and food systems requires support and collaboration from all. The coalition of the willing that GFSI represents with its mission to have safe food for people everywhere should be formally recognized.

70.3.4 Accredited third-party certification serves food business operators as a mechanism and framework with tools to improve their food safety management systems by creating a food safety culture

GFSI has been one of the first global organizations to issue guidelines[j] for the food industry to develop a food fraud mitigation plan[k] in its food safety management systems in 2014 by including the mandatory requirements to develop a food fraud plan for a FBO to succeed in a food safety audit led by a GFSI recognized CPOs. These additional requirements that have been included in GFSI benchmarking requirements involve that a FBO must perform a food fraud vulnerability assessment and have a food fraud vulnerability control plan in place to mitigate the identified vulnerabilities. As a consequence, since 2014, each FBO succeeding on a food safety audit by one of the 12 GFSI recognized CPOs, has put in place a food fraud mitigation plan with 871 491[l] certificates delivered since the implementation of the food fraud position in 2014.

With increased food safety challenges and current trends in contamination-related issues, FBOs are left with no option but to continuously seek and implement new techniques and strategies to ensure the manufacturing and distribution of safe food. In its latest version of its benchmarking requirements, version 2020, GFSI has integrated a food safety culture approach by requesting audits performance by a GFSI recognized CPOs to provide evidence of the senior management's commitment to establish, implement, maintain, and continuously improve the Food Safety Management System. This shall include elements of food safety culture, at a minimum consisting of communication, training, feedback from employees, and performance measurement on food safety-related activities. The deployment of version 2020 of the benchmarking requirements has encouraged FBOs to engage, maintain and consolidate a food safety culture with better-informed food safety management systems.

70.3.5 Future direction

70.3.5.1 Global Food Safety Initiative government to business: a public-private forum to collaborate, co-create, and scale-up impact on food safety

The G2B forum has been created by GFSI as a non-competitive initiative and a non-profit global industry and regulators network providing a collaborative platform between all categories of stakeholders to provide solutions to the collective concerns of the public and private sector to reduce food safety risks.

The G2B Meeting provides since 2016 a unique forum where the private sector, government food safety officials, and IGOs can engage in open discussions around food safety trends, opportunities and challenges It provides a unique place where senior leaders of food safety agencies and from food safety regulators, IGOs who have demonstrated expertise on projects related to food safety, market access and capacity building and who have a direct influence on the policy, regulatory and standard-setting domain come together.

Since 2016, it has gathered more than 60 countries representing 50 jurisdictions and 30 companies from all continents. From 2022 the G2B will focus on collaborating with UN agencies regarding food safety strategies (FAO, WHO, and WFP) in proposing concrete solutions via GFSI projects, tools, and programs for the industry to act as implementing partners in supporting those global food safety strategies,[m] GFSI will also be working with regulators on the use of information and communication technologies in audit activities and will be working with public stakeholders on its new capability building framework to ensure they have a role and responsibitlies in supporting and using the framework.

Endnotes

[a]GFSI Benchmarking requirements are based on CODEX Alimentarius.

[b]In September 2020, a survey was sent to 100 GFSI key users of the global markets program (buyers, foods business operators using the GMaP – mostly Global Markets awards winners, CPOs, CBs, NGOs), half of them responded that they were very dissatisfied with the program.

[c]GFSI Global Markets Programme and capability building work, stakeholders consultation summary - January 2022, Anne Gerardi - https://mygfsi.com/news_updates/reshaping-gfsis-global-markets-programme/.

[d]The Sustainable Development Goals are a collection of 17 interlinked global goals designed and adopted by all United Nations Member States in 2015, providing a *shared blueprint for peace and prosperity for people and the planet, now and into the future*. They recognize that ending poverty and other deprivations must go together with strategies that improve health and education, reduce inequality, and spur economic growth – all while tackling climate change and working to preserve our oceans and forests. The SDGs are intended to be achieved by the year 2030.

[e]OECD/FAO Agricultural outlook 2021–2030, Figure 1.7 Regional contributions to food demand growth 2011-20 and 2021-30 ttps://www.oecd-ilibrary.org/agriculture-and-food/data/oecd-agriculture-statistic-s_agr-data-en.

[f]OCDE/FAO (2021), OECD-FAO Agricultural Outlook 2021–2030, Éditions OCDE, Paris, https://doi.org/10.1787/19428846-en., chapter 1.3.3.

[g]Jaffee, Steven; Henson, Spencer; Unnevehr, Laurian; Grace, Delia; Cassou, Emilie. 2019. The Safe Food Imperative: Accelerating Progress in Low- and Middle-Income Countries. Agriculture and Food Series;. Washington, DC: World Bank. © World Bank.

[h]IPPC Secretariat. 2021. Summary for policymakers of the scientific review of the impact of climate change on plant pests – A global challenge to prevent and mitigate plant pest risks in agriculture, forestry and ecosystems. Rome. FAO on behalf of the IPPC Secretariat. https://doi.org/10.4060/cb4777en.

[i]FAO. 2020. Climate change: Unpacking the burden on food safety. Food safety and quality series No. 8. Rome. https://doi.org/10.4060/ca8185en

[j]https://mygfsi.com/press_releases/gfsi-position-paper-on-mitigating-the-public-health-risk-of-food-fraud/.

[k]In line with the GFSI's mission statement in 2014, GFSI declared that the additional requirements and food fraud definition ensure a focus on food safety, rather than other factors such as commercial gain. The requirements specify that companies must perform a food fraud vulnerability assessment and to have a food fraud vulnerability control plan in place to mitigate the identified vulnerabilities. The GFSI Board at that time stated that it *believes that the mitigation of food fraud is an integral part of a company's food safety management system.*

[l]GFSI sources, added number of certificates delievered each year since 2014.

[m]FAO coming new food safety strategy and WHO Global Strategy for Food Safety for 2022–2030.

References

1. Đuric' I. *Digital Technology and Agricultural Markets – Background Paper for The State of Agricultural Commodity Markets (SOCO) 2020.* Rome: FAO; 2020. Available from: https://doi.org/10.4060/cb0701en.

2. Baragwanath T. *Digital Opportunities for Demand-Side Policies to Improve Consumer Health and the Sustainability of Food Systems.* Paris: OECD Publishing; 2021, OECD Food, Agriculture and Fisheries Papers, No. 148. Available from: https://doi.org/10.1787/bec87135-en.

3. IPPC Secretariat. *Summary for Policymakers of the Scientific Review of the Impact of Climate Change on Plant Pests – A Global Challenge to Prevent and Mitigate Plant Pest Risks in Agriculture, Forestry and Ecosystems.* Rome: FAO on behalf of the IPPC Secretariat; 2021. Available from: https://doi.org/10.4060/cb4777en.

Section XV

Climate change, population demographics, urbanization, and economic growth: impact on food safety

Chapter 71

Food and nutrition security: challenges for farming, procurement, and consumption

Tessa Avermaete[1], Wannes Keulemans[2], Olivier Honnay[3], Gerard Govers[4], Barbara De Coninck[2] and Tjitske Anna Zwart[1]

[1]*Sustainable Food Economies Research Group, KU Leuven, Belgium,* [2]*Crop Biotechnics, KU Leuven, Belgium,* [3]*Ecology, Evolution and Biodiversity Conservation, KU Leuven, Belgium,* [4]*Geography and Tourism, KU Leuven, Belgium*

Abstract

Food security and nutrition security raise multiple questions at both the local and global levels. Experts have formulated three major challenges for the 21st century in this regard: the depletion of natural materials, the loss of environmental quality, and the assurance or guarantee of food supplies. Will we be able to produce enough food for an expanding global population? Will everyone have access to sufficient food? Will increasing food production not have to be paid for by deforestation and reduced biodiversity? Will increasing food production have an excessive impact on the environment? What kind of impact will climate change have on the production of food? What kind of potential do alternative production methods have? Should regions endeavor to establish independence with respect to their food needs? This chapter provides an overview of key elements of Food and Nutrition Security and points out key enablers for transition toward sustainable food systems.

Keywords: Food and nutrition security; sustainability; agriculture; sustainable intensification; health; biodiversity; climate change

71.1 Introduction

Food and nutrition security (FNS) raises multiple questions at both the local and global level. Experts have formulated three major challenges for the 21st century in this regard: the depletion of natural materials, the environment issue, and the assurance or guarantee of food supplies. Will we be able to produce enough food for an expanding global population? Will everyone have access to sufficient food? Will increasing food production not have to be paid for by deforestation and reduced biodiversity? Will food production come under threat from alternative agricultural products such as energy crops? Will increasing food production have an excessive impact on the environment? What kind of impact will climate change have on the production of food? In what way will food prices evolve? Will the globalization of the food chain continue and in what way will the role of the multinationals evolve? What kind of potential do alternative production methods have? Should regions endeavor to establish independence with respect to their food needs?

Currently, over 800 million people are faced with hunger and undernourishment. Perversely, at the same time, more than 1 billion people suffer from obesity, and diet-related, noncommunicable diseases due to unhealthy diets high in calories and heavily processed food.[1−4] Obesity does not only concern high-income countries, but increasingly also affects developing economies.

Enough food is produced to meet the needs of the entire global population. Issues of food insecurity thus are a consequence of the uneven distribution of food, and a failure to provide everybody with sufficient access to food, rather than a lack of food production.[5,6] The inequality in food distribution and resulting food security issues take place against the backdrop of a range of other environmental, economic, political, and social issues, which are impacted by and impact food production, processing, distribution, and consumption. These range from climate change,[2,3] a loss of biodiversity through poor agricultural practices,[7,8] and the depletion of natural resources,[9] to food waste and losses, an increase in the incidence of natural disasters, and an increasing demand for energy crops putting pressure on food prices. Future

Present Knowledge in Food Safety. DOI: https://doi.org/10.1016/B978-0-12-819470-6.00016-0

projections show that these issues will likely continue to challenge global food and nutrition security.[1–3]

The challenges and opportunities of our food system are both enormous and diverse. Climate change already has an impact on farming, in the South as well as in the North. The pressure of agriculture on the environment cannot be ignored. Biodiversity decreases. It is hard to motivate youngsters to start farming. And also on the consumption side, statistics illustrate that action is urgently needed. Against this tendency, diverse stakeholders in the chain call for a development toward a climate neutral food chain and a global sustainable food system that guarantees food security.

This chapter provides an overview of key elements of FNS. In the next section, we provide an outline of the concept of FNS. After this, we continue to look at FNS issues throughout food supply chains. Specifically, we focus on three "stages" in food supply chains: farming, procurement, and consumption, and the several FNS issues that arise in each of these stages. FNS implies sustainable food systems, that is, food systems that aim at achieving FNS and healthy diets while limiting negative environmental impacts and improving socio-economic welfare. Based on this background, we point out key enablers for transitions toward sustainable food systems. The chapter closes with an overview of research gaps and future directions.

71.2 Food and nutrition security

The concept of food security was coined for the first time during the 1974 World Food Conference. At first it was only seen as an issue of food supply. Over the years, however, more dimensions have been added to the definition.[10] Amartya Sen,[11] for example, insisted that access to food, use of food, and stable availability are crucial components of food security in addition to availability. This approach is now internationally recognized and was described at the World Food Summit[12] as follows: "Food security exists when each person at every moment has economic, social and physical access to sufficient, safe and nourishing food to meet their dietary needs and to live an active and healthy life."

More recently, experts warned that food security necessarily requires nutrition security, that is, access to an appropriate nutritious diet, coupled with a sanitary environment, adequate health services, and care to ensure a healthy and active life for all household members (Radhika and Hemantha, p. 35).[13] The fundamental connection between the two terms has resulted in the use of FNS, as a concept that emphasizes both the food and health requirements for populations.[14]

Specifically, four separate components of FNS can be distinguished: food availability, food access, food utilization, and stability of the other three dimensions over time.

71.2.1 Food availability, food access, food utilization, and stability

Food availability implies the physical existence of sufficient quality food. At the global level, food availability implies sufficient overall food production. At the national, regional, and local level, however, this component is much more sophisticated and includes a combination of domestic food production, intra- and international trade and commercial food imports and exports (including food aid), international, national, and local transport, storage capacity, logistics, and food stocks.

Food access results from the combination of economic endowments, physical access, and socio-cultural resources that allow the purchase or acquisition of appropriate food products for a nutritious diet. As centrally noted in the definition stemming from the 1996 FAO World Food Summit, FNS is fundamentally an issue of access to food. Food access is defined to consist of three elements. First, access relates to physical access to food, which may be difficult in some places. It also relates to allocation issues, which takes a range of forms due to varied reasons. For instance, in some cultures, men eat before women; aid agencies and emergency relief organizations need to decide priorities for who receives food and when; and food can be used as a political "weapon" to influence or even subjugate sections of society. Second, the affordability of food is a key element in food access. A major component in this regard is the price of food relative to the disposable income available for food purchasing. If prices rise faster than incomes, food insecurity can increase. A third key element is that of preference. Food preferences are determined by cultural and religious contexts, taste and appearance of food, convenience and cooking skills, health and ethical concerns, and also marketing and retail strategies. A food product may thus be safe and high in nutrients, but culturally inappropriate. Having to eat food we do not prefer can have psychological impacts, undermining overall well-being. However, there is no consensus on the extent to which the element of preference should be taken into account in food security debates.

Food utilization refers to how the body utilizes various nutrients in foodstuffs as well as food preparation and hygiene practices, sound eating habits, a diverse diet, and proper intra-household distribution of food. Food utilization is often primarily taken to mean the physiological nutritional value of food. Foods also need to be safe: free from toxins and other contaminants, and from pathogens and parasites. While many ultra-processed foods satisfy these conditions, excess consumption of such "empty calories" can also be termed "unsafe," as they may contribute to overweight and obesity, and concomitant diet-related diseases. Overall diets should therefore be sufficient in variety, quality, and quantity to avoid poor physical and mental health outcomes associated with hunger, stunting, wasting, and obesity. Finally, the social functions of food are often overlooked in food security debates. These are often deeply embedded in cultural norms, and contribute to notions of social- and self-identity, kinship, and family. Food often serves a real or symbolic function in religious or social ceremony; lack of the right types of food for such functions undermines the social function.

Finally, food security implies the stability of the other three dimensions over time, stressing the temporal element of food security. The widely cited FAO definition of food security states that people (i.e., a population, household, or individual) must have access to sufficient food at all times. They should not risk losing access to food because of shocks (e.g., an economic or political crisis, or an extreme weather event), cyclical events (e.g., seasonal food insecurity), or stresses (e.g., changes in demographics, climate or natural resource degradation). Many factors can therefore undermine food security, especially when they occur simultaneously. For instance, the increase in hunger over the last couple of years is attributed by FAO to the coincidence of conflict and climate change-induced weather shocks. At the same time, "stability" can be undesirable if a given food security situation is suboptimal. In some cases, the food system needs to be dynamic to address suboptimal performances.

71.2.2 Framing food and nutrition security

The public perception of FNS is shaped by insights and believes on the drivers and vulnerabilities of the food system performance and its resilience. In order to understand solutions that are put forward to enable more sustainable food systems, one needs to recognize and understand that various narratives and discourses exist on FNS.

A narrative takes specific vulnerabilities and hazards in the food system as point of departure for shaping potential solutions. Narratives are also present in the social media, influencing public perception and solutions, and leading to various discourses that encompass these views on reality. Over the past two decades, various narratives on FNS have been developed. Recently, there is a growing body of work on FNS framings that aim to gain an in-depth understanding of narrative formation and its policy implications.

Along with time, the focus has been enlarged from a narrow system/production-centered approach to a more encompassing people/access-centered approach, and the focus of analysis, also for measurement purposes, there has been as shift from "food security" to "food insecurity." The scientific and politic debate on the definitions addresses these two aspects, scale and dimensions of food security. Scale thereby refers to the level of analyses. In this context, one can observe a shift in interest from the international and national level toward FNS at the level of communities and even at the household level.

Discourses can be considered as external structures used by individuals, groups, and societies in order to organize, perceive, shape, and communicate about reality. Despite the multifaceted processes and the complexity that characterizes the FNS dynamics, solutions, and conceptualizations—envisaged from policy, academic spheres, and lobby groups—they have mostly revolved around oppositional narratives that reproduce old dichotomies and dialectics. These narratives have been identified under different flags such as the productivity (or efficiency) narrative and the sufficiency narrative,[15,16] or the bio-economy and eco-economy paradigms,[17] weak and strong ecological modernization,[18] and productivist or demand-led approaches.[19]

The food system is complex, and characterized by many feedback loops between parts of the food chain (production, processing, distribution, and consumption) and from the socio-economic and environmental outcomes of food production and consumption (such as food security and soil depletion) back to that production and consumption. The stakeholders in the food chain each have their own narratives and discourses in terms of FNS. A thorough understanding in discourses and the underlying arguments contributes to the dialog on FNS in general and the debate between proponents of—apparently—competing discourses in particular. Dealing with sustainable farming, for example, the ecological discourse and the technology discourse are emphasized while in when reflecting on citizen empowerment and local food strategies, the sovereignty discourse, and the social discourse is most relevant.

Whatever discourse or narrative on food and security is used, the globalized international frame is a reality that cannot be ignored. Indeed, the key drivers of change of our food system—such as climate change, population growth, unhealthy consumption patterns, biodiversity decline—are global and do not expand political and cultural borders.

71.3 Farming

FNS implies that enough food is produced to feed current and future generations. This goal can be aspired to in a variety of ways that can be distilled into three specific options: increasing production, reducing food waste, and introducing dietary changes, particularly a reduction in the consumption of meat. All three options will have to be deployed in unison. This section focuses on the first option: increasing production.

The challenges facing agriculture are varied and controversial. Radical efforts in the agricultural sector will have to be made to feed the growing world population.

Thereby, a number of preconditions will have to be accounted for, including limits to maximum production capacity, climate change, exhaustibility of natural reserves, and the impact of agriculture on the environment and society.

Global food production has seen a continuous increase in the last century, primarily as a result of innovation, and in particular technological innovation. Fundamental transformations have been realized through the use of artificial fertilizers, variety improvements (including genetic manipulation), herbicides, and pesticides. Wheat production in North West Europe illustrates how technology can impact productivity. After the World War II, and stimulated by Europe's Common Agricultural Policy, crop variety improvements and increased use of manure were applied in arable crop production. In less than 50 years, the productivity in the wheat sector doubled. Whereas a French farmer in the early 1960s would harvest 3 ton/ha, average wheat yields in France in 2020 exceed 8 ton/ha. Similar patterns can be observed for the productivity in sugar beet production and for the productivity of milk cows.

However, there is consensus that—at least in some regions—we have achieved the limits of the earth's carrying capacity. Climate change already affects farming, both in the North and in the South. Agriculture puts pressure on the use of natural resources. Biodiversity decreases, soil erosion removes valuable top soil, and water is a rising global issue.

71.3.1 Climate change and natural resources

Predicted climate change will also have an enormous influence on future agricultural production. The extent of this influence is difficult to estimate because the models used to do so comprise a large measure of uncertainty. Estimates of the expected increase in temperature by 2050 lie between 1°C and 3°C, and some sources even speak of 4°C. We can certainly expect significant differences between regions. It is clear that temperature increase will have an impact on the productivity of important agricultural crops. In many major producing regions, crops will be cultivated in a temperature that is higher than the optimum, with significant production loss as a result.[20] Important shifts are particularly expected in the domain of rainfall, with a decrease in total annual rainfall in Southern Europe (up to 20%) and an increase in Northern Europe (up to 10%). The global influence climate change will have on food production by 2050 is still not completely clear. Some prognoses suggest a clear decline in productivity in Africa, South America, Southern Europe, and the United States; even up to 50% in North Africa. In Northern Europe, North East Europe, Central Europe, and large parts of Central Asia, however, production is expected to increase significantly.[21] From the global perspective, the influence of climate change is expected to result in a decrease in food production if policies remain the same. Against the background of climate change, new and adapted varieties will certainly be an advantage. A great deal of importance is presently being attached to the refinement of various crop varieties with a view to increasing their resistance to drought and other forms of abiotic stress such as heat, frost, and flooding.

Climate change, in turn, has an impact on every type of natural resources, including those resources most relevant to agriculture: water, fossil energy, and fertilizers. In global terms, agriculture is far and away the primary user of the water that falls to earth in the form of rain. But this water is not used with much efficiency, especially in developing countries. In India, for example, the production of a ton of grain requires 10 times as much water as the same ton of grain in Western Europe. Agriculture is also profoundly dependent on fossil energy, for the production of fertilizers, crop protection products and in the form of fuel for machinery, etc. Sources suggest that primary production uses up 10 EJ (10×10^{18} J) of energy,[22] 6 EJ of which in the farm itself. This represents 2% of worldwide energy consumption. Of note, 20% of this consumption goes to the production of nitrogenous fertilizers. The global food chain (in addition to production, this includes processing, transport, and distribution/points of sale) consumes a lot more energy: 98 EJ. The fossil energy used to feed this demand is not inexhaustible. The same can be said for phosphorus, an important agricultural fertilizer. Phosphorus is harvested from phosphoric stone that is sourced primarily in Morocco. Global provisions are thus limited. Pessimistic prognoses suggest the reserves will be exhausted in 40 years, while more optimistic estimations suggest 400 years or more. Solar energy also deserves a mention here. Can it be adapted in such a way that it can be used for transport and storage and thus make a serious contribution to agriculture?

The present highly productive western agricultural system is facing its limits, especially with regard to the environmental aspect. In the past, for example, injudicious—read: excessive—use of fertilizers resulted in pollution of the surface water. Today, however, new fertilizing techniques facilitate the same production levels with less and more dedicated use of fertilizers. Livestock farming is also an important source of pollution, especially via methane emissions from ruminants such as cattle. Methane is a significant greenhouse gas, roughly 20 times stronger than CO_2. Farming, and livestock farming in particular, is said to account for roughly 30% of greenhouse gas emissions.[23]

A further problematic aspect of farming is related to the use of crop protection products that have contributed to the significant increases in production. Together with fertilization, mechanization, and the introduction of new varieties, crop protection was at the foundation of the postwar "green revolution." But crop protection products can have an undesired impact on the environment and the health of organisms not targeted by the product. For this reason, new products are only allowed on the market after they have been thoroughly evaluated by specialized government agencies for the safety of their use for humans, animals, and the environment. Yet crop protection products continue to appear in a bad light and social pressure has recently forced the banning of a large number of such products by European governments. The reduction of the number of available products, however, represents a serious threat. By alternating products in the past, disease and plague resistance levels were kept in check. This is much more difficult today. Fruit cultivation in Germany, for example, has seen the emergence of "super molds" that are difficult to combat. Rather than reducing the variety of crop protection products, therefore, a better strategy would be to reduce their deployment and thus spray less.

Now that the use of crop protection products has been forcibly and drastically reduced, improving the natural resistance of plants has become an important goal. Naturally resistant crops, moreover, are likely to offer considerable advantage in regions where the farmers have limited financial resources to dedicate to the purchase of crop protection products. Sensitivity to plant diseases can often be put down to the absence of a signal in the plant to defend itself. Such signals can be artificially stimulated via so-called "elicitors." The latter are produced naturally in resistant (not sensitive) plants in response to pathogenic infections, but they have been copied on an industrial scale and used with sensitive plants. The natural protection procedure will gain in importance in the years to come. In addition, refinement procedures can improve root systems, allowing plants to be more efficient in absorbing nutrients and water from the soil and thereby reducing the need for fertilizer use. All these evolutions will also have a positive effect on the environment.

The frequent use of crop protection products, intensive use of fertilizers, and—in particular—the use of more and more land for cultivation has also had a negative impact on biodiversity. This tendency would appear to have slowed down to some degree in western farming, but it remains a significant problem in regions where agricultural exploitation is intensifying.

71.3.2 Land use

Land is a natural resource that needs specific attention in the context of global food security. From a historical point of view, significant transformations have taken place in terms of agricultural acreage. The surface dedicated to agriculture has increased from 400 million ha in 1700, of which 200 million were used for crop production and 200 million for grass and grazing, to roughly 4750 million ha today, of which 1750 million ha are used for crops and 3000 million ha for animal grazing.

The 4750 million ha represent 28% of the earth's surface. This is more than a 10-fold increase with a shift toward grazing and pasture for animals. In recent years, the acreage dedicated to agriculture has remained stable, in part as a result of growth in the agriculture surface area at the cost of forestation (especially tropical rainforests in Latin America, Africa, and East Asia) and in part as a result of a decrease in acreage dedicated to cultivation in the industrialized nations (Europe and North America).

At a global scale, deforestation has stabilized. In the period 1900–2000, the deforestation took place at a rate of 16 million ha per year that is about 0.3% of the current land used for agriculture. In the period from 2000 to 2010, approximately 13 million ha of land were cut. Deforestation hence slows down, though in some countries—such as Brazil—large areas of tropical forest disappear, a process which is stimulated by political decisions.

In Europe, the United States and some developing countries—like Vietnam—the opposite tendency can be observed. In France, forest acreage more than doubled in the 20th century.[24] Two factors drive this transition, and they are both directly related to farming. On the one hand, farming becomes more intensive. This implies that less land is needed to keep up the production. On the other hand, farming has become more globally and market driven. Farmers specialize in those products that are best suited for their land. In this sense, they abandon marginal land, which can used for reforestation.

Given both the growing global population and the need to safeguard biodiversity, the question raises on how we should organize the agricultural land. There are, generally spoken, two discourses, known as land-sharing and land-sparing. Land-sparing allows for focusing agricultural activities on those portions of the landscape best suited to supporting production functions: access to water, fertile soils and proximity to market. Land-sparing allows maintaining or increasing natural habitats. A land-sharing approach recognizes the contribution of conservation efforts to supporting agricultural production such as pollination and pest control services, and in securing the multiple benefits provided by these landscapes.

Although a great level of nuance is needed and choices between intensive farming, extensive farming or a combination of both depends highly on local conditions, scientific insights support the land-sparing. The key argument thereby concerns the decrease in biodiversity of cultivated land, even if the production methods applied are considered environmentally friendly (e.g., extensive or organic farming). Moreover, these environmentally friendly types of farming overall lead to production losses. Maintaining production levels implies increase of farming land.

Focusing on land use, the impact of livestock production needs to be mentioned. Roughly 40% of the acreage dedicated to grain crops is used for cultivating animal feed, although livestock food conversion is many times less efficient than direct consumption by human beings. Estimates anticipate a doubling of meat consumption between 2010 and 2050. It is clear that we do not have the acreage necessary to meet this expected growth in demand.

71.3.3 Toward sustainable intensification

There is an overall consensus on the need for a more sustainable management of natural resources in order to ensure FNS for all, with agriculture playing a key role in such management. We are currently witnessing a global decrease in biodiversity, which, in turn, has an impact on food production. Several pathways have been formulated to respond to these challenges.

One pathway concerns a more efficient crop management. Increase in yield within the sustainability borders of the planet implies, besides other measures, no further land use changes, safeguarding and even expanding natural habitats, and adequate crop protection. This idea is conceptualized as sustainable intensification, which looks at whole landscapes, territories, and ecosystems to optimize resource utilization and management. Farmers must produce more from the same area of land and use fewer inputs while producing greater yields. Such a transition is both possible and necessary.

Sustainable intensification requires an evidence-based approach on farming practices. The example of a recent study on "farming without plant protection products," carried out for the European Commission, illustrates that the scientific evidence on sustainable intensification is not always in line with the public opinion.[25] Consumers generally expect the minimization or avoidance of the use of plant production products (PPP) to be more sustainable, especially the use of chemical plant protection products is considered unsustainable. However, it remains an open question whether it is possible to reduce the use of PPP without yield reduction. There are several indications that, for specific crops, a reduction in PPP is feasible. The general tendency is that reduction seems possible in the case of (very) high actual PPP use, but not in the case of low use.

Apart from improved and more targeted uses of PPPs, several other innovations fit in the process toward sustainable intensification. Precision farming, including remote sensing with unmanned aerial vehicles, can also contribute to more targeted application and reduction of PPP use. Furthermore, important contributions will come from the breeding of more resistant varieties, both by classical breeding and by new breeding techniques, such as precision mutation breeding using the CRISPR-Cas approach or by genetic transformation.

71.4 Procurement

From farm to fork is often a long process, whereby food passes through the diverse links in the food chain. It is beyond the scope of this chapter to deal with all the steps in the food chain. Alternatively, we set out the position of two players in food procurement: supermarkets and alternative food networks (AFNs) and discuss their pros and cons in the context of FNS.

71.4.1 Supermarkets

In past decades, systems of food procurement and provisioning have changed considerably. Innovations relating to the cooling, transportation, and processing of food have enabled the concentration, centralization, and consolidation of food retailers. As a consequence, supermarkets, especially Transnational Retail Corporations (TNCs), now take a central position within the global agrofood system.[26] Especially in Western societies, supermarkets are now the single most important access point of food.[9,27] Though in large parts of Asia, Africa, and Latin America, "traditional," nonchain, and informal markets remain important points of access to food, also in these regions the importance of supermarket-based retailing is growing.[4]

The expansion of supermarkets may provide both opportunities and threats for global FNS. On the one hand, the expansion of supermarkets can play an important role in providing global FNS by enabling and facilitating physical and economic access to food. For example, supermarkets can offer fresh and healthy food at more competitive prices than smaller grocery stores, because of the global systems of provisioning connected to supermarket-based retailing. Thus playing an important role in creating equitable access to (fresh and nutritious) food and thus offering an opportunity for improving the nutritional quality of diets to all layers of society.[4,28,29]

On the other hand, the supermarketization of food procurement has been argued to threaten global FNS. A growing body of literature has addressed the way in which supermarkets tend to be more present in wealthy than in socio-economically disadvantaged areas and neighborhoods. People in poorer neighborhoods tend to be more dependent on smaller, more expensive, convenience, and fast-food shops, typically selling less healthy foods at higher prices. These areas have therefore also been referred to as "food deserts." Moreover, evidence exists that supermarkets in poorer areas tend to offer less healthy foods than in wealthier areas. Consequently, residents of these neighborhoods have poor access to healthy and affordable food. This suggests that the spread of supermarkets has not equitably increased access to affordable, healthy, and nutritious foods.[30,31]

The concept of food deserts has mostly been addressed in the United States, where evidence of the existence of food deserts is now extensive. Similar, though less clear, patterns have been identified in other parts of the world, such as Canada, Europe,[32] Asia, and Africa.[28] Also, some nuance is warranted, as shown by Wertheim-Heck[33] and Battersby and Crush[30] as in these contexts an understanding is needed of the roles played not only by supermarket-based retailing, but also by informal and traditional food markets in the building of food and nutrition (in)security.

71.4.2 Alternative food networks

A variety of initiatives have emerged that aim to address the negative environmental, social, political, and economic side-effects that are often associated with the expansion of modernized, supermarket-based, industrial, and global systems of production and provisioning. These—often citizen-led—initiatives are mostly referred to as AFNs. This term refers to a diversity of initiatives ranging from farmers' markets, food basket, and self-harvest systems, to organic agriculture and community gardens.[34,35] Since the 1990s, there has been an expanding body of literature on AFNs, with a strong focus on Europe and Northern America,[36] though more recently AFNs have also been studied in the context of developing economies (e.g., Wertheim-Heck[33]). This body of literature has moved from an initial mostly positive appraisal of the impacts of AFNs, to an increasingly critical scholarship.[35] Yet, the way in which AFNs relate and may contribute to FNS has only been addressed recently and findings are sparse.[10] Overall, we find that, although AFNs may contribute to FNS in some ways, their overall impact remains small because of their small sizes.[37] It should also be mentioned that because of the many different kinds of AFNs that exist, the way in which they contribute to FNS may vary widely. The discussion below is therefore not conclusive. Rather it is meant to open up a discussion about the potential role to be played by AFNs in assuring FNS. The findings also mainly address this issue in Western societies as AFN literature in developing economies remains sparse.

One main aspect in which AFNs may contribute to FNS is by making *available and creating access* to specific types of food, that are normally hard to access within a specific context. For example, food cooperatives may provide access to fresh fruits and vegetables to low-income families that normally do not have access to them. Other types of AFNs, for example, food buying groups or food basket schemes may be a way to access locally produced and organic vegetables in a context where it is not easy to gain access to such produce in another way. Critical scholars have, however, also highlighted that AFNs tend to offer produce against higher prices than through mainstream channels. Dispersed distribution and relatively small volumes may drive up prices further. Consequently, AFNs may be rather elitist and attract more wealthy groups, unless specific effort is made to do otherwise (e.g., in the food cooperatives mentioned earlier).[10,35] Also, restricted opening hours for picking up produce may restrict access to consumers with restricted or flexible time-schedules.[38] Furthermore, based on a comparative case-study in, Cerrada-Serra et al.[10] mention that many AFNs do not tend to offer a full food basket. Especially during winter, AFNs may face difficulties to provide a varied offer to its consumers. Producers need to find the balance between offering an attractive wide range of different products and the higher production costs it entails.

Acquiring food through an AFN tends to require a change not only in how food is accessed, but also how it is *used and prepared.* Accessing food through an AFN may therefore require a change in skills and knowledge. Also, in many AFNs, consumers are not able to choose the type or amount of products they receive. Some authors highlight this as an advantage, since in this way AFNs introduce consumers to new, or more fresh produce, and it encourages innovation and creativity in cooking practices.[38] As such, an AFN may work as a site for learning. However, many consumers feel more comfortable buying only foodstuffs that they recognize and know how to cook. This highlights the importance of the key role that knowledge plays in the utilization dimension of FNS, and the different types of knowledge required to participate.

The *stabilization* aspect of FNS relates to multiple aspects. First, the stability of AFNs may be compromised by two general aspects that tend to characterize the way in which AFNs function: (1) a heavy reliance on voluntary work. Though this can be considered a positive aspect that allows for a reduction in operating costs, there is an inherent risk related to volunteers' burnout or drop-out that raises important questions around the viability of these initiatives; and (2) how over-reliance on public subsidies and on other organizations can compromise the financial sustainability of AFNs and their food security outcomes.[10]

71.5 Consumption

FNS implies healthy and sustainable food diets. The definition of the FAO (2010) on sustainable diets reads as follows: "Sustainable diets are those diets with low environmental impacts which contribute to food and nutrition security and to healthy life for present and future generations. Sustainable diets are protective and respectful of biodiversity and ecosystems, culturally acceptable, accessible, economically fair and affordable; nutritionally adequate, safe and healthy; while optimizing natural and human resources" (FAO, 2010, Sustainable Diets and Biodiversity).

Building on the definition of the FAO, several components contribute to a sustainable diet. Lairon[39] distinguishes six components of a sustainable diet: (1) food and nutrient needs, food security, and accessibility; (2) well-being, health; (3) biodiversity, environment, and climate; (4) equity and fair trade; (5) eco-friendly, local, seasonal foods; (6) cultural heritage, skills.

A more simplified way is the distinction between three components: environment, healthy, and fairness.

71.5.1 Environmental footprint

The environmental component, also referred to as the footprint of food, is extremely complex. It implies knowledge and data on all phases of the food chain, from field to fork. A complete picture of the footprint of a food diet requires insights on all the ingredients that are part of that diet. The most common methodology behind such calculation is life cycle assessment (LCA). LCA is a tool for an aggregated description on emissions, waste, and the resources use from soil to kitchen per unit of different food items. LCA on food is based on a large number of hypothesis. In this context, comparison of footprint outcomes needs to be dealt with very carefully and rough estimations and comparisons are often misleading.

The farming system, that is, primary production, is an important component of the footprint of food, and hence of the sustainability of diets. Certain food systems are thereby considered more sustainable than others. Low-input farming is, for example, framed as more sustainable than high-input farming. In the previous section, we emphasized that it is a misconception that extensive farming is per definition more sustainable then intensive farming.

Furthermore, the type of food produced plays an important role. Overall, plant-based products have a lower environmental impact as compared to animal-based products. The production of meat from ruminants (such as beef from cattle) puts a significantly higher impact on the environment and on the use of natural resources as compared to meat from other animals or milk production. Also the way meat is produced matters for its environmental impact.

The impact of grain, potatoes, and rice is—for an equal number of calories produced—far below the impact of calories produced from animals. However, a healthy diet also implies sufficient protein intake. Tuomisto and Roy[40] calculated the environmental impact of different protein sources. They used the footprint, land area needed for the total production, as unit of analyses. Their results show that the highest environmental impact per unit of protein for livestock and sheep. Pork, chicken, eggs, milk, and tofu have comparable impacts. Soy bean, beans, and Quom have the lowest environmental impact per unit protein.

Although media often put the focus on primary production in the public debate on sustainability, there are many more aspects of the environmental impact of food. Important elements that need to be accounted for are logistics, food processing, food packaging, and food waste along the chain. All links in the chain needs to be included to measure the environmental impact of food. As an example, ecologically friendly produced vegetables, transported over long distances by plane, have a high environmental impact. Similarly, local food, stored in extremely hygienic conditions over long period of time, may still have a high environmental impact.

71.5.2 Healthy diets

A second component of sustainable food diets is health. Statistics show that, at local and global levels, the ideal situation is still a long way to go. Over 800 million people suffer from malnutrition. For most regions, the situation improves continuously, with the exception of Sub-Saharan Africa. Taking into account both soil fertility and climate change, it is clear that this region is extremely vulnerable in terms of food security.

Most rapidly health issue in terms of food in the 21st century is not malnutrition, but overconsumption. Obesity has reached an epidemic size. On a yearly basis, at least 2.8 million people die from causes related to overweight or obesity. While in the past, overconsumption was especially related to high-income countries, it becomes the longer the more relevant in upcoming economies—such as China and Brazil—and in developing countries. This holds especially true for urban areas.

Bahdar et al.[41] focused in their research on the production side in relation to healthy diets. They explored whether global food production is nutritionally balanced by comparing the diet that nutritionists recommend versus global agricultural production statistics. Results show that the global agricultural system currently overproduces grains, fats, and sugars while production of fruits and vegetables and protein is not sufficient to meet the nutritional needs of the current population. Correcting this imbalance could reduce the amount of arable land used by agriculture by 51 million ha globally but would increase total land used for agriculture by 407 million ha and increase greenhouse gas emissions. For a growing population, our calculations suggest that the only way to eat a nutritionally balanced diet, save land, and reduce greenhouse gas emissions is to consume and produce more fruits and vegetables as well as transition to diets higher in plant-based protein.

Given the benefits of healthy diets for both people and planet, the question remains how to change the current tendency of overconsumption. There circulate a broad range of misconception and disinformation on healthy diets. This trend is further fed by the raise of self-declared food experts and the popularity of diets that are not evidence-based and which in the short or the long run worsen rather than improve healthy choices. Information and sensitize are certainly needed.

However, information and campaigns are not sufficient to change food consumption behavior. Action and good practices are needed. A good example is the case of Finland, which was confronted in the 1960s and 1970s with a high mortality rate caused by heart and vascular diseases. A combination of various policy interventions (such as the introduction of new foods, obligatory changes in food composition, and information campaigns) resulted in a decrease of the mortality rate.[42]

At the policy level, there have also been several cases of taxation of unhealthy food. In October 2011, Denmark was the first country to introduce a fat tax. Advocates of the fat tax claim that the government had not prepared the installation of the tax while opponents claim that a fat tax will never be the solution to reach more healthy food consumption behavior.

Apart from the responsibilities in the fight against obesity, one can expect that no measure will succeed in rapidly changes food consumption patterns. The transition toward healthy diets is a long process, in which external factors play a key role.

71.5.3 Fair food

Fair trade is a large concept that, as a whole, implies that everyone involved in the food chain receives a fair price for his or her work. It is most often used in the context of primary food producers in developing countries. However, the economic situation of farmers worldwide is under pressure and the concept of fair trade is increasingly also used for food products with primary production in high-income countries.

Fair food also implies foremost fair trade practices, which relates to the standards. The use of international standards, such as social and environmental standards, contributes to such transparency in trading practices. Regulation on food—from farm to fork—differs across countries and nations. This wide range of regulations and restrictions for actors in the food chain hinders trade. Fair trade thereby implies a transparent communication.

International trading practices compose a real burden for many small farmers in developing countries. One can think of the costs related to certification, risks of costs related to adapting the production methods to international standards and instability of yields. Several international networks focus specifically on producers in developing countries, such as World Fair Trade Organization (WFTO) and European Fair Trade Association (EFTA). Their focus is on the export of food from developing countries to developed countries. These organizations engage active in supporting producers, raising awareness and in campaigning for changes in rules and practices of conventional international trade. The success of these international networks is visible all across the world and gave rise to a Fair Trade movement, fair trade communities, and their key ideas are the pillars of many nongovernmental organizations.

As price competition on the global food market increases and environmental concerns increase, the concept of fair trade has become increasingly relevant for all farmers and not just for smallholders in developing countries. Farmers are most often price takers and their economic position is weak, both upstream and downstream in the food chain. They are therefore the first victims of fluctuations on the international food market. Moreover, farmers are confronted with the impact of climate change, which leads to uncertain production levels. Closely related to both the price fluctuations and the unstable yields, risk management becomes an important component of the farm business. Diversification, adequate yield protection measures, smart farming, and precision farming are examples of a farmers' risk management. More recently, the popularity of citizen' initiatives in which risks of farmers are shared with consumers gain importance.

71.6 Research to support a sustainable food system and FNS

71.6.1 The need for science-based quantitative data

A first remark concerning research and sustainability is the fact that there is a huge need for *science-based quantitative data on all aspects of sustainability and FNS.* There is a lot of subjective perception and belief that is not supported by good scientific data. Typical examples are organic farming and agro-ecology. Adepts of organic farming claim that its production system is more sustainable, as is also stated in many papers but in most cases not by quantitative data, sometimes just by principles or by misleading or incomplete arguments. As stated in a previous section and confirmed by solid published data, the perception of organic farming does not take into account all units: land use, climate change, biodiversity, eutrophication, acidification, and ecosystem services.

In literature data are sometimes conflicting as is the case for figures on food waste. According to FAO reports about one-third of the food produced in wasted. This is an extremely high figure, taken into account that to total food waste in the EU is about 20% and in Flanders 11%.[43] There are two main reasons for these conflicting data: the difference between food losses and food waste (avoidable losses) that is mixed up in some publications and the fact that the quality of the data depends on the party that delivers these data.

Another misconception that is based on nonscientific and inadequate data found in UN reports on the right on food,[44] wherein more extensive farming is the way to solve the food problem in Sub-Saharan Africa. The preoccupation is based on believe and not on science. It is clear that there is at this moment not enough manure and compost to fertilize the crop fields to provide enough food to feed the population. Since an increase of the population is expected by around 300%, one can expect that the undernutrition will only increase to really dramatic proportions by the choice for low-input farming as was described in the rapports.

A frequently happened phenomenon is neglecting data or the consequences of the interpretation of data. Starting form a healthy diet, it is clear that there is an overconsumption and an overproduction of animal proteins, at least in the United States and Europe. It is therefore inconsequent that in the F2F document of the European Commission, the reduction of red meat is advised, but not the reduction of the livestock production. This reduction will have a very considerable positive impact of the climate change, one of the most important objectives mentioned in the report.

So there is a real gap between questionable data and solid scientific-based data, as there is also a gap between the existing of good data and the use or denial of these data.

71.6.2 Focus of the research on the biggest challenges and knowledge gaps

There is a huge need for data to solve the problems related to the most important challenges toward a sustainable food chain and nutrition security and to close knowledge gaps.

The most crucial point for sustainability is to close the yield gap. In only a few cases, this production gap is well described. We need more concrete data on the level of this gap in specific situations at different levels (from local to global), the causes of the gaps and how to solve them, taking into account the specific context, including socio-cultural aspects. The increase of sustainable intensification must be achieved by minimal inputs (fertilizers, pesticides, etc.) and research must concentrate on this. Biotechnology, mechanization, and precision agriculture will help to achieve this goal.

The contribution of agriculture in climate mitigation and the adaptation of agriculture to climate change are the most challenging aspects in agricultural research. Climate mitigation is related to intensification when the spared land will be forested. Adaptation is not evident since we have to focus more on the irregularity of temperature and rainfall and not on average changes.

Another knowledge gap is the exact impact of (intensive) agriculture on biodiversity. Although there is a big public concern about biodiversity, there is little good science in this respect, but a lot of preoccupation and biased research. We need also more research on how the landscape has to be organized in relation to biodiversity: land sparing, land sharing, mixed forms, etc. and for which specific local condition, as was done by Finch et al.[45] for two regions in the United Kingdom.

We need to invest in research for alternative protein sources to save land and to contribute to lower the climate changes and impacts on biodiversity. The same holds for the search for more nutritional foods that can be produced with less inputs.

To stimulate a sustainable food system, external costs has to be calculated in food prices at the consumer level. These external costs are related to impact of food production on ecosystems services, but this holds also for processing, transport, retail, and packing. This will increase food prices and the government has to be aware on the impact of these food prices on the accessibility to food for lower-income classes.

An important contribution to sustainability is the reduction of food waste, including the need for quantification of waste in all steps of the food chain. This is crucial information to study how and to which extend the problem of food waste can be reduced in a realistic way.

And finally a most crucial aspect is how to bring all this knowledge to governmental bodies, politicians, stakeholders, consumers, and the public. It seems also very important that sustainability of the food chain and the food consumption gets a place in education and extension. This knowledge is one of the most important critical success factors for a transition to a sustainable food system.

71.7 Enabling transition toward sustainable food systems

Despite the research gaps, innovation and current know-how are available to create more sustainable food systems. In a metastudy, Herrero et al.[46] report 75 developments in (bio)technology that could be incorporated in the agricultural system in the future and could promote its sustainability. The developments were ranked from research that has just started (e.g., nano pesticides, nano drones, engineering of photosynthesis) to developments that can already be implemented (e.g., vertical farming, the production of insects for proteins, disease-resistant varieties via gene technology, 3D printing). It is clear that several of these developments can promote sustainability, for example, through reduced and more targeted input of pesticides and fertilizers. Several technologies are being developed to detect diseases at a very early stage allowing fewer pesticide applications. Spectral images can be used to determine which fertilization a plant needs at what time, which makes precision fertilization possible. The development of alternative feed products and additives will completely change the outlook for livestock farming, which will significantly reduce greenhouse gas emissions and land use. Herrero et al.[46] also define essential elements for accelerating the systemic transformation of food systems: developing transition pathways, transforming mindsets, enabling social license, changing policies and regulations, designing market incentives, safeguarding against undesirable effects, ensuing stable finance and building trust. This leads to a final and very important note: the need to create an environment in which stakeholders in the food chain understand each other. A dialogue implies a common language, clear definitions, arguments based on scientific evidence and respect. In this sense, it is important to recognize the role of education and extension to enable critical reflections and future-proof innovations.

In this contribution, we focused mainly on sustainable food production and less on other aspects of the food chain, such as supply, processing industry, retail, and consumer behavior. Of course sustainability is also an issue for these players in the food chain.

71.7.1 Prerequisites for a sustainable food system

There are several key factors to enable the transition to a sustainable for system, a prerequisite for FNS and safety and below a short overview is presented of the most important ones.

It is extremely important to define the challenges with the highest impacts to enable a sustainable food system and also the related problems to reach this sustainability. Several challenges are discussed in this contribution and there is more extended information in several international reports.[47]

The start of the problem analysis must be based on correct and scientific-based data and not on perceptions or slogans. Quantitative data are most important for this analysis and for the calculations of the impact of the solutions for the identified problems.

The above information has to be distributed to all stakeholders in the food chain, the decision makers, governments and their administration, and the public sector, including educations. All actors share the same science-based information.

All actors will develop in consultation a common strategy toward a sustainable food system; at the end the responsible body (government) must take the final decisions, based on the best choice for the society and not necessary on the agenda(s) of the individual stakeholder (s) with the strongest lobby. The strategy should be considered at different levels: local, regional, country, continent, globally.

Governments should facilitate the transition process in all aspects, including subsidies and regulations, if necessary at the different levels mentioned earlier and taking into account the measures with the highest impact.

To reach sustainability and fair prices, external costs related to environment, climate, and transport have to be taken into attention.

A multidisciplinary approach and the public acceptance and support are important prerequisites. Transparency and information are essential in this respect.

71.7.2 Critical success factors

This leads to a final and very important note: the need to create an environment in which stakeholders in the food chain understand each other. A dialogue implies a common language, clear definitions, and arguments based on scientific evidence and respect. In this sense, it is important to recognize the role of education and extension to enable critical reflections and future proof innovations.

Acknowledgment

This chapter was developed within the RUSTICA and COCOREADO projects. Both projects have received funding from the European Union's Horizon 2020 research and innovation programme under grant agreement N. 101000527 and N. 101000573, respectively.

References

1. FAO. *The Future of Food and Agriculture: Alternative Pathways to 2050*. Rome: FAO; 2018.
2. IPCC. *An IPCC Special Report on Climate Change, Desertification, Land Degradation, Sustainable Land Management, Food Security, and Greenhouse Gas Fluxes in Terrestrial Ecosystems*. Intergovernmental Panel on Climate Change; 2019.
3. Willet W, Rockström J, Loken B, et al. Food in the anthropocene: the EAT–Lancet Commission on healthy diets from sustainable

food systems. *Lancet*. 2019;393:447–492. Available from: https://doi.org/10.1016/S0140-6736(18)31788-4.

4. Timmer C. The impact of supermarkets on nutrition and nutritional knowledge: a food policy perspective. In: de Pee S, Taren D, Bloem M, eds. *Nutrition and Health in a Developing World*. Humana Press; 2017:737–751. https://doi.org/10.1007/978-3-319-43739-2.
5. Hospes O, Brons A. Food system governance: a systematic literature review. In: Kennedy A, Liljeblad J, eds. *Food Systems Governance: Challenges for Justice, Equality and Human Rights*. Routledge; 2016:13–42.
6. Searchinger T, Waite R, Hanson C, Ranganathan J, Dumas P, Matthews E. *World Resources Report: Creating a Sustainable Food Future: A Menu of Solutions to Feed Nearly 10 Billion by 2050*. World Resources Institute; 2019.
7. Balmford A, Amano T, Bartlett H, et al. The environmental costs and benefits of high-yield farming. *Nat Sustain*. 2018;1:477–485. Available from: https://doi.org/10.1038/s41893-018-0138-5.
8. Tilman D, Clark M, Williams D, Kimmel K, Polasky S, Packer C. Future threats to biodiversity and pathways to their prevention. *Nature*. 2017;546:73–81. Available from: https://doi.org/10.1038/nature22900.
9. Chkanikova O. *Sustainable Supply Chain Management in Food Retailing: Insights Into Corporate Practice of Managing Supplier Relationships*. Lund: International Institute for Industrial Environmental Economics, Lund University; 2016.
10. Cerrada-Serra P, Moragues-Faus A, Zwart T, Adlerova B, Ortiz-Miranda D, Avermaete T. Exploring the contribution of alternative food networks to food security. A comparative analysis. *Food Security*. 2018;1–18. Available from: https://doi.org/10.1007/s12571-018-0860-x.
11. Sen A. Ingredients of famine analysis: Availability and entitlements. *Q J Econ*. 1981;96(3):433–464.
12. World Food Summit. Rome Declaration on World Food Security and World Food Summit Plan of Action, 13-17 November. World Food Summit: Rome, Italy; 1996. ISBN 9251039399.
13. Radhika Ch., Hemantha U. Research study on nutrition security and equity in its access in watershed development programmes. Research reports series 107. National Institute of Rural Development & Panchayati Raj, 2017. ISBN 978-93-84503-81-9.
14. Weingartner L. Paper I. The concept of food and nutrition security. In: Klennert K, ed. *Achieving food and nutrition security: Actions to meet the global challenge: A training course reader*. Feldafing: German Society for International Cooperation; 2005:3–28. ISBN 3-937235-71-X.
15. Freibauer A, Mathijs E, Brunori G, et al. *Sustainable Food Consumption and Production in a Resource-Constrained World*. European Commission – Standing Committee on Agricultural Research (SCAR); 2011.
16. Huber J. Towards industrial ecology: sustainable development as a concept of ecological modernization. *J Environ Policy Plan*. 2000;2(4):269–285.
17. Kitchen L, Marsden T. Creating sustainable rural development through stimulating the eco-economy: beyond the eco-economic paradox? *Sociologia Ruralis*. 2009;49:273–293.
18. Horlings LG, Marsden TK. Towards the real green revolution? Exploring the conceptual dimensions of a new ecological modernisation of agriculture that could "feed the world. *Global Environ Change*. 2011;21(2):441–452.
19. Sonnino R, Moragues-Faus A, Maggio A. Sustainable food security: an emerging research and policy agenda. *Int J Sociol Agric Food*. 2014;21(1):173–188.
20. Schlenker W, Roberts MJ. Nonlinear effects of weather on corn yields. *Rev AgrEcon*. 2006;28:391–398.
21. Foley J, Ramankutty N, Brauman K, et al. Solutions for a cultivated planet. *Nature*. 2011;478:337–342. Available from: https://doi.org/10.1038/nature10452.
22. Woods J, Williams A, Hughes JK, Black M, Murphy R. Energy and the food system. *Phil Trans R Soc B*. 2010;365:2991–3006. Available from: https://doi.org/10.1098/rstb.2010.0172.
23. Tubiello FN, Salvatore M, Rossi S, Ferrara A, Fitton N, Smith P. The FAOSTAT database of greenhouse gas emissions from agriculture. *Environ. Res. Lett*. 2013;8:015009.
24. Lambin EF, Meyfroidt P. Global Land Use Change, Economic Globalization, and the Looming Land Scarcity. *Proceedings of the National Academy of Sciences*. 2011;108:3465–3472. Available from: https://doi.org/10.1073/pnas.1100480108.
25. Keulemans W, Bylemans D, De Coninck B. Farming without plant protection products: can we grow without using herbicides, fungicides and insecticides? *Strasbourg (France): European Parliament*. 2019;44. Available from: https://doi.org/10.2861/05433.
26. Fuchs D, Kalfagianni A, Arentsen M. Retail power, private standards, and sustainability in the global food system. In: Clapp J, Fuchs D, eds. *Corporate Power in Global Agrifood Governance*. The MIT Press; 2009:29–60.
27. Oosterveer P. Restructuring food supply: sustainability and supermarkets. In: Spaargaren G, Oosterveer P, Loeber A, eds. *Food Practices in Transition: Changing Food Consumption, Retail and Production in the Age of Reflexive Modernity*. Routledge; 2012:153–176.
28. Peyton S, Moseley W, Battersby J. Implications of supermarket expansion on urban food security in Cape Town, South Africa. *Afr Geogr Rev*. 2015;34(1):36–54.
29. Zwart TA, Wertheim-Heck SCO. Retailing local food through supermarkets: Cases from Belgium and the Netherlands. J Clean Prod. 2012;300:126948. ISSN: 0959-6526, Available from: https://doi.org/10.1016/j.jclepro.2021.126948.
30. Battersby J, Crush J. Africa's urban food deserts. *Urban Forum*. 2014;25:143–151.
31. Howerton G, Trauger A. "Oh honey, don't you know?" The social construction of food access in a food desert. *ACME: Int J Crt Geogr*. 2016;16(4):740–760.
32. Helbich M, Schadenberg B, Hagenauer J, Poelman M. Food deserts? Healthy food access in Amsterdam. *Appl Geogr*. 2017;83:1–12.
33. Wertheim-Heck S. *We Have to Eat, Right? Food Safety Concerns and Shopping for Daily Vegetables in Modernizing Vietnam* [Ph.D. thesis]. Wageningen, NL: Wageningen University; 2015.
34. Forssell S, Lankoski L. The sustainability promise of alternative food networks: an examination through "alternative" characteristics. *Agric Human Values*. 2015;32(1):63–75.
35. Tregear A. Progressing knowledge in alternative and local food networks: critical reflections and a research agenda. *J Rural Stud*. 2011;27:419–430.

36. Michel-Villarreal R, Hingley M, Canavari M, Bregoli I. Sustainability in Alternative Food Networks: A Systematic Literature Review. *Sustainability*. 2019;11:859. Available from: https://doi.org/10.3390/su11030859.
37. Dixon J, Richards C. On food security and alternative food networks: understanding and perfomring food security in the context of urban bias. *Agric Human Values*. 2016;33(1):191–202.
38. Crivits M, Paredis E. Designing an explanatory practice framework: local food systems as a case. *J Cons Cult*. 2013;13(3):306–336. Available from: https://doi.org/10.1177/1469540513484321.
39. Lairon D. Nutritional Quality and Safety of Organic Food. A Review. *Agronomy for Sustainable Development*. 2010;30:33–41. Available from: https://doi.org/10.1051/agro/2009019.
40. Tuomisto H, Roy A. Could cultured meat reduce environmental impact of agriculture in Europe. In Conference Proceedings: M.S. Corson, H.M.G. van der Werf, editors. Proceedings of the 8th international conference on life cycle assessment in the agri-food sector (LCA Food 2012). Rennes (France): INRA; 2012, p. 611–615.
41. Bahadur KCK, Fraser E, Dias G, Zundel T, Pascoal S. Pathways Leading to a More Sustainable and Healthy Global Food System. *Solution Journal*. 2016;10–12. September-October 2016.
42. Puska P, Vartiainen E, Nissinen A, Laatikainen T, Jousilahti P. Background, principles, implementation, and general experiences of the North Karelia project. Glob Heart. 2016;11(2):173–178. Available from: https://doi.org/10.1016/j.gheart.2016.04.010.
43. Departement Landbouw en Visseri. (2021). Landbouwrapport 2020 (LARA), Brussel.
44. De Schutter, O. (2014). The transformative potential of the right to food, Final report drawing conclusions from his mandate, presented to the 25th Session of the UN Human Rights Council http://www.srfood.org/images/stories/pdf/officialreports/20140310_finalreport_en.pdf.
45. Finch T, Green RE, Massimino D, Peach WJ, Balmford A. Optimising nature conservation outcomes for a given region-wide level of food production. *J Appl Ecol*. 2020;57:985–994. Available from: https://doi.org/10.1111/1365-2664.13594.
46. Herrero M, Thornton PK, Mason-D'Croz D, et al. Innovation can accelerate the transition towards a sustainable food system. *Nature Food*. 2020;1(5):266–272. Available from: https://doi.org/10.1038/s43016-020-0074-1. ISSN 2662-1355.
47. STOA. Science and Technology Options Assessment. Annual Report 2013. *European Parliamentary Research Service*. 2013. Available from: https://doi.org/10.2861/53582.

Chapter 72

Climate change: food safety challenges in the near future

Fumiko Kasuga
National Institute for Environmental Studies, Tsukuba-City, Japan

Abstract
Exponential increases in various human activities in the Anthropocene era are indicated to have led to rapid alteration in the environment such as climate change and ecosystem impairment. Scientists are seriously discussing the planetary health and threshold for climate stabilization and for safe human life. Food system including agriculture is one of major drivers to climate change, and at the same time, climate change has significant impacts on human health through food system. This chapter discusses various impacts of climate change as most pressing food safety challenges at present and in the near future. Temperature rise is increasing chance of people to be exposed to foodborne hazards, and multiple pathways are demonstrated to mediate climate change and increasing adverse health impact through food safety. Evidence-based food safety risk management is necessary, and inter- and trans-disciplinary researches with cross-sectorial collaboration should be promoted to address these challenges.

Keywords: Climate change; ecosystem change; food safety; food system; planetary health; transdisciplinary research

Chapter points

Environmental change

1. Human pressure on ecosystem is causing rapid environmental changes and ecosystem impairment, which have significant impacts on human health through heat, extreme climate disasters, disturbance of mediate species of zoonosis and vector-borne diseases, and also human societal changes.
2. Climate change, together with unsustainable practices in fisheries and agriculture and overexploitation of natural resources, is projected to worsen the rapid decrease in biodiversity.

Climate change and food safety

1. Climate change has direct effect on human health by enhanced growth of microorganisms contaminating food.
2. Extreme weather events, such as heavy rain and flooding, may spread pathogens in the pasture and also facilitate the entry of chemical contaminants into the food chain, for example, via overflow resulting in the discharge of untreated storm water and wastewater.
3. Higher water temperatures may result in increased concentrations of methylmercury in fish and mammals due to potential increase in metabolic rates and increased mercury uptake.
4. Climate change will harm human immunological status with heat stress and malnutrition by depletion of food yields, nutritional changes in the crops, and damages of food system infrastructures.
5. Climate change will alter susceptibility of livestock to disease/infestation, which could result in increased fecal shedding of foodborne pathogens. The use of pesticide, fertilizers, and veterinary medicines would be affected by changes in pest pressure and resultant shift of agricultural practices due to climate change, and the residue levels of those chemicals in food are concerned.
6. Environmental and climate crises are triggering human displacement. Forced migration and resultant loss of properties and life foundation, changes in food sources and nutrition would cause major health failure, both physically and mentally.
7. Food System Shock, extreme crop productivity shock events, may cause socioeconomic inequalities and political instability, and could trigger significant claims of insurance, due to political violence, business interruption, and others.

Research gaps and future directions

1. Both mitigation measures to stop carbon emission to slow down climate change, based on the planned roadmap and timeline, and adaptation efforts to adjust to already altered environment should be taken together,

Present Knowledge in Food Safety. DOI: https://doi.org/10.1016/B978-0-12-819470-6.00019-6

with sound science, sufficient consultation with the suffered communities.

2. Digitalization, artificial intelligence, big data, and precision agriculture can be strong tools to adapt food system to climate change and to take integrated measures in the complicated environmental and societal changes.
3. Evidence- and science-based approaches, risk-based systems thinking including risk analysis framework for food safety, and target-oriented approaches should be integrated in addressing climate change and its impact on food safety.
4. Science is a powerful and common tool to support decision making; however, more collaboration with various disciplines of science and with wider range of stakeholders, namely interdisciplinary and transdisciplinary researches, is necessary locally and globally.

72.1 Introduction

Due to countermeasures against COVID-19 taken by many governments and industries in the world, daily global CO_2 emissions decreased by 17% (−11% to −25% for $\pm 1\sigma$) by early April 2020 compared with the mean 2019 levels,[1] and were estimated to be 7% reduction by the end of 2020.[2] However, experts projected that the average atmospheric CO_2 concentration over the year 2020 was higher than that in 2019.[2] In the meantime, the world witnessed enormous numbers of bush fires in Amazon, Australia, Siberia, California, and elsewhere in 2019 and 2020.[3] Intergovernmental Panel on Climate Change (IPCC) pointed out melting of ice sheets and glaciers in Greenland, Arctic, and Antarctic is observed.[4] In the Paris Agreement, which was adopted in December 2015, its goal was agreed to limit global warming to well below 2.0°C, preferably to 1.5°C, compared to preindustrial levels, to strengthen the global response to the threat of climate change, in the context of sustainable development and efforts to eradicate poverty.[5] Many governments swiftly started actions; however, IPCC warned with high confidence that global warming was likely to reach 1.5°C between 2030 and 2052 if it continues to increase at the current rate,[6] and they now use more determined words in its 6th Assessment Report, such that: "It is unequivocal that human influence has warmed the atmosphere, ocean and land" and "Global warming of 1.5°C and 2°C will be exceeded during the 21st century unless deep reductions in carbon dioxide (CO_2) and other greenhouse gas emissions occur in the coming decades."[7]

Exponential increases in various human activities since 1950 (in the Anthropocene era) were clearly demonstrated as major drivers for inducing exponential increases in various elements in the environment ("Great Acceleration").[8] Socioeconomic trends include fertilizer consumption and water use, as related factors to food production, and transportation which is related to food transport. Earth system trends include atmospheric concentration of carbon dioxide, surface temperature and marine acidification as well as tropical forest loss, domesticated land, marine fish capture, shrimp aquaculture, and atmospheric concentrations of methane[9] and nitrous oxide,[10] which are strongly indicated to be linked to agriculture such as livestock industries and waste. Group of Earth system scientists has proposed a concept of Planetary Boundaries which define a safe operating space for humanity[11] by consolidating numerous scientific evidences on biophysical processes which regulate the stability of the Earth system. Global environmental change is pushing the safe space toward the boundaries, with several Earth system processes already stepping beyond the boundaries, into the dangerous zone. Those processes are genetic biodiversity and nitrogen and phosphorous flows, all of which are closely linked to food production. Food consumption was estimated to contribute to 10.3% for the assumed 2020 baseline of CO_2 emission (5.6 out of 54.1 billion tons CO_2 equivalent).[12] Steffen and his colleagues[13] also alerted that the crossing the planetary threshold could induce a failure of stabilization of the climate and, if cascade effect takes place, could cause continued warming toward a "Hothouse Earth" status with very high global average temperature.

Food system including agriculture is a major driver to climate change, and at the same time, climate change has significant impacts on food production and agriculture.[14] "Climate change will influence the fate, transport, transmission, viability, and multiplication rate of pathogens in the food chain."[15]. However, it is not fully understood how climate change is affecting human health via food safety. This chapter discusses various impacts of climate change as one of most pressing food safety challenges in the near future and already present.

72.2 Environmental change

72.2.1 Human pressure on ecosystem change

Environmental changes and ecosystem impairment bring significant changes in the habitats of wild animals and plants, and give great threats to human health. Inspired by Millennium Ecosystem Assessment,[16] the Rockefeller Foundation—Lancet Commission on planetary health identified climate change, stratospheric ozone depletion, land degradation and desertification, forest clearance and land cover change, wetlands loss and damage, biodiversity loss, freshwater depletion and contamination, urbanization, damage to coastal reefs and ecosystems, as examples of environmental changes and ecosystem impairment induced by human pressure on ecosystem.[17]

Then the Lancet Commission illustrated the impacts of environmental change on human health in three layers: direct (such as heat stress from climate change), secondary (due to the alteration of natural systems), or indirect or tertiary effects (due to social disruption).

Direct health effects include floods, heatwaves, water shortage, landslides, and other climate disasters, exposure to ultraviolet radiation or pollutants.

Secondary or ecosystem-mediated health effects indicate infectious disease risk, reduced food yields and resultant undernutrition and stunting, depletion of natural medicines, personal and community mental health, and esthetic or cultural impoverishment. As the background of the changes in infectious disease risk indicated in the second layer, climate change has an impact on the growth of pathogenic bacteria, on distribution of waterborne pathogens, such as *Vibrio* spp. and toxic algae, on migration routes of birds that career zoonotic diseases, and on distribution of vehicle mosquitos and other insects that mediate vector-borne pathogens. Details are discussed in later sections.

Finally, the Commission suggested, as the third layer, indirect, deferred, and displaced health effects by diverse health consequences of livelihood loss, population displacement (including slum dwelling), conflict, inappropriate adaptation, and mitigation.

72.2.2 Biodiversity loss

The Intergovernmental Science-Policy Platform on Biodiversity and Ecosystem Services (IPBES) pointed out in its Global Assessment Report on Biodiversity and Ecosystem Services[18] that an average of around 25% of species in assessed animal and plant groups, namely around 1 million species face extinction, unless actions are taken to reduce the biodiversity loss. Unsustainable practices in fisheries, aquaculture, and agriculture are often associated with land-/sea-use change and overexploitation of natural resources. Climate change is projected to become increasingly important as a direct driver of changes in nature and its contributions to people in the next decades. And climate change is lowering the threshold of resistance of biome against pressure from human economic and agricultural activities, and is worsening the rapid decrease in biodiversity. IPBES's Assessment Report estimates that the fraction of species at risk of climate-related extinction is 5% at 2°C warming and rises to 16% at 4.3°C warming.[18]

Large-scale wildfires in Amazon, Australia, Siberia, middle to west United States, peatland in Indonesia, and many other places were triggered by natural or human ignition, such as burning for agriculture, and fires spread widely and for long time due to raised temperature and dry air. And in the end, they facilitate biodiversity loss. Around 9000 km^2 in the Amazon was burnt in the number of fires across Brazil, Bolivia, and Peru in 2019 due to human-driven deforestation, logging, and exploitation[3].

The combination of deforestation, widespread use of fire for clearing and climate change is pushing tropical forest ecosystem in Amazon toward an ecological tipping point, and is concerned finally to a savannah system.[19] This potential shift is concerned seriously, also because the Amazon forest is the world's largest carbon sink, while its capture and storage of carbon dioxide has been decreasing over the past decades.[20] Gatti et al.[21] found that Southeastern Amazonia acts as a net carbon source to the atmosphere, not carbon sink, through their investigation from 2010 to 2018, and suggested intensification of the dry season and an increase in deforestation as the main cause. It should be noted that food production system in the Amazon for global consumption is one of the major drivers to the ignition of fires in the area.

Deforestation destroys and changes habitats for mammals which can mediate zoonosis. It could increase occasions of encounter of human being with such animals and could be the origin of emerging zoonosis, such as COVID-19.

Biodiversity provides rich ecosystem for agricultural and fishery environment; therefore loss of biodiversity brings a serious loss in diverse food resources and vulnerable status of agriculture.

72.3 Climate change and food safety

WHO alerted that climate sensitive risk factors and illnesses would be one of the largest contributors to the food-related disease and mortality.[22] Under the assumption that climate change continues as projected, the IPCC predicted (with very high confidence) that, until the middle of the century, the global risk of adverse health outcomes would increase because of additional intense heatwaves and fires, and an increased risk of food- and waterborne diseases.[23]

Impacts of climate change on food safety can be categorized in a way similar to the Lancet Commission report on planetary health[17]: direct (such as heat stress from climate change), secondary (due to the alteration of natural systems), and indirect or tertiary effects (due to social disruption).

Individual foodborne hazards, both biological and chemical, that are discussed in this subchapter and potential impact of climate change on those hazards are listed in Table 72.1, using a similar format provided by US Global Change Research Program (USGCRP)[15] and Balbus et al.[24]

72.3.1 Direct effect of climate change on the foodborne pathogens and spoilage organisms

Direct effects of climate change are increasing risk of pathogen proliferation in food and water due to temperature

TABLE 72.1 Foodborne hazards impacted by climate change

Foodborne hazards	Major food sources	Health outcomes and symptoms	Specific climate drivers, and/or direct and indirect effects of climate change on human health	References
Microorganisms				
Enteric viruses: enteroviruses; rotaviruses; noroviruses; hepatitis A and E	Drinking water, Shellfish	Vomiting, nonbloody diarrhea with abdominal pain, nausea, aches, low-grade fever. Severe outcomes may include paralysis and infection of the heart or other organs.	Extreme weather events (such as heavy precipitation and flooding)Noroviruses favoring colder/dryer conditions	15
Listeria monocytogenes	Soft cheese, milk, meats, smoked seafood, originally linked with contaminated soil and environment	Fever, muscle aches, and rarely diarrhea. Intensive infection can lead to miscarriage, stillbirth, premature delivery, or lifethreatening infections (meningitis).	Extreme weather events (such as heavy precipitation and flooding)	15,25
Campylobacter spp.	Raw and undercooked poultry, beef, sheep and pig meat, unpasteurized milk	Diarrhea, cramping, abdominal pain, nausea, and vomiting. Serious cases can be lifethreatening.	Changes in the timing or length of seasons, precipitation and flooding	15,25
Salmonella spp. (nontyphoidal)	Raw and undercooked beef, pig, sheep and poultry meat, unpasteurized milk, raw eggs	Diarrhea, fever, cramping, abdominal pain, nausea, and vomiting. Serious cases can be lifethreatening.	Extreme weather events, change in the timing or length of seasons Heavy rainfall and floods causing contamination of pastures	14,15,25
Vibrio vulnificus and *Vibrio parahaemolyticus*	Fish, Shellfish	Gastroenteritis (*V. parahaemolyticus, V. cholerae*), septicemia (bloodstream infection) through ingestion or wounds (*V. vulnificus*).	Sea surface temperature, extreme weather events, sea level rise, precipitation patterns via changes in coastal salinity	15
Escherichia coli	Beef, contaminated vegetables	Diarrhea including bloody diarrhea, fever, cramping, abdominal pain, nausea, and vomiting. Serious cases can be lifethreatening.	Extreme weather events, changes in the timing or length of seasons	15,25
Protozoan parasites: *Cryptosporidium, Giardia*	Drinking water	Gastrointestinal illness.	Temperature changes, heavy precipitation, and flooding	15
Zoonotic foodborne pathogens including some of those above	–	–	Warmer temperature results in increased susceptibility of animals to diseases and subsequent fecal shedding of pathogens	26
–	–	–	–	–
Toxic algal blooms and mycotoxins	–	–	–	–

(*Continued*)

TABLE 72.1 (Continued)

Foodborne hazards	Major food sources	Health outcomes and symptoms	Specific climate drivers, and/or direct and indirect effects of climate change on human health	References
Algae: Toxigenic marine species of *Alexandrium, Pseudo-nitzschia, Dinophysis, Gambierdiscus*	Shellfish Fish	Gastrointestinal and neurologic illness caused by shellfish poisoning (paralytic, amnesic, diarrhetic, neurotoxic) or fish poisoning (ciguatera).	Temperature (increased water temperature), ocean surface currents, ocean acidification, hurricanes (*Gambierdiscus* spp.)	24
Cyanobacteria (multiple freshwater species producing toxins including microcystin)	Drinking water	Liver and kidney damage, gastroenteritis (diarrhea and vomiting).	Temperature, precipitation patterns	24
Mycotoxins (e.g., Aflatoxins/ Deoxynivalenol/ Fmonisins/Fusarins/ Ochratoxin A)	Fungi-infected crops and nuts	Impaired development in children, immune suppression, known carcinogens.	Influenced by temperature and humidity. Mycotoxin contamination of crops is anticipated to increase due to drought stress, temperature stress, stress induced by pest attack, increases in arthropod vectors, poor nutrient status. Changes in the geographical range of crops produced could provide opportunity for new fungus–plant associations to arise, so mycotoxins currently not considered a threat to public health (e.g., sterigmatocystin, cyclopiazonic acid, moniliformin) may become important.	14,24,25
Hydrogen cyanide	Cassava	–	Changing biology of plants as a defense against herbivore attack	14
Chemicals	–	–	–	–
Arsenic	Natural contamination	–	Microbial communities and water chemistry of freshwater systems can affect the distribution of arsenic species in surface water. Increased irrigation results in greater contamination of food crops.	24
Persistent organic pollutants (dioxins, PCBs, DDT)	Waste sites, combustion, electrical equipment, forest fires	–	Changes in crop types, cultivation methods, farming environment, and in atmospheric transport—use of DDT may increase due to increased need for malaria control. Thawing of ice caps will release persistent organic compounds. Increases in	22,24

(*Continued*)

TABLE 72.1 (Continued)

Foodborne hazards	Major food sources	Health outcomes and symptoms	Specific climate drivers, and/or direct and indirect effects of climate change on human health	References
			flooding events will remobilize soil- and sediment-associated POPs and transport them to uncontaminated areas.	
Methylmercury	Contaminated soils and sediments	–	Increased concentrations of methylmercury in fish and mammals due to potential increase in metabolic rates and increased mercury uptake at higher water temperatures.	24,27
Pesticides	Agriculture	–	Outbreaks of a wider variety of insects and pathogens will result in increased pesticide use and changes in application timings. Geographical shifts in agriculture will mean that cropping patterns change and types of pesticide use change.	24,26
Fertilizers	Agriculture	–	Use patterns of fertilizers will happen to cope with new pests and diseases.	26
Veterinary medicines	Agriculture	–	Residues of pesticides and veterinary medicines in plant and animal products would be affected by changes in pest pressure and resultant shift of agricultural practices due to climate change. The proliferation of animal diseases due to climate-related changes may result in an increased use of veterinary drugs that could lead to increased releases to the environment.	22,24
Antimicrobial resistance in human and animal pathogens	Aquaculture and livestock	–	Increased residue levels of veterinary drugs in foods of animal origin poses an increased concerns of antimicrobial resistance.	28,29
Microbial pathogens, biochemical oxygen demand, suspended solids, and other pollutants in wastewater	–	–	Heavy precipitation and floodings spreading the contamination from industrial wastes and sewage overflows	30,31

rise and increased humidity. WHO[22] summarized that climate change was likely to affect the persistence and occurrence of foodborne pathogens including zoonotic ones—bacteria, viruses, parasites, harmful algae, fungi, and their vectors and toxins they produce. FAO issued a comprehensive report on climate change and food safety[32] by updating its publications in the past,[33,34] and provided precise perspective on how climate change would affect food safety hazards, which were categorized similarly to WHO, that is, foodborne pathogens and parasites, algal blooms, heavy metals, methylmercury, pesticides, and mycotoxins. The risk of waterborne diseases would be raised if climate disasters cause floods or other contamination more frequently.

EFSA's large-scale expert elicitation research has also identified potential effect of climate change on human health, in both impact and frequency, through plant diseases, biotoxin contaminations originated from harmful fungus and algae.[26] Its report showed an increasing growth rate of pathogenic bacteria living in the marine environment and those involved in fecal contamination of waters, for example, *Vibrio* spp., at higher water temperatures. An outbreak of *Vibrio parahaemolyticus* in 2004 was linked to significantly warmer temperature of coastal waters in Alaska from 1997 to 2004.[35] The emergence of *Vibrio vulnificus* was suspected to be associated with high water temperatures.[36] Increased number of *Vibrio* cases per year in the past decades in the Baltic Sea region had been linked to increases in sea surface temperature.[37] The EFSA report also introduced field and laboratory experiments which showed more active production of the toxic rather than nontoxic fractions of freshwater cyanobacteria populations at higher temperature, suggesting an increased exposure of humans and farmed animals to cyanotoxins in the warmer scenarios.

WHO alerted that the higher temperature and moisture will induce fungal growth and formation of mycotoxin on crops, which can cause both acute toxic effects and chronic health problems (including cancer) in humans and livestock.[22] It is suggested that the fungal growth also increases the loss of productivity and portion of crops to be disposed, which would induces malnutrition in the population.

Higher temperatures can increase the number of pathogens already present on produce.[38] Climate change will influence the viability, transmission, and proliferation rate of pathogens throughout the food chain, and will lead to changes in the geographic distribution, seasonal occurrence, and survivability of certain pathogens. Changes in temperature and humidity will not affect foodborne pathogens equally. Some pathogens, such as *Salmonella*, *Escherichia coli*, and *Campylobacter*, are considered to be more sensitive to climate change.[15]

Elevated temperatures and moisture increase pre- and postharvest contamination of molds and mycotoxin production, in particular if crops are not dried and stored properly at low humidity.[15]

72.3.2 Secondary effect of climate change on food safety via changes in ecosystem

The impact of climate on food safety occurs through multiple pathways. Secondary or ecosystem-mediated effects also include changes in migration routes of birds that career zoonotic diseases, and in distribution of vehicle mosquitos and other insects that mediate vector-borne pathogens.

Extreme weather events, such as heavy rain and flooding, may facilitate the entry of chemical contaminants into the food chain.[39] US EPA has been concerned that the capacity of combined sewer systems, which collect and cotreat storm water and municipal wastewater, can be exceeded during high intensity rainfall events. The overflow can result in the discharge of untreated storm water and wastewater directly into receiving streams with high concentrations of microbial pathogens, biochemical oxygen demand, suspended solids, and other pollutants.[31] Such events were actually observed and details were reported at Hurricane Sandy in 2012.[30]

Higher water temperatures may result in increased concentrations of methylmercury in fish and mammals[27] due to potential increase in metabolic rates and increased mercury uptake at higher water temperatures.

The EFSA report[26] indicates that extreme climate would alter the risk of pathogen infections and diseases in animals due to the emergence of more resistant bacteria, as some bacteria have evolved stress tolerant mechanisms when exposed to difficult environmental conditions. Climate change was indicated to allow entrance of new vectors that may carry foodborne pathogens to new ecological zones.

Crises of water quality and quantity are intimately linked with climate change. The impact mainly comes from extreme events of flooding and drought and is compounded by existing inequalities.[40]

72.3.3 Indirect or tertiary effects of climate change on food safety through human and social factors

Indirect or tertiary effects of climate change on food safety largely reflect human, societal, and behavioral factors, and also are influenced via systems and institutional alterations.

72.3.3.1 Human physiological factors

Human immunological status will be harmed by climate change with heat stress, and malnutrition by depletion of food yields, nutritional changes in the crops, damages of food system infrastructures by extreme weather events, and others, causes chronic damages to immunological system. Sometimes, exposure to multiple climate change threats may occur simultaneously, resulting in compounding or cascading health impacts.[15]

For most developed countries, nutritional quality and food safety are the primary health concerns. In addition to pathways mentioned above, it should be recognized that there is a direct "fertilization" effect of carbon dioxide on plant photosynthesis. Higher concentrations of CO_2 stimulate growth and carbohydrate production in plants; however, they can also lower the levels of protein and essential minerals in a number of crops, such as wheat, rice, and potatoes, and lead to negative implications for human nutrition.[41]

72.3.3.2 Factors in food supply chain

Climate change affects food safety through food supply chain system—before, during, and after the harvest, and at transport/storage, manufacturing, cooking, and consumption stages. Sometimes, climate change can create unprecedented or unanticipated health problems or health threats in places where they have not previously happened.[15]

EFSA[26] expressed their concerns that climate change would drive numerous generic issues that affect food safety. They included alteration of susceptibility to disease/infestation of livestock, as extremes of heat, cold, precipitation, storms, wind, and surges, and drought could result in increased susceptibility of animals to several diseases and subsequent fecal shedding of foodborne pathogens. They also pointed out several other concerned changes related to food, such as transport pathways in the environment; fate and toxicity of toxic compounds and exposure to them; use patterns of pesticide and fertilizers to cope with new pests and diseases as well as reduced nutrients availability and crop productivity; and food hygiene along the entire food chain processes.

WHO also concerned that residues of pesticides and veterinary medicines in plant and animal products would be affected by changes in pest pressure and resultant shift of agricultural practices due to climate change. Increased residue levels of veterinary drugs in foods of animal origin pose an increase in antimicrobial resistance in human and animal pathogens.[22,28,29] In addition, the risk of food contamination with heavy metals and persistent organic pollutants following changes in crop types, cultivation methods, farming environment, and in atmospheric transport was considered to increase also due to climate changes. WHO also indicated that the risk in food safety was related to that of food security, as people tended to take less healthy diets and consume more "unsafe foods" when they had insufficient food.

72.3.3.3 Human behavior

The summertime peaks of several major foodborne illnesses may be related not only to warmer temperatures causing pathogen growth but also to human behavioral change, such as increased outdoor activities during summer time.[15] Food hygiene practices are not always well employed when food is prepared outdoors and the risk of foodborne diseases is higher in such situations. Climate change may increase such opportunities in some regions.

Trade-off should also be considered when people prefer more sustainable food products in their life. New trends in food system and "healthy diet" will change food safety risk. Eat Lancet Commission described a global technological and management changes in food production and reducing food loss and waste, and concluded that a major global shift to eating plant-based diets and increased consumption of dairy food is needed to improve human health, reduce environmental impacts and keep planetary boundaries within a safe operating space for humanity.[42] Introducing of new dietary practices in wider scale with pretty rapid manner should be combined with careful management of food safety aspects throughout the food supply chain. When we try to reduce food loss and waste, we have to be aware that the base amount of wasted food would have been increased if molds grow faster in food storage due to temperature rise.

72.3.3.4 Societal factors

Climate disasters in short term and climate change in longer term could damage the established public health system in general, which could lead to food safety failure both in production and in consumption. IPCC predicted that poor regions would face an increased risk of undernutrition, compared with conditions with no climate change, resulting from diminished food production (with high confidence).[23]

As also summarized in Table 72.1, increased temperature could alter pathogens' growth and distribution in the farming area, and extreme weather, such as heavy precipitation and flooding, can cause contamination of pastures by pathogens, as they are transferred by rainwater and floods. In addition, farmers have to modify and adjust farming practices according to climate change, which may result in increased use of chemicals and veterinary drugs in livestock and agriculture due to potential changes in animal health status and in increased exposures to pests.[22,24,26] Similar concerns have been raised for aquaculture.

Effects of climate change on agricultural practices and food production are extensively discussed in the context of food security in Chapter 74 of this book.[43]

Environmental and climate crises are triggering human displacement. It was reported that weather-related disasters caused an in-country migration, or displacement, of 16.1 million people globally in 2018.[44] "Not only are human displacement scenarios influenced by water, energy and food systems, but they also influence the water, energy and food nexus. The impact of migration on food, water and energy security seems obvious at the place of origin, transit and destination, especially in case of forced migration."[45] Forced migration induced by climate extremes and disasters, and resultant loss of properties and life foundation, reduction of quality of life, changes in food sources and nutrition, culture and community changes would cause major health failure, both physically and mentally.

The report "Food System Shock: The Insurance Impacts of Acute Disruption to Global Food Supply" published by an insurance group Lloyd's[46] demonstrated a quantitative foresight analysis on potential consequences of extreme crop productivity shock events. Scenarios were developed on systematic weaknesses in the global food system to see the potential results when major system breakdowns take place due to extreme climatic events. They described not only the direct impacts on agriculture but also the potential shocks to global infrastructure and political stability, highlighting a shock to the global food supply could trigger significant claims of insurance, due to political violence, business interruption, and others. Political conflicts, especially wars are serious threats to environment and sustainability[47] and lead to serious damage to food system including food safety.

It is important to note that even though every citizen in a country is at risk to the health impacts associated with climate change, some populations, including those with low income, some communities of color, immigrant groups, indigenous peoples, children and pregnant women, senior adults, people with disabilities, and preexisting or chronic medical conditions are disproportionally vulnerable.[15]

72.4 Research gaps and future directions

Under climate change with rapidly changing various environmental elements, human health is impacted via multiple ways, and food safety takes part in the processes. It is critical to take food safety into consideration when holistic approaches are taken to turn toward sustainability in our daily life and socioeconomic systems.

The Lancet Commission on planetary health alerts that the current generations have been mortgaging the health of future generations to realize economic and development gains in the present, and concludes that "to support a world population of 9–10 billion people or more, resilient food and agricultural systems are needed to address both under- and overnutrition, reduce waste, diversify diets, and minimize environmental damage."[17] To reduce food safety risk due to climate change, immediate and multiple measures should be taken.

72.4.1 Mitigation

Food system is not only affected by climate change but also has significant impacts on the environmental change, as it is demonstrated that the atmospheric concentrations of major greenhouse gasses, methane,[9] and nitrous oxide[10] are linked to livestock industries, fertilizer use in agriculture, and industrial waste. To reduce future food safety risk linked to climate change, food system itself should be reviewed and improved with the mitigation measures to reduce greenhouse gas emissions throughout the food supply chain.

72.4.2 Adaptation

In parallel to mitigation actions, climate change adaptation is helpful to adjust ongoing societal systems to rapid changing environment and to reduce adverse health impact. Adaptation measures are in principle taken at local or national levels to reflect climate and environmental nature on site. National and regional platforms have been developed for sharing information among communities, help designing local adaptation plans and supporting adaptation businesses, such as Climate Change Adaptation Information Platform (A-PLAT), jointly developed by Ministry of Environment, National Institute for Environmental Studies (NIES), Japan and Center for Climate Change Adaptation (CCCA), and Asia-Pacific Climate Change Adaptation Information Platform (AP-PLAT). A-PLAT (https://ap-plat.nies.go.jp/index.html) provides climate change impacts on individual industry sectors, although mostly qualitative.

72.4.3 Cross-sectorial collaboration for food system and food safety

Under the COVID-19 pandemic, multiple, interlinked factors related to the pathogen, ecosystem, and human society, such as smart adaptation and genetic evolution of the virus, rapid change in land use, invasion of human life into wildlife, direct contact with wild animals at the market in the middle of big cities, and very rapid and frequent international travels, are recognized as root causes of the disease.[48,49] At the initial stage of the disease, weakness of global trade and value chain systems was observed. COVID-19 is not the last pandemic. To prepare for the next global-scale disasters, paradigm shift of business operations, including food business, is required, with the cross sectorial, holistic approaches to address such multilayered, complex causal factors.

COVID-19 has brought and highlighted socioeconomic inequalities in various communities in the world. Capacity development and international collaboration for global health have been more strongly recognized. It applies to food safety arena, especially in the developing countries.

Digitalization, artificial intelligence, and big data can be strong tools to adapt food system to climate change and to take integrated measures in the complicated environmental and societal changes. Precision agriculture by using Internet of things networks and other advanced digital technology is already in place in the world. Use of big data, digital management of food safety, and dynamic risk management system are discussed deeply with practical suggestions.[50]

Green recovery; environmental, social, and governance investment; and green finance are now the major trends in finance business. The role of finance and insurance sectors is significant in adding impact and motivation on various business sectors including food and agriculture to reduce carbon emission and, accordingly, to slow down climate change and other environmental changes. Food safety should also be considered in such entire business model to address climate change.

As climate change is shifting the food safety landscape, stronger and transparent collaborations are needed among all the relevant actors in the food chain, by adopting forward-looking approaches in the food safety,[32] which applies to collaboration with existing and new partners to address climate change more effectively.

72.4.4 Evidence- and science-based approaches

Policy makers and customers need more scientific evidence for the decision making and their choice of daily consumption and behavior to avoid health risk from infectious diseases and also from foodborne diseases. Industries shift to science-based approaches also in the context of accountability and transparency.

USGCRP[15] described that such needs can be benefited from research activities that: (1) synthesize and assess efforts to identify and respond to current and projected food safety concerns and their impacts on human health within the existing and future food safety infrastructure; (2) develop, test, and expand integrated assessment models to enhance understanding of climate and weather variability, particularly extreme events, and the role of human responses, including changes in farming technology and management, on health risks within the food chain; and (3) examine the impacts of rising CO_2 and climate change on human and livestock nutritional needs, as well as the impacts of changing nutritional sources on disease vulnerability.

Science community has responsibility to contribute to such activities.

72.4.5 Risk-based strategies

Food safety management framework has evolved from understanding and identifying hazards for food safety to analyzing risk. Risk analysis framework has been adopted by Codex Alimentarius Commission,[51] and risk management, risk assessment, and risk communication are in practice in many countries. Facing various confusions related to identifying SARS-CoV-2 virus or (part of) its genome on surface of food and food package, International Commission on Microbiological Specifications for Foods (ICMSF) delivered an opinion on COVID-19 and food safety, emphasizing the difference between hazard and risk.[52] In the context of food safety in climate change, we need to note this difference and develop strategies based on the risk.

72.4.6 Target-oriented approaches

ICMSF proposed food safety risk management metrics, food safety objectives (FSOs) and performance objectives, which have been adopted by the Codex Alimentarius Commission.[51,53] FSO should be set for the time of consumption, a target level at the consumption of the food. It is not easy in general to set a quantitative level, but once it is determined, every stakeholder can have individual goals to achieve in their own business and with their own roles. In the context of food safety under climate change, target-oriented debates will be useful by sharing common goals of level of protection, reduction, and agreement.

72.4.7 Collaborative activities within academia and with nonacademia—interdisciplinary and transdisciplinary researches

Food safety researches inherently need collaboration with nonacademic sectors in the society, such as food producers, consumers, food business workers, laboratory workers, and relevant authorities. Such collaboration has not been always common in other scientific disciplines. However, to address complex global challenges including climate change, people have recognized necessity of interdisciplinary and transdisciplinary researches, and therefore research platforms for collaboration such as Future Earth was created.[54]

To minimize food safety risk from climate change and other environmental changes, even more collaboration with various disciplines of science and wider range of stakeholders is needed from locally to globally.

References

1. Le Quéré C, et al. Temporary reduction in daily global CO_2 emissions during the COVID-19 forced confinement. *Nat Clim Change*. 2020;10:647–653. Available from: https://doi.org/10.1038/s41558-020-0797-x.

2. Friedlingstein P, et al. Global carbon budget 2020. *Earth Syst Sci Data*. 2020;12:3269–3340. Available from: https://doi.org/10.5194/essd-12-3269-2020.
3. Future Earth. Global Fires. <https://futureearth.org/publications/issue-briefs-2/global-fires/>; 2020a.
4. Intergovernmental Panel on Climate Change (IPCC). Special Report on the Ocean and Cryosphere in a Changing Climate (SROCC); 2019.
5. United Nations. Paris agreement; 2015.
6. Intergovernmental Panel on Climate Change (IPCC). Special Report on Global Warming of 1.5°C; 2018.
7. Intergovernmental Panel on Climate Change (IPCC). Climate change 2021: the physical science basis. In: Masson-Delmotte V, Zhai P, Pirani A, Connors SL, Péan C, Berger S, Caud N, Chen Y, Goldfarb L, Gomis MI, Huang M, Leitzell K, Lonnoy E, Matthews JBR, Maycock TK, Waterfield T, Yelekçi O, Yu R, Zhou B, eds. Contribution of Working Group I to the Sixth Assessment Report of the Intergovernmental Panel on Climate Change; 2021.
8. Steffen W, et al. The trajectory of the Anthropocene: the great acceleration. *Anthr Rev*. 2015;2:81–98. Available from: https://doi.org/10.1177/2053019614564785.
9. Saunois M, et al. The global methane budget 2000–2017. *Earth Syst Sci Data*. 2020;12(1561–1623). Available from: https://doi.org/10.5194/essd-12-1561-2020.
10. Tian H, et al. A comprehensive quantification of global nitrous oxide sources and sinks. *Nature*. 2020;586:248–256. Available from: https://doi.org/10.1038/s41586-020-2780-0.
11. Steffen W, et al. Planetary boundaries: guiding human development on a changing planet. *Science*. 2015;347:1259855. Available from: https://doi.org/10.1126/science.1259855.
12. Falk J, et al. Exponential Roadmap 1.5. Sweden: Future Earth. <https://exponentialroadmap.org/wp-content/uploads/2020/03/ExponentialRoadmap_1.5.1_216x279_08_AW_Download_Singles_Small.pdf>; 2019.
13. Steffen W, et al. Trajectories of the earth system in the Anthropocene. *PNAS*. 2018;115(33):8252–8259. Available from: http://www.pnas.org/cgi/doi/10.1073/pnas.1810141115.
14. Mbow C, Rosenzweig C, Barioni LG, et al. Food security. In: Shukla PR, Skea J, Calvo Buendia E, Masson-Delmotte V, Pörtner H-O, Roberts DC, Zhai P, Slade R, Connors S, van Diemen R, Ferrat M, Haughey E, Luz S, Neogi S, Pathak M, Petzold J, Portugal Pereira J, Vyas P, Huntley E, Kissick K, Belkacemi M, Malley J, eds. Climate Change and Land: An IPCC Special Report on Climate Change, Desertification, Land Degradation, Sustainable Land Management, Food Security, and Greenhouse Gas Fluxes in Terrestrial Ecosystems; 2019.
15. U.S. Global Change Research Program (USGCRP). In: Crimmins A, Balbus J, Gamble JL, Beard CB, Bell JE, Dodgen D, Eisen RJ, Fann N, Hawkins MD, Herring SC, Jantarasami L, Mills DM, Saha S, Sarofim MC, Trtanj J, Ziska L, eds. The Impacts of Climate Change on Human Health in the United States: A Scientific Assessment. Washington, DC: U.S. Global Change Research Program; 312 pp. <https://doi.org/10.7930/J0R49NQX>; 2016.
16. Millennium Ecosystem Assessment. *Ecosystems and Human Well-being: Synthesis*. Washington, DC: Island Press; 2005.
17. Whitmee S, Haines A, Beyrer C, et al. Safeguarding human health in the Anthropocene epoch: report of The Rockefeller Foundation–Lancet Commission on planetary health. *Lancet*. 2015;6736:1973–2028. Available from: https://doi.org/10.1016/S0140-6736(15)60901-1.
18. Intergovernmental Science-Policy Platform on Biodiversity and Ecosystem Services (IPBES). The global assessment report on biodiversity and ecosystem services. <https://ipbes.net/global-assessment>. ISBN No: 978-3-947851-13-3>; 2019.
19. Lovejoy TE, Nobre C. Amazon tipping point. *Sci Adv*. 2018;4(2). eaat2340.
20. Brienen RJ, et al. Long-term decline of the Amazon carbon sink. *Nature*. 2015;519(7543):344–348.
21. Gatti LV, Basso LS, Miller JB, et al. Amazonia as a carbon source linked to deforestation and climate change. *Nature*. 2021;595:388–393. Available from: https://doi.org/10.1038/s41586-021-03629-6.
22. World Health Organization. Food Safety Climate Change and the Role of WHO. <https://www.who.int/foodsafety/publications/all/Climate_Change_Document.pdf>; 2019.
23. Intergovernmental Panel on Climate Change (IPCC). Climate change 2014: Impacts, adaptation, and vulnerability. Part A: global and sectoral aspects. In: Field CB, Barros VR, Dokken DJ, Mach KJ, Mastrandrea MD, Bilir TE, Chatterjee M, Ebi KL, Estrada YO, Genova RC, Girma B, Kissel ES, Levy AN, MacCracken S, Mastrandrea PR, White LL, eds. Contribution of Working Group II to the Fifth Assessment Report of the Intergovernmental Panel on Climate Change. Cambridge, United Kingdom and New York, NY, USA Cambridge University Press; 2014:1132 pp.
24. Balbus JM, et al. Global climate change, implications of global climate change for the assessment and management of human health risks of chemicals in the natural environment. *Environ Toxicol Chem*. 2013;32(1):62–78.
25. International Commission on Microbiological Specifications for Foods (ICMSF). *Microorganisms in Foods 6, 2nd edition: Microbial Ecology of Food Commodities*. New York: Kluwer Academic & Plenum Publishers; 2005. ISBN: 0-306-48675-X.
26. European Food Safety Authority (EFSA), Maggiore A, Afonso A, Barrucci F, De Sanctis G. Climate change as a driver of emerging risks for food and feed safety, plant, animal health and nutritional quality. *Climate Change Food Saf*. 2020;17(6). Available from: https://doi.org/10.2903/sp.efsa.2020.EN-1881. EFSA supporting publication 2020: EN-1881. 146 pp.
27. Carrie J, et al. Increasing contaminant burdens in an arctic fish, Burbot (*Lota lota*), in a warming climate. *Environ Sci Technol*. 2010;44:316–322. Available from: http://doi.org/10.1021/es902582y.
28. Cooper KM, et al. Potential impacts of climate change on veterinary medicinal residues in livestock produce: an island of Ireland perspective. *Trends Food Sci Technol*. 2015;44:21–35. Available from: http://doi.org/10.1016/j.tifs.2014.03.007.
29. World Health Organization. Antimicrobial Resistance: Global Report on Surveillance. 257 pp. World Health Organization, Geneva. <http://www.who.int/drugresistance/documents/surveillancereport/en/>; 2014.
30. Kenward, A., Yawitz, D., Raja U. (2013): Sewage overflows from Hurricane Sandy. Climate Central. <https://semspub.epa.gov/work/02/210346.pdf>.
31. U.S. EPA. A Screening Assessment of the Potential Impacts of Climate Change on Combined Sewer Overflow (CSO) Mitigation in the Great Lakes and New England Regions (Final Report).

Washington, DC: U.S. Environmental Protection Agency; 2008. EPA/600/R-07/033F.

32. FAO. Climate Change: Unpacking the Burden on Food Safety. Food Safety and Quality Series No. 8. Rome: FAO. <https://doi.org/10.4060/ca8185en>; 2020.
33. FAO. In: Jaykus LA, Woolridge M, Frank JM, Miraglia M, McQuatters-Gollop A, Tirado C, Clarke R, Friel M, contributors. *Climate Change: Implications for Food Safety*. Rome: FAO. <http://www.fao.org/3/i0195e/i0195e00.pdf>; 2008:49 pp.
34. FAO. The State of Food and Agriculture 2016: Climate Change, Agriculture and Food Security. Rome: FAO. <http://www.fao.org/3/a-i6030e.pdf>; 2016:194 pp.
35. McLaughlin JB, et al. Outbreak of *Vibrio parahaemolyticus* gastroenteritis associated with Alaskan oysters. *N Engl J Med*. 2005;353:1463–1470. Available from: http://doi.org/10.1056/NEJMoa051594.
36. Paz S, et al. Climate change and the emergence of *Vibrio vulnificus* disease in Israel. *Environ Res*. 2007;103:390–396. Available from: http://doi.org/10.1016/j.envres.2006.07.002.
37. Vezzulli L, Grande C, Reid PC, et al. Climate influence on *Vibrio* and associated human diseases during the past half-century in the coastal North Atlantic. *Proc Natil Acad Sci USA*. 2016;113(34): E5062–E5071. Available from: https://doi.org/10.1073/pnas.1609157113.
38. International Commission on Microbiological Specifications for Foods (ICMSF). *Microorganisms in Foods 5: Characteristics of Microbial Pathogens*. London: Blackie Academic & Professional; 1996. ISBN: 041247350X.
39. Foulds SA, et al. Flood-related contamination in catchments affected by historical metal mining: an unexpected and emerging hazard of climate change. *Sci Total Environ*. 2014;476–477: 165–180. Available from: http://doi.org/10.1016/j.scitotenv.2013.12.079.
40. Future Earth, The Earth League, WCRP. 10 new insights in climate science 2020. Stockholm. <https://futureearth.org/10-insights-2020>; 2021.
41. Loladze I. Hidden shift of the ionome of plants exposed to elevated CO_2 depletes minerals at the base of human nutrition. *eLife*. 2014;3:e02245. Available from: http://doi.org/10.7554/eLife.02245.
42. Willett W, Rockström J, Loken B, et al. Food in the Anthropocene: the EAT–Lancet Commission on healthy diets from sustainable food systems. *Lancet Commission*. 2019;393(10170):447–492. Available from: https://doi.org/10.1016/S0140-6736(18)31788-4.
43. Avermaete T, et al. Food and nutrition security: challenges for farming, procurement and consumption. In: Present Knowledge in Food Safety – A Risk-Based Approach Throughout the Food Chain; (in press).
44. The Internal Displacement Monitoring Centre (IDMC). Global Report on Internal Displacement. <https://www.internal-displacement.org/publications/2019-global-report-on-internal-displacement>; 2019.
45. Nagabhatla N. Water-Migration Nexus and the Human Displacement Discourse. The Water-Energy-Food Nexus Blog Series. Future Earth. <https://futureearth.org/2019/01/14/water-migration-nexus-and-the-human-displacement-discourse/>; 2019 Accessed 11.05.21.
46. Lloyd's. Food System Shock: The Insurance Impacts of Acute Disruption to Global Food Supply. <https://www.lloyds.com/~/media/files/news-and-insight/risk-insight/2015/food-system-shock/food-system-shock_june-2015.pdf>; 2016. Accessed 22.05.21.
47. Kasuga F. Science as a common language for contribution to sustainability and peace. *Sustain Sci*. 2021;16:1229–1231. Available from: https://doi.org/10.1007/s11625-021-00972-5.
48. Asayama S, et al. Are we ignoring a black elephant in the Anthropocene? Climate change and global pandemic as the crisis in health and equality. *Sustain Sci*. 2020;. Available from: https://doi.org/10.1007/s11625-020-00879-7.
49. Future Earth. Policy Brief: COVID-19—A Global Health Concern Requiring Science-Based Solutions. <https://futureearth.org/2020/06/26/policy-brief-covid-19-a-global-health-concern-requiring-science-based-solutions/>; 2020b.
50. Donaghy, et al. Big data impacting dynamic food safety risk management in the food chain. *Front Microbiol*. 2021;12. Available from: https://doi.org/10.3389/fmicb.2021.668196.
51. Codex Alimentarius Commission (2016): Procedural Manual, 24th ed. Rome Joint FAO/WHO Food Standards Programme, ISBN 978-92-5-108928-6. <http://www.fao.org/3/a-i5079e.pdf>.
52. International Commission on Microbiological Specifications for Foods (ICMSF). ICMSF opinion on SARS-CoV-2 and its relationship to food safety. <https://www.icmsf.org/wp-content/uploads/2020/09/ICMSF2020-Letterhead-COVID-19-opinion-final-03-Sept-2020.BF_.pdf>; 2020.
53. International Commission on Microbiological Specifications for Foods (ICMSF). A simplified guide to understanding and using food safety objectives and performance objectives. In: Boisrobert CE, Stjepanovic A, Ho S, Lelieveld HLM, eds. *Ensuring Global Food Safety*. New York: Academic Press; 2010:91–98.
54. Future Earth. Our history. <https://futureearth.org/about/history/>; n.d.

Index

Note: Page numbers followed by "*f*," "*t*," and "*b*" refer to figures, tables and boxes, respectively.

B

C

E

F

H

M

N

S

T

U

X

Y

Z

www.ingramcontent.com/pod-product-compliance
Lightning Source LLC
Chambersburg PA
CBHW081326300325
24303CB00028B/753